Cancer Chemotherapy and Biotherapy

PRINCIPLES AND PRACTICE

FOURTH EDITION

Cancer Chemotherapy and Biotherapy

PRINCIPLES AND PRACTICE

FOURTH EDITION

EDITORS

■ **BRUCE A. CHABNER, M.D.**

Professor of Medicine
Chief, Hematology/Oncology
Clinical Director, Cancer Center
Massachusetts General Hospital
Boston, Massachusetts

■ **DAN L. LONGO, M.D.**

Scientific Director
National Institute on Aging
National Institutes of Health
Gerontology Research Center
Baltimore, Maryland

LIPPINCOTT WILLIAMS & WILKINS
A **Wolters Kluwer** Company

Philadelphia • Baltimore • New York • London
Buenos Aires • Hong Kong • Sydney • Tokyo

Acquisitions Editor: Jonathan Pine
Managing Editor: Lisa Kairis
Production Editor: Dave Murphy
Manufacturing Manager: Ben Rivera
Associate Director of Marketing: Adam Glazer
Art Director: Doug Smock
Compositor: TechBooks
Printer: Edwards Brothers

© 2006 by **LIPPINCOTT WILLIAMS & WILKINS**
530 Walnut Street
Philadelphia, PA 19106 USA
LWW.com

Copyright © 1990, 1996, 2001 by Lippincott Williams & Wilkins

Printed in the USA

Library of Congress Cataloging-in-Publication Data

Cancer chemotherapy and biotherapy : principles and practice / [edited by]
  Bruce A. Chabner, Dan L. Longo.—4th ed.
    p. ; cm.
  Includes bibliographical references and index.
  ISBN 0-7817-5628-6 (alk. paper)
  1. Cancer—Chemotherapy. 2. Cancer—Immunotherapy. 3. Antineoplastic
agents. 4. Biological response modifiers.
  [DNLM: 1. Neoplasms—drug therapy. 2. Antineoplastic Agents—therapeutic
use. 3. Biological Products—therapeutic use. QZ 267 C21515 2006] I. Chabner,
Bruce. II. Longo, Dan L. (Dan Louis), 1949–
RC271.C5C32219 2006
616.99′4061—dc22   2005022888

Care has been taken to confirm the accuracy of the information presented and
to describe generally accepted practices. However, the authors, editors, and
publisher are not responsible for errors or omissions or for any consequences from
application of the information in this book and make no warranty, expressed or
implied, with respect to the currency, completeness, or accuracy of the contents of
the publication. Application of this information in a particular situation remains
the professional responsibility of the practitioner.

The authors, editors, and publisher have exerted every effort to ensure that drug
selection and dosage set forth in this text are in accordance with current
recommendations and practice at the time of publication. However, in view of
ongoing research, changes in government regulations, and the constant flow of
information relating to drug therapy and drug reactions, the reader is urged to
check the package insert for each drug for any change in indications and dosage
and for added warnings and precautions. This is particularly important when the
recommended agent is a new or infrequently employed drug.

Some drugs and medical devices presented in this publication have Food and
Drug Administration (FDA) clearance for limited use in restricted research settings.
It is the responsibility of the health care provider to ascertain the FDA status of
each drug or device planned for use in their clinical practice.

To purchase additional copies of this book, call our customer service
department at (800) 638-3030 or fax orders to (301) 824-7390. International
customers should call (301) 714-2324.

Visit Lippincott Williams & Wilkins on the Internet: at LWW.com. Lippincott
Williams & Wilkins customer service representatives are available from 8:30 am to
6 pm, EST.

10 9 8 7 6 5 4 3 2 1

Contents

Preface

All substances are poisonous, there is none that is not a poison; the right dose differentiates a poison from a remedy.

—*Paracelsus* (1538 AD)

For physicians who daily care for patients with cancer, Paracelsus was clairvoyant. Cancer therapy has developed its unique ambiance: seriously toxic measures, often without positive results, but undertaken in hopes of averting a potentially fatal outcome. Bone marrow transplantation probably represents the epitome of this state of affairs, but, with the exception of hormonal therapies, prior to the current decade, most cancer treatments fulfilled this forbidding description. On the basis of remarkable events of the past few years, both in supportive care and in the development of new and less toxic therapies, the times may be changing.

Research in both the public and private sectors is adding new tools, both drugs and biological compounds, at a rapid rate and their application is exerting discernible effects on survival in patients with the most common forms of malignancy including the common solid tumors; lung cancer, colon cancer, and breast cancer.

Advances that affect patient survival are clear. Adjuvant therapy reduces recurrence rates in colon cancer and breast cancer by 40%, and the quality of adjuvant therapy, with the addition of new drugs (such as taxanes and biologicals) such as Herceptin is constantly improving. While this is clear progress, it remains disappointing that in some instances we treat 100 patients, all of whom tend to experience some toxic effects of treatment, in order to benefit 10 to 20. Thus, the majority of patients experience risk without benefit, because most were either never destined to relapse, or relapse despite treatment. In addition to finding new and better ways to attack cancers, a major challenge we face is determining whether we might be able to identify and distinguish patients who benefit from therapy from those who do not, based on patient or tumor characteristics knowable before treatment is delivered. Further, we face the challenge of selecting specific therapies based on molecular or genetic features of the tumor. This selection will not only improve treatment, but will also lower the over-all cost of cancer therapy, a matter of growing national concern.

Agents with novel mechanisms of action are demonstrating activity in a variety of clinical settings. At least two classes of agents that inhibit the epidermal growth factor receptor (EGFR) are now approved for use in certain settings. Cetuximab is a monoclonal antibody that blocks the receptor at the cell surface and gefitinib is a small molecule that interferes with the receptor's kinase activity intracellularly. Both have been approved for use in advanced solid tumors after failure of primary therapy. The hope that we might select patients for these therapies based on expression or mutation of EGFR remains to be proven, but early studies suggested that tumors expressing a mutated form of EGFR might be more responsive to gefitinib than tumors expressing wild-type EGFR. This observations must be confirmed in prospective trials. While the contribution of EGFR receptor antagonists is modest at this point, other Her receptor family inhibitors are making a clear contribution. Herceptin, an anti-her2/neu antibody, has won a significant role in the therapy of both advanced and primary Her 2+ breast cancers, in conjunction with chemotherapy.

The field of anti-angiogenic drugs has shown great promise for enhancing therapy for solid tumors. Antibody to vascular endothelial growth factor (VEGF), bevacizumab, extends progression free survival in renal cancer and improves response rates to chemotherapy in metastatic colorectal cancer and lung cancer, and is being tested for its ability to boost the efficacy of adjuvant chemotherapy and radiation therapy in selected tumor types. The success of bevacizumab is remarkable and was not necessarily predictable. While a role for VEGF in neo-vascularization and metastasis is well defined, one might have been skeptical that efforts to absorb all of the autocrine and paracrine secretion of this growth factor in the tumor with a systemically administered antibody was an effective way of interfering with VEGF action. Indeed, it may be shown later that VEGF receptor blockers, such as Su –11248 (Sugen/Pfizer) and Bay43-9006 (Bayer) are more effective than antibody, or are synergistic with antibody. These agents are hitting targets distinct from those attacked by other cancer chemotherapy agents and, most interestingly, the antibodies seem syngergistic with chemotherapy, whether through improving drug delivery or by lowering the threshold for apoptosis.

Some of the new agents work clinically, but we are not sure of their mechanism of action. Bortezomib is believed to interfere with proteasome activity. The proteasome is responsible for degrading cellular proteins, usually those marked for turnover by ubiquitinylation. We are not completely sure how tumor cells are killed by interfering with protein turnover; many hypotheses have been generated. However, it is clear that myeloma and other lymphoid malignancies are susceptible to the effects of bortezomib and ongoing work is trying to clarify how this agent can be rationally combined with others that have distinct mechanisms of action.

Some new agents hit familiar old targets but have advantages over older agents. The drug capecitabine, which requires metabolic activation to 5-fluorouracil, is orally bioavailable, has a long half-life in plasma, and appears to be at least equal in efficacy to infusional 5-fluorouracil plus leucovorin regimens in colon cancer and is active in breast cancer, as well. Because the last step in its activation is by an enzyme found mainly in cancer cells, thymidine phosphorylase, the therapeutic index appears to be increased compared to 5-fluorouracil. A new formulation of paclitaxel complexed to microalbumin (abraxane) seems to have less toxicity than paclitaxel formulated with cremaphor and may be more effective at penetrating tumor masses than the standard paclitaxel formulation.

Several newer agents that interfere with the biology of the estrogen receptor have opened new possibilities for hormonal therapy of breast cancer. It is not entirely clear what situations are best managed with aromatase inhibitors or tamoxifen. Tamoxifen has been proven to reduce cancer incidence by nearly 50% when used as a chemoprevention agent in high risk women. Aromatase inhibitors have not yet been validated as chemopreventive agents, but seem to be more active than tamoxifen in adjuvant therapy of ER+, PR+ breast cancer. In high risk women, should aromatase inhibitors be assumed to be effective preventive agents based on their superiority to tamoxifen in adjuvant studies? Extrapolation from one setting to another would seem to be reasonable; however, some data suggest that women with tumors that are ER+, PR− fare better when treated with adjuvant tamoxifen than with aromatase inhibitors. Given subsets of women in whom each class of agent may be more effective than the other, it isn't possible at this point to know whether the aromatase inhibitors are better chemopreventive agents than tamoxifen. Furthermore, large studies have suggested that 2–5 years of tamoxifen followed by 3–5 years of an aromatase inhibitor may be more effective at minimizing breast cancer recurrence than either tamoxifen or an aromatase inhibitor alone. With so much information unknown and optimal practices undefined, it is important to base therapeutic decisions on clinical trial results in the precise situation your patient is in rather than to hope that the results obtained in a large study are applicable to a patient who would not have been eligible for the study. Are there important differences among the aromatase inhibitors? If so, we haven't found them yet.

New biologic therapies are continuing to be approved for use in cancer patients. The targeting of radionuclides to tumors using monoclonal antibodies is called radioimmunotherapy. Two radionuclides, iodine-131 and yttrium-90, targeted to B cells and B-cell tumors by an anti-CD20 antibody are now in clinical use.

Advances are continuing to be made in supportive care and the prevention and amelioration of toxicity. For example, a new neurokinin receptor blocker, aprepitant, augments the control of cisplatin-induced nausea and vomiting and promises to improve the tolerability of many chemotherapeutic regimens.

This is a brief but impressive list of advances in the past five years. Learning to use all the new tools and integrating their use with those we already have is an enormous task In this new edition of our book, we have sought to provide the wisdom of widely recognized experts. The facts contained herein can form a framework from which clinical decisions can be made. However, the facts are not a substitute for excellent clinical judgment. The practice of medicine in general and oncology in particular cannot appropriately be reduced to recipes and algorithms that are universally applicable to every patient. Each physician has to develop a sense of what the agents can and cannot do based on first-hand experience. We hope the information in this book can form the starting point for the development of clinical skills that subsequent experience will embellish. We are happy to hear your thoughts about how this book could be made more useful to you.

Acknowledgment

Many devoted people made possible this Fourth Edition of *Cancer Chemotherapy and Biotherapy: Principles and Practice* published under the Lippincott, Williams & Wilkins banner. Jonathan W. Pine, Jr., Senior Executive Editor, and Lisa Kairis, Senior Managing Editor, provided constant encouragement, monitored outstanding manuscripts, and watched the calendar, keeping us on track as never before. They were greatly helped by our Editorial Assistants, Renee Johnson and Pat Duffey, whose diligence and spreadsheets kept us on time and under budget. We want to thank the contributing authors, who were extraordinarily conscientious, making our editorial task much easier. We all felt a sense of mission about this book, as we do about our field in general.

There are others we wish to recognize. Our many fellows and colleagues in the field of medical oncology, many of whom have contributed to this book, have always been the sustaining force behind our work and have only added to our passion to cure this disease. We were fortunate to share this passion with our close colleagues in the Medicine Branch, National Cancer Institute, Bob Young, Vince DeVita, and George Canellos, and with our fellow faculty members at the Massachusetts General Hospital and Harvard, and at the National Institutes of Health. Our patients give us the courage to continue seeking better treatments, in spite of failures and disappointments. With the benefit of decades of experience, we have seen remarkable progress, but for most of those patients, the benefits came too late.

Finally and most importantly, we owe much to our wives and children, who, despite their own careers and family concerns, never lose interest in what we do, and recognize that it is much more than a job.

Contributors

GHEATH ALATRASH, DO, PhD
Department of General Internal Medicine
The Cleveland Clinic Foundation
Cleveland, Ohio

CARMEN J. ALLEGRA, MD
Chief Medical Officer
Network for Medical Communication and
    Research
North Potomac, Maryland

KENNETH ANDERSON, MD
Division of Hematologic Oncology
Department of Medical Oncology
Dana-Farber Cancer Institute
Harvard Medical School
Boston, Massachusetts

STEVEN D. AVERBUCH, MD, MSc
Senior Medical Director
U.S. Drug Development
Astrazeneca Pharmaceuticals, LP
Wilmington, Delaware

TRACY T. BATCHELOR, MD
Chief
Division of Neuro-Oncology
Department of Neurology
Massachusetts General Hospital
Associate Professor of Neurology
Harvard Medical School
Boston, Massachusetts

LAWRENCE S. BLASZKOWSKY, MD
Instructor of Medicine
Department of Hemotology and Oncology
Massachusetts General Hospital
Boston, Massachusetts

ERNEST C. BORDEN, MD
Director
Center for Drug Discovery and
    Development
Taussig Cancer Center
The Cleveland Clinic Foundation
Learner Research Institute
Cleveland, Ohio

ANGELA BRADBURY, MD
Fellow
Department of Medicine
University of Chicago Medical Center
Section of Hematology/Oncology
Chicago, Illinois

RONALD M. BUKOWSKI, MD
Professor
Department of Medical Onocology and Hematology
Director
Experimental Therapeutics Program
Taussig Cancer Center
The Cleveland Clinic Foundation
Cleveland, Ohio

BRUCE A. CHABNER, MD
Professor of Medicine
Harvard Medical School
Clinical Director
Massachusetts General Hospital Cancer Center
Boston, Massachusetts

JEFFREY W. CLARK, MD
Assistant Professor of Medicine
Associate Physician
Medical Director, Clinical Research
Operations Office
Tucker Gosnell Gastrointestinal Cancer Center
Massachusetts General Hospital
Boston, Massachusetts

A. DIMITRIOS COLEVAS, MD
Senior Investigator
Investigational Drug Branch
Cancer Therapy Evaluation Program
National Cancer Institute, Bethesda, Maryland

JERRY M. COLLINS, PhD
Associate Director
Developmental Therapeutics Program
National Cancer Institute
Bethesda, Maryland

O. MICHAEL COLVIN, MD
Director Emeritus
Duke Comprehensive Cancer Center
Duke University Medical Center
Durham, North Carolina

JANET E. DANCEY, MD, FRCPC
Cancer Therapy Evaluation Program
National Cancer Institute
Bethesda, Maryland

ROBERT B. DIASIO, MD
Professor of Medicine and Pharmacology
Department of Pharmacology and Toxicology
University of Alabama at Birmingham
Birmingham, Alabama

ROSS C. DONEHOWER, MD
Professor of Medicine
Department of Oncology
Johns Hopkins University School of Medicine
Baltimore, Maryland

JAMES H. DOROSHOW, MD
Director
Division of Cancer Treatment and Diagnosis
National Cancer Institute
Bethesda, Maryland

GLENN DRANOFF, MD
Associate Professor
Department of Medicine
Harvard Medical School
Department of Medical Oncology
Dana-Farber Cancer Institute
Boston, Massachusetts

CHARLES ERLICHMAN, MD
Professor of Oncology
Department of Medical Oncology
Mayo Medical School
Mayo Clinic and Mayo Foundation
Rochester, Minnesota

JAMES H. FINKE, PhD
Staff Scientist
Department of Immunology
Lerner Research Institute
Taussig Cancer Center
The Cleveland Clinic Foundation
Cleveland, Ohio

JEANNE FOURIE, PhD
Postdoctoral Fellow
University of Alabama at Birmingham
Department of Pharmacology and Toxicology and Wallace
   Tumor Institute
Comprehensive Cancer Center
Birmingham, Alabama

HENRY S. FREIDMAN, MD
James B. Powell, Jr. Professor of Neuro-Oncology
The Brain Tumor Center at Duke
Duke University Medical Center
Durham, North Carolina

ALISON M. FRIEDMANN, MD
Assistant Professor
Division of Pediatric Hematology/Oncology
Massachusetts General Hospital
Boston, Massachusetts

ROCIO GARCIA-CARBONERO, MD
Consultant in Medical Oncology
Department of Hematology-Oncology
Hospital Clinico Universitario de Valencia
Valencia, Spain

FRANÇOIS GOLDWASSER, MD, PhD
Unite d'oncologie Medicale
Groupe Hospitalier Cochin
Paris, France

WILLIAM J. GRADISHAR, MD, FACP
Professor of Medicine
Division of Hematology/Oncology
Robert H. Lurie Comprehensive Cancer Center
Feinberg School of Medicine
Northwestern University
Chicago, Illinois

JEAN L. GREM, MD, FACP
Professor of Medicine
Department of Internal Medicine
University of Nebraska Medical Center
Omaha, Nebraska

KENNETH R. HANDE, MD
Professor of Medicine and Pharmacology
Vanderbilt University School of Medicine
Nashville, Tennessee

TERU HIDESHIMA, MD
Division of Hematologic Oncology
Department of Medical Oncology
Dana-Farber Cancer Institute
Harvard Medical School
Boston, Massachusetts

MELINDA HOLLINGSHEAD, DVM, PhD
Chief
Biological Testing Branch
Developmental Therapeutics Program
Division of Cancer Treatment and Diagnosis
National Cancer Institute
Fredrick, Maryland

S. PERCY IVY, MD
Senior Investigator
Investigational Drug Branch
Cancer Therapy Evaluation Program
National Cancer Institute
Rockville, Maryland

ROY B. JONES, PhD, MD
Professor
Blood and Marrow Transplantation
University of Texas MD Anderson Cancer Center
Houston, Texas

CARL H. JUNE, MD
Professor of Pathology and Laboratory Medicine
University of Pennsylvania School of Medicine
Director
Translational Research
Abramson Cancer Center
Philadelphia, Pennsylvania

RICHARD P. JUNGHANS, MD
Boston University School of Medicine
Roger Williams Medical Center
Boston, Massachusetts

JOSEPH G. JURCIC, MD
Assistant Member
Leukemia Service
Department of Medicine and Molecular Pharmacology
and Chemistry Program
Memorial Sloan-Kettering Cancer Center
New York, New York

BENNETT KAUFMAN, PhD
PSI International, Inc.
Fairfax , Virginia

PAULA M. KROSKY, PhD
Science Applications International Corporation
Fredrick National Cancer Institute
Frederick, Maryland

JOANNE KURTZBERG, MD
Professor of Pediatrics and Pathology
Director
Pediatric Blood and Marrow Transplant Program
Director
Carolinas Cord Blood Bank at Duke
Durham, North Carolina

DAVID J. KUTER, MD, DPhil
Chief of Hematology
Massachusetts General Hospital
Associate Professor of Medicine
Harvard Medical School
Boston, Massachusetts

JOHN S. LAZO, PhD
Professor and Chair
Department of Pharmacology
University of Pittsburg School of Medicine
Pittsburg, Pennsylvania

PETER F. LEBOWITZ, MD
Assistant Professor of Medicine
Lombardi Comprehensive Cancer Center
Georgetown University, Washington, DC

DANIEL J. LINDNER, MD, PhD
Associate Professor
Department of Molecular Medicine
Learner college of Medicine
Case Western Reserve, Tussig Cancer Center
The Cleveland Clinic Foundation, Cleveland, Ohio

DAN L. LONGO, MD
Scientific Director
National Institute on Aging
National Institutes of Health
Gerontology Research Center
Baltimore, Maryland

PAUL A. MASCI, DO
Division of Medical Oncology/Hematology
The Cleveland Clinic Foundation
Cleveland, Ohio

CONSTANTINE S. MITSIADES, MD, PhD
Department of Adult Oncology
Dana-Farber Cancer Institute
Harvard Medical School
Boston, Massachusetts

BRIAN P. MONAHAN, MD, FACP
Chair and Associate Professor of Medicine
Director of the Division of Hematology/Oncology
F. Edward Hebert School of Medicine
Uniformed Services, University of the Health Sciences
Bethesda, Maryland.

MACIEJ M. MRUGALA, MD, PhD
Clinical Fellow
Division of Neuro-Onocology
Department of Neurology
Massachusetts General Hospital
Stephen E & Catherine Pappas Center for Neuro-Oncology
Harvard Medical School
Boston, Massachusetts

DEBORAH A. MULFORD, MD
Assistant Member
Leukemia Service
Department of Medicine
Memorial Sloan-Kettering Cancer Center
New York, New York

LEN NECKERS, PhD
Urologic Oncology Branch
National Cancer Institute
Bethesda, Maryland

KEES NOOTER, MD
Division of Medical Oncology
Erasmus University Medical Center
Rotterdam, The Netherlands

OWEN A. O'CONNOR, MD, PhD
Assistant Attending Physician
Department of Medicine
Memorial Sloan Kettering Cancer Center
New York, New York

LUIS PAZ-ARES, MD, PhD
Consultant in Medical Oncology
Division of Medical Oncology
Hospital Universitario Doce de Octubre
Madrid, Spain

WILLIAM P. PETROS, PharmD, FCCP
Professor of Basic Pharmaceutical Services
School of Pharmacy
West Virginia University Health Sciences Center
Associate Director
Mary Babb Randolph Cancer Center
Morgantown, West Virginia

YVES G. POMMIER, MD, PhD
National Cancer Institute
National Institutes of Health
Bethesda, Maryland

EDDIE REED, MD
Director
Division of Cancer Prevention and Control
National Center for Chronic Disease Prevention and Helath
    Promotion
The Centers for Disease Control and Prevention
Atlanta, Georgia

FREDERIC J. REU, MD
Center for Drug Discovery and Development
Taussig Cancer Center
The Cleveland Clinic Foundation
Learner Research Institute
Cleveland, Ohio

PAUL RICHARDSON, MD
Division of Hematologic Oncology
Department of Medical Oncology
Dana-Farver Cancer Institute
Harvard Medical School
Boston, Massachusetts

THOMAS G. ROBERTS, JR, MD, MSocSci
Division of Hematology/Oncology
Massachusetts General Hospital
Harvard Medical School
Boston, Massachusetts
Program on the Pharmaceutical Industry
Massachusetts Institute of Technology
Cambridge, Massachusetts, Boston, Massachusetts

RACHEL P. ROSOVSKY, MD
Instructor in Medicine
Harvard Medical School
Boston, Massachusetts

ERIC K. ROWINSKY, MD, FACP
Chief Medical Officer
Senior Vice President
ImClone Systems, Inc., New York

DAVID P. RYAN, MD
Assistant Professor of Medicine
Harvard Medical School
Clinical Director
Tucker Gosnell Gastrointestinal Cancer Center
Massachusetts General Hospital
Boston, Massachusetts

EDWARD A. SAUSVILLE, MD, PhD, FACP
Professor
Department of Medicine
University of Maryland
Associate Director
Greenebaum Cancer Center
Baltimore, Maryland

ORIT SCHARF, PhD
PSI International, Inc.
Fairfax , Virginia

DAVID A. SCHEINBERG, MD, PhD
Chairman
Molecular Pharmacology and Chemistry
Sloan Kettering Institute
New York, New York

RICHARD L. SCHILSKY, MD
Professor
Department of Medicine
Associate Dean for Clinical Research
University of Chicago
Chicago, Illinois

GEORGE SGOUROS, MD
Associate Professor
Johns Hopkins University
School of Medicine
Baltimore, Maryland

ROBERT H. SHOEMAKER, PhD
Chief
Screening Technologies Branch
Developmental Therapeutics Program
Division of Cancer Treatment and Diagnosis
National Cancer Institute
Fredrick, Maryland

MATTHEW R. SMITH, MD, PhD
Assistant Professor
Harvard Medical School
Assistant Physician
Department of Hematology and Oncology
Massachusetts General Hospital
Boston, Massachusetts

ALEX SPARREBOOM, PhD
Staff Scientist
Clinical Pharmacology Research Core
National Cancer Institute
Bethesda, Maryland

JEFFREY G. SUPKO, PhD
Associate Professor of Medicine
Harvard Medical School
Director
Clinical Pharmacology Laboratory
Massachusetts General Hospital Cancer Center
Boston, Massachusetts

SANDRA M. SWAIN, MD
Chief
Cancer Therapeutics Branch
National Cancer Institute
Bethesda, Maryland

RICHARD SWERDLOW, PhD
PSI International, Inc.
Fairfax , Virginia

CHARLES S. TANNENBAUM, PhD
Project Scientist
Department of Immunology
Lerner Research Institute
The Cleveland Clinic Foundation
Cleveland, Ohio

KEVIN L. TAYLOR, PhD
Technology Specialist
Invitrogen Corporation
Carlsbad, California

KENNETH D. TEW, PhD, DSc
John C. West Chair in Cancer Research
Chairman
Department of Cell and Molecular Pharmacology
    and Experimental Therapeutics
Medical University of South Carolina
Charleston, South Carolina

LUCY VERESHCHAGINA, PhD
PSI International, Inc.
Fairfax, Virginia

JAAP VERWEIJ, MD, PhD
Division of Medical Oncology
Erasmus University Medical Center
Rotterdam, The Netherlands

EDWIN W. WILLEMS, MD
Division of Medical Oncology
Erasmus University Medical Center
Rotterdam, The Netherlands

ANAADRIANA ZAKARIJA, MD
Instructor of Medicine
Division of Hematology/Oncology
Feinberg School of Medicine
Northwestern University
Chicago, Illinois

WILLIAM C. ZAMBONI, PharmD
Assistant Professor of Pharmaceutical Sciences
    and Medicine
University of Pittsburgh Cancer Institute
Pittsburgh, Pennsylvania

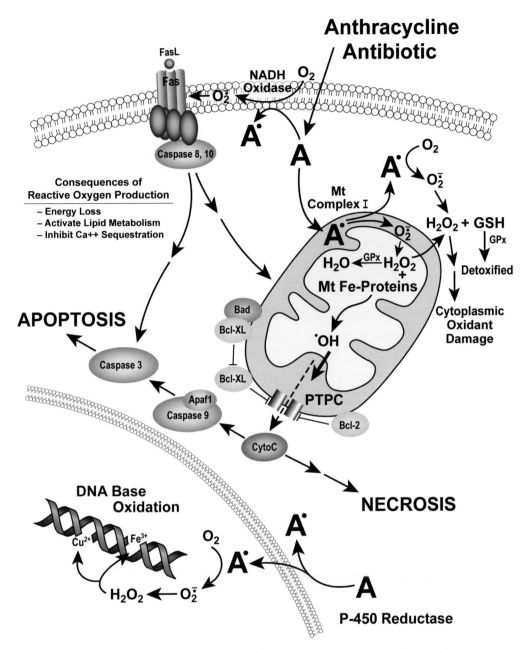

Figure 18.4 Anthracycline antibiotic cell death program. Anthracycline antibiotics can be metabolized at the cell surface, at complex I of the mitochondrial electron transport chain, in the cytosol, or at the nuclear envelop by flavin-containing dehydrogenases, leading to the production of reactive oxygen species with the potential to alter intracellular iron stores at multiple intracellular sites. This free-radical cascade can initiate both apoptotic and necrotic death programs associated with mitochondrial membrane injury, DNA base oxidation, altered calcium sequestration, energy loss, and altered proliferative potential. The effects of anthracycline-enhanced reactive oxygen production are modulated by intracellular antioxidant enzymes (glutathione peroxidase, catalase) and anti-apoptotic proteins. Mt, mitochondrial.

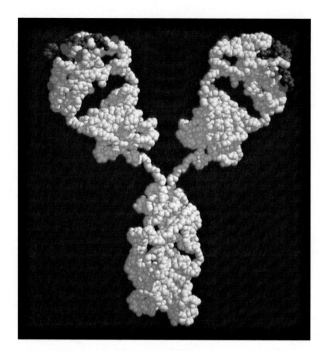

Figure 31.2 Space-filling model of human immunoglobulin G1 antibody with complementarity-determining regions in color representing anti–Tac-H; human myeloma protein Eu with complementarity-determining regions grafted from murine anti-Tac. (Photo provided courtesy of Dr. C. Queen.)

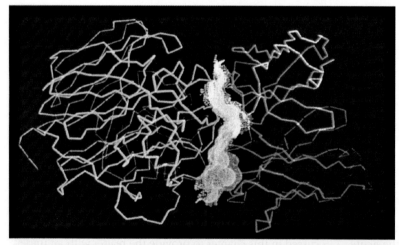

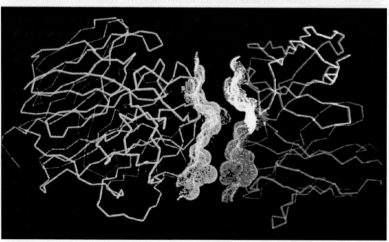

Figure 31.3 Antigen-antibody binding surface juxtaposition. The variable (V) region (Fv) of antibody (*right*) binds to influenza virus protein neuraminidase (*left*) in the top panel. The V_H (*red*) and V_L (*blue*) regions are separately colored to show their respective binding contributions. The bottom panel offsets the two molecules by 8 Å to show the complementarity of surfaces that promotes the binding interaction. The stippled surface of the neuraminidase defines the antigen "epitope." (Photo provided courtesy of Drs. P.M. Colman and W.R. Tulip, CSIRO Australia.)

Clinical Strategies for Cancer Treatment: The Role of Drugs

1

Bruce A. Chabner

Cancer treatment requires the cooperative efforts of multiple medical specialties. Although surgeons traditionally have been the first specialists to treat the cancer patient, newer modalities have created important roles for the radiotherapist and medical oncologist in the initial management of cancer patients, and responsibility for care of the majority of patients with metastatic cancer is in the hands of these specialists. The array of alternatives for the treatment of cancer is constantly expanding. With the demonstration of effectiveness of new drugs and new biologics, and with the evolution of more effective strategies for integrating chemotherapy, surgery, and radiation, the development of a treatment plan becomes increasingly complex. The plan must be based on a thorough understanding of the potential for beneficial response and an awareness of the acute and later toxicities of each component of the treatment regimen.

As a general rule, the medical oncologist is urged to use standard regimens as described in the *Physician Data Query* (*PDQ*) system of the National Cancer Institute (NCI).[a] *PDQ* contains information on state-of-the-art treatments for each pathologic type of cancer, as well as a listing of experimental protocols for each disease. An important alternative to "standard" therapy is the clinical trial, which should be considered for every eligible patient. Such trials offer alternative treatment that is thought by a panel of experts to be at least as effective as the recognized standard of care. In phase III (randomized) trials, a standard regimen is compared with a new one that may represent an improvement. With either choice, standard therapy or a clinical trial, the medical oncologist must understand the potential benefits and risks of using specific drugs or combinations of drugs, or combinations of drugs and biologics, often integrated with surgery and irradiation. All these considerations enter into the choice of a treatment plan. Steps in the treatment decision-making process are discussed in this chapter to provide the reader with an understanding of the overall role of drugs in cancer treatment.

DETERMINANTS OF TREATMENT PLANNING

The first and primary determinant of treatment is the histologic diagnosis. Malignant neoplasms occur in over 100 different pathologic forms, each with a characteristic natural history, pattern of progression, and responsiveness to treatment. Thus, the *histologic diagnosis*, usually made by surgical biopsy or excision of a primary tumor, is of critical importance as a first step in treatment planning. The clinical oncologist must be alert to the possibility of atypical presentations of treatable and even curable tumors, such as

---

[a]*PDQ* is available to physicians at most medical libraries, at many hospitals, through the Internet, or through private computer software vendors. Access to *PDQ* is also available directly from the NCI through the NCI Information Associates Program. For information about accessing *PDQ*, call the Information Associates Program Customer Service Desk at 1-800-NCI-7890 (or call 301-816-2083 outside the United States).

germ cell tumors of the testis and breast cancer, and must ask for special immunohistologic or molecular tests to rule in or rule out a potentially curable tumor type. For example, germ cell tumors may arise occasionally in the thoracic or abdominal cavity in the absence of a primary testicular tumor; still, these unusual presentations retain an excellent response to appropriate chemotherapy. Treatment in cases lacking a precise histologic diagnosis is usually directed against the most responsive tumor type within the realm of possible diagnoses, such as testicular carcinoma in a patient with poorly differentiated carcinoma of uncertain origin, and occasionally produces durable responses.[1]

In certain cases—for example, lung carcinoma or the non-Hodgkin's lymphomas—accurate *subtyping* of tumors is important because the subtypes of these diseases have different patterns of clinical response to treatment. Subtyping may require the characterization of cell surface immunologic markers (e.g., to distinguish T-cell and B-cell lymphomas), the identification of specific intracellular secretory granules or enzymatic markers, such as dopa decarboxylase in small cell carcinoma of the lung, or the S100 antigen to rule out malignant melanoma. Molecular or genetic analysis may reveal important prognostic information for subtyping leukemias, lymphomas, and lung cancers.[2] Epidermal growth factor receptor mutations identify a unique subgroup of patients with non-small cell lung cancer highly responsive to the epidermal growth factor receptor (EGFR) inhibitor (Iressa).[3] The essential point is that the precise identity of a tumor is the single most important determinant of treatment choice and patient management. In premenopausal women with stage I breast cancer (less than 2 cm primary, node negative), adverse tumor features, such as a high S-phase (DNA synthetic phase) fraction, absence of estrogen or progesterone receptors, or high expression of the *c-erbB-2/HER-2-neu* oncogene, may guide the selection of drugs for adjuvant therapy, such as dose-intensive adjuvant chemotherapy and herceptin. *Her-2-neu* positive metastatic disease is also best treated with herceptin and chemotherapy.[4]

While gene array studies have provided significant insight into subgroups of cancer with favorable or unfavorable prognosis, or with a high propensity for metastasis,[4] they have not yet demonstrated the ability to guide specific choice of therapies. Gene profiles that interrogate drug resistance markers for cytotoxic or hormonal therapy[5–7] may provide this guidance in the future. Molecular analysis of target molecules such as receptor tyrosine kinases and signaling pathways will undoubtedly be useful in developing a functional classification of human tumors that will in guide the selection of therapy for most kinds of cancer.[8]

Staging

The next step in treatment planning is to determine the extent of disease, and specifically whether the tumor is curable by local treatment measures such as surgery or radiation therapy. The process of determining the extent of disease is termed *staging* and plays an important role in making therapeutic choices for diseases that are responsive to multiple types of treatment. For example, non-Hodgkin's lymphomas with "indolent" histology are curable with radiotherapy in a majority of cases when the tumor is confined to a single lymph node region (stage I), but are rarely curable, even with aggressive early chemotherapy, when more extensive lymph node involvement or dissemination to extranodal sites is present. Immediate treatment of stage I disease with radiation is indicated, whereas, paradoxically, no immediate therapy may be indicated for patients with advanced disease.

Individualizing Treatment Choice

The choice of specific therapies depends on histology, molecular and immunologic subtype, stage, and an additional factor, the patient's probable tolerance for the side effects of the various possible treatments. Although chemotherapy cures a substantial fraction of patients with diffuse large cell lymphoma, not all patients with this diagnosis are suitable candidates for intensive treatment. Severely debilitated patients and those with underlying medical problems—for example, heart disease, renal failure, diabetes, or chronic obstructive pulmonary disease—might well suffer severely disabling or fatal complications from potentially curative regimens, as indicated in Table 1.1. In such cases, the physician and patient may choose a less toxic, palliative regimen. The ultimate decision must be based on a thorough understanding of the disease process under consideration, the *clinical* pharmacology of the drugs in question, and the potential benefits and risks of alternative forms of treatment, such as chemotherapy, radiotherapy, or surgery.

Finally, possessing the information about histology, stage, and other tumor-related variables and about the patient's age and baseline health, the oncologist must decide whether a realistic opportunity exists for curative treatment. A decision to treat with curative intent demands a high degree of adherence to drug dosage and scheduling requirements, as specified in the standard or experimental regimen, and an acceptance of treatment-related toxicity. When cure is not a realistic expectation, a decision to treat must be based on an expectation for prolongation of the patient's life or an improvement in the quality of life. In these cases, treatment-related side effects may be minimized by dosage adjustments or treatment delays, when necessary, but at the cost of antitumor efficacy. When the probability for benefit is low, chemotherapy should be offered only after frank and thorough discussion of the likely outcome. In such cases, experimental phase I or phase II drugs may be a more attractive alternative in the setting of a clinical trial.

TABLE 1.1		
TOXICITY OF CHOP REGIMEN FOR TREATING DIFFUSE LARGE CELL LYMPHOMA		
Drugs	**Toxicity**[a]	**Risk Factors**
Cyclophosphamide	Hair loss, myelosuppression, hemorrhagic cystitis, secondary leukemia	Underlying infection
Doxorubicin hydrochloride (Adriamycin)	Cardiomyopathy, myelosuppression, hair loss	History of heart disease, prior chest irradiation
Vincristine sulfate (Oncovin)	Peripheral and autonomic neuropathy	Liver dysfunction, other neurotoxic drugs, inherited or acquired peripheral neuropathy
Prednisone	Glucose intolerance, immune suppression, bone and muscle loss	Diabetes, underlying infection

[a]In general, elderly patients are at increased risk of toxicity because of underlying medical problems and altered rates of drug elimination.

DRUGS IN CANCER TREATMENT

Drugs are now used at some time during the course of the illness of most cancer patients. Cytotoxic drugs can cure some disseminated cancers (Table 1.2) and can be effective in decreasing tumor volume, alleviating symptoms, and even prolonging life in many other types of metastatic cancer. *Adjuvant* chemotherapy regimens are used in patients who have had primary tumors resected and who, although possibly cured by surgery, are at significant risk of recurrence. Adjuvant therapy has been shown in randomized trials to delay tumor recurrence and prolong survival in patients with breast cancer, colorectal cancer, non-small cell lung cancer, osteosarcoma, and other tumors. *Neoadjuvant* chemotherapy is used to reduce the bulk of primary tumors before surgical resection or irradiation of locally extensive head and neck carcinomas, esophageal cancer, non-small cell lung cancer, osteosarcoma and soft tissue sarcomas, bladder cancer, and locally advanced breast cancer. This approach can improve the probability of total surgical resection, decrease local recurrence, and allow organ preservation. Furthermore, the initial clinical response of the tumor mass can serve as an indication to continue therapy after surgery.

The design of drug treatment regimens is based on a number of considerations. These include (a) prior knowledge of the responsiveness of the pathologic category of tumor to specific drugs, (b) an understanding of the biochemical mechanisms of the drugs' cytotoxic activity as well as the mechanisms of resistance to the drugs, and (c) knowledge of the drugs' pharmacokinetic behavior and of patterns of normal organ toxicity. Some chemotherapy regimens have been designed to minimize emergence of drug resistance, based on the predictions of theoretical models of drug resistance. The biologic and pharmacokinetic features of individual drugs are considered in detail in succeeding chapters, but the impact of these and other factors, such as cell kinetics and drug mechanism of action and mechanism of resistance, on trial design is reviewed briefly at this juncture to provide a framework for understanding the use of individual agents.

Kinetic Basis of Drug Therapy

The objective of cancer treatment is to reduce the tumor cell population to zero cells. Chemotherapy experiments using rapidly growing transplanted tumors in mice have established the validity of the *fractional cell kill hypothesis*, which states that a given drug concentration applied for a defined time period will kill a constant fraction of the cell population, independent of the absolute number of cells. Regrowth of tumor occurs during the drug-free interval between cycles. Thus, each treatment cycle kills a specific fraction of the remaining cells. The results of treatment are a direct function of (a) the dose of drug administered and (b) the number and frequency of repetitions of treatment.

Most current chemotherapy regimens are based on cytokinetic considerations and use cycles of intensive therapy repeated as frequently as allowed by the tolerance of dose-limiting tissues, such as bone marrow or gastrointestinal tract. The object of these cycles is to reduce the absolute number of remaining tumor cells to zero (or less than one) through the multiplicative effect of successive fractional cell kills. (For example, given 99% cell kill per cycle, a tumor burden of 10^{11} cells will be reduced to less than one cell with six cycles of treatment: $[10^{11} \text{ cells}] \times [0.01]^6 < 1$.)

The fractional cell kill hypothesis was defined initially in animal models of leukemia and was applied most successfully in human leukemia and lymphoma.[9] The fundamental assumption of constant fractional cell kill per cycle

---

TABLE 1.2

CURABILITY OF DISSEMINATED CANCER WITH DRUGS

Disease	Therapy	Probable Cure Rate
Adults		
Hodgkin disease (stage III or IV)	Combination chemotherapy	50% or higher
Testicular carcinoma (stage III)	Combination chemotherapy followed by surgery	90% or higher
Gestational choriocarcinoma	Methotrexate sodium ± dactinomycin (actinomycin D)	90%
Ovarian carcinoma	Platinum-containing combination chemotherapy	10%
Acute myelogenous leukemia	Combination chemotherapy	50%
Hairy cell leukemia	Cladribine	80–90%
Acute lymphocytic leukemia	Combination chemotherapy plus cranial irradiation	50% or higher
Intermediate- and high-grade non-Hodgkin lymphomas	Combination chemotherapy	50% or higher
Wilms' tumor and sarcomas	Surgery, chemotherapy, and irradiation	50%
Burkitt's lymphoma	Combination chemotherapy	80%

with constant dosing is unlikely to be valid for the more heterogeneous, slowly growing solid tumors in humans. Most clinical neoplasms are recognized at a stage of decelerating growth, which may be due to poor tumor vascularity with resulting hypoxia or poor nutrient supply, or to other unidentified factors. These tumors contain a high fraction of slowly dividing or noncycling cells (termed G_0 cells). Antineoplastic agents, particularly the antimetabolites and antitumor antibiotics, are most effective against rapidly dividing cells and some are *phase-specific* (i.e., most effective in killing cells in a specific phase in the cell cycle). The initial kinetic features of a large, poorly vascularized tumor are unfavorable for treatment with most antimetabolites, which kill most effectively in the S phase. Drugs that attack DNA integrity, such as alkylators and adduct forming platinum derivatives retain activity against nondividing or slowly dividing cells, and are often used to reduce tumor bulk. An initial reduction in cell numbers produced by surgery, radiotherapy, or non–cell cycle-specific drugs improves blood flow, pushes the slowly dividing cells into more rapid cell division, and may recruit nondividing cells into the cell cycle, where they become increasingly susceptible to therapy with cell cycle-specific agents. Thus, an initially slowly responding tumor may become more responsive to therapy after surgical debulking or with continued treatment, and fractional cell kill may actually increase with sequential courses of treatment.

Biochemical heterogeneity of human tumors introduces additional complexity to the simple hypothesis that multiple cycles of fractional cell kill translate into tumor cure. Isoenzyme typing and karyotypic analysis of tumors demonstrate that most human tumors studied thus far have evolved clonally from a single malignant cell.[10] Techniques for in vitro cloning of solid tumors have shown, however, that this original homogeneity does not persist during later stages of tumor growth; in fact, both experimental and human tumors are composed of cell types with differing biochemical, morphologic, and drug-response characteristics.[11] This heterogeneity results from the inherent genetic instability of malignant cells. Indeed, mutations in cell-cycle checkpoint control genes, such as *p53*, and in DNA repair genes, such as the *MSH* genes in familial colon cancer, may be the initial event in malignant transformation of many tumor types, establishing a fundamentally mutable clone from which diverse subclones evolve. Thus, gene amplifications, deletions, or other alterations of genes coding for target proteins that control drug response and cell cycle lead to heterogeneity of the tumor cell population and probably account for outgrowth of resistant tumor cells during relapse of formerly sensitive tumors. This has been clearly demonstrated in the isolation of Gleevec-resistant cells from selected patients with chronic myelogenous leukemia prior to treatment.[12] When cells are subjected to the selective pressure of drug treatment, sensitive tumor cells are destroyed, but subpopulations of resistant cells survive and proliferate. With the possible exceptions of treatment of chronic myelogenous leukemia with Gleevec, gestational choriocarcinoma treated with methotrexate, cyclophosphamide treatment for African Burkitt lymphoma, and cladribine treatment for hairy cell leukemia, single-agent chemotherapy has rarely produced long-term survival or cure of advanced malignancies. The most successful drug treatment regimens have combined multiple agents with different mechanisms of action.

Prediction of Drug Response to Individual Agents

The selection of drugs for treating specific types of cancer is largely based on the results of previous clinical trials and is often empirical. To avoid the needless toxicity of ineffective agents, especially in diseases with only modest rates of response, predicting sensitivity for the specific tumor and patient at hand would be desirable. Various experimental systems for testing tumor cells or tumor fragments for response to panels of drugs have been studied intensively in the hope that they would accurately predict response in patients. Although some of these tests have been accurate in predicting resistance to various drugs in populations of highly resistant patients, with the possible exception of cell-based assays for resistance in acute lymphoblastic leukemia[7] and ovarian cancer,[13] limited data exist to justify their routine use.

Biochemical tests for the presence of a specific enzyme critical to the response of an antimetabolite (such as deoxycytidine kinase for cytosine arabinoside, or thymidylate synthase for the fluoropyrimidines) or the presence of a specific cytoplasmic receptor, such as the estrogen receptor for hormonal therapy of breast cancer, can discriminate responders from nonresponders. A few of these tests—most notably the test for estrogen receptor or *HER-2-neu* expression in breast cancer—have become cornerstones for therapeutic decision-making; other tests offer considerable promise. A study of non-small cell lung cancer showed that expression of components of the DNA repair pathway correlated with patient survival after platinum-based treatment.[14] Similarly, high concentrations of dihydrofolate reductase have been associated with resistance to methotrexate, as is a failure to transport or polyglutamate the drug.[15,16] High levels of the DNA repair enzyme O^6-alkylguanine alkyl transferase predict resistance to nitrosoureas, dacarbazine, and temozolomide, which damage DNA by alkylating the O^6 position of guanine.[17] The latter test may prove useful in predicting which patients will benefit from pretreatment with O^6-benzyl guanine, an irreversible inhibitor of the alkyl transferase enzyme that is in clinical testing. Mutations in mismatch DNA repair are associated experimentally with cisplatin resistance.[18] None of these molecular biochemical tests have been studied prospectively in a sizable patient population to prove their value in selecting routine treatment with cytotoxic drugs. In each case, other potentially important changes are known to occur in experimental examples of resistance to the various drugs.

Molecularly targeted drug discovery offers the hope of identifying new drugs tailored specifically to the mutations critical for malignant transformation and tumor progression, with limited toxicity to normal tissues lacking the molecular target. One such target, the tyrosine kinase, results from the bcr-abl translocation in chronic myelocytic leukemia.[18] Gleevec, an inhibitor of the BCR-abl

kinase, has striking activity in chronic and blastic phases of chronic myelocytic leukemia.[19] Because it also inhibits the c-kit tyrosine kinase, it was used against gastrointestinal stromal tumors, which exhibit high levels of expression of this receptor; it proved to be particularly active against gastrointestinal stromal tumors that have mutated and constitutively activated c-kit.[20]

The epidermal growth factor receptor has also become the object of targeted drug discovery. Antibodies or small molecules that bind to and inhibit this receptor show potent tumor inhibitory activity against epithelial tumors that overexpress the EGFR. In addition Erbitux, a monoclonal antibody against EGFR, shows synergy with irinotecan against relapsed colon cancer.[21] The synergy is believed to result from blockade of a critical growth factor signal, an event that lowers the tumor cell threshold for apoptosis. As mentioned previously, mutations and deletions that activate EGFR predict for response to Iressa.[3] Other interactions between cytotoxic drugs and signal pathway inhibitors, leading to synergistic cell kill, have been described for antiangiogenic drugs against colon cancer and the *HER-2-neu* receptor inhibitor, herceptin, with taxanes or anthracyclines against breast cancer. This general principle of drug-signal inhibitor interaction will undoubtedly be further exploited in treating cancers that present biologic targets related to overexpressed growth factor pathways. The reader is referred to the chapter on molecularly targeted therapies for a more detailed discussion of this subject.

PHARMACOKINETIC DETERMINANTS OF RESPONSE

Although the outcome of cancer chemotherapy depends in large part on the inherent sensitivity of the specific tumor being treated, the chances for success, even in patients with sensitive tumors, can be compromised by failure to consider important pharmacokinetic factors such as drug absorption, metabolism, and elimination in designing protocols that determine the dose, schedule, and route of drug administration.

Not only may protocol design affect pharmacokinetics and response, but even among patients with apparently normal hepatic and renal function, considerable variability is seen in peak drug concentration, area under the concentration $\times$ time curve (AUC).[22] The origin of this variability is uncertain. Clearly, pharmacogenetics (polymorphisms in expression of drug-metabolizing enzymes) plays an important role in determining the rate of elimination and thus the toxicity of some drugs, including irinotecan hydrochloride (by glucuronyl transferases), 6-mercaptopurine (by thiopurine methyl transferase), and 5-fluorouracil (by dihydropyrimidine dehydrogenase).[23] Genetic polymorphisms may also influence the susceptibility of tumors to cytotoxic and targeted drugs. In addition, differences in hepatic P-450 isoenzyme activity, protein binding of drug, and age-related changes in renal tubular function all contribute to this variability. The fact remains that most pharmacokinetic studies show at least a long range of drug concentration and AUC for a given dose of drug.

Pharmacokinetic factors are important not only in designing general protocol but also in determining specific modifications of dosage in individual patients. Dosage may be increased or decreased based on observed patterns of toxicity or lack of same and, in some cases, may be based on direct drug concentration measurements. Renal or hepatic dysfunction leads to delayed drug elimination, which sometimes results in overwhelming toxicity. To avoid such toxicity, dosages of certain agents must be modified based on estimates of renal or hepatic function.

Interindividual variations are not predictable solely on the basis of renal or hepatic function, however, and direct measurement of plasma drug concentrations can provide a better guide for dosage adjustment to ensure adequate and safe drug exposure, as shown by studies of maintenance therapy in children with acute lymphocytic leukemia and who receive methotrexate and 6-mercaptopurine.[24] One important source of the interindividual variability in pharmacokinetics is the variable oral absorption of a number of agents, including hexamethylmelamine, etoposide, methotrexate (in doses of more than 15 mg/m^2), 6-mercaptopurine, 5-fluorouracil (5-FU), busulfan in high-dose therapy, and phenylalanine mustard, and even the targeted drug, Gleevec. This problem has been documented by pharmacokinetic studies, and may lead to a poor therapeutic result. Drug concentration monitoring may provide a valuable guide to delayed elimination of agents such as methotrexate.[24] Monitoring allows dosage adjustment of the cytotoxic drug in later cycles and early institution or prolongation of rescue procedures. Reliable assays are available for many antineoplastic agents; most assays use high-pressure liquid chromatography, a technique available in most cancer centers. A few, such as the assays for methotrexate, have established importance as guides to the prediction of drug toxicity in high-dose therapy (Table 1.3). The utility of various assays is indicated in the discussion of individual agents in subsequent chapters.

COMBINATION CHEMOTHERAPY

Rationale for Combination Chemotherapy

Although the first effective drugs for treating cancer were brought to clinical trial in the 1940s, initial therapeutic results were disappointing. Impressive regressions of acute lymphocytic leukemia and adult lymphomas were obtained with single agents such as nitrogen mustard, antifolates, corticosteroids, and the vinca alkaloids, but responses were only partial and of short duration. When complete remissions were obtained, as in acute lymphocytic leukemia, they lasted less than 9 months, and relapse was associated with resistance to the original drug. The introduction of cyclic combination chemotherapy for acute lymphocytic leukemia of childhood in the late 1950s marked a turning point in the effective treatment of neoplastic disease. Such combinations are now a standard component of most treatment strategies for advanced cancer. The superior results of combination chemotherapy compared with single-agent treatment derive from the following considerations. First, initial resistance to any given single agent is frequent, even in the most responsive tumors; for example, in patients with Hodgkin's disease, the complete response rates to alkylating agents or procarbazine do not exceed 20%, and virtually all patients relapse. Second, initially responsive tumors rapidly acquire resistance after drug exposure, probably owing to selection of preexisting resistant tumor cells from a heterogeneous tumor cell population. Some anticancer drugs themselves increase the rate of mutation to resistance in experimental studies, as does hypoxia.[25] The use of multiple agents, each with cytotoxic activity in the disease under consideration but with different mechanisms of action, allows independent cell killing by each agent. Cells resistant to one agent might still be sensitive to the other drugs in the regimen.

TABLE 1.3
DRUG MONITORING IN CANCER THERAPY

Agent	Assay	Use
Methotrexate (MTX) sodium	HPLC	Aids in early detection of patients at high risk of toxicity. MTX level >5.10^7 mol/L at 48 hr alerts to need for increased leucovorin calcium dose for prolonged period. For toxic reactions, tailor leucovorin dosage to plasma MTX level. (See Antifolates, Chapter 6.) CSF MTX level aids in differential diagnosis of neurotoxicity. High level favors drug reaction.
6-Mercaptopurine	HPLC	Determines 6-MP nucleotide levels in red blood cells after oral therapy to assure appropriate metabolism.

CSF, cerebrospinal fluid; HPLC, high-pressure liquid chromatography.

Patterns of cross-resistance must be taken into consideration in formulating drug combinations. Resistance to many agents may result from unique and specific mutations, for example as may occur in the target enzymes of antimetabolites or targeted agents such as Gleevec.[12] Mutations that alter binding of inhibitors of topoisomerase II, an enzyme that promotes DNA strand breaks in the presence of anthracyclines and epipodophyllotoxins, may mediate resistance to each of these agents.[26] In other cases, a single mutational change may lead to multidrug resistance. Table 1.4 describes cross-resistance patterns for some of the well-defined mechanisms of multidrug resistance. The most thoroughly studied and undoubtedly one of the more important mechanisms of multidrug resistance is increased expression of the MDR-1 gene. This gene codes for the P-170 membrane glycoprotein, which promotes the efflux of vinca alkaloids, anthracyclines, taxanes, actinomycin D, epipodophyllotoxins, and other natural products. This protein occurs constitutively in many normal tissues, including epithelial cells of the kidney, large bowel, and adrenal gland,[27] and has been identified in tumors derived from these tissues, as well as in posttreatment lymphomas, leukemias, non-small cell lung cancer, multiple myeloma, and other cancers.[28] P-170–mediated resistance results from decreased intracellular drug levels and can be reversed experimentally by administration of calcium-channel blockers, amiodarone, quinidine, and derivatives of cyclosporine, as well as by a variety of aprotic polar solvents. At this time, evidence suggests that P-170 contributes to clinical drug resistance in multiple myeloma, non-Hodgkin's lymphomas, pediatric sarcomas, and acute nonlymphocytic leukemia.[27] Many clinical trials investigating the use of agents reversing multidrug resistance have been initiated, but the results of these trials are inconclusive. Many MDR inhibitors also inhibit hepatic clearance of doxorubicin hydrochloride, which significantly complicates the design and interpretation of these studies.[28]

TABLE 1.4
MECHANISMS OF RESISTANCE

Mechanism of Resistance	Drug Involved	Pharmacologic Defect
Decreased drug uptake	Methotrexate sodium	Decreased expression of the folate transporter
Decreased drug activation	Cytosine arabinoside Fludarabine phosphate Cladribine	Decreased deoxycytidine kinase
	Methotrexate	Decreased folylpolyglutamyl synthetase
Increased drug target	Methotrexate 5-fluorouracil Gleevec	Amplified DHFR Amplified TS Amplified bcr-abl kinase
Altered drug target	Etoposide Doxorubicin Gleevec	Altered topo II Altered DHFR Altered bcr-abl kinase
Increased detoxification	Alkylating agents	Increased glutathione or glutathione transferase
Enhanced DNA repair	Alkylating agents Platinum Analogs	Increased nucleotide excision repair
	Nitrosoureas Procarbazine Temozolomide	Increased O^6-alkyl-guanine alkyl transferase
Defective recognition of DNA adducts	Cisplatin	Mismatch repair defect
Increased drug efflux	Doxorubicin Etoposide Vinca alkaloids Paclitaxel Topotecan	Increased MDR expression or MDR gene amplification
Defective checkpoint function and apoptosis	Most anticancer drugs	p53 mutations

DHFR, dihydrofolate reductase; MDR, multidrug resistance; topo II, topoisomerase II; TS, thymidylate synthase.

A second mechanism for multidrug resistance involves the family of multidrug resistance proteins (MRPs), which, in experimental tumors, promotes drug efflux and confers resistance to anthracyclines, etoposide, and vinca alkaloids. Members of the MRP family may also mediate efflux of methotrexate, 6-mercaptopurine, camptothecin derivatives, and others.[29] Multiple members of the MRP gene family have been identified, and, again, their role in clinical drug resistance remains uncertain. The MRP family of genes is widely expressed in epithelial tumors,[27] and their potential for mediating multiagent resistance deserves further study.

Finally, classic alkylating agents (cyclophosphamide, melphalan hydrochloride, nitrogen mustard) may share cross-resistance related to enhanced DNA repair mediated by nucleotide excision repair enzymes and by increased levels of intracellular nucleophilic thiols, such as glutathione. There is clinical evidence that increased expression of nucleotide excision repair components correlates with a poor outcome in ovarian cancer treated with platinum-based regimens.[30] Not all alkylating agents share cross-resistance. As mentioned earlier, resistance to the nitrosourea, procarbazine, and dacarbazine classes of alkylators is mediated by increased levels of a different enzyme, O^6-alkyl- guanine alkyl transferase. Thus, there is a clear rationale for combining different alkylators in a single regimen. Undoubtedly, most resistant tumors have acquired a variety of mechanisms for avoiding the toxic effects of chemotherapy.

The acquisition of drug resistance is widely believed to be the product of random mutations in a tumor cell population. A corollary to this hypothesis is the concept that the probability of de novo drug resistance in any tumor population increases with increasing number of cells and number of cell divisions. More than 20 years ago, Goldie et al.[31] proposed a mathematical model based on the random-mutation hypothesis. It suggested several important considerations in protocol design to minimize treatment failure due to acquired drug resistance: (a) Treatment should begin as early as possible when the malignant cell population is at its smallest. (b) To avoid selection of doubly resistant mutants by sequential chemotherapy, multiple mutually non–cross-resistant drugs should be used together. (c) To achieve maximal kill of both sensitive and moderately resistant cells, cytotoxic drugs should be administered as frequently as possible and in doses well above the minimally cytotoxic doses. The Goldie-Coldman model serves to explain the success of combination therapies against hematologic malignancies such as non-Hodgkin's lymphoma and Hodgkin's disease.[32] However, randomized trials comparing new and more elaborate regimens, based on the Goldie-Coldman hypothesis, with older, empirically designed four-drug regimens have failed to demonstrate any improvement in the cure rates of either non-Hodgkin's lymphoma[33] or Hodgkin's disease.[34] Although these studies do not negate the basic tenants of Goldie-Coldman, they do suggest that the assumptions made to allow the formal mathematical modeling were overly simple. For instance, the model assumes that resistance develops to individual agents, one at a time, and thus does not account for multidrug resistance patterns. Multidrug resistance and broad resistance to apoptosis as conferred by inactivation of *p53* or overexpression of *bcl-2* are not considered. It is my opinion, unconfirmed, that a "model" can not substitute for the design of drug combinations based on a precise understanding of the molecular basis for drug resistance for each agent in the regimen.[12]

A third consideration supports combination chemotherapy. If drugs have nonoverlapping patterns of normal organ toxicity, each can be used in full dosage, and the effectiveness of each agent will be fully maintained in the combination. Drugs such as vincristine sulfate, prednisone, bleomycin sulfate, hexamethylmelamine, L-asparaginase, high-dose methotrexate/leucovorin calcium, and biologics, all lacking bone marrow toxicity, are particularly valuable in combination with traditional myelosuppressive agents. Based on these principles, curative combinations have been devised for diseases that are not curable with single-agent treatment, including acute lymphocytic leukemia (vincristine, prednisone, doxorubicin, and L-asparaginase), Hodgkin's disease (mechlorethamine, Oncovin [vincristine], procarbazine, and prednisone [MOPP] and Adriamycin (doxorubicin), bleomycin, vinblastine, and dacarbazine [ABVD]), diffuse large cell lymphoma (the combination of cyclophosphamide, doxorubicin, vincristine, and prednisone) and testicular carcinoma (bleomycin, cisplatin, and vinblastine or etoposide).

Schedule Development in Combination Therapy: Kinetic and Biochemical Considerations

The detailed scheduling of drugs in multidrug regimens was based initially on both practical and theoretical considerations. Intermittent cycles of treatment were used to allow periods of recovery of host bone marrow, gastrointestinal tract, and immune function, with the expectation that recovery of the tumor cell population would be slower than that of the injured normal tissues. This strategy allowed retreatment with full therapeutic doses as frequently as possible in keeping with the fractional cell kill hypothesis. A commonly used strategy is to incorporate myelotoxic agents on day 1 of each cycle, while delivering nonmyelosuppressive agents, such as bleomycin, vincristine, prednisone, or high-dose methotrexate with leucovorin rescue, in the period of bone marrow suppression (e.g., on day 8 of a 21-day cycle) to provide continuous suppression of tumor growth while allowing maximum time for marrow recovery. High-dose methotrexate with leucovorin rescue has proved to be particularly useful in this capacity during the "off period" because of its minimal effect on white blood cell and platelet counts.

Cytokinetic considerations also influence the specific sequencing of drugs in combination regimens. S-phase–specific drugs, such as cytosine arabinoside and methotrexate, are capable of killing cells only when they are present during the period of DNA synthesis. Experimentally, these agents are most effective if administered during the period of rapid recovery of DNA synthesis that follows a period of suppression of DNA synthesis. Thus, an initial phase of cytoreduction with drugs that are not cell cycle-phase–specific, such as the bifunctional alkylating agents, reduces tumor bulk and recruits slowly dividing cells into active DNA synthesis. These drugs can then be followed within the same cycle of treatment by cell cycle-phase–specific agents such as methotrexate or the fluoropyrimidines, which kill cells during periods of DNA synthesis.

Although most of the common anticancer regimens use intermittent bolus delivery of drugs, in recent years advantages of constant-infusion chemotherapy have been suggested. Early clinical trials have suggested improved therapeutic ratios for several drugs, including doxorubicin, 5-FU, etoposide, ifosfamide, and cytosine arabinoside.[35,36] Constant exposure of cells to cell cycle-phase–specific agents such as antimetabolites or cytosine arabinoside allows a greater fraction of the tumor cell population to cycle through the sensitive phase than is likely to occur with intermittent bolus therapy. The orally administered fluoropyrimidine, capecitabine, provides prolonged, low concentration exposure of tumors to the active metabolite of 5-fluorouracil, FdUMP. An additional consideration is the experimental evidence suggesting that constant exposure of agents such as natural products, resistance to which is mediated by p-170, may overwhelm the pump, which allows the killing of otherwise resistant cells.[37] Finally, infusional regimens may change the toxicity of cancer drugs. For example, the cardiotoxicity associated with anthracyclines is more closely correlated with the peak concentration than with AUC. Liposomal preparations of doxorubicin and daunorubicin provide the same advantage of prolonged exposure to drug, low peak concentrations, and decreased cardiotoxicity as does continuous intravenous infusion of the same agents.[38]

Additional Considerations in Combination Chemotherapy: Drug Resistance and Drug Interactions with Targeted, Anti-apoptotic Agents

Drug resistance, either apparent with initial treatment or emerging at the time of relapse after an initial response, inevitably occurs in all but the few cancer types that are curable with chemotherapy (Table 1.2). A panoply of potential mechanisms conferring resistance to cancer cells has been described (Table 1.4). As has become increasingly obvious, resistance is, in most cases, a complex process involving multiple mechanisms that may emerge in parallel or in series. With the appreciation of this complexity has come increasing skepticism that strategies aimed at reversal of discrete pathways conferring resistance to specific drugs or drug classes will have a major impact on the treatment of the common solid tumors. On the other hand, recent research suggests that a very common process conferring resistance to many, if not virtually all, chemotherapeutic agents is the suppression or inactivation of apoptosis, or programmed cell death. Inactivation of apoptotic mechanisms can be mediated by inactivation of the *p53* tumor suppressor gene (also termed a *death pathway gene*) or by inappropriate overexpression of genes that suppress apoptosis. The *p53* gene is mutated in almost 50% of human cancers at diagnosis, and in an even higher percentage of tumors at the time of emergence of drug resistance.[39] Thus, genes intimately involved with the fundamental processes of malignant transformation are now known to contribute directly to drug resistance.

Apoptosis is an active, energy-requiring, and protein synthesis-dependent process whereby cells, in response to specific signals, undergo an orderly, programmed series of intracellular events that lead to death. This process is a necessary component of normal development in all multicellular organisms and is required for the maintenance of normal function of many proliferating or renewable tissues such as the lymphatic system. Suppression of apoptosis is a common feature of neoplastic transformation. It may be the result of either overexpression of antiapoptotic genes such as *bcl-2*, or activation of growth factor pathways such as EGF epithelial cancers or *HER-2-neu* in breast cancer. Overexpression of *bcl-2* is linked to the pathogenesis of B-cell lymphomas.[40] Activation of other protective factors such as NF-K$_B$ and the PI-3 kinase pathway in response to DNA damage suppresses cytotoxicity of chemotherapy drugs and radiation.[41] Lowe et al[42] elegantly demonstrated that, in the presence of normal *p53*, transformation of normal mouse embryo fibroblasts (MEF) with the adenovirus E1A transforming gene (functionally equivalent to loss of *c-myc* regulation) created a cell line with supersensitivity to doxorubicin, 5-FU, and etoposide, as well as x-irradiation, and that the cells died through the process of apoptosis. MEF cells lacking the *p53* gene were resistant to doxorubicin, 5-FU, and etoposide, as well as x-irradiation. This experiment may explain the selectivity of chemotherapeutic agents for malignant cells over nonmalignant cells with similar proliferative rates and, reinforcing the results of other studies linking loss of cell-cycle control to resistance to chemotherapeutic agents,[43] offer an explanation for the high rate of inherent resistance of many *p53*-mutated solid tumors to chemotherapeutic agents (Fig. 1.1). Furthermore, these results suggest potential targets for effectively bypassing the elaborate defense machinery available to the cancer cell. Peptidomimetic drugs that activate proapoptotic

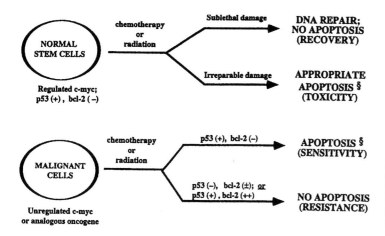

Figure 1.1 Effect of c-*myc* regulation, *p53*, and *bcl*-2 on sensitivity of normal and malignant cells proliferating at comparable rates. (The dose of drug or radiation causing apoptosis of normal stem cells with regulated c-*myc* is much higher than the dose causing apoptosis of malignant cells with normal *p53*, but unregulated c-*myc* or analogous oncogene.)

molecules have shown interesting ability to promote death of tumor cells in mice.[44]

Dose-Intensification Strategies

Dose intensification has received increasing emphasis in recent years as a strategy for overcoming resistance to chemotherapy. Citron and colleagues[45] have shown that the intensity of conventional treatment, that is, the dose per time unit, is an important consideration in adjuvant therapy of breast cancer. By decreasing the interval between treatments, using a "dose-dense" regimen, they found improvement in relapse-free survival. A steep dose-response effect for drug-responsive tumors has long been known, and the importance of delivering maximum tolerated doses in potentially curable diseases has been emphasized repeatedly. The concept of *dose intensity*, defined as the milligram per square meter of delivered drug per week of therapy, has been used by Levin and Hryniuk[46] in retrospective comparisons of published response rates obtained with different chemotherapeutic regimens (using the published protocol doses rather than actual delivered doses) in breast cancer, colon cancer, and ovarian cancer trials. They concluded that a dose-response correlation exists for 5-FU in colon cancer, doxorubicin in breast cancer, and cisplatin in ovarian cancer. Similarly, retrospective analyses of MOPP or related regimens in Hodgkin's disease have concluded that delivered doses of vincristine, as well as of alkylators and procarbazine, correlate with response rates and disease-free intervals.[47] These studies have been criticized because they are retrospective (i.e., an alternative and very plausible interpretation is that tumor-related or patient-related factors that are associated with inability to tolerate full chemotherapy doses also predict for poor response) and, in addition, in the case of the studies by Levin and Hryniuk,[46] because of the rather general assumptions the authors made regarding drug equivalency, which allowed numerical dose-intensity assignments to regimens containing different drugs.

The dose-response relationships discerned from acute leukemia trials[48] are probably applicable to other diseases, despite the lack of randomized studies. That is, in potentially curable cancers, readily tolerable ("standard") doses of effective combination chemotherapy drugs are sufficient for a subset of patients with sensitive tumors, whereas higher and, in some cases, very high doses may be necessary for the subset of patients with relative drug resistance. The challenge is to develop reliable de novo predictive markers (such as, potentially, *bcl*-2 overexpression or mutations in *p53* or K-*ras* genes) for each tumor to determine which patients will benefit from the higher doses. In the absence of such markers, treating every potentially curable patient with maximally tolerated doses, as established by the published or experimental protocol, is important. The following dosing principles have been used for the treatment of Hodgkin's disease,[49] but we believe they are broadly applicable to other potentially curable cancers: (a) Do not modify planned doses or schedules of chemotherapy in anticipation of toxicity that has not yet happened, nor for short-term, non–life-threatening toxicity, such as emesis or mild neuropathy. (b) Because significant individual variation may exist in the pharmacokinetics of drugs or in the sensitivity of the bone marrow (and other normal organs) to drug-related toxicity, the granulocyte count should be used as an in vivo biologic assay of the individual dosage limits of those agents with predominant myelotoxicity. If 100% of the planned doses do not produce a nadir granulocyte count of less than $1,000/mm^3$, the doses of the myelotoxic drugs are probably too low for that patient and should be increased in subsequent cycles to achieve a significant but tolerable level of myelotoxicity. (As a guideline, we aim for granulocyte nadirs in each cycle of between 500 and 1,000 per mm^3.) (c) Tumor response should be assessed at regular intervals throughout therapy. If evidence is seen of lack of response or of tumor regrowth, an alternative, non–cross-resistant regimen should be started.

The use of recombinant hematopoietic growth factors can mitigate the bone marrow toxicity of chemotherapy. Two recombinant agents, granulocyte colony-stimulating factor and granulocyte-macrophage colony-stimulating factor, are effective in decreasing the duration of granulocyte nadir after myelotoxic chemotherapy, although neither affects thrombocytopenia. Other factors that may have roles in ameliorating both the platelet and granulocyte toxicities, such as thrombopoietin, are under investigation.

High Dose Chemotherapy

Marrow-ablative dosages of chemotherapy are used to increase tumor cell kill. It is then possible rescue the host with either autologous bone marrow or peripheral blood stem cells, or stem cells, or marrow from a histocompatible donor. During the past 20 years, this approach has been investigated in many centers as salvage therapy for patients with relapsed leukemias, Hodgkin's and non-Hodgkin's lymphomas, as well as some solid tumors. Rescue with marrow from a human leukocyte antigen-compatible donor has the advantage of being free of malignant cells. Marrow donated by a second person contains T lymphocytes, however, which may cause graft-versus-host disease, a potentially lethal complication. On the other hand, evidence exists that a "graft-versus-tumor" effect may be more beneficial in prolonging remissions, in comparison with syngeneic or autologous marrow rescue. The drugs used in these programs have myelosuppression as the primary dose-limiting toxicity and are used in doses above the lethal dose to bone marrow in the absence of marrow reinfusion but below the limits of nonhematologic toxicity. Alkylators such as busulfan, ifosfamide, and cyclophosphamide are prominent in most ablative regimens because characteristically their extra myeloid toxicity occurs at twofold to sevenfold higher dosage than the myeloablative dosage. Some high-dose toxicities, such as cystitis, can be prevented through the use of mesna, a disulfide that inactivates alkylating mioeties in the acid environment of urine. Total-body, total-lymphoid, or limited-field radiation has been used frequently as an adjunct to chemotherapy. Hematopoietic growth factors and peripheral blood stem cells have been used in conjunction with high-dose chemotherapy and marrow reinfusion to shorten the duration of marrow aplasia and reduce infection complications.

Randomized trials comparing high-dose regimens with best conventional therapy generally have not proven the value of dose escalation in patients with metastatic breast cancer.[50] High-dose regimens with allogeneic bone marrow transplant appear to be very effective in some younger patients with acute myeloid leukemia and in chronic myelogenous leukemia, whereas autologous bone marrow transplant or peripheral blood stem cell transplant regimens appear to be effective in drug-responsive Hodgkin's disease in first or second relapse and in intermediate-grade and high-grade non-Hodgkin's lymphoma in first relapse. Reported trials generally have consisted of relatively small numbers of highly selected patients, however, and follow-up in most cases is still brief. One should remember that both early and late toxicities of high-dose chemotherapy bone marrow transplant regimens, both allogeneic and autologous, may be serious.[51] Acute pulmonary toxicity and vascular occlusive disease with liver failure contribute to acute mortality due to a high-dose regimen. Later, acute lung toxicity, and secondary acute leukemia and myelodysplasia are seen with increasing frequency.[52] The risk of treatment-related death from allogeneic programs may be as high as 15 to 40%, depending on the age and underlying health of the patient.

Drug Interactions in Combination Chemotherapy

Specific drug interactions, both favorable and unfavorable, must be considered in developing combination regimens. These interactions may take the form of pharmacokinetic, cytokinetic, or biochemical effects of one drug that influences the effectiveness of a second component of a combination. Patterns of overlapping toxicity are a primary concern. Drugs that cause renal toxicity, such as cisplatin, must be used cautiously in combination with other agents (such as methotrexate or bleomycin) that depend on renal elimination as their primary mechanism of excretion. Regimens that use cisplatin before methotrexate, as in the treatment of head and neck cancer, must incorporate careful monitoring of renal function, pretreatment plasma volume expansion, and dose adjustment for methotrexate to ensure that altered methotrexate excretion does not lead to severe drug toxicity. The sequence of drug administration may be critical; in many experimental systems, administration of paclitaxel before cisplatin gives additive or synergistic results, whereas the opposite sequence yields antagonism and increased toxicity.[53] Taxol delays the clearance of doxorubicin and increases the risk of cardiotoxicity.[54] Extensive interactions between P-450 inducers such as phenytoin or phenobarbital and P-450 substrates such as irinotecan, paclitaxel, or vincristine lead to marked increases in drug clearance and the need for upward dosage adjustment (see Chapter 21). The potential for important interactions between cancer drugs and other medications must be kept in mind during the routine care of cancer patients.

Biochemical interactions also may be important considerations in determining the choice of agents and their sequence of administration. Both synergistic and antagonistic interactions have been described. A chemotherapeutic drug may be modulated by a second agent that has no antitumor activity in its own right but that enhances the intracellular activation or target binding of the primary agent or inhibits the repair of lesions produced by the primary drug. The best example of this synergy is the use of leucovorin (5-formyltetrahydrofolate), which itself has no cytotoxic effect but which enhances the affinity of the binding of 5-FU to its target enzyme, thymidylate synthase, by forming a ternary complex among the enzyme, 5-FU, and folate.[55] This combination is more effective clinically than 5-FU alone in colorectal cancer. A number of such combinations have reached the clinic and are described in greater detail in subsequent chapters.

Combination of Chemotherapy with Radiotherapy or Biologic Agents

A further innovation in the use of antineoplastic drugs is to combine drugs with irradiation or biologic agents. Many clinical protocols have been designed to take advantage of the well-documented synergy between irradiation and drugs such as cisplatin, paclitaxel and 5-FU.

The design of integrated chemotherapy-radiotherapy trials presents special problems because of the synergistic effects of the two therapies on both normal and malignant tissue. The normal tissue of greatest concern is the bone marrow, although the heart, lungs, and brain may also be affected by such interactions.[56] Radiation given to the pelvic or midline abdominal areas produces a decline in blood counts, myelofibrosis, and a decrease in bone marrow reserve. This can severely compromise the ability to deliver myelotoxic chemotherapy, even months or years after the radiation. The use of conformal irradiation, administered through multiple portals, can preserve a greater portion of the marrow-bearing tissue. For some toxicities, the sequence of administration may be crucial. For example, mediastinal irradiation after combination chemotherapy for massive mediastinal Hodgkin's disease has proven to be practicable and effective. Because the initial chemotherapy results in significant shrinkage of the mediastinal tumor, smaller radiation portals can be used to encompass the residual tumor completely, with proportionately less resultant radiation pneumonitis. In small cell carcinoma of the lung confined to the thorax, simultaneous administration of radiotherapy and chemotherapy has produced better results than either therapy alone or in sequence.[57] Similarly, simultaneous radiation and chemotherapy is superior to radiotherapy alone in adjuvant therapy for cervical cancer[58] and rectal cancer.[59] Thus, although considering the cumulative toxicities of chemotherapy and radiation on bone marrow and other vulnerable tissues in the radiation field is essential, the net benefits of simultaneous irradiation and chemotherapy often outweigh the disadvantages.

Many chemotherapeutic agents greatly potentiate the effects of irradiation and may lead to synergistic toxicity for organs usually resistant to radiation damage. Doxorubicin sensitizes both normal and malignant cells to radiation damage, possibly because both doxorubicin and x-rays produce free-radical damage to tissues. Doxorubicin adjuvant chemotherapy given in conjunction with irradiation to the left chest wall increases the risk of increased cardiac toxicity.[60] Similarly, bleomycin and radiation cause synergistic pulmonary toxicity. When more than one effective chemotherapy regimen is available, the choice must be informed by consideration of these possible mutually potentiating toxicities.

A final consideration in the combined use of radiotherapy and chemotherapy is the carcinogenicity of both. The most important late side effect of cancer treatment among patients who are cured of their primary tumors is a secondary solid tumor induced by ionizing radiation. In studies of patients cured of Hodgkin's disease, the risk for secondary solid tumors begins to increase significantly after 10 years and continues to increase steadily into the second and third decades. The cumulative risk for all secondary radiation-induced (i.e., occurring within the radiation portal) solid tumors is approximately 15% at 15 years and may be as high as 20% at 25 years. On the other hand, little evidence exists that concomitant chemotherapy increases this risk of secondary solid tumors. The most important chemotherapy-related second malignancy is leukemia due to DNA alkylating or metalating agents. Among the most potently leukemogenic agents are the mustard-type alkylators, nitrosoureas, and procarbazine. The risk for leukemia increases with cumulative dose of alkylators, a fact that must be considered when long-term or high-dose alkylator use is contemplated. Leukemia has been reported after therapy for Hodgkin's disease, non-Hodgkin's lymphoma, breast cancer (adjuvant therapy), ovarian cancer, multiple myeloma, and other kinds of cancer (see Chapter 5). The most thoroughly studied group of patients consists of long- term survivors of Hodgkin's disease after MOPP chemotherapy. The cumulative risk for leukemia or myelodysplasia after MOPP is approximately 3% at 10 years. The risk for secondary myeloid malignancy decreases rapidly thereafter and approaches the age-related baseline 10 years after MOPP. Although earlier reports suggested a further increased risk for myeloid malignancy when radiation was added, either before or after MOPP, many analyses of large numbers of patients treated with both radiation and MOPP have not demonstrated any significant increased risk of acute myelogenous leukemia due to radiation.[61] One should mention that the risk for myeloid leukemia is not increased after ABVD therapy for Hodgkin disease. A qualitatively different type of secondary nonlymphocytic leukemia is associated with topoisomerase II inhibitors, including etoposide, teniposide, and doxorubicin.[62] Characteristically, acute myelogenous leukemia associated with topoisomerase II inhibitor therapy has a much shorter latency period than does alkylator-induced leukemia, is frequently of the myelomonocytic or monocytic FAB subtypes (M-4 or M-5, respectively), and is frequently associated with reciprocal chromosomal translocations involving band 11q23. The risk of this type of leukemia is associated with higher total cumulative dose of the topoisomerase II inhibitor and with a weekly or twice-weekly schedule. In addition, the risk may be increased when the topoisomerase II agent is combined with high-dose alkylators or with agents that inhibit DNA repair.

In summary, cancer chemotherapeutic agents have had a profound influence on the treatment and survival of patients with cancer. Because these agents have the potential for causing severe or disabling toxicity and yet must be used at maximal dosages to ensure full therapeutic benefit, the physician is literally walking a therapeutic tightrope and must constantly balance gain against likely toxicities. In this effort, every advantage afforded by knowledge of the patient, the disease, and the therapy must be used to achieve maximum benefit. The foregoing discussion should make it apparent that an intimate knowledge of drug action, drug disposition, and drug interactions, as well as late drug effects, is essential to the design and application of effective cancer chemotherapy. The essential information for this task is presented in the following chapters on individual drugs and is summarized in the initial tables that describe key features of each agent. This information can only enhance the chances of success in the difficult but rewarding task of treating cancer.

REFERENCES

1. Greco FA, Vaughn WK, Hainsworth JD. Advanced poorly differentiated carcinoma of unknown primary site: recognition of a treatable syndrome. Ann Intern Med 1986;104:547–553.
2. Kwiatkowski DJ, Harpole DH, Godleski J, et al. Molecular-pathologic substaging in 244 stage I non-small cell lung cancer patients: clinical implications. J Clin Oncol 1998;16:2468–2477.
3. Lynch TJ, Bell DW, Sordella R, et al. Activating mutations in the epidermal growth factor receptor underlying responsiveness of non-small-cell lung cancer to Gefitinib. N Engl J Med 2004; 350:2129–2139.
4. Ramaswamy S, Ross KN, Lander ES, Golub TR. A molecular signature of metastasis in primary solid tumors. Nature Genetics 2003;33:49–54.
5. Szakacs G, Annereau JP, Lababidi S, et al. Predicting drug sensitivity and resistance: profiling ABC transporter genes in cancer cells. Cancer Cell 2004;6:129–137.
6. Ma XJ, Wang Z, Ryan PD, et al. A two-gene expression ratio predicts clinical outcome in breast cancer patients treated with tamoxifen. Cancer Cell 2004;5:607–617.
7. Holleman A, Cheok MH, Den Boer ML, et al. Gene-expression patterns in drug-resistant acute lymphoblastic leukemia cells and response to treatment. N Engl J Med 2004;351:533–542.
8. Roberts TG Jr, Chabner BA. Beyond fast track for drug approvals. N Engl J Med. 2004 Jul 29;351(5):501–505.
9. Skipper HE, Schabel FM Jr, Mellett LB, et al. Implications of biochemical, cytokinetic, pharmacologic, and toxicologic relationships in the design of optimal therapeutic schedules. Cancer Chemother Rep 1970;54:431–450.
10. Fialkow PJ. Clonal origin of human tumors. Biochim Biophys Acta 1976;458:283–321.
11. Shapiro JR, Shapiro WR. Clonal tumor cell heterogeneity. Prog Exp Tumor Res 1984;27:49–66.
12. Deininger MW, Druker BJ. SRCircumventing imatinib resistance. Cancer Cell 2004;6:108–110.
13. Holloway RW, Mehta RS, Finkler NJ, et al. Association between in vitro platinum resistance in the EDR assay and clinical outcomes for ovarian cancer patients. Gyn Oncol 2002;87:8–16.
14. Gurubhagavatula S, Liu G, Park S, et al. XPD and XRCC1 genetic polymorphisms are prognostic factors in advanced non-small-cell lung cancer patients treated with platinum chemotherapy. J Clin Oncol 2004; 22:2594–2601.
15. Curt GA, Carney DN, Cowan KH, et al. Unstable methotrexate resistance in human small-cell carcinoma associated with double-minute chromosomes. N Engl J Med 1983;308:199–202.
16. Gorlick R, Goker E, Trippett T, et al. Defective transport is a common mechanism of acquired methotrexate resistance in acute

lymphocytic leukemia and is associated with decreased reduced folate carrier expression. Blood 1997;89:1013–1018.
17. Scudiero DA, Meyer SA, Clatterbuck BE, et al. Sensitivity of human cell strains having different abilities to repair O^6-methyl guanine in DNA to inactivation by alkylating agents including chloroethyl nitrosoureas. Cancer Res 1984;44:2467–2474.
18. Fedier A, Fink D. Mutations in DNA mismatch repair genes: implications for DNA damage signaling and drug sensitivity. Int J Oncol 2004;24:1039–1047.
19. Druker B. Perspectives on the development of a molecularly targeted agent. Cancer Cell 2002;1:31–36.
20. Demetri GD, von Mehren M, Blanke CD, et al. Efficacy and safety of imatinib mesylate in advanced gastrointestinal stromal tumors. N Engl J Med 2002;347:472–480.
21. Cunningham D, Humblet Y, Siena S, et al. Cetuximab monotherapy and cetuximab plus irinotecan in irinotecan-refractory metastatic colorectal cancer. N Engl J Med 2004;351:337–345.
22. Hande K, Messenger M, Wagner J, et al. Inter- and intrapatient variability in etoposide kinetics with oral and intravenous drug administration. Clin Cancer Res 1999;5(10):2742–2747.
23. Watters JW, Kraja A, Meucci MA, et al. Genome-wide discovery of loci influencing chemotherapy cytotoxicity. PNAS 2004;101: 11809–11814.
24. Pui CH, Cheng C, Leung W, et al. Extended follow-up of long-term survivors of childhood acute lymphoblastic leukemia. N Engl J Med 2003;349:640–649.
25. Rice GC, Hoy C, Schimke RT. Transient hypoxia enhances the frequency of DHFR gene amplification in Chinese hamster ovary cells. Proc Natl Acad Sci U S A 1986;83:5978–5982.
26. Sugimoto Y, Tsukahara S, Oh-hara T, et al. Decreased expression of DNA topoisomerase I in camptothecin-resistant tumor cell lines as determined by monoclonal antibody. Cancer Res 1990; 50:6925–6930.
27. Ross DD, Doyle LA. Mining our ABCs: Pharmacogenomic approach for evaluating transporter function in cancer drug resistance. Cancer Cell 2004;6:105–107.
28. Marie JP, Zittoun R, Sikic BI. Multidrug resistance (mdr1) gene expression in adult acute leukemias: correlation with treatment outcomes and in vitro drug sensitivity. Blood 1991;78:586–592.
29. Lee K, Belinsky MG, Bell DW, et al. Isolation of MOAT-B, a widely expressed multidrug resistance-associated protein/ canalicular multispecific organic anion transporter-related transporter. Cancer Res 1998;58:2741–2747.
30. Taniguchi T, Tischkowitz M, Ameziane N, et al. Disruption of the Fanconi anemia–BRCA pathway in cisplatin-sensitive ovarian tumors. Nat Med 2003;9:568–574.
31. Goldie JH, Coldman AJ, Gudanskas GA. Rationale for the use of alternating non-cross-resistant chemotherapy. Cancer Treat Rep 1982;66:439–449.
32. DeVita VT, Hubbard SM, Longo DL. The chemotherapy of lymphomas: looking back, moving forward—The Richard and Hinda Rosenthal Foundation Award Lecture. Cancer Res 1987;47: 5810–5824.
33. Gordon LI, Harrington D, Andersen J, et al. Comparison of a second-generation combination chemotherapeutic regimen (m-BACOD) with a standard regimen (CHOP) for advanced diffuse non-Hodgkin's lymphoma. N Engl J Med 1992;327:1342–1349.
34. Connors JM, Klimo P, Adams G, et al. Treatment of advanced Hodgkin's disease with chemotherapy—comparison of MOPP/ ABV hybrid regimen with alternating courses of MOPP and ABVD: a report from the National Cancer Institute of Canada clinical trials group. J Clin Oncol 1997;15:2762.
35. Anderson H, Hopwood P, Prendiville J, et al. A randomized study of bolus versus continuous pump infusion of ifosfamide and doxorubicin with oral etoposide for small cell lung cancer. Br J Cancer 1993;67:1385–1390.
36. De Gramont A, Bosset JF, Milan C, et al. Randomized trial comparing monthly low-dose leucovorin and fluorouracil bolus with bimonthly high-dose leucovorin and fluorouracil bolus plus continuous infusion for advanced colorectal cancer: a French intergroup study. J Clin Oncol 1997;15:808–815.
37. Cowens JW, Creaven PJ, Greco WR, et al. Initial clinical (phase I) trial of TLC-D-99 (doxorubicin encapsulated in lyposomes). Cancer Res 1993;53:2796–2802.

38. Bottini A, Bersiga A, Brizzi M. p53 but not bcl-2 immunostaining is predictive for poor clinical complete response to primary chemotherapy in breast cancer patients. Clin Cancer Res 2000; 6:2751–2758.

39. Lai GM, Chen YN, Mickley LA, et al. P-glycoprotein expression and schedule dependence of Adriamycin cytotoxicity in human colon carcinoma cell lines. Int J Cancer 1991;49:696–703.

40. Korsmeyer SJ. *Bcl-2* initiates a new category of oncogenes: regulators of cell death. Blood 1992;80:879–886.

41. Green DR, Bissonnette RP, Cotter TG. Apoptosis and cancer. PPO Updates 1994;8:37–52.

42. Lowe SW, Ruley HE, Jacks T, et al. *p53*-dependent apoptosis modulates the cytotoxicity of anticancer agents. Cell 1993;74:957–967.

43. Kohn KW, Jackman J, O'Connor PM. Cell cycle control and cancer chemotherapy. J Cell Biochem 1994;54:440–452.

44. Denicourt C, Dowdy SF. Medicine: Targeting Apoptotic Pathways in Cancer. Science 2004;305:1411–1413.

45. Citron ML, Berry DA, Cirrincione C, et al. Randomized trial of dose-dense versus conventionally scheduled and sequential versus concurrent combination chemotherapy as postoperative adjuvant treatment of node-positive primary breast cancer: first report of Intergroup Trial C9741/Cancer and Leukemia Group B Trial 9741. J Clin Oncol 2003;21:2226.

46. Levin L, Hryniuk WM. Dose intensity analysis of chemotherapy regimens in ovarian carcinoma. J Clin Oncol 1987;5:756–767.

47. Longo DL, Young RC, Wesley M, et al. Twenty years of MOPP therapy for Hodgkin's disease. J Clin Oncol 1986;4:1295–1306.

48. Greco FA, Vaughn WK, Hainsworth JD. Advanced poorly differentiated carcinoma of unknown primary site: recognition of a treatable syndrome. Ann Intern Med 1986;104:547–553.

49. Kaufman D, Longo DL. Hodgkin's disease. Crit Rev Oncol Hematol 1992;13:135–187.

50. Stadtmauer EA, O'Neill A, Goldstein LJ, et al., and the Philadelphia Bone Marrow Transplant Group. Conventional-dose chemotherapy compared with high-dose chemotherapy plus autologous hematopoietic stem-cell transplantation for metastatic breast cancer. N Engl J Med 2000;342:1069–1076.

51. Socié G, Stone JV, Wingard JR, et al. Long term survival and late deaths after allogeneic bone marrow transplantation. N Engl J Med 1999;341:14–21.

52. Howe R, Micallef INM, Inwards DJ, et al. Secondary myelodysplastic syndrome and acute myelogenous leukemia are significant complications following autologous stem cell transplantation for lymphoma. Bone Marrow Transpl 2003;32:317–324.

53. Liebmann J, Fisher J, Teague D, et al. Sequence dependence of paclitaxel (Taxol®) combined with cisplatin or alkylators in human cancer cells. Oncol Res 1994;6:25–31.

54. Holmes FA and Rowinsky EK. Pharmacokinetic profiles of doxorubicin in combination with taxanes. Semin Oncol 2001; 28(Suppl 12):8–14.

55. Sotos GA, Grogan L, Allegra CJ. Preclinical and clinical aspects of biomodulation of 5-fluorouracil. Cancer Treat Rev 1994;20:11–49.

56. Pihkala J, Saarinen UM, Lundstrom U, et al. Myocardial function in children and adolescents after therapy with anthracyclines and chest irradiation. Eur J Cancer 1996;32A:97–103.

57. Bunn PA, Lichter AS, Makuch RW, et al. Chemotherapy alone or chemotherapy plus chest radiation therapy in limited- stage small-cell lung cancer. Ann Intern Med 1987;106:655–662.

58. Rose PG, Bundy BN, Watkins EB, et al. Concurrent cisplatin-based chemoradiation improves progression-free and overall survival in advanced cervical cancer: results of a randomized Gynecologic Oncology Group study. N Engl J Med 1999;340:1144–1153.

59. Fisher B, Wolmark N, Rockette H, et al. Postoperative adjuvant chemotherapy or radiation therapy for rectal cancer: results from NSABP protocol R-01. J Natl Cancer Inst 1988;80:21–29.

60. Shapiro CL, Harrigan Hardenbergh P, Gelman R, et al. Cardiac effects in adjuvant doxorubicin and radiation therapy in breast cancer patients. J Clin Oncol 1998;16:3493–3501.

61. Lavey RS, Eby NL, Prosnitz LR. Impact on second malignancy risk of the combined use of radiation and chemotherapy for lymphomas. Cancer 1990;66:80–88.

62. Pui CH, Ribeiro RC, Hancock ML, et al. Acute myeloid leukemia in children treated with epipodophylotoxins for acute lymphoblastic leukemia. N Engl J Med 1991;321:1682–1687.

2

Preclinical Aspects of Cancer Drug Discovery and Development

Paula Krosky   *Melinda Hollingshead*   *Robert Shoemaker*
Edward A. Sausville

This chapter provides an overview of the preclinical phase of the development of any anticancer drug, which encompases three overall stages. The first stage is the discovery of a new molecule with therapeutic potential and the selection of the optimal candidate or limited set of candidates for further evaluation. These studies ideally would allow an assessment of how the new molecule differs from currently available therapeutic agents. In the second stage, early preclinical development is directed at increasing confidence that the drug lead will actually function as a useful therapeutic agent in humans. These studies focus predominantly on eliciting activity in animal models of cancer, and ideally correlate the degree of antitumor activity with the pharmacology of the drug. Late preclinical development, the final stage, leads to the completion of regulatory requirements for entry into initial human clinical trials, particularly safety testing at various doses in animal species. Within the past 10 years, the approach to the discovery and development of cancer drugs has undergone a marked change, from focusing mainly on empirical antiproliferative activity as a basis for initial interest in a compound, to selecting drug candidates on the basis of their capacity to modulate molecular targets that are important in cancer pathophysiology.

CANCER DRUG TARGET SELECTION

Our current understanding of cancer cell biology leads to the view that by the time a cancer is clinically manifest in a patient, a number of genetic lesions have occurred in the tumor, resulting in discrete sets of abnormalities that may differ in detail from tumor to tumor, but exist as categories of molecular defects common to essentially all tumor types. This idea, articulated elegantly by Hanahan and Weinberg,[1] points to deregulated proliferation-control pathways, loss of tumor suppressor gene function, loss of functions that would promote tumor cell programmed death (apoptosis), acquisition of limitless replication potential through telomere-replicating strategies, activation of host angiogenesis, and the capacity to invade into normal stroma as attributes of all tumors. To these features must be added the capacity of tumors to thwart the host immune system (e.g., Uttenhoeve et al.[2]). Each of the molecules creating the altered cellular state that underlies tumor cell biology as compared with normal could conceivably be a target for cancer drug discovery and development. Indeed, extensive efforts to define potential targets with altered expression patterns in tumors have been made available through publicly funded (e.g., the Cancer Genome Anatomy Project; see http://www.ncbi.nlm.nih.gov/ncicgap/) and privately maintained databases. These catalogs of genes expressed differentially in tumors are the starting point for current drug discovery and development campaigns. A major question is, how might these targets be prioritized?

One point of view is that those molecules consistently mutated in the course of the development of a cancer in a patient are defined by nature as important in the pathophysiology of that tumor. These molecules may come to attention not only by point mutations in their coding sequence, but by their proximity to frequently observed chromosomal breakpoints or regions of DNA amplification in tumors. Examples of molecules of this type that have been already validated as cancer drug targets include the p210[bcr/abl] oncoprotein of chronic myelogenous leukemia[3] and the *HER-2-neu* tyrosine kinase[4] that is frequently detected by genomic amplification in breast carcinoma. Approved drugs directed at these targets include imatinib and the monoclonal antibody trastuzumab, respectively. In seeming validation of this way of thinking, patients enjoying the best clinical response to the epidermal growth factor receptor tyrosine kinase inhibitor gefitinib have recently been demonstrated to possess with high frequency a mutated, activated form of the agent's target kinase.[5,6] Extending this general approach, the most important targets for cancer drug discovery would be those that can be clearly defined as being mutated in the course of carcinogenesis, or are "downstream" from a mutated molecule and transmit the effects of this mutation to a pathway. These would be exemplary of *pathogenic* targets because the targets can be reasonably construed as relating to the pathogenesis of the neoplastic process.

Ontologic targets relate to the normal tissue of origin of the tumor. Examples of validated targets of this type include the estrogen or androgen receptors in breast or prostate cancer, respectively, and the CD20 cell surface determinant of non-Hodgkin's lymphoma. *Pharmacologic* targets relate to the handling or response to a drug itself. For example, dihydropyrimidine dehydrogenase is a target whose degree of activity modulates susceptibility and toxicity of fluorinated pyrimidines, or dexrazoxane modulates levels of free iron and thus alters the cardiotoxic potential of anthracyclines. *Stromal* or *microenvironmental* targets include the large array of molecules responsible for sculpting tumor stroma and supporting cell framework including mediators of angiogenesis. The recent regulatory approval of bevacizumab, a monoclonal antibody to vascular endothelial growth factor (VEGF),[7] has validated this category of target and promises to be the harbinger of significant discovery efforts around targets of this class. Immunologic strategies, including immunomodulating cytokines or even vaccines, might be considered as special cases ultimately directed at the tumor microenvironment.

The argument for a particular target is strengthened when a phenotype related to tumor behavior can be modulated in cell models (antisense, small interfering RNA, dominant negatives, or ribozyme approaches) or in animal models (knock-outs or transgenics) by genetic approaches to altering the presence or function of a tumor target. For example, topoisomerase IIIβ knock-out mice exhibit premature senescence, which suggests that the use of a topoisomerase poison, such as Camptosar (irinotecan), would encourage rapidly dividing cells toward senescence.[8]

Other practical criteria that influence the suitability for selection of a molecular target for a drug discovery campaign include the availability (and cost) of reagents to allow screening of leads and the identification of an assay format that is amenable to high-throughput screening (HTS). Finally, the size of the patient population (market) and availability of effective treatments for a particular cancer are usually considered before investing resources toward a new target.

ANTICANCER DRUG SCREENING

Initial recognition of a lead compound can come from a purely molecularly targeted screen, directed against a purified enzyme or a cell engineered to overexpress or underexpress a particular target, or from a cell- or animal-model–based antiproliferative screen, against naturally occurring or engineered tumor cells. Each screening model has its distinct advantages and disadvantages. The molecular targeted approach may yield a drug candidate with clear selectivity for a particular target, but then target modulation must be documented in a cellular context, hopefully with evidence of useful antitumor activity. Ideally, constant evidence of effects "on target" can be an important aid to lead optimization. Cell-based screens have the advantage that drug candidates defined by this route select themselves for the ability to distribute across plasma membranes and survive in the intracellular milieu. On the other hand, their mechanism of action must be determined prior to efficient lead optimization, and cell-based screens are less frequently amenable to high-throughput approaches. In contrast, molecular targeted screens have the attraction of being very amenable to the screening of large collections of molecules.

Figure 2.1 illustrates the generic process of high-throughput, molecular targeted screening. The process requires initial identification and validation of a target, followed by development and characterization of an assay suitable for HTS. This assay is then used to screen chemical collections or "libraries" to identify active samples that are the focus of additional testing to establish potency, selectivity, and other features important for further development. Screening is typically conducted in a "campaign" mode, with primary screening data from a particular library evaluated after the whole library has been tested. Criteria for activity are frequently established such that a "hit rate" on the order of 1% is obtained. Thus, for a library of 100,000 samples, 1,000 of the most active samples would be selected for confirmatory testing. Efficient testing usually demands that the primary screen is conducted at a single concentration. Confirmatory testing may be done using the same protocol or may be done in concentration-response fashion to facilitate subsequent consideration of screening leads in the context of potency.

SOURCES OF DIVERSITY FOR LEAD IDENTIFICATION

A crucial issue in any screening project for the purpose of searching for new anticancer drugs is the acquisition of

Generic Process for High-Throughput Molecular Targeted Drug Discovery

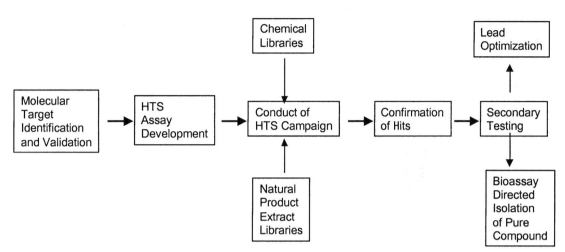

Figure 2.1 Generic process for high-throughput molecular targeted drug discovery.

compound libraries. Whether the initial screen is a target-based biochemical screen or an empirical antiproliferation screen, the greater the structural diversity in the set of molecules examined, the more likely a novel inhibitor will be identified. Historically, natural products—defined here as extracts from plants, microbial, and animal sources—have provided an excellent source of bioactive molecules with novel structures and mechanisms of action. In cancer treatment, natural products constitute several major therapeutic classes including the vinca alkaloids, camptothecins, and taxanes. Natural product extracts as sources for cancer drug discovery have been extensively reviewed[9] and are not discussed further here. More recently, collections or libraries of synthetic compounds have gained prominence in anticancer drug discovery efforts.

Again, there are distinct advantages to each type of compound source. Synthetic compound libraries are either already existing as single compounds or are usually amenable to assignment of activity to a unique chemical structure by a facile deconvolution algorithm. On the other hand, they are limited by the pharmacophore(s) around which the library has been constructed. Although natural product extracts have the possibility of remarkable diversity and stereochemically unique scaffolds, in some cases they require reacquisition from rather exotic ecological niches, optimization of fermentation or extraction approaches, and deconvolution of the active molecule(s) in the extract before the lead can be meaningfully pursued. These strengths and limitations, must be remembered when selecting sources for screening endeavors.

The number and variety of synthetic compounds available for screening endeavors has been magnified by the use of combinatorial chemistry. The method of deliberately

synthesizing more than one compound as a result of a single reaction began approximately 20 years ago with the synthesis by Geysen et al.[10] of multiple peptides on polyethylene rods. These early endeavors, confined to the synthesis of small peptide libraries, were of limited value to cancer drug discovery because peptides tend not to enter cells and generally are not suitable drug candidates. Subsequent advances in the field included more efficient ways to track the compounds, use of a greater number of scaffolds on which to construct libraries, and use of a wider variety of reagents and amenable reaction conditions. Now, combinatorial chemistry provides an efficient method of exploring chemical space in a focused manner and, when applicable, an excellent means of rapidly defining structure activity relationships around active compounds. Virtually all pharmaceutical companies use combinatorial chemistry at some point in their drug discovery and development programs. The precise position at which combinatorially derived molecules should be employed in a drug discovery and development campaign is a matter of current discussion in the field. "Brute force" screening of millions of compounds not previously enriched for likely valuable molecules has been of little convincing value. On the other hand, combinatorial approaches could greatly enhance the efficiency with which the potential of a lead structure with initial evidence of value is optimized.

Advances in computer-based analysis of the physical properties and interactions of a novel, active compound have provided powerful tools for the pursuit of new anticancer drugs. Medicinal chemists traditionally have used parameters such as steric bulk, hydrogen-bonding ability, and hydrophobic interactions in the design of new drugs. The target pharmacophore now can be further refined by supplementing the information from these physical properties with biologic factors such as the structural biochemistry of the target enzyme or receptor, the nature of the ligand, and the mechanism of the target-ligand interaction when defining the target pharmacophore. Moreover, computer programs such as the Universal Library (Sphinx pharmaceuticals, Durham, NC), Icepick (Axys pharmaceuticals, San Francisco, CA), and Matrix (ComGenex, Inc., Budapest, Hungary) can create "virtual libraries," which can be evaluated for how thoroughly biochemical, functional space and chemical, diversity space are covered before the proposed structures are synthesized. The use of computer models to design and filter novel structures can be a very efficient mechanism to increase the odds of identifying a potent and selective inhibitor of a well-defined target.

COMPOUND LIBRARIES

Over the years, collections of pure compounds and natural product extracts have coalesced into libraries, some of which are publicly available and arrayed into 96-well plates or 384-well plates in anticipation of HTS. Popular commercial libraries are available from ChemBridge Corp. (San Diego, CA), Maybridge (Cornwall, England), and Sigma-Aldrich (St. Louis, MO; notably the Library of Pharmacologically Active Compounds or LOPAC). The National Cancer Institute (NCI) compound repository is comprised of approximately 600,000 samples obtained by the Developmental Therapeutics Program (DTP) over the past 50 years for use in anticancer drug screening. However, approximately half of the database was submitted under confidentiality agreements that preclude disclosure of information regarding structure or biologic activity. Data for the fraction of the repository for which disclosable information is available, the NCI Open Source Repository (OSR), of approximately 250,000 samples can be obtained at the DTP website (http://dtp.nci.nih.gov). Additional smaller collections of compounds are available from an assortment of other suppliers.

A major challenge for all suppliers of compounds is authentication of the structure and quantification of the purity of library materials. Most collections show evidence of the toils of time, storage conditions, and questionable provenance. Most samples in the NCI compound repository were donated by academic chemists or industrial organizations, and were accepted without further chemical characterization. Samples were stored at room temperature unless other conditions were specified by the supplier. As a result, the samples in this collection range in quality from those with a very high degree of sample integrity (purity and authenticity of structure) to those with little or none of the substance indicated by the supplier and reflected in the database records. It is often easier to verify the structure and purity of selected "active" compounds than it is to characterize an entire biolibrary.

Numerous algorithms exist by which the diversity of a set of compound structures can be measured; however, little agreement is found regarding the best approach. In general, these software programs partition libraries into a uniform array of blocks or cells on the basis of descriptor coordinates, and the number of cells is proportional to the level of diversity. Some algorithms define atom pair fingerprints, which indicate the presence or absence of pairs of atom types separated by a defined number of bonds, and use them to describe and differentiate each structure. Other algorithms cluster structures into groups; the Jarvis-Patrick clustering algorithm requires that each member of a cluster have in common a predefined number of chemical neighbors.[11] The similar Hodes clustering model has been used by the NCI to assess structural novelty of new compounds submitted for screening.[12] Often, the goal of these computer algorithms is to define a library of the smallest number of compounds that covers the greatest diversity of space. Using these approaches, large collections of compounds can be winnowed into smaller sublibraries. However, detractors point out that by using these, for the most part, unproven tools and limiting the compounds screened, one risks decreasing the chance of finding drug leads. On the other hand, the economics of HTS calls for prudent use of reagents and encourages the use of such approaches.

A detailed analysis of the NCI OSR was conducted recently, with special emphasis on the uniqueness of the library relative to commercial libraries and other databases.[13] Substantial chemical diversity is present in the NCI repository, which has generated of a subset of the OSR containing approximately 140,000 compounds arrayed into multiwell plates. The inventory for most of the remaining compounds is simply too small for these compounds to be provided for routine screening campaigns. Notwithstanding, the plated version of the NCI OSR is a unique publicly available (see http://dtp.nci.nih.gov) resource that includes many compounds that cannot be found elsewhere.

In an attempt to provide the structural diversity of the OSR in a smaller package, a further subset of the compounds was selected using Chem-X (Chemical Design, Ltd., Oxfordshire, UK), a program that addresses coverage of three-dimensional space. The goal was to distill the broad set of structures in the larger OSR into a more easily manipulated set of compounds for initial application to screening campaigns. Additional information on the resulting approximately 2,000-member NCI "Diversity Set" may be found at the DTP website. Subsequent analysis of the two-dimensional structural diversity of this subset of compounds was performed by plotting the compounds onto a self-organizing map of "clusters" constructed from information about all of the compounds in the OSR. Although the Diversity Set does have representation spanning the entire map of structural space, it could potentially be more homogenously distributed across the different clusters of structures present in the OSR, and it substantially overrepresents several clusters.[14] The NCI currently is selecting a second generation of the Diversity Set that will be optimized for coverage of the chemical space defined by the self-organizing map. Despite these concerns, the current Diversity Set has found application in pilot-scale screening to support HTS assay development and has yielded interesting lead compounds from a variety of molecular targeted screens.[15–17]

As with the larger libraries that are commercially available, questions regarding the quality of the compounds with the Diversity Set arise. To address these issues, a chemical analysis of the Diversity Set was performed recently by DTP. A relatively high-throughput high-performance liquid chromatography/mass spectrometry method was devised that accommodates the majority of chemical species. By this analysis, approximately 1,600 of the 1,990 samples in the Diversity Set were shown to contain a mass ion corresponding to the database structure. Purity ranged from >95% to approximately 15% for samples yielding a correct mass ion. Some of the samples for which structural authenticity could not be confirmed have a structure indicated by the database for which this high-throughput analytical approach is not appropriate. Thus, these compounds may have "failed" for technical reasons. Structural authenticity of approximately 300 samples was not supported by this analysis. Detailed information for individual samples is available at the DTP website to allow interpretation of screening results obtained with the Diversity Set.

HIGH-THROUGHPUT SCREENING ASSAY DESIGN

To screen for modulators of a given molecular target, the activity of the protein or the system must be linked to a readily detectable readout. Commonly used types of screening assays can be loosely divided into two categories: separation-based, in which starting material must be removed before the product can be detected, and homogeneous, in which separation of the starting material and the product is not required. Examples of separation-based protocols include filter-binding assays in which the product is selectively retained by the filter (usually an ion-exchange media) and precipitation assays during which one component is selectively precipitated and removed by a glass fiber filter. When used as a screening assay, enzyme-linked immunosorbent assays are generally considered to be separation based. Some techniques that are classified as homogeneous assays include fluorescence polarization, fluorescent resonance energy transfer, scintillation proximity, and luminescent proximity (APLHA Screen). Other homogeneous assays measure changes in light absorbance (UV/vis), in the activity of luciferase, or in the expression of green fluorescent or other related proteins. In general, the throughput of samples with homogeneous assays is much higher than with separation-based assays because the latter require more extensive manipulation of the samples.

Within these categories, the assays can be further divided into cell-based and in vitro (cell-free). Cell-based assays measure the ability of a compound to affect a target within the milieu of an intact cell, whereas cell-free assays measure inhibition of a purified protein. A strength of cell-based assays is the ability to detect inhibitors of an entire targeted pathway (as opposed to a particular step in a pathway). Limitations of cell-based assays include the need to subsequently define the identity of the actual target within the pathway, interference from toxic compounds, and inability to test compounds that cannot penetrate the cell (although this latter feature can also be viewed as an advantage). In comparison, cell-free screening assays are limited neither by cell permeability of compounds nor by nontargeted compound toxicity. When possible, it can be very informative to screen a selected target in both cell-based and in vitro assay systems because their strengths are complementary.

COMMON ISSUES IN HIGH-THROUGHPUT SCREENING IMPLEMENTATION

A major restriction to the development of new HTS assays has been the acquisition and standardization of reagents. Even with substantial miniaturization, many molecularly targeted screens require much more target protein (and/or many more cells) than is needed for basic research on the target. It is essential that sufficient reagents are available for the entire screening effort to avoid batch-to-batch variation. Also, many of the newer, highly sensitive technologies, although affordable on a small scale, become prohibitively expensive when screening large libraries. The availability and cost of reagents can be the pivotal factor in deciding whether to screen a selected target.

An ideal assay plate design includes untreated, negative control wells and wells with compound or condition known to affect the target (positive controls). These provide clear definition of the maximum and minimum signal on an individual plate and, therefore, the window in which compound activity can be measured. However, when studying a newly identified and incompletely characterized target, a specific inhibitor (or activator) may not be known. For some targets, a more generic method of inhibition can be used in the absence of a specific inhibitor (for example, EDTA inhibits most metal-dependent enzymes.) The reproducibility among the control wells within a plate and the reproducibility of the control wells among the plates within a set are indicative of the quality of the screen; this will be addressed later.

Once a new screening assay has been designed and standardized, it is important to characterize its performance by completing pilot-scale screens. For DTP screens, the NCI

Training Set of 230 compounds routinely is tested at least twice, and the correlation between the two sets of data provides a quantitative measure of the reproducibility of the assay.[14] Sometimes intriguing lead structures can emerge from pilot-scale screening efforts; for example, a recent screen of the NCI Diversity Set for inhibitors of the HIF1α pathway identified several camptothecin analogs, the activities of which have been confirmed in secondary testing.[17]

EXAMPLES FROM NCI DTP SCREENS

The DTP website contains searchable and downloadable primary HTS data (Diversity Set) from screens targeting Met signaling, hypoxic cell signaling, the CEBPα transcription factor, and HIV-1 nucleocapsid/nucleic acid interaction. The first three of these utilized cell-based assays, whereas the latter was a cell-free assay. Figures 2.2 and 2.3 illustrate the character of the HTS data from the standpoint of frequency of active samples and the potential to utilize one screen as a selectivity "counterscreen" for another. Screening data from these two campaigns can be combined and compared to assess selectivity of the active compounds. The plot shown in Figure 2.4 demonstrates facile identification of samples that were active in both screens and thus of reduced interest as screening leads. For example, the single data point in the lower right corner of Figure 2.4, which had striking induction in the CEBPα-luciferase reporter assay and notable inhibition in the HIF-1α-luciferase reporter assay, was a quinocarmycin analog that appears to activate CEBP as a stress response and to inhibit HIF by generation of DNA damage.

CHEMOINFORMATICS

Lead Identification and Development

The goal of any molecularly targeted screen is to identify inhibitors (or activators, in some cases) of a particular protein or pathway, and it is a sine qua non of such exercises to distinguish real "hits" from false-positives. Two primary factors to consider are the overall quality of the screening data and the definition of a hit. The most common metric to quantify the quality of screening data is known as Z' and is defined by the following equation[18]:

$$Z' = 1 - \left[\frac{(3\sigma_{c+} - 3\sigma_{c-})}{\mu_{c+} - \mu_{c-}} \right]$$

In this equation, μ is the mean value of the positive and negative controls for the assay and σ is the standard deviation of these values. Assays for which $Z' > 0.5$ are considered acceptable for HTS. There are three commonly used strategies for selecting active compounds for secondary analysis: (a) to select all compounds displaying a particular level, or range of activity; (b) to select all compounds with activity that falls outside a designated level of deviation from the mean; and (c) to select a particular number of compounds defined by the institutional limitations for follow-up. In practice, the third strategy is employed, to some degree, with all screens because there are always practical limits on follow-up capabilities. Consistency among control samples and a manageable number of hits are evidence of a well-designed screen and increases the probability of identifying high-quality lead compounds.

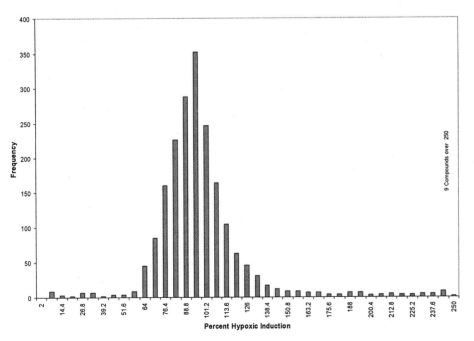

HIF-1 Diversity Set Frequency Distribution

Figure 2.2 Distribution of activity observed in primary HTS of the NCI Diversity Set (1 μM) for inhibition of induction of hypoxic cell signaling. The majority of samples tested were without inhibitory activity, with a modal activity around 100%. A minority of inhibitory samples are observed in the left-hand tail of distribution. This tail also includes toxic and nonselective inhibitors of transcription that were resolved in secondary testing. Data and details of the screening protocol are available on the DTP website. Overall results are described in Rapisarda et al.[17]

C/EBPa Diversity Set Frequency Distribution

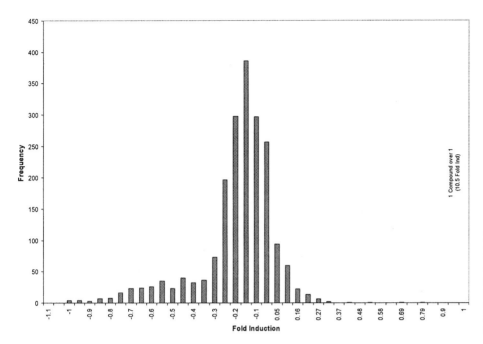

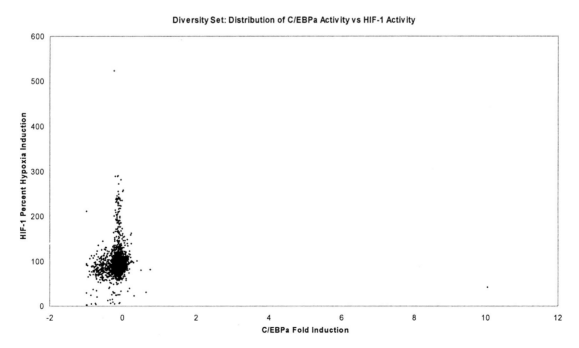

Figure 2.3 Distribution of activity observed in primary HTS of the NCI Diversity Set (1 μM) for induction of CEBPα-luciferase reporter. Only a very small number of samples in the right side of the distribution demonstrated activity equal to 50% or more of the positive control (retinoic acid). Data and details of the screening protocol are available on the DTP website.

The process for culling hits is multifold and usually begins by confirming compound identity and activity and demonstrating a dose-response relationship. Ideally, the proposed mechanism of action of compounds identified in in vitro assays is corroborated in cell-based assays and vice versa. Often, confirmed active compounds subsequently are filtered through one or more algorithms designed to recognize druglike molecules and purge compounds known to be toxic, reactive, and/or to affect multiple molecular targets nonselectively. Filtering software packages are available from several companies, including Leadscope, Inc. (Columbus, OH), Accerlys, Inc. (Burlington, MA), Bioreason, Inc.

Diversity Set: Distribution of C/EBPa Activity vs HIF-1 Activity

Figure 2.4 Plot of inhibitory activity in the HIF-1α HTS of the NCI Diversity Set versus activation of the CEBPα-luciferase reporter. Compounds in the lower right quadrant meet the indicated criteria for activity (reduction of HIF-1α signaling to 50% or less of the control value and induction of the CEBPα-luciferase reporter to at least 50% of the level of the positive control compound).

Results of Chemo- and Bio-informatic Analysis

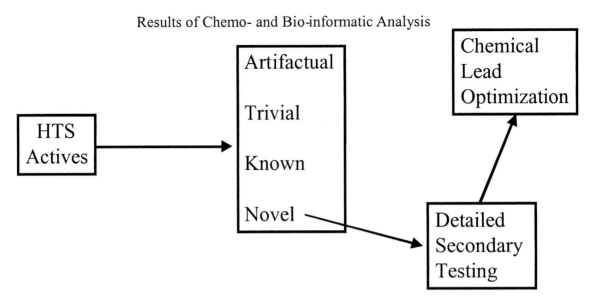

Figure 2.5   Results of chemoinformatic and bioinformatic analysis.

(Santa Fe, NM), and Golden Helix, Inc. (Bozeman, MT). Eventually, the active, desirable compounds are used as the basis for lead optimization and development. At a practical level, this process can be viewed as an informatic triage of the screening data in which active compounds or classes are partitioned into categories, as illustrated in Figure 2.5.

Pharmacokinetic Considerations

At some point during the culling process, the pharmacologic demands of absorption, distribution, metabolism, and excretion must be considered. A common criticism and limitation of HTS is that such screening assays are usually designed to find the compound that is most potent and most selective against a particular target, without regard to solubility, bioavailability, and/or toxicity. Historically, considerable effort in drug discovery programs has been spent refining drug leads that subsequently fail in the development process because of toxicity, lack of in vivo efficacy, or poor pharmacokinetic properties.

The development of predictive, inexpensive, in vitro assays and computer models to quantify pharmacologic properties are helping to alleviate this lead development bottleneck and substantially enhancing the multidisciplinary character of drug discovery. For example, assays such as those developed by Exelexis, Inc. (San Francisco, CA) use parameters including partition coefficients, P-glycoprotein efflux, P-450 induction and metabolism, and protein binding to predict the pharmacokinetics of novel compounds. These assays have been standardized to the greatest extent possible with the use of in vivo data from animals and humans. There are numerous, commercially available software packages that rely entirely on "well-trained" computer algorithms to predict compound absorption (GastroPlus [Simulations Plus, Inc., Lancaster, CA] and iDEA pk Express

[LION Bioscience Inc., Cambridge, MA]), subcompartment penetration, plasma protein binding, metabolism (MetabolExpert [CompuDrug International Inc., Sedona, AZ], META [Multicase, Beachwood, OH], and Meteor LHASA, Dept. of Chem, Leeds, UK), and drug-drug interactions (Q-DIPS Dr Pascal Bonnabry, Geneva, Switzerland). The use of these and other similar model systems is permitting analysis of the pharmacologic properties of a larger number of compounds earlier in the development process; it is hoped that this will reduce the rates of compound failure.

Ideally, initial pharmacologic studies in animals would provide confidence that the area under the concentration $\times$ time curve (AUC) achievable in animals approximates the drug exposure that is necessary in tumor cells propagated in vitro to achieve an effect on the target molecule leading to an expected tumor-modulating effect. This is most frequently assessed as proliferation, but could also be related to AUCs causing a decrease in clonogenic potential in semisolid media, an assay that has been related to tumorigenic or metastatic capacity.

NATIONAL CANCER INSTITUTE CELL-BASED SCREENING SYSTEMS

Anticancer drug screening began at the NCI about 50 years ago in response to Congressional interest in removing barriers to anticancer drug discovery and development. NCI screening initially was an empirical process in which test samples were administered to mice bearing transplantable tumors. The L1210 and P388 mouse leukemia models proved to be highly sensitive and evolved into prescreening models supplemented with secondary testing in solid mouse tumors and xenografts. Detailed historical information on the in vivo screening program can be found in

Zubrod.[19] Additional details, as well as the rationale for transition to in vitro human tumor cell models, can be found in Shoemaker and Sausville.[20]

This latter model, comprising 60 tumor cell lines representing multiple histologic tumor types, was operated as a primary antitumor drug screen for over a decade and was particularly noteworthy for the information-rich character of the screening data. A recent review has described in detail the value of this screen for characterizing mechanisms of growth inhibition and cytotoxicity.[21] Consideration of the 60-cell screening data for a new chemotype, even one selected on the basis of an a priori defined molecular target, can reveal important aspects of the action of the new molecule. This includes its utilization of previously described detoxification mechanisms such as the P-glycoprotein efflux pump, the relation of compound action to conventional cytotoxics, or tying the compound action to the presence or function of molecular targets or pathways in tumor cells. These interpretations of the 60-cell screening data utilize the COMPARE , neural network, cluster analysis, and self-organizing map algorithms.[21–23] However, the potential of the 60 tumor cell line screen has been limited by the labor-intensive nature of cell production, plating, drug addition, and end point processing. This, in addition to the growing number of attractive molecular targets for drug discovery, has led to development of an infrastructure for high-throughput molecular targeted screening at the NCI, much of which has been previously described.

IN VIVO EFFICACY TESTING

At the completion of the primary screening process, including confirmation of hits, definition of lead structures and their structural optimization (ideally using information derived from binding of the lead to its intended target molecule), a limited set of well-understood compounds should have been characterized for preliminary pharmacology and chemical stability in the physiologic milieu. Sufficient quantity should be available to allow detailed understanding of their actions in animal models of tumor cell growth, or in vivo efficacy evaluations. Historically, this testing has been empirically utilized with compounds tested at maximum tolerated doses on fixed schedules established for individual tumor models.[24] In the era of molecular targeted drug development, customization of in vivo model testing for individual agents is becoming more common, using tumor cells selected to overexpress or underexpress the drug's target. Indeed, the availability of a pharmacodynamic assay that can support testing to establish an optimal dose for target modulation can be crucial to development of a new agent. Data relating antitumor activity to pharmacodynamic and pharmacokinetic effects potentially can be followed from the preclinical arena to the earliest clinical testing. Lack of target modulation in the clinic or failure to obtain or maintain adequate drug levels

would be an early indication of lack of therapeutic potential. Conversely, clear evidence of target modulation at drug levels associated with preclinical activity can argue strongly for accelerated clinical development. Recent examples of approved drug molecules that have utilized modulation of their intended molecular target through the development process as key evidence supporting and informing their continued development include the proteosome inhibitor bortezomib[25] and the epidermal growth factor antagonist gefitinib.[26]

A common concern is how valid are various animal models of cancer drug action in projecting ultimate clinical activity. Recently, Johnson et al.[27] have examined the utility of subcutaneous xenografts in athymic mice in this regard for cytotoxic agents introduced between 1980 and 1990. It is clear that such models are relatively poor in predicting activity on a disease-by-disease basis. For example, activity in breast cancer xenografts poorly predicts ultimate activity in human breast cancer. On the other hand, activity in many different models does predict a higher likelihood of activity in some human clinical population. Specifically, activity of the agent in >33% of the models tested predicted an approximately 50% likelihood of clinical activity in at least one human tumor type. In contrast, cytotoxic agents with <33% of the tumor models affected had essentially no evidence of clinical activity. Careful consideration of the achievable pharmacology in humans in designing experiments in mice can clearly increase the predictive value of the murine experiments.[28] Whether these statistics can be improved by selection of models created to depend on the function of the molecular target of the action of a drug remains to be seen, and is the object of much current research interest.

PRACTICAL ASPECTS OF IN VIVO EFFICACY TESTING

A variety of animal models for evaluating anticancer therapies have been described. Although each model has its protagonists, no single model is ideal for all applications. Thus, one must determine what information is desired from the in vivo study to make an informed choice regarding which model(s) to use. Table 2.1 lists the types of critical information needed from efficacy studies.

Initial Detection of Antitumor Activity: The Hollow Fiber Assay

The desire to implement a high throuput, low-cost, in vivo prescreen so that lead compounds could be prioritized for efficacy testing in the xenograft models led to development of the hollow fiber assay.[29] This assay has emerged as the initial in vivo screen by the NCI for lead compounds with cytostatic or cytocidal potential. Compounds with activity in the hollow fiber assay are considered for testing

---

TABLE 2.1

INFORMATION TO BE GAINED FROM IN VIVO EFFICACY TESTING

Initial detection of antiproliferative activity
Is there efficacy at sublethal doses?
How do metabolism and excretion impact efficacy?
What administration route(s) is/are effective?
What dose and schedule are optimal?
Are toxic phenomena associated with an efficacious dose?
How do analogs and prodrugs compare in efficacy?
Which physiologic compartment does the compound reach?

---

in human tumor xenografts after compound mechanism of action, formulation, and pharmacokinetic issues are considered. The hollow fiber assay allows screening of ≥50 compounds per week in a 10-day assay that uses <500 mg of compound while testing for growth suppression of less than 10^6 tumor cells.[29,30] The assay as practiced at NCI evaluates the activity of a test agent against a standard panel of 12 cell lines consisting of 2 lines each from the breast, colon, lung, melanoma, CNS, and ovarian tumor histology subpanels. For the standard assay, compounds are evaluated at two dose levels based on the maximum tolerated dose (MTD) determined in mouse toxicity assays. The high test dose is set at $(1.5 \times \text{MTD})/4$ and the low dose is 67% of the high test dose. Hollow fiber cultures of each cell line are prepared in vitro and implanted subcutaneously and intraperitoneally into mice. Because compound delivery is accomplished through intraperitoneal injection, the anticellular activity can be assessed in a same site (intraperitoneally/intraperitoneally) and a distant site (subcutaneously/intraperitoneally) modality in the same mouse. The mice are treated with vehicle or test agent for 4 days, and the fibers are retrieved for evaluation of viable cell mass using a formazan dye conversion assay. The percent net growth of each cell line is calculated by comparison with a set of control fibers assessed for viable cell mass on the day of implantation.

Rodent Tumor Models: Additional Considerations

A variety of tumor models have been described in rodents, with those of greatest interest occurring in rats and mice. This results partly from their relatively low body weights, which minimize the amount of chemotherapeutic needed, and the fact that their physiology is the best understood of the rodent species and there are many inbred strains available. Murine leukemias, grown in the peritoneal cavity and producing morbidity as an end point, have been used for many years. Use of the L1210 and P388 leukemias in drug screening efforts was reviewed by Waud.[31] In addition to the leukemias, a variety of solid tumors are available for

modeling antitumor activity. These include tumors of varying histologic types and implant sites. These tumor systems have been thoroughly reviewed by Corbett et al.[32]

Human Tumor Xenograft Models

There is much in the literature regarding human tumor xenograft models that rely on immunocompromised mice as hosts for tumors of various histologies.[24,33–36] These models can be divided into subgroups based on the site at which the tumor cells are inoculated, as well as the end point measured by the assay. Tumors have been successfully generated following tumor cell inoculation into the peritoneal cavity, the subcutaneous tissues, the vascular network via cardiac or tail vein puncture, under the renal capsule, and various other organ sites.

One of the simplest xenograft models involves direct injection of tumor cells into the peritoneal cavity with subsequent administration of test agent by one of several routes. In most cases, the end point for these intraperitoneal xenograft assays is host morbidity. This results from ascites and intraperitoneal tumor formation and dissemination of the tumor to distant organs, for example, the brain, for some tumor cell lines. Because there is no requirement for daily tumor measurements, these assays are less labor-intensive and less cost-prohibitive than other xenograft models. Unfortunately, not all cells are amenable to growth in the peritoneal cavity, so the desired cell line must be assessed for its growth potential. An intraperitoneal tumor is difficult to observe until ascites are present, so it is important to standardize the assay so that all of the inoculated mice do produce viable tumor growth. It is also of value to determine the minimum inoculum required to give the desired end point in all of the test mice (e.g., time to ascites development). The NCI in vivo screening program has found the HL-60 promyelocytic leukemia, U251 glioblastoma, LOX melanoma, and several other ovarian, leukemic, and lymphoma cell lines acceptable for subcutaneous tumor models (M Hollingshead, unpublished data). With these models, direct administration of the test agent into the peritoneal cavity offers the greatest potential for activity for most compounds because they do not have to achieve effective plasma concentrations or distribute to the target tissues. This approach is often referred to as a "same-site" model because the target (tumor cells) and the test agent are placed into close proximity. Although this does not address issues such as agent uptake, distribution, metabolism, and excretion, it does allow an initial assessment of the in vivo potential of the test article. The occurrence of protein binding, local cellular uptake, rapid systemic absorption and distribution, metabolism, and host toxicity can be preliminarily assessed in these same-site models. Nonetheless, activity only in a same-site model is less valuable than activity that occurs after a molecule traverses several phamacologic compartments.

TABLE 2.2
SUBCUTANEOUS XENOGRAFT EFFICACY PARAMETERS

Number of tumor-free mice at end of experiment
Optimal percent treated/control based on median tumor weight
Median days to tumor reaching specified weight or doubling volumes
Growth delay at a specified tumor weight or doubling volume
Net log cell kill
Number of complete and partial tumor regressions
Toxicity-related deaths
Treatment-related weight loss

Subcutaneous Xenograft Tumors

The subcutaneous xenograft model is commonly used for chemotherapeutic assessment as the tumor growth can be monitored visually throughout the experiment. For these assays, tumor cells are placed under the skin of immunocompromised mice (e.g., SCID, nu/nu, NIH-III, SCID/bg, SCID/NOD) and the cells are monitored for growth by daily observation. When tumors are detected at the inoculation site, daily measurement of the tumor volume can be accomplished with calipers. Generally, the tumor length and width are measured, and the tumor volume is calculated using one of several formulas.[37] The NCI assumes the tumor is a prolate ellipsoid so the volume = [tumor length (mm) $\times$ tumor width (mm)^2]/2. Assuming a unit volume of 1, then the volume in cubic millimeters is equal to the tumor weight in milligrams. The tumor weights versus time can be plotted to produce tumor growth curves that are compared between control and experimentally treated mice to ascertain whether treatment has an impact on tumor growth. Parameters for measuring compound efficacy in these subcutaneous xenograft models have been described elsewhere. The parameters used in the NCI drug-screening program are given in Table 2.2, and a summary of the implementation features of various models are summarized in Table 2.3.

Orthotopic Implants

One of the deficiencies of the subcutaneous xenograft model is its failure to produce the metastatic lesions that ultimately kill many cancer patients.[38,39] There are a few subcutaneous xenograft models that do produce metastatic lesions (e.g., LOX melanoma, SK-MEL-28 melanoma, MDA-MB-435 breast, DU-145 prostate), but they are the exception rather than the rule.

Fidler and colleagues[40] and Fidler[41] demonstrated that the occurrence of metastatic lesions is not the result of a random event. Rather, they are selective, and the metastatic event consists of a series of steps that depend on the tumor cell injection site. Fidler demonstrated that a tumor implanted orthotopically, for example, into the organ of origin, behaved more like the clinical disease and was thus a better model for human cancer than the subcutaneous models. This concept has proven useful for studying tumor biology and therapies because orthotopic implantation generates tumors that produce metastatic lesions similar to those seen in man.[42–44] To further extend the importance of orthotopic xenografts, Fidler and coworkers[45] demonstrated differences in drug sensitivity between orthotopically and subcutaneously implanted tumor tissue. Although tissues of any origin can be implanted orthotopically, those most commonly used are breast, colon, brain, melanoma, and lung tumors. Building on the concept of orthotopic implantation, Hoffman[46] developed and patented the MetaMouse. This model differs from other orthotopic models in that the implanted tumor material consists of surgically attached pieces of tumor rather than cell suspensions or simple trocar-implanted tumor fragments. The tumor fragments used in the MetaMouse are obtained directly from human patients or from human tumor xenografts grown subcutaneously on immunocompromised mice. Giavazzi[47] and Hoffman[39] have reviewed orthotopic models and the resulting metastatic lesions.

Metastatic Models

Metastasis, the process by which tumor cells leave their tissue of origin and colonize distant tissues, has become a target for new antineoplastic therapies. The metastatic process consists of multiple events that result from invasion of the tissue and of vascular and lymphatic components adjacent to the primary tumor. This process is initiated by basement membrane invasion resulting from proteolysis and cell motility. Following tumor cell intravasation into the circulation, tumor cell emboli are trapped in distant capillary beds in which extravasation can occur.[48] A small percentage of these embolic tumor cells may survive to produce tumors.[49] Another critical component in these events is the tumor vasculature, as it provides the tumor with nutrients for growth as well as provides a pathway by which tumor cells can gain entry to distant tissues. Each step in the metastatic process may be viewed as a potential target to interrupt tumor spread.[50] Unfortunately, the in vivo tumor models currently available do not assess the individual targets but rely on demonstration of an effect downstream of these targets, an antitumor effect. This can be measured with standard subcutaneous xenograft models if the target is applicable, such as antiangiogenic agents. If the target is not relevant in the subcutaneous models, such as basement membrane proteolysis, then the orthotopic models are an option. These models are generally metastatic, so an effect on one or more steps in the metastatic process should reduce the number of detectable tumor nodules at the metastatic site(s).

TABLE 2.3
TYPES OF MURINE IN VIVO EFFICACY MODELS

Model	Host Immune Status	Assay Length	Relative Cost	Difficulty	End point
Murine IP	Competent	10 days	Low	Low	Survival leukemia
Murine solid tumor	Competent	10–30 days	Low	Moderate	Tumor size
Human IP	Deficient	15–90 days	Moderate	Low	Survival xenograft
Human SC	Deficient	15–90 days	Moderate	Moderate	Tumor size xenograft
Orthotopic	Either	weeks to months	Low to moderate	Moderate	Morbidity, survival, metastasis
Disseminated tumor	Either	14–90 days	Low to moderate	Moderate	Morbidity, survival, metastasis
Transgenic	Either	weeks to months	High	High	Morbidity, survival, metastasis

Intravenous Tumor (Disseminated Tumor)

Disseminated tumor models in which intravenously injected tumor cells colonize the lungs and other tissues offer another method for evaluating agents effective in the later stages of metastasis. Perhaps the best known of the disseminated tumor models is the murine melanoma, B16-BL6.[51] The B16-BL6 melanoma is able to metastasize from a primary subcutaneous site as well as following intravenous injection. Thus, the same tumor cell can be used to assess both upstream and downstream events in the metastatic process. This model has been utilized successfully to evaluate a matrix metalloproteinase inhibitor designed to inhibit basement membrane degradation.[52] Although not as well characterized as B16-BL6, there are human xenograft models in which intravenously administered cells produce disseminated disease in immune-deficient mice, particularly SCID mice. Examples of human tumor cell lines producing this effect are LOX melanoma, SK-MEL-28 melanoma, K562 chronic myelogenous leukemia, AS-283 AIDS-related lymphoma, and A549 lung tumor.[53] Problems with the disseminated models include the need for reproducible intravenous inoculations in rodents and the inability to identify the exact cause for reductions in lung or other organ colonization.

Antiangiogenic Agents

The impact of inhibiting angiogenesis on tumor growth and metastasis has led to the development of specific antiangiogenic assays in addition to the standard tumor growth-inhibition assays. Various in vitro assays can assess the impact of a therapeutic agent on endothelial cell proliferation, migration, and cord formation.[54] These assays help delineate the mechanism of action for a potential therapeutic, but they may not show activity with all agents. Compounds whose effects are mediated through a secondary mechanism, such as cytokine induction, would not demonstrate effects in these in vitro assays. For in vivo studies, many laboratories use the chicken chorioallantoic membrane as a substrate to assess antiangiogenic agents.[55] This is a more complex assay than the in vitro assays, but it does lack several features of human neoplasia. These differences include (a) it is not mammalian, (b) it is embryonic, (c) it does not simulate the tumor angiogenesis microenvironment, (d) it is only semiquantitative, and (e) some researchers believe that it may not measure clinically relevant activity.

Various in vivo models are described that measure the growth of blood vessels into an exogenously administered substrate. Although various substrates have been described,[54] the most commonly used is Matrigel to which various angiogenic agents, e.g. VEGF, bFGF, have been added.[56] Matrigel (BD Biosciences, San Jose, CA) is a basement membrane extract in which new blood vessels develop following injection into the subcutaneous tissue of rodents. By quantitating the number of vessels and/or the hemoglobin content, the angiogenesis response can be defined. Of note, Matrigel can be used to support xenogeneic tumor cells for injection into mice because it protects the tumor cells, provides a physiologic support, and may provide a medium into which vascular components can migrate.

The corneal angiogenesis assay provides another tumor-independent assay.[57,58] For this assay, controlled-release pellets containing angiogenic agents, for example, basic fibroblast growth factor (bFGF) or VEGF, are placed into corneal micropockets and vessel growth is quantified in the presence or absence of treatment with putative antiangiogenic agents. This approach was used in the initial assessment of the antiangiogenic potential of TNP-470 and thalidomide, two purported antiangiogenic compounds taken into clinical trials

Molecular Targets and Transgenic Animals

One current interest in cancer therapeutics involves modulation of various molecular targets in neoplastic cells. These targets include oncogenes, which promote unregulated cell growth (e.g., *ras, fos, myc, sis, erb*) and tumor suppressor genes that suppress tumor growth (e.g., *p53*).

Although a large number of targets have been defined, the importance of each of them is an area of current research. The interest in these targets has led to a two-pronged strategy to develop animal models to validate these molecular targets, both as important tumorigenicity targets and as chemotherapeutic targets. One approach is to transform cells with oncogenes so that the effect of the oncogene on cellular activity can be assessed both in vitro and in vivo. If the nontransformed cell line is tumorigenic, then the in vivo activity of a compound against the transformed and nontransformed cells can be compared using methods described earlier. Another approach is the generation of transgenic mice bearing one or more mutations. In many instances these transgenic mice develop spontaneous tumors at a defined age.

The impact of chemotherapeutic agents on tumor development and growth may be assessed following treatment at various times relative to the predicted tumor occurrence. The range of models available has recently been reviewed.[59] As an example of their value, Barrington et al.[60] reported that L-744,832, a farnesyltransferase inhibitor, is *p53*-independent utilizing transgenic mice expressing one or more oncogenes in the presence or absence of *p53*. These transgenic mice offer an exciting approach to manipulating potential treatment targets; however, their use for routine in vivo screening is often limited by the time required for tumor development and the amount of compound necessary to treat for a protracted period of time. Additionally, the number of mice developing tumors may be <50%, so extremely large treatment groups are necessary to obtain statistically relevant results. For example, a transgenic model in which only 30% of mice develop tumors may require hundreds of test animals to achieve statistical validity. It is recommended that a statistician be consulted to aid in determining the appropriate treatment group size for a given tumor model prior to embarking on a chemotherapy trial.

NEW IMAGING TECHNOLOGIES IN EFFICACY STUDIES

Highly sensitive imaging techniques for quantitating fluorescent and bioluminescent signals in live rodents are providing new approaches to model development efficacy. Tumor cell lines or transgenic mice engineered to express green fluorescent protein, luciferase, or other fluorescent/bioluminescent markers can be imaged in vivo. This allows small numbers of tumor cells to be visualized and quantitated following orthotopic implantation. Furthermore, small metastatic lesions, not obvious in classic tumor models, can be visualized in essentially all tissue sites. Transgenic mice can be engineered to express these signals when tumors are initiated or when other promoters are activated. This provides a means to progressively monitor otherwise "hidden" events. Even though these technologies are in the early phases of validation, they offer possibilities for significant enhancement of rodent tumor models.[61] Although these techniques are amenable to rodent models, they do not currently offer a potential for translating into direct human clinical endpoints. However, commercial availability of rodent positron emission tomography, magnetic resonance imaging, and computed tomography scanners is opening a pathway to techniques that can be directly translated into human studies. This is important not only for improving diagnostic imaging models, but for assessing the impact of treatment on tumor blood flow, tumor mass, and other clinically relevant end points.

PRECLINICAL PHARMACOLOGY AND TOXICOLOGY STUDIES

Following clear demonstration of antitumor activity in an appropriate range of animal models, the next phase of a drug's preclinical development addresses its effects on the host organism, independent of the presence of tumor. The goal of preclinical toxicology studies for anticancer drugs is to determine in appropriate species the maximally tolerated dose (MTD), the nature of dose-limiting toxicity (DLT), demonstration of schedule-dependent toxicity, and the reversibility of that toxicity.[62–66] This results in the ability to estimate a "safe" starting dose for initial clinical trials, which for small organic molecules is one-tenth the MTD, or one-third the toxic dose low (TDL) in nonrodents. The TDL is defined as the highest toxic dose that, when doubled corresponds to a nonlethal dose. Thus, one-sixth is used with the highest nonlethal dose. In no case is a dose that just begins to elicit reversible toxicity utilized to define the starting dose.

Toxicologic evaluations are typically divided into preliminary or "range-finding" studies, which assess clinical characteristics of drugs administered at a range of doses selected to bracket those that are effective and those that are toxic. More detailed investigational new drug (IND)-directed toxicology evaluations focus on the actual proposed clinical use schedule and seek to define a nontoxic, just toxic, and overtly toxic series of doses during which animals are followed for the appearance and reversibility of clinical signs, along with studies of clinical chemistry, hematology, and histopathology of all organs.[63] These studies are currently required by the Food and Drug Administration (FDA) to utilize two species, including at least one nonrodent species, and to utilize the proposed clinical dose and schedule.[64–66] In contrast, evaluation of "biologicals" including antibodies, immunotoxins, and vaccines, generally utilize only the most relevant animal species, exposed to the agent using the anticipated clinical route and schedule.

Previously, toxicology evaluations utilized "standard" protocols; for example, the standard NCI toxicology protocols from 1980 to 1988 included determination of the LD10 on day 1 and day 1 through day 5 dosing schedules, followed by assessment of safety and DLT when administered at the LD10 on a day 1 and day 1 through day 5 schedule.[65] The current development paradigm, in contrast, is "agent-directed" and targets the most effective route and schedule of administration.[63–66] For example, twice weekly, or continuous infusion for periods as long as 28 days are now routine initial phase 1 schedules.

Preclinical analytical studies routinely define a suitable assay for study of bulk and formulated drug stability and a separate assay for the drug in biologic fluids. Pharmacologic studies are conducted to determine the pharmacokinetics in rats and dogs after single intravenous doses and by the route and schedule that mimics what was efficacious in animal models. Toxicokinetic studies, referring to the relationship between plasma drug levels and the elicitation of toxicity in animals, are conducted as part of the toxicology studies. Additional studies that increase confidence that the drug will perform well in clinical trials provide demonstration that one can obtain efficacious drug levels in vivo, with correlation of drug plasma levels, and/or AUC with safety and toxicity. It should be noted that the toxicologic studies previously described are required for all drugs, whereas the development of pharmacology assays are only pursued if possible. Not all antineoplastic agents have been amenable to assay at the time of entry into clinical trial (especially many highly potent natural products), so pharmacology information is desirable, but not legally essential for clinical study.

INITIATION OF CLINICAL STUDIES

The regulatory requirements for use of an agent vary with the type of use. To enter early clinical trials (e.g., phase 1 or 2), documentation that the proposed schedule may be safely given is the goal of FDA review. To allow marketing of the agent, FDA must determine that the agent is safe and effective. The latter is customarily defined by behavior in phase 3 trials, in which the test agent is compared with standard or no therapy. An increasingly popular strategy is to attempt to gain "accelerated approval" for an agent to treat a dire or life-threatening disease. In that event, phase 2 data may be sufficient to allow such accelerated approval if the following end points were obtained: unequivocal evidence of tumor diminution or clear documentation of preserved performance status in the absence of a "response" including favorable outcome of "quality of life" indicators. In the event of accelerated approval, postmarketing stipulations to assure continued judgment of likely benefit are defined.

To allow inception of phase 1 dose-escalation trials, following completion of toxicologic evaluations, reversible toxicity must be demonstrated to be likely after the first manifestation of a drug's adverse effects (as opposed to poorly predictable and irreversible toxicity). The drug is then ready for entry into the clinic, provided that a reliable and workable formulation of the agent has been defined. To allow commencement of the clinical trial, an IND application must be approved by the FDA. The components of an IND include cover sheet (Form 1571); table of contents; introductory statement; general investigative plan; investigator's brochure; initial clinical protocol; chemistry, manufacturing, and control (this extremely important section provides for the precise description and chemical characteristics of the drug under study, how it was made, and how it is to be labeled); toxicology data; pharmacology data (if available); previous human experience; and miscellaneous (including potential for abuse, and results of radiotracer experiments). Responsibilities of the sponsor of phase 1 studies include submission of the IND application, assuring qualifications of investigators, writing and securing local Institutional Review Board (IRB) approval of protocols, shipping investigational agents and maintaining detailed shipping records corresponding to lots sent, assessing adverse drug reactions and submitting them in a timely fashion to FDA, preparing an annual report of the IND activities to the FDA, monitoring quality of the data through periodic audits, assuring that the use and disposition of the investigational agent is properly accounted for at the study sites, assuring informed consent is obtained for each patient entering into the study, tracking amendments made to protocols after inception of clinical studies, and informing investigators of new information pertinent to the trial. These regulations are contained in 21 CFR 312.50.

REFERENCES

1. Hanahan D, Weinberg RA. The hallmarks of cancer. Cell 2000; 100:57–70.
2. Uttenhoeve C, Pilotte L, Théate I, et al. Evidence for a tumoral immune resistance mechanism based on tryptophan degradation by indoleamine 2,3-dioxygenase. Nature Med 2003;9: 1269–1274.
3. O'Brien SG, Guilhot F, Larson RA, et al. Imatinib compared with interferon and low-dose cytarabine for newly diagnosed chronic myelogenous leukemia. N Engl J Med 2003;348:994–1004.
4. Vogel CL, Cobleigh MA, Tripathy D, et al. Efficacy and safety of trastuzumab as a single agent in first-line treatment of HER2-over-expressing metastatic breast cancer. J Clin Oncol 2002;20: 719–726.
5. Paez JG, Janne PA, Lee PC, et al. EGFR mutations in lung cancer: correlation with clinical response to gefitinib therapy. Science 2004;304:1458–1461.
6. Lynch TJ, Bell DW, Sordella R, et al. Activating mutations in the epidermal growth factor receptor underlying responsiveness of non-small-cell lung cancer to gefitinib. N Engl J Med 2004;350: 2129–2139.
7. Hurwitz H, Fehrenbacher L, Novotny W, et al. Bevacizumab plus irinotecan, fluorouracil, and leucovorin for metastatic colorecal cancer. N Engl J Med 2004;350:2335–2342.
8. Kwan KY, Wang JC. Mice lacking DNA topoisomerase IIIbeta develop to maturity but show a reduced mean lifespan. Proc Natl Acad Sci U S A 2001;98:5717–5721.
9. Cragg GM, Newman DJ. Antineoplastic agents from natural sources: achievements and future directions. Expert Opin Investig Drugs 2000;9:2783–2797.

10. Geysen HM, Meloen RH, Barteling SJ. Use of peptide synthesis to probe viral antigens for epitopes to a resolution of a single amino acid. Proc Natl Acad Sci U S A, 1984;81:3998–4002.

11. Jarvis RA, Patrick EA. Clustering using a similarity measure based on shared near neighbors. IEEE Trans Comput 1973;C22:1025–1034.

12. Hodes L. Clustering a large number of compounds. 1. Establishing the method on an initial sample. J Chem Inf Comput Sci 1989;29:66–71.

13. Voigt JH, Bienfait B, Wang S, et al. Comparison of the NCI open database with seven large chemical structural databases. J Chem Inf Comput Sci 2001;41:702–712.

14. Shoemaker RH, Scudiero DA, Melillo G, et al. Application of high-throughput, molecular-targeted screening to anticancer drug discovery. Curr Top Med Chem 2002;2:229–246.

15. Stephen AG, Worthy KM, Towler E, et al. Identification of HIV-1 nucleocapsid protein: nucleic acid antagonists with cellular anti-HIV activity. Biochem Biophys Res Commun 2002;296:1228–1237.

16. Lazo JS, Aslan DC, Southwick EC, et al. Discovery and biological evaluation of a new family of potent inhibitors of the dual specificity protein phosphatase Cdc25. J Med Chem 2001;44:4042–4049.

17. Rapisarda A, Uranchimeg B, Scudiero DA, et al. Identification of small molecule inhibitors of hypoxia-inducible factor 1 transcriptional activation pathway. Cancer Res 2002;62:4316–4324.

18. Zhang JH, Chung TD, Oldenburg KR. A simple statistical parameter for use in evaluation and validation of high throughput screening assays. J Biomol Screen 1999;4:67–73.

19. Zubrod CG. Origins and development of chemotherapy research at the National Cancer Institute. Cancer Treat Rep 1984;68:9–19.

20. Shoemaker RH, Sausville EA. New drug development. In: Souhami RL, Tannock I, Honenberger P, et al., eds. Oxford Textbook of Oncology. Oxford: Oxford University Press, 1999: 781–788.

21. Holbeck SL. Update on NCI in vitro drug screen utilities. Eur J Cancer 2004;40:785–793.

22. Paull KD, Shoemaker RH, Hodes L, et al. Display and analysis of patterns of differential activity of drugs against human tumor cell lines: development of mean graph and COMPARE algorithm. J Natl Cancer Inst 1989;81:1088–1092.

23. Rabow AA, Shoemaker RH, Sausville EA, et al. Mining the National Cancer Institute's tumor-screening database: identification of compounds with similar cellular activities. J Med Chem 2002;45:818–840.

24. Plowman J, Dykes DJ, Hollingshead MG, et al. Human tumor xenograft models in NCI drug development. In: Teicher BA, ed. Anticancer Drug Development Guide: Preclinical Screening, Clinical Trials, and Approval., Totowa, NJ: Humana Press, 1997:101–125.

25. AdamsJ, Kauffman M: Development of the proteosome inhibitor Velcade. (Bortezomib). Cancer Invest 2004;2:304–11.

26. El-Rayes BF, LoRusso PM: Targeting the epidermal growth factor receptor. Br J Cancer 2004;91:418–24.

27. Johnson JI, Decker S, Zaharevitz D, et al. Relationships between drug activity in NCI preclinical in vitro and in vivo models and early clinical trials. Br J Cancer 2001;84:1424–1431.

28. Peterson JK, Houghton PJ. Integrating pharmacology and in vivo cancer models in preclinical and clinical drug development. Eur J Cancer 2004;40:837–844.

29. Hollingshead MG, Alley MC, Camalier RF, et al. In vivo cultivation of tumor cells in hollow fibers. Life Sci 1995;57:131–141.

30. Decker S, Hollingshead M, Bonomi CA, et al. The hollow fibre model in cnacer drug screening: the NCI experience. Eur J Cancer 2004;40:821–826.

31. Waud WR. Murine L1210 and P388 Leukemias. In: Teicher BA, ed. Anticancer Drug Development Guide: Preclinical Screening, Clinical Trials, and Approval. Totowa, NJ: Humana Press, 1997: 59–74.

32. Corbett T, Valeriote F, LoRusso P, et al. In vivo methods for screening and preclinical testing use of rodent solid tumors for drug discovery. In: Teicher BA, ed. Anticancer Drug Development Guide: Preclinical Screening, Clinical Trials, and Approval. Totowa, NJ: Humana Press, 1997:75–99.

33. Fiebig HH, Maier A, Burger AM. Clonogenic assay with established human tumour xenografts: correlation of in vitro to in vivo activity as a basis for anti-cancer drug discovery. Eur J Cancer 2004;40:802–820.

34. Giovanella BC, Stehlin JS. Heterotransplantation of human malignant tumors in "nude" thymusless mice. I. Breeding and maintenance of "nude" mice. J Natl Cancer Inst 1973;51:615–619.

35. Leonessa F, Green D, Licht T, et al. MDA435/LCC6 and MDA435/LCC6MDR1: ascites models of human breast cancer. Br J Cancer 1996;73:154–161.

36. McLemore TL, Abbott BJ, Mayo JG, et al. Development and application of new orthotopic in vivo models for use in the US National Cancer Institute's drug screening program. In: Wu B-q, Zheng J, eds. Immune-Deficient Animals in Experimental Medicine. 6th International Workshop of Immune-Deficient Animals. Beijing: Basel, 1989:334–343.

37. Clarke R. Issues in experimental design and endpoint analysis in the study of experimental cytotoxic agents in vivo in breast cancer and other models. Breast Cancer Res Treat 1997;46:255–278.

38. Fine DL, Shoemaker R, Gazdar A, et al. Metastasis models for human tumors in athymic mice: useful models for drug development. Cancer Detect Prev Suppl 1987;1:291–299.

39. Hoffman RM. Patient-like models of human cancer in mice. Curr Perspec Molec Cell Oncol 1992;1:311–326.

40. Fidler IJ, Wilmanns C, Staroselsky A, et al. Modulation of tumor cell response to chemotherapy by the organ environment. Cancer Metastasis Rev 1994;13:209–222.

41. Fidler IJ. Rationale and methods for the use of nude mice to study the biology and therapy of human cancer metastasis. Cancer Metastasis Rev 1986;5:29–49.

42. Giavazzi R, Jessup JM, Campbell DE, et al. Experimental nude mouse model of human colorectal cancer liver metastases. J Natl Cancer Inst 1986;77:1303–1308.

43. Mohammad RM, Al-Katib A, Pettit GR, et al. An orthotopic model of human pancreatic cancer in severe combined immunodeficient mice: potential application for preclinical studies. Clin Cancer Res 1998;4:887–894.

44. Berry KK, Siegal GP, Boyd JA, et al. Development of a metastatic model for human endometrial carcinoma using orthotopic implantation in nude mice. Intl J Oncol 1994;4:1163–1171.

45. Wilmanns C, Fan D, O'Brian CA, et al. Orthotopic and ectopic organ environments differentially influence the sensitivity of murike colon carcinoma cells to doxorubicin and 5-fluroaracil Int J Cancer 1992;52:98–104.

46. Hoffman RM. Fertile seed and rich soil. In: Teicher BA, ed. Anticancer Drug Development Guide: Preclinical Screening, Clinical Trials, and Approval. Totowa, NJ: Humana Press, 1997:127–144.

47. Giavazzi R. Metastic models. In: Boven E, Winograd B, eds. The Nude Mouse in Oncology Research. Boca Raton, FL: CRC Press, 1991:117–132.

48. Dickson RB, Johnson MD, Maemura M, et al. Anti-invasion drugs. Breast Cancer Res Treat 1996;38:121–132.

49. Fidler IJ. Selection of successive tumour lines for metastasis. Nat New Biol 1973;242:148–149.

50. Zetter BR. Angiogenesis and tumor metastasis. Annu Rev Med 1998;49:407–424.

51. Talmadge JE, Fidler IJ. Cancer metastasis is selective or random depending on the parent tumour population. Nature 1982;297:593–594.

52. Chirivi RG, Garofalo A, Crimmin MJ, et al. Inhibition of the metastatic spread and growth of B16-BL6 murine melanoma by a synthetic matrix metalloproteinase inhibitor. Int J Cancer 1994;58:460–464.

53. Guilbaud N, Kraus-Berthier L, Saint-Dizier D, et al. Antitumor activity of S 16020-2 in two orthotopic models of lung cancer. Anticancer Drugs 1997;8:276–282.

54. Taraboletti G, Giavazzi R. Modelling approaches for angiogenesis. Eur J Cancer 2004;40:881–889.

55. Schlatter P, Konig MF, Karlsson LM, et al Quantitative study of intussusceptive capillary growth in the chorioallantoic membrane (CAM) of the chicken embryo. Microvasc Res 1997;54:65–73.

56. Passaniti A, Taylor RM, Pili R, et al. A simple, quantitative method for assessing angiogenesis and antiangiogenic agents using reconstituted basement membrane, heparin, and fibroblast growth factor. Lab Invest 1992;67:519–528.

57. Muthukkaruppan V, Auerbach R. Angiogenesis in the mouse cornea. Science 1979;205:1416–1418.

58. Kenyon BM, Voest EE, Chen CC, et al. A model of angiogenesis in the mouse cornea. Invest Ophthalmol Vis Sci 1996;37:1625–1632.

59. Hansen K, Khanna C. Spontaneous and genetically engineered animal models: use in preclinical cancer drug development. Eur J Cancer 2004;40:858–880.

60. Barrington RE, Subler MA, Rands E, et al. A farnesyltransferase inhibitor induces tumor regression in transgenic mice harboring multiple oncogenic mutations by mediating alterations in both cell cycle control and apoptosis. Mol Cell Biol 1998;18:85–92.

61. Hollingshead MG, Bonomi CA, Borgel SD, et al. A potential role for imaging technology in anticancer efficacy evaluations. Eur J Cancer 2004;40:890–898.

62. Grieshaber CK. Agent-directed preclinical toxicology for new antineoplastic drugs. In: Valeriote FA, Corbett H, eds. Cytotoxic Anticancer Drugs: Models and Concepts for Drug Discovery and Development. Boston: Kluwer Academic Publishers, 1992: 247–260.

63. Tomaszewski JE, Smith AC. Safety testing of antitumor agents. In: Williams PD, Hottendorf GH, eds. Comprehensive Toxicology, Toxicity Testing and Evaulation., Oxford: Elservier Science Ltd., 1997:299–309.

64. DeGeorge JJ, Ahn CH, Andrews PA, et al. Regulatory considerations for preclinical development of anticancer drugs. Cancer Chemother Pharmacol 1998;41:173–185.

65. Lowe MC, Davis RD. The current toxicology portocol of the National Cancer Institute. In: Hellman D, Carter S, eds. Fundamentals of Cancer Chemotherapy. New York: McGraw Hill, 1987:228–235.

66. Tomaszewski JE. Multi-species toxicology approaches for oncology drugs: the US perspective. Eur J Cancer 2004;40:907–913.

Pharmacokinetics

3

Jerry Collins   Jeffrey G. Supko

It has become generally accepted that the biologic effects of a drug are related to the time course of the concentration of the administered compound or an active metabolite in the bloodstream. The realization of this association has evolved as advances were made in the discipline of pharmacokinetics, which is defined as the study of rate processes involved in the absorption of drug from the administration site into the bloodstream, its subsequent distribution to extravascular regions throughout the body, and its eventual elimination from the body. From a broader perspective, pharmacokinetics may be thought of as the effect that the body has on a drug, whereas the pharmacologic effects that a drug has on the body are the realm of pharmacodynamics.

In anticancer chemotherapy, the general goal of killing tumor cells or inhibiting their proliferation and metastasis is clearly defined. However, in most cases we are severely limited by an inability to deliver drugs in a manner that separates antitumor effects from normal tissue toxicity. Much remains to be learned about the differences between normal and tumor tissues that can be exploited therapeutically. Thus, although pharmacokinetics is a tool that can be used to evaluate the feasibility of a drug delivery strategy based on intended pharmacodynamic effects, it is not a replacement for knowledge of exploitable differences between host and tumor.

Studies to characterize the pharmacokinetic behavior of a drug have become integral to the preclinical and clinical development of new anticancer agents. One group[1] has even suggested that "it is now inconceivable to perform clinical research in cancer chemotherapy without obtaining adequate pharmacokinetic data." Some of the usual objectives for undertaking a pharmacokinetic study in the context of a phase I or II clinical trial in cancer patients are: (a) initial characterization of the pharmacokinetic behavior of new chemotherapeutic agents in humans, (b) assessing whether or not an administration schedule provides a potentially effective pattern of systemic exposure to drug,

(c) determining the magnitude of intrapatient and interpatient variability in pharmacokinetic parameters, (d) assessing the influence of patient characteristics on drug disposition, (e) establishing predictive correlations between biologic effects and pharmacokinetic parameters, and (f) determining whether combining drugs results in pharmacokinetic interactions. In addition, pharmacokinetic drug level monitoring has been used to improve therapy through dose individualization, to evaluate patient compliance during chronic therapy, and to assess whether alterations in drug disposition or metabolism are associated with the development of toxicity or the lack of effect.

The fundamental obstacle to greater success in the application of pharmacokinetics and clinical drug level monitoring to anticancer therapy is our limited knowledge of pharmacodynamics. A complete understanding of the actions of a drug necessarily requires discerning the nature of the association between its pharmacokinetic behavior and pharmacodynamic effects. Relationships between pharmacokinetics and the severity of toxicity have been established for many anticancer drugs. However, pharmacokinetic associations accounting for the therapeutic effects of a chemotherapeutic agent are more difficult to establish because of the multiplicity of factors involving the host and tumor that influence response, as noted above, as well as the time lapse from initiating treatment to the first indications of a therapeutic response. Nevertheless, elucidating the pharmacokinetic behavior of an anticancer drug may benefit efforts to determine the dose, route of administration, and schedule that maximizes the potential for therapeutic effectiveness while minimizing the likelihood of serious toxic effects.

The intention of this chapter is to provide readers with a fundamental understanding of clinical pharmacokinetics and its practical application to the development and use of anticancer chemotherapy. Numerous texts with widely varying levels of complexity and focus are available for those interested in a more comprehensive discourse of the subject, ranging from easily understood introductions to the discipline[2] to more advanced texts with a mathematical approach.[3]

ACQUISITION AND ANALYSIS OF PHARMACOKINETIC DATA

Sample Collection and Drug Concentration Measurement

Pharmacokinetic studies involve collecting serial specimens of blood and other biologic fluids, such as urine, at predetermined time intervals from subjects following administration of the drug. Plasma is the blood component in which drugs are most commonly measured during pharmacokinetic studies, although determinations are also made in serum and, less frequently, whole blood. The concentration of drug present in the study samples is measured using an appropriate bioanalytical method. Technical advances in separation and detection methods, especially the maturation of high-performance liquid chromatography coupled to mass spectrometry into a technique suitable for routine use, have provided a greatly improved basis for drug concentration measurement during the past decade. Review articles surveying the current techniques used for assaying drugs in biologic fluids regularly appear in the literature.[4]

Many anticancer drugs are difficult to measure because of inherent instability, either spontaneously degrading or being degraded by enzymes in blood or tissues. It is therefore important to recognize that the quality of data derived from any pharmacokinetic study ultimately depends on the reliability of the assay used to measure the drug, as well as the manner by which samples were processed and stored prior to analysis. The majority of bioanalytical methods used for pharmacokinetic studies measure the total concentration of drug, that is, free drug plus that which is reversibly associated with plasma proteins. However, the reversible binding of a drug to plasma proteins, such as albumin and α_1-acid glycoprotein, needs to be considered in the interpretation of total drug concentrations.[5] Only the free or unbound drug is pharmacologically active. Protein binding is usually assessed experimentally by ultrafiltration or equilibrium dialysis.

The Plasma Concentration-Time Profile

Except for cases in which a drug is given by bolus intravenous injection, the plasma concentration-time (CxT) profile of any drug exhibits an initial region of increasing concentration, the achievement of a peak or maximum concentration (C_{max}), followed by a continual decline in concentration (Fig. 3.1A). The concentration of drug in plasma increases as long as the rate of input into systemic circulation exceeds the rate of loss due to distribution into other extracellular fluids, intracellular spaces, and tissues throughout the body, and elimination from the body. The C_{max} is achieved when the rate of drug input is equivalent to the rate of loss from plasma, which occurs at the instant that an intravenous injection or short infusion is terminated. During a continuous intravenous infusion, plasma levels of the drug increase at a progressively decreasing rate and eventually become constant, indicative of achieving steady-state conditions, if the infusion is continued for a sufficiently long time (Fig. 3.1C).

Figure 3.1 shows the same CxT data plotted on graphs with semilog axes (panel A) and rectangular coordinate axes (panel B). Presenting pharmacokinetic drug CxT profiles on semilog graphs provides a better visual depiction of the entire data set than a coordinate plot because plasma levels of a drug frequently differ by several orders of magnitude during the course of the observation period. Furthermore, the concentration of many drugs in systemic circulation decays in an apparent first-order manner, exemplified by a terminal region in the plasma profile in which the logarithm of the drug concentration is a linear function of time. Thus, a semilog plot provides some immediate inferences regarding the nature of the pharmacokinetic behavior of a drug.

The pattern of decay in the plasma concentration of a drug that exhibits first-order kinetics comprises one or more exponential phase. In the case of a plasma profile with drug concentrations that decline in a single log-linear phase, the entire body appears to be kinetically homogenous, with equilibrium of the drug between plasma and other fluids or tissues into which it distributes being very rapidly achieved, before the first blood specimen has been acquired. Polyexponential behavior results from distinguishable differences in the reversible transfer of drug from plasma to various regions or compartments of the body. Thus, for example, the presence of two exponential decay phases implies that the body behaves as if it is composed of two kinetically distinct compartments, comprising plasma and tissues with which equilibrium is rapidly established, and a second compartment comprising all other regions of the body into which drug distributes more slowly.

For some purposes, a mathematical equation or model is necessary to interpret pharmacokinetic data, but often questions may be answered without a formal model construction. Recently, there has been a growing trend toward analyzing pharmacokinetic data by empirical approaches that consider only the concentration of drug in the sampled fluid and require few assumptions about model structure. In these techniques, which include model-independent analysis[6] and noncompartmental analysis,[7] the various exponential decay phases are usually referred to simply as the initial, intermediate, and terminal disposition phase. Regardless of the particular method of analysis employed,

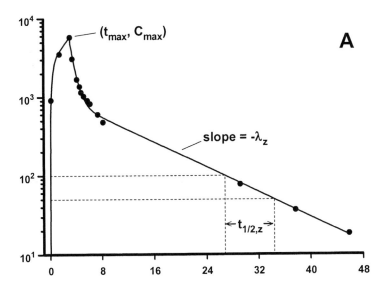

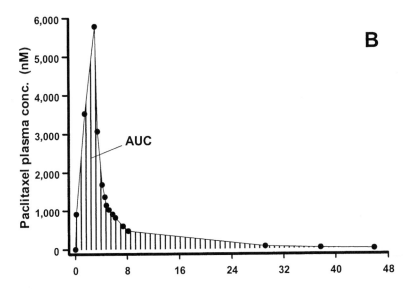

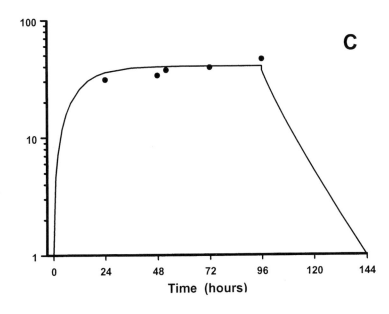

Figure 3.1   A. Plasma concentration-time profile for a 175 mg/m^2 dose of paclitaxel administered as a 3-hour continuous intravenous infusion shown on a graph with log-linear axes. Pharmacokinetic variables that can be estimated by visual inspection are indicated: maximum drug concentration (C_{max}), the time at which the peak concentration (t_{max}) occurs, and the biological half-life ($t_{1/2,z}$). **B.** Presentation of the same data shown in the upper panel on rectangular coordinate axes. The shaded area corresponds to the area under the curve (AUC). **C.** Time course of paclitaxel in plasma when given as a 96-hour continuous intravenous infusion at a rate of 25 mg/m^2 per day. The steady-state plasma concentration of the drug is approximately 40 nM.

the ultimate objective is the same, which is to estimate values of descriptive pharmacokinetic parameters from the CxT data.

Physiologic Pharmacokinetic Models

For pharmacologists interested in developing an understanding of drug disposition in individual tissue compartments, models that incorporate physiologic compartments are of considerable interest. These models require measurements of actual physiologic parameters, such as volumes and blood flow rates, as well as drug concentrations in various compartments, and therefore are based primarily on data from experimental animals. Entry into specific areas such as the central nervous system may be of critical importance in the use of drugs, and physiologic models can allow comparisons of CxT profiles for various schedules and routes of administration. Physiologic models have been constructed for many anticancer drugs. Models have been published for the most important drugs in clinical practice, among which are methotrexate (MTX),[8] 5-fluorouracil (5-FU),[9] cisplatin,[10] and doxorubicin.[11]

In the most general form, physiologic pharmacokinetic models are overly complex and require too large a database for routine clinical use. However, they provide a basis for understanding a drug's kinetic behavior that can be incorporated into simpler models, either physiologic or hybrid, assimilating both empiric observations and physiologic information. Physiologic modeling goes beyond the usual goals of empiric pharmacokinetic modeling to allow for incorporation of data into the model that has been obtained in other species or in vitro. The compartments comprising a physiologic pharmacokinetic model have an anatomic basis, and the transfer processes in the model have a physiologic or pharmacologic identity. Each organ is modeled separately; then, the model connections are provided by blood flow. The structure for the physiologic model for cytarabine is presented in Figure 3.2.[12]

PHARMACOKINETIC PARAMETERS

Area Under the Curve

Noncompartmental analysis is considerably simpler than any equation-defining method of pharmacokinetic data analysis. All calculations and data manipulations can be performed by most spreadsheet software programs. The observed plasma CxT data is numerically integrated, most commonly by the trapezoidal method. In its simplest application, each successive set of data points, beginning with time zero, is used to define a trapezoid, the area of which is readily calculated. The cumulative sum of the areas of all such trapezoids affords an estimation of the area under the CxT curve to the last sample with a measurable drug concentration ([C_t] $AUC_{0 \to t}$). The slope of the

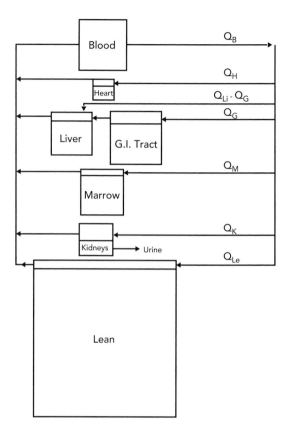

Figure 3.2 Physiologic pharmacokinetic model for cytosine arabinoside. GI, gastrointestinal. (Reprinted with permission from Dedrick RL, Forrester DD, Cannon JN, et al. Pharmacokinetics of 1-β-D-arabinofuranosylcytosine (ARA-C) deamination in several species. Biochem Pharmacol 1973;22:2405–2417.)

terminal log-linear phase of the CxT profile ($-\lambda_z$) is then determined by linear regression using log-transformed concentration values (see Fig. 3.1A). The area under the curve from time zero to infinity (AUC) can then be calculated as

$$AUC = AUC_{0 \to t} + C_t/\lambda_z \qquad [3.1]$$

Although the AUC is not a pharmacokinetic parameter per se, because its magnitude depends on the administered dose of drug, it represents an important quantitative measure of total systemic drug exposure, as illustrated in Figure 3.1B. In addition, knowledge of the AUC is required to calculate values of pharmacokinetic parameters, as described in the following section.

Total Body Clearance

The total body clearance (CL) of a drug is formally defined as the volume of plasma from which drug is completely removed per unit time. It is readily calculated as

$$CL = D_{iv}/AUC \qquad [3.2]$$

where D_{iv} is the dose of the drug given by intravenous injection or infusion. CL reflects the combined contribution of all processes by which drug is removed from the body, as represented by the equation

$$CL = CL_R + CL_{NR} \qquad [3.3]$$

where CL_R and CL_{NR} designate renal and nonrenal clearance, respectively.[13] Renal clearance is usually the only route of drug elimination that can be directly and quantitatively determined in patients by noninvasive procedures. All other mechanisms of drug elimination that cannot be readily estimated, including biliary excretion of unchanged drug, metabolism, nonenzymatic irreversible reactions with endogenous molecules, and spontaneous chemical degradation, are grouped together as CL_{NR}. CL has units of volume per time (e.g., milliliters per minute, Liter per hour) and is frequently normalized to the body weight or body surface area of subjects (e.g., milliliters per minute per kilogram, liter per hour per square meter) under the presumption of minimizing interpatient variability in the magnitude of the parameter. However, this practice has recently become a topic of considerable controversy because the underlying presumption of a relationship between unnormalized clearance values and body surface area does not exist for a significant number of anticancer drugs.[14] The CL values are often compared with glomerular filtration rate and hepatic blood flow, average values of which are approximately 125 mL/min (4.6 liter/hr per square meter) and 1,500 mL/min (56 liter/hr per square meter), respectively, in normal adults.[15,16] Although often informative, these comparisons can be extremely misleading unless the extent of plasma protein binding has been taken into account because only the free fraction of drug that is not bound to plasma proteins is usually subject to organ-mediated excretion or metabolism.

Apparent Volume of Distribution

The total body apparent volume of distribution, V_z, is strictly a proportionality constant relating the total amount of drug in the body to plasma concentration. It may be calculated by the equation

$$V_z = CL/\lambda_z \qquad [3.4]$$

and has units of volume, typically expressed in terms of milliliters or liters normalized to body weight or body surface area (e.g., milliliters per kilogram, liters per square meter). V_z is designated as an apparent volume because it is a hypothetical value that is not directly related to any real physiologic space. Nevertheless, it is an informative parameter, providing an indication of the relative extent of drug distribution from plasma. Specifically, for a given amount of drug in the body, the fraction present in plasma decreases as its distribution into peripheral tissues increases, leading to greater values of V_z.[17] Therefore, the effective lower limit of V_z is the plasma volume, which is approximately 4.5% of body weight (i.e., 45 mL/kg, 1.7 liter/m^2) for a normal adult. There really is no upper limit, as V_z can assume extremely large values in cases where the half-life of the terminal disposition phase is long relative to that of the preceding disposition phase, and drug levels decrease by several orders of magnitude before the terminal phase is achieved. For example, some anticancer agents, such as the anthracyclines, have V_z values exceeding 1,000 liters/m^2 (27 times body weight).

Biologic Half-Life

The biologic half-life of a drug ($t_{1/2,z}$) is the time required for its plasma concentration to decrease by 50% any time during the terminal log-linear phase in the CxT profile (see Fig. 3.1A). It is only applicable to drugs that exhibit apparent first-order pharmacokinetics (see later discussion). As indicated by the relationship

$$t_{1/2,z} = 0.693 \cdot V_z / CL \qquad [3.5]$$

$t_{1/2,z}$ reflects both the ability of the body to eliminate the drug as well as the extent to which the drug distributes throughout the body. Nevertheless, there is a recurrent tendency in the anticancer drug literature to place undue emphasis on the value of $t_{1/2,z}$ as an indicator of drug elimination. The $t_{1/2,z}$ has an important practical application in that steady-state conditions during administration of a drug by continuous intravenous infusion or a multiple dosing regimen are achieved when the duration of treatment exceeds 4 times the value of $t_{1/2,z}$.

Linear and Nonlinear Pharmacokinetics

The majority of clinically used anticancer agents exhibit linear or first-order pharmacokinetics, whereby plasma concentrations of the drug decline in an exponential manner following intravenous administration. A distinguishing and defining characteristic of linear pharmacokinetics is that the plasma concentration of drug at a given time after dosing is directly proportional to the administered dose. Thus, the AUC increases proportionately with the dose and values of the pharmacokinetic parameters (i.e., CL, V_z) and are independent of the dose. When a drug is predominantly eliminated by a potentially saturable process, such as hepatic metabolism or active tubular secretion, departures from linear pharmacokinetic behavior may become evident if sufficiently high doses can be administered to patients. As illustrated in Figure 3.3, classic nonlinear pharmacokinetics is indicated by a change in the appearance of the plasma profile from exponential character at lower doses to the appearance of a distinct downward curvature in the semilog plot of the plasma profile at higher doses.[18] In addition, the apparent CL exhibits a progressive decrease in magnitude as the dose is escalated. A clear example of this phenomenon was reported recently for high-dose cytarabine given by continuous intravenous infusions in which small changes in the infusion rate produced disproportionately large increases in the steady-state drug concentration in plasma.[19]

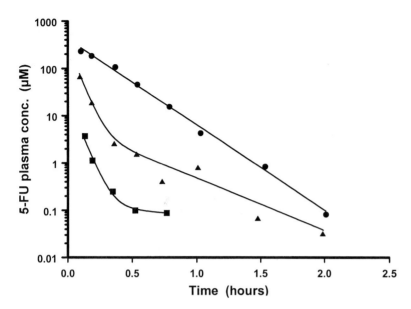

Figure 3.3 Plasma profiles of 5-flourouracil determined at doses of 25 mg/m^2(■), 125 mg/m^2 (▲), and 375 mg/m^2 (●) illustrating the effect of classic nonlinear pharmacokinetics. Values of the apparent total body clearance decreased progressively from 142 liter/hr per square meter for the 25 mg/m^2 dose to 47 liter/hr per square meter at 125 mg/m^2 and 30 liter/hr per square meter at 375 mg/m^2. There would be no significant difference between the clearance determined at different doses if the pharmacokinetic behavior of the drug was linear.

DRUG ELIMINATION

Renal and Hepatic Excretion

Establishing the major pathways of drug elimination in patients is also an important objective of clinical pharmacokinetic studies. Disease states that compromise the function of a major drug-eliminating organ, such as the kidneys or liver, can enhance a patient's sensitivity to the toxic effects of the drug as a result of increased drug exposure. For this reason, patients with significant organ impairment are usually excluded from initial phase I studies to avoid possibly confounding sources of toxicity.

Renal excretion is a quantitatively significant route of elimination for many relatively small compounds, with molecular weights less than about 300, that are also highly to moderately hydrophilic,[20] if they are not substantially metabolized. Larger compounds and those with a more lipophilic character tend to be predominantly eliminated by biliary excretion, either directly or after metabolism. Determining CL_R involves measuring the amount of unchanged drug present in the urine (A_e) collected during one or more defined time intervals (Δt) following intravenous drug administration. It may be calculated by either of the following equations

$$CL_R = A_e/AUC_{0\to t} \qquad [3.6]$$

$$CL_R \approx (\Delta A_e/\Delta t)/C_{mid} \qquad [3.7]$$

depending on whether urine has been continuously collected and pooled from the beginning of dose administration throughout the time that plasma specimens were obtained, or during one or more discrete time intervals after dosing. In the second equation, C_{mid} is the plasma concentration of drug at the midpoint of the urine collection interval. The amount of unchanged drug in feces cannot be taken as a direct indication of biliary excretion because of the potential for drug metabolism by the gastrointestinal microflora.[21]

In cases in which renal or biliary excretion are significant pathways of drug elimination, a predictive correlation may exist between clinical indicators of renal or hepatic function, such as serum creatinine and bilirubin levels, respectively, and CL. Establishing these relationships serves as the basis for defining guidelines pertaining to the minimal organ function required for patient eligibility in phase II studies and devising an empirical algorithm for dosage adjustment, including those documented in Table 3.1.[22] (See also "Eliminating Organ Dysfunction.")

Drug Metabolism

Metabolism represents a quantitatively important route of elimination for most anticancer agents. Xenobiotic biotransformation reactions may be broadly categorized into two classes, designated phase I and phase II. The principal phase I reactions are oxidation, reduction, and hydrolysis. Phase II reactions involve the conjugation or coupling of endogenous molecules, including glucuronide, sulfate, amino acid, methyl and glutathione moieties to the parent drug or a precursory phase I metabolite. Hepatic oxidation mediated by the cytochromes P$_{450}$ (CYP450), a large family of heme-containing isozymes, undoubtedly plays the greatest overall role in drug metabolism among the phase I reactions.[23] The CYP450 enzymes are most abundantly expressed in the liver, but they are also present in the kidney, lung, and gastrointestinal epithelium. The predominant enzyme in this family, CYP3A4, catalyzes the oxidation of a multitude of structurally diverse compounds.[24–26] These include imatinib, gefitinib, docetaxel, etoposide, ifosfamide, vincristine, and paclitaxel. In addition to hepatic metabolism, some important phase I reactions are mediated

TABLE 3.1

PREDOMINANT ELIMINATION MECHANISMS AND DOSE ADJUSTMENT RECOMMENDATIONS FOR ANTICANCER DRUGS

Major Route of Elimination	Anticancer Agent	Dose Adjustment for Organ Dysfunction[a]
Renal excretion	Bleomycin	b
	Carboplatin, Cisplatin	b
	Etoposide	b
	Fludarabine	b
	Hydroxyurea	b
	Methotrexate	b
	Pentostatin	b
	Topotecan	b
Hepatic metabolism CYP450	Busulfan	c
	Chlorambucil	no
	Cyclophosphamide[b]	no
	Ifosfamide[b]	no
	Imatinib	e
	Irinotecan	no
	Paclitaxel	c
	Thio-TEPA	no
	Vinca alkaloids	c
Conjugation	Etoposide	c
	SN-38	
Ubiquitous enzymes	Cytarabine	no
	Gemcitabine	no
	6-Mercaptopurine	d
Nonenzymatic hydrolysis	BCNU[b]	no
	Mechlorethamine	no
	Melphalan	no
Biliary excretion	Doxorubicin	no
	Irinotecan	no
	Vinca alkaloids	c

[a] b, Decrease dose in proportion to the reduction in creatinine clearance below 60 mL/min. c, Serum bilirubin: 1.5–3.0 mg/100 mL, 50% dose reduction; >3.0 mg/100 mL, 75% dose reduction. d, Patients with S-methyl transferase deficiency. e, Insufficient data to determine if dose reduction is necessary in hepatic dysfunction.
[b]Enzymatic or spontaneous chemical reactions required for drug activation.

by ubiquitous enzymes found in virtually all tissues of the body, such as dihydropyrimidine dehydrogenase, which catalyzes the reduction of 5-FU, and cytidine deaminase, which inactivates cytarabine.[27,28] Glucuronide conjugation catalyzed by uridine diphosphate glucuronosyl-transferases (UGT) is the most commonly encountered phase II reaction. In contrast to phase I metabolism, which may yield a biologically active product, glucuronidation almost exclusively represents a detoxification mechanism that inactivates a compound and facilitates its excretion through enhanced hydrophilicity and recognition by biliary canicullar efflux proteins.[29] Glucuronidation is a clinically important route of elimination for 7-ethyl-10-hydroxycamptothecin

(SN-38), the active metabolite of irinotecan, as the extent of its glucuronidation has been associated with the risk of severe diarrhea for the weekly treatment schedule of irinotecan.[30]

Chemical Degradation

Chemical degradation can be a significant elimination mechanism for drugs that are susceptible to hydrolysis, such as many of the alkylating agents. Nonenzymatic reactions between drugs and endogenous molecules can also contribute prominently to elimination. For example, platinum alkylating agents form covalent adducts with serum albumin.[31]

FACTORS CONTRIBUTING TO PHARMACOKINETIC VARIABILITY

Obtaining an indication of interpatient variability in the values of pharmacokinetic parameters and related variables are important objectives of phase I trials. This information has considerable practical utility with regard to clinical drug development. These findings provide the basis for assessing the ability to reliably predict the C_{max} and AUC of a drug following the administration of any given dose to patients who have not been previously studied. The recommended dose of cytotoxic anticancer drugs is typically close to the maximum tolerated dose, and dose-limiting toxicities are often related in some manner to the levels of drug achieved in plasma. Thus, the margin of safety of these agents very much depends on the consistency of their pharmacokinetic behavior between patients. Conversely, the existence of a high degree of interpatient pharmacokinetic variability can result in unpredictable episodes of toxicity at the maximum tolerated dose, which may make it difficult to establish a potentially effective and safe dose. Although rarely employed in these circumstances, drug level monitoring to establish the optimal dosing regimen in individual patients may be warranted.

Patient Characteristics

Clinically significant associations between CL and patient characteristics such as age, sex, and race have been identified for many anticancer drugs. For example, it has been shown that the CL of 5-FU in females is significantly lower than in males and that formation of the glucuronide metabolite of SN-38 by UGT is subject to pharmacogenetic variations related to both race and gender.[32,33] These factors are now being examined extensively during the clinical evaluation of new anticancer drugs.

Currently, more than half of all cancers are presented by patients over 60 years old. However, relatively few elderly patients are entered into early-stage clinical trials because of referral patterns and investigator bias. As a consequence, the pharmacokinetic behavior of most anticancer drugs has not been adequately characterized in elderly patients.[34] There is a very high degree of heterogeneity in older cancer patients as a result of natural changes in body composition, including decreased muscle mass, increasing adipose tissue, and decreased renal function that occur with advancing age. Normal aging is accompanied by a 25 to 35% decrease in liver volume and a 35 to 40% decrease in hepatic blood flow.[35,36] Thus, the CL of drugs with a high hepatic extraction ratio, which is limited by liver blood flow, may be decreased in the elderly.[37,38] Age-associated changes in the function of some drug-metabolizing enzymes have been identified but their clinical significance remains uncertain.[39,40]

At the other end of the age spectrum, experience has shown that safe and effective doses of anticancer agents for children very often cannot be based simply on body weight or body surface area scaling of an adult dosage.[41] Age-related changes in the enzymatic and excretory systems that are involved in drug elimination can have a profound effect on pharmacokinetics.[42] Thus, the rational use of drugs in pediatric patients that are known to be eliminated primarily by hepatic metabolism in adults may depend on thoroughly characterizing its pharmacokinetics and metabolism in children of various ages. Similarly, the potential for interaction of a new agent, that is a potential substrate or inhibitor of hepatic CYP450 enzymes, with other drugs that may be concurrently administered to pediatric patients also warrants careful evaluation.

Eliminating Organ Dysfunction

Physiologic conditions that affect hepatic or renal function, including blood flow to the liver or kidneys, can have a dramatic effect on the pharmacokinetic behavior of a drug in individual patients.[43] Powis[44] reviewed the effects of both renal and hepatic dysfunction for anticancer drugs. The estimation of creatinine clearance from serum creatinine concentration is a conveniently measured indicator of renal function. Hepatic function is more difficult to quantify. Serum transaminase and bilirubin concentrations provide indirect but somewhat useful information on hepatic function. Empirical guidelines for dose reduction in patients with underlying renal or hepatic dysfunction are devised by establishing relationships between these biochemical parameters and CL. In general, these adjustments would be expected to be less precise than adjustments based on drug-level measurements. Occasionally, there is a close relationship between a renal function indicator and plasma pharmacokinetics. Egorin et al[45] have elegantly applied such correlations for dose adjustments of carboplatin (Fig. 3.4) and hexamethylene bisacetamide.[46] In fact, individualizing the dose of carboplatin to target a specific AUC value based on estimated creatinine clearance in patients has

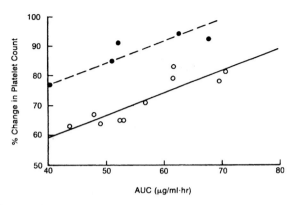

Figure 3.4 Relationship between thrombocytopenia and plasma levels of carboplatin. AUC, area under the concentration × time curve. (Reprinted with permission from Egorin MJ, Van Echo DA, Olman EA, et al. Prospective validation of a pharmacologically based dosing scheme for the *cis*-diamminedichloroplatinum(II) analog diamminecyclobutanedicarboxylatoplatinum. Cancer Res 1985; 46:6502–6506.)

become a routine clinical practice.[47] Table 3.1 summarizes the recommended dose modifications for the standard anticancer drugs.

Drug Interactions

Essentially all treatment protocols include combinations of drugs, encompassing two or more anticancer drugs, as well as various other drugs related to general symptomatic and supportive therapy of the patient. Many adjuvant medications that are routinely used in the management of cancer patients can potentially affect the pharmacokinetics of chemotherapeutic agents by either inhibiting or enhancing metabolic elimination (Table 3.2). Because cytotoxic anticancer drugs are usually administered at their maximum tolerated doses, there is a substantially greater risk for pharmacokinetic interactions resulting in clinically significant toxicity than exists with drugs for most other indications. Accordingly, the administration of an anticancer agent together with another drug that has the potential to modulate the activity of an enzyme that represents a major pathway of its elimination should be avoided whenever possible. Another consideration that should be recognized is that highly variable pharmacokinetics are frequently exhibited by drugs predominantly eliminated by hepatic metabolism.[48] It is becoming increasingly apparent that genetic polymorphisms and mutations affecting key drug-metabolizing enzymes may account for aberrant pharmacokinetics in a minority of patients, or an otherwise high degree of interpatient variability.[49]

The serious adverse reactions caused by administration of ketoconazole to patients taking terfenadine,[50] which had been widely used and considered to be a relatively safe antihistamine, provide a cautionary note for potential interactions with anticancer drugs because of their

TABLE 3.2
CLINICALLY SIGNIFICANT PHARMACOKINETIC DRUG INTERACTIONS INVOLVING ANTICANCER AGENTS

Chemotherapeutic Agent	Interacting Drug	Effect on Clearance of Anticancer Agent	Probable Mechanism
Cyclophosphamide	Phenobarbital	↑	CYP450 enzyme induction
Doxorubicin	Cyclosporin A	↓	Inhibit biliary excretion
Etoposide	Phenytoin	↑	CYP450 enzyme induction
Irinotecan		↑	
Paclitaxel		↑	
6-Mercaptopurine	Allopurinol	↓	Inhibit xanthine oxidase
	Methotrexate	↓	
Methotrexate	Aspirin	↓	Inhibit tubular secretion
	Probenecid	↓	
Paclitaxel	Verapamil	↓	Inhibit CYP450 metabolism or biliary excretion
Topotecan	Cisplatin	↓	Inhibit tubular secretion
Vinblastine	Erythromycin	↓	Inhibit CYP450 metabolism

much narrower therapeutic index. Another common drug, cimetidine, is reported to inhibit the metabolism of cyclophosphamide[51] and hexamethylmelamine.[52] On the other hand, anticancer drugs are reported to interfere with the absorption of noncancer drugs, such as digoxin.[53] Balis[54] has reviewed the literature of drug interactions related to anticancer drugs. When evaluating drug-drug interactions, recent findings with paclitaxel illustrate the difficulties generated by interspecies differences in metabolic pathways.[55]

Chemotherapeutic agents that are metabolized by the hepatic CYP450 system, especially members of the CYP3A subfamily, are particularly prone to pharmacokinetic interactions from the multitude of drugs and compounds of dietary origin that are inhibitors or inducers of CYP450.[56] A particularly serious example is the use of the dietary supplement, St. John's wort. This product induces drug-metabolizing enzymes and produces lack of drug efficacy.[57] Repeated daily administration of glucocorticoids, commonly used as antiemetics, can induce the expression of hepatic CYP450 and thereby enhance the CL of anticancer drugs that are CYP3A4 substrates.[58] In addition to hepatic drug-metabolizing enzymes, there are examples of pharmacokinetic interactions resulting from effects directed on other enzyme systems, excretory pathways, and even drug absorption. Salicylates can reduce the renal tubular secretion of MTX.[59,60] Morphine and its derivatives can alter the rate and extent of absorption of orally administered cytotoxic drugs by reducing gastrointestinal motility.[61] As discussed in a subsequent chapter, some antiseizure drugs that are frequently used in the clinical management of patients with brain tumors have been shown to significantly enhance the clearance of many anticancer agents by inducing CYP450 enzymes.

Dose Individualization

The existence of a high degree of interpatient pharmacokinetic variability can result in unpredictable episodes of toxicity and make it difficult to establish a potentially effective and safe dose for the population. For the individual, clinical monitoring and pharmacokinetics offer the possibility of tailoring drug delivery to the particular patient's needs. The standard doses derived from group studies do not allow for interindividual variability. However, doses may be adjusted on the basis of direct measurements of drug concentration in the individual patient, indicators of renal or hepatic dysfunction, or interactions of the anticancer drug with concomitant medications. Under these circumstances, it may also be beneficial to individualize doses of the drug based on plasma levels of the compound afforded by a test dose or a biochemical parameter that is predictive of CL.[62] Although this technique is rarely employed, dose individualization has significantly improved the outcome and minimized toxicity for children with B lineage ALL treated with MTX.[63]

DOSING REGIMENS

For the average patient, or the general population, pharmacokinetics can help answer the fundamental questions in delivery of drugs: (a) What route of administration? (b) How much to give (dose)? (c) How often to administer (schedule)? These questions are answered using empiric observation (what works best in an experimental or clinical setting) as well as biochemical, cell kinetic, and pharmacokinetic considerations.

Routes of Drug Administration

The choice of drug administration *route* is based primarily on the ability to formulate an acceptable dose preparation for intravenous, oral, intramuscular, intrathecal, or subcutaneous use and pharmacokinetic assessment of the pattern of systemic drug exposure that they provide. Although current trends point toward the preferential development of orally administered drugs, cytotoxic anticancer drugs are still most commonly given by the intravenous route as this provides complete control over the actual dosage delivered to the systemic circulation and the rate at which it is presented. This results in maximum safety because the variability in systemic drug exposure between and within patients achieved with direct intravenous administration is typically much lower than that resulting from oral administration. Furthermore, for agents given by continuous intravenous infusion, drug delivery can be readily terminated, if necessary, because of the occurrence of an acute adverse reaction during administration.

All routes of administration other than intravenous, including oral, subcutaneous, intramuscular, intraperitoneal, and intrathecal delivery, involve an absorption process whereby dissolved drug molecules are transferred from the site of administration into the vasculature. Accordingly, drug given by an extravascular route is conceptualized as being outside the body until gaining access to the systemic circulation. Oral dosage forms are presently available for an increasing number of anticancer drugs including hydroxyurea, MTX, etoposide, idarubicin, gefitinib and imatinib. In the future, oral administration will undoubtedly attain greater prevalence from the clinical development of cytostatic antiproliferative agents that require chronic dosing for efficacy.

The bioavailability of a drug given by any extravascular route is defined as the rate and extent of absorption into systemic circulation. The absolute systemic availability (F) of a drug is ascertained by determining the AUC in the same patient following intravenous and extravascular administration of the agent, with an adequate time interval period between the two treatments. For the same dose given intravenously and extravascularly,

$$F = (AUC_{ev}/AUC_{iv}) \cdot (D_{iv}/D_{ev}) \qquad [3.8]$$

where D is the dose. In studies where an agent is administered exclusively by the oral route, CL and F are indeterminable, as explicitly indicated by the relationship

$$D_{ev}/AUC_{ev} = CL/F \qquad [3.9]$$

Many factors influence oral bioavailability, including release of the drug from the dosage form, dissolution of drug within the gastrointestinal tract, drug stability under conditions encountered in the gastrointestinal tract, transport of dissolved drug across the intestinal epithelium into the vasculature, and the extent of first-pass hepatic metabolism. Mercaptopurine is an example of a drug with very low and erratic bioavailability,[64] whereas imatinib is a drug with consistently high bioavailability.[65]

Absorption through the lipid-bilayer cell membrane of the intestinal mucosa is determined by molecular size, lipid solubility, and the presence of transport systems. As cancer chemotherapy shifts increasingly towards oral drug delivery, the importance of many general carrier systems, such as the "ABC" transporters, is becoming more widely appreciated alongside such specialized carriers as the folate transport mechanisms for antifolates. The physiologic state of the intestinal tract may be affected adversely by disease or by previous drug therapy. Vomiting induced by chemotherapeutic drugs such as cisplatin may lead to loss of a major portion of an oral dose. In addition to intestinal absorption, presystemic metabolism and biliary excretion may prevent orally administered drugs from reaching the systemic circulation in an active form. Presystemic metabolism, also known as the "first-pass effect," is a unique concern for the oral route because a drug is exposed to metabolism both in the gastrointestinal mucosa and in the liver, which it enters through the portal vein before returning to the heart.[66]

A tumor may grow in a region of the body, such as the central nervous system, that is not penetrated readily by systemically administered drugs. Accordingly, several unusual routes of administration have been implemented to maximize delivery of drugs to the site of the tumor and to reduce the deleterious effects associated with ordinary systemic administration. At least two of these routes have become accepted therapeutic practice: intrathecal delivery for meningeal leukemia[67] and intravesical delivery for transitional-stage bladder carcinoma. As discussed in detail in Chapter 21, intrathecal administration has been used primarily to obtain adequate drug levels in the cerebrospinal fluid to eradicate cancer cells that are otherwise protected from effective therapy. Intra-arterial drug administration, especially hepatic arterial delivery, is another route that has been actively investigated but has not emerged as standard therapy.

Peritoneal dialysis continues to be evaluated as a delivery vehicle for anticancer drugs when disease is localized to the abdomen.[68] The pharmacokinetic rationale suggests that tumor tissue may be exposed to high local concentrations, whereas systemic levels are no greater than normally encountered with intravenous therapy. In an analogous fashion to intrathecal delivery, only cells in close contact with the peritoneal fluid will benefit from this mode of drug delivery. The intraperitoneal route has been the subject of many pilot studies and formal phase I and phase II trials by our group and others. Some promising pharmacologic results have been obtained and more definitive therapeutic trials are in progress. Three randomized phase III trials totaling approximately 3,000 patients with ovarian cancer have shown an advantage for intraperitoneal delivery compared with intravenous delivery for both time to disease recurrence/progression[69,70] and survival.[69,71]

Pharmacokinetic analysis can help to evaluate the potential usefulness of these approaches. Of course, the pharmacokinetic advantage of achieving greater drug exposure is not always associated with improved responses.

Dose

Dose is usually determined by an empiric phase I trial using a fixed treatment schedule, with stepwise evaluation of toxicity at progressively higher doses. In certain circumstances, dose also may be determined by setting pharmacologic objectives, such as a target drug concentration in a specific body compartment such as plasma, cerebrospinal fluid, or ascites. This type of regimen planning requires pharmacokinetic design and verification by drug level monitoring and has been used in only a few clinical oncologic settings, such as intrathecal chemotherapy with MTX and intraperitoneal therapy with MTX and 5-FU. Additional information on the relationship of drug concentration to tumor cell kill, as provided by in vitro assays, may provide a basis for more precise pharmacokinetic adjustment of dosage.

Pharmacologically guided dose escalation was developed as an alternative to the predetermined escalation procedures such as the modified Fibonacci method for phase I trials.[72] After the first group of patients has been treated with the starting dose in a phase I clinical trial, the rate of dose escalation is determined by the plasma levels of drug relative to target plasma levels measured in mice at the maximum tolerated dose. With this approach, investigators can estimate the difference between the target concentration and plasma levels produced by the current dose level. Such information provides the opportunity to intervene at an early stage in the phase I trial. Cautious escalation may be indicated if it is determined that plasma levels of the drug are close to the target. If the current plasma levels are substantially below the targeted value, then a more rapid escalation of the dose could generate considerable savings in time and clinical resources, and fewer patients will be exposed to doses that have little potential of being therapeutically effective. Although this procedure is conceptually attractive and found support in Europe and Japan, as well as the United States,[73–75] it has not been widely used, primarily because of logistical difficulties in its implementation.

Administration Schedule

The route and frequency of administration evaluated in the initial phase I trial of a cytotoxic anticancer agent is generally derived from the schedule that produces an optimal therapeutic effect against preclinical in vivo tumor models. There is an increasing interest in assessing the use of noncytotoxic compounds, such as cytostatic, differentiation-inducing, and antiangiogenic agents in the treatment of neoplastic diseases. However, accepted preclinical models

to evaluate and refine in vivo efficacy for many classes of candidate noncytotoxic antiproliferative drugs do not presently exist. Under these circumstances, it would be reasonable to base the treatment schedule evaluated in initial phase I trials on that required to achieve the pattern of systemic exposure to drug in laboratory animals that best approximates the concentration and duration of exposure necessary for optimal in vitro activity.

Past experience has repeatedly demonstrated that impressive preclinical antitumor activity is not a reliable predictor of clinical efficacy. A reasonable argument can also be advanced to support the hypothesis that a candidate drug has little likelihood of being therapeutically effective unless a clinically tolerable dosing regimen provides a pattern of systemic exposure to the drug that is at least comparable with that required for activity against appropriate in vivo or in vitro preclinical models. Accordingly, when considered together with toxicologic and physiologic response factors, pharmacokinetic data acquired during phase I studies can facilitate efforts to optimize dosing regimens. Alternatively, withdrawing an agent from continued clinical development may be an option that warrants serious consideration in situations in which the plasma concentrations achieved in patients treated at the maximum tolerated dose are considerably lower than target levels, given the availability of limited clinical resources and ethical considerations of entering patients into a phase II trial of a compound that has little prospect of being therapeutically effective.

The *schedule* of drug administration depends highly on pharmacokinetic considerations and requires a choice of the duration of administration (e.g., bolus intravenous injection versus prolonged intravenous infusion), frequency of repeated dosing, and the sequencing of multiple drugs or drugs and other treatment modalities such as radiation. Bolus intravenous injection provides maximal peak drug levels in plasma but a rapid decline thereafter as the drug is eliminated from the plasma compartment by metabolism or excretion. This very convenient dosing method is appropriate for drugs that are not cell cycle-phase–dependent and therefore do not have to be present during a specific phase of the cell cycle. Examples are the alkylating agents, such as chloroethylnitrosoureas, nitrogen mustards, and procarbazine, as well as other drugs that chemically interact with DNA.

Administration by prolonged intravenous infusion (i.e., 6 to 120 hours) is advantageous for agents that act preferentially in discrete phases of the cell cycle, such as S-phase–specific drugs (e.g., cytarabine, MTX, camptothecins), particularly if the drug is rapidly cleared from systemic circulation. Prolonged infusions have the additional advantage of providing a specific and constant plasma concentration of the drug, a desirable feature if information regarding the chemosensitivity of the tumor is available, as determined experimentally by various in vitro tests. Intermediate-length infusions (i.e., 1 to 4 hours) may provide a means to overcome the acute toxicities that are produced by exposing host organs to high peak drug levels. Particularly for neurotoxic or cardiotoxic compounds, rapid intravenous infusions may present unacceptable dangers, but intermediate-length infusions may reduce peak drug levels adequately while retaining some of the convenience of bolus dosing.

It may be desirable to achieve the steady-state concentration rapidly for a drug given as a continuous intravenous infusion, in which case a *loading dose* may be given by bolus injection at the same time that the infusion is started. The bolus dose is usually selected to achieve an initial concentration near the steady-state target value. In this way, the time lag to achieve the plateau in the CxT profile, which may be considerable for some drugs, is eliminated. As an alternative to administering a drug by continuous intravenous infusion, it may be possible to maintain reasonably constant plasma levels using a repeated bolus injection dosing regimen. There is an approach to steady-state conditions in which the peak and trough plasma concentrations increase successively during repeated doses before becoming constant. As with the continuous intravenous infusion, steady-state can be reached immediately with the proper choice of loading dose. The most common such schedule targets the peak concentration as twice the trough concentration. This design requires dosing once each half-life. An initial dose of twice the successive (maintenance) doses abolishes the time lag. As the dosing frequency increases, the ratio of peak-to-trough concentrations approaches 1, and the CxT curve appears more like that of a constant infusion. These same scheduling considerations also apply to the timing of oral drug delivery.

PHARMACOKINETIC-PHARMACODYNAMIC RELATIONSHIPS

The toxicities of anticancer drugs are often better correlated with a pharmacokinetic variable than the administered dose. Relationships between the severity of toxicity and the AUC are most commonly encountered. However, other variables such as the C_{max} and duration of time that the drug concentration in plasma exceeds a particular threshold level are also predictive of toxicity. For example, the time interval that plasma levels of paclitaxel remain above 50 nM is better correlated with neutropenia, the principal dose limiting toxicity, than either C_{max} or AUC.[76] The nature of these relationships can often be described by a sigmoidal E_{max} model but they may appear linear unless patients have been evaluated across a sufficiently broad range of doses.[77]

As previously indicated, therapeutic response ultimately depends on the delivery of drug from the bloodstream to the tumor in such a way that malignant cells are exposed to biologically effective concentrations of the active form of the agent for an adequate duration of time. The rate processes associated with drug distribution and elimination depend on the physicochemical properties of the drug and numerous physiologic factors. As is the case with any specific organ or tissue, the time course of the concentration of a compound within a solid tumor cannot be defined from experimental data restricted to measurements made in plasma, serum, or whole blood. Although there is undoubtedly some temporal relationship between drug concentrations in plasma and the tumor, elucidating the tumor CxT profile requires physical measurement of drug levels within the tumor itself. Whereas this cannot be easily accomplished in solid tumors, in most cases, hematologic malignancies are considerably more amenable to such studies because the cancer cells reside within the bloodstream itself, bone marrow or lymphatic tissues, which are considerably more accessible to drug. Consequently, efforts to determine whether adequate concentrations of the active form of a drug are achieved in cancer cells should be considered an important objective of phase I trials to evaluate new anticancer drugs in hematologic malignancies. The availability of this information will better facilitate the rational selection of drugs warranting further clinical evaluation. The emergence of noninvasive imaging techniques may provide some momentum for pharmacokinetic-pharmacodynamic (i.e., PK-PD) relationships in solid tumors.

CONCLUSION

There are numerous reasons for acquiring pharmacokinetic data during various stages in the clinical development of anticancer drugs. The therapeutic indices of many drugs used in the treatment of cancer are inherently narrow because they are used at doses close to the upper limit of tolerability. Furthermore, cancer patients frequently exhibit increased sensitivity to many medications because of compromised organ function or diminished overall tolerance from their underlying disease state, augmenting the potential for an undesirable pharmacokinetic interaction with the host of concurrent medications used in the clinical management of cancer patients. The chances for an adverse event resulting from inappropriate dosing of a chemotherapeutic agent to a cancer patient are, therefore, considerably greater than experienced with most other patient groups. Since the dose-limiting toxicities of a chemotherapeutic agent are very often related to some measure of systemic exposure to the drug, the margin of safety of a potentially effective dose depends on the consistency of its pharmacokinetic behavior among patients.

The ultimate goal of pharmacokinetics is to assist in the optimization of therapy. Although progress has been made in pharmacokinetic areas, the limiting step for optimization of therapy is inadequate knowledge of the relationship between drug CxT profiles and drug effects. Pharmacokinetics can serve as a useful tool to help elucidate pharmacodynamic relationships by determining which profiles are feasible and by helping design administration strategies. Also, because overall drug effect results from both kinetic and dynamic variables, studies can be designed to adjust doses individually so that kinetic differences between patients can be minimized and attention can be focused solely on drug dynamics. Finally, pharmacokinetics can serve a useful role in the process of drug development by assisting the overall integration of data between preclinical testing and early clinical trials.[78] Initial human studies rely heavily on toxicologic and pharmacologic data obtained in mice and dogs, and pharmacokinetics provides a convenient approach to comparative analysis.

REFERENCES

1. Donelli MG, D'Incalci M, Garattini S. Pharmacokinetic studies of anticancer drugs in tumor-bearing animals. Cancer Treat Rep 1984;68:381–400.
2. Notari, R. E. Biopharmaceutics and Clinical Pharmacokinetics. New York: Marcel Dekker, 1987.
3. Gilbaldi M, Perrier D, eds. Pharmacokinetics. 2nd Ed. New York: Marcel Dekker,1982.
4. Timmerman PM, de Vries R, Ingelse BA. Tailoring bioanalysis for PK studies supporting drug discovery. Curr Top Med Chem 2001;1:443–462.
5. Wright JD, Boudinot FD, Ujhelyi MR. Measurement and analysis of unbound drug concentrations. Clin Pharmacokinet 1996;30: 445–462.
6. Dunne A. An iterative curve stripping technique for pharmacokinetic parameter estimation. J Pharm Pharmacol 1986;38:97–101.
7. Gillespie WR. Noncompartmental versus compartmental modelling in clinical pharmacokinetics. Clin Pharmacokinet 1991;20: 253–262.
8. Dedrick RL, Myers CE, Bungay PM, et al. Pharmacokinetic rationale for peritoneal drug administration in the treatment of ovarian cancer. Cancer Treat Rep 1978;62:1–11.
9. Speyer JL, Sugarbaker PH, Collins JM, et al. Portal levels and hepatic clearance of 5-fluorouracil after intraperitoneal administration in humans. Cancer Res 1981;41:1916–1922.
10. Farris FF, King FG, Dedrick RL, et al. Physiologic model for the pharmacokinetics of cis-dichlorodiammineplatinum(II)(DDP) in the tumored rat. J Pharmacokinet Biopharm 1985;13:13–39.
11. Chan KK, Cohen JL, Gross JF, et al. Prediction of adriamycin disposition in cancer patients using a physiologic, pharmacokinetic model. Cancer Treat Rep 1978;62:1161–1171.
12. Dedrick RL, Forrester DD, Cannon JN, et al. Pharmacokinetics of 1-β-D-arabinofuranosylcytosine (ARA-C) deamination in several species. Biochem Pharmacol 1973;22:2405–2417.
13. Rowland M, Benet LZ, Graham GG. Clearance concepts in pharmacokinetics. J Pharmacokinet Biopharm 1973;1:123–136.
14. Sawyer M, Ratain M. Body surface area as a determinant of pharmacokinetics and drug dosing. Invest New Drugs 2001;19: 171–177.
15. Carlisle KM, Halliwell M, Read AE, et al. Estimation of total hepatic blood flow by duplex ultrasound. Gut 1992;33:92–97.
16. Cockcroft DW, Gault MH. Prediction of creatinine clearance from serum creatinine. Nephron 1976;16:31–41.
17. Gibaldi M, McNamara PJ. Apparent volumes of distribution and drug binding to plasma proteins and tissues. Eur J Clin Pharmacol 1978;13:373–380.
18. Collins JM, Dedrick RL, King FG, et al. Nonlinear pharmacokinetic models for 5-fluorouracil in man: intravenous and intraperitoneal routes. Clin Pharmacol Ther 1980;28:235–246.
19. Donehower RC, Karp JE, Burke PJ. Pharmacology and toxicity of high-dose cytarabine by 72-hour continuous infusion. Cancer Treat Rep 1986;70:1059–1065.
20. Besseghir K, Roch-Ramel F. Renal excretion of drugs and other xenobiotics. Ren Physiol 1987;10:221–241.
21. Ilett KF, Tee LB, Reeves PT, et al. Metabolism of drugs and other xenobiotics in the gut lumen and wall. Pharmacol Ther 1990; 46:67–93.
22. Balis FM, Holcenberg JS, Bleyer WA. Clinical pharmacokinetics of commonly used anticancer drugs. Clin Pharmacokinet 1983;8: 202–232.
23. Glue P and Clement RP. Cytochrome P450 enzymes and drug metabolism—basic concepts and methods of assessment. Cell Mol Neurobiol 1999;19:309–323.
24. von Moltke LL, Greenblatt DJ, Schmider J, et al. Metabolism of drugs by cytochrome P450 3A isoforms. Implications for drug interactions in psychopharmacology. Clin Pharmacokinet 1985; 29:33–43.
25. Gillum JG, Israel DS, Polk RE. Pharmacokinetic drug interactions with antimicrobial agents. Clin Pharmacokinet 1993;25:450–482.
26. Kivisto KT, Kroemer HK, Eichelbaum M. The role of human cytochrome P450 enzymes in the metabolism of anticancer agents: implications for drug interactions. Br J Clin Pharmacol 1995;40:523–530.
27. Chabot GG, Bouchard J, Momparler RL. Kinetics of deamination of 5-aza-2′-deoxycytidine and cytosine arabinoside by human liver cytidine deaminase and its inhibition by 3-deazauridine, thymidine or uracil arabinoside. Biochem Pharmacol 1983;32: 1327–1328.
28. Milano G, McLeod HL. Can dihydropyrimidine dehydrogenase impact 5-fluorouracil-based treatment? Eur J Cancer 2000;36: 37–42.
29. Clarke DJ, Burchell B. The uridine diphosphate glucronosyltransferase multigene family: function and regulation. In: Kauffman FC, ed. Handbook of Experimental Pharmacology, Conjugation-Deconjugation Reactions in Drug Metabolism and Toxicity. Berlin: Springer-Verlag, 1994:3–43.
30. Ratain MJ. Insights into the pharmacokinetics and pharmacodyamics of irinotecan. Clin Cancer Res 2000;6:3393–3394.
31. Ivanov AI, Christodoulou J, Parkinson JA, et al. Cisplatin binding sites on human albumin. J Biol Chem 1998;273:14721–14730.
32. Milano G, Etienne MC, Cassuto-Viguier E, et al. Influence of sex and age on fluorouracil clearance. J Clin Oncol 1992;10:1171–1175.
33. Innocenti F, Iyer L, Ratain MJ. Pharmacogenetics of anticancer agents: lessons from amonafide and irinotecan. Drug Metab Dispos 2001;29:596–600.
34. Lichtman SM, Skirvin JA. Pharmacology of antineoplastic agents in older cancer patients. Oncology 2000;14:1743–1752.
35. Geokas M, Haverback B. The aging gastrointestinal tract. Am J Surg 1969;117:881–892.
36. Bender A. the effect of increasing age on the distribution of peripheral blood flow in man. J Am Geriatr Soc 1965;13:192–198.
37. Bach B, Hansen J, Kampmann J, et al. Disposition of antipyrine and phenytoin correlated with age and liver volume in men. Clin Pharmacokinet 1981;6:389–396.
38. Durnas C, Loi C, Cusack, BJ. Hepatic drug metabolism and aging. Clin Pharmacokinet 1990;19:359–389.
39. Baker SD, Grochow LB. Pharmacology of cancer chemotherapy in the older person. Clin Geriatr Med 1997;13:169–183.
40. Kinirons MT, O'Mahony MS. Drug metabolism and ageing. Br J Clin Pharmacol 2004;57:540–544.
41. Anderson GD. Children versus adults: pharmacokinetic and adverse-effect differences. Epilepsia 2002;43(Suppl 3):53–59.
42. Hammerlein A, Derendorf H, Lowenthal DT. Pharmacokinetic and pharmacodynamic changes in the elderly. Clinical implications. Clin Pharmacokinet 1998;35:49–64.
43. Barre J, Houin G, Brunner F, et al. Disease-induced modifications of drug pharmacokinetics. Int J Clin Pharmacol Res 1983;3: 215–226.
44 Powis G. Effect of human renal and hepatic disease on the pharmacokinetics of anticancer drugs. Cancer Treat Rev 1982;9:85–124.
45. Egorin MJ, Van Echo DA, Olman EA, et al. Prospective validation of a pharmacologically based dosing scheme for the cis-diamminedichloroplatinum(II) analogue diamminecyclobutanedicarboxylatoplatinum. Cancer Res 1985;45:6502–6506.
46. Egorin MJ, Sigman LM, Van Echo DA, et al. Phase I clinical and pharmacokinetic study of hexamethylene bisacetamide

(NSC95580) administered as a five-day continuous infusion. Cancer Res 1987;47:617–623.

47. van den Bongard HJ, Mathot RA, Beijnen JH, et al. Pharmacokinetically guided administration of chemotherapeutic agents. Clin Pharmacokinet 2000; 39:345–367.

48. Shimada T, Yamazaki H, Mimura M, et al. Interindividual variations in human liver cytochrome P-450 enzymes involved in the oxidation of drugs, carcinogens and toxic chemicals: studies with liver microsomes of 30 Japanese and 30 Caucasians. J Pharmacol Exp Ther 1994;270:414–423.

49. Watters JW, McLeod HL, Cancer pharmacogenomics: current and future applications. Biochim Biophys Acta 2003;1603:99–111.

50. Peck CC, Temple R, Collins JM. Understanding consequences of concurrent therapies. JAMA 1993;269:1550–1552.

51. Dorr RT, Soble MJ, Alberts DS. Interaction of cimetidine but not ranitidine with cyclophosphamide in mice. Cancer Res 1986;46: 1795–1799.

52. Hande K, Combs G, Swingle R, et al. Effect of cimetidine and ranitidine on the metabolism and toxicity of hexamethylmelamine. Cancer Treat Rep 1986;70:1443–1445.

53. Bjornsson TD, Huang AT, Roth P, et al. Effects of high-dose cancer chemotherapy on the absorption of digoxin in two different formulations. Clin Pharmacol Ther 1986;39:25–28.

54. Balis FM. Pharmacokinetic drug interactions of commonly used anticancer drugs. Clin Pharmacokinet 1986;11:223–235.

55. Jamis-Dow CA, Klecker RW, Katki AG, et al. Metabolism of taxol by human and rat liver in vitro: a screen for drug interactions and interspecies differences. Cancer Chemother Pharmacol 1995; 36:107–114.

56. van Meerten E, Verweij J, Schellens JH. Antineoplastic agents. Drug interactions of clinical significance. Drug Saftey 1995;12: 168–182.

57. Markowitz JS, Donovan JL, DeVane CL, et al. Effect of St John's wort on drug metabolism by induction of cytochrome P450 3A4 enzyme. JAMA 2003;290:1500–1504.

58. McCune JS, Hawke RL, LeCluyse EL, et al. In vivo and in vitro induction of human cytochrome P4503A4 by dexamethasone. Clin Pharmacol Ther 2000;68:356–366.

59. Bannwarth B, Pehourcq F, Schaeverbeke T, et al. Clinical pharmacokinetics of low-dose pulse methotrexate in rheumatoid arthritis. Clin Pharmacokin 1996;30:194–210.

60. Evans WE, Christensen ML. Drug interactions with methotrexate. J Rheumatol 1985;12(Suppl 12):15–20.

61. Wood M. Pharmacokinetic drug interaction in anaesthetic practice. Clin Pharmacokinet 1991;21:285–307.

62 Kerr IG, Jolivet J, Collins JM, et al. Test dose for predicting high-dose methotrexate infusions. Clin Pharmacol Ther 1983;33:44–51.

63. Evans WE, Relling MV, Rodman JH, et al. Conventional compared with individualized chemotherapy for childhood acute lymphoblastic leukemia. N Engl J Med 1998;338:499–505.

64. Zimm S, Collins JM, Riccardi R, et al. Variable bioavailability of oral mercaptopurine: Is maintenance chemotherapy in acute lymphoblastic leukemia being optimally delivered? N Engl J Med 1983;308:1005–1009.

65. Peng B, Dutreix C, Mehring G, et al. Absolute bioavailability of imatinib (Glivec) orally versus intravenous infusion. J Clin Pharmacol 2004;44:158–62.

66. Rubin GM, Tozer TN. Theoretical considerations in the calculation of bioavailability of drugs exhibiting Michaelis-Menten elimination kinetics. J Pharmacokinet Biopharm 1984;12:437–450.

67. Blasberg R, Patlak CS, Fenstermacher JD. Intrathecal chemotherapy: brain tissue profiles after ventriculocisternal perfusion. J Pharmacol Exp Ther 1975;195:73–83.

68. Myers CE, Collins JM. Pharmacology of intraperitoneal chemotherapy. Cancer Invest 1983;1:395–407.

69. Markman M, Bundy BN, Alberts DS, et al. Phase III trial of standard-dose intravenous cisplatin plus paclitaxel versus moderately high-dose carboplatin followed by intravenous paclitaxel and intraperitoneal cisplatin in small-volume stage III ovarian carcinoma: an intergroup study of the Gynecologic Oncology Group, Southwestern Oncology Group, and Eastern Cooperative Oncology Group. J Clin Oncol 2001;19:921–923.

70. Alberts DS, Markman M, Armstrong D, et al. Intraperitoneal therapy for stage III ovarian cancer: a therapy whose time has come! J Clin Oncol 2002;20:3944–3946.

71. Alberts DS, Liu PY, Hannigan EV, et al. Intraperitoneal cisplatin plus intravenous cyclophosphamide versus intravenous cisplatin plus intravenous cyclophosphamide for stage III ovarian cancer. N Engl J Med 1996;335:1950–1955.

72. Collins JM, Zaharko DS, Dedrick RL, et al. Potential roles for preclinical pharmacology in phase I trials. Cancer Treat Rep 1986; 70:73–80.

73. EORTC Pharmacokinetics and Metabolism Group. Pharmacokinetically guided dose escalation in phase I clinical trials. Eur J Cancer Clin Oncol 1987;23:1083–1087.

74. Fuse E, Kobayashi S, Inaba M, et al. Application of pharmacokinetically guided dose escalation with respect to cell cycle phase specificity. J Natl Cancer Inst 1994;86:989–996.

75. Collins JM, Grieshaber CK, Chabner BA. Pharmacologically guided phase I trials based upon preclinical development. J Natl Cancer Inst 1990;82:1321–1326.

76. Gianni L, Kearns CM, Giani A, et al. Nonlinear pharmacokinetics and metabolism of paclitaxel and its pharmacokinetic/pharmacodynamic relationships in humans. J Clin Oncol 1995;13: 180–190.

77. Holford NH. Clinical pharmacokinetics and pharmacodynamics of warfarin. Understanding the dose-effect relationship. Clin Pharmacokinet 1986;11:483–504.

78. Collins JM. Pharmacology and drug development. J Natl Cancer Inst 1988;80:790–792.

Infertility After Cancer Chemotherapy

4

4

4

Angela Bradbury   *Richard L. Schilsky*

During the past 30 years, major strides have been made in the treatment of neoplastic disease with cytotoxic chemotherapy. Progress in understanding tumor cell biology and mechanisms of drug resistance, the introduction of new, effective antineoplastic drugs and technological advances that allow for more detailed and complete pharmacogenetic studies have all contributed to the successful application of cancer chemotherapy. Many patients with Hodgkin's disease, acute leukemia, non-Hodgkin's lymphoma, testicular cancer, and other tumors now regularly achieve sustained clinical remissions and cures. Moreover, adjuvant chemotherapy is now commonly employed for treatment of micrometastatic disease in clinically well patients with breast cancer, colorectal cancer, lung cancer, and soft tissue sarcoma and prolongs survival for many individuals. Thus, many more patients currently receive chemotherapy than ever before, and, of greater significance, many more individuals are cured of their tumors and survive to experience the potential late adverse effects of such treatment. Among these, infertility and mutagenesis are often of particular concern to cancer survivors who have new hopes and expectations for a return to normal lifestyle. This chapter will review the effects of cancer chemotherapy on the gonadal function, sexuality, and progeny of patients treated for malignant disease.

EFFECTS OF CANCER CHEMOTHERAPY ON GONADAL FUNCTION

Neoplastic disease and its treatment can potentially interfere with any of the cellular, anatomic, physiologic, or behavioral processes that comprise normal sexual function. The nature of the patient's illness, the extent of necessary surgery or radiation therapy, and the patient's relationship with spouse and family may all play an important role in reestablishing normal sexual interest and function following treatment for cancer. Further, many drugs used in the treatment of malignant disease have profound and often lasting effects on the testis and ovary. Germ cell production and endocrine function may both be altered, with the magnitude of the effect related to the age, pubertal status, and menstrual status of the patient as well as to the particular drug, dosage, or combination administered.

CHEMOTHERAPY EFFECTS IN MEN

The normal adult testis is an organ composed of diverse and highly specialized cell types, which may vary in their sensitivity to cytotoxic drugs. The exocrine function of the gland, spermatogenesis, proceeds in the seminiferous tubules, while the interstitial cells of Leydig carry out the primary endocrine function of the testis, testosterone production.[1]

The seminiferous tubules, which constitute 75% of the testicular mass, are lined by stratified epithelium composed of two cell types: spermatogenic cells and Sertoli cells. The spermatogenic cells are arranged in an orderly fashion: spermatogonia lie directly on the tubular basement membrane, and primary and secondary spermatocytes, spermatids, and maturing spermatozoa progress centrally toward the tubular lumen. Sertoli cells also lie on the basement membrane, and serve to regulate the release of mature spermatozoa from the germinal epithelium as well as to maintain the integrity of the blood-testis barrier.

Spermatogenesis is a dynamic and complex process that may be divided into three phases: (a) proliferation of spermatogonia to produce spermatocytes and to renew the germ cell pool, (b) meiotic division of spermatocytes to reduce the chromosome number in the germ cells by half, and (c) maturation of the spermatids to become spermatozoa.[2] Cytotoxic drugs could potentially effect this process in a number of ways: (a) a specific cell type within the germinal epithelium might be selectively damaged or destroyed; (b) the proliferative and meiotic phases of spermatogenesis might proceed normally, but sperm maturation might be abnormal, leading to functionally incompetent mature spermatozoa; or (c) chemotherapy might damage Sertoli cells, Leydig cells, or other supportive or nutritive constituents of the testis in such a way as to alter the particular microenvironment necessary for normal germ cell production.

Clinical Assessment

Testicular function in patients receiving cancer chemotherapy can be adequately evaluated with a careful physical examination, semen analysis, and determination of serum gonadotropin and testosterone levels (Table 4.1). Occasionally, testicular biopsy is necessary to complete the evaluation. Since the seminiferous tubules comprise such a large portion of the testicular mass, damage to the germinal epithelium frequently results in testicular atrophy, which is readily detected on physical examination. Impaired spermatogenesis is also manifest as a decrease in the number and/or motility of sperm present in the ejaculate and, since pituitary gonadotropin secretion is under feedback control by the testis, an increase in serum follicle stimulating hormone (FSH) level.[3,4] Leydig cell dysfunction may also occur and is detected by an increase in serum luteinizing hormone (LH) level, and if uncompensated, a fall in serum testosterone level. Subclinical abnormalities of Leydig cell function may occasionally be demonstrated by administration of LH-releasing hormone. An excessive rise in serum LH levels in this provocative test suggests the presence of abnormal Leydig cell function.[5-8]

Drug Effects on Spermatogenesis

Following cytotoxic chemotherapy, there appear to be common histopathologic changes that occur in the testis, independent of the type of drug employed, but related to the total dose administered. The primary testicular lesion caused by all antitumor agents studied thus far is depletion of the germinal epithelium lining the seminiferous tubules.[9-13] Testicular biopsy in most patients reveals complete germinal aplasia with only Sertoli cells left lining the tubular lumens. Occasionally, scattered spermatogonia, spermatocytes, or spermatids may be seen or there may be evidence for maturation arrest occurring at the spermatocyte stage. This latter finding appears most often in patients receiving short courses of chemotherapy with antimetabolites.[14]

Drugs Highly Toxic to Male Germ Cells

Chlorambucil

Among the anticancer drugs, alkylating agents most consistently cause male infertility. In particular, chlorambucil and cyclophosphamide deplete the testicular germinal epithelium in a dose-related fashion. Progressive oligospermia occurs in men with lymphoma who are treated with up to 400 mg of chlorambucil,[13] and those patients receiving cumulative doses in excess of 400 mg are uniformly azoospermic. Despite a high incidence of damage to the germinal epithelium, partial or full recovery of gonadal function may be possible for some individuals. Complete recovery of spermatogenesis has been reported in three of five previously azoospermic patients after therapy with chlorambucil at cumulative doses of 410 to 2600 mg.[15] In these patients, sperm counts were found to be normal at 33, 34, and 42 months following completion of chemotherapy. Two additional patients, who received the highest cumulative drug doses, demonstrated a partial return of spermatogenesis at 38 and 58 months after discontinuing treatment.[15]

Cyclophosphamide

Decreased sperm counts may occur in men treated with 50 to 100 mg of cyclophosphamide daily for courses as brief as 2 months, although azoospermia and germinal aplasia are infrequent until higher doses have been administered. Rivkees and Crawford[16] found that 80% of men treated with more than 300 mg/kg of single-agent cyclophosphamide developed gonadal dysfunction. As with chlorambucil, recovery of gonadal function is possible, although the probability of recovery appears to be related to the administered dose. In one study, all 26 men treated

TABLE 4.1

EVALUATION OF THE PATIENT WITH GERMINAL APLASIA

	Normal	Germinal Aplasia
Testicular size		
Length × width (cm)	5.0 × 3.0	3.7 × 2.3
Volume (mL)	16–30	8–15
Sperm count (10⁶/mL)	20–100	0
FSH (mIU/mL)	4–25	25–90
LH (mIU/mL)	4–20	8–25
LH response to LH–RH	Normal	Exaggerated
Testosterone (ng/dL)	250–1200	200–700

for 5 to 34 months with 50 to 100 mg of cyclophosphamide daily became azoospermic within 6 months of starting therapy.[17] Serial sperm counts demonstrated a return of spermatogenesis in 12 patients after a mean period of 31 months following discontinuation of cyclosphosphamide. Those patients demonstrating a recovery of spermatogenesis tended to receive lower initial drug doses. Other investigators found that 40% of men treated with cyclophosphamide-based regimens for sarcoma had recovery of spermatogenesis at 5 years, but only 10% had recovery when cumulative doses exceeded 7.5 g/m^2.[18]

Ifosfamide

Ifosfamide may be less toxic to the germinal epithelium than cyclophosphamide. One group reported recovery of spermatogenesis in 15 of 16 patients who received between 15 and 30 g/m^2 of ifosfamide.[19] Longhi et al[20] evaluated the effect of ifosfamide-based regimens in men with osteosarcoma. Although cisplatin, another gonadotoxic agent, was included in the treatment program, the investigators found that the likelihood of infertility was associated with the ifosfamide dose. The median ifosfamide dose in this study was 42g/m^2, with some men receiving up to 60 g/m^2. This group found a higher rate of azoospermia with ifosfamide-based regimens when compared with combinations that did not include ifosfamide. These studies suggest that ifosfamide, like other alkylating agents, has a dose-dependent effect on gonadal function.

Procarbazine

Several studies have suggested that procarbazine is particularly damaging to the germinal epithelium.[21,22] Animal studies have shown that procarbazine is severely toxic to the germinal epithelium in adult male monkeys and rats.[23,24] Human studies evaluating germinal damage after combination chemotherapy also suggest that procarbazine plays an important role in the development of chemotherapy-related infertility. In a report of 32 patients receiving combination chemotherapy for lymphoma, 31 patients developed increased serum FSH levels during their initial therapy, and of 15 patients studied, all had azoospermia. Sixteen patients were later evaluated for recovery of testicular function. Ten patients received regimens without procarbazine, and 7 of the 10 had normal serum FSH levels at 34 months post-treatment. In contrast, only one of six patients treated with a procarbazine-containing regimen demonstrated a decrease of serum FSH, or an increase in sperm count, during 52 months of follow-up.[21] In another study, patients treated with combination chemotherapy for non-Hodgkin's lymphoma appeared to have a lower incidence of gonadal dysfunction than those treated for Hodgkin's disease, despite receiving similar cumulative doses of cyclophosphamide and vincristine. Most of the patients with Hodgkin's disease also received procarbazine, whereas those treated for non-Hodgkin's lymphoma did not.[22] Although the patient numbers are small, these data suggest that the use of procarbazine in combination chemotherapy regimens may be associated with longer-lasting testicular damage than occurs with the use of alkylating agents alone.

Cisplatin

The effects of cisplatin alone on testicular function are difficult to discern, as the majority of men with testicular cancer have impaired spermatogenesis prior to therapy. Early studies reported that patients with testicular cancer treated with cisplatin-based combination chemotherapy uniformly became severely oligospermic or azoospermic soon after chemotherapy was initiated.[25–30] Subsequent studies have found that higher doses of cisplatin, or more cycles of chemotherapy, are associated with more profound and persistent decreases in sperm counts.[31,32] In a review of five published studies, DeSantis et al[19] determined that cumulative cisplatin doses less than 400 mg/m^2 were unlikely to cause azoospermia, whereas patients who received higher doses, or more than four cycles of chemotherapy, had a higher risk of impaired spermatogenesis when compared with controls. Likewise, other studies have found that almost all patients who receive cumulative cisplatin doses above 600 mg/m^2 have severe oligospermia or azoospermia.[33] As with other severely gonadotoxic agents, reversibility is possible even when there is severe azoospermia initially. Even after receiving a cumulative dose of 600 mg/m^2, 50% of men recovered spermatogenesis at 2 years and 80% had recovery at 5 years.[34]

Several groups have recently evaluated the gonadal toxicity of carboplatin. Although animal studies suggested a dose-related effect on spermatogenesis similar to cisplatin,[35] recent human studies suggest less germinal damage with carboplatin-based regimens. One group followed 22 patients with stage I seminoma who were treated with orchiectomy followed by single-agent carboplatin. After surgery, and prior to chemotherapy, 53% of the men had oligospermia and 35% were normospermic. At 2 years after therapy, 68% of men were normospermic, suggesting a significant recovery of spermatogenesis after therapy with single-agent carboplatin.[36] A second group found that patients who received carboplatin-based chemotherapy were 4.4 times more likely to recover spermatogenesis when compared with patients who received cisplatin-based therapy for testicular cancer.[37]

Vincristine

Although single-agent vincristine was thought to cause temporary and reversible damage to the germinal epithelium and to have an additive effect when combined with other highly gonadotoxic agents, a recent multivariate analysis suggests that vincristine itself may have a significant effect on fertility.[38] Vincristine does not appear to have significant germinal cell toxicity in animals. Vincristine is rarely administered as a single agent, and is often administered with other highly gonadotoxic agents, such as procarbazine. For this reason, it is difficult to assess the germinal toxicity of vincristine in humans. A recent study evaluated sperm counts in 55 males who received various chemotherapeutic regimens for different malignancies during childhood. The investigators employed multivariate methods to assess the effect of individual agents on future sperm quality. In this analysis, only vincristine and cyclophosphamide were shown to independently affect spermatogenesis, suggesting that vincristine may be more toxic to the germinal epithelium than previously suspected.[38]

Drugs with Low Toxicity to Male Germ Cells

Antimetabolites in conventional doses seem to have relatively few effects on spermatogenesis, although one study suggested that high-dose methotrexate (MTX, 250 mg/kg) may produce transient oligospermia in some patients.[39] This modest effect of MTX on spermatogenesis may result from the presence of a significant barrier to MTX passage from blood to seminiferous tubule.[40] Several reports have suggested that doxorubicin may be less toxic to the human testis than expected, based on animal studies. In both the mouse[41] and the rat,[42,43] doxorubicin produces severe germinal epithelial injury. Yet, clinical studies of the effects of doxorubicin-containing regimens on testicular function in men have revealed reversible testicular injury in the majority of patients under age 40.[44-47] Amsacrine, an acridine derivative with activity in acute leukemia, causes rapidly reversible azoospermia, suggesting that this drug produces little toxicity to stem cells in the human testis.[48] Recombinant interferon-α-2b, an active agent in the treatment of some chronic leukemias and solid tumors, seems to have no adverse effects on testicular function in men treated chronically for hairy cell leukemia.[49]

In considering individual agents, these data suggest that chemotherapeutic agents vary in toxicity to the germinal epithelium (Table 4.2). In addition, there appears to

TABLE 4.2
TOXICITY OF SINGLE AGENTS TO MALE GERM CELLS

Single Agent Drug	References
Drugs highly toxic to male germ cells	
Chlorambucil	13, 15
Cyclophosphamide	16–18
Ifosfamide	19, 20
Procarbazine	21–24
Cisplatin	19, 25–37
Vincristine	38
Drugs with low toxicity to male germ cells	
Methotrexate	40, 44
Doxorubicin	39, 41–43, 45–47
Interferon-α –2B	49

be a threshold dose for the development of testicular germinal aplasia for each particular drug. However, prospective studies of testicular function in large numbers of men receiving a variety of antitumor agents are needed to provide more reliable information concerning the threshold drug dose above which severe or irreversible testicular injury occurs. As newer agents are incorporated into standard cancer treatment programs, additional studies need to be completed to assess their effects on fertility.

Combination Chemotherapy and Disease-Specific Considerations

Hodgkin's Disease
As might be expected, combination chemotherapy regimens that include alkylating agents produce germinal aplasia and infertility in the majority of patients. This is clear in Hodgkin's disease, where the effects of MOPP (nitrogen mustard, vincristine, procarbazine, and prednisone) and a related regimen, MVPP (in which vinblastine replaces vincristine), have been extensively investigated. Sherins and DeVita[50] first reported the effects of combination chemotherapy on the fertility of 16 men with lymphoma in complete remission 2 months to 7 years after MOPP, CVP (cyclophosphamide, vincristine, and prednisone), or cyclophosphamide alone. All except three patients had azoospermia or severe oligospermia on semen analysis. Those patients with normal ejaculates and testis biopsies, of whom two received MOPP and one received CVP, had been off therapy for 2 to 7 years. Subsequent studies have confirmed that at least 80% of men receiving MOPP combination chemotherapy develop azoospermia, germinal aplasia, testicular atrophy, and elevated FSH levels.[8,51-54] Patients who receive COPP (cyclophosphamide, vinblastine, procarbazine, and prednisone) have significant gonadal dysfunction as well. In 92 men who received COPP, all developed azoospermia, and of the 19 who underwent testicular biopsy, all had evidence of germinal epithelial damage.[55] ChlVPP (chlorambucil, vincristine, procarbazine, and prednisolone) appears to be equally toxic as indicated in a study in which 11 of 13 patients remained azoospermic with no evidence of biochemical recovery 17 years after completing therapy.[56] Chapman et al[52] found that all 74 men who received cyclic combination chemotherapy for Hodgkin's disease were azoospermic after treatment, and only 4 of 74 recovered spermatogenesis after a median follow-up of 27 months. A decline in libido and decreased sexual activity also occurred during therapy and only partially recovered after treatment. Interpretation of this data is complicated by pretreatment azoospermia that occurs in at least 50% of men with advanced Hodgkin's disease.[52,57] In addition, a recent study found that 70% of men with Hodgkin's disease had dyspermia (defined as oligospermia, forward motility disturbances, or abnormal morphology) prior to treatment.

Although reversibility of gonadal dysfunction has been known to occur with single-agent therapy, patients who receive combination chemotherapy are likely to develop long-lasting and frequently permanent infertility. Sherins and DeVita[53] noted azoospermia and testicular germinal aplasia in patients as long as 4 years after completion of MOPP chemotherapy. Another group observed a return of spermatogenesis in only 4 of 64 men followed for 15 to 51 months after completion of MVPP chemotherapy.[5] Several other studies have confirmed these findings, and it seems reasonable to conclude that only about 10% of patients receiving MOPP or MVPP will ultimately have a return of spermatogenesis. In addition, recent evidence has shown that age is not protective because age at chemotherapy did not affect post-treatment sperm counts and recovery in patients who received combination chemotherapy for Hodgkin's disease and non-Hodgkin's lymphoma.[58,59]

A number of alternative combination chemotherapy regimens to MOPP have now been developed for the treatment of advanced Hodgkin's disease. Among these ABVD (Adriamycin, bleomycin, vinblastine, and dacarbazine) has been shown to be more efficacious and less toxic than the MOPP regimen. A comparison of these regimens revealed that azoospermia occurs in 100% of patients treated with MOPP, but in only 35% of patients receiving ABVD. In addition, recovery of spermatogenesis occurs rarely in patients treated with MOPP but nearly always in those treated with ABVD.[60-62] Hybrid regimens of MOPP or COPP and ABVD also produce persistent testicular dysfunction, with 60 to 80% of patients experiencing prolonged germinal damage.[57,61] Other regimens have been designed to reduce long-term toxicity and some may have less germinal toxicity. In a study evaluating patients with Hodgkin's disease treated with three cycles of mitoxantrone, vincristine, vinblastine, and prednisone, followed by radiation therapy, 90% developed severe oligospermia or azoospermia within 1 month of beginning chemotherapy, but sperm counts returned to normal in 63% of patients between 2.6 and 4.5 months after the completion of chemotherapy.[63] Another vincristine-based therapy, VEEP (vincristine, epirubicin, etoposide, and prednisolone) was designed to reduce treatment-related cardiotoxicity and infertility. In a phase II trial, 92% of patients had normal post-treatment sperm counts 2 years after completion of therapy.[64]

Non-Hodgkin's Lymphoma
Unlike patients with Hodgkin's disease, those with non-Hodgkin's lymphoma often have normal pretreatment sperm counts and motility.[65] Regimens containing modest doses of cyclophosphamide such as MACOP-B (MTX-leucovorin, Adriamycin, cyclophosphamide, vincristine, prednisone, and bleomycin) or VACOP-B (including vinblastine rather than MTX) have produced only transient azoospermia, with recovery of spermatogenesis in 100% of patients at a mean of 28 months after completion of chemotherapy.[65] However, with the standard cyclophosphamide regimens, sperm counts recovered in only two-thirds of patients at 7 years. Pryzant et al[66] found that 83% of men who received less than 9.5 g/m² of cyclophosphamide recovered a normal sperm count, and only 47% had recovery after cumulative doses greater than 9.5 g/m². Those who also received pelvic irradiation had more profound and longer-lasting gonadal damage. A small study evaluating 14 patients who received VAPEC-B (vincristine, doxorubicin, prednisolone, etoposide, cyclophosphamide, and bleomycin) for either Hodgkin's disease or non-Hodgkin's lymphoma reported only 1 case of azoospermia in a patient who also received pelvic radiation therapy.[67]

As new regimens are developed, they will need to be compared with standard regimens for efficacy. In addition, larger studies are necessary to confirm and compare the effects on spermatogenesis. This information may play an important role in treatment planning for young men with Hodgkin's disease and non-Hodgkin's lymphoma and who are concerned about preservation of fertility during and after treatment.

Testicular Cancer
As with patients with Hodgkin's disease, patients with testicular cancer have a high rate of oligospermia prior to treatment. Studies have shown that up to 50% of men with testicular cancer have oligospermia at diagnosis.[37,68,69] In addition, many patients undergo orchiectomy and retroperitoneal lymph node dissection, potentially contributing to future infertility. Studies have shown that patients who receive chemotherapy in addition to orchiectomy have a higher likelihood of azoospermia, oligospermia, and loss of testicular volume when compared with patients who receive orchiectomy alone.[26,28] Patients with testicular cancer treated with cisplatin-based combination chemotherapy uniformly become severely oligospermic or azoospermic soon after chemotherapy is initiated.[25-30,70] Despite this immediate gonadal injury, there appears to be a high degree of reversibility of testicular dysfunction, with as many as 50% of patients demonstrating resumption of spermatogensis within 2 years of completing chemotherapy. Among 98 patients with testicular germ cell tumors, 28 were treated with cisplatin-based chemotherapy and had profound decreases in sperm counts 1 year later, but a return to pretreatment levels 3 years after completion of chemotherapy, accompanied by a normalization of FSH values.[71] In a study with a median follow-up of 5 years, 27% of men who received PVB (cisplatin, vincristine, and bleomycin) were azoospermic. While some studies suggest that recovery of spermatogenesis is rare after 2 years,[28,72] there have been reports of recovery of spermatogenesis and fertility long after treatment. For example, a patient with malignant teratoma who underwent orchiectomy, chemotherapy, and pelvic irradiation was found to be azoospermic 8 years after completing treatment, but recovered fertility 6 years later, which was 14 years after completing treatment.[73] A recent study

evaluated 22 men with testicular cancer who were followed between 6 and 13 years after receiving six cycles of PVB. Although the majority of patients had no recovery in sperm counts, three patients had a significant recovery, despite early azoospermia.[74] Therefore, even though recovery beyond 2 years is rare, it does occur in isolated cases. Higher doses of chemotherapy generally induce longer-lasting oligospermia.[31] As previously described, patients who receive carboplatin-based therapy are more likely to recover spermatogenesis when compared with those who receive cisplatin-based therapy. Other predictors of recovery include normospermia prior to therapy and less than five cycles of chemotherapy.[37]

High-Dose Chemotherapy and Bone Marrow Transplantation

Recently, more information has become available regarding the impact of bone marrow transplantation-conditioning regimens on fertility. In general, conditioning regimens involving total body irradiation appear to severely affect fertility, and gonadal recovery occurs in a portion of patients receiving chemotherapy-only conditioning regimens. In men receiving a preparative regimen of high-dose cyclophosphamide alone, potential for recovery of spermatogenesis is reasonably high. In 72 men who received this treatment in Seattle, 65% had a normal FSH and normal sperm counts, and 94% had normal serum LH and testosterone levels.[75] Recovery of spermatogenesis was not age-related in this population. Recent studies evaluating different conditioning regimens found that 61 to 90% of men regain spermatogenesis within 3 years after single-agent cyclophosphamide.[76,77] Recovery of spermatogenesis was significantly lower in two studies that employed a busulfan-cyclophosphamide (Bu-Cy) conditioning regimen. Although early studies using 200 mg/kg of cyclophosphamide reported a dismal recovery rate of 17%,[76] more recent studies using a lower dose of cyclophosphamide (120 mg/kg + 16mg/kg busulfan) have reported higher rates of recovery, ranging from 50 to 84%.[77,78] Conditioning regimens combining cyclophosphamide with total body irradiation appear to severely affect gonadal function, with only 17% of patients recovering spermatogenesis and never earlier than 4 years post-treatment.[77]

Leukemia

There have been relatively few studies evaluating the gonadal effects of combination chemotherapy for acute lymphoblastic leukemia (ALL). An early study of 44 boys with ALL reported impaired spermatogenesis in 40% of patients and found that combinations including cyclophosphamide and cytosine arabinoside were associated with a higher likelihood of gonadal damage.[79] Quigley et al[80] also found severe germinal damage in 13 of 25 boys with ALL who received the modified LSA_2L_2 protocol, a regimen including both cyclophosphamide and cytosine arabinoside.

Despite these discouraging results, other ALL regimens have been associated with lower rates of gonadal damage. An aggressive eight-drug regimen that did not contain procarbazine was used in the treatment of adult ALL and was associated with preservation of fertility in the majority of patients.[81] More recently, Wallace et al[82] evaluated 37 men who received combination chemotherapy for ALL in childhood. Only six men had evidence of severe germinal damage at a median follow-up of 10 years. In addition, all six had received either cyclophosphamide or cyclophosphamide and cytosine arabinoside, supporting the hypothesis that ALL regimens excluding cyclophosphamide and cytosine arabinoside are less likely to cause permanent germinal aplasia.

Leydig Cell Dysfunction

Although the effect on spermatogenesis appears to be the most clinically relevant effect of cytotoxic chemotherapy, Leydig cell dysfunction may occur as well. Leydig cells remain morphologically intact after chemotherapy and basal serum LH levels generally remain normal, yet many patients have been found to have hypersecretion of LH in response to LH-releasing hormone, an indication of Leydig cell dysfunction.[5,8,55,83,84] In addition, the incidence of Leydig cell dysfunction appears to be associated with increasing age and more severe germinal damage.[84,85] As with germinal epithelial damage, there is evidence of partial recovery of Leydig cell function following treatment, although a recent study suggests that recovery beyond 5 years is unlikely.[85] The mechanism of Leydig cell failure is unclear. Even though it is possible that chemotherapy is directly toxic to the Leydig cells, germinal cell damage may indirectly affect Leydig cell function by decreasing testicular blood flow, disrupting paracrine control, or decreasing testicular volume, leading to structural changes in the testes.[84]

Despite recognition of these biochemical abnormalities, the clinical significance of these changes is unclear. Complete androgen deficiency has been associated with altered body composition, decreased sexual function, hot flushes, excessive sweating, fatigue, anxiety, depression, and reduced bone mineral density (BMD).[86–90]Mild-to-moderate testosterone deficiency has been less well studied, but may be associated with sexual dysfunction,[91,92] increased serum cholesterol,[93] and decreased BMD.[94] Howell et al [95] compared 36 men with mild Leydig cell dysfunction to similarly treated men without evidence of Leydig cell dysfunction. They found a significantly lower BMD, increased incidence of truncal fat distribution, but no change in lipid profiles in the group with mild androgen deficiency. Testosterone replacement in men with complete androgen deficiency has been shown to increase BMD, increase muscle mass, and decrease body fat.[96–99] These recent studies suggest that testosterone replacement may also be beneficial to the subset of men with moderate Leydig cell dysfunction. Further investigation is warranted to determine the incidence and clinical significance of mild androgen deficiency, as well as the role of replacement therapy.

Mutagenic Potential of Cancer Chemotherapy

In addition to the effects on fertility and Leydig cell function, cytotoxic treatment may be associated with chromosomal abnormalities in germ cells. These alterations may contribute to post-treatment infertility and may place subsequent generations at risk for carcinogenesis or developmental disorders. A study employing multicolor fluorescence in situ hybridization (FISH) suggests that up to 19% of sperm from healthy men may have chromosomal alterations.[100] The frequency of structural abnormalities of sperm in cancer patients receiving chemotherapy or radiation has been estimated at 9 to 40%, with more damage seen in patients who received multiple chemotherapeutic agents and longer durations of therapy.[101,102] Although many feel the rate of structural abnormalities is increased after exposure to chemotherapy, others have suggested that patients with cancer have a higher rate of sperm DNA abnormalities at baseline.[103–105] Until this controversy is resolved, there remains a concern that even men who have minimal germinal damage or recover germinal function may have underlying chromosomal changes that can be passed on to their progeny, resulting in genetic diseases including developmental abnormalities, metabolic abnormalities, or cancer.[106]

These concerns originate from animal studies, which have established the transgenerational effects of cytotoxic therapies. For example, dominant lethal mutations have been detected in zygotes after animals were treated with doxorubicin, melphalan, and chlorambucil.[107,108] The effects on the progeny of animals treated with cyclophosphamide, chlorambucil, doxorubicin, cisplatin, and procarbazine have included intrauterine death and developmental and morphologic abnormalities.[109–111] Despite the concerns generated from these studies, human studies to date have been inconclusive, and the significance to future generations remains unclear. Human epidemiologic studies have failed to show increased developmental abnormalities or carcinogenesis in the offspring of men who received chemotherapy.[112–117] Human studies evaluate men treated with chemotherapy who have conceived children after recovery of spermatogenesis, often well after treatment was completed, but animal studies appear to reflect the consequences of progeny conceived either during or shortly after exposure to cytotoxic therapy.[110] For this reason, many clinicians interpret the transgenerational human studies cautiously. Despite eight documented normal births to men who were receiving chemotherapy at the time of conception, it is reasonable to counsel men about the potential hazards to their future offspring. In addition, it is reasonable to recommend contraception for 6 months to 1 year after completion of treatment to allow for clearance of potentially affected germ cells from the reproductive tract.[106,111,118]

The absence of transgenerational effects may not apply to offspring conceived by specialized infertility techniques that utilize sperm collected during or soon after chemotherapy. It is likely that some natural selection occurs at the time of fertilization in vivo, decreasing the likelihood of fertilization by sperm with abnormal chromosomal material.[109] Sperm collected by advanced reproductive technology (ART) during chemotherapy or after completion of chemotherapy may not be subject to this natural selection.[106] The transgenerational animal studies support this potential, and Meistrich[111] discourages the use of sperm collection and cyropreservation during cancer treatment.

Assisted Reproductive Techniques for Men

Semen Cryopreservation

Pretreatment sperm banking is presently the only proven means of preserving fertility for men who are to receive combination chemotherapy for cancer. Although pretreatment sperm banking does not guarantee a successful conception in future years, advances in management of male factor infertility have made conception possible for many men who are not azoospermic.[119]

One of the significant challenges for preserving fertility in male patients with cancer has been poor quality semen, even prior to treatment. Studies have shown that approximately 50 % of male cancer patients have reduced sperm quality prior to chemotherapy.[52,57,120–124] Men with testicular cancer and Hodgkin's disease have significantly lower sperm motility and a higher incidence of azoospermia than men with other malignancies.[124,125] A review of patients from a single cryopreservation center found that 9.6% of men with testicular cancer and 18% of men with Hodgkin's disease were azoospermic prior to chemotherapy.[124] The cause of impaired spermatogenesis in male cancer patients prior to therapy is unknown. Hypotheses in testicular cancer include testicular fibrosis, orchidectomy, retroperitoneal lymph node dissection (RPLND), sperm antibodies, and elevated β-HCG and α-fetoprotein.[124] Postulated causes in Hodgkin's disease include elevated cytokines (IL-1, IL-6, TNF-α) or tumor-associated fever.[126] Although the majority of studies in untreated patients with Hodgkin's disease and testicular cancer have suggested that oligospermia does not correlate with age, stage, presence of symptoms or fever,[28,57,68,127–129] a recent study suggests that infertility is more frequent in patients with advanced Hodgkin's disease when compared with those with early stage disease.[130]

Despite a high rate of abnormal sperm quality, the majority of male cancer patients have adequate parameters for sperm storage.[131] The German Hodgkin Lymphoma Study Group found that 70% of their male patients had semen abnormalities prior to treatment, but only 8% had azoospermia and 13% had severe sperm abnormalities.[125] Other recent studies have found that only 12 to 17% of referred male cancer patients are unable to donate sperm for cryopreservation because of severe azoospermia prior to therapy.[124,132] In the past, minimal standards of sperm quality for crypreservation were used to maximize the chances of successful insemination. These included sperm concentration of at least 20×10^6 per milliliter, post-thaw motility greater than 40%, and post-thaw progression greater than 2+. It was thought that lower values were associated with a low probability of successful semen preservation, and ultimately of conception. Based on these critieria, many male cancer patients would be denied cryopreservation. In addition, cryopreservation itself has been known to decrease sperm motility.[68] More recent data suggest that despite poor semen quality at the time of cryopreservation, many cancer patients are able to have been able to conceive using advanced reproductive techniques.[133–137] Poor prefreeze semen quality has been associated with poor post-thaw outcome, but the association does not appear to be disease-related and the decline in semen quality does not appear to be different than in men without cancer.[128,138,139] Therefore, many groups recommend that suboptimal prefreeze sperm analysis should not be used to deny sperm banking, and cryopreservation should be offered to all male patients who have some motile spermatozoa in their sperm sample, even if the quality is below the required minimum standard for in vitro fertilization (IVF) (2×10^6).[131,133,138,139]

Although the technology of freezing, preserving, and thawing human semen has advanced considerably, ultimate conception rates using preserved semen have been limited by artificial insemination techniques. In the past, classic artificial insemination by husband (AIH) of the female partner using thawed spermatozoa was the only insemination technique available. AIH requires high numbers of spermatozoa and high-quality semen. Most early studies suggest that it is not very effective in subfertility secondary to sperm abnormalities.[140,141] More recent studies have reported better cumulative pregnancy rates with this technique in male cancer patients, ranging from 20 to 45%.[133] Despite success for some patients, the majority of male cancer patients have inadequate sperm quantity or quality for this procedure. IVF can be used with low spermatozoa quantity or when female factors prevent successful AIH. The fertilization rate with IVF for male factor infertility, and specifically male cancer patients, has been reported at 57 to 60 %.[135,142–144] The newest advance in fertilization technique is intracytoplasmic sperm injection (ICSI), a type of gamete micromanipulation. This procedure has revolutionized the treatment of male factor infertility and holds particular promise for azoospermic and oligospermic cancer survivors. ICSI involves the direct injection of a single spermatozoa into the cytoplasm of an oocyte in the context of in vitro fertilization. In the setting of male factor infertility, pregnancy rates of 52% have been reported with ICSI. The take-home-baby rate has been estimated at 22 to 37% per cycle, comparable with the 30% rate of successful pregnancy per cycle with natural conception.[145–147] Lass et al[124] described their experience at a tertiary-assisted conception center and reported successful pregnancies in all six cancer patients that returned for use of their cryopreserved sperm. Two were accomplished with AIH cycles, two with in vitro fertilization cycles, and two with ICSI.

Despite the increased success of semen cryopreservation with ICSI, the utility of sperm banking has been questioned by several authors because of the low percentage of later use to achieve pregnancy.[131,148,149] A survey of male cancer survivors found that only 24% of men completed sperm banking prior to cancer treatment.[150] In addition, of those who completed sperm collection, less than 10% returned to use their collected sperm for fertilization.[131,132,151] Regardless, many believe that sperm collection prior to therapy should still be pursued as the number of patients referred for cryopreservation has been increasing over the last several years, and the studies to date may be biased by a short period of follow-up.[132] In addition, a recent survey suggests that the low rate of referral may be related to a lack of discussion on the part of treating physicians. Of 201 men with a diagnosis of cancer in the preceding 2 years, 51% of men were interested in having children in the future, including 77% of childless men. On the other hand, only 51% recalled being given the option of semen cryopreservation and only 35% of respondents were not interested in having children in the future.[150] A companion study found that fewer than 50 % of practitioners were consistently discussing sperm banking with their male cancer patients.[150] The authors also found that men who were informed of fertility options by their oncologist, rather than by other means, were more likely to undergo sperm banking.[152] If lack of information is the primary reason for not pursuing sperm banking, increased attention to, and education regarding sperm cryopreservation may increase the number of referrals and later use of cryopreserved sperm.

Testicular Sperm Extraction

Although the majority of patients are able to have sperm collected prior to therapy, there are a proportion of male cancer patients who are azoospermic prior to therapy and therefore unable to undergo standard semen collection. In addition, many men fail to have sperm collected prior to therapy and find themselves azoospermic after treatment. For these patients, sperm may be obtained through newer technologies such as epididymal aspiration, testicular sperm extraction (TESE), or transrectal electroejaculation (TE). With TESE, testicular biopsy tissue is macerated, centrifuged, and examined for the presence of sperm. TESE is an important method of sperm recovery for patients who have undergone cytotoxic chemotherapy and have apparent germinal aplasia. Recovery rates with TESE in patients with either complete germinal aplasia or maturation arrest on biopsy have ranged from 45 to 76%, presumably because of adjacent areas of intact spermatogenesis.[153,154] The reported pregnancy rates with TESE and ICSI range from 30 to 40%, do not appear to be significantly altered by the source of sperm or the testicular history,[153,154] and are comparable with rates in men with nonobstructive azoospermia caused by non-neoplastic disorders.[154] As this technology is becoming more available, even men with long-standing azoospermia and absent sperm production may be able to father children. In addition, one group has suggested incorporating TESE prior to therapy in azoospermic men. Although a proportion of men who are azoospermic prior to therapy will regain spermatogenesis following therapy, many will remain azoospermic because of the therapy. Schrader et al[155] successfully collected spermatozoa in 14 of 31 azoospermic patients prior to therapy, 14 with a germ cell tumor and 17 with malignant lymphoma. These authors advocate pretreatment TESE in azoospermic men as it is difficult to predict who will regain fertility after therapy, there is a theoretical teratogenic risk to offspring, and pretreatment banking can reduce fertility-related concerns for the future. In addition, in men with tumor-associated azoospermia who were unable to undergo cryopreservation, TESE post-treatment was unsuccessful in over half of patients, likely because of cytotoxic germinal damage.[154-156]

Testicular Germ Cell Transplantation

Testicular germ cell transplantation is an additional experimental technique that may be available to male cancer patients in the future. This procedure was first developed in male mice, in which spermatogonial stem cells were transferred into the seminiferous tubules of busulfan-sterilized recipient animals.[157] Several animal studies have shown that spermatogonial stem cells can repopulate the seminiferous tubules with resumption of spermatogenesis and production of functional spermatozoa, leading to natural live births in the recipient animals.[157-159] Human application has just begun and remains experimental. One group has cryopreserved testicular cells in 12 patients with lymphoma prior to therapy. To date, seven of these patients have completed therapy and have undergone transplantation of their cryopreserved stem cells into the intratesticular rete testes. The outcomes of these transplants have not yet been published, but there is great hope that this will be feasible in humans.[157,160] Despite the great interest in testicular germ cell transplantation, there is a theoretical risk of disease transmission, especially in the setting of hematologic malignancies. This concern has been validated in an animal model in which all rats that received testicular germ cells from leukemic donors developed leukemia after testicular germ cell transplantation.[161] Tumor cell depletion techniques are currently being devel-

oped to address this limitation. If successful, testicular germ cell transplantation may be a viable option for male cancer patients hoping to preserve their reproductive potential.

Hormonal Manipulation To Prevent Male Infertility

The recognition that some chemotherapy regimens produce irreversible gonadal injury has prompted a search for means to protect the testis from the toxic effects of these drugs. Reducing the rate of spermatogenesis by interrupting the pituitary-gonadal axis has been proposed as a means of rendering the germinal epithelium relatively resistant to cytotoxic agents. Gonadotropin-releasing hormone (GnRH) analogs, both agonists and antagonists, have been shown to inhibit spermatogenesis in animals[162-164] and man.[165] In 1981, Glode et al[166] reported that treatment of mice with a GnRH analog resulted in protection of the testis from the damaging effects of cyclophosphamide. These findings stimulated the initiation of clinical trials to evaluate this approach in patients receiving cancer chemotherapy, but human trials to date have been largely unsuccessful.[167-170]

These failures in human studies have prompted new hypotheses, and recent studies suggest that the mechanism of hormonal therapy is stimulation of the surviving type A spermatogonia to differentiate, rather than to-protection of the germ cells through inhibition of spermatogenesis.[171-173] The animals studied had elevated FSH, LH, and intratesticular testosterone, but serum testosterone levels remained normal. These findings have led to the recent hypothesis that testosterone and FSH may inhibit spermatogonial differentiation in surviving germ cells. Further animal studies have shown that GnRH agonists and antagonists can prevent this block in differentiation through suppression of testosterone and FSH.[173-175] GnRH-treated rats had increased sperm counts and a significant increase in fertility.[176] The role of testosterone as a key inhibitor of differentiation has been shown in GnRH-treated animals. After treatment with GnRH, rats had the expected increase in spermatogenic differentiation. Animals were then administered exogenous androgens and spermatogonial differentiation declined in a dose-dependent fashion.[177,178]

Although these animal studies are very encouraging and much has been learned about the hormonal mechanisms controlling spermatogenesis, the relevance to humans remains unclear. The optimal timing and duration of hormonal therapy remains unclear and may be drug-dependent.[179] Meistrich suggests that future studies in humans should include frequent sperm samples and cryopreservation of sperm because the recovery of spermatogenesis was transient in some of the animal studies.[171] It appears that hormonal manipulation is likely to be most successful in a setting in which there is some survival of type A spermatogonia.[180] Therefore, human studies will need to start with cytotoxic agents and doses that do not completely deplete the germinal stem cell population.

CHEMOTHERAPY EFFECTS IN WOMEN

Oogenesis is the process of maturation of the primitive female germ cell to the mature ovum. This process occurs primarily during intrauterine life and involves multiple mitotic divisions to increase the number of germ cells, followed by the beginning of the first meiotic division, which will eventually reduce the diploid chromosome number to half before fertilization. At the time of birth, the oocytes are in the long prophase of their first meiotic division, and they remain in that state until the formation of a mature follicle before ovulation.[181]

In the postnatal ovary, most of the ongoing cellular growth and replication is related to the growth and development of follicles. Primordial follicles develop during gestation and consist of a primary oocyte covered by a layer of mesenchymal cells called granulosa cells. At the time of birth, the ovary may contain 150,000 to 500,000 primordial follicles, many of which subsequently become atretic. From childhood to menopause, follicular growth occurs as a continuous process, with ovulation occurring in a cyclic fashion.[182] The granulosa cells surrounding the primary oocyte proliferate, follicular fluid accumulates, and the ovum completes its first meiotic division to become a secondary oocyte. At this time, the follicle is known as a secondary or graafian follicle. The follicle continues to enlarge until the time of ovulation. Those follicles not undergoing ovulation become atretic and regress. During the reproductive life of a woman, only 300 to 400 oocytes mature and are extruded in the process of ovulation; the remainder undergo some form of atresia.

Assessment of Ovarian Function

The evaluation of chemotherapy effects on ovarian function is hampered by the relative inaccessibility of the ovary to biopsy. There is no readily available direct measurement of the female germ cell population analogous to semen analysis in men. Animal models to assess the effects of cytotoxic drugs on ovarian function have been developed only recently. Thus, one must rely primarily on menstrual and reproductive history and on determinations of serum hormone levels to assess the functional status of the ovary.

Follicular growth and maturation and estradiol production are under regulatory control of the pituitary and hypothalamus. Pituitary FSH stimulates granulosa cells to replicate and produce estradiol. The midcycle LH surge promotes ovulation and the ruptured follicle becomes the corpus luteum, which produces progesterone, thereby suppressing further LH secretion.[183] Drug-induced ovarian failure interrupts this delicate hormonal balance and results in abnormally low serum levels of estradiol and progesterone, markedly elevated levels of FSH and LH, amenorrhea, and symptoms of estrogen deficiency.

The primary histologic lesion noted in the ovaries of women receiving antineoplastic chemotherapy is ovarian fibrosis and follicle destruction.[184,185] Clinically, amenorrhea ensues and is accompanied by elevation of serum FSH and LH levels and a fall in serum estradiol. Vaginal epithelial atrophy and endometrial hypoplasia occur, and patients may complain of menopausal symptoms such as vaginal dryness and dyspareunia.

Drug Effects on Ovarian Function

The onset and duration of amenorrhea varies with the cytotoxic agent (Table 4.3) and appears to be both dose-related and age-related. Generally, younger patients are able to tolerate larger cumulative drug doses before amenorrhea occurs and have a greater likelihood of resumption of menses when therapy is discontinued.

Drugs Highly Toxic to Germ Cells

Alkylating Agents
Alkylating agents are the most frequent cause of ovarian dysfunction among the anticancer drugs. During the early clinical trials of busulfan, amenorrhea was a common side effect. Several investigators noted the onset of permanent amenorrhea among patients receiving busulfan in doses varying from 0.5 to 14.0 mg/day for at least 3 months.[186,187] The effects of cyclophosphamide on ovarian function in humans were first noted in the rheumatology literature as noted in a study showing that early cessation of menses and menopausal symptoms developed in 6 of 33 patients treated for rheumatoid arthritis with daily cyclophosphamide for 6 to 40 months.[188] One of these patients had elevated FSH levels consistent with primary ovarian failure.

TABLE 4.3

TOXICITY OF SINGLE AGENTS TO FEMALE GERM CELLS

Single Agent Drug	References
Drugs highly toxic to female germ cells	
Busulfan	186, 187
Cyclophosphamide	188–191
Melphalan	192
Drugs with moderate-to-low toxicity to female germ cells	
Methotrexate	39
5–FU	191, 192
Etoposide/vinca alkaloids	193, 194
Doxorubicin	195
Cisplatin	194, 196–198
Taxanes	199

Subsequently, several investigators documented the occurrence of amenorrhea, decreased urinary estrogens, and increased urinary gonadotropins in at least 50% of premenopausal women receiving 40 to 120 mg of cyclophosphamide daily for an average of 18 months.[189,190] Ovarian biopsy in some patients demonstrated arrest of follicular maturation and absence of ova.

Studies of the use of adjuvant chemotherapy for the prevention of recurrence of breast cancer suggest that the onset of amenorrhea and the resumption of menses are related to the age of the patient during chemotherapy and to the total dose administered.[191-193] Amenorrhea developed in 17 of 18 women treated with adjuvant cyclophosphamide for 13 to 14 months postoperatively.[194] Permanent cessation of menses occurred after a mean total dose of 5.2 g in all patients 40 years of age and older. Amenorrhea also developed in four of five women younger than age 40, but only after a mean cyclophosphamide dose of 9.3 g had been administered. Menses subsequently returned in two of these patients within 6 months of discontinuing therapy. Furthermore, a prospective study of ovarian function in premenopausal women receiving melphalan alone or in combination with 5-fluorouracil (5-FU) demonstrated the occurrence of amenorrhea in 22% of patients younger than age 39 but in 73% of patients older than age 40.[195] Time to the development of amenorrhea also appears to be age-related after adjuvant treatment with cyclophosphamide, MTX, and 5-FU (CMF).[196] In women younger than age 35, mean time to the onset of amenorrhea is 5.54 months; for women aged 35 to 45 years, the mean time is 2.31 months, and in women older than age 45, amenorrhea develops very quickly, with a mean onset of 1.01 months. It seems, then, that alkylating agent chemotherapy accelerates the onset of menopause, particularly in older patients, whereas younger patients may tolerate higher total doses before amenorrhea becomes irreversible. Other large studies examining the effects of CMF also have documented this age-related effect.[197-200] In addition, recent studies evaluating pulse intravenous cyclophosphamide in inflammatory diseases have confirmed the associations of age at treatment and cumulative dose with therapy-related ovarian failure. Women who receive intravenous cyclophosphamide before the age of 25 rarely experience permanent amenorrhea. Yet, rates of amenorrhea after age 31 range from 45 to 62% and have been reported as high as 83% after age 40.[201,202] Similar to the findings in adjuvant breast cancer therapy, there was an increased risk of amenorrhea associated with greater cumulative dose, although the difference was not statistically significant.[201]

Drugs with Moderate to Low Toxicity to Germ Cells

Although many other chemotherapeutic agents have been evaluated for long-term ovarian toxicity, most evidence comes from studying the effects of combination chemother-apy regimens. Therefore, it is often difficult to determine the contribution of individual agents.

In general, chemotherapeutic agents that are cell cycle-specific appear to have low gonadotoxicity in women. Many of these agents are toxic to reproductive germ cells in men, but they do not have the same toxicity in women. This is likely because there is constant cell division during spermatogenesis, and in women, there is intermittent cell division involving only a small number of primary oocytes with each menstrual cycle.

Antimetabolites

Among the antimetabolites, high-dose methotrexate and 5-FU have been evaluated and appear to have no immediate ovarian toxicity.[39] A study of single-agent 5-FU in nine patients with breast cancer found no evidence of ovarian failure.[194] In addition, Fisher et al[195] found no difference in the incidence of post-therapy amenorrhea in women who received 5-FU and melphalan compared with those who received melphalan alone.

Etoposide

The effects of oral etoposide on ovarian function were evaluated in one study of 22 patients receiving this agent. Age-related oligomenorrhea or amenorrhea occurred in 41% of patients after a mean cumulative etoposide dose of 5 g[204] In addition, Meirow[205] evaluated 168 women who received various combination regimens for lymphoma, leukemia, and breast cancer and found no association between vinca alkaloid administration and occurrence of amenorrhea.

Doxorubicin

Doxorubicin administration does not appear to have profound ovarian ablative effects. In women younger than age 35 who received adjuvant cyclophosphamide, doxorubicin, and 5-FU, 32% had temporary amenorrhea during treatment, and only 9% had permanent amenorrhea.[206]

Cisplatin

Although platinum chemotherapeutic agents have notable gonadal toxicity in men, the data in women are limited and contradictory. Many studies suggest that most women who receive platinum-based chemotherapy have temporary amenorrhea, but resume normal menstrual function. Low et al[207] evaluated 44 females, aged 10 to 35 years old, who received cisplatin-based therapy for malignant germ cell tumors of the ovary. While two-thirds of the patients experienced amenorrhea during therapy, 43 of 47 (91%) resumed normal menstrual patterns and 95% of those who attempted conception were successful. As described previously, Meirow[205] evaluated 168 patients who received combination chemotherapy for lymphoma, leukemia, or breast cancer for future risk of treatment-related ovarian failure. The author reported an odds ratio of 1.77 for cisplatin-containing therapy, although the results were not statistically significant. Other groups have reported persistent menstrual dysfunction in women after the administration of cisplatin-based therapies.[203,208,209] The inconsistencies in the literature may be explained by differences in defining treatment-related ovarian failure, the duration of follow-up, dose received, and age at administration. It is clear that further studies are needed to determine the true impact of platinum-based therapy on future fertility.

Taxanes

Although taxanes have become widely used in the treatment of breast cancer, there are little data regarding the ovarian toxicity of this class of chemotherapeutics. Early results of the BCIRG 001 trial reported that 51% of patients receiving TAC (docetaxel, Adriamycin, and cyclophosphamide) developed amenorrhea.[210] These results are preliminary, with short-term follow-up and an unclear definition of amenorrhea. Therefore, further studies are needed to draw definitive conclusions regarding the incidence of treatment-related ovarian failure following taxane therapy.

Combination Chemotherapy and Disease-Specific Considerations

Breast Cancer

Studies of adjuvant chemotherapy for breast cancer have yielded other important information regarding the effects of dose and treatment duration on menstrual cycles (Table 4.4). Evaluation of 95 premenopausal women who received cyclophosphamide, MTX, 5-FU, vincristine, and prednisone documented permanent amenorrhea in 70.5% of patients.[211] Women receiving chemotherapy for 12 weeks had a 55% incidence of amenorrhea, whereas 83% of women receiving a 36-week regimen were rendered amenorrheic. Breast cancer recurrence and mortality rates in women who experienced amenorrhea were lower than in those who continued to menstruate, even within each treatment group, suggesting a potential therapeutic benefit of ovarian ablation. However, the contribution of treatment-induced amenorrhea to the beneficial effects of adjuvant chemotherapy remains uncertain and controversial.

In counseling women with newly diagnosed breast cancer regarding the risk of chemotherapy-related amenorrhea or ovarian failure, age and risk of recurrence must be considered. Age at treatment is the primary factor in predicting chemotherapy-induced amenorrhea and is the most relevant consideration when counseling women with premenopausal breast cancer. Several studies have shown that younger women have a higher likelihood of resuming their menses and maintaining future fertility. For example, CMF has been associated with persistent amenorrhea in 21 to 71% of women under 40 years old, compared with 49 to 100% in those over 40 years old.[199] Other groups have found low rates of persistent amenorrhea (0 to 4%) in women under the age of 30 who received CMF or doxorubicin-based therapy, rates of 50% in women between 30 and 40 years old, and rates of 86% and higher in women over 40 years old.[212,213]

Although the choice of adjuvant therapy primarily depends on disease characteristics, it may be useful to consider the likelihood of amenorrhea with different adjuvant regimens in which subsequent fertility is of great importance to the patient. In general, studies suggest that the combination of cyclophosphamide, methotrexate and 5-FU (CMF) is the regimen with the highest likelihood of causing premature ovarian failure because up to two-thirds of premenopausal women who receive CMF will experience persistent amenorrhea.[199] An early study of doxorubicin-based adjuvant therapy reported persistent amenorrhea in 59% of women,[212] but more recent studies have found lower rates of persistent amenorrhea, ranging from 34 to 51% of premenopausal women treated with doxorubicin or epirubicin-based regimens.[199,210,214] As described previously, ovarian failure with taxane-containing regimens is not well studied, although the early results of the BCIRG

TABLE 4.4
RATES OF AMENORRHEA AFTER ADJUVANT REGIMENS FOR BREAST CANCER

Regimen		<40 Years Old	≥40 Years Old	References
CMF		40–61%	76–95%	198, 204
	≤30 Years Old	31–39 Years Old	≥40 Years Old	
Doxorubin –based regimens	None	33%	96%	212
		All Ages		
CAF/CEF		32.8–51%		199, 206, 214
AC		34%		206
AC/Taxol		51%		199
Melphalan/5-FU		9%		206

001 trial reported that 51% of patients receiving TAC developed amenorrhea.[210] Although the treatment is rarely used today, low rates of persistent amenorrhea (9%) have been reported with melphalan-based regimens.[199] These rates ignore the wide variability secondary to age at the onset of treatment, so the probability on basis of the age of the patient must also be carefully considered.

Hodgkin's Disease

The risk of ovarian failure after other combination chemotherapy for hematologic malignancies is also clearly related to the age of the patient at the time of treatment. Overall, at least 50% of women treated with MOPP or related regimens become amenorrheic.[215–222] The cessation of menses is accompanied by elevations of serum FSH and LH consistent with primary ovarian failure. Apart from age, no clear differences have been noted between those women who become amenorrheic during therapy and those who do not. In one study, follow-up of MOPP-treated patients for a median of 9 years after the completion of chemotherapy revealed that 46% had developed permanent amenorrhea.[217] Of these women, 89% were older than 25 years at the time of treatment. Moreover, the time of onset of amenorrhea seemed to be age-related; ovarian failure occurred within 1 year of discontinuing therapy in all patients 39 years of age or older, whereas in younger patients there was a gradual decrease in frequency of menses occurring more than several years after therapy. Another group found similar results with 76% of women who received MOPP or a related hybrid combination of chlorambucil, vinblastine, prednisolone, procarbazine, doxorubicin, vincristine, and etoposide developed amenorrhea during or immediately after treatment. Despite this, 10 women later regained normal menstrual periods and 16 had permanent amenorrhea. The mean age at treatment among the 10 with recovery was 25 years, and the mean age in the latter group was 36 years old, suggesting the importance of age at the time of therapy.[222] Another group reported persistent ovarian failure in 86% of women over 24 years old who received COPP (cyclophosphamide, vincristine, procarbazine, and prednisone), but a much lower rate of 28% in those who were under 24 years old at the time of treatment.[223] At present, it seems unlikely that those patients treated when younger than age 25 will experience any significant therapy-related ovarian dysfunction during the initial 5 to 10 years after the completion of therapy. As in men, ABVD chemotherapy may be less likely to produce premature ovarian failure, although longer follow-up is required to be certain. In a study comparing MOPP with ABVD, 50% of the patients who received MOPP and were over 30 years old developed prolonged amenorrhea. All the women who received MOPP under the age of 30 and all the women who received ABVD, regardless of age, had resumption of normal menstrual cycles.[60]

Non-Hodgkin's Lymphoma

Combination chemotherapy regimens for aggressive non-Hodgkin's lymphoma do not consistently cause premature ovarian failure, perhaps because procarbazine is rarely included in such regimens.[22] Of 10 women who received various combined modality regimens for non-Hodgkin's lymphoma, only 1 developed gonadal dysfunction. Similarly, among seven women aged 35 to 43 treated with MACOP-B or VACOP-B for aggressive non-Hodgkin's lymphoma, only one developed amenorrhea.[65]

Ovarian Germ Cell Tumors

Although malignant germ cell tumors of the ovary are rare, they principally occur during adolescence and early adulthood. With the advent of cisplatin-based chemotherapy regimens, high cure rates have been obtained, even in the setting of metastatic disease.[207] Fertility-sparing surgery has become the standard of care because evidence has shown that removal of the uninvolved ovary does not improve survival.[224] Many patients receive combination chemotherapy, and the regimens used appear to cause relatively little ovarian toxicity. In one study, 70% of women maintained regular menses after treatment with a variety of regimens containing drugs such as actinomycin D, vincristine, and cyclophosphamide.[225] Low et al[207] evaluated 47 females between the ages of 10 and 35 years old who received conservative surgery followed by chemotherapy for malignant germ cell tumors of the ovary. Forty-four of the patients received cisplatin-based regimens. Although two-thirds experienced amenorrhea during therapy, 43 of 47 (91%) resumed normal menstrual periods after completion of therapy. In addition, 95% of those who attempted to conceive children were successful. Tangir et al[203] found no difference in fertility outcomes between patients who received cyclophosphamide-based therapy versus cisplatin-based therapy. Other groups have reported similar results, and it appears that the majority of women who receive chemotherapy for germ cell tumors of the ovary will resume menstrual function.[226,227]

High-Dose Chemotherapy and Bone Marrow Transplantation

The risk of treatment-related ovarian failure after high-dose chemotherapy and bone marrow transplant appears to be largely related to age at the time of treatment. From the Seattle experience, cyclophosphamide-containing preparative regimens for allogeneic bone marrow transplantation induced reversible amenorrhea in women younger than 26 years of age, but permanent amenorrhea in 67% of women older than age 26.[228] Likewise, Schimmer et al[229] evaluated 17 premenopausal patients treated with a variety of conditioning regimens followed by autologous bone marrow transplant for predictors of ovarian failure. Of the 17 patients, only 5 (29%) had a return of normal menstrual cycles. The mean age of those with recovery of ovarian function was 19 years, and mean age of those with persistent amenorrhea was 30 years. In their analysis, younger age at treatment was a statistically significant predictor of future ovarian function. Univariate analysis suggested a trend toward total-body irradiation (TBI) as a predictor of permanent amenorrhea. In addition, the number of prior chemotherapy salvage regimens, or the number of regimens containing alkylating agents, did not predict for permanent amenorrhea. Other studies have suggested that regimens using TBI cause premature menopause in nearly all patients.[228] Chatterjee and Goldstone[230] found that 20 of 30 women who received conditioning regimens with chemotherapy only recovered normal menstrual patterns, and none of the 10 who received TBI recovered ovarian function. Others have found similar results, and it appears that most younger women, who receive chemotherapy-containing conditioning regimens will regain menstrual function, and the majority over age 26 years old will have treatment-related infertility.[65,205,231,232] Although most studies have found that the specific chemotherapy-conditioning regimen did not appear to affect future fertility, Singhal et al [233] reported a higher pregnancy rate among women who were conditioned with melphalan alone when compared with those who received other conditioning regimens. These authors suggested that this regimen is adequate for engraftment and may be less likely to cause treatment-related ovarian failure. Further studies are needed to confirm these results because variations in permanent ovarian failure among chemotherapy-conditioning regimens could be important to young women undergoing high-dose chemotherapy and bone marrow transplantation.

Estrogen Deficiency

Although infertility is a primary concern of many young women who receive cytotoxic therapy, women who develop premature ovarian failure may also be subject to the physical and emotional disorders that accompany estrogen deficiency. Depressed libido, irritability, sleep disturbances, and poor self-image all occur commonly in women with treatment-related amenorrhea.[216,234] Hormone replacement therapy may be of considerable benefit to patients with chemotherapy-induced amenorrhea, frequently producing dramatic relief of hot flashes, dyspareunia, and irritability. Another potential benefit of estrogen replacement therapy may be prevention of postmenopausal osteoporosis and diminished risk of premature atherosclerosis.

Mutagenic Potential of Cancer Chemotherapy in Women

As previously described, the mutagenic potential of cancer chemotherapy remains largely undefined. Some anecdotal reports suggest that there is no increased incidence of spontaneous abortion or fetal abnormalities in women

treated with chemotherapy in comparison with the general population.[206,235–238] Several larger series and reviews have generally confirmed this observation.[239–242] However, there are other reports suggesting an increase in structural congenital cardiac defects, spontaneous abortions, and other congenital anomalies in women previously treated with chemotherapy when compared with controls.[239,243] At present, it is impossible to define the risk of fetal wastage or abnormality in patients previously treated with cytotoxic drugs. Whether a specific fetal abnormality may occur more commonly than others, or whether a specific drug class, dose, or combination is more mutagenic than others remains unknown. Additional studies carried out over many years are required before the true risks to subsequent generations are known.

The mutagenic effects of chemotherapy on the offspring from oocytes obtained by advanced reproductive techniques soon after chemotherapy administration are unknown. Women considering ooctye retrieval soon after the completion of chemotherapy should be counseled regarding the theoretical risk of congenital malformation and early pregnancy loss. Based on the timing of cyclophosphamide-induced follicular injury in rats, Meirow[205] suggests that oocytes obtained in the 6 to 12 months following therapy may be compromised, and recommends that further studies are needed to better define the time period of greatest susceptibility.

Assisted Reproductive Techniques for Women

Embryo Cryopreservation

Prior to the development of embryo cryopreservation, no reliable techniques existed for women who wished to retain the ability to bear children following ovarian ablative chemotherapy. Embryo cryopreservation with later intrafallopian or intrauterine embryo transfer is the only successful clinical approach to postchemotherapy ovarian failure.[244] Before initiation of chemotherapy, women may have oocytes harvested and fertilized in vitro with husband or donor sperm. The embryos can be stored in liquid nitrogen and thawed for implantation at a later date when the patient's endometrium has been hormonally prepared. This option has been associated with pregnancy and take-home baby rates of 30 to 35% and 29%, respectively.[245] In women who did not have frozen zygotes or embryos stored before chemotherapy, donor ova are available for fertilization and implantation at specialized fertility centers.

Unfortunately, although successful, this procedure is not available for many women. First, embryo cryopreservation requires a partner at the time of harvest. Even though an anonymous sperm donor is an alternative, this is an unacceptable option for many women. In addition, embryo cryopreservation is not an option for prepubertal or pubertal girls. Secondly, the time involved in ovarian stimulation, monitoring, and oocyte retrieval requires a delay in beginning cancer treatment that many oncologists discourage. For this reason, some centers offer IVF only during breaks in treatment or after remission is achieved.[246,247] Lastly, ovarian stimulation increases levels of estradiol,[248,249] and studies have suggested that breast cancer cell proliferation and dissemination can be induced by estrogen.[250,251] For this reason, many oncologists believe that conventional stimulation programs are contraindicated in women with hormone-responsive malignancies such as breast cancer.

For women with breast cancer, an alternative to standard IVF is natural IVF, or oocyte retrieval without hyperstimulation. Unfortunately, unstimulated cycles generally only yield one or two metaphase II eggs. Hyperstimulation significantly increases the chance of a successful pregnancy and allows storage of multiple embryos for future transfer attempts. For this reason, alternative stimulation programs have recently been evaluated and may be available in the future. For example, tamoxifen has been used as an ovulation induction agent in Europe, similar to clomiphene in the United States. Oktay et al[249] recently developed and evaluated tamoxifen for ovarian stimulation in patients with breast cancer. This group compared their tamoxifen stimulation protocol with natural cycle IVF and reported a greater number of embryos available for cryopreservation in the tamoxifen-stimulation group. Only 3 of 5 women in the natural IVF program had embryo formation, while all 12 in the tamoxifen group had at least one embryo recovered. To date, only two women in the tamoxifen-stimulation group have attempted embryo transfer. Although one of these attempts resulted in a miscarriage at 8 weeks, the other woman had a successful twin birth. Aromatase inhibitors are now being investigated as an alternative to ovulation induction, as they are associated with lower mid-cycle estradiol levels.[249]

Cryopreservation of Oocytes

Embryo cryopreservation is the standard option, but oocyte cryopreservation would benefit prepubertal girls and women without a partner at the time of oocyte retrieval. Embryo cryopreservation became the procedure of choice because embryos survive cryopreservation better than oocytes. Animal studies have shown that freezing and thawing of unfertilized oocytes results in changes in the zona pellucida, leading to decreased rates of fertilization.[252] With advances and manipulation of cryopreservation media and conditions, oocyte freezing and storage have been partially successful in animals.[252-254] These techniques have been attempted in humans, and there are 26 pregnancies derived from cryopreserved oocytes reported in the literature.[255] Despite these successes, the overall pregnancy and delivery rates (4.7 and 3.1%, respectively) are too low for widespread clinical application. With continued advances, oocyte cryopreservation may become a valid reproductive option in the future.

Ovarian Tissue Cryopreservation and Transplantation

A technique that holds great promise for women anticipating treatment with potentially sterilizing chemotherapy is ovarian autografting. Already in clinical trials, the technique relies on the removal of oocyte-rich ovarian cortical tissue that is then slowly cooled and stored in a cryopreservative. At a later date, the tissue may be thawed and reimplanted near the fallopian tubes for potentially natural ovulation and fertilization. Ovarian tissue cryopreservation and transplantation offer several advantages over oocyte and embryo cryopreservation, including a greater number of immature oocytes, elimination of the need for hormonal stimulation and delays in therapy, and easier cryopreservation because follicles are small, lack a zona pellucida, and are metabolically inactive and undifferentiated. In addition, ovarian cryopreservation can be offered to prepubertal and pubertal girls.[256] In addition, this technique could provide an alternative to hormone replacement therapy for patients who develop premature ovarian failure. Gosden et al,[257] who pioneered this technique, reported successful pregnancies in sheep, and other groups have had similar success in various animals.[258] Although still investigational, applications with cryopreserved ovarian implants have begun in humans.[259-261] Cortical ovarian biopsies have been easily obtained in women via laparascopy without significant complications.[205] In addition, case reports and small series of successful ovarian autotransplants have been described. Ovarian tissue transplantation has restored ovarian hormonal function in a single patient, resulted in a normal ovulatory cycle in another, and shown evidence of follicular development after transplantation in a small series.[262,263] In addition, retrieval of a single oocyte has been described after hetertopic autologous ovarian transplant in one patient.[264] Despite these successes, this procedure is still in its infancy and pregnancies have not yet been reported. There are concerns with poor tissue survival as a result of ischemic-reperfusion injury, the longevity of ovarian tissue grafts, the ability to achieve follicular development within the graft, and malignant disease transmission via the autologous tissue graft. In addition, the optimal application for cryopreserved ovarian grafts is unclear. Although orthotopic autologous transplantation is the most obvious application, there are concerns for poor graft survival and follicular reserve. Heterotopic transplantation, involving grafting to a distant tissue site such as the arm or abdominal wall, may be an alternative, allowing for oocyte recovery prior to graft failure. Xenotransplantation, involving transplantation into an animal followed by later oocyte retrieval after adequate follicular development, could be an option to avoid malignant disease transmission.[265] Lastly, in vitro maturation followed by IVF has been demonstrated in a mouse model.[266] Although ovarian tissue transplantation remains investigational, it may become a management option for women with premature ovarian failure secondary to cytotoxic therapy.

Hormonal Manipulation in Women

Efforts to protect the ovary from the toxic effects of chemotherapy have focused on the use of oral contraceptives and GnRH agonists to induce ovarian suppression. Preliminary data reported by Chapman and Sutcliffe[267] suggested that ovarian follicles could be protected and normal menses could be preserved by the administration of oral contraceptives during chemotherapy. Only a small number of young women were studied, and follow-up was brief. More recent studies with longer follow-up have failed to demonstrate a protective effect of oral contraceptives.[220,221,268] Thus, the incomplete gonadal suppression induced by oral contraceptives may not be sufficient to protect ovarian follicles during cytotoxic therapy.[269]

Although GnRH analogs have not been proven to be protective of male germ cells, the studies in women have been more encouraging. The goal of this approach is to induce a dormant state in germ cells, suppressing cellular replication, and rendering the cells resistant to the cytotoxic effects of chemotherapy. GnRH analogs appear to partially protect ovarian follicles and fertility in rats and Rhesus monkeys from the damaging effects of cyclophosphamide,[270-273] with variable protective effects from x-irradiation.[274,275] However, preliminary clinical observations have failed to demonstrate a protective effect of the LHRH analog buserelin on ovarian function in women undergoing chemotherapy for Hodgkin's disease.[169] In contrast, GnRH agonists may have a protective effect in young women receiving chemotherapy for lymphoma.[269] Similarly, Blumenfeld et al[276] administered a GnRH agonist to 60 premenopausal women with lymphoma prior to chemotherapy and for 6 months during and after chemotherapy. Six months after the start of chemotherapy, only 3 of the 60 (5%) developed ovarian failure compared with 32 of 58 (55%) age-matched and disease-matched controls. Continued long-term, prospective follow-up of women maintaining normal menses during chemotherapy is necessary to determine the degree of risk of premature ovarian failure and early menopause in these individuals.

CHEMOTHERAPY EFFECTS IN CHILDREN

Over 70% of children now survive cancer that is diagnosed and treated in childhood.[277] Because discussion of remission rates, survival rates, and immediate toxicities tend to dominate initial dicussions regarding treatment options, consideration of future fertility is a quality of life aspect that is often neglected. Many regimens used as treatment for childhood cancer have significant gonadal toxicity. As a result, many survivors experience infertility

as adults. Any study of the effects of cytotoxic chemotherapy on gonadal function in children is particularly complex because of the variables introduced by the continuum of sexual development in this patient population. Thus, the effects of chemotherapy can be expected to vary according to when drugs are given and when their effects are evaluated relative to puberty.

Chemotherapy Effects in Boys

Early reports suggested differences in the sensitivity of the prepubertal, pubertal, and adult testis to alkylating-agent chemotherapy, concluding that the prepubertal testis is relatively unaffected by chemotherapy. For example, one group found serum FSH, LH, and testosterone levels normal for their age in 15 boys treated with cyclophosphamide during the prepubertal years or early puberty.[278] Another study evaluating gonadal function in boys undergoing combination chemotherapy (prednisone, vincristine, MTX, and 6-mercaptopurine) for ALL reported normal semen analyses in five of six patients after a median follow-up of 5.5 years.[279] Other investigators found an initial decrease in spermatogonia among patients undergoing chemotherapy for acute lymphoblastic leukemia, but reported improvement to normal levels over many years,[280,281] concluding that leukemia therapy has definite, although at least partially reversible, effects on the germinal epithelium of the prepubertal and intrapubertal boy. More recent data have contradicted the hypothesis that the prepubertal state offers protection against the gonadotoxic effects of chemotherapy. As early as 1976, Etteldorf et al[282] suggested that, even for the prepubertal patient, a dose-toxicity relationship may exist. These investigators evaluated eight boys, aged 7.5 to 13.0 years old, who received varying cumulative doses of cyclophosphamide. Those patients receiving 11.8 to 39.3 g of the drug were uniformly azoospermic with germinal aplasia as a finding on biopsy results, and those who received lower cumulative doses had normal sperm counts. More recently, Mustieles et al[283] evaluated 15 men who received polychemotherapy between ages 6 and 10 years old (12 were prepubertal) and reported only 1 patient with normal sperm counts after a mean follow-up of 6 years. Similarly, among 19 prepubertal boys receiving MOPP or more than 9 g/m^2 of cyclophosphamide, 12 were sterile at a mean follow-up of 9 years.[284] Other studies have confirmed that MOPP is uniformly toxic, even when administered during the prepubertal state, as almost all patients have evidence of azoospermia or oligospermia as adults.[285-288] These findings suggest that the prepubertal testis may be more tolerant of moderate doses of alkylating agents than is the adult testis, yet a threshold dose does seem to exist, above which germinal epithelial injury will result.[289,290]

Chemotherapy delivered to male patients during puberty appears to have profound effects on both germ cell production and endocrine function, similar to the effects seen in adult male cancer patients. Among 12 prepubertal and pubertal boys who received at least six cycles of MOPP for Hodgkin's disease at Stanford, all patients who provided semen for analysis had complete azoospermia as long as 11 years after treatment.[287] Two of these boys (aged 8 and 12 at diagnosis) had recovery of fertility and subsequently fathered children 12 and 15 years after therapy, but none of the boys treated during puberty recovered spermatogenesis. However, all boys attained normal sexual maturation, and androgen replacement was not necessary in any patient. In a review of childhood cancer patients, alkylating agents were the most likely drugs to cause azoospermia, with 68% of 93 male childhood cancer survivors azoospermic after therapy. Of the 57 patients who received cisplatin or cisplatin-based regimens, only 37% had long-term azoospermia. An even lower rate of gonadal toxicity was reported in the 31 patients who received nonalkylating agents (adriamycin, vincristine, methotrexate, and 6-mercaptopurine) as only 16% had future azoospermia.[291] Leydig cell dysfunction can also occur in some patients and may manifest as gynecomastia.

Although future fertility is not the most immediate concern when treating children or adolescent male cancer patients, improved survival rates have led to an increased appreciation for the long-term quality of life effects of chemotherapeutic treatment. For this reason, many authors suggest that clinicians address future infertility prior to instituting therapy. In addition, many authors advocate sperm collection and cryopreservation for peripubertal or postpubertal sexually mature adolescents. Although not routinely offered because of a presumption of inadequate collection in adolescent males, recent studies suggest there may be a role for sperm cryopreservation in adolescent cancer patients. Kleish et al[291] compared sperm concentrations, motility, and morphology in male cancer patients and found no significant differences in semen parameters from adolescent boys (14 to 17 years old), young adult males (17 to 20 years old), and adult males, suggesting feasibility of cryopreservation in adolescent male cancer patients. Postovsky et al[292] reported poor sperm collection in 27 male cancer patients aged 14 to 19 years old, with only 30% of attempts yielding a normal volume ejaculate and only 6.5 % of attempts producing semen with normal parameters. Similar inadequacies have been reported in male cancer patients in which 50 % of male cancer patients have reduced sperm quality prior to chemotherapy.[52,57,120–124] Despite this high rate of abnormal sperm quality, most male cancer patients have adequate parameters for sperm storage.[131] Successful sperm cryopreservation has been reported in more than 80% of male adolescent cancer patients.[293] Lastly, other mechanisms such as epididymal aspiration or testicular biopsy can be employed if adolescent ejaculates are suboptimal. In light of these findings and alternative collection procedures, Bahadur et al[293] suggest that all patients over 12 years old should be offered sperm cryopreservation prior to cytotoxic chemotherapy.

Although a feasible option for mature pubertal boys, semen cryopreservation is not an option for prepubertal male cancer patients because the prepubertal testes do not complete spermatogenesis and therefore do not have mature haploid spermatozoa. Prepubertal male cancer patients could potentially benefit from the development of gonadal tissue storage techniques, followed by autotransplant or in vitro maturation, sperm extraction, and ICSI. These techniques are still investigational but they may provide prepubertal boys receiving chemotherapy with an opportunity to remain fertile in adulthood.

Chemotherapy Effects in Girls

Early reports suggested no delay in menarche and no interruption of menses in girls treated with single-agent cyclophosphamide[278,290,294,295]; Arneil[288] reported normal ovarian histology at postmortem examination in six girls treated with cyclophosphamide for malignancy. However, the drug doses in these early studies were not clearly specified. More recent evidence suggests that damage to the germ cell pool does occur, although clinical manifestations may vary. Ovarian biopsy in girls treated for ALL showed a reduction in the number of follicles and cortical stromal fibrosis, with more severe changes noted in postmenarchal girls.[296] Others have noted absence or inhibition of follicle development after cytotoxic chemotherapy in girls dying from leukemia[297] and solid tumors.[298] As in adult female cancer patients, it is likely that the degree of gonadal damage depends on the specific cytotoxic agent, the cumulative dose, and the age of the patient at exposure.

Most studies that evaluated ovarian function in girls after exposure to chemotherapy have examined combination regimens. For this reason, it is difficult to make definitive conclusions regarding the contribution of individual agents. Nonetheless, the available information is useful to inform patients of the risk of ovarian failure when undergoing treatment for common childhood cancers. For example, studies evaluating combination chemotherapy for acute leukemia have generally found minimal ovarian damage. Siris et al[299] reported normal ovarian function in 80% of prepubertal to postmenarchal girls with acute leukemia who received intermittent cycles of prednisone, vincristine, MTX, and 6-mercaptopurine, and in some cases, cyclophosphamide. Although three patients developed secondary amenorrhea and elevated gonadotropins consistent with ovarian failure, menses subsequently returned in two other patients. In another study, premenarchal female patients with ALL had a high incidence of elevated sex-steroid levels after treatment, but most had normal pubertal development and no delay in the onset of menses.[80] Evaluation of 40 female survivors with ALL treated between ages 5 and 15 years old reported normal ovarian function in 90% of patients as only 4 patients had conclusive ovarian damage.[300] These results suggest that the majority of young girls who receive therapy for ALL maintain ovarian function and have normal pubertal development. However, with long-term follow-up, some patients may later experience premature menopause.[301] The effects of combination chemotherapy, including alkylating agents, on the prepubertal and pubertal ovary have also been studied in girls receiving treatment for Hodgkin's disease. Preliminary data suggested that ovarian function is likely to be preserved in most patients,[286,302] but more recent data from 32 female patients (aged 9 to 15) who received chemotherapy (chlorambucil, vinblastine, procarbazine, and prednisolone) for treatment of Hodgkin's disease found a higher rate of ovarian failure. Ten patients (31%) had evidence of symptomatic ovarian failure and six required hormone replacement therapy.[303] Preservation of fertility has been noted in a high proportion of long-term survivors of patients with childhood non-Hodgkin's lymphoma treated with regimens containing cyclophosphamide, vincristine, doxorubicin, and high-dose MTX.[304] However, in one study of 13 prepubertal girls receiving nitrosoureas or procarbazine, or both, for brain tumors, 9 showed biochemical evidence of primary ovarian failure (elevated basal FSH level or abnormal peak FSH response to GnRH stimulation), and only 3 had normal pubertal development and menarche.[305] Likewise, female children who receive high doses of busulfan as part of bone marrow transplant conditioning regimens appear to have high rates of ovarian failure.[306] Similar to adult women exposed to cytotoxic therapy, the age at administration may play a role in the risk of ovarian failure. Premenarchal girls appear to experience fewer menstrual irregularities and fewer elevations in gonadotropins than postmenarchal girls, consistent with the theory that younger females have a greater oocyte reserve than older girls.[307] Despite these data, counseling young female cancer patients and their parents regarding the likelihood of future infertility remains difficult as there is limited published experience, and long-term follow-up is necessary. Even though many girls will have normal pubertal development and continue to menstruate, it is likely that many will experience early menopause, potentially limiting their ability to have children by narrowing their window of fertility.[301]

As previously discussed, future fertility is usually not the most immediate concern when treating children or adolescent cancer patients. Nevertheless, improved survival rates have increased the need to consider the long-term quality of life effects of chemotherapy treatment, including fertility. In addition, advanced reproductive techniques have improved and are continuing to evolve. Although girls may not be candidates for embryo storage, postmenarchal mature adolescents could consider oocyte storage for future use with an established partner or a sperm donor. There are no traditional options for prepubertal girls, but there is great hope that ovarian tissue storage and transplantation will continue to develop and become a feasible option for the youngest female cancer patient.[308] Lastly, as discussed, many centers have ongoing trials evaluating the effectiveness of GnRH analogs for ovarian protection, providing an additional investigative option for young female cancer patients.[309]

REFERENCES

1. Walsh PC, Amelar RD. Embryology, anatomy and physiology of the male reproductive system. In: Amelar RD, Dublin L, Walsch,PC, eds. Male Infertility. Philadelphia: WB Saunders,1977: 3–32.
2. Clermont Y. Kinetics of spermatogenesis in mammals: seminiferous epithelium cycle and spermatogonial renewal. Physiol Rev 1972;52(1):198–236.
3. Schilsky RL, Sherins RJ. Gonadal dysfunction. In: DeVita,VT, Hellman S,.Rosenberg SA, eds. Cancer: Principles and Practice of Oncology. Philadelphia: JB Lippincott.. 1982:1713–1717.
4. Van Thiel DH, Sherins RJ, Myers GH, et al. Evidence for a specific seminiferous tubular factor affecting follicle-stimulating hormone secretion in men. J Clin Invest 1972;51:1009–1019
5. Chapman RM, Sutcliffe SB, Rees LH, et al. Cyclical combination chemotherapy and gonadal function. Retrospective study in males. Lancet 1979;1(8111):285–289.
6. Mecklenburg RS, Sherins RJ. Gonadotropin response to luteinizing hormone-releasing hormone in men with germinal aplasia. J Clin Endocrinol Metab 1974;38(6):1005–1008.
7. Waxman JH, Terry YA, Wrigley PF, et al. Gonadal function in Hodgkin's disease: long-term follow-up of chemotherapy. Br Med J Clin Res Ed 1982;285(6355):1612–1613.
8. Whitehead E, Shalet S, Blackledge G, et al. The effects of Hodgkin's disease and combination chemotherapy on gonadal function in the adult male. Cancer 1982;49:418–422.
9. Fairley KF, Barrie JU, Johnson W. Sterility and testicular atrophy related to cyclophosphamide therapy. Lancet 1972;1(7750): 568–569.
10. Kumar R, Biggart JD, McEvoy J, et al. Cyclophosphamide and reproductive function. Lancet 1972;1(7762):1212–1214.
11. Miller DG. Alkylating agents and human spermatogenesis. JAMA 1971;217:1662–1665.
12. Qureshi MS, Pennington JH, Goldsmith HJ, et al. Cyclophosphamide therapy and sterility. Lancet 1972;2(7790): 1290–1291.
13. Richter P, Calamera JC, Morganfeld MC, et al. Effect of chlorambucil on spermatogenesis in the human with malignant lymphoma. Cancer 1970;25:1026–1030.
14. Maquire LC, Dick FR, Sherman BM. The effects of antileukemia therapy on gonadal histology in adult males. Cancer 1981; 48:1967–1971.
15. Cheviakoff S, Calamera JC, Morgenfeld M, et al. Recovery of spermatogenesis in patients with lymphoma after treatment with chlorambucil. J Reprod Fertil 1973;33:155–157.
16. Rivkees SA, Crawford JD. The relationship of gonadal activity and chemotherapy-induced gonadal damage. JAMA 1988; 259:2123–2125.
17. Buchanan JD, Fairley KF, Barrie JU. Return of spermatogenesis after stopping cyclophosphamide therapy. Lancet 1975;2(7926): 156–157.
18. Meistrich ML, Wilson G, Brown BW, et al. Impact of cyclophosphamide on long-term reduction in sperm count in men treated with combination chemotherapy for Ewing and soft tissue sarcomas. Cancer 1992;70(11):2703–2712.
19. DeSantis M, Albrecht W, Holtl W, et al. Impact of cytotoxic treatment on long-term fertility in patients with germ-cell cancer. Int J Cancer 1999;83(6):864–865.
20. Longhi A, Macchiagodena M, Vitali G, et al. Fertility in male patients treated with neoadjuvant chemotherapy for osteosarcoma. J Pediatr Hematol Oncol 2003;25(4):292–296.
21. Roeser HP, Stocks AE, Smith AJ. Testicular damage due to cytotoxic drugs and recovery after cessation of therapy. Aust N Z J Med 1978;8(3):250–254.

22. Bokemeyer C, Schmoll HJ, van Rhee J, et al. Long-term gonadal toxicity after therapy for Hodgkin's and non-Hodgkin's lymphoma. Ann Hematol 1994;68(3):105–110.
23. Sieber SM, Correa P, Dalgard DW, et al. Carcinogenic and other adverse effects of procarbazine in nonhuman primates. Cancer Res 1978;38(7):2125–2134.
24. Johnson FE, Doubek WG, Tolman KC, et al. Testicular cytotoxicity of intravenous procarbazine in rats. Surg Oncol 1993;2(1):77–81.
25. Drasga RE, Einhorn LH, Williams SD, et al. Fertility after chemotherapy for testicular cancer. J Clin Oncol 1983;1(3):179–183.
26. Nijman JM, Schraffordt Koops H, Kremer J, et al. Gonadal function after surgery and chemotherapy in men with stage II and III nonseminomatous testicular tumors. J Clin Oncol 1987;5(4):651–656.
27. Leitner SP, Bosl GJ, Bajorunas D. Gonadal dysfunction in patients treated for metastatic germ-cell tumors [erratum appears in J Clin Oncol 1987;5(1):162]. J Clin Oncol 1986;4(10):1500–1505.
28. Hansen SW, Berthelsen JG, von der Maase H. Long-term fertility and Leydig cell function in patients treated for germ cell cancer with cisplatin, vinblastine, and bleomycin versus surveillance. J Clin Oncol 1990;8(10):1695–1698.
29. Stephenson WT, Poirier SM, Rubin L, et al. Evaluation of reproductive capacity in germ cell tumor patients following treatment with cisplatin, etoposide, and bleomycin. J Clin Oncol 1995;13(9):2278–2280.
30. Grossfeld GD, Small EJ. Long-term side effects of treatment for testis cancer. Urol Clin North Am 1998;25(3):503–15.
31. Stuart NS, Woodroffe CM, Grundy R, et al. Long-term toxicity of chemotherapy for testicular cancer—the cost of cure. Br J Cancer 1990;61(3):479–484.
32. Pont J, Albrecht W. Fertility after chemotherapy for testicular germ cell cancer. Fertil Steril 1997;68(1):1–5.
33. Petersen PM, Hansen SW, Giwercman A, et al. Dose-dependent impairment of testicular function in patients treated with cisplatin-based chemotherapy for germ cell cancer. Ann Oncol 1994;5(4):355–358.
34. Howell S, Shalet S. Gonadal damage from chemotherapy and radiotherapy. Endocrinol Metab Clin North Am 1998;27(4):927–943.
35. Kopf-Maier P. Effects of carboplatin on the testis. A histological study. Cancer Chemother Pharmacol 1992;29(3):227–235.
36. Reiter WJ, Kratzik C, Brodowicz T, et al. Sperm analysis and serum follicle-stimulating hormone levels before and after adjuvant single-agent carboplatin therapy for clinical stage I seminoma. Urology 1998;52(1):117–119.
37. Lampe H, Horwich A, Norman A, et al. Fertility after chemotherapy for testicular germ cell cancers. J Clin Oncol 1997;15(1):239–245.
38. Rautonen J, Koskimies AI, Siimes MA. Vincristine is associated with the risk of azoospermia in adult male survivors of childhood malignancies. Eur J Cancer 1992;28A(11):1837–1841.
39. Shamberger RC, Rosenberg SA, Seipp CA, et al. Effects of high-dose methotrexate and vincristine on ovarian and testicular functions in patients undergoing postoperative adjuvant treatment of osteosarcoma. Cancer Treat Rep, 1981;65(9–10):739–746.
40. Riccardi R, Vigersky R, Bleyer WA, et al. Studies of the blood-testis barrier to methotrexate in rats. Proc Am Soc Clin Oncol 1981;22:365.
41. Lu CC, Meistrich ML. Cytotoxic effects of chemotherapeutic drugs on mouse testis cells. Cancer Res 1979;39(9):3575–3582.
42. Russell LD, Russell JA. Short-term morphologic response of the rat testis to administration of five chemotherapeutic agents. Am J Anat 1991;192:142–168.
43. Lui R, LaRegina M, Johnson R. Testicular cytotoxicity of doxorubicin in rats. Proc Am Assoc Cancer Res 1985;26:371.
44. Shamberger, R.C., Sherins, R.J., and Rosenberg, S.A., The effects of postoperative adjuvant chemotherapy and radiotherapy on testicular function in men undergoing treatment for soft tissue sarcoma. Cancer, 1981;47(10):2368–74.
45. Meistrich ML, da Cunha MF, Chawla SP, et al. Sperm production following chemotherapy for sarcomas. Proc Am Assoc Cancer Res 1985;26:170.
46. Meistrich ML, Chawla SP, Da Cunha MF, et al. Recovery of sperm production after chemotherapy for osteosarcoma. Cancer 1989;63(11):2115–2123.
47. Bonadonna G, SantoroA. Chemotherapy in the treatment of Hodgkin's disease. Cancer Treat Rep 1982;9:21–35.
48. da Cunha MF, Meistrich MF, Haq MM, et al. Temporary effects of AMSA chemotherapy on spermatogenesis. Cancer 1982;49:2459–2462.
49. Schilsky RL, Davidson HS, Magid D. Gonadal and sexual function in male patients with hairy cell leukemia: lack of adverse effects of recombinant alpha-2 interferon treatment. Cancer Treat Rep 1987;71:179–181.
50. Sherins RJ, DeVita VT. Effects of drug treatment for lymphoma on male reproductive capacity. Ann Intern Med 1973;79:216–220.
51. Asbjornsen G, Molne K, Klepp O, et al. Testicular function after combination chemotherapy for Hodgkin's disease. Scand J Haematol 1976;16(1):66–69.
52. Chapman RM, Sutcliffe SB, Malpas JS. Male gonadal dysfunction in Hodgkin's disease. A prospective study. JAMA 1981;245:1323–1328.
53. Sherins RJ, DeVita VT. Effects of drug treatment for lymphoma on male reproductive capacity. Ann Intern Med 1973;79:216–220.
54. Wang C, Ng RP, Chan TK, et al. Effect of combination chemotherapy on pituitary gonadal function in patients with lymphoma and leukemia. Cancer 1980;45:2030–2037.
55. Charak BS, Gupta R, Mandrekar P, et al. Testicular dysfunction after cyclophosphamide-vincristine-procarbazine-prednisolone chemotherapy for advanced Hodgkin's disease. A long-term follow-up study. Cancer 1990;65(9):1903–1906.
56. Shafford EA, Kingston JE, Malpas JS, et al. Testicular function following the treatment of Hodgkin's disease in childhood. Br J Cancer 1993;68(6):1199–1204.
57. Viviani S, Ragni G, Santoro A, et al. Testicular dysfunction in Hodgkin's disease before and after treatment. Eur J Cancer 1991;27(11):1389–1392.
58. Dhabhar BN, Malhotra H, Joseph R, et al. Gonadal function in prepubertal boys following treatment for Hodgkin's disease. Am J Pediatr Hematol Oncol 1993;15(3):306–310.
59. Ben Arush MW, Solt I, Lightman A, et al. Male gonadal function in survivors of childhood Hodgkin and non-Hodgkin lymphoma. Pediatr Hematol Oncol 2000;17(3):239–245.
60. Santoro A, Bonadonna G, Valagussa P, et al. Long-term results of combined chemotherapy-radiotherapy approach in Hodgkin's disease: superiority of ABVD plus radiotherapy versus MOPP plus radiotherapy. J Clin Oncol 1987;5(1):27–37.
61. Kulkarni SS, Sastry PS, Saikia TK, et al. Gonadal function following ABVD therapy for Hodgkin's disease. Am J Clin Oncol 1997;20(4):354–357.
62. Tal R, Botchan A, Hauser R, et al. Follow-up of sperm concentration and motility in patients with lymphoma. Hum Reprod 2000;15(9):1985–1988.
63. Meistrich ML, Wilson G, Mathur K, et al. Rapid recovery of spermatogenesis after mitoxantrone, vincristine, vinblastine, and prednisone chemotherapy for Hodgkin's disease. J Clin Oncol 1997;15(12):3488–3495.
64. Hill M, Milan S, Cunningham D, et al. Evaluation of the efficacy of the VEEP regimen in adult Hodgkin's disease with assessment of gonadal and cardiac toxicity. J Clin Oncol 1995;13(2):387–395.
65. Muller U, Stahel RA. Gonadal function after MACOP-B or VACOP-B with or without dose intensification and ABMT in young patients with aggressive non-Hodgkin's lymphoma. Ann Oncol 1993;4(5):399–402.
66. Pryzant RM, Meistrich ML, Wilson G, et al. Long-term reduction in sperm count after chemotherapy with and without radiation therapy for non-Hodgkin's lymphomas. J Clin Oncol 1993;11(2):239–247.
67. Radford JA, Clark S, Crowther D, et al. Male fertility after VAPEC-B chemotherapy for Hodgkin's disease and non-Hodgkin's lymphoma. Br J Cancer 1994;69(2):379–381.
68. Hendry WF, Stedronska J, Jones CR, et al. Semen analysis in testicular cancer and Hodgkin's disease: pre- and post-treatment findings and implications for cryopreservation. Br J Urol 1983;55(6):769–773.

69. Meirow D, Schenker JG. Cancer and male infertility. Hum Reprod 1995;10(8):2017–2022.

70. Tseng A, Kessler R, Freiha F. Male fertility before and after treatment of testicular cancer. Proc Am Soc Clin Oncol 1984; 3:161.

71. Fossa SD, Aabyholm T, Vespestad S, et al. Semen quality after treatment for testicular cancer. Eur Urol 1993;23(1):172–176.

72. Kader HA, Rostom AY. Follicle stimulating hormone levels as a predictor of recovery of spermatogenesis following cancer therapy. Clin Oncol (Royal College of Radiologists)1991;3(1): 37–40.

73. Chakraborty PR, Neave F. Recovery of fertility 14 years following radiotherapy and chemotherapy for testicular tumor. Clin Oncol (Royal College of Radiologists) 1993;5:253.

74. Petersen PM, Hansen SW. The course of long-term toxicity in patients treated with cisplatin-based chemotherapy for non-seminomatous germ-cell cancer. Ann Oncol 1999;10(12): 1475–1483.

75. Sanders J, Sullivan K, Witherspoon R., et al. Long term effects and quality of life in children and adults after marrow transplantation. Bone Marrow Transplant 1989;4(Suppl 4):27–29.

76. Sanders JE, Hawley J, Levy W, et al. Pregnancies following high-dose cyclophosphamide with or without high-dose busulfan or total-body irradiation and bone marrow transplantation. Blood 1996;87(7):3045–3052.

77. Anserini P, Chiodi S, Spinelli S, et al. Semen analysis following allogeneic bone marrow transplantation. Additional data for evidence-based counselling. Bone Marrow Transplant 2002; 30(7):447–451.

78. Grigg AP, McLachlan R, Zaja J, et al. Reproductive status in long-term bone marrow transplant survivors receiving busulfan-cyclophosphamide (120 mg/kg). Bone Marrow Transplant 2000; 26(10):1089–1095.

79. Lendon M, Hann IM, Palmer MK, et al. Testicular histology after combination chemotherapy in childhood for acute lymphoblastic leukaemia. Lancet 1978;2(8087):439–441.

80. Quigley C, Cowell C, Jimenez M, et al. Normal or early development of puberty despite gonadal damage in children treated for acute lymphoblastic leukemia [comment]. N Engl J Med 1989; 321:143–151.

81. Evenson DP, Arlin Z, Welt S, et al. Male reproductive capacity may recover following drug treatment with the L–10 protocol for acute lymphocytic leukemia. Cancer 1984;53(1):30–36.

82. Wallace, W.H., Shalet, S.M., Lendon, M., et al. Male fertility in long–term survivors of childhood acute lymphoblastic leukaemia. International Journal of Andrology, 1991;14(5):312–9.

83. Chatterjee R, Mills W, Katz M, et al. Germ cell failure and Leydig cell insufficiency in post–pubertal males after autologous bone marrow transplantation with BEAM for lymphoma. Bone Marrow Transplant 1994;13(5):519–522.

84. Howell SJ, Radford JA, Ryder WD, et al. Testicular function after cytotoxic chemotherapy: evidence of Leydig cell insufficiency. J Clin Oncol 1999;17(5):1493–1498.

85. Gerl A, Muhlbayer D, Hansmann G, et al. The impact of chemotherapy on Leydig cell function in long term survivors of germ cell tumors. Cancer 2001;91(7):1297–1303.

86. Greenspan SL, Neer RM, Ridgway EC, et al. Osteoporosis in men with hyperprolactinemic hypogonadism. Ann Intern Med 1986; 104:777–582.

87. Finkelstein JS, Klibanski A, Neer RM, et al. Osteoporosis in men with idiopathic hypogonadotropic hypogonadism. Ann Intern Med 1987;106:354–361.

88. Katznelson L, Rosenthal DI, Rosol MS, et al. Using quantitative CT to assess adipose distribution in adult men with acquired hypogonadism. AJR. Am J Roentgenol 1998;170(2):423–427.

89. Bagatell CJ, Bremner WJ. Androgens in men—uses and abuses. N Engl J Med 1996;334:707–714.

90. Fossa SD, Opjordsmoen S, Haug E. Androgen replacement and quality of life in patients treated for bilateral testicular cancer. Eur J Cancer 1999;35(8):1220–1225.

91. Jonker–Pool G, van Basten JP, Hoekstra HJ, et al. Sexual functioning after treatment for testicular cancer: comparison of treatment modalities. Cancer 1997;80(3):454–464.

92. Howell SJ, Radford JA, Smets EM, et al. Fatigue, sexual function and mood following treatment for haematological malignancy:

the impact of mild Leydig cell dysfunction. Br J Cancer 2000; 82(4):789–793.

93. Goldberg RB, Rabin D, Alexander AN, et al. Suppression of plasma testosterone leads to an increase in serum total and high density lipoprotein cholesterol and apoproteins A-I and Br J Clin Endocrinol Metab 1985;60(1):203–207.

94. Holmes SJ, Whitehouse RW, Clark ST, et al. Reduced bone mineral density in men following chemotherapy for Hodgkin's disease. Br J Cancer 1994;70(2):371–375.

95. Howell SJ, Radford JA, Adams JE, et al. The impact of mild Leydig cell dysfunction following cytotoxic chemotherapy on bone mineral density (BMD) and body composition. Clin Endocrinol (Oxf) 2000;52(5):609–616.

96. Behre HM, Kliesch S, Leifke E, et al. Long–term effect of testosterone therapy on bone mineral density in hypogonadal men. J Clin Endocrinol Metab 1997;82(8):2386–2390.

97. Bhasin S, Storer TW, Berman N, et al. Testosterone replacement increases fat-free mass and muscle size in hypogonadal men. J Clin Endocrinol Metabol 1997;82(2):407–413.

98. Brodsky IG, Balagopal P, Nair KS. Effects of testosterone replacement on muscle mass and muscle protein synthesis in hypogonadal men—a clinical research center study. J Clin Endocrinol Metab 1996;81(10):3469–3475.

99. Katznelson L, Finkelstein JS, Schoenfeld DA, et al. Increase in bone density and lean body mass during testosterone administration in men with acquired hypogonadism. J Clin Endocrinol Metab 1996;81(12):4358–4365.

100. Bischoff FZ, Nguyen DD, Burt KJ, et al. Estimates of aneuploidy using multicolor fluorescence in situ hybridization on human sperm [erratum appears in Cytogenet Cell Genet 1995;69(3–4): 189]. Cytogenet Cell Genet 1994;66(4):237–243.

101. Genesca A, Miro R, Caballin MR, et al. Sperm chromosome studies in individuals treated for testicular cancer. Hum Reprod 1990;5(3):286–290.

102. Chatterjee R, Haines GA, Perera DM, et al. Testicular and sperm DNA damage after treatment with fludarabine for chronic lymphocytic leukaemia. Hum Reprod 2000;15(4):762–766.

103. Jenderny J, Jacobi ML, Ruger A, et al. Chromosome aberrations in 450 sperm complements from eight controls and lack of increase after chemotherapy in two patients. Hum Genet 1992; 90(1–2):151–154.

104. Martin RH, Rademaker AW, Leonard NJ. Analysis of chromosomal abnormalities in human sperm after chemotherapy by karyotyping and fluorescence in situ hybridization (FISH). Cancer Genet Cytogenet 1995;80(1):29–32.

105. Kobayashi H, Larson K, Sharma RK, et al. DNA damage in patients with untreated cancer as measured by the sperm chromatin structure assay. Fertil Steril 2001;75(3):469–475.

106. Morris ID. Sperm DNA damage and cancer treatment. International J Androl 2002;25(5):255–261.

107. Meistrich ML, Goldstein LS, Wyrobek AJ. Long–term infertility and dominant lethal mutations in male mice treated with adriamycin. Mutat Res 1985;152(1):53–65.

108. Generoso WM, Witt KL, Cain KT, et al. Dominant lethal and heritable translocation tests with chlorambucil and melphalan in male mice. Mutat Res 1995;345(3–4):167–180.

109. Brinkworth MH. Paternal transmission of genetic damage: findings in animals and humans. Int J Androl 2000;23(3): 123–135.

110. Hales BF, Robaire B. Paternal exposure to drugs and environmental chemicals: effects on progeny outcome. J Androl 2001;22(6): 927–936.

111. Meistrich ML., Potential genetic risks of using semen collected during chemotherapy [comment]. Hum Reprod 1993;8(1): 8–10.

112. Hawkins MM, Draper GJ, WinterDL. Cancer in the offspring of survivors of childhood leukaemia and non-Hodgkin lymphomas [comment]. Br J Cancer 1995;71(6):1335–1339.

113. Byrne J, Rasmussen SA, Steinhorn SC, et al. Genetic disease in offspring of long-term survivors of childhood and adolescent cancer [comment]. Am J Hum Genet 1998;62(1):45–52.

114. Meistrich ML, Byrne J. Genetic disease in offspring of long–term survivors of childhood and adolescent cancer treated with potentially mutagenic therapies. Am J Hum Genet 2002;70(4): 1069–1071.

115. Sankila R, Olsen JH, Anderson H, et al. Risk of cancer among offspring of childhood-cancer survivors. Association of the Nordic Cancer Registries and the Nordic Society of Paediatric Haematology and Oncology [comment]. N Engl J Med 1998; 338(19):1339–1344.

116. Hansen PV, Glavind K, Panduro J, et al. Paternity in patients with testicular germ cell cancer: pretreatment and post-treatment findings. Eur J Cancer 1991;27(11):1385–1389.

117. Babosa M, Baki M, Bodrogi I, et al. A study of children, fathered by men treated for testicular cancer, conceived before, during, and after chemotherapy. Med Pediatr Oncol 1994;22(1):33–38.

118. Carson SA, Gentry WL, Smith, A.L., et al., Feasibility of semen collection and cryopreservation during chemotherapy. Hum Reprod 1991;6(7):992–994.

119. Palermo GD, Cohen J, Alikani M, et al. Intracytoplasmic sperm injection: a novel treatment for all forms of male factor infertility. Fertil Steril 1995;63(6):1231–1240.

120. Chlebowski RT, Heber D. Hypogonadism in male patients with metastatic cancer prior to chemotherapy. Cancer Res 1982; 42(6):2495–2498.

121. Sanger WG, Armitage JO, Schmidt MA.Feasibility of semen cryopreservation in patients with malignant disease. JAMA 1980; 244(8):789–790.

122. Thachil JV, Jewett MA, Rider WD. The effects of cancer and cancer therapy on male fertility. J Urol 1981;126(2):141–145.

123. Berthelsen JG. Skakkebaek NE. Gonadal function in men with testis cancer. Fertil Steril 1983;39(1):68–75.

124. Lass A, Akagbosu F, Abusheikha N, et al. A programme of semen cryopreservation for patients with malignant disease in a tertiary infertility centre: lessons from 8 years' experience. Hum Reprod 1998;13(11):3256–3261.

125. Rueffer U, Breuer K, Josting A, et al. Male gonadal dysfunction in patients with Hodgkin's disease prior to treatment [comment]. Ann Oncol 2001;12(9):1307–1311.

126. Schrader M, Muller M, Sofikitis N, et al. Testicular sperm extraction prior to treatment in azoospermic patients with Hodgkin's disease [comment]. Ann Oncol 2002;13(2):333.

127. Redman JR, Bajorunas DR, Goldstein MC, et al. Semen cryopreservation and artificial insemination for Hodgkin's disease. J Clin Oncol 1987;5(2):233–238.

128. Shekarriz M, Tolentino MV Jr, Ayzman I, et al. Cryopreservation and semen quality in patients with Hodgkin's disease. Cancer 1995;75(11):2732–2736.

129. Fossa SD, Silde J, Theodorsen L, et al. Pre–treatment DNA ploidy of sperm cells as a predictive parameter of post-treatment spermatogenesis in patients with testicular cancer. Br J Urol 1994; 74(3):359–365.

130. Rueffer U, Breuer K, Josting A, et al. Male gonadal dysfunction in patients with Hodgkin's disease prior to treatment. Ann Oncol 2001;12(9):1307–1311.

131. Lass A, Akagbosu F, Brinsden P. Sperm banking and assisted reproduction treatment for couples following cancer treatment of the male partner. Hum Reprod Update 2001;7(4):370–377.

132. Ragni G, Somigliana E, Restelli L, et al. Sperm banking and rate of assisted reproduction treatment: insights from a 15-year cryopreservation program for male cancer patients. Cancer 2003; 97(7):1624–1629.

133. Sanger,WG, Olson JH, Sherman JK. Semen cryobanking for men with cancer—criteria change [comment]. Fertil Steril 1992; 58(5):1024–1027.

134. Rowland GF, Cohen J, Steptoe PC, et al. Pregnancy following in vitro fertilization using cryopreserved semen from a man with testicular teratoma. Urology 1985;26(1):33–36.

135. Cohen J, Edwards R, Fehilly C, et al. In vitro fertilization: a treatment for male infertility. Fertil Steril 1985;43(3):422–432.

136. Mahadevan MM, Trounson AO, Leeton JF. Successful use of human semen cryobanking for in vitro fertilization. Fertil Steril 1983;40(3):340–343.

137. Tournaye H, Camus M, Bollen N, et al. In vitro fertilization techniques with frozen-thawed sperm: a method for preserving the progenitive potential of Hodgkin patients. Fertil Steril 1991; 55(2):443–445.

138. Padron OF, Sharma RK, Thomas AJ Jr, et al. Effects of cancer on spermatozoa quality after cryopreservation: a 12-year experience. Fertil Steril 1997;67(2):326–331.

139. Agarwal A, Shekarriz M, Sidhu RK, et al. Value of clinical diagnosis in predicting the quality of cryopreserved sperm from cancer patients. J Urol 1996;155(3):934–938.

140. Hughes EG, Collins JP, Garner PR. Homologous artificial insemination for oligoasthenospermia: a randomized controlled study comparing intracervical and intrauterine techniques. Fertil Steril 1987;48(2):278–281.

141. Ho PC, Poon IM, Chan SY, et al. Intrauterine insemination is not useful in oligoasthenospermia. Fertil Steril 1989;51(4):682–684.

142. Khalifa E, Oehninger S, Acosta AA, et al. Successful fertilization and pregnancy outcome in in–vitro fertilization using cryopreserved/thawed spermatozoa from patients with malignant diseases. Hum Reprod 1992;7(1):105–108.

143. Audrins P, Holden CA, McLachlan RI, et al. Semen storage for special purposes at Monash IVF from 1977 to 1997 [comment]. Fertil Steril, 1999;72(1):179–181.

144. Rosenlund B, Sjoblom P, Tornblom M, et al. In–vitro fertilization and intracytoplasmic sperm injection in the treatment of infertility after testicular cancer. Hum Reprod 1998;13(2): 414–418.

145. Schlegel PN, Girardi SK. Clinical review 87: In vitro fertilization for male factor infertility. J Clin Endocrinol Metab 1997; 82(3):709–716.

146. Van Steirteghem AC, Liu J, Joris H, et al. Higher success rate by intracytoplasmic sperm injection than by subzonal insemination. Report of a second series of 300 consecutive treatment cycles. Hum Reprod 1993;8(7):1055–1060.

147. Van Steirteghem AC, Nagy Z, Joris H, et al. High fertilization and implantation rates after intracytoplasmic sperm injection [comment]. Hum Reprod 1993;8(7):1061–1066.

148. Milligan DW, Hughes R, Lindsay KS. Semen cryopreservation in men undergoing cancer chemotherapy—a UK survey. Br J Cancer 1989;60(6):966–967.

149. Radford J, Shalet S, Lieberman B. Fertility after treatment for cancer. Questions remain over ways of preserving ovarian and testicular tissue [comment]. BMJ 1999;319(7215):935–936.

150. Schover LR, Brey K, Lichtin A, et al. Knowledge and experience regarding cancer, infertility, and sperm banking in younger male survivors. J Clin Oncol 2002;20(7):1880–1889.

151. Kelleher S, Wishart SM, Liu PY, et al. Long–term outcomes of elective human sperm cryostorage. Hum Reprod 2001;16(12): 2632–2639.

152. Schover LR, Brey K, Lichtin A, et al. Oncologists' attitudes and practices regarding banking sperm before cancer treatment. J Clin Oncol 2002;20(7):1890–1897.

153. Tournaye H, Liu J, Nagy PZ, et al. Correlation between testicular histology and outcome after intracytoplasmic sperm injection using testicular spermatozoa [comment]. Hum Reprod 1996; 11(1):127–132.

154. Chan PT, Palermo GD, Veeck LL, et al. Testicular sperm extraction combined with intracytoplasmic sperm injection in the treatment of men with persistent azoospermia postchemotherapy. Cancer 2001;92(6):1632–1637.

155. Schrader,M, Mller M, Sofikitis N, et al. "Onco–tese": testicular sperm extraction in azoospermic cancer patients before chemotherapy—new guidelines? Urology 2003;61(2):421–425.

156. Schrader M, Muller M, Straub B, et al. Testicular sperm extraction in azoospermic patients with gonadal germ cell tumors prior to chemotherapy—a new therapy option. Asian J Androl 2002; 4(1):9–15.

157. Brinster RL, Zimmermann JW. Spermatogenesis following male germ–cell transplantation [comment]. Proc Nat Acad Sci U S A, 1994;91(24):11298–11302.

158. Avarbock MR, Brinster CJ, Brinster RL. Reconstitution of spermatogenesis from frozen spermatogonial stem cells [comment]. Nature Medicine 1996;2(6):693–696.

159. Ogawa T, Dobrinski I, Avarbock MR, et al. Xenogeneic spermatogenesis following transplantation of hamster germ cells to mouse testes. Biol Reprod 1999;60(2):515–521.

160. Brook PF, Radford JA, Shalet SM, et al. Isolation of germ cells from human testicular tissue for low temperature storage and autotransplantation. Fertil Steril 2001;75(2):269–274.

161. Jahnukainen K, Hou M, Petersen C, et al. Intratesticular transplantation of testicular cells from leukemic rats causes transmission of leukemia. Cancer Res 2001;61(2):706–710.

162. Heber D, Dodson R, Peterson M, et al. Counteractive effects of agonistic and antagonistic gonadotropin-releasing hormone analogs on spermatogenesis: sites of action. Fertil Steril 1984; 41(2):309–313.

163. Vickery BH, McRae GI, Briones W, et al. Effects of an LHRH agonist analog upon sexual function in male dogs. Suppression, reversibility, and effect of testosterone replacement. J Androl 1984;5(1):28–42.

164. Akhtar FB, Marshall GR, Wickings EJ, et al. Reversible induction of azoospermia in rhesus monkeys by constant infusion of a gonadotropin-releasing hormone agonist using osmotic minipumps. J Clin Endocrinol Metab 1983;56(3):534–540.

165. Linde R, Doelle GC, Alexander N, et al. Reversible inhibition of testicular steroidogenesis and spermatogenesis by a potent gonadotropin–releasing hormone agonist in normal men: an approach toward the development of a male contraceptive. New England Journal of Medicine, 1981;305(12):663–7.

166. Glode, L.M., Robinson, J., and Gould, S.F., Protection from cyclophosphamide–induced testicular damage with an analogue of gonadotropin–releasing hormone. Lancet 1981;1(8230): 1132–1134.

167. Johnson DH, Linde R, Hainsworth JD, et al. Effect of a luteinizing hormone releasing hormone agonist given during combination chemotherapy on posttherapy fertility in male patients with lymphoma: preliminary observations. Blood 1985;65(4): 832–836.

168. Kreuser ED, Hetzel WD, Hautmann R, et al. Reproductive toxicity with and without LHRHA administration during adjuvant chemotherapy in patients with germ cell tumors. Hormone Metab Res 1990;22(9):494–498.

169. Waxman JH, Ahmed R, Smith D, et al. Failure to preserve fertility in patients with Hodgkin's disease. Cancer Chemother Pharmacol 1987;19(2):159–162.

170. Krause W, Pfluger KH. Treatment with the gonadotropin-releasing-hormone agonist buserelin to protect spermatogenesis against cytotoxic treatment in young men. Andrologia 1989;21(3):265–270.

171. Meistrich ML, Wilson G, Huhtaniemi I. Hormonal treatment after cytotoxic therapy stimulates recovery of spermatogenesis. Cancer Res 1999;59(15):3557–3560.

172. Kangasniemi M, Huhtaniemi I, Meistrich ML. Failure of spermatogenesis to recover despite the presence of a spermatogonia in the irradiated LBNF1 rat. Biol Reprod 1996;54(6):1200–1208.

173. Shuttlesworth GA, de Rooij DG, Huhtaniemi I, et al. Enhancement of A spermatogonial proliferation and differentiation in irradiated rats by gonadotropin-releasing hormone antagonist administration. Endocrinology 2000;141(1):37–49.

174. Meistrich ML, Kangasniemi M. Hormone treatment after irradiation stimulates recovery of rat spermatogenesis from surviving spermatogonia. J Androl 1997;18(1):80–87.

175. Shetty G, Wilson G, Huhtaniemi I, et al. Gonadotropin-releasing hormone analogs stimulate and testosterone inhibits the recovery of spermatogenesis in irradiated rats. Endocrinology 2000; 141(5):1735–1745.

176. Meistrich MG, Shuttlesworth G, Huhtaniemi I, et al. GnRH agonists and antagonists stimulate recovery of fertility in irradiated LBNF1 rats. J Androl 2001;22(5):809–817.

177. Shetty G, Wilson G, Huhtaniemi I, et al. Testosterone inhibits spermatogonial differentiation in juvenile spermatogonial depletion mice. Endocrinology 2001;142(7):2789–2795.

178. Shetty G, Wilson G, Hardy MP, et al. Inhibition of recovery of spermatogenesis in irradiated rats by different androgens. Endocrinology 2002;143(9):3385–3396.

179. Udagawa K, Ogawa T, Watanabe T, et al. GnRH analog, leuprorelin acetate, promotes regeneration of rat spermatogenesis after severe chemical damage. Int J Urol 2001;8(11):615–622.

180. Howell SJ, Shalet SM. Pharmacological protection of the gonads. Med Pediatr Oncol 1999;33(1):41–45.

181. Mayer,DL, Odell WD. Physiology of reproduction. St. Louis: CV Mosby, 1971:20–27.

182. Peters H, Byskov AG, Himelstein-Braw R, et al. Follicular growth: the basic event in the mouse and human ovary. J Reprod Fertil 1975;45(3):559–566.

183. Chapman RM. Effect of cytotoxic therapy on sexuality and gonadal function. Semin Oncol 1982;9(1):84–94.

184. Sobrinho LG, Levine RA, DeConti RC. Amenorrhea in patients with Hodgkin's disease treated with antineoplastic agents. Am J Obstet Gynecol 1971;109(1):135–139.

185. Miller JJ 3rd, Williams GF, Leissring JC. Multiple late complications of therapy with cyclophosphamide, including ovarian destruction. Am J Med, 1971;50(4):530–535.

186. Louis J, Limarzi LR, Best WR. Treatment of chronic granulocytic leukemia and Myleran. Arch Intern Med 1957;97:299–308.

187. Galton DAG, Till M, Wiltshaw E. Busulfan: summary of clinical results. Ann N Y Acad Sci 1958;68:967.

188. Fosdick WM, Parsons JL, Hill DF. Long-term cyclophosphamide therapy in rheumatoid arthritis. Arthritis Rheumatism 1968;11 (2):151–161.

189. Warne GL, Fairley KF, Hobbs JB, et al. Cyclophosphamide-induced ovarian failure. N Engl J Med 1973;289(22):1159–1162.

190. Uldall PR, Kerr DN, Tacchi D. Sterility and cyclophosphamide. Lancet 1972;1(7752):693–694.

191. Dnistrian AM, Schwartz MK, Fracchia AA, et al. Endocrine consequences of CMF adjuvant therapy in premenopausal and postmenopausal breast cancer patients. Cancer 1983;51(5):803–807.

192. Samaan NA, deAsis DN Jr, Buzdar AU, et al. Pituitary-ovarian function in breast cancer patients on adjuvant chemoimmunotherapy. Cancer 1978;41(6):2084–2087.

193. Ravdin PM, Fritz NF, Tormey DC, et al. Endocrine status of premenopausal node-positive breast cancer patients following adjuvant chemotherapy and long-term tamoxifen. Cancer Res 1988; 48(4):1026–1029.

194. Koyama H, Wada T, Nishizawa Y, et al. Cyclophosphamide-induced ovarian failure and its therapeutic significance in patients with breast cancer. Cancer 1977;39(4):1403–1409.

195. Fisher B, Sherman B, Rockette H, et al. 1-phenylalanine mustard (L-PAM) in the management of premenopausal patients with primary breast cancer: lack of association of disease-free survival with depression of ovarian function. National Surgical Adjuvant Project for Breast and Bowel Cancers. Cancer 1979;44(3): 847–857.

196. Mehta RR, Beattie CW, Das Gupta TK. Endocrine profile in breast cancer patients receiving chemotherapy. Breast Cancer Res Treat,1992;20(2):125–132.

197. Goldhirsch A, Gelber RD, Castiglione M. The magnitude of endocrine effects of adjuvant chemotherapy for premenopausal breast cancer patients. The International Breast Cancer Study Group. Ann Oncol 1990;1(3):183–188.

198. Reichman BS, Green KB. Breast cancer in young women: effect of chemotherapy on ovarian function, fertility, and birth defects. J Nat Cancer Institute Monographs 1994;16:125–129.

199. Bines J, Oleske DM, Cobleigh MA. Ovarian function in premenopausal women treated with adjuvant chemotherapy for breast cancer [comment]. J Clin Oncol 1996;14(5):1718–1729.

200. Hensley ML. Reichman BS. Fertility and pregnancy after adjuvant chemotherapy for breast cancer. Crit Rev Oncol Hematol 1998; 28(2):121–128.

201. Huong du L, Amoura Z, Duhaut P, et al. Risk of ovarian failure and fertility after intravenous cyclophosphamide. A study in 84 patients. J Rheumatol 2002;29(12):2571–2576.

202. Boumpas DT, Austin HA 3rd, Vaughan EM, et al. Risk for sustained amenorrhea in patients with systemic lupus erythematosus receiving intermittent pulse cyclophosphamide therapy. Ann Intern Med 1993;119(5):366–369.

203. Wallace WH, Shalet SM, Crowne EC, et al. Gonadal dysfunction due to cis-platinum. Med Pediatr Oncol 1989;17(5):409–413.

204. Choo YC, Chan SY, Wong LC, et al. Ovarian dysfunction in patients with gestational trophoblastic neoplasia treated with short intensive courses of etoposide (VP-16-213). Cancer 1985;55(10):2348–2352.

205. Meirow D. Reproduction post-chemotherapy in young cancer patients. Molecular Cellular Endocrinol 2000;169(1–2):123–131.

206. Sutton R, Buzdar AU, Hortobagyi GN. Pregnancy and offspring after adjuvant chemotherapy in breast cancer patients. Cancer 1990;65(4):847–850.

207. Low JJ, Perrin LC, Crandon AJ, et al. Conservative surgery to preserve ovarian function in patients with malignant ovarian germ cell tumors. A review of 74 cases. Cancer 2000;89(2): 391–398.

208. Maneschi F, Benedetti-Panici P, Scambia G, et al. Menstrual and hormone patterns *in* women treated with high-dose cisplatin and bleomycin. Gynecol Oncol 1994;54(3):345–348.

209. Tangir J, Zelterman D, Ma W, et al. Reproductive function after conservative surgery and chemotherapy for malignant germ cell tumors of the ovary. Obstet Gynecol 2003;101(2):251–257.

210. Nabholtz J, Prenkowski T, Mackey J., et al. Phase III trial comparing TAC (docetaxel, doxorubicin, cyclophosphamide) with FAC (5–fluorouracil, doxorubicin, cyclophosphamide) in the adjuvant treatment of node-positive breast cancer (BC) patients: interim analysis of the BCIRG 001 study. Proceedings of the Annual Meeting of the American Society of Clinical Oncology, 2002,36A.

211. Reyno LM, Levine MN, Skingley P, et al. Chemotherapy induced amenorrhoea in a randomised trial of adjuvant chemotherapy duration in breast cancer. Eur J Cancer 1992;29A (1):21–23.

212. Hortobagyi GN, Buzdar AU, Marcus CE, et al. Immediate and long-term toxicity of adjuvant chemotherapy regimens containing doxorubicin in trials at M.D. Anderson Hospital and Tumor Institute. NCI Monographs 1986;1:105–109.

213. Valagussa P, Moliterni A, Zambetti M, et al. Long-term sequelae from adjuvant chemotherapy. Recent Results in Cancer Research 1993;127:247–255.

214. Levine MN, Bramwell VH, Pritchard KI, et al. Randomized trial of intensive cyclophosphamide, epirubicin, and fluorouracil chemotherapy compared with cyclophosphamide, methotrexate, and fluorouracil in premenopausal women with node-positive breast cancer. National Cancer Institute of Canada Clinical Trials Group [comment]. J Clin Oncol 1998;16(8):2651–2658.

215. Morgenfeld MC, Goldberg V, Parisier H, et al. Ovarian lesions due to cytostatic agents during the treatment of Hodgkin's disease. Surg Gynecol Obstet 1972;134(5):826–828.

216. Chapman RM, Sutcliffe SB, Malpas JS. Cytotoxic–induced ovarian failure in women with Hodgkin's disease. I. Hormone function. JAMA 1979;242:1877–1881.

217. Schilsky RL, Sherins RJ, Hubbard SM, et al. Long–term follow up of ovarian function in women treated with MOPP chemotherapy for Hodgkin's disease. Am J Med 1981;71(4):552–556.

218. Horning SJ, Hoppe RT, Kaplan HS, et al. Female reproductive potential after treatment for Hodgkin's disease. N Engl J Med 1981;304:1377–1382.

219. Andrieu JM, Ochoa-Molina ME. Menstrual cycle, pregnancies and offspring before and after MOPP therapy for Hodgkin's disease. Cancer 1983;52(3):435–438.

220. Whitehead E, Shalet SM, Blackledge G, et al. The effect of combination chemotherapy on ovarian function in women treated for Hodgkin's disease. Cancer 1983;52(6):988–993.

221. Specht L, Hansen MM, Geisler C. Ovarian function in young women in long-term remission after treatment for Hodgkin's disease stage I or II. Scand J Haematol 1984;32(3):265–270.

222. Clark ST, Radford JA, Crowther D, et al. Gonadal function following chemotherapy for Hodgkin's disease: a comparative study of MVPP and a seven-drug hybrid regimen. J Clin Oncol 1995;13(1):134–139.

223. Kreuser ED, Xiros N, Hetzel WD, et al. Reproductive and endocrine gonadal capacity in patients treated with COPP chemotherapy for Hodgkin's disease. J Cancer Res Clin Oncol 1987;113(3):260–266.

224. Creasman WT, Soper JT. Assessment of the contemporary management of germ cell malignancies of the ovary. Am J Obstet Gynecol 1985;153(8):828–834.

225. Gershenson DM. Menstrual and reproductive function after treatment with combination chemotherapy for malignant ovarian germ cell tumors. J Clin Oncol 1988;6(2):270–275.

226. Zanetta G, Bonazzi C, Cantu M, et al. Survival and reproductive function after treatment of malignant germ cell ovarian tumors. J Clin Oncol 2001;19(4):1015–1020.

227. Brewer M, Gershenson DM, Herzog CE, et al. Outcome and reproductive function after chemotherapy for ovarian dysgerminoma [comment]. J Clin Oncol 1999;17(9):2670–2675.

228. Sanders JE, Buckner CD, Leonard JM, et al. Late effects on gonadal function of cyclophosphamide, total-body irradiation, and marrow transplantation. Transplantation 1983;36(3):252–255.

229. Schimmer AD, Quatermain M, Imrie K, et al. Ovarian function after autologous bone marrow transplantation. J Clin Oncol 1998;16(7):2359–2363.

230. Chatterjee R, Goldstone AH. Gonadal damage and effects on fertility in adult patients with haematological malignancy undergoing stem cell transplantation. Bone Marrow Transplant 1996;17(1):5–11.

231. Hinterberger-Fischer M, Kier P, Kalhs P, et al. Fertility, pregnancies and offspring complications after bone marrow transplantation. Bone Marrow Transplant 1991;7(1):5–9.

232. Salooja N, Chatterjee R, McMillan AK, et al. Successful pregnancies in women following single autotransplant for acute myeloid leukemia with a chemotherapy ablation protocol. Bone Marrow Transplant 1994;13(4):431–435.

233. Singhal S, Powles R, Treleaven J, et al. Melphalan alone prior to allogeneic bone marrow transplantation from HLA-identical sibling donors for hematologic malignancies: alloengraftment with potential preservation of fertility in women. Bone Marrow Transplant 1996;18(6):1049–1055.

234. Mortimer JE, Boucher L, Baty J, et al. Effect of tamoxifen on sexual functioning in patients with breast cancer [comment]. J Clin Oncol 1999;17(5):1488–1492.

235. Johnson SA, Goldman JM, Hawkins DF. Pregnancy after chemotherapy for Hodgkin's disease. Lancet 1979;2(8133):93.

236. Li FP, Fine W, Jaffe N, et al. Offspring of patients treated for cancer in childhood. J Nat Cancer Institute 1979;62(5):1193–1197.

237. Van Thiel DH, Ross GT, Lipsett MB. Pregnancies after chemotherapy of trophoblastic neoplasms. Science 1970;169(952):1326–1327.

238. Kung FT, Chang SY, Tsai YC, et al. Subsequent reproduction and obstetric outcome after methotrexate treatment of cervical pregnancy: a review of original literature and international collaborative follow-up. Hum Reprod 1997;12(3):591–595.

239. Green DM, Zevon MA, Lowrie G, et al. Congenital anomalies in children of patients who received chemotherapy for cancer in childhood and adolescence [comment]. N Engl J Med 1991;325(3):141–146.

240. Aisner J, Wiernik PH, Pearl P. Pregnancy outcome in patients treated for Hodgkin's disease. J Clin Oncol 1993;11(3):507–512.

241. Dodds L, Marrett LD, Tomkins DJ, et al. Case-control study of congenital anomalies in children of cancer patients. BMJ 1993;307(6897):164–168.

242. Garber JE. Long-term follow-up of children exposed in utero to antineoplastic agents. Semin Oncol 1989;16(5):437–444.

243. Holmes GE, Holmes FF. Pregnancy outcome of patients treated for Hodgkin's disease: a controlled study. Cancer 1978;41(4):1317–1322.

244. Abdalla HI, Baber RJ, Kirkland A, et al. Pregnancy in women with premature ovarian failure using tubal and intrauterine transfer of cryopreserved zygotes. Br J Obstet Gynaecol 1989;96(9):1071–1075.

245. Pados G, Camus M, Van Waesberghe L, et al. Oocyte and embryo donation: evaluation of 412 consecutive trials. Hum Reprod 1992;7(8):1111–1117.

246. Brown JR, Modell E, Obasaju M, et al. Natural cycle in-vitro fertilization with embryo cryopreservation prior to chemotherapy for carcinoma of the breast. Hum Reprod 1996;11(1):197–199.

247. Lipton JH, Virro M, Solow H. Successful pregnancy after allogeneic bone marrow transplant with embryos isolated before transplant. J Clin Oncol 1997;15(11):3347–3349.

248. Blumenfeld Z, Avivi I, Ritter M, et al. Preservation of fertility and ovarian function and minimizing chemotherapy-induced gonadotoxicity in young women. J Soc Gynecol Invest 1999;6(5):229–239.

249. Oktay K, Buyuk E, Davis O, et al. Fertility preservation in breast cancer patients: IVF and embryo cryopreservation after ovarian stimulation with tamoxifen. Hum Reprod 2003;18(1):90–95.

250. Allred CD, Allred KF, Ju YH, et al. Soy diets containing varying amounts of genistein stimulate growth of estrogen-dependent (MCF-7) tumors in a dose-dependent manner. Cancer Res 2001;61(13):5045–5050.

251. Prest SJ, May FE, Westley BR. The estrogen-regulated protein, TFF1, stimulates migration of human breast cancer cells. FASEB J 2002;16(6):592–594.

252. Carroll J, Wood MJ, Whittingham DG. Normal fertilization and development of frozen-thawed mouse oocytes: protective action of certain macromolecules. Biol Reprod 1993;48(3):606–612.

253. Bos-Mikich A, Wood MJ, Candy CJ, et al. Cytogenetical analysis and developmental potential of vitrified mouse oocytes. Biol Reprod 1995;53(4):780–785.

254. Trounson A, Bongso A. Fertilization and development in humans. Curr Topics Devel Biol 1996;32:59–101.

255. Oktay K, Kan MT, Rosenwaks Z. Recent progress in oocyte and ovarian tissue cryopreservation and transplantation. Curr Opin Obstet Gynecol 2001;13(3):263–268.

256. Fabbri R, Venturoli S, D'Errico A, et al. Ovarian tissue banking and fertility preservation in cancer patients: histological and immunohistochemical evaluation. Gynecol Oncol 2003;89(2):259–266.

257. Gosden RG, Baird DT, Wade JC, et al. Restoration of fertility to oophorectomized sheep by ovarian autografts stored at –196 degrees C. Hum Reprod 1994;9(4):597–603.

258. Kim SS, Battaglia DE, Soules MR. The future of human ovarian cryopreservation and transplantation: fertility and beyond. Fertil Steril 2001;75(6):1049–1056.

259. Newton H, Aubard Y, Rutherford A, et al. Low temperature storage and grafting of human ovarian tissue. Hum Reprod 1996;11(7):1487–1491.

260. Newton H. The cryopreservation of ovarian tissue as a strategy for preserving the fertility of cancer patients. Hum Reprod Update 1998;4(3):237–247.

261. Law C. Freezing ovary tissue may help cancer patients preserve fertility. J Nat Cancer Inst 1996;88(17):1184–1185.

262. Radford JA, Lieberman BA, Brison DR, et al. Orthotopic reimplantation of cryopreserved ovarian cortical strips after high-dose chemotherapy for Hodgkin's lymphoma. Lancet 2001;357(9263):1172–1175.

263. Oktay K, Karlikaya G. Ovarian function after transplantation of frozen, banked autologous ovarian tissue. N Engl J Med 2000;342(25):1919.

264. Oktay K, Aydin BA, Economos K, et al. Restoration of ovarian function after autologous transplantation of ovarian tissue into the forearm [abstract]. Fertil Steril, 2000;74:79.

265. Shaw JM, Bowles J, Koopman P, et al. Fresh and cryopreserved ovarian tissue samples from donors with lymphoma transmit the cancer to graft recipients. Hum Reprod 1996;11(8):1668–1673.

266. Eppig JJ, O'Brien MJ. Development in vitro of mouse oocytes from primordial follicles. Biol Reprod 1996;54(1):197–207.

267. Chapman RM, Sutcliffe SB. Protection of ovarian function by oral contraceptives in women receiving chemotherapy for Hodgkin's disease. Blood 1981;58(4):849–851.

268. Longhi A, Pignotti E, Versari M, et al. Effect of oral contraceptive on ovarian function in young females undergoing neoadjuvant chemotherapy treatment for osteosarcoma. Oncol Rep 2003;10(1):151–155.

269. Blumenfeld Z, Haim N. Prevention of gonadal damage during cytotoxic therapy. Ann Med 1997;29(3):199–206.

270. Montz FJ, Wolff AJ, Gambone JC. Gonadal protection and fecundity rates in cyclophosphamide-treated rats. Cancer Res 1991;51(8):2124–2126.

271. Ataya KM, McKanna JA, Weintraub AM, et al. A luteinizing hormone-releasing hormone agonist for the prevention of chemotherapy-induced ovarian follicular loss in rats. Cancer Res 1985;45(8):3651–3656.

272. Ataya K, Ramahi-Ataya A. Reproductive performance of female rats treated with cyclophosphamide and/or LHRH agonist [comment]. Reprod Toxicol 1993;7(3):229–235.

273. Ataya K, Rao LV, Lawrence E, et al. Luteinizing hormone–releasing hormone agonist inhibits cyclophosphamide-induced ovarian follicular depletion in rhesus monkeys. Biol Reprod 1995;52 (2):365–372.

274. Jarrell J, YoungLai EV, McMahon A, et al. Effects of ionizing radiation and pretreatment with [D-Leu6,des-Gly10] luteinizing hormone-releasing hormone on developing rat ovarian follicles. Cancer Res 1987;47(19):5005–5008.

275. Jarrell JF, McMahon A, Barr RD, et al. The agonist (d-leu-6, des-gly-10)-LHRH-ethylamide does not protect the fecundity of rats exposed to high dose unilateral ovarian irradiation. Reprod Toxicol 1991;5(4):385–388.

276. Blumenfeld Z, Dann E, Avivi I, et al. Fertility after treatment for Hodgkin's disease. Ann Oncol 2002;13(Suppl 1):138–147.

277. Aslam I, Fishel S, Moore H, et al. Fertility preservation of boys undergoing anti-cancer therapy: a review of the existing situation and prospects for the future. Hum Reprod 2000;15(10):2154–2159.

278. Pennisi AJ, Grushkin CM, Lieberman E. Gonadal function in children with nephrosis treated with cyclophosphamide. Am J Dis Child 1975;129(3):315–318.

279. Blatt J, Poplack DG, Sherins RJ. Testicular function in boys after chemotherapy for acute lymphoblastic leukemia. N Engl J Med 1981;304(19):1121–1124.

280. Shalet SM, Hann IM, Lendon M, et al. Testicular function after combination chemotherapy in childhood for acute lymphoblastic leukaemia. Arch Dis Child 1981;56(4):275–278.

281. Wallace WH, Shalet SM, Lendon M, et al. Male fertility in long-term survivors of childhood acute lymphoblastic leukaemia. Int J Androl 1991;14(5):312–319.

282. Etteldorf JN, West CD, Pitcock JA, et al. Gonadal function, testicular histology, and meiosis following cyclophosphamide therapy in patients with nephrotic syndrome. J Pediatr 1976;88(2):206–212.

283. Mustieles C, Munoz A, Alonso M, et al. Male gonadal function after chemotherapy in survivors of childhood malignancy. Med Pediatr Oncol 1995;24(6):347–351.

284. Aubier F, Flamant F, Brauner R, et al. Male gonadal function after chemotherapy for solid tumors in childhood. J Clin Oncol 1989;7(3):304–309.

285. Heikens J, Behrendt H, Adriaanse R, et al. Irreversible gonadal damage in male survivors of pediatric Hodgkin's disease. Cancer 1996;78(9):2020–2024.

286. Ortin TT, Shostak CA, Donaldson SS. Gonadal status and reproductive function following treatment for Hodgkin's disease in childhood: the Stanford experience. Int J Radiat Oncol Biol Phys 1990;19(4):873–880.

287. Kirkland RT, Bongiovanni AM, Cornfield D, et al. Gonadotropin responses to luteinizing releasing factor in boys treated with cyclophosphamide for nephrotic syndrome. J Pediatr 1976;89(6):941–944.

288. Arneil GC. Cyclophosphamide and the prepubertal testis. Lancet 1972;2(7789):1259–1260.

289. Rapola J, Koskimies O, Huttunen NP, et al. Cyclophosphamide and the pubertal testis. Lancet 1973;1(7794):98–99.

290. Lentz RD, Bergstein J, Steffes MW, et al. Postpubertal evaluation of gonadal function following cyclophosphamide therapy before and during puberty. J Pediatr 1977;91(3):385–394.

291. Kliesch S, Behre HM, Jurgens H, et al. Cryopreservation of semen from adolescent patients with malignancies. Med Pediatr Oncol 1996;26(1):20–27.

292. Postovsky S, Lightman A, Aminpour D, et al. Sperm cryopreservation in adolescents with newly diagnosed cancer. Med Pediatr Oncol 2003;40(6):355–359.

293. Bahadur G, Ling KL, Hart R, et al. Semen quality and cryopreservation in adolescent cancer patients. Hum Reprod 2002;17(12):3157–3161.

294. Chiu, J. and Drummond, K.N., Long-term follow-up of cyclophosphamide therapy in frequent relapsing minimal lesion nephrotic syndrome. J Pediatr, 1974;84(6):825–830.

295. De Groot GW, Faiman C, Winter JS. Cyclophosphamide and the prepubertal gonad: a negative report. J Pediatr 1974;84(1):123–125.

296. Marcello MF, Nuciforo G, Romeo R, et al. Structural and ultra-structural study of the ovary in childhood leukemia after successful treatment. Cancer 1990;66(10):2099–2104.

297. Himelstein-Braw R, Peters H, Faber M. Morphological study of the ovaries of leukemic children. Br J Cancer 1978;38:82.

298. Nicosia SV, Matus-Ridley M, Meadows AT. Gonadal effects of cancer therapy in girls. Cancer 1985;55(10):2364–2372.

299. Siris ES, Leventhal BG, Vaitukaitis JL. Effects of childhood leukemia and chemotherapy on puberty and reproductive function in girls. N Engl J Med 1976;294(21):1143–1146.

300. Wallace WH, Shalet SM, Tetlow LJ, et al. Ovarian function following the treatment of childhood acute lymphoblastic leukaemia. Med Pediatr Oncol 1993;21(5):333–339.

301. Byrne J, Fears TR, Gail MH, et al. Early menopause in long-term survivors of cancer during adolescence. Am J Obstet Gynecol 1992;166(3):788–793.

302. Green DM, Brecher ML, Lindsay AN, et al. Gonadal function in pediatric patients following treatment for Hodgkin's disease. Med Pediatr Oncol 1981;9:235–44.

303. Mackie EJ, Radford M, Shalet SM. Gonadal function following chemotherapy for childhood Hodgkin's disease. Med Pediatr Oncol 1996;27(2):74–78.

304. Haddy TB, Adde MA, McCalla J, et al. Late effects in long–term survivors of high-grade non-Hodgkin's lymphomas. J Clin Oncol 1998;16(6):2070–2079.

305. Clayton PE, Shalet SM, Price DA, et al. Ovarian function following chemotherapy for childhood brain tumors. Med Pediatr Oncol 1989;17:92–96.

306. Cicognani A, Pasini A, Pession A, et al. Gonadal function and pubertal development after treatment of a childhood malignancy. J Pediatr Endocrinol Metab 2003;16(Suppl 2): 321–326.

307. Couto-Silva AC, Trivin C, Thibaud E, et al. Factors affecting gonadal function after bone marrow transplantation during childhood. Bone Marrow Transplant 2001;28(1):67–75.

308. Poirot,C, Vacher-Lavenu MC, Helardot P, et al. Human ovarian tissue cryopreservation: indications and feasibility. Hum Reprod 2002;17(6):1447–1452.

309. Pereyra Pacheco B, Mendez Ribas JM, Milone G, et al. Use of GnRH analogs for functional protection of the ovary and preservation of fertility during cancer treatment in adolescents: a preliminary report. Gynecol Oncol 2001;81:391–397.

Carcinogenesis of Anticancer Drugs

5

Lawrence S. Blaszkowsky   *Charles Erlichman*

Although the potential of antineoplastic agents to induce new malignancies was suggested by Haddow[1] in 1947 on the basis of the ability of chemical carcinogens to cause growth inhibition, convincing evidence for carcinogenic effects of these agents in humans has been reported only in the past 40 years. The major reasons for this belated recognition of the problem are the long latency periods seen for expression of drug-induced carcinogenicity in humans (3 to 4 years) and the brief survival of most patients treated with chemotherapy. Only in the past 4 decades have a sizable number of patients with advanced malignancy been cured by chemotherapy or been treated with adjuvant chemotherapy; thus, sufficient time has elapsed and sufficient numbers of individuals are now at risk for second tumors to be seen in clinically significant numbers. Although survival benefits will undoubtedly continue to accrue from the use of these agents and will probably outweigh the risks of second neoplasms, concern for this complication is likely to grow as the use of antineoplastic drugs gain wider use in adjuvant programs and in non-neoplastic conditions such as renal transplantation or autoimmune disease, in which long-term survival of a large fraction of the treated population is ensured. In these instances, the benefits and risks (including carcinogenicity) of antineoplastic agents must be considered.

Definition of the risk of carcinogenesis as the result of chemotherapy is a difficult task. Prediction of carcinogenicity at the experimental level depends on test systems that examine the ability of chemicals to cause mutation of bacteria or mammalian cells, malignant transformation of mammalian cells, chromosomal aberrations, or tumors in mice or rats. Such tests are subject to interspecies variability in drug metabolism and target-tissue kinetics, and to other host-specific factors that influence susceptibilities to tumor development. These factors make extrapolation of the quantitative risk to humans a difficult, if not impossible, task. Second, the immune status of the patient is believed to play an important role in determining carcinogenicity, as indicated by the increased risk of lymphoid and cutaneous neoplasms in patients receiving immunosuppressive therapy; in cancer patients, the immune system is suppressed both as a result of the neoplastic process and as a consequence of therapy. This immunosuppression undoubtedly influences the risk of carcinogenesis but is not duplicated in test systems. Finally, the assessment of risk in humans at present is based partly on analyses of retrospective series, which often give incomplete information regarding key parameters of treatment (dose, duration) and which lack a control or untreated population. Such a control population is particularly important in risk assessment because an increased incidence of second tumors, such as acute myelocytic leukemia in patients with Hodgkin's disease, may exist in the absence of treatment. More recently, analyses of randomized trials that compare adjuvant chemotherapy regimens with no additional treatment have been undertaken with respect to incidence of second malignancies.[2–6] The information derived from these studies clarifies some of the confounding variables mentioned.

With these limitations in mind, this chapter considers available information concerning the carcinogenic potential of antitumor agents. This discussion examines the common pharmacologic properties shared by antineoplastic agents and classic carcinogens, specific predictions of carcinogenicity based on nonhuman test systems, and clinical evidence for an increased risk of second neoplasms in patients receiving these agents.

RELATIONSHIP OF ANTINEOPLASTIC AGENTS TO CHEMICAL CARCINOGENS

The chemical induction of cancer in animals is thought to involve a multistage process with a long latency period. This process can be initiated by a variety of chemical structures that have at least one common thread in their mode of action: an interaction with DNA.[7–9] Initiation results from irreversible genetic alterations, such as mutations or deletions in DNA.[10] One of the most carefully studied systems of tumor induction is the induction of skin cancer in mice and rabbits by alkylating agents, polycyclic hydrocarbons, and ethyl carbamate (Fig. 5.1). Repeated applications of these agents over long periods result in the development of benign or malignant tumors. Exposure to these compounds in limited doses, however, causes morphologic changes in the epithelium but does not result in tumors unless this stage of initiation is followed by the introduction of a promoter, such as a phorbol ester, an ingredient of croton oil. Promoters are not carcinogenic by themselves but lead to tumor production if applied after the initiating agent. Treatment with a specific promoter before exposure to the initiating agent does not result in tumor formation. This stage of promotion occurs over weeks and months and is reversible in its early stages. Promotion involves changes not in DNA structure but in the expression of the genome mediated through promoter-receptor interaction. The binding of promoter to receptor alters the expression of genes downstream. For example, estrogens and androgens may act as promoters by binding to the estrogen and androgen receptors, respectively, in liver or mammary tissue.

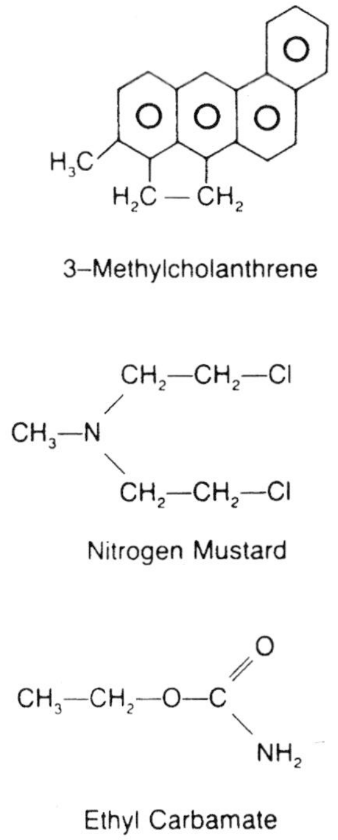

Promoters such as phorbol-12-myristate-13-acetate have a variety of biologic actions; they alter differentiation, cause changes in cell surface glycopeptides, alter various metabolic activities, and suppress immune surveillance of tumors by cytotoxic macrophages and natural killer cells.[11] The final stage of progression is irreversible and is characterized by karyotypic instability and malignant growth. Thus, carcinogenesis is a multistep process that may be arrested at intermediate stages, that requires a long latency period for induction, and that can be influenced by, if it does not require, a promoting agent.

The existence or identity of an associated promoter has not been established for well-documented carcinogens in humans. For cancer patients, induction of second tumors may require not only an initiator (a DNA damaging agent), but also a promoter, a function that may be fulfilled by a second chemotherapeutic agent, by radiotherapy, or by a disease-related abnormality in metabolism or immune function.

Chemical carcinogens show a diversity of structures but share important metabolic features. Most are inert and require microsomal metabolic activation to positively charged (or electrophilic) intermediates that react with DNA bases. The primary sites for attack of DNA are relatively electron-rich (or nucleophilic) sites, such as the N-7 position of guanine[12,13] (see Chapter 11). This characteristic of carcinogens—namely, microsomal metabolism to an electrophilic intermediate that attacks DNA—is shared by certain antineoplastic agents such as cyclophosphamide, procarbazine, and mitomycin C and is essential in the antineoplastic action of these drugs. Other agents, such as L-phenylalanine mustard and nitrogen mustard, do not require metabolic activation to form alkylating species. Carcinogenicity has also been ascribed to ionizing irradiation, which produces free radicals, such as superoxide or hydroxyl radicals. A number of antitumor drugs have the same ability to promote formation of reactive oxygen intermediates; such agents include those that possess quinone functional groups (doxorubicin hydrochloride and plicamycin [mithramycin]) and those that bind electron-donating heavy metals (such as bleomycin sulfate and hydroxyurea). Four antineoplastic agents suspected as carcinogens and their probable carcinogenic intermediates are given in Figure 5.2; the varied chemical features of their reactive intermediates are illustrated.

Host factors, including enzymes such as glutathione S-transferases (GST), detoxify potentially mutagenic and toxic DNA-reactive electrophiles. Functional polymorphisms of GSTP1 (codon 105 Val allele) are associated with a higher risk of treatment (chemotherapy)-related acute myelogenous leukemia (AML), and not to radiation-induced or de novo AML. This risk is particularly relevant in patients receiving agents that are substrates for GSTP1.[14] For example, in a report of 44 patients with breast cancer who had received chemotherapy and/or radiation therapy and subsequently developed AML/MDS (myelodysplasia), 55%

3–Methylcholanthrene

Nitrogen Mustard

Ethyl Carbamate

Figure 5.1   Chemical structures of three carcinogenic agents.

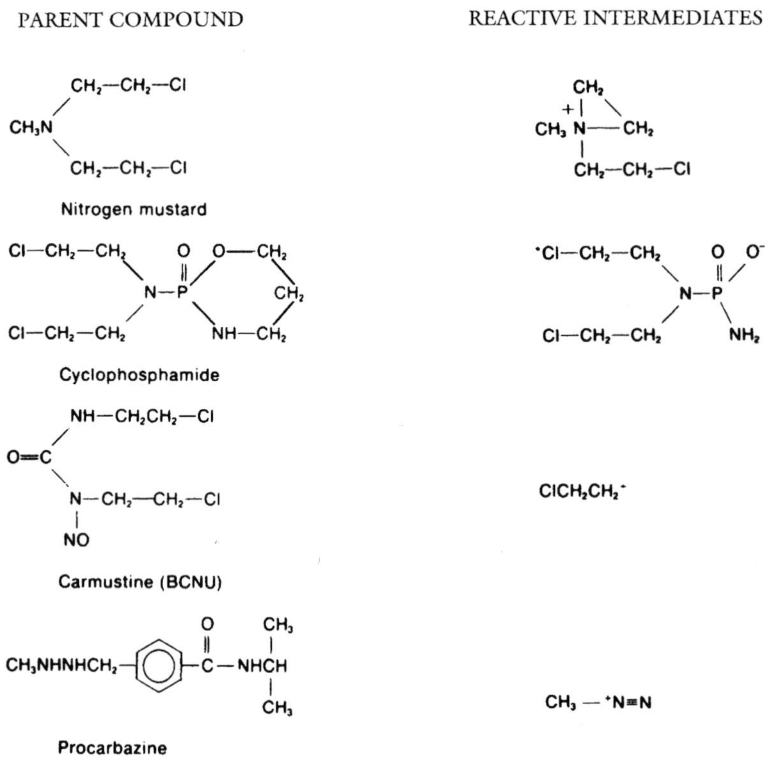

PARENT COMPOUND   REACTIVE INTERMEDIATES

Figure 5.2 Antineoplastic agents with reactive intermediates.

had combined deletions of the glutathione S-transferase polymorphisms GSTM1 and GSTT1; both polymorphisms are associated with diminished enzymatic activity. This is in contrast to 8.8% of patients in the control group with AML/MDS. An insufficient detoxification of cyclophosphamide is the proposed mechanism.[15] Other polymorphisms of drug-metabolizing enzymes, including cytochrome P450 3A4, NAD(P)H:quinine oxidoreductase and myeloperoxidase, may be markers of susceptibility to genotoxicity.[16] Direct genotoxicity may not be the sole explanation for drug-induced carcinogenesis. Short and long interspersed elements (SINEs and LINEs) comprise one-quarter of the human genome and are spread throughout the genome through retrotransposition. In retrotransposition, an element is transcribed into RNA and then converted back to DNA by reverse transcription. The copied DNA is then reinserted into a new location. Genotoxic agents and gamma irradiation have recently been shown to induce SINE transcription and reverse transcriptase activity. This observation suggests that genotoxic exposure may lead to genomic mutation through both DNA damage and through potentially mutagenic mobile elements in the genome.[17]

The identification of oncogenes and suppressor genes has added another variable to the equation. Their role in carcinogenesis is being pursued aggressively, and several possible mechanisms of actions have been proposed. The loss of one allele in a tumor suppressor gene such as p53 can potentially increase the risk of a drug-induced mutation in the other allele and development of the malignant phenotype. Oncogenes can be activated by a variety of mechanisms summarized in Table 5.1. Point mutations, chromosomal translocations, and gene amplification can alter expression of these genes. Just as altered oncogene expression and mutation occur with exposure to potential carcinogens, exposure to carcinogenic antitumor drugs likely alters oncogene expression and increases the risk of second malignancies. Most Nitrosomethylurea-induced mammary tumors contain an activated *ras* oncogene with a substitution of adenine for guanine in the 12th codon. This change is consistent with methylation of the oxygen in the 6 position of guanine, which would result in the replacement of guanine by adenine on DNA replication.[18] Such studies bring together environmental and genetic factors in cancer causation.

TABLE 5.1
ONCOGENE ACTIVATION

Alteration	Effect
Base mutation in coding sequence	New gene product with altered activity
Base deletion in noncoding sequence	Altered regulation of normal gene product
Chromosomal translocation	Altered message and level of expression
Gene amplification	Increased gene expression

Adapted with permission from Pitot HC. The molecular biology of carcinogenesis. Cancer 1993;72:962–970.

TESTING OF ANTINEOPLASTIC AGENTS FOR CARCINOGENIC POTENTIAL

In view of the damaging effects of many antineoplastic agents on DNA and the suggestive clinical evidence of their carcinogenicity, application of methods for determining carcinogenic potential before widespread use of new agents in humans has become imperative. An ideal test system would be simple, rapid, inexpensive, and yet specific for carcinogens and sensitive to modestly potent agents. Unfortunately, the various methods available, ranging from in vitro bacterial mutagenesis assays to long-term studies in rodents, all have recognized drawbacks.[19]

Five types of test systems for carcinogen exposure are available. Mutagenesis assays such as the Ames test attempt to quantify the frequency with which a chemical induces mutational events based on the assumption that mutagenicity correlates with the likelihood of causing cancer in animals. The underlying premise is that carcinogenesis is the product of a mutational event that can be expressed in the short term as a change in biochemical features of a test organism. Cytogenetic studies attempt to correlate drug-induced chromosomal aberrations such as sister chromatid exchanges (SCEs) with carcinogenicity. Although certain characteristic karyotypic changes are associated with specific malignancies, such as the Ph^1 chromosome with chronic myelogenous leukemia, cytogenetic abnormalities have proven neither necessary nor sufficient causes of neoplastic transformation. Tests of oncogenesis in tissue culture are based on the hypothesis that agents that produce neoplastic transformation in culture are likely to be carcinogenic in the whole animal. Like the Ames assay of bacterial mutagenesis, this system entails the assumption that the drug concentration, duration of exposure, and metabolism of the suspected carcinogen are relevant to the in vivo situation, but this assumption is of uncertain validity, and metabolic information is not available for many of the compounds tested. Carcinogenicity studies explore the tumorigenic potential in animals and attempt to predict the risk in humans. In vivo mammalian studies are usually conducted in rodents over extended periods and at great expense. The primary drawbacks of this system are the known species, sex, and age dependencies of drug metabolism in rodents and the lack of pharmacologic information that would allow an extrapolation of results from rodents to humans. The fifth approach, a measure of carcinogen exposure, uses detection of carcinogen-macromolecular adducts or somatic gene mutation in either target tissue or peripheral blood elements in animals or in man.

Mutagenesis Assays

Among the many mutagen-testing systems, the Ames test satisfies the requirements of simplicity and rapid return of results, and in addition, appears to possess high specificity for carcinogens, although certain exceptions have been identified. This test uses specific strains of *Salmonella typhimurium* that are histidine-requiring mutants.[20] Exposure of these strains to the suspected mutagen in a histidine-free medium leads to growth of revertant mutants if the appropriate mutation is induced. Small amounts of chemicals (less than 1 mg) can be used, and results are obtained in approximately 2 days. For agents that require metabolic activation (as do many carcinogens), rat or human liver microsomes can be added to the test plates.

In extensive testing of a wide variety of agents previously documented to be carcinogens and noncarcinogens, 90% of the known carcinogens gave positive results in the Ames assay, and 87% of the noncarcinogens were inactive.[21,22] These findings suggest that the system has a high degree of specificity and sensitivity. Many of the antineoplastic agents in use today have been examined in the Ames system,[23–26] and some of the results are incorporated in Table 5.2. Most antimetabolites and the vinca alkaloids give negative results in both the Ames test and in vivo systems, whereas alkylating agents and many antitumor antibiotics give

TABLE 5.2

RESULTS OF TESTING ANTINEOPLASTIC AGENTS IN THREE SYSTEMS FOR CARCINOGENICITY

Agent	Ames Test	SCEs	Animal Studies
Mechlorethamine hydrochloride	+	+	+
Cyclophosphamide	+	+[a]	+
Melphalan	+	+	+
Thiotriethylene phosphoramide (thiotepa)	+	+	+
Chlorambucil	NR	+	+
Procarbazine hydrochloride	−	+[a]	−
Lomustine (CCNU)	NR	+[b]	−
Doxorubicin hydrochloride	+	+	+
Streptozotocin	+	NR	+
Bleomycin sulfate	−	+[c]	−
Dactinomycin (actinomycin D)	−	±	+
Mitomycin C	+	+	+
Dacarbazine (DTIC)	NR	−[b]	+
Cisplatin	+	+	NR
5-Fluorouracil	−	NR	NR
6-Mercaptopurine	+	−	+
Cytosine arabinoside (ara-C)	−	NR	−
Vincristine sulfate	−	±	−
Vinblastine sulfate	−	NR	+
Pemetrexed	−	NR	−
Oxaliplatin	+	NR	NR
Methotrexate sodium		+	

[a]Drug must be activated.
[b]Test done on patient lymphocytes after treatment with agent.
[c]Concentration giving positive results also causes significant numbers of other chromosomal aberrations.
+, positive result reported in at least one study; −, no positive result reported; ±, slight decrease over control (which is of unknown significance); NR, no result reported.

positive results in both assay systems. Both procarbazine hydrochloride and dactinomycin (actinomycin D), however, are carcinogenic in animals but give negative results in the Ames test. In the case of procarbazine, this discrepancy may be due to the failure of the test system to simulate the metabolism of procarbazine as it occurs in vivo. The agent 6-mercaptopurine, which has been reported to be carcinogenic in animals, shows weakly mutagenic results in the Salmonella system.

From the foregoing analysis, the Ames test would appear to be an excellent screening procedure but one with obvious false-negative results. An analysis of the Ames test results by Rinkus and Legator[27] indicates that the false-negative rate is particularly high for specific chemical classes. At least seven classes of agents known to contain carcinogenic compounds are poorly detected in the Ames system, including azo compounds, carbonyl, hydrazine, chloroethylene, steroid, and antimetabolite structures. In some cases, known carcinogens such as urethane, probably cannot be metabolized to their carcinogenic form in the test system.

Another assay approach based on mutations measures the mutation frequency in the hypoxanthine-guanine phosphoribosyltransferase (HGPRT) gene.[28] This technique can be used in vitro in mammalian cells and in vivo in patient samples. Assessment of mutation frequency at baseline and after treatment, and comparison between control groups and populations treated with chemotherapy have been carried out.[29,30] Whether these assays are predictive of increased malignant risk is yet to be determined.

In vivo mutational assays have been developed using transgenic rodent models.[31] These models are composed of an altered genomic sequence that is inheritable, often the *Escherichia coli* lacI (lac repressor) or lacZ (β-galactosidase) genes. Animals are treated with the potentially carcinogenic agent and after sufficient time has passed to fix DNA adducts as mutations, genomic DNA is extracted, and the target gene is isolated by such methods as magnetic affinity capture. The transgenic model allows for rapid assessment of tissue-specific mutation after chemical treatment. This may focus subsequent clinical monitoring on specific organs. As with other in vivo studies, factors such as drug pharmacokinetics, DNA repair, animal age, diet, strain, sex, drug dose, and dosing duration influence the results.

Assay of Sister Chromatid Exchanges

Chromosomal damage resulting from exposure to chemical substances in vitro or in vivo has been used as an index of mutagenic or carcinogenic potential for many years but has required significant skill in recognizing the many different possible aberrations. Assay of SCE, a type of chromosomal study that detects the exchange of small DNA fragments between sister chromatid pairs, has considerable appeal because relatively few cells need to be exam-

ined, exchanges can be visualized easily, and the system is sensitive to small amounts of chemicals. The exchange is symmetric and does not alter the overall chromosomal morphology.[32]

The ability of various chemotherapeutic agents to induce SCE indicates that this technique might be useful as an assay for mutagenesis and ultimately carcinogenesis, but limitations of its potential have also become clear.[32,33] Ionizing radiation, known to be a potent mutagen and carcinogen, causes only slight increments in SCE; these changes are minimal in comparison with other chromosomal damage, including breaks, deletions, and other aberrations induced at the same dose level. On the other hand, ultraviolet light evokes dramatic increases in SCE frequency. Alkylating agents and some DNA intercalators induce a high frequency of SCE in addition to other chromosomal damage. Cyclophosphamide induces SCEs only after microsomal activation.[34] Among the antimetabolites, methotrexate, which is not carcinogenic in laboratory animals, or humans, has been reported to induce SCE, but 6-mercaptopurine, a suspected carcinogen, does not cause these chromosomal abnormalities.[35]

The use of SCE has particular appeal because the effects of chemotherapeutic agents can be assessed in vivo by performing this test on peripheral lymphocytes from patients receiving antineoplastic therapy. Studies of lymphocytes from patients before and at intervals after chemotherapy have shown a marked increase in SCEs after the administration of lomustine (CCNU), dacarbazine, and mitomycin.[36–38] Whether such increases in SCE frequency reflect the likelihood of carcinogenicity is still unclear.

Cell Culture Systems

Cell culture systems also have been advocated for the testing of carcinogenicity. Morphologic transformation of cells in culture and the ability of these cells to produce tumors when implanted in animals have been the primary criteria used for carcinogenicity. Three major test systems, which use hamster embryo cells, fibroblasts from the ventral prostate, or 3T3-like cells, have been applied to the screening of environmental carcinogens.[39–40] Using all three lines, investigators have shown a good quantitative correlation between transformation in vitro and in vivo carcinogenesis, although the number of antineoplastic agents tested has been limited. Mammalian cell culture systems, however, are subject to many of the same problems as those of bacterial mutagenesis assays discussed previously, including the need to activate compounds to reactive intermediates. An additional problem pertinent to these three systems is the use of cells of nonhuman and nonepithelial origin. Finally, tumors resulting from the implantation of transformed cells are sarcomas, and thus may not reflect the potential of the tested agent to cause tumors in epithelial cells or in humans.

The results of testing antineoplastic drugs in cell transformation systems have not correlated well with tests of carcinogenicity in experimental animals.[41,42] Carcinogenic alkylating agents (melphalan and thiotriethylene phosphoramide [thiotepa]) increased the transformation frequency of C3H/10T1/2 cells, and dactinomycin and bleomycin showed a concentration-dependent increase in transformation frequency. These results are consistent with the known carcinogenicity of these agents. However, methotrexate also caused a concentration-dependent increase in transformation but at a relatively low frequency, whereas two other antimetabolites, 5-fluorodeoxyuridine and arabinosylcytosine, produced transformation in synchronized cells exposed during the S phase of the cell cycle. None of these antimetabolites has proved to be carcinogenic in animals or humans.

Cultured human tissue and cells may be used for carcinogenesis studies.[43] Studies in these systems overcome some of the drawbacks of using nonhuman systems. Drug metabolism to the ultimate carcinogen, uptake of drug into human cells, the identification of specific DNA adducts, and the presence of DNA repair systems more closely approach the in vivo situation. However, since aspects of each of these processes differ among various human tissues, it is uncertain that any one test system can predict for results in people.

Animal Studies

The classic yardstick for assessing carcinogenicity has been the ability of the suspected agent to induce tumors in laboratory animals. These studies, although the most direct and reliable source of experimental information, are fraught with difficulties, including high cost, interspecies variability in susceptibility to carcinogens, and the long time required to obtain results. In addition, efforts must be made to design protocols of drug administration that mimic the intensity and duration of exposure found in humans, a problem compounded by differences in drug metabolism and pharmacokinetics in humans and rodents. A definite advantage of the bioassay system in intact animals is the preservation of the role of the immune system in determining the outcome. This factor is obviously missing in any of the in vitro assays.

The results of various bioassays of antineoplastic agents are recorded in Table 5.2.[44–47] Some results are conflicting and seem to depend on the age, sex, and species of animal used in the test. In general, however, most alkylating agents and antitumor antibiotics are carcinogenic in animals, whereas antimetabolites, including methotrexate, cytosine arabinoside (ara-C), and hydroxyurea, give negative results. Drug combinations have received only limited testing in bioassay systems.[48] Tests of the combination of prednisone and azathioprine, commonly used in organ transplantation, showed a decrease in time before tumor appearance compared with azathio-prine alone. With other combinations (e.g., prednisone plus CCNU, ara-C plus CCNU, and prednisone, vincristine sulfate, and cyclophosphamide), the median time before tumor appearance was longer than with the alkylating agent alone. Of the 10 combinations studied, 4 resulted in slightly higher tumor incidence than controls, whereas 6 caused fewer tumors than did the individual drugs.

Molecular and Biochemical Assays

Advances in the detection of carcinogen-molecular adducts and somatic gene mutations have opened the opportunity to study carcinogen exposure in humans.[49,50] The polymerase chain reaction and DNA sequencing enable rapid assessment of oncogene and tumor suppressor gene mutations in small patient samples. The use of ^{32}P-postlabeling thin-layer chromatography and autoradiography assays, enzyme-linked immunosorbent assays, synchronous fluorescence spectroscopy, and gas chromatography/mass spectroscopy has made it feasible to detect low levels of adducts in human samples. Carcinogen-DNA adducts, exposure to chemicals, and carcinogenicity have been correlated with each other; but in the past, the low levels of adducts present in human samples limited the conventional assay systems. Enzyme immunoassays combined with synchronous fluorescence spectroscopy have increased sensitivity and specificity for polycyclic aromatic hydrocarbon–DNA adducts. High-pressure liquid chromatography or immunoaffinity chromatography in combination with ^{32}P-postlabeling assay or immunoassay can be used to detect alkyl adducts in the human tissue with assay detection limits ranging from 1 to 600 adducts per 10^8 nucleotides, depending on assay and tissue examined. Such assays make it feasible to perform epidemiologic studies in patients receiving chemotherapy.

Proteomics may ultimately prove to be a more reliable and cost-effective tool to predict carcinogenicity. Studies have identified proteomic changes that occur as cells become cancerous.[51–53] Consequently, the identification of such changes of the proteome on exposure of the cell to the investigational agent, would raise concern regarding its oncogenic potential.

CLINICAL STUDIES IMPLICATING ANTINEOPLASTIC AGENTS IN CARCINOGENESIS

Although experimental evidence demonstrating the carcinogenic potential of many antineoplastic agents was abundant, the clinical evidence of this problem was slower to appear. The fact that the rate of development of "secondary" cancers in patients with malignant lymphoma, pediatric cancers, ovarian cancer, and breast cancer is higher than that seen in an age-matched normal population has become clear. Many good reviews of this topic are now available in the medical literature.[54–57] Reports of second tumors in patients with prior histories of cancer comes from a variety of sources. Initial reports were mainly anecdotal and thus did not allow an analysis of factors that might be important. Data reported more recently have come from hospital-based, national, and international tumor registries and from longer follow-up of chemotherapy and hormonal therapy studies. The use of longer-term clinical trial data has the advantage that the initial cohort and treatment are tightly controlled. This provides a better analysis of how different drugs and treatments would impact the risk of second cancers. The use of clinical trial data for this purpose is somewhat limited by patient numbers, which rarely exceed 1,000. Registries, on the other hand, can have several thousand or tens of thousands of patients and thus allow a better assessment regarding less common second cancers such as acute leukemia or sarcoma.

Determining treatment and outcome from registries can be labor-intensive, however. One method that is used to identify treatment factors involved in the development of new cancers from a registry is referred to as a "nested" case-control study. In this approach, patients in the registry who develop a second cancer are compared with others who did not. These comparisons have provided a better estimate of the risks and the factors that influence the development of second cancers. Clinical information about the total dosages of drugs, concomitant therapy, and the duration of treatment is important in estimating risk. For some drugs such as the alkylating agents or etoposide, a threshold exists above which the risk of neoplasia rises sharply. Such thresholds have been previously identified in experimental carcinogenesis and in the induction of SCEs. Duration of treatment may also have a bearing, because a brief but intense exposure to a cytotoxic agent may be less carcinogenic than long-term low-dose exposure.

Another issue in assessing the true risk of second cancers from cytotoxic agents is the existence of other factors that may also influence their development. An underlying increased incidence of second malignancy is found independent of therapy in patients with retinoblastoma, Wilms' tumor, multiple myeloma, Hodgkin's disease, and other tumors such as those associated with the hereditary nonpolyposis colorectal cancer syndrome. Other therapies used to treat the cancer, particularly radiation therapy, also impact the development of secondary cancers. An increase in solid tumors after therapy for Hodgkin's disease and testicular cancer is most likely related to radiation rather than chemotherapy. In many reports, combination treatment regimens or regimens using irradiation and chemotherapy were used. Thus, the carcinogenic effects cannot necessarily be ascribed to one compound of the regimen with certainty, although the use of the nested case-control method may allow conclusions to be drawn regarding the carcinogenicity of different components of the regimen.

Interpretation of studies in this area must also take into consideration the statistical methods used to assess relative risk.[58] The use of a person-years-of-risk analysis assumes that the yearly incidence of second malignancies is constant for the entire follow-up period and does not allow for the fact that a patient must live a certain time through the latency period for the occurrence of a second malignancy. Such an analysis allows a reasonable estimate of the carcinogenic effects of a single therapy, but its use when comparing two treatments biases results against the treatment that leads to a longer survival. Many studies compare the risk of cancer in the treated group with that of an age-matched cohort in the normal population to determine a relative risk. For a tumor that is uncommon in this age-matched population, an increase in the relative risk of fivefold to 10-fold sounds impressive but may only translate into a problem for fewer than 1% of patients who received therapy. On the other hand, small increases in relative risk for the more common solid tumors such as lung or breast cancer translate into a much greater problem in terms of absolute risk. This is the case with treatments for Hodgkin's disease as described later. One method that is useful in determining the overall impact of a secondary cancer in a population is to describe it in terms of the number of new cancers that occur per 10,000 patients treated.

Based on information currently available, one can attempt to categorize antineoplastic agents into high, moderate, low, and unknown risk groups on the basis of their oncogenic potential in humans (Table 5.3). The primary basis for this classification is reports of second malignancy in patients treated for both hematologic and solid tumors, with additional information coming from trials of cytotoxic agents in patients with immune diseases or after organ transplantation. Given that the latency period for the development of secondary cancers can range from 1 year (e.g., for etoposide-induced leukemias) to 20 years for solid tumors, the risk for many newer agents such as paclitaxel, docetaxel, irinotecan hydrochloride, gemcitabine hydrochloride, pemetrexed and oxaliplatin cannot yet be properly determined. Furthermore, the impact of the new targeted agents such as imatinib, gefitinb, and erlotinib on formation of secondary malignancies is unclear. Neither of the epidermal growth factor receptor tyrosine kinase inhibitors gefitinib nor erlotinib have demonstrated genotoxic potential with in vitro or in vivo assays. Imatinib, the tyrosine kinase inhibitor targeting C-kit, has been shown to induce benign and malignant tumors of preputial/clitoral gland, kidney and urinary bladder in rats. This has not been demonstrated in humans.[59] A true assessment of agents primarily used in palliative therapy is also difficult because most patients may not survive long enough for problems such as second cancers to manifest.

The development of a new cancer can occur many years after treatment of the initial cancer. This means that large numbers of patients and long follow-up are required to define the risk of carcinogenesis and to understand which

TABLE 5.3

CATEGORIZATION OF ANTINEOPLASTIC AGENTS ACCORDING TO CARCINOGENIC RISK IN HUMANS

High Risk	Moderate Risk	Low Risk	Unknown
Melphalan	Doxorubicin hydrochloride	Vinca alkaloids	Bleomycin sulfate
Mechlorethamine hydrochloride	Thiotriethylene phosphoramide (thiotepa)	Methotrexate sodium	Taxanes
Nitrosoureas		Cytosine arabinoside (ara-C)	Busulfan
Etoposide			Gemcitabine hydrochloride
Teniposide			Irinotecan hydrochloride
Azathioprine			Mitoxantrone hydrochloride
	Cyclophosphamide	5-Fluorouracil	Pemetrexed
	Procarbazine hydrochloride	L-Asparaginase	Oxaliplatin
	Dacarbazine (DTIC)	Carboplatin	
	Cisplatin		

drugs and schedules are the probable causes. Some investigators have used preneoplastic lesions as markers of carcinogenicity to provide an earlier estimate of the risk. For example, a small group of patients with breast cancer who had been randomized previously to receive adjuvant chemotherapy or oophorectomy underwent cytologic and colposcopic screening of the uterine cervix.[60] The results were compared with those for 79 controls with no known breast malignancy. Significantly more breast cancer patients who had received chemotherapy had cervical intraepithelial neoplasia ($P < .01$) than did controls; the proportion of breast cancer patients in the oophorectomy group who had cervical intraepithelial neoplasia did not differ significantly from the proportion in the control group. The incidence of chromosome abnormalities and structural chromosome changes in ovarian cancer patients treated with melphalan was higher than in a control group.[61] For patients receiving both melphalan and radiation therapy, the frequency of chromosomal aberrations was even higher. Whether these chromosomal changes act as a marker for subsequent development of secondary leukemia is not yet known. In children with hematologic cancer who had previously received chemotherapy and cranial irradiation, the total-body mole counts were compared with those of their siblings. The median number of moles was 20.0 in the patient group ($n = 79$) and 11.0 in the healthy siblings ($n = 88$).[62] In another study, a total-body count of melanocytic nevi in children receiving treatment for hematologic cancer was carried out before therapy and repeated 3 years later. Total-body nevus counts were significantly increased 3 years after treatment.[63] To what degree these results predict subsequent cancer development is yet unknown. With increasing knowledge of progression from benign to neoplastic growth in diseases such as colorectal and

pancreatic cancer, however, assessment of precursor lesions may be a useful way to evaluate risk.

SECOND MALIGNANCIES IN SPECIFIC POPULATIONS OF CANCER PATIENTS

Pediatric Patients

Long-term survival is now possible for many patients with pediatric malignancies. This group of patients is followed closely for the development of late complications from treatment. Some pediatric tumors such as retinoblastoma have been associated with genetic abnormalities that may predispose to other cancers.[64] Overall, the risk of developing a second cancer 20 years after childhood cancer has been estimated at 8 to 20%.[65,66] The Childhood Cancer Survivor Study analyzed the risk of second malignancies in 14,000 five-year survivors who received their treatment between 1970 and 1986. The relative risk for a second malignancy was as follows: non-Hodgkin's lymphoma, 3.2; leukemia, 5.7; and Hodgkin's disease, 9.7.[67] One consistent finding has been an association between treatment with the epipodophyllotoxins, etoposide, or teniposide, and secondary AML, often with monocytic features. One series examined 205 children with acute lymphoblastic leukemia (ALL) who were treated with a four-drug induction consisting of prednisone, L-asparaginase, vincristine, and daunorubicin hydrochloride followed by maintenance therapy with oral 6-mercaptopurine, methotrexate, L-asparaginase, etoposide, and cytarabine. The etoposide was given twice weekly. The risk of secondary AML at 4 years was $5.9 \pm 3.2\%$. Because none of these children received alkylating agent therapy or irradiation, etoposide was most likely responsible for these secondary leukemias.[68] Risk factors for secondary AML in 734 consecutively treated children with ALL who attained complete remission and received maintenance treatment with epipodophyllotoxins were reported by Pui et al.[69] Secondary AML was diagnosed in 21 of the 734 patients, and the overall cumulative risk at 6 years was 3.8% (range, 2.3 to 6.1%). For the subgroups treated twice weekly or weekly with etoposide or teniposide, the risk of AML at 6 years was 12.3%, whereas for the subgroups treated with these drugs only during remission induction, or every 2 weeks during maintenance treatment, the risk was 1.6%. In their analysis, the schedule of the epipodophyllotoxin administration was important, whereas the cumulative dose of drug did not appear to influence the risk of secondary leukemia. At the Dana-Farber Cancer Institute, no epipodophyllotoxin was used in their regimens. They reviewed 752 children with ALL who entered complete remission after induction therapy. Only two had developed AML after a median follow-up of 4 years.[70] In a review of all ALL patients treated at the Dana-Farber Cancer Institute, the risk of a second malignancy was 2.7%, but the risk of other adverse events, including relapse, death, or induction failure, was 31%.[71] Clinical and cytologic findings in epipodophyllotoxin-induced leukemia are a short latency period (mean, 24 to 36 months) between the completion of treatment and the development of AML, a Fab M-4 or M-5 subtype, a translocation of the MLL gene at chromosome band 11q23, and a poor response to treatment.[72] Studies have shown an association between the breakpoints in the MLL gene and DNA topoisomerase II cleavage sites that are stimulated by etoposide. Secondary leukemia due to alkylating agents is characterized by a different phenotype with a longer latency period, antecedent myelodysplasia, and deletions of chromosomes 5 or 7.[54]

In view of this apparent increased risk of leukemia with epipodophyllotoxins, the National Cancer Institute Cancer Therapy Evaluation Program has instituted a monitoring plan for secondary leukemias after treatment with these agents. One report[73] from this program analyzed 12 cooperative group clinical trials (11 in the pediatric population) that used cumulative doses of etoposide ranging from less than 1.5 g/m^2 to more than 3.0 g/m^2.[74] The risk of developing a secondary leukemia at 6 years was 3.3%, 0.7%, and 2.2% in the dose ranges of less than 1.5 g/m^2, 1.5 to 2.99 g/m^2, and more than 3.0 g/m^2, respectively. Their overall conclusions were that, at doses of less than 5 g/m^2, only a minor risk of secondary leukemia is found. The risk of leukemia in patients receiving etoposide is probably influenced by other agents used in the regimens, particularly alkylating agents and other topoisomerase inhibitors. Relatively high rates of secondary leukemia have been reported in small series after the use of intensive treatments for pediatric tumors with poor prognosis that included both topoisomerase II inhibitors and alkylating agents.[75]

The development of secondary solid tumors in pediatric cancer patients is an issue of growing concern. The Roswell Park Cancer Institute reviewed the courses of 1,406 patients younger than 20 years of age who were treated over a 30-year period.[76] The actuarial risk of a second malignant tumor 25 years after diagnosis was 5.6%. Prior therapy with carmustine and doxorubicin were the only factors that were significantly associated with the risk of a second malignant tumor. In Italy, a registry of all patients with childhood cancer who achieved complete remission was followed for a median time of 52 months after treatment. Twenty secondary malignancies occurred, which included nine hematologic malignancies (four AML, two chronic myelogenous leukemia, three non-Hodgkin's lymphoma), eight central nervous system tumors (all in patients given central nervous system radiation), and three other solid tumors.[77] Others have reported the occurrence of unusual tumors such as squamous cell cancers of the skin occurring in teenagers who have previously received therapy for AML.[78] The risk of specific types of second tumors appears to be a function of the types of treatment used, the sites of irradiation, and undoubtedly, the nature of the underlying malignancy.

In a follow-up of 674 patients treated in the German Ewing's sarcoma studies, the cumulative risk of a second malignancy was 0.7%, 2.9%, and 4.7% after 5, 10, and 15 years, respectively. The time until the development of myelodysplasia/leukemia was 17 to 96 months and until development of solid tumors was 82 to 136 months.[79] Of 397 patients with Ewing's sarcoma treated at the Mayo Clinic, 26 patients (6.5%) had 29 malignancies. The mean age was 16 years and the interval from diagnosis of the sarcoma and a second malignancy averaged 9.5 years (range, 1 to 32.5 years). The cancers consisted of 12 sarcomas, 9 carcinomas, and 8 hematologic malignancies. The hematologic malignancies occurred at a mean of 4.8 years (range, 1.7 to 12.9 years) and sarcomas occurred after a mean of 10.9 years (range, 1.5 to 32.5 years).[80] The importance of the development of second malignancy must be interpreted in relation to the risks of failure of therapy of the primary cancer. In the analysis of the German Ewing's sarcoma trials, second malignancies accounted for only 3 of the 328 deaths in this population; the remainder were due to Ewing's sarcoma.

The Memorial Sloan Kettering Cancer Center (MSKCC) group reported 14 second malignancies in 509 patients with osteosarcoma treated on 6 different clinical trials. Chemotherapy agents included high-dose methotrexate, doxorubicin, bleomycin, cyclophosphamide, dactinomycin, vincristine, cisplatin, and ifosfamide. The median age at diagnosis of the osteosarcoma was 16.6 years (range, 3.1 to 74.4 years), and time interval from osteosarcoma diagnosis and secondary malignancy was 5.5 years (range, 1.3 to 13.1 years). The most common secondary malignancy was in the CNS (four anaplastic gliomas, one meningioma, high-grade glioma and a maxillary astrocytoma). There were two cases of AML and one case each of MDS, Non-Hodgkins lymphoma (NHL), high-grade pleomorphic sarcoma, leiomyosarcoma, fibrosarcoma, breast cancer, and mucoepidermoid carcinoma. The overall 5- and 10-year cumulative incidences of secondary malignancies were 1.4 ± −1.1% and 3.1 ± −1.8%. The standardized incidence ratio for the cohort was 4.6% (95% confidence interval [CI], 2.53–7.78; $P = 0.00001$).[81]

A review from Stanford of 694 children with Hodgkin's disease showed a risk of both solid tumors and hematologic malignancies similar to that reported for adults with this disease (discussed later). Of note, the actuarial risk at 20 years in men was 10.6% and in women it was 15.4% because of the additional risk of breast cancers occurring within the radiation field.[82] Similar observations were made by the Late Effects Study Group, which found the relative risk for second tumors in children treated for Hodgkin's disease to be 18.5. The cumulative risk of any second malignancy was 10.6% at 20 years, increasing to 26.3% at 30 years. Solid malignancies occurred in 7.3% at 20 years and 23.5% at 30 years and breast cancer was the most common malignancy, with a standardized incidence ratio of 56.7. Forty-seven percent received mantle radiation alone and 57% received combined modality therapy. The incidence of breast cancer at age 40 was 13.9%, rising to 20.1% at age 45.[83] The risk of breast cancer is increased when the patient is of pubertal age at the time of radiation, and when the dose of radiation is higher.[84,85] Risk of leukemia was associated with use of alkylating agents and advanced stage at diagnosis. The second most common solid tumor developing in patients who have received radiation for Hodgkin's disease is thyroid cancer, with a relative risk of 36.[67,83] The risk of other epithelial malignancies such as colorectal and gastric cancer also seem to be increased, and occur at a younger age than the general population.[83] Knowledge of these predispositions to secondary malignancies and toxicities have resulted in modification of the treatment in the pediatric population.[86]

Overall, the risk of AML peaks a few years after therapy, whereas the risk of a solid tumor increases with the length of follow-up. It is still too early to assess what additional risk this population will experience when they enter an age group in which the development of cancer is more common. In this setting, a modest increase in relative risk could translate into a substantial increase in the overall absolute risk of cancer. This has already been observed to some degree in the population treated for Hodgkin's disease.

Patients with hereditary retinoblastoma have a high incidence of second malignancies, in part because of their genetic predisposition, but this is exacerbated by the treatment. In a long-term follow-up study of 1604 1-year survivors of retinoblastoma diagnosed between 1914 and 1984, the relative risk of developing a second malignancy in the hereditary retinoblastoma population was 30. The cumulative risk of secondary malignancy diagnosis after 50 years was 51% in the hereditary retinoblastoma group and

5% in the nonhereditary group. The 50-year cumulative risk of a secondary malignancy in the previously radiated group was 58%, compared with 27% in those not receiving radiation therapy. Although second malignancies occurred at any radiation dose, there was a dose-response relationship, with a 12-fold increase at doses of 60 Gy or higher. These tumors are primarily soft tissue sarcomas and osteosarcomas and possess the RB1 mutations see in the primary tumor.[87]

Children treated for Wilms' tumor have an eightfold increased risk of developing a secondary malignancy: leukemia, lymphomas, and solid tumors. Treatment-related AML was diagnosed 1 to 6 years following initial therapy, as were lymphomas. Solid tumors consisted of sarcomas and cancers of the breast, thyroid, colon, liver, and parotid, in addition to brain, at a latency period of 3 to 21 years. Abdominal radiation therapy increased the risk twofold.[88]

Patients with Ovarian Cancer

Advanced ovarian cancer was treated initially with alkylating agents such as melphalan.[89] Several reports have implicated alkylating agents (particularly melphalan and cyclophosphamide used as single agents) as a causative factor in the high incidence of AML in this group of patients.[90–93] A review of 5,455 cases of ovarian cancer revealed a 36.1-fold increased risk of acute leukemia compared with an age-matched control group. For patients surviving at least 2 years after the institution of therapy, the risk was 174.4-fold higher than that in the controls.[94] Many patients with acute leukemia identified in this series also received radiotherapy alone or in combination with alkylating agents. Thus, determining which agent was responsible for the leukemia was impossible. An analysis of a large cohort of patients with ovarian cancer treated with melphalan or cyclophosphamide revealed a 93-fold increased risk of AML in women treated with chemotherapy.[95] The risk was highest 5 to 6 years after the initiation of therapy and decreased thereafter. A dose-response relationship was apparent for melphalan and was suggested for cyclophosphamide. Melphalan was more likely to induce secondary leukemia than was cyclophosphamide. In an international collaborative group of cancer registries and hospitals, 114 cases of leukemia were identified after ovarian cancer.[96] Chemotherapy alone was associated with a relative risk for leukemia of 12 compared with surgery alone, whereas radiotherapy alone did not produce a significant increase in risk. The risk of leukemia was greatest 4 to 5 years after chemotherapy and was increased for at least 8 years. Cyclophosphamide, chlorambucil, melphalan, thiotepa, and treosulfan were independently associated with significantly increased risks of leukemia. Chlorambucil and melphalan were the most leukemogenic. These studies support the clinical impression that a dose-response effect may exist, that the carcinogenic potential of all alkylating agents is not necessarily the same, and that the latency period is approximately 5 years. They also suggest that the risk for secondary leukemia does decrease after a period. The largest analysis of second tumors in ovarian cancer was done on nine population registries of the National Cancer Institute and Connecticut Tumor Registry.[97] Researchers examined 32,251 women with ovarian cancer and found a relative risk of second cancers of 1.28 (95% CI, 1.21–1.35), with an excess of leukemia (relative risk [RR] = 4.1) and colorectal (RR = 1.4), bladder (RR = 2.1), and breast (RR = 1.2) cancers. The association with rectal and breast cancer was probably related to genetic predisposition; the risk of leukemia, to alkylating agents; and the risk of sarcomas and abdominal tumors, to previous radiation.

Ovarian cancer is now treated primarily with platinum-based regimens, and melphalan and chlorambucil are rarely used. The leukemogenic potential of cisplatin is assumed to be less than that for other alkylating agents. Anecdotal reports exist of patients developing acute non-lymphocytic leukemia (ANLL) after cisplatin therapy, but the relative risk of developing ANLL after cisplatin is not yet well known.[98,99] The newest agents for the treatment of ovarian cancer are paclitaxel and topotecan hydrochloride. It is too early to assess the carcinogenic potential of the topoisomerase I inhibitors and taxanes.

Patients with Breast Cancer

Breast cancer is another malignancy responsive to various cytotoxic and hormonal agents that are associated with an increased risk of secondary malignancies.[100] Among patients receiving adjuvant chemotherapy for breast cancer, no increased risk of leukemia was identified in a group of 1,265 patients who received postoperative thiotepa (with or without radiotherapy), compared with untreated controls.[101] The ongoing prospective adjuvant studies in breast cancer have addressed this question more definitively.[2,3,102] The results of the National Surgical Adjuvant Breast and Bowel Program database analysis indicate that risk of leukemia in patients receiving melphalan-based adjuvant chemotherapy increases fivefold. An initial analysis of the Milan studies of cyclophosphamide, methotrexate, and 5-fluorouracil (CMF) adjuvant chemotherapy revealed no increased incidence of leukemia or other second malignancies.[103] A more recent analysis of 2,465 patients with localized breast cancer treated in Milan from 1973 to 1990 revealed a 15-year cumulative risk of second cancers of 8.4% after local treatment only, 6.4% after CMF therapy, and 5.1% after doxorubicin-based chemotherapy. The relative risk for women receiving CMF treatment was 1.29.[104] An analysis of 1,113 patients in Sweden treated with adjuvant CMF or radiation therapy did not demonstrate any increase in second cancers in the first 10 years of follow-up.[105] Patients receiving chemotherapy actually had a lower rate of such cancers than those receiving radiation therapy.

The typical features of AML secondary to alkylating agent exposure include a latency period of 4 to 7 years,

during which MDS often becomes apparent, deletions of the long arms 5 and/or 7 or loss of the whole chromosome, and an unfavorable response to chemotherapy. There is also a higher incidence of p53 mutations and microsatellite instability observed in therapy-induced myelodysplastic syndrome.[106] Case reports have described the occurrence of a different type of AML with monocytic features associated with a translocation at 11q23 (the locus of the MLL gene) in patients who have received epirubicin hydrochloride-containing combination therapy for breast cancer.[107] These cases occur after a brief latency period of 1 to 3 years rather than the more prolonged interval preceding AML induced by alkylating agents and are similar, if not identical, to the cases of leukemia associated with etoposide, another topoisomerase II inhibitor.[73]

The M.D. Anderson Cancer Center reviewed data on 1,474 patients treated on six adjuvant or neoadjuvant trials that included 5-fluorouracil, doxorubicin, and cyclophosphamide.[108] The median follow-up was only 8 years, which is too short to evaluate risk of solid tumors. The 10-year estimated acute leukemia rate was 2.5% in patients who received both chemotherapy and radiation, and 0.5% in the chemotherapy-only group. This suggests that any leukemogenic risk from the use of anthracycline therapy is increased. A population-based cohort of 3,093 women in whom with breast cancer diagnosed were studied for the development of acute leukemia. Women who received chemotherapy and radiation had a standardized incidence ratio of 28.5. A dose-dependent increase in risk was observed in women treated with mitoxantrone and that the risk of leukemia was lower in the women receiving anthracyclines.[109] Curtis et al.[110] reviewed the Surveillance, Epidemiology, and End Results database of 21,708 patients with breast cancer and found an 11.5 relative risk of developing secondary leukemias in patients treated with alkylating agents with or without radiation therapy as an adjuvant after a median follow-up of 4.2 years. In an attempt to assess the contributions of adjuvant radiotherapy, melphalan, or cyclophosphamide, Curtis and colleagues also reported a case-control study in a cohort of 82,700 women in whom breast cancer had been diagnosed.[111] Results indicate a 2.4-fold increase in relative risk of leukemia after radiotherapy alone, a 10-fold increase after chemotherapy alone, and a 17.4-fold increase after a combination of the two. Melphalan was 10-fold more leukemogenic than cyclophosphamide, with little increase seen in the risk of leukemia after cumulative doses of cyclophosphamide of less than 20 g. The results from these analyses are consistent with data from the treatment of other malignancies. They do not rule out the possibility that second solid tumors that have a much longer latency period than leukemias may still develop.[112] It has been suggested that postmastectomy irradiation increases the risk of lung cancer in smokers, and it is well established that radiation to the breast increases the risk of sarcomas, particularly angiosarcoma.[113–115]

Adjuvant therapy with tamoxifen citrate is now well established to improve relapse-free survival and overall survival in selected patients with breast cancer. A number of large studies randomizing women to receive tamoxifen or placebo after surgery have been completed. Longer follow-up on these patients has provided evidence about the influence of tamoxifen on the subsequent development of other malignancies. The short-term and long-term adverse effects of tamoxifen have been thought to be the result of its estrogenic effects. In postmenopausal women, tamoxifen treatment leads to endometrial hyperplasia and polyps.[116] Tamoxifen also stimulates the growth of endometrial cancer in vitro.[117] An association is found between tamoxifen and the development of endometrial cancer. A relative risk of 6.4 was found in a Scandinavian study in which 40 mg per day was used and was continued for 5 years.[118] Other studies using lower tamoxifen dosages and a shorter duration of treatment have reported lower relative risks.[119] Some have not reported any increased risk of endometrial cancer.

Not all studies, however, prospectively collected information on second primaries.[120] The National Surgical Adjuvant Breast and Bowel Program reviewed 2,843 patients randomized to receive tamoxifen or placebo in their B-14 study.[121] The relative risk of endometrial cancer in the tamoxifen-treated group was 7.5, and the overall annual hazard rate for the development of endometrial cancer was 1.6 per 1,000. In a meta-analysis of 32 randomized trials of tamoxifen versus a similar control arm including data from 52,929 patients, there was a significantly increased risk of developing endometrial cancers (RR = 2.7; 95% CI, 1.94–3.75) and gastrointestinal cancers (RR = 1.31; 95% CI, 1.01–1.69).[122] If the estrogenic effects of tamoxifen cause endometrial cancer, those tumors that develop should be of low grade and have a relatively good prognosis. This assumption has been confirmed in some of the studies reported.[123] Other studies have shown a distribution of grade and stage similar to that seen in nonhormonally induced cancers.[124] In an analysis of 3,457 women with breast cancer, 53 subsequently developed endometrial cancer.[125] Of these women, 15 had received tamoxifen and 38 had not. The number of high-grade cancers increased significantly in the tamoxifen-treated women, who also were more likely to die of their endometrial cancer. In a Japanese study, however, 825 women with primary breast cancer were followed prospectively with annual gynecologic examinations.[126] Thirteen cases of endometrial cancer were discovered, but the incidence was no different in women who were and who were not taking tamoxifen. In a review of the Stockholm randomized trial of 2 years of adjuvant tamoxifen in postmenopausal women (n = 4,914; median follow-up of 9 years), an increased risk of endometrial cancer (RR = 4.1) and a decreased risk of contralateral breast cancers were noted.[127] In addition, an increase in colorectal (RR = 1.9) and gastric (RR = 3.2) cancers was associated with the use of tamoxifen.

In summary, most studies have demonstrated that adjuvant tamoxifen leads to a higher rate of endometrial cancer. The highest relative risks are associated with higher dosages and a longer duration of therapy. The histopathologic features of tamoxifen-associated endometrial cancer are less clear because each reported series had only small numbers of such cancers. Tamoxifen can induce liver cancer in laboratory animals, but no increased incidence of primary liver cancer has been seen in the adjuvant breast studies. These tumors could well be missed because any tumor developing in the liver probably would be presumed to be a recurrence of the previous breast cancer.

Several studies have reported a reduction in the development of cancers in the contralateral breast with tamoxifen use.[127–131] Either this could represent a reduction in the incidence of other breast cancers or could just be a manifestation of a reduction in the incidence of recurrence of the initial cancer within the contralateral breast. Reports have also appeared of reductions in cardiovascular mortality and increases in thromboembolic events when women take tamoxifen. An analysis of the impact of adjuvant tamoxifen on mortality was undertaken using published risks of endometrial cancers and thromboembolic events, as well as reductions in contralateral breast cancer and cardiovascular mortality.[132] This analysis concluded that the overall impact of tamoxifen was favorable, with between 3 and 41 deaths avoided per 1,000 patients treated, depending on the age of the women being treated. The importance of breast cancer as a source of morbidity and mortality in women and the observations of reductions in contralateral breast cancers with adjuvant tamoxifen, have led to two breast cancer prevention trials in which healthy women were randomized to receive tamoxifen or placebo. In a prevention trial, the increased risks of adverse events such as second malignancies are more of a concern. This was all taken into account when these trials were developed; however, some reservations have been expressed about exposing women to an increased risk of endometrial cancer.[133] No intervention is without risk; whether long-term tamoxifen usage leads to an overall health benefit to women can only be truly answered by these prevention trials.

Patients with Multiple Myeloma

Multiple myeloma, a disease commonly treated with single-agent alkylators such as melphalan, also has been associated with a high incidence of AML.[134–136] Because myeloma itself involves a bone marrow element, the possibility exists that a common process may be responsible for both diseases. However, the reported incidence of leukemia in patients with myeloma who do not receive alkylating therapy is no greater than expected for an age-matched population.[137] This suggests that the alkylating agents have contributed to the high incidence of leukemia. This contention is supported by a prospective trial of alkylating therapy for myeloma, which found that the actuarial risk of developing acute leukemia was 17.4% at 50 months, 214 times that expected.

Patients with Malignant Lymphoma

The incidence of second malignancies among patients with malignant lymphoma was no higher than expected during the era before intensive therapy.[138] The use of combination chemotherapy and combined radiotherapy and chemotherapy has been associated with a high incidence of second malignancies, specifically AML and solid tumors.[139-143] Many of these patients, however, would not have survived long enough to be exposed to the risk of a second malignancy before the introduction of intensive therapy. Many lymphoma patients have defective immune function, which may predispose them to a higher risk of cancer on exposure to an inciting agent. Mechlorethamine hydrochloride and procarbazine, components of nitrogen mustard, vincristine, procarbazine and prednisone (MOPP) combination chemotherapy for Hodgkin's disease, are potent carcinogens in animals.[46] A case-control study of 1,939 patients treated for Hodgkin's disease in the Netherlands assessed factors influencing the development of acute leukemia.[144] The cumulative dose of mechlorethamine was the most important factor. The use of lomustine was also associated with secondary leukemia, as was a requirement for a second course of chemotherapy. Overall, patients receiving chemotherapy had a 40-fold greater risk of leukemia than those receiving radiation therapy alone, whereas the use of combined-modality therapy did not increase the risk of leukemia beyond that seen with chemotherapy. Other analyses have similarly confirmed the importance of mechlorethamine, procarbazine, and nitrosoureas in the risk of second leukemia after treatment for lymphoma.[145,146] These studies also demonstrated that chemotherapy that did not include these three agents had a negligible risk of secondary leukemia.

Although many reports have been concerned with an increased risk of acute leukemia, solid tumors occur more frequently in patients with malignant lymphoma after intensive therapy.[147-150] Approximately one of patients with Hodgkin's disease develops a second cancer within 15 years of primary treatment.[148,151] Three-fourths of these are solid tumors, and the remainder are equally divided between leukemia and lymphoma. One hundred thirteen second cancers were seen in 2,846 British patients treated for Hodgkin's disease from 1970 to 1987.[152] The relative risk compared with that of the general population for leukemia and non-Hodgkin's lymphoma was 16, but the chance of developing colon, lung, and thyroid cancer, as well as osteogenic sarcoma, was also higher. In a German series of over 1,500 patients with Hodgkin's disease treated with radiation therapy, with or without chemotherapy, from 1940 to 1991, the cumulative risk for malignancy was 1.5%, 4.2%, 9.4%, and 21% at 5, 10, 15, and 20 years, respectively.[153] At the 20-year period, the risk for solid tumors, lymphoma, and leukemia was 19%, 1.9%, and 0.6%, respectively. Three-fourths of the solid tumors occurred within the radiation field. In patients receiving both chemotherapy and radiation therapy, the regimen of doxorubicin, bleomycin, vinblastine sulfate, and dacarbazine (ABVD) was associated with the highest risk. In another German report of 5,411 patients treated on one of three clinical trials for early, intermediate, and advanced Hodgkin's disease, 36 patients developed AML and 10 patients developed MDS. After a median observation time of 55 months, the incidence of AML/MDS was 1%. The prognosis was universally poor.[154]

In an intergroup trial of ABVD versus MOPP/ABV in 856 patients, secondary malignancies occurred in 18 patients receiving ABVD, 28 receiving MOPP/ABV, and 2 were initially treated with ABVD but subsequently received MOPP-containing regimens and radiation therapy before developing leukemia.[155] A case-control study that compiled data on 19,046 patients with Hodgkin's disease treated between 1965 and 1994 demonstrated an increased risk of lung cancer for those receiving radiation at doses exceeding 5 Gy. In patients who were treated with alkylating agents and no radiation therapy, the risk of lung cancer was fourfold and the risk increased with the number of cycles administered.[156] The risk of gastric cancer is increased twofold to 11-fold, and is highest for patients receiving combined modality therapy.[156] Arseneau et al.[142] reported a 23-fold increased risk of sarcoma after combined-modality therapy in patients with Hodgkin's disease. The overall risk of second malignancies increased 2.8-fold with intensive chemotherapy. In 885 women treated for Hodgkin's disease from 1961 to 1990, the relative risk of developing and dying from breast cancer was increased fourfold to fivefold.[147] Although this is primarily the result of upper mantle irradiation, the concurrent use of chemotherapy further increased the relative risk.

Because combined-modality therapy exposes patients to a higher risk of neoplasm, a long-term assessment of its benefits and risks continues to be necessary. One interesting analysis examined 313 patients with early-stage Hodgkin's disease who received either full-dose radiation therapy or chemotherapy followed by a lower dose of involved-field radiation.[157] The relative risk of a second cancer was 1.5 (95% CI, 0.6–3.5; P value not significant) in the combined-modality group but was 3.3 (95% CI, 2.2–5.3; $P < .001$) in the group receiving full-dose radiation.

Longer follow-up of patients receiving combination chemotherapy and radiotherapy for Hodgkin's disease has suggested that the increased risk of leukemia in this patient population may peak at between 3 and 9 years, followed by a decline thereafter.[65,139,158-160] The risks for the development of solid tumors increase over time.[160] Although the relative risk is highest for the development of leukemia and lymphoma, the twofold to threefold increase seen in the more common solid tumors accounts for most of the absolute increase in cancer cases in these patients.

Patients with non-Hodgkin's lymphoma are also at risk for developing second malignancies. The Groupe d'Etude des Lymphomes de l'Aduite (GELA) reported a 7-year cumulative incidence rate of 2.75% in 2,837 patients receiving doxorubicin, cyclophosphamide, vindesine, bleomycin and prednisone (ACVBP). Sixty-four of the 81 malignancies were solid tumors and 17 were hematologic malignancies. Age was the only risk factor on multivariate analysis. Considering all tumors, there was no increased risk of second cancers; however, in the male population there was an excess of lung cancer and MDS/AML, and in the female population there was an excess of MDS/AML.[161] Up to 10% of patients with non-Hodgkin's lymphoma treated with either conventional-dose chemotherapy or high-dose chemotherapy and autologous stem cell transplantation may develop treatment-related MDS/AML within 10 years of primary therapy.[162]

Patients with Essential Thrombocythemia

Essential thrombocythemia (ET) is a relatively indolent disease that is not typically appreciated to transform into acute leukemia. The leukemogenic potential of hydroxyurea (HU) has long been questioned. In a study of 114 patients with ET, 56 patients were randomized to receive HU and 58 patients to no receive cytotoxic therapy; however, 50% of the control group subsequently did receive HU. Fifteen patients had received busulfan prior to randomization. At a median follow-up of 73 months, seven patients (13%) in the HU group ultimately developed AML/MDS or a solid tumor, compared with one (1.7%) in the control group ($P = 0.032$). Three of the 77 patients (3.9%) who had only received HU and 5 of the 15 patients (33%) who had previously received busulfan developed neoplasia.[163]

Patients with Gastrointestinal Cancer

Analysis of randomized trials of adjuvant methyl-CCNU in the management of patients with gastrointestinal cancers performed by Boice et al.[4] has added more information regarding the leukemogenic potential of this treatment. The results of this analysis indicated that a 12.4 relative risk of leukemia exists in patients treated with methyl-CCNU. This risk seems to be dose-dependent when cumulative dose is considered. The latency period varies from 6 to 69 months and may continue to rise beyond that. Because the current data do not suggest a benefit in survival with such therapy, the leukemogenic risk has led to the removal of methyl-CCNU from adjuvant treatment regimens. The most important drug in adjuvant regimens for colorectal cancer is 5-fluorouracil, and it has not been associated with an increased risk of second cancers.

Patients with Testicular Cancer

More than 20 years have passed since cisplatin-based chemotherapy was first used for the treatment of advanced testicular cancer. This treatment has led to a large increase in the number of patients cured with chemotherapy, and reports about the long-term consequences of this therapy are only beginning to appear. In a group of 1,909 patients in The Netherlands diagnosed between 1971 and 1985, 78 second cancers occurred, or 1.6 times the number expected.[164] Significant increases were seen in gastrointestinal cancers (RR = 2.6) and leukemia (RR = 5.1). In this analysis, radiation therapy was the main contributing factor; patients treated with chemotherapy did not have an increased rate of second malignancies and actually had a decrease in the incidence of cancer in the contralateral testis. In a Norwegian series, the use of chemotherapy plus infradiaphragmatic radiation did increase the relative risk of second cancers over that seen with infradiaphragmatic radiation alone (RR = 1.3 versus 2.4).[165] The highest risk was seen in patients who received both infradiaphragmatic and supradiaphragmatic radiation. An update of the Norwegian experience confirmed a modest increase in relative risk from the use of combined-modality therapy.[166] The use of modern cisplatin-containing chemotherapy alone did not appear to increase the risk of a second cancer.

In a cohort of 1,025 German patients treated between 1970 and 1990, 224 received surgery only, 332 had radiation therapy, and 413 received chemotherapy, which in 293 cases included etoposide.[167] The incidence of secondary neoplasms increased in patients receiving radiation therapy but not in those who received chemotherapy. The median follow-up in this review was relatively short (61 months). In a more recent review from France of 131 patients with seminoma, the relative risk of second tumors was not increased by infradiaphragmatic radiation. It was increased threefold, however, in patients receiving both infradiaphragmatic and supradiaphragmatic radiation, and it was increased 26-fold in the small number of patients who received chemotherapy plus radiation.[168]

No increases in second cancers have been reported after the use of cisplatin, vinblastine, and bleomycin (PVB) for testicular cancer.[169] Etoposide is now used rather than vinblastine because a randomized trial demonstrated the improved effectiveness of cisplatin, etoposide, and bleomycin over PVB.[170] The association between etoposide and secondary leukemia in the pediatric population led to a more detailed scrutiny of this relationship in patients with testicular cancer. Among 315 patients at Indiana University receiving etoposide, two cases of acute leukemia (0.63%) occurred.[171] Of 340 patients treated with etoposide at Memorial Sloan-Kettering Cancer Center, two cases of acute leukemia also were seen.[172] The overall conclusion of these and other reviews of etoposide use is that the dosages used in most germ cell cancer protocols are associated with a slightly increased risk of acute leukemia that is acceptable, given the benefits of etoposide-based therapy in treating this disease.[173] It has been hypothesized that the total dose of epipodophyllotxin determines the risk of secondary AML, but researchers at the Cancer Therapy Evaluation Program (CTEP) have shown no such effect in patients receiving up to 5 g/m² of etoposide.[174]

The largest review of second neoplasms in patients with testicular cancer includes data for almost 29,000 men in 16 different tumor registries.[175] Overall, 1,406 second cancers were identified, yielding a relative risk of 1.43. An excess number of tumors were reported, including leukemias (RR = 3.07 to 5.20), melanoma (RR = 1.69), lymphoma (RR = 1.88), and a variety of gastrointestinal tumors (RR = 1.27 to 2.21). An analysis of the relationship between treatment and these new tumors revealed that the gastrointestinal tumors were associated with radiation therapy, whereas the secondary leukemia was associated with both radiation and chemotherapy.

Patients Receiving High-Dose Therapies

High-dose chemotherapy with autologous bone marrow transplantation (ABMT) or peripheral blood stem cell transplantation is being used with increased frequency for treating patients with hematologic malignancies and breast cancer. In this setting, very high doses of drugs are given over a short period of time, in contrast to the more conventional method of giving lower doses over a period of 4 to 12 months. The agents used differ slightly depending on the institution and tumor being treated, but commonly the oxazaphosphorine nitrogen mustards (cyclophosphamide and ifosfamide), carboplatin, and etoposide are used. The doses delivered with marrow rescue are threefold to sixfold higher than can be given with such support; thus, the total dose of drug delivered is similar to that given when such drugs are used in conventional regimens. In addition, patients frequently receive total body irradiation (TBI) as part of their preparative regimen. Myelodysplastic syndrome (MDS) and ANLL have been reported in patients who receive allogeneic, autologous, or peripheral blood transplantation for a variety of malignancies.[176,177] Most patients who have an ABMT, however, also receive other chemotherapy before this procedure, which confounds estimation of risk. A review of all 649 patients who received ABMT or peripheral blood stem cell transplantation at the University of Chicago from 1985 to 1997 revealed seven cases (1%) of MDS, ALL, or ANLL that were thought to be therapy-related.[178] These occurred in five patients with Hodgkin's disease, one patient with non-Hodgkin's lymphoma, and one patient with breast cancer. The median latency period between initial standard-dose treatment of the cancer and development of leukemia/MDS was approximately 5 years, whereas the interval was less than 2 years from the high-dose therapy. In a retrospective analysis of 262 patients undergoing ABMT for non-Hodgkin's lymphoma at the Dana-Farber Cancer Institute from 1982 to 1991, the overall incidence of post-transplant MDS or AML was 7.6%, with a median onset of 31 months after transplant or 69 months after initial treatment of lym-

phoma. Variables predicting for development of MDS included prolonged interval between initial treatment and the transplant, increased duration of exposure to chemotherapy, and use of radiation therapy before transplant.[179] Both of these studies suggest that conventional chemotherapy before the high-dose therapy was the more likely cause.

In a situation in which high-dose therapy is given repeatedly, however, the risk of secondary leukemia may become prohibitive. In a series of 86 patients with poor-risk solid tumors treated with repeated high doses of cyclophosphamide/ifosfamide, etoposide, and doxorubicin, the risk of ANLL at 24 months increased 5,000-fold.[180] Cytogenetic analysis was consistent with leukemias induced both by alkylators and by etoposide. The risk of subsequent development of treatment-related MDS or AML may be greater for patients transplanted with CD34 + peripheral stem cells following chemotherapy priming, compared with patients receiving cells from the bone marrow without priming.[181] The type and doses of alkylating agent used pretransplantation in addition to the dose of total body irradiation as part of the conditioning regimen may influence the risk of treatment-related MDS/AML. In a case-control study of 56 patients with MDS/AML and 168 matched controls within a cohort of 2,739 patients receiving autotransplants for Hodgkin's disease or non-Hodgkin's lymphoma, mechlorethamine less than 50 mg/m² and more than 50 mg/m² had a relative risk of 2.0 and 4.3, respectively, and chlorambucil given for fewer than 10 months and more than 10 months had a relative risk of 3.8 and 8.4, respectively, when compared with cyclophosphamide-based therapy. Total body irradiation at doses of 12 Gy or less had no influence on the development of AML/MDS, but doses of 1.2 Gy were associated with a relative risk of 4.6. Peripheral blood stems cells were associated with a nonsignificant risk of MDS/AML with relative risk of 1.8.[182]

Autologous stem cell transplant has been used for patients with breast cancer. As in other malignancies, the risk of AML/MDS appears to depend on the pretransplant chemotherapy. In a retrospective analysis of 364 patients with lymph node-positive breast cancer and who underwent autologous stem cell transplant, only one (0.27%) developed AML. The AML, which was FAB M4 with an 11q23 translocation, was diagnosed 18 months after receiving three cycles of epirubicin and cyclophosphamide.[183] The Netherlands Working Party on Transplantation in Solid Tumors reported similar results. Eight hundred eighty-five patients were randomized to two cycles of 5-fluorouracil, epirubicin, and cyclophosphamide (FEC) versus high-dose chemotherapy and autologous stem cell transplantation after completing three cycles of FEC. The high-dose chemotherapy regimen consisted of cyclophosphamide, thiotepa, and carboplatin. At a median follow-up of 57 months, 15 patients in the conventional therapy arm and 21 patients in the high-dose chemotherapy arm developed a second malignancy. One patient in the conventional dose group had a diagnosis of MDS/AML.[184] The Eastern Cooperative Oncology Group reported very different results. Five hundred eleven patients received six cycles of cyclophosphamide, doxorubicin, and 5-fluorouracil (CAF) and then randomized to no further therapy versus high-dose chemotherapy and stem cell transplantation. The high-dose chemotherapy consisted of cyclophosphamide and thiotepa. Similar to The Netherlands Study, there were more second malignancies in the high-dose chemotherapy group, 9 versus 15; however, no patients in the conventional therapy group had a diagnosis of MDS/AML, whereas 9 patients in the high-dose chemotherapy group developed MDS/AML.[185]

The University of Minnesota reported on the development of second malignancies in 3,372 patients who underwent stem cell transplants for various diseases from January 1974 through March 2001. There were 147 post-transplant malignancies in 137 patients; 24 of the malignancies were either nonmelanoma skin cancer or carcinoma in situ. This represented an 8.1-fold increased risk of post-transplant malignancy. The standardized incidence ratio (SIR) was 300 for MDS/AML, 54.3 for non-Hodgkin's lymphoma including post-transplant lymphoproliferative disorder, 14.8 for Hodgkin's disease, and 2.8 for solid tumors. For MDS/AML, the cumulative incidence plateaued at 1.4% by 10 years following transplant, but the cumulative incidence of developing a solid tumor did not plateau and was 3.8% at 20 years post-transplant.[186] A higher incidence of solid malignancies was reported by the City of Hope in their analysis of 2,129 patients who had undergone bone marrow transplant for hematologic malignancies. The estimated cumulative probability for developing a solid cancer was 6.1% at 10 years. The risk was particularly elevated for liver cancer with an SIR of 27.7, cancer of the oral cavity with SIR of 17.4, and cervical cancer with SIR of 13.3. Both patients with liver cancer had hepatitis C infection and all patients with squamous cell carcinoma of the skin had chronic graft-versus-host disease. The risk was highest for survivors who were younger than 34 years at the time of transplant. Cancers of the thyroid, liver, and oral cavity occurred primarily in patients who had received total body irradiation.[187] The development of solid tumors over a prolonged period warrants close long-term monitoring of these patients.

Patients who receive allogeneic transplants are also demonstrated to have an increased risk of solid tumors.[177] One advantage in analyzing this population is the existence of good registries for many of the patients. In an analysis of 19,229 patients at 235 centers, the relative risk of solid tumors at 10 years was 8.3; the cumulative incidence was 2.2% at 10 years and 6.7% at 15 years. Solid tumors with a notable increase in risk included tumors of the skin, oral cavity, central nervous system, connective tissue, and liver. A younger age and higher dose of total-body irradiation predicted for a higher relative risk. The increased risk of skin and oral cavity tumors was primarily related to the presence of graft-versus-host disease. Osteosarcomas have been reported in four patients undergoing bone marrow transplant for ALL (three patients) and sickle cell disease (one patient). All four patients received alkylating agents and three received total body irradiation. The osteosarcoma arose at an age (adolescence) and site (around the knee) typical for the disease.[188]

Patients Receiving Cyclophosphamide Therapy

Bladder toxicity associated with the use of the oxazaphosphorine nitrogen mustards cyclophosphamide and ifosfamide has been long recognized.[189] The acute cystitis is likely related to toxic metabolites and can be limited by the concomitant use of mesna. An increased number of reports have now been published of bladder cancer in patients who received long-term cyclophosphamide therapy.[190,191] The most common situations in which this occurs are in some pediatric protocols, in low-grade lymphomas, and in immunosuppressive therapy. A review of a cohort of 6,171 medium-term or long-term survivors of non-Hodgkin's lymphoma revealed 48 cases of urothelial cancer.[191] Overall, a 4.5-fold increase in risk of bladder cancer was estimated from the use of cyclophosphamide; however, the cumulative dose was critical in determining risk. In patients who received more than 50 g of cyclophosphamide, the risk increased 15-fold, which translated to an absolute risk of 7% within 15 years of treatment. The long-term use of cyclophosphamide is now less common in treating pediatric and adult cancers; however, the risk of secondary urothelial cancer may be an important consideration in decisions about therapy in immunologic diseases.

Patients Receiving Immunosuppressive Agents

Cytotoxic agents such as azathioprine and cyclophosphamide are also immunosuppressive agents and have been used in the treatment of rheumatoid arthritis, scleroderma, Wegener's granulomatosis, nephrotic syndrome, and glomerulonephritis, as well as in the control of rejection in renal transplantation.[192-194]

Accumulated experience with these and other immunosuppressive agents suggests a different mechanism of tumor induction from that observed in patients treated for neoplastic conditions. Patients treated with immunosuppressive agents have a high incidence of malignant lymphomas, often with evidence of the presence of Epstein-Barr virus, which show a predilection for primary sites in the brain; this may be from long-term immunosuppression resulting in decreased immune surveillance. This state resembles the chronic immunodeficiency of certain inherited disorders, such as Wiskott-Aldrich syndrome, which is also associated with a high incidence of lymphomas.[195]

Nucleoside analogs are known to be potent immunosuppressors. They have been used in hematologic malignancies such as chronic lymphocytic leukemia (CLL) and hairy cell leukemia (HCL). A review of 2,014 patients treated by National Cancer Institute protocols with fludarabine for relapsed or refractory CLL, and 2'-deoxycoformycin (DCF) and 2-chlorodeoxyadenosine (CdA) for HCL. Although comparison with the SEER database demonstrated an increased incidence of secondary malignancies for fludarabine and CdA compared with that of a normal population, the values were consistent with the increase already associated with these diseases. Consequently, these cytotoxic/immunosuppressive agents do not appear to increase the risk of secondary malignancies in CLL and HCL.[196]

Further evidence supporting the contention that long-term immunosuppression contributes to neoplastic induction is found in the experience of inadvertent engraftment of human tumors in donor kidneys. In one case, immunosuppression led to the development of a tumor of donor origin, but tumor rejection occurred rapidly after cytotoxic therapy ceased. Immunosuppression is not an entirely satisfactory explanation for the high incidence of lymphomas in transplant patients because long-term alkylating-agent therapy leads to nonlymphocytic leukemia in patients with multiple myeloma or ovarian carcinoma. Continued investigations into the role of immune surveillance in carcinogenesis are necessary to define the mechanisms responsible for the development of neoplasms in immunosuppressed patients. The complex interaction of various factors (such as the interleukins and interferons) is being defined. How antineoplastic drugs interact with these factors must be defined before the impact of antineoplastic agents on immune surveillance is known.

CONCLUSION

Both clinical and laboratory studies have implicated alkylating agents and epipodophyllotoxins as potent carcinogens. Strong evidence exists for carcinogenicity in laboratory systems for the antitumor antibiotics and procarbazine; the clinical evidence suggests less of a risk. Antimetabolites as a group are much less hazardous, likely because of fewer interactions with DNA. Newer agents such as the topoisomerase I inhibitors and the taxanes have not been used for a sufficient duration to allow estimation of any carcinogenic risk. Long-term immunosuppression with azathioprine has led to an increased incidence of lymphoid malignancies, perhaps by an entirely different mechanism than those producing mutagenic effects. The combined use of chemotherapy and radiotherapy definitely increases the risk of tumor induction. All of this, however, must be interpreted in the context of the need to successfully treat a potentially lethal primary cancer.

The available data suggest that certain guidelines should be followed in the design, use, and follow-up of chemotherapy (and radiation therapy) for patients with potentially curable diseases. A careful surveillance must be conducted for secondary neoplasms during long-term follow-up of these patients. An attempt should be made to establish the quantitative risk of neoplasia for any regimen that proves curative, and efforts should be made to limit the use of the more highly carcinogenic agents. On the basis of present information, caution is required when using alkylating agents or epipodophyllotoxins. Careful prospective and retrospective studies should be aimed at establishing whether a total-dose threshold exists for carcinogenicity of suspected carcinogens in humans and whether modification of the schedule of administration affects this risk. Pharmacogenetic factors may soon play a role in determining the most appropriate therapy to reduce the risk of secondary malignancies. Finally, further attention should be directed to the development of new agents that do not have mutagenic or cytotoxic actions, but that exert regulatory actions on cell growth and differentiation.

REFERENCES

1. Haddow A. Mode of action of chemical carcinogens. Br Med Bull 1947;4:331–342.
2. Lerner HJ. Acute myelogenous leukemia in patients receiving chlorambucil as long-term adjuvant chemotherapy for stage II breast cancer. Cancer Treat Rep 1978;62:1135–1138.
3. Fisher B, Rockette H, Fisher ER, et al. Leukemia in breast cancer patients following adjuvant chemotherapy or postoperative radiation: the NSABP experience. J Clin Oncol 1985;3:1640–1658.
4. Boice JD, Greene MH, Killen JY, et al. Leukemia after adjuvant chemotherapy with semustine (methyl-CCNU). N Engl J Med 1986;314:119–120.
5. Kapadia SB, Krause JR, Ellis LD, et al. Induced acute non-lymphocytic leukemia following long-term chemotherapy. Cancer 1980;45:1315–1321.
6. Rizzo SC, Ricevuti G, Gamba G, et al. Multimodal treatment in operable breast cancer. BMJ 1981:283–437.
7. Miller A. Carcinogenesis by chemicals: an overview— G.H.A. Clowes Memorial Lecture. Cancer Res 1970;30:559–576.
8. Farber E. Carcinogenesis—cellular evolution as a unifying thread: presidential address. Cancer Res 1973;33:2537–2550.
9. Miller EC. Some current perspectives on chemical carcinogenesis in humans and experimental animals: presidential address. Cancer Res 1978;38:1479–1496.
10. Pitot HC. The molecular biology of carcinogenesis. Cancer 1993;72:962–970.
11. Keller R. Suppression of natural antitumor defense mechanisms by phorbol esters. Nature 1979;282:729–731.
12. Price CC, Gaucher GM, Koneru P, et al. Mechanism of action of alkylating agents. Ann N Y Acad Sci 1969;163:593–600.
13. Singer B. Sites in nucleic acids reacting with alkylating agents of differing carcinogenicity or mutagenicity. J Toxicol Environ Health 1977;2:1279–1295.
14. Alban, JM, Wild, C, Rollinson, S, et al. Polymorphism in glutathione S-transferase P1 is associated with susceptibility to chemotherapy-induced leukemia. PNAS 2001;98:11592–11597.
15. Haase, D, Binder, Bunger, J et al. Increased risk for therapy-associated hematologic malignancies in patients with carcinoma of the breast and combined homozygous gene deletions of glutathione transferases M1 and T1. Leukemia Res 2002;226:249–254.
16. Kelly KM, Perentis JP. Polymorphisms of drug metabolizing enzymes and markers of genotoxicity to identify patients with

Hodgkin's lymphoma at risk of treatment-related complications. Ann Oncol 2002;13(Suppl1):34–39.

17. Hagan CR, Rubin CM. Mobile genetic element and genotoxic cancer therapy: potential clinical implications. Am J PharmacoGenomics 2002;2:25–35.

18. Zarbl H, Sukumar S, Arthur AV, et al. Direct mutagenesis of ha-ras-1 oncogenes by N-nitroso-N-methylurea during initiation of mammary carcinogenesis in rats. Nature 1985;315:382–385.

19. Nath J, Krichna G. Fundamental and applied genetic toxicology. In: Craig E, Stitzel RE, eds. Modern Pharmacology with Vlinical Applications. Boston: Little, Brown and Company, 1997:69–77.

20. McCann J, Ames BN. A simple method of detecting environmental carcinogens as mutagens. Ann N Y Acad Sci 1976;271:5–13.

21. McCann J, Choi E, Yamasaki E, et al. Detection of carcinogens as mutagens in the Salmonella/microsome test: assay of 300 chemicals. Proc Natl Acad Sci U S A 1975;72:5135–5139.

22. McCann J, Ames BN. Detection of carcinogens as mutagens in the Salmonella/microsome test: assay of 300 chemicals [discussion]. Proc Natl Acad Sci U S A 1975;73:950–954.

23. Seino Y, Nagao M, Yahagi T, et al. Mutagenicity of several classes of antitumor agents to Salmonella typhimurium TA98, TA100, and TA92. Cancer Res 1978;38:2148–2156.

24. Brundrett RB, Colvin M, White EH. Comparison of mutagenicity, antitumor activity, and chemical properties of selected nitrosoureas and nitrosoamides. Cancer Res 1979;39:1328–333.

25. Genther CS, Schoeny RS, Loper JC. Mutagenic studies of folic acid antagonists. Antimicrob Agents Chemother 1977;12:84–92.

26. Benedict WF, Baker MS, Haroun L, et al. Mutagenicity of cancer chemotherapeutic agents in the Salmonella/ microsome test. Cancer Res 1977;37:2209–2213.

27. Rinkus SJ, Legator MS. Chemical characterization of 465 known or suspected carcinogens and their correlation with mutagenic activity in the Salmonella typhimurium system. Cancer Res 1979;39:3289–3318.

28. Albertini RJ, Castle KL, Borcherding WR. T-cell cloning to detect the mutation 6-thioguanine-resistant lymphocytes present in human peripheral blood. Proc Natl Acad Sci U S A 1982;79:6617–6621.

29. Hirota H, Kubota M, Hashimoto H, et al. Analysis of hprt gene mutation following anti-cancer treatment in pediatric patients with acute leukemia. Mutat Res 1993;319:113–120.

30. Hirota H, Kirota M, Adachi A, et al. Somatic mutation at T-cell antigen receptor and glycophorin A loci in pediatric leukemia patients following chemotherapy: comparison with HPRT locus mutation. Mutat Res 1994;315:95–103.

31. Musalis JC, Monteforte JA, Winegar RA. Transgenic animal models for detection of in vivo mutations. Annu Rev Pharmacol Toxicol 1995;35:145–164.

32. Kato H. Spontaneous and induced sister chromatid exchanges as revealed by the BUdr-labeling method. Int Rev Cytol 1977;49:55–97.

33. Perry P, Evans HJ. Cytological detection of mutagen-carcinogen exposure by sister chromatid exchange. Nature 1977;258:121–125.

34. Guerrero PR, Rounds DE, Hall TC. Bioassay procedure for the detection of mutagenic metabolites in human urine with the use of sister chromatid exchange analysis. J Natl Cancer Inst 1979;62:805–809.

35. Banerjee A, Benedict WF. Production of sister chromatid exchanges by various cancer chemotherapeutic agents. Cancer Res 1979;39:797–799.

36. Lambert B, Ringborg U, Harper E, et al. Sister chromatid exchanges in lymphocyte cultures of patients receiving chemotherapy for malignant disorders. Cancer Treat Rep 1979;62:1413–1419.

37. Lambert B, Ringborn U, Linblad A, et al. The effects of DTIC, melphalan, actinomycin D and CCNU on the frequency of sister chromatid exchanges in peripheral lymphocytes of melanoma patients. In: Jones, Salmon SE, eds. Adjuvant Therapy of Cancer II. New York: Grune & Stratton, 1979:55–62.

38. Ohtsuru M, Ishi Y, Takai S, et al. Sister chromatid exchanges in lymphoctyes of cancer patients receiving mitomycin C treatment. Cancer Res 1980;40:477–480.

39. Heidelberger C. Chemical oncogenesis in culture. Cancer Res 1973;18:317–366.

40. Heidelberger C. Chemical carcinogenesis. Cancer 1977;40:430–433.

41. Benedict WF, Banerjee A, Gardner A. Induction of morphological transformation in mouse C3H/10T1/2 clone 8 cells and chromosomal damage in hamster A(T1)C1-3 cells by cancer chemotherapeutic agents. Cancer Res 1977;37:2202–2208.

42. Jones PA, Benedict WF, Baker MS. Oncogenic transformation of C3H/10T1/2 clone 8 mouse embryo cells by halogenated pyrimidine nucleosides. Cancer Res 1976;36:101–107.

43. Gabrielson EW, Harris CC. Use of cultured human tissues and cells in carcinogenesis research. J Cancer Res Clin Oncol 1985;110:1–10.

44. Schamhl D, Habs M. Experimental carcinogenesis of antitumor drugs. Cancer Treat Rev 1978;5:175–184.

45. Weisburger JH, Griswald DP, Prejean JD, et al. The carcinogenic properties of some of the principal drugs used in clinical cancer chemotherapy: recent results. Cancer Res 1975;52:1–17.

46. Weisburger EK. Bioassay program for carcinogenic hazards of cancer chemotherapeutic agents. Cancer 1977;40:1935–1949.

47. Solcia E, Ballerini L, Bellini O, et al. Mammary tumors induced in rats by Adriamycin and daunomycin. Cancer Res 1978;38:1444–1446.

48. Sieber SM, Adamson RH. Toxicity of antineoplastic agents in man: chromosomal aberrations, antifertility effects, congenital malformations and carcinogenic potential. Cancer Res 1978;22:57–155.

49. Harris C. Chemical and physical carcinogenesis: advances and perspectives for the 1990s. Cancer Res 1991;151:5023S–5044S.

50. Sugamiua H, Weston A, Caporaso NE. Biochemical and molecular epidemiology of cancer. Biomed Environ Sci 1991;4:73–92.

51. Harris RA, Yang A, Stein RC, et al. Cluster analysis of an extensive human breast cancer cell line protein expression map database. Proteomics 2002;2:2122–2223.

52. Pucci-Minafra I, Fontana S, Cancemi P, et al. Proteomic patterns of cultured breast cancer cells and epithelial mammary cells. Ann N Y Acad Sci 2002;963:122–139.

53. Wu W, Tang X, Hu W, et al. Identification and validation of metastasis associated proteins in head and neck cancer cell lines by two-dimensional electrophoresis and mass spectrometry. Clin Exp Metastasis 2002;19:319–326.

54. Smith MA, McCaffrey RP, Karp JE. The secondary leukemias: challenges and research directions. J Natl Cancer Inst 1996;88:407–418.

55. Bokemeyer C, Schmoll HJ. Treatment of testicular cancer and the development of secondary malignancies. J Clin Oncol 1995;13:283–292.

56. Van Leeuwen F. Second cancers. In: DeVita VT Jr, Hellman S, Rosenberg SA, eds. Cancer: Principles and Practice of Oncology. 6th Ed. Philadelphia: Lippincott, 2001:2939–2964.

57. Travis, LB. Therapy associated solid tumors. Acta Oncologica 2002;41:323–333.

58. Makuch R, Simon R. Recommendations for the analysis of the effect of treatment on the development of second malignancies. Cancer 1979;44:250–253.

59. Gleevec [package insert]. Novartis Pharmaceuticals Corp; East Hanover, NJ 2005.

60. Hughes RG, Colquhoun M, Alloub M, et al. Cervical intraepithelial neoplasia in patients with breast cancer: a cytological and colposcopic study. Br J Cancer 1993;67:1082–1085.

61. Islam MQ, Kopf I, Levan A, et al. Cytogenetic findings in 111 ovarian cancer patients: therapy-related chromosome aberrations and heterochromatic variants. Cancer Genet Cytogenet 1993;65:35–46.

62. De Wit PE, de Vaan GA, de Boo TM, et al. Prevalence of naevocytic naevi after chemotherapy for childhood cancer. Med Pediatr Oncol 1990;18:336–338.

63. Baird EA, McHenry PM, MacKie RM. Effect of maintenance chemotherapy in childhood on numbers of melanocytc naevi. Br J Med 1992;305:35–36.

64. Li FP, Abramson DH, Tarone RE, et al. Hereditary retinoblastoma, lipoma and second primary cancer. J Natl Cancer Inst 1997;89:83–84.

65. Tucker MA, D'Angi GJ, Boice JD, et al. Bone sarcomas linked to radiotherapy and chemotherapy in children. N Engl J Med 1987;317:588–593.

66. Tucker MA, Meadows AT, Boice JD, et al. Leukemia after therapy with alkylating agents for childhood cancer. J Natl Cancer Inst 1987;78:459–464.

67. Neglia JP, Friedman DL, Yasui Y, et al. Second malignant neoplasms in five-year survivors of childhood cancer: childhood cancer survivor study. J Natl Cancer Inst 2001;93:618–629.

68. Winick NJ, McKenna RW, Shuster JJ, et al. Secondary acute myeloid leukemia in children with acute lymphoblastic leukemia treated with etoposide. J Clin Oncol 1993;11:209–217.

69. Pui CH, Ribeiro RC, Hancock ML, et al. Acute myeloid leukemia in children treated with epipodophyllotoxins for acute lymphoblastic leukemia. N Engl J Med 1991;325:1682–1687.

70. Kreissman SG, Gelber RD, Cohen HJ, et al. Incidence of secondary acute myelogenous leukemia after treatment of childhood acute lymphoblastic leukemia. Cancer 1992;70:2208–2213.

71. Kimball Dalton VM, Gelber RD, Li F, et al. Second malignancies in patients treated for childhood acute lymphoblastic leukemia. J Clin Oncol 1998;16:2848–2853.

72. Felix CA. Secondary leukemias induced by topoisomerase-targeted drugs. Biochim Biophys Acta 1998;1400:233–255.

73. Smith MC, Rubinstein L, Ungerleider RS. Therapy-related acute myeloid leukemia following treatment with epipodophyllotoxins: estimating the risk. Med Pediatr Oncol 1994;23:86–98.

74. Smith MA, Rubinstein L, Anderson JR, et al. Secondary leukemia or myelodysplastic syndrome after treatment with epipodophyllotoxins. J Clin Oncol 1999;17:569–577.

75. Kushner BH, Cheung NKV, Kramer K, et al. Neuroblastoma and treatment related myelodysplasia/leukemia: the MSKCC experience. J Clin Oncol 1998;16:3880–3889.

76. Green DM, Zevon MA, Reese PA, et al. Second malignant tumors following treatment during childhood and adolescence for cancer. Med Pediatr Oncol 1994;22:1–10.

77. Jankovic M, Fraschini D, Amici A, et al. Outcome after cessation of therapy in childhood acute lymphoblastic leukaemia. Eur J Cancer 1993;29A:1839–1843.

78. Morland BJ, Radford M. Cutaneous squamous cell carcinoma following treatment for acute lymphoblastic leukaemia. Med Pediatr Oncol 1993;21:150–152.

79. Dunst J, Ahrens S, Paulussen M, et al. Second malignancies after treatment for Ewing's sarcoma: a report of the CESS- studies. Int J Radiat Oncol Biol Phys 1998;42:379–384.

80. Fuchs, B, Valenzuela, RG Petersen, IA, et al. Ewings sarcoma and the development of secondary malignancies. Clin Orthop Relat Res 2003;415:82–89.

81. Aung L, Gorlick RG, Shi W, et al. Second malignant neoplasms in long-term survivors of osteosarcoma: Memorial Sloan-Kettering Cancer center experience. Cancer 2002;95:1728–1734.

82. Wolden SL, Lamborn KR, Cleary SF, et al. Second cancers following pediatric Hodgkin's disease. J Clin Oncol 1998;16:536–544.

83. Bhatia S, Yasui Y, Robison LL, et al. High risk of subsequent neoplasms continue with extended follow-up of childhood Hodgkin's disease: report from the Late Effects Study Group. J Clin Oncol 2003;21:4386–4394.

84. Travis LB, Hill DA, Dores GM, et al. Breast cancer following radiotherapy and chemotherapy among young women with Hodgkin disease. JAMA 2003;290:465–470.

85. Horwich A, Swerdlow AJ. Second primary breast cancer after Hodgkin's disease. Br J Cancer 2004;90:294–298.

86. Schellong G, Potter R, Bramswig J, et al. High cure rates and reduced long-term toxicity in pediatric Hodgkin's disease: the German-Austrian multicenter trial DAL-HD-90-The German-Austrian Pediatric Hodgkin's Disease Study Group. J Clin Oncol 1999;17:3736–3744.

87. Wong FL, Boice JD, Abramson DH, et al. Cancer incidence after retinoblastoma:radiation dose and sarcoma risk. JAMA 1997;278:1262–1267.

88. Breslow NE, Takashima JR, Whitton JA, et al. Second malignant neoplasms following treatment for Wilms' tumor: a report from the National Wilms tumor Study Group. J Clin Oncol 1995;13:1851–1859.

89. Bagley CM, Young RC, Canellos GP, et al. Treatment of ovarian carcinoma: possibilities for progress. N Engl J Med 1972;287:856–862.

90. Einhorn N. Acute leukemia after chemotherapy (melphalan). Cancer 1978;41:444–447.

91. Sotrel G, Jafari K, Lash AF, et al. Acute leukemia in advanced ovarian carcinoma after treatment with alkylating agents. Obstet Gynecol 1976;47:67S–71S.

92. Morrison J, Yon JL. Acute leukemia following chlorambucil therapy of advanced ovarian and fallopian tube carcinoma. Gynecol Oncol 1978;6:115–120.

93. Casciato DA, Scott JL. Acute leukemia following prolonged cytotoxic agent therapy. Medicine 1979;53:32–47.

94. Reimer PR, Hoover R, Fraumeni J, et al. Acute leukemia after alkylating-agent therapy of ovarian cancer. N Engl J Med 1977;297:177–181.

95. Greene MH, Harris EL, Gershenson DM, et al. Melphalan may be a more potent leukemogen than cyclophosphamide. Ann Intern Med 1986;105:360–367.

96. Kaldor JM, Day NE, Pettersson F, et al. Leukemia following chemotherapy for ovarian cancer. N Engl J Med 1990;322:1–6.

97. Travis LB, Curtis RE, Boice JD, et al. Second malignant neoplasms among long-term survivors of ovarian cancer. Cancer Res 1996;56:1564–1570.

98. Sprance HE, Hempling RE, Piver MS. Leukemia following cis-platin-based chemotherapy for ovarian carcinoma. Eur J Gynecol Oncol 1992;13:131–137.

99. Reed E, Evans MK. Acute leukemia following cisplatin-based chemotherapy in a patient with ovarian cancer. J Natl Cancer Inst 1990;82:431–432.

100. Carbone PP, Bauer M, Baud P, et al. Chemotherapy of disseminated breast cancer: current status and prospects. Cancer 1977;39:2916–2922.

101. Chan PYM, Sadoff L, Winkley JH. Second malignancies following first breast cancer in prolonged thio-TEPA adjuvant chemotherapy. In: Salmon SE, Jones SE, eds. Adjuvant Therapy of Cancer. Amsterdam: North-Holland, 1977:597–607.

102. Fisher B, Glass A, Redmond C, et al. L-phenylalanine mustard (L-PAM) in the management of primary breast cancer: an update of earlier findings and a comparison with those utilizing L-PAM plus 5-fluorouracil (5-FU). Cancer 1977;39:2883–2903.

103. Valagussa P, Tancini G, Bonadonna G. Second malignancies after CMF for resectable breast cancer. J Clin Oncol 1987;5:1138–1142.

104. Valagussa P, Moliterni A, Terenziani M, et al. Second malignancies following CMF-based adjuvant chemotherapy in resectable breast cancer. Ann Oncol 1994;5:803–808.

105. Arriagada R, Rutqvist LE. Adjuvant chemotherapy in early breast cancer and incidence of new primary malignancies. Lancet 1991;338:535–538.

106. Ben Yehuda, D, Krichevsky, S, Caspi, O, et al. Microsatellite instability and p53 mutations in therapy-related leukemia suggest mutator phenotype. Blood 1996;88:4296–4303.

107. Pederson-Bjergaard J, Siqsgaard T, Nielsen D, et al. Acute monocytic or myelomonocytic leukemia with balanced chromosome translocations to band. 11q23 after therapy with 4 epidoxorubicin and cisplatin or cyclophosphamide for breast cancer. J Clin Oncol 1992;10:1444–1451.

108. Diamandidou E, Buzdar AU, Smith TL, et al. Treatment-related leukemia in breast cancer patients treated with fluorouracil-doxorubicin-cyclophosphamide combination adjuvant chemotherapy: the University of Texas M.D. Anderson Cancer Center experience. J Clin Oncol 1996;14:2722–2730.

109. Chaplain G, Milan C, Sgro et al. Increased risk of acute leukemia after adjuvant chemotherapy for breast cancer: a population based study. J Clin Oncol 2000;18:2836–2842.

110. Curtis RE, Boice JD, Moloney WC, et al. Leukemia following chemotherapy for breast cancer. Cancer Res 1990;50:2741–2746.

111. Curtis RE, Boice JD, Stovall M, et al. Risk of leukemia after chemotherapy and radiation treatment for breast cancer. N Engl J Med 1990;326:1745–1751.

112. Henne T, Schmahl D. Occurrence of second primary malignancies in man—a second look. Cancer Treat Rev 1985;12:77–94.

113. Neugut AI, Murray T, Santos J, et al. Increased risk of lung cancer after bresat cancer radiation therapy in cigarette smokers. Cancer 1994;73:1615–1620.

114. Yap J, Chuba PJ, Thomas R, et al. Sarcoma as a second malignancy after treatment for breast cancer. Int J Rad Oncol Biol Phys 2002;52:1231–1237.
115. Brady MS, Garfein CF, Petrek JA, et al. Post-treatment sarcoma in breast cancer patients. Ann Surg Oncol 1994;1:66–72.
116. Rutqvist LE. Long-term toxicity of tamoxifen. Cancer Res 1993;127:257–266.
117. Satyaswaroop PG, Zaino RJ, Marbel R. Estrogen-like effects of tamoxifen on human endometrial carcinoma transplanted into nude mice. Cancer Res 1984;44:4006–4010.
118. Fornander T, Rutqvist LE, Cedermark B, et al. Adjuvant tamoxifen in early breast cancer: occurrence of new primary cancers. Lancet 1989;1:117–120.
119. Andersson M, Storm HH, Mouridsen HT. Incidence of new primary cancers after adjuvant tamoxifen therapy and radiotherapy for early breast cancer. J Natl Cancer Inst 1991;83:1013–1017.
120. Ribeiro G, Swindell R. The Christie Hospital adjuvant tamoxifen trial. Monogr Natl Cancer Inst 1992;11:121–125.
121. Fisher B, Costantino JP, Redmond CK, et al. Endometrial cancer in tamoxifen-treated breast cancer patients: findings from the National Surgical Adjuvant Breast and Bowel Project (NSABP) B-14. J Natl Cancer Inst 1994;86:527–537.
122. Braithwaite RS, Cchlebowski RT, Lau J, et al. Meta-analysis of vascular and neoplastic events associated with Tamoxifen. Journal of General Internal Medicine 2003;18:37–47.
123. Seoud MA, Johnson J, Weed JC. Gynecological tumors in tamoxifen-treated women with breast cancer [review]. Obstet Gynecol 1993;82:165–169.
124. Fornander T, Hellstrom AC, Moberger B. Descriptive clinico-pathologic study of 17 patients with endometrial cancer during or after adjuvant tamoxifen in early breast cancer. J Natl Cancer Inst 1993;85:1850–1855.
125. Magriples U, Naftolin F, Schwartz PE, et al. High-grade endometrial carcinoma in tamoxifen-treated breast cancer patients. J Clin Oncol 1993;11:485–490.
126. Katase K, Sugiyama Y, Hasumi K, et al. The incidence of subsequent endometrial carcinoma with tamoxifen use in patients with primary breast cancer. Cancer 1998;82:1698–1703.
127. Rutqvist LE, Johansson H, Signomklao T, et al. Adjuvant tamoxifen therapy for early stage breast cancer and second primary malignancies. J Natl Cancer Inst 1995;87:645–651.
128. Fisher B, Costantino J, Redmond C, et al. A randomized clinical trial evaluating tamoxifen in the treatment of patients with node negative breast cancer. N Engl J Med 1989;320:479–484.
129. Stewart HJ. The Scottish trial of adjuvant tamoxifen in node-negative breast cancer: Scottish Cancer Trials Breast Group. Monogr Natl Cancer Inst 1992;11:117–120.
130. Rutqvist LE, Cedermark B, Glas U, et al. Contralateral primary tumors in breast cancer patients in a randomized trial of adjuvant tamoxifen therapy. J Natl Cancer Inst 1991;83:1299–1306.
131. Rubagotti A, Perrotta A, Casella C, et al. Risk of new primaries after chemotherapy and/or tamoxifen treatment for early breast cancer. Ann Oncol 1996;7:239–244.
132. Ragaz J, Coldman A. Survival impact of adjuvant tamoxifen on competing causes of mortality in breast cancer survivors. J Clin Oncol 1998;16:2018–2024.
133. Friedman MA, Trimble EL, Abrams JS. Tamoxifen: trials, tribulations, and tradeoffs. J Natl Cancer Inst 1994;86:478–479.
134. Rosner F, Grunwald H. Multiple myeloma terminating in acute leukemia. Am J Med 1974;57:927–939.
135. Kyle RA, Pierre RV, Bayard ED. Multiple myeloma and acute leukemia associated with alkylating agents. Arch Intern Med 1975;135:185–192.
136. Bergsagel DE, Bailey AJ, Langley GR, et al. The chemotherapy of plasma-cell myeloma and the incidence of acute leukemia. N Engl J Med 1979;301:743–748.
137. Sieber SM. Cancer chemotherapeutic agents and carcinogenesis. Cancer Chemother Rep 1975;59:915–918.
138. Moertel CG, Hagedorn AB. Leukemia or lymphoma and coexistent primary malignant lesions: a review of the literature and study of 120 cases. Blood 1957;12:788.
139. Tucker MA, Coleman CN, Cox RS, et al. Risk of second cancers after treatment for Hodgkin's disease. N Engl J Med 1988;318:76–81.
140. Krikorian JG, Burke JS, Rosenberg SA, et al. Occurrence of non-Hodgkin's lymphoma after therapy for Hodgkin's disease. N Engl J Med 1979;300:452–458.
141. Canellos GP, Arseneau JC, De Vita VT, et al. Second malignancies complicating Hodgkin's disease in remission. Lancet 1975;1:947–949.
142. Arseneau JC, Canellos GP, Johnson R, et al. Risk of new cancers in patients with Hodgkin's disease. Cancer 1977;40:1912–1916.
143. Rodriguez MA, Fuller LM, Zimmerman SO, et al. Hodgkin's disease: study of treatment intensities and incidences of second malignancies. Ann Oncol 1993;4:125–131.
144. Van Leeuwen FE, Chorus AM, van den Belt-Dusebout AW, et al. Leukemia risk following Hodgkin's disease: relation to cumulative dose of alkylating agents, treatment with teniposide combinations, number of episodes of chemotherapy, and bone marrow damage. J Clin Oncol 1994;12:1063–1073.
145. Brusamolini E, Anselm AP, Klersy C, et al. The risk of acute leukemia in patients treated for Hodgkin's disease is significantly higher after combined modality programs than after chemotherapy alone and is correlated with the extent of radiotherapy and type and duration of chemotherapy: a case-control study. Haematologica 1998;83:812–823.
146. Travis LB, Curtis RE, Stovall M, et al. Risk of leukemia following treatment for non-Hodgkin's lymphoma. J Natl Cancer Inst 1994;86:1450–1457.
147. Hancock SL, Tucker MA, Hoppe RT. Breast cancer after treatment of Hodgkin's disease. J Natl Cancer Inst 1993;85:25–31.
148. Sont JK, van Stiphout WA, Noordijk EM, et al. Increased risk of second cancers in managing Hodgkin's disease: the 20-year Leiden experience. Ann Hematol 1992;65:213–218.
149. Henry-Amar M. Second cancers after treatment of Hodgkin's disease: experience at the International Database on Hodgkin's disease (IDHD). Bull Cancer 1992;79:389–391.
150. Abrahamsen JF, Andersen A, Hannisdal E, et al. Second malignancies after treatment of Hodgkin's disease: the influence of treatment, follow-up time, and age. J Clin Oncol 1993;11:255–261.
151. Boice JD. Second cancer after Hodgkin's disease—the price of success? J Natl Cancer Inst 1993;85:4–5.
152. Swerdlow AJ, Douglas AM, Vaughn Hudson G, et al. Risk of second primary cancers after Hodgkin's disease by type of treatment. Br J Med 1992;304:1137–1143.
153. Slanina J, Heinemann F, Henne E, et al. Second malignancies after the therapy of Hodgkin's disease: the Freiburg collective 1940 to 1991. Strahlenther Onkol 1999;175:154–161.
154. Josting A, Wiedenmann S, Franklin J, et al. Secondary myeloid leukemia and myelodysplastic syndromes in patients treated for Hodgkin's disease: a report from the German Hodgkin's lymphoma study group. J Clin Oncol 2003;21:3440–3446.
155. Duggan, D, Petroni, G, Johnson, J, et al. Randomized comparison of ABVD and MOPP/ABV hybrid for the treatment of advanced Hodgkin's disease: report of an intergroup trial. J Clin Oncol 2003;21:607–614.
156. Travis, LB, Gospodarowicz, M, Curtis, RE, et al. Lung cancer following chemotherapy and radiotherapy for Hodgkin's disease. J Natl Cancer Inst 2002;94:182–192.
157. Salloum E, Doria R, Schubert W, et al. Second solid tumors in patients with Hodgkin's disease cured after radiation or chemotherapy plus adjuvant low-dose radiation. J Clin Oncol 1996;14:2435–2443.
158. Blayney DW, Longo DL, Young RC, et al. Decreasing risk of leukemia with prolonged follow-up after chemotherapy and radiotherapy for Hodgkin's disease. N Engl J Med 1987;316:710–714.
159. Meadows AT, Baum E, Fossati-Bellani F, et al. Second malignant neoplasms in children: an update from the Late Effects Study Group. J Clin Oncol 1985;3:532–538.
160. Glanzmann C, Veraguth A, Lutolf UM. Incidence of second solid cancer in patients after treatment of Hodgkin's disease. Strahlenther Onkol 1994;170:140–146.
161. Andre M, Mounier N, Leleu X, et al. Second cancers and late toxicities after treatment of aggressive non-Hodgkin lymphoma with the ACVBP regimen: a GELA chort study on 2837 patients. Blood 2004;103:122–128.

162. Armitage JO, Carbone PP, Connors JM, et al. Treatment realated myelodysplasia and acute leukemia in non-Hodgkin's lymphoma patients. J Clin Oncol 2004;21:897–906.

163. Finazzi G, Ruggeri M, Rodeghiero F et al. Second malignancies in patients with essential thrombocythaemia treated with busulphan and hydroxyurea: long-term follow-up of a randomized clinical trial. Br J Haematol 2002;116:923–924.

164. Van Leeuwen FE, Stiggelbout AM, van den Belt AW, et al. Second cancer risk following testicular cancer. J Clin Oncol 1993;11:415–424.

165. Fossa SD, Langmark F, Aass N, et al. Second non-germ cell malignancies after radiotherapy of testicular cancer with or without chemotherapy. Br J Cancer 1990;61:639–643.

166. Wanderas EJ, Fossa SD, Tretli S. Risk of subsequent non–germ cell cancer after treatment of germ cell cancer in 2006 Norwegian male patients. Eur J Cancer 1997;33:253–262.

167. Bokemeyer C, Schmoll HJ. Secondary neoplasms following treatment of malignant germ cell tumors. J Clin Oncol 1993;11:1703–1709.

168. Bachaud JM, Berthier F, Souile M, et al. Second non-germ cell malignancies in patients treated for state I–II testicular seminoma. Radiother Oncol 1999;50:191–197.

169. Nichols CR, Hoffman R, Einhorn LJ, et al. Hematologic malignancies associated with primary mediastinal germ cell tumors. Ann Intern Med 1985;102:603–609.

170. Williams SD, Birch R, Einhorn LH, et al. Treatment of disseminated germ-cell tumors with cisplatin, bleomycin and either vinblastine or etoposide. N Engl J Med 1987;316:1435–1440.

171. Nichols CR, Breeden ES, Loehrer PJ, et al. Secondary leukemia associated with a conventional dose of etoposide: review of serial germ cell tumor protocols. J Natl Cancer Inst 1993;85:36–40.

172. Bajorin DF, Motzer RJ, Rodriguez E, et al. Acute nonlymphocytic leukemia in germ cell tumor patients treated with etoposide-containing chemotherapy. J Natl Cancer Inst 1993;85:60–62.

173. Kollmannsberger C, Beyer J, Droz JP, et al. Secondary leukemia following high cumulative doses of etoposide in patients treated for advanced germ cell tumors. J Clin Oncol 1998;16:3386–3391.

174. Smith, MA, Rubinstein, L, Anderson, JR, et al. Secondary leukemia or myelodysplastic syndrome after treatment with epipodophyllotxins. J Clin Oncol 1999;17:569–77.

175. Travis LB, Curtis RE, Storm H, et al. Risk of second malignant neoplasms among long-term survivors of testicular cancer. J Natl Cancer Inst 1997;89:1429–1439.

176. Oddou S, Vey N, Viens P, et al. Second neoplasms following high-dose chemotherapy and autologous transplantation for malignant lymphomas. Leuk Lymphoma 1998;31:187–194.

177. Curtis RE, Rowlings PA, Deeg HJ, et al. Solid cancers after bone marrow transplantation. N Engl J Med 1997;336:897–904.

178. Sobecks RM, Le Beau MM, Anastasi J, et al. Myelodysplasia and acute leukemia following high-dose chemotherapy and autologous bone marrow or peripheral blood stem cell transplantation. Bone Marrow Transplant 1999;23:1161–1165.

179. Stone RM, Neuberg D, Soiffer R, et al. Myelodysplastic syndrome as a late complication following autologous bone marrow transplantation for non-Hodgkin's lymphoma. J Clin Oncol 1994;12:2535–2542.

180. Kushner BH, Heller G, Cheung N, et al. High risk of leukemia after short-term dose-intensive chemotherapy in young patients with solid tumors. J Clin Oncol 1998;16:3016–3020.

181. Pedersen-Bjergaard J, Andersen KM, Christiansen DH. Therapy-related acute myeloid leukemia and myelodysplasia after high-dose chemotherapy and autologogous stem cell transplant. Blood 2000;95:3273–3279.

182. Metayer C, Curtis RE, Vose J, et al. Myelodysplastic syndrome and acute myeloid leukemia after autotransplantation for lymphoma: a multicenter case-control study. Blood 2003;101:1015–1023.

183. Kroger N, Zander AR, Martinelli G, et al. Low incidence of secondary myelodysplasia and acute myeloid leukemia after high-dose chemotherapy as adjuvant therapy for breast cancer patients: a study by the Solid Tumors Working Party of the European Group for Blood and Marrow Transplantation. Ann Oncol 2003;14:554–558.

184. Rodenhuis S, Bontenbal M, Beex LVAM, et al. High-dose chemotherapy with hematopoietic stem-cell rescue for high-risk breast cancer. N Engl J Med 2003;349:7–16.

185. Tallman MS, Gray R, Robert NJ, et al. Conventional adjuvant chemotherapy with or without high-dose chemotherapy and autologous stem-cell transplantation in high-risk breast cancer. N Engl J Med 2003;349:17–26.

186. Baker KS, DeFor TE, Burns LJ, et al. New malignancies after blood or marrow stem-cell transplantation in children and adults: incidence and risk factors. J Clin Oncol 2003;21:1352–1358.

187. Bhatia S, Louie AD, Bhatia R, et al. Solid cancers after bone marrow transplantation. J Clin Oncolo 2001;19:464–471.

188. Bielack SS, Rerin JS, Dickerhoff R, et al. Osteosarcoma after allogeneic bone marrow transplantation. A report of four cases from the Cooperative Osteosarcoma Study Group (COSS). Bone Marrow Transplantation 2003;31:353–359.

189. Siu LL, Moore MJ. Evidence based guidelines: use of mesna in the prevention ofifosfamide induced urotoxicity. Support Care Cancer 1998;6:144–152.

190. Inagaki T, Ebisuno S. Cyclophosphamide induced urinary bladder and renal pelvic tumor: a case report. Nippon Hinyokika Gakkai Zasshi 1998;89:674–677.

191. Travis LB, Curtis RE, Glimelius B, et al. Bladder and kidney cancer following cyclophosphamide therapy for non- Hodgkin's lymphoma. J Natl Cancer Inst 1995;87:524–530.

192. Roberts MM, Bell R. Acute leukemia after immunosuppressive therapy. Lancet 1976;2:768–770.

193. Penn I. Second malignant neoplasms associated with immunosuppressive medication. Cancer 1976;37:1024–1032.

194. Steinberg AD, Plotz PH, Wolff SM, et al. Cytotoxic drugs in treatment of nonmalignant disease. Ann Intern Med 1972;76:619–642.

195. Penn I. Occurrence of cancer in immune deficiencies. Cancer 1974;34:858–866.

196. Cheson BD, Vena DA, Barrett J, et al. Second malignancies as a consequence of nucleoside analog therapy for chronic lymphoid leukemias. J Clin Oncol 1999;17:2454–2460.

Antifolates

6

Brian P. Monahan   *Carmen J. Allegra*

The folate-dependent enzymes represent attractive targets for antitumor chemotherapy because of their critical role in the synthesis of the nucleotide precursors of DNA (Fig. 6.1). In 1948, Farber and associates[1] were the first to show that aminopterin, a four-amino analog of folic acid, could inhibit the proliferation of leukemic cells and produce remissions in acute leukemia cases. Their findings ushered in the era of antimetabolite chemotherapy and generated great interest in the antifolate class of agents. Since then, the clinical value of antifolate compounds has been proven in the treatment of a variety of hematologic and nonhematologic malignancies. Their clinical application has also extended to the treatment of non-neoplastic disorders, including rheumatoid arthritis,[2] psoriasis,[3] bacterial and plasmodia infections,[4] and opportunistic infections.[5] The antifolates are one of the best understood and most versatile of all the cancer chemotherapeutic drug classes (Table 6.1).

MECHANISM OF ACTION

Substitution of an amino group for the hydroxyl at position 4 of the pteridine ring is the critical change in the structure of antifolate compounds that leads to their antitumor activity. This change transforms the molecule from a substrate to a tight-binding inhibitor of dihydrofolate reductase (DHFR), a key enzyme in intracellular folate homeostasis. The critical importance of DHFR stems from the fact that folic acid compounds are active as coenzymes only in their fully reduced tetrahydrofolate form. Two specific tetrahydrofolates play essential roles as one-carbon carriers in the synthesis of DNA precursors. The cofactor 10-formyltetrahydrofolate provides its one-carbon group for the de novo synthesis of purines in reactions mediated by glycineamide ribonucleotide (GAR) transformylase and aminoimidazole carboxamide ribonucleotide (AICAR) transformylase. A second cofactor, 5,10-methylenetetrahy-

drofolate (CH_2-FH_4), donates its one-carbon group to the reductive methylation reaction, converting deoxyuridylate to thymidylate (Fig. 6.1). In addition to contributing a one-carbon group, 5,10-methylenetetrahydrofolate is oxidized to dihydrofolate, which must then be reduced to tetrahydrofolate by the enzyme DHFR for it to rejoin the pool of active reduced-folate cofactors. In actively proliferating tumor cells, inhibition of DHFR by methotrexate (MTX) or other 2,4-diamino antifolates leads to an accumulation of folates in the inactive dihydrofolate form, with variable depletion of reduced folates.[6-12] Folate depletion, however, does not fully account for the metabolic inhibition associated with antifolate treatment because the critical reduced-folate pools may be relatively preserved even in the presence of cytotoxic concentrations of MTX. Additional factors may contribute to MTX-associated cytotoxicity, including metabolism of the parent compound to polyglutamated derivatives and the accumulation of dihydrofolate polyglutamates as a consequence of DHFR inhibition.[6,7,13-15] Methotrexate and dihydrofolate polyglutamates represent potent direct inhibitors of the folate-dependent enzymes of thymidylate and purine biosynthesis.[16-21] Thus, inhibition of DNA biosynthesis by 2,4-diamino folates is a multifactorial process consisting of both partial depletion of reduced-folate substrates and direct inhibition of folate-dependent enzymes. The relative roles of each of these mechanisms in determining antifolate-associated metabolic inhibition may depend on specific cellular factors that vary among different cancer cell lines and tumors.

CHEMICAL STRUCTURE

Various heterocyclic compounds with the 2,4-diamino configuration have antifolate activity and include pyrimidine analogs such as pyrimethamine and trimethoprim[18-25]; classical pteridines such as aminopterin and

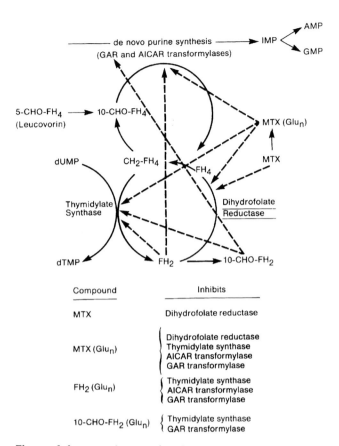

Figure 6.1 Sites of action of methotrexate (MTX), its polyglutamated metabolites (MTX[(Glu$_n$]), and folate byproducts of the inhibition of dihydrofolate reductase, including dihydrofolate (FH$_2$) and 10-formyldihydrofolate (10-CHO-FH$_2$). Also shown are 5,10-methylenetetrahydrofolate (CH$_2$-FH$_4$), the folate cofactor required for thymidylate synthesis, and 10-formyltetrahydrofolate (10-CHO-FH$_4$), the required intermediate in the synthesis of purine precursors. AICAR; aminoimidazole carboxamide ribonucleotide; AMP, adenosine monophosphate; dUMP, deoxyuridylate; dTMP, thymidylate; GAR; glycineamide ribonucleotide; GMP, guanosine monophosphate; IMP, inosine monophosphate. (From DeVita VT, Hellman S, Rosenberg SA, eds. Cancer: Principles and Practice of Oncology. Philadelphia: JB Lippincott, 1989:349–397.)

	TABLE 6.1

KEY FEATURES OF METHOTREXATE SODIUM (MTX)

Mechanism of action	Inhibition of dihydrofolate reductase leads to partial depletion of reduced folates
	Polyglutamates of MTX and dihydrofolate inhibit purine and thymidylate biosynthesis
Metabolism	Converted to polyglutamates in normal and malignant tissues. 7-Hydroxylation in liver
Pharmacokinetics	$t_{1/2}\alpha = 2-3$ h; $t_{1/2}\beta = 8-10$ hr
Elimination	Primarily as interact drug in urine
Drug interactions	Toxicity to normal tissues rescued by leucovorin calcium
	L-Asparaginase blocks toxicity and antitumor activity
	Pretreatment with MTX increases 5-fluorouracil and cytosine arabinoside nucleotide formation
	Nonsteroidal anti-inflammatory agents decrease renal clearance and increase toxicity
Toxicity	Myelosuppression
	Mucositis, gastrointestinal epithelial denudation
	Renal tubular obstruction and injury
	Hepatotoxicity
	Pneumonitis
	Hypersensitivity
	Neurotoxicity
Precaution	Reduce dose in proportion to creatinine clearance
	Do not administer high-dose MTX to patients with abnormal renal function
	Monitor plasma concentrations of drug, hydrate patients during high-dose therapy (see Tables 6.2 and 6.4)

$t_{1/2}$, half-life

CELLULAR PHARMACOLOGY AND MECHANISMS OF RESISTANCE

In this section, the sequence of events that leads to the cytotoxic action of MTX is considered, beginning with drug movement across the cell membrane, followed by its intracellular metabolism to the polyglutamate derivatives, binding to DHFR and other folate-dependent enzymes, effects on intracellular folates, and, finally, inhibition of DNA synthesis.

Transmembrane Transport

Folate influx into mammalian cells proceeds via two distinct transport systems: (a) the reduced-folate carrier (RFC) system, and (b) the folate receptor (FR) system (Fig. 6.2).[31–34] The proliferative or kinetic state of tumor cells influences the rate of folate and MTX transport. In general, rapidly

MTX[2]; and compounds with replacement of the nitrogen at either the 5 or 8 position, or both, with a carbon atom, such as the quinazolines (trimetrexate, piritrexim)[22,23] and 10-ethyl-10-deazaaminopterin (10-EDAM, Edatrexate).[24] Investigators have designed antifolate analogs directed at targets other than DHFR, including those folate-dependent enzymes required for the de novo synthesis of purines and thymidylate synthase. A host of potent thymidylate synthase (TS) inhibitors such as 10-propargyl-5,8-dideazafolate (PDDF, CB3717)[26] and closely related compounds raltitrexed (ZD1694, Tomudex) and ZD9331,[27] pemetrexed (LY231514, Alimta),[28] 1843U89,[29] and 5,8-dideazatetrahydrofolic acid (DDATHF, lometrexol) and LY231514,[30] both inhibitors of GAR transformylase, have been investigated.

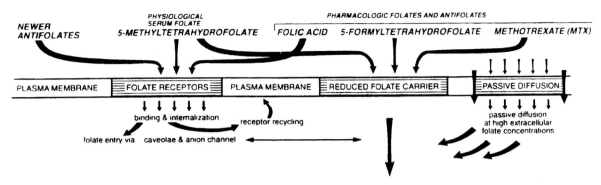

Figure 6.2 Transport systems identified for the physiologic folates and various antifolates. (Adapted from Antony AC. The biological chemistry of folate receptors. Blood 1992;79:2807–2820.)

dividing cells have a greater rate of MTX uptake and a lower rate of drug efflux than cells that are either in the stationary phase or that are slowly growing.[35] The RFC system, with its large transport capacity, transports folic acid inefficiently (K_t [transport coefficient] = 200 μmol/L) and is a primary transport mechanism of the reduced folates and antifolates like MTX (K_t = 0.7 to 6.0 μmol/L), at pharmacologic drug concentrations.[36–38] The RFC system also transports the naturally occurring reduced folates, including the rescue agent 5-formyltetrahydrofolate (leucovorin).[32,33,39–42] Studies have mapped the RFC gene to the long arm of chromosome 21, and this site encodes a protein with predicted molecular size of 58 to 68 kd.[43–44] Several mutations in the RFC have been identified in drug-resistant cell lines, including glutamic acid residue 45, that have been associated with MTX resistance.[45,46,47] In cells grown under relatively acidic conditions, as may be expected in watershed areas of solid tumor masses, even cell lines with absent RFC have been demonstrated to transport MTX via an RFC-independent pathway[48].

In the second folate transport mechanism, FRs mediate the internalization of folates via a high-affinity membrane-bound 38-kd glycoprotein. The FR gene family encodes three homologous glycoproteins that share a similar folate-binding site. The α and β FRs are anchored to the plasma membrane by a carboxyl-terminal glycosylphosphatidylinositol tail and transport the reduced folates and MTX at a lower capacity than the RFC system. The function of the FR is unknown. The FRs are expressed in normal tissues and, at high levels, on the surface of some epithelial tumors such as ovarian cancer.[49,50] The FR system has a 10-fold to 30-fold higher affinity for folic acid and the reduced folates (K_a [dissociation constant] = 1 to 10 μmol/L) than for MTX. In addition, MTX polyglutamates demonstrate a 75-fold increased affinity for FR compared with the monoglutamate form of MTX.[51] Variation in exogenous folate concentrations and normal physiologic conditions, such as pregnancy, can alter the tissue expression of FR. Intracellular levels of homocysteine, which increase under folate-deficient conditions, appear to be the critical modu-lator of the translational up-regulation of FRs.[52] Under conditions of relative folate deficiency, elevated levels of homocysteine stimulate the interaction between heterogeneous nuclear ribinucleoprotein E1 with an 18 base-pair region in the 5'-untranslated region of the FR mRNA resulting in increased translational efficiency, and therefore elevated cellular levels of FR protein. This mechanism serves as an example, in addition to thymidylate synthase and dihydrofolate reductase, of translational efficiency as a mechanism for protein level regulation in the folate biosynthetic pathways.

The FR isoforms (α, β, γ) are independently expressed in mammalian cells and normal human tissues.[53] FR-α is expressed in human epithelial neoplasms (ovarian cancer and nasopharyngeal KB carcinoma cells) where it is up-regulated by folate depletion and down-regulated in folate-replete medium.[31,37] Elwood et al.[54] and other colleagues[55,56] have shown that FR-α is expressed in a complex manner involving promoters upstream from exons 1 and 4 and differential messenger RNA (mRNA) splicing of 5' exons. FR-β is expressed in human placenta and nonepithelial tumors. FR-γ, found in hematopoietic and lymphatic cells and tissues, lacks a glycosylphosphatidylinositol membrane anchor and is secreted. Although human FR-α, FR-β, and FR-γ share 70% amino acid sequence homology, they differ in binding affinities for stereoisomers of folates.[57]

Although the precise mechanism of FR-mediated folate uptake remains controversial,[58] two separate pathways for FR-mediated folate uptake have been reported: (a) the classic receptor-mediated internalization of the ligand-receptor complex through clathrin-coated pits with subsequent formation of secondary lysosomes, and (b) a mechanism of small molecule uptake, termed potocytosis,[59–61] in which receptor complexes accumulate within distinct subdomains of the plasma membrane known as caveolae that internalize to form intracellular vesicles.[62] Once internalization has occurred, acidification within the vesicle causes the folate- receptor complex to dissociate and translocate across the cell membrane. Although questions remain as to the relative importance of the FR and RFC transport systems in the uptake of antifolates during chemotherapy, studies suggest that the RFC system is the more relevant transporter of MTX in mammalian cells, even in cells expressing high levels of FR.[63,64]

Both in vitro and in vivo experimental systems have identified defective transport as a common mechanism of intrinsic or acquired resistance to MTX. A number of MTX-resistant cell lines with functional defects in the RFC have now been described.[65-68] An MTX-resistant human lymphoblastic CCRF-CEM/MTX cell line maintained in physiologic concentrations of folate (2 nmol/L) lacked the RFC protein and, for this reason, were resistant to MTX[69]. These cells retained the folate-binding protein, however, and were able to use this transport process to maintain growth even in nanomolar concentrations of folic acid. This study is of particular interest because the concentration of folate used was in the physiologic range, and thus this mechanism of transport-mediated resistance may have direct clinical relevance.

Zhao et al. have characterized a mutated murine RFC (RFC1) with increased affinity for folic acid and decreased affinity for MTX, which suggests that amino acids in the first predicted transmembrane domain, in particular glutamic acid residue 45, play an important role in determining the spectrum of affinities for, and mobility of, RFC1. This domain is also a cluster region for mutations that occur when cells are placed under selective pressure with antifolates that use RFC1 as the major route of entry into mammalian cells.[70,71] Of interest, however, is that of 121 samples of malignant cells from patients with ALL, none contained a mutation of glutamic acid residue 45.[72] To identify clinical MTX resistance on the basis of impaired transport, a sensitive competitive displacement assay using the fluorescent analog of MTX was developed.[73] An analysis of 17 patients with acute lymphoblastic leukemia (ALL) revealed that blast cells from two of four patients in relapse after initial treatment with MTX-based combination chemotherapy demonstrated defective MTX transport. In 40 patients with newly diagnosed ALL, low RFC expression at diagnosis was found to correlate with a significantly reduced event-free survival.[74] These studies offer evidence that impaired transport may play a role in the development of clinical MTX resistance in patients with ALL. Using semiquantitative reverse-transcription polymerase chain reaction techniques, Guo et al.[75] investigated MTX resistance in tumors obtained from patients with high-grade osteosarcoma. In this study, 17 of 26 tumor samples (65%) derived from patients with poor response to chemotherapy had decreased RFC expression. Poor response to MTX-based chemotherapy was also observed in osteosarcoma samples with low levels of RFC at diagnosis.[76] These authors concluded that impaired transport of MTX may be a common mechanism of intrinsic resistance in osteosarcoma. An interesting use of the RFC as both a selectable and suicide gene in gene therapy has been recently described.[77] Transduction of bone marrow cells with RFC resulted in selection of transfected cells following exposure to trimetrexate, presumably from the increased cellular folate levels and enhanced sensitivity to MTX exposure. Such technology may be useful for enriching cells transduced with various genes that may have therapeutic value. For an in-depth analysis of RFC activity as it relates to transport-mediated MTX resistance, the reader is referred to recent reviews on this subject.[78,79]

Significant differences in the characteristics of antifolate drug transport have prompted interest in the development of new analogs. The nonglutamated antifolates such as trimetrexate and piritrexim, as well as the glutamyl esters of MTX, do not require active cellular transport and demonstrate activity against transport-resistant mutants.[80,81] The compound 10-EDAM is more avidly accumulated in tumor cells than in normal bone marrow or intestinal epithelium and has broader therapeutic activity and less marrow toxicity than MTX in experimental systems.[25,82]

In contrast to MTX, which has a relatively poor affinity for the folate-binding proteins, several antifolate inhibitors such as CB3717, raltitrexed, DDATHF, pemetrexed (LY231514), and BW1843U89 rely heavily on the high-affinity folate binding proteins for cellular transport.[83,84] Because several of these compounds are efficiently transported by either folate transport system, they may be less susceptible to the emergence of clinical resistance resulting from alterations in membrane transport. Although pemetrexed is transported by both the RFC and FR systems, recent investigations have uncovered an alternative route with a high affinity for this agent in particular.[85,86] This alternative transport system provides a mechanism for continued drug sensitivity even in cells that may have low levels of FR and absent RFC. Homofolate is a DHFR inhibitor that is primarily transported by the folate-binding proteins and has extremely potent activity against malignant cells overexpressing this protein, and thus may be useful for the treatment of human solid tumors that have developed MTX resistance either because of down-regulation or alterations of the RFC system.[87] In addition, low-folate conditions that up-regulate FR expression may have clinical relevance. Research has demonstrated that mice maintained on a low-folate diet had higher FR expression on their normal tissues and experienced significantly greater toxicity with the antifolate lometrexol, which suggests the potential for a human corollary in cancer patients with poor nutritional intake.[88]

Trimetrexate and piritrexim have demonstrated only modest activity against human solid tumors.[89,90] Trimetrexate combined with leucovorin calcium has significant activity against the pulmonary pathogen *Pneumocystis carinii*, whose DHFR enzyme is highly sensitive to this combination.[5,91] The compound 10-EDAM has clinical activity against a variety of human solid tumors. Its dose-limiting toxicity is mucositis rather than the myelosuppression normally associated with MTX therapy.[92] Phase II testing has shown this agent to be active in the treatment of non–small cell lung cancers, soft tissue sarcomas, and breast cancers, with overall response rates of 17%, 14%, and 41%, respectively.[93–95]

For many years, at least two poorly defined efflux mechanisms for MTX and the folates have been described including a bromosulfophthalein and probenecid sensitive pathway.[96–98] Recent investigations have identified the multidrug resistance-associated protein family of ATP-binding cassette transporters (MRP-1, -2, -3 and -4) as responsible for cellular MTX efflux with MRP-1 probably representing the primary route.[99–102] Overexpression of this efflux pump has been associated with MTX resistance, and the use of inhibitors such as probenecid have been shown to reverse antifolate resistance.[103] Interestingly, it has also been demonstrated that loss of MRP-1 expression may result in antifolate resistance through the expansion of intracellular folate pools, a condition that is well known to be associated with MTX resistance.[104] In addition to the MRP family of proteins, the breast cancer resistance protein has also been shown to be associated with the cellular efflux of MTX and MTX polyglutamates with 2 or 3 glutamic acid residues and overexpression of this protein has also been associated with MTX resistance.[105–107]

Intracellular Transformation

Naturally occurring folates exist within cells in a polyglutamated form. The polyglutamation of folate substrates is facilitated by folylpolyglutamyl synthetase (FPGS), an enzyme that adds up to four to six glutamyl groups in γ peptide linkage. This reaction serves three main purposes for folates: (a) it facilitates the accumulation of intracellular folates in vast excess of the monoglutamate pool that is freely transportable into and out of cells, (b) it allows selective intracellular retention of these relatively large anionic molecules and thus prolongs intracellular half-life, and (c) it enhances folate cofactor affinity for several folate-dependent enzymes. The MTX polyglutamates are more potent inhibitors of DHFR, TS, AICAR transformylase, and GAR transformylase than is MTX-Glu$_1$[13,14] Methotrexate and the other glutamyl-terminal analogs also undergo polyglutamation in normal liver cells, bone marrow myeloid precursors,[108,109] human fibroblasts, and a variety of leukemic and carcinoma cell lines.[109,110–112]

The efficiency of the polyglutamation reaction depends on the particular folate substrate and may vary widely among the antifolate compounds. The polyglutamation of MTX occurs over 12 to 24 hours of exposure, at which time most intracellular drug exists in the polyglutamate form.[110,113] In the few studies of polyglutamate formation in vivo, 80% or more of MTX in both normal and malignant tissues was shown to exist in the form of polyglutamates.[114,115] Human liver retains MTX polyglutamates for several months after drug administration.[116] Thus, the selective retention and depot formation in excess of free

monoglutamate, as seen with physiologic folates, appears to characterize MTX polyglutamates as well.

FPGS is a 62-kd magnesium-, adenosine triphosphate–, and potassium-dependent protein.[117–120] The most avid substrate for this enzyme is dihydrofolate (K_m [binding affinity] = 2 μmol/L) > tetrahydrofolate (K_m = 6 μmol/L) > 10-formyltetrahydrofolate or 5-methyltetrahydrofolate > aminopterin > leucovorin > MTX. Because of the relatively slow rate of formation of MTX polyglutamates compared with the naturally occurring folates, reductions in FPGS activity or cellular glutamate levels that have little effect on folate polyglutamate pools may have critical effects on the level of MTX polyglutamates and on the ultimate cytotoxicity of MTX. Some have postulated that the relatively inefficient metabolism of 5-methyltetrahydrofolate (the predominant folate present in human serum) to its polyglutamate form may be responsible for the folate depletion that occurs in vitamin B$_{12}$ deficiency. Lack of B$_{12}$ would inhibit methionine synthetase, which is responsible for the demethylation of 5-methyltetrahydrofolate to tetrahydrofolate, an excellent substrate for FPGS. The accumulation of MTX polyglutamates in liver reduces the polyglutamation of natural folates in that tissue and may, in part, account for the chronic hepatotoxicity associated with MTX. The intracellular content of polyglutamate derivatives represents a balance between the activity of two different enzymes, FPGS and γ-glutamyl hydrolase (GGH, conjugase).[121] The latter, a γ-glutamyl-specific peptidase, removes terminal glutamyl groups and returns MTX polyglutamates to their parent monoglutamate form. Models based on leukemic cells from patients with ALL suggest that the terminal one or two glutamic acid residues are most commonly cleaved by hydrolase.[122]

Yao et al.[123] isolated and cloned the complementary DNA (cDNA) for GGH, which codes for an enzyme of 318 amino acids and has a molecular weight of 36 kD. Although it may be expected that overexpression of hydrolase may result in MTX resistance, particularly with brief drug exposures, such was not the case in several human cell line models in which hydrolase was overexpressed.[124]

MTX polyglutamates exist essentially only within cells and enter or exit cells sparingly.[111,125] The diglutamate form has an uptake velocity of one-fifteenth that of MTX,[126] whereas higher glutamates have even slower transport rates.[111,125] Thus, MTX polyglutamates are selectively retained in preference to parent drug as extracellular levels of MTX fall.

Several parameters influence a cell's ability to polyglutamate MTX. Paramount among these factors is the rate of cell growth[112,127] and the level of intracellular folates.[127,128] Enhancement of cell proliferation with growth factors such as insulin, dexamethasone, tocopherol, and estrogen in hormone-responsive cells increases polyglutamation, whereas deprivation of essential amino acids[129] results in inhibition of polyglutamation. MTX and L-asparaginase are frequently used in combination for the treatment of acute leukemia. Conversion of MTX to polyglutamate forms can be markedly inhibited by preexposure to L-asparaginase, presumably through amino acid deprivation with resultant growth arrest.[130] Increasing intracellular folate pools through exposure of cells to high concentrations of leucovorin or 5-methyltetrahydrofolate results in a decrease in MTX polyglutamation.[128] Conversely, the process is enhanced in human hepatoma cells either by incubating cells with MTX in folate-free medium or by first depleting the intracellular folates by "permeabilizing" cell membranes in a folate-free environment.[127]

An important factor in the selective nature of MTX cytotoxicity may derive from diminished polyglutamate formation in normal tissues relative to that in malignant tissues. Although little metabolism to polyglutamates is observed in normal murine intestinal cells in vivo, most murine leukemias and Ehrlich ascites tumor cells efficiently convert MTX to higher polyglutamate forms in tumor-bearing animals.[38,131] Additionally, normal human and murine myeloid progenitor cells form relatively small amounts of MTX polyglutamates compared with leukemic cells.[108,109]

In addition to increasing its retention within cells, polyglutamation of MTX enhances its inhibitory effects on specific folate-dependent enzymes. The pentaglutamates have a slower dissociation rate from DHFR than does MTX[132] and a markedly enhanced inhibitory potency for TS (K_i = 50 nmol/L), AICAR transformylase (K_i = 57 nmol/L),[163] and, to a lesser extent, GAR transformylase (K_i = 2 μmol/L) in the presence of monoglutamated folate substrates.[12,133] The well-described incomplete depletion of physiologic folate cofactors by MTX suggests that direct enzymatic inhibition by MTX polyglutamates may contribute to MTX cytotoxicity. These effects may also explain the competitive nature of leucovorin rescue and the relatively selective rescue of normal versus malignant tissues, in that rescue may depend on the ability of leucovorin and its derived tetrahydrofolates to compete with MTX polyglutamates at sites other than DHFR.

The ability of antifolate analogs to undergo polyglutamation is one of several properties that influences cytotoxic potency. Aminopterin is a better substrate for FPGS than is MTX, and is a more potent cytotoxic agent. A fluorinated MTX analog, PT430, is a weak substrate for FPGS and has little cytotoxic activity.[134] The ability to generate polyglutamates has been correlated with sensitivity to MTX and to other antifolate agents that undergo polyglutamation, including pemetrexed and raltatrexed, and is frequently found to be defective in drug-resistant human and murine tumor cell lines.[134-138]

Although defective polyglutamation may coexist with other metabolic alterations, examples of pure polyglutamation defects have been described in human leukemia cell lines (CCRF-CEM)[139] and in human squamous cancer cell lines derived from head and neck tumors, and have appear to cause of MTX resistance secondary to decreased

levels of FPGS.[140,141] Faessel et al.[142] evaluated the combined action among polyglutamylatable and nonpolyglutamylatable antifolates directed against various folate-dependent enzymes in human ileocecal HCT-8 cells in vitro and determined that polyglutamation played a critical role in fostering synergy between inhibitors of DHFR and inhibitors of other folate-requiring enzymes. Further evidence for the role of polyglutamation as a determinant of drug sensitivity stems from investigations using other antifolates such as the GAR transformylase inhibitor DDATHF. Polyglutamates of DDATHF were readily formed in cultured human leukemia cell lines and were found to be retained for prolonged periods in drug-free conditions. The FPGS-deficient CCRF-CEM cell line generated few DDATHF polyglutamates and was insensitive to drug exposure.[143] Polyglutamation has been investigated as a determinant of response to MTX in clinical chemotherapy. In a study of six human small cell carcinoma cell lines that had demonstrated resistance in vitro after clinical treatment with MTX, two were resistant on the basis of a low capacity to form MTX polyglutamates.[144] One of seven samples from MTX-resistant leukemic patients demonstrated a decreased ability to form MTX polyglutamates as the sole explanation for resistance.[67] Investigating the reduced accumulation of long-chain MTX polyglutamates in ALL patients, Longo et al.[125] found a decrease in the binding affinity (K_m) of MTX to FPGS from blast cells of patients with acute myelogenous leukemia (AML) as opposed to ALL. This difference in affinity resulted in a predominance of MTX-Glu$_1$ species in AML cells, and MTX Glu$_{3-5}$ in ALL cells. No corresponding disparity in binding affinity was found when the equivalently cytotoxic antifolate TS inhibitors raltitrexed and BW1843U89, which exhibited similar levels of accumulation of the higher polyglutamate forms, were examined. A more recent study suggests that the evaluation of GGH and folylpolyglutamate synthetase activity at the time of clinical diagnosis may be used as a predictor of the extent of MTX polyglutamation and, therefore, of response to MTX therapy and outcome in patients with acute leukemias.[145] Hyperdiploid status in childhood ALL is a good prognostic feature, and patients exhibiting hyperdiploid lymphoblasts show higher levels of synthesis of cytotoxic MTX polyglutamates than patients exhibiting aneuploid or diploid lymphoblasts. Investigators have found a higher concentration of MTX long-chain polyglutamates in T than in B lymphoblasts and an increased level of expression of FPGS mRNA in B-lineage cells.[146,147] These findings suggest that the higher response rates observed in patients with B-cell ALL may result from increased levels of FPGS activity that, in turn, facilitate enhanced intracellular formation of more cytotoxic MTX polyglutamates. However, in a study involving 52 children with B-cell ALL, MTX accumulation and polyglutamation did not appear to have prognostic significance in the context of prolonged oral MTX therapy.[148] This study supports the notion that, under the conditions of continuous drug exposure, the activity of MTX may not depend on cellular polyglutamation to sustain intracellular levels. In fresh tumor specimens from patients with soft tissue sarcomas, 12 of 15 patients were determined to be naturally resistant to MTX as a result of impaired polyglutamation.[149,150]

Binding to Dihydrofolate Reductase

The physical characteristics of binding of NADPH (reduced form of nicotinamide adenine dinucleotide phosphate [NADP]) and MTX to DHFR have been established by x-ray crystallographic studies, nuclear magnetic resonance spectroscopy, amino acid sequencing of native and chemically modified enzyme, and site-directed mutagenesis. Enzyme from microbial, chicken, and mammalian sources have been studied[151–156]; strong amino acid sequence homology is found at positions involved in substrate cofactor and inhibitor binding.[157] In general, a long hydrophobic pocket binds MTX and is formed in part by the isoleucine-5, alanine-7, aspartate-27, phenylalanine-31 (Phe-31), phenylalanine-34 (Phe-34), and other amino acid residues. Several particularly important interactions contribute to the binding potency of the 4-amino antifolates: (a) hydrogen bonding of the carbonyl oxygen of isoleucine-5 to the 4-amino group of the inhibitor; (b) a salt bridge between aspartate and the N-1 position of MTX, which is not involved in binding to the physiologic substrates; (c) hydrophobic interactions of the inhibitor with DHFR, particularly with Phe-31 and Phe-34; (d) hydrogen bonding of the 2-amino group to aspartate-27 and to a structurally consistent bound water molecule; and (e) hydrogen binding of the terminal glutamate to an invariant arginine-70 residue. Investigations have identified the importance of the interactions of MTX with Phe-31 and Phe-34 because mutations in these positions result in a 100-fold and 80,000-fold decrease in MTX affinity for the enzyme, respectively.[158] Mutation of arginine-70 results in a decrease in MTX affinity by >22,000-fold but does not alter the binding affinity of trimetrexate, which lacks the terminal glutamate moiety. This finding supports the essential role of arginine-70 in the binding of inhibitors that preserve the terminal glutamate structure.[159] Mutations outside the enzyme active site also may result in marked reductions in folate and antifolate affinities.[160] In addition, the physiologic substrate dihydrofolate is bound to the enzyme in an inverted, or "upside down," configuration compared with the inhibitor MTX.[155,161] The reader is referred to more detailed reviews of this subject for consideration of substrate and cofactor binding characteristics and mutated DHFR cDNA studies.[153–156,162–165]

Optimal binding of MTX to DHFR depends on the concentration of NADPH. NADH (reduced form of nicotinamide adenine dinucleotide) may also act as a cosubstrate for DHFR but, unlike NADPH, it does not promote binding of MTX to the enzyme.[166] Thus, the intracellular ratios of NADPH/NADP and NADPH/ NADH may play an important role in the selective action of MTX to the extent that the cosubstrate ratios may differ in malignant and in normal tissues.[131,166] In the presence of excess NADPH, the binding affinity of MTX for DHFR has been estimated to lie between 10 and 200 pmol/L,[167,168] although this affinity is significantly affected by pH, salt concentration, and the status of enzyme sulfhydryl groups. Under conditions of low pH and with a low ratio of inhibitor to enzyme, binding is essentially stoichiometric, that is, one molecule of MTX is bound to one molecule of DHFR.

Binding of MTX to DHFR isolated from bacterial and mammalian sources in the presence of NADPH generates a slowly formed ternary complex. The overall process has been termed slow, tight-binding inhibition and involves an initial rapid but weak enzyme-inhibitor interaction followed by a slow but extremely tight-binding isomerization to the final complex.[153,165,169] The final isomerization step probably involves a conformational change of the enzyme with subsequent binding of the para-aminobenzoyl moiety to the enzyme.[154] Other folate analogs, such as aminopterin, follow the same slow, tight-binding kinetic process, in contrast to the pteridines and pyrimethamine, which behave as classic inhibitors of the bacterial enzymes. Trimethoprim is considered to be a classic, albeit weak, inhibitor of mammalian DHFR. Of note, it does not undergo an isomerization process to the ternary complex form.[165]

In the therapeutic setting, MTX acts as a tight-binding but reversible inhibitor. Under conditions of high concentrations of competitive substrate (dihydrofolate) and at neutral intracellular pH, a considerable excess of free drug is required to fully inhibit the enzyme. Both in tissue culture and in cell-free systems, tritium-labeled MTX bound to intracellular enzyme can be displaced by exposure of cells to unlabeled drug, dihydrofolate,[7,170,171] or reduced folates such as leucovorin and 5-methyltetrahydrofolate,[131] which indicates a slow but definite "off rate" or dissociation of MTX from the enzyme.[131,172] Thus, an excess of free, or unbound, drug is required to maintain total inhibition of DHFR.[173]

The polyglutamates of MTX have similar potency in their tight-binding inhibition of mammalian DHFR[110,165,174] and possess a slower rate of dissociation from the enzyme than the parent compound. In pulse-chase experiments using intact human breast cancer cells, MTX pentaglutamate was found to have a dissociation half-life of 120 minutes compared with 12 minutes for the parent compound. Cell-free experiments using purified preparations of mammalian enzyme indicate that MTX polyglutamation has a modest effect in enhancing binding and catalytic inhibition (twofold to sixfold) of DHFR.[12,165,168,175] As with MTX, enzyme-bound MTX polyglutamates may also be displaced by reduced folates[131] and high concentrations of dihydrofolate,[176,177] albeit at a slower rate than MTX.

These observations indicate that, in the absence of free drug, a small fraction of intracellular DHFR, either through new synthesis or through dissociation from the inhibitor, becomes available for catalytic activity and is adequate to allow for continued intracellular metabolism. The requirement for excess free drug to inhibit enzyme activity completely is important in understanding the clinical effects and toxicity of this agent, and is fundamental to the relationship between pharmacokinetics and pharmacodynamics.

Resistance to MTX as a result of decreased DHFR binding affinity for MTX has been described in murine leukemic cells,[160,178,179] Chinese hamster ovary[180] and lung[181] cells, and murine and hamster lung fibroblast cells.[182,183] These mutant enzymes may have several thousand–fold reduced binding affinity for MTX and, in general, are less efficient in catalyzing the reduction of dihydrofolate than is wild-type DHFR.

Drug-sensitive Chinese hamster lung cells have been found to express two different forms of DHFR encoded by distinct alleles.[184,185] The two species differ in molecular weight and isoelectric point (21,000 versus 20,000 and 6.7 versus 6.5) and result from a single amino acid substitution of asparagine for aspartic acid at position 95. Either allele may be predominantly expressed in various subclones of the parent cell line. This observation raises the possibility that distinct naturally occurring DHFR alleles

may exist in a variety of tissues and, to the extent that they may confer differential sensitivity to MTX, this DHFR genetic polymorphism of the host may serve as a mechanism by which cells may become clinically MTX resistant.

DHFR with reduced affinity for MTX may represent a clinically important mechanism of MTX resistance, as this phenomenon was observed in the leukemic cells of 4 of 12 patients with resistant AML.[186] MTX-resistant mutant DHFR has been used as a means to protect and/or select transduced hematopoietic progenitor cells and several laboratories have developed vectors to efficiently transduce human progenitor cells with the hope that such technology could be used to enable the use of higher, and hopefully more effective, doses of chemotherapeutic agents to treat human malignancies.[187,188] A common finding in MTX-resistant cells is an increase in the expression of DHFR protein with no associated change in the enzyme's affinity for MTX. Elevations in DHFR may persist for many generations of cell renewal in tumor cells from resistant patients. In resistant murine leukemic cells, the increased DHFR activity results from reduplication of the DHFR gene (Fig. 6.3), a process that has been shown to occur by exposing murine and human leukemia and carcinoma cells in culture to stepwise increases in the concentration of MTX.[181,184,189–191] Gene reduplication may take the form of a homogeneously staining region (HSR) on chromosomes or nonintegrated

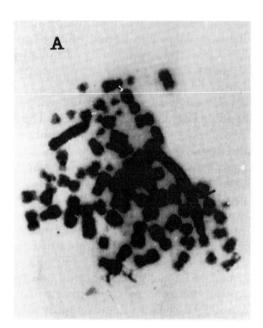
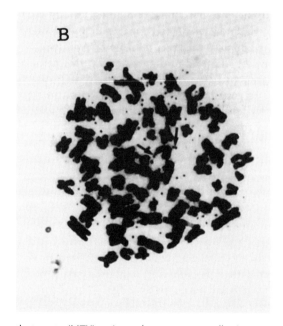

Figure 6.3 **A.** Marker chromosomes found in methotrexate (MTX)-resistant breast cancer cells. A human breast cancer cell line, MCF-7, resistant to MTX was isolated by growing cells in gradually increasing drug concentrations. These cells are resistant to drug concentrations more than 200-fold higher than those that kill wild-type cells and contain more than 30-fold increases in dihydrofolate reductase (DHFR). The arrow indicates a marker chromosome with a greatly expanded homogenously staining region. (Courtesy of National Cancer Institute, Bethesda, MD) **B.** Metaphase plate of a small cell lung cancer carcinoma cell line taken from a patient with clinical MTX resistance. The prominent double-minute chromosomes (arrows) were associated with amplification of the drug target enzyme, DHFR. (From Curt GA, Carney DN, Cowan KH, et al. Unstable methotrexate resistance in human small-cell carcinoma associated with double minute chromosomes. N Engl J Med 1983;308:199–202.)

pieces of DNA known as double-minute chromosomes (Fig. 6.3B). Although HSRs appear to confer stable resistance to the cell, double-minute chromosomes are unequally distributed during cell division,[183,190] and in the absence of the continued selective pressure of drug exposure, the cells revert to the original low-DHFR genotype. Evidence exists that gene amplification occurs initially in the form of double-minute chromosomes because this is the predominant abnormality in low-level drug-resistant cells, whereas HSRs occur in highly resistant cells that contain multiple gene copies.[183,190,191] Other investigations suggest the opposite sequence wherein chromosomal breaks result in HSRs, which are then processed to DMs or not, depending on how different cell types handle extra chromosomal sequences.[192] Another mechanism of gene amplification has been identified in an MTX-resistant HeLA 10B3 cell line in which were found submicroscopic extrachromosomal elements (amplisomes) containing amplified DHFR genes. These amplisomes appeared early in the development of MTX resistance and were not found to be integrated into the chromosome, nor were they associated with double- minute chromosomes. Although these amplisomes were lost in the absence of the selective pressure of MTX, they disappeared at a much slower rate than would be predicted from simple dilution of nonreplicating elements.

Although MTX resistance through DHFR gene amplification becomes apparent only after the prolonged selective pressure of drug exposure, studies indicate that highly MTX-resistant cells may be generated by gene amplification within a single cell cycle.[193] Early S-phase cells exposed transiently to agents that block DNA synthesis (e.g., hydroxyurea) may undergo reduplication of multiple genes synthesized during early S phase, including DHFR, after removal of the DNA synthetic inhibitor. This finding has broad implications for the rapid development of drug resistance in patients treated with MTX and other inhibitors of DNA synthesis. Exposure of cells to a variety of chemical and physical agents unrelated to MTX including hypoxia, alkylating agents,[194] ultraviolet irradiation,[194,195] phorbol esters,[194–196] cis-diamminedichloro-platinum,[197] doxorubicin,[198] and 5-fluorodeoxyuridine[199] may induce MTX resistance through DHFR gene amplification, with subsequent increases in DHFR protein. The induction of MTX resistance by a variety of chemical and physical agents may explain de novo MTX resistance in certain human tumors, given the constant presence of a host of environmental carcinogens. Unlike malignant cells, amplification of DNA has not been reported in normal cells of patients undergoing therapy with cytotoxic agents or in cell lines of normal cells.[200]

In addition to gene amplification, more subtle mechanisms exist for increasing DHFR expression. Molecular analysis of the DHFR gene encoding for overexpressed DHFR protein has occasionally revealed significant differences in non–protein coding regions that may impact mRNA expression.[184] The E2F-1 transcription factor has been shown to promote the transcription of DHFR as well as thymidylate synthase mRNA and has been correlated with the messenger RNA levels of these two enzymes in tumor samples of patients with osteosarcoma.[201] Exposure of human breast cancer cells to MTX results in an acute increase (up to fourfold) in the cellular DHFR content.[202] The expression of DHFR protein in this setting appears to be controlled at the level of mRNA translation, as no acute associated change occurs in the amount of DHFR mRNA or DHFR gene copy number after MTX exposure nor are alterations seen in DHFR enzyme stability. Using an RNA gel mobility shift assay, human recombinant DHFR protein was shown to specifically bind to its corresponding DHFR mRNA.[203] Incubation of DHFR protein either with the normal substrates dihydrofolate or NADPH, or with MTX, completely represses its binding to the target DHFR mRNA. In an in vitro translation system, this specific interaction between DHFR and its message is associated with inhibition of translation. These studies provide evidence for a translational autoregulatory mechanism underlying the control of DHFR expression. The presence of either excess MTX or dihydrofolate prevents DHFR protein from performing its normal autoregulatory function, thereby allowing for increased DHFR protein synthesis. Thus, the ability to regulate DHFR expression at the translational level allows normal cellular function to be maintained in the setting of an acute cellular stress and represents a unique mechanism whereby cells can react to and overcome the inhibitory effects of MTX and antifolate analogs. In further attempts to characterize DHFR autoregulation, Bertino et al.[204] used a series of truncated DHFR mRNA probes to investigate whether the enzyme directly contacts its cognate mRNA. A resultant DHFR protein/RNA interaction was found in an approximately 100–base-pair portion in the protein-coding region that contains two putative stem-loop structures. In addition, the binding of MTX prevented the DHFR/RNA interaction to DHFR, which thereby relieved translational autoregulation.

Although various in vitro and in vivo model systems have clearly demonstrated an association between DHFR gene amplification and MTX resistance, the clinical significance of gene amplification remains uncertain. Tumor samples from patients resistant to MTX have been evaluated, and several clinical specimens have been found to possess elevated levels of DHFR enzyme in association with DHFR gene amplification.[205] A small cell lung carcinoma cell line isolated from a patient clinically resistant to high-dose MTX was found to have amplification of the DHFR gene and increased expression of DHFR protein.[205,206] This amplification was associated with the presence of double-minute chromosomes (Fig. 6.3B). After serial passage in drug-free media, cells lost the double-minute chromosomes on which the amplified genes resided and regained drug sensitivity. Clinical MTX resistance attributable to DHFR amplification was also investigated in two patients with acute leukemia and in one patient with ovarian cancer. In all three cases, amplification of DHFR gene copies (twofold to threefold) with increased DHFR protein (threefold to sixfold) was observed, and the increase in DHFR gene copy number was postulated to be directly associated with the development of MTX resistance. Matherly et al.[207] found a markedly greater frequency of DHFR overexpression in T-cell ALL than in B-precursor ALL in children. The authors speculated that this difference in DHFR expression was associated with the poorer prognosis of T-cell ALL treated with standard doses of antimetabolites, implying that higher-dose MTX consolidation therapy may be particularly needed in this population.

Consequences of Dihydrofolate Reductase Enzyme Inhibition

The critical cellular events associated with MTX inhibition of DHFR are illustrated in Figure 6.1. Thymidylate synthase catalyzes the sole biochemical reaction resulting in the oxidation of tetrahydrofolates. Continued activity of this enzymatic reaction in the presence of DHFR inhibition results in rapid accumulation of intracellular levels of dihydrofolate polyglutamates. This accumulation is temporally associated with a depletion of several critical reduced-folate pools, most notably 5-methyltetrahydrofolate. In several in vitro cell systems studied to date, however, the reduced-folate cofactors required for de novo purine and thymidylate synthesis (10-formyltetrahydrofolate and 5,10-methylenetetrahydrofolate) are relatively preserved in the presence of cytotoxic concentrations of MTX.[7–10,12,208] In studies using human breast cancer cells, purified normal human myeloid precursor cells, and murine leukemia cells, exposure to lethal concentrations of MTX resulted in a 70 to 80% preservation of 10-formyltetrahydrofolate pools compared with untreated controls (Fig. 6.4). Additional studies using human breast cancer cells, promyelocytic leukemia cells, normal human myeloid progenitor cells, and Krebs ascites cells and L1210 murine leukemia cells grown in the peritoneal cavity of mice confirm a partial preservation of 5,10- methylenetetrahydrofolate pools (50 to 70%) during MTX exposures that produce profound TS inhibition and cytotoxicity.[11,12] Subsequent computer modeling of the intracellular human folate pools based on experimental data confirm the importance of direct inhibition of the various folate-dependent enzymes in the metabolic inhibition associated with MTX exposure.[20] To determine the importance of the inhibitory effects of MTX polyglutamates as distinct from the effects of folate depletion and direct dihydrofolate inhibition, several investigators have examined the change in folate pools associated with exposure to trimetrexate, an antifolate that is not polyglutamated but remains a potent inhibitor of DHFR.[20,209–211] Results of these studies are conflicting. In murine leukemia cells, folate pools were relatively preserved and dihydrofolate polyglutamates seemed to serve an essential role in meta-

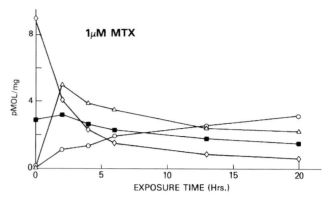

Figure 6.4 Effects of 1 μmol/L methotrexate (MTX) on intracellular folate pools in human breast cancer cells (MCF-7). (Δ, dihydrofolate; o, 10-formyldihydrofolate; ■, 10-formyltetrahydrofolate; ◇, 5-methyltetrahydrofolate.) (From Allegra CJ, Fine RL, Drake JC, et al. The effect of methotrexate on intracellular folate pools in human MCF-7 breast cancer cells. Evidence for direct inhibition of purine synthesis. J Biol Chem 1986;261:6478–6485.)

bolic inhibition. In contrast, folate depletion appeared to be the more critical event in rat hepatoma cells. Presumably, intrinsic differences between these cell lines with regard to the levels of TS, folate pools, and intracellular folate regulation may determine the relative roles of direct enzyme inhibition versus substrate depletion in the metabolic inhibitory effects of MTX. Although partial depletion of reduced-folate cofactors undoubtedly contributes to the inhibition of metabolic pathways, the accumulated dihydrofolate and MTX polyglutamates appear also to play a critical role as direct inhibitors of folate-dependent enzymes in both de novo purine and thymidylate synthesis.

Reduced-folate (leucovorin) rescue of MTX-treated cells may be anticipated to result in an accumulation of reduced folates that would compete with and overcome direct enzymatic inhibition rather than simply replete tetrahydrofolate levels (vide infra). This feature may, in large part, explain the competitive nature of leucovorin rescue observed in vitro and clinically. Also, selectivity of the cytotoxic effects of MTX and selectivity of leucovorin rescue may depend on the extent to which various normal and malignant cells generate dihydrofolate and MTX polyglutamates.

An additional factor that influences the folate pool changes associated with MTX exposure and, hence, cellular sensitivity to MTX is the level or activity of TS. Inhibition of TS by 5-fluorodeoxyuridylate or by depletion of its substrate deoxyuridylate diminishes sensitivity to MTX. TS activity in human leukemia, lung carcinoma, and colon carcinoma influences MTX sensitivity; specifically, low levels of TS activity are usually associated with MTX resistance.[67,144] In cells with low levels of TS, the slow rate of oxidation of 5,10-methylenetetrahydrofolate to dihydrofolate creates less dependence on DHFR to regenerate tetrahydrofolates. Under conditions of low cellular TS activity, a block in DHFR by MTX exposures produces minimal accumulation of inhibitory dihydrofolate and minimal depletion of tetrahydrofolates.

Mechanisms of Cell Death

As a consequence of the multiple effects of antifolates on nucleotide biosynthesis, several mechanisms of cell death are possible. Deoxythymidine triphosphate and deoxypurine nucleotides are required for both the synthesis of DNA and its repair. Inhibition of thymidylate and purine synthesis leads to a cessation of DNA synthesis. A close correlation is found between DNA strand breaks and cell death in Ehrlich ascites tumor cell exposed to MTX[212]; because the breaks occurred in mature DNA, the authors attributed them to ineffective repair mechanisms from lack of nucleotides. This work was supported by similar experimental findings in a mutant murine cell line lacking TS activity and grown in thymidine-deplete media[213] and in a Chinese hamster ovary cell line in which DNA damage was prevented by the use of thymidine and hypoxanthine.[214] Another hypothesis that attempts to explain MTX cytotoxicity concerns the increase in intracellular dUMP pools that occurs as a consequence of inhibition of de novo thymidylate synthesis. Clearly, the high concentrations of dUMP may ultimately lead to misincorporation of dUMP and deoxyuridine triphosphate into cellular DNA.[215] An enzyme, uracil-DNA-glycosylase, specifically excises uracil bases from DNA, a process that may be responsible for the fragments of DNA observed in antifolate-treated cells with high levels of uracil incorporation.[216,217] These studies implicate the presence of lesions expected in DNA undergoing excision repair of misincorporated uracil nucleotides. Further evidence for the importance of uracil misincorporation derives from a study of seven cell lines that varied widely in deoxyuridine triphosphatase activity.[218] An inverse correlation between deoxyuridine triphosphatase activity and MTX toxicity was found, which suggests that the level of deoxyuridine triphosphate misincorporation into DNA is an important factor in MTX cytotoxicity. Although these studies offer insights into the consequences of uracil misincorporation into DNA, they do not explain the marked toxicity of MTX-thymidine combinations, which must act through an antipurine effect. Probably both uracil nucleotide misincorporation (with subsequent excision repair) and the combined effects of purine and pyrimidine depletion result in the formation of DNA strand breaks. Although the induction of DNA strand breaks is central to the activity of MTX, it is the cellular response to these breaks that ultimately determines whether a cell incurring a given level of DNA damage dies.[219–221]

Using a tetracycline-inducible expression system in an osteosarcoma cell line (SaOs-2), Li et al.[222] found that p21/waf1-induced cells exhibited greater sensitivity to doxorubicin hydrochloride, raltitrexed, and MTX than noninduced cells and that this condition was associated with increased apoptosis. The SaOs-2 cells lack both p53 and a functional retinoblastoma protein. Overexpression of p21/waf1 protein was associated with diminished E2F-1 phosphorylation, which resulted in an increase in E2F-1 binding activity and enhanced expression of E2F-responsive genes (DHFR and TS). The authors suggested that this mechanism may mediate sensitivity to anticancer drugs by contributing to increased $S–G_2$ cell-cycle arrest or delay and increased cell susceptibility to apoptosis. Clearly, the identification of the critical cell death effectors will enable the development of more potent and, it is hoped, more selective therapeutic strategies.

A novel antiproliferative mechanism associated with MTX exposure has been described as resulting from the potent inhibition of isoprenylcysteine carboxyl methyltransferase (Icmt).[223] Inhibition of Imct results from the elevated levels of S-adenosylhomocysteine that occur with MTX exposure. Icmt is responsible for the Ras methylation, which is necessary for its proper function and, inhibition of this methylation process results in proliferative arrest. The relative extent to which this process contributes to the antiproliferative effects of MTX is not clear.

Pharmacokinetic and Cytokinetic Determinants of Cytotoxicity

At least two pharmacokinetic factors—drug concentration and duration of cell exposure—are critical determinants of cytotoxicity. In tissue culture and in intact animals, extracellular drug concentrations of 10 nmol/L are required to inhibit thymidylate synthesis in normal bone marrow. This same drug concentration is associated with depletion of bone marrow cellularity when maintained for 24 hours or longer. The rate of cell loss from murine bone marrow increases with increasing drug concentrations up to 10 μmol/L[224] (Fig. 6.5). Similar findings have been reported in studies with murine tumor cells. Compared with drug concentration, the duration of exposure to MTX is a more critical factor in determining cell death, provided the minimal threshold concentration for cytotoxicity is exceeded. For a given dose of drug, cell loss is directly proportional to the time period of exposure but doubles only with a 10-fold increase in drug concentration.[225] This relationship is likely the result of the S-phase specificity of MTX. With longer duration of exposure, more cells are allowed to enter the vulnerable DNA-synthetic phase of the cell cycle.

Time and concentration correlates of cytotoxicity for human tumor cells have also been studied. Hryniuk and Bertino[226] found variable inhibition of thymidine incorporation into DNA of human leukemic cells in short-term culture when these cells were exposed to 1 μmol/L MTX for 1 hour or less. In leukemia cell lines, the duration of exposure appears to play a far more important role than absolute drug concentration. A marked increase in toxicity (30-fold) was appreciated only when the duration rather than drug concentration was increased,[225] provided both parameters were changed by similar increments.

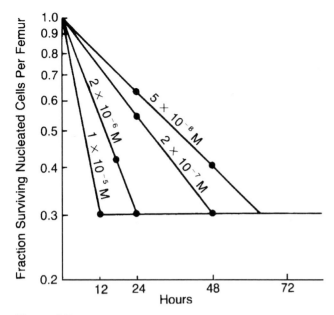

Figure 6.5 Nucleated cells per femur remaining after constant infusion of methotrexate sodium into mice to achieve indicated drug concentration for various periods. (From Pinedo HM, Zaharko DS, Bull J, et al. The relative contribution of drug concentration and duration of exposure to mouse bone marrow toxicity during continuous methotrexate infusion. Cancer Res 1977;37:445–450.)

In addition to pharmacokinetic and cytokinetic factors, physiologic compounds in the cellular environment may profoundly affect the cytotoxicity of MTX. Most prominent among these factors are the naturally occurring purine bases, purine nucleosides, and thymidine. In bone marrow and intestinal epithelium, the de novo synthesis of both thymidylate and purines is inhibited by concentrations of MTX above 100 nmol/L, but cells can survive this block when bone marrow is supplied with 10 μmol/L thymidine and a purine source (adenosine, inosine, or hypoxanthine) at similar concentrations. Thymidine alone is incapable of completely reversing the cytotoxic effect of MTX.[227] The purine salvage pathways in normal bone marrow appear to be highly efficient, however, and the endogenous concentrations of purines in this tissue are high, albeit variable.[228] Plasma thymidine levels in humans have been reported to be approximately 0.2 μmol/L,[229] whereas the concentration of the purine bases and nucleosides is somewhat higher (0.5 μmol/L).[230] Thus, under basal conditions, the concentrations of purines and thymidine would appear inadequate to rescue cells. Clinical investigations using the nucleoside transport inhibitor dipyridamole, however, have demonstrated an increase in toxicity when combined with MTX, which suggests that physiologic concentrations of nucleosides may affect the toxicity and potentially the antitumor activity of MTX.[231] Recent work has demonstrated that physiologic levels of endogenous nucleosides and nucleobases are adequate to sensitize even highly resistant osteosarcoma cell lines to the cytotoxic effects of MTX.[232] Pharmacologic interventions, such as allopurinol

treatment (which elevates circulating hypoxanthine concentrations) and chemotherapy, with subsequent tumor lysis, may further raise levels of the circulating nucleosides and ameliorate toxicity to tumor or host tissues.

A third determinant of antifolate cytotoxic action is the concentration of reduced folate in the circulation. Methyltetrahydrofolate (the predominant circulating folate cofactor), when present in sufficient concentration, can readily reverse MTX toxicity,[233] as can leucovorin. Circulating levels of 5-methyltetrahydrofolate are approximately 0.01 μmol/L and of little pharmacologic relevance. Exogenous administration of reduced folates, however, is able to reverse MTX toxicity in a competitive manner. Leucovorin is commonly used after MTX administration to reduce or prevent toxicity and is effective when given within 24 to 36 hours after MTX treatment. The concentration of leucovorin required to prevent MTX toxicity increases as the drug concentration increases (Fig. 6.6).[227] The reasons for this competitive relationship are only partly understood. However, given the current knowledge of direct enzymatic inhibition of the folate-dependent enzymes in de novo purine and thymidylate synthesis by intracellular metabolites formed after MTX treatment, several possibilities exist. Competition may occur at the level of membrane transport because both MTX and the reduced folates share a common transmembrane transport system. When given concurrently with MTX, leucovorin decreases the rate of MTX polyglutamation. An important consideration in leucovorin rescue is its effect on intracellular reduced-folate pools. Competitive concentrations of reduced folate are required to overcome inhibition by dihydrofolate and MTX polyglutamates as folate-dependent enzymes such as TS and AICAR transformylase. In addition, by raising intracellular concentrations of dihydrofolate, leucovorin indirectly increases substrate competition with MTX for the inhibited DHFR enzyme. In support of this latter mechanism as the basis for leucovorin rescue are studies that show nearly quantitative conversion of leucovorin to dihydrofolate and the ability of dihydrofolate to (a) compete with MTX and MTX polyglutamates for DHFR binding in intact human cancer cells, (b) reactivate DHFR, and (c) rescue cells from MTX cytotoxicity.[7,171,177,234] Furthermore, an important factor in the clinical efficacy of leucovorin rescue relates to the timing and dose of leucovorin.[235] Because leucovorin is capable of reversing the cytotoxic effects of MTX on host and malignant cells, the minimum dose of leucovorin needed to rescue host cells should be used. In patients with head and neck cancer randomized to receive standard-dose MTX and either leucovorin or placebo rescue starting 24 hours later,[236] both overall toxicity and response rate were significantly lower in patients treated with MTX and leucovorin. This study emphasizes that careful consideration must be given to the dose and timing of leucovorin when used in combination with MTX to avoid rescue of both cancerous and normal tissues.

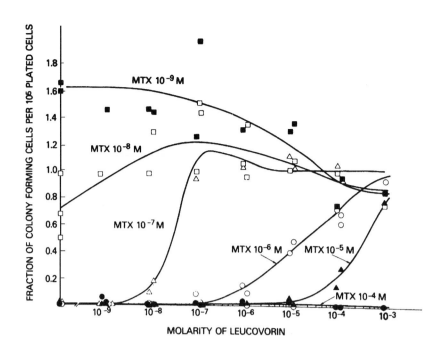

Figure 6.6 Effect of various combinations of leucovorin calcium and methotrexate sodium (MTX) on formation of granulocyte colonies in vitro by mouse bone marrow. Values are normalized to control value for marrow incubated without either drug. (MTX concentrations: ■, 10^{-9} mol/L; □, 10^{-8} mol/L; Δ, 10^{-7} mol/L; ○, 10^{-6} mol/L; ▲, 10^{-5} mol/L; ●, 10^{-4} mol/L.) (From Pinedo HM, Zaharko DS, Bull JM, et al. The reversal of methotrexate cytotoxicity to mouse bone marrow cells by leucovorin and nucleosides. Cancer Res 1976;36:4418–4424.)

METHOTREXATE ASSAY

Two methods are commonly used for the rapid assay of MTX and include one that is based on tight binding of drug to DHFR and another that depends on antibody-drug interactions. Both methods provide extremely sensitive measurement of MTX levels >10 nmol/L in biologic fluids. Significant differences are seen, however, in the time required to perform them and in their specificity for parent compound as opposed to metabolites (Table 6.2).

The first widely used method, the enzyme inhibition assay, measures MTX concentration by determining the ability of a clinical sample to inhibit DHFR activity. Although the enzyme inhibition assay is time-consuming, automation and microcomputer technology may allow for a more efficient use of this very sensitive and specific assay.[237]

A competitive binding assay that uses DHFR as the binding protein is available and preserves the specificity for parent compound that is observed in the enzyme inhibition assay. In the binding assay, MTX in a biologic sample competes for DHFR binding sites with a known quantity of radiolabeled drug. Multiple samples can be run simultaneously and results can be reported on the same day.[238] Trimethoprim, which is commonly used in the oncologic population in combination with sulfonamides for the treatment and prophylaxis of *P.carinii* pneumonia and bacterial infections, cross-reacts with MTX in this assay and may lead to spuriously elevated results when the bacterial enzyme is used.[239] This cross-reaction may be avoided by using a mammalian source of DHFR (e.g., bovine) that does not bind trimethoprim at clinically achievable serum concentrations.

Radioimmunoassays and fluorescence-polarization immunoassays for MTX are also available for routine clinical use, and employ antibodies generated by an MTX-bovine serum albumin complex.[240] These assays are as sensitive (0.01 to 800 µmol/L) and as rapid as the competitive DHFR binding procedure but have somewhat different specificity.

TABLE 6.2
METHOTREXATE ASSAY METHODS

Assay	Advantages	Disadvantages
DHFR inhibition	Sensitive, no cross-reaction with metabolites	Time-consuming
Competitive DHFR binding	Sensitive, no cross-reaction with metabolites, rapid	Not automated
Immunoassay		
Fluorescence polarization	Sensitive, rapid, automated	Cross-reacts with metabolites
Enzyme multiplied	Rapid, automated	Relatively insensitive, cross-reacts with metabolites
High-pressure liquid chromatography	Methotrexate and metabolites individually quantitated	Time consuming, expensive

DHFR, dihydrofolate reductase.

The immunoassay antibodies cross-react with one MTX metabolite, 2,4-diamino-N_{10}-methyl pteroic acid (DAMPA) (40%), but not with 7-hydroxymethotrexateMTX (7-OH-MTX) (1%). At later time points after drug administration, DAMPA is found in plasma in relatively high concentrations (equal to or greater than that of MTX) and thus produces spuriously elevated values for the parent compound[241] that are on average twofold to fourfold higher than the DHFR binding method. A variant of the radioimmunoassay (enzyme-multiplied immunoassay), based on antibody inhibition of an enzyme-MTX complex, is the most rapid assay available but also cross-reacts with DAMPA[242] and has a sensitivity limit of approximately 0.2 µmol/L. This limitation is critical when evaluating patient samples beyond 48 hours, when MTX concentrations may be at the limit of the assay's sensitivity. Prudent use of hydration and continued leucovorin can be guided only by accurate measurements of MTX concentrations down to the nontoxic level (approximately 10 nmol/L).[243]

High-pressure liquid chromatography (HPLC) can be used to separate and quantitate MTX and its various metabolites.[241,244] Although the sensitivity of HPLC is primarily limited by the ultraviolet detection systems commonly used (0.2 µmol/L), its sensitivity may be markedly enhanced by serum concentration methods,[244,245] electrochemical detection,[246] or post column derivatization and fluorescence detection. Although HPLC technology is generally too cumbersome for routine clinical monitoring, its use is required when high sensitivity and specificity along with an ability to measure individual MTX metabolites are required. Reports have compared the two more commonly used assay techniques, enzyme-multiplied immunoassay and fluorescence-polarization immunoassay, with HPLC and in over 100 patient plasma samples tested found a high concordance among all three methods.[247] Thus, several assays are available for the accurate and rapid measurement of MTX levels in patient samples. The final selection of an assay to be used in the clinical setting may ultimately depend on the requirements for sensitivity, specificity, identification of specific MTX metabolites, and cost and time constraints.

PHARMACOKINETICS

Although the pharmacologic properties of MTX are now better understood at the biochemical and molecular levels, clinical exploitation of this knowledge depends on a detailed understanding of the time profile of drug concentration in extracellular and intracellular spaces and the complex relationship of drug levels to effects on specific tissues. Although antifolate pharmacokinetics is well understood, the important second step—that is, definition of the relationship between drug concentration and effect (pharmacodynamics)—requires continued investigation.

The first attempts to define the distribution and disposition of MTX in a comprehensive manner were reported by Zaharko et al.[248] These authors developed a detailed model for MTX pharmacokinetics that accurately predicted drug-derived radioactivity in various tissue compartments for a 4-hour period after drug administration. The primary elements of that model were (a) elimination of MTX by renal excretion, (b) an active enterohepatic circulation, (c) metabolism of at least a small fraction of drug within the gastrointestinal tract by intestinal flora, and (d) multiple drug half-lives in plasma, the longest of which was found to be approximately 3 hours. Each of these elements has been observed in humans, although a longer terminal half-life is now appreciated, estimated to be between 8 and 27 hours, depending on the assay method used.[248] HPLC has also disclosed extensive metabolism of MTX in both mice and humans.

Absorption

MTX is absorbed from the gastrointestinal tract by a saturable active transport system.[249] Although small doses are well absorbed, absorption is incomplete at higher doses. Bioavailability for doses of 50 mg/m^2 or greater may be enhanced by subdividing the dose rather than delivering as a single large dose.[249,250] An investigation of the oral bioavailability of MTX given to 15 patients with acute leukemia (6 to 28 mg/m^2) revealed a longer absorptive phase and a lower fractional absorption of the drug for doses >12 mg/m^2 (2.5 hours and 51%, respectively) than for doses less than 12 mg/m^2 (1.5 hours and 87%, respectively).[251]

Drug absorbed in the intestine enters the portal circulation and thus must pass through the liver, where hepatocellular uptake, polyglutamation, and storage all occur; orally administered drug is further subject to degradation (deglutamylation) by intestinal flora to DAMPA, a metabolite that is inactive pharmacologically but that cross-reacts in commonly used radioimmunoassay systems for MTX. Drugs taken orally are also subject to the variability of intestinal absorption created by drug-induced epithelial damage, motility changes, and alterations in flora. One or all of these factors may be responsible for the highly variable nature of MTX pharmacokinetics observed in children receiving small doses of MTX (20 mg/m^2) by mouth.[252] For these reasons, MTX is usually given by systemic routes.

Distribution

The volume of distribution of MTX approximates that of total body water. The drug is loosely bound to serum albumin, with approximately 60% binding at concentrations at or above 1 µmol/L in plasma.[253] Weak organic acids such as aspirin[254] can displace MTX from plasma proteins, but the clinical significance of this displacement process has not been proven.

MTX penetrates slowly into third-space fluid collection, such as pleural effusions[255] or ascites,[256] reaching steady-state plasma concentrations in approximately 6 hours. It also exits slowly from these compartments, producing a concentration gradient of several-fold in favor of the loculated fluid at later time points. The clearance of MTX from peritoneal fluid is approximately 5 mL/minute, substantially less than its clearance from the plasma compartment, which equals or exceeds glomerular filtration (120 mL/minute). In brief, the mechanism responsible for drug accumulation in closed fluid spaces relates to the limited permeability of the peritoneal surface to both charged and high-molecular-weight compounds[257]; thus, only small amounts of drug are able to cross the peritoneal membrane and enter the portal circulation. Drug either not retained or metabolized in the liver passes into the systemic circulation and is then excreted rapidly in the urine.

Third-space retention of intravenously administered drug is associated with a prolongation of the terminal drug half-life in plasma, owing presumably to the slow reentry of sequestered drug into the bloodstream.[256] This effect must be considered when treating patients with ascites or pleural effusions. Although no strict guidelines exist for dose adjustment in patients with third-space accumulations, evacuation of this fluid before treatment and close monitoring of plasma drug concentrations in such patients is strongly advisable.

Fossa et al.[258] have described unexpectedly high levels of MTX in patients with bladder cancer receiving MTX-based combination chemotherapy who had previously undergone cystectomy and ileal conduit diversion, presumably because of drug resorption from the ileal conduit. Thus, special care must be given to patients with ileal conduit diversions who are at increased risk for delayed MTX elimination and subsequent MTX toxicity.

Plasma Pharmacokinetics

After the initial distribution phase, which lasts a relatively few minutes, at least two phases of drug disappearance from plasma are observed in laboratory animals and humans. Conventional doses of 25 to 100 mg/m² produce peak plasma concentrations of 1 to 10 µmol/L, whereas high-dose infusion regimens using 1.5 g/m² or more yield peak levels of 0.1 to 1 mmol/L.[251] Whether plasma concentrations are strictly proportional to dose is unclear. The initial phase of drug disappearance from plasma has a half-life of 2 to 3 hours, with no apparent variation as doses are increased to the high-dose range. This phase extends for the first 12 to 24 hours after drug administration and is largely determined by the rate of renal excretion of MTX. Prolongation of this phase, as well as of the terminal phase of drug disappearance from plasma, is observed in patients with renal dysfunction, in whom half- life is approximately proportional to the serum creatinine.[259] Bressolle and colleagues[260] studied the effects of moderate renal insufficiency on pharmacokinetics of MTX in patients with rheumatoid arthritis. Intramuscular MTX was administered to four separate groups of patients segregated according to creatinine clearance: less than 45, 45 to 60, 61 to 80, and more than 80 mL/minute. Noting an increased elimination half-life and reduced total clearance that correlated with the degree of renal impairment, the authors concluded that individual renal function testing was preferred over a general decrease of the MTX dose based only on observed serum creatinine. In patients with normal creatinine clearance, the half-life of the initial phase of drug disappearance increases with advancing age of the patient, which lends additional variability to plasma levels, disappearance kinetics, and toxicity.

The final phase of drug disappearance has a considerably longer half-life of 8 to 10 hours[256,258]; this half-life may further lengthen in patients with renal dysfunction or with third-space fluid such as ascites. After conventional doses of 25 to 200 mg/m², this terminal phase begins at drug concentrations above the threshold for toxicity to bone marrow and gastrointestinal epithelium. Thus, any prolongation of the terminal half-life is likely to be associated with significant toxicity.

The use of constant-infusion MTX has received increasing consideration because it offers the advantage of providing predictable blood and cerebrospinal fluid (CSF) concentrations for a specific period of time. Bleyer[261] has used the following formulas for achieving a desired plasma concentration in patients with normal renal function:

(a) Priming dose (in mg/m²) = 15 × plasma MTX concentration (in µmol/L)

(b) Infusion dose (in mg/m²/hour) = 3 × plasma MTX concentration (in µmol/L)

An approximate correction for renal function may be made by reducing the infusion doses in proportion to the reduction in creatinine clearance, based on a normal creatinine clearance of 60 mL/minute per square meter. The terminal elimination phase of MTX increases from 3 to 5 hours in proportion to the duration of the constant infusion over the range of 24 to 72 hours.[262] This variation probably represents slow tissue release of poorly effluxable MTX polyglutamates that form in cells in a time-dependent and dose-dependent manner.

The plasma pharmacokinetics of MTX may independently predict relapse in children treated during the maintenance phase of ALL with intermediate drug doses (1 g/m²). In a study of 108 children, a rapid drug clearance (84 to 132 mL/minute per square meter) was associated with a 40% risk of relapse, whereas those children with relatively slow drug clearance (45 to 72 mL/minute per square meter) had a significantly decreased (P_2 = .01) risk of relapse (25%).[263] Steady-state MTX concentrations of less than 16 µmol/L were also associated with a lower probability of remaining in remission (P < .05) than in patients with concentrations in excess of 16 µmol/L.[264] These associations were further supported by the finding of a systemic clearance of 123 mL/minute per square meter in 25 children who relapsed with ALL versus 72 mL/minute per square meter in 33 children who remained in continuous remission.[265] These results suggest that dose should be increased in children with rapid drug clearance and low steady-state MTX levels.[266]

Renal Excretion

The bulk of drug is excreted in the urine in the first 12 hours after administration, with renal excretion varying from 44% to virtually 100% of the administered dose.[258, 267] The higher figure is likely to be true for patients with normal renal function. MTX clearance by the kidney has exceeded creatinine clearance in some patients studied.[268]

During high-dose infusion, rapid drug excretion may lead to high MTX concentrations in the urine. These concentrations, approaching 10 mmol/L, exceed the solubility of the drug below pH 7.0 (Table 6.3) and are believed to be responsible for intrarenal precipitation of drug and renal failure. Thus, in high-dose regimens, hydration and alkalinization of the urine are recommended to avoid renal toxicity (Table 6.4). To ensure adequate intrarenal dissolution of MTX during high-dose therapy (0.7 to 8.4 g/m^2), a 20-fold greater urine flow is required at pH 5.0 (2 to 42 mL/minute per square meter) than at pH 7.0 (0.1 to 1.2 mL/minute per square meter).[269] Intensive hydration does not affect the clearance of MTX or the plasma pharmacokinetics, aside from its effects on the prevention of renal damage.[270]

The exact mechanism of MTX excretion in the human kidney has not been fully elucidated. In dog and monkey models, active secretion of MTX takes place in the proximal renal tubule, with reabsorption in the distal tubule.[271] As noted earlier, the high clearance values in excess of creatinine clearance suggest that active tubular secretion of MTX occurs in humans. MTX excretion is inhibited by weak organic acids such as aspirin,[215] piperacillin,[272,273] penicillin G,[274] oxacillin,[275] ciprofloxacin,[276] and probenecid, an inhibitor of organic acid secretion.[272] The cephalosporins, including ceftriaxone, ceftriazone, ceftazidime and sulfamethoxazole, enhance the renal elimination of MTX, probably through competition for tubular reabsorption.[273,274] Simultaneous folic acid administration blocks MTX reabsorption, which suggests that leucovorin might accelerate MTX excretion in high-dose rescue regimens.

In high-dose MTX therapy, despite interindividual variation in pharmacokinetics, blood levels of drug may be accurately predicted by a preliminary determination of drug clearance using a small test dose (10 to 50 mg/m^2).[268,277] Pharmacokinetic measurements made after delivery of this test dose provide a basis for calculating high-dose infusion rates according to the following formula (units of conversion must be carefully considered):

$$\text{Clearance (mL/minute)} = \text{dose (50 mg/m}^2\text{)}/ \frac{\text{area under concentration}}{} \times \frac{\text{time curve}}{}$$

$$\text{Infusion rate} = \frac{\text{plasma MTX concentration (in }\mu\text{mol/L)}}{} \times \text{MTX clearance}$$

Thus, the desired infusion rate is the product of the target steady-state concentration multiplied by the MTX clearance rate, as determined from the test dose.[268]

Extrapolation from the test dose of 50 mg/m^2 to a high-dose infusion schedule has proven to be reliable as long as renal function remains normal during the infusion period. The test dose technique has also been used to identify the subset of patients with impaired MTX elimination who are at increased risk for toxicity.[278]

Hepatic Uptake and Biliary Excretion

MTX undergoes uptake, storage, and metabolism in the liver, but the relative contribution of each of these processes to drug pharmacokinetics is unclear.

MTX is actively transported into hepatocytes by an uptake system that appears to have several components.[279,280] In the hepatocyte, MTX is converted to polyglutamate forms that persist for several months after drug administration.[281] The parent drug also undergoes excretion into the biliary tract and is reabsorbed into the systemic circulation from the small intestine. Dactinomycin (actinomycin D) strongly inhibits biliary secretion of MTX, with little effect on hepatic uptake, and causes a marked increase in intrahepatic levels of the drug.[282] Although this pharmacokinetic effect has not been examined in detail in humans; the possibility exists that the combination of MTX and dactinomycin may increase MTX levels in liver and enhance its hepatic toxicity.

The effects of conjugated and unconjugated bile salts on the enterohepatic circulation of MTX have been investigated in vivo in perfused rat intestinal preparations.[283] This study demonstrated a saturable intestinal transport mechanism ($K_t = 0.98$ μmol/L). The unconjugated bile salt deoxycholate and the conjugated salt taurocholate significantly diminished MTX absorption. Folic acid, 5-methyltetrahydrofolate, and the organic anions rose bengal and sulfobromophthalein, also inhibited transport. These compounds might be useful in altering both systemic and specific hepatic toxicities associated with MTX by promoting MTX excretion in the stool.

TABLE 6.3
AQUEOUS SOLUBILITY OF METHOTREXATE AND METABOLITES

Agent	Solubility (mg/mL)		
	pH 5.0	pH 6.0	pH 7.0
Methotrexate	0.39	1.55	9.04
7-Hydroxy methotrexate	0.13	0.37	1.55
2,4-diamino-N_{10}-methyl pteroic acid	0.05	0.10	0.85

TABLE 6.4
HIGH-DOSE METHOTREXATE SODIUM (MTX) THERAPY

Hydration and Urinary Alkalinization

Administer 2.5–3.5 L/m^2/d of IV fluids starting 12 hr before and for 24–48 hr after administration of MTX drug infusion. Sodium bicarbonate 45–50 mEq/L IV fluid to ensure that urine pH is >7.0 at the time of drug infusion.

Commonly Used Drug Infusion Regimens

MTX Dose	Duration (hr)	Fluid (L/24 hr)	Bicarbonate (mEq/24 hr)	Leucovorin Calcium Rescue	Onset of Rescue (hr after Start of MTX)
1.5–7.5 g/m^2	6.0	3/m^2	NS	15 mg IV q3hr × then 15 mg PO q6hr × 7	18
8–12 g/m^2	4.0	1.5–2.0/m^2	2–3/kg	10 mg PO q6hr × 10	20
3.0–7.5 g/m^2	0.3	3/m^2	288	10 mg/m^2 IV × 1, then 10 mg/m^2 PO q6hr × 12	24
1 g/m^2	24.0	2.4/m^2	48/m^2	15 mg/m^2 IV q6hr × 2, then 3 mg/m^2 PO q12hr × 3	36
1.0–7.5 g/m^2	0.5	3/m^2	288	10 mg/m^2 IV × 1, then 10 mg/m^2 PO q6hr × 11	24

IV, intravenously; NS, not specified; PO, per os.
Adapted from Ackland SP, Schilsky RL. High-dose methotrexate: a critical reappraisal. J Clin Oncol 1987;5:2017–2031.

Monitor Points

MTX drug levels above 5×10^{-7} mol/L at 48 hr after the start of MTX infusion require continued leucovorin rescue.[a] A general guideline for leucovorin rescue is as follows:

MTX Level	Leucovorin Dosage
5×10^{-7} mol/L	15 mg/m^2 q6h × 8
1×10^{-6} mol/L	100 mg/m^2 q6h × 8
2×10^{-6} mol/L	200 mg/m^2 q6h × 8

[a]MTX drug levels should be measured every 24 hr and the dosage of leucovorin adjusted until the MTX level is $<5 \times 10^{-8}$ mol/L.

Widely divergent estimates have been made of the relative importance of biliary excretion of MTX in humans. Lerne et al.,[284] using tritium-labeled MTX, found only 0.41% of an administered dose in the bile of a patient with a biliary fistula. Subsequent studies have variously estimated that 6.7 to 9%[285] or 20%[267] of an administered dose enters the biliary tract. Calvert and co-workers[267] used the highly specific DHFR inhibition assay to measure biliary concentrations of MTX and found that biliary levels were 2,500-fold to 10,000-fold higher than simultaneous concentrations in the plasma. Despite these high concentrations in bile, less than 10% of an intravenous dose of MTX is eliminated in the feces. In the presence of diminished renal function, the enterohepatic circulation may become an important determinant of drug elimination.[286] Under these conditions, intestinal binding to prevent reabsorption of the drug with activated charcoal[287] or the anion-exchange resin cholestyramine,[288] which has a 5.4-fold greater binding capacity than charcoal, may be used to enhance the nonrenal excretion of MTX.

METHOTREXATE METABOLISM

The introduction of high-dose MTX regimens has led to the identification of at least two MTX metabolites in humans. Jacobs et al.[289] identified 7-OH-MTX in the urine of patients receiving high-dose infusions; 7-OH-MTX constituted 20 to 46% of material excreted in the urine in the interval between 12 and 24 hours after the start of the infusion. The fraction of drug in the form of this metabolite was estimated to be as high as 86% in the period from 24 to 48 hours. A second metabolite, DAMPA, has also been identified in plasma and urine, and, at later times, this metabolite makes up an important fraction of drug-derived material, comprising a mean of 25% of material excreted in the interval from 24 to 48 hours.[241] Both of these metabolites are known to accumulate in plasma, and at 24 to 48 hours after high-dose MTX administration, they account for most of the MTX-derived material found in plasma and may give spuriously high MTX values when using certain assays

Regarding the sites of MTX metabolism, 7-OH-MTX is probably formed through the action of the liver enzyme aldehyde oxidase where levels of the 7-OH-MTX metabolite have been found to be 700-fold higher in bile than in serum.[290] The extent to which polyglutamated 7-OH-MTX is formed in malignant but not in normal cells may be important in the selective action of MTX because the 7-OH polyglutamates have measurable effects on several critical intracellular pathways. The polyglutamates of 7-OH-MTX are inhibitors of the folate-dependent enzymes AICAR transformylase and TS, with potency similar to that of MTX polyglutamates (K_i = 3 and 0.4 µmol/L, respectively).[291] These metabolites can bind to DHFR[109,153] but are relatively weak inhibitors (K_i = 9 nmol/L) of this enzyme compared with MTX.[165,175,292] Unlike with the inhibition of certain folate-dependent enzymes, polyglutamation has relatively minor effects on the potency of DHFR inhibition by 7-OH-MTX.[165,292] Exposure of murine leukemia cells to high concentrations of 7-OH-MTX (100 µmol/L) resulted in only mild inhibition of cell growth.[208] Despite primary metabolism of MTX to the 7-OH-MTX metabolite by the liver, no dosage adjustment of MTX appears to be necessary for patients with hepatic dysfunction.

The pteroic acid metabolite DAMPA is probably formed by the action of bacterial carboxypeptidases in the gastrointestinal tract. Enzymes specific for glutamate terminal peptide bonds have been characterized.[293] DAMPA is also produced by the enzymatic cleavage of MTX in a rescue regimen initially tested in the treatment of brain tumors.[294] In this protocol, high-dose systemic MTX is followed by the infusion of the bacterial enzyme carboxypeptidase G1, which degrades MTX in the systemic circulation but leaves drug intact in the brain and CSF.

The role of these metabolites in producing MTX toxicity or influencing therapeutic activity is uncertain. Both 7-OH-MTX and the pteroic acid metabolite are less soluble than the parent drug (Table 6.3). Jacobs and colleagues[289] demonstrated that 7-OH-MTX constituted more than 50% of precipitated intrarenal material in their study of MTX-induced renal failure in monkeys, but the role of either metabolite in the clinical syndrome of MTX-associated nephrotoxicity in humans is unproven.

TOXICITY

Primary Toxic Effects

The primary toxic effects of folate antagonists are myelosuppression and gastrointestinal mucositis. The incidence of these and other toxicities depends on the specific dose, schedule, and route of drug administration and is summarized in Table 6.5. The intestinal and oral epithelia are somewhat more sensitive than granulocyte and platelet precursors in that drug schedules that produce intense mucositis (particularly those with prolonged, low drug concentrations) may cause little marrow suppression. The threshold plasma concentration of MTX required to inhibit DNA synthesis in bone marrow has been estimated to be 10 nmol/L, whereas gastrointestinal epithelium is inhibited at 5 nmol/L plasma concentrations.[295] This greater sensitivity of gastrointestinal epithelium is believed to result from greater accumulation and persistence of MTX in intestinal epithelium than in bone marrow.[296] Mucositis usually appears 3 to 7 days after drug administration and precedes the onset of a fall in white blood count or platelet

count by several days. In patients with compromised renal function, small doses on the order of 25 mg may provide cytotoxic blood levels for up to 3 to 5 days and may result in serious bone marrow toxicity. Myelosuppression and mucositis usually are completely reversed within 2 weeks, unless drug excretion mechanisms are severely impaired.

Methylenetetrahydrofolate reductase (MTHFR) is a critical enzyme in folate metabolism that regulates the metabolism of folate, methionine and homocysteine. A C-to-T polymorphism of this enzyme at amino acid residue 677 results in a marked reduction in the activity of the enzyme particularly in individuals homozygous for this polymorphism. Multiple clinical studies in patients undergoing therapy with MTX for the management of rheumatoid arthritis, leukemia, ovarian cancer, and in the setting of bone marrow transplantation have reported a consistently elevated level of homocysteine following MTX exposure and a marked increase in the level of toxicity associated with MTX in patients homozygous for the 677C to T polymorphism.[297–301] These studies suggest that either assessment for the TT genotype or the occurrence of marked elevations in serum hymocycteine levels following MTX exposure may be useful as markers for predicting high-grade MTX toxicity.

The introduction of high-dose MTX regimens with leucovorin rescue[302] has been associated with a spectrum of clinical toxicities that has required more careful monitoring of drug pharmacokinetics in individual patients. These regimens use otherwise lethal doses in a 6- to 36-hour infusion, followed by a 24- to 48-hour period of multiple leucovorin doses to terminate the toxic effect of MTX. Several of the more commonly used high-dose regimens and their related pharmacokinetics are presented in Table 6.4. For each regimen, successful rescue by leucovorin depends on the rapid elimination of MTX by the kidneys. Early experience with high-dose regimens, however, indicated that MTX itself may have acute toxic effects on renal function during the period of drug infusion, which can lead to delayed drug clearance, ineffective rescue by leucovorin, and a host of secondary toxicities, including severe myelosuppression, mucositis, and epithelial desquamation.[258] During the early clinical trials of high-dose MTX, a number of toxic deaths were recorded.[303]

The cause of drug-induced renal dysfunction, which is usually manifested as an abrupt rise in serum blood urea nitrogen and creatinine with a corresponding fall in urine output, is thought to arise from the precipitation of MTX and possibly its less soluble metabolites, 7-OH-MTX and DAMPA, in acidic urine.[289] A direct toxic effect of antifolates on the renal tubule, however, has been suggested by the observation that aminopterin, an equally soluble compound that is used at one-tenth the dose of MTX, is also associated with renal toxicity; however, a direct nephrotoxic role of MTX has not been substantiated in clinical investigations.[304] Jacobs et al.[289] were able to reproduce the syndrome of MTX-induced renal failure in a monkey model system and demonstrated precipitation of both

TABLE 6.5

TOXICITIES ASSOCIATED WITH VARIOUS DOSES/ROUTES OF METHOTREXATE SODIUM ADMINISTRATION

Dose	Myelotoxicity	Nephrotoxicity	Hepatotoxicity	Mucositis	Pulmonary Toxicity	Neurotoxicity
Intermediate IV (50–100 mg/m^2)	+++	+	+ (transaminasemia)	++	±	−
High-dose IV with leucovorin calcium (100–12,000 mg/m^2)	+	+++ (requires urinary alkalinization and hydration)	++ (transaminasemia)	++	±	++ (acute and chronic)
Low-dose PO, daily dose (5–25 mg/m^2)	−	−	+++ (up to 25% cirrhosis)	−	±	−
Low-dose PO, pulse therapy (5–25 mg/m^2)	−	−	++ (rarely cirrhosis)	−	+	−
Intrathecal	−	−	−	−	−	++ (acute, subacute, and chronic)

+, some toxicity; ++, moderate toxicity; +++, high toxicity; −, no toxicity; ±, possible toxicity.
IV, intravenously; PO, per os.

MTX and 7-OH-MTX in the renal tubules. Both of these compounds have limited solubility under acid pH conditions. To prevent precipitation, most centers use vigorous hydration (2.5 to 3.5 L of fluid per square meter per 24 hours, beginning 12 hours before MTX infusion and continuing for 24 to 48 hours), with alkalinization of the urine (45 to 50 mEq of sodium bicarbonate per liter of intravenous fluid). The MTX infusion should not begin until urine flow exceeds 100 mL/hour and urine pH is 7.0 or higher, and these parameters should be carefully monitored during the course of drug infusion (Table 6.4).

With this regimen, the incidence of renal failure and myelosuppression has been markedly reduced. No change in the rate of MTX excretion or alteration of plasma pharmacokinetics results from the intense hydration used in the preparatory regimen previously described[270]; thus, these safety measures should have no deleterious effect on the therapeutic efficacy of the regimen. Despite careful attention to the details of hydration and alkalinization, occasional patients can develop serious or even fatal toxicity.[303] Almost all of these toxic episodes are associated with delayed MTX clearance from plasma and can be predicted by routine monitoring of drug concentration in plasma at appropriate times after drug infusion.[305] In an analysis of 790 patients treated with high-dose MTX for osteosarcoma, the incidence of delayed MTX clearance (>5umol/L at 24 hours postinfusion) was 1.6% per cycle of treatment.[306] The specific time for monitoring, and the guidelines for distinguishing between normal and dangerously elevated levels, must be determined for each regimen and for each assay procedure. In general, a time point well into the final phase of drug disappearance, such as 24 or 48 hours after the start of infusion, should be chosen (Table 6.4). The use of ketoprofen and other nonsteroidal anti-inflammatory

drugs (NSAIDs) has been associated with severe MTX toxicity.[307] A review of 118 cases of single-agent, high-dose MTX therapy revealed four cases of fatal toxicity associated with the use of NSAIDs. Patients treated with NSAIDs demonstrated a marked prolongation of serum MTX half-life that was postulated to be caused by decreased renal elimination secondary to inhibition of renal prostaglandin synthesis or competitive inhibition of human organic anion transporters (hOAT) responsible for MTX uptake in the kidney.[308,309]

Early detection of elevated concentrations of MTX allows institution of specific clinical measures. Continuous medical supervision is warranted until the severity and duration of myelosuppression can be determined. Leucovorin in increased doses is required and must be continued until plasma MTX concentration falls below 50 nmol/L. Because of the competitive relationship between MTX and leucovorin, the leucovorin dose must be increased in proportion to the plasma concentration of MTX. Small doses of leucovorin are unable to prevent toxicity in patients with elevated drug levels, even when leucovorin is continued beyond 48 hours.[305] As a general rule, a reasonable course is to treat with leucovorin at a dosage of 100 mg/m^2 every 6 hours for patients with MTX levels of 1 μmol/L and to increase this dosage in proportion to the MTX level up to a maximum of 500 mg/m^2 (Table 6.4). Subsequent leucovorin dosage adjustments should be based on repeated plasma MTX levels taken at 24-hour intervals. The results of in vitro studies indicate that leucovorin alone may not be able to rescue patients with plasma MTX concentrations above 10 μmol/L.

The absorption of oral leucovorin is saturable such that the bioavailability of the compound is limited above total doses of 40 mg. The fractional absorption of a 40-mg dose is 0.78, whereas that of 60- and 100-mg doses is 0.62 and 0.42, respectively. For this reason, leucovorin is usually administered intravenously to assure its absorption.

Because of the variable effectiveness of leucovorin in preventing toxicity in patients with levels of 10 µmol/L or greater at 48 hours, alternative methods of rescue have been proposed. Both intermittent hemodialysis and peritoneal dialysis are ineffective in removing significant quantities of MTX. However, continuous flow hemodialysis has been effective in reducing plasma MTX concentration and preventing toxicity in patients with MTX-induced failure.[309a] The use of charcoal hemoperfusion columns is capable of removing MTX and other antineoplastic drugs from whole blood and has been applied successfully in a few patients; however, platelet adherence to these columns may lead to thrombocytopenia.

Abelson and co-workers[294] used a bacterial enzyme, carboxypeptidase G1, which inactivates MTX by removal of its terminal glutamate, to destroy circulating MTX. The regimen of high-dose MTX followed by intravenous carboxypeptidase was well tolerated, but this form of enzymatic rescue carries a risk of hypersensitivity to the bacterial enzyme. Bertino et al.[310] have demonstrated the feasibility of attaching the enzyme to hollow fiber tubing, which can then be used in an extracorporeal shunt for drug removal and thus avoid immune sensitization. One potential disadvantage of carboxypeptidase G1, however, is its relatively high affinity for natural folates as well as MTX. DeAngelis and colleagues[311] conducted a pilot study to determine the efficacy of carboxypeptidase G2 (CPG2) rescue after high-dose MTX in patients with recurrent cerebral lymphoma. All patients had at least a 2-log decline in plasma MTX levels within 5 minutes of CPG2 administration, whereas CSF MTX concentrations remained elevated for 4 hours after CPG2. No MTX or CPG2 toxicity was observed, and anti-CPG2 activity antibodies were not detected in any patient. The authors concluded that CPG2 rescue was a safe and effective alternative to leucovorin rescue after high-dose MTX chemotherapy. Additional utility of CPG2 as a safe and effective means for preventing severe MTX toxicity was demonstrated in several reports of patients with delayed MTX clearance.[312,313] In an NCI study on the use of CPG2 in pediatric patients who developed nephrotoxicity while receiving high-dose MTX, Widemann et al.[314] found that CPG2 and thymidine rescue was well tolerated and resulted in a rapid and effective reduction in the plasma MTX concentration with only mild-to-moderate MTX-related toxicity.

Preliminary reports have described the successful prevention of MTX toxicity in humans using 6- to 40-hour infusions of the antifolate followed by a 72-hour infusion of thymidine at a rate of 8 g/m^2 per day.[229,315,316] Patients receiving a bolus dose of MTX, 3 g/m^2, were successfully rescued by thymidine infusion (1 g/m^2 per day); the infusion was begun 24 hours after MTX administration and continued until MTX concentration in the plasma reached 50 nmol/L.[317]

In the experimental setting, MTX toxicity can also be blocked by drugs that prevent cell progression into the S phase of the cell cycle. The antagonistic effect of L-asparaginase on MTX toxicity is a representative example; through depletion of the amino acid asparagine, L-asparaginase, inhibits protein synthesis and prevents entry of cells into the DNA-synthetic phase of the cell cycle.[318] Rescue regimens[319] that use high doses of MTX (up to 400 mg/m^2), followed within 24 hours by 20,000 to 40,000 U per m^2 of L-asparaginase, produce minimal bone marrow toxicity and mucositis, and appear to have some effectiveness in patients refractory to low-dose MTX alone. Yap et al.[319] reported a complete remission rate of 62% (13 of 21 cases) in adult patients with ALL who had failed initial therapy with conventional induction regimens.

Drugs that inhibit the TS reaction, thereby preventing alterations in the composition of the intracellular folate pools and negating the effect of DHFR enzyme inhibition, also prevent MTX toxicity. This effect has been studied in detail and seems to explain the antagonism of fluoropyrimidine pretreatment followed by MTX.[320]

Poor nutritional status has been associated with an increased risk of toxicity from MTX.[321,322] Poorly nourished patients appear to have an approximately twofold decrease in their clearance of MTX. The reason for this delayed drug clearance appears to be a protracted enterohepatic circulation. Providing dietary protein in the form of polypeptides (rather than amino acids) either alone or in combination with cholestyramine treatment to bind intestinal MTX may be useful in avoiding excess toxicity associated with nutritional deficiencies.

Other Toxicities

Hepatotoxicity

In addition to its inhibitory effects on rapidly dividing tissues, MTX has toxic effects on nondividing tissues not easily explained by its primary action on DNA synthesis. Long-term MTX therapy is associated with portal fibrosis, which may, on occasion, progress to frank cirrhosis. Chronic liver disease has occurred most frequently in patients with psoriasis or rheumatoid arthritis or in children with acute leukemia who have received maintenance therapy over a period of several years. The incidence of cirrhosis has been estimated to be 10% in MTX-treated patients with psoriasis but may reach as high as 25 to 30% in those patients treated for 5 years or longer with continuous daily therapy.[323] Cirrhosis does not always progress with continued antifolate treatment. Of 11 patients with psoriasis who showed cirrhotic changes on liver biopsy and continued to receive treatment, only 3 showed progression on subsequent biopsy, and 3 had no pathologic findings on a follow-up biopsy.[323] The use of "pulsed" weekly therapy rather than continuous daily treatment appears to lessen the incidence of MTX-associated hepatotoxicity.[324,325] Several studies suggest that the incidence of hepatic cirrhosis is no different in patients with rheumatoid arthritis treated with MTX pulse therapy than in untreated patients despite long-term therapy (longer than 5 years).[326,327] Evidence of hepatic toxicity was detected on liver biopsy in 76% of 29 patients receiving weekly (7.5-mg) pulse therapy with MTX for rheumatoid arthritis; however, only 1 patient had severe fibrosis.[326] These patients had been treated for an average of approximately 2.5 years (1,500 mg total dose). Abnormal elevations in serum transaminases have been found in up to 70% of patients treated with long-term weekly MTX; however, the enzyme elevations were poor predictors of liver damage.[328] In three series of patients who underwent liver biopsy while being treated with long-term weekly MTX, 17 to 30% had fibrotic changes but 0 to 3% demonstrated cirrhosis.[328,329]

Acute elevations of liver enzymes are commonly observed after high-dose MTX administration and usually return to normal within 10 days. The frequency and severity of liver enzyme elevations appear to be directly related to the number of MTX doses received.[330] Liver biopsy in such patients has revealed fatty infiltration but no evidence of hepatocellular necrosis or periportal fibrosis. The late occurrence of cirrhosis in patients treated with high-dose MTX has not been reported.

Pneumonitis

Treatment with MTX is associated with a poorly characterized, self-limited pneumonitis, with fever, cough, and an interstitial pulmonary infiltrate.[331,332] Eosinophilia has not been a consistent finding, either in the peripheral blood or in open lung biopsy specimens. Lung biopsies have revealed a variety of findings, from simple interstitial edema and a mononuclear infiltrate to noncaseating granulomas. The possibility that MTX pneumonitis may not represent a hypersensitivity phenomenon has been raised because of the failure of some patients to react to reinstitution of MTX therapy. However, bronchoalveolar lavage in three patients with presumptive MTX-induced lung damage revealed a predominance of T8 suppressor lymphocytes. In contrast to peripheral lymphocytes obtained from MTX-treated patients with no lung damage, lymphocytes from the study patients elaborated leukocyte inhibitory factor in response to MTX exposure.[333] This study supports an immunologic basis for MTX-related lung damage. The possibility exists, however, that many case reports of "MTX lung" in fact represent unrecognized viral infections or allergic reactions to unsuspected allergens. With the use of long-term weekly low-dose MTX therapy for rheumatoid arthritis, however, a number of cases of MTX-associated lung damage have been reported.[334,335] A review of 168 patients treated with MTX for rheumatoid arthritis uncovered 9 cases (5%) of probable MTX-associated lung toxicity.[336] Using a retrospective combined-cohort review and abstraction from the medical literature,

Kremer and colleagues[337] characterized the clinical features of MTX-associated lung injury in patients with rheumatoid arthritis. Clinical symptoms of MTX toxicity in the cohort included the subacute development of shortness of breath (93%), cough (82%), and fever (69%), with resultant death in 5 of 27 patients. The authors concluded that early symptom recognition and the cessation of MTX administration could avoid the serious and sometimes fatal outcome of this MTX-associated toxicity. Corticosteroids have been used in a small number of patients who ultimately recovered,[338] but the utility of this approach has yet to be established. Alarcon et al.[339] found that the strongest predictors of MTX-induced lung injury in rheumatoid arthritis patients included older age, presence of diabetes, rheumatoid pleuropulmonary involvement, presence of hypoalbuminemia, and prior use of disease-modifying antirheumatic drugs.

Hypersensitivity

True anaphylactic reactions to MTX are rare. Two cases of acute hypersensitivity reaction to MTX have been described.[340] In the first case, the patient experienced acute cardiovascular collapse, which was reproduced on rechallenge of the patient with MTX. In the second case, the acute reaction consisted of facial edema, rash, and generalized pruritus, and again was elicited on rechallenge. Both patients were receiving bacille Calmette-Guérin in conjunction with MTX at the time of these reactions, and thus may have developed a heightened sensitivity to MTX. Three cases of toxic erythema and desquamation of the hands were reported in patients receiving high doses (1.5 g/m^2) of MTX for the treatment of non-Hodgkin's lymphoma.[341] This toxic reaction was associated with severe mucositis and was ameliorated by MTX dose reductions on subsequent treatment.

Reversible oligospermia with testicular failure has been reported in men treated with high-dose MTX.[342] No alterations in follicle-stimulating hormone, luteinizing hormone, estradiol, or progesterone have been observed in women exposed to MTX.

PHARMACOKINETICS AND TOXICITY OF METHOTREXATE IN THE CENTRAL NERVOUS SYSTEM

Because of its high degree of ionization at physiologic pH, MTX penetrates into the CSF with difficulty. During a constant intravenous drug infusion,[343] the ratio of venous MTX concentration to CSF concentration is approximately 30:1 at equilibrium. Thus, plasma levels in excess of 30 μmol/L would be required to achieve the concentration of 1 μmol/L that is thought to be necessary for killing of leukemic cells. Protocols for prophylaxis against meningeal leukemia and lymphoma using systemic high-dose infusions of MTX have demonstrated that high-dose MTX infusions are a reasonable treatment alternative to intrathecal prophylaxis. Overt meningeal leukemia increases the CSF:plasma ratio and experience supports the use of MTX at a loading dose of 700 mg/m2 followed by a 23-hour infusion of 2,800 mg/m^2, with leucovorin rescue as an excellent treatment alternative for patients with carcinomatous meningitis capable of achieving the requisite CSF levels of 1 μmol/L.[344,345] In children with ALL, a diminished CSF:plasma ratio has been found to be a useful predictor of CNS relapse.[346]

Direct intrathecal injection of MTX has been used for the treatment and prophylaxis of meningeal malignancy. The readers are referred to a comprehensive review on this topic.[347] Drug injected into the intrathecal space distributes in a total volume of approximately 120 mL for patients over 3 years of age. Thus, a maximal total dose of 12 mg is advised for all patients over 3 years, with lower doses indicated for younger children. Bleyer[261] has recommended a dose of 6 mg for age 1 or younger, 8 mg for ages 1 to 2, and 10 mg for ages 2 to 3. The peak CSF concentration achieved by this schedule is approximately 100 μmol/L. Lumbar CSF drug concentrations decline in a biphasic pattern with a terminal half-life of 7 to 16 hours. This terminal phase of disappearance may be considerably prolonged in patients with active meningeal disease and in older-age patients.[347,348] Injection of radiolabeled MTX into the ventricular space of rabbits demonstrated rapid but variable distribution of MTX in the gray matter adjacent to the CSF, which suggests a mechanism for the various syndromes associated with MTX neurotoxicity.[349] MTX is cleared from spinal fluid by bulk resorption of spinal fluid (i.e., "bulk flow"), a process that may be prolonged by increases in intracranial pressure and the administration of acetazolamide. A second component of resorption involves the active transport of this organic anion by the choroid plexus. A prolongation of the terminal half-life is also found in patients who develop drug-related neurotoxicity, although a causal relationship between abnormal pharmacokinetics and neurotoxicity has not been firmly established.

MTX administered into the lumbar space distributes poorly over the cerebral convexities and into the ventricular spaces.[343] The concentration gradient between lumbar and ventricular CSF may exceed 10:1. Although this uneven distribution has no documented role in determining clinical relapse of patients treated for meningeal leukemia, awareness of this potential problem has led to clinical trials using direct intraventricular injection of MTX via an Ommaya reservoir. Bleyer and colleagues[350] have demonstrated that a concentration × time regimen in which 1 mg MTX was injected into the Ommaya reservoir every 12 hours for 3 days yielded continuous CSF levels above 0.5 μmol/L and achieved therapeutic results equivalent to those with the conventional intralumbar injection of 12 mg every 4 days. Moreover, this concentration × time

regimen was associated with a considerable reduction in neurotoxic side effects, presumably owing to the avoidance of high peak levels of drug associated with higher MTX doses. Glantz et al.[351] reported on the use of high-dose intravenous MTX as the sole treatment for nonleukemic meningitis. Sixteen patients with solid tumor neoplastic meningitis received high-dose intravenous MTX (8 g/m^2 over 4 hours) with leucovorin rescue. Compared with a reference group of patients receiving standard intrathecal MTX, the high-dose intravenous group exhibited cytotoxic CSF and serum MTX concentrations that were maintained much longer than with intrathecal dosing. In addition, median survival in the high-dose intravenous MTX group was 13.8 months versus 2.3 months for the intrathecal reference group ($P = .003$).

Three different neurotoxic syndromes have been observed after treatment with intrathecal MTX.[350] The most common and most immediate neurotoxic side effect is an acute chemical arachnoiditis manifested as severe headache, nuchal rigidity, vomiting, fever, and inflammatory cell pleocytosis of the spinal fluid. This constellation of symptoms appears to be a function of the frequency and dose of drug administered, and may be ameliorated either by reduction in dose or by a change in therapy to intrathecal cytosine arabinoside. A less acute but more serious neurotoxic syndrome has been observed in approximately 10% of patients treated with intrathecal MTX. This subacute toxicity appears during the second or third week of treatment, usually in adult patients with active meningeal leukemia, and is manifested as motor paralysis of the extremities, cranial nerve palsy, seizures, or coma. Because MTX pharmacokinetics is abnormal in these patients, the suspicion is that this subacute neurotoxicity may be the result of extended exposure to toxic drug concentrations.[347] Finally, a more chronic demyelinating encephalopathy has been observed in children months or years after intrathecal MTX therapy. The primary symptoms of this toxicity are dementia, limb spasticity, and, in more advanced cases, coma. Computerized axial tomography (CT) has revealed ventricular enlargement, white matter changes, cortical thinning, and diffuse intracerebral calcification in children who have received prophylactic intrathecal MTX.[352,353] Most of these patients had also received cranial irradiation (>2,000 rad) and all had received systemic chemotherapy.

Treatment with repeated courses of high-dose intravenous MTX may also result in encephalopathy.[354] In these patients, symptoms of dementia and paresis may develop in the second or third month after treatment and may also be associated with diffuse cortical hypodensities on CT scan. A second form of cerebral dysfunction associated with high-dose MTX is an acute transient dysfunction, which has been described in 4 to 15% of treated patients.[355-357] The syndrome consists of any combination of paresis, aphasia, behavioral abnormalities, and seizures. The neurologic events occur an average of 6 days after the MTX dose and completely resolve, usually within 48 to 72 hours.

Patients may have received any number of MTX doses before the onset of this neurotoxic event, and some patients may have repeat episodes with subsequent MTX doses. In general, CSF and head CT scans are normal, but low-density lesions have been noted in some cases.[358] The electroencephalogram may represent the only abnormal study and shows a diffuse or focal slowing. No clinical evidence exists to support the use of leucovorin, either acutely after intrathecal MTX or over the long term in patients who develop neurotoxic symptoms. Although leucovorin can enter the CSF, its penetration appears to be poor.[359,360] A comparison of neurologic toxicities was undertaken in a randomized trial involving 49 children with acute leukemia treated with either intrathecal MTX plus radiation or high-dose systemic MTX for central nervous system prophylaxis.[361] Long-term toxicities were similar with either treatment option, and overall decreases in intelligence quotients were found to be clinically significant in 61% of the children. In addition, 58% of the patients treated with systemic therapy had abnormal electroencephalograms and 57% of those treated with intrathecal MTX and radiation experienced somnolence syndrome. Mahoney and colleagues[362] described the incidence of acute neurotoxicity in 1,304 children with lower risk B-precursor lymphoid leukemia treated as part of the Pediatric Oncology Group trial. After remission induction, patients were randomized into one of three 24-week intensification schedules (intermediate-dose MTX or divided-dose oral MTX with or without intravenous mercaptopurine and extended intrathecal therapy). Overall, acute neurotoxicity occurred in 7.8% (95 of 1,218) of eligible patients, and the authors found that intensification with repeated intravenous MTX and low-dose leucovorin rescue was associated with a higher risk of acute neurotoxicity and leukoencephalopathy, especially in patients who received concomitant triple intrathecal therapy (MTX, dexamethasone, and cytosine arabinoside).

The etiology of the MTX-associated neurotoxicity is unknown. Vascular events in the form of vasospasm or emboli have been proposed to explain these neurologic abnormalities, and studies have suggested alterations in brain glucose metabolism after MTX treatment.[363] Investigators from St. Jude Children's Research Hospital found that the incidence of seizures in children treated for acute leukemia with MTX were related to acute elevations in serum homocysteine levels following MTX treatment.[364] Of interest, these investigators did not find an association between seizures and MTHFR genotype. Long-term exposure of rat cerebellar explants to 1 μmol/L MTX resulted in axonal death 2 weeks after drug exposure and loss of myelin sheaths in 5 weeks, which suggests a direct toxic effect of MTX on axonal cells.[365] DHFR is present in brain tissue, but its biochemical role in the cerebral cortex, the primary site of MTX neurotoxicity, is uncertain. Several studies have demonstrated the ability of cranial radiation to increase blood-brain barrier permeability to serum proteins and MTX.[366] Because radiation and MTX are frequently used together, this interaction may be an important mechanism for enhanced toxicity. Inadvertent overdose of intrathecal MTX generally has a fatal outcome. Immediate lumbar puncture with CSF removal along with ventriculolumbar perfusion has been successfully used to avert catastrophe in such situations.[367]

CLINICAL DOSAGE SCHEDULES

A variety of dosage schedules and routes of administration are used clinically, including high-dose therapy with the addition of leucovorin rescue. The selection of an appropriate schedule depends largely on the specific disease being treated, on other antineoplastic agents or radiation to be used in combination regimens, on the patient's tolerance for host toxicity, and on other factors that might alter pharmacokinetics. Parenteral schedules are preferred for induction therapy regimens in which maximal concentrations and duration of exposure are desirable in an effort to achieve complete remission. High-dose MTX regimens and leucovorin rescue offer the advantage of minimal bone marrow toxicity. This regimen, however, can safely be used only in patients with normal renal and hepatic function and under conditions in which no large extracellular accumulations of fluid are present. As emphasized previously, high-dose regimens should be instituted only when plasma monitoring is available to determine the adequacy of drug clearance and the risk of serious toxicity. Furthermore, because leucovorin may rescue tumor cells as well as normal cells, the optimal dose, schedule, and clinical utility of high-dose MTX with leucovorin rescue needs to be more carefully defined.

OTHER ANTIFOLATES

Pemetrexed

Thymidylate synthase (TS) represents a logical target for new drug development using folate analogs, and pemetrexed (LY231514, Alimta), a pyrrolo(2,3-d)pyrimidine-based antifolate analog, is a potent inhibitor of TS. Pemetrexed is avidly transported into cells via the reduced-folate carrier (RFC) and possibly by a unique transporter identified in mesothelioma cell lines.[368,368a] It is metabolized to the polyglutamated forms, which are potent inhibitors of several folate-dependent enzymatic reactions. The multitargeting effect of pemetrexed was seen in studies by Shih et al.[368] who suggested that, at higher concentrations, pemetrexed and its polyglutamates not only act as TS inhibitors, depleting dTTP pools, but also inhibit other key folate-requiring enzymes, including glycinamide ribonucleotide formyltransferase, and to a lesser extent DHFR, 5-aminoimidazole-4-carboxamide ribonucleotide formyltransferase, and C1-tetrahydrofolate synthase. The combined inhibitory effects of pemetrexed give rise to a cellular level end-product reversal pattern that is different from those of other inhibitors such as MTX and the quinazoline antifolates. In addition, pemetrexed has less effect on the folate and nucleotide pools as compared with MTX.[369] In studies evaluating the effects of folic acid on modulating the toxicity and antitumor efficacy of pemetrexed in human tumor cell lines adapted to growth in low-folate medium, folic acid was shown to be 100- to 1,000-fold less active than folinic acid at protecting cells from pemetrexed-induced cytotoxicity.[370] Further, folic acid supplementation was demonstrated to preserve the antitumor activity of pemetrexed while reducing toxicity in mice. In patients with mesothelioma, pemetrexed as a single agent produced a response rate of 14%. In patients, severe toxicity was correlated with high serum concentrations of hemocysteine, an indicator of folate deficiency. In an additional 15% of patients, B_{12} deficiency was thought to be responsible for pemetrexed toxicity. Of interest, the addition of vitamin B_{12} (1 mg intramuscularly) and folic acid (1 mg/day for 2 weeks beginning 2 weeks prior to pemetrexed) resulted in an improved toxicity profile and improved efficacy in patients with mesothelioma treated with pemetrexed.[371,372] In a randomized phase III investigation of 456 patients with mesothelioma, comparing cisplatin with the combination of cisplatin plus pemetrexed, the patients treated with the doublet enjoyed a significantly improved response rate (41 versus 17%), time to disease progression (5.7 versus 3.9 months), and overall survival (12.1 versus 9.3 months) when compared with single-agent cisplatin therapy. Pemetrexed has been demonstrated to have activity in several solid tumors including non–small cell lung cancer, in which it was shown to have a 16% response rate in untreated patients.[373] A phase III trial with 571 patients randomized patients with advanced and refractory non–small cell lung cancer to either pemetrexed or docetaxel and showed that both drugs resulted in identical efficacy outcomes, but the pemetrexed was associated with a significantly improved toxicity profile.[374] Aside from myelosuppression and intestinal toxicity, pemetrexed causes a rash in 40% of patients. The rash is suppressed by the administration of dexamethasome, 4 mg 2 times a day, on days 1, 0, and +1.

Nolatrexed

Nolatrexed (AG337 , THYMITAQ) is a nonclassic inhibitor of TS specifically designed to avoid potential resistance mechanisms that can limit the activity of the classic antifolate antimetabolites.[375] Nolatrexed is a lipophilic molecule designed using x-ray structure-based methods to interact at the folate cofactor binding site of the TS enzyme. TS was suggested as the locus of action of nolatrexed by the ability of thymidine to antagonize cell growth inhibition and the direct demonstration of TS inhibition in whole cells using a

tritium-release assay.[376] Nolatrexed is characterized as a non–glutamate-containing molecule that does not require facilitated transport for uptake and does not undergo, nor require, intracellular polyglutamylation for activity. L1210 cells treated with nolatrexed exhibited S-phase cell-cycle arrest and a pattern of nucleotide pool modulations, including a reduction in thymidine triphosphate levels, consistent with inhibition of TS.[376] Rafi et al.[375] measured plasma concentrations of deoxyuridine (dUrd) in patients receiving doses of nolatrexed at levels of more than 600 mg/m^2 and found elevation in plasma dUrd levels (60 to 290%), which implied that TS inhibition was being achieved in patients. In all cases, dUrd concentrations quickly returned to pretreatment levels after the end of the infusion; this suggested that TS inhibition was not maintained, presumably because of the brief intracellular half-life of the nonpolyglutamated parent compound. A phase I trial evaluating intravenous administration of nolatrexed found dose-limiting myelosuppression and a high incidence of thrombotic phenomena.[377] A second trial evaluating 5-day oral administration of nolatrexed showed rapid absorption with a median bioavailability of 89%; dose-limiting toxicities were gastrointestinal. The authors concluded that nolatrexed could be safely administered as an oral preparation at a dosage of 725 mg/m^2 per day for 5 days.[378] Using this dose and schedule, in 139 untreated patients with head and neck cancer, nolatrexed was found to have similar activity as MTX.[379]

Raltitrexed

Raltitrexed (ZD1694, Tomudex) is a water-soluble TS inhibitor that appears to have an acceptable toxicity profile, convenient dosing schedule, and antitumor activity in colorectal, breast, pancreatic, and a variety of other solid cancers.[380–383] This drug is a second-generation agent designed to overcome the major toxicity associated with its predecessor, CB3717, namely, poorly predictable nephrotoxicity. Yin and colleagues[384] conducted in vitro studies on the human A253 head and neck squamous carcinoma cell line to evaluate the downstream molecular alterations induced by the potent and sustained inhibition of TS by raltitrexed. TS inhibition by raltitrexed resulted in a time-dependent induction of megabase DNA fragmentation followed by a secondary 50- to 300-kilobase DNA fragmentation, which may correlate with reduced expression of p27 and increase in cyclin E and cdk2 kinase activity. Cunningham[382] reviewed the results of three large controlled studies that suggest that raltitrexed is an effective alternative to 5-fluorouracil–based therapy in patients with advanced colorectal cancer, and that raltitrexed has the advantage of a predictable toxicity profile, minimization or avoidance of mucositis, and convenient dosing schedule. The data concerning progression-free survival and survival are not consistent, however, with at least one large study demonstrating inferiority with respect to therapy with 5-fluorouracil and leucovorin. Raltitrexed has also been used in combination with either oxaliplatin or irinotecan for the treatment of patients with advanced colorectal cancer. These combinations have been associated with acceptable toxicity, response rates in the 35 to 45% range, and overall median survivals of approximately 15 months.[385,386] As has been found to be the case for 5-fluorouracil, intratumoral thymidylate synthase levels have also been demonstrated to predict for responsiveness to raltitrexed as well as overall survival with low levels of thymidylate synthase being associated with higher response rates and longer survival when compared to patients with higher enzyme levels.[387]

ZD9331

ZD9331 is a potent quinazoline antifolate inhibitor of TS that does not require polyglutamation for activity. The lack of required polyglutamation of ZD9331, which is in contrast to raltitrexed, may allow for antitumor activity in cells with low FPGS activity. ZD9331 is transported into cells predominantly by the RFC system and competes with both MTX and folinic acid for cellular uptake. Clinical investigations suggest single-agent activity in patients with refractory lung, ovarian and breast cancers.[388]

Antibody-Directed Enzyme Therapy

Antibody-directed enzyme therapy (ADEPT) systems separate cytotoxic and targeting functions by binding to cell surface markers expressed specifically on malignant cells and activating molecules, including antifolate compounds like MTX at the target cell. This targeted binding and activation theoretically minimizes generalized toxicity secondary to nonspecific delivery of cytotoxic drug. Studies done by Springer et al.[389] delivered an antibody-CPG2 enzyme before the nontoxic prodrug CMDA. Once delivered, CMDA was converted to a cytotoxic drug by the action of the localized conjugate at the tumor site. In addition, prodrugs of quinazoline antifolate TS inhibitors (ZD1694 and ICI198583) have been designed and synthesized for use in ADEPT systems. The α-linked L-dipeptide prodrugs were designed to be activated to their corresponding TS inhibitors at the tumor site by prior administration of a monoclonal antibody conjugated to the enzyme carboxypeptidase A. Activation of the α-linked L-alanine dipeptides with carboxypeptidase A led to a cytotoxicity enhancement of 10- to 100-fold.[390] ADEPT holds the potential of providing an effective and relatively nontoxic treatment of cancer.[391]

REFERENCES

1. Farber S, Diamond LK, Mercer RD, et al. Temporary remission in acute leukemia in children produced by folic acid antagonist 4-amethopteroylglutamic acid (aminopterin). N Engl J Med 1948;238:787.
2. Hoffmeister RT. Methotrexate therapy in rheumatoid arthritis: 15 years' experience. Am J Med 1983;75:69–73.
3. Rees RB, Bennett JH, Maibach HI, et al. Methotrexate for psoriasis. Arch Dermatol 1967;95:2–11.
4. Calabresi P, Chabner BA. Chemotherapy of neoplastic diseases. In: Gilman AG, Rall TW, Dies DS, et al., eds. The pharmacologic Basis of Therapeutics. 8th Ed. New York: Pergamon Press, 1990:1202.
5. Allegra CJ, Chabner BA, Tuazon CU, et al. Trimetrexate for the treatment of Pneumocystis carinii pneumonia in patients with the acquired immunodeficiency syndrome. N Engl J Med 1987;317:978–985.
6. Allegra CJ, Fine RL, Drake JC, et al. The effect of methotrexate on intracellular folate pools in human MCF-7 breast cancer cells. Evidence for direct inhibition of purine synthesis. J Biol Chem 1986;261:6478–6485.
7. Matherly LH, Barlowe CK, Phillips VM, et al. The effects of 4-amino-antifolates on 5-formyltetrahydrofolate metabolism in L1210 cells. J Biol Chem 1987;262:710–717.
8. Baram J, Allegra CJ, Fine RL, et al. Effect of methotrexate on intracellular folate pools in purified myeloid precursor cells from normal human bone marrow. J Clin Invest 1987;79:692–697.
9. Kesavan V, Sur P, Doig MT, et al. Effects of methotrexate on folates in Krebs ascites and L1210 murine leukemia cells. Cancer Lett 1986;30:55–59.
10. Bunni M, Doig MT, Donato H, et al. Role of methylenetetrahydrofolate depletion in methotrexate-mediated intracellular thymidylate synthesis inhibition in cultured L1210 cells. Cancer Res 1988;48:3398–3404.
11. Seither RL, Trent DF, Mikulecky DC, et al. Folate-pool interconversions and inhibition of biosynthetic processes after exposure of L1210 leukemia cells to antifolates. Experimental and network thermodynamic analyses of the role of dihydrofolate polyglutamylates in antifolate action in cells. J Biol Chem 1989;264:17016–17023.
12. Priest DG, Bunni M, Sirotnak FM. Relationship of reduced folate changes to inhibition of DNA synthesis induced by methotrexate in L1210 cells in vivo. Cancer Res 1989;49:4204–4209.
13. Allegra CJ, Hoang K, Yeh GC, et al. Evidence for direct inhibition of de novo purine synthesis in human MCF-7 breast cells as a principal mode of metabolic inhibition by methotrexate. J Biol Chem 1987;262:13520–13526.
14. Baram J, Chabner BA, Drake JC, et al. Identification and biochemical properties of 10-formyldihydrofolate, a novel folate found in methotrexate-treated cells. J Biol Chem 1988;263:7105–7111.
15. Kumar P, Kisliuk RL, Gaumont Y, et al. Inhibition of human dihydrofolate reductase by antifolyl polyglutamates. Biochem Pharmacol 1989;38:541–543.
16. Allegra CJ, Chabner BA, Drake JC, et al. Enhanced inhibition of thymidylate synthase by methotrexate polyglutamates. J Biol Chem 1985;260:9720–9726.
17. Allegra CJ, Drake JC, Jolivet J, et al. Inhibition of phosphoribosylaminoimidazolecarboxamide transformylase by methotrexate and dihydrofolic acid polyglutamates. Proc Natl Acad Sci U S A 1985;82:4881–4885.
18. Baggott JE, Vaughn WH, Hudson BB. Inhibition of 5-aminoimidazole-4-carboxamide ribotide transformylase, adenosine deaminase and 5′-adenylate deaminase by polyglutamates of methotrexate and oxidized folates and by 5-aminoimidazole-4-carboxamide riboside and ribotide. Biochem J 1986;236:193–200.
19. Chu E, Drake JC, Boarman D, et al. Mechanism of thymidylate synthase inhibition by methotrexate in human neoplastic cell lines and normal human myeloid progenitor cells. J Biol Chem 1990;265:8470–8478.
20. Morrison PF, Allegra CJ. Folate cycle kinetics in human breast cancer cells. J Biol Chem 1989;264:10552–10566.
21. Lyons SD, Sant ME, Christopherson RI. Cytotoxic mechanisms of glutamine antagonists in mouse L1210 leukemia. J Biol Chem 1990;265:11377–11381.
22. O'Dwyer PJ, Shoemaker DD, Plowman J, et al. Trimetrexate: a new antifol entering clinical trials. Invest New Drugs 1985;3:71–75.

23. Sigel CW, Macklin AW, Woolley JL Jr, et al. Preclinical biochemical pharmacology and toxicology of piritrexim, a lipophilic inhibitor of dihydrofolate reductase. J Natl Cancer Inst Monogr 1987;5:111–120.

24. Sirotnak FM, DeGraw JI, Schmid FA, et al. New folate analogs of the 10-deaza-aminopterin series. Further evidence for markedly increased antitumor efficacy compared with methotrexate in ascitic and solid murine tumor models. Cancer Chemother Pharmacol 1984;12:26–30.

25. Kamen BA, Eibl B, Cashmore A, et al. Uptake and efficacy of trimetrexate (TMQ, 2,4-diamino-5-methyl-6-[(3,4,5-trimethoxyanilino) methyl] quinazoline), a non-classical antifolate in methotrexate-resistant leukemia cells in vitro. Biochem Pharmacol 1984;33:1697–1699.

26. Jones TR, Calvert AH, Jackman AL, et al. A potent anti- tumor quinazoline inhibitor of thymidylate synthetase, biological properties and therapeutic results in mice. Eur J Cancer 1981;17:11–19.

27. Cheng YC, Dutschman GE, Starnes MC, et al. Activity of the new antifolate N10-propargyl-5,8-dideazafolate and its polyglutamates against human dihydrofolate reductase, human thymidylate synthetase, and KB cells containing different levels of dihydrofolate reductase. Cancer Res 1985;45:598–600.

28. Grindey GB, Shih C, Bernett CJ, et al. A novel pyrrolopyrimidine antifolate that inhibits thymidylate synthase (TS). Am Assoc Cancer Res 1992:2451.

29. Humphreys J, Smith G, Waters K, et al. Antitumor activity of the novel thymidylate synthase inhibitor 1843U89 in cells resistant to antifolates by multiple mechanisms. Am Assoc Cancer Res 1993:1625.

30. Beardsley GP, Taylor EC, Grindley GB, et al. Deaza derivatives of tetrahydrofolic acid: a new class of folate antimetabolite. In: Cooper BA, Whitehead VM, eds. Chemistry and Biology of Pteridines. Berlin: Walter deGruyter, 1986:953.

31. Antony AC, Kane MA, Portillo RM, et al. Studies of the role of a particulate folate-binding protein in the uptake of 5-methyltetrahydrofolate by cultured human KB cells. J Biol Chem 1985; 260:14911–14917.

32. Kamen BA, Capdevila A. Receptor-mediated folate accumulation is regulated by the cellular folate content. Proc Natl Acad Sci US A 1986;83:5983–5987.

33. Fan J, Vitols KS, Huennekens FM. Biotin derivatives of methotrexate and folate. Synthesis and utilization for affinity purification of two membrane-associated folate transporters from L1210 cells. J Biol Chem 1991;266:14862– 14865.

34. Brigle KE, Westin EH, Houghton MT, et al. Characterization of two cDNAs encoding folate-binding proteins from L1210 murine leukemia cells. Increased expression associated with a genomic rearrangement. J Biol Chem 1991;266:17243–17249.

35. Chello PL, Sirotnak FM, Dorick DM. Alterations in the kinetics of methotrexate transport during growth of L1210 murine leukemia cells in culture. Mol Pharmacol 1980;18:274–280.

36. Knight CB, Elwood PC, Chabner BA. Future directions for antifolate drug development. Adv Enzyme Regul 1989;29:3–12.

37. Kane MA, Portillo RM, Elwood PC, et al. The influence of extracellular folate concentration on methotrexate uptake by human KB cells. Partial characterization of a membrane- associated methotrexate binding protein. J Biol Chem 1986;261:44–49.

38. Price EM, Freisheim JH. Photoaffinity analogues of methotrexate as folate antagonist binding probes. 2. Transport studies, photoaffinity labeling, and identification of the membrane carrier protein for methotrexate from murine L1210 cells. Biochemistry 1987;26:4757–4763.

39. Henderson GB, Tsuji JM, Kumar HP. Transport of folate compounds by leukemic cells. Evidence for a single influx carrier for methotrexate, 5-methyltetrahydrofolate, and folate in CCRF-CEM human lymphoblasts. Biochem Pharmacol 1987;36:3007–3014.

40. Antony AC. The biological chemistry of folate receptors. Blood 1992;79:2807–2820.

41. Sirotnak FM, Goutas LJ, Jacobsen DM, et al. Carrier-mediated transport of folate compounds in L1210 cells. Initial rate kinetics and extent of duality of entry routes for folic acid and diastereomers of 5-methyltetrahydrohomofolate in the presence of physiological anions. Biochem Pharmacol 1987;36:1659–1667.

42. Matherly LH, Czajkowski CA, Angeles SM. Identification of a highly glycosylated methotrexate membrane carrier in K562 human erythroleukemia cells up-regulated for tetrahydrofolate cofactor and methotrexate transport. Cancer Res 1991;51: 3420–3426.

43. Moscow JA, Gong M, He R, et al. Isolation of a gene encoding a human reduced folate carrier (RFC1) and analysis of its expression in transport-deficient, methotrexate-resistant human breast cancer cells. Cancer Res 1995;55:3790–3794.

44. Prasad PD, Ramamoorthy S, Leibach FH, et al. Molecular cloning of the human placental folate transporter. Biochem Biophys Res Commun 1995;206:681–687.

45. Zhao R, Gao F, Wang PJ etal. Role of the amino acid 45 residue in reduced folate carrier function and ion-dependent transport as characterized by site-directed mutagenesis. Mol Pharmacol 2000;57(2):317–323.

46. Zhao R, Wang PJ, Gao F, etal. Residues 45 and 404 in the murine reduced folate carrier may interact to alter carrier binding and mobility. Biochim Biophys Acta 2003;1613(1–2):49–56.

47. Sharina IG, Zhao R, Wang Y, et al. Mutational analysis of the functional role of conserved arginine and lysine residues in transmembrane domains of the murine reduced folate carrier. Mol Pharmacol 2001;59(5):1022–1028.

48. Zhao R, Gao F, Hanscom M, et al. A prominent low-pH methotrexate transport activity in human solid tumors: contribution to the preservation of methotrexate pharmacologic activity in HeLa cells lacking the reduced folate carrier. Clin Cancer Res 2004;10(2):718–727.

49. Campbell IG, Jones TA, Foulkes WD, et al. Folate-binding protein is a marker for ovarian cancer. Cancer Res 1991;51:5329–5338.

50. Coney LR, Tomassetti A, Carayannopoulos L, et al. Cloning of a tumor-associated antigen: MOv18 and MOv19 antibodies recognize a folate-binding protein. Cancer Res 1991;51:6125–6132.

51. Elwood PC, Kane MA, Portillo RM, et al. The isolation, characterization, and comparison of the membrane-associated and soluble folate-binding proteins from human KB cells. J Biol Chem 1986;261:15416–15423.

52. Shen F, Ross JF, Wang X, et al. Identification of a novel folate receptor, a truncated receptor, and receptor type beta in hematopoietic cells: cDNA cloning, expression, immunoreactivity, and tissue specificity. Biochemistry 1994;33:1209–1215.

53. Roberts SJ, Petropavlovskaja M, Chung KN, et al. Role of individual N-linked glycosylation sites in the function and intracellular transport of the human alpha folate receptor. Arch Biochem Biophys 1998;351:227–235.

54. Elwood PC, Nachmanoff K, Saikawa Y, et al. The divergent 5′ termini of the alpha human folate receptor (hFR) mRNAs originate from two tissue-specific promoters and alternative splicing: characterization of the alpha hFR gene structure. Biochemistry 1997;36:1467–1478.

55. Roberts SJ, Chung KN, Nachmanoff K, et al. Tissue-specific promoters of the alpha human folate receptor gene yield transcripts with divergent 5′ leader sequences and different translational efficiencies. Biochem J 1997;326:439–447.

56. Sun XL, Murphy BR, Li QJ, et al. Transduction of folate receptor cDNA into cervical carcinoma cells using recombinant adeno-associated virions delays cell proliferation in vitro and in vivo. J Clin Invest 1995;96:1535–1547.

57. Shen F, Zheng X, Wang J, et al. Identification of amino acid residues that determine the differential ligand specificities of folate receptors alpha and beta. Biochemistry 1997;36: 6157–6163.

58. Wu M, Fan J, Gunning W, et al. Clustering of GPI-anchored folate receptor independent of both cross-linking and association with caveolin. J Membr Biol 1997;159:137–147.

59. Anderson RG, Kamen BA, Rothberg KG, et al. Potocytosis: sequestration and transport of small molecules by caveolae. Science 1992;255:410–411.

60. Kamen BA, Smith AK, Anderson RG. The folate receptor works in tandem with a probenecid-sensitive carrier in MA104 cells in vitro. J Clin Invest 1991;87:1442–1449.

61. Chang WJ, Rothberg KG, Kamen BA, et al. Lowering the cholesterol content of MA104 cells inhibits receptor-mediated transport of folate. J Cell Biol 1992;118:63–69.

62. Smart EJ, Mineo C, Anderson RG. Clustered folate receptors deliver 5-methyltetrahydrofolate to cytoplasm of MA104 cells. J Cell Biol 1996;134:1169–1177.

63. Spinella MJ, Brigle KE, Sierra EE, et al. Distinguishing between folate receptor-alpha-mediated transport and reduced folate carrier-mediated transport in L1210 leukemia cells. J Biol Chem 1995;270:7842–7849.

64. Westerhof GR, Rijnboutt S, Schornagel JH, et al. Functional activity of the reduced folate carrier in KB, MA104, and IGROV-I cells expressing folate-binding protein. Cancer Res 1995;55:3795–3802.

65. Schuetz JD, Matherly LH, Westin EH, et al. Evidence for a functional defect in the translocation of the methotrexate transport carrier in a methotrexate-resistant murine L1210 leukemia cell line. J Biol Chem 1988;263:9840–9847.

66. Assaraf YG, Schimke RT. Identification of methotrexate transport deficiency in mammalian cells using fluoresceinated methotrexate and flow cytometry. Proc Natl Acad Sci U S A 1987;84:7154–7158.

67. Rodenhuis S, McGuire JJ, Narayanan R, et al. Development of an assay system for the detection and classification of methotrexate resistance in fresh human leukemic cells. Cancer Res 1986;46:6513–6519.

68. Schuetz JD, Westin EH, Matherly LH, et al. Membrane protein changes in an L1210 leukemia cell line with a translocation defect in the methotrexate-tetrahydrofolate cofactor transport carrier. J Biol Chem 1989;264:16261–16267.

69. Jansen G, Westerhof GR, Kathmann I, et al. Identification of a membrane-associated folate-binding protein in human leukemic CCRF-CEM cells with transport-related methotrexate resistance [published erratum appears in Cancer Res 1995;55(18):4203]. Cancer Res 1989;49:2455–2459.

70. Zhao R, Assaraf YG, Goldman ID. A mutated murine reduced folate carrier (RFC1) with increased affinity for folic acid, decreased affinity for methotrexate, and an obligatory anion requirement for transport function. J Biol Chem 1998;273:19065–19071.

71. Zhao R, Assaraf YG, Goldman ID. A reduced folate carrier mutation produces substrate-dependent alterations in carrier mobility in murine leukemia cells and methotrexate resistance with conservation of growth in 5-formyltetrahydrofolate. J Biol Chem 1998;273:7873–7879.

72. Gifford AJ, Haber M, Witt TL etal. Role of the E45K-reduced folate carrier gene mutation in methotrexate resistance in human leukemia cells. Leukemia 2002;16(12):2379–2387.

73. Trippett T, Schlemmer S, Elisseyeff Y, et al. Defective transport as a mechanism of acquired resistance to methotrexate in patients with acute lymphoblastic leukemia. Blood 1992;80:1158–1162.

74. Levy AS, Sather HN, Steinherz PG etal. Reduced folate carrier and dihydrofolate reductase expression in acucte lymphocytic leukemia may predict outcome: a Children's Cancer Group Study. J Pediatr Hematol Oncol 2003;25(9):688–695.

75. Guo W, Healey JH, Meyers PA, et al. Mechanisms of methotrexate resistance in osteosarcoma. Clin Cancer Res 1999;5:621–627.

76. Ifergan I, Meller I, Issakov J etal. Reduced folate carrier protein expression in osteosarcoma: implications for the prediction of tumor chemosensitivity. Cancer 2003;98(9):1958–1966.

77. Liu S, Song L, Bevins R, et al. The murine-reduced folate carrier gene can act as a selectable marker and a suicide gene in hematopoietic cells in vivo. Hum Gene Ther 2002;13(14):1777–1782.

78. Moscow JA. Methotrexate transport and resistance. Leuk Lymphoma 1998;30:215–224.

79. Matherly LH, Goldman DI. Membrane transport of folates. Vitam Horm 2003;66:403–456.

80. Taylor IW, Slowiaczek P, Friedlander ML, et al. Selective toxicity of a new lipophilic antifolate, BW301U, for methotrexate-resistant cells with reduced drug uptake. Cancer Res 1985;45:978–982.

81. Mini E, Moroson BA, Franco CT, et al. Cytotoxic effects of folate antagonists against methotrexate-resistant human leukemic lymphoblast CCRF-CEM cell lines. Cancer Res 1985;45:325–330.

82. Schmid FA, Sirotnak FM, Otter GM, et al. Combination chemotherapy with a new folate analog: activity of 10- ethyl-10-deaza-aminopterin compared to methotrexate with 5-fluorouracil and alkylating agents against advanced metastatic disease in murine tumor models. Cancer Treat Rep 1987;71:727–732.

83. Jansen G, Schornagel JH, Westerhof GR, et al. Multiple membrane transport systems for the uptake of folate-based thymidylate synthase inhibitors. Cancer Res 1990;50:7544–7548.

84. Westerhof GR, Jansen G, van Emmerik N, et al. Membrane transport of natural folates and antifolate compounds in murine L1210 leukemia cells: role of carrier- and receptor-mediated transport systems. Cancer Res 1991;51:5507–5513.

85. Wang Y, Zhao R, Goldman ID. Decreased expression of the reduced folate carrier and folylpolyglutamate synthetase is the basis for acquired resistance to the pemetrexed antifolate (LY231514) in an L1210 murine leukemia cell line. Biochem Pharmacol 2003;65(7):1163–1170.

86. Zhao R, Hanscom M, Chattopadhyay S, et al. Selective Preservation of pemetrexed pharmacological activity in HeLa cells lacking the reduced folate carrier: association with the presence of a secondary transport pathway. Cancer Res 2004;64(9):3313–3319.

87. Henderson GB, Strauss BP. Growth inhibition by homofolate in tumor cells utilizing a high-affinity folate binding protein as a means for folate internalization. Biochem Pharmacol 1990;39:2019–2025.

88. Mendelsohn LG, Gates SB, Habeck LL, et al. The role of dietary folate in modulation of folate receptor expression, folylpolyglutamate synthetase activity and the efficacy and toxicity of lometrexol. Adv Enzyme Regul 1996;36:365–381.

89. Lin JT, Cashmore AR, Baker M, et al. Phase I studies with trimetrexate: clinical pharmacology, analytical methodology, and pharmacokinetics. Cancer Res 1987;47:609–616.

90. Laszlo J, Brenckman WD Jr, Morgan E, et al. Initial clinical studies of piritrexim. J Natl Cancer Inst Monogr 1987;5:121–125.

91. Allegra CJ, Kovacs JA, Drake JC, et al. Activity of antifolates against Pneumocystis carinii dihydrofolate reductase and identification of a potent new agent. J Exp Med 1987;165:926–931.

92. Currie VE, Warrell RP Jr, Arlin Z, et al. Phase I trial of 10- deaza-aminopterin in patients with advanced cancer. Cancer Treat Rep 1983;67:149–154.

93. Casper ES, Christman KL, Schwartz GK, et al. Edatrexate in patients with soft tissue sarcoma. Activity in malignant fibrous histiocytoma. Cancer 1993;72:766–770.

94. Vandenberg TA, Pritchard KI, Eisenhauer EA, et al. Phase II study of weekly edatrexate as first-line chemotherapy for metastatic breast cancer: a National Cancer Institute of Canada Clinical Trials Group study. J Clin Oncol 1993;11:1241–1244.

95. Kuriakose P, Gandara DR, and Perez EA. Phase I trial of edatrexate in advanced breast and other cancers. Cancer Invest 2002;20(4):473–749.

96. Henderson GB, Zevely EM. Inhibitory effects of probenecid on the individual transport routes which mediate the influx and efflux of methotrexate in L1210 cells. Biochem Pharmacol 1985;34:1725–1729.

97. Henderson GB, Tsuji JM. Methotrexate efflux in L1210 cells. Kinetic and specificity properties of the efflux system sensitive to bromosulfophthalein and its possible identity with a system which mediates the efflux of 3′,5′-cyclic AMP. J Biol Chem 1987;262:13571–13578.

98. Henderson GB, Tsuji JM, Kumar HP. Characterization of the individual transport routes that mediate the influx and efflux of methotrexate in CCRF-CEM human lymphoblastic cells. Cancer Res 1986;46:1633–1638.

99. Zeng H, Liu G, Rea PA, et al. Transport of amphipathic anions by human multidrug resistance protein 3. Cancer Res 2000;60(17):4779–4784.

100. Zeng H, Chen ZS, Belinsky MG, et al. Transport of methotrexate (MTX) and folates by multidrug resistance protein (MRP) 3 and MRP1: effect of polyglutamation on MTX transport. Cancer Res 2001;61(19):7225–7232.

101. Chen ZS, Lee K, Walther S, et al. Analysis of methotrexate and folate transport by multidrug resistance protein 4 (ABCC4): MRP4 is a component of the methotrexate efflux system. Cancer Res 2002;62(11):3144–3150.

102. Assaraf YG, Rothem L, Hooijberg JH, et al. Loss of multidrug resistance protein 1 expression and folate efflux activity results i a highly concentrative folate transport in human leukemia cells. J Biol Chem 2003;278(9):6680–6686.

103. Sirotnak FM, Wendel HG, Bornmann WG, et al. Co-administration of probenecid, an inhibitor of a cMOAT/MRP-like plasma membrane ATPase, greatly enhanced the efficacy of a new 10-deazaaminopterin against human solid tumors in vivo. Clin Cancer Res 2000;6(9):3705–3712.

104. Stark M, Rothem L, Jansen G, et al. Antifolate resistance associated with loss of MRP1 expression and function in Chinese hamster ovary cells with markedly impaired export of folate and cholate. Mol Pharmacol 2003;64(2):220–227.

105. Volk EL, Farley KM, Wu Y, et al. Overexpression of wild-type breast cancer resistance protein mediates methotrexate resistance. Cancer Res 2002;62(17):5035–5040.

106. Volk EL, Schneider E. Wild-type breast cancer resistance protein (BCRP/ABCG2) is a methotrexate polyglutamate transporter. Cancer Res 2003;63(17):5538–5543.

107. Chen ZS, Robey RW, Belinsky MG, et al. Transpor of methotrexate polyglutamates, and 17beta-estradiol 17-(beta-D-glucuronide) by ABCG2: effects of acquired mutations as R482 on methotrexate transport. Cancer Res 2003;63(14):4048–4054.

108. Koizumi S, Curt GA, Fine RL, et al. Formation of methotrexate polyglutamates in purified myeloid precursor cells from normal human bone marrow. J Clin Invest 1985;75:1008–1014.

109. Fabre I, Fabre G, Goldman ID. Polyglutamylation, an important element in methotrexate cytotoxicity and selectivity in tumor versus murine granulocytic progenitor cells in vitro. Cancer Res 1984;44:3190–3195.

110. Schilsky RL, Bailey BD, Chabner BA. Methotrexate polyglutamate synthesis by cultured human breast cancer cells. Proc Natl Acad Sci U S A 1980;77:2919–2922.

111. Jolivet J, Schilsky RL, Bailey BD, et al. Synthesis, retention, and biological activity of methotrexate polyglutamates in cultured human breast cancer cells. J Clin Invest 1982;70:351–360.

112. Kennedy DG, Van den Berg HW, Clarke R, et al. The effect of the rate of cell proliferation on the synthesis of methotrexate poly-gamma-glutamates in two human breast cancer cell lines. Biochem Pharmacol 1985;34:3087–3090.

113. Jolivet J, Chabner BA. Intracellular pharmacokinetics of methotrexate polyglutamates in human breast cancer cells. Selective retention and less dissociable binding of 4-NH2- 10-CH3-pteroylglutamate4 and 4-NH2-10-CH3-pteroylglutamate5 to dihydrofolate reductase. J Clin Invest 1983;72:773–778.

114. Winick NJ, Kamen BA, Balis FM, et al. Folate and methotrexate polyglutamate tissue levels in rhesus monkeys following chronic low-dose methotrexate. Cancer Drug Deliv 1987;4:25–31.

115. Shane B. Folylpolyglutamate synthesis and role in the regulation of one-carbon metabolism. Vitam Horm 1989;45:263–335.

116. Gewirtz DA, White JC, Randolph JK, et al. Formation of methotrexate polyglutamates in rat hepatocytes. Cancer Res 1979;39:2914–2918.

117. Clarke L, Waxman DJ. Human liver folylpolyglutamate synthetase: biochemical characterization and interactions with folates and folate antagonists. Arch Biochem Biophys 1987;256:585–596.

118. Cichowicz DJ, Shane B. Mammalian folylpoly-gamma-glutamate synthetase. 1. Purification and general properties of the hog liver enzyme. Biochemistry 1987;26:504–512.

119. Cichowicz DJ, Shane B. Mammalian folylpoly-gamma-glutamate synthetase. 2. Substrate specificity and kinetic properties. Biochemistry 1987;26:513–521.

120. McGuire JJ, Hsieh P, Franco CT, et al. Folylpolyglutamate synthetase inhibition and cytotoxic effects of methotrexate analogs containing 2,omega-diaminoalkanoic acids. Biochem Pharmacol 1986;35:2607–2613.

121. Galivan J, Johnson T, Rhee M, et al. The role of folylpolyglutamate synthetase and gamma-glutamyl hydrolase in altering cellular folyl- and antifolylpolyglutamates. Adv Enzyme Regul 1987;26:147–155.

122. Panetta JC, Wall A, Pui CH, et al. Methotrexate intracellular disposition in acute lymphoblastic leukemia: a mathematical model of gamma-glutamyl hydrolase activity. Clin Cancer Res 2002;8(7):2423–2429.

123. Yao R, Schneider E, Ryan TJ, et al. Human gamma- glutamyl hydrolase: cloning and characterization of the enzyme expressed in vitro. Proc Natl Acad Sci U S A 1996;93:10134–10138.

124. Cole PD, Kamen BA, Gorlick R, et al. Effects of overexpression of gamma-glutamyl hydrolase on methotrexate metabolism and resistance. Cancer Res 2001;61(11):4599–4604.

125. Longo GS, Gorlick R, Tong WP, et al. Disparate affinities of antifolates for folylpolyglutamate synthetase from human leukemia cells. Blood 1997;90:1241–1245.

126. Sirotnak FM, Chello PL, Piper JR, et al. Growth inhibitory, transport and biochemical properties of the gamma- glutamyl and gamma-aspartyl peptides of methotrexate in L1210 leukemia cells in vitro. Biochem Pharmacol 1978;27:1821–1825.

127. Galivan J, Nimec Z, Balinska M. Regulation of methotrexate polyglutamate accumulation in vitro: effects of cellular folate content. Biochem Pharmacol 1983;32:3244–3247.

128. Jolivet J, Faucher F, Pinard MF. Influence of intracellular folates on methotrexate metabolism and cytotoxicity. Biochem Pharmacol 1987;36:3310–3312.

129. Jolivet J, Cole DE, Holcenberg JS, et al. Prevention of methotrexate cytotoxicity by asparaginase inhibition of methotrexate polyglutamate formation. Cancer Res 1985;45:217–220.

130. Sur P, Fernandes DJ, Kute TE, et al. L-asparaginase-induced modulation of methotrexate polyglutamylation in murine leukemia L5178Y. Cancer Res 1987;47:1313–1318.

131. Matherly LH, Fry DW, Goldman ID. Role of methotrexate polyglutamylation and cellular energy metabolism in inhibition of methotrexate binding to dihydrofolate reductase by 5-formyltetrahydrofolate in Ehrlich ascites tumor cells in vitro. Cancer Res 1983;43:2694–2699.

132. Allegra CJ, Drake JC, Jolivet J, et al. Inhibition of folate-dependent enzymes by methotrexate polyglutamates. In: Goldman ID, ed. Proceedings of the Second Workshop on Folyl and Antifolyl Polyglutamates. New York: Praeger, 1985:348–359.

133. Galivan J, Inglese J, McGuire JJ, et al. Gamma-fluoromethotrexate: synthesis and biological activity of a potent inhibitor of dihydrofolate reductase with greatly diminished ability to form poly-gamma-glutamates. Proc Natl Acad Sci U S A 1985;82:2598–2602.

134. Samuels LL, Moccio DM, Sirotnak FM. Similar differential for total polyglutamylation and cytotoxicity among various folate analogues in human and murine tumor cells in vitro. Cancer Res 1985;45:1488–1495.

135. Matherly LH, Voss MK, Anderson LA, et al. Enhanced polyglutamylation of aminopterin relative to methotrexate in the Ehrlich ascites tumor cell in vitro. Cancer Res 1985;45:1073–1078.

136. Cowan KH, Jolivet J. A methotrexate-resistant human breast cancer cell line with multiple defects, including diminished formation of methotrexate polyglutamates. J Biol Chem 1984;259:10793–10800.

137. Mauritz R, Peters GJ, Priest DG, et al. Multiple mechanisms of resistance to methotrexate and novel antifolates in human CCRF-CEM leukemia cells and their implications for folate homeostasis. Biochem Pharmacol 2002;63(2):105–115.

138. Liani E, Rothem L, Bunni MA, et al. Loss of folylpoly-gamma-glutamate synthetase activity is a dominant mechanism of resistance to polyglutamation-dependent novel antifolates in multiple human leukemia sublines. Int J Cancer 2003;103(5):587–599.

139. Pizzorno G, Mini E, Coronnello M, et al. Impaired polyglutamylation of methotrexate as a cause of resistance in CCRF-CEM cells after short-term, high-dose treatment with this drug. Cancer Res 1988;48:2149–2155.

140. Pizzorno G, Chang YM, McGuire JJ, et al. Inherent resistance of human squamous carcinoma cell lines to methotrexate as a result of decreased polyglutamylation of this drug. Cancer Res 1989;49:5275–5280.

141. McCloskey DE, McGuire JJ, Russell CA, et al. Decreased folylpolyglutamate synthetase activity as a mechanism of methotrexate resistance in CCRF-CEM human leukemia sublines. J Biol Chem 1991;266:6181–6187.

142. Faessel HM, Slocum HK, Jackson RC, et al. Super in vitro synergy between inhibitors of dihydrofolate reductase and inhibitors of other folate-requiring enzymes: the critical role of polyglutamylation. Cancer Res 1998;58:3036–3050.

143. Pizzorno G, Sokoloski JA, Cashmore AR, et al. Intracellular metabolism of 5,10-dideazatetrahydrofolic acid in human leukemia cell lines. Mol Pharmacol 1991;39:85–89.

144. Curt GA, Jolivet J, Carney DN, et al. Determinants of the sensitivity of human small-cell lung cancer cell lines to methotrexate. J Clin Invest 1985;76:1323–1329.

145. Longo GS, Gorlick R, Tong WP, et al. Gamma-glutamyl hydrolase and folylpolyglutamate synthetase activities predict polyglutamylation of methotrexate in acute leukemias. Oncol Res 1997;9:259–263.

146. Galpin AJ, Schuetz JD, Masson E, et al. Differences in folylpolyglutamate synthetase and dihydrofolate reductase expression in human B-lineage versus T-lineage leukemic lymphoblasts: mechanisms for lineage differences in methotrexate polyglutamylation and cytotoxicity. Mol Pharmacol 1997;52:155–163.

147. Panetta JC, Yanishevski Y, Pui CH, et al. A mathematical model of in vivo methotrexate accumulation in acute lymphoblastic leukemia. Cancer Chemother Pharmacol 2002;50(5):419–428.

148. Mantadakis E, Smith AK, Hynan L etal. Methotrexate polyglutamation may lack prognostic significance in children with B-cell precursor acute lymphoblastic leukemia treated with intensive oral methotrexate. J Pediatr Hematol Oncol 2002;24(8):736–642.

149. Li WW, Lin JT, Tong WP, et al. Mechanisms of natural resistance to antifolates in human soft tissue sarcomas. Cancer Res 1992;52:1434–1438.

150. Li WW, Lin JT, Schweitzer BI, et al. Intrinsic resistance to methotrexate in human soft tissue sarcoma cell lines. Cancer Res 1992;52:3908–3913.

151. Matthews DA, Alden RA, Bolin JT, et al. X-ray structural studies of dihydrofolate reductase. In: Kisliuk RL, Brown GM, eds. Chemistry and Biology of Pteridines. New York: Elsevier/North Holland, 1979:465.

152. Matthews DA, Alden RA, Bolin JT, et al. Dihydrofolate reductase: x-ray structure of the binary complex with methotrexate. Science 1977;197:452–455.

153. Appleman JR, Howell EE, Kraut J, et al. Role of aspartate 27 in the binding of methotrexate to dihydrofolate reductase from Escherichia coli. J Biol Chem 1988;263:9187– 9198.

154. Taira K, Benkovic SJ. Evaluation of the importance of hydrophobic interactions in drug binding to dihydrofolate reductase. J Med Chem 1988;31:129–137.

155. Oefner C, D'Arcy A, Winkler FK. Crystal structure of human dihydrofolate reductase complexed with folate. Eur J Biochem 1988;174:377–385.

156. Cody V, Ciszak E. Computer graphic modeling in drug design—conformational analysis of antifolate binding to avian dihydrofolate reductase: crystal and molecular structures of 2,4-diamino-5-cyclohexyl-6-methylpyrimidine and 5-cyclohexyl-6-methyluracil. Anticancer Drug Des 1991;6:83–93.

157. Freisheim JH, Kumar AA, Blankenship D. Structure-function relationships of dihydrofolate reductases: sequence homology considerations and active center residues. In: Kislink RL, Brown GM, eds. Chemistry and Biology of Pteridines. New York: Elsevier/North Holland, 1979:419.

158. Schweitzer BI, Srimatkandada S, Gritsman H, et al. Probing the role of two hydrophobic active site residues in the human dihydrofolate reductase by site-directed mutagenesis. J Biol Chem 1989;264:20786–20795.

159. Thompson PD, Freisheim JH. Conversion of arginine to lysine at position 70 of human dihydrofolate reductase: generation of a methotrexate-insensitive mutant enzyme. Biochemistry 1991;30:8124–8130.

160. Dicker AP, Waltham MC, Volkenandt M, et al. Methotrexate resistance in an in vivo mouse tumor due to a non- active-site dihydrofolate reductase mutation. Proc Natl Acad Sci U S A 1993;90:11797–11801.

161. Bystroff C, Kraut J. Crystal structure of unliganded Escherichia coli dihydrofolate reductase. Ligand-induced conformational changes and cooperativity in binding. Biochemistry 1991;30:2227–2239.

162. Zhao SC, Banerjee D, Mineishi S, et al. Post-transplant methotrexate administration leads to improved curability of mice bearing a mammary tumor transplanted with marrow transduced with a mutant human dihydrofolate reductase cDNA. Hum Gene Ther 1997;8:903–909.

163. Flasshove M, Banerjee D, Leonard JP, et al. Retroviral transduction of human CD34+ umbilical cord blood progenitor cells with a mutated dihydrofolate reductase cDNA. Hum Gene Ther 1998;9:63–71.

164. Mareya SM, Sorrentino BP, Blakley RL. Protection of CCRF-CEM human lymphoid cells from antifolates by retroviral gene transfer of variants of murine dihydrofolate reductase. Cancer Gene Ther 1998;5:225–235.

165. Appleman JR, Prendergast N, Delcamp TJ, et al. Kinetics of the formation and isomerization of methotrexate complexes of recombinant human dihydrofolate reductase. J Biol Chem 1988;263:10304–10313.

166. Kamen BA, Whyte-Bauer W, Bertino JR. A mechanism of resistance to methotrexate. NADPH but not NADH stimulation of methotrexate binding to dihydrofolate reductase. Biochem Pharmacol 1983;32:1837–1841.

167. Jackson RC, Hart LI, Harrap KR. Intrinsic resistance to methotrexate of cultured mammalian cells in relation to the inhibition kinetics of their dihydrofolate reductases. Cancer Res 1976;36:1991–1997.

168. Kumar P, Kisliuk RL, Gaumont Y, et al. Interaction of polyglutamyl derivatives of methotrexate, 10-deazaaminopterin, and dihydrofolate with dihydrofolate reductase. Cancer Res 1986;46:5020–5023.

169. Blakley RL, Cocco L. Role of isomerization of initial complexes in the binding of inhibitors to dihydrofolate reductase. Biochemistry 1985;24:4772–4777.

170. White JC. Reversal of methotrexate binding to dihydrofolate reductase by dihydrofolate. Studies with pure enzyme and computer modeling using network thermodynamics. J Biol Chem 1979;254:10889–10895.

171. Allegra CJ, Boarman D. Interaction of methotrexate polyglutamates and dihydrofolate during leucovorin rescue in a human breast cancer cell line (MCF-7). Cancer Res 1990; 50:3574–3578.

172. Cohen M, Bender RA, Donehower R, et al. Reversibility of high-affinity binding of methotrexate in L1210 murine leukemia cells. Cancer Res 1978;38:2866–2870.

173. White JC, Loftfield S, Goldman ID. The mechanism of action of methotrexate. III. Requirement of free intracellular methotrexate for maximal suppression of (14C)formate incorporation into nucleic acids and protein. Mol Pharmacol 1975;11:287–297.

174. Galivan J. Evidence for the cytotoxic activity of polyglutamate derivatives of methotrexate. Mol Pharmacol 1980;17:105–110.

175. Drake JC, Allegra CJ, Baram J, et al. Effects on dihydrofolate reductase of methotrexate metabolites and intracellular folates formed following methotrexate exposure of human breast cancer cells. Biochem Pharmacol 1987;36:2416–2418.

176. Boarman DM, Baram J, Allegra CJ. Mechanism of leucovorin reversal of methotrexate cytotoxicity in human MCF-7 breast cancer cells. Biochem Pharmacol 1990;40:2651–2660.

177. Kruger-McDermott C, Balinska M, Galivan J. Dihydrofolate-mediated reversal of methotrexate toxicity to hepatoma cells in vitro. Cancer Lett 1986;30:79–84.

178. Goldie JH, Dedhar S, Krystal G. Properties of a methotrexate-insensitive variant of dihydrofolate reductase derived from methotrexate-resistant L5178Y cells. J Biol Chem 1981;256:11629–11635.

179. McIvor RS, Simonsen CC. Isolation and characterization of a variant dihydrofolate reductase cDNA from methotrexate- resistant murine L5178Y cells. Nucleic Acids Res 1990;18:7025–7032.

180. Flintoff WF, Essani K. Methotrexate-resistant Chinese hamster ovary cells contain a dihydrofolate reductase with an altered affinity for methotrexate. Biochemistry 1980;19:4321–4327.

181. Melera PW, Davide JP, Hession CA, et al. Phenotypic expression in Escherichia coli and nucleotide sequence of two Chinese hamster lung cell cDNAs encoding different dihydrofolate reductases. Mol Cell Biol 1984;4:38–48.

182. Melera PW, Lewis JA, Biedler JL, et al. Antifolate-resistant Chinese hamster cells. Evidence for dihydrofolate reductase gene amplification among independently derived sublines overproducing different dihydrofolate reductases. J Biol Chem 1980;255:7024–7028.

183. Haber DA, Schimke RT. Unstable amplification of an altered dihydrofolate reductase gene associated with double- minute chromosomes. Cell 1981;26:355–362.

184. Cowan KH, Goldsmith ME, Levine RM, et al. Dihydrofolate reductase gene amplification and possible rearrangement in estrogen-responsive methotrexate-resistant human breast cancer cells. J Biol Chem 1982;257:15079–15086.

185. Melera PW, Davide JP, Oen H. Antifolate-resistant Chinese hamster cells. Molecular basis for the biochemical and structural heterogeneity among dihydrofolate reductases produced by drug-sensitive and drug-resistant cell lines. J Biol Chem 1988;263:1978–1990.

186. Dedhar S, Hartley D, Fitz-Gibbons D, et al. Heterogeneity in the specific activity and methotrexate sensitivity of dihydrofolate reductase from blast cells of acute myelogenous leukemia patients. J Clin Oncol 1985;3:1545–1552.

187. Takebe N, Nakahara S, Zhao SC, et al. Comparison of methotrexate resistance conferred by a mutated dihydrofolate reductase cDNA in two different retroviral vectors. Cancer Gene Ther 2000;7(6):910–919.

188. Meisel R, Bardenheuer W, Strehblow C, et al. Efficient protection from methotrexate toxicity and selection of transduced human hematopoietic cells following gene transfer of dihydrofolate reductase mutants. Exp Hematol 2003;31(12):1215–1222.

189. Hamlin JL, Biedler JL. Replication pattern of a large homogenously staining chromosome region in antifolate-resistant Chinese hamster cell lines. J Cell Physiol 1981;107:101–114.

190. Brown PC, Beverley SM, Schimke RT. Relationship of amplified dihydrofolate reductase genes to double minute chromosomes in unstably resistant mouse fibroblast cell lines. Mol Cell Biol 1981;1:1077–1083.

191. Meltzer PS, Cheng YC, Trent JM. Analysis of dihydrofolate reductase gene amplification in a methotrexate-resistant human tumor cell line. Cancer Genet Cytogenet 1985;17:289–300.

192. Singer MJ, Mesner LD, Friedman CL, et al. Amplification of the human dihydrofolate reductase gene via double minutes is initiated by chromosome breaks. Proc Natl Acad Sci USA 2000;97(14):7921–7926.

193. Hoy CA, Rice GC, Kovacs M, et al. Over-replication of DNA in S phase Chinese hamster ovary cells after DNA synthesis inhibition. J Biol Chem 1987;262:11927–11934.

194. Fanin R, Banerjee D, Volkenandt M, et al. Mutations leading to antifolate resistance in Chinese hamster ovary cells after exposure to the alkylating agent ethylmethanesulfonate. Mol Pharmacol 1993;44:13–21.

195. Sharma RC, Schimke RT. Enhancement of the frequency of methotrexate resistance by gamma-radiation in Chinese hamster ovary and mouse 3T6 cells. Cancer Res 1989;49:3861–3866.

196. Barsoum J, Varshavsky A. Mitogenic hormones and tumor promoters greatly increase the incidence of colony-forming cells bearing amplified dihydrofolate reductase genes. Proc Natl Acad Sci U S A 1983;80:5330–5334.

197. Newman EM, Lu Y, Kashani-Sabet M, et al. Mechanisms of cross-resistance to methotrexate and 5-fluorouracil in an A2780 human ovarian carcinoma cell subline resistant to cisplatin. Biochem Pharmacol 1988;37:443–447.

198. Rice GC, Ling V, Schimke RT. Frequencies of independent and simultaneous selection of Chinese hamster cells for methotrexate and doxorubicin (Adriamycin) resistance. Proc Natl Acad Sci U S A 1987;84:9261–9264.

199. Schuetz JD, Gorse KM, Goldman ID, et al. Transient inhibition of DNA synthesis by 5-fluorodeoxyuridine leads to overexpression of dihydrofolate reductase with increased frequency of methotrexate resistance. J Biol Chem 1988;263:7708–7712.

200. Wright JA, Smith HS, Watt FM, et al. DNA amplification is rare in normal human cells. Proc Natl Acad Sci U S A 1990;87:1791–1795.

201. Sowers R, Toguchida J, Qin J etal. MRNA expression levels of E2F transcription factors correlate with dihydrofolate reductase, reduced folate carrier, and thymidylate synthase mRNA expression in osteosarcoma. Mol Cancer Ther 2003;2(6):535–541.

202. Cowan KH, Goldsmith ME, Ricciardone MD, et al. Regulation of dihydrofolate reductase in human breast cancer cells and in mutant hamster cells transfected with a human dihydrofolate reductase minigene. Mol Pharmacol 1986;30:69–76.

203. Chu E, Takimoto CH, Voeller D, et al. Specific binding of human dihydrofolate reductase protein to dihydrofolate reductase messenger RNA in vitro. Biochemistry 1993;32:4756–4760.

204. Ercikan-Abali EA, Banerjee D, Waltham MC, et al. Dihydrofolate reductase protein inhibits its own translation by binding to dihydrofolate reductase mRNA sequences within the coding region. Biochemistry 1997;36:12317–12322.

205. Curt GA, Carney DN, Cowan KH, et al. Unstable methotrexate resistance in human small-cell carcinoma associated with double minute chromosomes. N Engl J Med 1983;308:199–202.

206. Curt GA, Jolivet J, Bailey BD, et al. Synthesis and retention of methotrexate polyglutamates by human small cell lung cancer. Biochem Pharmacol 1984;33:1682–1685.

207. Matherly LH, Taub JW, Wong SC, et al. Increased frequency of expression of elevated dihydrofolate reductase in T-cell versus B-precursor acute lymphoblastic leukemia in children. Blood 1997;90:578–589.

208. Seither RL, Rape TJ, Goldman ID. Further studies on the pharmacologic effects of the 7-hydroxy catabolite of methotrexate in the L1210 murine leukemia cell. Biochem Pharmacol 1989;38:815–822.

209. Rhee MS, Balinska M, Bunni M, et al. Role of substrate depletion in the inhibition of thymidylate biosynthesis by the dihydrofolate reductase inhibitor trimetrexate in cultured hepatoma cells. Cancer Res 1990;50:3979–3984.

210. Rhee MS, Coward JK, Galivan J. Depletion of 5,10-methylenetetrahydrofolate and 10-formyltetrahydrofolate by methotrexate in cultured hepatoma cells. Mol Pharmacol 1992;42:909–916.

211. Trent DF, Seither RL, Goldman ID. Compartmentation of intracellular folates. Failure to interconvert tetrahydrofolate cofactors to dihydrofolate in mitochondria of L1210 leukemia cells treated with trimetrexate [published erratum appears in Biochem Pharmacol 1991;42(12):2405]. Biochem Pharmacol 1991;42:1015–1019.

212. Li JC, Kaminskas E. Accumulation of DNA strand breaks and methotrexate cytotoxicity. Proc Natl Acad Sci U S A 1984;81: 5694–5698.

213. Hori T, Ayusawa D, Shimizu K, et al. Chromosome breakage induced by thymidylate stress in thymidylate synthase-negative mutants of mouse FM3A cells. Cancer Res 1984;44:703–709.

214. Borchers AH, Kennedy KA, Straw JA. Inhibition of DNA excision repair by methotrexate in Chinese hamster cells following exposure to ultraviolet irradiation or ethylmethanesulfonate. Cancer Res 1990;50:1786–1789.

215. Goulian M, Bleile B, Tseng BY. Methotrexate-induced misincorporation of uracil into DNA. Proc Natl Acad Sci U S A 1980;77: 1956–1960.

216. Grafstrom RH, Tseng BY, Goulian M. The incorporation of uracil into animal cell DNA in vitro. Cell 1978;15:131–140.

217. Curtin NJ, Harris AL, Aherne GW. Mechanism of cell death following thymidylate synthase inhibition: 2′-deoxyuridine-5′-triphosphate accumulation, DNA damage, and growth inhibition following exposure to CB3717 and dipyridamole. Cancer Res 1991;51:2346–2352.

218. Beck WR, Wright GE, Nusbaum NJ, et al. Enhancement of methotrexate cytotoxicity by uracil analogues that inhibit deoxyuridine triphosphate nucleotidohydrolase (dUTPase) activity. Adv Exp Med Biol 1986;195:97–104.

219. Bertino JR, Goker E, Gorlick R, et al. Resistance mechanisms to methotrexate in tumors. Oncologist 1996;1:223–226.

220. Li W, Fan J, Hochhauser D, et al. Lack of functional retinoblastoma protein mediates increased resistance to antimetabolites in human sarcoma cell lines. Proc Natl Acad Sci U S A 1995;92: 10436–10440.

221. Goker E, Waltham M, Kheradpour A, et al. Amplification of the dihydrofolate reductase gene is a mechanism of acquired resistance to methotrexate in patients with acute lymphoblastic leukemia and is correlated with p53 gene mutations. Blood 1995;86:677–684.

222. Li WW, Fan J, Hochhauser D, et al. Overexpression of p21waf1 leads to increased inhibition of E2F-1 phosphorylation and sensitivity to anticancer drugs in retinoblastoma-negative human sarcoma cells. Cancer Res 1997;57:2193–2199.

223. Winter-Vann AM, Kamen BA, Bergo MO, et al. Targeting ras signaling through inhibition of carboxyl methylation: an unexpected property of methotrexate. Proc Natl Acad Sci USA 2003; 100(11):6529–6534.

224. Pinedo HM, Zaharko DS, Bull J, et al. The relative contribution of drug concentration and duration of exposure to mouse bone marrow toxicity during continuous methotrexate infusion. Cancer Res 1977;37:445–450.

225. Cherry LM, Hsu TC. Restitution of chromatid and isochromatid breaks induced in the G2 phase by actinomycin D. Environ Mutagen 1982;4:259–265.

226. Hryniuk WM, Bertino JR. Treatment of leukemia with large doses of methotrexate and folinic acid: clinical- biochemical correlates. J Clin Invest 1969;48:2140–2155.

227. Pinedo HM, Zaharko DS, Bull JM, et al. The reversal of methotrexate cytotoxicity to mouse bone marrow cells by leucovorin and nucleosides. Cancer Res 1976;36:4418–4424.

228. Howell SB, Mansfield SJ, Taetle R. Thymidine and hypoxanthine requirements of normal and malignant human cells for protection against methotrexate cytotoxicity. Cancer Res 1981;41:945–950.

229. Howell SB, Ensminger WD, Krishan A, et al. Thymidine rescue of high-dose methotrexate in humans. Cancer Res 1978;38: 325–330.

230. Rustum YM. High-pressure liquid chromatography. I. Quantitative separation of purine and pyrimidine nucleosides and bases. Anal Biochem 1978;90:289–299.

231. Willson JK, Fischer PH, Remick SC, et al. Methotrexate and dipyridamole combination chemotherapy based upon inhibition of nucleoside salvage in humans. Cancer Res 1989;49: 1866–1870.

232. Cole PD, Smith AK, Kamen BA. Osteosarcoma cells, resistant to methotrexate due to nucleoside and nucleobase salvage, are sensitive to nucleoside analogs. Cancer Chemother Pharmacol 2002;50(2):111–116.

233. Novelli A, Mini E, Liuffi M, et al. Clinical data on rescue of high-dose methotrexate with N^5-methyltetrahydrofolate in human solid tumors. In: Periti P, ed. High-Dose Methotrexate Pharmacology, Toxicology and Chemotherapy. Firenze, Italy: Giuntina, 1978:299.

234. Matherly LH, Barlowe CK, Goldman ID. Antifolate polyglutamylation and competitive drug displacement at dihydrofolate reductase as important elements in leucovorin rescue in L1210 cells. Cancer Res 1986;46:588–593.

235. Bernard S, Etienne MC, Fischel JL, et al. Critical factors for the reversal of methotrexate cytotoxicity by folinic acid. Br J Cancer 1991;63:303–307.

236. Browman GP, Goodyear MD, Levine MN, et al. Modulation of the antitumor effect of methotrexate by low-dose leucovorin in squamous cell head and neck cancer: a randomized placebo-controlled clinical trial. J Clin Oncol 1990;8:203–208.

237. Yap AK, Luscombe DK. Rapid and inexpensive enzyme inhibition assay of methotrexate. J Pharmacol Methods 1986;16: 139–150.

238. Myers CE, Lippman ME, Elliot HM, et al. Competitive protein binding assay for methotrexate. Proc Natl Acad Sci U S A 1975;72:3683–3686.

239. Hande K, Gober J, Fletcher R. Trimethoprim interferes with serum methotrexate assay by the competitive protein binding technique. Clin Chem 1980;26:1617–1619.

240. Pesce MA, Bodourian SH. Evaluation of a fluorescence polarization immunoassay procedure for quantitation of methotrexate. Ther Drug Monit 1986;8:115–121.

241. Donehower RC, Hande KR, Drake JC, et al. Presence of 2,4-diamino-N10-methylpteroic acid after high-dose methotrexate. Clin Pharmacol Ther 1979;26:63–72.

242. Oellerich M, Engelhardt P, Schaadt M, et al. Determination of methotrexate in serum by a rapid, fully mechanized enzyme immunoassay (EMIT). J Clin Chem Clin Biochem 1980;18:169–174.

243. Allegra CJ, Drake JC, Bell BA, et al. Measuring levels of methotrexate [letter]. N Engl J Med 1985;313:184.

244. So N, Chandra DP, Alexander IS, et al. Determination of serum methotrexate and 7-hydroxymethotrexate concentrations. Method evaluation showing advantages of high-performance liquid chromatography. J Chromatogr 1985;337:81–90.

245. Stout M, Ravindranath Y, Kauffman R. High-performance liquid chromatographic assay for methotrexate utilizing a cold acetonitrile purification and separation of plasma or cerebrospinal fluid. J Chromatogr 1985;342:424–430.

246. Palmisano F, Cataldi TR, Zambonin PG. Determination of the antineoplastic agent methotrexate in body fluids by high-performance liquid chromatography with electrochemical detection. J Chromatogr 1985;344:249–258.

247. Slordal L, Prytz PS, Pettersen I, et al. Methotrexate measurements in plasma: comparison of enzyme multiplied immunoassay technique, TDx fluorescence polarization immunoassay, and high pressure liquid chromatography. Ther Drug Monit 1986;8:368–372.

248. Zaharko DS, Dedrick RL, Bischoff KB, et al. Methotrexate tissue distribution: prediction by a mathematical model. J Natl Cancer Inst 1971;46:775–784.

249. Chungi VS, Bourne DW, Dittert LW. Drug absorption VIII: kinetics of GI absorption of methotrexate. J Pharm Sci 1978;67: 560–561.

250. Stuart JF, Calman KC, Watters J, et al. Bioavailability of methotrexate: implications for clinical use. Cancer Chemother Pharmacol 1979;3:239–241.

251. Balis FM, Savitch JL, Bleyer WA. Pharmacokinetics of oral methotrexate in children. Cancer Res 1983;43:2342–2345.

252. Balis FM, Holcenberg JS, Poplack DG, et al. Pharmacokinetics and pharmacodynamics of oral methotrexate and mercaptopurine in children with lower risk acute lymphoblastic leukemia: a joint children's cancer group and pediatric oncology branch study. Blood 1998;92:3569–3577.

253. Steele WH, Lawrence JR, Stuart JF, et al. The protein binding of methotrexate by the serum of normal subjects. Eur J Clin Pharmacol 1979;15:363–366.

254. Liegler DG, Henderson ES, Hahn MA, et al. The effect of organic acids on renal clearance of methotrexate in man. Clin Pharmacol Ther 1969;10:849–857.

255. Wan SH, Huffman DH, Azarnoff DL, et al. Effect of route of administration and effusions on methotrexate pharmacokinetics. Cancer Res 1974;4:3487–3491.

256. Chabner BA, Stoller RG, Hande K, et al. Methotrexate disposition in humans: case studies in ovarian cancer and following high-dose infusion. Drug Metab Rev 1978;8:107–117.

257. Torres IJ, Litterst CL, Guarino AM. Transport of model compounds across the peritoneal membrane in the rat. Pharmacology 1978;17:330–340.

258. Fossa SD, Heilo A, Bormer O. Unexpectedly high serum methotrexate levels in cystectomized bladder cancer patients with an ileal conduit treated with intermediate doses of the drug. J Urol 1990;143:498–501.

259. Kristenson L, Weismann K, Hutters L. Renal function and the rate of disappearance of methotrexate from serum. Eur J Clin Pharmacol 1975;8:439–444.

260. Bressolle F, Bologna C, Kinowski JM, et al. Effects of moderate renal insufficiency on pharmacokinetics of methotrexate in rheumatoid arthritis patients. Ann Rheum Dis 1998;57:110–113.

261. Bleyer WA. The clinical pharmacology of methotrexate: new applications of an old drug. Cancer 1978;41:36–51.

262. Howell SB, Tamerius RK. Achievement of long duration methotrexate exposure with concurrent low dose thymidine protection: influence of methotrexate pharmacokinetics. Eur J Cancer 1980;16:1427–1432.

263. Evans WE, Crom WR, Stewart CF, et al. Methotrexate systemic clearance influences probability of relapse in children with standard-risk acute lymphocytic leukaemia. Lancet 1984;1: 359–362.

264. Evans WE, Crom WR, Abromowitch M, et al. Clinical pharmacodynamics of high-dose methotrexate in acute lymphocytic leukemia. Identification of a relation between concentration and effect. N Engl J Med 1986;314:471–477.

265. Borsi JD, Moe PJ. Systemic clearance of methotrexate in the prognosis of acute lymphoblastic leukemia in children. Cancer 1987;60:3020–3024.

266. Pearson AD, Amineddine HA, Yule M, et al. The influence of serum methotrexate concentrations and drug dosage on outcome in childhood acute lymphoblastic leukaemia [see comments]. Br J Cancer 1991;64:169–173.

267. Calvert AH, Bondy PK, Harrap KR. Some observations on the human pharmacology of methotrexate. Cancer Treat Rep 1977;61:1647–1656.

268. Monjanel S, Rigault JP, Cano JP, et al. High-dose methotrexate: preliminary evaluation of a pharmacokinetic approach. Cancer Chemother Pharmacol 1979;3:189–196.

269. Sasaki K, Tanaka J, Fujimoto T. Theoretically required urinary flow during high-dose methotrexate infusion. Cancer Chemother Pharmacol 1984;13:9–13.

270. Romolo JL, Goldberg NH, Hande KR, et al. Effect of hydration on plasma-methotrexate levels. Cancer Treat Rep 1977;61:1393–1396.

271. Huang KC, Wenczak BA, Liu YK. Renal tubular transport of methotrexate in the rhesus monkey and dog. Cancer Res 1979;39:4843–4848.

272. Iven H, Brasch H. Influence of the antibiotics piperacillin, doxycycline, and tobramycin on the pharmacokinetics of methotrexate in rabbits. Cancer Chemother Pharmacol 1986;17:218–222.

273. Iven H, Brasch H. The effects of antibiotics and uricosuric drugs on the renal elimination of methotrexate and 7-hydroxymethotrexate in rabbits. Cancer Chemother Pharmacol 1988;21:337–342.

274. Iven H, Brasch H. Cephalosporins increase the renal clearance of methotrexate and 7-hydroxymethotrexate in rabbits. Cancer Chemother Pharmacol 1990;26:139–143.

275. Titier K, Lagrange F, Pehourcq F, et al. Pharmacokinetic interaction between high-dose methotrexate and oxacillin. Ther Drug Monit 2002;24(4):570–572.

276. Dalle JH, Auvrignon A, Vassal G etal. Interaction between methotrexate and ciprofloxacin. J Pediatr Hematol Oncol 2002;4(4):321–322.

277. Kerr IG, Jolivet J, Collins JM, et al. Test dose for predicting high-dose methotrexate infusions. Clin Pharmacol Ther 1983;33:44–51.

278. Favre R, Monjanel S, Alfonsi M, et al. High-dose methotrexate: a clinical and pharmacokinetic evaluation. Treatment of advanced squamous cell carcinoma of the head and neck using a prospective mathematical model and pharmacokinetic surveillance. Cancer Chemother Pharmacol 1982;9:156–160.

279. Gewirt DA, White JC, Goldman ID. Transport, binding and polyglutamation of methotrexate (MTX) in freshly isolated hepatocytes. Am Assoc Cancer Res 1979:147.

280. Strum WB, Liem HH. Hepatic uptake, intracellular protein binding and biliary excretion of amethopterin. Biochem Pharmacol 1977;26:1235–1240.

281. Jacobs SA, Derr CJ, Johns DG. Accumulation of methotrexate diglutamate in human liver during methotrexate therapy. Biochem Pharmacol 1977;26:2310–2313.

282. Strum WB, Liem HH, Muller-Eberhard U. Effect of chemotherapeutic agents on the uptake and excretion of amethopterin by the isolated perfused rat liver. Cancer Res 1978;38:4734–4736.

283. Said HM, Hollander D. Inhibitory effect of bile salts on the enterohepatic circulation of methotrexate in the unanesthetized rat: inhibition of methotrexate intestinal absorption. Cancer Chemother Pharmacol 1986;16:121–124.

284. Lerne PR, Creaven PJ, Allen LM, et al. Kinetic model for the disposition and metabolism of moderate and high-dose methotrexate in man. Cancer Chemother Rep 1975;59:811–817.

285. Shen DD, Azarnoff DL. Clinical pharmacokinetics of methotrexate. Clin Pharmacokinet 1978;3:1–13.

286. Steinberg SE, Campbell CL, Bleyer WA, et al. Enterohepatic circulation of methotrexate in rats in vivo. Cancer Res 1982;42:1279–1282.

287. Breithaupt H, Kuenzlen E. Pharmacokinetics of methotrexate and 7-hydroxymethotrexate following infusions of high-dose methotrexate. Cancer Treat Rep 1982;66:1733–1741.

288. Erttmann R, Landbeck G. Effect of oral cholestyramine on the elimination of high-dose methotrexate. J Cancer Res Clin Oncol 1985;110:48–50.

289. Jacobs SA, Stoller RG, Chabner BA, et al. 7-Hydroxymethotrexate as a urinary metabolite in human subjects and rhesus monkeys receiving high dose methotrexate. J Clin Invest 1976;57:534–538.

290. Bremnes RM, Slordal L, Wist E, et al. Formation and elimination of 7-hydroxymethotrexate in the rat in vivo after methotrexate administration. Cancer Res 1989;49:2460–2464.

291. Sholar PW, Baram J, Seither R, et al. Inhibition of folate-dependent enzymes by 7-OH-methotrexate. Biochem Pharmacol 1988;37:3531–3534.

292. Clendeninn NJ, Drake JC, Allegra CJ, et al. Methotrexate polyglutamates have a greater affinity and more rapid on-rate for purified human dihydrofolate reductase than MTX. Proc Am Assoc Cancer Res 1985:232.

293. McCullough JL, Chabner BA, Bertino JR. Purification and properties of carboxypeptidase G1. J Biol Chem 1971;246:7207–7213.

294. Abelson HT, Ensminger W, Rosowsky A, et al. Comparative effects of citrovorum factor and carboxypeptidase G1 on cerebrospinal fluid-methotrexate pharmacokinetics. Cancer Treat Rep 1978;62:1549–1552.

295. Chabner BA, Young RC. Threshold methotrexate concentration for in vivo inhibition of DNA synthesis in normal and tumorous target tissues. J Clin Invest 1973;52:1804–1811.

296. Sirotnak FM, Moccio DM. Pharmacokinetic basis for differences in methotrexate sensitivity of normal proliferative tissues in the mouse. Cancer Res 1980;40:1230–1234.

297. Toffoli G, Russo A, Innocenti F etal. Effect of methylenetetrahydrofolate reductase C677T polymorphism on toxicity and homocysteine plasma level after chronic methotrexate treatment of ovarian cancer patients. Int J Cancer 2003;103(3):294-299.

298. Chiusolo P, Reddiconto G, Casorelli I, et al. Preponderance of methylenethtrahydrofolate reductase C677T homozygosity among leukemia patients intolerant to methotrexate. Ann Oncol 2002;13(12):1915–1918.

299. Ulrich CM, Yasui Y, Storb R, et al. Pharmacogenetics of methotrexate: toxicity among marrow transplantation patients varies with the methylenetetrahydrofolate reductase C677T polymorphism. Blood 2001;98(1):231–234.

300. Urano W, Taniguchi A, Yamanaka H, et al. Polymorphisms in the methylenetetrahydrofolate reductase gene were associated with both the efficacy and the toxicity of methotrexate used for the treatment of rheumatoid arthritis, as evidenced by single locus haplotype analysis. Pharmacogenetics 2002;12(3):183–190.

301. Van Ede AE, Laan RF, Blom HJ, et al. The C677T mutation in the methylenetetrahydrofolate reductase gene: a genetic risk factor for methotrexate-related elevation of liver enzymes in rheumatoid arthritis patients. Arthritis Rheum 2001;44(11):2525–2530.

302. Ackland SP, Schilsky RL. High-dose methotrexate: a critical reappraisal. J Clin Oncol 1987;5:2017–2031.

303. Von Hoff DD, Penta JS, Helman LJ, et al. Incidence of drug-related deaths secondary to high-dose methotrexate and citrovorum factor administration. Cancer Treat Rep 1977;61:745–748.

304. Hempel L, Misselwitz J, Fleck C etal. Influence of high-dose methotrexate therapy on glomerular and tubular kidney function. Med Pediatr Oncol 2003;40(6):348–354.

305. Stoller RG, Hande KR, Jacobs SA, et al. Use of plasma pharmacokinetics to predict and prevent methotrexate toxicity. N Engl J Med 1977;297:630–634.

306. Bacci G, Ferrari S, Longhi A, et al. Delayed methotrexate clearance in osteosarcoma patients treated with multiagent regimens of neoadjuvant chemotherapy. Oncol Rep 2003;10(4):851–857.

307. Thyss A, Milano G, Kubar J, et al. Clinical and pharmacokinetic evidence of a life-threatening interaction between methotrexate and ketoprofen. Lancet 1986;1:256–258.

308. Takeda M, Khamdang S, Narikawa S, et al. Characterization of methotrexate transport and its drug interactions with human organic anion transporters. J Pharmacol Exp Ther 2002;302(2):666–671.

309. Nozaki Y, Kusuhara H, Endou H, et al. Quantitative evaluation of the drug-drug interactions between methotrexate and nonsteroidal anti-inflammatory drugs in the renal uptake process based on the contribution of organic anion transporters and reduced folate carrier. J Pharmacol Exp Ther 2004;309(1):226–234.

309a. Wall, S.M., Johansen, M.J., Molony, D.A., DuBose, T.D., Jr., Jaffe, N., and Madden, T. Effective clearance of methotrexate using high-flux hemodialysis membranes. Am J Kidney Dis 1996;28:846–854.

310. Bertino JR, Condos S, Horvath C, et al. Immobilized carboxypeptidase G1 in methotrexate removal. Cancer Res 1978;38:1936–1941.

311. DeAngelis LM, Tong WP, Lin S, et al. Carboxypeptidase G2 rescue after high-dose methotrexate. J Clin Oncol 1996;14: 2145–2149.

312. Mohty M, Peyriere H, Guinet C, et al. Carboxypeptidase G2 rescue in delayed methotrexate elimination in renal failure. Leuk Lymphoma 2000;37(3-4):441–443.

313. Krause AS, Weihrauch MR, Bode U, et al. Carboxypeptidase-G2 rescue in cancer patients with delayed methotrexate elimination after high-dose methotrexate therapy. Leuk Lymphoma 2002;43(11):2139–2143.

314. Widemann BC, Balis FM, Murphy RF, et al. Carboxypeptidase-G2, thymidine, and leucovorin rescue in cancer patients with methotrexate-induced renal dysfunction. J Clin Oncol 1997;15: 2125–2134.

315. Schornagel JH, Leyva A, Bucsa JM, et al. Thymidine prevention of methotrexate toxicity in head-and-neck cancer. In Pinedo HM, ed. Clinical Pharmacology of Antineoplastic Drugs. Amsterdam: Elsevier/North Holland, 1978:83.

316. Van den Bongard HJ, Mathjt RA, Boogerd W, et al. Successful rescue with leucovorin and thymidine in a patient with high-dose methotrexate induced acute renal failure. Cancer Chemother Pharmacol 2001;47(6):537–540.

317. Howell SB, Herbst K, Boss GR, et al. Thymidine requirements for the rescue of patients treated with high-dose methotrexate. Cancer Res 1980;40:1824–1829.

318. Capizzi RL. Schedule-dependent synergism and antagonism between methotrexate and L-asparaginase. Biochem Pharmacol 1974;23:151.

319. Yap BS, McCredie KB, Benjamin RS, et al. Refractory acute leukaemia in adults treated with sequential colaspase and high-dose methotrexate. BMJ 1978;2:791–793.

320. Moran RG, Mulkins M, Heidelberger C. Role of thymidylate synthetase activity in development of methotrexate cytotoxicity. Proc Natl Acad Sci U S A 1979;76:5924–5928.

321. Rajeswari R, Shetty PA, Gothoskar BP, et al. Pharmacokinetics of methotrexate in adult Indian patients and its relationship to nutritional status. Cancer Treat Rep 1984;68:727–732.

322. Mihranian MH, Wang YM, Daly JM. Effects of nutritional depletion and repletion on plasma methotrexate pharmacokinetics. Cancer 1984;54:2268–2271.

323. Zachariae H, Kragballe K, Sogaard H. Methotrexate induced liver cirrhosis. Studies including serial liver biopsies during continued treatment. Br J Dermatol 1980;102:407–412.

324. Dahl MG, Gregory MM, Scheuer PJ. Methotrexate hepatotoxicity in psoriasis—comparison of different dose regimens. BMJ 1972;1:654–656.

325. Podurgiel BJ, McGill DB, Ludwig J, et al. Liver injury associated with methotrexate therapy for psoriasis. Mayo Clin Proc 1973;48:787–792.

326. Willkens RF, Clegg DO, Ward JR, et al. Liver biopsies in patients on low-dose pulse methotrexate for the treatment of rheumatoid arthritis [abstract]. In: Sixteenth International Congress on Rheumatology. Sydney, Australia: 1985:88.

327. Mackenzie AH. Hepatotoxicity of prolonged methotrexate therapy for rheumatoid arthritis. Cleve Clin Q 1985;52:129–135.

328. Scully CJ, Anderson CJ, Cannon GW. Long-term methotrexate therapy for rheumatoid arthritis. Semin Arthritis Rheum 1991;20:317–331.

329. Phillips CA, Cera PJ, Mangan TF, et al. Clinical liver disease in patients with rheumatoid arthritis taking methotrexate. J Rheumatol 1992;19:229–233.

330. Weber BL, Tanyer G, Poplack DG, et al. Transient acute hepatotoxicity of high-dose methotrexate therapy during childhood. J Natl Cancer Inst Monogr 1987;5:207–212.

331. Clarysse AM, Cathey WJ, Cartwright GE, et al. Pulmonary disease complicating intermittent therapy with methotrexate. JAMA 1969;209:1861–1868.

332. Sostman HD, Matthay RA, Putman CE, et al. Methotrexate-induced pneumonitis. Medicine (Baltimore)1976;55:371–388.

333. Akoun GM, Mayaud CM, Touboul JL, et al. Use of bronchoalveolar lavage in the evaluation of methotrexate lung disease. Thorax 1987;42:652–655.

334. Kremer JM, Phelps CT. Long-term prospective study of the use of methotrexate in the treatment of rheumatoid arthritis. Update after a mean of 90 months. Arthritis Rheum 1992;35:138–145.

335. Searles G, McKendry RJ. Methotrexate pneumonitis in rheumatoid arthritis: potential risk factors. Four case reports and a review of the literature. J Rheumatol 1987;14:1164–1171.

336. Carson CW, Cannon GW, Egger MJ, et al. Pulmonary disease during the treatment of rheumatoid arthritis with low dose pulse methotrexate. Semin Arthritis Rheum 1987;16:186–195.

337. Kremer JM, Alarcon GS, Weinblatt ME, et al. Clinical, laboratory, radiographic, and histopathologic features of methotrexate-associated lung injury in patients with rheumatoid arthritis: a multicenter study with literature review [see comments]. Arthritis Rheum 1997;40:1829–1837.

338. Hargreaves MR, Mowat AG, Benson MK. Acute pneumonitis associated with low dose methotrexate treatment for rheumatoid arthritis: report of five cases and review of published reports. Thorax 1992;47:628–633.

339. Alarcon GS, Kremer JM, Macaluso M, et al. Risk factors for methotrexate-induced lung injury in patients with rheumatoid arthritis. A multicenter, case-control study. Methotrexate Lung Study Group. Ann Intern Med 1997;127:356–364.

340. Goldberg NH, Romolo JL, Austin EH, et al. Anaphylactoid type reactions in two patients receiving high dose intravenous methotrexate. Cancer 1978;41:52–55.

341. Doyle LA, Berg C, Bottino G, et al. Erythema and desquamation after high-dose methotrexate. Ann Intern Med 1983;98: 611–612.

342. Shamberger RC, Rosenberg SA, Seipp CA, et al. Effects of high-dose methotrexate and vincristine on ovarian and testicular functions in patients undergoing postoperative adjuvant treatment of osteosarcoma. Cancer Treat Rep 1981;65:739–746.

343. Shapiro WR, Young DF, Mehta BM. Methotrexate: distribution in cerebrospinal fluid after intravenous, ventricular and lumbar injections. N Engl J Med 1975;293:161–166.

344. Tatef ML, MargolinKA, Doroshow JH, et al. Pharmacokinetics and toxicity of high-dose intravenous methotrexate in the treatment of leptomeningeal carcinomatosis. Cancer Chemother Pharmacol 2000;46(1):19–26.

345. Bleyer WA, Drake JC, Chabner BA. Neurotoxicity and elevated cerebrospinal-fluid methotrexate concentration in meningeal leukemia. N Engl J Med 1973;289:770–773.

346. Morse M, Savitch J, Balis F, et al. Altered central nervous system pharmacology of methotrexate in childhood leukemia: another sign of meningeal relapse. J Clin Oncol 1985;3:19–24.

347. Blaney SM, Balis FM, Poplack DG. Current pharmacological treatment approaches to central nervous system leukaemia. Drugs 1991;41:702–716.

348. Ettinger LJ, Chervinsky DS, Freeman AI, et al. Pharmacokinetics of methotrexate following intravenous and intraventricular administration in acute lymphocytic leukemia and non-Hodgkin's lymphoma. Cancer 1982;50:1676–1682.

349. Grossman SA, Reinhard CS, Loats HL. The intracerebral penetration of intraventricularly administered methotrexate: a quantitative autoradiographic study. J Neurooncol 1989;7:319–328.

350. Bleyer WA, Poplack DG, Simon RM. "Concentration · time" methotrexate via a subcutaneous reservoir: a less toxic regimen for intraventricular chemotherapy of central nervous system neoplasms. Blood 1978;51:835–842.

351. Glantz MJ, Cole BF, Recht L, et al. High-dose intravenous methotrexate for patients with nonleukemic leptomeningeal cancer: is intrathecal chemotherapy necessary? J Clin Oncol 1998;16:1561–1567.

352. Peylan-Ramu N, Poplack DG, Blei CL, et al. Computer assisted tomography in methotrexate encephalopathy. J Comput Assist Tomogr 1977;1:216–221.

353. Paakko E, Vainionpaa L, Lanning M, et al. White matter changes in children treated for acute lymphoblastic leukemia. Cancer 1992;70:2728–2733.

354. Shapiro WR, Allen JC, Horten BC. Chronic methotrexate toxicity to the central nervous system. Clin Bull 1980;10:49–52.

355. Jaffe N, Takaue Y, Anzai T, et al. Transient neurologic disturbances induced by high-dose methotrexate treatment. Cancer 1985;56:1356–1360.

356. Fritsch G, Urban C. Transient encephalopathy during the late course of treatment with high-dose methotrexate. Cancer 1984; 53:1849–1851.

357. Walker RW, Allen JC, Rosen G, et al. Transient cerebral dysfunction secondary to high-dose methotrexate. J Clin Oncol 1986; 4:1845–1850.

358. Kubo M, Azuma E, Arai S, et al. Transient encephalopathy following a single exposure of high-dose methotrexate in a child with acute lymphoblastic leukemia. Pediatr Hematol Oncol 1992;9:157–165.

359. Allen J, Rosen G, Juergens H, et al. The inability of oral leucovorin to elevate CSF 5-methyl-tetrahydrofolate following high dose intravenous methotrexate therapy. J Neurooncol 1983; 1:39–44.

360. Mehta BM, Glass JP, Shapiro WR. Serum and cerebrospinal fluid distribution of 5-methyltetrahydrofolate after intravenous calcium leucovorin and intra-Ommaya methotrexate administration in patients with meningeal carcinomatosis. Cancer Res 1983;43:435–438.

361. Ochs J, Mulhern R, Fairclough D, et al. Comparison of neuropsychologic functioning and clinical indicators of neurotoxicity in long-term survivors of childhood leukemia given cranial radiation or parenteral methotrexate: a prospective study. J Clin Oncol 1991;9:145–151.

362. Mahoney DH Jr, Shuster JJ, Nitschke R, et al. Acute neurotoxicity in children with B-precursor acute lymphoid leukemia: an association with intermediate-dose intravenous methotrexate and intrathecal triple therapy—a Pediatric Oncology Group study. J Clin Oncol 1998;16:1712–1722.

363. Phillips PC, Dhawan V, Strother SC, et al. Reduced cerebral glucose metabolism and increased brain capillary permeability following high-dose methotrexate chemotherapy: a positron emission tomographic study. Ann Neurol 1987;21:59–63.

364. Kishi S, Griener J, Cheng C, et al. Homocysteine, pharmacogenetics, and neurotoxicity in children with leukemia. J Clin Oncol 2003;21(16):3084–3091.

365. Gilbert MR, Harding BL, Grossman SA. Methotrexate neurotoxicity: in vitro studies using cerebellar explants from rats. Cancer Res 1989;49:2502–2505.

366. Livrea P, Trojano M, Simone IL, et al. Acute changes in blood-CSF barrier permselectivity to serum proteins after intrathecal methotrexate and CNS irradiation. J Neurol 1985;231:336–339.

367. Spiegel RJ, Cooper PR, Blum RH, et al. Treatment of massive intrathecal methotrexate overdose by ventriculolumbar perfusion. N Engl J Med 1984;311:386–388.

368. Shih C, Chen VJ, Gossett LS, et al. LY231514, a pyrrolo[2,3-d]pyrimidine-based antifolate that inhibits multiple folate-requiring enzymes. Cancer Res 1997;57:1116–1123.

368a. Wang Y, Zhao R, Chattopadhyay S, et al. A novel folate transport activity in human mesothelioma cell lines with high affinity and specificity for the new-generation antifolate, Pemetrexed. Cancer Res 2002, 62:6434–6437.

369. Shih C, Habeck LL, Mendelsohn LG, et al. Multiple folate enzyme inhibition: mechanism of a novel pyrrolopyrimidine-based antifolate LY231514 (MTA). Adv Enzyme Regul 1998; 38:135–152.

370. Worzalla JF, Shih C, Schultz RM. Role of folic acid in modulating the toxicity and efficacy of the multitargeted antifolate, LY231514. Anticancer Res 1998;18:3235–3239.

371. Scagliotti GV, Shin DM, Kindler HL, et al. Phase II study of pemetrexed with and without folic acid and vitamin B12 as front-line therapy in malignant pleural mesothelioma. J Clin Oncol 2003;21(8):1556–1561.

372. Vogelzang NJ, Rusthoven JJ, Symanowski J, et al. Phase III study of pemetrexed in combination with cisplatin versus cisplatin alone in patients with malignant pleural mesothelioma. J Clin Oncol 2003;21(14):2636–2644

373. Clarke SJ, Abatt R, Goedhals L, et al. Phase II trial of pemetrexed disodium (Alimta, LY231514) in chemotherapy-naive patients with advanced non-small-cell lung cancer. Ann Oncol 2002;13(5):737–741.

374. Hanna N, Shepherd FA, Fossella FV, et al. Randomized phase III trial of pemetrexed versus docetaxel in patients with non-small-cell lung cancer previously treated with chemotherapy. J Clin Oncol 2004;22(9):1589–1597.

375. Rafi I, Taylor GA, Calvete JA, et al. Clinical pharmacokinetic and pharmacodynamic studies with the nonclassical antifolate thymidylate synthase inhibitor 3, 4-dihydro-2- amino-6-methyl-4-oxo-5-(4-pyridylthio)-quinazoline dihydrochloride (AG337) given by 24-hour continuous intravenous infusion. Clin Cancer Res 1995;1:1275–1284.

376. Webber S, Bartlett CA, Boritzki TJ, et al. AG337, a novel lipophilic thymidylate synthase inhibitor: in vitro and in vivo preclinical studies. Cancer Chemother Pharmacol 1996;37: 509–517.

377. Creaven PJ, Pendyala L, Meropol NJ, et al. Initial clinical trial and pharmacokinetics of Thymitaq (AG337) by 10-day continuous infusion in patients with advanced solid tumors. Cancer Chemother Pharmacol 1998;41:167–170.

378. Hughes AN, Rafi I, Griffin MJ, et al. Phase I studies with the nonclassical antifolate nolatrexed dihydrochloride (AG337, THYMITAQ) administered orally for 5 days. Clin Cancer Res 1999;5:111–118.

379. Pivot X, Wadler S, Kelly C, et al. Result of two randomized trials comparing nolatrexed (Thymitaq) versus methotrexate in patients with recurrent head and neck cancer. Ann Oncol 2001; 12(11):1595–1599.

380. Zalcberg JR, Cunningham D, Van Cutsem E, et al. ZD1694: a novel thymidylate synthase inhibitor with substantial activity in the treatment of patients with advanced colorectal cancer. Tomudex Colorectal Study Group. J Clin Oncol 1996;14: 716–721.

381. Cunningham D, Zalcberg J, Smith I, et al. "Tomudex" (ZD1694): a novel thymidylate synthase inhibitor with clinical antitumour activity in a range of solid tumours. "Tomudex" International Study Group. Ann Oncol 1996;7:179–182.

382. Cunningham D. Mature results from three large controlled studies with raltitrexed ("Tomudex"). Br J Cancer 1998;77:15–21.

383. Van Cutsem E, Cunningham D, Maroun J, et al. Raltitrexed: current clinical status and future directions. Ann Oncol 2002; 13(4):513–522.

384. Yin MB, Guo B, Panadero A, et al. Cyclin E-cdk2 activation is associated with cell cycle arrest and inhibition of DNA replication induced by the thymidylate synthase inhibitor Tomudex. Exp Cell Res 1999;247:189–199.

385. Santini D, Massacesi C, D'Angelillo RM, et al. Raltitrexed plus weekly oxaliplatin as a first-line chemotherapy in metastatic colorectal cancer: a multicenter non-randomized phase II study. Med Oncol 2004;21(1):59–66.

386. Feliu J, Salud A, Escudero P, et al. Irinotecan plus raltitrexed as first-line treatment in advanced colorectal cancer: a phase II study. Br J Cancer 2003;90(8):1502–1507.

387. Farrugia DC, Ford HE, Cunningham D, et al. Thymidylate synthase expression in advanced colorectal cancer predicts for response to raltitrexed. Clin Cancer Res 2003;9(2):792–801.

388. Hainsworth J, Vergote I, Janssens J. A review of phase II studies of ZD9331 treatment for relapsed or refractory solid tumours. Anticancer Drugs 2003;14(Suppl1):S13 –19.

389. Springer CJ, Poon GK, Sharma SK, et al. Analysis of antibody-enzyme conjugate clearance by investigation of prodrug and active drug in an ADEPT clinical study. Cell Biophys 1994;25: 193–207.

390. Springer CJ, Bavetsias V, Jackman AL, et al. Prodrugs of thymidylate synthase inhibitors: potential for antibody directed enzyme prodrug therapy (ADEPT). Anticancer Drug Des 1996;11:625–636.

391. Syrigos KN, Epenetos AA. Antibody directed enzyme prodrug therapy (ADEPT): a review of the experimental and clinical considerations. Anticancer Res 1999;19:605–613.

5-Fluoropyrimidines

Jean L. Grem

7

The 5-fluorinated pyrimidines were rationally synthesized by Heidelberger et al.[1] on the basis of the observation that rat hepatomas use radiolabeled uracil more avidly than nonmalignant tissues, a finding that suggested differences in the enzymatic pathways used for uracil metabolism. Fluorouracil (5-FU) has become particularly useful in the treatment of gastrointestinal (GI) adenocarcinomas and squamous cell carcinomas arising in the head and neck. Synergistic interaction of 5-FU and related fluoropyrimidines with other antitumor agents, irradiation, and physiologic nucleosides, and enhanced activity of 5-FU activity by leucovorin (LV), have also invoked interest.

STRUCTURE AND CELLULAR PHARMACOLOGY

The chemical structures of the initial two 5-fluoropyrimidines to enter clinical trials are shown in Figure 7.1. The simplest derivative, 5-FU (molecular weight [MW] = 130), has the slightly bulkier fluorine atom substituted at the carbon-5 position of the pyrimidine ring in place of hydrogen. The key features of 5-FU are outlined in Table 7.1. Activation to the nucleotide level is essential to antitumor activity. The ribonucleoside derivative 5-fluorouridine (FUrd) has been used exclusively in preclinical studies. The deoxyribonucleoside derivative 5-fluoro-2′-deoxyuridine (FdUrd, MW = 246) is commercially available (floxuridine, FUDR) and is primarily used for hepatic arterial administration.

Transport

5-FU shares the same facilitated-transport system as uracil, adenine, and hypoxanthine. In human erythrocytes, 5-FU and uracil exhibited similar saturable (K [(binding affinity] ~4 mmol/L; V_{max} 500 pmol/sec per 5 μL cells) and nonsaturable (rate constant approximately 80 pmol/sec per 5 μL cells) components of influx. The system is neither temperature-dependent nor energy-dependent.[2,3] 5-FU permeation is pH-dependent. Ionization of the hydroxyl group attached to the fourth carbon (pK [ionization constant of acid] = 8.0) markedly depresses its transmembrane passage. 5-FU entry into erythrocytes via nonfacilitated diffusion and a facilitated nucleobase transport system clearly differs from that used by pyrimidine nucleosides.[3] In rat hepatoma cells, maximal accumulation of free intracellular 5-FU occurs within 200 seconds[2]; total intracellular 5-FU increases thereafter as the result of formation of nucleotides and RNA incorporation.

FdUrd is a nucleoside. There are at least four major nucleoside transport (NT) systems in mammalian cells that vary in substrate specificity, sodium dependance, and sensitivity to nitrobenzylthioinosine.[4] Two basic classes of human NT systems are present: equilibrative (bidirectional) and concentrative (sodium-dependent, unidirectional). Human equilibrative NT (ENT-1) and concentrative NT (CNT-1) are selective for pyrimidines; the former is present in most cell types, including cancer cells, and the latter is present in liver, kidney, intestine, choroid plexus, and some tumor cells. In Ehrlich ascites cells, intracellular FdUrd reaches equilibrium with extracellular drug within 15 seconds.[5] Total intracellular drug continues to accumulate thereafter from rate-limiting phos-phosphorylation to form fluorodeoxyuridylate (5-fluoro-2′-deoxyuridine-5′monophosphate, FdUMP) and other nucleotides.

Metabolic Activation

Activation of 5-FU to the ribonucleotide level may occur through one of two pathways, as outlined in Figure 7.2[6–15]: direct transfer of a ribose phosphate to 5-FU from 5-phosphoribosyl-1-pyrophosphate (PRPP) as catalyzed by orotic acid phosphoribosyl transferase (OPRTase); the addition of a ribose moiety by uridine (Urd) phosphorylase followed by phosphorylation by Urd kinase. Sequential

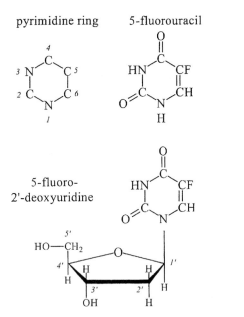

Figure 7.1 Structures of pyrimidine ring, 5-fluorouracil, and 5-fluoro-2'-deoxyuridine.

action of uridine/cytidine monophosphate kinase (UMP/CMP kinase) and pyrimidine diphosphate kinase result in the formation of fluorouridine diphosphate (FUDP) and fluorouridine triphosphate (FUTP); the latter is incorporated into RNA by the action of RNA polymerase.

The pathway catalyzed by OPRTase may be of primary importance for 5-FU activation in healthy tissues because its inhibition by a nucleotide metabolite of allopurinol diminishes toxicity to bone marrow and GI mucosa,[7,12,14] but it is also the dominant route of 5-FU activation in many murine leukemias.[6] Other cancer cell lines appear to activate the drug by the action of Urd phosphorylase and Urd kinase.[7-14] Although one activation pathway may appear to predominate in a given cancer cell under certain conditions, both pathways can often be used.

In the presence of a 2'-deoxyribose-1-phosphate (dR-1-P) donor, 5-FU is converted to FdUrd by thymidine (dThd) phosphorylase.[15,16] dThd kinase then forms FdUMP, a potent inhibitor of thymidylate synthase (TS). FdUMP can be also be formed by ribonucleotide reductase-mediated conversion of FUDP to fluorodeoxyuridine diphosphate (FdUDP), followed by dephosphorylation to FdUMP. FdUMP and FdUDP are substrates for thymidine monophosphate and diphosphate kinases, respectively, resulting in the formation of fluorodeoxyuridine triphosphate (FdUTP). FdUTP can be incorporated into DNA by DNA polymerase.

Physiologic Urd metabolites are largely present in vivo as nucleotide sugars that are necessary for the glycosylation of proteins and lipids, which plays an important role in cytoplasmic and cell membrane metabolism. 5-FU nucleotide sugars, such as FUDP-glucose, FUDP-hexose,

FUDP-N-acetylglucosamine, and FdUDP-N-acetylglucosamine, have been detected in mammalian cells.[17-19] The extent to which 5-FU nucleotide sugars are incorporated into proteins and lipids and any possible metabolic consequences are unclear.

Catabolic enzymes also play important roles in nucleoside metabolism. Acid and alkaline phosphatases nonspecifically remove phosphate groups to convert nucleotides to nucleosides. 5'-Nucleotidases also remove a phosphate group from the nucleotide. Nucleosidases break the glycosyl linkage to release a free base. Pyrophosphatases remove two phosphate groups from the 5'-position of the nucleotide, with release of a monophosphate. The pyrimidine phosphorylases catalyze the reversible conversion of pyrimidine base to nucleoside. FdUrd serves as a substrate for both Urd and dThd phosphorylases in a tissue-dependent manner, yielding 5-FU.[15,16] dThd phosphorylase is homologous to platelet-derived endothelial growth factor, which is involved in angiogenesis.

MECHANISM OF ACTION

Inhibition of Thymidylate Synthase

At least two primary mechanisms of action appear capable of causing cell injury: inhibition of TS and incorporation into RNA. FdUMP binds tightly to TS and prevents formation of thymidylate (thymidine 5'-monophosphate, dTMP), the essential precursor of thymidine 5'-triphosphate (dTTP), which is required for DNA synthesis and repair. The functional TS enzyme comprises a dimer of two identical subunits, each of MW $\sim$30 kd (bacterial) or $\sim$36 kd (human). Each subunit has a nucleotide-binding site and two distinct folate binding sites, one for 5,10-methylenetetrahydrofolate (5,10-CH FH$_4$) monoglutamate or polyglutamate, and one for dihydrofolatepolyglutamates. FdUMP competes with the natural substrate 2'-deoxyuridine monophosphate (dUMP) for the TS catalytic site.[20,21] During methylation of dUMP, transfer of the folate methyl group to dUMP occurs by elimination of hydrogen attached to the pyrimidine carbon-5 position (Fig. 7.3). This elimination cannot occur with the more tightly bound fluorine atom of FdUMP, and the enzyme is trapped in a slowly reversible ternary complex (Fig. 7.4). The "thymineless state" that ensues is toxic to actively dividing cells. Toxicity can be circumvented by salvage of dThd in cells that contain dThd kinase. The circulating concentrations of dThd in humans are not thought to be sufficient (approximately 0.1 μmol/L) to afford protection.[22] The plasma levels of dThd are approximately 10-fold higher in rodents, which complicates preclinical evaluation of the antitumor activity of various TS inhibitors.

The reduced-folate cofactor is required for tight binding of the inhibitor to TS. The natural cofactor for the TS

TABLE 7.1

KEY FEATURES OF 5-FLUOROURACIL

Mechanism of action:	Incorporation of fluorouridine triphosphate into RNA interferes with RNA synthesis and function.
	Inhibition of thymidylate synthase by fluorodeoxyuridylate (FdUMP) leads to depletion of thymidine 5' monophosphate and thymidine 5' triphosphate, and accumulation of deoxyuridine monophosphate and deoxyuridine triphosphate.
	Incorporation of fluorodeoxyuridine triphosphate and deoxyuridine triphosphate into DNA may affect DNA stability. Genotoxic stress triggers programmed cell death pathways.
Metabolism:	Converted enzymatically to active nucleotide forms intracellularly.
	DPD catalyzes the initial, rate-limiting step in 5-fluorouracil (5-FU) catabolism.
Pharmacokinetics:	Primary half-life is 8–14 minutes after IV bolus.
	Nonlinear pharmacokinetics from saturable catabolism: Total-body clearance decreases with increasing doses; clearance is faster with infusional schedules.
	Volume of distribution slightly exceeds extracellular fluid space.
Elimination:	Approximately 90% is eliminated by metabolism (catabolism → anabolism).
	<3% and < 10% unchanged drug excreted by kidneys with infusional and bolus 5-FU.
	Reduction of 5-FU to dihydrofluorouracil by DPD is rate-limiting. Thereafter: dihydrofluorouracil → fluoroureidopropionic acid → fluoro-β-alanine.
	5-FU and its catabolites undergo biliary excretion.
Pharmacokinetic drug Interactions:	Interference with 5-FU catabolism markedly prolongs its half-life.
	Inhibitors of DPD:
	Thymidine and thymine
	Uracil (component of uracil and ftorafur)
	5-chloro-2,4-dihydroxypyridine (component of ftorafur, 5-chloro-2,4-dihydroxypyridine, and potassium oxonate)
	3-cyano-2,6-dihydroxypyridine (component of emitefur, 3-{3-[6-benzoyloxy-3-cyano-2-pyridyloxycarbonyl]benzoyl}-1-ethoxymethyl-5-fluorouracil)
	(E)-5(2-bromovinyl)uracil (metabolite of sorivudine)
	Eniluracil
	Chronic administration of cimetidine (but not ranitidine) may decrease the clearance of 5-FU
	Dipyridamole increases 5-FU clearance during continuous i.v. infusion.
	Interferon-α may decrease 5-FU clearance in a dose- and schedule-dependent manner.
Biochemical drug interactions	Thymidine salvage via thymidine kinase repletes thymidine 5' triphosphate pools, decreases FdUMP formation, and antagonizes the DNA-directed toxicity of 5-FU and 5-fluoro-2'deoxyuridine; thymidine may increase fluorouridine triphosphate formation and its incorporation into RNA.
	Sequential methotrexate 5-FU increases 5-FU toxicity and increases fluorouridine triphosphate (FUTP) incorporation into RNA; may antagonize DNA-directed toxicity of 5-FU.
	Leucovorin increases intracellular pools of reduced folates; 5,10-methylenetetrahydrofolate polyglutamates enhance the stability of reduced folate-FdUMP–thymidylate synthase ternary complex; the magnitude and duration of thymidylate synthase inhibition is increased.
	Inhibitors of de novo pyrimidine synthesis (N-phosphonoacetyl-l-aspartic acid, brequinar) increase 5-FU anabolism to the ribonucleotide level and 5-FU–RNA incorporation; uridine triphosphate, cytidine triphosphate, deoxycytidine triphosphate, and deoxyuridine monophosphate depletion may enhance RNA- and DNA-directed toxicity of 5-FU
Toxicity:	Gastrointestinal epithelial ulceration
	Myelosuppression
	Dermatologic
	Ocular
	Neurotoxicity (cognitive dysfunction and cerebellar ataxia)
	Cardiac (coronary spasm)
	Biliary sclerosis (hepatic arterial infusion of FdUrd)
Precautions:	Nonlinear pharmacokinetics: difficulty in predicting plasma concentrations and toxicity at high doses.
	Patients with deficiency of DPD may have life-threatening or fatal toxicity if treated with 5-fluoropyrimidines.
	Duration of DPD inhibition with eniluracil may be prolonged (8-week washout period recommended).
	Patients receiving sorivudine should not receive concurrent 5-fluoropyrimidines (4-week washout period recommended).
	Older, female, and poor-performance–status patients have greater risk of toxicity.
	Closely monitor prothrombin time and INR in patients receiving concurrent warfarin DPD, dihydropyrimidine dehydrogenase.

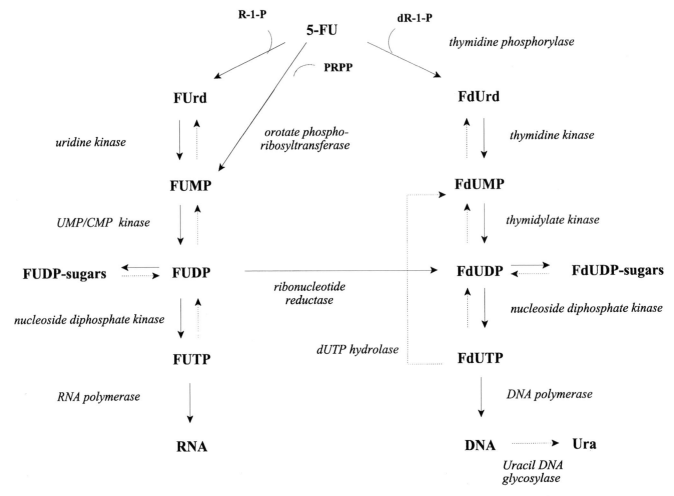

Figure 7.2 Intracellular activation of 5-fluorouracil (5-FU). dUTP, deoxyuridine triphosphate; FdUDP, fluorodeoxyuridine diphosphate; FdUMP, fluorodeoxyuridylate; FdUrd, 5-fluoro-2'-deoxyuridine; FdUTP, fluorodeoxyuridine triphosphate; FUDP, fluorouridine diphosphate; FUMP, fluorouridine monophosphate; FUrd, 5-fluorouridine; FUTP, fluorouridine triphosphate; PPRP, phosphoribosyl phosphate.

reaction, 5,10-CH FH, in its monoglutamate and polyglutamate forms, binds through its methylene group to the carbon-5 position of FdUMP. The polyglutamates of 5,10-CH FH$_4$ are much more effective in stabilizing the ternary complex.[23,24] Most other naturally occurring folates also promote FdUMP binding to the enzyme, but form a more readily dissociable complex. Polyglutamated forms of dihydrofolic acid (FH) promote extremely tight binding of FdUMP to the enzyme.[25,26] FH accumulates in cells exposed to methotrexate (MTX). Although MTX is a relatively weak inhibitor of TS in cell-free experiments, MTX polyglutamates are more potent inhibitors.[26] MTX polyglutamates decrease the rate of ternary complex formation among FdUMP, folate cofactor, and TS. The ability of MTX polyglutamates to inhibit ternary-complex formation is influenced by the glutamation state of the reduced-folate cofactor and is substantially reduced in the presence of 5,10-CH FH$_4$ pentaglutamate.[26] Similarly, in tissue culture, MTX-induced depletion of intracellular reduced folates

causes a marked reduction in the rate of formation of ternary complex.[25,27]

The kinetics of formation and dissociation of the ternary complex have been studied using bacterial enzyme.[28] After binding of inhibitor and 5,10-CH FH$_4$ to the first catalytic site in the free enzyme, the second site becomes exposed. The two binding sites seem to be nonequivalent in terms of their dissociation constants, with Kd values of $1.1 \times 10e\text{-}11$ and $2 \times 10e\text{-}10$ mol/L.[29] FdUMP binds less avidly to the mammalian enzyme, with a dissociation half-life ($t_{1/2}$) of 6.2 hours.[30]

Elucidation of the crystal structure of TS has permitted a complex kinetic and thermodynamic description of ternary complex formation.[31,32] The interaction proceeds by an ordered mechanism with initial nucleotide binding followed by 5,10-CH FH$_4$ binding to form a rapidly reversible noncovalent ternary complex. Enzyme-catalyzed conversions result in the formation of a covalent bond between carbon-5 of FdUMP and the one-carbon unit of the cofactor.

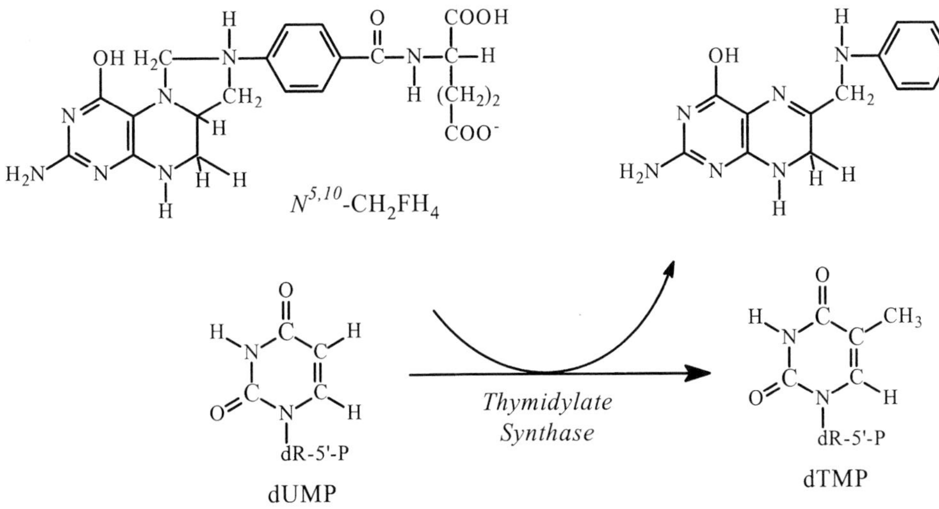

Figure 7.3 Synthesis of thymidylate from deoxyuridylate

The overall dissociation constant of 5,10-CH FH$_4$ from the covalent complex is approximately $1 \times 10e\text{-}11$ mol/L.

The three-dimensional conformation of free and bound TS has been characterized through molecular modeling and iterative crystallographic analysis of bacterial enzymes.[31–33] Although the MW and amino acid composition of the bacterial and mammalian enzymes differ, the primary sequence and the active site residues show high homology.[34] Thus, the bacterial ternary complex has served as a surrogate for the design of novel inhibitors of human TS.

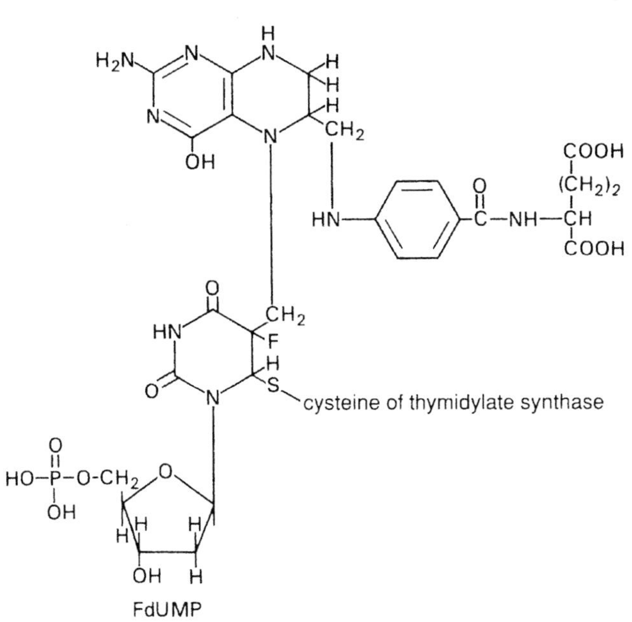

Figure 7.4 Interaction of fluorodeoxyuridylate (FdUMP) with thymidylate synthase.

Despite the high specificity and potency of TS inhibition by FdUMP and the well-established lethality of dTMP and dTTP depletion, inhibition of TS is not the sole cause of 5-FU toxicity. If 5-FU toxicity results from dTTP depletion, then dThd should reverse the toxic effects. Examples of complete protection from 5-FU cytotoxicity by dThd have been reported, but dThd shows variable effectiveness in rescuing cells exposed to 5-FU.[35,36] Murine lymphoma cells experience an early phase of toxicity during the initial 24 hours of 5-FU exposure, associated with S-phase accumulation.[35] Addition of dThd prevents the S-phase block induced by dTTP depletion and abolishes early growth inhibition. After 24 hours (approximately one cell-cycle length) of 5-FU incubation, dThd no longer prevents lethality, and toxicity is maximal for cells exposed during G$_1$ phase of the cell cycle; this phenomenon is attributed to progressive incorporation of 5-FU into RNA. In another model, a 3-hour incubation with 5-FU at 5 to 20 μmol/L produces a dThd-reversible toxicity, although dThd could not reverse toxicity associated with high 5-FU concentrations.[36]

Experimental evidence from in vivo studies supports the concept that 5-FU toxicity is at least partially independent of its effect on TS. Coadministration of 5-FU and dThd prevents the early inhibition of DNA synthesis, but markedly increases 5-FU toxicity to healthy tissues in the whole animal, increases the antitumor effect of 5-FU against various animal tumors, and increases [^{3}H]FUrd incorporation into RNA.[37–39] Other pharmacologic measures that increase FUTP formation and its RNA incorporation also increase its toxicity.[37,40]

RNA-Directed Effects

The contribution of RNA-directed toxicity to ultimate lethality varies greatly, depending on the type of cancer cell and the experimental conditions. 5-FU is extensively incorporated into nuclear and cytoplasmic RNA fractions, which may result in alterations in RNA processing and function, such as inhibiting the processing of initial pre-rRNA transcripts to the cytoplasmic rRNA species in a dose- and time-dependent manner (Table 7.2).[40-46]

Net RNA synthesis may be inhibited during and after fluoropyrimidine exposure in a concentration- and time-dependent fashion. In some cancer cell lines, a highly significant relationship exists between 5-FU incorporation into total cellular RNA and the loss of clonogenic survival.[8,47-49] 5-FU is incorporated into all species of RNA; substantial amounts of [³H]5-FU accumulate in low-MW (4S) RNA at lethal drug concentrations.[45] Although the analog replaces only a small percentage of uracil residues in RNA, the incorporated 5-FU residues appear to be stable and to persist in RNA for many days after drug administration.[36,50,51]

5-FU exposure affects mRNA processing and translation. Polyadenylation of mRNA is inhibited at relatively low concentrations of 5-FU,[52,53] and altered metabolism of specific proteins such as dihydrofolate reductase (DHFR) precursor mRNA has been reported.[54] Incorporation of 5-FU into RNA may affect quantitative and qualitative aspects of protein synthesis.[55-59]

In vitro-transcribed TS mRNA with 100% substitution of 5-FU leads to alteration in the secondary structure of mRNA, but no differences in the translational efficiency.[58] In another system, 100% substitution of uracil residues in human-TS complementary DNA (cDNA) with either FUTP or 5-bromouridine 5′-triphosphate (BrUTP) indicated that the translational rate is inhibited only in the presence of BrUTP-substituted cDNA.[59] The stability of the transcribed mRNA in a cell-free system is increased by threefold and 10-fold with FUTP and BrUTP, respectively, and nondenaturing gel electrophoresis shows different conformations for each of the substituted mRNA species.

TABLE 7.2

RNA-DIRECTED CYTOTOXIC EFFECTS OF 5-FLUOROURACIL (5-FU)

Decrease in net RNA synthesis.
Inhibition with RNA processing.
Inhibition of messenger RNA polyadenylation.
Alteration of the secondary structure of RNA.
5-FU residues in transfer RNA form covalent complex with enzymes involved in posttranslational modification of uracil residues.
Incorporation into uracil-rich small nuclear RNA species interferes with normal splicing.
Quantitative changes in protein synthesis.
Qualitative changes in protein synthesis.
Up-regulation of thymidylate synthase (TS) protein synthesis.
TS bound in ternary complex cannot bind to TS messenger RNA.
TS protein translation no longer repressed.

Changes in the structure and levels of small nuclear RNAs (snRNA) and small nuclear ribonuclear proteins (snRNP) result from 5-FU treatment.[60-65] With 8% replacement with 5-FU in HeLA cells, the levels of U2-snRNA and U2-snRNPs decrease in nuclear extracts.[62] The substitution of FUTP for uridine triphosphate (UTP) in a cell-free system (84% replacement of uracil residues by 5-FU) leads to pH-dependent missplicing of [³²P]-labeled human β-globin precursor mRNA; pH values favoring 5-FU ionization promote missplicing.[63]

The splicing reaction of precursor RNA exposed to either 1 mmol/L UTP or FUTP in *Tetrahymena* rRNA, an autocatalytic, self-splicing system with one intron and two exons, reveals that the rate and extent of formation of all RNA product species is decreased with 100% FUTP substitution.[64] Further, 5-FU substitution greatly increases the pH and temperature sensitivity of the process. Partial ionization of 5-FU residues at physiologic pH (pK 5-FU = 7.8 versus pK uracil = 10.1) may therefore destabilize the active conformation of RNA.[65]

Another potential locus of 5-FU action is inhibition of enzymes involved in posttranscriptional modification of RNA.[43,66-69] 5-FU exposure inhibits tRNA uracil 5-methyltransferase, which may result in decreased formation of modified Urd (pseudouridine) bases in tRNA.[66] In the presence of S-adenosylmethionine, 5-FU-substituted tRNA forms a stable covalent complex containing uracil 5-methyltransferase, 5-FU-tRNA, and the methyl group of S-adenosylmethionine, suggesting that irreversible inhibition of RNA methylation contributes to RNA-directed cytotoxicity.[67] 5-FU-substituted yeast glycine tRNAs form highly stable covalent complexes with pseudouridine synthase, which might interfere with the posttranscriptional modifications of many nucleotide positions in tRNA, rRNA, and snRNA that are otherwise converted to pseudouridine. 5-FU incorporation alters the biosynthesis of U2-snRNA with subsequent effects on snRNA-protein interactions.[69] Even low levels of 5-FU incorporation (5% replacement) inhibit the formation of pseudouridine.[69] Subtle changes in the structures of these essential splicing cofactors may thus have profound effects on snRNP-precursor mRNA interactions and interfere with precursor mRNA splicing.

Although 5-FU-associated cytotoxicity in cancer cells exposed in the presence of sufficient concentrations of dThd to circumvent TS inhibition is presumed to result from RNA-directed effects of 5-FU, it is paradoxical that significant incorporation of 5-FU into RNA may occur in some cancer cell lines in the absence of toxicity. The factors that influence whether 5-FU–RNA incorporation results in cytotoxicity are not clear. The rate of RNA incorporation and the species into which the fluoropyrimidine is incorporated may be more important determinants of cytotoxicity than the total amount incorporated. 5-FU and FUrd may be channeled into different ribonucleotide compartments and, ultimately, into distinct classes of RNA.[70]

In summary, the changes that result in altered pre-RNA processing and mRNA metabolism are not uniform for all RNA species after 5-FU exposure. Effects on precursor and mature rRNA, precursor and mature mRNA, tRNA, and snRNA species suggest inhibition of processing; incorporated 5-FU residues also inhibit enzymes involved in posttranscriptional modification of uracil. Many of the RNA-directed effects of 5-FU undoubtedly occur as a consequence of its fraudulent incorporation into various RNA species. However, rapid changes in mRNA levels suggest that at least some of these alterations may be mediated by other 5-FU-associated alterations in cellular metabolism or posttranslational modification.[71] The changes in certain key mRNAs resulting from 5-FU exposure may be relevant as a mechanism of cytotoxicity. 5-FU-mediated interference with the production of enzymes involved in DNA repair may have cytotoxic consequences, such as 5-FU-mediated inhibition of ERCC-1 mRNA expression in cisplatin-resistant cancer cells.[72] 5-FU and FUrd produce structural and functional alterations in uracil-rich snRNAs, and consequently in snRNPs with potential repercussions on cellular growth and metabolism. The RNA-directed effects of 5-FU are even more complex than previously appreciated, and some RNA effects may be independent of 5-FU incorporation into RNA.

DNA-Directed Cytotoxic Mechanisms

The biochemical consequences of TS inhibition and the potential effects on DNA integrity are summarized in Table 7.3. Inhibition of TS results in depletion of dTMP and dTTP, thus leading to inhibition of DNA synthesis and interference with DNA repair. Accumulation of dUMP

TABLE 7.3
DNA-DIRECTED CYTOTOXIC EFFECTS OF 5-FLUOROURACIL (5-FU)

Biochemical consequences of thymidylate synthase inhibition
Deoxyribonucleotide imbalance
Depletion of thymidine monophosphate and thymidine
  triphosphate
Accumulation of deoxyuridine monophosphate
Elevation of extracellular deoxyuridine
Formation of deoxyuridine triphosphate
Accumulation of deoxyadenosine triphosphate
Direct and indirect effects on DNA synthesis and integrity
Inhibition of net DNA synthesis
"Uracil" misincorporation into DNA (fluoro- and deoxyuridine
  triphosphate)
Interference with nascent DNA chain elongation
Altered stability of nascent DNA
Induction of single-strand breaks in nascent DNA
Interference with DNA repair
Induction of single- and double-strand breaks in parental DNA
Induction of programmed cell death

occurs behind the blockade of TS, and further metabolism to the deoxyuridine triphosphate (dUTP) level may occur.[73-75] Inhibition of TS is accompanied by elevated concentrations of deoxyuridine in the extracellular media in cell culture models and in plasma of rodents; monitoring changes in plasma deoxyuridine levels may, therefore, serve as an indirect reflection of TS inhibition.

FdUTP and dUTP are substrates for DNA polymerase, and their incorporation into DNA is a possible mechanism of cytotoxicity.[76-85] 5-FU cytotoxicity in some models correlates with the level of 5-FU-DNA.[80,81,84] Two mechanisms prevent incorporation of FdUTP and dUTP into DNA. The enzyme dUTP pyrophosphatase or dUTP hydrolase catalyses the hydrolysis of FdUTP to FdUMP and inorganic pyrophosphate.[86,87] The DNA repair enzyme uracil-DNA-glycosylase hydrolyzes the fluorouracil-deoxyribose glycosyl bond of the FdUMP residues in DNA, thereby creating an apyrimidinic site.[82,84,88] The bare deoxyribose 5'-monophosphate is subsequently removed from the DNA backbone by an AP (apurinic/apyrimidinic) endonuclease, creating a single strand break, which is subsequently repaired. With thymidine triphosphate depletion, however, the efficiency of the repair process is substantially weakened. Uracil-DNA-glycosylase is a cell cycle-dependent enzyme with maximal levels of activity at the G1 and S interface, such that excision of the fraudulent bases occurs before DNA replication. The activity of uracil-DNA-glycosylase inversely correlates with the level of FdUrd incorporation into DNA in human lymphoblastic cells.[80] Because the affinity of human uracil-DNA-glycosylase is much lower for 5-FU than for uracil, it is removed more slowly from DNA by this mechanism.[88] Recent studies suggest that FdUTP inhibits the activity of uracil-DNA-glycosylase.[89] Accumulation of deoxyadenosine triphosphate (dATP) accompanies TS inhibition.[90-92] The combined effects of deoxyribonucleotide imbalance (high dATP, low dTTP, high dUTP) and misincorporation of FdUTP into DNA may have several deleterious consequences affecting DNA synthesis, the integrity of nascent DNA, and induction of apoptosis.

A variety of DNA-directed effects have been described.[93-101] 5-FU treatment inhibits DNA elongation and decreases the average DNA chain length.[79,93,94] DNA strand breaks accumulate in 5-FU-treated cells and correlate with excision of [³H]5-FU from DNA.[93] 5-FU and FdUrd result in single- and double-stranded DNA breaks in HCT-8 cells in a concentration- and time-dependent fashion, a process that is enhanced by LV and limited by dThd.[95,96] FdUrd exposure may result in the formation of large (one to five-megabase) DNA fragments as a result of double-strand DNA breaks; the time course and extent of DNA megabase fragmentation correlates with loss of clonogenicity in HT29 cells.[97] The pattern of DNA fragmentation is distinct from that associated with gamma radiation, which produces random breaks. The pattern of high-MW DNA damage differs in SW620 cells, which are equally sensitive as HT29 cells to FdUrd-induced inhibition of TS, but require higher drug concentrations and longer exposures to achieve a comparable degree of DNA fragmentation and cytotoxicity. The basis is higher activity of dUTPase and failure to accumulate dUTP.[98] Simple dThd starvation of a TS-deficient murine cell line produces much smaller DNA fragments, 50 to 200 kb in length.[99]

Inhibition of protein synthesis by cycloheximide within 8 hours of FdUrd exposure dramatically reduces DNA double-strand breakage and lethality in murine FM3A cells, suggesting that FdUrd exposure triggers the synthesis of an endonuclease capable of inducing DNA strand breaks.[90] In rat prostate cancer cells with intact programmed cell-death pathways, FdUrd induces oligonucleosomal fragmentation of genomic DNA.[101]

Factors that regulate recognition of DNA damage and apoptosis contribute to 5-FU lethality. The oncogene *p53* plays a pivotal role in the regulation of cell-cycle progression and apoptosis and influences the sensitivity of murine embryonic fibroblasts to 5-FU.[102] Transfection and expression of the *bcl*-2 oncogene in a human-lymphoma cell line renders it resistant to FdUrd. TS inhibition, dTTP depletion, and induction of single-strand breaks in nascent DNA are similar in vector control cells and *bcl*-2-expressing cells.[103] In vector control cells, induction of double-stranded DNA fragmentation in parental DNA coincides with onset of apoptosis. The contribution of DNA damage to cell lethality varies among different malignant lines, and DNA fragmentation does not appear to contribute to 5-FU-mediated cytotoxicity in some cancer cell lines.[104,105]

In summary, TS inhibition, as seen in "pure" form with FdUrd treatment in the absence of dThd salvage, and 5-FU incorporation into RNA are capable of producing lethal effects on cells. DNA damage also contributes to cytotoxicity and can occur in the absence of detectable FdUTP incorporation into DNA. The combined effects of deoxyribonucleotide imbalance (high dATP, low dTTP, high dUTP) and misincorporation of FdUTP and dUTP into DNA result in a number of deleterious consequences affecting DNA synthesis and the integrity of nascent DNA. The pattern and extent of DNA damage induced by fluoropyrimidines in human colorectal cancer cells varies and may be affected by the activity of enzymes involved in DNA repair and by downstream pathways that are required to implement cellular destruction. It is now recognized that the genotoxic stress resulting from TS inhibition activates programmed cell-death pathways, resulting in induction of parental DNA fragmentation. Depending on the cell line in question, two different patterns of parental DNA damage may be noted: internucleosomal DNA laddering, the hallmark of classical apoptosis, and high-MW DNA fragmentation with segments ranging from approximately 50 kb to 1 to 3 megabases. Differences in the type and activity of endonucleases and DNA-degradative enzymes triggered in a given cell line most likely explain these disparate patterns of parental DNA fragmentation. In "apoptosis-competent"

cancer cell lines, such as HL60 promyelocytic leukemia cells, genotoxic stress results in rapid (within hours) induction of programmed cell death, with classic DNA laddering. In contrast, many cancer cell lines derived from epithelial tumors, including colon cancer, appear to undergo delayed programmed cell death. This phenomenon may reflect a "postmitotic" cell death, in which one or more rounds of mitosis are needed before cell death occurs.[106] In such cell lines, the duration of the genotoxic insult may determine whether induction of cytostasis or programmed cell death occurs. One possible explanation for delayed apoptosis is that originally sublethal damage to genes, which are essential for cell survival, may ultimately lead to cell death with subsequent rounds of DNA replication.

Factors operating downstream from TS clearly influence the cellular response to genotoxic stress, such as overexpression of the cellular oncoproteins *bcl*-2 and mutant *p53*. Disruption of the signal pathways that sense genotoxic stress or lead to induction of programmed cell death, or both, may render a cancer cell inherently resistant to 5-FU. In some cancer cell lines, thymine-less death may be mediated by Fas and Fas-ligand interactions.[107,108] Fas is a cell-surface receptor that belongs to the tumor necrosis factor-receptor superfamily. Binding of Fas by Fas-ligand activates caspase 8, thus initiating a proapoptotic cascade. Cancer cell lines that are insensitive to Fas-mediated apoptosis are insensitive to 5-FU, suggesting that modulation of their expression may influence sensitivity to 5-FU.[107–110] Although induction of programmed cell death is generally thought to be a consequence of DNA-directed events, 5-FU-mediated induction of apoptosis in intestinal crypt cells with an intact *p53* pathway appears to be a consequence of RNA-directed effects.[111] Although induction of apoptosis is the final common pathway for cell death, DNA- and RNA-directed effects of 5-FU may provide the triggering stimulus.

As previously mentioned, base excision repair plays an essential role in removing incorporated 5-FU and uracil residues from DNA, resulting in single-strand DNA breaks. Because BER involves mutliple proteins, deficiencies in one of the components such as uracil DNA glycosylase, XRCC1 or DNA polymerase-β, may negatively modulate the toxic effects of TS inhibitors.[112]

Microsatellite instability (MSI) is a manifestation of genomic instability in human cancers that have a decreased overall ability to faithfully replicate DNA, and is a surrogate phenotypic marker of underlying functional inactivation of the human DNA mismatch repair genes (MMR).[113] Functional loss of a MMR gene results from inactivation of both alleles via some combination of coding region mutations, loss of heterozygosity, and/or promoter methylation, which leads to gene silencing. In vitro studies suggest that MMR-proficient cells are more sensitive to 5-FU or FdUrd than MMR-deficient cells.[114,115] The MSI phenotype has been associated with a better prognosis in stage-for-stage matched tumors in primary colorectal cancer,[116] but data are conflicting as to whether MSI status influences benefit from 5-FU-based adjuvant therapy.

Relative Importance of RNA- versus DNA-Directed Effects

The relative contributions of DNA- and RNA-directed mechanisms to the cytotoxicity of 5-FU are influenced by the specific patterns of intracellular drug metabolism, which vary among different healthy and tumor tissues. 5-FU concentration and duration of exposure play pivotal roles in determining the basis of cytotoxicity. The improved response rates observed with LV modulation of bolus 5-FU therapy, the correlation between high TS expression in tumor tissue and insensitivity to 5-FU-based therapy, and the clinical activity of the antifolate-based TS inhibitors provide strong evidence that TS is an important therapeutic target. In some models, RNA-directed effects have been predominant, with prolonged duration of exposure, and are not necessarily cell-cycle dependent, whereas DNA-directed effects have been important during short-term exposure of cells in S phase. In different models, contrary results have been observed. The mechanism of insensitivity differs in human colon cancer cells selected for resistance to either short-term, high-concentration 5-FU exposure (1,000 μmol/L for 4 hours, simulating bolus administration) or more prolonged, lower-concentration exposure (15 μmol/L for 7 days).[117] A subline resistant to short-term 5-FU exposure has decreased 5-FU-RNA incorporation, whereas the subline insensitive to protracted 5-FU exposure displays more rapid recovery from TS inhibition after drug exposure. The subline with RNA-directed resistance retains sensitivity to protracted exposure.[118]

In two human colon carcinoma cell lines, the determinants of cytotoxicity with prolonged (120-hour) exposure to 5-FU at pharmacologically relevant concentrations (0.1 to 1.0 μmol/L) suggested that DNA-directed effects (inhibition of TS and induction of single-strand breaks in nascent DNA) and the gradual and stable accumulation of 5-FU into RNA both contribute to 5-FU toxicity.[119] Thus, the primary mechanism of 5-FU cytotoxicity varies among cancer cell lines and can change within a given cell line by alterations in schedule or the circumstances of drug exposure (the presence or absence of potential modulators of toxicity). More than one mechanism of action may be operative, and each may contribute to cytotoxicity.

DETERMINANTS OF SENSITIVITY TO FLUOROPYRIMIDINES

Because of the complexity of fluoropyrimidine metabolism and the multiple sites of biochemical action, multiple factors may be associated with responsiveness to this class of antimetabolites (Table 7.4). Deletion of or diminished activity of the various activating enzymes may result in

TABLE 7.4
DETERMINANTS OF SENSITIVITY TO 5-FLUOROURACIL (5-FU)

Extent of 5-FU anabolism
  Cellular uptake FUrd and FdUrd require facilitated nucleoside transport)
  Activity of anabolic enzymes
  Availability of (deoxy)ribose-1-phosphate donors and phosphoribosyl phosphate
Activity of catabolic pathways
  Alkaline and acid phosphatases
  Dihydropyrimidine dehydrogenase
Thymidylate synthase (TS)
  Baseline activity of enzyme
  Affinity of TS for fluorodeoxyuridine monophosphate
  Stability of the ternary complex
  Intracellular reduced-folate content
  Transport across cell membranes
  Polyglutamation
    Folylpolyglutamate synthetase activity
    Folylpolyglutamate hydrolase activity
  Concentration of deoxyuridine monophosphate
  Up-regulation of TS protein expression with TS inhibition
Extent of fluorouridine triphosphate incorporation into RNA
    concentration of competing normal substrates (uridine triphosphate, cytidine 5' triphosphate)
Salvage pathways
  Thymidine rescue
  Uridine rescue
Extent of deoxyuridine triphosphate (dUTP) and FdUTP incorporation into DNA
  Ability to accumulate dUTP (dUTP hydrolase activity)
  Uracil-DNA-glycosylase activity
Activity of other enzymes involved in base-excision repair
Extent and type of DNA damage
  Single-strand breaks
  Double-strand breaks
  Newly synthesized DNA vs. parental DNA
  Activity of DNA repair enzymes
Cellular response to genotoxic stress
  Cytostasis vs. cell death
  Intact DNA damage recognition pathways
  Intact programmed cell death signaling pathways
  Duration of genotoxic stress

FdUrd, 5-fluoro-2'-deoxyuridine; FUrd, 5-fluoro-uridine.

resistance to 5-FU.[120–129] Conversely, elevated levels of certain activating enzymes have been associated with increased fluoropyrimidine sensitivity. Clones derived from murine leukemia selected for stable resistance to either 5-FU, FUrd, or FdUrd is each deficient in one enzyme involved in pyrimidine metabolism: decreased OPRT was associated with 5-FU resistance, whereas FdUrd and FUrd resistance was associated with deletion of dThd and Urd kinase, respectively.[122,123] Clones retained sensitivity to alternate fluoropyrimidines; thus, resistance to 5-FU may not preclude sensitivity to FdUrd, or vice versa.

In addition to the importance of these activating enzymes, the availability of ribose-1-phosphate, dR-1-P, and PRPP may influence activation and response.[8,9,130–133]

Inosine and deoxyinosine augment 5-FU activation to the ribonucleotide and deoxyribonucleotide levels by serving as a source of ribose-1-phosphate and dR-1-P.

The formation of 5-fluoropyrimidine nucleotides within target cells and the size of the competitive physiologic pools of UTP and dTTP also influence 5-FU cytotoxicity.[134-138] The extent of 5-FU incorporation into RNA depends on FUTP formation and the size of the competing pool of UTP. Strategies that increase FUTP formation generally increase incorporation of FUTP into RNA and enhance 5-FU toxicity. Modulators including 6-methylmercaptopurine riboside (MMPR), N-phosphonoacetyl-l-aspartic acid (PALA), pyrazofurin, MTX, and dThd may increase FUTP formation by virtue of inhibiting de novo purine or pyrimidine synthesis, thereby increasing PPRP levels. Through feedback inhibition, expansion of dTTP pools decreases FdUMP formation by two means: blocking phosphorylation of FdUrd by dThd kinase and inhibiting the reduction of FUDP to FdUDP. In contrast, expansion of UTP or cytidine triphosphate (CTP) pools inhibits formation of FUMP by Urd kinase. Changes in nucleotide pool size have been implicated in 5-FU resistance in Chinese hamster fibroblast and in murine S49 lymphoma sublines that have altered CTP synthase activity, increased CTP pools, and decreased UTP pools.[139,140]

Because RNA- and DNA-directed effects of 5-FU may differ in importance among different malignant cell lines, any single manipulation of 5-FU metabolism may produce conflicting results if different tumor models are compared. The development and application of sensitive assays that permit reliable measurement of FUTP, 5-FU-RNA levels, and TS inhibition in patient samples will help elucidate clinical determinants of sensitivity to fluorinated pyrimidines given by various schedules. RNA and DNA incorporation in tumor biopsy specimens taken 2, 24 or 48 hours from patients receiving bolus 5-FU (500 mg/m^2) was measured using gas chromatography/mass spectrometry after complete degradation of isolated RNA and DNA to bases. Maximal incorporation occurred 24 hours after 5-FU administration: 1.0 pmol/mg RNA ($n = 59$) and 127 fmol/mg DNA ($n = 46$). Incorporation into RNA, but not DNA, significantly correlated with intratumoral 5-FU levels. The extent of TS inhibition, but not RNA or DNA incorporation, correlated with response to 5-FU therapy.[141] Results of such studies in clinical samples from patients receiving various infusional schedules of 5-FU are not yet available.

Determinants of Thymidylate Synthase Inhibition

The ability of FdUMP to inhibit TS is influenced by several variables, including the concentration of enzyme, the amount of FdUMP formed and its rate of breakdown, the levels of the competing healthy substrate (dUMP) and 5,10-CH FH$_4$ cofactor, and the latter's extent of polygluta-

mation. The degree and persistence of TS inhibition is a crucial determinant of cytotoxicity. Blockade of TS can lead to a gradual expansion of the intracellular dUMP pool; resumption of DNA synthesis is a function of two factors: the rate of decrease of intracellular FdUMP and the rate of increase in dUMP, which competes with FdUMP for newly synthesized TS and for enzyme that has dissociated from the ternary complex.

FdUMP accumulates rapidly in both responsive L1210 leukemia and resistant Walker 256 carcinoma, but more rapid recovery of DNA synthesis in the insensitive line correlates with accelerated decline in intracellular free FdUMP concentrations.[134] Other studies have confirmed that a more rapid decline in FdUMP concentration may be characteristic of resistant neoplasms, perhaps because of the increased phosphatase activity.[117,120,135] The basis for resistance in some cells may be explained by the rate of nucleotide inactivation rather than slower formation of the active product.

Determination of TS content in tumor tissue may help to clarify the relationship between pretreatment TS levels and prognosis, response, or both, to 5-FU therapy. Biochemical assays permit measurement of dUMP, TS, the ternary complex, and free FdUMP.[136-138,142,143] The total content of TS is estimated by the [^{3}H]FdUMP-binding assay. TS catalytic activity is determined by a tritium release assay (using either [5-^{3}H]dUrd in intact cells or [5-^{3}H]dUMP in cytosolic preparations); during dTMP formation, the addition of a methyl group displaces the [^{3}H] from the carbon-5 of dUMP. Although these assays are extremely useful for preclinical studies, their application to clinical tumor samples is limited by the need for relatively large quantities of tissue (at least 50 mg) as well as fresh or frozen tumor tissue. Despite the limitations, these biochemical assays have yielded important information. Biopsies of liver metastases obtained 20 to 240 minutes after 500 mg/m^2 5-FU among 21 patients undergoing elective surgery, maximal TS inhibition occurred within 90 minutes and averaged 70 to 80% in tumor tissue.[144] Large variations in TS binding and catalytic activity were noted in primary colon tumors, but the overall enzyme levels were significantly higher than in adjacent healthy colonic tissue.[145]

Measurement of TS gene expression provides an alternative to directly assaying intracellular TS enzyme. Polymerase chain reaction (PCR)-based methods can quantitate the expression of TS in clinical tumor samples, and overexpression to TS in tumor biopsies correlates with insensitivity to 5-FU-based regimens.[146-148]

Monoclonal antibodies have been developed that are capable of detecting human TS in immunoprecipitation and enzyme-linked immunosorbent assays (ELISA) and by immunoblot analysis, which have high specificity and tight binding affinities.[149] Immunologic quantitation of TS in 10 5-FU-sensitive and resistant cell lines showed a good correlation with biochemical assays; the limit of sensitivity was

0.3 fmol protein in lysates.[150] TS protein content in 1-mg tumor biopsy specimens can be measured with an ultrasensitive ELISA and chemiluminescent technique with a lower limit of detection of 30 attamol.[151] A number of studies have reported a relationship between TS expression in clinical specimens and prognosis; a systematic review of such studies in colorectal cancer has been published.[152]

Quantitative and qualitative changes in TS have been identified in cells with innate or acquired resistance to fluoropyrimidines. Amplification of the TS gene, with corresponding elevation of enzyme content, has been found in lines resistant to 5-FU or FdUrd.[153–155] Resistant cell lines may have an altered TS protein with either decreased binding affinity for FdUMP or decreased affinity for 5,10-CH FH$_4$.[156–159] Error-prone PCR has been used to mutagenize the full-length human TS cDNA and then to selected mutants resistant to FdUrd. Mutations distributed throughout the linear sequence and three-dimensional structure of human TS, including those distant from the active site, conferred resistance.[160] Decreased stability of the ternary complex has been described in HCT 8 cancer cells with acquired resistance to 5-FU and LV.[161] The rate of LV uptake, expansion of the reduced-folate pool, and polyglutamate chain length distribution of 5,10-CH FH$_4$ were similar in both lines, suggesting that mutations in TS may account for the reduced formation and stability of the ternary complex.

Adequate reduced-folate pools are required to form and maintain a stable ternary complex. Administration of exogenous reduced folates enhances the cytotoxicity of 5-FU and FdUrd in preclinical models, and clinical administration of LV is used to elevate the reduced-folate content in the cancer cell.[162] Tumor cells transport LV intracellularly and convert the folates to more potent and stable polyglutamates.[163–166] Deficiency of the low-affinity, high-capacity folate transport system (impaired membrane transport) and reduced folylpolyglutamate synthetase activity (impaired polyglutamation) impair the ability of LV to expand the reduced-folate pools.

dTTP depletion after fluoropyrimidine exposure influences sensitivity; salvage of preformed dThd by dThd kinase can bypass FdUMP-mediated TS inhibition and represents a potential mechanism of resistance.[167,168] Coadministration of 5-FU with an inhibitor of nucleoside transport would theoretically prevent cellular entry of preformed dThd. In a human colon parental line (GC C) and a subline selected for dThd kinase deficiency, the cytotoxicity and cellular pharmacology of 5-FU were similar, although only the parental line could be rescued by exogenous dThd.[169]

In summary, to inhibit TS, 5-FU must reach the tumor and then be metabolized to FdUMP. Cell lines lacking the capacity for nucleoside transport are unresponsive to FdUrd but retain sensitivity to 5-FU.[170,171] Additional factors influence the ability of FdUMP to inhibit TS. The tumor cell must enter the vulnerable synthetic phase of the cell cycle during drug exposure. The intracellular reduced-folate content must be adequate to promote stable inhibition of TS. The ratio of endogenous dUMP to FdUMP pools can affect the duration of TS inhibition. In certain cell lines, however, dUMP accumulation is associated with increased formation of dUTP; incorporation of dUTP into DNA may subsequently contribute to cytotoxicity by enhancing DNA damage.

Regulation of Thymidylate Synthase

TS is required for DNA replication; its activity is higher in rapidly proliferating cells than in noncycling cells. When nonproliferating cells are synchronized and stimulated to enter the synthetic phase of the cell cycle, TS content may increase up to 20-fold.[172] In proliferating cancer cells, TS activity varies by fourfold to eightfold from resting to synthetic phase.[173] Increased expression of the TS gene at the G1-S boundary is controlled by posttranscriptional regulation; elements in the promoter region of the human TS gene may also regulate gene expression.[174,175]

5-FU exposure may be accompanied by an acute increase in TS content, which may in turn permit recovery of enzymatic activity, and the magnitude of the increase is influenced by drug concentration and time of exposure.[176–182] In NCI-H630 colon cancer cells, TS content increases up to 5.5-fold during 5-FU exposure and is regulated at the translational level.[181] TS protein binds to specific regions in its corresponding TS-mRNA, which contributes to the regulation of TS-mRNA translation.[182,183] Antisense oligodeoxynucleotides targeted at the AUG translational start site of TS-mRNA inhibit translation in rabbit reticulocyte lysate; transfection of KB31 nasopharyngeal cancer cells with a plasmid construct containing the TS antisense fragment decreases the expression of TS protein and enhances the sensitivity to FdUrd by eightfold.[184] Small interfering double-stranded RNA (siRNA) targeted against TS are effective inhibitors of TS protein expression, and may have therapeutic potential by themselves or in combination with TS inhibitor compounds.[185]

Reduced-folate content also influences TS expression. A functionally TS-negative mutant (TS-C1) that has normal levels of TS-mRNA transcripts and immunologically reactive TS protein has normal clonogenic growth in the presence of high folate levels, suggesting folate responsiveness of the TS-C1 mutant.[186,187] The mutant has greatly reduced affinity for the reduced-folate cofactor, and endogenous total reduced-folate pools were only 6% of the parental level. Exposure of TS-C1 cells to 20 μmol/L LV stimulated de novo dTMP synthesis by 6 hours, whereas over 80% of the TS activity was lost by 24 hours after LV removal.[187]

Importance of Schedule of Administration in Preclinical Models

Drug concentration and duration of exposure in vitro are important determinants of response to 5-FU.[36,51,188–190]

High drug concentrations (above 100 μmol/L) are generally required for cytotoxicity if the duration of exposure is brief (<6 hours), whereas prolonged exposure (>72 hours) to concentrations between 1 and 10 μmol/L results produces cytotoxicity among a various tumors.

CLINICAL PHARMACOLOGY OF 5-FLUOROURACIL

The pharmacokinetics of 5-FU are important because of the choices of routes and schedules of administration available for this drug. Regional approaches permit selective exposure of specific tumor-bearing sites to high local concentrations of drug. Pharmacokinetic studies have played an important role in assessing these therapeutic alternatives.

Clinical Pharmacology Assay Methods

5-FU has been assayed in biologic fluids using high-performance liquid chromatography (HPLC) and gas chromatography-mass spectrometry (GC-MS). Various methods are used to extract 5-FU from biologic fluids. In general, an initial deproteination step is performed by chemical or filtration techniques. Subsequent steps separate 5-FU from other constituents in biologic fluids that may interfere with 5-FU detection. A number of different HPLC assays have been described for the analysis of 5-FU, including reversed-phase, reversed-phase ion-pairing, and normal-phase chromatography. HPLC methods using ultraviolet detection of 5-FU are typically associated with limits of detection in the range of 0.2 to 1.0 μmol/L. Column or valve-switching techniques and the use of microbore-HPLC columns can further improve the limits of detection.

The nucleoside metabolites of 5-FU can be separated from parent drug on reversed-phase and ion-exchange columns, whereas separation of the nucleotide metabolites is obtained with either anion-exchange or reversed-phase ion-pairing methods. Preclinical studies describing intracellular metabolism generally typically use radiolabeled 5-FU; HPLC with inline liquid scintillation detection is used to quantify the metabolites.

Derivitization of 5-FU is required for GC-MS. Mass spectrometry generally provides much greater sensitivity than that achievable with HPLC, with limits of detection as low as 0.5 ng/mL (4 nmol/L) for a 1-mL plasma sample.[191,192] Recent advances in fluorine-19 magnetic resonance imaging (MRI) have permitted monitoring of the pharmacokinetics and cellular pharmacology of 5-FU, thus allowing noninvasive determination of 5-FU content in tissues.[193]

5-FU is unstable in whole blood and plasma at room temperature, and catabolism is much more rapid in whole blood than in plasma.[194,195] Blood samples should be placed on ice immediately; plasma should be quickly isolated. 5-FU is stable in plasma at 4°C for up to 24 hours and is stable for prolonged periods when stored at –20°C.

ABSORPTION AND DISTRIBUTION

Bioavailability of 5-FU by the oral route is erratic; <75% of a dose reaches the systemic circulation.[195–197] When administered by intravenous bolus or infusion, 5-FU readily penetrates the extracellular space, cerebrospinal fluid (CSF) and extracellular "third-space" accumulations. The volume of distribution (Vd) ranges from 13 to 18 L (8 to 11 L per m^2) after intravenous bolus doses of 370 to 720 mg per m^2, which slightly exceeds extracellular fluid space.[191,198]

Plasma Pharmacokinetics

The pharmacokinetic profile of 5-FU varies according to dose and schedule of administration. After intravenous bolus injection of 370 to 720 mg per m^2, peak plasma concentrations (Cp) of 5-FU are 300 to 1,000 μmol per L (Table 7.5).[191,198–201] Rapid metabolic elimination accounts for a primary $t_{1/2}$ of 8 to 14 minutes; 5-FU Cp fall below 1 μmol per L within 2 hours.

McDermott et al. reported triexponential elimination of intravenous bolus 5-FU with $t_{1/2}$ values of 2, 12, and 124 minutes.[202] A prolonged third elimination phase of 5-FU was noted by GC-MS after bolus administration with a $t_{1/2}$ of 5 hours: 5-FU Cp ranged from 36 to 136 nmol per L 4 to 8 hours after intravenous bolus doses of 500 to 720 mg/m^2 and may reflect tissue release.[191]

The clearance of 5-FU is much faster with continuous infusion (CI) than with bolus administration and increases as the dose rate decreases (Table 7.6).[192,197,203–208] As the duration of 5-FU infusion increases, the tolerated daily dose decreases. A recommended starting dose of single-agent 5-FU given by protracted CI is 300 mg/m^2; the achieved steady-state plasma levels (Css) are in the submicromolar range. With CI over 96 to 120 hours, a daily dose of 1,000 mg/m^2 produces a Css in the 1 to 3 μmol/L range, and an intermittent schedule is necessary. CI of 2,000 to 2,600 mg/m^2 5-FU daily given either for 72 hours every 3 weeks or for 24 hours weekly yields a Css of 5 to 10 μmol/L.

5-FU clearance varies considerably between individuals. The elimination kinetics of 5-FU are nonlinear.[191,195,196,202–214] The following are noted with increasing doses: a decrease in hepatic extraction ratio; an increase in bioavailability; an increase in plasma $t_{1/2}$; a decrease in total-body clearance; and an increase in 5-FU area under the curve (AUC). Although the change in 5-FU clearance or AUC with increasing 5-FU dosage on a given schedule may be linear over a certain dose range, with higher dosages these parameters may change disproportionately. This nonlinear behavior represents saturation of metabolic processes at higher drug concentrations, leading to difficulty in predicting plasma levels or toxicity at higher dosages.

TABLE 7.5
PHARMACOKINETICS OF 5-FLUOROURACIL GIVEN BY INTRAVENOUS BOLUS

Investigators	Dose (mg/m²)	No.	Half-Life (min)	Clearance (mL/min/m²)	Plasma Concentration (μmol/L)	AUC per Dose (μmol•min/L)
Grem et al.[198]	370	16	8.1 ± 0.4	862 ± 24	C_0 : 332 ± 27 15 min: 82 ± 6 60 min: 4 ± 1	3,761 ± 286
Macmillan et al.[199]	400	8	11.4 ± 1.5	744 ± 145	5 min: 469 ± 85 20 min: 100 ± 20 60 min: 13 ± 6	9,885 ± 1,569
Heggie et al.[200]	500	10	12.9 ± 7.3	594 ± 7.3	5 min: 420 ± 102 20 min: 114 ± 52 60 min: 10 ± 11	7,125 ± 2,371
van Gröeningen et al.[191]	500 600 720	15 18 7	9.8 ± 2.4 14.4 ± 2.5	558 404 349	Not stated	7,338 ± 1,708 12,000 ± 2,446 16,200 ± 2,446
Grem et al.[201]	425 490	11 13	9.8 ± 0.5 (all doses)	743 ± 81 713 ± 28	$C_{0'}$: 378 ± 46 393 ± 24	4,401 ± 363 5,304 ± 227

AUC, area under the concentration time curve; C_0, estimated initial concentration. *Note:* If either AUC or clearance was not provided, it was calculated from the following equation: intravenous dose/AUC = clearance. The molecular weight of 5-FU = 130.1.

Variation in 5-FU pharmacokinetics has been reported according to time of day. A 2.2-fold difference was noted in 5-FU Cp during a 5-day infusion of 1,000 mg/m² per day; the peak value averaged 4.5 μmol/L at 1:00 AM, whereas the minimum value averaged 2 μmol/L at 1:00 PM.[207] With CI of 300 mg/m² per day 5-FU, the peak 5-FU Cp was 0.22 μmol/L around noon; the trough 5-FU value, 0.04 μmol/L, occurred around midnight.[205] The discrepancy between the times of day at which peak and trough 5-FU levels occurred in these two studies suggests that other factors, perhaps

TABLE 7.6
PHARMACOKINETICS OF 5-FLUOROURACIL GIVEN BY CONTINUOUS INTRAVENOUS INFUSION

Investigators	Duration of Infusion	Daily Dose (mg/m²)	No.	Cpss (μmol/L)	Clearance (mL/min/m²)
Grem et al.[206]	Protracted	64–200	24	0.30 ± 0.04 (0.14–1.04)	3,050 ± 330
Anderson et al.[192]	Protracted	176–300	3	0.32 (0.05–0.57)	Not provided
Harris et al.[205]	Protracted	300	7	0.13 ± 0.01	Not provided
Yoshida et al.[204]	Protracted	190–600	19	1.15 ± 0.15 (0.08–2.40)	2,033
Petit et al.[207]	120 hr	450–966	7	2.6 ± 0.2	Not provided
Fleming et al.[208]	120 hr	1,000	57	2.1	2,523 ± 684
Fraile et al.[197]	96 hr	1,000–1,100	6	24–48 hr, 1.3 ± 0.1 72–96 hr, 1.8 ± 0.3	Not provided
Benz et al.[203]	24 hr	1,500	7	4 (1.94–5.63)	2,118 (1,235–3,471)
Erlichman et al.[209]	120 hr	1,250 1,500 1,750 2,000 2,250	15 6 14 25 17	3.4 ± 0.4 5.1 ± 1.0 6.4 ± 0.9 7.2 ± 0.7 7.5 ± 1.0	2,410 1,790 1,990 1,910 2,000
Remick et al.[210]	72 hr	1,655 2,875	6 8	5.4 ± 0.3 13.9 ± 0.5	1,750 ± 105 1,117 ± 37
Grem et al.[211]	72 hr	1,150–1,525 1,750 2,000 2,300 2,645	19 31 53 14 10	3.4 ± 0.5 5.0 ± 0.5 6.5 ± 0.9 8.8 ± 1.3 10.0 ± 2.1	3,011 ± 356 2,671 ± 563 2,651 ± 324 2,116 ± 572 2,247 ± 443
Grem et al.[226]	24 hr	2,300	12	6.6 ± 1.7	1,953 ± 453

Css, plasma concentration at steady state. *Note:* Plasma clearance converted from milliliter per minute assuming an average body surface area of 1.7 m² and from milliliter per kilogram assuming a conversion factor of 37 from kg to m².

geographic, seasonal, individual sleep and wake habits, and administration of other drugs may influence 5-FU clearance.

The diurnal and interindividual variations in 5-FU pharmacokinetics suggest that, to compare and assess pharmacokinetic parameters with clinical outcome or the effect of another drug, it is important to have each patient serve as his or her own control, obtain samples for pharmacokinetic studies at the same time of day and for consecutive daily schedules, on the same day of treatment, and to collect pharmacokinetic samples for all subjects within as narrow a time window as possible.

Correlations have been described between 5-FU pharmacokinetics and toxicity with intravenous bolus and infusion schedules (Table 7.7).[191,198,204,206,210,211,215-217] Serious clinical toxicity tends to increase with higher systemic exposure, reflected by total AUC with bolus injection and Css with 5-FU infusion. These findings suggest that pharmacokinetic monitoring may be used to adjust 5-FU doses to avoid or minimize serious clinical toxicity.[217,218] However, not all patients with relatively high 5-FU systemic exposure experience serious toxicity, and some patients have toxicity despite relatively low 5-FU systemic exposure, suggesting that other factors contribute. The relationship between antitumor activity and 5-FU pharmacokinetics is less clear.

FdUrd is generally given by CI. The achieved Css with protracted schedules have not been well defined because the predicted Cp are below the detection limits of HPLC assays; analysis by GC-MS has been hampered by the difficulty in preparing stable, volatile derivatives of FdUrd. With intravenous bolus FdUrd given weekly, the AUC of 5-FU is twofold to threefold greater than FdUrd, suggesting that FdUrd is acting in part as a precursor to 5-FU.[219] With 1,650 mg/m² given at the midpoint of a 2-hour infusion of 500 mg/m² LV, the median clearance was 3,500 mL/min.

Regional Administration of 5-Fluorouracil

The administration of 5-FU and FdUrd by intrahepatic arterial infusion (HAI) is a strategy to maximize the regional exposure while limiting systemic toxicity. Approximately 19 to 51% of infused 5-FU is cleared in its first pass through the liver, whereas FdUrd first-pass clearance exceeds 94%.[212] Systemic and hepatic metabolic clearances and extraction ratios decrease progressively with increasing 5-FU dose rates. Systemic exposure to 5-FU after HAI ranges from 12 to 52% of that after intravenous administration of dose rates equivalent to 0.37 to 10 g/m²; the regional advantage

TABLE 7.7

CORRELATION OF 5-FLUOROURACIL PHARMACOKINETIC PARAMETERS WITH CLINICAL TOXICITY

Reference	Dose (mg/m²/d)	Intra-venous Schedule	Parameter AUC, μmol/L/min; C_{ss}, μmol/L	Toxicity Grade	Incidence (%)	No. Patients	P Value (Test)
191	500–720	Bolus	AUC: ≤8,300	≥1	11	11	Not stated
			>8,300		71	28	
198	370	Bolus	AUC: <4,000	≥3	0	15	.03 (Wilcoxon rank sum)
			4,000–5,000		21	14	
			>5,000		43	7	
204	190–360	Protracted CI	Css: 0.8 ± 0.4[a]	≤2	100	9	<.05 (Bonferroni)
			1.5 ± 0.7[a]	≥3	100	10	
136 a	64–200	Protracted CI	C_{ss}: 0.24 ± 0.02[a]	# 1	100	19	.02 (Mann-Whitney)
			0.53 ± 0.14	2	100	5	
215	1,000	120 hr CI	AUC: <1,800	≥1	3	31	<.01 (not stated)
			≥1,800		78	32	
211	1,150–3,500	72 hr CI	≥3		Gastrointestinal toxicity/ ANC/platelet:		
			C_{ss}: ≤8.9		1/14/0	91	.02, .01, .007 (Fisher's exact)
			≥9.0		14/41/14	11	
216	185–3,600	72 hr CI	C_{ss}: ≤2.0	≥1	6	32	% Mucositis = 100 x (1–e– 0.114Css)
			2.1–4.0		28	32	
137			> 4.0		70	50	$r^2 = 0.88$
217 [b]	~1,000	96 hr CI	AUC 27,622 ± ±962[a]	0–2 heme toxicity		65	.035 (t-test)
			31,451 ± 1,358[a]	3-4		26	

AUC, area under the concentration time curve; CI, continuous infusion; Css, plasma concentration at steady state; ANC, absolute neutrophil count

a Mean ± SE. [b] AUC units are ng•hr/mL over 96 hr.

CI, continuous infusion; HAI, hepatic arterial infusion; LV, leucovorin CI, continuous infusion; HAI, hepatic arterial infusion.

relative to systemic exposure varies from sixfold at the lowest 5-FU doses to twofold at the highest doses.[214] Drug dose, blood flow, and the rate of administration influence the extent of hepatic removal and systemic exposure.[220]

Portal venous perfusion was based on the premise that although most large metastases obtain their blood supply predominantly from the arterial circulation, small metastases may be fed by the portal circulation. Mean tumor uptake of FdUrd in patients with established metastases was 15.5-fold greater after bolus administration of [³H]FdUrd into the hepatic artery compared with portal vein, whereas the uptake into healthy liver is similar.[221] These findings suggest that portal perfusion may be effective in the setting of micrometastatic disease, and this approach has been explored as adjuvant therapy for stage II and III colon cancer.

Low MW compounds such as 5-FU and FdUrd injected into the peritoneal cavity are absorbed primarily through the portal circulation, passing through the liver before reaching the systemic circulation. The rates of absorption and clearance from the peritoneal cavity depend on the drug's lipid solubility and MW, as well as the surface area of the peritoneum (which may be altered by tumor, adhesions, or other pathologic changes).

Peritoneal dialysate concentrations up to 5 mmol/L 5-FU maintained by intermittent exchanges of fluid are tolerated for up to 5 days.[222,223] Mean 5-FU clearance from the peritoneal cavity was 840 mL/min, about fivefold slower than systemic clearance; the ratio of intraperitoneal to systemic 5-FU levels was 300.[222] Higher intraperitoneal drug concentrations (>5 mmol/L) saturate hepatic clearance mechanisms, with increased systemic levels and significant myelosuppression. Mild-to-moderate abdominal pain and chemical peritonitis may occur, particularly with repeated dosing. 5-FU give intraperitoneally in escalating concentrations for 4 hours along with a fixed dose of cisplatin (90 mg/m²) every 28 days was associated with dose-limiting neutropenia with 5-FU concentrations of >20 mmol/L; other toxicities included nausea, vomiting and diarrhea.[224] Between dialysate concentrations of 5 and 24 mmol/L, the mean peritoneal levels of 5-FU ranged from 2.2 to 12.5 mmol/L, and peak Cp, which occurred 1 hour after intraperitoneal instillation, ranged from 6 to 60 μmol/L.

FdUrd 3 g given intraperitoneal in 2 L of 1.5% dialysate with a dwell time of up to 3 days was associated with excellent local tolerance; the major systemic toxicities, nausea and vomiting, were well controlled with antiemetics.[225]

Peritoneal FdUrd levels over the initial 4 hours were above 1,000 μg/mL (4 mmol/L); peritoneal 5-FU levels were also high 0.75 to 1.50 mmol/L. FdUrd Cp were below 2 μmol/L, whereas 5-FU Cp were much higher: 150 to 300 μmol/L. The AUC values extrapolated to infinity at the recommended dose indicate a pharmacologic advantage for FdUrd of about 2,700. The $t_{1/2}$ and clearance of FdUrd in peritoneal fluid was 97 minutes and 31 mL/min, compared with values of 7.5 minutes and 7,000 mL/min after 2 g FdUrd intravenous over 30 minutes.[225]

Topical 5-FU, 2 to 5% in a hydrophilic cream base or propylene glycol, is used by dermatologists for the treatment of multiple actinic keratoses of the face, intraepidermal carcinomas, superficial basal cell carcinoma, vaginal intraepithelial neoplasia, and genital condylomas. Local application of 5-FU has also been used after trabeculectomy in patients with uncontrolled glaucoma to improve intraocular pressure control.

Mechanisms of Drug Elimination

After bolus dosing of 5-FU, about 90% is eliminated by metabolism (catabolism > anabolism), and less than 10% is renally excreted.[200] With continuous infusion of 5-FU 2.3 g/m², less than 2% of 5-FU was excreted in the urine.[226] The initial rate-limiting step in 5-FU catabolism is reduction of the pyrimidine ring by dihydropyrimidine dehydrogenase (DPD) (Fig. 7.5). In the presence of the reduced form of nicotinamide adenine dinucleotide phosphate (NADPH), DPD converts pyrimidines, such as uracil and 5-FU, to the dihydropyrimidine form (dihydrouracil and dihydrofluorouracil [DHFU]). Kinetic studies of purified DPD from a number of mammalian tissues have shown that the affinity of uracil and 5-FU are similar (Km ranging from 1.8 to 5.5 μmol/L).[227–230] Saturation of DPD accounts for the dose-dependent pharmacokinetics. DPD is widely distributed in tissues throughout the body, including the liver, GI mucosa, and peripheral blood mononuclear cells (PBMCs).[231,232] Because of the size of the organ, the liver has the highest total content of DPD in the body and is a major site of 5-FU catabolism.

The clearance of 5-FU during CI exceeds hepatic blood flow (1,000 mL/min) by several-fold, suggesting that a substantial portion of 5-FU metabolism occurs in extrahepatic tissue. In clinical practice, the dosage of 5-FU is not usually reduced in the presence of hepatic dysfunction. Full-dose 5-FU has been given by HAI to patients with

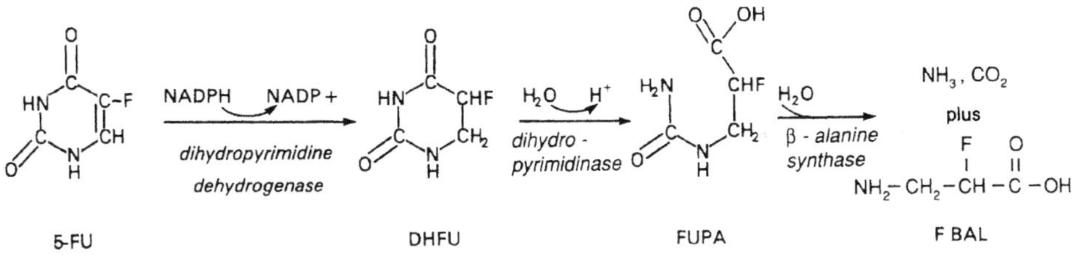

Figure 7.5 Catabolism of 5-fluorouracil (5-FU). DHFU, dihydrofluorouracil; FBAL, fluoro-β-alanine; FUPA, α-fluoroureido-propionic acid; NADP, nicotinamide adenine dinucleotide; NADPH, nicotinamide adenine dinucleotide phosphate.

extensive liver replacement and jaundice; improvement or resolution of jaundice may occur in some patients without undue systemic toxicity.[233,234] Patients with severe hepatic dysfunction in general have been excluded from randomized trials of HAI FdUrd and systemic 5-FU. The dosage of 5-FU need not be reduced automatically for hepatic dysfunction; however, a more conservative approach may be prudent in jaundiced patients with a poor performance status.

DHFU appears rapidly after intravenous bolus 5-FU. The pyrimidine ring is subsequently opened by dihydropyrimidinase forming 5-fluoroureido-propionic acid (FUPA); FUPA is then converted by β-alanine synthase to fluoro-β-alanine (FBAL), with the release of ammonia from the nitrogen-3 position and CO from the carbon-2 of the pyrimidine ring. In 10 patients receiving 500 to 700 mg/m^2 [^{3}H]5-FU, peak DHFU Cp of 10 to 30 μmol/L were seen 30 to 90 minutes later. FUPA reached maximum Cp (C_{max}) of 13 μmol/L at 90 minutes; FBAL C_{max} occurred between 60 to 90 minutes (60 μmol/L). The excretion of unchanged drug, FBAL, and FUPA in the urine occurred within the 6 hours; FBAL was the major metabolite.[200]

Significant biliary concentrations of 5-FU (11 to 259 μmol/L) have been detected during the first hour after intravenous bolus.[200] A conjugate of FBAL and cholic acid was seen within 30 minutes; peak values of 1 mmol/L were seen within 2 to 4 hours.[200,235]

After intravenous bolus administration of [^{3}H]FBAL in rats, tissue levels of FBAL were at least fivefold to 10-fold higher than the corresponding Cp for up to 8 days.[236] The radioactivity was present as free FBAL in all tissues except liver, in which FBAL undergoes enterohepatic circulation as FBAL-bile acid conjugates. FBAL accumulated in tissues that correspond to sites of 5-FU toxicity in humans, suggesting it might contribute to host toxicity.

Dihydropyrimidine Dehydrogenase Activity and 5-Fluorouracil-Associated Toxicity

Human DPD protein has been purified and its crystal structure has been elucidated.[229,230,237] DPD enzymatic activity has often been measured by incubating cellular lysates with excess NADPH and radiolabeled 5-FU, with separation of 5-FU and DHFU by HPLC and scintillation detection. This is a labor-intensive assay that has generally limited its availability to research laboratories. Although there appears to be a relationship between DPD activity and 5-FU clearance, the correlation is not tight in general study populations of cancer patients that have not been preselected for insensitivity to 5-FU-based therapy.[205,208,238] In contrast, profound DPD deficiency is more likely to be identified in patients who have experienced excessive toxicity with a 5-FU-based therapy.[239,240] Population studies that measured DPD activity in human peripheral blood mononuclear cells suggest a Gaussian distribution.[238,239,241–245] Although total DPD deficiency is relatively rare, a cut-point of 100 pmol/min

per milligram may designate patients with partial DPD deficiency at increased risk of toxicity with 5-FU-based therapy.[239,241] The wide interpatient variability in DPD activity in these studies is consistent with the broad interpatient variations in 5-FU clearance.

The human cDNA for DPD has been cloned, and the gene is localized to the centromeric region of human chromosome 1 between 1p22 and q21.[246,247] The structural organization of the human DPD gene indicates that it is approximately 150 kb in length and consists of 23 exons ranging in size from 69 to 1,404 base pairs.[248] Given the large size of the DPD protein, several different molecular defects have been described in different populations of DPD-deficient kindreds, including point mutations and deletions caused by exon skipping.[249–252] Familial studies suggest that total DPD deficiency is associated with an autosomal-recessive pattern of inheritance. However, childhood familial thymine-uraciluria in homozygous-deficient patients has a variable clinical phenotype, and not all subjects exhibit the abnormal phenotype.[251,253]

Pharmacokinetic interactions between 5-FU and several compounds are related to interference with 5-FU catabolism by DPD. Clinical studies using pharmacologic doses of dThd with 5-FU demonstrated marked slowing of 5-FU clearance.[254–256] The clearance of 5-FU was inversely related to the plasma level of thymine, which competitively inhibits the catabolism of 5-FU by DPD.[255] Pyrimidine nucleosides and bases competitively interfere with the catabolism of various substrates by DPD.[257] Chronic cimetidine therapy (1,000 mg daily in divided doses for 4 weeks) has been reported to decrease the clearance of 5-FU (555 mg/m^2 of intravenous bolus) by 28%.[258] Studies in rats and monkeys indicate that chronic cimetidine treatment decreases the clearance of 5-FU, apparently as a result of inhibition of DPD activity.[259] Cimetidine is an H$_2$-receptor antagonist; of note, ranitidine is chemically distinct and does not affect 5-FU clearance.

In Japan, shortly after the commercial release of 1-β-d-arabinofuranosyl-(E)-5-(2-bromovinyl) uracil (sorivudine), an oral antiviral agent with activity against herpes zoster, 15 patients died, and other patients experienced severe clinical toxicity while taking concomitant oral 5-FU prodrugs.[260–262] The basis for this interaction was shown to be production of (E)-5-(2-bromovinyl)uracil (BVU) by gut flora.[260] In the presence of NADPH, BVU forms a covalent complex with DPD, thereby inhibiting its activity. Rats treated with the combination of oral ftorafur and sorivudine had markedly elevated levels of 5-FU in plasma and in tissues; all animals died within 10 days with marked myelosuppression, atrophy of intestinal membrane mucosa, bloody diarrhea, and severe anorexia, which mirrored the clinical picture. Rats given sorivudine or ftorafur alone had minimal toxicity. Prolonged inhibition of DPD for up to 19 days has been documented in patients with herpes zoster taking sorivudine (40 mg once daily for 10 days).[261] Sorivudine is an investigational antiviral agent in

North America and Europe. Patients receiving sorivudine should not receive other fluoropyrimidines for at least 4 weeks after completing sorivudine therapy and should be monitored carefully thereafter.[262]

Impact of Schedule on Clinical Toxicities

The main toxic effects of 5-FU and FdUrd occur in rapidly dividing tissues (primarily gastrointestinal mucosa and bone marrow). The spectrum of toxicity associated with 5-FU and FdUrd (Tables 7.8 and 7.9) varies according to dose, schedule, and route. In general, bolus administration produces more myelosuppression than infusional schedules. The toxicity of infusional 5-FU depends on dose and duration.

A 5-day loading course (10 to 15 mg/kg per day) of intravenous bolus 5-FU followed by half-dosages every other day for 11 dosages or until toxicity supervened caused a 3% mortality rate.[263,264] Modification to a 5-day

loading course followed on recovery by single weekly dosages was associated with leukopenia, mucositis, nausea and vomiting, diarrhea, and dermatitis. Bolus FdUrd given daily for 5 days (30 mg/kg per day) followed by half-dosages every other day for 11 dosages or until toxicity supervened led to a similar toxicity profile to bolus 5-FU except for a higher incidence of nausea, vomiting and dermatitis.[263] Mucositis and diarrhea are dose-limiting with bolus 5-FU given intravenous daily for 5 days every 4 weeks, although neutropenia may also be problematic.[265] A single intravenous bolus dose given weekly is frequently associated with myelosuppression, diarrhea, and mucositis.[266]

CI of 5-FU has been given over durations ranging from 24 hours to several weeks. With infusion durations of 72 to 120 hours, 5-FU is generally given at 3- to 4-week intervals. The tolerated daily dosage decreases as the duration of infusion increases. Mucositis is usually dose-limiting with CI of 1000 or 750 mg/m^2 per day for 4 or 5 days, respec-

TABLE 7.8

RELATIONSHIP OF ROUTE AND SCHEDULE TO TOXICITY OF 5-FLUOROURACIL

Reference	Route/Schedule	Daily Dose: mg/m^2 (Exceptions Noted)	Toxicities
265, 273, 275	IV bolus daily for 5 days q 4 weeks	500 425 (+LV 20) 370–400 (+LV 200)	Myelosuppression, mucositis, diarrhea Ocular, dermatitis
266	IV bolus weekly (for 6 of 8 weeks)	750 500–600 (+LV 500/2-hr)	Myelosuppression, diarrhea mucositis, ocular
270–272	IV CI 24 hr q week	2,600 2,300–2,600 (+LV 50–500/24 hr)	Neurologic, diarrhea Mucositis, skin (hand-foot), myelosuppression
273	IV CI 48 hr q week	1,750/24 hr (3,500 total)	Diarrhea, mucositis, skin (hand-foot), myelosuppression, neurologic
210, 211	IV CI 72 hr q 3 weeks	2,300/24 hr (6,900 total) 2,000 (+LV 500/24 hr)	Mucositis Diarrhea, myelosuppression
197, 208	IV CI over 96–120 hr q 3 weeks	1,000/24 hr (4,000–5,000 total)	Mucositis, diarrhea, myelosuppression, dermatitis
267, 268	IV CI over 144 hr q 3 weeks	750/24 hr	Mucositis, skin (hand-foot), diarrhea
270, 274	IV CI over 24 hr daily for 4 weeks with 1 week rest	300 200 (+LV 20 q week)	Skin (hand-foot), mucositis, Diarrhea, myelosuppression
275	IV bolus + CI over 22-hr day 1,2 q 2 weeks	400 + 600/22 hr (+LV 200/2 hr)	Myelosuppression, diarrhea, mucositis, conjunctivitis
276	IV CI over 48 hr q 2 weeks	1,500–2,000 (+LV 500/2 hr day 1, 2)	Diarrhea, mucositis, myelosuppression, skin (hand-foot), neurologic
277	HAI CI over 24 hr daily for 14–21 days	750–1,100	Mucositis, diarrhea, upper gastrointestinal ulceration, myelosuppression, chemical hepatitis
278	HAI IV over 15 min CI over 22-hr day 1,2 q 2 weeks	400 1,600 (+LV 200/2 hr day 1, 2)	Diarrhea, cardiac, neurotoxicity
223, 224	IP installation for 32–120 hr q 28 days	5 mmol/L	Mucositis, diarrhea, peritonitis, myelosuppression
224	IP installation over 4 hr q 28 days	3,900 mg (15 mmol/L) (+cisplatin 90 mg/m^2)	Myelosuppression, nausea and vomiting, diarrhea, abdominal pain
	Topical daily	5% cream	Local inflammation

TABLE 7.9

TOXICITY ASSOCIATED WITH VARIOUS CLINICAL SCHEDULES OF 5-FLUORO-2'-DEOXYURIDINE

Reference	Route/Schedule	LV	Maximum Daily Dose		Toxicities
			mg/kg	mg/m²	
263	IV bolus x 5 day x q 4 week	No	30	1,110	Diarrhea, mucositis
219	IV bolus q week x 6 q 8 week	Yes (high)	45	1,650	Diarrhea
269	IV CI x 3 days	No	30	1,100	Diarrhea, mucositis, and myelosuppression
279	IV CI x 5–7 days q 3–4 weeks	No	0.75–1.00	28–37	Mucositis, diarrhea
285	IV CI x 5 days q 3 weeks	Yes (high)	0.3	11.1	Myelosuppression
280–281	IV CI x 14 days q 4 weeks	No	0.15	5.6	Diarrhea
		Yes (low)	0.075	2.8	
280–281	HAI x 14 days q 28 days	No	0.125–0.150	7.4–11.0	Chemical hepatitis, cholestatic jaundice, and biliary sclerosis, upper GI ulceration
225	i.p. 4 hr day x 3 q 3 weeks	No		3,000	Nausea and vomiting

CI, continuous infusion; 5-FU, 5fluorouracil; HAI, hepatic arterial infusion.

tively, although diarrhea and dermatitis occur; myelosuppression is generally mild to moderate.[197,207,267] With a 72-hour CI, 2,000 to 2,300 mg/m² per day is tolerated.[210,211] Mucositis (18% grade 3 to 4) is dose-limiting with CI of 750 mg/m² 5-FU daily for 7 days every 3 weeks, 14% of patients experience grade 2 or worse palmar-plantar erythrodysesthesia (hand-foot syndrome).[268] Intermittent doses up to 14 g (8 g/m²) over a 24-hour period have been tolerated, but this latter schedule is not currently in clinical use.[269] High-dose 5-FU infusion over 24-hours repeated weekly involves 2,600 mg/m²; neurotoxicity and GI toxicity are dose-limiting.[270–272] The 5-FU dosage is 1,750 mg/m² per day when given weekly over 48 hours; diarrhea and mucositis are generally dose-limiting.[273] With protracted CI of 5-FU, the recommended dosage is 300 mg/m² per day.[270,274] When initially developed, the intention was to continue the infusion indefinitely until toxicity supervened.[274] However, a daily-for-28-days schedule followed by a 1-week break is now more frequently used.[270] Mucositis and hand-foot syndrome are dose-limiting, whereas diarrhea is less common.

An every-2-week schedule of LV-modulated 5-FU given by combined bolus and CI was developed to exploit the potential for different mechanisms of action with bolus versus infusional 5-FU. A randomized study comparing the monthly schedule of low-dose LV and bolus 5-FU with a high-dose LV and 5-FU bolus plus CI every 2 weeks as first-line therapy of patients with metastatic colorectal cancer demonstrated a higher response rate (32.6% versus 14.4%, $P = .0004$) and median progression-free survival (27.6 versus 22 weeks, $P = .0012$) in favor of the every-2-week regimen.[275] The bimonthly regimen has been modified several times.[276]

The highest tolerated dose of FdUrd administered as a 14-day CI is 0.125 to 0.15 mg/kg per day (4.6 to 5.6 mg/m²

per day).[279–281] Diarrhea predominates, whereas mucositis is less common. Severe myelosuppression is uncommon with prolonged CI of either 5-FU or FdUrd. When considering comparable schedules of 5-FU and FdUrd, the tolerated doses of FdUrd given by CI for either 5 or 14 days are 90- and 50-fold lower, respectively.[282–285]

Myelosuppression

Serious myelosuppression is more common with intravenous bolus schedules of 5-FU and FdUrd. The greatest impact is on leukocytes and neutrophils, although anemia may also be problematic. Serious thrombocytopenia occurred with the loading schedules, but is uncommon with current schedules. Serial bone marrow aspirates examined in patients undergoing loading courses of 5-FU revealed alterations in metamyelocytes as early as 24 hours after the first dose of 5-FU; megaloblastic erythropoiesis was the dominant process in the bone marrow between days 5 and 7, and recovery of the marrow to normoblastic hematopoiesis was apparent within 3 to 5 days after discontinuing 5-FU.[286] Interference with conversion of dUMP to dTMP as a consequence of decreased activity of TS or DHFR formed the basis of the deoxyuridine suppression test, which was previously used to confirm the basis of the megaloblastic anemia. The acute megaloblastic changes seen with this bolus loading schedule are likely the result of inhibition of TS.

Gastrointestinal Toxicity

5-FU-associated GI toxicity can be severe and life-threatening. Mucositis may be preceded by a sensation of dryness that is followed by erythema, formation of a white, patchy membrane, ulceration, and necrosis. Similar lesions have been observed throughout the GI tract and in the stoma of colostomies. Enteric lesions may occur at any level, resulting in clinical symptoms of dysphagia, retrosternal burning, watery diarrhea, abdominal pain, and proctitis. The diarrhea can be bloody. Nausea, vomiting, and profuse diarrhea can lead to marked dehydration and hypotension. Disruption of the integrity of the gut lining may permit access of enteric organisms into the bloodstream, with the potential for overwhelming sepsis, particularly if the neutrophil nadir coincides with diarrhea. Radiographic changes on small bowel series have shown extensive or segmental narrowing of the ileum and thickening or effacement of the mucosal folds in the distal ileum.[287]

Before each dose, it is essential to question whether the patient has experienced mouth soreness, watery stools, or both. 5-FU should be withheld in cases of ongoing mucositis or diarrhea, even if mild, and subsequent dosages should be reduced when the patient has fully recovered. If diarrhea occurs, supportive care and vigorous hydration should be given as dictated by the severity of the toxic reaction. Antidiarrheal agents may provide symptomatic relief from secretory diarrhea. Loperamide is a standard therapy for uncomplicated diarrhea, but it is less effective in the setting of severe diarrhea. Aggressive management of complicated diarrhea requires intravenous fluids, octreotide, administration of antibiotics, and stool workup for blood, fecal leukocytes, and infectious causes of colitis.[288]

An oral hygiene program including chlorhexidine may be used to help reduce the severity of mucositis, and topical preparations such as anesthetics can provide local pain relief. A randomized, double-blind crossover study of allopurinol mouthwash in patients receiving 5-FU with LV daily for 5 days showed no amelioration of mucositis.[289] Mouth cooling (oral cryotherapy) with oral ice chips for 30 minutes starting immediately before bolus 5-FU reduces the severity of mucositis.[290]

Skin Toxicity

Dermatologic toxicity occurs with bolus and CI schedules.[291-293] Loss of hair, occasionally progressing to total alopecia, nail changes (onycholysis and pigmentation), dermatitis, and increased pigmentation and atrophy of the skin may occur. Manifestations vary from erythema alone to a maculopapular erythematous rash. 5-FU enhances the cutaneous toxicity of radiation; reactions typically occur within 7 days of radiation. Erythema followed by dry desquamation occurs, with vesicle formation in severe cases. Photosensitivity reactions may occur and can result in exaggerated sunburn reactions, residual tanning, or both, in the distribution of sunlight exposure. Hyperpigmentation over the veins into which 5-FU has been administered also occurs. Allergic contact dermatitis may occur with topical 5-FU. Actinic keratoses may develop an erythematous inflammatory reaction with systemic 5-FU. Hand-foot syndrome is particularly common

with CI schedules. Oral pyridoxine 50 to 150 mg daily and liberal application of lanolin-containing creams are often suggested to ameliorate this toxicity, but definitive data are lacking.

Neurotoxicity

5-FU may produce acute neurologic symptoms. A cerebellar syndrome has been most frequently reported and may be accompanied by ataxia, global motor weakness, bulbar palsy, bilateral oculomotor nerve palsy, and upper motor neuron signs.[294-299] Serious cognitive impairment, such as somnolence, coma, organic brain syndrome, and dementia, has also been seen. These symptoms are usually reversible after drug discontinuation. Neurologic toxicity has been seen on several 5-FU schedules, but is more prominent on schedules that feature high daily doses (bolus and 24- to 48-hour infusions) or with intensive daily schedules. Neurotoxicity has been prominent in some studies of 5-FU given with biomodulators including dThd, PALA, and allopurinol.[270,272,300-302]

Severe neurotoxic reactions, including coma, have been reported in patients with previously unrecognized complete deficiency of DPD after receiving conventional doses of 5-FU, and the time to recovery may be longer than in non-DPD-deficient patients.[303-305] Pharmacokinetic analysis of one patient confirmed a markedly prolonged $t_{1/2}$ of 5-FU; no catabolites were identified in serum, urine, or CSF; the neurotoxic reactions correlated with prolonged exposure to elevated 5-FU Cp.[303] A patient who was later found to be DPD-deficient developed severe neurotoxicity and remained in a comatose state for 4 days after bolus 5-FU/LV therapy; dramatic improvement in the neurologic status occurred after CI of dThd at 8 g/m^2 per day.[305]

An uncommon complication of 5-FU and levamisole therapy is cerebral demyelination reminiscent of multifocal leukoencephalopathy.[306,307,307a] The symptoms occur after several months of adjuvant therapy, and include a decline in mental status, ataxia, and loss of consciousness. MRI scans with gadolinium enhancement show prominent multifocal-enhancing white matter lesions, and cerebral biopsy shows morphologic features of an active, demyelinating disease. Myelin loss is associated with numerous dispersed and vasocentric macrophages, sparing of axons, and perivascular lymphocytic inflammation. Three patients improved after cessation of therapy and a short course of corticosteroids, but recovery was incomplete in two other patients. Because a similar phenomenon has not been reported in adjuvant studies involving 5-FU and LV or single-agent levamisole, the leukoencephalopathy may be unique to the combination.

A role for 5-FU catabolites is suggested by prolonged accumulation of [^{3}H]FBAL as noted in brain tissue of rats.[236] In a canine model, 5-FU administration with osmotic blood-brain barrier disruption produces neurotoxicity accompanied by foci of hemorrhagic necrosis and edema in brain tissue.[308] The administration of eniluracil, an inhibitor of DPD, protects dogs from neurotoxicity associated with a 72-hour CI of 5-FU.[309] Cats receiving either orally administered 5-FU or direct instillation of FBAL into the left ventricle have similar neuropathologic changes, and FBAL is more toxic than fluoroacetic acid, a potential metabolite of FBAL.[310] Because neurotoxicity is a prominent feature of 5-FU toxicity in DPD-deficient patients, who cannot produce catabolites, direct effects of the 5FU or its anabolites may contribute to neurotoxicity.

In rhesus monkeys, after a 10-mg intraventricular dose, 5-FU disappears from ventricular CSF in a monoexponential fashion with a $t_{1/2}$ of 51 minutes.[311] The peak ventricular 5-FU concentration is 10 to 15 mmol/L, and the AUC is >18 mmol/L per hour, but without evident toxicity. After intralumbar administration, however, delayed onset of bilateral hindlimb paralysis was seen. Necropsy revealed abnormalities ranging from demyelination of the lumbar and sacral cords to severe necrosis of the ventral horn of the sacral spinal cord, and provides further evidence of direct 5-FU neurotoxicity. In vitro, FdUrd is more toxic to glial cancer cells than is 5-FU, but it is far less toxic to cultured neurons than 5-FU.[312]

Cardiotoxicity

5-FU therapy may be complicated by cardiac toxicity characterized by chest pain, arrhythmia, and changes in electrocardiograms (ECGs) with bolus and infusional schedules.[313-317] Chest pain generally occurs in temporal association with 5-FU administration. The chest discomfort is often accompanied by ECG and serum enzyme changes indicative of myocardial ischemia. Some of these episodes have occurred in patients with a prior history of chest irradiation or cardiac disease, but coronary angiography performed subsequently showed no evidence of atherosclerotic disease, suggesting that coronary vasospasm might be involved. Cardiac shock and sudden death have also been reported. In a prospective multicenter cohort study of 483 patients receiving CI 5-FU, the incidence of suspected or documented cardiotoxic events was 1.9%; preexisting cardiac disease appeared to be a risk factor.[315] There is no unequivocally effective prophylaxis or treatment for this syndrome. Once 5-FU administration is discontinued, symptoms are usually reversible, although fatal events have been described. There is a high risk of recurrent cardiac symptoms when patients are reexposed to this drug; therefore, it seems prudent to discontinue 5FU.

The pathophysiology of fluorouracil-associated cardiac adverse events is controversial. [^{3}H]FBAL accumulates in cardiac tissue of rats for up to 8 days after a single dose.[236] Fluoroacetic acid, a known cardiotoxic poison, was detected by fluorine-19 MRI in the perfusates of isolated rat hearts.[318] Impurities such as fluoroacetaldehyde (which is metabolized into fluoroacetate) have been detected in the commercial formulation, and may result from degradation of 5-FU in the basic medium used to dissolve the drug.[318a] Fluoroacetate was detected in the urine of 15 patients treated with CI 5-FU, 6 of whom developed signs or symptoms of cardiac toxicity.[318a] Two patients who developed 5-FU-associated cardiac toxicity had high venous levels of endothelin-1, a potent naturally occurring vasoconstrictor, but whether this is cause or effect is unclear.[319]

Concentration-dependent vasoconstriction of smooth muscle in aortic rings freshly isolated from rabbits occurred in 23% and 54% of rings within minutes of exposure to 70 and 700 μmol/L 5-FU, but not with FdUrd.[320] Pretreatment with inhibitors of protein kinase C reduced 5-FU-induced vasoconstriction, whereas protein kinase C activators increased it. Nitroglycerin abolished 5-FU-associated vasoconstriction in vitro.

Ocular Toxicity

5-FU may cause significant ocular toxicity, such as ocular irritation, tearing, epiphora, blepharitis, conjunctivitis, keratitis, eyelid dermatitis, cicatricial ectropion, tear duct stenosis, punctal-canalicular stenosis, and blurred vision.[321,322] Excessive lacrimation is the most frequent ocular symptom, but ocular pruritus and burning also occur. Conjunctivitis is reversible with discontinuation of 5-FU early in the patient's course, but progression of the inflammatory response may require surgical correction of dacryostenosis and ectropion. In a randomized, crossover trial in 62 patients with 5-FU-associated ocular toxicity, ocular ice pack therapy lessened 5-FU-induced ocular toxicity to a clinically moderate degree.[323] Ocular toxicity often improves with dose reduction. Early ophthalmologic evaluation should be considered to avoid potentially permanent damage from fibrosis.

Pulmonary Toxicity with Systemic FdUrd

Three patients with renal cell cancer receiving FdUrd as a 14-day CI every 4 weeks developed nonproductive cough, dyspnea, and fever after a median of 15 months of therapy.[324] Chest radiographs showed interstitial disease; pulmonary function tests revealed a restrictive pattern. Lung biopsies showed interstitial inflammation. The patients improved after discontinuation of FdUrd and institution of oral prednisone therapy, but required maintenance low-dose steroids to preserve their pulmonary function. One patient rechallenged with intravenous FdUrd developed recurrent symptoms. Pulmonary toxicity has not been reported with single-agent 5-FU.

Toxicity of Hepatic Arterial Infusion

HAI of 5-FU or FdUrd is often used in patients with liver-only metastases to provide high local drug concentrations. Systemic toxicities are usually dose-limiting with HAI of 5-FU, presumably because more drug reaches the systemic circulation, and include oral mucositis, nausea, vomiting, and diarrhea.[277,278] Chemical hepatitis is usually mild. A strategy to limit systemic toxicity is to use continuous low-dose HAI of 5-FU.[325]

In contrast, systemic toxicities are uncommon with FdUrd, whereas hepatic toxicity is dose-limiting.[280,281,283,326–329] Peptic ulcers, gastritis, and duodenitis occurred in up to 25% of patients in older studies, but the incidence has been substantially reduced with improved surgical technique (ligation of distal vessels that supply the superior border of the distal stomach and proximal duodenum, verification of catheter position). Chemical hepatitis, evidenced by elevations of alkaline phosphatase, transaminases, and bilirubin occurs commonly with HAI FdUrd. Cholestatic jaundice is a serious complication of HAI FdUrd, may progress to biliary sclerosis, and is believed to result from perfusion of the blood supply of the gallbladder and upper bile duct, via the hepatic artery. In more severely affected patients, cholangiograms reveal characteristic radiographic changes: narrowing of the common hepatic duct and the lobar ducts, varying degrees of intrahepatic ductal stricture, and sparing of the common bile duct. Liver biopsy reveals canalicular cholestasis and focal pericholangitis. The hepatocytes appear normal, although reactive changes (hyperplasia, intracellular bile staining, and small clusters of neutrophils in association with aggregates of Kupffer's cells) are present. Some patients require cholecystectomy for acalculous cholecystitis; at surgery, the gallbladder appears shrunken, hypovascular, and densely fibrotic. The onset of biliary sclerosis can be delayed by decreasing the initial dose (median time to toxicity at 0.2 or 0.3 mg/kg per day is three or five cycles). Although FdUrd may be reinstituted at a lower dose after normalization of liver enzymes, most patients became progressively intolerant. The clinical picture may not improve after interruption of therapy.

Patients receiving HAI FdUrd should have careful monitoring of the liver enzymes; therapy should be interrupted if elevations of alkaline phosphatase or transaminases occur. Imaging studies should rule out tumor progression. A randomized trial comparing HAI of FdUrd (0.3 mg/kg per day for 14 of 28 days) with or without dexamethasone (20 mg total) showed the incidence of patients experiencing a more than a twofold increase in bilirubin was decreased from 30 to 9%.[327] The incidence of biliary sclerosis, 12%, seemed to be higher when low-dose LV was given concurrently with HAI FdUrd.[328] In a subsequent phase 2 study in which dexamethasone, 20 mg total dose, was added to FdUrd (0.30 mg/kg per day) and LV (15 mg/m² per day) as a 14-day HAI, the incidence of biliary sclerosis was only 3%.[329]

Catheter-related complications include arterial thrombosis, hemorrhage or infection at the arterial puncture site, and slippage of the catheter into the arterial supply of the duodenum or stomach, with necrosis of the intestinal epithelium, hemorrhage, and perforation. The occurrence of epigastric pain or vomiting should alert the clinician to promptly reassess the catheter position. In some patients, HAI may be impossible because of difficulties in catheter placement, thrombosis of the portal vein, or variations in vascular anatomy.

Age and Gender as Prognostic Factors for 5-Fluorouracil Clinical Toxicity

A number of clinical studies have reported significantly greater clinical toxicity in female and older patients treated with 5-FU-based therapy.[330–335] Among 334 patients treated in a trial comparing monthly bolus 5-FU with weekly bolus 5-FU and LV, the incidence of clinical toxicities of grade 3 to 4 severity was significantly higher in patients older than 70 years compared with younger patients, and in women compared with men.[330] Among 212 patients who received a monthly schedule of 5-FU and low-dose LV, the incidence of grade 3 to 4 leukopenia (21% versus 32% versus 40%) and mucositis (11% versus 26% versus 36%) increased with advancing age (<60 years, 60 to 69 years, and >70 years). Women had a higher incidence of grade 3 to 4 leukopenia than did men (39% versus 23%).[331] Women experienced more severe neutropenia, diarrhea, and stomatitis than men in an adjuvant rectal study comparing two cycles of either 5-FU, 5-FU and LV, 5-FU and levamisole, or 5-FU, LV, and levamisole before and after chemoradiation with 5-FU ± LV.[332] The Meta-Analysis Group in Cancer, using individual data from six randomized trials comparing infusional with bolus 5-FU, found that female patients, older patients, and those with poorer performance had a significantly higher risk of diarrhea, mucositis, nausea, and vomiting.[333] Hand-foot syndrome was 2.6-fold more common in patients receiving infusional 5-FU (34% versus 13%, $P < .0001$); female patients and older patients also had a higher risk of hand-foot syndrome. Grade 3 to 4 hematologic toxicity, mainly neutropenia, was sevenfold more common with bolus 5-FU therapy (31% versus 4%, $P < .0001$); poor performance status was a significant prognostic factor for serious hematologic toxicity.

The possible influence of age and gender on 5-FU clearance and DPD activity (in PBMCs or liver tissue) has yielded inconsistent results in different studies.[208,238,239,240,336–338] Even in trials that report a difference according to gender, there is considerable overlap in the values between men and women, and the correlation between either age and gender and 5-FU clearance or DPD activity is not tight. Other factors may also account for the increased toxicity in female and older patients. Age-related physiologic changes in the liver and kidneys, perhaps involving organ mass and function, and alterations in regional blood flow might account for the reduced elimination of metabolized drugs, such as 5-FU, in the older population.[339]

Because of the reports of increased clinical toxicity, it seems prudent to closely monitor blood counts and symptoms in older and female patients during 5-FU-based therapy with appropriate dose adjustments. It is not currently recommended that the dose of 5-FU be lowered a priori in these patient subsets.

Randomized Trials Comparing Various Fluoropyrimidine Routes and Schedules

A series of meta-analyses has been performed by the Advanced Colorectal Cancer Meta-Analysis Group (Table 7.10).[340–344] CI is superior to intravenous bolus 5-FU when given as a single agent; hand-foot syndrome is significantly more common with CI (34% versus 13%), and hematologic toxicity is much less frequent (4% versus 31%).[342] HAI of 5-FU or FdUrd consistently produced higher response rates in patients with liver metastases compared with systemic infusion of 5-FU or FdUrd.[343] Improvement in survival was significant only when considering data from two trials in which patients randomized to the control arm may have remained untreated. The rationale for the use of LV and MTX as modulators of 5-FU is addressed subsequently.

PROTECTION STRATEGIES

A number of approaches have been explored in an effort to ameliorate toxic reactions of 5-FU in the experimental host (Table 7.11).

Allopurinol

Allopurinol is converted to oxypurinol ribonucleotide, which inhibits orotidylate decarboxylase and causes a buildup in the pools of orotidylate and orotic acid (orotate), which blocks 5-FU activation by OPRT.[7,9] Because host tissues, but not all tumors, may depend on this activation pathway, coadministration of allopurinol diminishes host toxicity in some in vivo models. Antitumor responses are maintained in tumors that use Urd phosphorylase and Urd kinase to activate 5-FU to FUMP. Patients receiving CI 5-FU were able to tolerate twice the daily dose of 5-FU if given with allopurinol (2.2 versus 1.1 g/m^2 per day).[345] The granulocyte nadir in patients who received a single dose of 5-FU 1,200 mg/m^2 alone the first cycle (mean, 577 per µL) was 75% lower than that observed during the second cycle, in which allopurinol was added to 5-FU. Allopurinol appeared to increase the maximally tolerated dose of 5-FU by 1.5- fold.[301] Reduction of 5-FU toxicity by allopurinol has not been consistent. High-dose allopurinol given with bolus 5-FU on biweekly and daily-for-5-days schedules was associated with unacceptable neurotoxicity.[346,347] A randomized trial showed no protection afforded by allopurinol mouthwash from 5-FU-associated mucositis.[289] Allopurinol might potentially interfere with 5-FU activation in tumors that rely on the OPRT pathway. In a rat model, allopurinol decreased FdUMP formation in colon carcinoma tissue by less than twofold, but did not affect FdUMP levels in liver tissue.[176]

By consuming PRPP, purine bases (e.g., hypoxanthine and adenine) can reduce 5-FU toxicity in some cell lines that use the OPRT pathway. Coadministration of hypoxanthine or adenine with 5-FU promptly reduced PRPP levels to less than 20% of baseline and reversed 5-FU toxicity in L5178Y cells.[348,349] There is currently no clinical role for allopurinol or purine bases as modulators of 5-FU.

Uridine Rescue

Several preclinical studies demonstrate a selective rescue of healthy tissue from 5-FU toxicity by delayed Urd.[350–354] Delayed administration of pharmacologic doses of Urd (800 mg/kg every 2 hours for three doses followed 18 hours later by four doses every 2 hours) in tumor-bearing mice reduces 5-FU toxicity to the host without affecting its antitumor activity.[350] Urd administration expands UTP

TABLE 7.10

META-ANALYSES COMPARING ROUTES AND SCHEDULES OF 5-FLUOROPYRIMIDINE THERAPY

Reference	Comparison	No. of Patients	% Responding (*P* value)	Median Survival (months) (*P* value)
340	Bolus 5-FU	578	11.1	11
	Bolus 5-FU + leucovorin	803	22.5 (<1 × 10)-7	11.5
341	5-FU	570	10	9.1
	5-FU + methotrexate	608	19 (<.0001)	10.7 (.024)
343	IV 5-FU or FdUrd or supportive care	655 (391 got 5-FU or FdUrd)	14	11 (12 months + chemotherapy)
	HAI FdUrd	654	41 (< 1 × 10)–10	16 (.0009 vs. all controls) (0.14 vs. + IV chemotherapy)
342	Bolus 5-FU	551	13.6	11.3
	CI 5-FU	552	22.5 (.0002)	12.1 (.04)

TABLE 7.11
STRATEGIES TO REDUCE THE TOXICITY OF 5-FLUOROURACIL (5-FU) IN HEALTHY TISSUES

| Modulator | Evidence for Protection in Preclinical Models | | Reduction in Clinical Toxicity | Mechanism(s) |
	In vitro	In vivo		
Allopurinol	Yes	Yes	Mixed results	Oxypurinol ribonucleotide inhibits orotate decarboxylase; orotate buildup inhibits 5-FU activation by orotate phosphoribosyl transferase; decreased leukopenia observed in some trials.
Purine bases	Yes	Yes	Unknown	Depletion of phosphoribosyl phosphate decreases 5-FU activation via orotate phosphoribosyl transferase.
Uridine rescue	Yes	Yes	Yes	Delayed administration of pharmacologic doses of uridine increases the clearance of 5-FU from RNA and DNA and allows faster recovery from RNA and DNA synthetic inhibition (host effect > tumor effect in tumors with limited capacity to salvage uridine).
Variable-rate CI "chronomodulation"	NA	Yes	Yes	In preclinical models, toxicity of 5-FU and 5-fluoro-2'-deoxyuridine influenced by time of administration; circadian-modulated CI regimens may reduce clinical toxicity of 5-fluoro-2'-deoxyuridine given systemically or by HAI.
Thymidine	Yes	No	No	Thymidine used in vitro to replete deoxythymidine triphosphate pools via thymidine kinase salvage, thus antagonizing DNA-directed toxicity of 5FU.

CI, continuous infusion; HAI, hepatic arterial infusion; NA, not applicable.

pools and increases the clearance of [^{3}H]5-FU from RNA and DNA in tumor and healthy tissues.[351] Delayed administration of Urd doubles the tolerated dose of 5-FU given intraperitoneally once weekly, increases [^{3}H]5-FU incorporation into RNA by 2.2-fold and improves experimental antitumor effect.[354]

Delayed administration of Urd by CI (5 g/kg daily for 5 days subcutaneously) allows a threefold increase in 5-FU dose from 200 to 600 mg/kg and resulted in an improved therapeutic index in mice bearing B16 melanoma but not L1210 leukemia.[352] An improved therapeutic index results from 5-FU and delayed Urd rescue in mice bearing either murine colon carcinoma 26 or 38, with less severe hematologic toxicity and more rapid recovery.[353] The biochemical mechanism allowing selective Urd rescue of healthy tissues with retention of antitumor activity in these murine models is suspected to involve differences in Urd uptake and UTP-pool expansion, resulting in inhibition of further 5-FU-RNA formation and faster clearance of 5-FU from RNA. Tumors with limited capacity to salvage Urd represent the most logical model for selective protection.

In clinical trials, doses up to Urd 12 g/m^2 given over 1 hour intravenously were well tolerated and increased plasma Urd above 100 μmol/L for up to 8 hours. However, delayed administration of 5 to 6 g/m^2 24 and 48 hours after bolus 5-FU did not prevent myelosuppression.[355] CI of Urd produced dose-limiting febrile reactions.[356] An intermittent schedule of 3 g/m^2 over 3 hours, alternating with a 3-hour rest, over 72 hours was tolerable and resulted in peak and trough Urd levels in the 1 mmol/L and 100 to 300 μmol/L range, respectively.[357] This intermittent Urd schedule ame-

liorated leukopenia, but did not affect platelet toxicity.[357] Phlebitis of peripheral veins necessitates administration of Urd via a central venous catheter.

Preclinical studies suggested that adequate plasma levels of Urd could be achieved by oral administration.[358,359] However, clinical studies suggested that the bioavailability of oral Urd indicated was only 6 to 10% for single-dose levels of 8 to 12 g/m^2.[360]

Delayed administration of uridine as a modulator of 5-FU toxicity is currently being explored with triacetyluridine, an investigational Urd ester prodrug with high bioavailability. It remains to be resolved whether protection might be afforded to tumors with high levels of Urd kinase, and whether the timing of Urd rescue after 5-FU therapy might affect the rescue of healthy tissues versus tumor tissue.

Circadian-Dependent Toxicity of Fluoropyrimidines

In preclinical models, the time of administration of 5-FU and FdUrd influences host toxicity.[361-365] In mice, drug administration during the active phase produces greater hematologic toxicity, whereas treatment during the rest phase results in longer tumor growth delay and smaller tumor volume in a 5-FU-sensitive tumor.[362] The toxicity of an intraperitoneal bolus dose of FdUrd (1,200 mg/kg) administered at six different times was compared in rats. FdUrd was not lethal when administered at 12:00 PM (midpoint, resting phase), but killed 40% of rats when given at 4:00 AM (late, active phase).[365]

These observations may be explained by circadian-dependent changes in the rates of DNA and RNA synthesis and activities of enzymes such as dThd kinase and DPD, which are involved with 5-FU anabolism and catabolism.[366–369] Several studies in humans have also shown that DNA synthesis in bone marrow and intestinal mucosa follows a circadian pattern. The highest DNA synthetic rate in bone marrow occurs during the waking hours, with lowest DNA synthesis during the sleep span (12:00 AM to 4:00 AM).[370,371] 5-FU Cp during fixed-rate CI may vary in a diurnal fashion, and an inverse correlation was reported between 5-FU plasma levels and DPD activity.[205,207] Other studies that monitored either 5-FU Cp or DPD activity on several occasions, however, reported marked interindividual and intraindividual variations.[372–375] It is possible to impose a circadian profile on 5-FU pharmacokinetics through the use of programmable infusion pumps (Fig. 7.6).[373,374]

Several variable-rate infusion schedules have been explored in an effort to minimize host activity. When FdUrd was administered as either a fixed-rate infusion (0.15 mg/kg per day for 14 days) or a variable-rate infusion (15% of the total dose from 9:00 AM to 3:00 PM, 68% from 3:00 PM to 9:00 PM, 15% from 9:00 PM to 3:00 AM, 2% from 3:00 AM to 9:00 AM), the incidence and severity of diarrhea was significantly lower with the variable-rate infusion program.[375] Patients tolerated an average of 1.5- fold more FdUrd with minimal toxicity with variable-rate infusion.[376] Variable-rate HAI of FdUrd appears to be less toxic than does fixed-rate infusion.[377]

Levi et al.[378] developed a regimen involving a CI of 5-FU and LV (600 and 300 mg/m² per day for 5 days) given between 10:15 PM and 9:45 AM, with peak delivery at 4:00 AM, and oxaliplatin (20 mg/m² per day) given between 10:15 AM and 9:45 PM, with a peak at 4:00 PM, repeated every 21 days. A randomized trial comparing this regimen versus fixed-rate infusion of all three drugs concurrently over 24 hours daily in patients with metastatic colorectal cancer indicated a lower incidence of severe mucositis (18% versus 89%), higher median tolerated 5-FU dose (700 versus 500 mg/m²), and higher response rate (53% versus 32%) in favor of chronotherapy.[378] A second trial confirmed these results.[379] A randomized trial comparing chronomodulated 5-FU/LV (750/300 mg/m² daily for 4 days over 11.5 hours with a peak at 4:00 AM) and oxaliplatin (25 mg/m² daily for 4 days over 11.5 hours with a peak at 5:00 PM) with oxaliplatin 100 mg/m² over 2 hours on day 1 with LV 250 mg/m² intravenous over 2 hours followed by 5-FU 1500 mg/m² intravenous over 22 hours on days 1 and 2, with both regimens repeated every 14 days demonstrated comparable efficacy.[380]

It is not clear whether the reduction in clinical toxicity with the 4-day chronomodulated regimen is the results of having an intermittent 11.5-hour exposure to drug with a 12.5-hour drug-free interval each day as opposed to specific timing of peak drug infusion. Other investigators have recommended a variable-rate schedule in which two-thirds

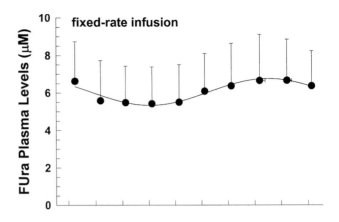

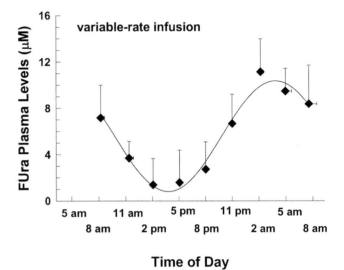

Figure 7.6 5-Fluorouracil (5-FU) plasma levels during fixed and variable-rate infusion. 5-FU plasma levels were measured at 3-hour intervals over the second day of a 72-hour infusion of 5-FU 1,750 mg/m² per day using either constant-rate infusion (top, *n* = 29) or a programmable infusion pump that delivered a smooth continuous sinusoidal variable infusion rate with a peak at 4 AM and a trough rate of 0 at 4 PM (bottom, *n* = 10). The data are shown as the mean and the standard deviation. (Reproduced with permission from the European Society for Medical Oncology from Grem JL, Yee LK, Schuler B, Hamilton JM et al. Phosphonacetyl-L-aspartate and calcium leucovorin modulation of fluorouracil administered by constant rate and circadian pattern of infusion over 72-hours in metastatic gastrointestinal adenocarcinoma. Ann Oncol 2002;12:1581–1587)

of the total daily dose of 5-FU would be administered during the evening hours.[381] Why different times for peak drug infusion are recommended in different trials is not clear. A general finding in the clinical trials evaluating variable-rate infusion schedules is that higher doses of 5-FU or FdUrd are tolerated, with reduced host toxicity.

Several key issues are unresolved. Do the major enzymes involved in 5-FU anabolism and catabolism in tumor tissue display circadian variation, and, if so, does the pattern differ from that of the healthy tissues? If the pattern of enzyme activity in tumor tissues parallels that of healthy tissues, then drug administration at a time intended to reduce host toxicity also may lead to decreased activation in tumor. Considering the clinical activity of the variable-rate infusion regimens, this may not be a major concern. However, given the diversity of human genetics, varying lifestyles with different sleep and wake cycles, geographic and seasonal changes that influence the duration of sunlight, the possible influences of other drugs, hormones, feeding and fasting, and rate of cell proliferation on circadian rhythms, the wide interpatient and intrapatient variability in diurnal profiles of 5-FU-plasma levels and DPD activity is perhaps to be expected.

BIOCHEMICAL STRATEGIES TO INCREASE THE CYTOTOXICITY OF 5-FLUOROURACIL

A number of important interactions have been demonstrated between 5-FU and other antineoplastic drugs or normal metabolites in experimental and clinical investigations (Table 7.12). These strategies include attempts to increase the conversion of 5-FU to its active metabolites, modulate its binding to TS, increase its incorporation into RNA or DNA, decrease the competing pools of normal nucleotides by blocking the de novo and salvage pathways of pyrimidine synthesis, decrease the catabolism of 5-FU and its metabolites, and combine 5-FU with other agents with complementary mechanisms of cytotoxicity. Several of these strategies have yielded convincing evidence of clinical benefit, whereas others have failed to improve the therapeutic index.

Sequential Methotrexate-Fluorouracil

5-FU and MTX both inhibit the synthesis of dTMP and dTTP by either binding of FdUMP to TS or depletion of intracellular reduced folates and the generation of toxic polyglutamates (Fig. 7.7). Several biochemical interactions are possible.[382] The reduced folate 5,10-CH FH, which is required for binding of FdUMP to TS, is oxidized to FH_2 in the TS reaction and cannot be resynthesized in the presence of MTX. Pretreatment of cells with MTX depletes 5,10-CH FH, which could interfere with FdUMP binding to TS.[26] Because depletion of reduced folates by MTX is only partial, however, this may be insufficient to affect the binding of FdUMP to TS. FH_2 polyglutamates, which accumulate in the presence of antifolates, may substitute for 5,10-CH FH_4 in the ternary complex with FdUMP and TS.[25] MTX pretreatment also results in accumulation of dUMP, which may compete with FdUMP for binding to TS.

MTX pretreatment augments FUTP formation. Above threshold concentrations of 0.1 to 1.0 μmol/L, MTX inhibits de novo purine synthesis, thus expanding the intracellular pool of PRPP. PRPP is then available for the conversion of 5-FU to FUMP by OPRT; FUTP formation, 5-FU-RNA incorporation, and cytotoxicity are thereby

increased, leading to cytotoxic synergism when MTX precedes 5-FU in L120 cells.[9] With cultured human cancer cells tumors, longer periods of incubation with MTX are required to produce expansion of the PPRP pools. Enhancement of 5-FU toxicity in some human cancer cells is greatest when exposure to ≥1 μmol/L MTX is maintained for 24 hours before 5-FU.[11,383,384] In MCF-7 breast cancer cells, in contrast, pretreatment with MTX did not enhance 5-FU activation.[384] The synergistic cytotoxicity of sequential MTX 5-FU in vitro requires medium containing serum with low concentrations of hypoxanthine and dThd because the addition of physiologic concentrations of hypoxanthine (1 to 10 μmol/L) and dThd (0.5 μmol/L) to dialyzed serum antagonizes the synergistic effects of sequential exposure.[385] Several in vivo models have shown improved antitumor activity when MTX is given 22 to 24 hours before bolus 5-FU, along with increased formation of 5-FU ribonucleotides and 5-FU-RNA incorporation.[386,387]

The reverse sequence of drug administration (5-FU followed by MTX) produces the least favorable antitumor effects in cell culture and *in vivo*.[9,382,387-389] The sequence-dependent antagonism is a consequence of antagonism of the antipurine effects of MTX by 5-FU. The antipurine action of MTX is believed to result from two factors: partial depletion of 10-formyl FH and buildup of FH, an inhibitor of de novo purine synthesis. Ongoing dTMP synthesis is required to deplete the cellular reduced-folate pool. Pretreatment with 5-FU inhibits TS, thereby blocking the conversion of reduced folates to FH. The reduced-folate pool is thus spared for purine synthesis, and the FH_2 pool does not expand.[389] When MTX precedes 5-FU, ongoing dTMP synthesis leads to depletion of reduced folates and accumulation of FH_2 pools, thus allowing blockade of purine biosynthesis.

In summary, despite potential interference with the formation of the ternary complex involving FdUMP, TS, and reduced folate, experimental sequences using MTX before 5-FU have produced more favorable results than have regimens using 5-FU first, presumably through enhancement of the RNA-directed toxicities of 5-FU. The dosage of MTX and the interval before 5-FU administration must be sufficient to allow the biochemical effects of MTX to become established. Pharmacodynamic studies suggest that PRPP levels are significantly increased 24 hours after MTX.[390] One randomized trial in colorectal cancer demonstrated that a 24-hour interval between MTX and 5-FU was superior to a 1-hour interval.[391] In contrast, a trial involving MTX, 5-FU, and LV in patients with head and neck cancer showed no advantage for an 18-hour interval compared with concurrent administration in terms of response rate, but host toxicity was greater with sequential MTX 5-FU and LV.[392] These results suggest that the ability of MTX to modulate 5-FU toxicity and the optimal time of administration may depend on the tissue type. A meta-analysis of eight randomized trials comparing MTX modulation of 5-FU

TABLE 7.12

STRATEGIES TO ENHANCE THE CYTOTOXICITY OF 5-FLUOROURACIL (5-FU) IN CANCER CELLS

Modulator	Evidence for Increased Cytotoxicity in Preclinical Models		Enhancement of Clinical Activity	Putative Mechanism(s)
	In Vitro	*In Vivo*		
Methotrexate	Yes	Yes	Yes: phase 3 trials	Sequential methotrexate 5-FU inhibits de novo purine synthesis, causing expansion of phosphoribosyl phosphate pools, increased formation of FUTP, and increased incorporation of FUTP into RNA.
Leucovorin	Yes	Yes	Yes: phase 3 trials	Expansion of 5,10-CH FH monoglutamate and polyglutamate pools increases the stability of the reduced folate-fluorodeoxyuridylate-TS ternary complex; enhances DNA-directed effects of 5-FU.
Thymidine	Yes	Yes	No: phase 1, 2 trials	Thymidine antagonizes the DNA-directed effects of 5-FU, but pharmacologic doses may increase 5-FU anabolism to FUTP and increase FUTP-RNA incorporation; thymidine and thymine competitively decrease 5-FU catabolism by dihydropyrimidine dehydrogenase, markedly prolonging the $t_{1/2}$ of 5-FU and increasing toxicity to the host.
N-(phospho-noacety l)-l-aspartic acid, brequinar	Yes	Yes	*N*-(phosphono-acetyl)-l-aspartic acid: No: random-ized phase II and III trials	Inhibition of *de novo* pyrimidine synthesis leads to depletion of uridine triphosphate and cytidine triphosphate pools, which compete with FUTP for RNA incorporation; less feedback inhibition of uridine kinase; decreased uridine triphosphate and cytidine triphosphate pools in turn result in decreased formation of deoxyuridine monophosphate and deoxycytidine triphosphate; increased phosphoribosyl phosphate pools and decreased production of orotic acid favor formation of fluorouridine monophosphate; increased FUTP incorporation into RNA; may increase RNA and DNA-directed toxicities of 5-FU.
IFN α,β,γ	Yes	Yes	IFN-α: No: phase III trials	Mechanism of interaction may differ in various cancer cell lines; IFN-α may increase fluorodeoxyuridylate formation, enhance DNA-damage, and potentiate natural killer cell–mediated cytotoxicity; IFN-γ may abrogate acute increase in TS content during 5-FU exposure, thus extending the extent and duration of TS inhibition; *in vivo*, IFN-α may affect 5-FU clearance in a dose and schedule-dependent manner in some individuals. 146 FUTP, fluorouridine triphosphate; IFN, interferon; TS, thymidylate synthase.
Cisplatin and analogs	Yes	Yes	Cisplatin: Yes: phase III trials, squamous cell cancers Oxaliplatin: Yes: phase III trials in colorectal cancer	Cisplatin may indirectly increase the FH_4 and $5,10-CH_2$ FH_4 pools; 5-FU may interfere with the repair of cisplatin-associated DNA damage. Oxaliplatin is active against DNA mismatch repair deficient cancer cells; clinical evidence of synergy between oxaliplatin and 5-FU in colorectal cancer; underlying mechanism uncertain.
Ionizing radiation	Yes	Yes	Yes: phase III trials: various squamous cell cancers and rectal cancer	Augmentation of DNA directed cytotoxicity.

with bolus 5-FU alone in patients with metastatic colorectal cancer documents a doubling of the response rate with MTX modulation (Table 7.10).[341]

When higher-than-standard doses of MTX are used, LV rescue is used to protect the patient, which may contribute to the improved activity of MTX, 5-FU, and LV regimens.

The strategy of LV rescue is based on the assumption that delayed administration of LV will be more likely to rescue healthy tissues than tumor tissues, although the potential for tumor protection remains a concern. Substitution of the lipophilic-antifolate trimetrexate for MTX in regimens involving sequential antifolate 5-FU with LV rescue has

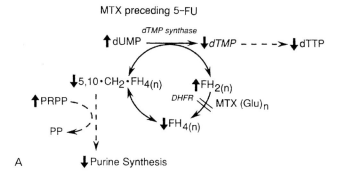

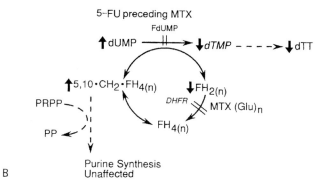

Figure 7.7 Interaction between 5-fluorouracil (5-FU) and methotrexate (MTX). A. MTX preceding 5-FU. DHFR, dihydrofolate reductase; dTMP, thymidine 5'-monophosphate; dTTP, thymidine 5'-triphosphate; dUMP, deoxyuridine monophosphate; FdUMP, fluorodeoxyuridylate; PP, pyrophosphate; PRPP, phosphoribosyl phosphate.

been recommended because trimetrexate and LV do not compete for transport or polyglutamation. Sequence-dependent synergism is seen with trimetrexate given before 5-FU in preclinical models.[392–394] Despite promising results in phase 2 studies in colorectal cancer with a regimen of trimetrexate, 5-FU and LV, no benefit of this three-drug combination was seen when compared with 5-FU and LV alone in two randomized clinical trials in previously untreated colorectal cancer.[395]

MODULATION OF FLUORINATED PYRIMIDINES BY FOLINIC ACID

The ability to form and maintain a stable ternary complex is a critical determinant of sensitivity to 5-FU and FdUrd. The concentration of reduced folate in equilibrium with the ternary complex inversely correlates with its rate of dissociation.[32,396–399] High levels of intracellular reduced folates are, therefore, necessary for the optimal binding and inhibition of TS by FdUMP. Enhanced inhibition of TS over a sustained period results in further depletion of dTTP pools, greater inhibition of DNA synthesis, increased DNA damage, and enhanced cytotoxicity. The endogenous reduced-folate levels are insufficient to promote maximal

inhibition of TS in many tumors; in 5-FU-sensitive tumors, in contrast, maximal FdUMP binding into the ternary complex occurs without exogenous LV.[397–401] LV (folinic acid, citrovorum factor, 5-formyltetrahydrofolate, 5-CHO-FH) has been used to expand intracellular reduced-folate pools and thereby permit maximal ternary-complex formation.[162] LV increases the in vitro and in vivo cytotoxicity of 5-FU in many, but not all, cancer cell types in a concentration and time-dependent manner.[27,95,96,163–165,186,401–411] LV concentrations below 1 μmol/L are insufficient to expand intracellular folate pools, and 10 μmol/L is often cited as the target concentration. As the duration of exposure increases, the concentration of LV required to optimally modulate total intracellular levels of 5,10-CH FH$_4$ and enhance fluoropyrimidine toxicity decreases. With brief exposures to 5-FU or FdUrd, several preclinical studies suggest the importance of giving LV before or concurrently with the fluoropyrimidine to permit metabolism of LV to 5,10-CH FH$_4$ polyglutamates, which are more effective in promoting ternary-complex formation.[398,402,403,406] Other investigators have argued that 5-FU should be given 30 to 40 minutes before LV to achieve peak concentrations of FdUMP and 5,10-CH FH$_4$ simultaneously.[399,409] The optimal concentration of LV and time of administration relative to 5-FU exposure may vary depending on the tumor model used. In two different human cancer cell lines, maximum ternary complex formation occurred when 5-FU exposure was delayed for either 4 hours or 18 hours after exposure to LV; the time of peak folate-polyglutamate formation coincided with the time of peak TS complex formation and total TS protein in each cell line.[403] The ability of LV to modulate cytotoxicity is also influenced by the duration of exposure to 5-FU.[404]

LV is chemically synthesized and consists of equal amounts of the diastereoisomers R- (or D-) and S- (or L-) 5-CHO-FH. The natural diastereoisomer is S-5-CHO- FH$_4$, which must be metabolized to exert its modulatory effects on 5-FU (Fig. 7.8). After intravenous administration, S-5-CHO-FH is rapidly cleared from plasma by conversion to its metabolite S-5-methyl-tetrahydrofolate (5-CH-FH) and by urinary excretion. 5-CHO-FH and 5-CH-FH$_4$ are transported across the cell membrane by a common saturable reduced-folate carrier and then undergo complex intracellular metabolism, including polyglutamation. An important determinant of sensitivity to LV modulation is variation in the intracellular metabolism of 5-CHO-FH$_4$ and 5-CH-FH to 5,10-CH FH$_4$ and its conversion to polyglutamates. In cell-free systems, 5,10-CH FH$_4$ with a five-chain length polyglutamate binds more tightly to TS than the monoglutamate (apparent Km, 0.6 versus 23 μmol/L for Glu-5 and Glu-1, respectively) and is 40-fold more potent in promoting ternary-complex formation.[24] The intracellular t$_{1/2}$ increases as the number of glutamate residues increases. 5,10-CH FH$_4$ with three or six glutamate residues was 18-fold and 200-fold more effective in stabilizing the ternary complex with TS purified from a human colon

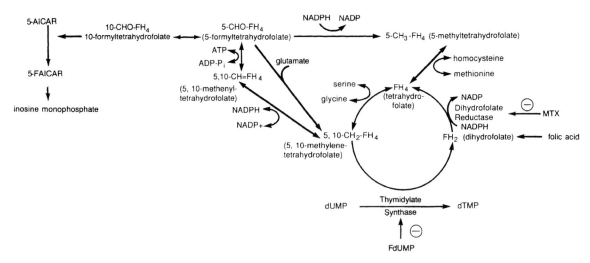

Figure 7.8 Interconversions of reduced folates. ADP, adenosine 5'-diphosphate; 5-AICAR, 5-aminoimidazole-4-carboxamide ribonucleotide; ATP, adenosine 5'-triphosphate; dTMP, thymidine 5'-monophosphate; dUMP, deoxyuridine monophosphate; 5-FAICAR, 5-formamidoimidazole-4-carboxamide ribonucleotide; FdUMP, fluorodeoxyuridylate; MTX, methotrexate; NADP, nicotinamide adenine dinucleotide; NADPH, nicotinamide adenine dinucleotide phosphate; –, inhibition.

cancer than the monoglutamate form.[407] The increase in total reduced-folate cofactor content is concentration-dependent; prolonged exposure is necessary to permit accumulation of the more potent longer chain length polyglutamates.[163–165,407,410] Cell lines with impaired ability to transport, metabolize, and polyglutamate reduced folates are relatively insensitive to LV modulation of 5-FU toxicity in proportion to the severity of the metabolic defect in folate metabolism.[161,166,410] Although exposure to higher doses of LV may not be necessary to promote optimal formation and stabilization of ternary complex in all cancer cell types, increasing the dosage and duration of LV exposure may sensitize certain tumors that are otherwise unaffected by low-dose or short-term exposure to LV. There appears to be no advantage to using the active stereoisomer compared with racemic LV.[162–164,412]

The combination of 5-FU and LV has been extensively tested in the clinic. Dose, route, and schedule of LV administration have varied. Pharmacokinetic studies have been performed for several LV regimens. With intravenous bolus injection of 50 mg racemic LV, plasma levels of bioactive reduced folates (S-5-CHO-FH and 5-CH-FH) remain above 1 μmol/L for 1 hour.[413] When the intravenous bolus dose is increased to 200 mg/m² and with a 2-hour infusion of 500 mg/m² LV, peak plasma levels of bioactive reduced folates exceed 40 μmol/L.[414,415] With CI of 500 mg/m² LV, the Css values of S-5-CHO-FH and 5-CH₃-FH are 4 to 5 μmol/L each.[416] Bioavailability studies after five different dosages ranging from 10 to 500 mg/m² showed that LV absorption with oral dosing was saturable. Accumulation of several metabolites was greater after intravenous than oral administration, and peak plasma levels of FH and 5,10-CH-FH exceeded 2 μmol/L after an intravenous dose of 500 mg/m².[417] Host-mediated biotransformation of LV

to the active metabolite occurs before tumor uptake, which may provide an added rationale for high-dose intravenous LV.

Numerous randomized phase 3 trials have evaluated the worth of LV-modulation of intravenous bolus 5-FU. The tolerated dose of 5-FU when given in combination with LV is lower than that for single-agent 5-FU, and increased GI epithelial toxicity is noted. A meta-analysis of nine randomized trials of 5-FU and LV compared with 5-FU alone in patients with advanced colorectal cancer indicated that 5-FU and LV therapy showed a highly significant benefit over single-agent 5-FU in terms of tumor response rate, although this did not translate into a survival advantage, but no apparent differences were noted between weekly and monthly (daily for 5 days) schedules in the meta-analysis of 5-FU and LV trials[340] (Table 7.10). Randomized trials comparing the monthly 5-FU and low-dose LV with weekly 5-FU high-dose LV schedules in advanced colorectal cancer and as adjuvant therapy reveal similar efficacy, with different toxicity profiles.[418]

Interferon with 5-Fluorouracil

Numerous in vitro studies have demonstrated that interferons (INFs) α, β and γ may interact with 5-FU or FdUrd in a greater than additive fashion to produce cytotoxicity in a variety of human cancer cell lines.[177,419–430] The type of IFN that maximally enhances fluoropyrimidine cytotoxicity differs among cell lines. Because of the ability of dThd to rescue cells from the additive effects of IFN, enhancement of the DNA-directed actions of 5-FU is implicated.[92,108,177,181,419,424,425] In several models, pretreatment with IFN for 24 to 48 hours followed by concurrent exposure to 5-FU and IFN produced optimal effects; other studies gave IFN concurrently with 5-FU for 24 to 72 hours. New protein synthesis appears to be a requirement for IFN-mediated augmentation of fluoropyrimidine toxicity in some studies.[108,422,423,426,428] In some leukemia and colon cancer cell lines, IFN increases FdUMP formation and enhances TS inhibition, apparently as the result of an increase in the activities of dThd phosphorylase.[420,421,422]

In other models, enhancement of 5-FU cytotoxicity by IFN is noted in the absence of an effect on 5-FU metabolism or the extent of TS inhibition; the locus of interaction appears to be at the level of DNA damage.[424,425,430] In H630 colon cancer cells, IFN-γ abrogates the 5-FU-induced increase in TS content by interfering with TS-mRNA translation, leading to enhanced inhibition of TS.[177,181] In HT29 colon cancer cells, the combination of IFN-γ,

IFN-γ and 5-FU led to more than additive cytotoxic effects.[430] More profound dTTP depletion occurred with the IFNs combination compared to 5-FU alone; this was not caused by enhanced TS inhibition. The exaggerated dTTP depletion was accompanied by greater imbalance in the ratio of dATP to dTTP pools, and more pronounced inhibition of DNA synthesis and damage to nascent and parental DNA.[430]

The underlying basis for enhancement of 5-FU toxicity by IFN is variable, and the implicated mechanisms appear to depend on the specific cancer cell line or tumor model studied. In addition to biochemical and molecular mechanisms, immunomodulatory effects may be operative in vivo.[426,427]

The potential impact of IFN-α on the activity of 5-FU plus or minus LV has been extensively evaluated in clinical trials using a variety of dosages and schedules. Although the response rates in phase 2 studies seemed much higher than expected with 5-FU or 5-FU and LV alone, meta-analysis of results from randomized trials in advanced colorectal cancer has failed to support a clinical benefit for IFN, although IFN definitely increases host toxicity, particularly with higher dosages[344] (Table 7.10).

The increased toxicity with IFN-α and 5-FU alone or with LV suggests no selective preference for tumor over host tissues. The basis for the enhanced clinical toxicity may, in part, be explained by alterations in dThd phosphorylase expression in host tissues and by a pharmacologic interaction between IFN-α and 5-FU. Several investigators have reported a decrease in 5-FU clearance by IFN-α, perhaps because of interference with the ability of DPD to catabolize 5-FU, particularly with consecutive daily dosing of IFN and 5-FU.[198,431–434] The correlation noted between higher 5-FU AUC or Css and increased GI toxicity in several of these studies suggests that the pharmacokinetic interaction of IFN-α with 5-FU contributes to the toxicity of the combination.[199,431,434]

Fluorouracil and Thymidine

Although dThd is known to reverse the cytotoxicity of low concentrations of 5-FU in vitro, high concentrations of 5-FU (above 10 μmol/L) may not be countered effectively by dThd in all cancer cells. Enhancement of 5-FU potency by pharmacologic doses of dThd has been observed in vivo.[37–39] Thymine, produced from the catabolism of dThd by dThd phosphorylase, competes with 5-FU for degradation by DPD, thus prolonging the plasma $t_{1/2}$ of 5-FU (Fig. 7.9). dThd is anabolized to dTMP via dThd kinase, which has several consequences. First, dThd can compete with FdUrd for dThd kinase, thereby decreasing FdUMP formation. Subsequent metabolism of dThd monophosphate to dTTP will expand the dTTP pools; dTTP, in turn, acts as a feedback inhibitor of dThd kinase and ribonucleotide reductase. Inhibition of the latter enzyme prevents FUDP conversion to FdUDP and consequently FdUMP, thus allowing enhanced FUTP formation and its incorporation into RNA. dThd acts as a donor of the deoxyribose moiety to promote the direct conversion of 5-FU to FdUrd by dThd phosphorylase; in some models, low concentrations of dThd may promote 5-FU incorporation into DNA.[80] Pharmacologic concentrations of dThd are intended to increase the RNA-directed effects of 5-FU while negating the DNA-directed toxicity.[37–39,435]

Clinical trials of the 5-FU and dThd combination confirmed enhanced 5-FU toxicity.[254–256,435,436] CI of dThd 8 g/day produces a Css of approximately 1 μmol/L; when given with 5-FU doses of 370 to 555 mg/m² daily for 5 days, severe myelosuppression and mucositis occurred.[436] Pretreatment of patients with dThd (7.5 to 45 g) 1 hour before 5-FU produced severe thrombocytopenia, leukopenia, mucositis, and diarrhea.[255] dThd markedly alters 5-FU plasma pharmacokinetics.[254–256]

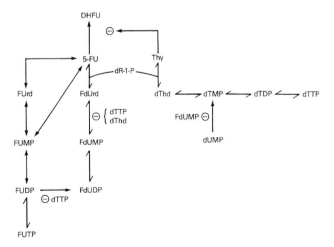

Figure 7.9 Interaction between 5-fluorouracil (5-FU) and thymidine (dThd). DHFU, dihydrofluorouracil; dR-1-P, deoxyribose-1-phosphate; dTDP, thymidine 5'-diphosphate; dThd, thymidine; dTMP, thymidine 5'-monophosphate; dTTP, thymidine 5'-triphosphate; dUMP, deoxyuridine monophosphate; FdUDP, fluorodeoxyuridine diphosphate; FdUMP, fluorodeoxyuridylate; FdUrd, 5-fluoro-2'-deoxyuridine; FUDP, fluorouridine diphosphate; FUMP, fluorouridine monophosphate; FUrd, 5-fluorouridine; FUTP, fluorouridine triphosphate; Thy, thymine; −, inhibition.

The clinical results do not indicate a differential effect on tumor cells as opposed to the host. Severe hematologic, GI, and CNS toxicity has been a feature of virtually all 5-FU/dThd regimens irrespective of dose or schedule. The increase in clinical toxicity with the combination of dThd and 5-FU required a more than 50% 5-FU dose reduction from conventional regimens, with no improvement in antitumor activity.

5-Fluorouracil and Inhibitors of de Novo Pyrimidine Biosynthesis

A number of inhibitors of the de novo synthesis of pyrimidines have been evaluated as modulators of 5-FU, including pyrazofurin and 6-azauridine, inhibitors of orotidylate decarboxylase; acivicin, an inhibitor of carbamoylphosphate synthetase and CTP synthase; PALA, an inhibitor of aspartate carbamoyltransferase; and brequinar, an inhibitor of dihydroorotate dehydrogenase (Fig. 7.10).[437–444] Inhibition of specific steps in the de novo pathway by these compounds causes reductions in pyrimidine nucleotide pools and promotes use of preformed pyrimidines, such as 5-FU. Inhibitors of orotate decarboxylase also elevate intracellular levels of orotic acid, which competitively inhibits the conversion of 5-FU to FUMP by OPRT.

PALA inhibits the second step in the de novo pathway of pyrimidine biosynthesis. PALA-mediated depletion of UTP and CTP results in diminished feedback inhibition of Urd-cytidine kinase activity, thereby favoring formation of FUMP through the salvage pathway and decreased competition with FUTP for RNA polymerase.[445] Inhibition of the de novo pathway increases the availability of PRPP and decreases formation of orotic acid, thus favoring the formation of FUMP via OPRT. Depletion of pyrimidine nucleotide pools decreases dUMP formation through the ribonucleotide reductase pathway, with less competition with FdUMP for TS binding. Finally, decreased deoxycytidine triphosphate pools might enhance the DNA-directed toxicity of 5-FU. A number of these biochemical effects have been noted in preclinical in vitro and in vivo models, and a common feature of PALA modulation is increased 5-FU incorporation into RNA.

Preclinical studies showing enhancement of 5-FU activity with low-dose PALA led to clinical interest in exploring lower, biochemically active dosages of PALA given with full-dose 5-FU. Pharmacodynamic studies have led to different recommendations regarding the PALA dosage, depending on the biochemical indicator used. In a phase 1 study of PALA given 24 hours before intravenous bolus 5-FU, the biochemical effects of PALA were monitored using a

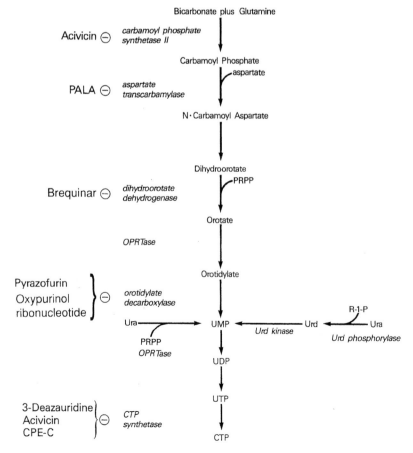

Figure 7.10   Sites of action of inhibitors of de novo pyrimidine biosynthesis. CPE-C, cyclopentenyl cytosine; CTP, cytidine triphosphate; OPRTase, orotate phosphoribosyl transferase; PALA, N-phosphonoacetyl-L-aspartic acid; PRPP, phosphoribosyl phosphate; R-1-P, ribose-1-phosphate; UDP, uridine diphosphate; UMP, uridine monophosphate; Ura, uracil; Urd, uridine; UTP, uridine triphosphate; –, inhibition.

surrogate healthy tissue end point: the effect on pyrazofurin-mediated urinary excretion of orotic acid and orotidine.[446] Because PALA (250 mg/m^2) was associated with a biochemical effect and allowed administration of full-dose bolus 5-FU, this dose was selected for subsequent clinical studies. Other studies that directly monitored ACTase activity suggested incomplete and transient inhibition by PALA 250 mg/m^2.[211,447]

Nonrandomized studies reported encouraging response rates in patients with colorectal cancer who were treated with PALA, 250 mg/m^2, given 24 hours before a 24-hour CI of 5-FU 2,600 mg/m^2 on a weekly schedule, but randomized trials failed to support a benefit of low-dose PALA.[270,272]

Hydroxyurea

Hydroxyurea, an inhibitor of ribonucleotide reductase, has been combined with 5-FU by virtue of its ability to decrease dUMP formation. In mice bearing L1210 leukemia, the combination of hydroxyurea (100 mg/kg daily intraperitoneally) and FdUrd (75 mg/day intraperitoneally on days 1 to 5, 8, 11, and 14) resulted in significantly longer survival compared with either drug alone at optimal dosages.[448] The combination of hydroxyurea and 5-FU has been explored clinically in the treatment of colorectal carcinoma, but several randomized trials have shown no apparent advantage.[449–451]

Combination with Purines and Pyrimidines

In cell lines that possess Urd phosphorylase, dThd phosphorylase, Urd kinase, and dThd kinase, simultaneous exposure of cancer cells to 5-FU and purines, such as inosine and deoxyinosine, or low concentrations (10 to 25 μmol/L) of pyrimidines, such as Urd and dUrd, may enhance 5-FU toxicity.[73,131,452–457] In a human colon cancer cell line, the addition of 25 μmol/L dUrd to 5-FU enhanced FdUMP and dUMP formation, the extent of DNA damage, and cytotoxicity.[73] Urd functions as a potent inhibitor of DPD (Ki [inhibition constant] 0.7 μmol/L for DPD isolated from hepatic tissue); at 10 μmol/L, Urd totally inhibits 5-FU catabolism by this enzyme,[456] which highlights the importance of sequence of administration and the drug concentration to the outcome.

Healthy tissues can catabolize FdUrd by either Urd phosphorylase or dThd phosphorylase. Some malignant cells are known to be deficient in dThd phosphorylase while retaining Urd phosphorylase. In such tumors, the combination of FdUrd with an inhibitor of Urd phosphorylase is predicted to prevent its catabolism to 5-FU and increase anabolism to FdUMP. In contrast, host tissues that contain dThd and Urd phosphorylases would retain the ability to catabolize FdUrd, despite inhibition of the latter enzyme. This hypothesis has been confirmed with benzylacyclouridine (BAU), an inhibitor of Urd phosphorylase.

BAU potentiates the cytotoxicity of FdUrd against human carcinoma cell lines in vitro and in vivo.[458,459] Delayed administration of BAU in combination with Urd reduces host toxicity from 5-FU; the combination of 5-FU and BAU, with or without Urd, was more effective than 5-FU alone against murine colon tumor 38 in vivo.[459]

5-Fluoropyrimidines as Biochemical Modulators of Other Halogenated Pyrimidines

The halogenated pyrimidines iododeoxyuridine (IdUrd) and bromodeoxyuridine (BdUrd) have been studied as radiosensitizers because their 5′-triphosphate metabolites are incorporated into DNA.[460] IdUrd has cytotoxic properties as a single agent. Iododeoxyuridine triphosphate (IdUTP) and bromodeoxyuridine triphosphate (BrdUTP) compete with dTTP for incorporation into DNA. Iododeoxyuridine and bromodeoxyuridine monophosphate are substrates for TS; this interaction results in cleavage of the iodine or bromine from the carbon-5 position.[461] Coadministration of an inhibitor of TS is expected to diminish the inactivation of iododeoxyuridine monophosphate and bromodeoxyuridine monophosphate, whereas depletion of dTTP should stimulate incorporation of IdUTP and BrdUTP into DNA. The success of this approach depends on duration of exposure and substrate competition for phosphorylation by dThd kinase. The activity of dThd kinase is dependent on feedback inhibitors, such as dTTP and IdUTP. 5-FU may be converted to FdUMP by alternate pathways not involving dThd kinase, thus avoiding potential competition with IdUrd or BdUrd. In several in vitro and in vivo models, 5-FU and FdUrd increase the DNA incorporation of IdUTP or BdUTP, resulting in increased cytotoxicity, radiosensitization, or both.[462–466] In a human bladder cancer cell line, enhancement of IdUrd-DNA incorporation and cytotoxicity requires exposure times of 4 to 24 hours.[463] In contrast, a concurrent 1-hour exposure to 3 μmol/L each of IdUrd and FdUrd is antagonistic, with decreased formation of FdUMP.[466] In HT 29 colon cancer cells, the increased radiosensitization appears to result from decreased dTTP pools accompanied by increased incorporation of IdUrd into DNA, and cell-cycle redistribution with an accumulation of cells in the G$_1$ and S phases.[465]

In early clinical trials, IdUrd was generally given by short intravenous infusions of 2 hours or less. The combination of FdUrd and IdUrd was associated with some tumor regressions, but toxicity was severe.[467–469] Prolonged CI of 1,000 mg/m^2 per day IdUrd for 14 days can be administered safely; at this dose, IdUrd Css of 3 μmol/L were achieved, and up to 11% substitution of dThd by IdUrd was observed in the DNA of peripheral granulocytes.[470–472] Selective incorporation of IdUrd into DNA of hepatic tumor was seen compared with healthy liver when IdUrd was given by either systemic CI or HAI.[473] IdUrd

(200 to 675 mg/m^2 per day) and FdUrd (0.6 to 3.5 mg/m^2 per day, 15 to 78% of the single-agent highest tolerated dose) were subsequently combined as a concurrent 14-day CI.[474] At a fixed dosage of IdUrd, increasing dosages of FdUrd did not appear to increase IdUrd Css or percent IdUrd substitution. With escalating doses of IdUrd and fixed doses of FdUrd, the Css for IdUrd rose proportionally, as did the percent IdUrd substitution, but no relevant enhancement of IdUrd incorporation into DNA by FdUrd was evident. Dose-limiting toxicities included thrombocytopenia, diarrhea, mucositis, and elevation of serum transaminases.[474] The addition of LV 200 mg/m^2 to a 14-day infusion of IdUrd reduced the highest tolerated dose to 400 mg/m^2 (Css 0.7 μmol/L), but did not enhance IdUrd-DNA incorporation in peripheral blood granulocytes.[475]

A 14-day HAI of 5-FU 300 mg/day was studied with escalating doses of IdUrd given as a 3-hour HAI on days 8 to 14.[476] With IdUrd 37 to 81 mg/m^2 per day, the systemic peak plasma levels of IdUrd (0.2 to 0.8 μmol/L) and iodouracil (0.4 to 1.8 μmol/per L) increased. Although 5-FU was undetectable during infusion of 5-FU alone, Cp of 0.5 μmol/L were seen during infusion of IdUrd doses of 37 mg/m^2 per day or more.[476] Hepatic toxicity was dose-limiting; biliary sclerosis was documented in one patient. Although tumor regression occurred in some cases, the use of this regimen is limited by hepatic toxicity, reminiscent of that seen with HAI of FdUrd.

Combination with Nucleoside Transport Inhibitors

Human colon carcinomas possess high levels of the enzymes necessary for nucleoside salvage, and dThd salvage represents a potential mechanism of resistance to 5-FU or FdUrd. Dipyridamole, nitrobenzylthioinosine, and dilazep inhibit the uptake and efflux of nucleosides, such as dThd, FdUrd, and dUrd, in a dose-dependent manner.[477–479] Because the effects of dipyridamole on nucleoside transport are rapidly reversible on drug removal, continuous exposure is necessary to modulate 5-FU toxicity. In HCT 116 colon cancer cells, dipyridamole and NBMPR increase FdUMP formation and the cytotoxicity of 5-FU.[478-480] Augmentation of 5-FU toxicity is concentration-dependent; free dipyridamole concentrations as low as 50 nmol/L modulated 5-FU toxicity, but optimal effects required 500 nmol/L.[478] Increased FdUMP levels result in part from blockade of the efflux of FdUrd and other deoxyribonucleosides, such as dUrd, which serve as donors of dR-1-P.[73,479] Expansion of dUMP pools with 5-FU is accompanied by increased production of alkaline-labile sites in newly synthesized DNA.[73] A direct correlation is noted between increased accumulation of dUTP and increased DNA fragility in cells treated with the antifolate TS inhibitor CB3717 and dipyridamole.[74] The interaction between nucleoside transport inhibitors and 5-FU and FdUrd is complex, and more than one mechanism may exist.

The combination of 5-FU with or without LV and dipyridamole has been explored in clinical trials. With 175 mg/m^2 dipyridamole orally every 6 hours, mean peak and trough free drug concentrations are 38 and 23 nmol/L, respectively, which are much lower than the optimal concentrations in cell culture models.[481,482] With CI of 285 mg/m^2 per day of dipyridamole for 3 days (the highest tolerated dose), the mean Css of total and free dipyridamole is 6.7 μmol/L and 24 nmol/L, respectively.[483] In paired patient courses of CI 5-FU, with or without dipyridamole, dipyridamole administration was associated with significantly lower 5-FU Css and a faster clearance.[210,216] Thus, the relatively high concentrations of free dipyridamole needed to optimally modulate 5-FU toxicity, metabolism, and DNA damage in tissue culture systems are not clinically achievable with systemic administration. The achievable Css of free dipyridamole with infusional or high-dose oral therapy may be sufficient to modulate the transport of dThd and other nucleosides in healthy tissues and some tumor tissues.[483,484] However, orally administered dipyridamole failed to improve the activity of a 5-FU and LV regimen in a randomized trial in patients with advanced colorectal cancer.[485]

Interaction of 5-Fluorouracil with Platinum Analogs

Synergism between cisplatin and 5-FU has been demonstrated in preclinical models in vitro and in vivo,[486–492] and preclinical studies point to enhancement of DNA-directed toxicity as the mechanism. In some models, the toxicity of 5-FU and cisplatin is abrogated by dThd but potentiated by LV.[486,489,490] In an ovarian cancer cell line, a 1-hour incubation with cisplatin (10 μmol/L) increased FH and CH FH$_4$ pools by 2.5-fold and increased ternary complex formation by the same magnitude.[486] The apparent basis is cisplatin-mediated inhibition of methionine uptake, which stimulates the endogenous synthesis of methionine from homocysteine and increases the conversion of 5-CH FH to FH, which is a precursor of 5,10-CH FH (Fig. 7.8). Cisplatin-mediated inhibition of intracellular L-methionine metabolism accompanied by expansion of the reduced folate pool has been confirmed in vivo.[492] Other effects of cisplatin on DNA integrity or interactions with cell surface nucleic acids and plasma membrane also may be important. Enhanced DNA damage and inhibition of the repair of cisplatin-induced DNA interstrand cross-links have been noted with the combination.[488,490]

In some models, concurrent exposure to both drugs is efficacious,[486,489] whereas other models report that preexposure to 5-FU before cisplatin administration is superior to the opposite sequence.[487,488,490] In a human squamous cancer cell line, optimal cytotoxicity was seen with a 24-hour preexposure to 5-FU, followed by cisplatin after a 24 to 48-hour drug-free interval; the removal of cisplatin-induced DNA interstrand cross-links was significantly reduced compared with cells exposed to cisplatin alone or to 5-FU followed immediately by cisplatin.[488] The lag time for 5-FU effects and the inability of dThd to reverse the interaction raised the possibility that RNA-directed effects might be involved. 5-FU inhibits ERCC1 and γ-glutamyl-cysteine synthetase mRNA expression in a cisplatin-resistant human squamous carcinoma cell line, suggesting that 5-FU-mediated interference with the expression of DNA repair enzymes might enhance DNA damage associated with cisplatin exposure.[72] Preexposure of NCI H548 colon cancer cells to 5-FU for 24 hours followed by cisplatin for 2 hours produced more than additive cytotoxicity and a greater degree of single-stranded-DNA fragmentation in parental and nascent DNA compared with the opposite sequence.[488]

Although phase 2 studies suggested a beneficial effect of 5-FU plus cisplatin in colorectal carcinoma, randomized studies comparing bolus or CI 5-FU with or without bolus cisplatin indicated that the clinical toxicity was increased without improvement in overall disease control.[493-495] Cisplatin is inactive as a single agent in colorectal cancer, and the necessary cellular events allowing a positive interaction are not present in this tumor type. In contrast, the combination of 5-FU and cisplatin has shown promising results in diseases in which both agents have single-agent activity, including squamous cell cancers arising in the anus, head and neck, esophagus, and cervix. The influence of sequence and timing of cisplatin and 5-FU administration in determining the extent of therapeutic effect, toxicity, or both, has not been carefully studied in clinical trials.

Oxaliplatin has also shown additive or synergistic cytotoxic properties with 5-FU in vitro and in vivo.[496-499] Decreased catabolism of 5-FU and down-regulation of thymidylate synthase expression are possible explanations for the synergy.[498,499] Unlike cisplatin, oxaliplatin has single-agent activity in colorectal cancer. Responses have been seen when oxaliplatin is added to a 5-FU-based regimen on which patients have had documented disease progression, suggesting clinical synergy. Randomized trials suggest a substantial improvement in the response rate when oxaliplatin is added to 5-FU and LV in advanced colorectal cancer and 3-year, disease-free survival as adjuvant therapy for colon cancer.[500,501]

5-Fluorouracil and Taxanes

Paclitaxel is a taxane derivative that binds to the β-subunit of tubulin in the microtubule and promotes the formation of extremely stable microtubules. Antagonism between paclitaxel and 5-FU has been described in vitro.[502-504] Sequential 24-hour exposures to paclitaxel followed by 5-FU were additive in four human cancer cell lines using the MTT assay, whereas the opposite sequence was subadditive in three of the four cell lines.[502] Concurrent exposure of BCap37 breast cancer cells and KB cells to 100 nmol/L paclitaxel and 10 μmol/L 5-FU inhibited the customary oligonucleosomal-DNA fragmentation seen with paclitaxel alone at 48 and 72 hours.[503] In this model, 5-FU diminishes the ability of paclitaxel to produce G_2-M blockade and prevents apoptosis.

In MCF-7 breast cancer cells, 24-hour exposures to 5-FU and paclitaxel in various sequences suggested that preexposure to 5-FU, followed by paclitaxel, resulted in marked antagonism, whereas sequential paclitaxel followed by 5-FU was optimal.[504] Concurrent or preexposure to paclitaxel did not affect [³H]5-FU metabolism, [³H]5-FU-RNA incorporation, or the extent of 5-FU-mediated TS inhibition. Paclitaxel led to G_2-M phase accumulation persisting for 24 hours after drug exposure, whereas a 24-hour 5-FU exposure produced S-phase accumulation. 5-FU preexposure diminished paclitaxel-associated G_2-M phase block, whereas subsequent exposure to 5-FU after paclitaxel did not. 5-FU exposure resulted in transient induction of *p53* and *p21*, which returned to basal levels 24 hours after drug removal. *p53* and *p21* protein content also markedly increased during paclitaxel exposure, accompanied by phosphorylation of *Bcl-2*. Pronounced DNA fragmentation was seen at 48 hours when cells were exposed to paclitaxel for an initial 24-hour period. Paclitaxel-associated DNA fragmentation was not prevented by concurrent or subsequent exposure to 5-FU. In this model, paclitaxel-mediated G_2-M phase arrest appeared to be a crucial step in induction of DNA fragmentation. The potential importance of sequence of taxane and 5-FU administration has not been explored in clinical trials.

Camptothecins and 5-Fluorouracil

In preclinical models, CPT-11 given 6 to 24 hours prior to 5-FU or other TS inhibitors is the most effective sequence compared with concurrent or reverse sequences.[505–510] Because active DNA synthesis is required to convert the formation of covalent SN-38-topoisomerase I-cleavable complexes to a cytotoxic lesion, inhibition of TS during or prior to formation of the SN-38 cleavable complex is antagonistic.

Interaction of 5-Fluorouracil with Ionizing Radiation

Heidelberger et al.[511] discovered that growth-inhibitory doses of radiotherapy in rodent tumors were made curative by the addition of 5-FU, and ineffective regimens of 5-FU became active by the addition of a single dose of radiotherapy. The synergistic interaction has been confirmed by other investigators.[512–521] Combined treatment with 5-FU and radiotherapy leads to concentration- and time-dependent enhancement of cell killing in HeLA and HT-29 cells.[513,514] Enhanced radiosensitization depends on 5-FU exposure for a period longer than the cell-doubling time. The optimal effects are observed when 5-FU continues for at least 48 hours after irradiation, with little or no synergy if 5-FU is given either before or for only 3 hours after irradiation. However, the optimal schedule for 5-FU radiosensitization in preclinical models varies depending on the model system used. In DU-145 prostate cancer cells, 5-FU modulation of radiosensitivity is apparent with either a 1-hour pulse of 100 μmol/L 5-FU plus irradiation at 30 minutes, or with continuous exposure to 4 μmol/L 5-FU and irradiation given either immediately before or 17 hours after 5-FU.[515]

In *p53* mutant HT-29 cells, time-dependent radiosensitization occurs after a 2-hour exposure to 0.5 μmol/L FdUrd.[518] TS is maximally inhibited at the end of FdUrd exposure, but TS inhibition persists for up to 32 hours after drug removal, accompanied by dTTP pool depletion. An increase in radiosensitivity, however, is not apparent until 16 hours after drug removal. The increase in radiation sensitivity parallels the gradual accumulation of cells in early S phase, a radiosensitive phase of the cell cycle. In another model, 8- or 24-hour preexposures to low concentrations of FdUrd enhance DNA damage by inhibiting repair of double-stranded breaks; the addition of LV and dipyridamole enhances FdUrd-mediated radiosensitization and the interference with DNA repair.[516,517] Although HT-29 and SW-620 colon cancer cells have the same *p53* mutation, the response to FdUrd-mediated radiosensitization is different.[520] Exposure to 100 nmol/L FdUrd for 14 hours produces comparable inhibition of TS activity by 75 to 80%, yet the radiosensitive HT-29 cell line progresses into S phase, whereas the insensitive cell line arrests at the G_1-S boundary. Although cyclin D protein levels do not change with FdUrd treatment in either cell line, cyclin E protein content increases by sevenfold to ninefold in both lines. Cyclin E-dependent kinase activity increases only in HT-29 cells, which may account for this cell line's progression into S phase.[520] These findings suggest that a G_1-S checkpoint that influences radiosensitization produced by FdUrd is not dependent on normal *p53* function.

In vivo, the combination of 5-FU, with or without LV, with radiation on several schedules has proven effective in increasing the delay in tumor regrowth.[511–514] The experimental evidence predominantly supports more prolonged exposure to fluoropyrimidines as optimal. The underlying mechanism(s) for this synergistic interaction may be influenced by schedule and duration of exposure. FdUMP-mediated inhibition of TS with resulting dTTP pool depletion, deoxyribonucleotide imbalance, increased DNA damage, inhibition of DNA repair, and accumulation of cells in S phase appear to be important features of radiosensitization. The RNA-directed effects of 5-FU might conceivably play a role, but have not been clearly implicated.

5-FU given alone or in combination with other agents during radiotherapy has demonstrated efficacy in patients with either squamous cell cancers arising in the anal canal, cervix, head and neck, and esophagus, or adenocarcinomas arising in the rectum.[522–525] Diverse schedules of 5-FU have been used, including bolus administration of 5-FU during

the first and final 3 days of radiation, 96- to 120-hour CI for the first and last week of radiation, and CI throughout the entire radiation treatment. A randomized trial in patients with high-risk rectal cancer comparing 5-FU given by intermittent bolus injections with protracted CI during postoperative radiation therapy to the pelvis demonstrated significant improvements in time to relapse and survival in favor of the infusional 5-FU arm.[525]

ORALLY BIOAVAILABLE 5'-FLUOROPYRIMIDINES

The structures of selected oral 5-FU-prodrugs are shown in Figure 7.11. Two of the drugs, ftorafur and doxifluridine, were initially tested with intravenous administration, whereas the other drugs were developed as a strategy to permit oral administration. Features of the oral 5-fluoropyrimidine drugs are shown in Table 7.13.

Ftorafur and UFT

Ftorafur [1-(2-tetrahydrofuranyl)-5-fluorouracil, tegafur; MW = 200] is a furan nucleoside that has clinical activity against adenocarcinomas and is less myelosuppressive, but more neurotoxic, than 5-FU. Ftorafur is a prodrug and is slowly metabolized to 5-FU by two major metabolic pathways.[526–531] One pathway is mediated by microsomal cytochrome P-450 oxidation at the 5'-carbon of the tetrahydrofuran moiety, resulting in the formation of a labile intermediate (5'-hydroxyftorafur) that spontaneously cleaves to produce succinaldehyde and 5-FU (Fig. 7.12).[528] Studies with human liver microsomes indicate that cytochromes P450 1A2, 2A6, and 2C8 contribute to the biotransformation of tegafur into 5-FU.[530] The second pathway occurs in the cytosol, and is thought to be mediated by thymidine phosphorylase.[529,531] Enzymatic cleavage of the N-1-C-2' bond to yield 5-FU and 4-hydroxybutanal; the latter undergoes further enzymatic conversion to form γ-butyrolactone (γ-BL), BL, or γ-hydroxybutyric acid (γ-HB); succinaldehyde is partially converted to these latter two compounds. In vivo, the liver is the major source of cytochrome P-450, with lower levels in the GI tract and much lower levels in the brain. In vitro studies with tissue homogenates from liver, GI tract, and the brain containing the soluble enzyme pathway have documented metabolism of ftorafur to 5-FU. Small amounts of 3'- and 4'-hydroxyl derivatives have been isolated from urine.[526,527] After intravenous bolus injection of 1 g/m^2, ftorafur and a major metabolite, dehydroftorafur, were detected in serum, whereas 5-FU was not.[532] The uniformly low 5-FU Cp in pharmacokinetic studies suggest that metabolic conversion of ftorafur to 5-FU occurs intracellularly, without subsequent redistribution via the systemic circulation.[533–535] Thus, 5-FU Cp may not accurately reflect the extent of this intracellular conversion.

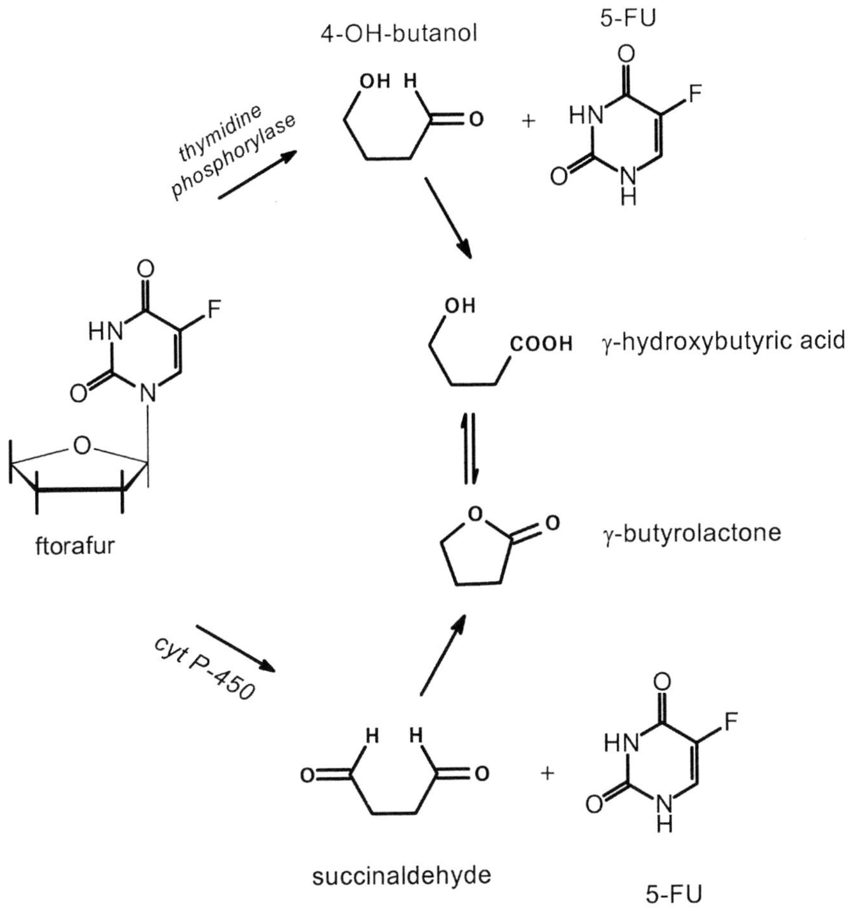

Figure 7.11 Structures of orally administered 5-fluoropyrimidine analogs. BOF-A2, emitefur, 3-{3-[6-benzoyloxy-3-cyano-2-pyridyloxycarbonyl]benzoyl}-1-ethoxymethyl-5-fluorouracil.

The pharmacokinetic behavior of ftorafur has been described for intravenous and oral routes of administration. After intravenous bolus injection, ftorafur undergoes an initial distribution phase, followed by a prolonged $t_{1/2}$ ranging from 6 to 16 hours.[526,527,533–536] The clearance is approximately 31 mL/min per square meter, and the Vd (15 to 30 L/m^2) approximates that of total-body water. After oral administration, absorption is virtually 100%. After 2 g/m^2 orally, ftorafur appears in plasma by 11 minutes, and C_{max} occurs at 3.2 hours.[535] Simultaneous sampling of blood from portal and peripheral veins indicates that ftorafur appears sooner in the portal vein; peak levels in the peripheral vein occur 1.7 hours later, consistent with rapid absorption and hepatic retention.

Ftorafur has been administered intravenously in doses of 1.50 to 2.25 g/m^2 daily for 4 or 5 days or single doses of 4 g/m^2 weekly.[537–542] The primary clinical toxicities with these schedules are GI symptoms (diarrhea, cramps, vomiting, and mucositis) and neurologic side effects (altered mental status, cerebellar ataxia, and, rarely, coma). The neurotoxicity has been attributed to the high concentrations of parent drug found in the CSF.[526,533,534] The ftorafur metabolite γ-hydroxybutyrate occurs physiologically in brain and CSF, has anesthetic properties, produces concentration-dependent CNS depression, and may contribute to neuro-

toxicity. A recommended oral dose is 1.5 g/m^2 daily for 14 to 21 days, although some investigators suggest that a less-intensive regimen of 0.8 to 1.0 g/m^2 daily (in divided doses) for 14 of 28 days is better tolerated.[539,540] GI side effects are predominant with the oral route, while neurotoxicity (dizziness and lethargy) occurs infrequently.

Phase 2 trials in a variety of solid tumors suggest that ftorafur has activity consistent with that expected with 5-FU.[537–541] Some patients failing 5-FU-containing regimens have responded to a protracted oral schedule of ftorafur.[540,542] A randomized trial indicated similar antitumor activity for single-agent ftorafur and 5-FU, whereas toxicity profiles differed.[542]

The option for oral administration has maintained interest in the use of ftorafur. Oral ftorafur has been combined with oral LV on a 21-day schedule; the recommended dose is 1,600 mg in three divided doses with 500 mg LV in five divided doses.[543] UFT, a combination of uracil and ftorafur (molar ratio of 4:1), entered into clinical trials in Japan in the early 1980s. Preclinical studies indicate that UFT results in significantly higher tumor-to-serum 5-FU ratios than observed with ftorafur alone.[532,544] UFT is usually given orally in divided doses daily for either 5 or 28 days. With oral doses ranging from 50 to 300 mg/m^2, maximum Cp of ftorafur and 5-FU occur between 0.6 and

TABLE 7.13
ORALLY ADMINISTERED 5-FLUOROPYRIMIDINES

Agents	Pharmacologic Effect	Common Clinical Schedules
UFT, 2-drug combination: uracil and ftorafur (4:1 molar ratio) Orzel = UFT + calcium leucovorin	Prodrug containing Uracil, a competitive inhibitor of DPD; Ftorafur is an oral fluorouracil prodrug.	UFT 300 mg/m (2 + LV 75–150 mg p.o. daily in 3 divided doses for 28 of 35 d or LV 500 mg/m^2 IV + UFT 195 mg/m (2 p.o. d 1 then oral LV 15 mg + UFT 195 mg/m^2 q 12 hr for 14 of 28 d
Eniluracil with oral 5-FU	Eniluracil is a mechanism-based inhibitor of DPD; It renders 5-FU bioavailability near 100%; It prevents formation of 5-FU catabolites.	Eniluracil 20 mg p.o. + 1 mg/m (2 5-FU p.o. twice daily for 28 of 35 d
S-1, 3-drug combination: Ftorafur 5-chloro-2,4-dihydroxypyridine	Ftorafur is an oral fluorouracil prodrug. 5-chloro-2,4-dihydroxypyridine is a potent, competitive inhibitor of DPD.	40 mg/m^2 (40–60 mg) p.o. twice daily for 28 of 42 d or 30 mg/m^2 p.o. twice daily for 28 of 35 d
Potassium oxonate 1:0.4:1 molar ratio	Potassium oxonate is a competitive inhibitor of orotate phosphoribosyl transferase (decreases 5-FU anabolism and gastrointestinal toxicity).	
Capecitabine (xeloda)	Oral 5-FU prodrug. Parent drug absorbed intact. Converted sequentially to 5'-deoxy-5-fluorocytidine, 5'-deoxy-5-fluorouridine, and 5-FU. 5-FU liberated by thymidine phosphorylase.	2,500 mg/m^2 p.o. daily in 2 divided doses for 14 of 21 d
BOF-A2 (emitefur) 1-ethoxymethyl-5-fluorouracil· 3-cyano-2,6-dihydroxypyridine	Masked oral 5-FU prodrug. Parental drug absorbed intact. 5-FU liberated by hepatic microsomal enzymes. 3-cyano2, 6dihydroxypyridine is a potent competitive inhibitor of DPD.	200 mg p.o. twice daily for 14 of 28 d or 200 mg/m^2 p.o. + LV 60 mg p.o. in 2 divided doses daily for 14 of 21 d

BOF-A2, emitefur, 3{3[6benzoyloxy3cyano2pyridyloxycarbonyl]benzoyl}-1-ethoxymethyl-5-fluorouracil; DPD, dihydropyrimidine dehydrogenase; 5-FU, 5-fluorouracil; LV, leucovorin; UFT, uracil and ftorafur.

2.1 hours; ftorafur levels (13.5 to 100 μmol/L) greatly exceed 5-FU levels (0.2 to 7.0 μmol/L), and ftorafur clearance is approximately 70 mL/min per square meter.[545] Intratumoral 5-FU levels were 2.3-fold higher than in healthy kidney tissue in patients undergoing nephrectomy for renal cell carcinoma 1 day after a 5-day course of twice-daily ftorafur.[546] Another study reported that the maximum 5-FU concentration in bladder cancer tissue was fourfold and 10-fold higher than in healthy bladder epithelium and peripheral blood, respectively.[547] An interesting preclinical study reported that (-HB and 5-FU, both metabolites of ftorafur and UFT, inhibit the angiogenesis induced by vascular endothelial growth factor.[548]

Combined phase 2 data from 438 patients revealed that UFT had activity in cancers arising in the stomach (28%), pancreas (25%), gallbladder and bile duct (25%), liver (19%), colon and rectum (25%), breast (32%), and lung (7%).[549] Hematologic toxicity was mild; GI toxicity included anorexia (24%), nausea and vomiting (12.5%), and diarrhea (12%).

Comparison of 5-FU pharmacokinetics with equimolar total daily doses of UFT and CI 5-FU indicated that during the first day, the Css and AUC(0-8h) were 1.8- and 1.7-fold higher with CI 5-FU.[550] By day 5, however, these parameters were comparable. With a 28-day schedule followed by a 2-week break, administration of UFT in three divided doses every 8 hours was much better tolerated than single-daily or twice-daily dosing.[551] Ftorafur clearance is saturable, resulting in disproportionate increases in the AUC and toxicities with increasing dose levels. A daily dose of 400 mg/m^2 given in three divided doses was recommended on this schedule. A phase 2 study of UFT (300 to 350 mg/m^2) orally plus LV (150 mg orally) in three divided doses daily for 28 days revealed a 42% response rate in 45 patients with previously untreated colorectal cancer.[552] With this schedule, GI toxicity (anorexia, nausea, vomiting, and diarrhea) is generally mild to moderate in severity. Hematologic toxicity is mild, and symptomatic hand-foot syndrome is uncommon. A different schedule used a single intravenous dose of LV

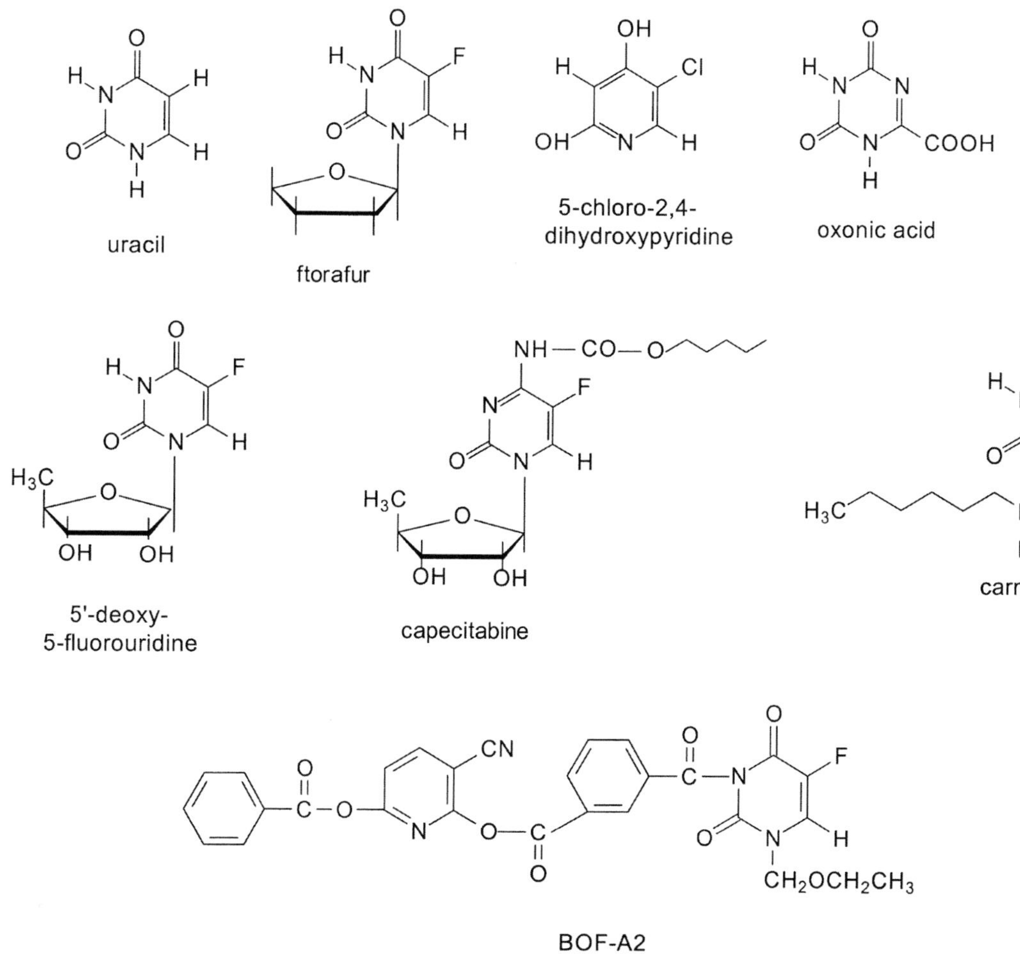

Figure 7.12 Metabolism of ftorafur. 5-FU, 5-fluorouracil.

(500 mg/m^2) followed by oral UFT (195 mg/m^2) on day 1, followed by oral LV (15 mg) and UFT (195 mg/m^2) every 12 hours on days 2 through 14, followed by a 2-week rest.[553] The response rate as first-line therapy in 75 patients with advanced colorectal cancer was 39%. The primary toxicity was GI, but was of grade 3 to 4 severity in only 3.5%; hematologic toxicity was minimal, and the regimen was safe in older patients.

The extent of TS inhibition was determined in tumor tissue taken from patients with gastric cancer assigned treatment with UFT alone (400 mg ftorafur per day) or with LV (30 mg/day) in divided doses every 12 hours for 3 days before gastrectomy, with the last dose 6 hours before surgery.[554] TS inhibition was significantly greater in eight patients treated with UFT and LV compared with that measured in nine patients receiving UFT alone (61% versus 32% inhibition).[554]

A bioavailability study compared the pharmacokinetics of UFT and LV in 18 patients after UFT alone, LV alone, or a combination of the two.[555] When LV was coadministered with UFT, there were no significant effects on tegafur,

uracil, or 5-FU C_{max} or AUC; no significant differences were seen in LV and 5-methyltetrahydrofolate plasma levels after LV alone or with UFT. As might be expected, interpatient variability in UFT and LV pharmacology was pronounced.

No randomized trials have directly evaluated the benefit of adding LV to UFT. In Western countries, a proprietary combination of UFT and oral calcium LV (Orzel) showed activity in phase 2 studies.[556] A monthly schedule was selected for randomized trials owing to the higher projected dose intensity (2,100 versus 1,365 mg/m^2 per week) and excellent safety profile. The results of two large phase 3 trials comparing UFT plus LV with the monthly schedule of bolus 5-FU plus LV in patients with metastatic colorectal cancer suggest comparable efficacy (response rates, 12% versus 15% and 11% versus 9%), but a more favorable safety profile with significantly fewer episodes of febrile neutropenia and infection.[557,558] Because the sponsor could not provide data supporting the contribution of each of the individual components of Orzel, it was not approved in the United States.

5'-Deoxy-5-Fluorouridine

The synthetic fluoropyrimidine 5'-deoxy-5-fluorouridine (5'-dFUrd, doxifluridine, Furtulon; MW = 246) has shown increased specificity for tumor cells as compared with healthy tissues in some preclinical models.[559–564] Because the 5'-carbon of the ribose moiety lacks a hydroxyl group, 5'-dFUrd cannot serve as a substrate for Urd kinase. Urd and dThd phosphorylase are potentially capable of liberating 5-FU by cleaving the glycosidic bond. 5-FU is thus released intracellularly and can undergo further metabolic activation.[559–565] Urd phosphorylase primarily cleaves pyrimidine ribonucleosides but also cleaves pyrimidine 2'- and 5'-deoxyribonucleosides. In contrast, dThd phosphorylase is thought to be relatively specific for pyrimidine 2'- and 5'-deoxyribonucleosides.[15,16,564–568] Urd phosphorylase is present in virtually all healthy and tumor tissues studied, whereas the activity of dThd phosphorylase is much more variable in human and rodent tumors.[15,16,469,562,567,568] Distinct differences exist between the enzymes isolated from human and mouse tissues in terms of biologic properties, substrate specificities, and their roles in the metabolism of endogenous pyrimidine nucleosides and their 5-fluorinated analogs.[565] Substrate specificity also varies between enzymes from different human tissues, suggesting the presence of isoenzymes. In human liver, dThd phosphorylase contributes from 99 to 100% of the phosphorolysis of 5'-dFUrd and FdUrd, whereas the contribution from dThd phosphorylase isolated from mouse liver (73% and 83%, respectively) or human placenta (86% and 93%) is lower.[565]

5'-dFUrd shows selective cytotoxicity against tumor tissues and relatively low toxicity against healthy tissues, presumably because of greater enzymatic activation in neoplastic tissues than in healthy tissues.[561,563] When 5'-dFUrd is used as the substrate, human and rodent tumor tissue (including esophagus, stomach, intestine, pancreas, breast, urinary bladder, and lung) usually contains higher specific activity of pyrimidine phosphorylase(s) than do healthy tissues from the same organs, suggesting potentially selective cytotoxicity.[562,564] In contrast, nonmalignant human liver tissue has much higher activity than healthy tissues of other digestive organs, but its activity is either comparable with or higher than that in malignant tissues from various origins.[564]

The cytotoxicity of 5'-dFUrd in vitro correlates with activity of the pyrimidine phosphorylases.[559–561] Comparison of the toxicity of 5'-dFUrd in human tumor cells and human bone marrow in vitro indicates that 5'-dFUrd, but not 5-FU or FdUrd, has selective tumor toxicity.[561] Several investigators have reported that the antitumor activity of 5'-dFUrd against human tumor xenografts does not correlate with the ability of tumor homogenates to convert [^{3}H]5'-dFUrd to 5-FU, suggesting that the liver may be the major site of metabolic activation of this prodrug in vivo.[563,564]

Pharmacokinetic studies after intravenous administration by either 30- or 60-minute infusions reveals nonlinear elimination: 5'-dFUrd metabolism is saturable at plasma levels above 40 to 50 μmol/L; a fall in clearance of the drug occurs with increasing dose.[569,570] With low doses (1 to 2 g/m^2 over 30 minutes), the disappearance of 5'-dFUrd follows first-order kinetics. With higher dosages (15 g/m^2), the C_{max} is about 175 μmol/L, with a primary $t_{1/2}$ of 25 minutes.[570] With rapid intravenous injection of 2 or 4 g/m^2, the clearance falls from 330 to 200 mL/min per square meter. The peak plasma levels of 5-FU are much lower than 5'-dFUrd levels, and the ratio is influenced by the infusion rate.[571–574] Urinary excretion is virtually 100%; unchanged drug and FBAL account for the majority of the compounds.[571,572] After intravenous bolus, the renal clearance of 5'-dFUrd (166 mL/min per square meter) exceeds the expected glomerular filtration rate, suggesting that 5'-dFUrd undergoes renal tubular secretion; however, there is no evidence that renal clearance is saturable.[570] The cumulative biliary excretion has been estimated to be 0.8% of the injected dosage; a FBAL-bile acid conjugate is the major biliary metabolite, and FBAL accounts for 10%.[572] When 5'-dFUrd is administered by CI over 5 days (0.75 to 4 g/m^2 per day), nonrenal clearance is not saturable; Css levels range from 0.7 to 26.5 μmol/L, and increase linearly with dose.[571] Nonrenal clearance averages 728 mL/min per square meter and is about seven times higher than renal clearance.

Initial phase 1 testing indicated that myelosuppression and stomatitis were dose-limiting at 4,000 mg/m^2 per day for 5 days intravenously; CNS toxicity and ECG changes were also noted.[574] With a 6-hour intravenous infusion weekly-for-3-weeks schedule of 5'-dFUrd, neurotoxicity is dose-limiting with 10 to 12.5 g/m^2 per week.[575] Nausea and vomiting, diarrhea, and cutaneous reactions occur with both schedules. A 5-day CI of 5'-dFUrd is well tolerated at daily doses of 3.5 g/m^2 or less, except for mild nausea; dose-limiting toxicities at 4 g/m^2 per day include neutropenia, thrombocytopenia, mucositis, and rash.[573]

Phase 2 studies using the weekly 6-hour infusion schedule demonstrated responses in breast cancer (36%) and colorectal cancer (22%).[575,576] eurologic toxicity (dizziness, ataxia, and alterations of consciousness) was prominent, occurring in 42% of the patients, with four lethal events. 5'-dFUrd is active in colorectal, breast, ovarian, and head and neck cancer when given by rapid intravenous infusion on a daily-for-5-days schedule, but was accompanied by a high incidence of dose-related neurotoxicity reminiscent of Wernicke-Korsakoff syndrome.[577–579] A small randomized trial comparing a 5-day course of either 5-FU (450 mg/m^2 per day) with 5'-dFUrd (4,000 mg/m^2 per day) was interrupted because of cardiac toxicity (chest pain, arrhythmias, and ventricular fibrillation) and neurotoxicity (48%) on the 5'-dFUrd arm.[577] The response rate favored the 5'-dFUrd arm (20% of 25 patients versus 7% of 27 patients with 5-FU). Cardiac toxicity was observed sporadically in other clinical trials.

Lengthening the infusion of 5′-dFUrd to 1 hour reduces the incidence and severity of neurotoxicity to 16 to 23%. Two randomized trials compared a 1-hour infusion of either 5′-dFUrd (4 g/m^2 per day) or 5-FU (450 or 500 mg/m^2 per day) daily for 5 days in advanced colorectal cancer.[580,581] The response rate was higher with 5′-dFUrd on both trials (23% of 31 and 5% of 112 patients, respectively) compared with 5-FU (7% of 30 and 1% of 110 patients, respectively), and the time to disease progression favored the 5′-dFUrd arm in one study (48 versus 39 weeks, $P = .02$); survival was not improved on either trial. The arms were not equitoxic; the 1-hour infusion of 5-FU was relatively nontoxic, and dose escalation was not allowed.

Unlike 5-FU, 5′-dFUrd is well absorbed by the oral route. An oral regimen of 5′-dFUrd 1,200 mg daily for 28 days is well tolerated, with mild-to-moderate diarrhea, nausea, and vomiting as the principal side effects; higher doses were complicated by a higher incidence of diarrhea.[582] Another commonly used oral regimen is l-LV 25 mg followed 2 hours later by 5′-dFUrd 1,200 mg/m^2 daily for 5 days followed by 5 days of rest. With this schedule, C_{max} values for 5′-FdUrd and 5-FU average approximately 67 and 6 µmol/L, respectively.[583] Among 62 previously untreated patients with colorectal cancer, 32% responded, as did 13% of patients with prior systemic-5-FU therapy.[583]

Capecitabine

Capecitabine [N (4-pentoxycarbonyl-5′-deoxy-5-fluorocytidine, Xeloda] is the first oral 5-FU prodrug to be approved in the United States, on the basis of its activity in patients with metastatic breast cancer whose disease is refractory to two earlier regimens.[584] This agent is absorbed intact as the parent drug through the GI mucosa. It then undergoes a three-step enzymatic conversion to 5-FU (Fig. 7.13). In the liver, 5′-deoxy-5-fluorocytidine (5′-dFCyd) formation is catalyzed by carboxylesterase (CES), which is mainly expressed in microsomes, but a cytosolic carboxylesterase, CES1A1, also contributes to formation of 5′-dFCyd.[585,586] Cytidine deaminase, a widely distributed enzyme, produces 5′-dFUrd, and dThd phosphorylase then generates 5-FU. Clinical studies have documented rapid GI absorption of the parent drug with efficient conversion to 5′-dFUrd; 5-FU Cp are low.[587–589]

Several preclinical studies have documented preferential accumulation of 5-FU in tumor tissue compared with healthy tissue.[590–594] Intracellular accumulation of 5-FU was studied in four human-cancer xenografts after administration of either oral capecitabine (1.5 mmol/kg) or intraperitoneal 5-FU (0.15 mmol/kg) at their maximum tolerated doses (MTD) on a daily for a 7-day schedule.[591] With capecitabine, the median AUC of 5-FU in tumor tissue was 250 nmol/hr per gram, 120-fold higher than the plasma AUC. After 5-FU, the median 5-FU AUC in tumor tissue was 12.2 nmol/hr per gram, a twofold increase over the plasma AUC. Despite the 10-fold higher dose of capecitabine, the 5-FU AUC in plasma was one-third of that observed with intraperitoneal 5-FU. This study provides strong evidence that 5-FU is preferentially formed in tumor tissue versus plasma after capecitabine administration.

Eighteen (75%) of 24 human cancer xenografts were sensitive to capecitabine.[592] Among 15 tumors with dThd-phosphorylase activity greater than 50 µg/mg per hour, 87% were sensitive, but 56% of tumors with lower enzyme activity were also sensitive.[592] However, tumors with relatively low ratios of dThd phosphorylase to DPD activity were more likely to be resistant, whereas tumors with higher ratios were uniformly sensitive. Thus, tumors with low dThd-phosphorylase activity may still retain sensitivity to capecitabine provided the activity of DPD is also low, whereas capecitabine might not be effective in tumors with higher dThd phosphorylase if the DPD activity is also high. Measurement of dThd phosphorylase and DPD by ELISA assay in 241 human tumor specimens indicated that the ratio of dThdPase:DPD was high (median ratio of >1.5) in esophageal, renal, breast, colorectal, and gastric cancers.[595]

The activities of carboxylesterase, cytidine deaminase, and dThd phosphorylase were measured in human tumor and adjacent healthy tissue surgically resected from patients with a variety of cancers.[590] Using capecitabine as the substrate, carboxylesterase activity was almost exclusively

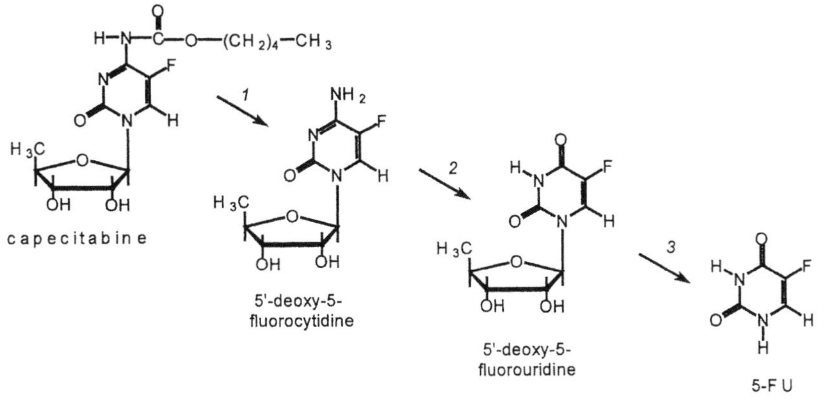

Figure 7.13 Activation of capecitabine. The enzymes are 1, carboxylesterase; 2, cytidine deaminase; 3, thymidine phosphorylase. 5-FU, 5-fluorouracil.

localized in human-liver and hepatocellular carcinoma, with minimal activity in other tumors and organs, including the intestinal tract and plasma. Homogenates prepared from most healthy and tumor tissues were able to deaminate 5'-dFCyd, although healthy liver had the highest activity. With 5'-dFUrd as substrate, dThd-phosphorylase activity was detected in all healthy tissues, with the highest activity in liver tissue. dThd-phosphorylase activities showed much greater variability in tumor tissue; with few exceptions, the activity was higher in tumor tissue obtained from 11 different sites of origin than that of the corresponding healthy tissues.

Two schedules have been evaluated in the clinic: a continuous schedule for 28 days (MTD 1,600 mg/m^2 orally daily), and a daily for 14 days every 3-weeks schedule (MTD 3,200 mg/m^2 orally daily).[587,590] Capecitabine is given as two equal doses approximately12 hours apart, taken within 30 minutes after a meal. The toxicity profile favors the daily for 14 of 21-day schedule, with a recommended total daily dose of 2,500 mg/m^2 orally. When given with low-dose oral LV (60 mg orally daily), the recommended total daily dose is 1,650 mg/m^2 for 14 of 21 days.[596] Dose-limiting toxicities include diarrhea, nausea, vomiting, and hand-foot syndrome; myelosuppression is uncommon. With more widespread use, capecitabine-associated cardiac, ocular, and neurologic toxicity has been reported.[597-599]

Preferential accumulation of 5-FU in primary colorectal tumors compared with adjacent healthy tissue has been documented after oral administration of capecitabine to patients. The ratio of 5-FU concentration in tumor tissue was about 3.2-fold higher than healthy tissue, and the mean tissue:plasma 5-FU concentration ratios exceeded 20 for colorectal tumor.[600] These results could be explained by the fourfold higher activity of dThd phosphorylase in colorectal tumor tissue. Another study reported the importance of the ratio of dThd phosphorylase and DPD levels in primary colorectal cancer as correlates of benefit to adjuvant 5'-dFUrd therapy.[601]

The pharmacokinetics of capecitabine and its metabolites have been measured using liquid chromatography mass spectrometry in studies by the pharmaceutical sponsor.[588,602–605] After an initial dose of 1,255 mg/m^2 (total daily dose 2,510 mg/m^2), peak Cp of parent drug, the two nucleoside metabolites, 5-FU and FBAL are reached about 2 hours after dosing. The $t_{1/2}$ is about 1 hour for all metabolites except for FBAL, which has an initial $t_{1/2}$ of 3 hours. The AUC of 5'-dFUrd is the greatest and exceeds the AUC (units = microgram × hour per milliliter) of 5-FU by 12-fold. Over the dosage range used clinically, there is no evidence of dose dependency in the pharmacokinetic parameters. No appreciable accumulation of either parent drug or metabolites is noted when comparing pharmacokinetic values from days 1 and 14, other than a 22% higher 5-FU AUC on day 14, suggesting a change in 5-FU clearance with time. The low Cp of 5-FU supports the notion that its formation primarily occurs within cells.

The clinical safety of capecitabine has been determined exclusively with capecitabine taken within 30 minutes after a meal. Comparison of capecitabine pharmacokinetics before and after food intake indicates a profound effect on the C_{max} of capecitabine and most of its metabolites. The AUC of capecitabine is 1.5-fold higher when taken before food; a moderate effect is also noted for 5'-dFCyd, with a 1.26-fold higher AUC before food, and food ingestion has only a minor influence on the AUC of the other metabolites.[602,603] This reinforces the recommendation to ingest capecitabine within 30 minutes following food. In patients with hepatic dysfunction, Cp of capecitabine, 5'-dFUrd, 5-FU, DHFU, and FBAL were higher than in those with normal function, while the opposite was found for 5'-dFCyd.[604] These effects did not appear to be clinically significant, and it is recommended that although caution should be used when treating patients with moderately impaired hepatic function, but there is no a priori need for dose reduction.[604] In a small study, the AUC of 5'-dFUrd was higher in those patients with impaired renal function, and this increased correlated with an excess risk of severe toxicity.[605] Based on these results, the sponsor recommends that patients with severe renal dysfunction should not be treated with capecitabine. In addition to the pharmacokinetic results, information from the clinical safety database led to the recommendation that patients with moderate renal impairment (30-50 mL/min based on a 24-hour urine collection) should be treated with 75% of the recommended standard starting dose to achieve systemic exposure comparable with that in patients with normal renal function.

Other analytic methods that have been developed to measure capecitabine and its metabolites in biologic samples, including liquid chromatography with mass selective detection for analysis of parent drug and nucleosides, gas chromatography/mass selective detection to measure 5-FU and FBAL, liquid chromatography with UV detection, flourine-19 magnetic resonance spectroscopy, and capillary electrophoresis.[606–609]

Two large randomized phase 3 trials comparing capecitabine with the monthly schedule of 5-FU and LV (425 mg/m^2 and 20 mg/m^2 daily for 5 days, respectively) in patients with advanced colorectal cancer have been conducted.[610,611] One trial involving 605 patients demonstrated a response rate in favor of capecitabine (23% versus 16%).[610] Grade 3 to 4 toxicities included hand-foot syndrome (18%) and diarrhea (15%) for capecitabine and neutropenia (26%), mucositis (16%), and diarrhea (14%) for 5-FU and LV. A second international trial using an identical design involved 602 patients; the response rate favored capecitabine (27% versus 18%).[611] Hand-foot syndrome and diarrhea of grade 3 to 4 severity occurred in 16% and 10% of capecitabine patients, whereas severe or worse neutropenia, mucositis, and diarrhea occurred in 20%, 13%, and 10% of patients receiving 5-FU and LV. Current strategies focus on combining capecitabine with agents that might induce thymidine phosphorylase in tumor tissue, such as ionizing radiation and cytokines.[612–615]

Eniluracil Combined With 5-Fluorouracil

The uracil analog eniluracil (776C85, 5-ethynyluracil) is an extremely potent mechanism-based inactivator of DPD, and is ninefold more potent than bromvinyluracil.[616] On binding of eniluracil to DPD (apparent K, 1.6 µmol/L), an unstable intermediate is formed, after which the drug becomes covalently linked to the enzyme through modification of an amino acid residue (Fig. 7.14).[616] Administration of eniluracil to animals and humans results in complete inhibition of DPD throughout the body, as evidenced directly by enzyme assays and indirectly by up to 100-fold elevations of plasma-uracil levels.[617–619] When given with eniluracil, renal excretion of 5-FU becomes the predominant route of elimination. Oral administration of 5-FU with eniluracil renders 5-FU completely bioavailable.

Although eniluracil appears to be nontoxic when given alone, it shifts the 5-FU dose toxicity-response curves to lower doses. The combination of eniluracil (1 mg/kg per day) with 5-FU at one-tenth the single-agent dose produced complete tumor regressions in rats that are sustained for at least 90 days posttherapy.[619] These results are superior to that seen with maximum 5-FU doses given either bolus daily for 5 days or with CI for 4 days, suggesting that the improved antitumor activity is not simply the result of prolonged 5-FU plasma exposure. To test the hypothesis that 5-FU catabolites may attenuate the antitumor activity of 5-FU, the antitumor activity of three regimens was compared in the rat model: 5-FU alone (100 mg/kg), eniluracil (1 mg/kg) followed by 5-FU (10 mg/kg), and eniluracil (10 mg/kg) followed by 5-FU (10 mg/kg) and DHFU (90 mg/kg). The regimen was repeated weekly for 3 weeks on all arms. The complete response rate was 13% with 5-FU alone, 94% with eniluracil plus 5-FU, and 38% with the three-drug combination, indicating that administration of DHFU interfered with the efficacy of eniluracil plus 5-FU.[620]

5-FU metabolism was monitored in an isolated rat liver perfusion model with fluorine-19 nuclear magnetic resonance spectroscopy during perfusion with 5-FU alone (15 mg/kg) or 5-FU preceded by eniluracil (0.5 mg/kg). Eniluracil produced a 27-fold decrease in the formation of

catabolites and a sevenfold increase in anabolite formation.[621] Eniluracil prevented the formation of the toxic catabolites FBAL, fluoroacetate, and 2-fluoro-3-hydroxypropionic acid, which have been implicated in 5-FU-associated neurotoxicity and cardiac toxicity. In mice bearing murine colon 38 tumors, ex vivo measurements of tissue extracts from liver, kidney, and tumor indicate a greater than 95% elimination of FUPA and FBAL signals in the tissues of mice that received 2 mg/kg of eniluracil before administration of 5-FU.[622] A prolonged presence of 5-FU and increased formation of fluoronucleotides was noted in healthy and tumor tissues. Eniluracil prevented neurotoxicity associated with a CI of 5-FU in a canine model, suggesting that eniluracil-mediated inhibition of DPD prevents the formation of potentially toxic catabolites.[309]

Clinical studies of oral eniluracil given once daily for 7 days at 0.74, 3.7, or 18.5 mg/m^2 indicated that DPD activity in PBMCs was inactivated within 1 hour and remained inhibited by 93 to 98% 24 hours after dosing.[623] Fourteen days after eniluracil, mean DPD activity was approximately 60% (0.74 mg/m^2), 70% (3.7 mg/m^2), and 125% (18.5 mg/m^2) relative to baseline values. Because lower dosages of eniluracil would be expected to produce faster recovery, these observations suggest potential interpatient variability in the duration of DPD inhibition.

Pharmacokinetic comparison of 5-FU (10 mg/m^2) given either intravenously or orally on day 2 with oral eniluracil (3.7 mg/m^2 orally) on days 1 and 2 (24 hours and 30 minutes before the 5-FU dose) indicated complete oral bioavailability of 5-FU.[624] The terminal $t_{1/2}$ of 5-FU was prolonged to 4.5 hours, and systemic clearance was reduced to 60 mL/min per square meter. The MTD of oral 5-FU was 25 mg/m^2 given on days 2 through 6 with eniluracil 3.7 mg/m^2 orally on days 1 through 7. In another trial, no toxicity was observed after oral eniluracil given at doses of 0.74, 3.7, and 18.5 mg/m^2 daily for 7 days.[623] After a 14-day washout period, eniluracil was given daily for 3 days with 5-FU 10 mg/m^2 intravenously on day 2; no toxicity was seen. With 50 mg of eniluracil on days 1 through 3 and either 10 mg/m^2 intravenously or 20 mg orally 5-FU on day 2, the $t_{1/2}$ of 5-FU averaged 4.9 and 6.1 hours, respectively. After a 14-day washout, patients received eniluracil orally on days 1 through 7 with escalating doses of either oral or intravenous 5-FU. Neutropenia and thrombocytopenia were dose-limiting; nonhematologic toxicities

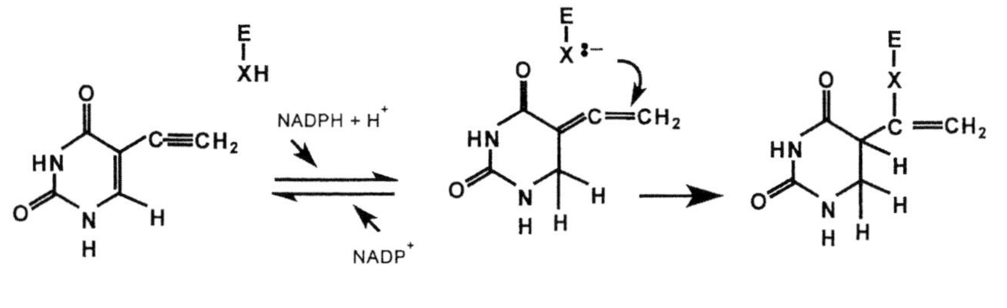

Figure 7.14 Interaction between eniluracil and dihydropyrimidine dehydrogenase. E, dihydropyrimidine dehydrogenase; NADP, nicotinamide adenine dinucleotide; NADPH, nicotinamide adenine dinucleotide phosphate.

(nausea, vomiting, diarrhea, anorexia, mucositis, and fatigue) occurred less frequently. When 5-FU was given on days 2 through 6 with 50 mg each of eniluracil and LV on days 1 through 7, the recommended dose of oral 5-FU was 15 mg/m^2, 28-fold lower than the customary dose of 5-FU and LV on a monthly schedule.

A 28-day schedule has been explored in which eniluracil and 5-FU were administered orally twice a day. The recommended doses of eniluracil and 5-FU are 10 and 1 mg/m^2 twice daily for 28 of 35 days.[625] For the majority of the subsequent phase 2 and 3 trials, a combination tablet that incorporates eniluracil and 5-FU in a dose ratio of 10 to 1 was used. Phase 2 trials indicated the 28-day regimen is active as first-line therapy in breast cancer (52% of 29 patients responded) and colorectal cancer (24% of 45 patients responded).[625,626] In contrast to the experience with CI 5-FU schedules and oral capecitabine, hand-foot syndrome was not observed.

Phase 3 trials that compared the oral 28-day schedule of eniluracil and 5-FU as first-line therapy for colorectal cancer with a daily for 5 days schedule of intravenous bolus 5-FU plus LV failed to demonstrate equivalence for oral eniluracil/5-FU, and clinical development has ceased.[627]

Some patients who received a subsequent 5-FU-type regimen 3 to 5 weeks after completing protocol therapy with the 28-day schedule of eniluracil and 5-FU experienced life-threatening or fatal toxicity, leading to the recommendation that a minimum of 8 weeks elapse between the last dose of eniluracil and subsequent therapy with another 5-fluoropyrimidine. In a phase 1 trial of oral eniluracil given days 1 to 3 with 5-FU given twice daily on day 2 (intended to simulate a weekly high-dose 24-hour CI schedule), pharmacodynamic studies suggested prolonged inhibition of DPD for up to 19 days after the last dose of eniluracil as reflected by DPD-catalytic activity in PBMCs and elevated uracil levels compared with baseline values.[628] Another study evaluated the pharmacodynamic effects of two schedules of eniluracil on a weekly schedule: 20 mg orally on days 1 to 3 with a single dose of 5-FU given day 2, or a single dose of eniluracil and 5-FU. DPD activity was profoundly depressed during oral therapy, and uracil levels were strikingly elevated with both schedules. With the daily-for-3-days schedule, DPD activity was similar to baseline values by 3 weeks after the earlier eniluracil dose, whereas it appeared to recover earlier in patients receiving the single-dose schedule, reaching baseline values by 2 weeks.[629] These latter studies raise a question as to whether the dose of eniluracil used in the pivotal studies may have been excessive.

Other Oral 5-Fluoropyrimidines

Several other oral 5-FU prodrugs are either commercially available outside the United States are undergoing clinical investigation.[630–634] Carmofur is 5-fluoro-N-hexyl-3,4-dihydro-2,4-dioxopyrimidine-1(2H)-carboxamide (MW 257).

S-1 is a three-drug preparation containing ftorafur; 5-chloro-2,4-dihydroxypyridine (CDHP), a competitive, reversible inhibitor of DPD that is about 180-fold more potent than uracil in vitro, and oxonic acid, which strongly inhibits the anabolism of 5-FU to FUMP by OPRTase; the molar ratio is 1.0 to 0.4 to 1.0. BOF-A2 (emitefur, 3-{3-[6-benzoyloxy-3-cyano-2-pyridyloxycarbonyl]benzoyl}-1-ethoxymethyl-5-fluorouracil; MW 558) contains 1-ethoxymethyl-5-fluorouracil, a masked 5-FU prodrug, and 3-cyano-2, 6-dihydroxypyridine (CNDP), a potent inhibitor of DPD. The features of these oral 5-FU prodrugs are highlighted in Table 7.13.

INTERFERENCE OF WARFARIN AND PHENYTOIN METABOLISM BY 5-FLUOROURACIL AND CAPECITABINE

Case reports have described prolongation of the prothrombin time in patients receiving either therapeutic and minidose warfarin in conjunction with 5-FU or capecitabine. In some cases, this effect has been associated with supraanticoagulation and bleeding complications. A retrospective study of 95 patients that employed infusional 5-FU regimens in conjunction with warfarin 1 mg daily to decrease the risk of catheter-associated thrombosis reported elevations of the institutional normalized ratio (INR) of more than 1.5 in 33% of patients; the INR was greater than 3.0 in 19%, and bleeding complications were observed in 8%.[635] Similarly, patients receiving phenytoin concurrently with 5-FU have experienced elevated phenytoin concentrations.[636] Both warfarin and phenytoin are principally metabolized by cytochrome P-450 2C9. Preclinical studies in rats suggest a probable explanation. Rats treated with a single intraperitoneal dose of 5-FU had decreased protein expression and catalytic activity of two constitutive CYP isozymes, CYP2C11 and CYP3A.[637] Rats given oral racemic warfarin during a 8-day intraperitoneal regimen of 5-FU had a significant decrease in the total serum clearance of S-warfarin, which was attributed to a significant decrease in the rate of formation of the oxidative metabolites of the potent S-enantiomer.[638] Administration of 5-FU for 7 days reduces phenytoin-p-hydroxylation activity and decreases the total clearance of phenytoin.[639] These findings indicate that patients receiving warfarin concurrently with either 5-FU or capecitabine should have their prothrombin time and INR values monitored frequently to allow dose adjustment of warfarin to prevent overanticoagulation.

REFERENCES

1. Heidelberger C, Chaudhuari NK, Daneberg P, et al. Fluorinated pyrimidines. A new class of tumor inhibitory compounds. Nature 1957;179:663–666.

2. Wohlhueter RM, McIvor RS, Plagemann PGW. Facilitated transport of uracil and 5-fluorouracil, and permeation of orotic acid into cultured mammalian cells. J Cell Physiol 1980;104: 309–319.

3. Domin BA, Mahony WB, Zimmerman TP. Transport of 5-fluorouracil and uracil into human erythrocytes. Biochem Pharmacol 1993;46:503–510.

4. Pastor-Anglada, M, Felipe A, Casado FJ. Transport and mode of action of nucleoside derivatives used in chemical and antiviral therapies. Trends Pharmacol Sci 1998;19,424–430.

5. Bowen D, Diasio RB, Goldman ID. Distinguishing between membrane transport and intracellular metabolism of fluorodeoxyuridine in Ehrlich ascites tumor cells by application of kinetic and high-performance liquid chromatographic techniques. J Biol Chem 1979;254:5333–5339.

6. Kessel D, Deacon J, Coffey B, et al. Some properties of a pyrimidine phosphoribosyltransferase from murine leukemia cells. Mol Pharmacol 1972;8:731–739.

7. Schwartz PM, Handschumacher RE. Selective antagonism of 5-fluorouracil cytotoxicity by 4-hydroxypyrazolopyrimidine (allopurinol) in vitro. Cancer Res 1979;39:3095–3101.

8. Cory J, Breland JB, Carter GL. Effect of 5-fluorouracil on RNA metabolism in Novikoff hepatoma cells. Cancer Res 1979;39: 4905–4913.

9. Cadman E, Davis L, Heimer R. Enhanced 5-fluorouracil nucleotide formation following methotrexate: biochemical explanation for drug synergism. Science 1979;205:1135–1137.

10. Houghton JA, Houghton RJ. 5-Fluorouracil in combination with hypoxanthine and allopurinol: toxicity and metabolism in xenografts of human colonic carcinomas in mice. Biochem Pharmacol 1980;29:2077–2080.

11. Benz C, Cadman E. Modulation of 5-fluorouracil metabolism and cytotoxicity by antimetabolite pretreatment in human colorectal adenocarcinoma HCT-8. Cancer Res 1981;41:994–999.

12. Houghton JA, Houghton PJ. Elucidation of pathways of 5-fluorouracil metabolism in xenografts of human colorectal adenocarcinoma. Eur J Cancer Clin Oncol 1983;19:807–815.

13. Finan PJ, Kiklitis PA, Chisholm EM, et al. Comparative levels of tissue enzymes concerned in the early metabolism of 5-fluorouracil in normal and malignant human colorectal tissue. Br J Cancer 1984;50:711–715.

14. Schwartz PM, Moir RD, Hyde CM, et al. Role of uridine phosphorylase in the anabolism of 5-fluorouracil. Biochem Pharmacol 1987;34:3585–3589.

15. Woodman PW, Sarrif AM, Heidelberger C. Specificity of pyrimidine nucleoside phosphorylases and the phosphorolysis of 5-fluoro-2' deoxyuridine. Cancer Res 1980;40:507–511.

16. Niedzwicki JG, El Kouni MH, Chu SH, et al. Structure activity relationship of ligands of the pyrimidine nucleoside phosphorylases. Biochem Pharmacol 1983;32:399–415.

17. Pogolotti AL, Nolan PA, Santi DV. Methods for the complete analysis of 5-fluorouracil metabolites in cell extracts. Anal Biochem 1981;117:178–186.

18. Peterson MS, Ingraham HA, Goulian M. 2'-Deoxyribosyl analogues of UDP-N-acetylglucosamine in cells treated with methotrexate or 5-fluorodeoxyuridine. J Biol Chem 1983;258: 10831–10834.

19. Peters GJ, Laurensse E, Lankelma J, et al. Separation of several 5-fluorouracil metabolites in various melanoma cell lines: evidence for the synthesis of 5-fluorouracil-nucleotide sugars. Eur J Cancer Clin Oncol 1984;20:1425–1431.

20. Santi DV, McHenry CS, Sommer A. Mechanisms of interactions of thymidylate synthetase with 5-fluorodeoxyuridylate. Biochemistry 1974;13:471–480.

21. Sommer A, Santi DV. Purification and amino acid analysis of an active site peptide from thymidylate synthetase containing covalently bound 5'-fluoro-2'-deoxyuridylate and methylene tetrachloride. Biochem Biophys Res Commun 1974;57:689–696.

22. Howell SB, Mansfield SJ, Taetle R. Significance of variation in serum thymidine concentration for the marrow toxicity of methotrexate. Cancer Chemother Pharmacol 1981;5:221–226.

23. Dolnick BJ, Cheng Y-C. Human thymidylate synthetase derived from blast cells of patients with acute myelocytic leukemia. J Biol Chem 1977;252:7697–7703.

24. Dolnick BJ, Cheng Y-C. Human thymidylate synthetase: II. Derivatives of pteroylmono- and polyglutamates as substrates and inhibitors. J Biol Chem 1978;253:3563–3567.

25. Fernandes DJ, Bertino JR. 5-Fluorouracil-methotrexate synergy: enhancement of 5-fluorodeoxyuridylate binding to thymidylate synthetase by dihydropteroylpolyglutamates. Proc Natl Acad Sci U S A 1980;77:5663–5667.

26. Allegra CJ, Chabner BA, Jolivet J. Enhanced inhibition of thymidylate synthase by methotrexate polyglutamates. J Biol Chem 1986;230:9720–9726.

27. Ullman B, Lee M, Martin DW Jr, et al. Cytotoxicity of 5- fluoro-2'-deoxyuridine: requirement for reduced folate cofactors and antagonism by methotrexate. Proc Natl Acad U S A 1978; 75:980–983.

28. Danenberg KD, Danenberg PV. Evidence for sequential interaction of the subunits of thymidylate synthetase. J Biol Chem 1979;254:4345–4348.

29. Murinson DS, Anderson T, Schwartz HS, et al. Competitive radioassay for 5-fluorodeoxyuridine 5'-monophosphate in tissues. Cancer Res 1979;39:2471–2479.

30. Washtien WL, Santi DV. Assay of intracellular free and macromolecular-bound metabolites of 5-fluorodeoxyuridine and 5-fluorouracil. Cancer Res 1979;39:3397–3404.

31. Hardy LW, Finer-Moore JS, Montfort WR, et al. Atomic structure of thymidylate synthase: target for rational drug design. Science 1987;235:448–455.

32. Santi DV, McHenry CS, Raines RT, et al. Kinetics and thermodynamics of the interaction of 5-fluoro-2'-deoxyuridylate. Biochemistry 1987;26:8606–8613.

33. Appelt K, Bacquet RJ, Bartlett CA, et al. Design of enzyme inhibitors using iterative protein crystallographic analysis. J Med Chem 1991;34:1925–1934.

34. Schoichet BK, Stroud RM, Santi DV, et al. Structure-based discovery of inhibitors of thymidylate synthase. Science 1993;259: 1445–1450.

35. Maybaum J, Ullman B, Mandel HG, et al. Regulation of RNA-and DNA-directed actions of 5-fluoropyrimidines in mouse T-lymphoma (S-49) cells. Cancer Res 1980;40:4209–4215.

36. Evans RM, Laskin JD, Hakala MT. Assessment of growth-limiting events caused by 5-fluorouracil in mouse cells and in human cells. Cancer Res 1980;40:4113–4122.

37. Spiegelman S, Sawyer R, Nayak R, et al. Improving the antitumor activity of 5-fluorouracil by increasing its incorporation into RNA via metabolic modulation. Proc Natl Acad Sci U S A 1980;77:4996–4970.

38. Santelli G, Valeriote F. In vivo enhancement of 5-fluorouracil cytotoxicity to AKR leukemia cells by thymidine in mice. J Natl Cancer Inst 1978;61:843–847.

39. Carrico CK, Glazer RI. Augmentation by thymidine of the incorporation and distribution of 5-fluorouracil into ribosomal RNA. Biochem Biophys Res Commun 1979;87:664–670.

40. Kufe DW, Egan EM. Enhancement of 5-fluorouracil incorporation into human lymphoblast ribonucleic acid. Biochem Pharmacol 1981;30:129–133.

41. Wilkinson DS, Tisty TD, Hanas RJ. The inhibition of ribosomal RNA synthesis and maturation in Novikoff hepatoma cells by 5-fluorouridine. Cancer Res 1975;35: 3014–3020.

42. Chaudhuri NK, Montag B, Heidelberger C. Studies on fluorinated pyrimidines: III. The metabolism of 5-fluorouracil-2-C14 and 5-fluoroorotic-2-C14 acid in vivo. Cancer Res 1958; 18:318–328.

43. Herrick D, Kufe DW. Lethality associated with incorporation of 5-fluorouracil into preribosomal RNA. Mol Pharmacol 1984;26:135–140.

44. Kanamaru R, Kakuta H, Sato T, et al. The inhibitory effects of 5-fluorouracil on the metabolism of preribosomal and ribosomal RNA in L-1210 cells in vitro. Cancer Chemother Pharmacol 1986;17:43–46.

45. Greenhalgh DA, Parish JH. Effect of 5-fluorouracil combination therapy on RNA processing in human colonic carcinoma cells. Br J Cancer 1990;61:415–419.

46. Ghoshal K, Jacob ST. Specific inhibition of pre-ribosomal RNA processing in extracts from the lymphosarcoma cells treated with 5-fluorouracil. Cancer Res 1994;54:632–636.

47. Ghoshal K, Jacob ST. An alternative molecular mechanism of action of 5-fluorouracil, a potent anticancer drug. Biochem Pharmacol 1997;53:1569–1575.

48. Kufe DW, Major PP. 5-Fluorouracil incorporation into human breast carcinoma RNA correlates with cytotoxicity. J Biol Chem 1981;256:9802–9805.

49. Glazer RI, Lloyd LS. Association of cell lethality with incorporation of 5-fluorouracil and 5-fluorouridine into nuclear RNA in human colon carcinoma cells in culture. Mol Pharmacol 1982;21:468–473.

50. Laskin JD, Evans RM, Slocum HK, et al. Basis for natural variation in sensitivity to 5-fluorouracil in mouse and human cells in culture. Cancer Res 1979;39:383–390.

51. Spears CP, Shani J, Shahinian AH, et al. Assay and time course of 5-fluorouracil incorporation into RNA of L1210/ 0 ascites cells in vivo. Mol Pharmacol 1985;27:302–307.

52. Carrico CK, Glazer RI. The effect of 5-fluorouracil on the synthesis and translation of poly(A) RNA from regenerating liver. Cancer Res 1979;39:3694–3701.

53. Tseng W-C, Medina D, Randerath K. Specific inhibition of transfer RNA methylation and modification in tissue of mice treated with 5-fluorouracil. Cancer Res 1978;38:1250–1257.

54. Will CL, Dolnick BJ. 5-Fluorouracil inhibits dihydrofolate reductase precursor mRNA processing and/or nuclear mRNA stability in methotrexate-resistant KB cells. J Biol Chem 1989;264:21413–21421.

55. Iwata T, Watanabe T, Kufe DW. Effects of 5-fluorouracil on globin mRNA synthesis in murine erythroleukemia cells. Biochemistry 1986;25:2703–2707.

56. Armstrong RD, Lewis M, Stern SG, et al. Acute effect of 5-fluorouracil on cytoplasmic and nuclear dihydrofolate reductase messenger RNA metabolism. J Biol Chem 1986;261:7366–7371.

57. Armstrong RD. RNA as a target for antimetabolites. In: Glazer RI, ed. Developments in Cancer Chemotherapy. Vol 2. Boca Raton, FL: CRC Press, 1989:154–174.

58. Takimoto CH, Voeller DB, Strong JM, et al. Effects of 5-fluorouracil substitution on the RNA conformation and in vitro translation of thymidylate synthase messenger RNA. J Biol Chem 1993;28:21438–21442.

59. Schmittgen TD, Danenberg KD, Horikoshi T, et al. Effect of 5-fluoro- and 5-bromouracil substitution on the translation of human thymidylate synthase mRNA. J Biol Chem 1994;269:16269–16275.

60. Armstrong RD, Takimoto CH, Cadman EC. Fluoropyrimidine-mediated changes in small nuclear RNA. J Biol Chem 1986;261:21–24.

61. Takimoto CH, Cadman EC, Armstrong RD. Precursor-dependent differences in the incorporation of fluorouracil in RNA. Mol Pharmacol 1986;29:637–642.

62. Sierakowska H, Shukla RR, Dominsksi A, et al. Inhibition of pre-mRNA splicing by 5-fluoro-, 5-chloro- and 5-bromouridine. J Biol Chem 1989;264:19185–19191.

63. Doong SL, Dolnick BJ. 5-Fluorouracil substitution alters pre-mRNA splicing in vitro. J Biol Chem 1988;263:4467–4473.

64. Danenberg PV, Shea LCC, Danenberg K. Effect of 5-fluorouracil substitution on the self-splicing activity of Tetrahymena ribosomal RNA. Cancer Res 1990;50:1757–1763.

65. Lenz H-J, Manno DJ, Danenberg KD, et al. Incorporation of 5-fluorouracil into U2 and U6 snRNA inhibits mRNA precursor splicing. J Biol Chem 1994;269:31962–31968.

66. Randerath K, Tseng W-C, Harris JS, et al. Specific effects of fluoropyrimidines and 5-azapyrimidines on modification of the 5 position of pyrimidines, in particular the synthesis of 5-methyluracil and 5-methylcytosine in nucleic acids. Cancer Res 1983;84:283–297.

67. Santi DV, Hardy LW. Catalytic mechanism and inhibition of tRNA (uracil-5-)methyltransferase: evidence for covalent catalysis. Biochemistry 1987;26:8599–8606.

68. Samuelsson T. Interactions of transfer RNA pseudouridine synthases with RNAs substituted with fluorouracil. Nucleic Acids Res 1991;19:6139–6144.

69. Patton JR. Ribonucleoprotein particle assembly and modification of U2 small nuclear RNA containing 5-fluorouridine. Biochemistry 1993;32:8939–9844.

70. Shani J, Danenberg PV. Evidence that intracellular synthesis of 5-fluorouridine-5′-phosphate from 5-fluorouracil and 5-fluorouridine is compartmentalized. Biochem Biophys Res Commun 1984;122:439–445.

71. Jin Y, Heck DE, DeGeorge G, et al. 5-Fluorouracil suppresses nitric oxide biosynthesis in colon carcinoma cells. Cancer Res 1996;56:1978–1982.

72. Fujishima H, Niho Y, Kondo T, et al. Inhibition by 5-fluorouracil of ERCC1 and gamma-glutamylcysteine synthetase messenger RNA expression in a cisplatin-resistant HST-1 human squamous carcinoma cell line. Oncol Res 1997;9:167–172.

73. Grem JL, Mulcahy RT, Miller EM, et al. Interaction of deoxyuridine with fluorouracil and dipyridamole in a human colon cancer cell line. Biochem Pharmacol 1989;38:51–59.

74. Curtin NJ, Harris AL, Aherne GW. Mechanism of cell death following thymidylate synthase inhibition: 2′-deoxy- 5′-triphosphate accumulation, DNA damage, and growth inhibition following exposure to CB3717 and dipyridamole. Cancer Res 1991;51:2346–2352.

75. Aherne GW, Hardcastle A, Raynaud F, et al. Immunoreactive dUMP and TTP pools as an index of thymidylate synthase inhibition; effect of tomudex (ZD1694) and a nonpolyglutamated quinazoline antifolate (CB30900) in L1210 mouse leukaemia cells. Biochem Pharmacol 1996;51:1293–1301.

76. Tanaka M, Yoshida S, Saneyoshi M, et al. Utilization of 5- fluoro-2′-deoxyuridine triphosphate and 5-fluoro-2′-deoxycytidine triphosphate in DNA synthesis by DNA polymerases alpha and beta from calf thymus. Cancer Res 1981;41: 4132–4135.

77. Ingraham HA, Tseng BY, Goulian M. Mechanism for exclusion of 5-fluorouracil from DNA. Cancer Res 1980;40:998–1001.

78. Herrick D, Major PP, Kufe DW. Effect of methotrexate on incorporation and excision of 5-fluorouracil residues in human breast carcinoma DNA. Cancer Res 1982;42:5015–5017.

79. Cheng Y-C, Nakayama K. Effects of 5-fluoro-2′-deoxyuridine on DNA metabolism in HeLa cells. Mol Pharmacol 1983;23: 171–174.

80. Tanaka M, Kimura K, Yoshida S. Enhancement of the incorporation of 5-fluorodeoxyuridylate into DNA of HL-60 cells by metabolic modulations. Cancer Res 1983;43:5145–5150.

81. Kufe DW, Scott P, Fram R, et al. Biologic effect of 5-fluoro- 2′-deoxyuridine incorporation in L1210 deoxyribonucleic acid. Biochem Pharmacol 1983;32:1337–1340.

82. Schuetz JD, Wallace HJ, Diasio RB. 5-Fluorouracil incorporation into DNA of CF-1 mouse bone marrow cells as a possible mechanism of toxicity. Cancer Res 1984;44:1358–1363.

83. Sawyer RC, Stolfi RL, Martin DS, et al. Incorporation of 5- fluorouracil into murine bone marrow DNA in vivo. Cancer Res 1984;44:1847–1851.

84. Caradonna DJ, Cheng YC. The role of deoxyuridine triphosphate nucleotidohydrolase, uracil-DNA glycosylase, and DNA polymerase alpha in the metabolism of FUdR in human tumor cells. Mol Pharmacol 1980;18:513–520.

85. Chu E, Lai GM, Zinn S, et al. Resistance of a human ovarian cancer line to 5-fluorouracil associated with decreased levels of 5-fluorouracil in DNA. Mol Pharmacol 1990;38:410–417.

86. Harris JM, McIntosh EM, Muscat GE. Structure/function analysis of a dUTPase: catalytic mechanism of a potential chemotherapeutic target. J Mol Biol 1999;2:275–287.

87. Canman CE, Lawrence TS, Shewach DS, et al. Resistance to fluorodeoxyuridine-induced DNA damage and cytotoxicity correlates with an elevation of deoxyuridine triphosphatase activity and failure to accumulate deoxyuridine triphosphate. Cancer Res 1993;53:5219–5224.

88. Mauro DJ, De Riel JK, Tallarida RJ, et al. Mechanisms of excision of 5-fluorouracil by uracil DNA glycosylase in normal human cells. Mol Pharmacol 1993;43:854–857.

89. Wurzer JC, Tallarida RJ, Sirover MA. New mechanism of action of the cancer chemotherapeutic agent 5-fluorouracil in human cells. J Pharmacol Exp Ther 1994;269:39–43.

90. Yoshioka A, Tanaka S, Hiraoka O, et al. Deoxyribonucleoside triphosphate imbalance—fluorodeoxyuridine-induced DNA double strand breaks in mouse FM3A cells and the mechanism of cell death. J Biol Chem 1987;262:8235–8241.

91. Houghton JA, Tillman DM, Harwood FG. Ratio of 2′-deoxyadenosine-5′-triphosphate/thymidine-5′-triphosphate influences the commitment of human colon carcinoma cells to thymineless death. Clin Cancer Res 1995;1:723–730.

92. Wadler S, Horowitz R, Mao X, et al. Effect of interferon of 5-fluorouracil-induced perturbations in pools of deoxynucleotide triphosphates and DNA strand breaks. Cancer Chemother Pharmacol 1996;38:529–535.

93. Schuetz JD, Collins JM, Wallace HJ, et al. Alteration of the secondary structure of newly synthesized DNA from murine bone marrow cells by 5-fluorouracil. Cancer Res 1986;46:119–123.

94. Jones S, Willmore E, Durkacz BW. The effects of 5-fluoropyrimidines on nascent DNA synthesis in Chinese hamster ovary cells monitored by pH-step alkaline and neutral elution. Carcinogenesis 1994;15:2435–2438.

95. Yin M, Rustum YM. Comparative DNA strand breakage induced by FUra and FdUrd in human ileocecal adenocarcinoma (HCT-8) cells: relevance to cell growth inhibition. Cancer Commun 1991;3:45–51.

96. Lonn U, Lonn S. Increased levels of DNA lesions induced by leucovorin-5-fluoropyrimidine in human colon adenocarcinoma. Cancer Res 1988;48:4153–4157.

97. Dusenbury CE, Davis MA, Lawrence TS, et al. Induction of megabase DNA fragments by 5-fluorodeoxyuridine in human colorectal tumor (HT29) cells. Mol Pharmacol 1991;39:285–289.

98. Canman CE, Tang H-Y, Normolle DP, et al. Variations in patterns of DNA damage induced in human colorectal tumor cells by 5-fluorodeoxyuridine. Implications for mechanisms of resistance and cytotoxicity. Proc Natl Acad U S A 1992;89:10474–10478.

99. Ayusawa D, Arai H, Wataya Y, et al. A specialized form of chromosomal DNA degradation induced by thymidylate stress in mouse FM3A cells. Mutat Res 1988;200:221–230.

100. Li Z-R, Yin M-B, Arredendo MA, et al. Down-regulation of c-myc gene expression with induction of high molecular weight DNA fragments by fluorodeoxyuridine. Biochem Pharmacol 1994;48:327–334.

101. Kyprianou N, Isaacs JT. "Thymineless" death in androgen-independent prostatic cancer cells. Biochem Biophys Res Commun 1989;165:73–81.

102. Lowe SW, Ruley HE, Jacks T, et al. p53-Dependent apoptosis modulates the cytotoxicity of anticancer agents. Cell 1993;74:957–967.

103. Fisher TC, Milner AE, Gregory CD, et al. Bcl-2 modulation of apoptosis induced by anticancer drugs: resistance to thymidylate stress is independent of classical resistance pathways. Cancer Res 1993;53:3321–3326.

104. Lonn U, Lonn S. The increased cytotoxicity in colon adenocarcinoma of methotrexate-5-fluorouracil is not associated with increased induction of lesions in DNA by 5-fluorouracil. Biochem Pharmacol 1986;35:177–181.

105. Parker WB, Kennedy KA, Klubes P. Dissociation of 5-fluorouracil- induced DNA fragmentation from either its incorporation into DNA or its cytotoxicity in murine T- lymphoma (S-49). Cancer Res 1987;47:979–982.

106. Darzynkiewicz Z. Methods in analysis of apoptosis and cell necrosis. In: Parker J, Stewart C, eds. The Purdue Cytometry CD-ROM. Vol 3. West Lafayette, IN: Purdue University, 1997.

107. Houghton JA, Harwood FG, Tillman DM. Thymineless death in colon carcinoma cells is mediated via Fas signaling. Proc Natl Acad U S A 1997;94:8144–8149.

108. Tillman DM, Petak I, Houghton JA. A fas-dependent component in 5-fluorouracil/leucovorin-induced cytotoxicity in colon carcinoma cells. Clin Cancer Res 1999;5:425–430.

109. Ciccolini J, Peillard L, Evrard A, et al. Enhanced antitumor activity of 5-fluorouracil in combination with 2′-deoxyinosine in human colorectal cell lines and human colon tumor xenografts. Clin Cancer Res 2000;6:1529–1535.

110. Longley DB, Allen WL, McDermott U, et al. The roles of thymidylate synthase and p53 in regulating Fas-mediated apoptosis in response to antimetabolites. Clin Cancer Res 2004;10:3562-3571.

111. Pritchard DM, Watson AJM, Potten CS, et al. Inhibition of uridine but not thymidine of p53-dependent intestinal apoptosis initiated by 5-fluorouracil: evidence for the involvement of RNA perturbation. Proc Natl Acad U S A 1997;94:1795–1799.

112. Li L, Berger SH, Wyatt MD. Involvement of base excision repair in response to therapy targeted at thymidylate synthase. Mol Cancer Ther 2004;3(6):747–753.

113. Goel A, Arnold CN, Boland CR: Multistep progression of colorectal cancer in the setting of microsatellite instability: new details and novel insights. Gastroenterology 2001;121:1497–1502, .

114. Meyers M, Wagner MW, Hwang HS, et al. Role of the hMLH1 DNA mismatch repair protein in fluoropyrimidine-mediated cell death and cell cycle responses. Cancer Res 2001;61(13): 5193–5201.

115. Arnold CN, Goel A, Boland CR. Role of hMLH1 promoter hypermethylation in drug resistance to 5-fluorouracil in colorectal cancer cell lines. Int J Cancer 2003;106(1):66–73.

116. Gryfe R, Kim H, Hsieh ET, et al. Tumor microsatellite instability and clinical outcome in young patients with colorectal cancer. N Engl J Med 2000;342:69–77.

117. Aschele C, Sobrero A, Faderan MA, et al. Novel mechanisms of resistance to 5-fluorouracil in human colon cancer (HCT- 8) sublines following exposure to two different clinically relevant dose schedules. Cancer Res 1992;52:1855–1964.

118. Sobrero AF, Aschele C, Guglielmi AP, et al. Synergism and lack of cross-resistance between short-term and continuous exposure to fluorouracil in human colon adenocarcinoma cells. J Natl Cancer Inst 1993;85:1937–1944.

119. Ren Q-F, Van Groeningen CJ, Geoffroy F, et al. Determinants of cytotoxicity with prolonged exposure to fluorouracil in human colon cancer cells. Oncol Res 1997;9:77–88.

120. Reichard P, Skold O, Klein G, et al. Studies on resistance against 5-fluorouracil: I. Enzymes of the uracil pathway during development of resistance. Cancer Res 1962;22:235–243.

121. Ardalan B, Cooney DA, Jayaram HN, et al. Mechanisms of sensitivity and resistance of murine tumors to 5-fluorouracil. Cancer Res 1980;40:1431–1437.

122. Mulkins MA, Heidelberger C. Isolation of fluoropyrimidine-resistant murine leukemic cell lines by one-step mutation and selection. Cancer Res 1982;42:956–964.

123. Mulkins MA, Heidelberger C. Biochemical characterization of fluoropyrimidine-resistant murine leukemic cell lines. Cancer Res 1982;42:965–973.

124. Piper AA, Fox RM. Biochemical basis for the differential sensitivity of human T- and B-lymphocyte lines to 5-fluorouracil. Cancer Res 1982;42:3753–3760.

125. Ardalan B, Villacorte D, Heck D, et al. Phosphoribosyl pyrophosphate pool size and tissue levels as a determinant of 5-fluorouracil response in murine colonic adenocarcinomas. Biochem Pharmacol 1982;31:1989–1992.

126. Au J L-S, Rustum YM, Minowad J, et al. Differential selectivity of 5-fluorouracil and 5′-deoxy-5-fluorouridine in cultured human B lymphocytes and mouse L1210 leukemia. Biochem Pharmacol 1983;32:541–546.

127. Yoshida M, Hoshi A. Mechanism of inhibition of phosphoribosylation of 5-fluorouracil by purines. Biochem Pharmacol 1984;33:2863–2867.

128. El-Assouli SM. The molecular basis for the differential sensitivity of B and T lymphocytes to growth inhibition by thymidine and 5-fluorouracil. Leuk Res 1985;9:391–398.

129. Peters GJ, Laurensse E, Leyva A, et al. Sensitivity of human, murine and rat cells to 5-fluorouracil and 5′-deoxy-5-fluorouridine in relation to drug-metabolizing enzymes. Cancer Res 1986;46:20–28.

130. Tamemasa O, Tezuka M. Additive formation of antineoplastic 5-fluorouracil nucleosides from 5-fluorouracil by Ehrlich ascites tumor extracts in the presence of ribose 1-phosphate/uridine or deoxyribose 1-phosphate/deoxyuridine. J Pharmacobiodyn 1982;5:720–726.

131. Beltz RE, Waters RN, Hegarty TJ. Enhancement and depression by inosine of the growth inhibitory action of 5- fluorouracil on cultured Jensen tumor cells. Biochem Biophys Res Commun 1983;112:235–241.

132. Washtien WL. Comparison of 5-fluorouracil metabolism in two human gastrointestinal tumor cell lines. Cancer Res 1984;44:909–914.

133. Iigo M, Yamaizumi Z, Nishimura S, et al. Mechanism of potentiation of antitumor activity of 5-fluorouracil by guanine

ribonucleotides against adenocarcinoma 755. Eur J Cancer Clin Oncol 1987;23:1059–1065.

134. Klubes P, Connelly K, Cerna I, et al. Effects of 5-fluorouracil on 5-fluorodeoxyuridine 5-monophosphate and 2- deoxyuridine 5'-monophosphate pools and DNA synthesis in solid mouse L1210 and rat Walker 256 tumors. Cancer Res 1978;38: 2325–2331.

135. Fernandes DJ, Cranford SK. Resistance of CCRF-CEM cloned sublines to 5-fluorodeoxyuridine associated with enhanced phosphatase activities. Biochem Pharmacol 1985;34: 125–132.

136. Moran RG, Spears CP, Heidelberger C. Biochemical determinants of tumor sensitivity to 5-fluorouracil: ultrasensitive methods for determination of 5-fluoro-2'-deoxyuridylate, 2'-deoxyuridylate, and thymidylate synthetase. Proc Natl Acad Sci U S A 1979;76:1456–1460.

137. Berger SH, Hakala MT. Relationship of dUMP and free FdUMP pools to inhibition to thymidylate synthase by 5- fluorouracil. Mol Pharmacol 1984;25:303–309.

138. Houghton JA, Weiss KD, Williams LG, et al. Relationship between 5-fluoro-2'-deoxyuridylate, 2'-deoxyuridylate, and thymidylate synthase activity subsequent to 5-fluorouracil administration, in xenografts of human colon adenocarcinomas. Biochem Pharmacol 1986;35:1351–1358.

139. Kaufman ER. Resistance to 5-fluorouracil associated with increased cytidine triphosphate levels in V79 Chinese hamster cells. Cancer Res 1984;44:3371–3376.

140. Aronow B, Watts T, Lassetter J, et al. Biochemical phenotype of 5-fluorouracil-resistant murine T-lymphoblasts with genetically altered CTP synthetase activity. J Biol Chem 1984;259: 9035–9043.

141. Noordhuis P, Holwerda U, Van Der Wilt CL, et al. 5-Fluorouracil incorporation into RNA and DNA in relation to thymidylate synthase inhibition of human colorectal cancers. Ann Oncol 2004;15(7):1025–1032.

142. Fernandes DJ, Cranford SK. A method for the determination of total, free, and 5-fluorodeoxyuridylate-bound thymidylate synthase in cell extracts. Anal Biochem 1984;142:378–385.

143. Yalowich JC, Kalman TI. Rapid determinations of thymidylate synthase activity and its inhibition in intact L1210 leukemia cells in vitro. Biochem Pharmacol 1985;34:2319–2324.

144. Spears CP, Gustavsson BG, Mitchell MS, et al. Thymidylate synthetase inhibition in malignant tumors and normal liver of patients given intravenous 5-fluorouracil. Cancer Res 1984; 44:4144–4150.

145. Peters GJ, van Groeningen CJ, Leurensse EJ, et al. Thymidylate synthase from untreated human colorectal cancer and colonic mucosa: enzyme activity and inhibition by 5-fluoro-2-deoxyuridine-5-monophosphate. Eur J Cancer 1991;27:263–267.

146. Horikoshi T, Danenberg KD, Staglbauer THW, et al. Quantitation of thymidylate synthase, dihydrofolate reductase, and DT-diaphorase gene expression in human tumors using the polymerase chain reaction. Cancer Res 1992;52:108–116.

147. Lenz H-J, Leichman CG, Danenberg KD, et al. Thymidylate synthase mRNA level in adenocarcinoma of the stomach: a predictor for primary tumor response and overall survival. J Clin Oncol 1985;14:176–182.

148. Leichman CG, Lenz H-J, Leichman L, et al. Quantitation of intratumoral thymidylate synthase expression predicts for disseminated colorectal cancer response and resistance to protracted-infusion fluorouracil and weekly leucovorin. J Clin Oncol 1997;15:3223–3229.

149. Johnston PG, Liang C-M, Henry S, et al. Production and characterization of monoclonal antibodies that localize human thymidylate synthase in the cytoplasm of human cells and tissue. Cancer Res 1991;51:6668–6676.

150. Johnston PG, Drake JC, Trepel J, et al. Immunological quantitation of thymidylate synthase using the monoclonal antibody TS 106 in 5-fluorouracil-sensitive and -resistant human cancer cell lines. Cancer Res 1992;52:4306–4312.

151. Johnston PG, Drake JC, Steinberg SM, et al. The quantitation of thymidylate synthase in human tumors using an ultrasensitive enzyme-linked immunoassay. Biochem Pharmacol 1993;12: 2483–2486.

152. Popat S, Matakidou A, Houlston RS. Thymidylate synthase expression and prognosis in colorectal cancer: a systematic review and meta-analysis. J Clin Oncol 2004;22(3):529–536

153. Berger SH, Jenh C-H, Johnson LF, et al. Thymidylate synthase overproduction and gene amplification in fluorodeoxyuridine-resistant human cells. Mol Pharmacol 1985;28:461–467.

154. Clark JL, Berger SH, Mittelman A, et al. Thymidylate synthase gene amplification in a colon tumor resistant to fluoropyrimidine chemotherapy. Cancer Treat Rep 1987;71:261–265.

155. Copur S, Aiba K, Drake JC, et al. Thymidylate synthase gene amplification in human colon cancer cell lines resistant to 5-fluorouracil. Biochem Pharmacol 1995;49:1419–1426.

156. Jastreboff MM, Kedzierska B, Rode W. Altered thymidylate synthetase in 5-fluorodeoxyuridine-resistant Ehrlich ascites carcinoma cells. Biochem Pharmacol 1985;32:2259–2267.

157. Bapat AR, Zarow C, Danenberg PV. Human leukemic cells resistant to 5-fluoro-2'deoxyuridine contain a thymidylate synthase with a lower affinity for nucleotides. J Biol Chem 1983; 258:4130–4136.

158. Berger SH, Barbour KW, Berger FG. A naturally occurring variation in thymidylate synthase structure is associated with a reduced response to 5-fluoro-2'-deoxyuridine in a human colon tumor cell line. Mol Pharmacol 1988;34:480–484.

159. Barbour KW, Berger SH, Berger SG. Single amino acid substitution defines a naturally occurring genetic variant of human thymidylate synthase. Mol Pharmacol 1990;37:515–518.

160. Kawate H, Landis DM, Loeb LA. Distribution of mutations in human thymidylate synthase yielding resistance to 5-fluorodeoxyuridine. J Biol Chem 2002;277(39):36304–36311.

161. Lu K, McGuire JJ, Slocum HK, et al. Mechanisms of acquired resistance to modulation of 5-fluorouracil by leucovorin in HCT-8 human ileocecal carcinoma cells. Biochem Pharmacol 1997;53:689–696.

162. Grem JL, Hoth DF, Hamilton JM, et al. Overview of current status and future direction of clinical trials with 5-fluorouracil in combination with folinic acid. Cancer Treat Rep 1987;71:1249–1264.

163. Zhang Z-G, Rustum YM. Effects of diastereoisomers of 5-formyl-tetrahydrofolate on cellular growth, sensitivity to 5-fluoro-2'-deoxyuridine, and methylenetetrahydrofolate polyglutamate levels in HCT-8 cells. Cancer Res 1991; 51:3476–3481.

164. Boarman DM, Allegra CJ. Intracellular metabolism of 5-formyltetrahydrofolate in human breast and colon cell lines. Cancer Res 1992;52:36–44.

165. Romanini A, Lin JT, Niedzwiecki D, et al. Role of folylpolyglutamates in biochemical modulation of fluoropyrimidines by leucovorin. Cancer Res 1991;51:789–793.

166. Wang F-S, Aschele C, Sobrero A, et al. Decreased folylpolyglutamate synthetase expression: a novel mechanism of fluorouracil resistance. Cancer Res 1993;53:3677–3680.

167. Cohen A, Ullman B. Role of intracellular dTTP levels in fluorodeoxyuridine toxicity. Biochem Pharmacol 1984;33: 3298–3301.

168. Grem JL, Fischer PH. Enhancement of 5-fluorouracil's anticancer activity by dipyridamole. Pharmacol Ther 1989;40:349–371.

169. Radparvar S, Houghton PJ, Germain G, et al. Cellular pharmacology of 5-fluorouracil in a human colon adenocarcinoma cell line selected for thymidine kinase deficiency. Biochem Pharmacol 1990;39:1759–1765.

170. Sobrero AF, Moir RD, Bertino JR, et al. Defective facilitated diffusion of nucleosides, a primary mechanism of resistance to 5-fluoro-2'-deoxyuridine in the HCT-8 human carcinoma. Cancer Res 1985;45:3155–3160.

171. Sobrero AF, Handschumacher RE, Bertino JR. Highly selective drug combinations for human colon cancer cells resistant in vitro to 5-fluoro-2'-deoxyuridine. Cancer Res 1985;45:3161–3163.

172. Jenh C-H, Rao LG, Johnson LF. Regulation of thymidylate synthase enzyme synthesis in 5-fluorodeoxyuridine-resistant mouse fibroblasts during the transition from the resting to growing state. J Cell Physiol 1985;122:149–154.

173. Cadman E, Heimer R. Levels of thymidylate synthetase during normal culture growth of L1210 cells. Cancer Res 1986;46: 1195–1198.

174. Johnson LF. Post transcriptional regulation of thymidylate synthase gene expression. J Cell Biochem 1994;54:378–392.

175. Horie N, Takeishi K. Identification of functional elements in the promoter region of the human gene for thymidylate synthase and nuclear factors that regulate the expression of the gene. J Biol Chem 1997;272:18375–18381.

176. Berne M, Gustavsson B, Almersjo O, et al. Concurrent allopurinol and 5-fluorouracil: 5-fluoro-2′-deoxyuridylate formation and thymidylate synthase inhibition in rat colon carcinoma in regenerating rat liver. Cancer Chemother Pharmacol 1987;20:193–197.

177. Chu E, Zinn S, Boarman D, et al. Interaction of interferon and 5-fluorouracil in the H630 human colon carcinoma cell line. Cancer Res 1990;50:5834–5840.

178. Van der Wilt CL, Pinedo HM, Smid K, et al. Elevation of thymidylate synthase following 5-fluorouracil treatment is prevented by the addition of leucovorin in murine colon tumors. Cancer Res 1992;52:4922–4928.

179. Parr AL, Drake JC, Gress RE, et al. 5-Fluorouracil-mediated thymidylate synthase induction in malignant and nonmalignant human cells. Biochem Pharmacol 1998;56:231–235.

180. Swain SM, Lippman ME, Chabner BA, et al. Fluorouracil and high-dose leucovorin in previously treated patients with metastatic breast cancer. J Clin Oncol 1989;7:890–899.

181. Chu E, Voeller DM, Johnston PG, et al. Regulation of thymidylate synthase in human colon cancer cells treated with 5-fluorouracil and interferon-gamma. Mol Pharmacol 1993;43:527–533.

182. Chu E, Koeller DM, Casey JL, et al. Autoregulation of human thymidylate synthase messenger RNA translation by thymidylate synthase. Proc Natl Acad U S A 1991;88:8977–8981.

183. Chu E, Voeller D, Koeller DM, et al. Identification of an RNA binding site for human thymidylate synthase. Proc Natl Acad USA 1993;90:517–521.

184. Ju J, Kane SE, Lenz HJ, et al. Desensitization and sensitization of cells to fluoropyrimidines with different antisenses directed against thymidylate synthase messenger RNA. Clin Cancer Res 1998;4:2229–2236.

185. Schmitz JC, Chen TM, Chu E. Small interfering double-stranded RNAs as therapeutic molecules to restore chemosensitivity to thymidylate synthase inhibitor compounds. Cancer Res 2004;64:1431–1435.

186. Houghton PJ, Germain GS, Hazelton VJ, et al. Mutant of human colon adenocarcinoma selected for thymidylate synthase deficiency. Proc Natl Acad Sci U S A 1989;86:1377–1381.

187. Houghton PJ, Rahman A, Will CL, et al. Mutations of the thymidylate synthase gene of human adenocarcinoma cells causes a thymidylate synthase-negative phenotype that can be attenuated by exogenous folates. Cancer Res 1992;52:558–565.

188. Calabro-Jones PM, Byfield JE, Ward JF, et al. Time-dose relationships for 5-fluorouracil cytotoxicity against human epithelial cancer cells in vitro. Cancer Res 1982;42:4413–4420.

189. Santelli G, Valeriote F. Schedule-dependent cytotoxicity of 5-fluorouracil in mice. J Natl Cancer Inst 1986;76:159–164.

190. Moran RG, Scanlon KL. Schedule-dependent enhancement of the cytotoxicity of fluoropyrimidines to human carcinoma cells in the presence of folinic acid. Cancer Res 1991;51:4618–4623.

191. van Gröeningen CJ, Pinedo HM, Heddes J, et al. Pharmacokinetics of 5-fluorouracil assessed with a sensitive mass spectrometric method in patients on a dose escalation schedule. Cancer Res 1988;48:6956–6961.

192. Anderson LW, Parker RJ, Collins JM, et al. Gas chromatographic-mass spectrometric method for routine monitoring of 5-fluorouracil in plasma of patients receiving low-level protracted infusions. J Chromatogr 1992;581:195–201.

193. Martino R, Malet-Martino M, Gilarad V. Fluorine nuclear magnetic resonance, a privileged tool for metabolic studies of fluoropyrimidine drugs. Curr Drug Metab 2000;1:271–303.

194. Murphy RF, Balis FM, Poplack DG. Stability of 5-fluorouracil in whole blood and plasma. Clin Chem 1987;33:2299–2300.

195. Almersjo OE, Gustavsson BG, Regardh CG, et al. Pharmacokinetic studies of 5-fluorouracil after oral and intravenous administration in man. Acta Pharmacol Toxicol 1980;46:329–336.

196. Christophidis N, Vajda FJE, Lucas I, et al. Fluorouracil therapy in patients with carcinoma of the large bowel: a pharmacokinetic comparison of various rates and routes of administration. Clin Pharmacokinet 1978;3:330–336.

197. Fraile RJ, Baker LH, Buroker TR, et al. Pharmacokinetics of 5-fluorouracil administered orally by rapid intravenous and by slow infusion. Cancer Res 1980;40:2223–2228.

198. Grem JL, McAtee N, Murphy RF, et al. A pilot study of interferon alfa-2a in combination with fluorouracil plus high-dose leucovorin in metastatic gastrointestinal carcinoma. J Clin Oncol 1991;9:1811–1820.

199. MacMillan WE, Wolberg WH, Welling PG. Pharmacokinetics of fluorouracil in humans. Cancer Res 1978;38:3479–3482.

200. Heggie GD, Sommadossi J-P, Cross DS, et al. Clinical pharmacokinetics of 5-fluorouracil and its metabolites in plasma, urine, and bile. Cancer Res 1987;47:2203–2206.

201. Grem JL, McAtee N, Murphy RF, et al. Phase I and pharmacokinetic study of recombinant human granulocyte-macrophage colony-stimulating factor given in combination with fluorouracil plus calcium leucovorin in metastatic gastrointestinal adenocarcinoma. J Clin Oncol 1994;12:560–568.

202. McDermott BJ, van der Berg HW, Murphy RF. Nonlinear pharmacokinetics for the elimination of 5-fluorouracil after intravenous administration in cancer patients. Cancer Chemother Pharmacol 1982;9:173–178.

203. Benz C, DeGregorio M, Saks S, et al. Sequential infusions of methotrexate and 5-fluorouracil in advanced cancer: pharmacology, toxicity, and response. Cancer Res 1985;45:3354–3358.

204. Yoshida T, Araki E, Iigo M, et al. Clinical significance of monitoring serum levels of 5-fluorouracil by continuous infusion in patients with advanced colonic cancer. Cancer Chemother Pharmacol 1990;26:352–354.

205. Harris BE, Song R, Soong SJ, et al. Relationship between dihydropyrimidine dehydrogenase activity and plasma 5-fluorouracil levels with evidence for circadian variation of enzyme activity and plasma drug levels in cancer patients receiving 5-fluorouracil by protracted continuous infusion. Cancer Res 1990;50:197–201.

206. Grem JL, McAtee N, Balis F, et al. A phase II study of continuous infusion 5-fluorouracil and leucovorin with weekly cisplatin in metastatic colorectal carcinoma. Cancer 1993;72:663–668.

207. Petit E, Milano G, Levi F, et al. Circadian rhythm-varying plasma concentration of 5-fluorouracil during a five-day continuous venous infusion at a constant rate in cancer patients. Cancer Res 1988;48:1676–1680.

208. Fleming RF, Milano G, Thyss A, et al. Correlation between dihydropyrimidine dehydrogenase activity in peripheral mononuclear cells and systemic clearance of fluorouracil in cancer patients. Cancer Res 1982;52:2899–2902.

209. Erlichman C, Fine S, Elhakim T. Plasma pharmacokinetics of 5-FU given by continuous infusion with allopurinol. Cancer Treat Rep 1986;70:903–904.

210. Remick SC, Grem JL, Fischer PH, et al. Phase I trial of 5-fluorouracil and dipyridamole administered by 72-hour concurrent continuous infusion. Cancer Res 1990;50:2667–2672.

211. Grem JL, McAtee N, Steinberg SM, et al. A phase I study of continuous infusion 5-fluorouracil plus calcium leucovorin in combination with n-(phosphonacetyl)-L-aspartate in metastatic gastrointestinal adenocarcinoma. Cancer Res 1993;53:4828–4836.

212. Ensminger WD, Rosowsky A, Raso VO, et al. A clinical pharmacological evaluation of hepatic arterial infusion of 5-fluoro-2′-deoxyuridine and 5-fluorouracil. Cancer Res 1978; 38:3784–3792.

213. Collins JM, Dedrick RL, King FG, et al. Nonlinear pharmacokinetic models for 5-fluorouracil in man: intravenous and intraperitoneal routes. Clin Pharmacol Ther 1980;28:235–246.

214. Wagner JG, Gyves JW, Stetson PL, et al. Steady-state nonlinear pharmacokinetics of 5-fluorouracil during hepatic arterial and intravenous infusions in cancer patients. Cancer Res 1986;46:1499–1506.

215. Thyss A, Milano G, Renee N, et al. Clinical pharmacokinetic study of 5-FU in continuous 5-day infusions for head and neck cancer. Cancer Chemother Pharmacol 1986;16:64–66.

216. Trump DL, Egorin MJ, Forrest A, et al. Pharmacokinetic and pharmacodynamic analysis of fluorouracil during 72-hour continuous infusion with and without dipyridamole. J Clin Oncol 1991;9:2027–2035.

217. Fety R, Rolland F, Barberi-Heyob M. Clinical impact of pharmacokinetically-guided dose adaptation of 5-fluorouracil: results from a multicentric randomized trial in patients with locally advanced head and neck carcinomas. Clin Cancer Res 1998; 4:2039–2045.

218. Santini J, Milano G, Thyss A, et al. 5-FU therapeutic monitoring with dose adjustment leads to an improved therapeutic index in head and neck cancer. Br J Cancer 1989;59:287–290.

219. Creaven PJ, Rustum YM, Petrelli NJ, et al. Phase I and pharmacokinetic evaluation of floxuridine/leucovorin given on the Roswell Park weekly regimen. Cancer Chemother Pharmacol 1994;34:261–265.

220. Goldberg JA, Kerr DJ, Watson DG, et al. The pharmacokinetics of 5-fluorouracil administered by arterial infusion in advanced colorectal hepatic metastases. Br J Cancer 1990;61:913–915.

221. Sigurdson ER, Ridge JA, Kemeny N. Tumor and liver drug uptake following hepatic artery and portal vein infusion. J Clin Oncol 1987;5:1836–1840.

222. Speyer JL, Collins JM, Dedrick RL, et al. Phase I and pharmacologic studies of 5-fluorouracil administered intraperitoneally. Cancer Res 1980;40:567–572.

223. Sugarbaker PH, Gianola FJ, Speyer JC, et al. Prospective, randomized trial of intravenous versus intraperitoneal 5-fluorouracil in patients with advanced primary colon or rectal cancer. Surgery 1985;98:414–422.

224. Schilsky RL, Choi KE, Grayhack J, et al. Phase I clinical and pharmacologic study of intraperitoneal cisplatin and fluorouracil in patients with advanced intra-abdominal cancer. J Clin Oncol 1990;8:2054–2061.

225. Muggia FM, Chan KK, Russell C, et al. Phase I and pharmacologic evaluation of intraperitoneal 5-fluoro-2'-deoxyuridine. Cancer Chemother Pharmacol 1991;28:241–250.

226. Grem JL, Harold N, Shapiro J, et al. A phase I and pharmacokinetic trial of weekly oral 5-fluorouracil given with eniluracil and low-dose leucovorin. J Clin Oncol 2000;18:3952–3963.

227. Shiotani T, Weber T. Purification and properties of dihydrothymine dehydrogenase from rat liver. J Biol Chem 1981; 256:219–224.

228. Podschun B, Cook PF, Schnackerz KD. Kinetic mechanism of dihydropyrimidine dehydrogenase in pig liver. J Biol Chem 1990;265:12966–12972.

229. Lu Z, Zhang R, Diasio RB. Purification and characterization of dihydropyrimidine dehydrogenase from human liver. J Biol Chem 1992;267:17102–17109.

230. Lu Z, Zhang R, Diasio RB. Comparison of dihydropyrimidine dehydrogenase from human, rat, pig, and cow liver: biochemical and immunological properties. Biochem Pharmacol 1993;46:945–952.

231. Naguib FN, El Kouni MH, Cha S. Enzymes of uracil catabolism in normal and neoplastic tissues. Cancer Res 1985;45: 5405–5412.

232. Ho DH, Townsend L, Luna MA, et al. Distribution and inhibition of dihydrouracil dehydrogenase activities in human tissues using 5-fluorouracil as a substrate. Anticancer Res 1986;6:781–784.

233. Ansfield FJ, Schroeder JM, Curreri AR. Five years clinical experience with 5-fluorouracil. JAMA 1962;181:295–299.

234. Ansfield FJ, Ramirez G, Davis HL, et al. Further clinical studies with intrahepatic arterial infusion with 5-fluorouracil. Cancer 1975;36:2413–2417.

235. Sweeny DJ, Barnes S, Heggie GD, et al. Metabolism of 5-fluorouracil to an n-cholyl-2-fluoro-β-alanine conjugate: previously unrecognized role for bile acids in drug conjugation. Proc Natl Acad Sci U S A 1987;84:5439–5443.

236. Zhang R, Soong S-J, Liu T, et al. Pharmacokinetics and tissue distribution of 2-fluoro-β-alanine in rats: potential relevance to toxicity pattern of 5-fluorouracil. Drug Metab Dispos 1992; 20:113–119.

237. Dobritzsch D, Schneider G, Schnackerz KD, et al. Crystal structure of dihydropyrimidine dehydrogenase, a major determinant of the pharmacokinetics of the anti-cancer drug 5-fluorouracil. Embo J 2001;20(4):650–660.

238. Etienne MC, Lagrange JL, Dassonville O, et al. Population study of dihydropyrimidine dehydrogenase in cancer patients. J Clin Oncol 1994;12:2248–2253.

239. Lu A, Zhang R, Diasio RB. Dihydropyrimidine dehydrogenase activity in human peripheral blood mononuclear cells and liver: population characteristics, newly identified deficient patients, and clinical implication in 5-fluorouracil chemotherapy. Cancer Res 1993;53:5433–5438.

240. Milano G, Etienne MC, Pierrefite V, et al. Dihydropyrimidine dehydrogenase deficiency and fluorouracil-related toxicity. Br J Cancer 1999;79:627–630.

241. Lu Z, Zhang R, Diasio RB. Population characteristics of hepatic dihydropyrimidine dehydrogenase activity, a key metabolic enzyme in 5-fluorouracil chemotherapy. Clin Pharmacol Ther 1995;58:512–522.

242. Lu Z, Zhang R, Carpenter JT, et al. Decreased dihydropyrimidine dehydrogenase activity in a population of patients with breast cancer: implication for 5-fluorouracil-based chemotherapy. Clin Cancer Res 1998;4:325–329.

243. McLeod HL, Sludden J, Murray GI, et al. Characterization of dihydropyrimidine dehydrogenase in human colorectal tumours. Br J Cancer 1998;77:461–465.

244. McMurrough J, McLeod HL. Analysis of the dihydropyrimidine dehydrogenase polymorphism in a British population. Br J Clin Pharmacol 1996;41:425–427.

245. Chazal M, Etienne MC, Renee N, et al. Link between dihydropyrimidine dehydrogenase activity in peripheral blood mononuclear cells and liver. Clin Cancer Res 1996;2:507–510.

246. Yokota H, Fernandez-Salguero P, Furuya H, et al. cDNA cloning and chromosome mapping of human dihydropyrimidine dehydrogenase, an enzyme associated with 5-fluorouracil toxicity and congenital thymine uraciluria. J Biol Chem 1994;269: 23192–23196.

247. Takai S, Fernandez-Salguero P, Kimura S, et al. Assignment of the human dihydropyrimidine dehydrogenase gene (DPYD) to chromosome region 1p22 by fluorescence in situ hybridization. Genomics 1994;24:613–614.

248. Johnson MR, Diasio RB, Albin N, et al. Structural organization of the human dihydropyrimidine dehydrogenase gene. Cancer Res 1997;57:1660–1663.

249. Ridge SA, Sludden J, Wei X, et al. Dihydropyrimidine dehydrogenase pharmacogenetics in patients with colorectal cancer. Br J Cancer 1998;77:497–500.

250. Fernandez-Salguero PM, Gonzalez FJ, Idle JR, et al. Lack of correlation between phenotype and genotype for the polymorphically expressed dihydropyrimidine dehydrogenase in a family of Pakistani origin. Pharmacogenetics 1997;7: 161–163.

251. Mattison LK, Soong R, Diasio RB. Implications of dihydropyrimidine dehydrogenase on 5-fluorouracil pharmacogenetics and pharmacogenomics. Pharmacogenomics 2002;3:485–492

252. Van Kuilenburg AB, De Abreu RA, van Gennip AH. Pharmacogenetic and clinical aspects of dihydropyrimidine dehydrogenase deficiency. Ann Clin Biochim 2003;40:41–45.

253. van Kuilenburg AB, Vreken P, Abeling NG, et al: Genotype and phenotype in patients with dihydropyrimidine dehydrogenase deficiency. Hum Genet 1999;104:1–9

254. Kirkwood JM, Ensminger W, Rosowsky A, et al. Comparison of pharmacokinetics of 5-fluorouracil and 5-fluorouracil with concurrent thymidine infusions in a phase I trial. Cancer Res 1980;40:107–113.

255. Woodcock TM, Martin DS, Damin LEM, et al. Clinical trials with thymidine and fluorouracil: a phase I and clinical pharmacologic evaluation. Cancer 1980;45:1135–1143.

256. Au JL-S, Rustum YM, Ledesma EJ, et al. Clinical pharmacological studies of concurrent infusion of 5-fluorouracil and thymidine in treatment of colorectal carcinomas. Cancer Res 1982;42:2930–2937.

257. Tuchman M, O'Dea RF, Ramnaraine MLR, et al. Pyrimidine base degradation in cultured murine C-130 neuroblastoma cells and in situ tumors. J Clin Invest 1988;81:425–430.

258. Harvey VJ, Slevin ML, Dilloway MR, et al. The influence of cimetidine on the pharmacokinetics of 5-fluorouracil. Br J Clin Pharmacol 1984;18:421–430.

259. Dilloway MR, Lant AF. Effect of H-receptor antagonists on the pharmacokinetics of 5-fluorouracil in the rat and monkey. Biopharm Drug Dispos 1991;12:17–28.

260. Okuda H, Watabe T, Kawaguchi Y, et al. Lethal drug interactions of sorivudine, a new antiviral drug, with oral 5-fluorouracil prodrugs. Drug Metab Dispos 1997;25:270–273.

261. Yan J, Tyring SK, McCrary MM, et al. The effect of sorivudine on dihydropyrimidine dehydrogenase activity in patients with acute herpes zoster. Clin Pharmacol Ther 1997;61:563–573.

262. Diasio RB. Sorivudine and 5-fluorouracil; a clinically significant drug-drug interaction due to inhibition of dihydropyrimidine dehydrogenase. Br J Clin Pharmacol 1998;46:1–4.

263. Curreri AR, Ansfield FJ, McIvor FA, et al. Clinical studies with 5-fluorouracil. Cancer Res 1958;18:478–484.

264. Ansfield R, Klotz J, Nealon T, et al. A phase III study comparing the clinical utility of four regimens of 5-fluorouracil. Cancer 1977;39:34–40.

265. Poon MA, O'Connell MJ, Moertel CG, et al. Biochemical modulation of fluorouracil: evidence of significant improvement of survival and quality of life in patients with advanced colorectal carcinoma. J Clin Oncol 1989;7:1407–1418.

266. Petrelli N, Douglass HD, Herrera L, et al. The modulation of fluorouracil with leucovorin in metastatic colorectal carcinoma: a prospective randomized phase III trial. J Clin Oncol 1991;7:1419–1426.

267. Seifert P, Baker L, Reed ML, et al. Comparison of continuously infused 5-fluorouracil with bolus injection in treatment of patients with colorectal adenocarcinoma. Cancer 1975;36:123–128.

268. Rougier P, Paillot B, LaPlanche A, et al. 5-Fluorouracil (5-FU) continuous intravenous infusion compared with bolus administration. Final results of a randomised trial in metastatic colorectal cancer. Eur J Cancer 1997;33:1789–1793

269. Sullivan RD, Young CW, Miller E, et al. The clinical effects of the continuous administration of fluorinated pyrimidines (5-fluorouracil and 5-fluoro-2'-deoxyuridine). Cancer Chemother Rep 1960;8:77–83.

270. Leichman CG, Fleming TR, Muggia FM, et al. Phase II study of fluorouracil and its modulation in advanced colorectal cancer: a Southwest Oncology Group study. J Clin Oncol 1995;13:1303–1311.

271. Kohne CH, Schoffski P, Wilke H, et al. Effective biomodulation by leucovorin of high-dose infusion fluorouracil given as a weekly 24-hour infusion: results of a randomized trial in patients with advanced colorectal cancer. J Clin Oncol 1998;16:418–426.

272. O'Dwyer PJ, Manola J Valone FH, et al. Fluorouracil modulation in colorectal cancer: lack of improvement with N-phosphonoacetyl-l-aspartic acid or oral leucovorin or interferon, but enhanced therapeutic index with weekly 24-hour infusion schedule—an Eastern Cooperative Oncology Group/Cancer and Leukemia Group B Study. J Clin Oncol 2001;19:2413–2421.

273. Aranda E, Diaz-Rubio E, Cervantes A, et al. Randomized trial comparing monthly low-dose leucovorin and fluorouracil bolus with weekly high-dose 48-hour continuous-infusion fluorouracil for advanced colorectal cancer: a Spanish Cooperative Group for Gastrointestinal Tumor Therapy (TTD) study. Ann Oncol 1998;9:727–731.

274. Lokich JJ, Ahlgren JD, Gullo JJ, et al. A prospective randomized comparison of continuous infusion fluorouracil with a conventional bolus schedule in metastatic colorectal carcinoma: a Mid-Atlantic Oncology Program Study. J Clin Oncol 1989;7:425–432.

275. de Gramont A, Bosset JF, Milan C, et al. Randomized trial comparing monthly low-dose leucovorin and fluorouracil bolus with bimonthly high-dose leucovorin and fluorouracil bolus plus continuous infusion for advanced colorectal cancer: a French intergroup study. J Clin Oncol 1997;15:808–815.

276. Beerblock K, Rinaldi Y, Andre T, et al. Bimonthly high dose leucovorin and 5-fluorouracil 48-hour continuous infusion in patients with advanced colorectal carcinoma. Groupe d'Etude et de Recherche sur les Cancers de l'Ovaire et Digestifs (GERCOD). Cancer 1997;79:1100–1105.

277. Ansfield F, Ramirez G, Skibba JL, et al. Intrahepatic arterial infusion with 5-fluorouracil. Cancer 1971;28:1147–1151.

278. Kerr DJ, Ledermann JA, McArdle CS, et al. Phase I clinical and pharmacokinetic study of leucovorin and infusional hepatic arterial fluorouracil. J Clin Oncol 1995;13:2968–2972.

279. Sullivan RD, Miller E. The clinical effects of prolonged intravenous infusion of 5-fluoro-2'-deoxyuridine. Cancer Res 1965;25:1025–1030.

280. Kemeny N, Daly J, Reichman B, et al. Intrahepatic or systemic infusion of fluorodeoxyuridine in patients with liver metastases from colorectal carcinoma. Ann Intern Med 1987;107:459–465.

281. Hohn D, Stagg R, Friedman M, et al. A randomized trial of continuous intravenous versus hepatic intraarterial floxuridine in patients with colorectal cancer metastatic to the liver: the Northern California Oncology Group trial. J Clin Oncol 1989;7:1646–1654.

282. Anderson N, Lokich J, Bern M, et al. A phase I clinical trial of combined fluoropyrimidines with leucovorin in a 14-day infusion. Demonstration of biochemical modulation. Cancer 1989;63:233–237.

283. Martin JK, O'Connell MJ, Wieand HS, et al. Intra-arterial floxuridine vs systemic fluorouracil for hepatic metastases from colorectal cancer. Arch Surg 1990;125:1022–1027.

284. Creaven PJ, Rustum YM, Petrelli NJ, et al. Phase I and pharmacokinetic evaluation of floxuridine/leucovorin given on the Roswell Park weekly regimen. Cancer Chemother Pharmacol 1994;34:261–265.

285. Vokes EE, Raschko JW, Vogelzang NJ, et al. Five day infusion of fluorodeoxyuridine with high-dose oral leucovorin: a phase I study. Cancer Chemother Pharmacol 1991;28:69–73.

286. Brennan MJ, Waitkevicius VK, Rebuck JW. Megaloblastic anemia associated with inhibition of thymine synthesis (observations during 5-fluorouracil treatment). Blood 1960;14:1535–1545.

287. Kelvin FM, Gramm HF, Gluck WL, et al. Radiologic manifestations of small-bowel toxicity due to floxuridine therapy. AJR Am J Roentgenol 1986;146:39–43.

288. Benson AB III, Ajana JA, Catalano RB, et al. Recommended guidelines for the treatment of cancer treatment-induced diarrhea. J Clin Oncol 2004;22:2918–2926.

289. Loprinzi CL, Cianflone SG, Dose AM, et al. A controlled evaluation of an allopurinol mouthwash as prophylaxis against 5-fluorouracil induced stomatis. Cancer 1990;65:1879–1882.

290. Mahood DJ, Kose AM, Loprinzi CL, et al. Inhibition of fluorouracil-induced stomatitis by oral cryotherapy. J Clin Oncol 1991;9:449–452.

291. DeSpain JD. Dermatologic toxicity of chemotherapy. Semin Oncol 1992;19:501–507.

292. Vukelja SJ, Bonner MW, McCollough M, et al. Unusual serpentine hyperpigmentation associated with 5-fluorouracil. Case report and review of cutaneous manifestations associated with systemic 5-fluorouracil. J Am Acad Dermatol 1991;25:905–908.

293. Pujol RM, Rocamora V, Lopez-Pousa A, et al. Persistent supravenous erythematous eruption. A rare local complication of intravenous 5-fluorouracil therapy. J Am Acad Dermatol 1998;39:839–842.

294. Riehl JL, Brown WJ. Acute cerebellar syndrome secondary to 5-fluorouracil therapy. Neurology 1964;14:961–967.

295. Moertel CG, Reitemeier RJ, Bolton CF, et al. Cerebellar ataxia associated with fluorinated pyrimidine therapy. Cancer Chemother Rep 1964;41:15–18.

296. Lynch HT, Droszcz CP, Albano WA, et al. "Organic brain syndrome" secondary to 5-fluorouracil toxicity. Dis Colon Rectum 1981;24:130–131.

297. Moore DH, Fowler WC Jr, Crumpler IS. 5-Fluorouracil neurotoxicity. Gynecol Oncol 1990;36:152–154.

298. Tuxen MK, Hansen SW. Neurotoxicity secondary to antineoplastic drugs. Cancer Treat Rev 1994;20:191–214.

299. Bygrave HA, Geh JI, Jani Y, et al. Neurological complications of 5-fluorouracil chemotherapy. Case report and review of the literature. Clin Oncol 1998;10:334–336.

300. O'Connell MJ, Powis G, Rubin J, et al. Pilot study of PALA and 5-FU in patients with advanced cancer. Cancer Treat Rep 1982;66:77–80.

301. Wooley PV, Ayoob MJ, Smith FP, et al. A controlled trial of the effect of 4-hydroxypyrazolopyrimidine (Allopurinol) on the toxicity of a single bolus dose of 5-fluorouracil. J Clin Oncol 1985;3:103–109.

302. Muggia FM, Camacho FJ, Kaplan BH, et al. Weekly 5-fluorouracil combined with PALA. Toxic and therapeutic effects in colorectal cancer. Cancer Treat Rep 1987;71:253–256.

303. Diasio RB, Beavers TL, Carpenter T. Familial deficiency of dihydropyrimidine dehydrogenase: biochemical basis for familial pyrimidinemia and severe 5-fluorouracil-induced toxicity. J Clin Invest 1998;81:47–51.

304. Harris BE, Carpenter JT, Diasio RB. Severe 5-fluorouracil toxicity secondary to dihydropyrimidine dehydrogenase deficiency. Cancer Res 68:499–501, 1991

305. Takimoto CH, Lu Z-H, Zhang R, et al. Severe neurotoxicity following 5-fluorouracil-based chemotherapy in a patient with dihydropyrimidine dehydrogenase deficiency. Clin Cancer Res 1996;2:477–481.

306. Hook CC, Kimmel DW, Kvols LK, et al. Multifocal inflammatory leukoencephalopathy with 5-fluorouracil and levamisole. Ann Neurol 1992;31:262–267.

307. Figueredo AT, Fawcet SE, Molloy DW, et al. Disabling encephalopathy during 5-fluorouracil and levamisole adjuvant therapy for resected colorectal cancer. A report of two cases. Cancer Invest 1995;13:608–611.

307a. Luppi G, Zoboli A, Barbieri F, et al. Multifocal leukoencephalopathy associated with 5-fluorouracil and levamisole adjuvant therapy for colon cancer. A report of two cases and review of the literature. The INTACC Intergruppo Nazionale Terpia Adiuvante Colon Carcinoma. Ann Oncol 1996;7:412–415.

308. Neuwelt EA, Barnet PA, Glasberg M, et al. Neurotoxicity of chemotherapeutic agents after blood-brain barrier modification neuropathological studies. Ann Neurol 1983;14:316–324.

309. Davis ST, Joyner SS, Baccanari DP, et al. 5-Ethynyluracil (776C85). Protection from 5-fluorouracil-induced neurotoxicity in dogs. Biochem Pharmacol 1994;48:233–236.

310. Okada R, Shibutani M, Matsuo T, et al. Experimental neurotoxicity of 5-fluorouracil and its derivatives is due to poisoning by the monofluorinated organic metabolites, monofluoroacetic acid and α-fluoro-β-alanine. Acta Neuropathol 1990; 81:66–73.

311. Berg SL, Balis FM, McCully CL, et al. Intrathecal 5-fluorouracil in the rhesus monkey. Cancer Chemother Pharmacol 1992;31: 127–130.

312. Yamada M, Nakagawa H, Fukushima M, et al. In vitro study on intrathecal use of 5-fluoro-2′-deoxyuridine (FdUrd) for meningeal dissemination of malignant brain tumors. J Neurooncol 1998;37:115–121.

313. Tsavaris N, Kosmas C, Vadiaka M, et al. Cardiotoxicity following different doses and schedules of 5fluorouracil administration for malignancy—a survey of 427 pattients. Med Sci Monit 2002;8:151–157.

314. Becker K, Erckenbrecht JF, Haussinger D, et al. Cardiotoxicity of the antiproliferative compound fluorouracil. Drugs 1999;57: 475–484.

315. Meyer CC, Calis KA, Burke LB, et al. Symptomatic cardiotoxicity associated with 5-fluorouracil. Pharmacotherapy 1997;17: 729–736.

316. Grandi AM, Pinotti G, Morandi E, et al. Noninvasive evaluation of cardiotoxicity of 5-fluorouracil and low doses of folinic acid. A one-year follow-up study. Ann Oncol 1997;8:705–708.

317. Wang WS, Hsieh RK, Chiou TJ, et al. Toxic cardiogenic shock in a patient receiving weekly 24-hr infusion of high-dose 5-fluorouracil and leucovorin. Jpn J Clin Oncol 1998;28:551–554.

318. Arrellano M, Malet-Martino M, Martine R, et al. The anti-cancer drug 5-fluorouracil is metabolized by the isolated perfused rat liver and in rats into highly toxic fluoroacetate. Br J Cancer 1998;77:79–86.

318a. Lemaire L, Malet-Martino MC, de Forni M, et al. Cardiotoxicity of commercial 5-fluorouracil stems from the alkaline hydrolysis of this drug. Br J cancer 1992;66:119–127.

319. Porta C, Moroni M, Ferrari S, et al. Endothelin-1 and 5-fluorouracil-induced cardiotoxicity. Neoplasma 1998;45:81–82.

320. Mosseri M, Fingert HJ, Varticovoski L, et al. In vitro evidence that myocardial ischemia resulting from 5-fluorouracil chemotherapy is due to protein kinase C-mediated vasoconstriction of vascular smooth muscle. Cancer Res 1993;53:3028–3033.

321. al-Tweigeri T, Nabholtz JM, Mackey JR. Ocular toxicity and cancer chemotherapy. A review. Cancer 1996;78:1359–1373.

322. Eiseman AS, Flanagan JC, Brooks AB, et al. Ocular surface, ocular adnexal, and lacrimal complications associated with the use of systemic 5-fluorouracil. Ophthal Plast Reconstr Surg 2003;19:216–224.

323. Loprinzi CL, Wender DB, Veeder MH, et al. Inhibition of 5-fluorouracil-induced ocular irritation by ocular ice packs. Cancer 1994;74:945–948.

324. Wong MK, Bjarnason GA, Hrushesky WJ, et al. Steroid- responsive interstitial lung disease in patients receiving 2′- deoxy-5-fluorouridine infusion chemotherapy. Cancer 1995;75:2558–2564.

325. Boyle FM, Smith RC, Levi JA. Continuous hepatic artery infusion of 5-fluorouracil for metastatic colorectal cancer localised to the liver. Aust N Z J Med 1993;23:32–34.

326. Hohn DC, Rayner AA, Economou JS, et al. Toxicities and complications of implanted pump hepatic arterial and intravenous floxuridine infusion. Cancer 1986;57:465–470.

327. Kemeny N, Seiter K, Niedzwiecki D, et al. A randomized trial of intrahepatic infusion of fluorodeoxyuridine with dexamethasone versus fluorodeoxyuridine alone in the treatment of metastatic colorectal cancer. Cancer 1992;69:327–334.

328. Kemeny N, Seiter K, Conti JA, et al. Hepatic arterial floxuridine and leucovorin for unresectable liver metastases from colorectal carcinoma. New dose schedules and survival update. Cancer 1994;73:1134–1142.

329. Kemeny N, Conti JA, Cohen A, et al. Phase II study of hepatic arterial floxuridine, leucovorin, and dexamethasone for unresectable liver metastases from colorectal carcinoma. J Clin Oncol 1994;12:2288–2295.

330. Stein BN, Petrelli NJ, Douglass HO, et al. Age and sex are independent predictors of 5-fluorouracil toxicity. Cancer 1995; 75:11–17.

331. Zalcberg J, Kerr D, Seymour L, et al. Haematological and non-haematological toxicity after 5-fluorouracil and leucovorin in patients with advanced colorectal cancer is significantly associated with gender, increasing age and cycle number. Tomudex International Study Group. Eur J Cancer 1998;34:1871–1875.

332. Tepper JE, O'Connell MJ, Petroni GR, et al. Adjuvant postoperative fluorouracil-modulated chemotherapy combined with pelvic radiation therapy for rectal cancer. Initial results of intergroup 0114. J Clin Oncol 1997;15:2030–2039.

333. Toxicity of fluorouracil in patients with advanced colorectal cancer. Effect of administration schedule and prognostic factors. Meta-analysis group in cancer. J Clin Oncol 1988;16:3537–3541.

334. Sloan JA, Goldberg RM, Sargent DJ, et al. Women experience greater toxicity with fluorouracil-based chemotherapy for colorectal cancer J Clin Oncol 2002;20:1491–1498.

335. Tsalic M, Bar-Sela G, Beny A, et al. Severe toxicity related to the 5-fluorouracil/leucovorin combination (the Mayo Clinic regimen): a prospective study in colorectal cancer patients. Am J Clin Oncol 2003;26:103–106.

336. Port RE, Daniel B, Ding RW, et al. Relative importance of dose, body surface area, sex and age for 5-fluorouracil clearance. Oncology 1991;48:277–281.

337. Milano G, Etienne MC, Cassuto-Viguier E, et al. Influence of sex and age on fluorouracil clearance. J Clin Oncol 1992;10: 1171–1175.

338. Etienne MC, Chatelut E, Pivot X, et al. Co-variables influencing 5-fluorouracil clearance during continuous venous infusion. A NONMEM analysis. Eur J Cancer 1998;34:92–97.

339. Wildiers H, Highley MS, de Bruijn EA, Van Oosterom AT. Pharmacology of anticancer drugs in the elderly population. Clin Pharmacokinet 2003;42:1213–1242

340. Modulation of fluorouracil by leucovorin in patients with advanced colorectal cancer. Evidence in terms of response rate. The advanced colorectal cancer meta-analysis project. J Clin Oncol 1992;10:896–903.

341. Meta-analysis of randomized trials testing the biochemical modulation of fluorouracil by methotrexate in metastatic colorectal cancer. The advanced colorectal cancer meta-analysis project. J Clin Oncol 1994;12:960–969.

342. Efficacy of intravenous continuous infusion of fluorouracil compared with bolus administration in advanced colorectal cancer. Meta-analysis group in cancer. J Clin Oncol 1998;16:301–308.

343. Reappraisal of hepatic arterial infusion in the treatment of nonresectable liver metastases from colorectal cancer. Meta- analysis group in cancer. J Natl Cancer Inst 1996;88:252–258.

344. Thirion P, Piedbois P, Buyse M, et al. Alpha-interferon does not increase the efficacy of 5-fluorouracil in advanced colorectal cancer. Br J Cancer 2001;84:611–620.

345. Fox RM, Woods RL, Tattersall MHN. Allopurinol modulation of high-dose fluorouracil toxicity. Cancer Treat Rev 1979;6 (Suppl):143–147.

346. Campbell TN, Howell SB, Pfeifle C, et al. High-dose allopurinol modulation of 5-FU toxicity. Phase I trial of an outpatient dose schedule. Cancer Treat Rep 1982;66:1723–1727.

347. Howell SB, Pfeifle CE, Wung WE. Effect of allopurinol on the toxicity of high-dose 5-fluorouracil administered by intermittent bolus injection. Cancer 1983;51:220–225.

348. Yoshida M, Hoshi A, Kuretani K. Prevention of antitumor effect of 5-fluorouracil by hypoxanthine. Biochem Pharmacol 1978;27:2979–2982.

349. Yoshida M, Hoshi A. Mechanism of inhibition of phosphoribosylation of 5-fluorouracil by purines. Biochem Pharmacol 1984;33:2863–2867.

350. Martin DS, Stolfi RL, Sawyer RC, et al. High-dose 5-fluorouracil with delayed uridine "rescue" in mice. Cancer Res 1982;42:3864–3870.

351. Sawyer RC, Stolfi RL, Spiegelman S, et al. Effect of uridine on the metabolism of 5-fluorouracil in the CD8F1 murine mammary carcinoma system. Pharm Res 1984;2:69–75.

352. Klubes P, Cerna I. Use of uridine rescue to enhance the antitumor selectivity of 5-fluorouracil. Cancer Res 1983;43: 3182–3186.

353. Peters GJ, van Dijk J, Laurensse E, et al. In vitro biochemical and in vivo biological studies of the uridine "rescue" of 5-fluorouracil. Br J Cancer 1988;57:259–265.

354. Nord LK, Stolfi RL, Martin DS. Biochemical modulation of 5-fluorouracil with leucovorin or delayed uridine rescue. Biochem Pharmacol 1992;43:2543–2549.

355. Leyva A, van Groeningen CJ, Kraal I, et al. Phase I and pharmacokinetic studies of high-dose uridine intended for rescue from 5-fluorouracil toxicity. Cancer Res 1984;44:5928–5933.

356. van Groeningen CJ, Leyva A, Kraal I, et al. Clinical and pharmacokinetic studies of prolonged administration of high-dose uridine intended for rescue from 5-FU toxicity. Cancer Treat Rep 1986;70:745–750.

357. van Groeningen CJ, Peters GJ, Leyva A, et al. Reversal of 5-fluorouracil-induced myelosuppression by prolonged administration of high-dose uridine. J Natl Cancer Inst 1989;81:157–162.

358. Martin DS, Stolfi RL, Sawyer RC. Utility of oral uridine to substitute for parenteral uridine rescue of 5-fluorouracil therapy, with and without a uridine phosphorylase inhibitor (5-benzylacyclouridine). Cancer Chemother Pharmacol 1989;24:9–14.

359. Klubes P, Geffen DB, Cysyk RL. Comparison of the bioavailability of uridine in mice after either oral or parenteral administration. Cancer Chemother Pharmacol 1986;17:236–240.

360. van Groeningen CJ, Peters GJ, Nadal JC, et al. Clinical and pharmacological study of orally administered uridine. J Natl Cancer Inst 1991;83:437–441.

361. Burns ER, Beland SS. Effect of biological time on the determination of the LD50 of 5-fluorouracil in mice. Pharmacology 1984;28:296–300.

362. Peters GJ, van Dijk J, Nadal JC, et al. Diurnal variation in the therapeutic efficacy of 5-fluorouracil against murine colon cancer. In Vivo 187;1:113–118.

363. van Roemeling R, Hrushesky WJM. Determination of the therapeutic index of floxuridine by its circadian infusion pattern. J Natl Cancer Inst 1990;82:386–393.

364. Minshull M, Gardner MLG. The effects of time of administration of 5-fluorouracil on leucopenia in the rat. Eur J Cancer Clin Oncol 1984;20:857–858.

365. Zhang R, Lu Z, Liu T, et al. Relationship between circadian-dependent toxicity of 5-fluorodeoxyuridine and circadian rhythms of pyrimidine enzymes. Possible relevance to fluoropyrimidine therapy. Cancer Res 1993;53:2816–2822.

366. Burns ER. Circadian rhythmicity in DNA synthesis in untreated and saline-treated mice as a basis for improved chemotherapy. Cancer Res 1981;41:2795–2802.

367. Burns ER, Beland SS. Induction by 5-fluorouracil of a major phase difference in the circadian profiles of DNA synthesis

368. Harris BE, Song R, He YJ, et al. Circadian rhythm of rat liver dihydropyrimidine dehydrogenase. Biochem Pharmacol 1988;37:4759–4762.

369. Zhang R, Lu Z, Liu T, et al. Circadian rhythm of rat spleen cytoplasmic thymidine kinase. Biochem Pharmacol 1993;45:1115–1119.

370. Smaaland R, Laerum OD, Lote K, et al. DNA synthesis in human bone marrow is circadian stage dependent. Blood 1991;77:2603–2611.

371. Buchi KN, Moore JG, Hrushesky WJM, et al. Circadian rhythm of cellular proliferation in human rectal mucosa. Gastroenterology 1991;101:410–415.

372. Grem JL, Yee LK, Venzon DJ, et al. Inter- and intraindividual variation in dihydropyrimidine dehydrogenase activity in peripheral blood mononuclear cells. Cancer Chemother Pharmacol 1997;40:117–125.

373. Takimoto CH, Yee LK, Venzon D, et al. High inter- and intrapatient variation in 5-fluorouracil plasma concentrations during a prolonged drug infusion. Clin Cancer Res 1999;5:1347–1352.

374. Metzger G, Massari C, Etienne MC, et al. Spontaneous or imposed circadian changes in plasma concentrations of 5-fluorouracil coadministered with folinic acid and oxaliplatin. Relationship with mucosal toxicity in patients with cancer. Clin Pharmacol Ther 1994;56:190–201.

375. von Roemeling R, Hrushesky WJM. Circadian patterning of continuous floxuridine infusion reduces toxicity and allows higher dose intensity in patients with widespread cancer. J Clin Oncol 1989;7:1710–1719.

376. Hrushesky WJM, von Roemeling R, Lanning TM, et al. Circadian-shaped infusions of floxuridine for progressive metastatic renal cell carcinoma. J Clin Oncol 1990;8:1504–1513.

377. Wesen C, Hrushesky WJM, von Roemeling R. Circadian modification of intra-arterial 5-fluoro-2'-deoxyuridine infusion rate reduces its toxicity and permits higher dose-intensity. J Infus Chemother 1992;2:69–75.

378. Levi FA, Zidani R, Vannetzel JM, et al. Chronomodulated versus fixed-infusion-rate delivery of ambulatory chemotherapy with oxaliplatin, fluorouracil, and folinic acid (leucovorin) in patients with colorectal cancer metastases. A randomized multi-institutional trial. J Natl Cancer Inst 1994;86:1608–1617.

379. Levi F, Zidani R, Misset JL. Randomised multicentre trial of chronotherapy with oxaliplatin, fluorouracil, and folinic acid in metastatic colorectal cancer. International organization for cancer chronotherapy. Lancet 1997;350:681–686.

380. Giacchetti S, Bjarnason G, Garufi C, et al. First line infusion of 5-fluorouracil, leucovorin and oxaliplatin for metastatic colorectal cancer : 4-day chronomodulated (FFL4-10) versus 2-day FOLFOX2. A multicenter randomized Phase III trial of the Chronotherapy Group of the European Organization for Research and Treatment of Cancer (EORTC 05963). Proc Am Soc Clin Oncol 2004;22(14Suppl): abstr 3526.

381. Bjarnason GA, Kerr IG, Doyle N, et al. Phase I study of 5-fluorouracil by a 14-day circadian infusion in metastatic adenocarcinoma patients. Cancer Chemother Pharmacol 1993; 33:221–228.

382. Bertino JR. Biomodulation of 5-fluorouracil with antifolates. Semin Oncol 1997;24(Suppl 18):52–56.

383. Benz C, Tillis T, Tattelman E, et al. Optimal scheduling of methotrexate and 5-fluorouracil in human breast cancer. Cancer Res 1982;42:2081–2086.

384. Donehower RC, Allegra JC, Lippman ME, et al. Combined effects of methotrexate and 5-fluoropyrimidines on human breast cancer cells in serum-free tissue culture. Eur J Cancer 1980;16:655–661.

385. Piper AA, Nott SE, Mackinnon WB, et al. Critical modulation by thymidine and hypoxanthine of sequential methotrexate-5-fluorouracil synergism in murine L1210 cells. Cancer Res 1983; 43:5101–5105.

386. Sawyer RC, Stolfi RL, Martin DS, et al. Inhibition by methotrexate of the stable incorporation of 5-fluorouracil into murine bone marrow DNA. Biochem Pharmacol 1989;38:2305–2311.

387. McSheehy PMJ, Prior MJW, Griffiths JR. Enhanced 5-fluorouracil cytotoxicity and elevated 5-fluoronucleotides in the rat walker

carcinosarcoma following methotrexate pre-treatment. A 19 F-MRS study in vivo. Br J Cancer 1992;65:369–375.

388. Tattersall MHN, Jackson RC, Connors TA, et al. Combination chemotherapy. The interaction of methotrexate and 5-fluorouracil. Eur J Cancer 1973;9:733–739.

389. Bertino JR, Sawicki WL, Linquist CA, et al. Schedule- dependent antitumor effects of methotrexate and 5-fluorouracil. Cancer Res 1977;37:327–328.

390. Kemeny N, Ahmed T, Michaelson R, et al. Activity of sequential low-dose methotrexate and fluorouracil in advanced colorectal carcinoma. Attempt at correlation with tissue and blood levels of phosphoribosylpyrophosphate. J Clin Oncol 1984;2:311–315.

391. Marsh JC, Bertino JR, Katz KH, et al. The influence of drug interval on the effect of methotrexate and fluorouracil in the treatment of advanced colorectal cancer. J Clin Oncol 1991;9:371–380.

392. Browman GP, Levine MN, Goodyear MD, et al. Methotrexate/fluorouracil scheduling influences normal tissue toxicity but not antitumor effects in patients with squamous cell head and neck cancer. Results from a randomized trial. J Clin Oncol 1988;6:963–968.

393. Elliot WL, Howeard CT, Kykes DJ, et al. Sequence and schedule-dependent synergy of trimetrexate in combination with 5-fluorouracil in vitro and in mice. Cancer Res 1989;15:5586–5590.

394. Romanini A, Li WW, Colofiore JR, et al. Leucovorin enhances cytotoxicity of trimetrexate/fluorouracil, but not methotrexate/fluorouracil, in CCRF-CEM cells. J Natl Cancer Inst 1992;84:1033–1038.

395. Punt CJ, Blanke CD, Zhang J, et al. Integrated analysis of overall survival in two randomised studies comparing 5-fluorouracil/leucovorin with or without trimetrexate in advanced colorectal cancer. Ann Oncol 2002;13(1):92–94.

396. Danenberg PV, Danenberg KD. Effect of 5,10-methylenetetrahydrofolate and the dissociation of 5-fluorodeoxyuridylate binding of human thymidylate synthetase. Evidence for an ordered mechanism. Biochemistry 1978;17:4018–4024.

397. Houghton JA, Maroda SJ, Phillips JO, et al. Biochemical determinants of responsiveness to 5-fluorouracil and its derivatives in xenografts of human colorectal adenocarcinomas in mice. Cancer Res 1981;41:144–149.

398. Houghton JA, Torrance PM, Radparvar S, et al. Binding of 5-fluorodeoxyuridylate to thymidylate synthase in human colon adenocarcinoma xenografts. Eur J Cancer Clin Oncol 1986;22:505–510.

399. Spears CP, Gustavsson BG, Fiosing R. Folinic acid modulation of fluorouracil. Tissue kinetics of bolus administration. Invest New Drugs 1989;7:21–36.

400. Evans RM, Laskin JD, Hakala MT. Effects of excess folates and deoxyinosine on the activity and site of action of 5-fluorouracil. Cancer Res 1981;41:3288–3295.

401. Yin M-B, Zakrzewski SF, Hakala MT. Relationship of cellular folate cofactor pools to the activity of 5-fluorouracil. Mol Pharmacol 1983;23:190–197.

402. Cao S, Frank C, Rustum YM. Role of fluoropyrimidine Schedule and (6R,S)leucovorin dose in a preclinical animal model of colorectal carcinoma. J Natl Cancer Inst 1996;88:430–436.

403. Drake JC, Voeller DM, Allegra CJ, et al. The effect of dose and interval between 5-fluorouracil and leucovorin on the formation of thymidylate synthase ternary complex in human cancer cells. Br J Cancer 1995;71:1145–1150.

404. Keyomarsi K, Moran R. Folinic acid augmentation of the effects of fluoropyrimidines on murine and human leukemic cells. Cancer Res 1986;46:5229–5235.

405. Matherly LH, Czaijkowski CA, Muench SP, et al. Role for cytosolic folate binding proteins in compartmentation of endogenous tetrahydrofolates and the formyltetrahydrofolate-mediated enhancement of 5-fluoro-2'-deoxyuridine antitumor activity in vitro. Cancer Res 1990;50:3262–3269.

406. Nadal JC, van Groeningen CJ, Pinedo HM, et al. In vivo potentiation of 5-fluorouracil by leucovorin in murine colon carcinoma. Biomed Pharmacother 1988;42:387–393.

407. Radparvar S, Houghton PJ, Houghton JA. Effect of polyglutamylation of 5,10-methylenetetrahydrofolate on the binding of 5-fluoro-2-deoxyuridylate to thymidylate synthase purified from a human colon adenocarcinoma xenograft. Biochem Pharmacol 1989;38:335–342.

408. Wright JE, Dreyfuss A, El-Magharbel I, et al. Selective expansion of 5,10-methylenetetrahydrofolate pools and modulation of 5-fluorouracil antitumor activity by leucovorin in vivo. Cancer Res 1989;49:2592–2596.

409. Carlsson G, Gustavsson BG, Spears CP, et al. 5-Fluorouracil plus leucovorin as adjuvant treatment of an experimental liver tumor in rats. Anticancer Res 1990;10:813–816.

410. Houghton JA, Williams LG, Cheshire PJ, et al. Influence of dose of [6RS]-leucovorin on reduced folate pools and 5-fluorouracil-mediated thymidylate synthase inhibition in human colon adenocarcinoma xenografts. Cancer Res 1990; 50:3940–3946.

411. Houghton JA, Williams WG, deGraaf SS, et al. Comparison of the conversion of 5-formyltetrahydrofolate and 5- methyltetrahydrofolate to 5,10-methylenetetrahydrofolates and tetrahydrofolates in human colon tumors. Cancer Commun 1989;1:167–174.

412. Bertrand R, Jolivet J. Lack of interference by the unnatural isomer of 5-formyltetrahydrofolate with the effects of the natural isomer in leucovorin preparations. J Natl Cancer Inst 1989;81:1175–1178.

413. Straw JA, Szapary D, Wynn WT. Pharmacokinetics of the diastereoisomers of leucovorin after intravenous and oral administration to normal subjects. Cancer Res 1984;44:3114–3119.

414. Machover D, Goldschmidt E, Chollet P, et al. Treatment of advanced colorectal and gastric adenocarcinomas with 5-fluorouracil and high-dose folinic acid. J Clin Oncol 1986;4:685–696.

415. Trave F, Rustum YM, Petrelli NJ, et al. Plasma and tumor tissue pharmacology of high dose intravenous leucovorin calcium in combination with fluorouracil in patients with advanced colorectal carcinoma. J Clin Oncol 1988;6:1181–1188.

416. Newman EA, Straw JA, Doroshow JH. Pharmacokinetics of diastereoisomers of (6R,S)-folinic acid (leucovorin) in humans during constant high-dose intravenous infusion. Cancer Res 1989;49:5755–5760.

417. Priest DG, Schmitz JC, Bunni MA, et al. Pharmacokinetics of leucovorin metabolites in human plasma as a function of dose administered orally and intravenously. J Natl Cancer Inst 1991; 83:1806–1812.

418. Haller DG, Catalano PJ, Macdonald JS, et al. Fluorouracil, leucovorin and levamisole adjuvant therapy for colon cancer. Five-year final report of INT-0089. Proc Am Soc Clin Oncol 1998; 17:265a.

419. Elias L, Crissman HA. Interferon effects upon the adenocarcinoma MCA 38 and HL-60 cell lines. Antiproliferative responses and synergistic interactions with halogenated pyrimidine antimetabolites. Cancer Res 1988;48:4868–4873.

420. Elias L, Sandoval JM. Interferon effects upon fluorouracil metabolism by HL-60 cells. Biochem Biophys Res Commun 1989;163:867–874.

421. Schwartz EL, Hoffman M, O'Connor CJ, et al. Stimulation of 5-fluorouracil metabolic activation by interferon-α in human colon carcinoma cells. Biochem Biophys Res Commun 1992; 182:1232–1239.

422. Schwartz EL, Baptiste N, O'Connor CJ, et al. Potentiation of the antitumor activity of 5-fluorouracil in colon carcinoma cells by the combination of interferon and deoxyribonucleosides results from complementary effects on thymidine phosphorylase. Cancer Res 1994;54:1472–1478.

423. Morita T, Tokue A. Biomodulation of 5-fluorouracil by interferon-alpha in human renal carcinoma cells. Relationship to the expression of thymidine phosphorylase. Cancer Chemother Pharmacol 1999;44:91–96.

424. Houghton JA, Adkins DA, Rahman A, et al. Interaction between 5-fluorouracil, [6R,S]leucovorin, and recombinant human interferon-α2a in cultured colon adenocarcinoma cells. Cancer Commun 1991;3:225–231.

425. Houghton JA, Morton CL, Adkins DA, et al. Locus of the interaction among 5-fluorouracil, leucovorin and interferon-α2a in colon carcinoma cells. Cancer Res 1993;53:4243–4250.

426. Neefe JR, Glass J. Abrogation of interferon-induced resistance to interferon-activated major histocompatibility complex-unre-

stricted killers by treatment of a melanoma cell line with 5-fluorouracil. Cancer Res 1991;51:3159–3163.

427. Reiter Z, Ozes ON, Blatt LM, et al. A dual antitumor effect of a combination of interferon-α or interleukin-2 and 5-fluorouracil on natural killer (NK) cell-mediated cytotoxicity. Clin Immunol Immunopathol 1992;62:103–111.

428. Koshiji M, Adachi Y, Taketani S, et al. Mechanisms underlying apoptosis induced by combination of 5-fluorouracil and interferon-gamma. Biochem Biophys Res Commun 1997; 240:376–381.

429. van der Wilt CL, Smid K, Aherne GW, et al. Biochemical mechanisms of interferon modulation of 5-fluorouracil activity in colon cancer cells. Eur J Cancer 1997;33:471–478.

430. Ismail A, Van Groeningen CJ, Hardcastle A, et al. Modulation of fluorouracil cytotoxicity by interferon-alpha and -gamma. Mol Pharmacol 1998;53:252–261.

431. Danhauser LL, Freimann JH Jr, Gilchrist TL, et al. Phase I and plasma pharmacokinetic study of infusional 5-fluorouracil combined with recombinant interferon alfa-2a in patients with advanced cancer. J Clin Oncol 1993;11:751–761.

432. Schuller J, Czejka M. Pharmacokinetic interaction of 5-fluorouracil and interferon alpha-2b with or without folinic acid. Med Oncol 1995;12:47–53.

433. Yee LK, Allegra CJ, Steinberg SM, et al. Decreased catabolism of 5-fluorouracil in peripheral blood mononuclear cells during therapy with 5-fluorouracil, leucovorin, and interferon α-2a. J Natl Cancer Inst 1992;84:1820–1825.

434. Grem JL, Quinn M, Ismail AS, et al. Pharmacokinetics and pharmacodynamic effects of 5-fluorouracil given as a one-hour intravenous infusion. Cancer Chemother Pharmacol 2001; 47:117–125.

435. O'Dwyer PJ, King SA, Hoth DF, et al. Role of thymidine in biochemical modulation. A review. Cancer Res 1987;47: 3911–3919.

436. Vogel SJ, Presant CA, Ratkin FA, et al. Phase I study of thymidine plus 5-fluorouracil infusions in advanced colorectal carcinoma. Cancer Treat Rep 1979;63:1–5.

437. Chen J-J, Jones ME. Effect of 6-azauridine on de novo pyrimidine biosynthesis in cultured Ehrlich ascites cells. J Biol Chem 1979;254:4908–4914.

438. Ahluwalia GS, Grem JL, Ho Z, et al. Metabolism and action of amino acid analog anti-cancer agents. Pharmacol Ther 1990; 46:243–271.

439. O'Dwyer PJ, Alonso MT, Leyland-Jones B. Acivicin. A new glutamine antagonist in clinical trials. J Clin Oncol 1984; 2:1064–1071.

440. Pizzorno G, Wiegand RA, Lentz SK, et al. Brequinar potentiates 5-fluorouracil antitumor activity in a murine model colon 38 tumor by tissue-specific modulation of uridine nucleotide pools. Cancer Res. 1992;52:1660–1665.

441. Moyer JD, Smith PA, Levy EJ, et al. Kinetics of n-(phosphonacetyl)-l-aspartate and pyrazofurin depletion of pyrimidine ribonucleotide and deoxyribonucleotide pools and their relationship to nucleic acid synthesis in intact and permeabilized cells. Cancer Res 1982;42:4525–4531.

442. Ardalan B, Glazer RI, Kensler TW, et al. Synergistic effect of 5-fluorouracil and n-(phosphonacetyl)-l-aspartate on cell growth and ribonucleic acid synthesis in human mammary carcinoma. Biochem Pharmacol 1981;30:2045–2049.

443. Liang C-M, Donehower RC, Chabner BA. Biochemical interactions between n-(phosphonacetyl)-L-aspartate and 5-fluorouracil. Mol Pharmacol 1982;21:224–230.

444. Martin DS, Stolfi RL, Sawyer RC, et al. Therapeutic utility of utilizing low doses of n-(phosphonacetyl)-l-aspartic acid in combination with 5-fluorouracil. A murine study with clinical relevance. Cancer Res 1983;43:2317–2321.

445. Grem JL, King SA, O'Dwyer PJ, et al. Biochemistry and clinical activity of n-(phosphonacetyl)-l-aspartate. A review. Cancer Res 1988;48:4441–4454.

446. Casper ES, Vale K, Williams LJ, et al. Phase I and clinical pharmacological evaluation of biochemical modulation of 5-fluorouracil with n-(phosphonacetyl)-l-aspartic acid. Cancer Res 1983;43:2324–2329.

447. Fleming RA, Capizzi RL, Muss HB, et al. Phase I study of N-(phosphonacetyl)-l-aspartate with fluorouracil and with or without dipyridamole in patients with advanced cancer. Clin Cancer Res 1996;2:1107–1114.

448. Moran RG, Danenberg PV, Heidelberger C. Therapeutic response of leukemic mice treated with fluorinated pyrimidines and inhibitors of deoxyuridylate synthesis. Biochem Pharmacol 1982;31:2929–2935.

449. Engstrom PF, MacIntyre JM, Mittelman A, et al. Chemotherapy of advanced colorectal carcinoma. Fluorouracil alone vs two drug combinations using fluorouracil, hydroxyurea, semustine, dacarbazine, razoxane, and mitomycin. A phase III trial by the Eastern Cooperative Oncology Group. Am J Clin Oncol 1984; 7:313–318.

450. Engstrom PF, MacIntyre JM, Schutt AJ, et al. Chemotherapy of large bowel carcinoma—fluorouracil plus hydroxyurea vs methyl-CCNU, oncovin, fluorouracil and streptozotocin. An Eastern Cooperative Oncology Group Study. Am J Clin Oncol 1985;8:358–361.

451. Di Costanzo F, Gasperoni S, Malacarne P, et al. High-dose folinic acid and 5-fluorouracil alone or combined with hydroxyurea in advanced colorectal cancer. A randomized trial of the Italian Oncology Group For Clinical Research. Am J Clin Oncol 1998;21:369–375.

452. Santelli J, Valeriote F. In vivo potentiation of 5-fluorouracil cytotoxicity against AKR leukemia by purines, pyrimidines and their nucleosides and deoxynucleosides. J Natl Cancer Inst 1980;64:69–72.

453. Iigo M, Kuretani K, Hoshi A. Relationship between antitumor effect and metabolites of 5-fluorouracil in combination treatment with 5-fluorouracil and guanosine in ascites sarcoma 180 tumor system. Cancer Res 1983;43:5687–5694.

454. Iigo M, Yamaizumi Z, Nishimura S, et al. Mechanism of potentiation of antitumor activity of 5-fluorouracil by guanine ribonucleotides against adenocarcinoma 755. Eur J Cancer Clin Oncol 1987;23:1059–1065.

455. Parker WB, Klubes P. Enhancement by uridine of the anabolism of 5-fluorouracil in mouse T-lymphoma (S-49) cells. Cancer Res 1985;45:4249–4256.

456. Tuchman M, Ramnaraine ML, O'Dea RF. Effects of uridine and thymidine on the degradation of 5-fluorouracil, uracil and thymine by rat liver dihydropyrimidine dehydrogenase. Cancer Res 1985;45:5553–5556.

457. Nabeya Y, Isono K, Moriyama Y, et al. Ribose-transfer activity from uridine to 5-fluorouracil in Ehrlich ascites tumor cells. Jpn J Cancer Res 1990;81:692–700.

458. Chu MYW, Naguib FNM, Iltzsch MH, et al. Potentiation of FdUrd antineoplastic activity by the uridine phosphorylase inhibitors benzylacyclouridine and benzyloxybenzylacyclouridine. Cancer Res 1984;44:1852–1856.

459. Darnowski JW, Handschumacher RE. Tissue-specific enhancement of uridine utilization and 5-fluorouracil therapy in mice by benzylacyclouridine. Cancer Res 1985;45: 5364–5368.

460. Pu T, Robertson JM, Lawrence TS. Current status of radiation sensitization by fluorinated pyrimidines. Oncology (Basel) 1995;9:707–735.

461. Garrett C, Wataya Y, Santi D. Thymidylate synthetase. Catalysis of dehalogenation of 5-bromo- and 5-iodo-2′-deoxyuridylate. Biochemistry 1979;18:2784–2798.

462. Heidelberger C, Griesback I, Ghobar A. The potentiation of 5-iodo-2′-deoxyuridine of the tumor-inhibitory activity of 5-fluoro-2′-deoxyuridine. Cancer Chemother Rep 1960;6: 37–38.

463. Benson AB, Trump DL, Cummings KB, et al. Modulation of 5-iodo-2′-deoxyuridine metabolism and cytotoxicity in human bladder cancer cells by fluoropyrimidines. Biochem Pharmacol 1985;34:3925–3931.

464. Mancini WR, Stetson PL, Lawrence TS, et al. Variability of 5-bromo-2′-deoxyuridine incorporation into DNA of human glioma cell lines and modulation with fluoropyrimidines. Cancer Res 1991;51:870–874.

465. Lawrence TS, Davis MA, Maybaum J, et al. Modulation of iodo-deoxyuridine-mediated radiosensitization by 5-fluorouracil in human colon cancer cells. Int J Radiat Oncol Biol Phys 1992; 22:449–503.

466. Vazquez-Padua MA, Risueno C, Fischer PH. Regulation of the activation of fluorodeoxyuridine by substrate competition and feedback inhibition in 647V cells. Cancer Res 1989;49: 618–624.

467. Calabresi P, Creasey WA, Prusoff WH, et al. Clinical and pharmacological studies with 5-iodo-2'-deoxyuridine. Cancer Res 1963;23:583–592.

468. Papac R, Jacobs E, Wong F, et al. Clinical evaluation of the pyrimidine nucleosides 5-fluoro-2'-deoxyuridine and 5- iodo-2'-deoxyuridine. Cancer Chemother Rep 1962;20:143–146.

469. Young CW, Ellison RR, Sullivan RD, et al. The clinical evaluation of 5-fluorouracil and 5-fluoro-2'-deoxyuridine in solid tumors in adults. Cancer Chemother Rep 1960;6:17–20.

470. Kinsella TJ, Russo A, Mitchell JB, et al. A phase I study of intravenous iododeoxyuridine as a clinical radiosensitizer. Int J Radiat Oncol Biol Phys 1985;11:1941–1946.

471. Kinsella TJ, Collins J, Rowland J, et al. Pharmacology and phase I/II study of continuous intravenous infusions of iododeoxyuridine and hyperfractionated radiotherapy in patients with glioblastoma multiforme. J Clin Oncol 1988;6:871–879.

472. Belanger K, Klecker RW Jr, Rowland J, et al. Incorporation of iododeoxyuridine into DNA of granulocytes in patients. Cancer Res 1986;46:6509–6512.

473. Speth PA, Kinsella TJ, Chang AE, et al. Selective incorporation of iododeoxyuridine into DNA of hepatic metastases versus normal human liver. Clin Pharmacol Ther 1988;44:369–375.

474. Speth PA, Kinsella TJ, Belanger K, et al. Fluorodeoxyuridine modulation of the incorporation of iododeoxyuridine into DNA of granulocytes. A phase I and clinical pharmacology study. Cancer Res 1988;48:2933–2937.

475. McGinn CJ, Kunugi KA, Tutsch KD, et al. Leucovorin modulation of 5-iododeoxyuridine radiosensitization. A phase I study. Clin Cancer Res 1986;2:1299–1305.

476. Remick SC, Benson AB, Weese JL, et al. Phase I trial of hepatic artery infusion of 5-iodo-2'-deoxyuridine and 5-fluorouracil in patients with advanced hepatic malignancy. Biochemically based combination therapy. Cancer Res 1989;49:6437–6442.

477. Pastor-Anglada M, Felipe A, Casado FJ. Transport and mode of action of nucleoside derivatives used in chemical and antiviral therapies. Trends Pharmacol Sci 1998;19:424-440.

478. Grem JL, Fischer PH. Augmentation of 5-fluorouracil cytotoxicity in human colon cancer cells by dipyridamole. Cancer Res 1985;45:2967–2972.

479. Grem JL, Fischer PH. Modulation of fluorouracil metabolism and cytotoxicity by nitrobenzylthioinosine. Biochem Pharmacol 1986;35:2651–2654.

480. Grem JL, Fischer PH. Alteration of fluorouracil metabolism in human colon cancer cells by dipyridamole with a selective increase in fluorodeoxyuridine monophosphate levels. Cancer Res 1986;46:6191–6199.

481. Budd GT, Jayaraj A, Grabowski D, et al. Phase I trial of dipyridamole with 5-fluorouracil and folinic acid. Cancer Res 1990;50:7206–7211.

482. Fischer PH, Willson JKV, Risueno C, et al. Biochemical assessment of the effects of acivicin and dipyridamole given as a continuous 72-hour intravenous infusion. Cancer Res 1988;48:5591–5596.

483. Bailey H, Wilding G, Tutsch KD, et al. A phase I trial of 5- fluorouracil, leucovorin, and dipyridamole given by concurrent 120-h continuous infusions. Cancer Chemother Pharmacol 1992;30:297–302.

484. Willson JKV, Fischer PH, Remick SC, et al. Methotrexate and dipyridamole combination chemotherapy based upon inhibition of nucleoside salvage in humans. Cancer Res 1989;49:1866–1889.

485. Köhne C-H, Hiddemann W, Schüller J, et al. Failure of orally administered dipyridamole to enhance the antineoplastic activity of fluorouracil in combination with leucovorin in patients with advanced colorectal cancer. A prospective randomized trial. J Clin Oncol 1995;13:1201–1208.

486. Scanlon KJ, Newman EM, Lu Y, et al. Biochemical basis for cisplatin and 5-fluorouracil synergism in human ovarian carcinoma cells. Proc Natl Acad Sci U S A 1986;83:8923–8925.

487. Pratesi G, Gianni L, Manzotti C, et al. Sequence dependence of the antitumor and toxic effects of 5-fluorouracil and cis-diamminedichloroplatinum combination on primary colon tumors in mice. Cancer Chemother Pharmacol 1988;20:237–241.

488. Esaki T, Nakano S, Tatsumoto T, et al. Inhibition by 5-fluorouracil of cis-diamminedichloroplatinum(II)-induced DNA interstrand cross-link removal in a HST-1 human squamous carcinoma cell line. Cancer Res 1992;52:6501–6506.

489. Tsai C-M, Hsiao S-H, Frey CM, et al. Combination cytotoxic effects of cis-diamminedichloroplatinum(II) and 5- fluorouracil with and without leucovorin against human non-small cell lung cancer cell lines. Cancer Res 1993; 53:1079–1084.

490. Johnston PG, Geoffroy F, Drake J, et al. The cellular interaction of 5-fluorouracil and cisplatin in a human colon carcinoma cell line. Eur J Cancer 1996;32A:2148–2154.

491. Araki H, Fukushima M, Kamiyama Y, Shirasaka T. Effect of consecutive lower-dose cisplatin in enhancement of 5-fluorouracil cytotoxicity in experimental tumor cells in vivo. Cancer Lett 200;160:185–191.

492. Shirasaka T, Shimamoto Y, Ohshimo H, et al. Metabolic basis of the synergistic antitumor activities of 5fluorouracil and cisplatin in rodent tumor cells models in vivo. Cancer Chemother Pharmacol 1993;32:167–172.

493. Lokich JJ, Ahlgren HD, Cantrell J, et al. A prospective randomized comparison of protracted infusional 5-fluorouracil with or without weekly bolus cisplatin in metastatic colorectal carcinoma. Cancer 1991;67:14–19.

494. Diaz-Rubio E, Jimeno J, Anton A, et al. A prospective randomized trial of continuous infusion 5-fluorouracil (5-FU) versus 5-FU plus cisplatin in patients with advanced colorectal cancer. A trial of the Spanish Cooperative Group for Digestive Tract Tumor Therapy (T.T.D.). Am J Clin Oncol 1992;15:56–60.

495. Hansen RM, Ryan L, Anderson T, et al. Phase III study of bolus versus infusion fluorouracil with or without cisplatin in advanced colorectal cancer. J Natl Cancer Inst 1996;88:668–674.

496. Raymond E, Buquet-Fagot F, Djelloul C, et al. Antitumor activity of oxaliplatin in combination with 5-fluorouracil and the thymidylate synthase inhibitor AG337 in human colon, breast and ovarian cancers. Anticancer Drugs 1997;8:876–885.

497. Fischel JL, Etienne MC, Formento P, et al. Search for the optimal schedule for the oxaliplatin/5-fluorouracil association modulated or not by folinic acid. Preclinical data. Clin Cancer Res 1998;4:2529–2535.

498. Fischel JL, Formento P, Ciccolini J, et al. Impact of the oxaliplatin-5-luorouracil-folinic acid combination on respective intracellular determinants of drug activity. Br J Cancer 2002;86:1162–1168.

499. Yeh K-H, Cheng A-L, Wan J-P, et al. Down-regulation of thymidylate synthase expression and its steady-state mRNA by oxaliplatin in colon cancer cells. Anti-Cancer Drugs 2004;15:371–376.

500. de Gramont A, Figer A, Seymour M, et al. Leucovorin and fluorouracil with or without oxaliplatin as first-line treatment in advanced colorectal cancer. J Clin Oncol 2000; 18:2938–2947.

501. Andre T, Boni C, Mounedji-Boudiaf L, Navarro M, Tabernero J, Hickish T, et al. Oxaliplatin, fluorouracil, and leucovorin as adjuvant treatment for colon cancer. N Engl J Med 2004; 350:2343–2351.

502. Kano Y, Akutsu M, Tsunoda S, et al. Schedule-dependent interaction between paclitaxel and 5-fluorouracil in human carcinoma cell lines in vitro. Br J Cancer 1996;74:704–710.

503. Johnson KR, Wang L, Miller MC III, et al. 5-Fluorouracil interferes with paclitaxel cytotoxicity against human solid tumor cells. Clin Cancer Res 1997;3:1739–1745.

504. Grem JL, Nguyen D, Monahan BP, et al. Sequence-dependent antagonism between fluorouracil and paclitaxel in human breast cancer cells. Biochem Pharmacol 1999;58:477–486.

505. Houghton JA, Cheshire PJ, Hallman II JD, et al. Evaluation of irinotecan in combination with 5-fluorouracil or etoposide in xenograft models of colon adenocarcinoma and rhabdomyosarcoma. Clin Cancer Res 1996;2:107–118.

506. Guichard S, Cussac D, Hennebelle I, et al. Sequence-dependent activity of the irinotecan-5FU combination in human colon-cancer model HT-29 in vitro and in vivo. Int J Cancer 1997; 73: 729–734.

507. Aschele C, Baldo C, Sobrero AF, et al. Schedule-dependent synergism between raltitrexed and irinotecan in human colon cancer cells in vitro. Clin Cancer Res 1998;4: 1323–1330.

508. Pavillard V, Formento P, Rostagno P, et al. Combination of irinotecan (CPT11) and 5-fluorouracil with an analysis of cellular determinants of drug activity. Biochem Pharmacol 1998; 56:1315–1322.

509. Mans DR, Grivicich I, Peters GJ, Schwartsmann G. Sequence-dependent growth inhibition and DNA damage formation by the irinotecan-5-fluorouracil combination in human colon carcinoma cell lines. Eur J Cancer 1999;35:1851–1861.

510. Azrak RG, Cao S, Slocum HK, et al. Therapeutic synergy between irinotecan and 5-fluorouracil against human tumor xenografts. Clin Cancer Res 2004;10:1121–1129.

511. Heidelberger C, Griesvach L, Montag BJ, et al. Studies on fluorinated pyrimidines. II. Effects on transplanted tumors. Cancer Res 1958;18:305–317.

512. Byfield JE, Calabro-Jones P, Klisak I, et al. Pharmacologic requirements for obtaining sensitization of human tumor cells in vitro to combined 5-fluorouracil or ftorafur and x-rays. Int J Radiat Oncol Biol Phys 1982;8:1923–1933.

513. Weinberg MJ, Rauth AM. 5-Fluorouracil infusions and fractionated doses of radiation. Studies with a murine squamous cell carcinoma. Int J Radiat Oncol Biol Phys 1987;13:1691–1699.

514. Ishikawa T, Tanaka Y, Ishitsuka H, et al. Comparative antitumor activity of 5-fluorouracil and 5′-deoxyfluorouridine in combination with radiation therapy in mice bearing colon 26 adenocarcinoma. Cancer Res 1989;80:583–591.

515. Smalley SR, Kimler BF, Evans RG. 5-Fluorouracil modulation of radiosensitivity in cultured human carcinoma cells. Int J Radiat Oncol Biol Phys 1991;20:207–211.

516. Bruso CE, Shewach DS, Lawrence TS. Fluorodeoxyuridine-induced radiosensitization and inhibition of DNA double-strand break repair in human colon cancer cells. Int J Radiat Oncol Biol Phys 1990;19:1411–1417.

517. Lawrence T, Heimburger D, Shewach DL. The effects of leucovorin and dipyridamole on fluoropyrimidine-induced radiosensitization. Int J Radiat Oncol Biol Phys 1991;20:377–381.

518. Miller EM, Kinsella TJ. Radiosensitization by fluorodeoxyuridine. Effects of thymidylate synthase inhibition and cell synchronization. Cancer Res 1992;52:1687–1694.

519. Davis MA, Tang HY, Maybaum J, et al. Dependence of fluorodeoxyuridine-mediated radiosensitization on S phase progression. Int J Radiat Biol 1995;67:509–517.

520. Lawrence TS, Davis MA, Loney TL. Fluoropyrimidine-mediated radiosensitization depends on cyclin E-dependent kinase activation. Cancer Res 1996;56:3203–3206.

521. Lawrence TS, Tepper JE, Blackstock AW. Fluoropyrimidine-radiation interactions in cells and tumors. Semin Radiat Oncol 1997;7:260–266.

522. Bartelink H, Roelofsen F, Eschwege F, et al. Concomitant radiotherapy and chemotherapy is superior to radiotherapy alone in the treatment of locally advanced anal cancer. Results of a phase III randomized trial of the European Organization for Research and Treatment of Cancer Radiotherapy and Gastrointestinal Cooperative Groups. J Clin Oncol 1997;15:2040–2049.

523. Morris M, Eifel PJ, Lu J, et al. Pelvic radiation with concurrent chemotherapy compared with pelvic and para-aortic radiation for high-risk cervical cancer. N Engl J Med 1999;340:1137–1143.

524. Cooper JS, Guo MD, Herskovic A, et al. Chemoradiotherapy of locally advanced esophageal cancer. Long-term follow-up of a prospective randomized trial (RTOG 85-01). Radiation Therapy Oncology Group. JAMA 1999;281:1623–1627.

525. O'Connell MJ, Martenson JA, Wieand HS, et al. Improving adjuvant therapy for rectal cancer by combining protracted infusion fluorouracil with radiation therapy after curative surgery. N Engl J Med 1994;33:502–507.

526. Au JL, Sadee W. The pharmacology of ftorafur. Recent Results Cancer Res 1981;76:100–114.

527. Benvenuto JA, Liehr JG, Winkler T, et al. Human urinary metabolites of 1-(tetrahydro-2-furanyl)-5-fluorouracil (ftorafur). Cancer Res 1980;40:2814–2870.

528. El Sayed YM, Sadee W. Metabolic activation of ftorafur. the microsomal oxidative pathway. Biochem Pharmacol 1982;31:3006–3008.

529. El Sayed YM, Sadee W. Metabolic activation of R,S-1-(tetrahydro-2-furanyl)-5-fluorouracil (ftorafur) to 5-fluorouracil by soluble enzymes. Cancer Res 1983;43:4039–4044.

530. Komatsu T, Yamazaki H, Shimada N, et al. Roles of cytochrome P450 1A2, 2A6, and 2C8 in 5-fluorouracil formation from tegafur, an anti-cancer prodrug, in human liver microsomes. Drug Metab Dispos 2000;28:1457–1463.

531. Komatsu T, Yamazaki H, Shimada N, et al. Involvement of microsomal cytochrome P450 and cytosolic thymidine phosphorylase in 5-fluorouracil formation from tegafur in human liver. Clin Cancer Res 2001;7:675–681.

532. Fuji S, Ikenaka K, Fukushima M, et al. Effect of uracil and its derivatives on antitumor activity of 5-fluorouracil and 1-(2-tetrahydrofuryl)-5-fluorouracil. Jpn J Cancer Res 1979; 69:763–772.

533. Benvenuto J, Lu K, Hall SW, et al. Metabolism of 1-(tetrahydro-2-furanyl)-5-fluorouracil (ftorafur). Cancer Res 1978;38:3867–3870.

534. Hall SW, Valdivieso M, Benjamin RS. Intermittent high single dose ftorafur. A phase I clinical trial with pharmacologic- toxicity correlations. Cancer Treat Rep 1977;61:1495–1498.

535. Antilla MI, Sotaniemi EA, Kaiaralcoma MI, et al. Pharmacokinetics of ftorafur after intravenous and oral administration. Cancer Chemother Pharmacol 1983;10:150–153.

536. Hornbeck CL, Griffiths JC, Floyd RA, et al. Serum concentrations of 5-FU, ftorafur, and a major serum metabolite following ftorafur chemotherapy. Cancer Treat Rep 1981;65:69–72.

537. Blokhina NG, Vozny EK, Garin AM. Results of treatment of malignant tumors with ftorafur. Cancer 1972;30:390–392.

538. Friedman MA, Ignoffo RJ. A review of the United States clinical experience of the fluoropyrimidine, ftorafur (NSC 148958). Cancer Treat Rev 1980;7:205–213.

539. Ansfield FJ, Kallas GJ, Singson JP. Phase I–II studies of oral tegafur (ftorafur). J Clin Oncol 1983;1:107–110.

540. Kajanti MJ, Pyrhönen SO, Maiche AG. Oral tegafur in the treatment of metastatic breast cancer. A phase II study. Eur J Cancer 1993;29A:863–866.

541. Palmeri S, Gebbia V, Russo A, et al. Oral tegafur in the treatment of gastrointestinal tract cancers. A phase II study. Br J Cancer 1990;61:475–478.

542. Bjerkeset T, Fjosne HE. Comparison of oral ftorafur and intravenous 5-fluorouracil in patients with advanced cancer of the stomach, colon or rectum. Oncology 1986;43:212–215.

543. Manzuik LV, Perevodchikova NI, Gorbunova VA, et al. Initial clinical experience with oral ftorafur and oral 6R,S-leucovorin in advanced colorectal carcinoma. Eur J Cancer 1993;29A:1793–1794.

544. Tang SG, Hornbeck CL, Byfield JE. Enhanced accumulation of 5-fluorouracil in human tumors in athymic mice by co-administration of ftorafur and uracil. Int J Radiat Oncol Biol Phys 1984;10:1687–1689.

545. Ho DH, Cobington WP, Pazdur R, et al. Clinical pharmacology of combined oral uracil and ftorafur. Drug Metab Dispos 1992;20:936–940.

546. Fujita K, Munakata A. Concentration of 5-fluorouracil in renal cells from cancer patients administered a mixture of 1-(2-tetrahydrofuryl)-5-fluorouracil and uracil. Int J Clin Pharmacol Res 1991;11:171–174.

547. Takayama H, Konami T, Konishi T, et al. Studies on 5-FU concentration in serum and bladder tumor tissue after oral administration of UFT. Acta Urol Jpn 1986;32:1449–1453.

548. Basaki Y, Chikahisa L, Aoyagi K, et al. gamma-Hydroxybutyric acid and 5-fluorouracil, metabolites of UFT, inhibit the angiogenesis induced by vascular endothelial growth factor. Angiogenesis 2001;4(3):163–173.

549. Ota K, Taguchi T, Kimura K. Report on nationwide pooled data and cohort investigation in UFT phase II study. Cancer Chemother Pharmacol 1988;22:333–338.

550. Ho DH, Pazdur R, Covington W, et al. Comparison of 5-fluorouracil pharmacokinetics in patients receiving continuous 5-fluorouracil infusion and oral uracil plus N1-(2′-tetrahydrofuryl)-5-fluorouracil. Clin Cancer Res 1998;4:2085–2088.

551. Muggia FM, Wu X, Spicer D, et al. Phase I and pharmacokinetic study of oral UFT, a combination of the 5-fluorouracil prodrug tegafur and uracil. Clin Cancer Res 1996;2:1461–1467.

552. Pazdur R, Lassere Y, Rhodes V, et al. Phase II trial of uracil and tegafur plus oral leucovorin. An effective oral regimen in the treatment of metastatic colorectal carcinoma. J Clin Oncol 1994;12:2296–2300.

553. Gonzalez Baron M, Feliu J, Garcia Giron C, et al. UFT modulated with leucovorin in advanced colorectal cancer. Oncopaz experience. Oncology 1997;54:24–29.

554. Ichikura T, Tomimatsu S, Okusa Y, et al. Thymidylate synthase inhibition by an oral regimen consisting of tegafur- uracil (UFT) and low-dose leucovorin for patients with gastric cancer. Cancer Chemother Pharmacol 1996;38:401–405.

555. Meropol NJ, Sonnichsen DS, Birkhofer MJ, et al. Bioavailability and phase II study of oral UFT plus leucovorin in patients with relapsed or refractory colorectal cancer. Cancer Chemother Pharmacol 1999;43:221–226.

556. Sulkes A, Benner SE, Canetta RM. Uracil-ftorafur. An oral fluoropyrimidine active in colorectal cancer. J Clin Oncol 1998;16: 3461–3475.

557. Carmichael J, Tadeusz P, Radstone D, et al. Randomized comparative study of tegafur/uracil and oral leucovorin versus parenteral fluorouracil and leucovorin in patients with previously untreated metastatic colorectal cancer. J Clin Oncol 2002;20: 3617–3627.

558. Douillard J-Y, Hoff PM, Skillings JR, et al. Multicenter phase III study of uracil/tegafur and oral leucovorin versus fluorouracil and leucovorin in patients with previously untreated metastatic colorectal cancer. J Clin Oncol 2002;20:3605–3616.

559. Eda H, Fujimoto K, Watanabe S-I, et al. Cytokines induce uridine phosphorylase in mouse colon 26 carcinoma cells and make the cells more susceptible to 5'-deoxy-5-fluorouridine. Jpn J Cancer Res 1993;84:341–347.

560. Eda H, Fujimoto K, Watanabe S-I, et al. Cytokines induce thymidine phosphorylase in tumor cells and make the cells more susceptible to 5'-deoxy-5-fluorouridine. Cancer Chemother Pharmacol 1993;32:333–339.

561. Armstrong RD, Cadman E. 5'-Deoxyfluorouridine selective toxicity for human tumor cells compared to human bone marrow. Cancer Res 1983;43:2525–2528.

562. Miwa M, Nishimura J, Kayamiyama T, et al. Conversion of 5'-deoxyuridine to 5-FU by pyrimidine nucleoside phosphorylase in normal and tumor tissues from rodents bearing tumors and cancer patients. Jpn J Cancer Chemother 1987;14:2924–2929.

563. Peters GJ, Braakhuis BJM, de Bruijn EA, et al. Enhanced therapeutic efficacy of 5'-deoxy-5-fluorouridine in 5-fluorouracil resistant head and neck tumours in relation to 5-fluorouracil metabolising enzymes. Br J Cancer 1989;59:327–334.

564. Nio Y, Kimura H, Tsubone M, et al. Antitumor activity of 5'-deoxy-5-fluorouridine in human digestive organ cancer xenografts and pyrimidine nucleoside phosphorylase activity in normal and neoplastic tissues from human digestive organs. Anticancer Res 1992;12:1141–1146.

565. el Khouni MH, el Kouni MM, Naguib NM. Differences in activities and substrate specificity of human and murine pyrimidine nucleoside phosphorylases. Implications for chemotherapy with 5 fluoropyrimidines. Cancer Res 1993;53:3687–3693.

566. el Khouni MH, Naguib FNM, Chu SH, et al. Effect of the n-glycosidic bond conformation and modifications in the pentose moiety on the binding of nucleoside ligands to uridine phosphorylase. Mol Pharmacol 1988;34:104–110.

567. Veres Z, Szabolcs A, Szinai I, et al. Enzymatic cleavage of 5- substituted-2'-deoxyuridines by pyrimidine nucleoside phosphorylases. Biochem Pharmacol 1986;35:1057–1059.

568. Vertongen F, Fondu P, Van den Heule B, et al. Thymidine kinase and thymidine phosphorylase activities in various types of leukemia and lymphoma. Tumour Biol 1984;5:303–311.

569. de Bruijn EA, van Oosterom AT, Tjaden UR, et al. Pharmacology of 5'-deoxy-5-fluorouridine in patients with resistant ovarian cancer. Cancer Res 1985;45:5931–5935.

570. Schaaf LJ, Dobbs BR, Edwards IR, et al. The pharmacokinetics of doxifluridine and 5-fluorouracil after single intravenous infusions of doxifluridine to patients with colorectal cancer. Eur J Clin Pharmacol 1988;34:439–443.

571. Malet-Martino MC, Servin P, Bernadou J, et al. Human urinary excretion of doxifluridine and metabolites during a 5-day

572. Martino R, Bernadou J, Malet-Martino MC, et al. Excretion of doxifluridine catabolites in human bile assessed by 19F NMR spectrometry. Biomed Pharmacother 1987;41:104–106.

573. Reece PA, Olver IN, Morris RG, et al. Pharmacokinetic study of doxifluridine given by 5-day stepped-dose infusion. Cancer Chemother Pharmacol 1990;25:274–278.

574. Abele R, Alberto P, Seematter RJ, et al. Phase I clinical study with 5'-deoxy-5-fluorouridine, a new fluoropyrimidine derivative. Cancer Treat Rep 1982;1307–1313.

575. Hurteloup P, Armand JP, Cappelaere P, et al. Phase II clinical evaluation of doxifluridine. Cancer Treat Rep 1986;70:1339–1340.

576. Fossa SD, Dahl O, Hoel R, et al. Doxifluridine (5'dFUR) in patients with advanced colorectal carcinoma. Cancer Chemother Pharmacol 1985;15:161–163.

577. Alberto P, Mermillod B, Germano G, et al. A randomized comparison of doxifluridine and fluorouracil in colorectal cancer. Eur J Cancer Clin Oncol 1998;24:559–563.

578. Alberto P, Jungi WF, Siegenthaler P, et al. A phase II study of doxifluridine in patients with advanced breast cancer. Eur J Cancer Clin Oncol 1988;24:565–566.

579. Heier MS, Fossa SD. Wernicke-Korsakoff-like syndrome in patients with colorectal carcinoma treated with high-dose doxifluridine. Acta Neurol Scand 1986;73:449–457.

580. Schuster D, Heim ME, Dombernowski P, et al. Prospective randomized phase III trial of doxifluridine versus 5-fluorouracil in patients with advanced colorectal cancer. Onkologie 1991;14: 333–337.

581. Bajetta E, Colleoni M, Rosso R, et al. Prospective randomised trial comparing fluorouracil versus doxifluridine for the treatment of advanced colorectal cancer. Eur J Cancer 1993;29A: 1658–1663.

582. Alberto P, Winkelmann JJ, Paschoud N, et al. Phase I study of oral doxifluridine using two schedules. Eur J Cancer Clin Oncol 1989;25:905–908.

583. Bajetta E, Colleoni M, Di Bartolomeo M, et al. Doxifluridine and leucovorin. An oral treatment combination in advanced colorectal cancer. J Clin Oncol 1995;13:2613–2619.

584. Dooley M, Goa KL. Capecitabine. Drugs 1999;58(1):69–76.

585. Tabata T, Katoh M, Tokudome S, et al. Bioactivation of capecitabine in human liver: involvement of the cytosolic enzyme on 5'-deoxy-5-fluorocytidine formation. Drug Metab Dispos 2004;32(7):762–767.

586. Tabata T, Katoh M, Tokudome S, et al. Identification of the cytosolic carboxylesterase catalyzing the 5'-deoxy-5-fluorocytidine formation from capecitabine in human liver. Drug Metab Dispos 2004 32():1103–1110.

587. Budman DR, Meropol NJ, Reigner B, et al. Preliminary studies of a novel oral fluoropyrimidine carbamate. Capecitabine. J Clin Oncol 1998;16:1795–1802.

588. Mackean M, Planting A, Twelves C, et al. Phase I and pharmacologic study of intermittent twice-daily oral therapy with capecitabine in patients with advanced and/or metastatic cancer. J Clin Oncol 1998;16:2977–2985.

589. Judson IR, Beale PJ, Trigo JM, et al. A human capecitabine excretion balance and pharmacokinetic study after administration of a single oral dose of 14C-labelled drug. Invest New Drugs 1999;17(1):49–56.

590. Miwa M, Ura M, Nishida M, et al. Design of a novel oral fluoropyrimidine carbamate, capecitabine, which generates 5-fluorouracil selectively in tumours by enzymes concentrated in human liver and cancer tissue. Eur J Cancer 1998;34:1274–1281.

591. Ishikawa T, Utoh M, Sawada N, et al. Tumor selective delivery of 5-fluorouracil by capecitabine, a new oral fluoropyrimidine carbamate, in human cancer xenografts. Biochem Pharmacol 1998;55:1091–1097.

592. Ishikawa T, Sekiguchi F, Fukase Y, et al. Positive correlation between the efficacy of capecitabine and doxifluridine and the ratio of thymidine phosphorylase to dihydropyrimidine dehydrogenase activities in tumors in human cancer xenografts. Cancer Res 1998;58:685–690.

593. Tsukamoto Y, Kato Y, Ura M, et al. Investigation of 5-FU disposition after oral administration of capecitabine, a triple-prodrug

of 5-FU, using a physiologically based pharmacokinetic model in a human cancer xenograft model: comparison of the simulated 5-FU exposures in the tumour tissue between human and xenograft model. Biopharm Drug Dispos 2001; 22(1):1–14.

594. Chung YL, Troy H, Judson IR, et al. Noninvasive measurements of capecitabine metabolism in bladder tumors overexpressing thymidine phosphorylase by fluorine-19 magnetic resonance spectroscopy. Clin Cancer Res 2004;10: 3863–3870.

595. Mori K, Hasegawa M, Nishida M, et al. Expression levels of thymidine phosphorylase and dihydropyrimidine dehydrogenase in various human tumor tissues. Int J Oncol 2000;17: 33–38.

596. Cassidy J, Dirix L, Bissett D, et al. A Phase I study of capecitabine in combination with oral leucovorin in patients with intractable solid tumors. Clin Cancer Res 1998;4:2755–2761.

597. Saif MW, Quinn MG, Thomas RR, et al. Cardiac toxicity associated with capecitabine therapy. Acta Oncol 2003;42:342–344.

598. Walkhorm B, Fraunfelder FT. Severe ocular irritation and corneal deposits associated with capecitabine use. New Eng J Med 2004;343:740–741.

599. Couch LS, Groteluschen DL, Stewart JA, et al. Capecitabine-related neurotoxicity presenting as trismus. Clin Colorectal Cancer 2003;3:121–123.

600. Schuller J, Cassidy J, Dumont E, et al. Preferential activation of capecitabine in tumor following oral administration to colorectal cancer patients. Cancer Chemother Pharmacol 2000;45: 291–297.

601. Nishimura G, Terada I, Kobayashi T, et al. Thymidine phosphorylase and dihydropyrimidine dehydrogenase levels in primary colorectal cancer show a relationship to clinical effects of 5'-deoxy-5-fluorouridine as adjuvant chemotherapy. Oncol Rep 2002;9:479–482.

602. Reigner B, Blesch K, Weidekamm E. Clinical pharmacokinetics of capecitabine. Clin Pharmacokinet 2001;40:85–104.

603. Reigner B, Verweij J, Dirix L, et al. Effect of food on the pharmacokinetics of capecitabine and its metabolites following oral administration in cancer patients. Clin Cancer Res 1998;4: 941–948.

604. Twelves C, Glynne-Jones R, Cassidy J, et al. Effect of hepatic dysfunction due to liver metastases on the pharmacokinetics of capecitabine and its metabolites. Clin Cancer Res 1999;5: 1696–1702.

605. Poole C, Gardiner J, Twelves C, et al. Effect of renal impairment on the pharmacokinetics and tolerability of capecitabine (Xeloda) in cancer patients. Cancer Chemother Pharmacol 2002;49:225–234.

606. Xu Y, Grem JL. Liquid chromatography-mass spectrometry method for the analysis of the anti-cancer agent capecitabine and its nucleoside metabolites in human plasma. J Chromatogr B Analyt Technol Biomed Life Sci 2003;783(1): 273–285.

607. Zufia L, Aldaz A, Giraldez J. Simple determination of capecitabine and its metabolites by liquid chromatography with ultraviolet detection in a single injection. J Chromatogr B Analyt Technol Biomed Life Sci 2004;809:51–58.

608. van Laarhoven HW, Klomp DW, Kamm YJ, et al. In vivo monitoring of capecitabine metabolism in human liver by 19fluorine magnetic resonance spectroscopy at 1.5 and 3 Tesla field strength. Cancer Res 2003;63:7609–7612.

609. Mader RM, Schrolnberger C, Rizovski B, et al. Penetration of capecitabine and its metabolites into malignant and healthy tissues of patients with advanced breast cancer. Br J Cancer 2003;88:782–787.

610. Hoff PM, Ansari R, Batist G, et al. Comparison of oral capecitabine versus intravenous fluorouracil plus leucovorin as first-line treatment in 605 patients with metastatic colorectal cancer: results of a randomized phase III study. J Clin Oncol 2001;19:2282–2292.

611. Van Cutsem E, Twelves C, Cassidy J, et al. Oral capecitabine compared with intravenous fluorouracil plus leucovorin in patients with metastatic colorectal cancer: results of a large phase III study. J Clin Oncol 2001;19:4097–4106

612. Endo M, Shinbori N, Fukase Y, et al. Induction of thymidine phosphorylase expression and enhancement of efficacy of capecitabine or 5'-deoxy-5-fluorouridine by cyclophosphamide in mammary tumor models. Int J Cancer 1999;83: 127–134.

613. Blanquicett C, Gillespie GY, Nabors LB, et al. Induction of thymidine phosphorylase in both irradiated and shielded, contralateral human U87MG glioma xenografts: implications for a dual modality treatment using capecitabine and irradiation. Mol Cancer Ther 2002;1:1139–1145.

614. Xiao YS, Tang ZY, Fan J, et al. Interferon-alpha 2a up-regulated thymidine phosphorylase and enhanced antitumor effect of capecitabine on hepatocellular carcinoma in nude mice. J Cancer Res Clin Oncol 2004;130:546–550.

615. Magne N, Fischel JL, Dubreuil A, et al. ZD1839 (Iressa) modifies the activity of key enzymes linked to fluoropyrimidine activity: rational basis for a new combination therapy with capecitabine. Clin Cancer Res 2003;9:4735–4742.

616. Porter DJ, Chestnut WG, Merrill BM, et al. Mechanism- based inactivation of dihydropyrimidine dehydrogenase by 5-ethynyluracil. J Biol Chem 1992;267:5236–5242.

617. Spector T, Harrington JA, Porter DJ. 5-Ethynyluracil (776C85). Inactivation of dihydropyrimidine dehydrogenase in vivo. Biochem Pharmacol 1993;46:2243–2248.

618. Baccanari DP, Davis ST, Knick VC, et al. 5-Ethynyluracil (776C85). A potent modulator of the pharmacokinetics and antitumor efficacy of 5-fluorouracil. Proc Natl Acad Sci U S A 1993;90:11064–11068.

619. Cao S, Rustum YM, Spector T. 5-Ethynyluracil (776C85). Modulation of 5-fluorouracil efficacy and therapeutic index in rats bearing advanced colorectal carcinoma. Cancer Res 1994; 54:1507–1510.

620. Spector T, Cao S, Rustum YM, et al. Attenuation of the antitumor activity of 5-fluorouracil by (R)-5-fluoro-5,6- dihydrouracil. Cancer Res 1995;55:1239–1241.

621. Arellano M, Malet-Martino M, Martino R, et al. 5-Ethynyluracil (GW776). Effects on the formation of the toxic catabolites of 5-fluorouracil, fluoroacetate and fluorohydroxypropionic acid in the isolated perfused rat liver model. Br J Cancer 1997;76: 1170–1180.

622. Adams ER, Leffert JJ, Craig DJ, et al. In vivo effect of 5- ethynyluracil on 5-fluorouracil metabolism determined by 19F nuclear magnetic resonance spectroscopy. Cancer Res 1999;59:122–127.

623. Schilsky RL, Hohneker J, Ratain MJ, et al. Phase I clinical and pharmacologic study of eniluracil plus fluorouracil in patients with advanced cancer. J Clin Oncol 1998;16:1450–1457.

624. Baker SD, Khor SP, Adjei AA, et al. Pharmacokinetic, oral bioavailability, and safety study of fluorouracil in patients treated with 776C85, an inactivator of dihydropyrimidine dehydrogenase. J Clin Oncol 1996;14:3085–3096.

625. Mani S, Hochster H, Beck T, et al. Multicenter phase II study to evaluate a 28-day regimen of oral fluorouracil plus eniluracil in the treatment of patients with previously untreated metastatic colorectal cancer. J Clin Oncol 2000;18:2894–2901.

626. Smith IE, Johnston SR, O'Brien ME, et al. Low-dose oral fluorouracil with eniluracil as first-line chemotherapy against advanced breast cancer: a phase II study. J Clin Oncol 2000; 18:2378–2384.

627. Schilsky RL, Levin J, West WH, et al. Randomized, open-label, phase III study of a 28-day oral regimen of eniluracil plus fluorouracil versus intravenous fluorouracil plus leucovorin as first-line therapy in patients with metastatic/advanced colorectal cancer. J Clin Oncol 2002;20:1519–1526.

628. Grem JL, Harold N, Shapiro J, et al. Phase I and pharmacokinetic trial of weekly oral fluorouracil given with eniluracil and low-dose leucovorin to patients with solid tumors. J Clin Oncol 2000;18:3952–3963.

629. Keith B, Guo XD, Zentko S, et al. Impact of two weekly schedules of oral eniluracil given with fluorouracil and leucovorin on the duration of dihydropyrimidine dehydrogenase inhibition. Clin Cancer Res 2002;8:1045–1050

630. Shirasaka T, Shimamato Y, Ohshimo H, et al. Development of a novel form of an oral 5-fluorouracil derivative (S-1) directed to the potentiation of the tumor selective cytotoxicity of

5-fluorouracil by two biochemical modulators. Anticancer Drugs 1996;7:548–557.

631. Fujii S, Fukushima M, Shimamoto Y, et al. Antitumor activity of BOF-A2, a new 5-fluorouracil derivative. Jpn J Cancer Res 1989; 80:173–181

632. Schöfski P. The modulated oral fluoropyrimidine prodrug S-1, and its use in gastrointestinal cancer and other solid tumors. Anti-Cancer Drugs 2004;15:85–106.

633. Sakamoto J, Kodaira S, Hamada C, et al. An individual patient data meta-analysis of long supported adjuvant chemotherapy with oral carmofur in patients with curatively resected colorectal cancer. Oncol Rep 2001;8:697–703.

634. Rich TA, Shepard RC, Mosley ST. Four decades of continuing innovation with fluorouracil: current and future approaches to fluorouracil chemoradiation therapy. J Clin Oncol 2004;22: 2214–2232.

635. Masci G, Magagnoli M, Zucali PA, et al. Minidose warfarin prophylaxis for catheter-associated thrombosis in cancer patients: can it be safely associated with fluorouracil-based chemotherapy? J Clin Oncol 2003;21:736–739.

636. Gilbar PJ, Brodribb TR. Phenytoin and fluorouracil interaction. Ann Pharmacother 2001;35:1367–1370.

637. Afsar A, Lee C, Riddick DS. Modulation of the expression of constitutive rat hepatic cytochrome P450 isozymes by 5-fluorouracil. Can J Physiol Pharmacol 1996;74: 150–156.

638. Zhou Q, Chan E. Effect of 5-fluorouracil on the anticoagulant activity and the pharmacokinetics of warfarin enantiomers in rats. Eur J Pharm Sci 2002;17:73-80.

639. Konishi H, Yoshimoto T, Morita K, et al. Depression of phenytoin metabolic capacity by 5-fluorouracil and doxifluridine in rats. J Pharm Pharmacol 2003;55:143–149.

Cytidine Analogues

8

David P. Ryan   Rocio Garcia-Carbonero
Bruce A. Chabner

Nucleoside analogs compete with their physiologic counterparts for incorporation into nucleic acids and have earned an important place in the treatment of acute leukemia. The most important of these are the arabinose nucleosides, a unique class of antimetabolites originally isolated from the sponge *Cryptothethya crypta*[1] but now produced synthetically.[2] They differ from the physiologic deoxyribonucleosides by the presence of a 2'-OH group in the *cis* configuration relative to the *N*-glycosyl bond between cytosine and the arabinose sugar (Fig. 8.1). Several arabinose nucleosides have useful antitumor and antiviral effects. The most active cytotoxic agent of this class is cytosine arabinoside (ara-C, cytarabine). A related nucleoside, adenine arabinoside, has antitumor and antiviral action,[3] and its analog, 2-fluoro-ara-adenosine monophosphate, has strong activity in lymphomas and in chronic lymphocytic leukemia.[4] Another member of the group is arabinosyl-5-azacytidine, a synthetic analog that failed in the clinic.[5]

CYTOSINE ARABINOSIDE

Ara-C is one of the most effective agents in the treatment of acute myelogenous leukemia[6] and is incorporated into virtually all standard induction regimens for this disease, generally in combination with an anthracycline (daunorubicin hydrochloride or idarubicin hydrochloride). Ara-C is also a component of consolidation and maintenance regimens in acute myelogenous leukemia after remission is attained. Clear clinical evidence now exists that a dose-response effect is present for ara-C, both as induction[7] and consolidation[8] therapy in acute myelogenous leukemia. High-dose ara-C confers particular benefit in patients with certain cytogenetic abnormalities related to the core binding factor that regulates hematopoiesis (t8:21, inv 16, del 16, t16:16)[9] (Table 8.1). Ara-C is also active against other

hematologic malignancies, including non-Hodgkin's lymphoma,[10] acute lymphoblastic leukemia,[11] and chronic myelogenous leukemia,[12] but has little activity as a single agent against solid tumors. This limited spectrum of activity has been attributed to the lack of metabolic activation of this agent in solid tumors and its selective action against rapidly dividing cells. The essential features of ara-C pharmacology are described in Table 8.2.

Mechanism of Action

Ara-C acts as an analog of deoxycytidine and has multiple effects on DNA synthesis. Ara-C undergoes phosphorylation to form arabinosylcytosine triphosphate (ara-CTP), which competitively inhibits DNA polymerase α in opposition to the normal substrate deoxycytidine 5'-triphosphate (dCTP).[13] This competitive inhibition has been demonstrated with crude DNA polymerase from calf thymus[13] and with purified enzyme from human leukemic cells,[14] as well as with enzyme from a variety of murine tumors.[15,16] Ara-CTP has an affinity for human leukemia cell DNA polymerase α in the range of 1×10^{-6} mol/L, and the inhibition is reversible in cell-free systems by the addition of dCTP or in intact cells by the addition of deoxycytidine, the precursor of dCTP.[17] When present at high intracellular concentrations, ara-CTP also inhibits DNA polymerase β.[18] The effects of ara-C on DNA polymerase activity extend not only to semiconservative DNA replication but also to DNA repair. Repair of ultraviolet light damage to DNA, a function that depends on polymerase α, is blocked more potently than the repair of photon-induced or γ radiation-induced strand breaks,[19,20] the repair of which is accomplished by a different polymerase. In addition to having an effect on eukaryotic DNA polymerases, ara-CTP is a potent inhibitor of viral RNA-directed DNA polymerase (K_i [inhibition constant] = 0.1 μmol/L).

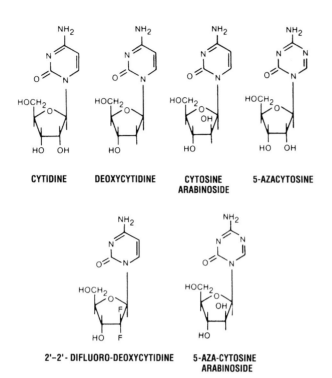

Figure 8.1   Structure of cytidine analogs.

More important than the effects of ara-C on DNA synthesis, however, is its incorporation into DNA, a feature that correlates closely with cytotoxicity[21,22] (Fig. 8.2). In fact, a preponderance of evidence suggests that this is the major cytotoxic lesion in ara-C–treated cells. Drugs that prevent ara-C incorporation into DNA, such as aphidicolin, also block its cytotoxicity.[23] A given level of ara-C incorporation can be achieved by various combinations of concentrations (C) and times (T) of exposure that yield a specific C × T product. A linear relationship exists between picomoles of ara-C incorporated and the log of cell survival for a wide range of drug concentrations and durations of exposure. Thus, drug toxicity is a direct function of incorporation into DNA, and the latter varies directly with the C × T product.[24] Once it is incorporated into DNA, tumor cells excise ara-C slowly,[25] and the incorporated ara-C inhibits template function and chain elongation.[23,26,27] In experiments with purified enzyme and calf thymus DNA, the consecutive incorporation of two ara-C or two arabinosyl-5-azacytidine (ara-5–aza-C) residues effectively stopped chain elongation by DNA polymerase α.[14] At high concentrations of ara-C, one finds a greater than expected proportion of ara-C residues at the 3′-terminus, which confirms a direct effect on chain termination.[25] These observations support the hypothesis that ara-C incorporation into DNA is a prerequisite for drug action and is responsible for cytotoxicity.

Ara-C also causes an unusual reiteration of DNA segments.[28] Human lymphocytes exposed to ara-C in culture synthesize small reduplicated segments of DNA, which results in multiple copies of limited portions of DNA. These reduplicated segments increase the possibility of recombination, crossover, and gene amplification; gaps and breaks are observed in karyotype preparations after ara-C treatment. The same mechanism, reiteration of DNA synthesis after its inhibition by an antimetabolite, may explain the high frequency of gene reduplication induced by methotrexate sodium, 5-fluorouracil, and hydroxyurea (see Chapters 6, 7, and 10). In summary, although ara-C has multiple effects on DNA synthesis, the most important effect seems to be its incorporation into DNA.

TABLE 8.1

COMPLETE REMISSION (CR) DURATION BY CYTOGENETIC GROUP ACCORDING TO CYTOSINE ARABINOSIDE (ARA-C) DOSE RANDOMIZATION

Cytogenetic Group	Ara-C Dose	No. of Patients	Median Time of CR (months)	% 5-year CR Estimate (95% CI)	% Cure Estimate
Group CBF[a]	3 g/m²	18	NR	78 (59–97)	66
	400 mg/m²	20	NR	57 (34–80)	52
	100 mg/m²	19	14.3	16 (0–32)	23
Group NL[b]	3 g/m²	45	18.2	40 (25–54)	47
	400 mg/m²	48	21.4	37 (13–51)	32
	100 mg/m²	47	12.5	20 (8–32)	12
Group other[c]	3 g/m²	27	13.3	21 (5–37)	17
	400 mg/m²	31	10.6	13 (1–25)	10
	100 mg/m²	30	9.6	13 (026)	3

[a]Core binding factor type [t(8;21), t(16;16), inv(16), and del(16)].
[b]Normal karyotype.
[c]Other karyotype abnormalities.
CI, confidence interval; NR, not reached.

TABLE 8.2

KEY FEATURES OF CYTOSINE ARABINOSIDE (ARA-C) PHARMACOLOGY

Factor	Result
Mechanism of action	Inhibits DNA polymerase α, is incorporated into DNA, and terminates DNA chain elongation
Metabolism	Activated to triphosphate in tumor cells. Degraded to inactive ara-U by deamination
	Converted to ara-CDP choline derivative
Pharmacokinetics	Plasma: $t_{1/2}\alpha$ 7–20 min, $t_{1/2}\beta$ 2 hr; CSF: $t_{1/2}$ 2 hr
Elimination	Deamination in liver, plasma, and peripheral tissues—100%
Drug interactions	Methotrexate sodium increases ara-CTP formation
	Tetrahydrouridine, 3-deazauridine inhibits deamination
	Ara-C blocks DNA repair, enhances activity of alkylating agents
	Fludarabine phosphate increases ara-CTP formation
Toxicity	Myelosuppression
	Gastrointestinal epithelial ulceration
	Intrahepatic cholestasis, pancreatitis
	Cerebellar and cerebral dysfunction (high dose)
	Conjunctivitis (high dose)
	Hidradenitis
	Noncardiogenic pulmonary edema
Precautions	High incidence of cerebral-cerebellar toxicity with high-dose ara-C in the elderly, especially in those with compromised renal function

ara-CDP, arabinosylcytosine diphosphate; ara-CTP, arabinosylcytosine triphosphate; ara-U, uracil arabinoside; CSF, cerebrospinal fluid; $t_{1/2}$, half-life.

Other biochemical actions of ara-C have been described, including inhibition of ribonucleotide reductase[29] and formation of ara-CDP-choline, an analog of cytidine 5'- diphosphocholine (CDP-choline) that inhibits synthesis of membrane glycoproteins and glycolipids.[30] Ara-C also has the interesting property of promoting differentiation of leukemic cells in tissue culture, an effect that is accompanied by decreased c-*myc* oncogene expression.[31,32] These changes in morphology and oncogene expression occur at concentrations above the threshold for cytotoxicity and may simply represent terminal injury of cells. Molecular analysis of clinical bone marrow samples from patients in remission has revealed persistence of leukemic markers,[33] which suggests that differentiation may have occurred in response to ara-C in clinical use.

The molecular mechanism of cell death after ara-C exposure is unclear. Both normal and malignant cells undergo apoptosis in experimental models.[34,35] A complex system of interacting transduction signals ultimately determines whether a cell exposed to a cytotoxic agent is destined to die. Exposure of leukemic cells to ara-C stimulates the formation of ceramide, a potent inducer of apoptosis.[36] On the other hand, an increase in protein kinase C (PKC) activity is observed in leukemic cells in response to ara-C in vitro.[37] This is thought to be the result of ara-C induction of diacylglycerol, which in turn induces PKC activity. Because PKC activation is known to oppose apoptosis in hematopoietic cells, the lethal actions of ara-C may depend, at least partially, on its relative effects on the PKC and sphingomyelin pathways. Transcriptional regulation of gene expression is another key mechanism through which the growth and differentiation of mammalian cells are controlled. The induction of some transcription factors, such as AP-1 (a dimer of jun-fos or jun-jun proteins) and NF-kB, has been temporally associated with ara-C–induced apoptosis.[38,39] Whether increased expression of

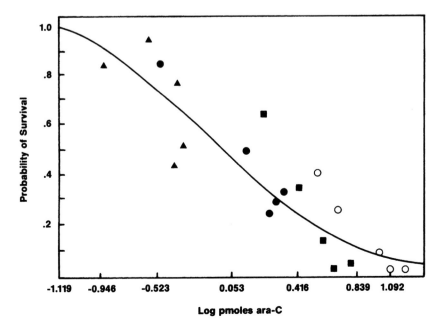

Figure 8.2 Relationship between acute myelogenous leukemia blast clonogenic survival and incorporation of tritium-labeled cytosine arabinoside (ara-C) in DNA at ara-C concentrations of 10^{-7} mol/L (▲), 10^{-6} mol/L (●), 10^{-5} mol/L (■), and 10^{-4} mol/L (○) during periods of 1, 3, 6, 12, and 24 hours. (From Kufe DW, Spriggs DR. Biochemical and cellular pharmacology of cytosine arabinoside. Semin Oncol 1985;12:34.)

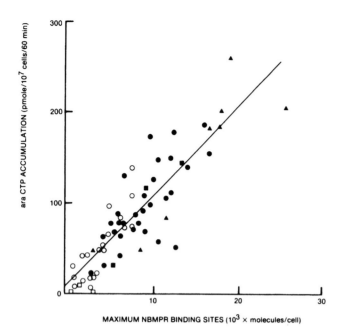

Figure 8.3 Correlation between accumulation of arabinosylcytosine triphosphate (ara-CTP) and nucleoside transport capacity measured by the maximal number of nitrobenzylthioinosine (NBMPR) binding sites on leukemic cells (r = 0.87; P < .0001). Ara-CTP accumulation was measured after incubation of cells with 1 μmol/L of tritium-labeled cytosine arabinoside for 60 minutes. (● acute myelogenous leukemia; ○ non-T-cell acute lymphoblastic leukemia; ▲, T-cell leukemia/lymphoma, lymphoblastic leukemia;■, acute undifferentiated leukemia; □, chronic lymphocytic leukemia. (From Wiley JS, Taupin J, Jamieson GP, et al. Cytosine arabinoside transport and metabolism in acute leukemias and T-cell lymphoblastic lymphoma. J Clin Invest 1985;75:632.)

these transcription factors plays a direct role in the molecular signaling that leads to anticancer drug-induced programmed cell death is not clear. The ability of PKC inhibitors to promote ara-C–induced apoptosis despite antagonizing c-*jun* up-regulation illustrates the fact that apoptosis can occur by a mechanism that does not involve the induction of c-*jun* expression.[40] Some have also reported that induction of pRb phosphatase activity by DNA-damaging drugs, including ara-C, is at least one of the mechanisms responsible for p53-independent, Rb-mediated G_1 arrest and apoptosis.[41] The resulting hypophosphorylated pRb binds to and inactivates the E2F transcription factor, which inhibits the transcription of numerous genes involved in cell-cycle progression.[42]

Cellular Pharmacology and Metabolism

Ara-C penetrates cells by a carrier-mediated process shared by physiologic nucleosides.[43,44] Several different classes of transporters for nucleosides have been identified in mammalian cells[45]; the most extensively characterized in human tumors is hENT1, the equilibrative transporter, identified by its binding to nitrobenzylthioinosine (NBMPR). The number of transport sites on the cell membrane is greater in acute myelocytic leukemia than in acute lymphocytic

leukemia cells and can be enumerated by incubation of cells with NBMPR. The hENT1 transporter is highly up-regulated in biphenotypic leukemia associated with the 11q23 MLL gene (4:11) translocation.[45a] A steady-state level of intracellular drug is achieved within 90 seconds at 37°C. Studies of Wiley et al.[44,46] and others[45,47,48] suggest that the NBMPR transporter plays a limiting role in the action of this agent in that the formation of the ultimate toxic metabolite ara-CTP is strongly correlated with the number of transporter sites on leukemic cells[46] (Fig. 8.3). At drug concentrations above 10 μmol/L, the transport process becomes saturated, and further entry takes place by passive diffusion.[49] hENT1 is strongly inhibited by various receptor tyrosine kinase inhibitors, an interaction that could limit ara-C use with targeted drugs.[49a]

As shown in Figure 8.4, ara-C must be converted to its active form, ara-CTP, through the sequential action of three enzymes: (a) deoxycytidine (CdR) kinase, (b) deoxycytidine monophosphate (dCMP) kinase, and (c) nucleoside diphosphate (NDP) kinase. Ara-C is subject to degradation by cytidine deaminase, forming the inactive product uracil arabinoside (ara-U); arabinosylcytosine monophosphate (ara-CMP) is likewise degraded by a second enzyme, dCMP deaminase, to the inactive arabinosyluracil monophosphate (ara-UMP). Each of these enzymes, with the exception of NDP kinase, has been examined in detail because of its possible relevance to ara-C resistance.

The first activating enzyme, CdR kinase, is found in lowest concentration (Table 8.3) and is believed to be rate-limiting in the process of ara-CTP formation. The enzyme is a 30.5-kd protein that phosphorylates deoxycytidine, deoxyguanosine, deoxyadenosine, ara-C, dideoxycytidine, fludarabine, gemcitabine, and other cytidine and purine

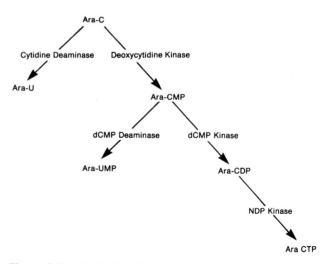

Figure 8.4 Metabolism of cytosine arabinoside (ara-C) by tumor cells. The conversion of arabinosyluracil monophosphate (ara-UMP) to a triphosphate has not been demonstrated in mammalian cells. ara-CMP, arabinosylcytosine monophosphate; ara-CDP, arabinosylcytosine diphosphate; ara-CTP, arabinosylcytosine triphosphate; ara-U, uracil arabinoside; dCMP, deoxycytidine monophosphate; NDP, nucleoside diphosphate.

analogs. The complementary DNA (cDNA) coding for CdR kinase has been cloned as well as cDNAs with specific mutations that lead to ara-C resistance in experimental cells.[50,51] The rate-limiting role of CdR kinase in ara-C activation is illustrated by the fact that transfection of malignant cell lines with retroviral vectors containing CdR kinase cDNA substantially increases their susceptibility to ara-C, 2-chloro-2′-deoxyadenosine, 2-fluoro-9-β-D-arabinofuranosyladenine, and less potently to gemcitabine.[52] Moreover, some investigators have demonstrated higher ara-C cytotoxicity in intradermal and intracerebral gliomas transduced with CdR kinase in rat models than in the same tumor models with no CdR kinase transduction.[53] This transduction of genes that sensitize tumor cells to prodrugs in vivo represents a potential strategy for cancer gene therapy.

CdR kinase activity is highest during the S phase of the cell cycle.[54] The K_m, or affinity constant, for ara-C is 20 μmol/L, compared with the higher affinity or 7.8 μmol/L for the physiologic substrate CdR.[55] This enzyme is strongly inhibited by dCTP but weakly inhibited by ara-CTP. This lack of "feedback" inhibition allows accumulation of the ara-C nucleotide to higher concentrations. Protein kinase C-α, the activity of which is increased after ara-C exposure, has been implicated in phosphorylation of deoxycytidine kinase, increasing its overall activity at concentrations of substrate greater than the K_m. This observation raises the possibility that ara-C at high doses may potentiate its own metabolism by induction of the PKC activator diacylglycerol.[56]

The second activating enzyme, dCMP kinase,[57] is found in several hundred-fold higher concentration than CdR kinase. Its affinity for ara-CMP is low (K_m = 680 μmol/L) but greater than the affinity for the competitive physiologic substrate dCMP. Because of its relatively poor affinity for ara-CMP, this enzyme could become rate-limiting at low ara-C concentrations. The third activating enzyme, the diphosphate kinase, appears not to be rate-limiting because the intracellular pool of arabinosylcytosine diphosphate (ara-CDP) is only a fraction of the ara-CTP pool.[58]

Opposing the activation pathway are two deaminases found in high concentration in some tumor cells as well as normal tissues. Cytidine deaminase is widely distributed in mammalian tissues, including intestinal mucosa, liver, and granulocytes.[59–62] It is found in granulocyte precursors and in leukemic myeloblasts in lower concentrations than in mature granulocytes, but even in these immature cells the deaminase level exceeds the activity of CdR kinase, the initial activating enzyme.[55,61] The second degradative enzyme, dCMP deaminase (Fig. 8.4), regulates the flow of physiologic nucleotides from the dCMP pool into the deoxyuridine monophosphate pool that is ultimately converted to deoxythymidine 5′-phosphate (dTMP) by thymidylate synthase.[63] The enzyme dCMP deaminase is strongly activated by intracellular dCTP (K_m = 0.2 μmol/L) and strongly inhibited by deoxythymidine triphosphate in concentrations of 0.2 μmol/L or greater. Ara-CTP weakly activates this enzyme (K_m = 40 μmol/L)[64] and thus would not promote degradation of its own precursor nucleotide, ara-CMP. The affinity of dCMP deaminase for ara-CMP is somewhat higher than that of dCMP kinase for the same substrate, but the activity of these competitive enzymes depends greatly on their degree of activation or inhibition by regulatory triphosphates (dCTP), and dCMP deaminase concentration in leukemic myeloblasts is slightly less than that of dCMP kinase (Table 8.3).

The balance between activating and degrading enzymes thus is crucial in determining the quantity of drug converted

TABLE 8.3

KINETIC PARAMETERS OF CYTOSINE ARABINOSIDE (ARA-C) METABOLIZING ENZYMES

Enzyme	Substrate	K_m (mol/L)	Activity in AML Cells (nmol/hr/ mg Protein at 37°C)
CdR kinase	Ara-C	2.6×10^{-5}	15.4 ± 16
	CdR	7.8×10^{-6}	
dCMP kinase	Ara-CMP	6.8×10^{-4}	$1,990 \pm 1,500$
	dCMP	1.9×10^{-3}	
dCDP kinase	Ara-CDP	?	Not known
	Other NDPs	?	
CR deaminase	Ara-C	8.8×10^{-5}	372 ± 614
	CdR	1.1×10^{-5}	
dCMP deaminase	Ara-CMP	Ara-CMP has higher K_m than	$1,250$ (5 patients)
	dCMP	dCMP; exact K_m not determined	

AML, acute myelogenous leukemia; Ara-C, ara-CDP, arabinosylcytosine diphosphate; ara-CMP, arabinosylcytosine monophosphate; CdR, deoxycy tidine; CR, cytidine; dCDP, deoxycytidine diphosphate; dCMP, deoxycytosine monophosphate; NDPs, nucleoside diphosphates.

to the active intermediate, ara-CTP. This enzymatic balance varies greatly among cell types.[55] Kinase activity is higher and deaminase activity lower in lymphoid leukemia than in acute myeloblastic leukemia. Enzyme activities vary also with cell maturity; deaminase increases dramatically with maturation of granulocyte precursors, whereas kinase activity decreases correspondingly.[61] Thus admixture of normal granulocyte precursors with leukemic cells in human bone marrow samples complicates the interpretation of enzyme measurements unless normal and leukemic cells are separated. In general, cytidine deaminase (D) activity greatly exceeds kinase (K) (the kinase:deaminase ratio averages 0.03) in human acute myeloblastic leukemia, whereas the enzyme activities are approximately equal in acute lymphoblastic leukemia and Burkitt's lymphoma. Thus, the biochemical setting seems to favor drug activation by lymphoblastic leukemia cells if these initial enzymes play a rate-limiting role.

In fact, this may not be the case. Chou et al.[58] found that human acute myeloblastic leukemia cells formed 12.8 ng of ara-CTP per 10^6 cells after 45 minutes of incubation with 1×10^{-5} mol/L ara-C. Acute lymphoblastic leukemia cells formed less ara-CTP, 6.3 ng/10^6 cells, and as expected, the more mature chronic myelocytic and chronic lymphocytic leukemia cells formed lesser amounts of ara-CTP (4.7 to 5.2 ng/10^6 cells). From this study and others,[46,48] the likelihood is that other factors, such as transport across the cell membrane, may limit ara-CTP formation.

In addition to its activation to ara-CTP, ara-C is converted intracellularly to ara-CDP-choline,[65] an analog of the physiologic CDP-choline lipid precursor. However, ara-C does not inhibit incorporation of choline into phospholipids of normal or transformed hamster embryo fibroblasts.[30] Ara-CMP does inhibit the transfer of galactose, N-acetylglucosamine, and sialic acid to cell surface glycoproteins. Further, ara-CTP inhibits the synthesis of cytidine monophosphate–acetylneuraminic acid, an essential substrate in sialylation of glycoproteins, although high ara-CTP concentrations (0.1 to 1 mmol/L) are needed to produce this effect.[66] Thus, ara-C treatment could alter membrane structure, antigenicity, and function.

Biochemical Determinants of Cytosine Arabinoside Resistance

The foregoing consideration of ara-C metabolism and transport makes it clear that a number of factors could affect ara-C response. Not surprisingly, many of these factors have been implicated in various preclinical models of ara-C resistance. The most frequent abnormality found in resistant leukemic cells recovered from mice treated with ara-C has been decreased activity of CdR kinase.[67,68] In cultured cells exposed to a mutagen and then to low concentrations of ara-C, some single-step mutants developed high-level resistance to ara-C through loss of activity of CdR kinase, whereas other resistant clones exhibited

markedly expanded dCTP pools, presumably through increased cytidine-5'-triphosphate (CTP) synthetase activity or through deficiency of dCMP deaminase.[69–72] As mentioned previously, specific mutations and deletions in the CdR kinase coding cDNAs derived from resistant cells have been described by Owens et al.[51]

The role of cytidine deaminase in experimental models of resistance is less clear. Retrovirus-mediated transfer of the cytidine deaminase cDNA into 3T3 murine fibroblast cells significantly increases drug resistance to ara-C and other nucleoside analogs such as 5-aza-2'-deoxycytidine and gemcitabine. This phenotype of increased cytidine deaminase activity and drug resistance is reversed by the cytidine deaminase inhibitor tetrahydrouridine.[73] Other genes, including proto-oncogenes, may affect ara-C response. Transfection of rodent fibroblasts and human mammary HBL 100 cells with c-H-ras conferred resistance to ara-C, an event attributed to decreased activity of CdR kinase.[74] On the other hand, N-ras or K-ras mutations strongly correlated with increased ara-C sensitivity in the screening of human tumor cell lines from the National Cancer Institute's in vitro drug screen.[75]

Although various metabolic lesions have been implicated as causing ara-C resistance in animals, their relevance to resistance in human leukemia is less certain. Studies have described specific biochemical changes in drug-resistant cells from patients with leukemia, including deletion of CdR kinase,[76] increased cytidine deaminase,[77] a decreased number of nucleoside transport sites,[46] and increased dCTP pools.[78] Other clinical investigators have not been able to correlate resistance with either CdR kinase or cytidine deaminase,[79,80] but with the exception of Wiley et al.,[46] who correlated clinical response with in vitro transport, few have examined transport. All studies have shown extreme variability in enzyme levels among patients with acute myelocytic or lymphocytic leukemia (Fig. 8.5). Thus, no agreement exists as to the specific changes responsible for resistance in human leukemia.

Although *specific biochemical lesions* associated with resistance in humans are unclear, the current understanding of ara-C action suggests that the ultimate formation of ara-CTP and the duration of its persistence in leukemic cells determine response.[58,81] Chou et al.[58] found greater ara-CTP formation in leukemic cells of responders when these cells were incubated in vitro with ara-C, but in other series of patients no correlation was seen between remission induction or duration of complete remission and ara-CTP formation.[82–84]

Preisler et al.[85] found a strong correlation between duration of remission and the ability of cells to *retain* ara-CTP in vitro after removal of ara-C from the medium (Table 8.4). Attempts to monitor ara-CTP formation in leukemic cells taken from patients during therapy have yielded useful information on rates of nucleotide formation and disappearance (the intracellular ara-CTP half-life is approximately 3 hours) but have not disclosed useful correlations

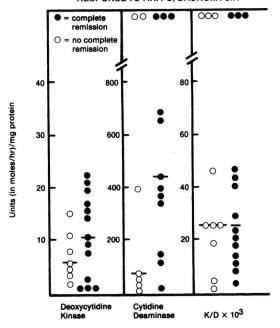

Figure 8.5 Response as a function of deoxycytidine kinase (K) and cytidine deaminase (D) activities and their ratio in patients with acute myelogenous leukemia. ara-C, cytosine arabinoside; K/D, kinase/deaminase ratio. (From Chang P, Wiernik PH, Reich SD, et al. Prediction of response to cytosine arabinoside and daunorubicin in acute nonlymphocytic leukemia. In: Mandelli F, ed. Therapy of Acute Leukemias: Proceedings of the Second International Symposium, Rome, 1977. Rome: Lombardo Editore, 1979:148.)

whether the genotoxic insult results in cell death. In this sense, overexpression of Bcl-2 and Bcl-X_L in leukemic blasts have been associated with in vitro resistance to ara-C–mediated apoptosis.[87] The intracellular metabolism of ara-C and its initial effects on DNA are not modified by Bcl-2 expression, which suggests that Bcl-2 primarily regulates the more distal steps in the ara-C–induced cell death pathway. Although the precise mechanism by which these proteins prevent ara-C–induced cytotoxicity remains to be elucidated, Bcl-2 and Bcl-X_L have been shown to antagonize ara-C–mediated cell death by a mechanism that prevents the activation of *Caenorhabditis elegans* deathlike proteases, such as Yama/CPP32 protease, which are involved in the execution of apoptosis.[87] The fact that antisense oligonucleotides directed against Bcl-2 increase the susceptibility of leukemic blasts to ara-C–induced apoptosis in vitro,[88] and that patients whose blasts express high levels of Bcl-2 respond poorly to ara-C–containing regimens,[89] further illustrates the potential role of Bcl-2 in ara-C resistance. Exceptions are seen, however, in which even high levels of Bcl-2 expression apparently fail to prevent cell death.

Phosphorylation of apoptotic or DNA damage response factors may also determine the outcome of ara-C exposure. Studies have shown that phosphorylation of Bcl-2 is required for its antiapoptotic function, and a functional role for PKC-α in Bcl-2 phosphorylation and suppression of apoptosis has been postulated,[90] although this observation has not been confirmed by others.[91] Altered phosphorylation of transcription factors also influences the cellular response to ara-C toxic insult. Ara-C–induced activation of PKC and mitogen-activated protein kinase (MAPK) has been reported to increase c-*jun* expression and phosphorylation,[37,92] and hyperphosphorylation of the AP-1 transcription factor has been associated with ara-C resistance in human myeloid leukemic cell lines in vitro.[93]

Clinical studies of determinants of ara-C response are complicated by the fact that ara-C is almost always given in

of ara-CTP levels with response.[84,86] Again, considerable variability has been observed in the rates of formation of ara-CTP, and this rate does not correlate well with plasma ara-C concentrations in individual patients (Fig. 8.6).

Although specific steps in ara-C activation and degradation exert a strong influence on its ultimate action, the cellular response to ara-C–mediated DNA damage also governs

TABLE 8.4

CORRELATION OF IN VITRO ARA-CTP POOLS AND RETENTION OF ARA-CTP 4 HOURS AFTER DRUG REMOVAL WITH DURATION OF COMPLETE RESPONSE OF PREVIOUSLY UNTREATED PATIENTS WITH ACUTE NONLYMPHOCYTIC LEUKEMIA[a]

	No. of Patients	Ara-CTP Retention at 4 Hr after Removal of ara-C (% of Peak ara-CTP)	Median Duration of CR (months)
All patients	80	18.4	21.4
>20% retention	36	42.0	44.8
<20% retention	44	13.9	12.2

[a]Patients were treated with protocol using ara-C (100 mg/m^2/day).
ara-C, cytosine arabinoside; ara-CTP, arabinosylcytosine triphosphate; CR, complete response.
Data from Preisler HD, Rustum Y, Priore RL. Relationship between leukemic cell retention of cytosine arabinoside triphosphate and the duration of remission in patients with acute non-lymphocytic leukemia. Eur J Cancer Clin Oncol 1985;21:23.

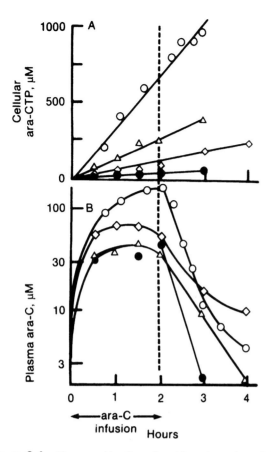

Figure 8.6 Pharmacokinetics of arabinosylcytosine triphosphate (ara-CTP) in leukemia cells and of cytosine arabinoside (ara-C) in plasma. Blood samples were drawn at the indicated times during and after infusion of ara-C, 3 g/m², to patients with acute leukemia in relapse. Symbols for each analysis are the same for individual patients. (From Plunkett W, Liliemark JO, Estey E, et al. Saturation of ara-CTP accumulation during high-dose ara-C therapy: pharmacologic rationale for intermediate- dose ara-C. Semin Oncol 1987;14[2(Suppl 1)]:159.)

combination with an anthracycline or an anthraquinone. Thus, a complete response or long remission duration does not necessarily imply sensitivity to ara-C. A lack of response does imply resistance to both agents in the combination, except for the not-infrequent cases in which failure can be attributed to infection or inability to administer full dosages of drug. With these limitations, the duration of complete response is probably the most appropriate and most important single yardstick of drug sensitivity because it reflects the fractional cell kill during induction therapy.

Cell Kinetics and Cytosine Arabinoside Cytotoxicity

In addition to biochemical factors that determine response, cell kinetic properties exert an important influence on the results of ara-C treatment. As an inhibitor of DNA synthesis, ara-C has its greatest cytotoxic effects during

the S phase of the cell cycle,[94] perhaps because of the requirement for its incorporation into DNA and the greater activity of anabolic enzymes during S phase. The duration of exposure of cells to ara-C is directly correlated with cell kill because the longer exposure period allows ara-C to be incorporated into the DNA of a greater percentage of cells as they pass through S phase (Fig. 8.7). The cytotoxic action of ara-C is not only cell-cycle phase–dependent but also affects the rate of DNA synthesis. That is, cell kill in tissue culture is greatest if cells are exposed during periods of maximal rates of DNA synthesis, as in the recovery period after exposure to a cytotoxic agent. In experimental situations it has been possible to schedule sequential doses of ara-C to coincide with the peak in recovery of DNA synthesis and thus to improve the therapeutic results.[95-97]

Burke and colleagues[96] and Vaughan and colleagues[98] have attempted to exploit kinetic patterns of leukemic cell recovery after ara-C by optimizing sequential doses of drug. Thus, retreatment 8 to 10 days after an initial dose of ara-C has yielded a promising improvement in the duration of unmaintained remission in adult patients with leukemia in uncontrolled studies.[98]

In humans, the influence of tumor cell kinetics on response is unclear. Although earlier studies showed that the complete remission rate seems to be *higher* in patients who have a high percentage of cells in S phase,[99] remissions are *longer* in patients with leukemias that have long cell-cycle time.[100]

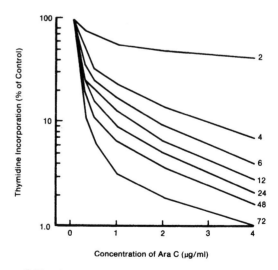

Figure 8.7 Thymidine incorporation into DNA of M19 human melanoma cells as a function of drug concentration and duration of exposure to cytosine arabinoside (ara-C). The exposure duration in hours is indicated by the numbers adjacent to the individual curves. The data indicate a near-linear relationship between inhibition of thymidine incorporation and drug concentration but a lesser dependence on time for intervals longer than 12 hours, perhaps because of the cell-cycle dependence of the drug. Thus, most replicating cells are exposed to ara-C during their period of DNA synthesis if the exposure time is 12 hours or longer.

Clinical Pharmacology—Assay Methods

A number of assay methods have been used to measure ara-C concentration in plasma.[101-105] The preferred method for assay of ara-C and its primary metabolite ara-U is high-pressure liquid chromatography, which has the requisite specificity and adequate (0.1 μmol/L) sensitivity.[106,107] An alternative method using gas chromatography–mass spectrometry combines high specificity with greater sensitivity (4 nmol/L) but requires derivatization of samples and thus prolonged performance time.[108] Because of the presence of cytidine deaminase in plasma, the deaminase inhibitor tetrahydrouridine must be added to plasma samples immediately after blood samples are obtained.

Pharmacokinetics

The important factors that determine ara-C pharmacokinetics are its high aqueous solubility and its susceptibility to deamination in liver, plasma, granulocytes, and gastrointestinal tract. Ara-C is amenable to use by multiple schedules and routes of administration and has shown clinical activity in dosages ranging from 3 mg/m² twice weekly to 3 g/m² every 12 hours for 6 days. Remarkably, over this wide dosage range, its pharmacokinetics remains quite constant and predictable.

Distribution

As a nucleoside, ara-C is transported across cell membranes by a nucleoside transporter and distributes rapidly into total-body water.[109,110] It crosses into the central nervous system (CNS) with surprising facility for a water-soluble compound and reaches steady-state levels at 20 to 40% of those found simultaneously in plasma during constant intravenous infusion.[102] At conventional doses of ara-C (100 mg/m² by 24-hour infusion), spinal fluid levels reach 0.2 μmol/L, which is probably above the cytotoxic threshold for leukemic cells. High doses of ara-C yield proportionately higher ara-C levels in the spinal fluid.[111-113]

Plasma Pharmacokinetics

The pharmacokinetics of ara-C are characterized by rapid disappearance from plasma owing to deamination, with some variability seen among individual patients.[102,104,108,110] Peak plasma concentrations reach 10 μmol/L after bolus doses of 100 mg/m² and are proportionately higher (up to 150 μmol/L) for doses up to 3 g/m² given over a 1- or 2-hour infusion[111,114] (Fig. 8.8). Thereafter, the plasma concentration of ara-C declines, with a half-life of 7 to 20 minutes. A second phase of drug disappearance has been detected after high-dose ara-C infusion, with a terminal half-life of 30 to 150 minutes, but the drug concentration during this second phase has cytotoxic potential only in patients treated with high-dose ara-C.[113,115] Seventy to eighty percent

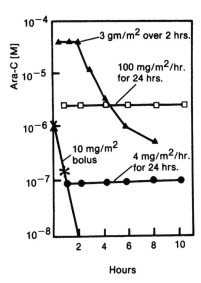

Figure 8.8 Cytosine arabinoside (ara-C) pharmacokinetics in plasma after doses of 3 g/m² given over 2 hours, 100 mg/m² per hour by continuous infusion for 24 hours, 4 mg/m² per hour (a conventional antileukemic dose) by continuous intravenous infusion, and 10 mg/m² subcutaneously or intravenously as a bolus.

of a given dose is excreted as ara-U,[102] which, within minutes of drug injection, becomes the predominant compound found in plasma. Ara-U has a longer half-life in plasma (3.2 to 5.8 hours) than does ara-C and may enhance the activation of ara-C through feedback inhibition of ara-C deamination in leukemic cells.[115]

The steady-state level of ara-C in plasma achieved by constant intravenous infusion remains proportional to dose for dose rates up to 2 g/m² per day. At this dosage, steady-state plasma levels approximate 5 μmol/L. Above this rate of infusion, the deamination reaction is saturated and ara-C plasma levels rise unpredictably, which leads to severe toxicity in some patients.[116] To accelerate the achievement of a steady-state concentration, one may give a loading dose of three times the hourly infusion rate before infusion.[110] Equivalent drug exposure (area under the curve) is achieved by subcutaneous or intravenous infusion of ara-C,[117] although one study has reported higher ara-CTP concentrations in leukemia cells after subcutaneous administration.[118]

Owing to the presence of high concentrations of cytidine deaminase in the gastrointestinal mucosa and liver, orally administered ara-C provides much lower plasma levels than does direct intravenous administration. Threefold to 10-fold higher doses must be given in animals to achieve an equal biologic effect. The oral route, therefore, is not routinely used in humans.

Ara-C may also be administered by intraperitoneal infusion for treatment of ovarian cancer.[119] After instillation of 100 μmol/L of drug, ara-C levels fall in the peritoneal cavity with a half-life of approximately 2 hours. Simultaneous plasma levels are 100- to 1,000-fold lower, presumably because of deamination of ara-C in liver before it reaches the systemic circulation. In 21-day continuous infusion, patients tolerated up to 100 μmol/L intraperitoneal concentrations but developed peritonitis at higher concentrations.[120]

Cerebrospinal Fluid Pharmacokinetics

After intravenous administration of 100 mg/m² of ara-C, parent drug levels reach 0.1 to 0.3 μmol/L in the cerebrospinal fluid (CSF), with a decline in levels thereafter characterized by a half-life of 2 hours. Proportionately higher CSF levels are reached by intravenous high-dose ara-C regimens; for example, a 3 g/m² infusion intravenously over 1 hour yields peak CSF concentrations of 4 μmol/L,[114] whereas the same dose over 24 hours yields peak CSF ara-C concentrations of 1 μmol/L.[116]

Ara-C is effective when administered intrathecally for the treatment of metastatic neoplasms. A number of dosing schedules for giving intrathecal ara-C have been recommended, but twice weekly or weekly schedules of administration are the most widely used. The dose of ara-C ranges from 30 to 50 mg/m². The dose is generally adjusted in pediatric patients according to age (15 mg for children below 1 year of age, 20 mg for children between 1 and 2 years, 30 mg for children between 2 and 3 years, and 40 mg for children older than 3 years). The clinical pharmacology of ara-C in the CSF following intrathecal administration differs considerably from that seen in the plasma following a parenteral dose. Systematically administered ara-C is rapidly eliminated by biotransformation to the inactive metabolite ara-U. In contrast, little conversion of ara-C to ara-U takes place in the CSF following an intrathecal injection. The ratio of ara-U to ara-C is only 0.08, a finding that is consistent with the very low levels of cytidine deaminase present in the brain and CSF. Following an intraventricular administration of 30 mg of ara-C, peak levels exceed 2 mmol/L, and levels decline slowly, with the terminal half-life being approximately 3.4 hours.[102] Concentrations above the threshold for cytotoxicity (0.1 μg/mL, or 0.4 μmol/L) are maintained in the CSF for 24 hours. The CSF clearance is 0.42 mL/minute, which is similar to the CSF bulk flow rate. This finding suggests that drug elimination occurs primarily by this route. Plasma levels following intrathecal administration of 30 mg/m² of ara-C are less than 1 μmol/L, which illustrates again the advantage of intracavitary therapy with a drug that is rapidly cleared in the systemic circulation.

Depocytarabine (DTC 101) is a depot formulation in which ara-C is encapsulated in microscopic Gelfoam particles (DepoFoam) for sustained release into the CSF so that the need for repeated lumbar punctures is avoided. The encapsulation of ara-C in DepoFoam results in a 55-fold increase in CSF half-life after intraventricular administration in rats, from 2.7 hours to 148 hours. Cytotoxic concentrations of free ara-C (>0.4 μmol/L) in CSF were maintained for more than 1 month following a single intrathecal dose administration of 2 mg of DTC 101 in rhesus monkeys. A phase I trial of DTC 101 given intraventricularly has been performed in patients with leptomeningeal metastasis. Free ara-C CSF concentration decreased biexponentially. After a dose of 50 mg of DTC, ara-C concentration was maintained above the threshold for cytotoxicity for an average of 12 ± 3 days. The maximum tolerated dosage was 75 mg administered every 3 weeks, and the dose-limiting toxicity was headache and arachnoiditis.[121] Preliminary results of a randomized study involving patients with lymphomatous meningitis demonstrate a possible prolongation of time to neurologic progression in patients treated with 50 mg of DTC 101 every 2 weeks compared with patients treated with standard intrathecal ara-C.[122] DTC appears to give equivalent results to standard intrathecal methotrexate, given every 4 days, for treatment of carcinomatous meningitis.[122a]

Alternate Schedules of Administration

Although ara-C is used most commonly in regimens of 100 to 200 mg/m² per day for 7 days, other high-dose and low-dose schedules have been used in treating leukemia. The more effective of these newer regimens have been high-dose schemes, usually 2 to 3 g/m² every 12 hours for six doses.[123] High-dose ara-C is used primarily in the consolidation phase for acute myelocytic leukemia.[8] The rationale for the higher-dose regimen initially rested on the assumption that ara-C phosphorylation is the rate-limiting intracellular step in the drug's activation and could be promoted by raising intracellular concentrations to the K_m of deoxycytidine kinase for ara-C, or approximately 20 μmol/L. Above this level, further increases in ara-C do not lead to increased ara-CTP because the phosphorylation pathways become saturated.[48,124]

Others have examined the clinical activity of low-dose ara-C, particularly in older patients with myelodysplastic syndromes.[125] These regimens have used dosages in the range of 3 to 20 mg/m² per day for up to 3 weeks. The rationale for low-dose regimens has been based primarily on the expectation that they would produce less toxicity; low concentrations of ara-C were also thought to promote leukemic cell differentiation (or apoptosis) in tissue culture. In isolated cases, the persistence of chromosomal markers for the leukemic cell line in remission granulocytes has been documented, findings that support differentiation.[126,127] In general, although the low-dose regimens produce less toxicity, particularly at the lower end of the dose spectrum, the therapeutic results have been disappointing in that less than 20% of patients achieve a clinical remission.[128] Continuous exposure of normal myeloid precursor cells to drug concentrations as low as 10 nmol/L inhibits proliferation, a further problem in MDS treatment.[129] After intravenous doses as low as 3 mg/m², peak plasma levels reach 100 nmol/L and remain above the inhibitory concentration (10 nmol/L) for 30 to 60 minutes. Thus, low-dose ara-C regimens have not avoided the myelosuppressive effects of standard schedules.

Toxicity

The primary determinants of ara-C toxicity are drug concentration and duration of exposure. Because ara-C is cell cycle phase-specific, the duration of cell exposure to the drug is critical in determining the fraction of cells killed.[130] In humans, single-bolus doses of ara-C as large as 4.2 g/m^2 are well tolerated because of the rapid inactivation of the parent compound and the brief period of exposure, whereas constant infusion of drug for 48 hours using total doses of 1 g/m^2 produces severe myelosuppression.[131]

Myelosuppression and gastrointestinal epithelial injury are the primary toxic side effects of ara-C. With the conventional 5- to 7-day courses of treatment, the period of maximal toxicity begins during the first week of treatment and lasts 14 to 21 days. The primary targets of ara-C are platelet production and granulopoiesis, although anemia also occurs. Little acute effect is seen on the lymphocyte count, although a depression of cell-mediated immunity is found in patients receiving ara-C.[132] Megaloblastic changes consistent with suppression of DNA synthesis are observed in both the white and red cell precursors.[133]

Gastrointestinal symptoms, including nausea, vomiting, and diarrhea, are frequent during the period of drug administration but subside quickly after treatment. Severe gastrointestinal lesions occur in patients treated with ara-C as part of complex chemotherapy regimens, and the specific contribution of ara-C is difficult to ascertain in these cases. All parts of the gastrointestinal tract are affected. Oral mucositis also occurs and may be severe and prolonged in patients receiving more than 5 days of continuous treatment. Clinical symptoms of diarrhea, ileus, and abdominal pain may be accompanied by gastrointestinal bleeding, electrolyte abnormalities, and protein-losing enteropathy. Radiologic evidence of dilatation of the terminal ileum, termed typhlitis, may be associated with progressive abdominal pain and bowel perforation. Pathologic findings include denudation of the epithelial surface and loss of crypt cell mitotic activity. Reversible intrahepatic cholestasis occurs frequently in patients receiving ara-C for induction therapy but requires cessation of therapy in fewer than 25% of patients.[134,135] It is manifested primarily as an increase in hepatic enzymes in the serum, together with mild jaundice, and rapidly reverses with discontinuation of treatment. Ara-C has been implicated as the cause of pancreatitis in a small number of patients.[136]

Toxicity of High-Dose Cytosine Arabinoside

High-dose ara-C significantly increases the incidence and severity of bone marrow and gastrointestinal toxic effects.[7] Hospitalization for fever and neutropenia is required in 71% of the treatment courses in patients receiving 3 g per m^2 per 12 hours given on alternative days for six doses, and platelet transfusions are required in 86%.[8] Treatment-related deaths,

primarily the result of infection, occurred in 5% of the patients treated with this schedule.[8] In addition, high-dose ara-C produces pulmonary toxicity, including noncardiogenic pulmonary edema, in approximately 10% of patients, and a surprisingly high incidence of *Streptococcus viridans* pneumonia is seen, especially in pediatric populations.[137-139] The pulmonary edema syndrome is frequently irreversible.

Cholestatic jaundice and elevation of serum glutamic-oxaloacetic transaminase, serum glutamic-pyruvic transaminase, and alkaline phosphatase, with underlying cholestasis and passive congestion on liver biopsy, are also frequently observed with the high-dose regimen.[140] These changes, however, are generally clinically unimportant and reversible. A more dangerous toxicity involving cerebral and cerebellar dysfunction occurs in 10% of patients receiving 3 g/m^2 for 6 doses[8] and in two-thirds of patients receiving 4.5 g/m^2 for 12 doses.[141] Age over 40 years, abnormal alkaline phosphatase activity in serum, and compromised renal function[142] are risk factors associated with an increased susceptibility to CNS toxicity, which is manifested as slurred speech, unsteady gait, dementia, and coma.[141] Patients with two or more of these risk factors treated with high-dose ara-C develop CNS toxicity in 37% of the cases, whereas the incidence is less than 1% when fewer than two of these criteria are present.[142] Symptoms of neurologic toxicity resolve within several days in approximately 20% of patients and gradually recede in approximately 40%; however, a permanent disability is present in the remaining 40%, and occasionally patients have died of CNS toxicity.[8] Progressive brainstem dysfunction[143] and an ascending peripheral neuropathy[144] also have been reported after high-dose ara-C.

Other bothersome toxicities complicate high-dose AraC. Conjunctivitis, responsive to topical steroids, also has been a frequent side effect of high-dose ara-C.[145] Rarely, skin rash[146] and even anaphylaxis have been noted.[147] Neutrophilic eccrine hydradenitis, an unusual febrile cutaneous reaction manifested as plaques or nodules during the second week after chemotherapy, is being reported with increasing frequency after high-dose ara-C.[148] Finally, reports have appeared sporadically in the literature of cardiac toxicity associated with ara-C, generally at high dosages. Findings have included arrhythmias, pericarditis, and congestive heart failure. None of these reports provide conclusive evidence for a cause-and-effect relationship.[149]

Toxicity of Intrathecal Cytosine Arabinoside

Ara-C given intrathecally is infrequently associated with fever and seizures occurring within 24 hours of administration, and arachnoiditis occurring within 4 to 7 days.[150] Rarely, it causes a progressive brainstem toxicity that may be fatal.[151] Intrathecal ara-C should be used with caution in patients who have previously experienced methotrexate neurotoxicity.

Although ara-C causes chromosomal breaks in cultured cells and in the bone marrow of patients receiving therapy,[152] it is not an established carcinogen in humans. The drug is teratogenic in animals.[153]

Drug Interactions

Ara-C has synergistic antitumor activity with a number of other antitumor agents in animal tumor models. These other agents include alkylating agents (cyclophosphamide[154] and carmustine [BCNU][155]), cisplatin,[156] purine analogs,[157,158] methotrexate,[159,160] and etoposide.[161] In the past, ara-C and 6-thioguanine (6-TG) were frequently combined in the treatment of acute leukemia. This interaction seems to be highly schedule-dependent. Ara-C, an inhibitor of DNA synthesis, blocks the incorporation of 6-TG into DNA; however, if ara-C is given 12 hours before 6-TG, enhanced incorporation of the purine analog is observed.[162] On the other hand, evidence exists that 6-TG, given before or with ara-C, enhances ara-C incorporation into DNA by blocking exonuclease activity.[163]

The basis for ara-C potentiation of alkylating agents and cisplatin is thought to be inhibition of repair of DNA-alkylator adducts. The hypothesis is consistent with the finding that ara-C exposure preceding cisplatin is synergistic—perhaps allowing for inhibition of repair[164]—whereas ara-C after cisplatin is not.[156]

Tetrahydrouridine (THU), a potent inhibitor of cytidine deaminase ($K_i = 3 - 10^{-8}$ mol/L),[62] also enhances ara-CTP formation in acute myelocytic leukemia cells in vitro but not in chronic lymphocytic leukemia cells, which lack deaminase activity.[165] THU enhances the growth-inhibitory effects of sublethal concentrations of ara-C in experiments with the sarcoma 180 cell line, which contains high amounts of cytidine deaminase.[166] Initial clinical evaluation of the combination indicates that THU in intravenous doses of 50 mg/m² markedly prolongs the plasma half-life of ara-C from 10 to 120 minutes and causes a corresponding enhancement of toxicity to bone marrow.[167,168] In combination with THU, the tolerable dosage of ara-C is reduced 30-fold to 0.1 mg/kg per day for 5 days. Whether the combination has greater therapeutic effects and a better therapeutic ratio than ara-C alone is unclear.

Inhibitors of ribonucleotide reductase—such as hydroxyurea,[169] 2,3-dihydro-1 *H*-imidazolo(1,2-*b*)pyrazole,[170] and thymidine triphosphate[171]—enhance ara-C toxicity by decreasing dCTP pools (Fig. 8.9). A decrease in dCTP should have several beneficial effects on ara-C activity. CdR kinase, the enzyme that converts ara-C to ara-CMP (Fig. 8.4), is inhibited by dCTP, whereas dCMP deaminase, which would convert ara-CMP to the inactive ara-UMP, is activated by dCTP; a decrease in dCTP pools should thus increase ara-CTP formation. Second, because ara-CTP and dCTP compete for the same active site on DNA polymerase, a decrease in dCTP pools should lead to a relative increase in the amount of ara-C incorporated into DNA.

Experimental studies have confirmed that synergy between ara-C and thymidine occurs in some but not all tumor cell lines[171,172] and experimental chemotherapy settings.[173,174] The combination of ara-C and thymidine has received limited clinical evaluation in patients with refractory leukemia and lymphoma, and the initial results have

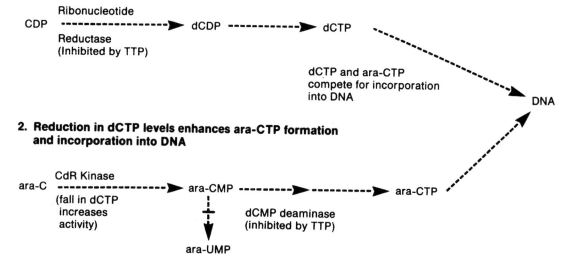

1. Thymidine triphosphate inhibits dCTP synthesis

CDP ----Ribonucleotide Reductase (Inhibited by TTP)----> dCDP ----------> dCTP

dCTP and ara-CTP compete for incorporation into DNA

DNA

2. Reduction in dCTP levels enhances ara-CTP formation and incorporation into DNA

ara-C ----CdR Kinase (fall in dCTP increases activity)----> ara-CMP --------> ara-CTP

ara-CMP --‖--> ara-UMP

dCMP deaminase (inhibited by TTP)

Figure 8.9 Interactions of thymidine and cytosine arabinoside (ara-C). ara-CMP, arabinosylcytosine monophosphate; ara-CTP, arabinosylcytosine triphosphate; ara-UMP, arabinosyluracil monophosphate; CDP, cytidine diphosphate; CdR, deoxycytidine; dCDP, deoxycytidine diphosphate; dCMP, deoxycytidine monophosphate; dCTP, deoxycytidine triphosphate; TTP, thymidine triphosphate.

not been favorable as only 7 of 26 patients in the largest study achieved remission.[174-176] Thymidine (75 g/m^2 per day) is extremely cumbersome to administer because of the massive fluid load required.[174,175] Tumor cells may develop resistance to both agents by a single-step mutation related to expansion of the dCTP pool as a result of increased de novo synthesis of pyrimidines.[69]

The conversion of ara-C to its active form, ara-CTP, is also augmented by pretreatment with methotrexate, according to studies of the murine lymphoma cell lines L1210 and L5178Y.[159,160] Simultaneous administration of ara-C and methotrexate is associated with greater retention of ara-CTP in tumor cells and better therapeutic results than achieved with schedules using ara-C alone or ara-C and methotrexate administered 24 hours apart.[177] The combination has not been evaluated in definitive clinical trials. Ara-C is commonly used in combination with daunorubicin or etoposide for the treatment of acute myelocytic leukemia. In experimental systems, minute (0.01 μmol/L) concentrations of ara-C cause an increase in levels of topoisomerase II, enhance the rate of protein-associated DNA strand breaks induced by etoposide,[161] and increase their cytotoxicity. Ara-C has no apparent direct effect on topoisomerase II activity.[178]

Ara-CTP formation, a requisite step for cytotoxicity, is markedly augmented by prior exposure of leukemic cells to fludarabine (fluoro-ara-adenine) phosphate, but this combination decreases the intracellular levels of fluoro-arabynosyl-adenine-triphosphate (F-ara-ATP).[157,179] Increased ara-CTP results from the inhibition of ribonucleotide reductase by fludarabine triphosphate. Approximately a 50% increase in leukemic cell ara-CTP is associated with pretreatment of chronic lymphocytic leukemia patients with fludarabine. Ara-C also may shorten the plasma half-life of fludarabine.[158] Clinical studies performed during treatment of patients with acute myelogenous leukemia demonstrated that the accumulation of ara-CTP in circulating leukemia blasts was increased by a median of twofold when fludarabine was infused 4 hours before ara-C. The augmentation depended on the cellular concentration of fludarabine triphosphate. Fludarabine at 15 mg/m^2 infused over 30 minutes consistently produced cellular fludarabine triphosphate levels that maximized ara-CTP accumulation in acute myelocytic leukemia blasts.[180]

Considerable interest has focused on the use of ara-C in combination with hematopoietic growth factors (HGFs). The theoretical gain of this combination would be that administration of HGFs before the administration of a cell-cycle–specific drug, such as ara-C, would recruit leukemia cells into the susceptible S phase of the cell cycle, which would thereby enhance cytotoxicity. In fact, several in vitro studies have shown that cytokines, particularly interleukin 3 and granulocyte-macrophage colony-stimulating factor, stimulate myeloid leukemia proliferation[181] and increase leukemic blast susceptibility to ara-C–induced apoptosis.[182] Growth regulatory molecules might also affect the therapeutic index by increasing the ara-CTP to dCTP ratio[183] and the ara-C incorporation into DNA.[184] Conflicting results have been observed in in vivo studies, however, and several randomized clinical trials have shown no advantage in response rate or survival in patients with acute myelocytic leukemia treated with HGFs in combination with ara- C compared with patients treated with ara-C alone.[185]

As resistance to a broad range of chemotherapeutic agents, including ara-C, may arise from defects in damage recognition and apoptosis pathways, a major field of investigations has been the modulation of signal transduction-apoptotic pathways. Staurosporine, a highly potent but nonspecific inhibitor of PKC (20 to 50 nmol/L), significantly potentiated ara-C–mediated apoptosis in human myeloid leukemia cell lines HL-60 and U937, but was ineffective when given alone at these concentrations.[186] In contrast, coadministration of another nonspecific PKC inhibitor, H7, and two highly selective PKC inhibitors, calphostin C and chelerythrine, also increased the extent of DNA fragmentation observed in ara-C–treated cells, but only at concentrations that were themselves sufficient to induce DNA damage.[186] Sustained exposure to bryostatin 1, a macrocyclic lactone PKC activator, also enhanced ara-C–mediated apoptosis. These apparently conflicting observations may be explained by the down-regulation of PKC expression that follows a period of sustained activation, or by effects of PKC activation on Bcl-2 phosphorylation.[91,187]

OTHER CYTIDINE ANALOGS

One objective of analog development in the general area of cytidine antimetabolites has been to find compounds that preserve the inhibitory activity of ara-C but are resistant to deamination. This goal is based primarily on the assumptions that the rapid metabolism of ara-C and its short half-life in plasma constitute an inconvenience because they require continuous infusion of drug rather than intermittent bolus administration, and that deamination may play a role in tumor cell resistance. As reviewed previously in this chapter, the evidence that nucleoside deamination is responsible for resistance is limited to the study of Steuart and Burke[77] and has not been confirmed by subsequent work. Nonetheless, a number of deaminase-resistant analogs have been developed, and several, including cyclo-cytidine (O^2,2'-cyclocytidine)[188] and N^4-behenoyl ara-C,[189] showed antileukemic activity in limited clinical trials, but had undesirable side effects.[190-192] Representative compounds are listed in Table 8.5.

A hybrid of ara-C and 5-azacytidine, 5-aza-cytosine arabinoside[193] (Fig. 8.1), is activated by the same pathway as ara-C and is incorporated into DNA, where it inhibits DNA synthesis. It is not deaminated and has broad activity against human xenografts in nude mice and against murine

TABLE 8.5

ALTERNATIVE FORMS OF CYTIDINE ANTIMETABOLITE CHEMOTHERAPY

	Rationale	Effect	Reference
Entrapment of ara-C in liposomes	Prevents deamination; preferential uptake by tumor cells	Acts as depot form of ara-C with slow release	194, 312
N^4-Palmitoyl-ara-C	Resistant to deaminase, highly lipid soluble, active orally	Greater ara-C nucleotide formation in vitro, longer $t_{1/2}$	313
2'-Azido-2'-deoxy-ara-C	Resistant to deaminase	Has antitumor activity	314
5'-(Cortisone-21-phosphoryl) ester of ara-C	Resistant to deaminase, combines two active drugs, targets to steroid receptor + cells	Less active than ara-C in vivo	315
5'-Acyl esters of ara-C (e.g., 5'-palmitate ester)	Lipid-soluble, depot form, resistant to deamination	Prolonged $t_{1/2}$, has antitumor activity, but clinical formulation difficult owing to poor aqueous solubility	316
N^4-Behenoyl-ara-C	Resistant to deamination	Active in human acute leukemia	190
Ara-C conjugate with poly-H^5-(2-hydroxyethyl)-L-glutamine	Slow release of ara-C in vivo	Increased in vivo activity in mice	317
Dihydro-5-azacytidine	Resistant to chemical degradation	—	318
5-Aza-arabinosylcytosine	Resistant to deamination	Broad solid tumor spectrum in mice	319
5-Aza-2'-deoxycytidine	Activated by deoxycytidine kinase	Antileukemic activity in humans	320
2'-2'-Difluorodeoxycytidine	Longer intracellular half-life, different mechanism of action	Broad solid tumor spectrum in experimental tumors	321

ara-C, cytosine arabinoside; $t_{1/2}$, half-life.

solid tumors, but it failed to demonstrate clinical activity. A related analog, 5-aza-2'-deoxycytidine (decitabine), is incorporated into DNA and, as does 5-azacytidine, inhibits DNA methylation and promotes differentiation.[194] In human K562 cells, decitabine was a more effective inducer of erythroid differentiation than its related analog 5-azacytidine, with less acute cell toxicity.[195] In addition, decitabine showed a greater antileukemic activity than ara-C when the two drugs were compared in vitro on a panel of human leukemia cell lines of different phenotypes,[196] and also in some animal tumor models.[197] Decitabine has entered human clinical trials. Encouraging antileukemic activity has been observed in patients with untreated and heavily pretreated acute myelocytic leukemia and acute lymphoblastic leukemia, and the drug has been shown to induce trilineage responses in patients with advanced myelodysplastic syndromes.[198,199] Its most frequent side effects are myelosuppression and moderate emesis, with no other major extrahematologic toxicities.[198,199]

5-Azacytidine

The success of ara-C as an antileukemic agent has encouraged the search for other cytidine analogs, particularly those that would not require activation by deoxycytidine kinase (the enzyme deleted in many ara-C–resistant tumors). Considering ribonucleosides with structural changes in the basic pyrimidine ring was logical because these would be activated in all likelihood by uridine-cytidine kinase, an entirely separate enzyme. Considerable enthusiasm greeted the introduction of 5-azacytidine, an analog of cytidine synthesized by Sorm and colleagues in 1963[200] and later isolated as a product of fungal cultures.[201] The compound was found to be toxic to both bacterial and mammalian cells. In clinical trials, however, its most important cytostatic action was exerted against myeloid leukemias and myelodysplasia (MDS),[202–205] Other actions of 5-azacytidine have awakened interest among biologists and clinicians, however, particularly its ability to inhibit DNA cytosine methylation and, as a consequence, to promote expression of "suppressed" genes. For example, the drug is able to promote the synthesis of fetal hemoglobin, an effect believed to be mediated by hypomethylation of the γ-globin gene in erythroid precursor cells.[206,207] The use of 5-azacytidine for gene demethylation in inherited diseases, a subject of considerable interest in molecular genetics, has been limited by its bone marrow toxicity and by concerns about carcinogenesis. The important features of the pharmacokinetics and clinical effects of 5-azacytidine are summarized in Table 8.6.

Structure and Mechanism of Action

The biochemistry and pharmacology of 5-azacytidine have been reviewed in depth by Glover and Leyland-Jones.[208] The analog 5-azacytidine differs from cytidine in the presence of a nitrogen at the 5 position of the heterocyclic ring (Fig. 8.10). This substitution renders the ring chemically unstable and leads to spontaneous decomposition of the compound in neutral or alkaline solution, with a half-life of approximately 4 hours. The product of this ring opening, N-formylamidinoribofuranosylguanylurea, may recyclyze

TABLE 8.6

KEY FEATURES OF 5-AZACYTIDINE PHARMACOLOGY

Factor	Result
Mechanism of action	Incorporated into DNA and RNA; prevents DNA methylation
Metabolism	Activated to a triphosphate
	Degraded to inactive, unstable 5-azauridine by cytidine deaminase
Pharmacokinetics and elimination	Plasma half-lives not known, but the drug is chemically unstable and is rapidly deaminated
Drug interactions	Tetrahydrouridine inhibits deamination, increases toxicity
Toxicity	Myelosuppression
	Nausea, vomiting after bolus dose
	Hepatocellular dysfunction
	Muscle tenderness, weakness
	Lethargy, confusion, coma
Precautions	Hepatic failure may occur in patients with underlying liver dysfunction
	Use with caution in patients with altered mental status

to form the parent compound but is also susceptible to further spontaneous decomposition to ribofuranosylurea.[209] This spontaneous chemical instability is important in the drug's use in two ways: (a) the ultimate antitumor activity of the drug has been attributed to its incorporation into nucleic acids and subsequent spontaneous decomposition, and (b) the preparation formulated for clinical application must be administered within several hours of its dissolution in dextrose and water or saline.[210] In buffered solutions such as Ringer's lactate and at acidic pH, the agent is considerably more stable, with a half-life of 65 hours at 25°C and 94 hours at 20°C.[211]

The mechanism of 5-azacytidine action has not been firmly established, although the balance of evidence suggests

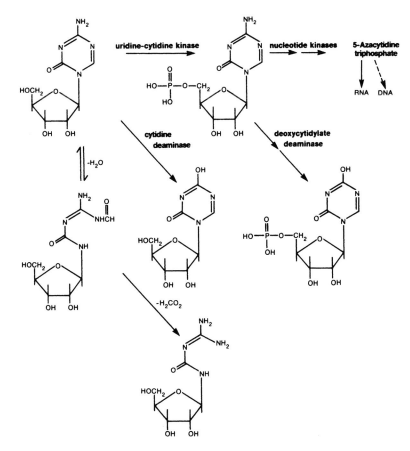

Figure 8.10 Metabolic activation and degradation of 5-azacytidine.

that, as a triphosphate, it competes with CTP for incorporation into RNA,[212] the primary event that leads to a number of different effects on RNA processing and function.[213] These effects include an inhibition of the formation of ribosomal 28 S and 18 S RNA from higher molecular-weight species,[214] defective methylation[215] and acceptor function of transfer RNA,[216] disassembly of polyribosomes,[217] and a marked inhibition of protein synthesis.[218]

Other effects of 5-azacytidine, however, may be more relevant to its antitumor activity. This analog is also incorporated into DNA,[219,220] although to a lesser extent than into RNA. The consequences of 5-azacytidine incorporation into DNA are not fully understood, but one important effect is the inhibition of DNA methylation. The methylation of cytosine residues in DNA inactivates specific genes, whereas treatment of cells with 5-azacytidine inhibits the function of DNA methyl transferase and leads to enhanced expression of a broad variety of genes, depending on the cell type studied.[221,222] Transferase inhibition occurs through formation of a covalent bond between the azacytidine base and a prolylcysteine dipeptide group on the enzyme[223] (Fig. 8.11).

Cellular Pharmacology

The analog 5-azacytidine readily enters mammalian cells by a facilitated nucleoside transport mechanism shared with the physiologic nucleosides uridine and cytidine.[220] The initial step in its activation consists of conversion to a monophosphate by uridine-cytidine kinase (Fig. 8.10), which is found in low concentration in human acute myelocytic leukemia cells,[209] has low affinity for 5-azacytidine ($K_m = 0.2$ to 11 mmol/L),[224,225] and probably represents the rate-limiting step in 5-azacytidine activation. Either uridine[226] or cytidine is capable of preventing 5-azacytidine toxicity in the whole animal and in tissue culture[227] by competitively inhibiting its phosphorylation. Deletion of uridine-cytidine kinase has been observed in mutant Novikoff hepatoma cells resistant to 5-azacytidine,[221] as well as in other resistant cell types.[228] Cytidine deaminase, found in 10-fold to 30-fold higher concentration than uridine-cytidine kinase in leukemic cells, degrades 5-azacytidine to 5-azauridine. The role of this enzyme in resistance to 5-azacytidine has not been defined.

Further activation of 5-azacytidine monophosphate (5-aza-CMP) to a triphosphate probably occurs by the enzyme dCMP kinase and nucleoside diphosphate kinase. One hour after exposure of cells to the drug, 60 to 70% of acid-soluble radioactivity was identified as 5-azacytidine triphosphate.[221]

Both drug concentration and duration of exposure are important determinants of 5-azacytidine cytotoxicity in tissue culture, a finding consistent with a preferential action on rapidly dividing cells. In tissue culture experiments it

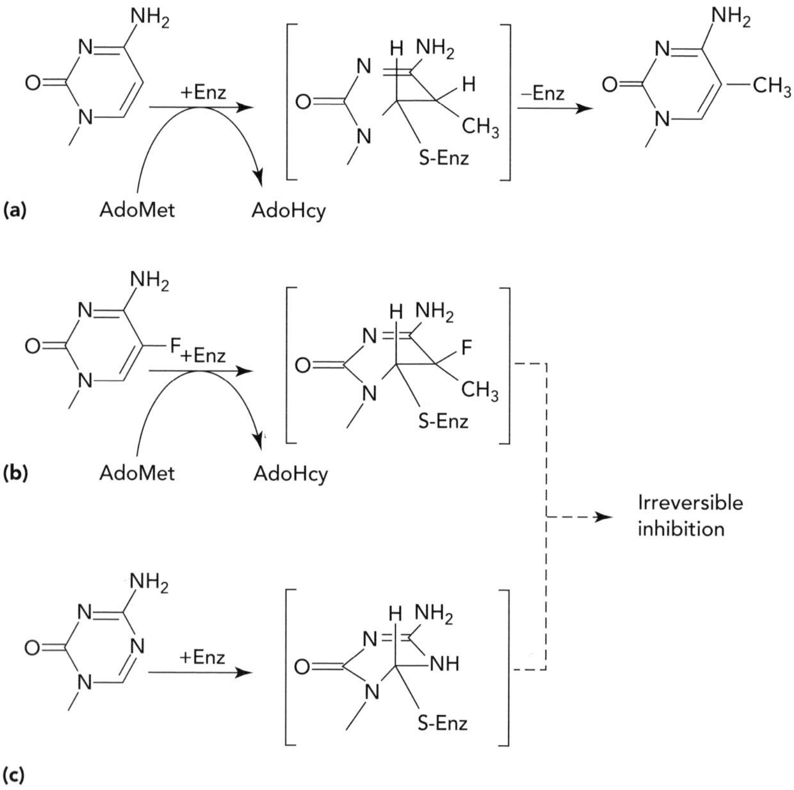

Figure 8.11 Formation of a 5,6-dihydropyrimidine intermediate during methylation of a target DNA containing (a) Cyt, (b) deoxy-5 flurocytidine; and (c) 5-azacytidine.

has greatest lethality for cells in the S phase of the cell cycle and relatively little effect against nondividing cells.[229,230] Dose-survival curves in vivo for L1210 and normal hematopoietic cells are both biphasic, however, which indicates perhaps the presence of more than a single site or mechanism of cytotoxic action.[231] A closely related analog, 5-aza-2′-deoxycytidine, causes an induction of p21[WAF1] and cell cycle arrest in G_1 at very low concentrations ($2–4 \times 10^{-8}$ m) while at levels of 10^{-7} m it induced phosphorylation of MAP kinase and G_2 arrest as well. At these higher doses, cells become apoptotic.[232]

In addition to its cytotoxic effects, 5-azacytidine has other biologic actions of possible importance in its clinical use. Through its inhibition of DNA methylation, it has been found to induce the synthesis of various proteins, including hepatic enzymes (tyrosine aminotransferase),[233] metallothionein,[234] β- and γ-globin,[206] histocompatibility proteins,[235,236] and T-cell surface markers.[237] It can reactivate repressed genes coding for thymidine kinase,[238] hypoxanthine-guanine phosphoribosyl transferase,[239] or DNA repair[240] and in doing so may convert drug-resistant cells to drug-sensitive, or vice versa. Probably through its effects on DNA methylation, 5-azacytidine is able to increase the immunogenicity of tumor cells,[235] induce senescence in cell lines,[241] and increase the phenotypic diversity of tumor cell lines in mice.[238] The drug has mutagenic and teratogenic effects,[229,242,243] but it is not known to be carcinogenic in humans.

Assay Methods

At present, no assay method specific for 5-azacytidine has been developed for clinical use. Future attempts to develop such methods will undoubtedly be complicated by the chemical instability of the drug, its very limited lipid solubility (which will complicate attempts at extraction and concentration from plasma), and the presence in serum of cytidine deaminase, an enzyme that hydrolyzes 5-azacytidine.

Clinical Pharmacology and Pharmacokinetics

The limited information available on 5-azacytidine pharmacokinetics in animals and humans is based on studies using drug labeled with radioactive carbon (^{14}C)[210,244–246] and provides an incomplete understanding of drug disposition because of the drug's extensive metabolism and chemical decomposition. After subcutaneous injection [^{14}C]5-azacytidine is well absorbed, as judged by radioactivity levels in plasma.[237] Radioactivity distributes into a volume approximately equal to or greater than total-body water (0.58 to 1.15 L/kg) with little plasma protein binding. Peak plasma levels of 0.1 to 1.0 mmol/L are reached by drug infusion at a rate of 2 to 6 mg/hour in adult patients. The primary half-life of radioactivity in plasma is approximately 3.5 hours after bolus intravenous injection but after 30 minutes, less than 2% of radioactivity is associated with intact drug.[210] Isolated measurements of radioactivity in the CSF indicate poor penetration of drug, with a CSF:plasma ratio of less than 0.1.

The identity of metabolites is unclear in humans. 5-Azacytidine is known to be susceptible to deamination by cytidine deaminase,[247,248] an enzyme found in high concentrations in liver, granulocytes, and intestinal epithelium and in lower concentration in plasma. A number of metabolic products have been identified in the urine of beagle dogs, including 5-azacytosine, 5-azauracil, and ring cleavage products.[244] The last-named product may result from decomposition of the parent compound or of its deamination product, 5-azauridine.

Toxicity

In patients with acute myelogenous leukemia, a number of schedules of administration have been used for 5-azacytidine,[202–205] including single weekly intravenous doses of up to 750 mg/m², daily doses of 150 to 200 mg/m² for 5 to 10 consecutive days, and continuous infusion of similar daily doses for up to 5 days (Table 8.7). With each of these

---

TABLE 8.7

5-AZACYTIDINE IN THE TREATMENT OF ACUTE MYELOGENOUS LEUKEMIA

Reference	Dosage (mg/m²/day)	Bolus (B) or Infusion (I)	Toxicity	CR Rate
203	150–200 × 5 days	B	N, V, D, M	5/14 (36%)
204	300–400 × 5 days	B	N, V, D, M	3/18 (17%)
205	150–200 × 5 days	I	M	11/45 (24%)
206	200–250 × 5 days	B	N, V, M, Neuro	5/18 (28%)

CR, complete remission; D, diarrhea; M, myelosuppression; N, nausea; Neuro, neuromuscular symptoms (see text); V, vomiting.

schedules, the primary toxicity has been leukopenia, although nausea and vomiting have been extremely bothersome for patients receiving the drug in bolus doses, which has led some investigators to favor continuous intravenous infusion.[204] The latter schedule is also supported by cell kinetic considerations, in view of the drug's greater activity in the S phase of the cell cycle and its very rapid metabolism in humans. The continuous infusion of 5-azacytidine requires fresh preparation of drug at frequent intervals, usually every 3 to 4 hours, because of the chemical instability of the agent. The response rate to 5-azacytidine in previously treated patients with acute myelocytic leukemia has varied from 17 to 36% and seems to be approximately equivalent for the bolus and continuous-infusion schedules.

In patients with MDS, a lower dose of 75 mg/m^2 per day for 7 days repeated every 28 days, yields a best response after the fifth cycle of therapy.[205] Maximal dosages, as shown in Table 8.7, produce profound leukopenia and somewhat lesser thrombocytopenia. Hepatotoxicity also has been observed, particularly in patients with preexisting hepatic dysfunction.[249] The lower doses in MDS cause an initial decrease in peripheral blood counts, with a subsequent rise with onset of response.

A syndrome of neuromuscular toxicity was observed by Levi and Wiernik[250] in patients receiving 200 mg/m^2 per day by intravenous bolus injection. Whether this peculiar reaction was related to the somewhat higher dosage of drug is unclear, but neurotoxicity has been reported only sporadically by other investigators using this agent.[204] Several less worrisome acute toxic reactions have been associated with 5-azacytidine, including transient fever, a pruritic skin rash, and, rarely, hypotension during or immediately after bolus intravenous administration.[203]

Low-dose 5-azacytidine has been used in experimental trials to raise fetal hemoglobin levels in patients with sickle cell anemia and thalassemia,[207] but concerns regarding carcinogenicity, as demonstrated in studies of rats exposed to the drug,[251] have discouraged routine use to treat these diseases and it has been largely replaced by hydroxyurea for this indication. When given as a continuous infusion of 2 mg/kg per day for 5 days, one cycle per month, the drug regularly produces a reticulocytosis of fetal hemoglobin-containing cells and an increase in hemoglobin content in blood of 2 to 3 g/100 mL.[252] On this schedule, little myelosuppression, nausea, or vomiting occur.

5-Azacytidine was approved for treatment of patients with MDS in 2004, based on the results of a randomized phase III trial comparing the drug to best supportive care. Thirty-five percent of patients achieved either a clear improvement in blood counts or decreased transfusion requirements, the transfusion benefits lasting a median of more than 330 days.[205] In an overview of published trials on 5-azacytidine in MDS, 6% achieved a complete response in bone marrow and peripheral blood.[253.]

Decitabine, a deoxynucleoside analog of 5-azacytidine, has a similar spectrum of activity against myeloid leukemias and MDS, a similar spectrum of toxicity (myelosuppresion), but no evidence of carcinogenicity in preclinical tests.[254] It inhibits DNA methyltransferase activity in a manner analogous to 5-azaC[223] becoming incorporated into DNA and forming a covalent link with the methyltransferase. It induces hemoglobin F synthesis in patients with sicle cell anemia. In seven patients, refractory to hydroxyurea, a schedule of 0.3 mg/kg per day for 5 days a week for 2 weeks, repeating every 6 weeks, raised Hb F levels from a baseline of 2% to a median of 14%, with a corresponding increase in total Hb of 1.5 g/dL.[255] These promising results have led to larger trials aimed at establishing its beneficial effects on clinical end points, such as painful crisis and hospitalization.

Decitabine in higher doses (45 mg/m^2 daily for 3 days every 6 weeks) produced a 49% response rate in patients with MDS, as judged by improvement in blood counts, but at the expense of severe myelosuppression, and a 7% mortality rate from infection.[256] In significantly higher doses (50 to 100 mg/m^2 twice daily for 5 days), it produced objective responses in 18 of 64 patients (28%) in blastic crisis of chronic myelogenous leukemia, including six complete hematologic remissions.[257] This regimen produced severe myelosuppression in most patients, with platelet recovery above 30,000 per milliliter occurring at a median of 27 days at the lowest doses given. Other toxicities included drug-related fever in 21%, and drug-related infection in 34%. The role of this drug in leukemia treatment is still uncertain.

GEMCITABINE

Gemcitabine (2,2-difluorodeoxycytidine, dFdC) is the most important cytidine analog to enter clinical trials since ara-C (Fig. 8.12). It has become incorporated into the standard first-line therapy for patients with pancreatic cancer, lung cancer, and transitional cell cancer of the bladder.[258–261] The drug was selected for development on the basis of its impressive activity against murine solid tumors and human xenografts in nude mice.[262] In tissue culture it is generally more potent than ara-C; the 50% inhibition concentration values for human leukemic cells range from 3 to 10 nmol/L for 48-hour exposure compared with 26 to 52 nmol/L for ara-C.[263] Although its metabolism to triphosphate status and its effects on DNA in general mimic those of ara-C, differences are found in kinetics of inhibition and additional sites of action of the newer compound, and clearly the spectrum of clinical activity is different.

Cellular Pharmacology, Metabolism, and Mechanism of Action

Gemcitabine retains many of the characteristics of ara-C. Its key features are shown in Table 8.2. Influx of gemcitabine through the cell membrane occurs via active nucleoside transporters,[264] and deoxycytidine kinase phosphorylates

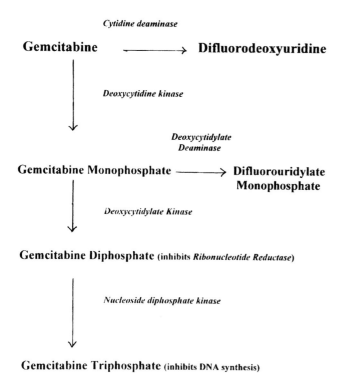

Gemcitabine $\xrightarrow{\text{\textit{Cytidine deaminase}}}$ **Difluorodeoxyuridine**

$\downarrow$ *Deoxycytidine kinase*

Gemcitabine Monophosphate $\xrightarrow{\text{\textit{Deoxycytidylate Deaminase}}}$ **Difluorouridylate Monophosphate**

$\downarrow$ *Deoxycytidylate Kinase*

Gemcitabine Diphosphate (inhibits *Ribonucleotide Reductase*)

$\downarrow$ *Nucleoside diphosphate kinase*

Gemcitabine Triphosphate (inhibits DNA synthesis)

Figure 8.12   Key steps in gemcitabine metabolism.

gemcitabine intracellularly to produce difluorodeoxycytidine monophosphate (dFdCMP), from which point it is converted to its diphosphate and triphosphate difluorodeoxycytidine (dFdCDP, dFdCTP) (Fig. 8.12).[265] Its affinity for deoxycytidine kinase is threefold lower than that of deoxycytidine itself, whereas it has a 50% lower affinity for cytidine deaminase than does deoxycytidine.[266] Cytidine deaminase conversion of gemcitabine to difluorodeoxyuridine (dFdU) represents the main catabolic pathway.[267] To a lesser extent, pyrimidine nucleoside phosphorylase clears gemcitabine by cleaving the pyrimidine base from the furanose ring.

As with ara-C, in vitro studies of gemcitabine suggest potent inhibition of DNA synthesis as its mechanism of action,[262,265,268] but kinetic studies indicate that the killing effects of gemcitabine are not confined to the S phase of the cell cycle, and the drug is as effective against confluent cells as it is against cells in log-phase growth.[269] The cytotoxic activity may be a result of several actions on DNA synthesis: dFdCTP competes with dCTP as a weak inhibitor of DNA polymerase[268]; dFdCDP is a potent inhibitor of ribonucleotide reductase, which results in depletion of deoxyribonucleotide pools necessary for DNA synthesis[270]; and dFdCTP is a substrate for incorporation into DNA and, after the incorporation of one more nucleotide, leads to DNA strand termination.[271] This "extra" nucleotide may be important in hiding the dFdCTP from DNA repair enzymes because incorporation of gemcitabine into DNA appears to be resistant to the normal mechanisms of DNA repair.[272] These effects on DNA synthesis represent the main action of gemcitabine, and evidence demonstrates that incorporation of dFdCTP into DNA is critical for gemcitabine-induced apoptosis.[273,274]

Several important differences exist between ara-C and gemcitabine (Fig. 8.13). First, dFdCTP has a biphasic elimination from leukemic cells with α half-life ($t_{1/2}\alpha$) of 3.9 hours and β half-life ($t_{1/2}\beta$) of 16 hours, whereas ara-CTP has a monophasic elimination with $t_{1/2} = 0.7$ hours.[265] Also, dFdCDP is a stronger inhibitor of ribonucleotide reductase (50% inhibition concentration of 4 μmol/L), and exposure to the drug blocks incorporation of labeled cytidine into the cellular pool of dCTP.[270] Further, dFdC causes a decrease in all intracellular deoxynucleotide triphosphates, consistent with inhibition of ribonucleotide reductase. The significance of ribonucleotide reductase inhibition is uncertain. Some cell lines selected for resistance to

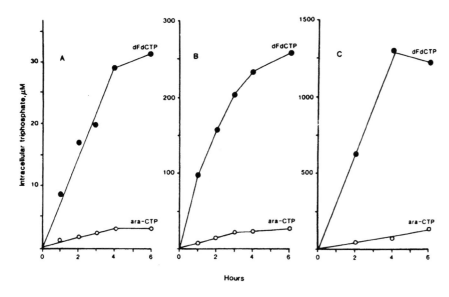

Figure 8.13   Accumulation of difluorodeoxycytidine triphosphate (dFdCTP) and arabinosylcytosine triphosphate (ara-CTP) as a function of time after incubation of cells with either dFdCTP or ara-C at drug concentrations of 1 μmol/L (A), 10 μmol/L (B), and 100 μmol/L (C). (Adapted from Heinemann V, Hertel LW, Grindey GB, et al. Comparison of the cellular pharmacokinetics and toxicity of 2',2'-difluorodeoxycytidine and 1-beta-D-arabinofuranosylcytosine. Cancer Res 1988;48:4024–4031.)

other inhibitors of this enzyme, such as hydroxyurea and deoxyadenosine, do not show cross-resistance to dFdC.[275] On the other hand, resistance to gemcitabine has been demonstrated through overexpression of ribonucleotide reductase.[276] Nevertheless, the significance of ribonucleotide reductase inhibition may be in the potentiating effects of deoxyribonucleotide depletion on other sites of gemcitabine action.[277] For example, deamination of dFdCMP by dCMP deaminase requires activation by dCTP. As dCTP pools become depleted by the effect of gemcitabine on ribonucleotide reductase, less deamination of gemcitabine diphosphate occurs and intracellular accumulation of gemcitabine metabolites increases. Furthermore, high intracellular concentration of dFdCTP appears to inhibit dCMP deaminase directly.[267]

The activity of dFdCTP on DNA repair mechanisms may allow for increased cytotoxicity of other chemotherapeutic agents, particularly platinum compounds. Cisplatin works by creating interstrand and intrastrand cross-links. A mechanism of resistance may be removal of these cross-links by nucleotide excision repair (NER). Preclinical studies of tumor cell lines show that cisplatin-DNA adducts are enhanced in the presence of gemcitabine.[278] In cisplatin-resistant tumor cell lines, which have increased expression of NER, the addition of gemcitabine inhibited the repair of cisplatin-induced DNA lesions and correlated with cytotoxic synergism.[274,278] Combined gemcitabine and cisplatin are standard agents in the treatment of lung cancer and transitional cell cancer.

Mechanisms of Resistance

Resistance to gemcitabine is not fully understood. In vitro studies have suggested several possible mechanisms. Gemcitabine resistance has been correlated with tumor levels of deoxycytidine kinase.[279] Induction of cytidine deaminase and high concentrations of heat-shock protein have also conferred gemcitabine resistance to cells.[280,281] Preclinical studies have also demonstrated that increased expression of ribonucleotide reductase may be associated with gemcitabine resistance.[282] Lastly, inhibition of nucleoside transporters can prevent the influx of gemcitabine through the cell membrane and the absense of transporters has been associated with reduced survival in patients with pancreatic cancer.[264,283] Resistance to gemcitabine has not been associated with increased P-glycoprotein expression.[284]

Pharmacokinetic Data

In animals, gemcitabine pharmacokinetics is largely determined by deamination, which proceeds more rapidly in mice than in rats or dogs.[285] Gemcitabine half-life in mice is 0.28 hours compared with 1.38 hours in dogs. In both species, the predominant elimination product is dFdU. Grunewald and colleagues[286] have found that, in both in vitro cell lines and cells taken from patients during treatment, maximal accumulation of dFdCTP occurs when plasma (or tissue culture) drug concentrations are in the range of 15 to 20 µmol/L, a level achieved during 3-hour infusions of 300 mg/m^2.

Abbruzzese et al.[287] performed a phase I study of gemcitabine given weekly as a 30-minute infusion on days 1, 8, and 15, followed by a 1-week rest in patients with refractory solid tumors. The maximum tolerated dose (MTD) was 1,000 mg/m^2 per week. The dose-limiting toxicity was myelosuppression characterized by thrombocytopenia with relative sparing of granulocytes. Pharmacokinetic analysis showed a $t_{1/2}$ of 8 minutes for the parent compound and a biphasic elimination of dFdU, with $t_{1/2}\alpha = 27$ minutes and $t_{1/2}\beta = 14$ hours. No relationship was found between degree of myelosuppression and any of the pharmacokinetic parameters. The area under the curve of plasma dFdC was proportional to the dose over a range of 10 to 1,000 mg/m^2 per week. Clearance was dose-independent but varied widely among individuals (39 to 1,239 L/hour per m^2 at a dose of 1,000 mg/m^2).

Although a higher gemcitabine dose of 2,200 mg/m^2 administered over 30 minutes on days 1, 8, and 15 can be safely given to less heavily treated or chemonaïve patients, no improvement in efficacy has been demonstrated.[288] This lack of dose responsiveness may be caused by the limited ability of cells to generate the active metabolite. In the case of ara-C, the ability of peripheral blood mononuclear cells to accumulate ara-CTP saturates at ara-C concentrations of greater than 10 µmol/L.[289] A similar series of studies with gemcitabine have demonstrated that activation of gemcitabine by deoxycytidine kinase to dFdCTP is saturated at infusion rates of approximately 10 mg/m^2 per minute.[285,290] This "dose-rate infusion" produced steady-state dFdC levels of 15 to 20 µmol/L in plasma. In leukemic patients, the maximum tolerated dose (MTD) for "dose-rate infusion" is 4,800 mg/m^2 infused over 480 minutes.[291,] Biphasic elimination of gemcitabine was seen in the leukemic cells at this infusion rate, and inhibition of DNA synthesis was proportional to the intracellular level of dFdCTP. Based on these results, a phase I study using constant dose-rate infusion of gemcitabine on days 1, 8, and 15 every 28 days was carried out in patients with metastatic solid tumors.[292] Although the first-cycle MTD was estimated to be 2,250 mg/m^2 over 225 minutes, the recommended phase II dose of gemcitabine administered as a dose-rate infusion is 1,500 mg/m^2 over 150 minutes because of the occurrence of cumulative neutropenia and thrombocytopenia at higher doses. The dose-rate infusion resulted in higher levels of dFdCTP in circulating leukemic cells than a fixed infusion duration of 30 minutes (Fig. 8.14).

In a proof-of-concept study, Tempero and colleagues[293] performed a randomized phase II study of constant dose-rate infusion at 10 mg/m^2 per minute versus dose-intense infusion over 30 minutes in patients with advanced pancreatic cancer. Patients were randomized to receive gemcitabine

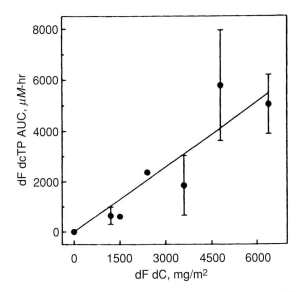

Figure 8.14 Relationship between dose of gemcitabine (difluorodeoxycytidine, dFdC) and area under the curve (AUC) of difluorodeoxycytidine triphosphate (dFdCTP) in circulating leukemia cells during gemcitabine infusion. Shown is the mean ± standard error of the mean of the AUC observed for patients at each dose during this phase I study of dose-rate infusion of gemcitabine in patients with leukemia. (Adapted from Grunewald R, Kantarjian H, Du M, et al. Gemcitabine in leukemia: a phase I clinical, plasma, and cellular pharmacology study. J Clin Oncol 1992;10:406–413.)

1,500 mg/m² over 150 minutes or 2,200 mg/m² over 30 minutes. Constant dose-rate infusion resulted in a twofold increase in intracellular gemcitabine triphosphate in peripheral blood mononulear cells compared with the standard 30-minute infusion. Furthermore, activity appeared to be enhanced with the constant dose-rate infusion because 1-year survival increased from 9% to 28%. Further studies utilizing the dose rate infusion schedule are underway.

Gemcitabine has been studied in children and the maximum tolerated dose of gemcitabine given as a 30-minute infusion weekly for 3 of 4 weeks is 1,200 mg/m². Myelosuppression is the dose-limiting toxicity, and pharmacokinetics in pediatric patients is similar to the adult population.[294]

Toxicity

The dose-limiting toxicity of gemcitabine is invariably hematologic, and the toxicity profile differs according to schedule. In general, the longer-duration infusions lead to greater myelosuppression. The MTD for a daily × 5 schedule every 21 days is 12 mg/m² per day or 60 mg/m² per cycle.[295] The MTD for twice-weekly doses of gemcitabine administered for 3 weeks with a 1-week rest period depends on the time of infusion. When the drug is administered over 5 minutes, the MTD is 150 mg/m², and when it is administered as a 30-minute infusion, the MTD is 75 mg/m².[296] For a 24-hour infusion given weekly in 3 of 4 weeks, the MTD is 180

mg/m² per dose.[297] The weekly dose schedule has gained popularity and is implemented as a 30-minute infusion in 3 of 4 weeks. The MTD for chemonaïve patients is 2,200 mg/m² per week, and the MTD for pretreated patients is 800 to 1,000 mg/m² per week.[287,288] A dose of 1,000 mg/m² per week, for 3 to 4 weeks, given over 30 minutes, is recommended for treatment of a variety of solid tumors.

The safety of gemcitabine has been evaluated in a database including 22 studies using the once-weekly treatment regimen.[298] Nine hundred seventy-nine patients received at least one dose of gemcitabine and were evaluable for toxicity. World Health Organization (WHO) grade 3 and 4 neutropenia occurred in 19.3% and 6% of patients, respectively. WHO grade 3 and 4 thrombocytopenia occurred in 4.1% and 1.1% of patients, respectively. Clinically significant consequences of hematologic toxicity were uncommon: only 1.1% of patients experienced WHO grade 3 infection and 0.7% of patients required platelet transfusions. Among nonhematologic toxicities, flulike symptoms including fever, headache, back pain, and myalgias occur in approximately 45% of patients. The duration of these symptoms was short, and less than 1% of patients discontinued therapy because of flulike symptoms. Asthenia is also common, occurring in 42% of patients. A transient, mild elevation in liver function test results (WHO grade 1 or 2 elevations in alanine aminotransferase) was detected in 41% of cycles.

Although severe nonhematologic reactions are rare, several specific syndromes complicating gemcitabine therapy are emerging. Thrombotic microangiopathy as manifested by hemolytic-uremic syndrome or thrombotic thrombocytopenic purpura has been reported as a complication of gemcitabine therapy,[299–301] and a review of the manufacturer's database estimated an overall incidence rate of 0.015%.[302] However, a large single institution review demonstrated 9 cases of gemcitabine-associated microangiopathy among a total of 2,586 cases of microangiopathy for an estimated incidence of 0.31%.[303] Patients who are treated for prolonged periods (i.e., longer than 1 year) may be at higher risk for developing hemolytic-uremic syndrome or thrombotic microangiopathy.

Severe pulmonary toxicity as manifested by acute respiratory distress syndrome, capillary leak syndrome, or interstitial pneumonitis has been reported in patients treated with gemcitabine.[304,305] A review of the Lilly world-wide database identified 91 patients with serious pulmonary toxicity for an estimated incidence of less than 0.1%.[306] Caution is warranted when combining gemcitabine with drugs known to cause pulmonary dysfunction, such as bleomycin. A study substituting gemcitabine for etoposide in the BEACOPP regimen in Hodgkin's lymphoma led to severe pulmonary toxicity, possibly as a result of interaction with bleomycin.[307]

A multicenter study evaluated the role of gemcitabine in patients with hepatic or renal dysfunction.[308] Patients with elevated bilirubin experienced increased toxicity and should receive reduced doses; whereas, patients with elevated transaminases did not experience increased toxicity. Patients with elevated creatinine appeared to be more sensitive to gemcitabine but did not require dose reductions.

Radiation Sensitization

Because of its inhibition of ribonucleotide reductase and DNA polymerase, gemcitabine may have strong radiosensitization effects. Preclinical studies of gemcitabine have shown potent radiosensitization effects in human colon, pancreatic, head and neck, and cervical cancer cell lines.[309–312] These effects parallel the intracellular depletion of deoxyadenosine triphosphate and are most prominent when gemcitabine is administered before radiation therapy. Interestingly, the radiosensitization effect had no correlation with dFdCMP incorporation into DNA, which suggests that the inhibition of ribonucleotide reductase is the key mechanism of action.[313] In vitro studies suggest that maximal enhancement of radiation sensitization occurs when gemcitabine is administered before radiation, and in vivo studies suggest that this effect is most pronounced when the time interval is 24 to 60 hours.[309,314,315] Gemcitabine radiosensitization may be best in mismatch repair-deficient cells when compared with mismatch repair-proficient cells.[316]

Despite the radiosensitization seen in preclinical studies, the initial phase I and II studies of gemcitabine and radiation therapy have not demonstrated markedly improved clinical activity, and are associated with increased toxicity. In a phase I trial of twice-weekly gemcitabine and concurrent radiation in patients with advanced pancreatic cancer, the MTD was 40 mg/m^2 administered over 30 minutes on Monday and Thursday of each week.[317] The dose-limiting toxicities were grade 3 neutropenia, thrombocytopenia, nausea, and vomiting. This regimen was subsequently evaluated in phase II study for patients with locally advanced pancreatic cancer, and the median survival was 7.9 months.[318] When given once weekly with radiation at doses of 300 to 500 mg/m^2 to patients with locally advanced pancreatic cancer, gemcitabine is associated with increased severe toxicity and similar survival when compared with historical conrols using flouropyrimidines with external beam radiation therapy.[319] An attempt to combine weekly gemcitabine with fluorouracil and external beam radiation therapy in patients with locally advanced pancreatic cancer was stopped when five of the first seven patients experienced dose-limiting toxicities at gemcitabine doses of 100 and 50 mg/m^2.[320]

The inability to deliver full-dose gemcitabine concurrent with radiation has been demonstrated in other tumor types as well. A phase II study of gemcitabine administered weekly with concurrent external beam radiation therapy in patients with unresectable head and neck cancer required dose de-escalation from 300 mg/m^2 per week to 50 mg/m^2 per week as the result of a high rate of mucosa-related toxicity.[321] A phase I study of weekly gemcitabine with concurrent radiotherapy in patients with locally advanced lung cancer established a maximally tolerated dose of 300 mg/m^2.[322] Dose-limiting toxicities included grade 3 esophagitis and grade 3 pneumonitis. Ongoing trials are continuing to define the toxicity of efficacy of gemcitabine when combined with external beam radiation therapy.

REFERENCES

1. Bergmann W, Feeney R. Contributions to the study of marine products: XXXII. The nucleosides of sponges. J Org Chem 1951;16:981.
2. Roberts WK, Dekker CA. A convenient synthesis of arabinosylcytosine (cytosine arabinoside). J Org Chem 1967; 32:84.
3. Lee WW, Benitez A, Goodman L, et al. Potential anticancer agents: XL. Synthesis of the beta-anomer of 9-(D-arabinofuranosyl) adenine. J Am Chem Soc 1960;82:2648.
4. Warrell RP, Berman E. Phase I and II study of fludarabine phosphate in leukemia: therapeutic efficacy with delayed central nervous system toxicity. J Clin Oncol 1986;4:74.
5. Dalal M, Plowman J, Breitman TR, et al. Arabinofuranosyl-5-azacytosine: antitumor and cytotoxic properties. Cancer Res 1986;46:831.
6. Ellison RR, Holland JF, Weil M, et al. Arabinosyl cytosine: a useful agent in the treatment of acute leukemia in adults. Blood 1968;32:507.
7. Bishop JF, Matthews JP, Young GA, et al. A randomized study of high-dose cytarabine in induction in acute myeloid leukemia. Blood 1996;87:1710.
8. Mayer RJ, Davis RB, Schiffer CA, et al. Intensive chemotherapy in adults with acute myeloid leukemia. N Engl J Med 1994;331:896.
9. Bloomfield CD, Lawrence D, Byrd JC, et al. Frequency of prolonged remission duration after high-dose cytarabine by cytogenetic subtype. Cancer Res 1998;58:4173.
10. Cadman E, Farber L, Berd D, et al. Combination therapy for diffuse leukocytic lymphoma that includes antimetabolites. Cancer Treat Rep 1977;61:1109.
11. Bryan JH, Henderson ES, Leventhal BG. Cytosine arabinoside and 6-thioguanine in refractory acute lymphocytic leukemia. Cancer 1974;33:539.
12. Guilhot F, Chastang C, Michallet M, et al. Interferon alfa-2b combined with cytarabine versus interferon alone in chronic myelogenous leukemia. N Engl J Med 1997;337:223.
13. Furth JJ, Cohen SS. Inhibition of mammalian DNA polymerase by the 5′-triphosphate of 9-β-D-arabinofuranosylcytosine and the triphosphate of 9-β-D-arabinofuranosyladenine. Cancer Res 1968;28:2061.
14. Townsend AJ, Cheng YC. Sequence-specific effects of ara-5- aza-CTP and ara-CTP on DNA synthesis by purified human DNA polymerases in vitro: visualization of chain elongation on a defined template. Mol Pharmacol 1987;32:330.
15. Kimball AP, Wilson MJ. Inhibition of DNA polymerase by β-D-arabinosylcytosine and reversal of inhibition by deoxycytidine-5′-triphosphate. Proc Soc Exp Biol 1968;127:429.
16. Graham FL, Whitmore GF. Studies in mouse L-cells on the incorporation of 1-β-D-arabinofuranosylcytosine into DNA and on inhibition of DNA polymerase by 1-β-D-arabinofuranosylcytosine-5′-triphosphate. Cancer Res 1970;30:2636.
17. Chu MY, Fischer GA. A proposed mechanism of action of 1-β-D-arabinofuranosylcytosine as an inhibitor of the growth of leukemic cells. Biochem Pharmacol 1962;11:423.
18. Yoshida S, Yamada M, Masaki S. Inhibition of DNA polymerase-α and -β of calf thymus by 1-β-D-arabinofuranosylcytosine-5′-triphosphate. Biochim Biophys Acta 1977;477:144.
19. Fram RJ, Kufe DW. Effect of 11-β-D-arabinofuranosyl cytosine and hydroxyurea on the repair of x-ray-induced DNA single-strand breaks in human leukemic blasts. Biochem Pharmacol 1985;34:2557.

20. Fram RJ, Kufe DW. Inhibition of DNA excision repair and the repair of x-ray-induced DNA damage by cytosine arabinoside and hydroxyurea. Pharmacol Ther 1985;31:165.

21. Kufe WE, Major PP, Egan EM, et al. Correlation of cytotoxicity with incorporation of araC into DNA. J Biol Chem 1980;255: 8997.

22. Fram RJ, Egan EM, Kufe DW. Accumulation of leukemic cell DNA strand breaks with adriamycin and cytosine arabinoside. Leuk Res 1983;7:243.

23. Kufe DW, Munroe D, Herrick D, et al. Effects of 1-β-D- arabinofuranosylcytosine incorporation on eukaryotic DNA template function. Mol Pharmacol 1984;26:128.

24. Kufe DW, Spriggs DR. Biochemical and cellular pharmacology of cytosine arabinoside. Semin Oncol 1985;12:34.

25. Major P, Egan E, Herrick D, et al. The effect of araC incorporation on DNA synthesis. Biochem Pharmacol 1982;31:2937.

26. Mikita T, Beardsley GP. Functional consequences of the arabinosylcytosine structural lesion in DNA. Biochemistry 1988;27: 4698.

27. Ross DD, Cuddy DP, Cohen N, et al. Mechanistic implications of alterations in HL-60 cell nascent DNA after exposure to 1-β-D-arabinofuranosylcytosine. Cancer Chemother Pharmacol 1992;31:61.

28. Woodcock DM, Fox RM, Cooper IA. Evidence for a new mechanism of cytotoxicity of 1-β-D-arabinofuranosylcytosine. Cancer Res 1979;39:418.

29. Moore EC, Cohen SS. Effects of arabinonucleotides on ribonucleotide reduction by an enzyme system from rat tumor. J Biol Chem 1967;242:2116.

30. Hawtrey AO, Scott-Burden T, Robertson G. Inhibition of glycoprotein and glycolipid synthesis in hamster embryo cells by cytosine arabinoside and hydroxyurea. Nature 1974;252:58.

31. Mitchell T, Sarabin E, Kufe D. Effects of 1-β-D-arabinofuranosylcytosine on proto-oncogene expression in human U-937 cells. Mol Pharmacol 1986;30:398.

32. Bianchi Scarra GL, Romani M, Civiello DA, et al. Terminal erythroid differentiation in the K-562 cell line by 1-β-D-arabinofuranosylcytosine: accompaniment by c-myc messenger RNA decrease. Cancer Res 1986;46:6327.

33. Vogelstein ER, Burke PJ, Schiffer CA, et al. Differentiation of leukemia cells to polymorphonuclear leukocytes in patients with acute nonlymphocytic leukemia. N Engl J Med 1986; 315:15.

34. Anilkumar TV, Sarraf CE, Hunt T, et al. The nature of cytotoxic drug-induced cell death in murine intestinal crypts. Br J Cancer 1992;65:552.

35. Gunji H, Kharbanda S, Kufe D. Induction of internucleosomal DNA fragmentation in human myeloid leukemia cells by 1-β-D-arabinofuranosylcytosine. Cancer Res 1991; 51:741.

36. Strum JC, Small GW, Pauig SB, et al. 1-β-D-arabinofuranosylcytosine stimulates ceramide and diglyceride formation in HL-60 cells. J Biol Chem 1994;269:15493.

37. Kharbanda S, Datta R, Kufe D. Regulation of c-jun gene expression in HL-60 leukemia cells by 1-β-D-arabinofuranosylcytosine. Potential involvement of a protein kinase C dependent mechanism. Biochemistry 1991;30:7947.

38. Brach MA, Kharbanda SM, Herrmann F, et al. Activation of the transcription factor kB in human KG-1 myeloid leukemia cells treated with 1-β-D-arabinofuranosylcytosine. Mol Pharmacol 1992;41:60.

39. Kharbanda SM, Sherman ML, Kufe DW. Transcriptional regulation of c-jun gene expression by arabinofuranosylcytosine in human myeloid leukemia cells. J Clin Invest 1990;86:1517.

40. Bullock G, Ray S, Reed J, et al. Evidence against a direct role for the induction of c-jun expression in the mediation of drug-induced apoptosis in human acute leukemia cells. Clin Cancer Res 1995;1:559.

41. Dou QP, An B, Will P. Induction of a retinoblastoma phosphatase activity by anticancer drugs accompanies p53-independent G_1 arrest and apoptosis. Proc Natl Acad Sci U S A 1995;92: 9019.

42. Ikeda M, Jakoi L, Nevins J. A unique role for the Rb protein in controlling E2F accumulation during cell growth and differentiation. Proc Natl Acad Sci U S A 1996;93:3215.

43. Plagemann PGW, Marz R, Wolhueter RM. Transport and metabolism of deoxycytidine and 1-β-D-arabinofuranosylcytosine into cultured Novikoff rat hepatoma cells, relationship to phosphorylation and regulation of triphosphate synthesis. Cancer Res 1978;38:978.

44. Wiley JS, Jones SP, Sawyer WH, et al. Cytosine arabinoside influx and nucleoside transport sites in acute leukemia. J Clin Invest 1982;69:479.

45. Belt JA, Noel DL. Isolation and characterization of a mutant of L1210 murine leukemia deficient in nitrobenzylthioinosine-insensitive nucleoside transport. J Biol Chem 1988;263:13819.

45a. Pui CH, Relling MV, Downing JR. Acute lymphoblastic leukemia. N Engl J Med. 2004; 350:1535–1548.

46. Wiley JS, Taupin J, Jamieson GP, et al. Cytosine arabinoside transport and metabolism in acute leukemias and T-cell lymphoblastic lymphoma. J Clin Invest 1985;75:632.

47. Tanaka M, Yoshida S. Formation of cytosine arabinoside-5′-triphosphate in cultured human leukemic cell lines correlates with nucleoside transport capacity. Jpn J Cancer Res 1987;78:851.

48. White JC, Rathmell JP, Capizzi RL. Membrane transport influences the rate of accumulation of cytosine arabinoside in human leukemia cells. J Clin Invest 1987;79:380.

49. Jamieson GP, Snook MB, Wiley JS. Saturation of intracellular cytosine arabinoside triphosphate accumulation in human leukemic blast cells. Leuk Res 1990;14:475.

49a. Damaraju VL, Damarjus S, Young JD, et al. Nucleoside anti-cancer drugs: The role of nucleoside transporters in resistance to cancer chemotherapy. Oncogene 2003;22:7524.

50. Chottiner EG, Shewach SDS, Datta NS, et al. Cloning and expression of human deoxycytidine kinase cDNA. Proc Natl Acad Sci U S A 1991;88:1531.

51. Owens JK, Shewach DS, Ullman B, et al. Resistance to 1-β-D-arabinofuranosylcytosine in human T lymphoblasts mediated by mutations within the deoxycytidine kinase gene. Cancer Res 1992;52:2389.

52. Hapke DM, Stegmann APA, Mitchell BS. Retroviral transfer of deoxycytidine kinase into tumor cell lines enhances nucleoside toxicity. Cancer Res 1996;56:2343.

53. Manome Y, Wen PY, Dong Y, et al. Viral vector transduction of the human deoxycytidine kinase cDNA sensitizes glioma cells to the cytotoxic effects of cytosine arabinoside in vitro and in vivo. Nat Med 1996;2:567.

54. Gandhi V, Plunkett W. Cell cycle-specific metabolism of arabinosyl nucleosides in K562 human leukemia cells. Cancer Chemother Pharmacol 1992;31:11.

55. Coleman CN, Stoller RG, Drake JC, et al. Deoxycytidine kinase: properties of the enzyme from human leukemic granulocytes. Blood 1975;46:791.

56. Wang L, Kucera GL. Deoxycytidine kinase is phosphorylated in vitro by protein kinase Cα. Biochim Biophys Acta 1994;1224:161.

57. Hande KR, Chabner BA. Pyrimidine nucleoside monophosphate kinase from human leukemic blast cells. Cancer Res 1978;38:579.

58. Chou T-C, Arlin Z, Clarkson BD, et al. Metabolism of 1-β-D-arabinofuranosylcytosine in human leukemic cells. Cancer Res 1977;37:3561.

59. Chou T-C, Hutchison DJ, Schmid FA, et al. Metabolism and selective effects of 1-β-D-arabinofuranosylcytosine in L1210 and host tissues in vivo. Cancer Res 1975;35:225.

60. Camiener GW, Smith CG. Studies of the enzymatic deamination of cytosine arabinoside: I. Enzyme distribution and specific specificity. Biochem Pharmacol 1965;14:1405.

61. Chabner B, Johns D, Coleman C, et al. Purification and properties of cytidine deaminase from normal and leukemic granulocytes. J Clin Invest 1974;53:922.

62. Stoller RG, Myers CE, Chabner BA. Analysis of cytidine deaminase and tetrahydrouridine interaction by use of ligand techniques. Biochem Pharmacol 1978;27:53.

63. Jackson RC. The regulation of thymidylate biosynthesis in Novikoff hepatoma cells and the effects of Amethopterin, 5- fluorodeoxyuridine, and 3-deazauridine. J Biol Chem 1978;253:7440.

64. Ellims P, Kao AH, Chabner BA. Deoxycytidylate deaminase: purification and kinetic properties of the enzyme isolated from human spleen. J Biol Chem 1981;256:6335.

65. Lauzon GJ, Paran JH, Paterson ARP. Formation of 1-β-D-arabinofuranosylcytosine diphosphate choline in cultured human leukemic RPMI 6410 cells. Cancer Res 1978; 38:1723.

66. Myers-Robfogel MW, Spatato AC. 1-β-D-Arabinofuranosylcytosine nucleotide inhibition of sialic acid metabolism in WI-38 cells. Cancer Res 1980; 40:1940.

67. Chu MY, Fischer GA. Comparative studies of leukemic cells sensitive and resistant to cytosine arabinoside. Biochem Pharmacol 1965;14:333.

68. Drahovsky D, Kreis W. Studies on drug resistance: II. Kinase patterns in P815 neoplasms sensitive and resistant to 1-β-D-arabinofuranosylcytosine. Biochem Pharmacol 1970;19:940.

69. De Saint Vincent BR, Dechamps M, Buttin G. The modulation of the thymidine triphosphate pool of Chinese hamster cells by dCMP deaminase and UDP reductase. J Biol Chem 1980; 255:162.

70. De Saint Vincent BR, Buttin G. Studies on 1-β-D-arabinofuranosyl cytosine–resistant mutants of Chinese hamster fibroblasts: III. Joint resistance to arabinofuranosyl cytosine and to excess thymidine—a semidominant manifestation of deoxycytidine triphosphate pool expansion. Somatic Cell Genet 1979;5:67.

71. De Saint Vincent BR, Buttin G. Studies on 1-β-D-arabinofuranosyl cytosine–resistant mutants of Chinese hamster fibroblasts: IV. Altered regulation of CTP synthetase generates arabinosylcytosine and thymidine resistance. Biochim Biophys Acta 1980;610:352.

72. Cohen A, Ullman B. Analysis of the drug synergism between thymidine and arabinosyl cytosine using mouse S-49 T lymphoma mutants. Cancer Chemother Pharmacol 1985;14:70.

73. Eliopoulos N, Cournoyer D, Momparler RL. Drug resistance to 5-aza-2'-deoxycytidine, 2',2'-difluorodeoxycytidine, and cytosine arabinoside conferred by retroviral-mediated transfer of human cytidine deaminase cDNA into murine cells. Cancer Chemother Pharmacol 1998;42:373.

74. Riva C, Khyari SE, Rustum Y, et al. Resistance to cytosine arabinoside in cells transfected with activated Ha-ras oncogene. Anticancer Res 1995;15:1297.

75. Koo H, Monks A, Mikheev A, et al. Enhanced sensitivity to 1-β-D-arabinofuranosylcytosine and topoisomerase II inhibitors in tumor cell lines harboring activated ras oncogenes. Cancer Res 1996;56:5211.

76. Tattersall MNH, Ganeshaguru K, Hoffbrand AV. Mechanisms of resistance of human acute leukaemia cells to cytosine arabinoside. Br J Haematol 1974;27:39.

77. Steuart CD, Burke PJ. Cytidine deaminase and the development of resistance to arabinosylcytosine. Nature New Biol 1971;233:109.

78. Chiba P, Tihan T, Szekeres T, et al. Concordant changes of pyrimidine metabolism in blasts of two cases of acute myeloid leukemia after repeated treatment with araC in vivo. Leukemia 1990;4:761.

79. Chang P, Wiernik PH, Reich SD, et al. Prediction of response to cytosine arabinoside and daunorubicin in acute nonlymphocytic leukemia. In: Mandelli F, ed. Therapy of Acute Leukemias: Proceedings of the Second International Symposium, Rome, 1977. Rome: Lombardo Editore, 1979:148.

80. Smyth JF, Robins AB, Leese CL. The metabolism of cytosine arabinoside as a predictive test for clinical response to the drug in acute myeloid leukaemia. Eur J Cancer 1976;12:567.

81. Estey E, Plunkett W, Dixon D, et al. Variables predicting response to high dose cytosine arabinoside therapy in patients with refractory acute leukemia. Leukemia 1987;1:580.

82. Ross DD, Thompson BW, Joneckis CC, et al. Metabolism of araC by blast cells from patients with ANLL. Blood 1986;68:76.

83. Rustum YM, Riva C, Preisler HD. Pharmacokinetic parameters of 1-β-D-arabinofuranosylcytosine and their relationship to intracellular metabolism of araC, toxicity, and response of patients with acute nonlymphocytic leukemia treated with conventional and high-dose araC. Semin Oncol 1987;14:141.

84. Estey EH, Keating MJ, McCredie KB, et al. Cellular ara-CTP pharmacokinetics, response, and karyotype in newly diagnosed acute myelogenous leukemia. Leukemia 1990;4:95.

85. Preisler HD, Rustum Y, Priore RL. Relationship between leukemic cell retention of cytosine arabinoside triphosphate and the duration of remission in patients with acute non-lymphocytic leukemia. Eur J Cancer Clin Oncol 1985;21:23.

86. Plunkett W, Iacoboni S, Keating MJ. Cellular pharmacology and optimal therapeutic concentrations of 1-β-D-arabinofuranosylcytosine 5'-triphosphate in leukemic blasts during treatment of refractory leukemia with high-dose 1-β-D-arabinofuranosylcytosine. Scand J Haematol 1986;34:51.

87. Ibrado AM, Uang Y, Fang G, et al. Overexpression of Bcl-2 or Bcl-xL inhibits araC-induced CPP32/Yama protease activity and apoptosis of human acute myelogenous leukemia HL-60 cells. Cancer Res 1996;56:4743.

88. Keith FJ, Bradbury DA, Zhu Y, et al. Inhibition of bcl-2 with antisense oligonucleotides induces apoptosis and increases the sensitivity of AML blasts to araC. Leukemia 1995;9:131.

89. Campos L, Rouault J, Sabido O, et al. High expression of bcl-2 protein in acute myeloid leukemia cells is associated with poor response to chemotherapy. Blood 1993;81:3091.

90. Ruvolo PR, Deng X, Carr BK, et al. A functional role for mitochondrial protein kinase Cα Bcl2 phosphorylation and suppression of apoptosis. J Biol Chem 1998;273:25436.

91. Wang S, Vrana JA, Bartimole TM, et al. Agents that down-regulate or inhibit protein kinase C circumvent resistance to 1-β-D-arabinofuranosylcytosine–induced apoptosis in human leukemia cells that overexpress Bcl-2. Mol Pharmacol 1997;52:1000.

92. Kharbanda S, Emoto Y, Kisaki H, et al. 1-β-D-arabinofuranosylcytosine activates serine/threonine protein kinases and c-jun gene expression in phorbol ester-resistant myeloid leukemia cells. Mol Pharmacol 1994;46:67.

93. Kolla SS, Studzinski GP. Constitutive DNA binding of the low mobility forms of the AP-1 and SP-1 transcription factors in HL60 cells resistant to 1-β-D-arabinofuranosylcytosine. Cancer Res 1994;54:1418.

94. Karon M, Chirakawa S. The locus of action of 1-β-D-arabinofuranosylcytosine in the cell cycle. Cancer Res 1970;29:687.

95. Young RC, Schein PS. Enhanced antitumor effect of cytosine arabinoside given in a schedule dictated by kinetic studies in vivo. Biochem Pharmacol 1973;22:277.

96. Burke PJ, Karp JE, Vaughan WP, et al. Recruitment of quiescent tumor by humoral stimulatory activity: requirements for successful chemotherapy. Blood Cells 1982;8:519.

97. Aglietta M, Colly L. Relevance of recruitment-synchronization in the scheduling of 1-β-D-arabinofuranosylcytosine in a slowgrowing acute myeloid leukemia of the rat. Cancer Res 1979;39:2727.

98. Vaughan WP, Karp JE, Burke PJ. Two-cycle-timed sequential chemotherapy for adult acute nonlymphocytic leukemia. Blood 1984;64:975.

99. Preisler HD, Azarnia N, Raza A, et al. Relationship between percent of marrow cells in S phase and the outcome of remission induction therapy for acute nonlymphocytic leukemia. Br J Haematol 1984;56:399.

100. Raza A, Preisler HD, Day R, et al. Direct relationship between remission duration in acute myeloid leukemia and cell cycle kinetics: a leukemia intergroup study. Blood 1990;76:2191.

101. Boutagy J, Harvey DJ. Determination of cytosine arabinoside in human plasma by gas chromatography with a nitrogen-sensitive detector and by gas chromatography-mass spectrometry. J Chromatogr 1978;146:283.

102. Ho DHW, Frei E III. Clinical pharmacology of 1-β-D-arabinofuranosylcytosine. Clin Pharmacol Ther 1971;12:944.

103. Mehta BM, Meyers MB, Hutchison DJ. Microbiologic assay for cytosine arabinoside (NSC-63878): the use of a mutant of *Streptococcus faecium* var. *durans* resistant to methotrexate (NSC-740) and 6-mercaptopurine (NSC-755). Cancer Chemother Rep 1975;59:515.

104. Van Prooijen HC, Vierwinden G, van Egmond J, et al. A sensitive bioassay for pharmacokinetic studies of cytosine arabinoside in man. Eur J Cancer 1976;12:899.

105. Piall EM, Aherne GW, Marks VM. A radioimmunoassay for cytosine arabinoside. Br J Cancer 1979;40:548.

106. Sinkule JA, Evans WE. High-performance liquid chromatographic assay for cytosine arabinoside, uracil arabinoside, and some related nucleosides. J Chromatogr 1983;274:87.

107. Liversidge GG, Nishihata T, Higuchi T, et al. Simultaneous analysis of 1-β-D-arabinofuranosyluracil and sodium salicylate

in biologic samples by high-performance liquid chromatography. J Chromatogr 1983;276:375.

108. Harris AL, Potter C, Bunch C, et al. Pharmacokinetics of cytosine arabinoside in patients with acute myeloid leukaemia. Br J Clin Pharmacol 1979;8:219.

109. Van Prooijen R, van der Kleijn E, Haanen C. Pharmacokinetics of cytosine arabinoside in acute leukemia. Clin Pharmacol Ther 1977;21:744.

110. Wau SH, Huffman DH, Azarnoff DL, et al. Pharmacokinetics of 1-β-d-arabinofuranosylcytosine in humans. Cancer Res 1974;34:392.

111. Lopez JA, Nassif E, Vannicola P, et al. Central nervous system pharmacokinetics of high-dose cytosine arabinoside. J Neurooncol 1985;3:119.

112. Slevin ML, Piall EM, Aherne GW, et al. Effect of dose and schedule on pharmacokinetics of high-dose cytosine arabinoside in plasma and cerebrospinal fluid. J Clin Oncol 1983;1:546.

113. Beithaupt H, Pralle H, Eckhardt T, et al. Clinical results and pharmacokinetics of high-dose cytosine arabinoside (HD ARA-C). Cancer 1982;50:1248.

114. Early AP, Preisler HD, Slocum H, et al. A pilot study of high-dose of 1-β-d-arabinofuranosylcytosine for acute leukemia and refractory-lymphoma: clinical response and pharmacology. Cancer Res 1982;42:1587.

115. Capizzi RL, Yang JL, Ching E, et al. Alterations of the pharmacokinetics of high-dose araC by its metabolite, high araU in patients with acute leukemia. J Clin Oncol 1983;1:763.

116. Donehower RC, Karp JE, Burke PJ. Pharmacology and toxicity of high-dose cytarabine by 72-hour continuous infusion. Cancer Treat Rep 1986;70:1059.

117. Slevin ML, Piall EM, Aherne GW, et al. Subcutaneous infusion of cytosine arabinoside: a practical alternative to intravenous infusion. Cancer Chemother Pharmacol 10;112:1983.

118. Liliemark JO, Paul CY, Gahrton CG, et al. Pharmacokinetics of 1-β-d-arabinofuranosylcytosine 5′-triphosphate in leukemic cells after intravenous and subcutaneous administration of 1-β-D-arabinofuranosylcytosine. Cancer Res 1985;45:2373.

119. Markman M. The intracavitary administration of cytarabine to patients with nonhematopoietic malignancies: pharmacologic rationale and results of clinical trials. Semin Oncol 1985;12 (Suppl 3):177.

120. Kirmani S, Zimm S, Cleary SM, et al. Extremely prolonged continuous intraperitoneal infusion of cytosine arabinoside. Cancer Chemother Pharmacol 1990;25:454.

121. Chamberlain MC, Khatibi S, Kim JC, et al. Treatment of leptomeningeal metastasis with intraventricular administration of Depot cytarabine (DTC 101). Arch Neurol 1993;50:261.

122. Howell SB, Glantz MJ, LaFollette S, et al. A controlled trial of Depocyt™ for the treatment of lymphomatous meningitis. Proc Am Soc Clin Oncol 1999;18:11a(abst 34).

122a. Cole, B.F., Glantz, M.J., Jaeckle, K.A., et al. Quality-of-life-adjusted survival comparison of sustained-release cytosine arabinoside versus intrathecal methotrexate for treatment of solid tumor neoplastic meningitis. Cancer 2003;97:3053.

123. Capizzi RL, Powell BL, Cooper MR, et al. Dose-related pharmacologic effects of high-dose araC and its use in combination with asparaginase for the treatment of patients with acute nonlymphocytic leukemia. Scand J Haematol 1986;34(Suppl 44):17.

124. Plunkett W, Iacoboni S, Estey E, et al. Pharmacologically directed araC therapy for refractory leukemia. Semin Oncol 1985;12(Suppl 3):20.

125. Wisch JS, Griffin JD, Kufe DN. Response of preleukemic syndromes to continuous infusion of low-dose cytarabine. N Engl J Med 1983;309:1599.

126. Tilly H, Bastard C, Bizet M, et al. Low-dose cytarabine: persistence of a clonal abnormality during complete remission of acute nonlymphocytic leukemia. N Engl J Med 1986;314:246.

127. Beran M, Hittelman WN, Andersson BS, et al. Induction of differentiation in human myeloid leukemia cells with cytosine arabinoside. Leuk Res 1986;10:1033.

128. Cheson BD, Jasperse DM, Simon R, et al. A critical appraisal of low-dose cytosine arabinoside in patients with acute nonlymphocytic leukemia and myelodysplastic syndromes. J Clin Oncol 1986;4:1857.

129. Raijmakers R, DeWitte T, Linssen P, et al. The relation of exposure time and drug concentration in their effect on cloning efficiency after incubation of human bone marrow with cytosine arabinoside. Br J Haematol 1986;62:447.

130. Skipper HE, Schabel FM Jr, Wilcox WS. Experimental evaluation of potential anticancer agents: XXI. Scheduling of arabinosyl cytosine to take advantage of its S-phase specificity against leukemia cells. Cancer Chemother Rep 1967;51:125.

131. Frei E III, Bickers JN, Hewlett JS, et al. Dose schedule and antitumor studies of arabinosyl cytosine (NSC 63878). Cancer Res 1969;29:1325.

132. Mitchell MS, Wade ME, DeConti RC, et al. Immunosuppressive effects of cytosine arabinoside and methotrexate in man. Ann Intern Med 1969;70:535.

133. Talley RW, Vaitkevicius VK. Megaloblastosis produced by a cytosine antagonist, 1-β-D-arabinofuranosyl cytosine. Blood 1963;21:352.

134. Slavin RE, Dias MA, Saral R. Cytosine arabinoside-induced gastrointestinal toxic alterations in sequential chemotherapeutic protocols. Cancer 1978;42:1747.

135. Goode UB, Leventhal B, Henderson E. Cytosine arabinoside in acute granulocytic leukemia. Clin Pharmacol Ther 1971;12:599.

136. Altman A, Dinndorf P, Quinn JJ. Acute pancreatitis in association with cytosine arabinoside therapy. Cancer 1982;49:1384.

137. Anderson BS, Luna MA, Yee C, et al. Fatal pulmonary failure complicating high-dose cytosine arabinoside therapy in acute leukemia. Cancer 1990;65:1079.

138. Weisman SJ, Scoopo FJ, Johnson GM, et al. Septicemia in pediatric oncology patients: the significance of viridans streptococcal infections. J Clin Oncol 1990;8:453.

139. Rudnick SA, Cadman EC, Capizzi RL, et al. High-dose cytosine arabinoside (HD ARA-C) in refractory acute leukemia. Cancer 1979;44:1189.

140. George CB, Mansour RP, Redmond J, et al. Hepatic dysfunction and jaundice following high-dose cytosine arabinoside. Cancer 1984;54:2360.

141. Herzig RH, Hines JD, Herzig GP, et al. Cerebellar toxicity with high-dose cytosine arabinoside. J Clin Oncol 1987;5:927.

142. Rubin EH, Anderson JW, Berg DT, et al. Risk factors for high-dose cytarabine neurotoxicity: an analysis of a cancer and leukemia group B trial in patients with acute myeloid leukemia. J Clin Oncol 1992;10:948.

143. Shaw PJ, Procopis PG, Menser MA, et al. Bulbar and pseudobulbar palsy complicating therapy with high-dose cytosine arabinoside in children with leukemia. Med Pediatr Oncol 1991;19:122.

144. Paul M, Joshua D, Rahme N, et al. Fatal peripheral neuropathy associated with axonal degeneration after high-dose cytosine arabinoside in acute leukemia. Br J Haematol 1991;79:521.

145. Castleberry RP, Crist WM, Holbrook T, et al. The cytosine arabinoside syndrome. Pediatr Oncol 1981;9:257.

146. Hopen G, Mondino BJ, Johnson BL, et al. Corneal toxicity with systemic cytarabine. Am J Ophthalmol 1981;91:500.

147. Rassiga AL, Schwartz HJ, Forman WB, et al. Cytarabine-induced anaphylaxis: demonstration of antibody and successful desensitization. Arch Intern Med 1980;140:425.

148. Flynn TC, Harris TJ, Murphy GF, et al. Neutrophilic eccrine hidradenitis: a distinctive rash associated with cytarabine therapy and acute leukemia. J Am Acad Dermatol 1984;11:584.

149. Reykdal S, Sham R, Kouides P. Cytarabine-induced pericarditis: a case report and review of the literature of the cardio-pulmonary complications of cytarabine. Leuk Res 1995;19:141.

150. Eden OB, Goldie W, Wood T, et al. Seizures following intrathecal cytosine arabinoside in young children with acute lymphoblastic leukemia. Cancer 1978;42:53.

151. Kleinschmidt-DeMasters BK, Yeh M. "Locked-in syndrome" after intrathecal cytosine arabinoside therapy for malignant immunoblastic lymphoma. Cancer 1992;70:2504.

152. Bell WR, Whang JJ, Carbone PP, et al. Cytogenetic and morphologic abnormalities in human bone marrow cells during cytosine arabinoside therapy. Blood 1966;27:771.

153. Dixon RL, Adamson RH. Antitumor activity and pharmacologic disposition of cytosine arabinoside (NSC 63878). Cancer Chemother Rep 1965;48:11.

154. Schabel FM Jr. In vivo leukemic cell kill kinetics and curability in experimental systems. In: The Proliferation and Spread of Neoplastic Cells. Baltimore: Williams & Wilkins, 1968:379.

155. Tyrer DD, Kline I, Vendetti JM, et al. Separate and sequential chemotherapy of mouse leukemia L1210 with 1-β-D-arabinofuranosylcytosine hydrochloride and 1,3-bis-(2-chloroethyl)-1-nitrosourea. Cancer Res 1968;27:873.

156. Kern DH, Morgan CR, Hildebrand-Zanki SU. In vitro pharmacodynamics of 1-β-D-arabinofuranosylcytosine: synergy of antitumor activity with cis-diamminedichloroplatinum(II). Cancer Res 1988;48:117.

157. Burchenal JH, Dollinger MR. Cytosine arabinoside in combination with 6-mercaptopurine, methotrexate, or fluorouracil in L1210 mouse leukemia. Cancer Chemother Rep 1967;51:435.

158. Gandhi V, Kemena A, Keating MJ, et al. Fludarabine infusion potentiates arabinosylcytosine metabolism in lymphocytes of patients with chronic lymphocytic leukemia. Cancer Res 1992;52:897.

159. Cadman E, Eiferman F. Mechanism of synergistic cell killing when methotrexate precedes cytosine arabinoside. J Clin Invest 1979;64:788.

160. Hoovis ML, Chu MY. Enhancement of the antiproliferative action of 1-β-D-arabinofuranosylcytosine by methotrexate in murine leukemic cells (L5178Y). Cancer Res 1973; 33:521.

161. Chresta CM, Hicks R, Hartley JA, et al. Potentiation of etoposide-induced cytotoxicity and DNA damage in CCRF- CEM cells by pretreatment with non-cytotoxic concentrations of arabinosyl cytosine. Cancer Chemother Pharmacol 1992;31:139.

162. LePage GA, White SC. Scheduling of arabinosylcytosine (araC) and 6-thioguanine (TG). Proc Am Assoc Cancer Res 1972;13:11.

163. Lee MYW, Byrnes JJ, Downey KM, et al. Mechanism of inhibition of deoxyribonucleic acid synthesis by 1-β-D-arabinofuranosyladenosine triphosphate and its potentiation by 6-mercaptopurine ribonucleoside 5′-monophosphate. Biochemistry 1980;19:213.

164. Swinnen LJ, Barnes DM, Fisher SG, et al. 1-β-D-arabinofuranosylcytosine and hydroxyurea: production of cytotoxic synergy with cis-diamminedichloroplatinum(II) and modifications in platinum-induced DNA interstrand crosslinking. Cancer Res 1989;49:1383.

165. Ho DHW, Carter CJ, Brown NS, et al. Effects of tetrahydrouridine on the uptake and metabolism of 1-β-D-arabinofuranosylcytosine in human normal and leukemic cells. Cancer Res 1980;40:2441.

166. Chabner BA, Hande KR, Drake JC. AraC metabolism: implications for drug resistance and drug interactions. Bull Cancer 1979;66:89.

167. Kreis W, Woodcock TM, Gordon CS. Tetrahydrouridine: physiologic disposition and effect upon deamination of cytosine arabinoside in man. Cancer Treat Rep 1977; 61:1347.

168. Wong PP, Currie VE, Mackey RW, et al. Phase I evaluation of tetrahydrouridine combined with cytosine arabinoside. Cancer Treat Rep 1979;63:1245.

169. Rauscher F III, Cadman E. Biochemical and cytokinetic modulation of L1210 and HL-60 cells by hydroxyurea and effect on 1-1-β-D-arabinofuranosylcytosine metabolism and cytotoxicity. Cancer Res 1983;43:2688.

170. Grant S, Bhalla K, Rauscher F III, et al. Potentiation of 1-β-D-arabinofuranosylcytosine metabolism and cytotoxicity by 2,3-dihydro-1H-imidazolo[1,2-b]pyrazole in the human promyelocytic leukemia cell, HL-60. Cancer Res 1983; 43:5093.

171. Harris AW, Reynolds EC, Finch LR. Effects of thymidine on the sensitivity of cultured mouse tumor cells to 1-β-D-arabinofuranosylcytosine. Cancer Res 1979;39:538.

172. Grant S, Lehman C, Cadman E. Enhancement of 1-β-D-arabinofuranosylcytosine accumulation with L1210 cells and increased cytotoxicity following thymidine exposure. Cancer Res 1980;40:1525.

173. Danhauser LL, Rustum YM. Effect of thymidine on the toxicity, antitumor activity and metabolism of 1-β-D-arabinofuranosylcytosine in rats bearing a chemically induced colon carcinoma. Cancer Res 1980;40:1274.

174. Fram R, Major P, Egan E, et al. A phase I-II study of combination therapy with thymidine and cytosine arabinoside. Cancer Chemother Pharmacol 1983;11:43.

175. Blumenreich MS, Chou TC, Andreeff M, et al. Thymidine as a kinetic and biochemical modulator of 1-β-D-arabinofuranosylcytosine in human acute nonlymphocytic leukemia. Cancer Res 1984;44:825.

176. Zittoun R, Zittoun J, Marquet J, et al. Modulation of 1-β-D-arabinofuranosylcytosine metabolism by thymidine in human acute leukemia. Cancer Res 1985;45:5186.

177. Roberts D, Peck C, Hillard S, et al. Methotrexate-induced changes in the level of 1-β-D-arabinofuranosylcytosine triphosphate in L1210 cells. Cancer Res 1979;39:4048.

178. Bakic M, Chan D, Andersson BS, et al. Effect of 1-β-D-arabinofuranosylcytosine on nuclear topoisomerase II activity and on the DNA cleavage and cytotoxicity produced by 4′-(9-acridinylamino)methanesulfon-m-anisidide and etoposide in m-AMSA-sensitive and -resistant human leukemia cells. Biochem Pharmacol 1987;36:4067.

179. Kemena A, Gandhi V, Shewach DS, et al. Inhibition of fludarabine metabolism by arabinosylcytosine during therapy. Cancer Chemother Pharmacol 1992;31:193.

180. Gandhi V, Estey E, Du M, et al. Minimum dose of fludarabine for the maximal modulation of 1-β-D-arabinofuranosylcytosine triphosphate in human leukemia blasts during therapy. Clin Cancer Res 1997;3:1539.

181. Karp JE, Burke PJ, Donehower RC. Effects of rhGM-CSF on intracellular araC pharmacology in vitro in acute myelocytic leukemia: comparability with drug-induced humoral stimulatory activity. Leukemia 1990;4:553.

182. Bhalla K, Tang C, Ibrado AM, et al. Granulocyte-macrophage colony-stimulating factor/interleukin-3 fusion protein (pIXY 321) enhances high-dose ara-C-induced programmed cell death or apoptosis in human myeloid leukemia cells. Blood 1992;80:2883.

183. Bhalla K, Holladay C, Arlin Z, et al. Treatment with interleukin-3 plus granulocyte-macrophage colony-stimulating factors improves the selectivity of araC in vitro against acute myeloid leukemia blasts. Blood 1991;78:2674.

184. Hiddemann W, Kiehl M, Zuhlsdorf M, et al. Granulocyte-macrophage colony-stimulating factor and interleukin-3 enhance the incorporation of cytosine arabinoside into the DNA of leukemic blasts and the cytotoxic effect on clonogenic cells from patients with acute myeloid leukemia. Semin Oncol 1992;19:31.

185. Stone RM, Berg DT, George SL, et al. Granulocyte-macrophage colony-stimulating factor after initial chemotherapy for elderly patients with primary acute myelogenous leukemia. N Engl J Med 1995;332:1671.

186. Grant S, Turner AJ, Bartimole TM, et al. Modulation of 1-β-D-arabinofuranosyl cytosine-induced apoptosis in human myeloid leukemia cells by staurosporine and other pharmacologic inhibitors of protein kinase C. Oncol Res 1994;6:87.

187. Jarvis WD, Povirk LF, Turner AJ, et al. Effects of bryostatin 1 and other pharmacological activators of protein kinase C on 1-β-D-arabinofuranosyl cytosine-induced apoptosis in HL-60 human promyelocytic leukemia cells. Biochem Pharmacol 1994;47:839.

188. Ho DHW. Biochemical studies of a new antitumor agent, O²,2′-cyclocytidine. Biochem Pharmacol 1974;23:1235.

189. Kodama K, Morozumi M, Saitoh K, et al. Antitumor activity and pharmacology of 1-β-D-arabinofuranosylcytose-5′- stearylphosphate: an orally active derivative of 1-β-D-arabinofuranosylcytosine. Jpn J Cancer Res 1989;80:679.

190. Ueda T, Nakamura T, Ando S, et al. Pharmacokinetics of N^4-behenoyl-of 1-β-D-arabinofuranosylcytosine in patients with acute leukemia. Cancer Res 1983;43:3412.

191. Chow TC, Burchenal JH, Fox JJ, et al. Metabolism and effects of 5-(β-D-ribofuranosyl)isocytosine in P815 cells. Cancer Res 1979;39:721.

192. Woodcock TM, Chou TC, Tan CTC, et al. Biochemical, pharmacological, and phase I clinical evaluation of pseudoisocytidine. Cancer Res 1980;40:4243.

193. Allen TM, Mehra T, Hansen C, et al. Stealth liposomes: an improved sustained release system for 1-β-D-arabinofuranosylcytosine. Cancer Res 1992;52:2431.

194. Covey JM, Zaharko DS. Comparison of the in vitro cytotoxicity (L1210) of 5-aza-2′-deoxycytidine with its therapeutic and toxic effects in mice. Eur J Cancer Clin Oncol 1985;21:109.

195. Attadia V, Saglio G, Fusco A, et al. Effects of 5-aza-2′-deoxycytidine on erythroid differentiation and globin synthesis of the human leukemic cell line K562. In: Momparler RL, de Vos D, eds. 5-Aza-2′-Deoxycytidine: Preclinical and Clinical Studies. Haarlem, The Netherlands: PHC, 1990:89.

196. Momparler RL, Onetto-Pothier N, Momparler LF. Comparison of the anti-leukemic activity of cytosine arabinoside and 5-aza-2′-deoxycytidine against human leukemic cells of different phenotype. Leuk Res 1990;14:755.

197. Richel DJ, Colly LP, Lurvink E, et al. Comparison of the anti-leukemic activity of 5-aza-2′-deoxycytidine and arabinofuranosyl-cytosine arabinoside in rats with myelocytic leukemia. Br J Cancer 1988;58:730.

198. Pinto A, Zagonel V. 5-aza-2′-deoxycytidine (Decitabine) and 5-azacytidine in the treatment of acute myeloid leukemias and myelodysplastic syndromes: past, present and future trends. Leukemia 1993;7:51.

199. Kantarjian HM, O'Brien SM, Estey E, et al. Decitabine studies in chronic and acute myelogenous leukemia. Leukemia 1997;11:S35.

200. Sorm F, Piskala A, Cihak A, et al. 5-Azacytidine, a new highly effective cancerostatic. Experientia 1964;20:202.

201. Hanka LJ, Evans JS, Mason DJ, et al. Microbiological production of 5-azacytidine: 1. Production and biological activity. Antimicrob Agents Chemother 1966;6:619.

202. Karon M, Sieger L, Leimbrock S, et al. 5-Azacytidine: a new active agent for the treatment of acute leukemia. Blood 1973;42:359.

203. McCredie KB, Bodey GP, Burgess MA, et al. Treatment of acute leukemia with 5-azacytidine (NSC-102816). Cancer Chemother Rep 1973;57:319.

204. Vogler WR, Miller DS, Keller JW. 5-Azacytidine (NSC-102816): a new drug for the treatment of myeloblastic leukemia. Blood 1976;48:331.

205. Silverman LR, Demakos EP, Peterson BL,, et al. Randomized controlled trial of azacitidine in patients with the myelodysplastic syndrome: a study of the cancer and leukemia group B. J Clin Oncol. 2002;20:2429–2440.

206. Galanello R, Stamatoyannopoulos G, Papayannopoulou T. Mechanism of Hb F stimulation by S-stage compounds: in vitro studies with bone marrow cells exposed to 5-azacytidine, araC, or hydroxyurea. J Clin Invest 1988;81:1209.

207. Lowrey CH, Nienhuis AW. Brief report: treatment with azacytidine of patients with end-stage β-thalassemia. N Engl J Med. 1993;329:845–848

208. Glover AB, Leyland-Jones B. Biochemistry of azacytidine: a review. Cancer Treat Rep 1987;71:959.

209. Beisler J. Isolation, characterization, and properties of a labile hydrolysis product of the antitumor nucleoside, 5-azacytidine. J Med Chem 1978;21:204.

210. Israili ZH, Vogler WR, Mingioli ES, et al. The disposition and pharmacokinetics in humans of 5-azacytidine administered intravenously as a bolus or by continuous infusion. Cancer Res 1976;36:1453.

211. Notari RE, De Young JL. Kinetics and mechanisms of degradation of the antileukemic agent 5-azacytidine in aqueous solutions. J Pharm Sci 1975;64:1148.

212. Vesely J, Cihak A. 5-Azacytidine: mechanism of action and biological effects in mammalian cells. Pharmacol Ther 1978;2:813.

213. Glazer RI, Peale AL, Beisler JA, et al. The effects of 5-azacytidine and dihydro-5-azacytidine on nucleic ribosomal RNA and poly(A) RNA synthesis in L1210 cells in vitro. Mol Pharmacol 1980;17:111.

214. Weiss JW, Pitot HC. Inhibition of ribosomal precursor RNA maturation by 5-azacytidine and 8-azaguanine in Novikoff hepatoma cells. Arch Biochem Biophys 1974;165:588.

215. Lee T, Karon MR. Inhibition of protein synthesis in 5-azacytidine-treated HeLa cells. Biochem Pharmacol 1976;25:1737.

216. Kalousek F, Raska K, Jurovik M, et al. Effect of 5-azacytidine on the acceptor activity of sRNA. Colln Czech Chem Commun 1966;31:1421.

217. Cihak A, Vesela H, Sorm F. Thymidine kinase and polyribosomal distribution in regenerating rat liver following 5-azacytidine. Biochim Biophys Acta 1968;166:277.

218. Cihak A, Vesely J. Prolongation of the lag period preceding the enhancement of thymidine and thymidylate kinase activity in regenerating rat liver by 5-azacytidine. Biochem Pharmacol 1972;21:3257.

219. Li LH, Olin EJ, Buskirk HH, et al. Cytotoxicity and mode of action of 5-azacytidine on L1210 leukemia. Cancer Res 1970; 30:2760.

220. Plagemann PGW, Behrens M, Abraham D. Metabolism and cytotoxicity of 5-azacytidine in cultured Novikoff rat hepatoma and P388 mouse leukemia cells and their enhancement by preincubation with pyrazofurin. Cancer Res 1978;38:2458.

221. Adams RL, Burdon RH. DNA methylation in eukaryotes. CRC Crit Rev Biochem 1982;13:349.

222. Jones PA, Taylor SM, Wilson V. DNA modification, differentiation, and transformation. J Exp Zool 1983;228:287.

223. Christman JK. 5-azacytidine and 5-aza-2′-deoxycytidine as inhibitors of DNA methylation: mechanistic studies and their implications for cancer therapy. Oncogene 2002;21:5483–5495.

224. Drake JC, Stoller RG, Chabner BA. Characteristics of the enzyme uridine-cytidine kinase isolated from a cultured human cell line. Biochem Pharmacol 1977;26:64.

225. Lee T, Karon M, Momparler RL. Kinetic studies on phosphorylation of 5-azacytidine with the purified uridine-cytidine kinase from calf thymus. Cancer Res 1974;34:2481.

226. Vadlamudi S, Padarathsingh M, Bonmassar E, et al. Reduction of antileukemic and immunosuppressive activities of 5-azacytidine in mice by concurrent treatment with uridine. Proc Soc Exp Biol Med 1970;133:1232.

227. Vadlamudi S, Choudry JN, Waravdekar VS, et al. Effect of combination treatment with 5-azacytidine and cytidine on the life span and spleen and bone marrow cells of leukemic (L1210) and nonleukemic mice. Cancer Res 1970;30:362.

228. Vesely J, Cihak A, Sorm F. Biochemical mechanisms of drug resistance: IV. Development of resistance to 5-azacytidine and simultaneous depression of pyrimidine metabolism in leukemic mice. Int J Cancer 1967;2:639.

229. Li LH, Olin EJ, Fraser TJ, et al. Phase specificity of 5-azacytidine against mammalian cells in tissue culture. Cancer Res 1970; 30:2770.

230. Lloyd HH, Dalmadge EA, Wikoff LJ. Kinetics of the reduction in viability of cultured L1210 leukemic cells exposed to 5-azacytidine (NSC-102816). Cancer Chemother Rep 1972;56:585.

231. Presant CA, Vietti TJ, Valeriote F. Kinetics of both leukemic and normal cell population reduction following 5-azacytidine. Cancer Res 1975;35:1926.

232. Lavelle D, DeSimone J, Hankewych M, et al. Decitabine induces cell arrest at the G1 phase via p21^{WAF1} and the G2/M phase via the p38 MAP kinase pathway. Leukemia Res 2003; 27:999–1007.

233. Cihak A, Lamar C, Pitot HC. Studies on the mechanism of the stimulation of tyrosine aminotransferase activity in vivo by pyrimidine analogs: the role of enzyme synthesis and degradation. Arch Biochem Biophys 1973;156:176.

234. Stallings RL, Crawford BD, Tobey RA, et al. 5-Azacytidine-induced conversion to cadmium resistance correlated with early S phase replication of inactive metallothionein genes in synchronized CHO cells. Somat Cell Mol Genet 1986;12:423.

235. Carlow DA, Kerbel RS, Feltis JT, et al. Enhanced expression of class I major histocompatibility complex gene (Dk) products on immunogenic variants of a spontaneous murine carcinoma. J Natl Cancer Inst 1985;75:291.

236. Bonal FJ, Pareja E, Martin J, et al. Repression of class I H-2K, H-2D antigens or GR9 methylcholanthrene-induced tumour cell clones is related to the level of DNA methylation. J Immunogenet 1986;13:179.

237. Richardson B, Kahl L, Lovett EJ, et al. Effect of an inhibitor of DNA methylation on T cells: I. 5-Azacytidine induces T4 expression on T8+ T cells. J Immunol 1986;137:35.

238. Liteplo RG, Alvarez E, Frost P, et al. Induction of thymidine kinase activity in a spontaneously enzyme-deficient murine tumor cell line by exposure in vivo to the DNA-hypomethylating agent 5-aza-2′-deoxycytidine: implications for mechanisms of tumor progression. Cancer Res 1985;45:5294.

239. Jones PA, Taylor SM, Mohandas T, et al. Cell cycle-specific reactivation of an inactive X-chromosome locus by 5-azadeoxycytidine. Proc Natl Acad Sci U S A 1982;79:1215.

240. Jeggo PA, Holliday R. Azacytidine-induced reactivation of a DNA repair gene in Chinese hamster ovary cells. Mol Cell Biol 1986;6:2944.

241. Holliday R. Strong effects of 5-azacytidine on the in vitro lifespan of human diploid fibroblasts. Exp Cell Res 1986;166:543.

242. Karon M, Benedict W. Chromatid breakage: differential effect of inhibitors of DNA synthesis during G_2 phase. Science 1972; 178:62.

243. Seifertova M, Vesely J, Cihak A. Enhanced mortality in offspring of male mice treated with 5-azacytidine prior to mating: morphological changes in testes. Neoplasma 1976;23:53.

244. Coles E, Thayer PS, Reinhold V, et al. Pharmacokinetics and excretion of 5-azacytidine (NSC-102816) and its metabolites. Proc Am Assoc Cancer Res 1974;16:91.

245. Chan KK, Staroscik JA, Sadee W. Synthesis of 5-azacytidine-6-^{3}C and -6-^{14}C. J Med Chem 1977;20:598.

246. Troetel WM, Weiss AJ, Stambaugh JE, et al. Absorption, distribution, and excretion of 5-azacytidine (NSC-102816) in man. Cancer Chemother Rep 1972;56:405.

247. Chabner BA, Drake JC, Johns DC. Deamination of 5-azacytidine by a human leukemia cell cytidine deaminase. Biochem Pharmacol 1973;22:2763.

248. Neil GL, Moxley TE, Kuentzel SL, et al. Enhancement by tetrahydrouridine (NSC-112907) of the oral activity of 5-azacytidine (NSC-102816) in L1210 leukemic mice. Cancer Chemother Rep 1975;59:459.

249. Bellet RE, Mastrangelo MJ, Engstrom PF, et al. Hepatotoxicity of 5-azacytidine (NSC-102816): a clinical and pathologic study. Neoplasma 1973;20:303.

250. Levi J, Wiernik P. A comparative clinical trial of 5-azacytidine and guanazole in previously treated adults with acute nonlymphocytic leukemia. Cancer 1976;38:36.

251. Huang M, Wang Y, Cogut SB, et al. Inhibition of nucleoside transport by protein kinase inhibitors. J Pharmacol Exp Ther. 2003;304:753–760.

252. Ley TJ, DeSimone J, Keller GH, et al. 5-Azacytidine selectively increases gamma-globin synthesis in a patient with beta + thalassemia. N Engl J Med 1982;307:1469.

253. Kaminskas E, Farrell AT, Wang YC, et al. FDA Drug approval summary: Azacytidine (5 azacytidine, Vidaza™) for injectable suspension. The Oncologist, in press.

254. Carr BI, Rahbar S, Asmeron Y, et al. Carcinogenicity and haemoglobin synthesis induction bycytidine analogues. Br J Cancer 1988;57:395–402.

255. DeSimone J, Koshy M, Dorn L, et al. Maintenance of elevated fetal hemoglobin levels by decitabine during dose interval treatment of sickle cell anemia. Blood 2002;99:3905–3908.

256. Wijermans P, Lubbert M, Verhoef G, et al. Low-dose 5-aza-2′-deoxycytidine, a DNA hypomethylating agent, for the treatment of high-risk myelodysplastic syndrome: a multicenter phase II study in elderly patients. J Clin Oncol 2000;18:956–962.

257. Kantarjian HM, O'Brien S, Cortes J, et al. Results of decitabine (5-aza-2′deoxycytidine) therapy in 130 patients with chronic myelogenous leukemia. Cancer 2003;93:522–528.

258. Burris HA 3rd, Moore MJ, Andersen J, et al. Improvements in survival and clinical benefit with gemcitabine as first-line therapy for patients with advanced pancreas cancer: a randomized trial. J Clin Oncol 1997;15:2403.

259. von der Maase H, Hansen SW, Robert JT, et al. Gemcitabine and cisplatin versus methotrexate, vinblastine, doxorubicin, and cisplatin in advanced or metastatic bladder cancer: results of a large, randomized, mutinational, multicenter pahse III study. J Clin Oncol 2000;18:3068–3077.

260. Schiller JH, Harrington D, Belani CP, et al. Comparison of four chemotherapy regimens for advanced non-small cell lung cancer. N Engl J Med 2002;346:92–98.

261. Lippe P, Tummarello D, Monterubbianesi MC, et al. Weekly gemcitabine and cisplatin in advanced non- small-cell lung cancer: a phase II study. Ann Oncol 1999;10:217.

262. Hertel LW, Boder GB, Kroin JS, et al. Evaluation of the antitumor activity of gemcitabine (2′,2′-difluoro-2-deoxycytidine). Cancer Res 1990;50:4417.

263. Bouffard DY, Laliberte J, Momparler RL. Comparison of antineoplastic activity of 2-2-difluoro-2-deoxycytidine and cytosine arabinoside against human myeloid and lymphoid leukemic cells. Anticancer Drugs 1991;2:49.

264. Mackey JR, Mani RS, Selner M, et al. Functional nucleoside transporters are required for gemcitabine influx and manifestation of toxicity in cancer cell lines. Cancer Res 1998;58:4349.

265. Heinemann V, Hertel LW, Grindey GB, et al. Comparison of the cellular pharmacokinetics and toxicity of 2′,2′-difluorodeoxycytidine and 1-beta-D-arabinofuranosylcytosine. Cancer Res 1988;48:4024.

266. Bouffard DY, Laliberte J, Momparler RL. Kinetic studies on 2′,2′-difluorodeoxycytidine (gemcitabine) with purified human deoxycytidine kinase and cytidine deaminase. Biochem Pharmacol 1993;45:1857.

267. Heinemann V, Xu YZ, Chubb S, et al. Cellular elimination of 2′,2′-difluorodeoxycytidine 5′-triphosphate: a mechanism of self-potentiation. Cancer Res 1992;52:533.

268. Gandhi V, Plunkett W. Modulatory activity of 2′,2′-difluorodeoxycytidine on the phosphorylation and cytotoxicity of arabinosyl nucleosides. Cancer Res 1990;50:3675.

269. Rockwell S, Grindey GB. Effect of 2′,2′-difluorodeoxycytidine on the viability and radiosensitivity of EMT6 cells in vitro. Oncol Res 1992;4:151.

270. Heinemann V, Xu YZ, Chubb S, et al. Inhibition of ribonucleotide reduction in CCRF-CEM cells by 2′,2′-difluorodeoxycytidine. Mol Pharmacol 1990;38:567.

271. Huang P, Chubb S, Hertel LW, et al. Action of 2′,2′-difluorodeoxycytidine on DNA synthesis. Cancer Res 1991; 51:6110.

272. Gandhi V, Legha J, Chen F, et al. Excision of 2′,2′-difluorodeoxycytidine (gemcitabine) monophosphate residues from DNA. Cancer Res 1996;56:4453.

272a. Iwasaki H, Huang P, Keating MJ, et al. Differential incorporation of ara-C, gemcitabine, and fludarabine into replicating and repairing DNA in proliferating human leukemia cells. Blood 1997;90:270.

273. Huang P, Plunkett W. Fludarabine- and gemcitabine- induced apoptosis: incorporation of analogs into DNA is a critical event. Cancer Chemother Pharmacol 1995;36:181.

274. Huang P, Plunkett W. Induction of apoptosis by gemcitabine. Semin Oncol 1995;22:19.

275. Cory AH, Hertel LW, Kroin JS, et al. Effects of 2′,2′-difluorodeoxycytidine (gemcitabine) on wild type and variant mouse leukemia L1210 cells. Oncol Res 1993;5:59.

276. Goan YG, Zhou B, Hu E, et al. Overexpression of ribonucleotide reductase as a mechanism of resistance to 2′,2′- difluorodeoxycytidine in human KB cancer line. Cancer Res 1999; 59: 4204.

277. Van Moorsel CJ, Pinedo HM, Veerman G, et al. Mechanisms of synergism between cisplatin and gemcitabine in ovarian and non-small-cell cancer cell lines. Br J Cancer 1999;80:981.

278. Lang LY, Li L, Jiang H, et al. Expression of ERCC! Antisense RNA abrogates gemcitabine-mediated cytotoxic synergism with cisplatin in human colon tumor cells defective in mismatch repair but proficient in nucleotide excision repair. Clin Cancer Res 2000;6:773.

279. Kroep JR, Loves WJP, van der Wilt CL, et al. Pretreatment deocycytidine kinase levels predict in vivo gemcitabine sensitivity. Moleculr Cancer Therapeutics 2002;1:371.

280. Sliutz G, Karlseder J, Tempfer C, et al. Drug resistance against gemcitabine and topotecan mediated by constitutive hsp70 overexpression in vitro: implication of quercetin as sensitiser in chemotherapy. Br J Cancer 1996;74:172.

281. Neff T, Blau CA. Forced expression of cytidine deaminase confers resistance to cytosine arabinoside and gemcitabine. Exp Hematol 1996;24:1340.

282. Davidson JD, Ma L, Flagella M, et al. An increase in the xpression of ribonucleotide reductase loarge subunit 1 is associated with gemcitabine resistance in non-small cell lung cancer cell lines. Cancer Res 2004;64:3761.

283. Spratlin J, Sangha R, Glubrecht D, et al. The absence of human equilibrative nucleoside transporter 1 is associated with reduced survival in patients with gemcitabine treated pancreas adenocarcinoma. Clin Cancer Res 2004;10:6956.

284. Waud WR, Gilbert KS, Grindey GB, et al. Lack of in vivo cross-resistance with gemcitabine against drug-resistant murine P388 leukemias. Cancer Chemother Pharmacol 1996;38:178.

285. Shipley LA, Brown TJ, Cornpropst JD, et al. Metabolism and disposition of gemcitabine, and oncolytic deoxycytidine analog, in mice, rats, and dogs. Drug Metab Dispos 1992;20:849.

286. Grunewald R, Abbruzzese JL, Tarassoff P, et al. Saturation of 2',2'-difluorodeoxycytidine 5'-triphosphate accumulation by mononuclear cells during a phase I trial of gemcitabine. Cancer Chemother Pharmacol 1991;27:258.

287. Abbruzzese JL, Grunewald R, Weeks EA, et al. A phase I clinical, plasma, and cellular pharmacology study of gemcitabine. J Clin Oncol 1991;9:491.

288. Fossella FV, Lippman SM, Shin DM, et al. Maximum-tolerated dose defined for single-agent gemcitabine: a phase I dose-escalation study in chemotherapy-naive patients with advanced non-small-cell lung cancer. J Clin Oncol 1997;15:310.

289. Plunkett W, Liliemark JO, Adams TM, et al. Saturation of 1-beta-D-arabinofuranosylcytosine 5'-triphosphate accumulation in leukemia cells during high-dose 1-beta-D-arabinofuranosylcytosine therapy. Cancer Res 1987;47:3005.

290. Grunewald R, Kantarjian H, Keating MJ, et al. Pharmacologically directed design of the dose rate and schedule of 2',2'-difluorodeoxycytidine (gemcitabine) administration in leukemia. Cancer Res 1990;50:6823.

291. Grunewald R, Kantarjian H, Du M, et al. Gemcitabine in leukemia: a phase I clinical, plasma, and cellular pharmacology study. J Clin Oncol 1992;10:406.

292. Touroutoglou N, Gravel D, Raber MN, et al. Clinical results of a pharmacodynamically-based strategy for higher dosing of gemcitabine in patients with solid tumors. Ann Oncol 1998;9:1003.

293. Tempero M, Plunkett W, Ruiz van Haperen V, et al. Randomized phase II comparison of dose-intense gemcitabine: thirty minute infusion and fixed sdose rate infusion in patients with pancreatic adenocarcinoma. J Clin Oncol 2003;21:3402.

294. Reid JM, Qu W, Safgren S, et al. Phase I trial and pharmacokinetics of gemcitabine in children with advanced solid tumors. J Clin Oncol 2002;22:2445.

295. O'Rourke TJ, Brown TD, Havlin K, et al. Phase I clinical trial of gemcitabine given as an intravenous bolus on 5 consecutive days [letter]. Eur J Cancer 1994;30A:417.

296. Poplin EA, Corbett T, Flaherty L, et al. Difluorodeoxycytidine (dFdC), gemcitabine: a Phase I study. Invest New Drugs 1992;10:165.

297. Anderson H, Thatcher N, Walling J, et al. A phase I study of a 24 hour infusion of gemcitabine in previously untreated patients with inoperable non-small-cell lung cancer. Br J Cancer 1996;74:460.

298. Aapro MS, Martin C, Hatty S. Gemcitabine—a safety review. Anticancer Drugs 1998;9:191.

299. Casper ES, Green MR, Kelsen DP, et al. Phase II trial of gemcitabine (2,2'-difluorodeoxycytidine) in patients with adenocarcinoma of the pancreas. Invest New Drugs 1994;12:29.

300. Brodowicz T, Breiteneder S, Wiltschke C, et al. Gemcitabine-induced hemolytic uremic syndrome: a case report [letter]. J Natl Cancer Inst 1997;89:1895.

301. Flombaum CD, Mouradian JA, Casper ES, et al. Thrombotic microangiopathy as a complication of long-term therapy with gemcitabine. Am J Kidney Dis 1999;33:555.

302. Fung MC, Storniolo AM, Nguyen B, et al. A review of hemolytic uremic syndrome in patients treated with gemcitabine therapy. Cancer 1999;85:2023.

303. Humphreys BD, Sharman JP, Henderson JM, et al. Gemcitabine-associated thrombotic microangiopathy. Cancer 2004;100:2664.

304. Pavlakis N, Bell DR, Millward MJ, et al. Fatal pulmonary toxicity resulting from treatment with gemcitabine. Cancer 1997;80:286.

305. Vander Els NJ, Miller V. Successful treatment of gemcitabine toxicity with a brief course of oral corticosteroid therapy. Chest 1998;114:1779.

306. Roychowdhury DF, Cassidy CA, Peterson P, and Arning M. A report on serious pulmonary toxicity associated with gemcitabine-based therapy. Invest New Drugs 2002;20:311.

307. Bredenfeld H, Franklin J, Nogova L, et al. Severe pulmonary toxicity in patients with advanced stage Hodgkin's Disease treated with a modified bleomycin, doxorubicin, cyclophosphamide, vincristine, procarbazine, prednisone, and gemcitabine (BEACOPP) regimen is probably related to the combination of gemcitabine and blemycin: a report of the Gemran Hodgkin's Lymphoma Study Group. J Clin Oncol 2004;22:2424.

308. Venook AP, Egorin MK, Rosner GL, et al. Phase I and pharmacokinetic trial of gemcitabine in patients with hepatic or renal dysfunction: Cancer and Leukemia Group B 9565. J Clin Oncol 2000;18:2780.

309. Shewach DS, Hahn TM, Chang E, et al. Metabolism of 2'- 2'-difluoro-2'-deoxycytidine and radiation sensitization of human colon carcinoma cells. Cancer Res 1994;54:3218.

310. Lawrence TS, Chang EY, Hahn TM, et al. Radiosensitization of pancreatic cancer cells by 2',2'-difluoro-2'-deoxycytidine. Int J Radiat Oncol Biol Phys 1996;34:867.

311. Mohideen MN, McCall A, Kamradt M, et al. Activity of gemcitabine and its radiosensitization of human cervical cancer cells [abstract]. Proc Annu Meet Am Soc Clin Oncol 1997; 16:A865.

312. Rosier JF, Beauduin M, Bruniaux M, et al. The effect of 2'-2' difluorodeoxycytidine (dFdC, gemcitabine) on radiation-induced cell lethality in two human head and neck squamous carcinoma cell lines differing in intrinsic radiosensitivity. Int J Radiat Biol 1999;75:245.

313. Shewach DS, Keena D, Rubsam LZ, et al. Mechanism of radiosensitization by 2',2'-difluorodeoxycytidine [abstract]. Proc Annu Meet Am Assoc Cancer Res 1996;37:A4196.

314. Shewach DS, Lawrence TS. Gemcitabine and radiosensitization in human tumor cells. Invest New Drugs 1996;14:257.

315. Milas L, Fujii T, Hunter N, et al. Enhancement of tumor radioresponse in vivo by gemcitabine. Cancer Res 1999;59:107.

316. Robinson BW, Im MM, Ljungman M, et al. Enhanced radiosensitization with gemcitabine in mismatch repair-deficient HCT116 cells. Cancer Res 2003;63:6935.

317. Blackstock AW, Bernard SA, Richards F, et al. Phase I trial of twice-weekly gemcitabine and concurrent radiation in patients with advanced pancreatic cancer. J Clin Oncol 1999;17:2208.

318. Blackstock AW, Tempero MA, Niedzwiecki D, et al. Cancer and Leukemia Group B 89805: phase II chemoradiation trial using gemcitabine in patients with locoregional adenocarcinoma of the pancreas. Proc Annu Meet Am Assoc Cancer Res 2001;A627.

319. Crane CH, Abbruzzese JL, Evans DB, et al. Is the therapeutic index better with gemcitabine-based chemoradiation than with 5-fluorouracil based chemoradiaition in locally advanced pancreatic cancer? Int J Radiat Oncol Biol Phys 2002;52:1293.

320. Talamonti MS, Catalono PJ, Vaughn DJ, et al. Eastern Cooperative Oncology Group phase I trial of protracted venous infusion fluorouracil plus weekly gemcitabine with concurrent radiation therapy in patients with locally advanced pancreatic cancer. J Clin Oncol 2000;18:3384.

321. Eisbruch A, Shewach DS, Bradford CR, et al. Radiation concurrent with gemcitabine for locally advanced head and neck cancer: a phase I trial and intracellular drug incorporation study. J Clin Oncol 2001;19:792.

322. Van Putten JW, Price A, van der Leest AH, et al. A phase I study of gemcitabine with concurrent radiotherapy in stage III, locally advanced non-small cell lung cancer. Clin Cancer Res 2003;9:2472.

Purine Antimetabolites

9

Kenneth R. Hande

GUANINE ANALOGS

(6-Mercaptopurine, 6-Thioguanine, and Azathioprine)

More than 50 years after its initial use, 6-mercaptopurine (6-MP) is still employed as primary therapy for children with acute lymphoblastic leukemia (ALL)[1]. 6-Thioguanine (6-TG) is given for remission induction and maintenance therapy of acute myelogenous leukemia. Azathioprine, a prodrug of 6-MP, is widely used as an immunosuppressant. These three drugs are closely related in structure (Fig. 9.1), metabolism, mechanism of action, and toxicity. Because of their similarities, they will be discussed together in this section. The key pharmacologic features of these drugs are summarized in Tables 9.1 through 9.3.

Mechanism of Action

6-MP is a structural analog of hypoxanthine with a substitution of a thiol for the naturally occurring 6-hydroxyl group (Fig. 9.1). 6-MP undergoes extensive hepatic and cellular metabolism after dosing.[2] Three major competing transformation routes are present, one anabolic and two catabolic. 6-MP is activated intracellularly by the enzyme hypoxanthine-guanine phosphoribosyl transferase (HGPRT) to form 6-thioinosine monophosphate (TIMP). TIMP inhibits de novo purine synthesis (Fig. 9.2). Sequential metabolism of TIMP to thioguanine monophosphate and then to 6-thioguanosine triphosphate (6-TGTP) occurs. 6-TGTP is incorporated into DNA and RNA. The quantity of 6-MP metabolite present in DNA correlates with cytotoxicity.[3] Incorporation of 6-TGTP into DNA triggers programmed cell death by a process involving the mismatch repair pathway.[4,5] Cytotoxicity depends on (a) incorporation of 6-TG into DNA, (b) miscoding during DNA replication, and (c) recognition of the abnormal base pairs by proteins of the postreplicative mismatch repair system.

Methylation of 6-MP contributes to its antiproliferation properties, probably through inhibition of de novo purine synthesis by methymercaptopurine nucleotides.[6]

6-TG is activated in a manner similar to that outlined for 6-MP.[7] Thioguanine is converted to 6-thioguanylic acid (TGMP) by HGPRT. TGMP is subsequently incorporated into RNA and DNA in its deoxytriphosphate form. Incorporation of fraudulent nucleotides into DNA is believed to be the primary mechanism of cytotoxicity,[8] triggering apoptosis by a process involving the mismatch repair pathway, similar to 6-MP.[5] Conversion of 6-TG into cytotoxic thioguanine nucleotides involves fewer metabolic steps than needed for 6-MP. Significantly higher cellular concentrations of thioguanine nucleotides are seen after 6-TG administration than with 6-MP.[9]

Azathioprine (Fig. 9.1) is rapidly cleaved by nonenzymatic mechanisms to 6-MP and methyl-4-nitro-5-imidazole derivatives (Fig. 9.2). Although incorporation of false nucleotides into DNA and inhibition of purine synthesis by 6-MP ribonucleotides are the probable mechanism for cytotoxicity, the mechanism by which azathioprine and mercaptopurine modify immune response is likely different. Azathioprine inhibits T-lymphocyte activity to a greater extent than B-lymphocytes. Formation of 6-thioguanine triphosphate (6-TGTP) binds to and inhibits Rac 1, a small GTP-binding protein. Rac proteins play a major role in T cell development, differentiation, and proliferation The activation of Rac1 targeted genes, such as mitogen-activated protein kinase (MEK), NF κ BI, and bcl-X_L, is suppressed by azathioprine leading to the mitochondrial pathway of apoptosis.[10]

Clinical Pharmacology

6-Mercaptopurine

6-MP is commercially available in 50-mg tablets, which also contain the inactive ingredients corn and potato starch, lactose, magnesium stearate, and stearic acid. An

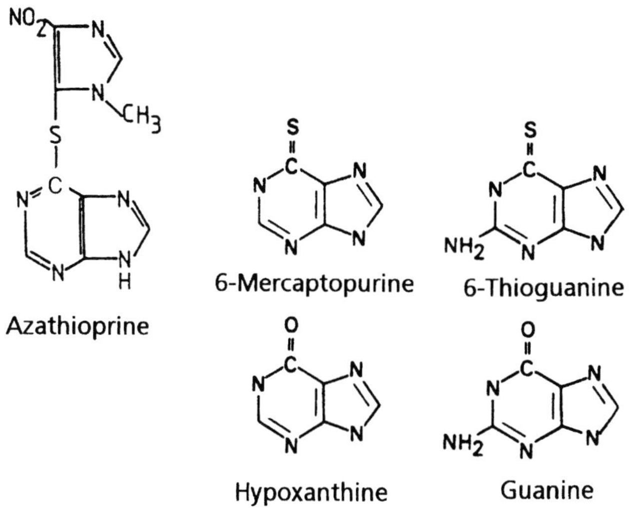

Figure 9.1 Structure of the naturally occurring purine, guanine, and related antineoplastic agents 6-mercaptopurine, 6-thioguanine and azathioprine.

intravenous preparation of 6-MP has been formulated for research purposes. 6-MP is relatively insoluble and unstable in alkaline solutions.

Plasma 6-MP, 6-TG, and metabolite concentrations as low as 0.1 µM can be measured using high-performance liquid chromatography techniques.[11] Using these assays, accurate kinetics of oral and intravenous preparations have been determined. Following oral administration of commonly used 6-MP doses (75 mg/m^2), peak plasma concentrations

of 0.3 to 1.8 µM are seen within a mean of 2.2 hours.[12] The volume of distribution exceeds that of total body water (0.9 L/kg). There is little penetration into the cerebrospinal fluid (CSF). With high-dose oral 6-MP (500 mg/m^2), plasma 6-MP concentrations of 5 to 12 µM are achieved.[13] In human leukemic cell culture models, concentrations of 1 to 10 µM are cytotoxic. Following intravenous dosing, the half-life of 6-MP is 50 to 100 minutes and plasma concentrations of 6-MP reach 25 µM and CSF concentrations 3.8 µM.[14] Only weak protein binding is noted with 6-MP (20% bound).

Oral absorption of 6-MP is incomplete and highly variable.[15] At a dose of 75 mg/m^2 6-MP, mean 6-MP bioavailability is 16% (range, 5 to 37%).[16] Clearance occurs primarily through two routes of metabolism. 6-MP is oxidized to the inactive metabolite, 6-thiouric acid, by xanthine oxidase (Fig. 9.2). 6-MP also undergoes S-methylation by the enzyme, thiopurine methyltransferase (TPMT), to yield 6-methyl mercaptopurine. The intestinal mucosa and liver contain high concentrations of the enzyme xanthine oxidase. The low bioavailability of 6-MP is the result of a large first-pass effect as drug is absorbed through the intestinal wall into the portal circulation and metabolized by xanthine oxidase. The use of concomitant allopurinol (an inhibitor of xanthine oxidase) increases 6-MP bioavailability by 500%.[17] Interestingly, allopurinol does not alter the plasma kinetics of intravenously administered 6-MP, although more 6-MP and less thiouric acid is excreted in the urine following allopurinol therapy.[18] Methotrexate, often used with 6-MP in maintenance treatment of acute lymphoblastic leukemia, is a weak inhibitor of xanthine

TABLE 9.1
KEY FEATURES OF 6-MERCAPTOPURINE

Factor	Result
Mechanism of Action	(1) Primary: Incorporation of metabolites into DNA causes miscoding during DNA replication. Correlates with cytotoxicity
	(2) Secondary: Inhibits de novo purine synthesis; incorporated into RNA.
Metabolism	Activation: conversion to thiopurine nucleotides
	Catabolism: to 6-thiouric acid by xanthine oxidase
	Catabolism: to 6-methylthiopurine by thiopurine methyltransferase (TPMT)
Pharmacokinetic:	T½: 50 minutes
	Poor (<25%) and variable oral bioavailability
Elimination	Metabolism, at conventional doses, by xanthine oxidase and TPMT
Drug Interactions	Allopurinol decreases 6-MG elimination and concomitant use requires dose reduction (75%)
Toxicity	(1) Myelosuppression
	(2) Mild gastrointestinal (nausea, vomiting)
	(3) Rare hepatotoxicity
Precautions	(1) Dose reductions with allopurinol
	(2) Persons with genetic deficiency of TPMT will have significantly increased toxicity (genetic screening available to test for TPMT deficiency)

TABLE 9.2
KEY FEATURES OF 6-THIOGUANINE

Factor	Result
Mechanism of Action	Incorporation of fraudulent nucleotides into DNA
Metabolism	Activation: conversion to thiopurine nucleotides
	Catabolism: to 6-thioxanthine by guanase
	Catabolism: to 2-amino-6-methyl thiopurine by thiopurine methyltransferase (TPMT)
Pharmacokinetics	T½: 90 minutes
	Poor (15-40%) and variable bioavailability
Elimination	Hepatic metabolism
Drug Interactions	None well defined
Toxicity	(1) Myelosuppression
	(2) Mild gastrointestinal (nausea, vomiting)
	(3) Rare hepatotoxicity
Precautions	Increased toxicity in individuals with genetic deficiency of TPMT

oxidase. Concomitant use of methotrexate results in a small increase in the bioavailability of 6-MP. However, the modest increase in bioavailability is thought not to be clinically significant.[15] The plasma concentration versus time profile of 6-MP differs in the same patient when studied on repeated occasions.[19]

High-dose, oral 6-MP (500 mg/m^2) has been used in an attempt to saturate the first-pass metabolism of 6-MP, thereby increasing bioavailability.[13] Even at a dose of 500 mg/m^2, 6-MP, xanthine oxidase is not saturated and no improvement in bioavailability is seen. Food intake and oral antibiotic reduce the oral absorption of 6-MP.[20,21]

As previously mentioned, two catabolic pathways for 6-MP metabolism exist that significantly affect drug activity: one via xanthine oxidase (just discussed) and a second via thiopurine methyltransferase (TPMT). Patient-to-patient variation in TPMT activity results in significant changes in 6-MP metabolism and drug toxicity. As seen in Figure 9.2, TPMT catalyzes the S-methylation of 6-MP to a relatively inactive metabolite, 6-methyl mercaptopurine (6CH$_3$MP). Interindividual TPMT activity is controlled by a common genetic polymorphism.[22] (See chapter-Diasio) The frequency distribution of TPMT activity in large population studies is trimodal. One in 200 to 300 subjects has absent enzyme activity; 10% of the population has intermediate activity, and the rest have high enzyme activity.[23] A number of polymorphic variants coding for varying levels of enzyme activity have been identified. A single genetic locus with two alleles is responsible for the trimodal distribution. Lymphoblasts from individuals heterozygous for the

TABLE 9.3
KEY FEATURES OF AZATHIOPRINE

Factor	Result
Mechanism of Action	Similar to 6-MP.
Metabolism	Rapidly converted to 6-MP by nonenzymatic mechanisms.
Pharmacokinetics	See 6-MP
Elimination	Rapid metabolism to 6-MP and with subsequent elimination similar to 6-MP
Drug interactions	Allopurinol decreases elimination. Concomitant use with allopurinol requires azathioprine dose reductions (≥75%).
Toxicity	(1) Myelosuppression
	(2) Gastrointestinal (nausea, vomiting)
	(3) Rare hepatotoxicity
Precautions	(1) Dose reduction with allopurinol required
	(2) Increased toxicity in individuals with genetic deficiency of thiopurine methyl-transferase

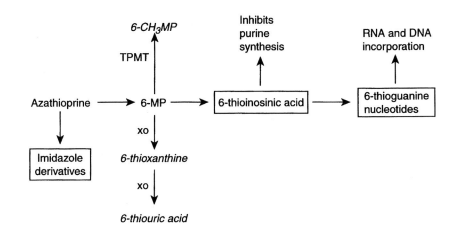

Figure 9.2 Mechanism of activation and catabolism of azathioprine and 6-MG. Active metabolites are indicated by surrounding boxes. Inactive (or less active) metabolites are indicated by italic print. CH₃MP, 6-methyl mercaptopurine; TPMT, thiopurine methyltransferase; XO, xanthine oxidase.

normal TMTP gene have lower TMPT activity than lymphoblasts from homozygous patients.[24] Patients with low TPMT activity are more susceptible to 6-MP and 6-TG–induced myelosuppression. Marked myelosuppression in patients receiving 6-MP, 6-TG, or azathioprine therapy may be a result of genetic deficiency in TPMT activity in that patient.[25] Patients with absence of TMPT activity should have the dose of 6-MP reduced, but not the dose of other chemotherapeutic agents given for their leukemia. There is a suggestion that Blacks may have less TPMT activity than Whites,[26] which could increase toxicity in that population. A reciprocal relationship between TPMT activity and the formation of 6-thiopurine nucleotides has been demonstrated. Several studies,[27-29] but not all,[16] have suggested that variability in oral absorption of 6-MP may affect the risk of relapse in children with ALL. Lennard et al.[30] have suggested that children with high TPMT activity are at greater risk of disease relapse as a result of decreased drug activation.

The TPMT gene has been cloned. Eight TPMT polymorphisms associated with reduced enzyme activity have been identified.[31] Variant TPMT alleles are present in 5 to 10% of persons in most populations.[32] In describing gene mutations, the convention has been adopted that the nonmutated gene is designated a TPMT 1 and mutated genes are assigned as TPMT 2-8 on the basis of the order in which they were first described. In White populations, the most common mutation genotype associated with low enzyme activity is TPMT 3, which accounts for more than 80% of heterozygotes.[33] Genetic testing using PCR-based methods can now identify TPMT-deficient and heterozygous patients.[34] This test, as opposed to direct measurement of TPMT activity in red blood cells, is not affected by prior blood transfusions to the patient. Although dosage reductions have been suggested for patients with hepatic and renal function impairment, there is no good data justifying such dose adjustments. Dose adjustment for patients homozygous for mutant TPMT are required.

6-Thioguanine

6-TG is available as 40-mg tablets for oral use. An intravenous preparation is investigational. As with 6-MP, the absorption of 6-TG in humans is variable and incomplete (mean bioavailability is 30%; range: 14 to 46%).[35] Peak plasma levels of 0.03-5 μM occur 2 to 4 hours after ingestion; the median drug half-life is 90 minutes but with wide variability reported.[36] Intravenously administered 6-TG has been evaluated. Clearance of drug (600 to 1,000 mL/min per square meter) appears to be dose-dependent, suggesting saturation of clearance at doses over 10 mg/m² per hour.[37] Plasma concentrations of 4 to 10 μM can be achieved.

The catabolism of 6-TG differs from that of 6-MP. Thioguanine is not a substrate for xanthine oxidase. Thioguanine is converted to 6-thioinosine (an inactive metabolite) by the action of the enzyme, guanase. Because thioguanine inactivation does not depend on the action of xanthine oxidase, an inhibitor of xanthine oxidase, such as allopurinol, will not block the detoxification of thioguanine. In humans, methylation of thioguanine, via thiopurine methyltransferase (TPMT), is more extensive than is that of 6-MP. The product of methylation, 2-amino-6-methylthiopurine, is substantially less active and less toxic than thioguanine.

Azathioprine

Azathioprine is rapidly degraded by nonenzymatic mechanisms to 6-MP. The metabolic pathways thereafter are identical to 6-MP.[38] In transplant patients taking 2 mg/kg per day azathioprine, peak 6-MP plasma concentrations (T$_{max}$<2 hours) are low (75 ng/mL) and plasma drug half-life is short (1.9 hours).[39] Plasma 6-MP concentrations exceed those of azathioprine within an hour of drug administration. Loss of renal function does not alter the plasma kinetics of either azathioprine or 6-MP.

Toxicity

6-Mercaptopurine

The dose-limiting toxicity of 6-MP is myelosuppression, occurring 1 to 4 weeks following the onset of therapy and reversible when the drug is discontinued. Platelets, granulocytes, and erythrocytes are all affected. Weekly monitoring of blood counts during the first 2 months of therapy is recommended. Myelosuppression following 6-MP therapy is related to TPMT phenotype. Most patients (65%) with excessive toxicity following 6-MP or azathioprine administration have TMPT deficiency or heterozygosity.[40,41]

6-MP is an immunosuppressant. Immunity to infectious agents or vaccines is subnormal in patients receiving 6-MP. Gastrointestinal mucositis and stomatitis are modest. Approximately one-quarter of treated patients experienced nausea, vomiting, and anorexia. Gastrointestinal side effects appear to be more common in adults than in children. Pancreatitis is seen in 3% of patients with long-term therapy.[41] Hepatotoxicity is noted infrequently and is usually mild and reversible.[42] The development of hepatotoxicity, in contrast to myelosuppression, is not associated with TPMT polymorphisms,[43] but is correlated with the dose of 6-MP given and with the formation of methylated metabolites of 6-MP (but not with 6-TG nucleotide formation).[44]

At very high doses ($>1,000$ mg/m^2), the limited solubility of 6-MP can cause precipitation of drug in the renal tubules with hematuria and crystalluria.[45] Mercaptopurine has potential teratogenic properties.[46] However, in a recent cohort analysis, differences in conception failures, congenital malformations, or incidence of neoplasia was not noted in patients taking 6-MP before or at the time of conception.[47]

Thioguanine

As with 6-MP, the primary toxicity of 6-TG is myelosuppression.[48] Blood counts should be frequently monitored because there may be a delayed effect during oral drug administration. Higher doses result in mucositis. Thioguanine produces gastrointestinal toxicities similar to 6-MP but less frequently. Jaundice and hepatic veno-occlusive disease have been reported.[49]

Azathioprine

Adverse effects from azathioprine are similar to those seen with 6-MP. These effects include leukopenia, diarrhea, nausea, abnormal liver function tests and skin rashes. Frequent monitoring of the complete blood count is warranted throughout therapy (weekly during the first 8 weeks of therapy). A hypersensitivity reaction, generally characterized by fever, chills, severe nausea, diarrhea, hypertension, and hepatic dysfunction, has been reported.[50] The mechanism for the hypersensitivity reaction is unclear. Chronic immunosuppressive therapy, including use of azathioprine,

results in an increased frequency of secondary infections and an increased risk of malignant tumors.[51] Acute myeloid leukemia associated with karyotypic changes of 7q-/-7 has been reported.[52] Risk of cancer development increases with longer duration of azathioprine use (<5 years, the relative risk [RR] = 1.3; 5 to 10 years, RR = 2.0; >10 years, RR = 4.4).

Toxicity from azathioprine, primarily myelosuppression and gastrointestinal intolerance, requires dose adjustment or discontinuation of treatment in up to 40% of patients. Several studies[53,54] indicate that patients heterozygous for mutant TPMT are at high risk for toxicity and dose modification. In a study by Black et al.,[53] all patients heterozygous for the TMPT 3A allele required discontinuation of therapy within 1 month. Molecular testing for TMPT may be a cost-effective way of identifying the 10% of the population at high risk for toxicity.[32]

Use and Drug Interactions

6-MP is a standard component of maintenance therapy for ALL. It has little role in therapy of solid tumors or remission induction in myeloid leukemias. 6-MP is also used to treat inflammatory bowel disease.

Azathioprine is used as an immunosuppressant in preventing rejection of organ transplants and in the therapy of illnesses believed autoimmune in character (such as lupus, rheumatoid arthritis, and ulcerative colitis).

As previously mentioned, allopurinol inhibits the catabolism of 6-MP and increases its bioavailability.[17] Oral doses of 6-MP and azathioprine should be reduced by at least 75% in patients also receiving allopurinol. Combined use of standard dose azathioprine (or 6-MP) with allopurinol will result in life-threatening toxicity.[55] Methotrexate causes a modest increase in 6-MP bioavailability but not to an extent significant enough to warrant dosage reduction.[15] Methotrexate increases 6-MP plasma concentrations slightly, but antagonizes thiopurine metabolite disposition in leukemia blasts resulting in lower thioguanine nucleotide incorporation.[56]

ADENOSINE ANALOGS

Adenosine deaminase (ADA) catalyzes the deamination of adenosine to inosine and deoxyadenosine to deoxyinosine. Congenital deficiency of ADA in men leads to lymphocyte dysfunction and severely impaired cellular immunity caused by an accumulation of deoxyadenosine, which is cytotoxic to lymphocytes. The cytotoxic effect of deoxyadenosine on lymphocytes prompted investigators to evaluate adenosine analogs in the treatment of lymphocytic malignancies. Adenosine analogs with documented clinical utility are fludarabine, pentostatin, and cladribine (2'-chlorodeoxyadenosine) (Fig. 9.3). Key pharmacologic features of the adenosine analogs are listed in Tables 9.4 through 9.6.

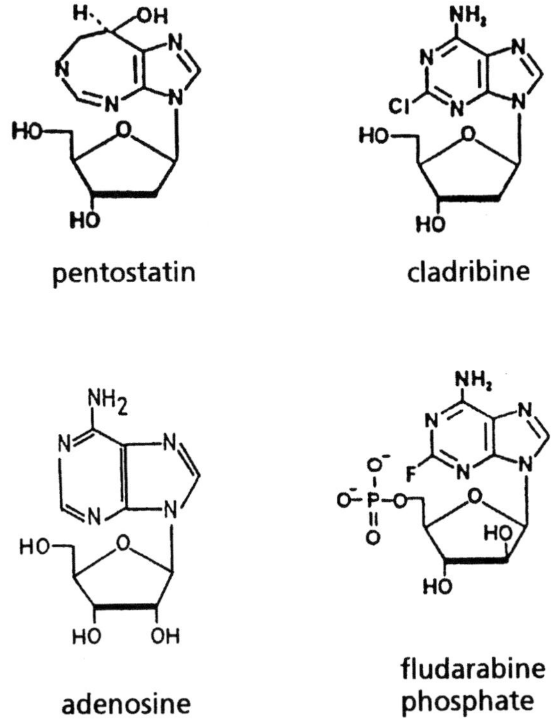

Figure 9.3 Structure of adenosine and the adenosine analogs fludarabine (9-arabinofuranosyl-2-fluoroadenosine monophosphate; F-ara-AMP), pentostatin (2-deoxycoformycin), and cladribine (2-chlorodeoxyadenosine).

Fludarabine

Fludarabine, a monophosphate analog of adenosine arabinoside (9-β-D-arabinofuranosyl-2-fluoroadenine monophosphate), is resistant to adenosine deaminase with good aqueous solubility allowing intravenous administration[57]

(Fig. 9.3). Key features of fludarabine are summarized in Table 9.4.

Mechanism of Action

After intravenous administration, fludarabine is rapidly and completely dephosphorylated in plasma to the nucleoside 9-β-D-arabinofuranosyl-2-fluoroadenine (F-ara-A) (Fig. 9.4).[58] F-ara-A enters cells via carrier-mediated transport[59] and is phosphorylated to its active form, F-ara-ATP. All cytotoxic mechanisms of action of fludarabine require the presence of fludarabine triphosphate (F-ara-ATP).[60] F-ara-ATP inhibits several intracellular enzymes important in DNA replication including DNA polymerase, ribonucleotide reductase, DNA primase, and DNA ligase I.[60,61] In addition, the monophosphate, F-ara-AMP, is incorporated into DNA. Once incorporated, F-ara-AMP is an effective DNA chain terminator[62] primarily at the 3' end of DNA. The amount of F-ara-AMP incorporated is linearly correlated with loss of clonagenicity. Excision of the 3'-terminal F-ara-AMP does not easily occur, and the presence of this false nucleotide leads to apoptosis.

Although the effects of fludarabine on DNA synthesis account for its activity in dividing cells, fludarabine is also cytotoxicity in diseases with very low growth fractions such as chronic lymphocytic leukemia (CLL) or indolent lymphomas. This raises the question as to how an "S-phase" agent is active in nondividing cells.[63] The specific mechanism(s) by which fludarabine induces cell death among quiescent cells is under investigation, but several proposed mechanisms of action include fludarabine's ability to inhibit RNA polymerases by incorporation into RNA, depletion of nicotinamide adenine dinucleotide (NAD) with resultant decrease in cellular energy stores, and interference with normal DNA repair processes.[64,65] The most

TABLE 9.4
KEY FEATURES OF FLUDARABINE

Factor	Result
Mechanism of Action	(1) Incorporation into DNA as a false nucleotide.
	(2) Inhibition of DNA polymerase, DNA primase and DNA ligase
	(3) DNA chain termination
Metabolism	(1) Rapid dephosphorylation in plasma to 2-fluoro-ara A (F-ara-A)
	(2) Activation of F-ara-A to F-ara-ATP (the active metabolite) within cells
Pharmacokinetics	(1) Rapid dephosphorylation to 2-F-ara A
	(2) T½ 2-F-ara-A = 6–30 hours in plasma; intracellular t½ of F-ara-ATP = 15 hours
Elimination	Primarily renal excretion of 2-F-ara-A
Drug interactions	Increases cytotoxicity of cytarabine and cisplatin
Toxicity	(1) Myelosuppression
	(2) Immunosuppression with resulting infections
	(3) Neurotoxicity at high doses
	(4) Rare: interstial pneumonitis and hemolytic anemia
Precautions	Dose reduction needed for patients with renal failure

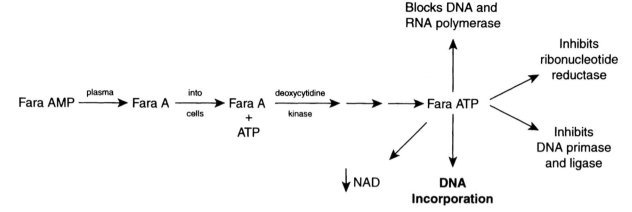

Figure 9.4 Activation of fludarabine. Fludarabine loses its phosphate group in plasma to fluoro adenine (F-ara-A). F-ara-A enters cells and is phorphorylated to F-ara-ATP, which is the active metabolite. NAD, nicotinamide adenine dinucleotide.

compelling evidence suggests fludarabine triggers apoptosis after incorporation into DNA during the DNA repair process.[65]

Clinical Pharmacology

Plasma concentrations of parent fludarabine and F-ara-A have been determined using high-performance liquid chromatography.[66] Following intravenous administration, parent drug (2-F-ara-AMP) undergoes rapid (2 to 4 minutes) and quantitative conversion to F-ara-A. The rapid conversion of fludarabine to F-ara-A is attributed to the action of 5'nucleotidase present in erythrocytes and endothelial cells. Peak plasma F-ara-A concentrations of 1 to 5 μmol/L are achieved after commonly used doses of 25 to 30 mg/m^2 per milligram fludarabine.[66,67] Wide variations in terminal drug half-life (7 to 33 hours) and area under the curve (AUC) are found. Drug clearance is linear, with no change with repeated doses. F-ara-A is excreted primarily in the urine (50 to 60%) with no metabolites detected.[60] Among patients with renal impairment, there is a significant decrease in clearance of 2-F-ara-A (Cl_T = 51.82 $\pm$ 6.70 mL/minute per square meter versus 73.53 $\pm$ 3.79 mL/minute per square meter) compared with patients with normal kidney function.[66,68] Lichtman et al.[68] have proposed that patients with a creatinine clearance (Cl_{cr}) of >70 mL/minute per1.73 m^2 should receive 25 mg/m^2 per day for 5 days of fludarabine, and patients with Cl_{cr} of 30 to 70 mL/minute per 1.73 m^2 should receive 20 mg/m^2 per day for 5 days, and those with Cl_{cr} of <30 mL/minute per 1.73 m^2 should receive 15 mg/m^2 per day for 5 days fludarabine.

Oral administration of fludarabine has been evaluated.[69] The AUC of F-ara-A increases linearly with increasing dose. Mean bioavailability averages 50 to 55% with large interpatient (30 to 80%), but minimal intraindividual variability. Absorption is not affected by meals.[70]

The triphosphate (F-ara-ATP) is the major intracellular metabolite of fludarabine and the only metabolite with known cytotoxic activity. Peak F-ara-ATP concentrations in circulating leukemic cells are achieved 4 hours after intravenous fludarabine administration.[67] F-ara-ATP has a relatively long intracellular half-life (15 hours), which may account for the efficacy of a daily administration schedule.[60] A linear relationship exists between plasma F-ara-A concentrations and intracellular F-ara-ATP in leukemic cells.[71]

Toxicity

The dose-limiting toxicities of fludarabine are myelosuppression and infectious complications from immunosuppression.[57] Toxicity is similar with oral and intravenous preparations.[69] Reversible leukopenia and thrombocytopenia have been reported following fludarabine administration with a median time to nadir of 13 days (range, 3 to 25 days) and 16 days (range, 2 to 32 days), respectively. Twenty percent to 50% of treated patients have a neutrophil count nadir less than 1,000/mm^3 at standard doses of 25 mg/m^2 per day for 5 days. Platelet nadirs of less than 50 to 100,000/mm^3 are seen in 20%.[72] Myelosuppression is more common when fludarabine is combined with other chemotherapeutic drugs, including rituximab.[73] Up to 25% of patients treated with fludarabine will have a febrile episode. Many will be fevers of unknown origin but one-third will have a serious documented infection.

Fludarabine is immunosuppressive. The immunosuppression by fludarabine is associated with inhibition of a key component of signal transduction of lymphocyte activation.[74] Therapy is associated with an increased risk of opportunistic infections. CD4 and CD8 T-lymphocytic subpopulations decrease to levels of 150 to 200/mm^3 after three courses of therapy.[75] Lymphopenia may persist for over 1 year. The most frequent infectious complications are respiratory. Infections with Cryptococcus, *Listeria monocytogenes, Pneumocystis carinii,* cytomegalovirus, herpes simplex virus, *Varicella zoster,* and mycobacterium, organisms associated with T-cell dysfunction, are seen.[76] Previous therapy, advanced disease, and neutropenia are risk factors. The incidence of infections complications and grade 3-4 myelosuppression is significantly greater in patients with a creatinine clearance <80 mL/minute, again suggesting dose modifications for patients with renal insufficiency.[77] Patient age is not an independent risk factor for fludarabine toxicity.

The development of autoimmune hemolytic anemia has been seen with fludarabine use.[78] Hemolysis has been noted following any treatment cycle, but is most common during cycles one through three (71% of cases). Acute tumor lysis is a rare complication in patients with CLL and indolent lymphomas treated with fludarabine.[79] Other reported fludarabine toxicities include mild nausea and vomiting, infection, peripheral sensorimotor neuropathy, and hepatocellular toxicity with elevations in serum transaminases. An irreversible neurotoxicity syndrome with cortical blindness, optic neuritis, encephalopathy, generalized seizures, and coma has been described.[80] This occurs in patients receiving high drug doses (>40 mg/m^2 per d for 5 days). However, mild, reversible neurotoxicity is seen at lower doses with increased frequency and severity with older age. Neurotoxicity is reported in 16% of patients. Pulmonary toxicity characterized by fever, cough, hypoxia, and diffuse interstitial pneumonitis has been reported in 5 to 10% of fludarabine-treated patients.[81] Patients with CLL are particularly at risk. Corticosteroid therapy is recommended. Therapy-related myeloid malignancies have been reported in patients receiving the combination of fludarabine and chlorambucil.[82]

Clinical Use

Fludarabine has demonstrated clinical activity in a variety of low-grade lymphoproliferative malignancies including CLL, hairy-cell leukemia, Waldenstrom's macroglobulinemia, and non-Hodgkin's lymphoma. Response rates from 32 to 57% have been reported among patients with refractory chronic lymphocytic leukemia treated with fludarabine. The median duration of disease control is 65 to 91 weeks. Among patients with previously untreated chronic lymphocytic leukemia, fludarabine has produced responses in more than 70% of patients, including complete responses in one-third. A median survival of 63 months has been reported. In CLL, patients treated with fludarabine have a higher complete response rate (20% versus 4%) than those receiving chlorambucil alone, as well as an increased partial response rate (43% versus 33%). However, no survival difference has been noted.[83] Fludarabine has been employed as a component of nonmyeloablative stem cell transplantation for lymphoma.[84]

Drug Interactions

Fludarabine is synergistic with cytosine arabinoside. Fludarabine increases intracellular accumulation of ara-C. Increased incorporation of ara-CTP into DNA occurs through modulation of dNTP pools by fludarabine. Fludarabine also acts with ara-C to inhibit DNA polymerase alpha.[85]

Pentostatin or Deoxycoformycin

Pentostatin or 2'-deoxycoformycin (dCF) is a purine analog originally prepared from a Streptomycin culture but now chemically synthesized. Pentostatin was identified as a potent ADA inhibitor[86] and subsequently evaluated as treatment for lymphocytic leukemias. No activity was seen in patients with acute leukemias, but patients with hairy cell leukemia and indolent lymphomas had impressive responses.[87] The key pharmacologic features of pentostatin are listed in Table 9.5.

TABLE 9.5
KEY FEATURES OF PENTOSTATIN (DEOXYCOFORMYCIN)

Factor	Result
Mechanism of Action	(1) Inhibits adenosine deaminase with subsequent accumulation of dATP pools
	(2) Inhibition of DNA replication and repair by dATP
Metabolism	Minimal
Pharmacokinetics	Clearance rate of 8 mL/min/m^2, which decreases with decreasing creatinine clearance
Elimination	Majority of drug is excreted unchanged in the urine
Drug interactions	None recognized
Toxicity	(1) Well tolerated at low doses
	(2) At high doses: nausea, immunosuppression, nephrotoxicity and CNS disturbances
Precautions	Dose reductions for patients with renal failure

Mechanism of Action

The specific mechanism for pentostatin cytotoxicity is believed to be the result of the accumulation of deoxyadenosine and dATP following ADA inhibition. Pentostatin binds tightly to ADA with a slow dissociation rate of 60 hours.[88] Abnormally high levels of deoxyadenosine triphosphate (dATP) achieved following ADA inhibition exert a negative feedback on ribonucleotide reductase, resulting in an imbalance in deoxynucleotide pools. This imbalance slows DNA synthesis and alters DNA replication and repair. S-adenosylhomocysteine hydrolase is also inhibited, blocking normal cellular methylation reactions.[87,88] These mechanisms are relevant to proliferating cells. The mechanism of action of pentostatin on nonproliferating cells is unclear.

Pentostatin enters cells via the nucleoside transport system[89] with a rate of cellular uptake that parallels that of other nucleosides. Pentostatin exerts tight-binding inhibition of ADA.[86] When administered in doses intended to produce total-body ADA inhibition in ALL, serious renal, pulmonary, and central nervous system toxicity is encountered. Thus, toxicity has limited the usefulness of this drug in conditions associated with high ADA activity, such as acute leukemias. However, pentostatin is active in hairy-cell leukemia, in which cellular ADA levels are lower.[90]

Clinical Pharmacology

Pentostatin is reasonably stable at neutral pH; however, care must be taken if the drug is extensively diluted with 5% dextrose in water as pentostatin's stability is compromised at pH ≤ 5.[91] Pentostatin has a large volume of distribution with little protein binding.[92] The terminal elimination half-life averages 6 hours.[93,94] Plasma levels of pentostatin 1 hour after administration exceed the ADA inhibitory concentration by approximately 10^6, supporting the recommendation for an intermittent infusion schedule. Only a small amount of pentostatin is metabolized; 40 to 80% of the drug is excreted in urine unchanged within 24 hours.[93,94] Plasma clearance averages 68 mL/minute per square meter and correlates with creatinine clearance. For patients with impaired renal function (creatinine clearance <60 mL/minute), drug half-life is prolonged (approximately 18 hours). Dose reductions are suggested for patients with renal function impairment. Patients with a creatinine clearance >60 mL/minute should receive a dose of 4 mg/m^2 every 14 days, patients with Cl$_{cr}$ of 41 to 60 mL/minute should receive 3 mg/m^2 every 2 weeks, and patients with a Cl$_{cr}$ of 20 to 40 mL/minute should receive a 2 mg/m^2 dose every 14 days.[95] Pentostatin is not orally bioavailable. Pentostatin crosses the blood-brain barrier with CSF concentrations 10 to 13% of serum drug concentrations.[96]

Toxicity

At commonly used doses (4 mg/m^2 every 2 weeks), pentostatin toxicity is modest and therapy is usually well tolerated.[97] In a large intergroup trial of 313 patients, grade 3-4 toxicity was uncommon.[98] Twenty-two percent of patients treated at 4 mg/m^2 every 2 weeks develop grade 3-4 neutropenia. Nausea and vomiting ($>$grade 3) occurs in 11% of patients. The most common nonmyelosuppressive drug toxicity is nausea (11% of patients at standard doses). Nausea and vomiting may be delayed (12 to 72 hours after administration). Mild-to-moderate lethargy (3% incident), rash, and reactivation of herpes zoster have been reported. Toxicity from higher doses of pentostatin (≥ 10 mg/m^2 per day) includes immunosuppression, conjunctivitis, renal impairment, hepatic enzyme elevation, and central nervous system disturbances.[96] Renal toxicity seen in early trials is minimized with the use of lower drug doses and adequate hydration. Nephrotoxicity occurs 10 to 20 days after drug administration. Cardiac complications in older patients have been described but appear to be uncommon.[99] Patients with poor performance status or impaired renal function have a higher incidence of life-threatening toxicity. An increased risk of opportunistic infections similar to fludarabine and cladribine is seen with pentostatin.[100] Initial concerns regarding an increased risk of second malignancies following use of pentostatin have not been confirmed.[101]

Clinical Use

Pentostatin, delivered in low doses, produces responses in over 90% of patients with hairy-cell leukemia, even those refractory to splenectomy and α-interferon therapy. Estimated disease-free survival at 5 and 10 years is over 85% and 65%, respectively.[102] Overall, 5- and 10-year survival is 90% and 80%, respectively.[102] Because of its activity in hairy-cell leukemia, pentostatin has also been evaluated in a number of other closely related disorders, including chronic lymphocytic leukemia, Waldenstrom's macroglobulinemia, refractory multiple myeloma, and adult T-cell lymphomas. It produces responses, but has no apparent advantage over standard therapies.

Cladribine or 2-Chlorodeoxyadenosine (Leustatin)

Mechanism of Action

Cladribine or 2-chlorodeoxyadenosine is a purine nucleoside analog with antineoplastic activity against low-grade lymphoproliferative diseases, childhood leukemias, and multiple sclerosis. Its important pharmacologic features are noted in Table 9.6.

TABLE 9.6

KEY FEATURES OF CLADRIBINE (2-CHLORODEOXADENOSINE)

Factor	Result
Mechanism of Action	(1) Activation to 2-CdATP that is incorporated into DNA producing DNA strand breaks
	(2) 2-CdATP inhibits ribonucleotide reductase
	(3) Triggers apoptosis by activating caspaces
Metabolism	Activation to 2-CdATP within cells
Pharmacokinetics	(1) Significant variability in cladribine plasma AUC
	(2) 40-50% oral bioavailability
	(3) 50% urinary excretion
Drug interactions	Increases toxicity of cytarabine
	More frequent rash when used with allopurinol
Toxicity	(1) Myelosuppression
	(2) Fever
	(3) Immunosuppression with resulting infection complications
	(4) Rash

Substitution of chlorine at the two position of deoxyadenosine produces 2-chlorodeoxyadenosine or cladribine (2-CdA) (Fig. 9.3), which is relatively resistant to enzymatic deamination by adenosine deaminase. Intracellular transport of 2-CdA occurs via nucleoside delivery mechanisms. Cladribine is a prodrug and requires intracellular phosphorylation for activation. The 5′-triphosphate metabolite (2-chloro-2′-deoxyadenosine 5-triphosphate, 2-CdATP) accumulates in cells rich in deoxycytidine kinase[103] (Fig. 9.5). 2-CdATP is incorporated into DNA, producing DNA strand breaks and inhibition of DNA synthesis.[104] Cladribine, incorporated into DNA promoter sequences, acts as a transcription antagonist.[105] High intracellular concentrations of 2-CdATP also inhibit DNA polymerases[106] and ribonucleotide reductase,[61] causing an imbalance in deoxyribonucleotide triphosphate pools with subsequent impairment of DNA synthesis and repair.

The mechanism for triggering apoptosis in nondividing cells by 2-CdATP is not clear. Cysteine proteases, referred to as caspaces, are active in apoptosis triggered by cladribine.[107] 2-CdATP interacts with cytochrome C and protease activating factor-1 (PAF-1) to initiate the caspase cascade leading to DNA degradation, even in the absence of cell division.[108] Cladribine resistance is most often caused by a deficiency in deoxycytidine kinase.[109] P53 mutations[110] and, to a significantly lesser extent, the presence of multidrug resistance protein 4,[111] also result in resistance to cladribine.

Clinical Pharmacology

Liquid chromatography is used to quantify cladribine and its primary metabolite, 2-chlorodeoxyadenosine.[112] Cladribine is a prodrug. It is activated within the cell to

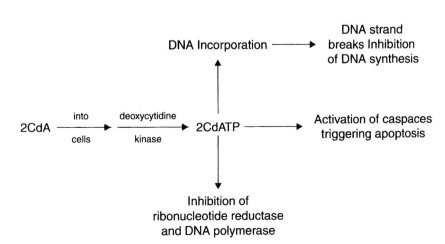

Figure 9.5 Activation of cladribine (2-chorodeoxyadenosine or 2 CdA).

cladribine nucleotides. Intracellular drug concentrations are several hundred-fold higher than plasma concentrations.[113] Cladribine nucleotides are retained in leukemic cells with a intracellular half-life of 9 to 30 hours. The long intracellular half-life supports the use of intermittent drug administration.[114] Unfortunately, no correlations have been found between the plasma AUC of cladribine or intracellular cladribine concentrations and the response to treatment.[115]

Following a 2-hour infusion of 0.12 mg/kg cladribine, peak serum concentrations of nearly 50 µg/mL are achieved.[114] A linear dose-concentration relationship is present up to doses of 2.5 mg/m^2 per hour. Cladribine clearance rates of 664 to 978 mL/hr per kilogram have been reported with significant interpatient variability ($\pm$50%). The drug is weakly bound to plasma protein (20%). Renal clearance accounts for 50% of total drug clearance, with 20 to 30% of drug excreted as unchanged cladribine within the first 24 hours.[114,116] Little information is available regarding dose adjustments for renal or hepatic insufficiency. However, given the high renal drug clearance, caution should be taken in using cladribine in patients with renal failure. Chloroadenine is the major metabolite formed. Renal excretion of chloroadenine accounts for clearance of 3% of administered cladribine.[114]

Bioavailability of subcutaneously administered cladribine is excellent (100%).[117] Oral administration has been evaluated with bioavailability of 40 to 50%. Increased metabolism to chloroadenine is seen following oral administration suggesting a first-pass effect.[112,117] Significant patient-to-patient variability ($\pm$28%) exists in the AUC achieved following administration of drug by any method.[114,116]

Toxicity

Cladribine's dose-limiting toxicity using a standard dosage of 0.7 mg/kg per cycle (usually as a continuous 7-day infusion at 0.1 mg/m^2 per day) is myelosuppression.[118] Nausea, alopecia, hepatic and renal toxicity rarely occur at this dose. Fever (temperature >100°F) is seen in two-thirds of patients treated with cladribine, mostly during the period of neutropenia. Myelosuppression and immunosuppression with development of opportunistic infections are the major adverse events.[100,119] Severe (grade 3-4) neutropenia and lymphopenia occur in half of treated patients. Neutrophil counts decrease 1 to 2 weeks after starting therapy and persist for 3 to 4 weeks.[119] Twenty percent of patients develop grade 3-4 thrombocytopenia. Infections occur in 15 to 40% of patients, often opportunistic infections, such as Candida or Aspergillis. Betticher et al.[120] have found that reducing the dose of 2CdA from 0.7 to 0.5 mg/kg per cycle decreases the grade 3 myelosuppression rate (33 to 8%) and the infection rate (30 to 7%) without a change in response rate.

Toxicities other than myelosuppression and infections are rare, but have been reported. Following high dose 2CdA (5 to 10 times the recommended therapeutic dose), renal failure, and motor weakness has been described. Autoimmune hemolytic anemia has been reported in patients with CLL who are receiving cladribine.[121] Eosinophilia, nausea, and fatigue have been noted.

Clinical Use and Drug Interactions

Cladribine's spectrum of activity is similar to other adenosine analogs (e.g., fludarabine). Patients with CLL, hairy-cell leukemia, low-grade non-Hodgkin's lymphomas, cutaneous T-cell lymphoma, Waldenstrom's macroglobulinemia systemic mastocytosis, and blast-phase chronic myelogenous leukemia have responded to cladribine therapy.[122,123] Subcutaneous and oral routes of drug administration have demonstrated activity.[124] A drug-drug interaction between cladribine and cytarabine has been reported. Pretreatment of patients with cladribine increases the intracellular accumulation of ara-CTP, the active metabolite of cytarabine, by 40%.[125] An increased frequency of drug rash has been noted when cladribine and allopurinol have been used concomitantly.[126]

ALLOPURINOL

Allopurinol has no antineoplastic activity. However, it is frequently used in patients with leukemia and lymphoma to prevent hyperuricemia and uric acid nephropathy. The clinical use of allopurinol in cancer chemotherapy and its potential interactions with various antitumor agents are summarized in this section. The key features of allopurinol are summarized in Table 9.7.

Mechanism of Action

Allopurinol (4-hydroxypyrazolo [3,4-d] pyrimidine) and its major metabolic product oxipurinol (4,6-dihydroxypyrazolo [3,4-d] pyrimidine) are analogs of hypoxanthine and xanthine, respectively. Both inhibit the enzyme xanthine oxidase and block the conversion of hypoxanthine and xanthine to uric acid (Fig. 9.6). Allopurinol binds to xanthine oxidase and undergoes internal conversion to oxipurinol, simultaneously reducing xanthine oxidase.[127] Oxipurinol inhibits xanthine oxidase by attaching at the active site of the enzyme in a stoichiometric fashion, one molecule of oxipurinol for each functionally active site of xanthine oxidase (K_I=5.4 $\times$ 10^{-10} M).

Allopurinol reduces serum uric acid concentrations not only by inhibiting xanthine oxidase but also by decreasing the rate of de novo purine biosynthesis. Administration of allopurinol to patients with primary gout causes an increase in serum xanthine and hypoxanthine concentrations.[128] Increased conversion of hypoxanthine to inosinic acid and subsequently to adenylic and guanylic acid occurs (Fig. 9.7). Adenylic and guanylic acid are allosteric

TABLE 9.7
KEY FEATURES OF ALLOPURINOL

Factor	Result
Mechanism of Action	(1) Limits conversion of xanthine and hypoxanthine to uric acid by inhibiting xanthine oxidase. (2) Causes feedback inhibition of de novo purine synthesis.
Metabolism	Rapid metabolic conversion to oxipurinol, which is the active metabolite
Pharmacokinetics	Allopurinol $t_{1/2}$: 0.7–1.6 hr Oxipurinol $t_{1/2}$: 14–28 hr
Elimination	Allopurinol - metabolism to oxipurinol Oxipurinol - renal excretion
Drug Interactions	(1) Prolongs half-life of 6-MP and azathioprine by decreasing rate of metabolic elimination. (2) May impair hepatic microsomal enzyme function.
Toxicity	(1) Rash (2) Hypersensitivity syndrome (TEN, renal failure, liver, hepatic failure) (3) Rare: xanthine nephropathy
Precautions	(1) Reduce doses of 6-MP or azathioprine. (2) Reduce allopurinol doses for renal insufficiency. (3) Stop drug for rash.

inhibitors of 5′phosphoribosyl-1-pyrophosphate (PRPP) aminotransferase, the critical enzyme involved in de novo purine synthesis. Total purine excretion (xanthine plus hypoxanthine plus uric acid) decreases by 30 to 40% after initiation of allopurinol therapy. Allopurinol and oxipurinol are also converted to their respective ribonucleotides. This leads to decreased intercellular concentrations of PRPP, which also contributes to decreased purine synthesis.[129] The effect of allopurinol on de novo purine synthesis is negligible in treatment of the tumor lysis syndrome, in which release of purines from DNA occurs.

Clinical Pharmacology

Allopurinol is available in 100- and 300-mg tablets and as an intravenous preparation.[130] Allopurinol is well absorbed orally (50 to 80% bioavailability).[131] After oral administration of 300 mg allopurinol, plasma oxipurinol concentrations of 10 to 40 μM (1.5 to 6.5 mg/L) are achieved within 1 to 3 hours.[132] Intravenous allopurinol achieves maximal plasma concentrations within 30 minutes. Kinetics of the active metabolite, oxipurinol, are similar following intravenous or oral administration.

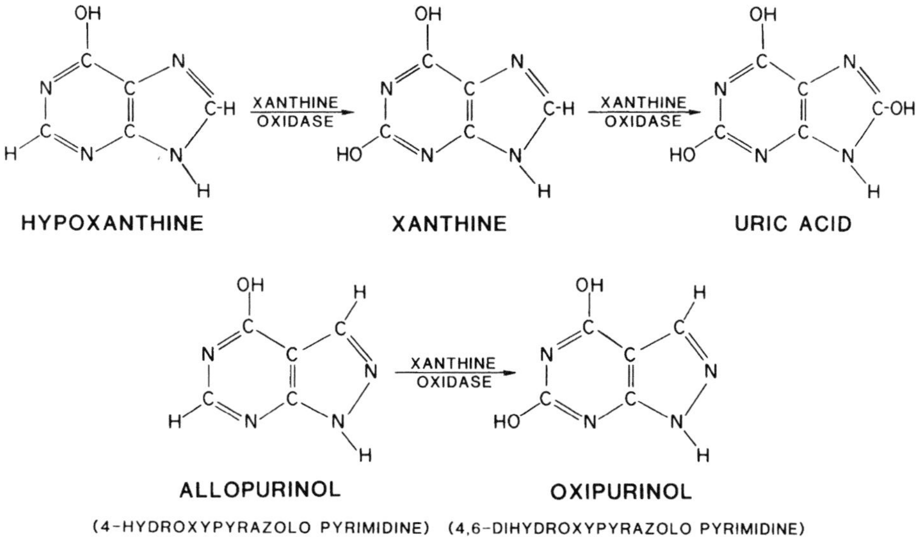

Figure 9.6 Metabolic pathway for the conversion of hypoxanthine and xanthine to uric acid and of allopurinol to oxipurinol.

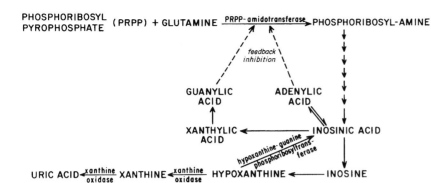

Figure 9.7 Feedback inhibition of de novo purine biosynthesis. Inhibition of xanthine oxidase by allopurinol causes an increase in serum hypoxanthine concentrations, which in turn causes increased concentrations of inosinic, xanthylic, adenylic, and guanylic acids. Guanylic and adenylic acids are inhibitors of phosphoribosylpyrophosphate aminotransferase (PRPP- aminotransferase), the initial step in de novo purine synthesis.

The plasma half-life of allopurinol is short (30 to 100 minutes) with rapid conversion of allopurinol to oxipurinol. The volume of distribution of both allopurinol and oxipurinol is roughly that of total body water with little binding of either drug to plasma proteins. A small amount of allopurinol is excreted directly in the urine (clearance rate, 13 to 19 mL/minute), but most of an administered dose of allopurinol is metabolized to oxipurinol. In patients with normal renal function, steady-state oxipurinol plasma concentrations are 15 mg/L (100 μM) at an allopurinol dose of 300 mg/day. This is in excess of the concentration needed to inhibit xanthine oxidase (25 μM). Impaired renal clearance of oxipurinol leads to a prolonged oxipurinol plasma half-life (14 to 28 hours).[133] Oxipurinol clearance and drug half-life are closely tied to creatinine clearance. Patients with renal failure have delayed oxipurinol excretion and require a dose reduction to prevent drug accumulation. Maintenance doses of allopurinol should be reduced to maintain serum oxipurinol levels comparable with those in patients with normal renal function.[133,134] Older patients (>70 years) have reduced oxipurinol clearance related to an age-dependent decline in renal function.[135]

Toxicity

Allopurinol therapy is well tolerated in most patients and produces few side effects. Skin rash is seen in 2% of patients taking allopurinol.[136] In patients allergic to allopurinol, oxipurinol may be tried as an alternative therapy for xanthine oxidase inhibition. However, cross-sensitivity between allopurinol and oxipurinol has been noted. In patients allergic to allopurinol, the drug should be avoided, if possible. However, desensitization to allopurinol has been successfully employed in allergic patients for whom no substitute is available.[137] Gastrointestinal intolerance, fever, and alopecia are rare complications of allopurinol therapy. A severe, potentially life-threatening hypersensitivity syndrome resulting from allopurinol use has been reported.[133,138] Patients usually have fever (87% of reported cases), eosinophilia (73%), skin rash (92%) including toxic epidermal neurolysis, renal dysfunction, and hepatic failure

(68%). Death has been reported in 21% of published cases. This hypersensitivity syndrome usually appears 2 to 4 weeks after the initiation of 300 to 400 mg/day allopurinol. Over 80% of patients developing this syndrome have underlying renal failure when allopurinol therapy is started. Steady-state concentrations of oxipurinol are elevated in this situation and may play a role in the development of the toxicity syndrome. It is hoped that adjustments of allopurinol doses for renal insufficiency will lower the risk for drug toxicity.[133]

Xanthine nephropathy is a rare complication of allopurinol therapy in cancer patients.[139] Even though xanthine precipitation is a potential complication of allopurinol therapy in patients who have massive tumor lysis, allopurinol treatment is beneficial to such patients. It enables them to excrete a larger total purine load. Because the solubility of a single purine, such as xanthine, hypoxanthine, or uric acid, is independent of the others, dividing the purine load among these three purines by the use of allopurinol will increase the total amount of purine that can be excreted in the urine. Xanthine concentrations in excess of 5 mg/dL may cause a falsely low uric acid measurement as determined by the uricase method.[140] Elevated xanthine concentrations do not affect uric acid measurements determined by the phosphotungstate colorimetric assay.

Clinical Uses and Drug Interactions

In the treatment of primary gout, allopurinol produces a fall in serum uric acid concentration and a decrease in urinary uric acid excretion 1 or 2 days following initiation of therapy and produces a maximal reduction in serum urate levels within 4 to 14 days. A once-daily dose of 300 mg of allopurinol is clinically as effective as three equally divided doses of 100 mg.[141] In patients who do not respond to 300 mg of allopurinol per day, dosages of 600 to 1,000 mg/day are usually effective in lowering serum uric acid concentrations.

With rapid tumor lysis following cancer treatment, there is a sudden rise in serum uric acid caused by cell destruction with release of preformed purines from degraded DNA. The rapid release of uric acid can result in renal failure because of the precipitation of urate crystals in the distal renal tubules where concentration and acidification are maximal. The development of hyperuricemia after treatment of many leukemias and lymphomas is so common that hydration and allopurinol therapy are recommended before chemotherapy for these diseases is begun. Doses of 300 mg to 400 mg/m^2 per day should be given for 2 to 3 days, with subsequent doses reduced to 300 to 400 mg/day. These doses prevent marked increases in uric acid excretion after chemotherapy,[142,143] although clinically significant tumor lysis is still seen in 5% of patients with high-grade lymphomas and laboratory evidence of lysis in 40%.

Xanthine oxidase catalyzes the conversion of both azathioprine and 6-MP to the inactive metabolite, 6-thiouric acid. Oral doses of 6-MP or azathioprine should be reduced by at least 65 to 75% when allopurinol is concomitantly used. White blood cell counts should be monitored frequently. Even with azathioprine dose reductions of 67%, myelosuppression is seen in over one-third of patients also treated with allopurinol.[144]

REFERENCES

1. Burchenal JH, Murphy ML, Ellison RR, et al. Clinical evaluation of a new antimetabolite, 6-mercaptopurine, in the treatment of leukemia and allied diseases. Blood 1953;8:965–999.
2. Lennard L. The clinical pharmacology of 6-mercaptopurine. Eur J Clin Pharmacol 1992;43:329–339.
3. Tidd DM, Patterson ARP. Distinction between inhibition of purine nucleotide synthesis and the delayed cytotoxic reaction of 6-mercaptopurine. Cancer Res 1974;34:733–737.
4. Waters TR, Swann PF. Cytotoxic mechanism of 6-thioguanine: L Mut S, the human mismatch binding heterodimer binds to DNA containing S^6-methythioguanine. Biochemistry 1997;36:2501–2506.
5. Swann PF, Waters TR, Moulton DC, et al. Role of postreplicative DNA mismatch repair in the cytotoxic action of thioguanine. Science 1996;273:1109–1011.
6. Dervieux T, Blanco JG, Krynetcki EY, et al. Differing contribution of thiopurine methyltransferase to mercaptopurine versus thioguanine effects in human leukemic cells. Cancer Research 2001;61:5810–5816.
7. Fairchild CR, Maybaum J, Kennedy KA. Concurrent unilateral chromatic damage and DNA strand breakage in response to 6-thioguanine treatment. Biochem Pharmacol 1986;35: 3533–3541.
8. Pan BF, Nelson JA. Characterization of the DNA damage in 6-thioguanine treated cells. Biochem Pharmacol 1990;40:1063–1069.
9. Erb N, Harms DO, Janka-Schaab G. Pharmacokinetics and metabolism of thiopurines in children with ALL receiving 6-thioguanine versus 6-mercaptopurine. Cancer Chemother Pharmacol 1998;42: 266–272.
10. Tiede I, Fritz G, Stand S, et al. C28-dependent RAC activation is the molecular target of azathioprine in primary human CD4 T lymphocytes. J Clin Invest 200;111:1133–1145.
11. Lavi L, Holcenberg JS. A rapid sensitive high performance liquid chromatography assay for 6-mercaptopurine metabolites in red blood cells. Anal Biochem 1985;144:514–521.
12. Zimm S, Collins JM, Riccardi R, et al. Variable bioavailability of oral mercaptopurine. Is maintenance chemotherapy in ALL being optimally delivered? N Eng J Med 1983;308:1005–1009.
13. Arndt CAS, Balis FM, McCully CL, et al. Bioavailability of low-dose vs high-dose 6-mercaptopurine. Clin Pharmacol Ther 1988;43:588–591.
14. Jacqz-Aigrain E, Nafa S, Medard Y, et al. Pharmacokinetics and distribution of 6-mercaptopurine administered intravenously in children with lymphoblastic leukaemia. Eur J Clin Pharmacol 1997;53:71–74.
15. Balis FM, Holcenberg JS, Zimm, S et al. The effect of methotrexate on the bioavailability of oral 6-mercaptopurine. Clin Pharmacol Ther 1987;41:384–387.
16. Balis FM, Holcenberg JS, Poplack DG, et al. Pharmacokinetics and pharmacodynamics of oral methotrexate and mercaptopurine in children with lower risk ALL; a joint Children's Cancer Group and Pediatric Oncology Branch study. Blood 1998;92:3569–3577.
17. Zimm S, Collins JM, O'Neill D, et al. Chemotherapy: Inhibition of first-pass metabolism in cancer interaction of 6-mercaptopurine and allopurinol. Clin Pharmacol Ther 1983;34:810–817.
18. Zimm S, Ettinger LJ, Holcenberg JS, et al. Phase I and clinical pharmacological study of mercaptopurine administered as a prolonged intravenous infusion. Cancer Res 1985;45:1869–1873.
19. Lafolie P, Hayder S, Bjork O, et al. Intraindividual variation in 6-mercaptopurine pharmacokinetics during oral maintenance therapy of children with ALL. Eur J Clin Pharmacol 1991;40:599–601.
20. Burton NK, Barnett MJ, Aherne GW, et al. The affect of food on the oral administration of 6-mercaptopurine. Cancer Chemother Pharmacol 1986;18:90–91.
21. Burton NK, Aherne GW. The effect of cotrimoxazole on the absorption of orally administered 6-mercaptopurine in the rat. Cancer Chemother Pharmacol 1986;16:81–84.
22. Weinshilboum RM. Methyltransferase pharmacogenetics. Pharmacol Ther 1989;43:77–90.
23. Holme SA, Duley JA, Sanderson J. Erythrocyte thiopurine methyl transferase assessment prior to azathioprine use in the UK. QJM 2002;95:439–444.
24. Coulthard SA, Howell C, Robson J, Hall AG. The relationship between thiopurine methyltransferase activity and genotype in blasts from patients with acute leukemia. Blood 1998;92:2856–2862.
25. Lennard L, VanLoon JA, Weinshilboum RM. Pharmacogenetics of acute azathioprine toxicity: Relationship to thiopurine methyltransferase genetic polymorphism. Clin Pharmacol Ther 1989;46:149–154.
26. Jones CD, Smart C, Titus A, et al. Thiopurine methyltransferase activity in a sample population of black subjects in Florida. Clin Pharmacol Ther 1993;53:348–353.
27. Koren G, Ferrazini G, Sulh H, et al. Systemic exposures to mercaptopurine as a prognostic factor in acute lymphocytic leukemia. N Engl J Med 1990;323:17–21.
28. Hayder S, Lafolie P, Bjork O, et al. 6-Mercaptopurine plasma levels in children with acute lymphoblastic leukemia: Relationship to relapse risk and myelotoxicity. Ther Drug Monit 1989;11:617–622.
29. Lennard L, Lilleyman JS. Variable 6-mercaptopurine metabolism and treatment outcome in childhood lymphoblastic leukemia. J Clin Oncol 1989;7:1816–1823.
30. Lennard L, Lilleyman JS, Van Loon JA, et al. Genetic variation in response to 6-mercaptopurine for childhood acute lymphoblastic leukemia. Lancet 1991;336:225–229.
31. Otterness D, Szumlanski C, Lennard L, et al. Human thiopurine methyltransferase pharmacogenetics: Gene sequence polymorphisms. Clin Pharmacol Ther 1997;62:60–73.
32. Evans WE. Thiopurine 5-methyltransferase: a genetic polymorphism that affects a small number of drugs in a big way. Pharmacogenetics 2002;12:421–423,
33. Tai HL, Krynetski EY, Yates CR, et al. Thiopurine 5-methyltransferase deficiency: two nucleotide transitions define the most prevalent mutant allele associated with loss of catalytic activity in Caucasians. Am J Hum Genet 1996;58:694–702.
34. Yates CR, Krynetski EY, Loennechen T, et al. Molecular diagnosis of thiopurine 5-methylltransferase deficiency: genetic basis for azathioprine and mercaptopurine intolerance. Ann Intern Med 1997;126:608–614.
35. LePage GA, Whitecar JP. Pharmacology of 6-thioguanine in man. Cancer Res 1971;31:1627–1631.
36. Brox LW, Birkett L, Belch A. Clinical pharmacology of oral thioguanine in acute myelogenous leukemia. Cancer Chemother Pharmacol 1981;6:35–638.

37. Kitchen BJ, Balis FM, Poplack DG, et al. A pediatric Phase I trial and pharmacokinetic study of thioguanine administered by continuous i.v. infusion. Clin Cancer Res 1997;3:713–717.

38. Liliemark J, Petterson B, Lafolie P, et al. Determination of plasma azathioprine and 6-mercaptoprine in patients with rheumatoid arthritis treated with oral azathioprine. Ther Drug Monit 1990;12:339–343.

39. Chan CLC, Erdmen GR, Gruber SA, et al. Azathioprine metabolism: Pharmacokinetics of 6-mercaptopurine, 6-thiouric acid and 6-thioguanine nucleotides in renal transplant patients. J Clin Pharm 1990;30:358–363.

40. Evans WE, Hon YY, Bomgaars, L et al. Preponderance of thiopurine S-methyltransferase deficiency and heterozygosity among patients intolerant to mercaptopurine or azathioprine. J Clin Oncol 2001;19:2293–2301.

41. Schwab M, Schaffeler E, Marx C, et al. Azathioprine therapy and adverse drug reactions in patients with inflammatory bowel disease: impact of thiopurine 5-methyltranferase polymorphism. Pharmacogenetics 2002;12:429–436.

42. Einhorn M, Davidson I. Hepatotoxicity of 6-mercaptopurine. JAMA 1964;188:802–806.

43. Gearry RB, Barclay ML, Burt MJ, et al. Thiopurine 5-methltransferase (TPMT) gene type does not predict adverse drug reactions to thiopurine drugs in patients with inflammatory bowel disease. Alimentary Pharmacol Ther 2003;18:395–400.

44. Nygaard U, Toft N, Schmiegelow K. Methylated metabolites of 6-mercaptopurine are associated with hepatotoxicity. Clin Pharmacol Ther 2004;75:274–281.

45. Duttera MJ, Caralla RL, Gallelli JF. Hematuria and crystalluria after high-dose 6-mercaptopurine administration. N Eng J Med 1972;287:292–294.

46. Polifka JE, Friedman, JM. Teratogen update: azathioprine and 6-mercaptopurine. Teratology 2002;65:240–261.

47. Francella A, Dyan H, Bodian C, et al. The safety of 6-mercaptopurine for childbearing patients with inflammatory bowel disease: a retrospective cohort study. Gastroenterology 2003;124:9–17.

48. Kovach JS, Rubin J, Creagan ET, et al. Phase I trial of parenteral 6-thioguanine given on 5 consecutive days. Cancer Res 1986;46:5959–5962.

49. Gill RA, Onstad GR, Cardmore JM, et al. Hepatic veno-occlusive disease caused by 6-thioguanine. Ann Intern Med 1982;96:58–60.

50. Fields CK, Robinson JW, Roy TM, et al. Hypersensitivity reaction to azathioprine. South Med J 1998;91:471–474.

51. Silman AJ, Petrie J, Hazelman B, et al. Lymphoproliferative cancer and other malignancy in patients with rheumatoid arthritis treated with azathioprine: A 20 year follow-up study. Ann Rheum Dis 1988;47:988–992.

52. Kwong AL, Au WY, Liang RH. Acute myeloid leukemia after azathioprine treatment for autoimmune disease association with -7/7q-. Cancer Genetics and Cytogenetics 1998;104:94–97.

53. Black AJ, McLeod HL, Capell HA, et al. Thiopurine methyltransferase genotype predicts therapy-limiting severe toxicity from azathioprine. Ann Intern Med 1998;129:716–718.

54. Lennard L, Welch JC, Lilleyman JS. Thiopurine drugs in the treatment of childhood leukaemia: the influence of inherited thiopurine methyltransferase activity on drug metabolism and cytotoxicity. Br J Clin Pharmacol 1997;44:455–461.

55. Kennedy DT, Hayney MS, Lake KD. Azathioprine and allopurinol: the price of an avoidable drug interaction. Ann Pharmacothera 1996;30: 951–954.

56. Dervieux T, Hancock ML, Pui CH, et al. Antagonism by methotrexate on mercaptopurine disposition in lymphoblastic during upfront treatment of acute lymphoblastic leukemia. Clin Pharmacol Ther 2003;73:506–516.

57. Adkins JC, Peters DH, Markham A. Fludarabine. An update of its pharmacology and use in the treatment of haematological malignancies. Drugs 1997;53:1005–1037.

58. Danhauser L, Plunkett W, Keating M, et al. 9-B-D-arabinofuranosyl-2-fluoroadenine 5′-monophosphate pharmacokinetics in plasma and tumor cells of patients with relapsed leukemia and lymphoma. Cancer Chemother Pharmacol 1986;18:145–152.

59. Molina-Arcas M, Bellosillo B, Casado FJ, et al. Fludarabine uptake mechanisms in B-cell chronic lymphocytic leukemia. Blood 2003;101:2328–2334.

60. Gandhi V, Plunkett W. Cellular and clinical pharmacology of fludarabine. Clin Pharmacokinet 2002;41:93–103.

61. Parker WB, Ashok RB, Shen SX, et al. Interaction of the 2-halogenated dATP analogs (F, Cl, and Br) with human DNA polymerase, DNA primase and ribonucleotide reductase. Mol Pharmacol 1988;34:485–489.

62. Kamiya K, Huang P, Plunkett W. Inhibition of the 3′→ 5′ exonucleases of human DNA polymerase epsilon by fludarabine-terminated DNA. J Biol Chem 1996;271:19428–19435.

63. Plunkett W, Begleiter A, Liliemark O, et al. Why do drugs work in CLL? Leuk Lymphoma 1996;22(Suppl 2):1–11.

64. Pettitt A. Mechanism of action of purine analogs in chronic lymphocytic leukaemia. Br J Hematol 2003;121:692–702.

65. Sandoval A, Consoli U, Plunkett W. Fludarabine-mediated inhibition of nucleotide excision repair induces apoptosis in quiescent human lymphocytes. Clin Cancer Res 1996;2:1731–1741.

66. Malspeis L, Grever MR, Staubus AE, et al. Pharmacokinetics of 2-F-ara-A (9-B-D-arabinofuranosyl-2-fluoroadenine) in cancer patients during the phase I clinical investigation of fludarabine phosphate. Sem Oncol 1990;17(Suppl 8):18–32.

67. Danhauser L, Plunkett W, Liliemark J, et al. Comparison between the plasma and intracellular pharmacology of 1-(-D-arabinofuranosyl-2-fluoroadenine 5′-monophosphate in patients with relapsed leukemia. Leukemia 1987;1:638–643.

68. Lichtman SM, Etcubanas E, Budman D, et al. The pharmacokinetics and pharmacodynamics of fludarabine phosphate in patients with renal impairment: a perspective dose adjustment study. Cancer Invest 2002;20:904–913.

69. Posker GL, Figgitt DP. Oral fludarabine. Drugs 2003;63: 2317–2323.

70. Oscier D, Orchard JA, Culligan D, et al. The bioavailability of oral fludarabine phosphate is unaffected by food. Hematol J 2001;2:316–321.

71. Gandhi V, Estey E, Du M, et al. Maximum dose of fludarabine for maximal modulation of arabinosyl -cytosine triphosphate in human leukemic blast cells during therapy. Clin Cancer Res 1997;3:1539–1545.

72. Sorensen JM, Vena DA, Fallavollita A, et al. Treatment of refractory chronic lymphocytic leukemia with fludarabine phosphate via the group C protocol mechanism of the National Cancer Institute: five-year follow-up report. J Clin Oncol 1997;15:458–465.

73. Byrd JC, Peterson BL, Morrison VA, et al. Randomized Phase II study of fludarabine with concurrent versus sequential treatment with rituximab in symptomatic untreated patients with B-cell chronic lymphocytic leukemia: results from the CALGB 9712. Blood 2003;101:6–14.

74. Frank DA, Mahajan S, Ritz J. Fludarabine-induced immunosuppression is associated with inhibitor of STAT 1 signaling. Nat Med 1999;5:444–447.

75. Keating MJ, O'Brien S, Lerner S, et al. Long-term follow-up of patients with chronic lymphocytic leukemia (CLL) receiving fludarabine regimens as initial therapy. Blood 1998;92:1165–1171.

76. Anaissie EJ, Kontoyiannis DP, O'Brien S, et al. Infections in patients with chronic lymphocytic leukemia treated with fludarabine. Ann Intern Med 1998;129:559–566.

77. Mortell RE, Peterson BL, Cohen HJ, et al. Analysis of age, estimated creatinine clearance and pretreatment hematologic parameters as predictors of fludarabine toxicity in patients treated for chronic lymphocytic leukemia. Chemother Pharmacol 2002; 50:37–45.

78. Weiss RB, Freiman J, Kweder SL, et al. Hemolytic anemia after fludarabine therapy for chronic lymphocytic leukemia. J Clin Oncol 1998;16:1885–1889.

79. Cheson BD, Frame JN, Vena D, et al Tumor lysis syndrome: an uncommon complication of fludarabine therapy of chronic lymphocytic leukemia. J Clin Oncol 1998;16:2313–2320.

80. Cheson BD, Vena DA, Foss FM, et al. Neurotoxicity of purine analogs: a review. J Clin Oncol 1994;12:2216–2228.

81. Helman DL, Byrd JL, Alex NC, et al. Fludarabine-related pulmonary toxicity: a distinct clinical entity in chronic lymphoproliferative syndromes. Chest 2002;127:785–790.

82. Morrison VA, Rai KR, Peterson BL, et al. Therapy-related myeloid leukemias are observed in patients with chronic lymphocytic leukemia after treatment with fludarabine and chlorambucil;

results of an inter group study: Cancer and Leukemia Group B 9011. J Clin Oncol 2002;20:3878–3884.

83. Rai K, Peterson B, Applebaum F, et al. Fludarabine compared with chlorambucil as primary therapy for active chronic lymphocytic leukemia. N Engl J Med 2000;343:1750–1757.

84. Khouri IF, Champlin RE. Nonmyeloablative stem cell transplantation for lymphoma. Sem Oncol 2004;31:22–26.

85. Gandhi V, Huang P, Chapman AJ, et al. Incorporation of fludarabine and 1-beta-D-arabinofuranosylcytosine 5′-triphosphates by DNA polymerase alpha: affinity, interaction and consequences. Clin Cancer Res 1997;3:1347–1355.

86. Agarwal RP. Inhibitors of adenosine deaminase. Pharmacol Ther 1982;17:399–429.

87. O'Dwyer PJ, Wagner B, Leyland-Jones B, et al. 2′-Deoxycoformycin (Pentostatin) for lymphoid malignancies. Ann Intern Med 1988;108:733–743.

88. Jackson RC, Leopold WR, Ross DA. The biochemical pharmacology of (2′R)-chloropentostatin, a novel inhibitor of adenosine deaminase. Adv Enzyme Regul 1986;25:125–139.

89. Wiley JS, Smith CL, Jamieson GP. Transport of 2′deoxycoformycin in human leukemic and lymphoma cells. Biochem Pharmacol 1991;42:708–710.

90. Johnston JB, Glazer RI, Pugh L, et al. The treatment of hairy-cell leukaemia with 2′-deoxycoformycin. Br J Haematol 1986;63:525–534.

91. Al-Razzak KA, Benedetti AE, Waugh WN, et al. Chemical stability of pentostatin (NSC-218321), a cytotoxic and immunosuppressant agent. Pharmaceutical Res 1990;7:452–460.

92. Kane BJ, Kuhn JG, Roush MK. Pentostatin: an adenosine deaminase inhibitor for the treatment of hairy cell leukemia. Ann Pharmacother 1992;26:939–946.

93. Smyth JF, Paine RM, Jackman AL, et al. The clinical pharmacology of the adenosine deaminase inhibitor 2′deoxycorformycin. Cancer Chemother Pharmacol 1980;5: 93–101.

94. Major PP, Hgarwal RP, Kufe DW. Clinical pharmacology of deoxycoformycin. Blood 1981;58:91–96.

95. Lathia C, Fleming G, Mayer M, et al. Pentostatin pharmacokinetics and dosing recommendations in patients with mild renal impairment. Cancer Chemother Pharmacol 2002;50:121–126.

96. Major PP, Agarwal RP, Kufe DW. Deoxycoformycin: neurological toxicity. Cancer Chemother Pharmacol 1981;5:193–196.

97. Margolis J, Grever MR. Pentostatin; Nipent: a review of potential toxicity and its management. Sem Oncol 2000;27(Suppl)5:9–14.

98. Grever M, Kopecky K, Foucar MK, et al. Randomized comparison of pentostatin versus interferon alfa 2A in previously untreated patients with hairy cell leukemia: an intergroup study. J Clin Oncol 1995;13:974–982.

99. Grem JL, King SA, Chun HG, et al. Cardiac complications observed in elderly patients following 2′deoxycoformycin therapy. Am J Hematol 1991;38:245–247.

100. Samonis G, Kontoyiannis DP. Infectious complications of purine analog therapy. Current Opin Infect Disease 2001; 14:409–413.

101. Cheson BD, Vena DA, Barrett J, et al. Second malignancies as a consequence of nucleoside analog therapy for chronic lymphoid leukemias. J Clin Oncol 1999;17:2454–2460.

102. Flinn IW, Kopecky KJ, Foucar MK, et al. Long-term follow-up of remission duration mortality and second malignancy in hairy cell leukemia patients treated with pentostatin. Blood 2000;96:2981–2986.

103. Kawasaki H, Carrera CJ, Piro LO, et al. Relationship of deoxycytidine kinase and cytoplasmic 5′ nucleotidase to the chemotherapeutic efficacy of 2-chlorodeoxyadenosine. Blood 1993;81:597–601.

104. Seto S, Carrera CJ, Kubota M, et al. Mechanism of deoxyadenosine and 2-chlorodeoxyadenosine toxicity to nondividing human lymphocytes. J Clin Invest 1985;75:377–383.

105. Hartman WR, Hantosh P. The antileukemic drug 2-chlorodeoxyadenosine: an intrinsic transcription antagonist. Mol Pharmacol 2004;65:227–234.

106. Hentosh P, Kools R, Blakley RL. Incorporation of 2-halogen-2′-deoxyadenosine 5-triphosphosphates into DNA during replication by human polymerases alpha and beta. J Bio Chem 1990;265:4033–4040.

107. Ceruti S, Beltrami E, Matarrese P, et al. A key role for caspase-2 and caspase-3 in apoptosis induced by 2′chloro-2-deoxyadenosine (cladribine) and 2-chloro adenosine in human astrocytoma cells. Mol Pharmacol 2003;63:1437–1447.

108. Leoni LM, Chao Q, Cottam HB, et al. Induction of an apoptotic program in cell free extracts by 2-chloro-2′deoxyadenosine 5′ triphosphate and cytochrome C. Proc Natl Acad Sci U S A 1998;95:9567–9571.

109. Mansson E, Spaskoukoskaja T, Sallstrom, J et al. Molecular and biochemical mechanisms of fludarabine and cladribine resistance in a human promyelocytic cell line. Cancer Res 1999; 59:5956–5963.

110. Galnarini CM, Voorzanger N, Faletten N, et al. Influence of P53 and P21 (WAFI) expression on sensitivity of cancer cells to cladribine. Biochem Pharmacol 2003;65:121–129.

111. Reid G, Wielinga P, Zelcer N, et al. Characterization of the transporter of nucleoside analog drugs by the human multidrug resistant proteins MRP4 and MRP5. Sem Oncol 2003;30:243–247.

112. Lindemalm S, Lilemark J, Julinsson G, et al. Cytotoxicity and pharmacokinetic of cladribine metabolite 2-chloroadenine in patients with leukemia. Cancer Lett 2004;210:171–177.

113. Liliemark J, Juliusson G. Cellular pharmacokinetics of 2-chloro-2′-deoxyadenosine nucleotides: comparison of intermittent and continuous intravenous infusion and subcutaneous and oral administration in leukemia patients. Clin Cancer Res 1995; 1:385–390.

114. Liliemark J. The clinical pharmacokinetics of cladribine. Clin Pharmacokinet 1997;32:120–131.

115. Albertioni F, Lindemalm S, Reichelova V, et al. Pharmacokinetics of cladribine and its 5′monophosphate and 5′ triphosphate in leukemic cells of patients with chronic lymphocytic leukemia. Clin Cancer Res 1998;4:653–658.

116. Kearns CM, Blakley RL, Santana VM, et al. Pharmacokinetics of cladribine (2-chlorodeoxyadenosine) in children with acute leukemia. Cancer Res 1994;54:1235–1239.

117. Lilliemark J, Albertioni F, Hansen M, et al. On the bioavailability of oral and subcutaneous 2-chloro2′-deoxyadenosine in humans: alternative routes of administration. J Clin Oncol 1992;10: 1514–1518.

118. Piro LD, Carrera CJ, Carson DA, et al. Lasting remission in hairy-cell leukemia induced by a single infusion of 2-chlorodeoxyadenosine. N Engl J Med 1990;322: 1117–1121.

119. Cheson BD. Infectious and immunosuppressive complications of purine analog therapy. J Clin Oncol 1995;13:2431–2448.

120. Betticher DC, von Rohr A, Ratschiller D, et al. Fewer infections, but maintained antitumor activity with lower-dose *vs* standard-dose cladribine in pretreated low-grade non-Hodgkin's lymphoma. J Clin Oncol 1998;16:850–858.

121. Chasty RC, Myint H, Oscier DG, et al. Autoimmune haemolysis in patients with B-CLL treated with chlorodeoxyadenosine (CDA). Leuk Lymphoma 1998;29:391–398.

122. Saven A, Lemon RH, Kosty M, et al. 2-Chlorodeoxyadenosine activity in patients with untreated chronic lymphocytic leukemia. J Clin Oncol 1995;13:570–574.

123. Byrd JC, Peterson B, Piro L, et al. A Phase II study of cladribine treatment for fludarabine refractory B cell chronic lymphocytic leukemia. Results form CALGB study q9211. Leukemia 2003; 17:323–327.

124. Juliusson G, Christiansen I, Hansen MM, et al. Oral cladribine as primary therapy for patients with B-cell chronic lymphocytic leukemia. J Clin Oncol 1996;14:2160–2166.

125. Crews KR, Gandhi V, Srivostava DK, et al. Interim comparison of a continuous infusion versus a short daily infusion of cytarabine given in combination with cladribine for pediatric acute myeloid leukemia. J Clini Oncol 2002;20:4217–4224.

126. Chubar Y, Bennett M. Cutaneous reations in hairy cell leukemia treated with 2-chlorodeoxyadenosine and allopurinol. Br J Hematol 2003;122:768–770.

127. Spector T. Inhibition of urate production by allopurinol. Biochem Pharmacol 1977;26:355–358.

128. Caskey CT, Ashton DM, Wyngaarden JB. Enzymology of feedback inhibition of glutamine phosphoribosylpyrophosphate aminotransferase by purine ribonucleotide. J Biol Chem 1964; 239:2570–2579.

129. Fox IH, Wyngaarden JB, Kelley WN. Depletion of erythrocyte phosphoribosylpyrophosphate in man; a newly observed effect of allopurinol. N Engl J Med 1970;283:1177–1182.

130. Smalley RV, Guaspari A, Haase-Statz S, et al. Allopurinol:intravenous use for prevention of hyperuricemia. J Clin Oncol 2000;18:1758–1763.

131. Guerra P, Frias J, Ruiz B, et al. Bioequivalence of allopurinol and its metabolite oxipurinol in two tablet formulations. Pharm Ther 2001;26:113–119.

132. Hande KR, Reed E, Chabner BA. Allopurinol kinetics. Clin Pharmacol Ther 1978;23:598–605.

133. Hande KR, Noone RM, Stone WJ. Severe allopurinol toxicity; description and guidelines for prevention in patients with renal insufficiency. Am J Med 1984;76:47–56.

134. Kumar A, Edward N, White MI, et al. Allopurinol, erythema multiform and renal insufficiency. BMJ 1996;312:173–174.

135. Turnheim K, Krivanek P, Oberbauer R. Pharmacokinetics and pharmacodynamices of allopurinol in elderly and young subjects. Br J Clin Pharmacol 1999;48:501–509.

136. Boston Collaborative Drug Surveillance Program. Excess of ampicillin rash associated with allopurinol or hyperuricemia. N Engl J Med 1972;286:505–507.

137. Fam AG, Lewtas J, Stein J, et al. Desensitization to allopurinol in patients with gout and cutaneous reactions. Am J Med 1992; 93:299–302.

138. Plum HJ, van Deuren M, Wetzels JFM. The allopurinol hypersensitivity syndrome. Neth J Med 1998;52:107–110.

139. Green ML, Fujimoto WY, Seegmiller JE. Urinary xanthine stones - a rare complication of allopurinol therapy. N Engl J Med 1969; 280:426–427.

140. Hande KR, Perini R, Putterman G, et al. Hyperxanthinemia interferes with serum uric acid determinations by the uricase method. Clin Chem 1979;25:1492–1494.

141. Rodnan GP, Robin JA, Tolchin SF, et al. Allopurinol and gouty hyperuricemia. JAMA 1975;231:1143–1147.

142. Feusner J, Farber MS. Role of intravenous allopurinol in the management of acute tumor lysis syndrome. Sem Oncol 2001;285:13–18

143. Hande KR, Garrow GC. Acute tumor lysis syndrome in patients with high-grade non-Hodgkins lymphoma. Am J Med 1993;94: 133–139.

144. Cummins D, Sekar M, Halil O, et al. Myelosuppression associated with azathioprine-allopurinol interaction after heart and lung transplantation. Transplantation 1996;61:1661–1662.

Hydroxyurea

10

Luis Paz-Ares   *Ross C. Donehower*   *Bruce A. Chabner*

Hydroxyurea (HU), one of the simplest of the anticancer drugs, has won a supportive role in the treatment of myeloproliferative disease because of its ability to suppress proliferation of myeloid, erythroid, and platelet precursors, but its value is limited by its failure to induce bone marrow remission, and the equally rapid reversibility of its effect. However, it has other notable clinical properties, including the ability to induce β-globin synthesis in patients with sickle cell anemia and thalassemia. It has been an invaluable probe for the laboratory study of its intracellular target, ribonucleotide reductase (RR), the rate-limiting step in the de novo synthesis of deoxyribonucleotide triphosphates (dNTPs). Other actions, including the generation of nitroxyl radicals and radiosensitizing effects, have potential clinical applications. The key features of this drug are shown in Table 10.1.

HU (Fig. 10.1) was originally synthesized in Germany in 1860,[1] and was found to have inhibitory effects on granulocyte production.[2] Following evaluation in the National Cancer Institute's screening system, in which it displayed myelosuppressive and antileukemic activity,[3,4] it entered clinical trials in the 1960s, and was soon recognized as a potent myelosuppressive agent with a novel mechanism of action and few side effects, properties that have earned it a limited role in cancer chemotherapy. Other inhibitors of RR have since been evaluated in the clinic, including compounds of the thiosemicarbazone series and guanazole,[5,6] but have no special therapeutic advantage and greater toxicity. The principle use of HU at present is in controlling lineage proliferation in chronic myelogenous leukemia (CML), polycythemia vera (PV), and essential thrombocythemia (ET). It has little ability to induce bone marrow remission, but provides excellent control of and prevents complications of high peripheral blood counts.[7]

HU was once a primary agent with interferon-α in first-line therapy against CML,[8-10] but has been largely replaced by the targeted agent, Gleevec, and it now used primarily for acute control of white cell count at presentation or during blastic transformation. In PV, it effectively prevents thrombosis resulting from elevated hematocrit and high platelet count,[11] and it similarly lessens the incidence of thrombosis in ET in patients with platelet counts above 1.5 million.[12] Because both PV and ET are chronic, slowly progressive diseases, there is concern that HU may increase the risk of leukemic conversion, a risk that has not been substantiated thus far.[13,14] In younger patients with PV, who have the prospect of long-term treatment, prophylactic phlebotomy may be favored, and in patients with ET, anagrolide and interferon- are alternatives to HU.

A major current use of HU is in the prevention of complications of sickle cell anemia. In patients with sickle cell anemia, HU increases the production of fetal hemoglobin, ameliorates symptoms, and reduces the incidence of painful crisis and hospitalization.[15,16] In vitro incubation of HU with erythroid progenitors induces fetal hemoglobin β-globin production.[17] Whether the induction of fetal hemoglobin represents a response to inhibition of DNA synthesis in red cell progenitors or a specific alteration of γ-globin gene transcription is uncertain.[17] Recent evidence suggests that nitroxy radicals produced by decomposition of HU may directly stimulate γ-globin gene transcription.[18] Convincing evidence now exists that induction of fetal hemoglobin is not the only, and perhaps not the major, contributor to the drug's efficacy. The benefit from HU may be partly from its ability to suppress both erythropoiesis and myelopoiesis, and its effects on red cell adhesion to vessel walls.[19] A marked decrease in the endothelial adhesion of a patient's red blood cells is observed after 2 weeks of HU therapy, coincident with a decrease in absolute reticulocyte levels, but before fetal hemoglobin levels start to rise. A strong inverse correlation between neutrophil count and crisis rate has also been noticed.[20] In terms of clinical efficacy, a randomized, double-blind study has demonstrated that long-term treatment with HU decreases the incidence of painful crisis by 44% in adult patients with sickle cell disease.[21] HU treatment also reduced the frequency of acute chest syndrome and hospitalization, and also reduced the need for

TABLE 10.1	
KEY FEATURES OF HYDROXYUREA	

Mechanism of action:	Inhibitor of ribonucleotide reductase by inactivation of the tyrosyl free radical on the M-2 subunit.
	Regulation of gene expression.
Pharmacokinetics:	Nonlinear at high doses.
	Bioavailability of essentially 100%.
	Elimination half-life of 3.5–4.5 hr.
	Rapid distribution to tissues and extracellular fluid compartments.
Elimination/metabolism:	Renal excretion predominates, although interpatient variability is significant.
	Several enzyme systems capable of metabolism of HU exist, but the extent of metabolism in humans is not known.
Drug interactions:	Increases metabolism of AraC to active metabolite and the incorporation of arabinosylcytosine triphosphate into DNA.
	Enhances the effects of other antimetabolites.
	Increases the phosphorylation of antiviral nucleosides and favors their incorporation into viral DNA.
	Enhances effects of ionizing radiation.
Toxicity:	Myelosuppression, with white blood cells affected to a greater extent than platelets or red blood cells.
	Gastrointestinal effects (nausea, vomiting, changes in bowel habits, ulceration).
	Dermatologic effects (pigmentation, leg ulcers, erythema, rash, atrophy).
	Renal effects, rare.
	Hepatic effects, occasionally severe.
	Neurologic effects, rare.
	Acute interstitial lung disease, rare.
Precautions:	Decrease dosage in renal failure until patient tolerance demonstrated.
	When given with concomitant radiotherapy, anticipate increased tissue reaction.
	Use with caution when combined with AraC or other antimetabolites.
	Use with caution in pregnant or lactating women.

blood transfusion. These results establish HU as the first clinically acceptable drug shown to decrease crises in sickle cell disease. Studies have shown that HU appears to be as effective in children with sickle cell disease[22] and in patients with sickle cell–β-thalassemia and sickle cell–hemoglobin C disease,[23] although only a small number of patients have been treated and the studies were uncontrolled.[24]

HU may serve as an important model for agents that contribute to inhibition of the replication of HIV by a mechanism other than targeting of a viral enzyme or a structural protein. The ability of HU to decrease intracellular levels of dNTPs first led Lori[25] to propose using the compound to inhibit HIV replication. Subsequent studies have confirmed this effect and have focused on the anti-HIV

mechanism of action of HU and its synergistic interactions with other antiretroviral compounds, particularly the nucleoside reverse transcriptase inhibitors such as didanosine.[26] Currently available clinical data, including those from several uncontrolled studies and four randomized trials, reveal that HU has little activity as a single agent, but produces a pronounced inhibition of HIV replication when combined with didanosine or with didanosine plus stavudine in patients who have not been heavily pretreated. Importantly, HU appears to maintain the activity of the nucleoside reverse transcriptase inhibitors even in the presence of genotypic mutations of HIV that is characteristically associated with resistance.[26]

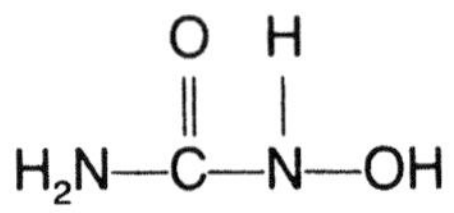

The anti-HIV effect of HU is not consistently accompanied by an increase in the CD4$^+$ lymphocyte count. The lack of such an increase has been attributed to the cytostatic activity of the drug and has uncertain clinical relevance. The antiviral activity of HU is induced at low doses, typically 1,000 mg/day orally, that cause minimal toxicity. Questions about the role of the compound in the treatment of HIV infection that remain to be answered include

$$H_2N—\overset{\overset{\displaystyle O}{\|}}{C}—\overset{\overset{\displaystyle H}{|}}{N}—OH$$

Figure 10.1 Structure of hydroxyurea.

its effectiveness in boosting immune function, the most appropriate dosage regimen, the timing of individual doses, its role in salvage therapy, and the risk associated with long-term use.

MECHANISM OF ACTION AND CELLULAR PHARMACOLOGY

The primary site of cytotoxic action for HU is inhibition of the RR enzyme system. This highly regulated enzyme system is responsible for the conversion of ribonucleotide diphosphates to the deoxyribonucleotide form, which can subsequently be used in either de novo DNA synthesis or DNA repair.[27] HU can be shown to inhibit RR in vitro,[28] and the extent of inhibition of DNA synthesis observed in HU-treated cells correlates closely with the size of the decreased deoxyribonucleotide pools.[29] This enzyme has an important role as a rate-limiting reaction in the regulation of DNA synthesis. In human and other mammalian cells, this unique enzyme consists of two different subunits, usually referred to as M-1 and M-2.[30] Protein M-1 is a dimer with a molecular weight of 170 kd and contains the binding site for the substrates as well as the allosteric effector sites.[30,31] This subunit is responsible for the complex regulation of the enzyme by cellular nucleotide pools. Although considerable variability exists among enzymes from various tissue sources, the general regulatory effects are summarized in Table 10.2.[31] The reduction of all substrates is inhibited and the enzyme complex dissociates in the presence of deoxyadenosine triphosphate.[32] Protein M-1 is present at a relatively constant level throughout the cell cycle, except in cells in G_0 or those that have undergone terminal differentiation, in which it is markedly decreased.[33] The gene coding for this protein can be mapped to chromosome 11.[33] Protein M-2 is the catalytic subunit of the enzyme and exists as a dimer with a molecular weight of 88

kd. This unique protein contains stoichiometric amounts of iron and a stable organic free radical localized to a tyrosine residue. The fully conserved tyrosyl radical is essential to enzyme activity, and is localized in proximity to and stabilized by the binuclear nonheme iron complex.[34,35] The cellular concentration of M-2 protein is variable throughout the cell cycle; it peaks in S phase, which suggests that functional enzyme activity depends on the concentration of M-2 protein.[36] The M-2 subunit sequences have been mapped to chromosome 2 in human cells and seem to be in the same amplification unit as the gene for ornithine decarboxylase.

HU enters cells by passive diffusion. The inhibition of RR occurs as a result of inactivation of the tyrosyl free radical on the M-2 subunit, with disruption of the enzyme's iron-binding center.[37] The fact that this inhibition can be partially reversed in vitro by ferrous iron and that cytotoxicity can be enhanced by iron-chelating agents[38] emphasizes the importance of the nonheme iron cofactor in this process. HU selectively kills cells in S phase, and within an S-phase population of cells, those that are most rapidly synthesizing DNA are most sensitive.[39] The cytotoxic effects of HU correlate with dose or concentration achieved, as well as with duration of drug exposure.[40] Following HU exposure, cells progress normally through the cell cycle until they reach the G_1-S interface. Rather than being prevented from entering S phase, as was once thought, cells enter S phase at a normal rate but are accumulated there as a result of the inhibition of DNA synthesis.[41] Cells undergo apoptosis in a process mediated by both *p53* and non-*p53* pathways.

Jiang et al.[42] have demonstrated that HU may be transformed in vivo to nitric oxide (NO), which is a known RR inhibitor. The possibility therefore exists that the RR inhibition observed after HU exposure may be both direct and mediated through the NO metabolite. Indeed, HU-borne NO may be the intermediate effector in other actions of the drug, such as its induction of fetal hemoglobin.[18]

Several of the enzymes involved in DNA polymerization and DNA precursor synthesis are assembled in a replitase complex during S phase of the cell cycle to channel metabolites to enzymes sequentially during the synthetic process.[43] Replitase contains DNA polymerases, thymidine kinase, dihydrofolate reductase, nucleoside-5' phosphate kinase, thymidylate synthase, and RR. Cross-inhibition is a phenomenon observed with enzymes of the replitase complex, in which inhibition of one enzyme in the complex leads to inhibition of a second, unrelated enzyme. This occurs only in intact cells and only in S phase. Evidence suggests that this is the result of a direct allosteric, structural interaction from a remote site within the complex because disruptions of deoxyribonucleotide pools do not explain the findings.[44] HU appears to be able to inhibit DNA polymerases, thymidylate synthase, and thymidine kinase by this mechanism under certain conditions.

TABLE 10.2
REGULATORY EFFECTS OF NUCLEOTIDE TRIPHOSPHATE ON RIBONUCLEOTIDE REDUCTASE

Substrate	Activators	Inhibitors
CDP	ATP	dATP, dGTP
UDP		dUTP, dTTP, dATP
ADP	dGTP, GTP	dATP, dTTP
GDP	dTTP	dATP, dGTP

ADP, adenosine diphosphate; ATP, adenosine triphosphate; CDP, cytidine diphosphate; dATP, deoxyadenosine triphosphate; dGTP, deoxyguanosine triphosphate; dTTP, deoxythymidine triphosphate; dUTP, deoxyuridine triphosphate; GDP, guanosine diphosphate; GTP, guanosine triphosphate; UDP, uridine diphosphate.

A potentially important consequence of HU action is the acceleration of the loss of extrachromosomally amplified genes that are present in double-minute chromosomes.[45] Evidence indicates that such acentric extrachromosomal elements are common in the gene amplification process. Exposure to HU at clinically achievable concentrations leads to enhanced loss of both amplified oncogenes and drug-resistance genes.[46] Strategies for use of this phenomenon clinically are under consideration.

MECHANISMS OF CELLULAR RESISTANCE

The principal mechanism by which cells achieve resistance to HU is elevation in cellular RR activity. As previously noted, the cellular levels of the M-1 subunit do not change during the cell cycle, whereas levels of the M-2 catalytic subunit increase during DNA synthesis. The site of action of HU specifically involves the M-2 subunit, and the increased RR activity seen in resistant cells is principally the result of overexpression of this protein.[47] Transfection of the human M-2 gene into drug-sensitive KB cells confers resistance by increasing the enzyme activity, and subsequently the dNTP intracellular pools.[48] Transfection of the M-1 gene does not result in a decreased sensitivity to HU, although transfected cells resist dNTP inhibition of RR activity, probably because of an alteration of the function of effector binding sites. Several different molecular mechanisms can contribute to the increased RR activity in HU-resistant cells. A number of cell lines have amplifications of the gene coding for M-2 protein accompanied by an elevation in M-2 messenger RNA and M-2 protein levels.[49] It also seems that posttranscriptional modifications, such as an increase in initiation factor 4E, can occur during drug selection, which results in an increased translational efficiency. An increase in M-2 protein biosynthetic rate can then occur with no further increase in messenger RNA levels.[50]

In most studies, HU resistance has been associated with parallel decreased sensitivity to other RR inhibitors and often to other antimetabolites.[51] Interestingly, some inhibitors of the M-2 subunit, including the new compound Triapine (3-aminopyridine-2-carboxaldehyde thiosemicarbazone, or 3-AP), retain their antitumor effect in HU-resistant cell lines.[5] In addition, some of these cell lines with increased RR activity display an increased sensitivity to nucleotide analogs such as 6-thioguanine (via increased conversion to the deoxynucleotide and enhancement of its incorporation into DNA)[52] or gemcitabine (via increased drug uptake by the cells).[53]

DRUG INTERACTIONS

HU has been studied both in the laboratory and in the clinic as a modulator of cytosine arabinoside (AraC)

metabolism and cytotoxicity. It causes a significant increase in formation of arabinosylcytosine triphosphate and AraC incorporation into DNA[54] in HU-treated cells. The assumption was that this was the result of the decreased pools of the competitor, deoxycytidine triphosphate, expected after HU exposure. In some cell lines, deoxycytidine levels fall as well, increasing AraC conversion to ara-CMP.[54] The phosphorylation of nucleoside analogs such as gemcitabine, fludarabine, and cladribine also increases in the presence of HU. No randomized clinical trial has purely assessed the contribution of HU to combination therapy with AraC. A controlled phase 3 trial, however, has shown the superiority of interferon-α and HU plus AraC over interferon-α and HU in patients with newly diagnosed CML.[55] HU also has been shown to increase the toxicity of fludarabine in a small clinical pilot study.

The major clinical interest in HU in the treatment of solid tumors has been in combination with 5-fluorouracil. Synergy has been demonstrated in experimental tumor models, presumably based on the ability of HU to lower cellular pools of deoxyuridine monophosphate, the competitive substrate for inhibition of thymidylate synthase by 5-fluorodeoxyuridylate.[56] A number of clinical trials of this combination have been performed, but its role remains uncertain. These two G_1-S arresting agents, 5-fluorouracil and HU, have been shown in vitro to interfere with the cytotoxic effects of antimitotic agents (vinblastine sulfate, colchicine, nocodazole) that produce mitotic arrest and apoptosis.[57] The antimetabolites perturb the ability of the antimitotic drugs to induce bcl-2 phosphorylation and c-raf-1 activation, and to increase the p21$^{WAF1/CIP1}$ protein levels, and prevents the majority of cells from progressing to the G_2-M phase.

HU has been evaluated in both clinical and laboratory studies in combination with chemotherapy agents that produce DNA damage, such as alkylating agents, cisplatin, and inhibitors of topoisomerase II.[56] Although synergy has been observed in preclinical testing, the clinical role for such combinations remains speculative. Synchronization in the G_1-S phase drives cells to a condition of increased sensitivity to radiation. Besides, HU exerts a radiosensitizing action through other mechanisms because it selectively kills cells in the S phase of the cell cycle and significantly affects DNA repair mechanisms after radiation damage.

CLINICAL PHARMACOLOGY

HU is generally administered orally, and doses are titrated in response to changes in peripheral white blood cell counts. Although significant interpatient variability is observed, peak concentrations of 0.1 to 2.0 mmol/L are achieved 1.0 to 1.5 hours after doses of 15 to 80 mg/kg.[58] Oral bioavailability is excellent (80 to 100%), and comparable plasma concentrations are seen after oral and intravenous dosing.[58-61] (Table 10.3) After attainment of peak plasma concentrations, HU disappears rapidly from plasma. The elimination half-life ranges from 3.5 to 4.5 hours.[60] Data available from a comprehensive population pharmacokinetic study of multiple oral and intravenous dosing are best described by a one-compartment model with parallel Michaelis-Menten metabolism and first-order renal excretion.[60,61] Renal clearance at standard doses is 60 to 90 mL/minute in an average patient, and pharmacokinetics are nonlinear with dose. The volume of distribution is described by the formula 0.186 (body weight) + 25.4 L. Other studies using a unique dose level (1,000 or 2,000 mg daily) described a correct fit by a one- or two-compartment linear model.[58]

Several high-dose 24- to 120-hour continuous-infusion regimens for HU administration, with or without initial loading, have been evaluated.[66,67] Continuous infusion of 1 g/hr for 24 hours is capable of sustaining plasma concentrations in excess of 1 mmol/L. Doses of 0.5 g/m² per day were tolerated for 12 weeks, 1 g/m² per day was tolerated for 5 weeks, 1.66 g/m² per day was tolerated for 3 weeks, and 2.5 g/m² per day was tolerated for 1 week.[68] Based on the available data, from the standpoint of pharmacokinetics and bioavailability, administering HU parenterally has

no clear advantages, except in those patients with impaired gastrointestinal function.

Although precise guidelines are not available, the prudent course is to modify dosages for patients with abnormal renal function until individual tolerance can be assessed. Unfortunately, pharmacokinetic studies of patients with altered renal function have not been performed to provide guidelines. The full extent and significance of HU metabolism in humans has not been established. Data from several experimental animal systems suggest that the metabolism of HU does occur, but none of these conversions has been demonstrated conclusively in humans. HU is degraded by urease, an enzyme found in intestinal bacteria.[69] Hydroxylamine (NH_2OH), a product of this reaction, has not been identified in humans. Acetohydroxamic acid is found in the plasma of patients receiving HU therapy,[70] however, and may represent the product of a reaction between hydroxylamine and acetylcoenzyme A, a major thioester in mammalian tissues. The conversion of HU to urea in mice has also been reported.[71] An enzyme system capable of this conversion is found in mouse liver, with the greatest activity localized in the mitochondrial subcellular fraction. Similar activity has not been demonstrated in human liver.

HU distributes rapidly to tissues. Studies using radiolabeled HU in rats and mice demonstrate that the drug is

TABLE 10.3
SUMMARY OF PHARMACOKINETIC PARAMETERS OF HYDROXYUREA

Study	Dose	Route	N	PK Model	F (%)	$t_{1/2}$ (hr)	V_d (L/kg)	C_{max}, C_{min} (mmol/L)	Clearance
Tracewell et al.[62]	1,520 mg/m² q6hr 84–315 mg/m² (48–72 hr infants)	PO, IV	8 46	Nonlinear[a]	79.2	1.6–4.2[b]	0.186 × body weight (kg) + 25.4		CL_R = 90.8 mL/min CL_{NR}
									v_{max} = 97 μmol/L/hr K_m = 0.32 mmol/L
Veale et al.[63]	1,000 mg/hr q6hr 1,000 mg/hr (48 hr infants)	PO IV	9 9					$C_{ss,av}$ = 1.730 $C_{max,ss}$ = 2 $C_{min,ss}$ = 1 $C_{ss,av}$ = 0.045	CL = 126.8 mL/min
Villani et al.[64]	500 mg q12hr	PO	9	Linear One-compartment		2.5		$C_{max,ss}$ = 0.135 $C_{min,ss}$ = 0.0085	CL/F = 0.18 L/kg/hr
Rodriguez et al.[65]	2,000 mg	PO and IV	29	Linear Two-compartment	108	3.32 3.39	Vss = 19.71 mg/m2		CL/F = 124 mL/min CL = 106 mL/min

[a]One-compartment pharmacokinetic model with parallel Michaelis-Menten metabolism and first-order renal excretion.
[b]$t_{1/2}$ was concentration-dependent (nonlinear pharmacokinetics).
C_{max}, maximum plasma concentration; $C_{max,ss}$, maximum plasma concentration at steady state; C_{min}, minimum plasma concentration; $C_{min,ss}$, minimum plasma concentration at steady state; $C_{ss,av}$, average steady-state plasma concentration; CL, clearance; CL_R, renal clearance; CL_{NR}, nonrenal clearance; F, bioavailability; K_m, binding affinity; N, number of patients; PK, pharmacokinetic; $t_{1/2}$, half-life; V_d, volume of distribution; v_{max}, maximum volume; V_{ss}, steady-state volume.

found in body tissues in quantities proportional to weight 30 to 60 minutes after injection.[72] The drug readily enters cerebrospinal fluid and third-space collections of fluid such as ascites or pleural effusions. Ratios for simultaneous plasma and cerebrospinal fluid concentrations of 4:1 to 9:1 and for plasma and ascites concentrations of 2:1 to 7.5:1 have been observed.[73] The significance of these ratios is uncertain because they were single points taken at arbitrary times after drug administration, and the time course of disappearance from these extravascular sites was not evaluated.

TOXICITY

The dose-limiting toxicity of HU is myelosuppression.[61,66] This is the direct result of inhibition of DNA synthesis in bone marrow, and megaloblastic changes can be detected in granulocyte and erythroid precursors within 48 hours of the first dose. In patients with nonhematologic malignancies, the peripheral white blood cell count begins to fall in 2 to 5 days. Patients with leukemia or myeloproliferative syndromes have a more rapid fall in white blood cell counts. The rapidity of the effect on the circulating leukemia cell population and the brief duration of its action have been the basis for the use of HU in patients with acute myelogenous leukemia who present with markedly elevated peripheral blood blast counts, or in patients with dangerously elevated platelet counts, as in cases of essential thrombocythemia. Whether this provides an advantage over the prompt institution of standard AraC–containing leukemia therapy has not been demonstrated conclusively.

All patients on dosages of 80 mg/kg per day become leukopenic within 14 days, whereas the incidence is 70% for patients receiving half that dose. Intermittent dosing with the higher doses decreases the hematologic toxicity, but the impact on therapeutic effect has not been fully evaluated. Reversal of the HU effect on peripheral white blood cell counts occurs rapidly, but the nadir in platelet count may occur 7 to 10 days later. Treatment of the myeloproliferative syndromes usually begins with much lower dosages of 0.5 to 2.0 g/day, which are titrated to the clinical response.

The gastrointestinal side effects of nausea, vomiting, anorexia, and either diarrhea or constipation rarely require discontinuation of therapy at the dosages that are commonly used clinically. Oral mucositis and ulceration of the gastrointestinal tract are less common, but may be higher in patients receiving concomitant radiation and HU than in those receiving either therapy alone.

Patients who have taken HU for an extended period may develop one of several dermatologic changes, including hyperpigmentation, erythema of the face and hands, a more diffuse maculopapular rash, or dry skin with atrophy.[74] Changes in the nails may include atrophy or the formation of multiple pigmented nail bands. More severe skin reactions include an ulcerative dermatitis resembling lichen planus.[75] Skin ulcerations, usually on the legs, may occur in patients undergoing long-term treatment for myeloproliferative diseases.[76] Healing or improvement of these ulcers requires cessation of treatment. Topical GM-CSF reportedly accelerates healing.[77] When concomitant radiation therapy is given, patients receiving HU seem to have an increased tissue reaction and may have a recurrence or "recall" of erythema or hyperpigmentation in previously irradiated areas.[78] Alopecia has been seen rarely.

A number of other, less frequent, drug-related effects have been either reported anecdotally or mentioned briefly in the clinical studies already discussed. Transient abnormalities of renal function have been noted in a number of studies, and include elevations of serum urea nitrogen and creatinine, proteinuria, and an active urine sediment. Renal failure or severe, prolonged periods of kidney dysfunction have not been reported. Liver function test abnormalities, on the other hand, have been more significant, and occasionally the patient has progressed to clinical jaundice. A more typical pattern has been transient elevation of hepatocellular enzymes.[79] Headache, drowsiness, confusion, and dizziness also have been reported but are of uncertain significance. The frequency of sensorial neuropathy, rarely seen with single-agent HU therapy, is significant in regimens combining HU with didanosine, stavudine, or both.[80] Several cases of acute interstitial lung disease and alveolitis have been reported.[81] Drug-induced fever has also been noted.[82]

Because of the mechanism of action of HU, of particular concern are the effects on growth and development and its mutagenic potential (teratogenic and carcinogenic), especially in patients with nonmalignant diseases, who frequently need long-term drug administration. Although the number of studies is limited and the median follow-up is short, no growth failures or chronic organ damage has been observed in children with sickle cell disease who are treated with HU. A single study has demonstrated an increased incidence of chromosomal abnormalities in patients treated with HU.[83] HU treatment, especially when HU is combined with other agents, is associated with an incidence of leukemia of 3 to 12% in patients with myeloproliferative syndromes. This risk is possibly higher than in patients not treated with cytotoxic drugs and appears to be proportional to the intrinsic leukemogenic risk of the underlying condition (higher in polycythemia vera [PV] than in essential thrombocythemia [ET]). To date, no secondary leukemia has occurred in patients with sickle cell disease who have been treated with HU.[23]

Because of the limited available data, HU should be considered to have uncertain carcinogen potential and should be used with caution to treat nonmalignant diseases. HU is a potent teratogen in all animal species tested so far, and qualifies as a universal teratogen; it should not be used in women of childbearing age unless the possibility of pregnancy can be excluded. However, a number of patients who conceived while receiving HU for a variety of hematologic conditions completed normal pregnancies after discontinuation of the drug.[84] The reader is referred to Chapter 4 ("Infertility after Cancer Chemotherapy") and Chapter 5 ("Carcinogenesis of Anticancer Drugs") for further discussion of these side effects.

REFERENCES

1. Dresler WFC, Stein R. Uber den Hydroxylharnstoff. Justus Liebigs Ann. Chemie 150:242–252, 1869.
2. Rosenthal F, Wislicki L, Koller L. Uber die Beziehungen von schwersten Blutgiften zu Abbauprodukten des Eiweisses: ein Beitrag zum Entstehungmechanismus der pernizosen Anemie. Klin Wochenschr 1928;7:972–977.
3. Tarnowski GS, Stock CC. Chemotherapy studies on the RC and S790 mouse mammary carcinomas. Cancer Res 1958;18:201.
4. Stearns B, Losee KA, Bernstein J. Hydroxyurea: a new type of potential antitumor agent. J Med Chem 1963;6:1–45.
5. Finch RA, Liu MC, Cory AH, et al. Triapine (3-aminopyridine-2-carboxaldehyde thiosemicarbazone; 3-AP): an inhibitor of ribonucleotide reductase with antineoplastic activity. Adv Enzyme Regul 1999;39:3–12.
6. Yakar D, Holland JF, Ellison RR, et al. Clinical pharmacological trial of guanazole. Cancer Res 1973;33:972–975.
7. Kennedy BJ, Yarbro JW. Metabolic and therapeutic effects of hydroxyurea in chronic myelogenous leukemia. JAMA 1966;195:1038–1043.
8. Frutchman SM, Mack K, Kaplan ME, et al. From efficacy to safety: a Polycythemia Vera Study Group Report on hydroxyurea in patients with polycythemia vera. Semin Hematol 1997;34:17–23.
9. Cortelazzo S, Finazzi G, Ruggieri M, et al. Hydroxyurea for patients with essential thrombocythemia and a high risk of thrombosis. N Engl J Med 1995;332:1126–1136.
10. Hehlmann R, Heimpel H, Hasford J, et al. Randomized comparison of busulfan and hydroxyurea in chronic myelogenous leukemia: prolongation of survival by hydroxyurea. The German CML Study Group. Blood 1993;82:4064–4077.
11. Ohnishi K, Ohno R, Tomonaga M, et al. A randomized trial comparing interferon-α with busulfan for newly diagnosed chronic myelogenous leukemia in chronic phase. Blood 1995;86:906–916.
12. Silver RT, Woolf SH, Hehlmann R, et al. An evidence-based analysis of the effect of busulfan, hydroxyurea, interferon and allogenic bone marrow transplantation in treating the chronic phase of chronic myeloid leukemia: developed for the American Society of Hematology. Blood 1999;94:1517–1536.
13. Lofvenberg E, Nordenson I, Wahlin A. Cytogenetic abnormalities and leukemia transformation in hydroxyurea- treated patients with Philadelphia chromosome negative myeloproliferative disease. Cancer Genet Cytogenet 1990; 49:57–67.
14. Murphy S, Peterson P, Iland H, et al. Experience of the Polycythemia Vera Study Group with essential thrombocythemia: a final report on diagnostic criteria, survival, and leukemic transition to treatment. Semin Hematol 1997;34:29–39.
15. Brockman RW, Shaddix S, Laster WR Jr, et al. Inhibition of ribonucleotide reductase, DNA synthesis, and L1210 leukemia by guanazole. Cancer Res 1970;30:2358–2368.
16. Fibach E, Burke KP, Schechter AN, et al. Hydroxyurea increases fetal hemoglobin in cultured erythroid cells derived from normal individuals and patients with sickle cell anemia or beta-thalassemia. Blood 1993;81:1630–1635.
17. Galanello R, Stamatoyannopoulos G, Papayannopoulou T. Mechanism of Hb F stimulation by S-stage compounds: in vitro studies with bone marrow cells exposed to 5-azacytidine, ARA-C, or hydroxyurea. J Clin Invest 1988;81:1209–1216.
18. Cokic VP, Smith RD, Beleslin-Cokic BB, et al. Hydroxyurea induces fetal hemoglobin by the nitric oxide-dependent activation of soluble guanylyl cyclase. J Clin Invest. 2003;111(2):231–9.
19. Adragna NC, Fonseca P, Lauf PK. Hydroxyurea affects cell morphology, cation transport, and red blood cell adhesion in cultured vascular endothelial cells. Blood 1994;83:533–560.
20. Charache S, Barton FB, Moore RD, et al. Hydroxyurea and sickle cell anemia: clinical utility of a myelosuppressive "switching agent." Medicine 1996;75:300–326.
21. Charache S, Terrin ML, Moore RD, et al. Effect of hydroxyurea on the frequency of painful crises in sickle cell anemia. N Engl J Med 1995;332:1317–1322.
22. Kinney TR, Helms RW, O'Branski EE, et al. Safety of hydroxyurea in children with sickle cell anemia: results of the HUG-KIDS study, a phase I/II trial. Blood 1999;94:1550–1554.
23. Voskaridou E, Kalotychou V, Loukopoulos D. Clinical and laboratory effects of long-term administration of hydroxyurea to patients with sickle cell/β-thalassemia. Br J Hematol 1995; 89:479–484.
24. Steinberg MH. Management of sickle cell disease. N Engl J Med 1999;340:1021–1030.
25. Lori F. Hydroxyurea and HIV: 5 years later—from antiviral to immune-modulation effects. AIDS 1999;13:1433–1442.
26. Lori F, Malykh AG, Foli A. Combination of a drug targeting the cell with a drug targeting the virus controls human immunodeficiency virus type I resistance. AIDS Res Hum Retroviruses 1997;13:1403–1409.
27. Thelander L, Reichard P. Reduction of ribonucleotides. Annu Rev Biochem 1979;48:133–158.
28. Elford HL. Effect of hydroxyurea on ribonucleotide reductase. Biochem Biophys Res Commun 1968;33:129–135.
29. Nicander B, Reichard P. Relations between synthesis of deoxyribonucleotides and DNA replication in 3T6 fibroblasts. J Biol Chem 1986;260:5376–5381.
30. Thelander L, Eriksson S, Akerman M. Ribonucleotide reductase from calf thymus. J Biol Chem 1980;255:7426–7432.
31. Eriksson S, Thelander L, Akerman M. Allosteric regulation of calf thymus ribonucleotide diphosphate reductase. Biochemistry 1979;18:2948–2952.
32. Cory JG, Fleischer AE, Munro JB III. Reconstitution of the ribonucleotide reductase in mammalian cells. J Biol Chem 1978; 253:2898–2901.
33. Mann GJ, Musgrove EA, Fox RM, et al. Ribonucleotide reductase M1 subunit in cellular proliferation, quiescence, and differentiation. Cancer Res 1988;48:5151–5156.
34. Graslund A, Ehrenberg A, Thelander L. Characterization of the free radical of mammalian ribonucleotide reductase. J Biol Chem 1982;257:5711–5715.
35. Thelander M, Graslund A, Thelander L. Subunit M2 of mammalian ribonucleotide reductase. J Biol Chem 1985; 260:2737–2741.
36. Engstrom Y, Eriksson S, Jildevik I, et al. Cell cycle-dependent expression of mammalian ribonucleotide reductase. J Biol Chem 1985;260:9114–9116.
37. Nyholm S, Thelander L, Graslund A. Reduction and loss of the iron center in the reaction of the small subunit of mouse ribonucleotide reductase with hydroxyurea. Biochemistry 1993;32: 11569–11574.
38. Satyamoorthy K, Chitnis M, Basrur V. Sensitization of P388 murine leukemia cells to hydroxyurea cytotoxicity by hydrophobic iron-chelating agents. Anticancer Res 1986;6:329–333.
39. Ford SS, Shackney SE. Lethal and sublethal effects of hydroxyurea in relation to drug concentration duration of drug exposure in sarcoma 180 in vitro. Cancer Res 1977;37:2628–2637.
40. Moran RE, Straus MJ. Cytokinetic analysis of L1210 leukemia after continuous infusion of hydroxyurea in vivo. Cancer Res 1979;39:1616–1622.
41. Cress AE, Gerner EW. Hydroxyurea inhibits ODC induction, but not the G_1 to S-phase transition. Biochem Biophys Res Commun 1979;87:773–780.
42. Jiang R, Zhang JL, Satoh Y, Sairenji T. Mechanism for induction of hydroxyurea resistance and loss of latent EBV genome in hydroxyurea-treated Burkitt's lymphoma cell line Raji. J Med Virol. 2004; 73(4):589–595.
43. Reddy GP, Pardee AB. Inhibitor evidence for allosteric interaction in the replitase multienzyme complex. Nature 1983;304: 114–120.

44. Plucinski TM, Fager RS, Reddy GP. Allosteric interaction of components of the replitase complex is responsible for enzyme cross-inhibition. Mol Pharmacol 1990;38:86–88.

45. Von Hoff DD, Waddelow T, Forseth B, et al. Hydroxyurea accelerates loss of extrachromosomally amplified genes from tumor cells. Cancer Res 1991;51:6273–6279.

46. Nevaldine BH, Rizwana R, Hahn PJ. Differential sensitivity of double minute chromosomes to hydroxyurea treatment in cultured methotrexate-resistant mouse cells. Mutation Res 1999;406:55–62.

47. McClarty GA, Tonin PN, Srinivasan PR, et al. Relationships between reversion of hydroxyurea resistance in hamster cells and the coamplification of ribonucleotide reductase M2 component, ornithine decarboxylase and P5-8 genes. Biochem Biophys Res Commun 1988;154:975–981.

48. Zhou BS, Hsu NY, Pan BC, et al. Overexpression of ribonucleotide reductase in transfected human KB cells increases their resistance to hydroxyurea: M2 but not M1 is sufficient to increase resistance to hydroxyurea in transfected cells. Cancer Res 1995;55:1328–1333.

49. Choy BK, McClarty GA, Chan AK, et al. Molecular mechanisms of drug resistance involving ribonucleotide reductase: hydroxyurea resistance in a series of clonally related mouse cell lines selected in the presence of increasing drug concentrations. Cancer Res 1988;48:7524–7531.

50. Abid MR, Li Y, Anthony C, et al. Translational regulation of ribonucleotide reductase by eukaryotic initiation factor 4E protein synthesis to the control of DNA replication. J Biol Chem 1999;274:35991–35998.

51. Wong SJ, Myette M, Wereley JP, et al. Increased sensitivity of hydroxyurea-resistant leukemic cells to gemcitabine. Clin Cancer Res 1999;5:439–453.

52. Yen Y, Grill SP, Dutschman GE, et al. Characterization of a hydroxyurea-resistant human KB cell line with supersensitivity to 6-thioguanine. Cancer Res 1994;54:3689–3691.

53. Kubota M, Takimoto T, Tanizawa A, et al. Differential modulation of 1-β-D-arabinofuranosylcytosine metabolism by hydroxyurea in human leukemic cell lines. Biochem Pharmacol 1988;37:1745–1749.

54. Robichaud NJ, Fram RJ. Potentiation of ara-C induced cytotoxicity by hydroxyurea in LoVo colon carcinoma cells. Biochem Pharmacol 1987;36:1673–1677.

55. Guilhot F, Chastang C, Michallet M, et al. Interferon alfa-2b combined with cytarabine versus interferon alone in chronic myelogenous leukemia. N Engl J Med 1997; 337:223–229.

56. Schilsky RL, Ratain MJ, Vokes EE, et al. Laboratory and clinical studies of biochemical modulation by hydroxyurea. Semin Oncol 1992;19:84–89.

57. Johnson KR, Young KK, Fan W. Antagonistic interplay between antimitotic and G_1-S arresting agents observed in experimental combination therapy. Clin Cancer Res 1999;5:2559–2565.

58. Villani P, Maserati R, Regazzi MB, et al. Pharmacokinetics of hydroxyurea in patients infected with human immunodeficiency virus type I. J Clin Pharmacol 1996;36:117–121.

59. Creasey WA, Capizzi RL, DeConti RC. Clinical and biochemical studies of high-dose intermittent therapy of solid tumors with hydroxyurea. Cancer Chemother Rep 1970;54:191–194.

60. Tracewell WG, Trump DL, Vaughan WP, et al. Population pharmacokinetics of hydroxyurea in cancer patients. Cancer Chemother Pharmacol 1995;35:417–422.

61. Belt RJ, Haas CD, Kennedy J, et al. Studies of hydroxyurea administered by continuous infusion. Cancer 1980;46:455–462.

62. Veale D, Cantwell BM, Kerr N, et al. Phase I study of high-dose hydroxyurea in lung cancer. Cancer Chemother Pharmacol 1988;1:53–56.

63. Rodriguez GI, Kuhn JG, Weiss GR, et al. A bioavailability and pharmacokinetic study of oral and intravenous hydroxyurea. Blood 1998;91:1533–1541.

64. Smith DC, Vaughan WP, Gwilt PR, et al. A phase I trial of high-dose continuous infusion hydroxyurea. Cancer Chemother Pharmacol 1993;33:139–143.

65. Blumenreich MS, Kellihan MJ, Joseph UG, et al. Long-term intravenous hydroxyurea infusions in patients with advanced cancer: a phase I trial. Cancer 1993;71:2828–2832.

66. Fishbein WN, Carbone PP. Hydroxyurea: mechanism of action. Science 1963;142:1069–1070.

67. Adamson RH, Ague SL, Hess SM, et al. The distribution, excretion, and metabolism of hydroxyurea-[14]C. J Pharmacol Exp Ther 1965;150:322–334.

68. Colvin M, Bono VH Jr. The enzymatic reduction of hydroxyurea to urea by mouse liver. Cancer Res 1970; 30:1516–1519.

69. Fishbein WN, Carbone PP, Freireich EJ, et al. Clinical trials of hydroxyurea in patients with cancer and leukemia. Clin Pharmacol Ther 1964;5:574–580.

70. Lerner JH, Beckloff GL. Hydroxyurea administered intermittently. JAMA 1965;192:1168–1170.

71. Kennedy BJ, Smith LR, Goltz RW. Skin changes secondary to hydroxyurea. Arch Dermatol 1975;111:183–187.

72. Renfro L, Kamino H, Raphael B, et al. Ulcerative lichen planus-like dermatitis associated with hydroxyurea. J Am Acad Dermatol 1991;24:143–145.

73. Sirieix ME, Debure C, Baudot N, et al. Leg ulcers and hydroxyurea: forty-one cases. Arch Dermatol 1999;135:818–820.

74. Stagno F, Guglielmo P, Consoli U, et al. Successful healing of hydroxyurea-related leg ulcers with topical granulocyte- macrophage colony-stimulating factor. Blood 1999; 94:1479–1480.

75. Sears ME. Erythema in areas of previous irradiation in patients treated with hydroxyurea. Cancer Chemother Rep 1965;40:31–32.

76. Heddle R, Calvert AF. Hydroxyurea-induced hepatitis. Med J Aust 1980;1:121.

77. Moore RD, Wong WM, Keruly JC, et al. Incidence of neuropathy in HIV-infected patients on monotherapy versus those on combination therapy with didanosine stavudine and hydroxyurea. AIDS 2000;14:273–278.

78. Kavuru MS, Gadsden T, Lichtin A, et al. Hydroxyurea-induced acute interstitial lung disease. South Med J 1994;87:767–769.

79. Cheung AYC, Browne B, Capen C. Hydroxyurea-induced fever in cervical carcinoma: case report anTd review of the literature. Cancer Invest 1999;17:245–248.

80. Kaung DT, Swartzendruber AA. Effect of chemotherapeutic agents in chromosomes of patients with lung cancer. Dis Chest 1969;55:98–100.

81. Diav-Citrin O, Hunnisett L, Sher G, et al. Hydroxyurea use during pregnancy: a case report in sickle cell disease and review of the literature. Am J Hematol 1999;60:148–150.

Antimicrotubule Agents

11

Eric K. Rowinsky

Microtubules are highly strategic subcellular targets of anticancer therapies, and antimicrotubule agents are mainstay constituents of both curative and palliative therapeutic regimens. Over the last several decades, an increasing number of structurally complex, naturally occurring alkaloids or synthetic compounds that disrupt microtubules have also been identified.[1-5] The natural product antimicrotubule agents have wide chemical diversity, and it is notable from an evolutionary standpoint that the microtubule seems to be a preferred, self-protective target of many marine and plant species alike. These organisms produce highly potent, structurally diverse compounds that are capable of binding to nearly identical sites on microtubules and induce almost identical actions. Despite their early promise and diversity, only two antimicrotubule agents, vincristine (VCR) and vinblastine (VBL), were widely used until the late 1980s. However, the identification of other classes of antimicrotubule agents with novel mechanisms of cytotoxic action and spectra of antitumor activity, such as the taxanes, epothilones, semisynthetic vinca analogs, and estramustine phosphate, has resulted in a resurgence of interest in the microtubule as an important target in cancer chemotherapy.

MICROTUBULE STRUCTURE

Microtubules are composed of molecules of tubulin, each of which is a heterodimer consisting of two tightly linked, closely related globular polypeptide subunits.[1-5] These protein subunits, α-tubulin and β-tubulin, each consist of approximately 450 amino acids with a molecular weight of 50,000 daltons and are encoded by small families of related genes.[1,2,4,6,7] When tubulin molecules assemble into microtubules, they form linear "protofilaments" with the dimers aligned side by side around a hollow central core, and the β subunit of one dimer in contact with the α-tubulin subunit of the next, as shown in Figure 11.1. The

protofilaments are aligned in parallel with the same "polarity," that is, one end, termed the plus end, at which assembly is rapid and one end, termed the minus end, at which growth is slow or net disassembly occurs. A third, less abundant, member of the tubulin superfamily, γ-tubulin, comprises the microtubule-organizing center (MTOC) or centrosome.[8]

The functional diversity of microtubules is achieved through the binding of various regulatory proteins such as microtubule-associated proteins (MAPs), expression of various tubulin isotopes, and post-translational modifications of tubulin. There are at least six isotypes of α-tubulin and seven isotypes of β-tubulin, which are distinguished by slightly different amino acid sequences, encoded by different genes, and expressed at varying degrees in different cells and tissues.[9,10] Nevertheless, they are similar proteins from a functional standpoint and copolymerize in vitro.[9,10] The intrinsic dynamicity of microtubules is also influenced by the isotypic composition of tubulin, and the sensitivity of microtubules to both microtubule depolymerizing and polymerizing agents relates, in part, to the composition of both tubulin isotypes, post-translation modifications on tubulin, and MAPs.[10-12] Both α-tubulin and β-tubulin can be modified post-translationally by acetylation, detyrosination/tyrosination, and removal of the penultimate glutamic-acid residue of α-tubulin, which occur only on microtubule polymers, modify the behavior and stability of microtubules, and account, in part, for the distinct functional differences of microtubules in various tissues.[9,13] The C-terminal amino acid sequence of β-tubulin is the most variable in terms of both amino acid composition and post-translational modifications, which may also partially account for tissue-dependent functional diversity. Modified regions of polymerized tubulin provide sites for the binding of MAPs, which regulate the dynamic behavior and stability of cytoplasmic microtubules.[12] The major classes of MAPs, which can be isolated with microtubules from tubulin-rich brain tissue, include tau (molecular weights, 40,000 to 60,000 daltons) and

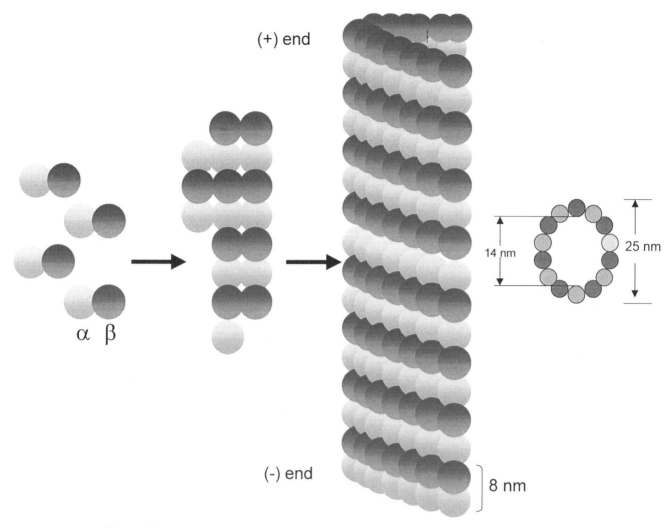

Figure 11.1 Heterdimers of α-tubulin and β-tubulin assemble to form a short microtubule nucleus. Nucleation is followed by elongation of the microtubule at both ends to form a cylinder that is composed of tubulin heterodimers arranged head-to-tail in 13 protofilaments. Each microtubule has an end where net addition of heterodimers takes place, called the plus (+) end, with β-tubulin facing the solvent, and a minus end (–) with α-tubulin facing the solvent.

high-molecular weight (200,000 to 300,000 daltons) proteins whose members include MAP1, MAP1c (an ATPase), MAP2, MAP4, and the motor proteins dynein (a GTPase) and kinesin (an ATPase). Both classes of MAPs have two binding domains, one of which binds to microtubules. Because this domain also binds to free tubulin molecules simultaneously, MAPs facilitate the initial nucleation step of tubulin polymerization. The other domain appears to be involved in linking the microtubule to other cellular components. Some MAPs, such as the dyneins and kinesins, function as microtubule motors, transmitting chemical energy to mechanical sliding force and moving various solutes and subcellular organelles along the microtubule.[1,7,10–12,14] Motor protein function is critical to many types of dynamic cellular processes such as mitosis, premeiosis, and organelle transport. In addition to the MAPs, other regulatory proteins, such as survivin, stathmin, TOG, MCAK, MAP4, EB1, dynactin I, RAC1, and RHIT regulate microtubule function.[7, 12]

MICROTUBULE FUNCTION

Although microtubules are primarily recognized as being principal components of the mitotic spindle apparatus that separates the duplicate set of chromosomes, they also play critical roles in many interphase functions such as maintenance of cell shape and scaffolding, intracellular transport, secretion, neurotransmission, and possibly the relay of signals between cell surface receptors and the nucleus.[15–18] Furthermore, the integrity of microtubule structures is required for cells to pass through various cell cycle checkpoints, and the lack of integrity appears to trigger programmed cell death or apoptosis.[19]

The unique functions of microtubules are related to their polymerization dynamics, which involve an equilibrium between α-β-tubulin heterodimer subunits and the microtubule polymer.[1,2,7,15,16] Tubulin polymerization occurs by a nucleation-elongation mechanism, in which the slow formation of a short microtubule "nucleus" is followed by rapid elongation of the microtubule at its ends by the reversible, noncovalent addition of α-β-tubulin heterodimers (Fig. 11.1). In essence, the microtubule polymer is in a complex and dynamic equilibrium with the intracellular pool of α-β-tubulin heterodimers, which incorporates free heterodimers into the polymerized structure and simultaneously releases heterodimers into the soluble tubulin pool. Microtubule assembly and disassembly occur simultaneously at both ends of the microtubule and these processes are in dynamic equilibrium, the direction of which is determined by several factors, including the concentration of free tubulin and various chemical mediators that promote assembly (e.g., Mg^{2+}, guanosine triphosphate [GTP]) and inhibition of assembly (Ca^{2+}).[12,13 20-23] The assembly process uses energy provided by the hydrolysis of GTP. Tubulin binds GTP with high affinity, and as tubulin-GTP is added to the ends of growing microtubules, GTP is gradually hydrolyzed to guanosine diphosphate (GDP) and P_i. The P_i ultimately dissociates from the microtubule, leaving a microtubule core that consists of tubulin bound to GDP. The GDP nucleotide remains nonexchangeable until the tubulin subunit dissociates from the microtubule. Although tubulin polymerization and dissociation, and consequently microtubule elongation and shortening, occur simultaneously at each end, the net changes in length at the more kinetically dynamic plus end are much larger over time than those at the minus end. If the polymerization reaction is followed in vitro, an initial lag phase is noted, after which microtubules form rapidly until a plateau phase is reached. In the intact cell, microtubules usually grow from a specific nucleating site or the MTOC, which, in most cases, is the centrosome.

Dynamic instability gives rise to a dynamically changing cytoplasm. At any instant, cytoplasmic microtubules are either rapidly growing or catastrophically dissociating. Microtubules undergo long periods of slow lengthening, short periods of rapid shortening, and periods of attenuated dynamics. During rapid polymerization, the high concentration of free tubulin results in net assembly until a plateau phase is reached, at which time a critical concentration of tubulin is attained and the rates of both polymerization and depolymerization are balanced. Two fundamental processes govern microtubule dynamics in vivo. The first, known as *treadmilling*, is the net growth at one end of the microtubule and the net shortening at the opposite end.[21,24] Treadmilling plays a role in many microtubule functions, most notably the polar movement of the chromosomes during the anaphase stage of mitosis. The second dynamic behavior, termed *dynamic instability*, is a process in which the plus ends of individual microtubules switch spontaneously between states of slow sustained growth and rapid shortening.[25,26] The transition between microtubule growth and shortening is regulated, in part, by the presence or absence of the region of GTP-containing-tubulin at the microtubule end. A microtubule can grow as long as it maintains a stabilizing "cap" of tubulin-GTP

or tubulin-GDP-P_i. Once the GTP cap is lost from the plus end, the end loses subunits more rapidly.[27] Depolymerizatin occurs approximately 100-fold faster at a GDP cap than a GTP cap, and therefore, once rapid depolymerization occurs, the GTP cap is difficult to regain. On the other hand, the minus end is bound tightly to the MTOC, which interferes with both assembly and disassembly of the subunits. In essence, the capping process represents an adaptation that results in microtubule stability at the capped end. The rate of dynamic instability is accelerated during some processes, such as mitosis, which results in the formation and attachment of the mitotic spindles to the chromosomes. The rate and magnitude of both dynamic instability and treadmilling are much slower in purified tubulin than in cells, and it is clear that these mechanisms can be altered by MAPs and other regulatory proteins, variable expression of tubulin isotypes, post-translational tubulin modifications, and the expression of tubulin mutations.[2,28]

In the nonmitotic phases of the cell cycle, microtubules radiate from the MTOC, which is located centrally near the nucleus and consists of a centrosome, a lattice of MAPs, γ-tubulin, and a pair of centrioles. The minus ends of the microtubules are positioned in or near the centrosome, whereas the plus ends extend out toward the cell periphery. The centrosome duplicates before mitosis and the two centrosomes then separate into the poles of the forming mitotic spindle. The microtubules of the interphase array depolymerize and, as the nuclear envelope breaks down and releases the now condensed chromosomes, a spindle-shaped array of newly assembled microtubules is organized. In essence, the interphase microtubule network disassembles at the onset of mitosis and is replaced by a new population of spindle microtubules that are much more dynamic than the microtubules that comprise the interphase cytoskeleton.[28-30] In most cells, mitosis progresses rapidly and the highly dynamic microtubules that comprise the mitotic spindle render them sensitive to the vinca alkaloids, taxanes, and other antimicrotubule agents.[2,29-31]

Dynamic instability and treadmilling are vital to the assembly and function of the mitotic spindle, and the high dynamaticity of mitotic spindle microtubules is required for the precise alignment of the chromosomes and their attachment to the spindle during metaphase, as well as chromosome separation during anaphase. These processes enable microtubules, which emanate from each of the two spindle poles to make vast growing and shortening excursions, essentially probing the cytoplasm, until they become attached to a chromosome at the kinetochore. Attachment of the plus end of the microtubules to the kinetochore of the chromosomes selectively "caps" or stabilizes this end of the mitotic spindle microtubules that emanate from the centrosomes. If even a single chromosome is unable to achieve a bipolar attachment to the spindle, perhaps from drug-induced suppression of microtubule dynamics, the cell will not traverse beyond aprometaphase/metaphase-like state, which eventually triggers apoptosis. Although mitotic spindles form in the presence of low concentrations of antimicrotubule agents, mitosis cannot progress beyond the mitotic cell cycle checkpoint at the metaphase/anaphase transition or is delayed in this stage.[27,31] Such perturbations in mitotic spindle dynamics may delay cell cycle progression at critical mitotic checkpoints, ultimately triggering apoptosis.[19,28-31] In the unperturbed normal state, oscillations of the duplicated chromosomes, dynamic instability, and microtubule treadmilling, in which there is addition of tubulin to the spindle at the kinetochore and loss of tubulin at the spindle poles, exert considerable tension on the chromosomes in metaphase.[22] Both tension and oscillations are required for the proper function of the mitotic spindle and progression from metaphase to anaphase. In the next mitotic stage, anaphase, microtubules that are attached to the chromosomes undergo shortening, while another subpopulation of microtubules called interpolar microtubules lengthen, resulting in polar movement of the chromosomes. Suppression of spindle-microtubule treadmilling and dynamic instability by antimicrotubule agents reduce spindle tension and impedes progression from metaphase to anaphase, triggering cell death.[19,28-30,32]

VINCA ALKALOIDS

The vinca alkaloids are naturally occurring or semisynthetic nitrogenous bases that are present in minute quantities in the pink periwinkle plant *Catharanthus roseus* G. Don (formerly *Vinca rosea* Linn). The early medicinal uses of *C. roseus* for controlling hemorrhage, scurvy, toothaches, and diabetes and for the healing of chronic wounds led to the screening of these compounds for their hypoglycemic activity, which turned out to be of little importance compared with their anticancer properties.[33,34] Although many vinca alkaloids have been investigated clinically, only VCR,

VBL, and vinorelbine (VRL) are approved for use in the United States. A third widely studied vinca alkaloid, vindesine (VDS, desacetyl VBL carboxyamide), a semisynthetic derivative and human metabolite of VBL, was introduced in the 1970s. It has been used in combination with other agents, particularly the platinating agents and/or mitomycin C (or both), to treat non–small cell lung cancer, but it is also active in several hematologic and solid malignancies.[17,33-36] Although VDS demonstrated notable activity against several tumor types, particularly non–small cell lung cancer, it has been available only for investigational purposes in the United States and has not demonstrated a unique role in cancer therapeutics. The semisynthetic VBL derivative VRL (5'-norhydro-VBL), which is structurally modified on its catharanthine nucleus, is approved in the United States as either a single agent or in combination with cisplatin to treat non–small cell lung cancer and has been also registered for advanced breast cancer in many other countries.[17,33,35-41] In addition to demonstrating broad antitumor activity as a single agent and the possibility that it is not completely cross-resistant with VCR and VBL, VRL can be administered orally, in contrast to other available vinca alkaloids. The key features of these vinca alkaloids are given in Tables 11.1 and 11.2. Although the clinical development of other vinca alkaloids, such as vinleurosine and vinrosidine, have been abandoned because of unpredictable toxicity, a novel bifluorinated vinca analog, vinflunine, appears to have unique antitumor and toxicologic profiles and has demonstrated impressive activity in bladder and other cancer.[17,33,35-42]

Despite the minor structural differences between VCR and VBL, their antitumor and toxicologic profiles differ vastly. VCR is used more commonly in pediatric oncology than in adults with cancer, most likely owing to the higher level of sensitivity of pediatric malignancies and better tolerance of therapeutic VCR doses in children. VCR is an

TABLE 11.1
KEY FEATURES OF THE VINCA ALKALOIDS

	Vincristine Sulfate	Vinblastine Sulfate	Vindesine Sulfate	Vinorelbine Tartrate
Mechanism of action	Low concentrations inhibit microtubule dynamics (dynamic instability and treadmilling) High concentrations inhibit polymerization of tubulin			
Standard dosage (mg/m^2)	1–1.4 every 3 weeks	6–8 every week	3–4 every 1–2 weeks	15–30 every 1–2 weeks
Pharmacokinetics and disposition	See Table 11.2			
Principal toxicity	Peripheral neuropathy	Neutropenia	Neutropenia	Neutropenia
Other common toxicities	Constipation, SIADH	Thrombocytopenia	Peripheral neuropathy (moderate)	Peripheral neuropathy (moderate)
		Alopecia	Alopecia	Constipation
		Peripheral neuropathy (mild)		Nausea and vomiting
		SIADH		Diarrhea
Precautions	Patients with abnormal liver function should be treated with caution. See section on dosage and schedule for specific dosing guidelines.			

SIADH, syndrome of inappropriate antidiuretic hormone secretion.

TABLE 11.2

PHARMACOKINETIC PARAMETERS OF THE VINCA ALKALOIDS[124_126, 32,134,154]

	Vincristine Sulfate	Vinblastine Sulfate	Vindesine Sulfate	Vinorelbine Tartrate
Standard adult dosage range (mg/m^2/week)	1.0–1.4	6–8	3–4	15–30
Optimal pharmacokinetic model	Triexponential	Triexponential	Triexponential	Triexponential
Elimination half-lives				
α (min)	<5	<5	<5	<5
β (min)	50–155	53–99	55–99	49–168
γ (h)	23–85	20–64	20–24	18–49
Clearance (L/hr/kg)	0.16	0.74	0.25	0.4–1.29
Primary mechanism of disposition	Hepatic metabolism and biliary excretion	Hepatic metabolism and biliary excretion	Hepatic metabolism and biliary excretion	Hepatic metabolism and biliary excretion

essential part of the combination chemotherapeutic regimens used for acute lymphocytic leukemia and plays an important role in the treatment of both Hodgkin's and non-Hodgkin's lymphomas. VCR-based combination regimens, particularly those in which the agent is administered as a protracted infusion or as daily bolus injections in combination with doxorubicin and dexamethasone (known as VAD) and occasionally other agents, are commonly used to treat multiple myeloma.[43] VCR also plays a role in the treatment of Wilms' tumor, Ewing's sarcoma, neuroblastoma, oligodendroglioma, medulloblastoma, and rhabdomyosarcoma in children, and in treating small cell lung cancer in adults.[17] VBL has been an integral component of therapeutic regimens for germ cell malignancies and advanced lymphoma and has been used in combination with other agents to treat Kaposi's sarcoma and bladder, brain, and non–small cell lung and breast cancers.[17,33] In addition to the clinically relevant antitumor activity of VRL in non–small cell and breast cancers, VRL has demonstrated activity in advanced ovarian carcinoma and lymphoma, but a unique role in the treatment of these cancers has not been defined. It has also been reported that VRL as single-agent treatment confers high therapeutic indices to older patients with advanced breast and lung cancers.[38,40]

Structures

The vinca alkaloids have a large dimeric asymmetric structure composed of a dihydroindole nucleus (vindoline), which is the major alkaloid in the periwinkle, linked by a carbon-carbon bond to an indole nucleus (catharanthine), which is found in much lower quantities in the plant (Fig. 11.2). VCR and VBL are structurally identical except for the substituent (R_1) attached to the nitrogen of the vindoline nucleus, where VCR possesses a formyl group and VBL has a methyl group. These small structural differences impart major clinical differences. VBL and VDS differ in two substituents (R_2 and R_3) attached to the

vindoline nucleus, whereas the catharanthine ring of VRL is modified.

Mechanism of Action

The vinca alkaloids induce cytotoxicity by interacting with tubulin.[6, 44-54] However, they are also capable of many other biochemical and biologic actions that may or may not be related to their effects on microtubules, including competition for transport of amino acids into cells;inhibition of purine, RNA, DNA, and protein syntheses;disruption of lipid metabolism;elevation of oxidized glutathione;inhibition of glycolysis;alterations in the release of antidiuretic hormone;inhibition of release of histamine by mast cells and enhanced release of epinephrine;inhibition of calcium-calmodulin–regulated cyclic adenosine monophosphate phosphodiesterase;and disruption in the integrity of the cell membrane and membrane function.[15–17,33,38]

Despite their diverse biologic properties, the cytotoxic activity of the vinca alkaloids is primarily the result of their ability to disrupt microtubules, particularly microtubules comprising the mitotic spindle apparatus. In support of this mechanism of action, there is a strong relationship between cytotoxicity and the dissolution of the mitotic spindle and accumulation of mitotic figures.[47] Furthermore, the accumulation of mitotic figures correlates with both drug concentration and duration of treatment. Although the vinca alkaloids are generally classified as "antimitotics," this mechanism may not be the sole mechanism of cytotoxicity in vivo because they also disrupt interphase microtubules involved in chemotaxis, migration, intracellular transport, movement of organelles, secretory processes, membrane trafficking, and transmission of growth factor signals from the cell surface receptor to the nucleus.[15,17] In addition, the vinca alkaloids disrupt the structural integrity of platelets and other cells, which are rich in tubulin and depend on microtubules for structure.[48] Therefore, the fact that the vinca alkaloids induce morphologic changes and cytotoxicity in

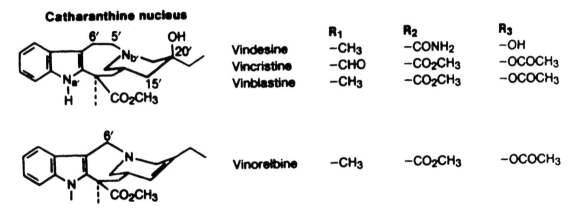

Figure 11.2 Structural modifications of the vindoline nucleus and catharanthine nucleus in various vinca alkaloids. (Reprinted with permission from Rahmani R, Zhou XJ. Pharmacokinetics and metabolism of vinca alkaloids. In: Workman P, Graham MA, eds. Cancer Surveys, Pharmacokinetics and Cancer Chemotherapy, vol 17. Plainview, NY: Cold Spring Harbor Laboratory Press, 1993:269.)

normal and malignant cells in both mitosis and interphase is not surprising.[15,49-51]

The vinca alkaloids bind rapidly, avidly, and reversibly to sites on tubulin (known as the vinca domain), which appear to be the same binding sites for other agents such as the complex plant alkaloid maytansine.[6,33,44,45,53,54] However, the binding sites are distinct from those of the taxanes, GTP and GDP, and the site on the tubulin heterodimer shared by colchicine, podophyllotoxin, steganacin, combretastatin, and many synthetic compounds.[6] Unlike colchicine, the vinca alkaloids bind directly to microtubules without first forming a complex with soluble tubulin, and they do not copolymerize with the tubulin lattice of the microtubule.[3,6,55,56]

The vinca alkaloids bind to microtubules at two binding sites, each with different affinities. These agents bind to tubulin at the microtubule ends with high affinity (K_d, 1 to 2 μmol) and considerably lower affinity (K_d, 0.25 to 0.3 mmol) to tubulin sites located along the sides of the microtubule surface.[3,21] There are approximately 1 to 17 high-affinity binding sites per microtubule located at the ends of each microtubule in bovine brain (from a potential number of 17,000 tubulin dimers per average 10-μm microtubule), whereas the density of the low-affinity, high-capacity binding site is 1.4 to 1.7 sites per heterodimer.[54,57] The binding of the vinca alkaloids to high-affinity sites is responsible for the substoichiometric and

potent suppression of tubulin exchange that occur at low drug concentrations (<1 μmol). At low concentrations, treadmilling is disrupted, but microtubule mass is not affected. Furthermore, low concentrations of the vinca alkaloids perturb dynamic instability in an "end-dependent" fashion. Dynamic instability is strongly enhanced at the minus ends (kinetic destabilization), whereas dynamic instability is inhibited at the plus end. In essence, these actions increase the time that microtubules spend in a state of attenuated activity, neither growing nor shortening, the end result of which is a potent block at the metaphase/anaphase transition in mitosis.[2]

At high stoichiometric concentrations (μmol), these actions are accompanied by microtubule depolymerization as the result of effects on low affinity sites. Binding of the vinca alkaloids to the low affinity sites induces tubulin to self-associate into nonmicrotubule tubulin polymers and ordered aggregates through a self-propagation pathway. Self-propagation occurs as vinca alkaloid binding progressively weakens the lateral interactions between protofilaments, induces conformation changes in tubulin, and exposes new sites. The exposure of new sites further increases the binding affinity of the vinca alkaloids and, in turn, likely results in the formation of vinca alkaloid-tubulin spiral aggregates, protofilaments, and paracrystalline structures, ultimately leading to the disintegration of microtubules. The proposal has been made that MAPs stabilize

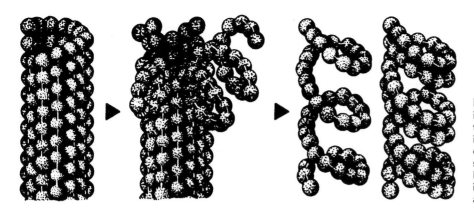

Figure 11.3 Model of the vinca alkaloid-induced disassembly of microtubules containing microtubule-associated protein into spiraled protofilaments composed of one or two spirals. (Reprinted with permission from Donoso JA, Haskins KM, Himes RH. Effect of microtubule proteins on the interaction of vincristine with microtubules and tubulin. Cancer Res 1979;39:1604.)

the longitudinal interactions between dimers in the protofilaments as they splay apart after binding the vinca alkaloid, as illustrated in Figure 11.3.[58]

The vinca alkaloids potently block mitosis at the metaphase/anaphase transition. Following nuclear envelop breakdown, the vinca alkaloids block mitotic spindle formation and reduce the tension at the kinetochores of the chromosomes. Although chromosomes may condense, they remain scattered in the cells. The chromosomes separate along their lengths, but still remain attached at their centromeres.[55,59] Mitotic progress is delayed in a metaphase-like state with chromosomes "stuck" at the spindle poles, unable to move to the spindle equator. The cell-cycle signal to the anaphase-promoting complex, which is required for the cell to transition from metaphase to anaphase is blocked and the cells eventually undergo apoptosis. However, cyclin B concentrations may remain high and cell cycle progression to interphase in the absence of anaphase or cytokinesis may occur, resulting in chromatin decondensation and formation of multilobed nuclei.[55] At low concentration, the vinca alkaloids may induce mitotic arrest, which does not involve microtubule depolymerization. Nevertheless, the disruption of spindle microtubule dynamics without microtubule depolymerization may ultimately lead to apoptosis, which involves the inactivation of antiapoptotic proteins and induction of apoptotic genes (see "Mechanism of Action" and "Mechanism of Resistance" in "Taxanes" section).[19,54] The induction of apoptosis, however, does not depend on the presence of an intact p53 checkpoint;sensitivity of isogenic cell lines differing only in p53 status are the same.[60] The loss of p21, a protein that controls entry into mitosis at the G_2-M checkpoint, enhances sensitivity of tumor cells to both vinca alkaloids and taxanes, possibly by hastening entry of drug-damaged cells into mitosis.[19,61]

The relationships between the inhibitory effects of vinca alkaloids on cell proliferation, mitotic arrest, mitotic spindle disruption, and depolymerization of microtubules have been characterized in a series of elegant studies.[44,62] Although the antiproliferative effects of the vinca alkaloids are noted over a wide range of drug concentrations, the concentration that inhibits cell proliferation is directly related to the concentration that induces metaphase arrest.

The inhibition of proliferation and blockage of cells in metaphase at the lowest effective drug concentrations occur with little or no microtubule depolymerization or disorganization of the mitotic spindle apparatus. With increasing drug concentrations, the organization of microtubules and chromosomes in arrested mitotic spindles deteriorates in a manner that is common to all derivatives. The cumulative body of data indicates that the antiproliferative effects of the vinca alkaloids at their lowest effective concentrations are caused by alterations in the dynamics of tubulin addition and loss at the ends of mitotic spindle microtubules rather than by simple depolymerization of the microtubules. Similar effects have been demonstrated with nocodazole, podophyllotoxin, and the taxanes.[32,62,63]

In addition to their direct cytotoxic effects on tumor cells, the vinca alkaloids, taxanes, and other antimicrotubule agents inhibit angiogenesis with surprising potency. In vitro, 0.1 to 1.0 pmol/L VBL blocked endothelial proliferation, chemotaxis, and spreading on fibronectin, all essential steps in angiogenesis.[64] In combination with antivascular endothelial growth factor receptor antibodies, low doses of VBL significantly augment antitumor activity, even in tumors resistant to direct cytotoxic effects of the drug.[65] In these experiments, the combination of drug and antibody produced early and marked endothelial necrosis and tumor regression. However, the relative contribution of these antiangiogenic effects to the clinical antitumor activity of the vinca alkaloids is unclear.

Mechanistic and Functional Differences

With regard to effects on microtubule dynamics, the naturally occurring vinca alkaloids VCR and VBL, the semisynthetic analog VRL, and the bifluorinated analog vinflunine impart similar actions, but they have distinguishing features as well.[66,67] For example, vinflunine appears to be more active than the other vinca alkaloids against several murine and human tumor xenografts even though it has a significantly lower affinity to tubulin and a lower potential to induce vinca alkaloid-tubulin spiral polymers.[42,68] However, the effects of vinflunine and VRL on microtubule dynamics differ from than those induced by VBL and VCR in that they decrease the growth rate and duration of time growing, but decrease the time spent in attenuation to a greater extent. In contrast, VBL and VCR decrease the shortening rate and increase the time spent in attenuation.

The explanation for the differential effects of the vinca alkaloids on both normal tissues and tumors is not clear. VCR, the most potent of the analogs in humans and the most neurotoxic, has the greatest affinity for tubulin.[69] However, although the vinca alkaloids may demonstrate similar potencies against preparations of tubulin derived from any given tissue, the differential sensitivities of various tissues to the vinca alkaloids are the result of many factors.[5,46,58,67,70–76] One possible contributing factor is tubulin isotype composition, which varies among tissues. Differential tubulin isotype expression may influence the intracellular accumulation of the vinca alkaloids and other antimicrotubule agents that avidly bind tubulin.[9,10,77] In addition, differences in the type and concentration of MAPs, which may influence drug interactions with tubulin, and variability in cellular permeation and retention may influence the formation and stability of complexes formed between the vinca alkaloids and tubulin.[15,46,66,69–71,78,79] For example, the higher cellular retention of VCR compared with VBL in cultured leukemia cells may explain why VCR is more potent than VBL during short treatment periods, whereas the drugs are equitoxic with more prolonged exposures.[70, 75,76,79–81] The magnitude of intracellular GTP concentrations may also influence the type of interactions between the vinca alkaloids and tubulin, and variability in VCR retention among tumors and normal tissues may be related to differences in GTP hydrolysis.[76,79–81] Other factors that might account for differences in vinca alkaloid sensitivities between various tissues include differences in cellular pharmacology and pharmacokinetics, which will be discussed in subsequent sections.

Cellular Pharmacology

Although the vinca alkaloids are rapidly taken up into cells and then accumulate intracellularly, intracellular/extracellular concentration ratios range from 5- to 500-fold depending on the cell type.[70,72,78,81,82] In murine leukemia cells, the intracellular concentrations of VCR are 5- to 20-fold higher than the extracellular concentrations, and this ratio has been reported to range from 150- to 500-fold for other vinca alkaloids in human and murine leukemia cell lines.[75,83] In isolated human hepatocytes, VRL is more rapidly taken up and metabolized than other vinca alkaloids.[71,82–85] Although the vinca alkaloids are retained in cells for long periods of time and thus may have prolonged cellular effects, there are marked differences in cellular retention between these agents.[85–89] For example, VBL is retained to a much greater degree than either VCR or VDS. Overall, the most important determinant of drug accumulation and retention is lipophilicity, although a number of factors undoubtedly play a role.[82,83] Drug uptake and retention also appear to be determined by tissue-specific

and drug-specific factors, as illustrated by studies indicating that the accumulation and retention of VRL in neurons are much less than other vinca alkaloids.[80] The mechanisms responsible for the intracellular accumulation of the vinca alkaloids and other antimicrotubule agents are not fully known but likely involve binding to cellular tubulin.[44] Differential uptake of drugs in different tumor types may also result from diverse expression of tubulin isotypes with different binding characteristics, different uptake, efflux pump mechanisms, and intracellular reservoirs for drug accumulation.

It was originally believed that the vinca alkaloids entered cells by both energy-dependent and temperature-dependent transport processes; however, temperature-independent, nonsaturable mechanisms, analogous to simple diffusion, most likely account for most transport, and temperature-dependent saturable processes are less important.[15,18,82,90] Although the drug concentration and duration of treatment are important determinants of both drug accumulation and cytotoxicity, the duration of drug exposure above a critical threshold concentration is perhaps the most important determinant of cytotoxicity.[71,84] Cytotoxicity is directly related to the extracellular concentration of drug when the duration of treatment is kept constant; for prolonged exposure to VCR, the concentration yielding 50% inhibition lies in the range of 1 to 5 nmol/L (Fig. 11.4).[84,91]

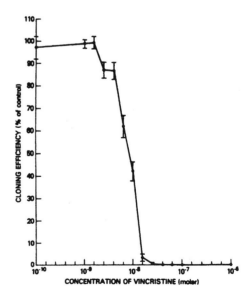

Figure 11.4 Cytotoxicity of vincristine (VCR) for L1210 murine leukemia cells as measured by cloning efficiency. Cells were placed in soft agar containing VCR at the specified concentration; the number of colonies was counted 14 days later and expressed as a percentage of the number of colonies that developed from unexposed (control) cells. (Reprinted with permission from Jackson DV, Bender RA. Cytotoxic thresholds of vincristine in a murine and human leukemia cell line in vitro. Cancer Res 1979;39:4346.)

Mechanisms of Resistance

Resistance to the vinca alkaloids develops rapidly in vitro in the presence of the agents and arises by at least two different mechanisms. In most experimental models, drug resistance is associated with decreased drug accumulation and retention, but the clinical relevance of this phenomenon is not known. The first mechanism is pleiotropic or multidrug resistance (MDR), which can be innate or acquired. Although a large number of proteins that mediate MDR, the best-characterized ones are the ATP-binding cassette (ABC) transporters that belong to the largest known transporter gene family and translocate a variety of substrates across cellular compartments. These intracellular and extracellular membrane-spanning proteins transport endobiotics and xenobiotics and confer resistance to the vinca alkaloids and other structurally bulky, natural product chemotherapeutic agents in vitro.[92] The best studied ABC transporters with respect to conferring resistance to the vinca alkaloids are the permeability glycoprotein (P-gp), or the *MDR1* encoded gene product MDR1 (ABC Subfamily B1;ABCB1), and the multidrug resistance protein (MRP) (ABC Subfamily C2;ABCB1).[85,92–99]

MDR1 is a 170-kD P-gp energy-dependent transmembrane transport pump that regulates the efflux of a large range of amphiphatic hydrophobic substances, resulting in decreased drug accumulation. Pgp forms a channel in the membrane through which drugs are transported, and drug resistance is proportional to the amount of Pgp.[93] Pgp is constitutively overexpressed by various normal tissues, including renal tubular epithelium, colonic mucosa, adrenal medulla, and other epithelial tissues.[86] The efflux protein is also commonly expressed in human cancers, particularly those derived from tissues in which it is constitutively expressed (e.g., kidney and colon cancers). It is also found in post-treatment lymphomas, leukemias, and multiple myeloma.

MDR1 confers varying degrees of cross-resistance to other structurally bulky natural products, such as the taxanes, anthracyclines, epipodophyllotoxins, dactinomycin (actinomycin D), and colchicine.[92–99] These cells may have homogeneously stained chromosomal regions or double-minute chromosomes, which indicates the presence of an amplified gene that codes for P-gp.[87,88] The specific Pgp associated with resistance to the vinca alkaloids shows slight antigenic and amino acid sequence differences and a different peptide map after digestion than does Pgp from cells selected for resistance to colchicine or paclitaxel.[96,97] In fact, two forms of the protein are produced by a single clone of VCR-resistant cells, and these forms undergo post-translational *N*-glycosylation and phosphorylation, which leads to further structural diversity. This diversity may explain the greater degree of resistance for the specific agent used compared with the resistance to other drugs conferred by MDR, and it also may explain the variable patterns of resistance among cells of the MDR type. The composition of membrane gangliosides in cancer cells

resistant to the vinca alkaloids has also been shown to differ from that of wild-type cells. The clinical ramifications of this resistance mechanism are not known. However, in one study in childhood acute lymphoblastic leukemia, VCR resistance measured in vitro did not correlate with P-gp overexpression.[99]

Resistance to the vinca alkaloids is also conferred by MRP1, which is a 190-kD membrane-spanning protein that shares 15% amino acid homology with MDR1.[89,92,100–102] MRP1 expression has been found in many types of tumors and has been implicated as a component of the MDR phenotype in cancers of the lung, colon, breast, bladder, and prostate, as well as leukemia.[87–89,92,100–102] MRP1 has been shown to transport glutathione conjugates of several types of compounds, including alkylating agents, as well as etoposide and doxorubicin but only confers resistance to the latter agents. The MRP1 resistance profile also includes the vinca alkaloids and methotrexate.[89,92,100–102] The clinical significance of the role of MRP1 in transporting conjugated forms of certain chemotherapy agents has not been determined. Although many other ABC transporters have been characterized in vitro and several enhance cellular resistance to the vinca alkaloids, their roles in conferring inherent or acquired resistance to the vinca alkaloids in the clinic are even less clear than those of MDR1 and MRP1.

Another important feature of MDR1 and MRP in vitro is that drug resistance is reversible after treatment with various agents that have distinctly different structural and functional characteristics, such as the calcium-channel blockers, calmodulin inhibitors, detergents, progestational and antiestrogenic agents, antibiotics, antihypertensives, antiarrhythmics, antimalarials, and immunosuppressives.[92] These agents bind directly to Pgp, thereby blocking the efflux of the cytotoxic drugs and increasing intracellular drug concentrations. Therefore, the role of MDR modulators has been a source of great contemporary interest, but the interpretation of clinical studies of resistance modulation has been confounded by the fact that MDR modulators, particularly MDR1 reversal agents, also enhance drug uptake in normal cells, decrease biliary elimination and drug clearance, and lead to enhanced toxicity.[103–105] Overall, strategies aimed at reversing resistance to the vinca alkaloids in the clinic with pharmacologic modulators of both MDR1 and MRP, have been disappointing, most likely because of the placticity of *MDR1*, which is capable of producing a large number of alternate resistance proteins in response to environmental stress.[92] Nevertheless, the characterization of the genetics and role of the ABC transporters in normal organ function and the disposition of chemotherapeutic agents have led to the delineation of genetic polyporphisms that may impact upon pharmacokinetics and drug toxicity.

Structural alterations in α- or β-tubulin, resulting from either genetic mutations and consequential amino acid substitutions or posttranslational modifications, including phosphorylation and acetylation, have been identified in tumor cells with acquired resistance to the vinca alkaloids.[10,44,57,58,106,107] The consequences of functionally significant differences in α- and β-tubulins are "hyperstable" microtubules that are collaterally sensitive to the taxanes and similar tubulin stabilizing natural products (see "Mechanisms of Resistance, Taxanes"). Although the means by which tubulin alterations confer resistance to the vinca alkaloids is not clear, the phenomenon is not apparently due to decreased drug-binding affinity of the altered tubulin.[108–111] Instead, alterations in α- and β-tubulins promote resistance to agents that inhibit microtubule assembly by increasing microtubule stability, perhaps by promoting longitudinal interdimer and intradimer interactions and/or lateral interactions between protofilaments.[112]

Resistance to the vinca alkaloids has also been demonstrated to be related to overexpression of the β-III isotype of β-tubulin.[113] Some have also speculated that changes in the GTP- binding domain of tubulin may be the structural basis for this type of resistance.[109] Another important feature of this type of resistance to the vinca alkaloids is that collateral sensitivity is conferred to the taxanes, which inhibit microtubule disassembly.

Clinical Pharmacology

Analytical Assays

Information about the pharmacology of the vinca alkaloids in humans has been limited in the past by lack of sensitive, specific, and reliable analytic assays capable of measuring the minute plasma concentrations that result from the administration of milligram quantity doses of these agents. Pharmacologic studies were performed initially with radiolabeled drugs;however, interpretation of the results has been confounded by the chemical instability of these agents. Several vinca alkaloids, particularly VCR and VBL, may undergo spontaneous degradation under mild conditions, forming degradative products that can be separated using high-pressure liquid chromatography (HPLC).[114] Therefore, investigators have used radiolabeled compounds coupled to HPLC for further separation to define the plasma disposition of the vinca alkaloids.[115–120] The extent to which the formation of degradative products occurs in vivo, however, is not known.

Radioimmunoassay and enzyme-linked immunosorbent assay (ELISA) methods using specific antisera are capable of detecting picomolar drug concentrations.[17] Because polyclonal antisera raised against the vinca alkaloids cannot distinguish between the parent compounds and related derivatives, these assays may not provide sufficient quantitative information about degradation products and metabolites. However, more refined radioimmunoassay and ELISA methods using monoclonal antibodies have considerably greater sensitivity and specificity.[17]

Technical advances in extraction and chromatographic detection (electrochemical and fluorescence) have made HPLC and gas chromatography the most feasible means of separating the vinca alkaloids from their metabolites. Tandem mass spectrometry used in conjunction with HPLC has enhanced the sensitivity of chromatographic methods.[121–123]

Pharmacokinetics

General

The vinca alkaloids are most commonly administered intravenously as a bolus injection or brief infusion, and their pharmacokinetic behavior in plasma optimally fits open three-compartment models.[17] Pharmacokinetic characteristics include large volumes of distribution, high clearance rates, long terminal half-lives ($t_{1/2}$), hepatic metabolism, and biliary/fecal excretion. At conventional adult dosages, peak plasma concentrations (C_{peak}), which persist for only a few minutes, range from 100 to 500 nmol, and plasma levels remain above 1 to 2 nmol for long durations.[124,125] Pertinent pharmacokinetic parameters are summarized in Table 2. There is also large interindividual and intraindividual variability in their pharmacologic behavior, which has been attributed to many factors, including differences in protein and tissue binding, hepatic metabolism, and biliary clearance.[91] In comparative studies of VCR, VBL, and VDS, VCR has had the longest terminal $t_{1/2}$ and the lowest clearance rate, VBL has had the shortest terminal $t_{1/2}$ and the highest clearance rate, and VDS has had intermediate values.[125,126] The proposal has been made that the longer terminal $t_{1/2}$ and lower clearance rate of VCR account in part for its greater propensity to induce neurotoxicity, but there appear to be other determinants of tissue sensitivity as discussed in "Mechanistic and Functional Differences."[125]

Although prolonged infusion schedules may avoid excessively toxic C_{peak} values and increase the duration of drug exposure in plasma above biologically relevant threshold concentrations for any given tumor, there is little, if any, evidence to support the notion that prolonged infusion schedules are more effective than bolus schedules. This approach has primarily been directed at achieving plasma concentrations for relevant periods, since the duration of exposure to relevant concentrations is a principal determinant of cytotoxicity in vitro;however, rapid, high, and avid distribution and binding of the vinca alkaloids to peripheral tissues, owing to the ubiquitous nature of tubulin, is likely responsible for the efficacy of short administration schedules.

Vincristine

After conventional doses of VCR (1.4 mg/m²) given as brief infusions, peak plasma levels approach 400 nmol/L.[17,36,115,116,125–128] VCR binds extensively to both plasma proteins (reported values in the range of 48 to 75%) and formed blood elements, particularly platelets, which contain high concentrations of tubulin and led, in the past, to the use of VCR-loaded platelets for treating disorders of platelet consumption, such as idiopathic thrombocytopenia purpura.[17,113] The platelet count has been inversely related to drug exposure.[17,128] In dogs and rodents, the spleen accumulates VCR to a greater extent than any other tissue.[17,115,130] Poor drug penetration across the blood-brain barrier has been documented in most studies.[17] The low penetration of VCR across the blood-brain barrier and other tumor sanctuary sites can be attributed to its large size and the fact that it is an avid substrate for the ABC transporters, which maintain the integrity of these blood-tissue barriers.[17,36,74,115,116,119,125–128] Pharmacologic inhibition of MDR, however, may allow entry of VCR into the brain.[115,119,130,131] In humans, VCR concentrations in cerebrospinal fluid are 20- to 30- fold lower than in plasma and do not exceed 1.1 nmol/L.[131]

After standard doses of VCR administered intravenously as a bolus injection, plasma disposition is triphasic, with $t_{1/2\alpha}$ values of less than 5 minutes because of extensive and rapid tissue binding. Consequently, the apparent volumes of distribution (V_d) are high (mean central V_d, 0.328 ± 0.1061 L/kg and $V_{d\gamma}$ [V_d for the terminal γ phase] of 8.42 ± 3.17 L/kg), which indicates extensive tissue binding.[125] Beta $t_{1/2}$ ($t_{1/2\beta}$) values range from 50 to 155 minutes, and gamma $t_{1/2}$ ($t_{1/2\gamma}$) values are even more variable, ranging from 23 to 85 hours, which suggests slow clearance from the tissue compartment.[17,118,125,128] Considerable interest has arisen in using protracted VCR administration schedules, because prolonged infusions may closely simulate the optimal in vitro conditions required for cytotoxicity.[84,91,128,131] For example, VCR concentrations of 100 to 400 nmol/L are achieved only briefly after bolus injection, and levels generally decline to less than 10 nmol/L in 2 to 4 hours. Exposure to 100 nmol/L VCR for 3 hours is required to kill 50% of L1210 murine or CEM human lymphoblastic leukemia cells, whereas treatment durations of 6 to 12 hours are required to achieve this degree of cytotoxicity at 10 nmol/L, and no lethal effects occur at VCR concentrations below 2 nmol/L.[84] A 0.5-mg intravenous bolus injection of VCR followed by a continuous infusion at dosages of 0.5 to 1.0 mg/m² per day for 5 days results in steady-state VCR concentrations ranging from 1 to 10 nmol/L, and terminal $t_{1/2}$ after discontinuation of the infusions ranging from 10.5 hours (1.0 mg/m²) to 21.7 hours (0.5 mg/m²).[128] Although peak VCR plasma concentrations achieved with prolonged infusions are lower than levels achieved with bolus injections, more prolonged schedules are associated with a greater duration of drug exposure above a critical threshold concentration.[128] However, this reasoning involves relating drug exposure in plasma to cytotoxicity and the drug exposure in tumors is likely disproportionately higher because of extensive tissue distribution, avid tissue binding, and slow clearance from tissue compartments.

VCR is metabolized and excreted primarily by the hepatobiliary system.[73,74,115,116] Within 72 hours after the administration of radiolabeled VCR, approximately 12% of the radioactivity is excreted in the urine (at least 50% of which consists of metabolites), and approximately 70 to 80% is excreted in the feces (40% of which consists of metabolites).[36,83,115,116,119,120,124–126,128,131,132] VCR is rapidly excreted into bile with an initial bile to plasma concentration ratio of 100:1 that declines to 20:1 at 72 hours posttreatment.[115] Metabolites accumulate rapidly in the bile, so that only 46.5% of the total biliary product is the parent compound.[115] As many as 6 to 11 metabolites have been detected in both humans and animals.[130,133–135] The structures of most, however, most have not been identified. The metabolites 4-deacetylVCR and N-deformylVCR have been isolated from human bile, whereas 4-deacetylVCR, and both 4'-deoxy-3'-hydroxyVCR and 3',4'- epoxyVCR N-oxide have been identified after incubation of VCR with bile.[114,120,127,133] The nature of the metabolites identified to date, as well as the results of metabolic studies in vitro, indicate that is VCR is metabolized principally by the hepatic cytochrome P-450 mixed function oxidase CYP3A.[36,83,126,133–136] The importance of CYP3A in drug disposition is also supported by observations of enhanced clearance with phenytoin and carbamazepine that induce CYP3A4, and increased toxicity with CYP3A inhibitors, particularly itraconazole.[134,135] In addition, transfection of tumor cells with CYP3A4 increases resistance to VBL, whereas cancer cells selected for VBL resistance may show increased CYP3A4 activity.[136] There has been conflicting, albeit sparse, evidence indicating that VCR C_{peak} values or systemic exposure are directly related to the degree of neurotoxicity.[33]

Vinblastine

The pharmacologic behavior of VBL also reflects its extensive tissue binding and resembles that of VCR. Although plasma protein binding has been reported to range from 43 to 99.7%, it most likely approaches the high end of this range.[118,137] VBL binds extensively to formed blood elements, with 50% of radiolabeled drug bound to platelets, red blood cells, and white blood cells within 20 minutes after an intravenous injection.[140] Extensive platelet binding is most likely the result of the high concentrations of tubulin in platelets.

Plasma disappearance fits a triexponential model with a rapid distribution phase ($t_{1/2\alpha}$ <5 minutes) from rapid tissue binding.[118] VBL is more avidly sequestered in tissues than VCR, as demonstrated by retention of 73% of radioactivity in the body 6 days after an injection of the radiolabeled agent.[118] Values for $t_{1/2\alpha}$ and $t_{1/2\beta}$ have been reported to range from 53 to 99 minutes and 20 to 24 hours, respectively.[17,118,125] High steady-state levels and long terminal $t_{1/2}$ values have been reported after 5-day infusions of VBL: 1.1 nmol/L at 1 mg/m² per day ($t_{1/2}$, 28 days);3.3 nmol/L at 1.7 mg/m² per day ($t_{1/2}$, 3 days);and 6.6 nmol/L at 2 mg/m² per day ($t_{1/2}$, 6 days).[17,141]

The principal mode of VBL disposition is hepatic metabolism and biliary excretion. Over a 9-day period after treatment of dogs with radiolabeled VBL, 30 to 36% of radioactivity is recovered in bile and 12 to 17% is found in urine.[142] Fecal excretion of the parent compound is relatively low, which indicates that metabolism is significant. In vitro studies indicate that the cytochrome P-450 CYP3A isoform is primarily responsible for drug biotransformation.[143] At least one metabolite, desacetylvinblastine (VDS), which may be as active as the parent compound, has been identified in both dogs and humans.[118,142] Small quantities of VDS also have been detected in both urine and feces.

Vindesine

Similar to the other vinca alkaloids, plasma disposition of VDS is characterized by a triexponential process.[17,118,119,125,144,145] VDS is also rapidly distributed to peripheral tissues except for sanctuary sites that are protected by ABC transporters (e.g., brain and testes). $T_{1/2\alpha}$ values for VDS are less than 5 minutes and values for $t_{1/2\beta}$ and $t_{1/2\gamma}$ range from 55 to 99 minutes and 20 to 24 hours, respectively. Clearance is low, which indicates that drug accumulation may occur with short-interval, repetitive dosing schedules. The large V_d, low renal clearance rate, and long terminal $t_{1/2}$ of VDS also suggest that it undergoes extensive tissue binding and delayed elimination. Although peak plasma VDS concentrations that range from 0.1 to 1.0 μmol/L are achieved with bolus injections, levels typically decline to <0.1 μmol/L in 1 to 2 hours after treatment. Plasma levels achieved with bolus injection are approximately 16-fold higher than levels achieved with prolonged infusions; however, optimal steady-state VDS concentrations for cytotoxicity (0.01 to 0.1 μmol/L) are readily achieved with prolonged infusion schedules (1.2 to 2.0 mg/m^2 per day for 2 to 5 days).[128,134,140,144,146–148]

The liver is the main organ involved in VDS metabolism and disposition, and CYP3A appears to be the principal P-450 CYP isoform involved in drug biotransformation.[83,117,130,149] VDS concentrations in bile are much higher than simultaneously measured plasma levels, and biliary and renal clearance rates have been reported to be 29 and 12 mL/minute, respectively.[130] Renal excretion accounts for only 1 to 13% of drug disposition.[17,134,147]

Vinorelbine

The pharmacologic behavior of VRL is similar to that of the other vinca alkaloids, and the decline of plasma concentrations following rapid injection have been characterized by biexponential and triexponential models.[36,41,53,83,132,150] After intravenous administration, there is a rapid decay of VRL concentrations followed by a much slower elimination phase ($t_{1/2\gamma}$, 18 to 49 hours). Plasma protein binding has been reported to range from 80 to 91%, with binding primarily to α_1-acid glycoprotein, albumin, and lipoproteins, and platelet binding is also extensive.[17,53,44,83,151] The unbound fraction has been reported to range from 0.09 to 0.20.[53]

VRL is widely distributed, and high concentrations are found in virtually all tissues (tissue to plasma ratios of 20 to 80), except brain.[53,54,83,135,152] The wide distribution of VRL reflects the agent's lipophilicity, which is among the highest of the vinca alkaloids. In fact, drug concentrations in human lung have been demonstrated to be 300-fold greater than plasma levels and 3.4- to 13.8-fold higher than lung concentrations achieved with VDS and VCR, respectively. Plasma protein binding in the range of 80 to 90% has been reported. As with other vinca alkaloids, drug disposition principally occurs in the liver, and 33 to 80% of the drug is excreted in the feces, whereas urinary excretion represents only 16 to 30% of total drug disposition, most of which is unmetabolized VLR.[39,,53,83,132,153,154] Studies in humans indicate that 4-O-deacetyl-VRL and 3,6- epoxy-VRL are the principal metabolites, and several minor hydroxy-VRL metabolites have been identified.[53,44,154] Although most metabolites are inactive, the deacetyl-VRL metabolite may be as active as VRL but this finding is of minor clinical significance because concentrations of this metabolite are minute. The CYP3A isoenzyme appears to be principally involved in biotransformation.[53,54]

In one study the total body clearance of VRL (1.2 L/hour per kilogram) and $t_{1/2\gamma}$ values of approximately 26 hours were found to be the same in older and younger patients, provided that patients have normal hepatic function.[155] Clearance has been found to be adversely affected in patients who have liver metastases that replace more than 75% of the organ; clearance can be predicted in such patients by the monoethylglycinexylidide clearance test, which assesses CYP3A4 function.[156] Although VRL clearance is not accurately predicted by bilirubin concentrations in serum, markedly elevated levels have been associated with significant reductions in clearance in the few patients studied.

VRL is active when given orally. In animal studies, 100% of total radioactivity is absorbed after the ingestion of tritium-labeled VRL, whereas human studies using powder-filled, liquid-filled, and gelatin-filled capsules have shown that the bioavailability of the parent compound is 43% for the powder-filled and 27% for the liquid-filled capsules; the bioavailability of the gel-filled capsule was negligibly affected by food.[41,157,158] C_{peak} values are achieved within 1 to 2 hours after oral treatment, and interindividual variability is moderate.

Drug Interactions

Pharmacokinetic interactions of the vinca alkaloids and other drugs have not been studied in detail. Methotrexate accumulation in tumor cells is enhanced in vitro by the presence of VCR or VBL, an effect mediated by a vinca alkaloid-induced blockade of drug efflux; however, the minimal concentrations of VCR required to achieve this effect in myeloblasts (0.1 μmol/L) is realized only momentarily during clinical treatment, and even higher concentrations are needed to enhance MTX uptake in lymphoblasts.[159–161] The schedule of VCR followed by MTX has not demonstrated synergism in the L1210 murine leukemia cells.[162] Cytotoxic synergy is noted with the sequence of MTX followed by VCR; however, but this interaction is not likely the result of the enhancement of MTX uptake. Thus, very little justification exists for routine use of VCR pretreatment in high-dose MTX protocols. The vinca alkaloids also inhibit the cellular influx of the epipodophyllotoxins in vitro, resulting in less cytotoxicity, but the clinical ramifications are unknown.[163] L-Asparaginase may reduce the hepatic clearance of the vinca alkaloids, particularly VCR, which may result in increased toxicity. To minimize the possibility of this interaction, VCR should be given 12 to 24 hours before L-asparaginase. The use of mitomycin C in combination with the vinca alkaloids has been associated with pulmonary toxicity as described in "Toxicity, Pulmonary."

Treatment with the vinca alkaloids has precipitated seizures associated with subtherapeutic plasma phenytoin concentrations, most likely due to induction of CYP3A.[164,165] Reduced plasma phenytoin levels have been noted from 24 hours to 10 days after treatment with both VCR and VBL. As previously discussed, administration of the vinca alkaloids with erythromycin, itraconazole, and other inhibitors of CYP3A may also lead to severe toxicity.[133–135,137,138,166,167,168] Concomitantly administered drugs, such as pentobarbital and H_2-receptor antagonists, may also influence VCR clearance by modulating hepatic cytochrome P-450 metabolic processes.[161] Another potential drug interaction may occur in patients who have Kaposi's sarcoma related to acquired immunodeficiency syndrome and are receiving concurrent treatment with 3' azido-3'-deoxythymidine (AZT) and the vinca alkaloids, as the vinca alkaloids may inhibit glucuronidation of AZT to its 5'-O-glucuronide metabolite.[167] Based on a report of a constellation of severe toxicities, including inappropriate secretion of antidiuretic hormone (SIADH), bilateral cranial nerve palsies, peripheral neuropathy, cranial nerve palsies, heart failure and cardiovascular effects following VCR treatment in pediatric patient with acute lymphocytic leukemia who had been receiving treatment with nifedipine and itraconazole, it is possible that these medications may enhance the neurologic and cardiovascular effects of the vinca alkaloids.[133,168] Lastly, the significant interindividual and intraindividual variability of VCR pharmacokinetics in children has been attributed to the variable induction of P-450 metabolism because of concurrent use of P-450-inducing corticosteroids.[168]

Doses and Schedules

The vinca alkaloids are most commonly administered by direct intravenous injection or through the side-arm tubing of a running intravenous infusion. Experienced oncology personnel should administer these agents because drug extravasation causes severe soft tissue injury.

Vincristine

VCR is routinely administered to children weighing more than 10 kg (body surface area ≥ 1 m^2) as a rapid (bolus)

intravenous injection at a dose of 1.5 to 2.0 mg/m^2 weekly, whereas 0.05 to 0.065 mg/kg weekly is commonly used in smaller children ($<$10 kg or body surface area $<$1 m^2). For adults, the conventional weekly dose is 1.4 mg/m^2 weekly. A restriction of the absolute single dose of VCR to 2.0 mg/m^2, which is commonly referred to as *capping*, has been adopted, based on early reports of substantial neurotoxicity at higher doses. This restriction is largely empirical, and available evidence suggests that the practice of capping should be reconsidered.[164] The fact that the cumulative dose may be a more critical factor than single dose has readily been appreciated;however, significant interpatient variability exists, and some patients are able to tolerate much higher VCR doses with little or no toxicity.[171,172] This may be because of large interindividual differences in drug exposure, which may vary as much as 11-fold.[173,174] Moreover, the safety and efficacy of treatment regimens that do not employ capping at 2.0 mg have been documented in adults.[164,175] In any case, VCR dosage modifications should be based on toxicity, particularly peripheral and autonomic neuropathy. However, dosage should not be reduced for mild peripheral neurotoxicity, particularly if the agent is being used in a potentially curative setting. Instead, doses should be modified for manifestations indicative of more serious neurotoxicity, including severe symptomatic sensory changes, motor and cranial nerve deficits, and ileus, until toxicity resolves. In clearly palliative situations, dose reductions, lengthened dosing intervals, or selection of an alternative agent may be justified in the event of moderate neurotoxicity. A routine prophylactic regimen, consisting of stool softeners, dietary bulk, and laxatives, to prevent the consequences of severe autonomic toxicity, particularly severe constipation, is also recommended.

Based on in vitro data indicating that the duration of VCR exposure above a critical threshold concentration is an important determinant for cytotoxicity, prolonged infusion schedules have been evaluated.[17,128,134] After a 0.5-mg/m^2 intravenous injection of VCR, total daily VCR doses of 0.25 to 0.50 mg/m^2 as a 5-day infusion are generally well tolerated.[17] In children, the administration of VCR as a 5-day infusion has permitted a twofold increase in the dose that can be safely administered without major toxicity compared with bolus schedules.

VCR is a potent vesicant and should not be administered intramuscularly, subcutaneously, or intraperitoneally. Direct intrathecal injection of VCR or other vinca alkaloids, which has occurred as an inadvertent clinical mishap, induces a severe myeloencephalopathy characterized by ascending motor and sensory neuropathies, encephalopathy, and rapid death (see "Toxicity, Miscellaneous").[176,177] Administration of VCR 0.4 mg/day as a 5-day infusion by the hepatic intraarterial route also has been associated with profound toxicity, including disorientation and diarrhea.[178]

Although the issue has not been evaluated carefully, the major role of the liver in the disposition of VCR implies that dose modifications should be considered for patients with hepatic dysfunction.[174] However, firm guidelines for dose modifications have not been established. A 50% dosage reduction is recommended for patients with plasma total bilirubin levels between 1.5 and 3.0 mg/dL and at least a 75% dosage reduction for serum total bilirubin levels above 3.0 mg/dL. Dosage reductions for renal dysfunction are not indicated.[179]

Vinblastine

Although VBL has been administered intravenously on various schedules, the most commonly used schedule administers a bolus injection at a dose of 6 mg/m² per day in cyclic combination-chemotherapy regimens. Approved initial dose recommendations for weekly dosing are 2.5 and 3.7 mg/m² for children and adults, respectively, followed by gradual dose escalation in increments of 1.8 and 1.25 mg/m², respectively, each week based on hematologic tolerance. The recommendation is also that maximal weekly doses of 18.5 and 12.5 mg/m² in adults and children, respectively, should not be exceeded;however, these doses are substantially higher than most patients can tolerate because of myelosuppression, even on less frequent treatment schedules. Because the severity of the leukopenia that may occur with identical VBL doses varies widely, VBL probably should not be given more frequently than once each week. Oral administration may result in unpredictable toxicity.[180]

Five-day continuous infusions of VBL have been used at dosages ranging from 1.5 to 2.0 mg/m² per day, which achieve plasma concentrations of approximately 2 nmol/L. In one study of VBL on this administration schedule, patients who were more likely to respond to treatment had longer terminal-phase $t_{1/2}$ values.[181] Little, if any, evidence exists, however, to support the notion that prolonged infusion schedules are more effective than bolus schedules.

Although specific guidelines have not been established, VBL dosages should be modified for patients with hepatic dysfunction, especially biliary obstruction, because of the importance of the liver in drug disposition (see "Doses and Schedules, Vincristine"). Dosage reductions in patients with renal dysfunction are not indicated.[179]

Vindesine

VDS has been administered intravenously on many schedules, including weekly and biweekly bolus and prolonged infusion schedules. The agent also has been given in fractionated doses as either an intermittent or a continuous infusion over 1 to 5 days. VDS is most commonly administered as a single intravenous dose of 2 to 4 mg/m² every 7 to 14 days, which is associated with antitumor activity and a tolerable toxicity profile.[17] Intermittent or continuous-infusion schedules usually administer VDS dosages of 1 to 2 mg/m² per day for 1 to 2 days or 1.2 mg/m² per day for 5 days every 3 to 4 weeks.[17,124] More prolonged schedules (up to 21 days) also have been evaluated.

Specific dosing guidelines have not been established for patients with hepatic or renal dysfunction; however, the pharmacologic similarities of VDS and other vinca alkaloids and the increased toxicity of VDS noted in patients with abnormal liver function mandate dosage reduction for patients with severe hepatic dysfunction, especially biliary obstruction (see "Doses and Schedules, Vincristine"). Dosage modifications are not indicated for renal dysfunction.[179]

Vinorelbine

VRL is most commonly administered intravenously at a dose of 30 mg/m² on a weekly or biweekly schedule as a slow injection through a side-arm port into a running infusion (alternatively, a slow bolus injection followed by flushing the vein with 5% dextrose or 0.9% sodium chloride solutions) or as a short infusion over 20 minutes.[182] It appears that the more rapid infusions produce less local venous toxicity.[182] An acceptable oral formulation, however, is not yet available. Other dosing schedules that have been evaluated include long-term oral administration of low doses and intermittent high-dose and prolonged intravenous infusion schedules.[182] Like the other vinca alkaloids, VRL clearance is impaired in patients with hepatic dysfunction, and dosage reductions should be considered in this setting.[156] Recommendations include a 50% dosage reduction for serum total bilirubin concentrations between 1.5 and 3 mg/dL and a 75% dosage reduction for patients with plasma total bilirubin concentrations above 3.0 mg/dL. Dosage reductions are not recommended for patients with renal insufficiency.

Toxicity

The principal toxicities of the vinca alkaloids differ dramatically despite their structural and pharmacologic similarities. Peripheral neurotoxicity is the predominant toxicity of VCR, whereas myelosuppression predominates with VBL, VDS, and VRL. Nevertheless, peripheral neurotoxicity is often noted following cumulative treatment with VBL, VDS, and VRL, inadvertent high-dose treatment, and settings or patients who are inordinately susceptible (see "Neurologic"). On the other hand, VCR can cause myelosuppression under the similar conditions. Several potential explanations for the selective effects in various normal and neoplastic tissues are discussed in "Mechanism of Action, Vinca Alkaloids", in this chapter.

Neurologic

The vinca alkaloids, particularly VCR, induce neurotoxicity characterized by a peripheral, symmetric mixed sensory-motor, and autonomic polyneuropathy.[33,36,53,170,183–186] The primary neuropathologic effects are axonal degeneration and decreased axonal transport as a result of the interference with axonal microtubule function. Initially, only symmetric sensory impairment and paresthesias in a length-dependent manner (distal extremities first) usually are encountered. Neuritic pain and loss of deep tendon reflexes may develop with continued treatment, which may be followed by foot drop, wrist drop, motor dysfunction, ataxia, and paralysis. Back, bone, and limb pains occasionally occur. Nerve conduction velocities are usually normal, although diminished amplitude of sensory and motor nerve action potentials and prolonged distal latencies, suggesting axonal degeneration, may be noted.[33,36,53,183–185] Cranial nerves may be affected rarely, resulting in hoarseness, diplopia, jaw pain, and facial palsies. The uptake of VCR into the brain is low, and central nervous system effects, such as confusion, mental status changes, depression, hallucinations, agitation, insomnia, seizures, coma, SIADH, ataxia, athetosis, and visual disturbances, are rare.[33,74,119,120,187,188] Acute, severe autonomic neurotoxicity is uncommon but may arise as a consequence of high-dose therapy (>2 mg/m^2) or in patients with altered hepatic function. Autonomic toxicities include abdominal cramping, paralytic ileus (see "Gastrointestinal, Toxicity, Vinca Alkaloids"), urinary retention (see "Genitourinary"), cardiac autonomic dysfunction, orthostatic hypotension, and arterial hypotension and hypertension (see "Cardiovascular").[170,185,186,187–191] Laryngeal paralysis may also occur.[192]

In adults, the neurotoxic effects of VCR may begin with cumulative doses as little as 5 to 6 mg, and manifestations may be profound after cumulative doses of 15 to 20 mg. Children appear to be less susceptible than adults, but older persons are particularly prone. However, the apparent influence of age may, in fact, be the result of previously inadequate dose calculation by body weight in children and adults and by body surface area in infants.[193,194] In infants, VCR doses are calculated now according to body weight. Patients with antecedent neurologic disorders, such as Charcot-Marie-Tooth disease, hereditary and sensory neuropathy type 1, Guillain-Barré syndrome, and childhood poliomyelitis, are highly predisposed.[195–197] Hepatic dysfunction or obstructive liver disease increases the risk of developing severe neuropathy because of impaired drug metabolism and delayed biliary excretion.

The only known treatment for VCR neurotoxicity is discontinuation of the drug or reduction of the dose or frequency of treatment.[170,198,199] Although a number of antidotes, including thiamine, vitamin B$_{12}$, folinic acid, and pyridoxine, have been used, these treatments have not been clearly shown to be effective.[33,126,170,198,199] Folinic acid (not folic acid) has been shown to protect mice against an otherwise lethal dose of VCR and has been used successfully in several cases of VCR overdosage in humans;however, it has not been studied prospectively.[200,201] Concurrent administration of a mixture of gangliosides with VCR also has been reported to reduce the peripheral neurotoxicity produced with standard dosages of VCR.[202] Another agent used to prevent neurotoxicity for which results are encour-

aging, is glutamic acid on the basis of its ability to enhance microtubule formation in vitro, as well as its possible competition with VCR for carrier-mediated membrane transport.[199,203] In a randomized clinical trial, coadministration of glutamic acid and VCR reduced the incidence of paresthesia and loss of the Achilles tendon reflex.[203] However, glutamic acid has not been shown to ameliorate VCR-related gastrointestinal and hematologic toxicities. The adrenocorticotropic hormone analogue ORG 2766 has also been shown to protect against VCR-induced neuropathy, both in an animal model and in cancer patients in a placebo-controlled pilot study, but the relative younger age of the patients in the experimental arm as compared with that of the the placebo group may have accounted for this result.[33] Nerve growth factor, insulin-like growth factor I, and amifostine have been anecdotally reported to alter the natural course of drug-induced neurotoxicity.[37]

The manifestations of neurotoxicity are similar for the other vinca alkaloids;however, they are typically less common and severe.[17,33,36,53,126] Severe neurotoxicity is observed infrequently with both VBL and VDS. VRL has been shown to have a lower affinity for axonal microtubules than either VCR or VBL, which seems to be confirmed by clinical observations.[68,204] Mild-to-moderate peripheral neuropathy, principally characterized by sensory effects, occurs in 7 to 31% of patients, and constipation and other autonomic effects are noted in 30% of subjects, whereas severe toxicity occurs in 2 to 3%. Muscle weakness and discomfort at tumor sites may also occur. In a study in patients with non–small cell lung cancer who were treated with either VRL alone, VRL plus cisplatin, or VDS plus cisplatin, the rate of severe neurotoxicity was lower in both the single-agent VRL and VRL plus cisplatin arms than in the VDS plus cisplatin arm.[205] Furthermore, the addition of cisplatin did not increase the incidence of severe toxicity in excess of that observed with VRL alone.

Hematologic

Neutropenia is the principal dose-limiting toxicity of VBL, VDS, and VRL. Thrombocytopenia and anemia are usually less common and less severe. The onset of neutropenia is usually 7 to 11 days after treatment, and recovery is generally by days 14 to 21. Myelosuppression is not typically cumulative. Hematologic toxicity of clinical relevance is uncommon after VCR treatment but may be a major manifestation following inadvertent administration of high dosages. VCR also may increase circulating platelets because of the endoreduplication of megakaryocytes.[206]

Gastrointestinal

Gastrointestinal toxicities, aside from those caused by autonomic dysfunction, may be caused by all the vinca alkaloids.[17,33,36,53,126,207] Gastrointestinal autonomic dysfunction, as manifested by bloating, constipation, ileus, and abdominal pain, occur most commonly with VCR or high doses of the other vinca alkaloids. Paralytic ileus, intestinal necrosis, and perforation have been reported.[208] Poor intestinal transit may result in the impaction of stool in the upper colon. An empty rectum may be noted on digital examination, and an abdominal radiograph may be useful in diagnosing this condition. This condition may be responsive to high enemas and laxatives. A routine prophylactic regimen to prevent constipation is therefore recommended for all patients receiving VCR. Paralytic ileus also may occur, particularly in pediatric patients. The ileus, which may mimic a "surgical abdomen," usually resolves with conservative therapy alone after termination of treatment. Patients who receive high dosages of VCR or have hepatic dysfunction may be especially prone to develop severe gastrointestinal complications as a result of autonomic neurotoxicity. Although success with drugs used prophylactically to minimize toxicity, including lactulose, caeruluin, metaclopramide, and the cholecystokinin analog sincalide, has been reported anecdotally, these agents also may alter the pharmacokinetic behavior of the vinca alkaloids by affecting biliary excretion and/or enterohepatic recirculation, which may ultimately result in increased drug clearance.[17] Mucositis, stomatitis, and pharyngitis occur more frequently with VBL than with VRL or VDS and is least common with VCR. Nausea, vomiting, and diarrhea may also occur to a lesser extent. Asymptomatic and transient elevations in liver function test results, particularly alkaline phosphatase levels, have been noted. Pancreatitis has also been reported with VRL.[207]

Cardiovascular

Hypertension and hypotension, presumably resulting from autonomic neurotoxicity, have been observed.[189,190] The vinca alkaloids alone or in combination-chemotherapy regimens, particularly those that also include cisplatin and bleomycin, have been implicated rarely in causing acute cardiac ischemia and massive myocardial infarctions.[209] The underlying mechanism for these effects is not known. Hypertension is the most common cardiovascular effect of VBL. Raynaud's phenomenon may be a lingering effect, especially in patients treated with the combination of VBL, cisplatin, and bleomycin (PVB).[210] In one study, symptomatic Raynaud's phenomenon developed in 44% of patients with germ cell malignancies who were treated with PVB, and an even higher percentage developed abnormal vasoconstrictive responses to cold stimuli.[210] This toxicity occurs less frequently when etoposide is substituted for VBL. The calcium-channel–blocking agent nifedipine has been reported to ameliorate the symptoms of Raynaud's phenomenon induced by VBL.[211]

Pulmonary

Respiratory reactions, characterized by dyspnea, have been reported in approximately 5% of patients, particularly when vinca alkaloids are combined with mitomycin C.[212,213] These respiratory reactions may be classified into two types. One type is an acute reaction with bronchospasm, resembling an allergic reaction. The second type is a subacute reversible reaction associated with cough and dyspnea and occasionally with interstitial infiltrates. This reaction typically occurs within 1 hour after treatment. The use of steroids has been felt to be beneficial in severe cases, and several patients have been retreated without sequelae. No evidence exists that VRL causes chronic pulmonary toxicity.

Genitourinary

VCR-induced autonomic neurotoxicity may produce bladder atony, thereby causing polyuria, dysuria, incontinence, and urinary retention.[190] Therefore, the suggestion has been made that other drugs that are known to cause urinary retention, particularly in the older population, should be discontinued if possible for several days after treatment with VCR.

Extravasation

All vinca alkaloids are potent vesicants and may cause severe tissue damage if extravasation occurs. Injection-site reactions, including erythema, pain, and venous discoloration, are common;however, severe local toxicity is uncommon (< 2%). The risk of phlebitis increases if veins are not adequately flushed after treatment. If extravasation is suspected, treatment should be discontinued, and aspiration of any residual drug remaining in the tissues should be attempted.[51,214–217] Animal experiments have demonstrated that cold packs may increase toxicity, and hot packs may limit damage. The application of local heat immediately for 1 hour four times daily for 3 to 5 days and the injection of hyaluronidase, 150 to 1500 units (15 units/mL in 6 mL of 0.9% sodium chloride solution) subcutaneously, through six clockwise injections in a circumferential manner using a 25-gauge needle (changing the needle with each injection) into surrounding tissues is the treatment of choice in minimizing both discomfort and latent cellulitis. The use of calcium leucovorin, diphenydramine, hydrocortisone, isoproterenol, sodium bicarbonate, and vitamin A cream have been ineffective in animal models.[216] An immediate surgical consultation to consider early debridement is recommended. Discomfort and signs of phlebitis may also occur along the course of an injected vein, with resultant sclerosis. The risk of phlebitis may increase if the vein is not adequately flushed after treatment.

Endocrine

All the vinca alkaloids have been implicated as a cause of SIADH by directly affecting the hypothalamus, neurohypophyseal tract, or posterior pituitary. Patients who are receiving intensive hydration are particularly prone to severe hyponatremia secondary to SIADH, which may result in generalized seizures.[17,33,36,53,126] This entity has been associated with elevated plasma levels of antidiuretic hormone and usual remits in 2 to 3 days. Hyponatremia generally responds to fluid restriction, as with hyponatremia associated with SIADH from other causes.

Miscellaneous

Alopecia occurs in a small proportion of patients. An acute necrotizing myopathy has also been observed.[218] Hand-foot syndrome is a rare toxicity of VRL.[219] VBL may cause photosensitivity reactions, possibly as a result of corneal irritation.

The inadvertent intrathecal administration of the vinca alkaloids causes an ascending myeloencephalopathy that is usually fatal. Reports of immediate cerebrospinal fluid withdrawal and lavage with Ringer's lactate solution supplemented with fresh-frozen plasma (15 mL/L) at a rate of 55 mL/hour for 24 hours has provided somewhat encouraging results, in that two affected patients survived with significant paraplegia, but intact cerebral function.[176, 177] To prevent this mistake, pharmacy, nursing, and physicians should be trained not to administer intrathecal methotrexate and intravenous VCR in a single setting, and the drugs should not be delivered together to staff. [220]

TAXANES

The taxanes are perhaps the most important additions to the chemotherapeutic arsenal in the late twentieth century.

The prototypical taxane, paclitaxel, and docetaxel, a potent semisynthetic analog, have demonstrated antitumor activity of major impact. Paclitaxel was discovered as part of a National Cancer Institute program in which extracts of thousands of plants were screened for anticancer activity.[221] In 1963, a crude extract with antitumor activity was isolated from the bark of the Pacific yew, *Taxus brevifolia*, a slowly growing evergreen found in the old-growth forests of the Pacific Northwest, and paclitaxel was identified as the active constituent of the extract by Wall and Wani in 1971.[222-225] Interest in the agent accelerated in 1979 after researchers described its unique mechanism of action on microtubules.[222-225] Paclitaxel is also isolated from other members of the Taxus genus and produced by *Taxomyces andreanae*, a fungal endophyte isolated from the inner bark of the Pacific yew. Although paclitaxel originally came from the bark of the scarce Pacific yew, alternate sources, including nonbark biomass, ornamental species, and, most importantly, partial synthesis from a readily available precursor, 10-deacetylbaccatin III, derived from the needles of more abundant yew species such as the European yew, *Taxus baccata*, are producing sufficient quantities of the drug to meet commercial demand. Docetaxel, which is also derived semisynthetically from 10-deacetylbaccatin III, is slightly more water soluble than paclitaxel and a more potent antimicrotubule agent in vitro.[226] The key features of the taxanes are displayed in Tables 11.3 and 11.4, respectively.

The most impressive clinical activity of the taxanes has been in patients with ovarian and breast cancers.[221,226-229] Paclitaxel initially received regulatory approval for the treatment of patients with ovarian cancer after failure of first-line or subsequent chemotherapy.[221] It was next incorporated

TABLE 11.3
KEY FEATURES OF THE TAXANES

	Paclitaxel	Docetaxel
Mechanism of action	Low concentrations inhibit microtubule dynamics (dynamic instability and treadmilling). High concentrations inhibit depolymerization of tubulin	
Standard dosage (mg/m^2)	175 over 3 hours every 3 weeks 135–175 over 24 hours every 3 weeks 80 over 1 hour weekly	60-100 over 1 hour every 3 weeks (75 is the most common dose used) 36 over 1 hour weekly
Pharmacokinetics and disposition	See Table 11.4	
Principal toxicity	Myelosuppression	Myelosuppression
Other common toxicities	Alopecia Peripheral neurotoxicity HSRs	Alopecia Peripheral neurotoxiicty Rashes and nail disorders HSRs (mild to moderate)
Premedication	Corticosteroids, H$_1$- and H$_2$-histamine antagonists before each treatment to prevent HSR (see "Administration")	Corticosteroids with each treatment to prevent fluid retention;H$_1$-histamine antagonists recomemended to HSRs.
Precautions:	Patients with abnormal liver function should be treated with caution. See section on dosage and schedule for specific dosing guidelines.	

HSRs, hypersensitivity reactions.

TABLE 11.4

PHARMACOKINETIC PARAMETERS OF THE TAXANES[331,337,353,357]

	Paclitaxel		Docetaxel	
	1-hour infusion	**3-hour infusion**	**1-hour infusion**	**1-hour infusion**
Dosage (mg/m^2/week)	**100 (weekly)**	**175 (every 3 weeks)**	**35 (weekly)**	**75 (every 3 weeks)**
Optimal pharmacokinetic model	Triexponential	Triexponential;saturable elimination and distribution above 175 mg/m^2	Triexponential	Triexponential
C$_{peak}$ (_mol/L)	3.37	4.3	1.9	2.3
Clearance (L/hr/m^2)	244	12.7	29.1	25.8
Vd$_{ss}$ (L/m^2)	—	99	—	67
T$_{1/2\gamma}$ (hr)	—	18.8	61.3	91.7
Protein binding (%)	>95%;albumin and α_1-acid glycoprotein		>80to 95%;α1–acid glycoprotein, albumin, and lipoproteins	
Primary mechanism of disposition	Hepatic metabolism and biliary excretion		Hepatic metabolism and biliary excretion	

C$_{peak}$, peak plasma concentration; T$_{1/2\gamma}$, terminal phase half-life;Vd$_{ss}$, volume of distribution at steady-state.

into first-line treatment with a platinum compound in patients with suboptimally debulked stage III or IV ovarian cancer;the regimen demonstrated a survival advantage over standard treatment and received regulatory approval for this induction.[221,228] Regulatory approval was subsequently granted for patients with advanced breast cancer after failure of combination chemotherapy or at relapse within 6 months of adjuvant chemotherapy.[221,227] Recently, the combination of gemicitabine and paclitaxel demonstrated superior survival to paclitaxel alone in the first-line metastatic breast cancer setting, and received regulatory approval.[230] Additionally, regulatory approval for treating patients with stage II breast cancer following standard doxorubicin-based adjuvant chemotherapy after the early results of a phase 3 study suggested that the addition of the taxane conferred superior progression-free and overall survival;however, a survival advantage was not apparent with longer follow-up.[227,231] Intriguing results have been noted following treatment of patients with stage II breast cancer with alternative taxane-containing regimens, particularly "dose-dense" regimens, but randomized studies to determine the effects of these approaches on survival are being carried out.[227,231] Paclitaxel also received approval in the United States for second-line treatment of Kaposi's sarcoma associated with AIDS and in combination with cisplatin as primary treatment of non–small cell lung cancer.[233,234]

Although docetaxel initially received regulatory approval for the treatment of patients with metastatic breast cancer that progressed on or relapsed after anthracycline-based chemotherapy, the indication was next broadened to a general second-line indication and, more recently, as first-line chemotherapy for locally advanced or metastatic breast cancer in combination with capecitabine.[226,227] More recently, regulatory approval was granted for docetaxel's use in combination with cyclophosphamide and doxorubicin in the adjuvant treatment of patients with local breast cancer following definitive local treatment.[227] In non–small cell lung cancer, docetaxel initially received regulatory approval for treatment of unresectable, locally advanced or metastatic disease after demonstrating increased survival after failure of cisplatin-based therapy, and, more recently, regulatory approval was granted for docetaxel in combination with cisplatin as first-line treatment for such patients. Both paclitaxel and docetaxel have demonstrated notable activity in patients with hormone-refractory prostate cancer (HRPC) and regulatory approval was recently granted for docetaxel in combination with prednisone for this indication as the regimen has a survival advantage compared to mitoxantrone and prednisone.[235–237,239] It is important to note that the antitumor spectra for paclitaxel and docetaxel are identical, with activity noted in many other diverse cancers including head and neck, esophageal, gastric, endometrial, bladder, small cell lung, and germ cell carcinomas, and lymphoma and melanoma. The extent to which apparent differences in response rates, other end points, and regulatory indications granted between docetaxel and paclitaxel reflect differences in study design, dose, schedule, or inherent drug activities cannot be determined at this juncture.

Structures

The structures of paclitaxel, docetaxel, and their precursor 10-deacetylbaccatin III are shown in Figure 11.5. The taxanes are complex alkaloid esters, consisting of a 15-member taxane ring system linked to an unsualy four-member oxetane ring at positions C-4 and C-5.[238,239] The taxane rings of both paclitaxel and docetaxel, but not 10-deacetylbaccatin III, are linked to an ester at the C-13 position. Structure-function studies suggest that taxane

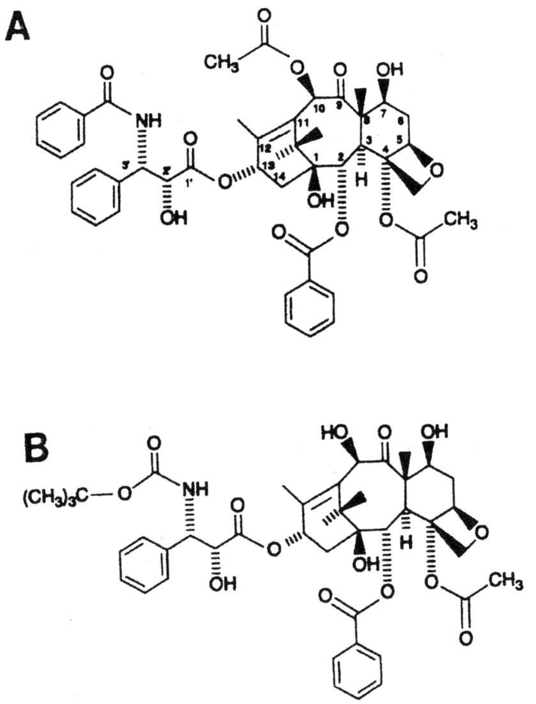

A

B

Figure 11.5 Structures of the taxanes: paclitaxel **(A)** and docetaxel **(B)**.

analogs without this ester linkage interact minimally with mammalian tubulin, although they still stabilize microtubules of the amoeba *Physarum polycephalum*. Furthermore, the moieties at the C-2′ and C-3′ positions are essential for the unqiue antimicrotubule action of the taxanes. Acetyl substitution at C-2′ results in a substantial loss of activity. Neither the acetyl group at C-10 nor the phenyl group at C-5′ are required for in vitro activity, and the structures of paclitaxel and docetaxel differ in linkages at these positions.[238,240]

Mechanisms of Action

The unique mechanism of action for paclitaxel was initially defined by Schif and colleagues[223,224] and Manfredi and colleagues[225] in 1979. The taxanes bind poorly to soluble tubulin, however, these agents bind directly and with high affinity to tubulin along the length of the microtubule. The binding sites are distinct from exchangeable GTP, colchicine, podophyllotoxin, and the vinca alkaloids, and the taxanes do not inhibit the binding of these agents to their respective sites. Photoaffinity studies have indicated that paclitaxel binds to the N-terminal 1-31 amino acids and residues 217-233 of the β-tubulin subunit, and the paclitaxel pharmacophore has been characterized.[240–242] Cystallographic models of the β-tubulin *N*-terminus indicate that His 227 and Asp 224 are critical to binding the C-2 benzoyl side chain of paclitaxel, and modeling data also indicate that both paclitaxel and docetaxel bind to the interior surface of the microtubule lumen.[7,243,244]

Other antimicrotubule natural products with similar mechanisms of action, such as the epothilones and eleutherobins, occupy the same binding sites, albeit with an altered core and side chain.[242,244] Paclitaxel binds reversibly to microtubules reassembled in vitro with high affinity (K_d, 10 nmol), whereas the binding affinity for docetaxel, which is slightly more water soluble, is approximately 1.9-fold higher.[2,3,4,7,225,246,247] It has been reported that tubulin assembly induced by docetaxel also proceeds with a critical protein concentration that is 2.1-fold lower than that of paclitaxel.[246] However, these differences, along with the higher potency of docetaxel, do not necessarily mean that docetaxel has a higher therapeutic index as greater potency may also portend more severe toxicity at identical drug concentrations in vivo. Furthermore, preclinical and clinical studies have been inconsistent about whether the taxanes are completely cross-resistant, possibly because these studies used dose schedules that are not equivalent.[249–251]

In contrast to the vinca alkaloids, the taxanes disrupt microtubule dynamics by reducing the critical tubulin concentration required for microtubule assembly and promoting both the nucleation and elongation phases of the polymerization reaction, which, in essence, stabilizes the microtubule against depolymerization and enhances polymerization.[2,3,5,18,30,32,223–225,251–255,257,258] Nevertheless, the vinca alkaloids and taxanes seem to produce similar disruptive effects on the spindle apparatus. Binding of the taxanes to their binding site on the inside of the microtubule stabilizes the microtubules and enhances tubulin polymerization, presumably by inducing a conformation change in tubulin, that, by an unknown mechanism, increases its affinity for neighboring tubulin molecules.[2] In essence, these actions profoundly alter the tubulin dissociation rate constants at each end of the microtubule without affecting the association rate constants, thereby suppressing both treadmilling and dynamic instability. There is one paclitaxel binding site on each tubulin molecule of the microtubule, and the ability of paclitaxel to enhance polymerization is associated with nearly 1:1 stoichiometric binding of paclitaxel to tubulin in microtubules. At submicromolar concentrations that are readily achieved in the clinic, binding is stoichiometric and tubulin polymerization is enhanced. However, substoichiometric concentrations suppress microtubule dynamics without increasing the amount of polymerized tubulin.[225,253] The taxanes induce tubulin self-assembly into microtubules in the cold and in the absence of exogenous GTP and MAPs, which are normally required for these processes[223–252] Furthermore, taxane-treated microtubules are highly stable, resisting depolymerization by cold, calcium ions, dilution, and depolymerizing agents. This stability inhibits the dynamic reorganization of the microtubule network, which is essential for many vital cell functions in mitosis and interphase.

The stoichiometry of taxane binding to microtubules in vitro greatly influences the nature of the perturbations of these agents on tubulin dynamics. Both stoichiometric and substoichiometric drug binding inhibit the proliferation of cells, principally by inducing a sustained mitotic block at the metaphase/anaphase boundary. At low concentrations (10 to 50 nmol/L), the binding of small numbers of paclitaxel molecules to microtubules reduce the rate and extent of microtubule shortening at their assembly (plus) ends.[2,3,18,27,252] At higher concentrations (10 to 100 nmol/L), however, paclitaxel preferentially suppresses tubulin dynamics and induces a modest increase in microtubule length at the plus ends with negligible effect on dynamics at the minus ends.[236] At paclitaxel concentrations ranging from 100 nmol/L to 1 μmol/L, which are readily achieved in cancer patients, growing and shortening rates are suppressed to the same extent, and microtubules remain in a state of attenuation. At very high concentrations (1 to 20 μmol/L), which are likely achieved intracellularly following administration of standard doses, the binding of paclitaxel to microtubules is saturated at a stoichiometry of 1 mole drug/mole tubulin, and the mass of microtubule polymer increases sharply as tubulin is recruited into the microtubules. In HeLa cells, mitosis is half-maximally blocked at 8 nmol/L paclitaxel, whereas polymer mass is half-maximally increased at 80 nmol/L, and there is no increase in microtubule polymer mass below 10 nmol/L.[251] The taxanes inhibit tubulin dissociation at both microtubule ends, but the ends remain free for tubulin addition.[208,256] The taxanes also inhibit microtubule treadmilling.[3,52] Most studies with docetaxel indicate that it suppresses tubulin dynamics similar to paclitaxel, but the structural aspects of abnormal microtubules induced by paclitaxel and docetaxel may differ. In one report, for example, paclitaxel induced the formation of microtubules with predominantly 12 protofilaments, whereas 13 protofilaments are usually evident in docetaxel-induced microtubules.[246]

The taxanes delay or block mitosis at the metaphase/anaphase boundary similar to the vinca alkaloids. At low concentrations (<10 nmol/L), mitosis is blocked with no concomitant increase in microtubule mass. Alterations in spindle organization also resemble those induced by the vinca alkaloids, suggesting that mitotic arrest is principally due to perturbations in microtubule dynamics. At higher concentrations (>100 nmol/L), microtubule mass is increased, mitosis is blocked, and large and dense spindle asters containing prominent bundles of stabilized microtubules are formed. With increasing taxane concentrations, the spindles become monopolar and the chromosomes condense, but do not congress.[18,224] Similar to the vinca alkaloids, even substoichiometric taxane concentrations, which are sufficient to induce mitotic arrest without increasing microtubule mass, may induce apoptosis (see "Drug Resistance, Taxanes").[219,32,259-269]

Although the precise mechanisms by which microtubule disturbances lead to apoptosis are not clear, the taxanes interact with numerous substances and regulatory molecules. Microtubule disruption induces the tumor suppressor gene *p53* and inhibitors of cyclin-dependent

kinases (e.g., p21/Waf-1), and modulates several protein kinases.[19,32,259-269] As a consequence, cells are arrested in G_2/M, after which time they may either undergo apoptosis or traverse through G_2/M and divide.[270] Several different mechanisms that potentially link the mitotic arrest induced by the taxanes and other antimicrotubule agents to the initiating event in the intrinsic pathway of apoptosis have been characterized. These initiating events include activation of the pro-apoptotic molecules Bax and Bad and inactivation of the antiapoptotic regulators Bcl-2 and Bcl_{xL}.[271-273] Various kinases have been implicated in the phosphorylation of Bcl-2 induced by the taxanes and other antimicrotubule agents, including Jun N-terminal kinase (JNK) and its proapoptitic effector Bim, c-Raf, extracellular signal regulated kinase (ERK) 1/2, cyclin-dependent kinase (CDK)-1, cAMP-dependent protein kinase A, and protein kinase Cα.[19,272] Phosphorylation (inactivation) of Bcl-2 family members and phosphorylation of pro-apoptotic molecules (activation) stimulate the intrinsic pathway of apoptosis and downstream effector caspases.[270,274] Although the precise mechanism by which Bcl-2 is inactivated following drug treatment has not been elucidated, paclitaxel has been shown to bind to the 'loop domain' of Bcl-2, but it does not appear that Bcl-2 phosphorylation plays a pre-eminent role in inducing apoptosis in all types of cancer.[275] The antimitotic effects of the taxanes and other antimicrotubule agents may be linked to apoptosis though other modulatory events such as the phosphorylation of the proapoptotic protein Bad by activating CDK1.[273]

The taxanes also perturb interphase microtubules in nonproliferating cells. Taxanes induce the formation of microtubule bundles, which resemble hoops and ribbons.[274] Paclitaxel has also been reported to induce transcription factors and enzymes that mediate proliferation, apoptosis, and inflammation.[262,273-275] The taxanes enhance the effects of ionizing radiation in vitro at clinically achievable concentrations (<50 nmol/L) and in vivo, which may related to the inhibition of cell-cycle progression in the G_2 phase, which is the most radiosensitive phase of the cell cycle.[276-282] In angiogenesis inhibition assays, they also inhibit parameters indicative of angiogenesis at concentrations below those that induce cytotoxicity, but the contribution of these effects on malignant angiogenesis to the overall antitumor actions of the taxanes is not clear.[283-285]

The taxanes have been demonstrated to induce many other cellular effects that may or may not relate to their disruptive effects on microtubule dynamics. Although the taxanes primarily block cell-cycle traverse in the mitotic phases, the agents prevents G_0 to S phase transition in both normal and malignant cells.[276,286] Explanations that have been proposed to account for the nonmitotic actions of the taxanes include disruptive effects on tubulin in the cell membrane, the interphase cytoskeleton, and microtubules that are involved in growth factor signaling.[17,287]

The taxanes also inhibit specific functions in nonmalignant tissues, which may be mediated through their disruptive effects on microtubule dynamics.[20] For example, paclitaxel inhibits relevant morphologic and biochemical processes in human neutrophils, including chemotaxis, migration, spreading, polarization, hydrogen peroxide generation, and killing of phagocytized microorganisms.[17] In addition, paclitaxel antagonizes the effects of microtubule-disrupting drugs on lymphocyte function and cAMP metabolism, and inhibits the proliferation of stimulated human lymphocytes.[17] Paclitaxel mimics the effects of endotoxic bacterial lipopolysaccharide on macrophages, which results in a rapid decrement in tumor necrosis factor-α (TNF-α) receptors and TNF-α release.[277,288] The agent also induces expression of the gene for TNF-α, but these activities are not related to paclitaxel's disruptive effects on microtubule assembly, which raises the issue of the role of cytokines in the antitumor activities of the taxanes.[277] Additionally, paclitaxel has been demonstrated to inhibit chorioretinal fibroblast proliferation and contractility in an in vitro model of proliferative vitreoretinopathy, as well as neointimal smooth muscle cell proliferation after angioplasty in a rat model.[289,290] Cardiac arterial stents coated with paclitaxel received regulatory approval in the United States and elsewhere in 2003 because of a significantly decreased incidence of restenosis from fibroblast proliferation and intimal hyperplasia.[291] Finally, paclitaxel inhibits secretory functions in many specialized cells, such as insulin secretion in isolated rat islets of Langerhans, protein secretion in rat hepatocytes, and the nicotinic receptor-stimulated release of catecholamines from chromaffin cells of the adrenal medulla.[17]

Mechanisms of Resistance

The MDR phenotype, which is mediated by several members of the ABC transporter family and confers cross-resistance to a wide range of xenobiotics (as discussed previously in "Mechanisms of Resistance, Vinca Alkaloids") is the best characterized mechanism of resistance to the taxanes. The most important ABC transporters with respect to conferring taxane resistance is P-gp or the *MDR1* encoded gene product MDR1 (ABC Subfamily B1;ABCB1) and MDR2 (ABC Subfamily ABCB4).[92,254,292] In contrast to the vinca alkaloids, ABCC1 (MRP1) and ABCC2 (MRP2) do not appear to be involved in taxane transport.[293,294] Low-level taxane resistance also appears to be conferred by the bile salt export protein (BSEP, also known as ABCC11).[92] Early clinical observations of the antitumor profile of the taxanes, particularly in women with breast cancer who respond to the taxanes following the development of progressive disease while receiving treatment with the anthracyclines, indicate that cross-resistance to the taxanes and anthracycline is incomplete, but the role of MDR as a major cause of anthracycline resistance is not clear. Similar to the vinca alkaloids, cells with taxane resistance and the MDR phenotype can be reversed by many classes of drugs, including the calcium channel blockers, tamoxifen, cyclosporine A, and antiarrhythmic agents.[92,295,296] In fact, plasma concentrations of the principal component of the vehicles used

to formulate paclitaxel and docetaxel, polyoxyethylated castor oil and polysorbate-80, respectively, can also reverse taxane resistance.[297,298] However, the plasma concentrations of polyoxyethylated castor oil achieved with paclitaxel on clinically relevant dose schedules are sufficient to reverse MDR, whereas sufficient modulatory concentrations of polysorbate-80 are not achieved with docetaxel. Strategies aimed at reversing taxane resistance with various transporter substrates in the clinic have resulted in low impact at best; however, the interpretation of these results is confounded by the effects of these agents, particularly those that are MDR substrates, on taxane clearance and toxicity.[295,296,298,299] Nevertheless, MDR modulators, including verapamil, cyclosporine A, VX-710, the nonimmunomodulatory cyclosporine analogue PSC 833, and other agents that do not affect taxane pharmacokinetics and toxicity, do not appear to significantly enhance antitumor activity.[92,296,299]

Several taxane-resistant mutant cell lines that have structurally altered α-tubulin and β-tubulin proteins and an impaired ability to polymerize into microtubules have been identified (discussed previously in "Mechanisms of Resistance, Vinca Alkaloids").[9,109–111,129,262,300–304] Mutants with "hypostable" microtubules exhibit collateral sensitivity to the vinca alkaloids. Paclitaxel-resistant Chinese hamster ovary cells with mutated β-tubulin alleles that encode the putative taxane binding sites, specifically, leucine moieties at positions 215, 217, and 228 mutated to histidine, arginine, or phenylalanine, have been described.[305,306] Low-level expression led to resistance, whereas high-level expression of any of these mutations caused impairment of assembly, cell-cycle arrest, and failure to proliferate.[306]

A number of cell lines resistant to tubulin-binding agents, including the taxanes, have been shown to have alterations in tubulin content, tubulin isotype profiles, and tubulin polymerization dynamics.[262,302,304,307,308] For example, paclitaxel-resistant tumors have been demonstrated to have significantly higher levels of class I, III, and IVa isotypes of β-tubulin.[19,112,304,309] Higher intratumoral levels of the β-III isotype, which is a minor component of cellular β-tubulin that increases the dynamic instability of microtubules, impedes microtubule assembly, and confers resistance to taxanes, has been demonstrated in tumor biopsies sampled from patients with taxane-resistant malignancies and cell lines with acquired drug resistance.[129,310] Further proof that β-III tubulin levels relate to taxane resistance is provided by experiments that demonstrate that antisense oligonucleotides to β-tubulin class III RNA decrease protein expression and increase drug sensitivity in taxane resistant cells.[311] Others have found that mutations affecting the β-tubulin class I genes lead to drug resistance.[19]

Mutations of tubulin isotype genes, gene amplifications, and isotype switching have also been reported in taxane-resistant cell lines.[109,262,263,303,306,308,312–314] Although clinical data from patients with non–small cell lung cancer indicate that mutations in β-tubulin are associated with taxane resistance, these observations have not been confirmed, and several reports have failed to demonstrate that β-tubulin to be a clinically relevant determinant of paclitaxel resistance in breast and ovarian cancers.[19,312,313] Furthermore, the positive findings may have been caused by amplification of pseudogenes.[19,312,313] Higher levels of class III β-tubulin RNA levels have also been reported in non–small cell lung cancers of patients who did not respond to taxance-based treatment, which is in line with in vitro findings.[315,316]

Growth factor signaling may contribute to taxane resistance by raising the cell's threshold for apoptosis induced by the taxanes and other antimicrotubule agents. For example, insulin-like growth factor I has been demonstrated to protect responsive breast cancer cell lines from anthracyclines and taxanes, possibly by activating the phosphatidylinositol 3-kinase (PI3K) pathway and inducing phosphorylation (inactivation) of antiapoptotic factors.[317] Other mediators that may influence the cell's threshold for drug-induced apoptosis include p53, erbB2, auora 2-kinase, survivin, and BRAC1. The centromere-associated serine/threonine kinase, aurora 2-kinase, which is involved in centrosome separation, biopolar spindle formation, and chromosomal kinetochore attachment to the mitotic spindle, appears to override the mitotitc assembly checkpoint and induce taxane resistance.[19] In addition, the overexpresssion of survivin, a member of the inhibitor of apoptosis family of proteins, inhibits caspase activity and apoptosis induced by antimicrotubule agents.[19] The disruption of the tumor-suppressor gene, BRAC1, which is implicated in maintaining genomic stability through DNA repair and involved in hereditary breast and ovarian cancers, appears to play a role in conferring resistance to paclitaxel and the inducible expression of BRAC1 may enhance paclitaxel-induced apoptosis.[19] The mutational loss of the p53 tumor suppressor does not confer resistance to paclitaxel and other microtubule polymerizing agents in contrast to DNA disruptive agents.[19] Also, there was no relationship evident between paclitaxel sensitivity and p53 status in the National Cancer Institute's 60-tumor type-specific drug screening panel.[19] Additionally, cells lacking wild-type p53 display increased sensitivity to paclitaxel.[19] MAPs have been implicated in mechanisms of resistance to apoptosis induced by the taxanes and other antimicrotubule agents, as illustrated by the observation that MAP4, which is negatively regulated by wild-type *p53*, increases sensitivity to paclitaxel.[318,319] The suppression of dynamic instability by low concentrations of microtubule polymerizing agents may also enhance the nuclear accumulation of p53 and the induction of proapoptotic p53–up-regulated modulator of apoptosis.[19] This may represent a p53-dependent mechanism of apoptosis induced by antimicrotubule agents in cells that harbor functional p53.[19] Finally, overexpression of p21, a downstream effector of p53, appears to impede cell cycle traverse in G_2, thereby blocking progression into the more drug-vulnerable mitotic phase and decreasing taxane sensitivity.[320,321]

Transfection of cells with erbB-2, a member of the epidermal growth factor receptor family that is amplified and overexpressed in approximately 30% of breast cancers, increases taxane resistance, and high expression of erbB-2 in vitro relates to taxane resistance.[322,323] Overexpression of erbB2 can also inhibit CDK1 either by inducing p21, which participates in the G2/M checkpoint and contributes to resistance to apoptosis induced by antimicrotubule agents, or directly phosphorylating (inactivating) CDK1, which may block taxane-mediated entry into mitosis and apoptosis.[19] Consistent with this relationship, down-regulation of erbB2 by the anti–erbB2 antibody trastuzimab sensitizes breast cancer cells to the taxanes, and the treatment of women with erbB2 overexpressing breast cancer with traztuzimab combined with paclitaxel increases survival compared to paclitaxel alone.[322,324] Nevertheless, the presence of *erbB2* amplification was demonstrated not to adversely influence response to first-line chemotherapy with either epirubicin-paclitaxel or epirubicin-cyclophosphamide.[325] Furthermore, the taxane-containing regimen may preferentially benefit women with erbB2-expressing breast cancer.

Clinical Pharmacology

Analytical Assays

The earliest analytical assays used to measure paclitaxel concentrations in biologic samples were biochemical assays that exploited the ability of paclitaxel to induce tubulin to form cold-resistant polymers that hydrolyze GTP at 0°C;however, such as assays lacked requisite sensitivitiy (0.1 μmol/L) to measure low plasma concentrations achieved in clinical trials and were too cumbersome for monitoring large numbers of clinical samples.[326] Immunologic assays, including indirect competitive inhibition enzyme immunoassays and ELISAs that were developed for detecting taxanes in plant extracts were highly sensitive (0.3 nmol/L) and amenable to high-throughput procedures, but the degree of cross-reactivity of the antibodies to the taxanes, their metabolites, and other moieties are not known.[327] The earliest chromatographic separation methods, including HPLC with ultraviolet detection, had variable extraction efficiencies, suboptimal lower limits of sensitivity (≥50 nmol/L), and other assay performance characteristics, which rendered them inadequate for monitoring plasma levels in patients receiving low doses or prolonged infusions. More sensitive HPLC assays, particularly those using tandem mass spectroscopy and solid phase extraction, can detect paclitaxel and docetaxel concentrations in the low nanomolar to picomolar range in minute quanties of plasma ((0.05 mL) and several are capable of simultaneously measuring metabolites.[298,328,329]

Pharmacokinetics

The oral bioavailability of both paclitaxel and docetaxel is poor, owing in part to the constitutive overexpression of

P-gp and other ABC transporters by enterocytes and/or first-pass metabolism in the liver and/or intestines. Nevertheless, biologically relevant plasma concentrations can be achieved if the taxanes are administered orally with oral modulators of ABC transporters and/or cytochrome P-450 mixed-function oxidases such as cyclosporin.[298,330] Rapid, avid, and protracted drug distribution and binding to all tissues except for central nervous system tissue result in large volumes of distribution, high clearance rates, short distribution $t_{1/2}$ values, and long terminal $t_{1/2}$ values.

Paclitaxel

The pharmacokinetics of paclitaxel on both long and short administration schedules have been characterized (Table 3). In early studies that principally evaluated prolonged (6- and 24-hour) schedules, substantial interpatient variability was noted, and nonlinear, dose-dependent behavior was not observed.[330] In these studies, drug disposition was characterized as a biphasic process, with values for alpha and beta $t_{1/2}$ values averaging 20 minutes and 6 hours, respectively. However, more recent studies of shorter administration schedules, especially a 3-hour infusion, indicate that the pharmacokinetic behavior of paclitaxel is nonlinear.[298,331–334] Nonlinearity occurs with all administration schedules, but it is more apparent with shorter infusions that result in higher plasma paclitaxel concentrations that more saturate both drug elimination and tissue distribution processes. Both saturable distribution and elimination may be, in part, responsible for paclitaxel's nonlinear behavior. Tissue distribution becomes saturated at lower drug concentrations (achieved with paclitaxel doses <175 mg/m^2 over 3 hours) compared with elimination processes that are effectively saturated at higher concentrations (achieved with paclitaxel doses >175 mg/m^2 over 3 hours). The use of shorter infusion schedules also results in higher plasma concentrations of paclitaxel's polyoxyethylated castor oil vehicle, which may be responsible for an appearance of nonlinearity, termed pseudononlinearity.[335, 336] A true nonlinear profile may have several important clinical implications, particularly regarding dose modifications at doses associated with nonlinearity because dose escalation may result in a disproportionate increase in drug exposure and hence toxicity, whereas dose reductions may result in a disproportionate decrease in drug exposure, thereby decreasing antitumor activity. Interestingly, shorter paclitaxel infusion schedules are also associated with reduced clearance of the polyoxyethylated castor oil vehicle and reduced exposure to unbound paclitaxel, which may explain the lower incidence of hematologic toxicity and higher incidence of hypersensitivity reactions with shorter infusions.[337]

The volume of distribution of paclitaxel is much larger than that of total body water, which is likely the result of extensive drug distribution and binding to plasma proteins and other tissue elements, particularly tubulin. In addition,

plasma protein binding is high (>95%) and readily reversible.[298] At clinically-relevant concentrations (0.1 to 0.6 μmol/L), protein binding is concentration-independent, which may be attributable to nonspecific hydrophobic binding. Despite extensive binding to plasma proteins, paclitaxel is readily eliminated from the plasma compartment, a finding that suggests lower-affinity, reversible binding. Albumin and α_1-acid glycoprotein contribute equally to the binding, with a minor contribution from lipoproteins.[338,339] None of the drugs that are commonly administered with paclitaxel, including ranitidine, dexamethasone, diphenhydramine, doxorubicin, 5-fluorouracil, and cisplatin, appear to substantially alter protein binding.[338] Drug binding to platelets is extensive and saturable, whereas binding to red blood cells is insignificant.[368] Animal distribution studies with radiolabeled paclitaxel indicate extensive drug uptake and retention by virtually all tissues, except "tumor sanctuary sites" such as the central nervous system and testes.[340]

In addition, clearance is significantly related to body surface area, providing a rationale for dosing based on this measurement.[341] In humans, peak plasma concentrations achieved with 3- to 96- hour infusions (>0.05 to 10 μmol/L) and drug concentrations in third-space fluid collections, such as ascites (>0.1 μmol/L), are capable of inducing significant biologic effects in vitro, but drug penetration into the unperturbed central nervous system is negligible.[298,331–334,336,337,341]

Paclitaxel disposition occurs predominately by cytochrome P-450 mixed function oxidase metabolism in the liver followed by the excretion of both paclitaxel and metabolites into the bile.[330,331 342–347] Ninety-eight percent of radioactivity is recovered from feces collected for 6 days after rats are treated with radiolabeled paclitaxel, and approximately 71% of an administered dose of paclitaxel is excreted in the feces over 5 days as either parent compound or metabolites in humans, with 6α- hydroxypaclitaxel being the largest component and accounting for 26% of the dose. Only 5% is unchanged paclitaxel. Renal clearance of paclitaxel and metabolites is minimal, accounting for 14% of the administered dose.[298] In humans, cytochrome P-450 mixed-function oxidases, specifically the isoenzymes CYP2C8 and CYP3A4, are responsible for the bulk of drug disposition. All human paclitaxel metabolites that have been identified are hydroxylated derivatives with intact side chains at taxane ring positions C-2 and C-13, whereas low concentrations of baccatin III, which lacks the side chain at position C-13, are found in rat bile.[343,348] The major metabolites in human plasma and bile include 6α- hydroxypaclitaxel, a product of CYP2C8;p-hydroxyphenyl-C3'-paclitaxel, a product of CYP3A4;and a dihydroxymetabolite (6α- and C3'-dihydroxypaclitaxel). There is considerable interindividual variability in the qualitative and quantitative aspects of taxane metabolism, which can be attributed to pharmacogenetic differences in P-450 metabolism and concurrent medications that variably alter metabolism.[298,334,346,348] The metabolites are much less active against L1210 leukemia than paclitaxel, but several are as active as paclitaxel in stabilizing microtubules against disassembly in a cell-free system. One possible explanation for this discrepancy is that the cell does not take up these hydroxylated metabolites, which are more polar than paclitaxel.

Several pharmacokinetic parameters indicative of drug exposure have been related to the various principal toxicities of paclitaxel, the most important of which is the relationship between the severity of neutropenia and the duration of drug exposure above biologically relevant plasma concentrations ranging from 0.05 to 0.1 μmol/L.[298,331,333,334,347,349] However, a prospective analysis of pharmacokinetic determinants of outcome in patients with advanced non–small cell lung cancer treated with cisplatin combined with paclitaxel at either 135 or 250 mg/m^2 over 24 hours showed that the magnitude of the steady-state plasma paclitaxel concentration correlated poorly with antitumor activity, disease-free survival, and overall survival.[350] In randomized trials evaluating the effects of paclitaxel dose on outcome in patients with advanced ovarian, non–small cell lung, breast, and head and neck, doses above 175 mg/m^2 resulted in neither increased progression-free or overall survival

Docetaxel

The pharmacokinetics of docetaxel on a 1-hour schedule are linear at doses of 115 mg/m^2 or less and optimally fit a three-compartment model.[226,351–357] Terminal $t_{1/2}$ values ranging from 11.1 to 18.5 hours have been reported. In one population study, plasma concentration data were optimally fit by a three-compartment model, and the following pharmacokinetic parameters were generated: $t_{1/2\gamma}$ of 12.4 hours, clearance of 1 L/hr per square meter, and steady-state volume of distribution of 74 L/m^2.[354,355,357] The most important determinants of docetaxel clearance were the body surface area, hepatic function, and plasma α1–acid glycoprotein concentration, whereas age and albumin level had significant influences on clearance. As with paclitaxel, plasma protein binding is high (>85 to 95%), and binding is primarily to α1–acid glycoprotein, albumin, and lipoproteins.[226,351–357] Higher free fraction values relate to low α1–acid glycoprotein concentrations and may portend greater toxicity. As with paclitaxel, docetaxel is widely distributed and avidly bound in all tissues except the central nervous system.[355,357,358] In both dogs and mice treated with radiolabeled drug, fecal excretion accounts for 70 to 80% of total radioactivity, whereas urinary excretion accounts for 10% or less.[385,387] In rats and dogs, tissue-distribution studies using [^{14}C]docetaxel have demonstrated a rapid initial distribution phase of plasma radioactivity with an apparent $t_{1/2}$ of 10 minutes.[355] In mice, autoradiographic studies indicate that docetaxel rapidly accumulates in almost all tissues except for the central nervous

system.[355] Immediately after treatment, tissue uptake of radioactivity is highest in the liver, bile, and intestines, a finding that is consistent with substantial hepatobiliary extraction and excretion. High levels of radioactivity are also found in the stomach, which indicates the possibility of gastric excretion, as well as in the spleen, bone marrow, myocardium, skeletal muscles, and pancreas.

The hepatic cytochrome P-450 mixed-function oxidase isoenzyme CYP3A, the activity of which, in adults, is represented by the combined activities of CYP3A4, CYP3A5, CYP3A7, and CYP3A43 is responsible for the bulk of docetaxel metabolism.[386,387,390] However, CYP3A4, and CYP3A5, to a lesser extent, confer the highest relative contributions to overall CYP3A activity and are primarily involved in biotransformation that, in contrast to paclitaxel, principally affects the C13 side chain and not the taxane ring.[359–361] CYP2B, and CYP1A also appear to play major roles in biotransformation. The main metabolic pathway consists of oxidation of the tertiary butyl group on the side chain at the C-13 position of the taxane ring, as well as cyclization of the side chain all metabolites appear to maintain their 10-deacetylbaccatin III or 7-epi isomer structural backbones. These metabolites seem to be much less active than docetaxel.

The main pharmacokinetic determinants of toxicity, particularly the principal toxicity neutropenia, are drug exposure and the time that plasma concentrations exceed biologically relevant concentrations.[357,359–361] A population pharmacodynamic analysis of determinants of outcome in phase 2 trials of docetaxel in patients with metastatic breast cancer revealed that the most important positive determinants of a response and progression-free survival are low pretreatment plasma concentration of α1–acid glycoprotein, number of prior chemotherapeutic regimens, and number of disease sites, whereas both drug exposure and the pretreatment plasma concentration of α1–acid glycoprotein were strong positive determinants of time to progression in patients with advanced lung cancer.[352] Conversely, the pretreatment plasma level of α1–acid glycoprotein was negatively, albeit significantly, related to the probability of experiencing both severe neutropenia and febrile neutropenia. α1–Acid glycoprotein has also been demonstrated to be a principal determinant of interindividual variability in docetaxel clearance and one of the main predictors of docetaxel clearance.[298,352]

Drug Interactions

Both sequence-dependent pharmacokinetic and toxicologic interactions between paclitaxel and several other chemotherapy agents have been noted, but the number of clinically significant drug-drug interactions has been surprisingly low in light of the importance of cytochrome P-450 pathways in drug disposition.[298,362] The sequence of cisplatin followed by paclitaxel (24-hour schedule) induces more profound neutropenia than the reverse sequence, which is explained by a 33% reduction in the clearance of paclitaxel after cisplatin.[362-364] The least toxic sequence—paclitaxel before cisplatin—was demonstrated to induce more cytotoxicity in vitro;therefore, this drug sequence was selected for clinical development.[362-364] As expected, however, sequence dependence does not appear to be a clinically relevant phenomenon on shorter schedules. Treatment with paclitaxel on either a 3- or 24-hour schedule followed by carboplatin was demonstrated to produce equivalent neutropenia and less thrombocytopenia as compared with carboplatin as a single agent, which is not explained by pharmacokinetic interactions.[365,366] Although sequence dependence has not been noted with combinations of carboplatin and paclitaxel, which induce less thrombocytopenia than comparable single-agent doses of carboplatin, other paclitaxel-based chemotherapy combinations, most notably those involving the anthracyclines, are associated with this phenomena.[362-367] Both neutropenia and mucositis are more severe when paclitaxel on a 24-hour schedule is administered before doxorubicin, compared with the reverse sequence, which is most likely caused by an approximately 32% reduction in the clearance rates of both doxorubicin and doxorubicinol when doxorubicin is administered after paclitaxel.[368,369] Although neither sequence-dependent pharmacologic interactions nor toxicologic interactions between doxorubicin and paclitaxel on a shorter (3-hour) schedule have been noted, pharmacologic interactions occur with both sequences, and combined treatment with paclitaxel (3-hour schedule) and doxorubicin as a bolus infusion has been associated with a higher incidence of cardiotoxicity than would have been expected from an equivalent cumulative doxorubicin dose given without paclitaxel (see "Cardiac").[368-370] The precise etiology for these interactions is unclear. The pharmacokinetic interactions may not be of sufficient magnitude to account for the enhanced cardiotoxicity of the combination and there are experimental data indicating that paclitaxel enhances the metabolism of doxorubicin to cardiotoxic metabolites, such as doxorubicinol, in cardiomyoctes.[370] Docetaxel does not appear to influence doxorubicin pharmacokinetics, but there are experimental data suggesting that, as with paclitaxel, docetaxel can enhance the metabolism of doxorubicin to toxic species in the human heart.[370] Similar decrements in the clearance of epirubicin and its metabolites have been noted in studies of paclitaxel combined with epirubicin, but cardiotoxicity does not appear to be enhanced.[371] Competition for the hepatic or biliary P-gp transport of the anthracyclines with paclitaxel or its polyoxyethylated castor oil vehicle (or both) is an alternate explanation.[297,349,362] Interestingly, similar effects have not been noted with docetaxel, which is not formulated in polyoxyethylated castor oil. Hematologic toxicity has also been more profound with the sequence of cyclophosphamide before paclitaxel (24-hour schedule) than the reverse sequence.[372] In human tumor xenografts, both paclitaxel and docetaxel have been demonstrated to induce thymidine phosphorylase activity, which may increase the metabolic activation of the oral fluoropyrimidine prodrug capecitabine.[373]

Drug interactions may also result from the effects of other classes of drugs on the cytochrome P-450–dependent metabolism of the taxanes. Various inducers of cytochrome P-450 mixed-function oxidases, such as the anticonvulsants phenytoin and phenobarbital, accelerate the metabolism of both paclitaxel and docetaxel in human microsomes in vitro and in both children and adults who are concurrently receiving treatment with these anticonvulsants, as manifested by rapid drug clearance and tolerance of high drug doses.[277,298,343-346,359,360,362,374-377] There is preclinical evidence to suggest that docetaxel has markedly reduced propensity to cause drug interactions that may entail hepatic CYP3A4 induction.[378] Conversely, many types of agents that inhibit cytochrome P-450 mixed-function oxidases, such as orphenadrine, erythromycin, cimetidine, testosterone, ketoconazole, fluconazole, midazolam, polyoxyethylated castor oil, and corticosteroids, interfere with the metabolism of paclitaxel and docetaxel in human microsomes in vitro;however, the inhibitory concentrations of these agents exceed those achieved in clinical practice, and the clinical relevance of these findings is not known.[27,298,359,343-346,359,360,374-377] With regard to potential interactions between ketoconazole and the taxanes, inconsistent conclusions have been reached although docetaxel exposure has been demonstrated to be increased in a high proportion of patients receiving concurrent ketoconazole.[379] Besides the potent inhibitors of CYP3A listed previously, other well-established inhibitors and inducers of CYP3A, including grapefruit juice and herbal products (e.g., St. John's wort and Echinacea), may potentially induce pharmacokinetic interactions with the taxanes. Although there has been concern that the use of different H_2-receptor antagonists with variable cytochrome P-450 inhibitory activities as components of premedication regimens may differentially affect drug clearance and hence toxicity, neither toxicologic nor pharmacologic differences between the agents were noted in a randomized clinical trial.[380] As previously discussed (see "Pharmacokinetics"), the considerable interindividual variability in the relative amounts of paclitaxel metabolites may, in part, be the result of isoenzyme activity and induction or inhibition as a result of drug interactions.[346,348,376] For example, prolonged treatment with corticosteroids induces CYP3A4 and leads to increased dihydroxypaclitaxel, whereas biricodar, an inhibitor of MDR-1 and multidrug resistance protein, inhibits the same enzyme, delays clearance, and significantly lowers the maximum tolerated dosage.[296,348] In addition, interactions between warfarin and the taxanes, possibly because of protein binding displacement effects, have been reported.[381]

Concern has also arisen that H_2-histamine antagonist premedications may be an important source of drug interactions. Use of these agents with the taxanes may produce variable pharmacologic and toxicologic effects because these agents differentially inhibit cytochrome P-450 metabolism, with cimetidine being the most potent inhibitor. However, H_2 histamine antagonists do not appear to alter the metabolism and pharmacologic disposition of the taxanes in animal and in vitro studies.[382,383] In addition, the results of a clinical trial in which patients were randomized to receive either cimetidine or famotidine premedication before their first course of paclitaxel and then crossed over to the alternate premedication during their second course have failed to show significant toxicologic and pharmacologic differences between these H_2 histamine antagonists.[380]

Dose and Schedule

Paclitaxel

The development of effective premedication regimens associated with a decreased incidence of major hypersensitivity reactions led to evaluations of paclitaxel on a broad range of schedules. Although paclitaxel, 135 mg/m^2 over 24 hours was initially approved for patients with refractory and recurrent ovarian cancer, regulatory approval was subsequently obtained for paclitaxel, 175 mg/m^2 on a 3-hour schedule. In patients with advanced breast and ovarian cancers, the cumulative body of randomized study results indicates that both schedules are equivalent, particularly with regard to event-free survival and overall survival, although response rates have occasionally been higher with the 24-hour infusion. However, weekly "dose-dense" regimens have also been associated with intriguing activity.[231,384–389]

Based on in vitro studies, which indicated that the duration of exposure above a biologically relevant threshold is one of the most important determinants of cytotoxicity, more protracted infusion schedules were evaluated.[221,384] Although intriguing results were initially obtained with a 96-hour infusion schedule in patients with advanced breast cancer and non-Hodgkin's lymphoma, there is no clear evidence that protracted schedules are superior to shorter schedules with regard to efficacy, and toxicities, particularly myelosuppression and mucositis, appear to more somewhat greater.[384,386,388,389,390] The lack of clearly superior results with protracted schedules in vivo is likely because of the extensive and rapid distribution of the taxanes to peripheral tissues and, more importantly, the avid and protracted tissue binding of these agents, whereas the agents are washed out from cells in tissue culture. There has also been considerable interest in intermittent schedules, particularly those in which paclitaxel is administered as a 1-hour infusion weekly, which results in substantially less myelosuppression than every 3-week schedules.[231,385,387,391,392] Furthermore, there have been reports of impressive and superior activity of weekly compared with every 3-week schedules in several disease settings, particularly in treatment of metastatic breast cancer patients.[387,393]

However, there is no convincing evidence that weekly treatment results in robust activity in tumors unresponsive to the taxanes on every 3-week schedules. Nevertheless, the weekly schedule may be advantageous for patients who are at high risk of developing severe myelosuppression, but there appears to be a higher incidence of neuromuscular effects. Paclitaxel is generally administered every 3 weeks at a dose of 175 mg/m^2 over 3 hours. Alternatively, 135 to 175 mg/m^2 over 24 hours every 3 weeks is a less common dose-schedule. Several phase 3 studies in patients with advanced lung, head and neck, ovarian, and breast cancers have consistently failed to show that paclitaxel doses greater than 135 to 175 mg/m^2 on a 24-hour schedule or greater than 175 mg/m^2 on a 3-hour schedule confer superior efficacy than conventional doses.[384,394,395] The following doses have been recommended on less conventional schedules: 200 mg/m^2 over 1 hour as either a single dose or three divided doses every 3 weeks;140 mg/m^2 over 96 hours every 3 weeks;and 80 to 100 mg/m^2 weekly. The most common schedules evaluated in patients with AIDS-associated Kaposi's sarcoma are paclitaxel, 135 mg/m^2 over 3 or 24 hours every 3 weeks, and 100 mg/m^2 every 2 weeks.[396] Following intracavitary administration, paclitaxel concentrations in the peritoneal and pleural cavities are several orders of magnitude greater than plasma concentrations, which are biologically relevant, and the results of a single randomized trial indicate that the administration of intraperitoneal paclitaxel in conjuction with carboplatin and paclitaxel administered intravenously confers a survival advantage in previously untreated women with optimally debulked advanced ovarian cancer.[397–399]

The following premedication is recommended to prevent major hypersensitivity reactions: dexamethasone, 20 mg orally or intravenously, 12 and 6 hours before treatment;an H_1-receptor antagonist (such as diphenhydramine, 50 mg intravenously) 30 minutes before treatment;and an H_2-receptor antagonist (such as cimetidine, 300 mg;famotidine, 20 mg;or ranitidine, 150 mg intravenously) 30 minutes before treatment. A single dose of a corticosteroid (dexamethasone, 20 mg intravenously) administered 30 minutes before treatment also appears to confer somewhat effective prophylaxis of major hypersensitivity reactions, however, the relative merits of this schedule is not known.[400,401] Contact of paclitaxel with plasticized polyvinyl chloride equipment or devices must be avoided because of the risk of patient exposures to plasticizers that may be leached from polyvinyl chloride infusion bags or sets. Paclitaxel solutions should be diluted and stored in glass or polypropylene bottles or suitable plastic bags (polypropylene or polyolefin) and administered through polyethylene-lined administration sets that include an in-line filter with a microporous membrane not greater than 0.22 μm.

The extensive involvement of hepatic metabolism and biliary excretion in the disposition of paclitaxel, similar to that of other anticancer drugs, such as the vinca alkaloids, in which dose modifications are required indicates that doses should be modified in patients with hepatic dysfunction. Although official recommendations have not been formulated, prospective evaluations indicate that patients with moderate-to-severe elevations in serum concentrations of hepatocellular enzymes or bilirubin (or both) are more likely to develop severe toxicity than patients without hepatic dysfunction.[402,403] Therefore, it is prudent to reduce paclitaxel doses by at least 50% in patients with moderate or severe hepatic excretory dysfunction (hyperbilirubinemia) or significant elevations in hepatic transaminases. Renal clearance contributes minimally to overall clearance (5 to 10%), and even patients with severe renal dysfunction do not appear to require dose modification.[404] Based on the pharmacologic behavior, particularly the wide distributive properties of the taxanes, dose modifications are not required solely for peripheral edema and third-space fluid collections.

Docetaxel

Docetaxel is most commonly administered at a dose of 75 mg/m^2 over 1 hour every 3 weeks but regulatory approval was granted in the United States for a dose range of 60 to 100 mg/m^2 over 1 hour in patients with breast and non–small cell lung cancers, respectively;much less data are available for patients treated at 60 mg/m^2.[226,405] The most common dose schedule of docetaxel used as a single-agent and in combination regimens is 75 mg/m^2 over 1 hour. Although some untreated or minimally pretreated patients generally tolerate docetaxel at a dose of 100 mg/m^2 without severe toxicity, tolerance is poorer in more heavily pretreated patients in whom 75 mg/m^2 is a much more reasonable from a toxicologic perspective.[405] Hematologic toxicity is much less than with conventional dose schedules; however, weekly administration schedules have been associated with a higher incidence of cumulative asthenia and neurotoxicity, particularly with docetaxel doses exceeding 36 mg/m^2 per week.[391,392] Despite the use of a polysorbate 80 formulation instead of polyoxyethylated castor oil, which is used to formulate paclitaxel, an unacceptably high rate of major hypersensitivity reactions and profound fluid retention in patients who did not receive premedication has led to the development of several effective premedication regimens, the most popular of which is dexamethasone, 8 mg orally twice daily for 3 or 5 days starting 1 or 2 days, respectively, before docetaxel, with or without both H$_1$-receptor and H$_2$-receptor antagonists given 30 minutes before docetaxel.[406,407]

In a retrospective review of docetaxel pharmacokinetics and toxicity in patients without hyperbilirubinemia, clearance was reduced by approximately 25% in patients with elevations in serum concentrations of both hepatic transaminases (1.5-fold or greater) and alkaline phosphatase (2.5-fold or greater), regardless of whether the elevations are the result of hepatic metastases.[352,353] Therefore,

dose reductions by at least 25% are recommended for such patients. However, greater dose reductions (50% or greater) may be required in patients who have moderate or severe hepatic excretory dysfunction (hyperbilirubinemia).[402] As with paclitaxel (discussed previously in "Dose, and Schedule, Paclitaxel"), there is no rationale for dose modification solely for renal deficiency or third-space fluid accumulation (or both). Also similar to the case with paclitaxel, glass bottles or polypropylene or polyolefin plastic products should be used for preparation and storage, and docetaxel should be administered through polyethylene-lined administration sets.

Toxicity

Despite having similar structural features, the toxicity spectra of paclitaxel and docetaxel do not completely overlap. Myelosuppression, primarily neutropenia, is the principal toxicity of both agents, but the types and frequencies of several nonhematologic side effects are different.

Paclitaxel

Hematologic

Neutropenia is the principal toxicity of paclitaxel. The onset is usually on days 8 to 10, and recovery is generally complete by days 15 to 21 on every 3-week dosing regimens. A critical pharmacologic determinant of the severity of neutropenia is the duration that plasma drug concentrations are maintained above biologically relevant levels (0.05 to 0.1 μmol/L as discussed earlier in "Pharmacokinetics"), which may explain why neutropenia is more severe with more protracted infusions.[331,332,347] This does not imply that shorter infusions should always be used, because the optimal dose and schedule have not been determined for clinical settings. Instead, the results of randomized clinical studies do not indicate that there is an optimal schedule for any particular tumor, although treatment with higher doses or "equitoxic doses" should be considered if shorter schedules are used.[384] Notwithstanding these differences, the main clinical determinant of the severity of neutropenia is the extent of prior myelotoxic therapy.

Neutropenia is noncumulative, and the duration of severe neutropenia, even in heavily pretreated patients, is usually brief. At paclitaxel doses exceeding 175 mg/m^2 on a 24-hour schedule and 225 mg/m^2 on a 3-hour schedule, nadir neutrophil counts are typically less than 500/μL for fewer than 5 days in most courses, even in untreated patients. Even patients who have received extensive prior therapy can usually tolerate paclitaxel doses of 175 to 200 mg/m^2 over 3 or 24 hours. More frequent administration schedules, particularly weekly treatment schedules with doses of 80 to 100 mg/m^2, are associated with less severe neutropenia and at least equivalent or greater antitumor activity in a number of tumor types, as compared with single-dose schedules (see "Dose, and Schedule"). Severe effects on platelets and red blood cells are unusual, except in heavily pretreated patients.

Hypersensitivity

The incidence of major hypersensitivity reactions (HSRs) in early trials was approximately 30%, but declined to 1 to 3% following development of effective prophylaxis.[221,408-410] Major reactions, which are characterized by dyspnea with bronchospasm, urticaria, hypotension, chest, abdominal and backpain, usually occur within the first 10 minutes after the first (and less frequently after the second) treatment and resolve completely after stopping treatment and occasionally occur after treatment with antihistamines, fluids, and vasopressors. Patients who have major reactions have been rechallenged successfully after receiving high doses of corticosteroids, but this approach has not always been successful.[411-413] Rechallenge appears to be most successful in patients who experience severe hypersensitivity manifestations within minutes of starting treatment, if the infusion is immediately discontinued, and if treatment resumes within approximately 30 minutes, which is likely the result of profound and persistent depletion of histamines and other mediators at the time of rechallenge.[411-413] Although the incidence of minor hypersensitivity reactions (HSRs), such as flushing and rash, is about 40%, major reactions do not generally occur after minor HSRs. Based on the resemblence of the HSRs to those caused by radio-contrast dyes, they are probably caused by a nonimmunologically mediated release of histamine or other vasoactive substances, owing to the taxane moiety or, more likely, its polyoxyethylated castor oil vehicle, possibly through complement activation.[414] The vehicle is the suspected culprit because it induces histamine release and similar manifestations in dogs, and other drugs formulated in it, such as cyclosporine A and vitamin K, induce similar reactions. Although the incidence of major HSRs is reduced with lower administration rates and longer infusion durations, the rates of major HSRs are low on both 3- and 24-hour schedules when patients are premedicated with corticosteroids and both H_1-receptor and H_2-receptor antagonists (see "Administration, Dose, and Schedule").[409] In an assessment of the relative safety of two different paclitaxel schedules (3- and 24-hour infusions), the rates of major reactions were low and similar (2.1% versus 1.0%) with premedication.

Peripheral Neurotoxicity

Paclitaxel induces a peripheral neuropathy characterized by sensory symptoms, such as numbness in a symmetric glove-and-stocking distribution.[242,408,415-417] The most common findings on neurologic examination loss are of sensation and deep tendon reflexes. Neurophysiologic studies support a primary disruption of neuronal microtubules resulting in axonal degeneration and demyelination as the primary pathogenic mechanism;however, manifestations suggestive of microtubule disruption resulting in a neuronopathy may be noted, particularly at higher doses or when combined with other neurotoxic agents.[242,408,415-417] Severe neurotoxicity is uncommon when paclitaxel is given alone at doses below 200 mg/m^2 on a 3- or 24-hour schedule every 3 weeks or below 100 mg/m^2 on a continuous weekly schedule, but almost all "low-risk" patients experience mild or moderate effects. Patients with preexisting neuropathy caused by prior exposure to other neurotoxic agents, diabetes mellitus, congenital conditions, or alcholism, even when manifestations are subclinical, are more prone to paclitaxel-induced neuropathy. Symptoms may begin as soon as 24 to 72 hours after treatment with higher doses ($\geq$250 mg/m^2) but usually occur only after multiple courses at 135 to 250 mg/m^2 every 3 weeks. Neurotoxicity is generally more pronounced when paclitaxel is administered on short infusion schedules, indicating that peak plasma concentration is a principal determinant. The combination of paclitaxel on a 3-hour schedule and cisplatin is particularly neurotoxic, and regimens consisting of paclitaxel and carboplatin produce less neurotoxicity than paclitaxel-cisplatin regimens. Motor and autonomic dysfunction may occur, especially at high doses and in patients with preexisting neuropathies caused by diabetes mellitus and alcoholism. Glutamate has been reported to reduce the severity of peripheral neuropathy from high doses of paclitaxel. Anecdotal reports, experimental models, and/or insufficiently powered randomized trials have suggested that the sulfahydryl group scavenger drugs, pyridoxine, and anticonvulsants reduce the neurotoxic effects of paclitaxel, but there is no convincing evidence that any specific measure is effective at ameliorating existing manifestations or preventing the development or worsening of neurotoxicity.[407,408,418,419] Transient myalgia and arthralgia of uncertain etiology, usually noted 24 to 48 hours after therapy and apparently dose-related, are also common, and a myopathy has been described in patients receiving high doses with cisplatin. Several investigators have reported that treatment with corticosteroids, specifically prednisone 10 mg twice daily for 5 days beginning 24 hours after treatment, is effective at reducing myalgia and arthralgia, and gabapentin, glutamate, and potentially antihistamines could be used for management or prevention.[408,419] Optic nerve disturbances, manifested by scintillating scotoma, may also occur.[420,421] Acute encephalopathy, which can progress to coma and death, has been reported after treatment with high doses (600 mg/m^2 or greater).[422] A transient acute encephalopathy has also been observed, rarely, within several hours following paclitaxel in patients who received prior cranial irradiation.[423]

Cardiac

Paclitaxel treatment has been associated with cardiac rhythm disturbances, most of which were identified using cardiac monitoring, the clinical relevance of these effects is not known.[407,408,424-426] The most common disturbance, transient, asymptomaic bradycardia, was noted in 29% of patients in one trial in which patients underwent cardiac monitoring, and, in the absence of hemodynamic effects, is not an indication for discontinuing paclitaxel.[408,424,426] More important bradyarrhythmias, such as Mobitz type I (Wenckeback syndrome), Mobitz type II, and third-degree heart block, have been noted, but the incidence in a large National Cancer Institute database was only 0.1%.[426] Most episodes have been asymptomatic and almost all documented events involved patients in early trials in which continuous cardiac monitor was routinely performed, indicating that second-degree and third-degree heart block are likely underreported. However, these bradyarrhythmias are probably caused by paclitaxel, as related taxanes affect cardiac automaticity and conduction, and similar disturbances have occurred in humans and animals after ingesting various species of yew plants.[426]

Myocardial infarction, cardiac ischemia, atrial arrhythmias, and ventricular tachycardia have been noted, but whether there is a causal relationship between paclitaxel and these events is uncertain. There is no evidence that chronic, long-term treatment with paclitaxel causes progressive cardiac dysfunction. Routine cardiac monitoring during paclitaxel therapy is not necessary, but is advisable for patients who may not be able to tolerate bradyarrhythmias, such as those with atrioventricular conduction disturbances or ventricular dysfunction. Although patients with a wide range of cardiac abnormalities and cardiac histories were broadly and empirically restricted from participating in early clinical trials, paclitaxel treatment has been reported to be well tolerated in a small series of patients with gynecologic cancer and with major cardiac risk factors.[424] However, repetitive treatment of patients with the combined regimen of paclitaxel on a 3-hour schedule and doxorubicin as a brief infusion is associated with a higher frequency of congestive cardiotoxicity than would be expected to occur with the same cumulative doxorubicin dose given without paclitaxel, as discussed in "Drug Interactions."[349,369,370] In one study of previously untreated women with advanced breast cancer who were treated with escalating doses of paclitaxel as a 3-hour infusion and doxorubicin, 60 mg/m^2 to a cumulative dose of 480 mg/m^2, which would be predicted to result in a less than 5% incidence of congestive cardiotoxicity in patients treated with doxorubicin alone, the incidence of congestive cardiotoxicity was approximately 25%.[349] However, the incidence of cardiotoxicity was less than 5% when similar patients received identical schedules of paclitaxel and doxorubicin, but the cumulative doxorubicin dose did not exceed 360 mg/m^2. Both experimental and early clinical results suggest that dexrazoxane reduces the cardiotoxicity of the doxorubicin and paclitaxel combination.[427,428] The incidence of congestive heart failure was also significantly higher in patients treated with the combination of trastuzumab and paclitaxel than paclitaxel alone;therefore, cardiac function should be monitored.[429]

Miscellaneous

Drug-related gastrointestinal effects, such as vomiting and diarrhea, are uncommon. Higher paclitaxel doses or protracted (96-hour) infusional administration may cause mucositis.[390,422,430] Rare cases of neutropenic enterocolitis and gastrointestinal necrosis have been noted, particularly in patients given high doses of paclitaxel in combination with doxorubicin or cyclophosphamide.[431,432] Severe hepatotoxicity and pancreatitis have also been noted rarely.[219,433] Acute bilateral pneumonitis has been reported in fewer than 1% of patients treated on a 3-hour schedule in one series, and both interstitial and parenchymal pulmonary toxicity have been reported, but clinically significant pulmonary effects are uncommon.[434,435] In contrast to the vinca alkaloids, the agent is not a potent vesicant but extravasation of large volumes can cause moderate soft tissue injury. Inflammation at the injection site and along the course of an injected vein may occur. Paclitaxel also induces reversible alopecia of the scalp in a dose-related fashion, and loss of all facial and body hair is usually because of cumulative therapy. Nail disorders have been reported, particularly in patients treated on weekly schedules.[436] Recall reactions in previously irradiated sites have also been noted.

Docetaxel

Hematologic

Following treatment with docetaxel administered over 1 hour every 3 weeks, the onset of neutropenia, the principal toxicity of docetaxel, is usually noted by day 8 and complete resolution typically occurs by days 15 to 21.[226,407,436] At a dose of 100 mg/m^2 administered over 1 hour, neutrophil counts are commonly below 500/μL and the incidence of neutropenic sequalae is high.[226,405] Although severe neutropenia at 75 mg/m^2 is common, the duration of severe neutropenia and incidence of complications are lower than the higher dose. As with paclitaxel, neutropenia is significantly less when lower doses are administered on a weekly schedule (see "Dose, and Schedule"). The most important determinant of neutropenia is the extent of prior treatment. Significant thrombocytopenia and anemia are uncommon with docetaxel alone.

Hypersensitivity

Despite not being formulated in polyoxyethylated castor oil, HSRs were reported in approximately 31% of patients receiving docetaxel without premedications in early phase 2 studies.[226,407,437] As with paclitaxel, major reactions characterized by dyspnea, bronchospasm, and hypotension typically occur during the first two courses and within minutes after the start of treatment. Signs and symptoms generally resolve within 15 minutes after cessation of treatment, and docetaxel is usually able to be reinstituted without sequelae, occasionally after treatment with an H_1-receptor antagonist. Fortunately, however, most events are minor and rarely result in discontinuation of treatment.[407] Both the incidence and severity of HSRs appear to be reduced by premedication with corticosteroids and H_1-receptor and H_2-receptor antagonists (discussed later in "Administration, Dose, and Schedule"), but the corticosteroid premedication regimen is principally administered to prevent fluid retention. As with paclitaxel, patients who experience major reactions have been retreated successfully after the resolution of symptoms and after treatment with corticosteroids and H_1-receptor antagonists. Furthermore, there are several anecdotal reports of patients treated successfully with docetaxel following severe HSRs as the result of taking paclitaxel, but it is not known whether these reactions would have occurred if the patients had been retreated with paclitaxel.[407,438]

Fluid Retention

Docetaxel induces a unique fluid retention syndrome characterized by edema, weight gain, and third-space fluid collection.[226,392,406,407,439] Fluid retention is cumulative and does not appear to be caused by hypoalbuminemia or cardiac, renal, or hepatic dysfunction. Instead, increased capillary permeability appears to be responsible for this phenomenon.[439] Capillary filtration studies in patients who were not receiving corticosteroid premedication have revealed a two-stage process, with progressive congestion of the interstitial space by proteins and water starting between the second and fourth course, followed by insufficient lymphatic drainage.[439] In early studies in which premedication was not used, fluid retention was not usually significant at cumulative docetaxel doses below 400 mg/m²;however, the incidence and severity of fluid retention increased sharply at cumulative doses of 400 mg/m² or greater and often resulted in the delay or termination of treatment. Premedication with corticosteroids with or without H_1-receptor and H_2-receptor antagonists has been demonstrated to reduce the overall incidence of fluid retention and increase the number of courses and cumulative docetaxel dose before the onset of this toxicity (see "Dose, and Schedule").[406,437] Fluid retention typically resolves slowly after docetaxel is stopped, but complete resolution occurs several months after treatment in patients with severe toxicity. Aggressive and early treatment with progressively more potent diuretics starting with potassium-sparing diuretics has been used to manage fluid retention.[406,407,439] The incidence of fluid retention appears to be lower in studies using lower doses (60 to 75 mg/m²) of docetaxel during each course, but this may be because of the administration of lower overall cumulative doses, and the effects of lower doses on antitumor activity are unknown.

Dermatologic

Skin toxicity may occur in as many as 50 to 75% of patients; however, premedication may reduce the overall incidence of this effect.[226,407,440,441] An erythematous pruritic maculopapular rash that affects the forearms, hands, or feet is typical. Other cutaneous effects include desquamation of the hands and feet, that may respond to pyridoxine or cooling, and onychodystrophy characterized by brown discoloration, ridging, onycholysis, soreness, and brittleness and loss of the nail plate.[440–443] Skin and nail changes appear to be most prominent in patients treated with high cumulative doses over long periods, particularly on weekly administration schedules.[392]

Neurotoxicity

Docetaxel produces neurotoxicity, which is qualitatively similar to that of paclitaxel.[226,407,444] Patients typically complain of paresthesia and numbness, but peripheral motor effects may also occur. Both neurosensory and neuromuscular effects are generally less frequent and less severe with docetaxel as compared with paclitaxel, and preferential use of docetaxel should be considered in high-risk patients in whom taxane treatment is indicated.[226,407,444,445] Nevertheless, mild-to-moderate peripheral neurotoxicity occurs in approximately 40% of untreated patients, and patients who had received prior cisplatin appear to be particularly susceptible, with the incidence approaching 74% in one trial.[226,391,392,407,437] Severe toxicity has been unusual after repetitive treatment with docetaxel doses less than 100 mg/m², except in patients with antecedent neurotoxicity and relavent disorders, such as alcohol abuse and diabetes mellitus. Transient arthralgia and myalgia are occasionally noted within days after treatment. Malaise or asthenia have been prominent complaints in patients who have been treated with large cumulative doses, particularly when docetaxel is administered on a continuous weekly schedule.[226,391,392,407,437]

Miscellaneous

Stomatitis is more common with docetaxel than paclitaxel, but still occurs infrequently. Nausea, vomiting, and diarrhea have also been observed infrequently, but severe manifestations are rare. Empiric use of antiemetic premedication does not appear to be warranted. Mild-to-moderate conjunctivitis, which is responsive to topical corticosteroids, and canalicular stenosis causing lacrimation may also occur, particularly with weekly schedules.[446] Nausea, vomiting, and diarrhea have also been observed, but severe gastrointestinal toxicity is rare. Similar to paclitaxel, docetaxel is not a potent vesicant and infusion site reactions are uncommon. Other rare events reported that may or may not be drug-related included arrythmias, confusion, erythema multiforme, neutropenic enterocolitis, hepatitis, ileus, interstial pneumonia, seizures, pulmonary fibrosis, hepatitis, radiation recall, and visual disturbances.[392] Cardiovascular manifestations, such as angina, arrhythmia, conduction disturbances, congestive heart failure, hypertension, and hypotension, have been noted rarely following treatment, but these events have not been linked convincingly to docetaxel.

Estramustine Phosphate

Estramustine, a conjugate of the alkylating agent nor-nitrogen mustard that is linked to 17β-estradiol by a carbamate ester bridge, is administered as the oral prodrug estramustine phosphate, which is rapidly dephosphorylated by gastrointestinal tract phosphatases to produce estramustine. Estramustine was synthesized so that the 17β-estradiol component would bind to, and accumulate in estrogen receptor–bearing breast cancer cells, and selectively deliver the nor-nitrogen mustard alkylating moiety, after degradation of the carbamate ester. Estramustine was subsequently demonstrated to be capable of inducing cytotoxicity in estrogen receptor–negative cancer cells, and drug binding was not inhibited by 1,000-fold excess concentrations of estradiol.[447] Furthermore, no significant anticancer activity was noted in early clinical trials involving patients with breast cancer, and, thereafter, it was determined that DNA alkylation and DNA damage did not occur in vitro at concentrations that induce cytotoxicity.[447–449] This led to radiolabeled drug distribution studies in rats that showed that estramustine did not distribute to tissues that expressed the estrogen receptor.[450] Instead, drug accumulated in the ventral prostate, which was mediated by a prostate tissue-specific protein called the *estramustine-binding protein* (EMBP) that has a heterodimeric structure and a molecular weight of 46,000 daltons.[450,451] This finding, as well as the demonstration of anticancer activity in patients with prostate cancer that were refractory to the estrogen analog diethylsilbesterol, led to evaluations of estramustine in patients with HRPC and regulatory approval for this indication.[451,452] Although estramustine has been associated with activity as a single agent, antitumor activity has been most prominent with estramustine phosphate combined with other antimicrotubule agents including vinca alkaloids, taxanes, and epothilones. The combination of estramustine and docetaxel has demonstrated decrements in prostate specific antigen in approximately 50% of HRPC patients.[453, 454] In a randomized phase 3 trial, in which patients with HRPC were treated with either docetaxel plus estramustine phosphate or a standard regimen consisting of mitoxantrone plus prednisone, both overall and progression-free survival were superior in patients treated with the estramustine-based regimen.[237,239,455]

Mechanism of Action

Estramustine's principal mechanism of antineoplastic action involves perturbations in microtubule dynamics. Estramustine depolymerizes both microtubules and microfilaments, binds to and disrupt MAPs, and inhibit cell growth at high concentrations, which ultimately result in mitotic arrest and apoptosis.[456–458] The agent binds to β-tubulin ($K_d \approx 23$ μmol) at a site distinct from the colchicine and vinca alkaloid binding sites, and its binding affinity to β-tubulin is isotype-dependent.[3,456,459] Although the phosphorylated form binds to MAPs and estramustine itself binds to other cellular proteins besides tubulin, the drug's interaction with tubulin appears to be principally responsible for its anticancer activity.[459–461] Estramustine reduces the rates of both microtubule lengthening and shortening, inhibits dynamic instability and polymerization of MAP-free microtubules, and modestly increases microtubule mass.[459,462–464] Although estramustine may affect microtubules comprising the interphase cytoskeleton, it principally affects those comprising the mitotic spindle apparatus and induces arrest in G_2/M. Similar to the vinca alkaloids and taxanes, mitotic arrest is often followed by apoptosis. The aforementioned antimicrotubule effects of estramustine are mediated by the intact conjugate and not the individual nor-nitrogen or estradiol moieties.[459]

The tissue-selective accumulation and actions of estramustine and its metabolite, estromustine appear to depend on the presence, distribution, and magnitude of EMBP.[465,466] This is supported by the finding that the magnitude of G_2/M arrest directly relates to intracellular concentrations of EMBP after estramustine treatment in vitro.[465–467] In addition to prostate cancer, EMBP and related binding proteins have been identified in malignant brain tumors, but the therapeutic relevance of this finding is not clear.[468–470] Because estramustine phosphate blocks cell cycle traverse in G_2/M, crosses the blood-brain barrier, and accumulates in both gliomas and astrocytomas, the potential for estramustine to selectively sensitize brain malignancies to irradiation is being investigated.[471,472]

Three distinct mechanisms of resistance have been characterized in cancer cell lines that have been selected for resistance to estramustine including alterations in β-tubulin isotype expression, MAP expression, and ATP-dependent drug efflux. With regard to differential β-tubulin isotype expression, higher ratios of $β_{III}$- and $β_{IVa}$-tubulin relative to other β-tubulin isotypes have been demonstrated in prostate cancer cell lines with acquired resistance to estramustine.[3,304,473] Estramustine binds less avidly to microtubules with higher $β_{III}$-tubulin isotype content compared to other β-tubulin isotypes, and tumor cells with high levels of $β_{III}$-tubulin appear to be less prone to the inhibitory and destabilizing effects of estramustine on microtubule dynamics.[3,304,473] However, in studies in which the gene encoding $β_{III}$-tubulin has been transfected into prostate cancer cells with resultant overexpression of $β_{III}$-tubulin, resistance to estramustine and other antimicrotubule agents is not conferred.[473,474] Overexpression of the MAP tau is another mechanism of acquired resistance to estramustine that has been demonstrated in prostate cancer cell lines.[475] However, the extent to which alterations in tau or other altered MAPs contribute to clinical estramustine resistance is not known. Although estramustine is a substrate for the drug efflux pump characterized by the MDR phenotype,

P-gp overexpression does are not appear confer resistance to estramustine.[473,476–478] In fact, estramustine may competitively inhibit P-gp function, reducing the efflux of cytotoxic agents that are substrates for P-gp.[473,476,478] In addition, cells with amplifications of the ABC2 transporter gene demonstrate a magnitude of estramustine resistance that is proportional to the level of ABC2 gene amplification.[473,479]

Pharmacology

The bioavailability of oral estramustine phosphate, which undergoes rapid and complete dephosphorylation to estramustine within the gastrointestinal tract (Fig. 11.6), has been reported to range from 37 to 75%.[473,479–481] The principal route of estramustine elimination is by rapid oxidative metabolism at C17 to yield estromustine, which is the main metabolite in the plasma.[473,482] Estromustine concentrations in plasma peak within 2 to 4 hours after oral administration, and the mean elimination half-life of estromustine is 14 hours.[480,483] The pharmacokinetic behavior of estromustine in plasma is dose proportional following oral administration of estramustine phosphate in its therapeutic dose range. In patients treated orally with estramustine phosphate 560 mg/day, peak plasma concentrations average 227 ng/mL for estromustine, 23 ng/mL for estramustine, 95 ng/mL for estrone, and 9.3 ng/mL for estradiol.[482]

Significant first-pass hepatic metabolism occurs after oral administration of estramustine phosphate, and further hydrolysis of estromustine and its carbamate linker in the liver results in the formation of estrone and the release of the alkylating group. Following oral and intravenous administration of radiolabeled estramustine phosphate in humans, estromustine and estramustine are principally excreted in the feces, and only small amounts of conjugated estrone and estradiol are excreted in the urine (<1%).[473,480–483] Although the pathways responsible for hepatic metabolism of estramustine, estromustine, and the estrogen metabolites have not been fully elucidated, hepatic CYP1A2 and CYP3A4 P-450 isoenzymes are largely responsible for oxidative metabolism of estradiol- and estrone-like steroids in hepatic microsome studies.[473,484]

An intravenous formulation of estramustine phosphate, which is available only for investigational use in the United States, results in 10- to 15-fold higher peak plasma concentrations of estramustine phosphate, estramustine, and estromustine than those achieved following oral administration.[455,473,480–484] The parenteral formulation is also associated with markedly less interpatient variability in pharmacokinetics.[455,480–484] The absence of first-pass hepatic metabolism with parenteral administration results in lower clearance rates; the terminal half-lives of elimination for estramustine phosphate, estromustine, and estramustine average 3.7, 110, and 64 hours, respectively, following intravenous administration.[483] The reduced clearance of intravenous estramustine results in the accumulation of estromustine, estramustine, estradiol, and estrone in the plasma of patients treated on weekly intravenous dosing regimens.[455]

Drug Interactions

Coadministration of calcium-rich foods, particularly dairy products, impairs the gastrointestinal absorption of estramustine phosphate as the result of the formation of poorly absorbable calcium complexes.[485] Therefore, it is recommended that patients fast for at least 2 hours before oral administration of estramustine phosphate and avoid calcium-rich food and antacids.

The clearance rates of docetaxel and paclitaxel have been reported to be significantly reduced by estramustine phosphate.[238] Although the mechanism by which this occurs is not known, the potential inhibitory effects of estramustine on taxane-metabolizing CYP3A4 isoenzyme have been proposed to account for this potential drug-drug interaction.[238,453,484] Therefore, recommended doses

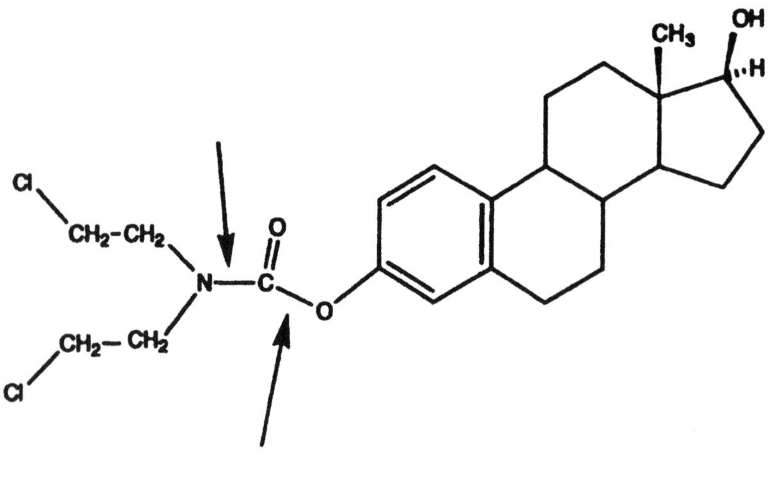

Figure 11.6 Structure of estramustine. Arrows show the bonds that separate the estrogenic portion of the molecule from the nitrogen mustard. (Reprinted with permission from Tew KD, Glusker JP, Hartley-Asp B, et al. Preclinical and clinical perspectives on the use of estramustine as an antimitotic drug. Pharmacol Ther 1992;56:323.)

of docetaxel and paclitaxel in combination with estramustine phosphate are less than single agent doses, despite the fact that the taxanes and estramustine phosphate essentially have non-overlapping toxicities.

Toxicity

Because of nausea and vomiting, which are the principal toxicities encountered with oral estramustine phosphate, patients may require modification of dose-schedule or termination of treatment. However, these toxicities are readily managed with standard antiemetic medications. Diarrhea has also been observed in patients treated with estramustine phosphate for protracted periods. Myelosuppression is usually not significant in patients treated with estramustine phosphate as a single agent.

Common estrogenic side effects of treatment with estramustine phosphate include gynecomastia, nipple tenderness, and fluid retention. Physicians should exercise caution in prescribing estramustine phosphate to patients with a history of congestive heart failure because of the risk for fluid retention and edema that can result in a decompensated cardiac state. Thromboembolic complications, including venous thrombosis, pulmonary emboli, and cerebrovascular and coronary thrombotic events, which may occur in up to 10% of patients, represent the most serious toxicities of estramustine phosphate. The cardiovascular effects of oral estramustine phosphate have been attributed to high intrahepatic concentrations of estrogenic metabolites, which result in reduced antithrombin III levels and hypercoagulability.[486] Transient elevations in hepatic transaminases has been reported in approximately 33% of patients. In a phase 3 study, in which patients with advanced prostate carcinoma were randomized to treatment with either estramustine phosphate or diethylstilbestrol, the rates of hepatic toxicity were similar on both treatment arms.[487] Clinically significant acute hypocalemia, which has been proposed to be the result of an avid uptake of calcium in osteoblastic metastases (i.e., tumor calcium sink), increased uptake of calcium by healing bone lesions and/or the unmasking of a subclinical vitamin D-deficient state, is uncommon.[488,489] Asymptomatic reductions in serum calcium concentrations have been reported in up to 20% of patients.

Patients treated with estramustine phosphate by the intravenous route complain infrequently of the acute onset of perianal and/or perineal pain, which can be minimized by administering the agent over a more protracted infusion duration (60 to 90 minutes).[484]

Administration, Dose, and Schedule

The recommended daily dose of estramustine phosphate, which is available as a 140-mg capsule, is 14 mg/kg of body weight in three to four divided daily doses; however, patients are usually treated in the daily dosing range of 10 to 16 mg/kg. The agent should be ingested with water at least 1 hour before or 2 hours after meals. Patients are generally treated for 30 to 90 days before assessment of therapeutic benefit. Chronic oral therapy can be maintained for months or even years. Abbreviated 1-, 3-, and 5-day courses of oral estramustine phosphate have been proposed for use in combination the taxanes and other chemotherapeutics. Such schedules appear to reduce the gastrointestinal toxicity associated with chronic oral administration.[238,490,491] In studies with docetaxel using this abbreviated schedule, the recommended dose of estramustine is 280 mg three times daily ($\approx$ 600 mg/m^2 per day) for 5 days.[453]

Novel Antimicrotubule Agents in Early Clinical Development

The clinical success of the taxanes has led to a search for other drugs that enhance tubulin polymerization, yielding several promising compounds that may confer a therapeutic advantage over the taxanes, including the epothilones (isolated from myxobacterium *Sorangium cellulosum*), discodermolide (isolated from the Caribbean sponge *Discodermia dissoluta*), eleutherobin (isolated from the soft coral *Eleutherobia* sp), laulimalides (isolated from the marine sponge *Cacospongia mycofijiensis*), and sarcodictyins (isolated from the Mediterranean stoloniferan coral *Sarcodictyon roseum* (Fig. 11.7). Some of these compounds compete with paclitaxel for binding to microtubules and appear to bind at or near the taxane site (epothilones, discodermolide, eleutherobins and sarcodictyins), but others, such as laulimalide, seem to bind to unique sites on microtubules.[2,3,243] Eleutherobin, discodermolide, and laulimalide are especially potent, with K_i values in the 5 to 40 nM range.[2–4] All of the aforementioned compounds possess either low level or no substrate affinity for P-gp and other ABC transporters, and retain various degrees of activity against taxane-resistant cells in vitro, but the clinical implications of these characteristics are not clear.

Of the aforementioned compounds, the epothilones are the furthest along in development. Not only do they promote tubulin polymerization and induce mitotic arrest, but several epothilones possess much greater cytotoxic potency than either paclitaxel or docetaxel, with IC$_{50}$ values in the submolar or low nanomolar range.[2–4,492–494] Similar to the taxanes, they induce tubulin polymerization in the absence of GTP and/or MAPs, resulting in microtubules that are relatively long, rigid, and resistant to destabilization by cold temperature and calcium. In contrast to the taxanes and vinca alkaloids, overexpression of P-gp minimally affects the cytotoxicity of epothilones A and B.[2,3,492] Furthermore, various point mutations in β-tubulin, which confer resistance to the taxanes in vitro, do not necessarily confer resistance to the epothilones.[492,495] Several epothilone B analogs, including ixabepilone (BMS-247550)

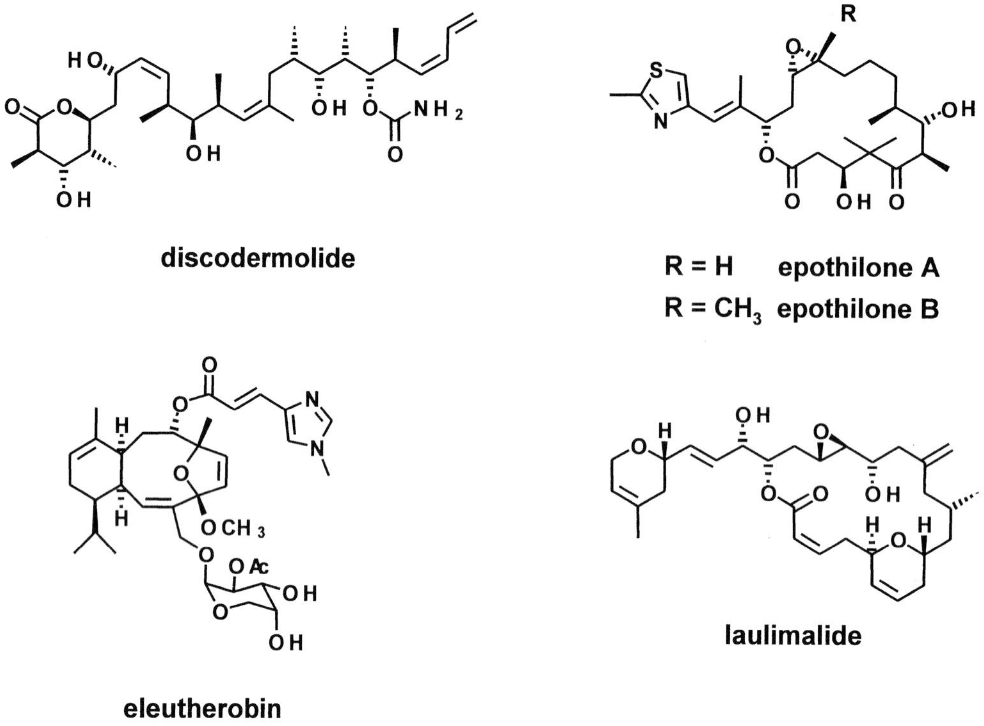

Figure 11.7   Structures of discodermolide, epotholones A and B, eleutherobin, and laulimalides

and patupiline (EPO906), are currently undergoing clinical evaluation.[492,493,496–498] The principal mode of disposition for ixabepilone is via cytochrome P450 metabolism and biliary excretion, whereas patupiline is metabolized via carboxyesterases.[492,496–498] The pharmacologic characteristics are typified by marked tissue uptake, avid and protracted tissue binding, and long terminal half-lives of elimination.[492] Furthermore, their principal toxicities differ, namely diarrhea for patupiline and both myelosuppression and neurotoxicity for ixabepilone.[492] In early clinical trials, responses have been noted in patients with advanced carcinomas of the breast, lung, prostate, and ovary, some of whom experienced recurrent disease following or during treatment with the taxanes.[492,496,498] However, the magnitude of their activity in taxane-refractory malignancies needs to be addressed. Of note, patupiline has shown evidence of antitumor activity in advanced colorectal and renal carcinomas, which are almost always inherently resistant to antimicrotubule agents, but the magnitude of appreciable activity in cancers with primary or acquired resistance to the taxanes is negligible.[5,492,496–498] An epotholone D, desoxyepotholone B (KOS862) that has demonstrated at least equivalent potency and less toxicity than the taxanes and epotholone B analogs in preclinical studies, is in early clinical development.[494,499]

Similar to the epothilones A and B, discodermolide-induced tubulin polymers are stable to treatment with calcium and are composed of short microtubules instead of tubulin spirals.[500,501] In addition to low-level to complete cross-resistance to P-gp overexpressing cancer cells, paclitaxel and epothilone-resistant human tumor cells that express mutant β-tubulin, retain sensitivity to discodermolide.[500–503] Furthermore, discodermolide and paclitaxel have demonstrated synergistic cytotoxicity in vitro, suggesting that their tubulin binding sites and microtubule effects are not identical.[504,505] However, unforeseen pulmonary toxicity has been seen in early clinical studies of a completely synthetic discodermolide (XAA296).[506] The marine soft coral–derived natural products, sarcotidicytins A and B and eleutherobin, also promote tubulin polymerization in a manner analogous to that of paclitaxel.[2,3,507,508] The marine-derived, microtubule-stabilizing cytotoxins laulimalide and isolaulimalide appear to be poor substrates for ABC transporters such as P-gp.[2–4,508,509] Because eleutherobin, epothilones A and B, and discodermolide, competitively inhibit [³H]paclitaxel binding to microtubules, a common pharmacophore was sought and identified, which may enable the development of hybrid constructs with more desirable biological characteristics.[243]

Other natural products and semisynthetic antimicrotubule compounds under evaluation interact with tubulin in the vinca alkaloid-binding or colchicine-binding domains. Among the most potent are the dolastatins, which constitute a series of oligopeptides isolated from the sea hare, *Dolabela auricularia*. Two of the most potent dolastatins, dolastatin-10 and dolastatin-15, noncompetitively inhibit the binding of vinca alkaloids to tubulin, inhibit tubulin polymerization and tubulin-dependent GTP hydrolysis, stabilize the colchicine-binding activity of tubulin, and possess cytotoxic activity in the picomolar to low nanomolar range. Dolastatin-10 and semisynthetic dolastatin analogs (ILX-651 and well as TZT-1027), which binds in the vinca domain, are undergoing preclinical development and clinical evaluation.[2–4,510]

Phomopsin A, halichondrin B, homohalichondrin B, and spongistatin 1, which competitively inhibit vinca alkaloid binding to tubulin are being evaluated in preclinical or early clinical evaluations.[511,512,513] E7389, a macrocyclic ketone analog of the marine natural product halichondrin B originally isolated from the marine sponge *Halicondrin okadai*, and two less complex synthetic marocyclic ketone analogs, ER-076349 and ER-086526 are in early clinical evaluations.[511] These compounds bind to tubulin, inhibit tubulin polymerization, disrupt mitotic spindle formation, induce mitotic arrest, and possess growth inhibitory properties in the subnanomolar range and marked activity in preclinical studies. Several biochemical correlates of apoptosis are also observed following E7389 treatment, including phosphorylation of the antiapoptotic protein Bcl-2, cytochrome c release from mitochondria, proteolytic activation of caspase-3 and -9, and cleavage of the caspase-3 substrate poly(ADP-ribose) polymerase. The agent is currently in phase 1 to 2 evaluations in patients with advanced solid malignancies.

Also in clinical development is HTI-286, a synthetic form of hemiasterlin, which is is a natural product derived from marine sponges.[513] Hemiasterlin and its analogs bind to the vinca-peptide site in tubulin, disrupt normal microtubule dynamics, and, at stoichiometric amounts, depolymerize microtubules. HTI-286 is a much weaker substrate for P-gp than the vinca alkaloids and taxanes.[513] It has excellent in vivo antitumor activity in human xenograft models, including tumors that express P-gp. The agent is cross-resistant with other vinca peptide-binding agents, including hemiasterlin A, dolastatin-10, and vinblastine (7- to 28-fold), and DNA-damaging drugs, including doxorubicin and mitoxantrone (16- to 57-fold), but is minimally cross-resistant with the taxanes, epothilones, or colchicine (onefold to fourfold). However, resistance appears to be at least partially mediated by mutation of α-tubulin and by an ATP-binding cassette drug pump distinct from P-glycoprotein, ABCG2, MRP1, or MRP3.

Most efforts targeting the tumor vasculature are aimed at the development of agents that inhibit the process of angiogenesis, but recently, several antimicrotubule agents have been demonstrated to rapidly shut down existing tumor vasculature.[514] Since the late 1990s, the combretastatins and *N*-acetylcolchicinol-*O*-phosphate, compounds that resemble colchicine and bind to the colchicine domain on tubulin, have undergone extensive development as antivascular agents. Several of them (combretastatin-A-43-*O*-phosphate, combrestatin A-1-phosphate (CA-1-P), ZD6126 and AVE8062A are in clinical trials.[515] Although objective antitumor activity in preliminary evaluations have been noted, cardiovascular toxicity has been problematic.

Targeting Mitotic Kinesins and Kinases

Although tubulin is the most abundant protein component of the mitotic spindle apparatus, many additional proteins, such as mitotic kinesins, play critical roles in the mechanics of mitosis and in progression through the premitotic cell cycle checkpoint. Kinesins are motor proteins that translate chemical energy released by the hydrolysis of adenosine triphosphate (ATP) into mechanical force for movement along microtubules, transport of a wide variety of cargoes, and the intracellular organization of the mitotic spindle and other microtubule-containing structures.[514,516,517]

The mitotic kinesins are a subgroup of kinesin motor proteins that function exclusively in mitosis in proliferating cells.[518] During mitosis, different, highly specialized mitotic kinesins play critical roles in various aspects of mitotic spindle assembly, including the establishment of spindle bipolarity, spindle pole organization, chromosome alignment and segregation, and regulation of microtubule dynamics. The establishment of mitotic spindle bipolarity is among the earliest events in spindle assembly and it requires the function of a specific kinesin motor protein KSP (also known as Eg5), which has no known role outside of mitosis.[519] The expression profiles of KSP mRNA in normal tissues are consistent with preferential expression of KSP in proliferating cells relative to normal adjacent tissue and postmitotic neurons. As essential elements in mitotic spindle assembly and function, KSP and mitotic kinesins provide attractive targets for intervention into the cell cycle. CK0106023 (SB-715992) a polycyclic, nitrogen containing heterocycle and allosteric inhibitor of KSP motor domain ATPase with a Ki of 12 nM, is a very potent KSP inhibitor that causes mitotic arrest. It is entering clinical trials.[193,520] The compound, which is 10,000-fold more selective for KSP relative to other members of the kinesin superfamily, has been shown to block assembly of a functional mitotic spindle, thereby causing cell cycle arrest in mitosis and subsequent cell death.[519,521] In tumor-bearing mice, the agent exhibited antitumor activity comparable to or exceeding that of paclitaxel, and caused the formation of monopolar mitotic figures identical to those produced in cultured cells.[520]

A host of mitotic kinases are also being assessed as strategic targets for anticancer therapeutic development. For example, the aurora kinases (A, B, C) are essential for the regulation of chromosome segregation and cytokinesis during mitosis and aberrant expression and activity of these kinases occur in a wide range of human tumors, and lead to aneuploidy and tumorigenesis.[522] Recently, a highly potent and selective small-molecule inhibitor of the aurora kinases, VX-680, that blocks cell-cycle progression and induces apoptosis in a diverse range of human tumor types.[522] This compound causes profound inhibition of tumor growth in a variety of in vivo xenograft models, leading to regression of leukemia, colon and pancreatic tumors at well-tolerated doses, and is entering clinical trials.

REFERENCES

1. Gelfand VI, Bershadsky AD. Microtubule dynamics: mechanism, regulation, and function. Annu Rev Cell Biol 1991;7:93.
2. Jordan MA, Wilson L. Microtubules as a target for anticancer drugs. Nat Rev Cancer 2004;4:253.
3. Jordan MA. Mechanism of action of antitumor drugs that interact with microtubules and tubulin. Curr Med Chem Anti-Cancer Agents 2002;2:1.
4. Kavallaris M, Verrills NM, Hill BT. Anticancer therapy with novel tubulin-interacting drugs. Drug Resist Updates 2001;4:392.
5. Pinz H. Recent advances in the field of tubulin polymerization inhibitors. Expert Rev Anticancer Ther 2002;2:695.
6. Correia JJ, Lobert S. Physiochemical aspects of tubulin-interacting antimitotic drugs. Curr Pharm Des 2001;7:1213.
7. Nogales E, Whittaker M, Milligan RA, Downing KH. High-resolution model of the microtubule. Cell 1999;96:78.
8. Zheng Y, Jung MK, Oakley BR. Gamma-tubulin is present in Drosophila melanogaster and Homo sapiens and is associated with the centrosome. Cell 1991;65:817.
9. Luduena RF. Multiple forms of tubulin: different gene products and covalent modifications. Int Rev Cytol 1998;178:207.
10. Raff EC. The role of multiple tubulin isoforms in cellular microtubule function. In: Hyams JF, Lloyd CD, eds. Microtubules. New York: Wiley-Liss 1993;89.
11. Khan A, Luduena F. Different effects of vinblastine on the polymerization of isotypicallly purified tubulins from bovine brain. Invest New Drugs 2003;21:3.
12. Olmsted JB. Microtubule-associated proteins. Annu Rev Cell Biol 1986;2:421.
13. Schulze E, Asai DJ, Bulinski JC, et al. Post-translational modification and microtubule stability. J Cell Biol 1987;105:2167.
14. Vale RD. Microtubule motors: many new models off the assembly line. Trends Biochem Sci 1992;17:300.
15 Beck WT. Alkaloids. In: Fox BW, Fox M, eds. Antitumor Drug Resistance. Berlin: Springer-Verlag 1984;589.
16. Crossin KL, Carney DH. Microtubule stabilization by Taxol inhibits initiation of DNA synthesis by thrombin and epidermal growth factor. Cell 1981;27:341.
17. Rowinsky EK, Donehower RC. The clinical pharmacology and use of antimicrotubule agents in cancer chemotherapeutics. Pharmacol Ther 1992;52:35.
18. Wilson L, Jordan MA. Pharmacological probes of microtubule function. In: Hyams JF, Lloyd CD, eds. Microtubules. New York: Wiley-Liss 1993.
19. Bhalla KN. Microtubule-targeted anticancer agents and apoptosis. Oncogene 2003;22:9075.
20. Carlier M-F. Role of nucleotide hydrolysis in the polymerization of actin and tubulin. Cell Biophys 1998;12:105.
21. Farrell KW, Jordan MA, Miller HP, et al. Phase dynamics at microtubule ends: the coexistence of microtubule length changes and treadmilling. J Cell Biol 1987;104:1035.
22. Mandelkow E-M, Mandelkow E. Microtubule oscillations. Cell Motil Cytoskeleton 1992;22:235.
23. Mitchison TJ. Localization of exchangeable GTP binding site at the plus end of microtubules. Science 1993;261:1044.
24. Margolis RL, Wilson L. Microtubule treadmilling: what goes around comes around. Bioessays 1998;20:830.
25. Erickson HP, O'Brien ET. Microtubule dynamic instability and GTP hydrolysis. Annu Rev Biophys Biomol Struct 1992;21:145.
26. Mitchison T, Kirschner M. Dynamic instability of microtubule growth. Nature 1984;312:237.
27. Wilson L, Jordan MA. Microtubule dynamics: taking aim at a moving target. Chem Biol 1995;2:569.
28. Alli E, Bash-Babula J, Yang J-M, et al. Effect of stathmin on the sensitivity to antimicrotubule drugs in human breast cancer. Cancer Res 2002;62:6864.
29. Zhai Y, Kronebusch PJ, Simon PM, et al. Microtubule dynamics at the G2/M transition: abrupt breakdown of cytoplasmic microtubules at nuclear envelope breakdown and implications for spindle morphogenesis. J Cell Biol 1996;135:201.
30. Yvon A-M, Wadsworth P, Jordan MA. Taxol suppresses dynamics of individual microtubules in living human tumor cells. Mol Biol Cell 1999;10:947.
31. Wilson L, Panda D, Jordan MA. Modulation of microtubule dynamics by drugs: a paradigm for the actions of cellular regulators. Cell Struc Funct 1999;24:329.
32. Jordan MA, Wendell KL, Gardiner S, et al. Mitotic block induced in HeLa cells by low concentrations of paclitaxel (Taxol) results in abnormal mitotic exit and apoptotic cell death. Cancer Res 1996;56:816.
33. Johnson IS, Armstrong JG, Gorman M, et al. The vinca alkaloids: a new class of oncolytic agents. Cancer Res 1963;23:1390.
34. Johnson IS. Historical background of vinca alkaloid research and areas of future interest. Cancer Chemother Rep 1968;52:455.
35. Dancey J, Steward WP. The role of vindesine in oncology—recommendations after 10 years' experience. Anticancer Drugs 1995;6:625.
36. Joel S. The comparative clinical pharmacology of vincristine and vindesine: Does vindesine offer any advantage in clinical use? Cancer Treat Rev 1996;21:513.
37. Gridelli C, De Vivo R. Vinorelbine in the treatment of non-small cell lung cancer. Curr Med Chem 2002;9:879.
38. Domenech GH, Vogel CL. Single agent vinorelbine as first-line chemotherapy in elderly patients with advanced breast cancer. Anticancer Res 2003;23:1657.
39. Budman DR. Vinorelbine (Navelbine): a third-generation vinca alkaloid. Cancer Invest 1997;15:475.
40. Curran MP, Plosker GL. Vinorelbine: a review of its use in elderly patients with advanced non-small cell lung cancer. Drugs Aging 2002;19:695.
41. Rowinsky EK, Noe DA, Lucas VS, et al. A phase I, pharmacokinetic and absolute bioavailability study of oral vinorelbine (Navelbine) in solid tumor patients. J Clin Oncol 1994;12:1754.
42. Kruczynski A, Hill BT. Vinflunine, the latest Vinca alkaloid in clinical development. A review of its preclinical anticancer properties. Crit Rev Oncol Hematol 2001;40:159.
43. Dimopoulos MA, Pouli A, Zervas K, et al. Prospective randomized comparison of vincristine, doxorubicin and dexamethasone (VAD) administered as intravenous bolus injection and VAD with liposomal doxorubicin as first-line treatment in multiple myeloma. Ann Oncol 2003;14:1039.
44. Donoso RJ, Jordan MA, Farrell KW, et al. Kinetic stabilization of the microtubule dynamic instability in vitro by vinblastine. Biochemistry 1993;32:185.
45. Himes RH, Kersey RN, Heller-Bettinger I, et al. Action of the vinca alkaloids, vincristine and vinblastine, and desacetyl vinblastine amide on microtubules in vitro. Cancer Res 1976;36:3798.
46. Tucker RW, Owellen RJ, Harris SB. Correlation of cytotoxicity and mitotic spindle dissolution by vinblastine in mammalian cells. Cancer Res 1977;37:4346.
47. White JG. Effect of colchicine and Vinca alkaloids on human platelets: I. Influence on platelet microtubules and contractile function. Am J Pathol 1968;53:281.
48. Bruchovsky N, Owen AA, Becker AJ, et al. Effects of vinblastine on the proliferative capacity of L cells and their progress through the division cycle. Cancer Res 1965;25:1232.
49. Schrek R, Stefani SS. Toxicity of microtubular drugs to leukemic lymphocytes. Exp Mol Pathol 1981;34:369.
50. Schrijvers DL. Extravasation: a dreaded complication of chemotherapy. Ann Oncol 2003;14(Suppl 3):iii26.
51. Schrek R. Cytotoxicity of vincristine to normal and leukemic cells. Am J Clin Pathol 1974;62(1):2004.
52. Johnson SA, Harper P, Hortobagyi GN, Pouillart P. Vinorelbine: an overview. Cancer Treat Rev 1996;22:127.
53. Jordan MA, Thrower D, Wilson L. Mechanism of inhibition of cell proliferation by the vinca alkaloids. Cancer Res 1991;51:2212.
54. Himes RH. Interactions of the catharanthus (vinca) alkaloids with tubulin and microtubules. Pharmacol Ther 1991;51:256.

55. Jordan MA, Margolis RL, Himes RH, et al. Identification of a distinct class of vinblastine binding sites on microtubules. J Mol Biol 1986;187:61.

56. Jordan MA, Wilson L. Kinetic analysis of tubulin exchange at microtubule ends at low vinblastine concentrations. Biochemistry 1990;29:2730.

57. Singer WD, Jordan MA, Wilson L, et al. Binding of vinblastine to stabilized microtubules. Mol Pharmacol 1989;36:366.

58. Donoso JA. Effect of microtubule proteins on the interaction of vincristine and microtubules and tubulin. Cancer Res 1979;39:1604.

59. Palmer CG, Livengood D, Warren AK, et al. The action of the vincaleukolastine on mitosis in vitro. Experl Cell Res 1960;20:198.

60. Fan S, Cherney B, Reinhold W, et al. Disruption of p53 function in immortalized human cells does not affect survival or apoptosis after taxol or vincristine treatment. Clin Cancer Res 1998;4:1047.

61. Blagosklonny MV, Robey R, Bates S, et al. Pretreatment with DNA-damaging agents permits selective killing of checkpoint-deficient cells by microtubule-active drugs. J Clin Invest 2000;105:533.

62. Jordan MA, Thrower D, Wilson L. Effects of vinblastine, podophyllotoxin and nocodazole on mitotic spindles. Implications for the role of microtubule dynamics in mitosis. J Cell Sci 1992;102:401.

63. Wilson L, Miller HP, Farrell KW, et al. Taxol stabilization of microtubules in vitro: dynamics of tubulin addition and loss at opposite microtubule ends. Biochemistry 1985;24:5254.

64. Vacca A, Iurlaro M, Ribatti D, et al. Antiangiogenesis is produced by nontoxic doses of vinblastine. Blood 1999;94:4143.

65. Klement G, Baruchel S, Rak J, et al. Continuous low-dose therapy with vinblastine and VEGF receptor-2 antibody induces sustained tumor regression without overt toxicity. J Clin Invest 2000;105:R15.

66. Ngan V, Bellman K, Hill B, et al. Novel actions of the antitumor drugs vinflunine and vinorelbine on microtubules. Mol Pharmacol 2001;60:225.

67. Jordan MA, Himes RH, Wilson L. Comparison of the effects of vinblastine, vincristine, vindesine, and vinepidine on microtubule dynamics and cell proliferation in vitro. Cancer Res 1985;45:2741.

68. Lobert S, Correia JJ. Energetics of vinca alkaloid interactions with tubulin. Methods Enzymol 2000;323:77.

69. Lobert S, Vulevic B, Correria JJ. Interaction of vinca alkaloids with tubulin: a comparison of vinblastine, vincristine, and vinorelbine. Biochemistry 1996;35:6806.

70. Bowman LC, Houghton JA, Houghton PJ. Formation and stability of vincristine-tubulin complex in kidney cytosols. Role of GTP and GTP hydrolysis. Biochem Pharmacol 1988;37:1251.

71. Ferguson PJ, Cass CE. Differential cellular retention of vincristine and vinblastine by cultured human promyelocytic leukemia HL-60/C-1 cells: the basis of differential toxicity. Cancer Res 1985;45:5480.

72. Bleyer WA, Frisby SA, Oliverio VT. Uptake and binding of vincristine by murine leukemia cells. Biochem Pharmacol 1975;24:633.

73. Rahmani R, Zhou XJ, Placidi M, et al. In vivo and in vitro pharmacokinetics and metabolism of vinca alkaloids in rat. I. Vindesine (4-deacetyl-vinblastine 3-carboxyamide). Eur J Drug Metab Pharmacokinet 1990;15:49.

74. Zhou XJ, Martin M, Placidi M, et al. In vivo and in vitro pharmacokinetics and metabolism of vinca alkaloids: II. Vinblastine and vincristine. Eur J Drug Metab Pharmacokinet 1990;15:323.

75. Ferguson PJ, Phillips JR, Steiner M, et al. Differential activity of vincristine and vinblastine against cultured cells. Cancer Res 1984;45:5480.

76. Houghton JA, Williams LG, Houghton PJ. Stability of vincristine complexes in cytosols derived from xenografts of human rhabdomyosarcoma and normal tissues of the mouse. Cancer Res 1985;45:3761.

77. Sullivan KF. Structure and utilization of tubulin isotypes. Annu Rev Cell Biol 1988;4:687.

78. Bowman LC, Houghton JA, Houghton PJ. GTP influences the binding of vincristine in human tumor cytosols. Biochem Biophys Res Commun 1986;135:695.

79. Gout PW, Noble RL, Bruchovsky N, Beer CT. Vinblastine and vincristine growth-inhibitory effects correlate with their retention by cultured Nb2 node lymphoma cells. Int J Cancer 1984;34:245.

80. Ferguson PJ, Philips JR, Seiner M, et al. Biochemical effects of Navelbine on tubulin and associated proteins. Cancer Res 1984;44:3307.

81. Lengfeld AM, Dietrich J, Schultze-Maurer B. Accumulation and release of vinblastine and vincristine in HeLa cells: light microscopic, cinematographic, and biochemical study. Cancer Res 1982;42:3798.

82. Zhou XJ, Placidi M, Rahmani R. Uptake. Uptake and metabolism of vinca alkaloids by freshly isolated human hepatocytes in suspension. Anticancer Res 1994;14:1017.

83. Rahmani R, Zhou XJ. Pharmacokinetics and metabolism of vinca alkaloids . In: Workman P, Graham M, eds. Plainview, NY: Cold Spring Harbar Laboratory Press 1993:269.

84. Jackson DV, Bender RA. Cytotoxic thresholds of vincristine in a murine and human leukemia cell line in vitro. Cancer Res 1979;39:4346.

85. Inaba M, Fujikura R, Sakurai Y. Active efflux common to vincristine and daunorubicin in vincristine-resistant P388 leukemia. Biochem Pharmacol 1981;30:1863.

86. Greenberger LM, Williams SS, Horwitz SB. Biosynthesis of heterogeneous forms of multidrug resistance associated glycoproteins. J Biol Chem 1987;262:13685.

87. Choi K, Chen C, Kriegler M, et al. An altered pattern of cross-resistance in multidrug-resistant human cells results from spontaneous mutations in the mdr1 (P-glycoprotein) gene. Cell 1988;53:519.

88. Peterson RHF, Meyers MB, Spengler BA. Alterations of plasma membrane glycopeptides and gangliosides of Chinese hamster cells accompanying development of resistance to daunorubicin and vincristine. Cancer Res 1983;43:222.

89. Pieters R, Hongo T, Loonen AH, et al. Different types of non-P-glycoprotein mediated multiple drug resistance in children with relapsed acute lymphoblastic leukaemia. Br J Cancer 1992;65:691.

90. Fojo AT, Ueda K, Slamon DJ, et al. Expression of a multidrug-resistance gene in human tumors and tissues. Proc Natl Acad Sci USA 1987;84:265.

91. Beck WT, Mueller TJ, Tanzer LR. Altered cell surface membrane glycoproteins in Vinca alkaloid-resistant human leukemic lymphoblasts. Cancer Res 1979;39:2070.

92. Cornwell MM, Tsuruo T, Gottesman MM, et al. ATP-binding properties of P-glycoprotein from multidrug-resistant KB cells. FASEB J 1987;1:51.

93. Nooter K, Westerman AM, Flens MJ, et al. Expression of the multidrug resistance-associated protein (MRP) in human tissues and adult solid cancers. Clin Cancer Res 1995;1:1301.

94. Beck WT, Cirtain MC, Lefko JL. Energy-dependent reduced drug binding as a mechanism of Vinca alkaloid resistance in human leukemia lymphoblasts. Mol Pharmacol 1983;24:485.

95. Bender RA, Kornreich WD, Wodinsky I. Correlates of vincristine resistance in four murine tumor cell lines. Cancer Lett 1982;15:335.

96. Lockhart A, Tirona G, Kim B. Pharmacogenetics of ATP-binding cassatte transporters in cancer and chemotherapy. Mol Ther 2003;2:695.

97. Safa AR, Glover CJ, Meyers MB, et al. Vinblastine photoaffinity labeling of a high molecular weight surface membrane glycoprotein specific for multidrug-resistant cells. Biochemistry 1987;262:13685.

98. Grant CE, Validmarsson G, Hipfner R, et al. Overexpression of multidrug resistance associated protein (MRP) increases resistance to natural product drugs. Cancer Res 1994;54:356.

99. Scheper RJ, Broxterman HJ, Scheffer GL. Overexpression of a Mr 110000 vesicular protein in non-P-glycoprotein-mediated multidrug resistance. Cancer Res 1993;53:1475.

100. Kruh GD, Gaughan KT, Godwin A, et al. Expression pattern of MRP in human tissues and adult solid tumor cell lines. J Natl Cancer Inst 1995;87:1256.

101. Hipner DR, Deeley RG, Cole SP. Structural, mechanistic, and clinical aspects of MRP1. Biochim Biopsy Acta 1999;1461:359.

102. Zaman GJ, Floens JM, van Leusden MR, et al. The human multidrug resistance-protein MRP is a plasma membrane drug-efflux pump. Proc Natl Acad Sci USA 1994;91:8822.

103. Betrand Y, Capdeville R, Balduck N, et al. Cyclosporin A used to reverse drug resistance increases vincristine neurotoxicity. Am J Hematol 1992;40:158.

104. Pinkerton CR. Multidrug resistance reversal in childhood malignancies: potential for a real step forward? Eur J Cancer 1996; 32A:641.

105. List AF, Kopecky KJ, Willman CL, et al. Benefit of cyclosporine modulation of drug resistance in patients with poor-risk acute myeloid leukemia: a Southwest Oncology Group Study. Blood 2004;98:3212.

106. Amos LA, Baker TS. The three dimension structure of tubulin protofilaments. Nature 1979;279:607.

107. Rai SS, Wolf J. Localization of critical histidyl residues required for vinblastine-induced tubulin polymerization and for microtubule assembly. J Biol Chem 1998;273:31131.

108. Minotti AM, Barlow SB, Cabral F. Resistance to antimitotic drugs in Chinese hamster ovary cells correlates with changes in the level of polymerized tubulin. J Biol Chem 1991;266:3987.

109. Cabral FR, Barlow SB. Resistance to the antimitotic agents as genetic probes of microtubule structure and function. Pharmacol Ther 1991;52:159.

110. Cabral FR, Barlow SB. Mechanisms by which mammalian cells acquire resistance to drugs that affect microtubule assembly. FASEB J 1989;3:1593.

111. Cabral FR, Brady RC, Schiber MJ. A mechanism of cellular resistance to drugs that interfere with microtubule assembly. Ann N Y Acad Sci 1986;466:748.

112. Hari M, Wang Y, Veeraraghavan S. Mutations in alpha- and beta-tubulin that stabilize microtubules and coner resistance to colcemid and vinblastine. Mol Cancer Ther 2003;2:597.

113. Ranganathan S, Dexter DW, Benetatos CA, et al. Cloning and sequencing of human βIII-tubulin cDNA: induction of betaIII isotype in human prostate carcinoma cells by acute exposure to antimicrotubule agents. Biochim Biophys Acta 1998;1395:237.

114. Sethi VS, Thimmaiah KN. Structural studies of the degradation products of vincristine dihydrogen sulfate. Cancer Res 1985;45: 4386.

115. Castle MC, Margileth DA, Oliverio VT. Distribution and excretion of [3H]vincristine in the rat and the dog. Cancer Res 1976;36:3684.

116. Bender RA, Castle MC, Margileth DA, et al. The pharmacokinetics of [3H]-vincristine in man. Clin Pharmacol Ther 1977;22: 430.

117. Culp HW, Daniels WD, McMahon RE. Disposition and tissue levels of [3H]-vindesine in rats. Cancer Res 1977;37:3053.

118. Owellen RJ, Hartke CA, Hains FO. Pharmacokinetics and metabolism of vinblastine in humans. Cancer Res 1977;37:2597.

119. Owellen RJ, Root MA, Hains FO. Pharmacokinetic of vindesine and vincristine in humans. Cancer Res 1977;37:2603.

120. Jackson DV, Castle MC, Bender RA. Biliary excretion of vincristine. Clin Pharmacol Ther 1978;24:101.

121. Ramirez J, Ogan K, Ratain MJ. Determination of vinca alkaloids in human plasma by liquid chromatography/atmospheric pressure chemical ionization mass spectrometry. Cancer Chemother Pharmacol 1997;39:286.

122. Van Tellingen O, Beijnen JH, Nooyen WJ. Analytical methods for the determination of vinca alkaloids in biological specimens: a survey of the literature. J Pharm Biomed Anal 1991;9:1077.

123. Ylinen M, Suhonen P, Naaranlahti T, et al. Gas chromatographic-mass spectrometric analysis of major indole alkaloids of Catharanthus roseus. J Chromatogr 1990;505:429.

124. Rahmani R, Bruno R, Iliadis A, et al. Clinical pharmacokinetics of the antitumor drug Navelbine (5′-noranhydrovinblastine). Cancer Res 1987;47:5796.

125. Nelson RL, Dyke RW, Root MA. Comparative pharmacokinetics of vindesine, vincristine, and vinblastine in patients with cancer. Cancer Treat Rev 1980;7(Suppl):17.

126. Gidding CE, Kellie SJ, Kamps WA, et al. Vincristine revisited. Crit Rev Oncol Hematol 1999;29:267.

127. Sethi VS, Jackson DV, White CT, et al. Pharmacokinetics of vincristine sulfate in adult cancer patients. Cancer Res 1981;41:3551.

128. Jackson DV Jr. The periwinkle alkaloids. In: Lokich JJ, ed. Cancer Chemotherapy by Infusion. Chicago: 1990:155.

129. Ferrara F, Annunziata M, Pollio F, et al. Vincristine as treatment for recurrent episodes of thrombotic thrombocytopenic purpura. Ann Hematol 2002;81:7.

130. Owellen RJ, Donigian DW. 3H-Vincristine: preparation. and preliminary pharmacology. J Med Chem 1972;15:894.

131. Jackson DV, Sethi VS, Spurr CL, et al. Pharmacokinetics of vincristine in the cerebrospinal fluid of humans. Cancer Res 1981;41:1466.

132. Jehl F, Quoix E, Leveque D, et al. Pharmacokinetic and preliminary metabolic fate of Navelbine in humans as determined by high performance liquid chromatography. Cancer Res 1991; 51:2073.

133. Sethi VS, Castle MC, Surratt P, et al. Isolation and partial characterization of human urinary metabolites of vincristine sulfate. Proc Am Assoc Cancer Res 1981;22:173.

134. Villikka K, Kivistö KT, Mäenpää H, et al. Cytochrome P450-inducing antiepileptics increase the clearance of vincristine in patients with brain tumors. Clin Pharmacol Ther 1999;66:589.

135. Gillies J, Hung KA, Fitzsimons E, et al. Severe vincristine toxicity in combination with itraconazole. Clin Lab Haematol 1998;20:123.

136. Yao D, Ding S, Burchell B, et al. Detoxication of vinca alkaloids by human P450 CYP3A4-mediated metabolism: implications for the development of drug resistance. J Pharmacol Exp Ther 2000;294:387.

137. Steele WH, Barber HE, Dawson AA, et al. Protein binding of prednisone and vinblastine in the serum of normal subjects. Br J Clin Pharmacol 1982;13:595.

138. Hebden HF, Hadfield JR, Beer CT. The binding of vinblastine by platelets in the rat. Cancer Res 1970;30:1417.

139. Young JA, Howell S, Green MR. Pharmacokinetics and toxicity of 5-day continuous infusion of vinblastine. Cancer Chemother Pharmacol 1994;12:43.

140. Creasey WA, Marsh JC. Metabolism of vinblastine (VBL) in the dog. Proc Am Assoc Cancer Res 1973;14:57.

141. Zhou-Pan XR, Seree E, Zhou XJ, et al. Involvement of human liver cytochrome P450 3A in vinblastine metabolism: drug interactions. Cancer Res 1993;53:5121.

142. Ohnuma T, Norton L, Andrejczuk A, et al. Pharmacokinetics of vindesine given as an intravenous bolus and 24-hour infusion in humans. Cancer Res 1985;45:464.

143. Nelson RL, Dyke RW, Root MA. Clinical pharmacokinetics of vindesine. Cancer Chemother Pharmacol 1979;2:243.

144. Rahmani R, Martin M, Favre R, et al. Clinical pharmacokinetics of vindesine: repeated treatments by intravenous bolus injections. Eur J Cancer Clin Oncol 1984;20:1409.

145. Rahmani R, Kleisbauer JP, Cano JP, et al. Clinical pharmacokinetics of vindesine infusion. Cancer Treat Rep 1985; 69:839.

146. Jackson DV Jr, Sethi VS, Long TR, et al. Pharmacokinetics of vindesine bolus and infusion. Cancer Chemother Pharmacol 1994; 13:114.

147. Hande K, Gay J, Gober J, et al. Toxicity and pharmacology of bolus vindesine injection and prolonged vindesine infusion. Cancer Treat Rev 1980;7:25.

148. Zhou XJ, Zhou-Pan XR, Gauthier T, et al. Human liver microsomal cytochrome P450 3A isoenzymes mediated vindesine biotransformation: metabolic drug interactions. Biomed Pharmacol 1993;4:853.

149. Levêque D, Jehl F. Clinical pharmacokinetics of vinorelbine. Clin Pharmacokinet 1996;31:184.

150. Urien S, Bree F, Breillout F, et al. Vinorelbine high-affinity binding to human platelets and lymphocytes: distribution in human blood. Cancer Chemother Pharmacol 1988;23:247.

151. Levêque D, Quoiz E, Dumont P, et al. Pulmonary distribution of vinorelbine in patients with non-small lung cancer. Cancer Chemother Pharmacol 1993;33:176.

152. Rahmani R, Gueritte F, Martin M, et al. Comparative pharmacokinetics of antitumor vinca alkaloids: intravenous bolus injections of Navelbine and related alkaloids to cancer patients and rats. Cancer Chemother Pharmacol 1986;16:223.

153. Levêque D, Merle-Melet M, Bresler L, et al. Biliary elimination and pharmacokinetics of vinorelbine in micropigs. Cancer Chemother Pharmacol 1993;32:487.

154. Krikorian A, Rahmani R, Bromet M, et al. Pharmacokinetics and metabolism of Navelbine. Semin Oncol 1989;16(Suppl 4):21.

155. Sorio R, Robieux I, Galligioni E, et al. Pharmacokinetics and tolerance of vinorelbine in elderly patients with metastatic breast cancer. Eur J Cancer 1997;33:301.

156. Robieux I, Sorio R, Borsatti E, et al. Pharmacokinetics of vinorelbine in patients with liver metastases. Clin Pharmacol Ther 1996;59:32.

157. Bugat R, Variol P, Roche H, et al. The effects of food on the pharmacokinetic profile of oral vinorelbine. Cancer Chemother Pharmacol 2002;50:285.

158. Zhou XJ, Zhou-Pan XR, Favre R, et al. Relative bioavailability of two oral formulations of navelbine in cancer patients. Biopharm Drug Dispos 1994;15:577.

159. Bender RA, Bleyer WA, Frisby SA. Alteration of methotrexate uptake in human leukemia cells by other agents.. Cancer Res 1975;35:1305.

160. Zager RF, Frisby SA, Oliverio VT. The effects of antibiotics and cancer chemotherapeutic agents on the cellular transport and antitumor activity of methotrexate in L1210 murine leukemia. Cancer Res 1973;33:1670.

161. Chan JD. Pharmacokinetic drug interactions of vinca alkaloids. Summary of case reports. Pharmacotherapy 1998;18:1304.

162. Bender RA, Nichols AP, Norton L, et al. Lack of therapeutic synergism of vincristine and methotrexate in L1210 murine leukemia in vivo. Cancer Treat Rep 1978;62:997.

163. Yalowich JC. Effect of microtubule inhibition on etoposide accumulation and DNA damage in human K562 cells in vitro. Cancer Res 1987;47:1010.

164. Bollini R, Riva R, Albani R, et al. Decreased phenytoin levels during antineoplastic therapy: a case report. Epilepsia 1983;24:75.

165. Jarosinski PF, Moscow JA, Alexander MS, et al. Altered phenytoin clearance during intensive chemotherapy for acute lymphoblastic leukemia. J Pediatr 1988;112:996.

166. Tobe SW, Siu LL, Jamel SA, et al. Vinblastine and erythromycin: an unrecognized serious drug interaction. Cancer Chemother Pharmacol 1995, 35:188.

167. Rajaonarison JF, Lacarelle B, Catalin J, et al. Effect of anticancer drugs on the glucuronidation of 3'azido-3'-deoxythymidine in human liver microsomes. Drug Metab Dispos 1993;21:823.

168. Sathiapalan RK, El-Soth H. Enhanced vincristine neurotoxicity from drug interactions: case report and review of literature. Pediatr Hematol Oncol 2001;18:543.

169. Sulkes A, Collins JM. Reappraisal of some dosage adjustment guidelines. Cancer Treat Rep 1987;71:229.

170. Quasthoff S, Hartung HP. Chemotherapy-induced peripheral neuropathy. J Neurol 2002;249:9.

171. Peltier AC, Russell JW. Recent advances in drug-induced neuropathies. Curr Opin Neurol 2002;15:633.

172. Costa G, Hreshchyshyn MM, Holland JF. Initial clinical studies with vincristine. Cancer Chemother Rep 1962;24:39.

173. Holland JF, Scharlan C, Gailani S, et al. Vincristine treatment of advanced cancer: a cooperative study of 392 cases. Cancer Res 1973;33:1258.

174. Desai ZR, Van den Berg HW, Bridges JM, et al. Can severe vincristine neuropathy be prevented? Cancer Chemother Pharmacol 1982;8:211.

175. Van den Berg HW, Desai ZR, Wilson R, et al. The pharmacokinetics of vincristine in man: reduced drug clearance associated with raised serum alkaline phosphatase and dose-limiting elimination. Cancer Chemother Pharmacol 1982;8:215.

176. Sweet DL, Golumb HM, Ultmann JE, et al. Cyclophosphamide, vincristine, methotrexate with leukovorin rescue, and cytarabine (COMLA) combination sequential chemotherapy for advanced diffuse histiocytic lymphoma. Ann Intern Med 1980;92:785.

177. Slyter H, Liwnicz B, Herrick MK, et al. Fatal myeloencephalopathy caused by intrathecal vincristine. Neurology 1980;30:867.

178. Dyke RW. Treatment of inadvertent intrathecal administration of vincristine. N Engl J Med 1989;321:1270.

179. Jackson DV Jr, Richards F, Spurr CL, et al. Hepatic intra-arterial infusions of vincristine. Cancer Chemother Pharmacol 1984;13:120.

180. Kinzel PE, Dorr RT. Anticancer drug renal toxicity and elimination: dosing guidelines for altered renal function. Cancer Treat Rev 1995;21:33.

181. Falkson G, Van Dyk JJ, Falkson FC. Oral vinblastine sulfate (NSC 49842) in malignant disease. S Afr Cancer Bull 1968;2:78.

182. Zeffrin J, Yagoda A, Kelsen D, et al. Phase I-II trial of 5-day continuous infusion of vinblastine sulfate. Anticancer Res 1984;4:411.

183. Cvitkovic E, Izzo J. The current and future place of vinorelbine in cancer therapy. Drugs 1982;44(Suppl 2):34.

184. Legha SS. Vincristine neurotoxicity. Pathophysiology and management. Med Toxicol 1986;1:421.

185. Bradley WG, Lassman LP, Pearce GW. The neuromyopathy of vincristine in man: clinical electrophysiological and pathological studies. J Neurol Sci 1970;10:107.

186. Casey EB, Jellife AM, Le Quesne PM, et al. Vincristine neuropathy, clinical and electrophysiological observations. Brain 1973;96:69.

187. Greig NH, Soncrant TT, Shetty HU, et al. Brain uptake and anticancer activities of vincristine and vinblastine are restricted by their low cerebrovascular permeability and binding to plasma constituents in rats. Cancer Chemother Pharmacol 1990;26:263.

188. Carpentieri R, Lockhart LH. Ataxia and athetosis as side effects of chemotherapy with vincristine in non-Hodgkin's lymphomas. Cancer Treat Rep 1978;62:561.

189. Hironen HE, Saknu TT, Heinonen E, et al. Vincristine treatment of acute lymphoblastic leukemia induces transient autonomic cardioneuropathy. . Cancer 1988;64:801.

190. Gottlieb RJ, Cuttner J. Vincristine-induced bladder atony. Cancer 1971;28:674.

191. Carmichael SM, Eagleton L, Ayers CR, et al. Orthostatic hypotension during vincristine therapy. Arch Intern Med 1970;126:290.

192. Burns BV, Shotton JC. Vocal fold palsy following vinca alkaloid treatment. J Laryngol Otol 1998;112:485.

193. Woods WG, O'Leary M, Nesbit ME. Life-threatening neuropathy and hepatotoxicity in infants during induction therapy for acute lymphoblastic leukemia. J Pediatr 1981;98:642.

194. Orejana-Garcia AM, Pascual-Huerta J, Perez-Melero A. Charcot-Marie-Tooth disease and vincristine. J Am Podiatr Med Assoc 2003;93:229.

195. Olek MJ, Bordeaux B, Leshner RT. Charcot-Marie-Tooth disease type I diagnosed in a 5-year old boy after vincristine neurotoxicity, resulting in maternal diagnosis. J Am Osteopath Assoc 1999;99:165.

196. McGuire SA, Gospe SM Jr, Dahl G. Acute vincristine neurotoxicity in the presence of hereditary motor and sensory neuropathy type I. Med Pediatr Oncol 1989;17:520.

197. Trobaugh-Lotrario AD, Smith AA, Odom L. F. Vincristine neurotoxicity in the presence of hereditary neuropathy. Med Pediatr Oncol 2003;40:39.

198. Desai ZR, Van den Berg HW, Bridges JM, et al. Can severe vincristine neurotoxicity be prevented? Cancer Chemother Pharmacol 1982;8:211.

199. Boyle FM, Wheeler HR, Shenfield GM. Glutamate ameliorates experimental vincristine neuropathy. J Pharmacol Exp Ther 1996;279:410.

200. Jackson DV Jr, McMahan RA, Pope EK, et al. Clinical trial of folinic acid to reduce vincristine neurotoxicity. Cancer Chemother Pharmacol 1986;17:281.

201. Grush OC, Morgan SK. Folinic acid rescue for vincristine toxicity. Clin Toxicol 1979;14:71.

202. Helmann K, Hutchinson GE, Henry K. Reduction of vincristine toxicity by Cronassial. Cancer Chemother Pharmacol 1987;20:21.

203. Jackson DV, Wells HB, Atkins JN, et al. Amelioration of vincristine neurotoxicity by glutamic acid. AmJ Med 1988;84:1016.

204. Binet S, Fellous A, Lataste H, et al. In situ analysis of the action of Navelbine on various types of microtubules using immunofluorescence. Semin Oncol 1989;16(Suppl 4):5.

205. Le Chevalier T, Brisgand D, Douillard J-Y, et al. Randomized study of vinorelbine and cisplatin versus vindesineand cisplatin versus vindesine and cisplatin versus vinorelbine alone in non-small cell lung cancer: results of a European multicenter trial including 612 patients. J Clin Oncol 1994;12:360.

206. Bunn PA, Ford SS, Shackney SE. The effects of colcemide on hematopoiesis in the mouse. . J Clin Invest 1975;58:1280.

207. Tester W, Forbes W, Leighton J. Vinorelbine-induced pancreatitis: a case report. J Natl Cancer Inst 1997;89:1631.

208. Sharma RK. Vincristine and gastrointestinal transit. Gastroenterology 1988;95:1435.

209. Subar M, Muggia FM. Apparent myocardial ischemia associated with vinblastine administration. CancerTreat Rep 1986;70:690.

210. Hansen SW, Helweg-Larsen S, Trajoborg W. Long-term neurotoxicity in patients treated with cisplatin, vinblastine, and bleomycin for metastatic germ cell cancer. J Clin Oncol 1989;7:1457.

211. Hantel A, Rowinsky EK, Donehower RC. Nifedipine and oncologic Raynaud's phenomenon. Ann Intern Med 1988;108:767.

212. Ballen KK, Weiss ST. Fatal acute respiratory failure following vinblastine and mitomycin administration for breast cancer. Am J Med Sci 1988;295:558.

213. Hohneker JA. A summary of vinorelbine (Navelbine) safety data from North American clinical trials. Semin Oncol 1994;21(Suppl 10):42.

214. Dorr RT, Alberts DS. Vinca alkaloid skin toxicity: antidote and drug disposition studies in the mouse. J Natl Cancer Inst 1985;74:113.

215. Bellone JD. Treatment of vincristine extravasation. JAMA 1981;245:343.

216. Dorr T. Antidotes to vesicant chemotherapy extravasation. Blood Rev 1990;4:41.

217. Pattison J. Managing cytotoxic extravasation. Nurs Times 2002;98:32.

218. Blain PG. Adverse effects of drugs on skeletal muscle. Adverse Drug React Bull 1984;104:384.

219. Hoff PM, Valero V, Ibrahim N, et al. Hand-foot syndrome following prolonged infusion of high doses of vinorelbine. Cancer 1998;85:965.

220. Stenfanou A, Dooley M. Simple method to eliminate the risk of inadvertent intrathecal vincristine administration. J Clin Oncol 2003;21:2044.

221. Rowinsky EK, Donehower RC. Drug Therapy: paclitaxel (Taxol). N Engl J Med 1995;332:1004.

222. Wani MC, Taylor HL, Wall ME, et al. Plant antitumor agents: VI. The isolation and structure of Taxol, a novel antileukemic and antitumor agent from Taxus brevifolia. J Am Chem Soc 1971;93:2325.

223. Schiff PB, Fant J, Horwitz SB. Promotion of microtubule assembly in vitro by taxol. Nature 1979;22:665.

224. Schiff PB, Horwitz SB. Taxol stabilizes microtubules in mouse fibroblast cells. Proc Natl Acad Sci USA 1980;77:1561.

225. Manfredi JJ, Parness J, Horwitz SB. Taxol binds to cellular microtubules. J Cell Biol 1982;94:688.

226. Cortes JE, Pazdur R. Docetaxel. J Clin Oncol 1995;13:2643.

227. Nowak AK, Wilcken NR, Stockler MR, et al. Systematic review of taxane-containing versus non-taxane-containing regimens for adjuvant and neoadjuvant treatment of early breast cancer. Lancet Oncol 2004;5:372.

228. McGuire WP, Hoskins WJ, Brady MF, et al. Cyclophosphamide and cisplatin compared with paclitaxel and cisplatin in patients with stage III and IV ovarian cancer. N Engl J Med 1996;334:1.

229. Katsumata N. Docetaxel: an alternative taxane in ovarian cancer. Br J Cancer 2003;89(Suppl 3):S9.

230. Moinpour C, Wu J, Donaldson G, et al. Gemcitabine plus paclitaxel (GT) versus paclitaxel (T) as first-line treatment for anthracycline pre-treated metastatic breast cancer (MBC): quality of life (QoL) and pain palliation results from the global phase III study. Proc Am Soc Clin Oncol 2004;22:14S.

231. Citron ML, Berry DA, Cirrincione C, et al. Randomized trial of dose-dense versus conventionally scheduled and sequential versus concurrent combination chemotherapy as postoperative adjuvant treatment of node-positive primary breast cancer: first report of Intergroup Trial C9741/Cancer and Leukemia Group B Trial 9741. J Clin Oncol 2003;21:1432.

232. Henderson IC, Berry D, Demetri G, et al. Improved outcomes from adding sequential Paclitaxel but not from escalating Doxorubicin dose in an adjuvant chemotherapy regimen for patients with node-positive primary breast cancer. J Clin Oncol 2003;21:976-83.

233. Jie C, Tulpule A, Zheng T, et al. Treatment of epidemic AIDS-related Kaposi's sarcoma. Curr Opin Oncol 1997;9:433.

234. Bonomi P, Kim K, Fariclough D, et al. Comparison of survival and quality of life in advanced non-small cell lung cancer

patients treated with two dose levels of paclitaxel combined with cisplatin versus etoposide with cisplatin: results from an Eastern Cooperative Oncology Group trial. J Clin Oncol 2000;18:623.

235. Eisenberger MA, De Wit R, Berry W, et al. A multicenter phase III comparison of docetaxel (D) + prednisone (P) and mitoxantrone (MTZ) + P in patients with hormone-refractory prostate cancer (HRPC). Proc Am Soc Clin Oncol 2004;22:14S.

236. Petrylak DP, Macarthur RB, O'Connor J, et al. Phase I trial of docetaxel with estramustine in androgen-independent prostate cancer. J Clin Oncol 1999;17:958.

237. Petrylak DP, Tangen C, Hussain M, et al. SWOG 99-16: Randomized phase III trial of docetaxel (D)/estramustine (E) versus mitoxantrone(M)/prednisone(p) in men with androgen-independent prostate cancer (AIPCA). Proc Am Soc Clin Oncol 2004;22:145.

238. Lataste H, Senilh V, Wright M, et al. Relationships between the structures of Taxol and baccatine III derivatives and their in vitro action of the disassembly of mammalian brain and Pysarum amoebal microtubules. Proc Natl Acad Sci USA 1984;81:4090.

239. Gueritte-Voegelein F, Guenard D, Lavelle F, et al. Relationships between the structures of Taxol analogues and their antimitotic activity. J Med Chem 1991;34:992.

240. Rao S, Krauss NE, Heerding JM, et al. 3´-(p-Azidobenzamido)taxol photolabels the N-terminal 31 amino acids of b-tubulin. J Biol Chem 1994;269:3132.

241. Rao S, Orr GA, Chaudhary AG, et al. Characterization of the Taxol binding site on the microtubule: 2-(m-azidobenzoyl)taxol photolabels a peptide (amino acids 217-231) of beta tubulin. J Biol Chem 1995;270:20235.

242. Ojima I, Chakravarty S, Inoue T, et al. A common pharmacophore for cytotoxic natural products that stabilize microtubules. Proc Natl Acad Sci U S A 4-13-1999;96:4256.

243. Nogales E, Wofl SG, Downing KH. Structure of the alpha beta tubulin dimer by electron crystallography. Nature 1998;391:199.

244. Jordan A, Hadfield JA, Lawrence NJ, et al. Tubulin as a target for anticancer drugs which interact with the mitotic spindle. Med Res Rev 1998;18:259.

245. He L, Yang CP, Horwitz SB. Mutations in beta-tubulin map to domains involved in regulation of microtubule stability in epothilone-resistant cell lines. Mol Cancer Ther 2001;1:3.

246. Diaz JF, Andreu JM. Assembly of purified GDP-tubulin into microtubules induced by taxol and taxotere: reversibility, ligand stoichiometry and competition. Biochemistry 1993;32:2747.

247. Caplow M, Shanks J, Ruhlen R. How taxol modulates microtubule disassembly. J Biol Chem 1994;269:23399.

248. Vanhoerfer U, Cao S, Harstrict A, et al. Comparative antitumor efficacy of docetaxel and paclitaxel in nude mice bearing human tumor xenografts that overexpress the multidrug resistant protein. Ann Oncol 1997;8:1221.

249. Valero V, Jones SE, Von Hoff DD, et al. A phase II study of docetaxel in patients with paclitaxel-resistant metastatic breast cancer. J Clin Oncol 1998;16:3362.

250. Ravdin P, Erban J, Overmoyer B, et al. Phase III comparison of docetaxel (D) and paclitaxel (P) in patients with metastatic breast cancer (MBC). Proc Eur Cancer Conference 2003;12:670.

251. Jordan MA, Toso RJ, Thrower D, et al. Mechanism of mitotic block and inhibition of cell proliferation by taxol at low concentrations. Proc Natl Acad Sci USA 1993;90:9552.

252. Derry WB, Wilson L, Jordan MA. Substoichiometric binding of taxol suppresses microtubule dynamics. Biochemistry 1995;34:2203.

253. Horwitz SB, Cohen D, Rao S, et al. Taxol: mechanisms of action and resistance. Monogr Natl Cancer Inst 1993;15:63.

254. Chen J-G, Horwitz SB. Differential mitotic responses to microtubule-stabilizing and -destabilizing drugs. Cancer Res 62:1935.

255. Abal M, Andreu JM, Barasoain I. Taxanes microtubule and centrosome targets, and cell cycle dependent mechanisms of action. Curr Cancer Drug Targets 2003;3:193.

256. Derry WB, Wilson L, Jordan MA. Low potency of taxol at microtubule minus ends: implications for its antimitotic and therapeutic mechanism. Cancer Res 1998;58:1177.

257. Jordan MA, Wilson L. Use of drugs to study the role of microtubule assembly dynamics in living cells. Methods Enzymol 1998;298:252.

258. Ringel I, Horwitz SB. Studies with RP56976 (Taxotere): a semi-synthetic analogue of taxol. J Natl Cancer Inst 1991;83:288.

259. Bhalla K, Ibrado AM, Tourkina E, et al. Taxol induces internucleosomal DNA fragmentation associated with programmed cell death in human myeloid leukemia cells. Leukemia 1993;7:563.

260. Poruchynsky MS, Wang EE, Rudin CM, et al. Bcl-xL is phosphorylated in malignant cells following microtubule disruption. Cancer Res 1998;58:3331.

261. Wang LG, Liu XM, Kreis W, et al. The effect of antimicrotubule agents on signal transduction pathways of apoptosis: a review. Cancer Chemother Pharmacol 1999;44:355.

262. Dumontet C, Sikic B. Mechanism of action and resistance to antitubulin agents: microtubule dynamics, drug transport, and cell death. J Clin Oncol 1999;17:1061.

263. Zhang CC, Yang JM, Bash-Babula J, et al. DNA damage increases sensitivity to vinca alkaloids and decreases sensitivity to taxanes through p53-dependent repression of microtubule-associated protein 4. Cancer Res 1999;59:3663.

264. Strobel T, Swanson L, Korsmeyer S, et al. BAX enhances paclitaxel-induced apoptosis through a p53-independent pathway. Proc Natl Acad Sci USA 1996;93:14094.

265. Scatena CD, Stewart ZA, Mays D, et al. Mitotic phosphorylation of Bcl-2 during normal cell cycle progression and Taxol-induced cell growth arrest. J Biol Chem 1998;273:30777.

266. Torres K, Horwitz SB. Mechanisms of Taxol-induced cell death are concentration dependent. Cancer Res 1998;58:3620.

267. Fernlini C, Raspaglio G, Mozzetti S. Bcl-2 down-regulation is a novel mechanism of paclitaxel resistance. Mol Pharmacol 2003;64:51.

268. Moss PJ, Fitzpatrick FA. Taxane-mediated gene induction is independent of microtubule stabilization: induction of transcription regulators and enzymes that modulate inflammation and apoptosis. Proc Natl Acad Sci USA 1998;95:3896.

269. Griffon-Etienne G, Boucher Y, Brekken C, et al. Taxane-induced apoptosis decompresses blood vessels and lowers interstitial fluid pressure in solid tumors: clinical implications. Cancer Res 1999;59:776.

270. Ganansia-Leymarie V, Bischoff P, Bergerat JP. Signal transduction pathways of taxanes-induced apoptosis. Curr Med Chem Anti-Cancer Agents 2003;291.

271. Blagosklonny MV, Schulte TW, Nguyen P, et al. Taxol-induction of p21 WAF1 and p53 requires c-raf-1. Cancer Res 1995;55:4623.

272. Blagosklonny MV. Unwinding the loop of Bcl-2 phosphorylation. Leukemia 2001;15:869.

273. Konishi Y, Lehtinen M, Donovan N, et al. Cdc2 phosphorylation of BAD links the cell cycle to the cell death machinery. Mol Cell 2002;9:1005.

274. Moos PJ, Fitzpatrick FA. Taxane-mediated gene induction is independent of microtubule stabilization: induction of transcription regulators and enzymes that modulate inflammation and apoptosis. Proc Natl Acad Sci U S A 1998;95:3896.

275. Rodi DJ, Janes RW, Sanganee HJ, et al. Screening of a library of phage-displayed peptides identifies human bcl-2 as a taxol-binding protein. J Mol Biol 1999;285:197.

276. Rowinsky EK, Donehower RC, Jones RJ, et al. Microtubule changes and cytotoxicity in leukemic cell lines treated with taxol. Cancer Res 1988;48:4093:4093.

277. Burkhart CA, Berman JW, Swindell CS, et al. Relationship between taxol and other taxanes on induction of tumor necrosis factor-a gene expression and cytotoxicity. Cancer Res 1994;54:5779.

278. Creane M, Seymour CB, Colucci S. Radiobiological effects of docetaxel (Taxotere): a potential radiation sensitizer. I. Int J Radiat Biol 1999;75:731.

279. Fettel MR, Grossman SA, Fisher J, et al. Pre-irradiation paclitaxel in glioblastoma multiforme (GBM): efficacy, pharmacology, and drug interactions. J ClinOncol 1997;15:3121.

280. Tishler RB, Geard CR, Hall EJ, et al. Taxol sensitizes human astrocytoma cells to radiation. Cancer Res 1992;52:3595.

281. Mason KA, Hunter NR, Milas M, et al. Docetaxel enhances tumor radioresponse in vivo. Clin Cancer Res 1997;3:2431.

282. Niero A, Emiliani E, Monti G, et al. Paclitaxel and radiotherapy: sequence-dependent efficacya preclinical model. Clin Cancer Res 1999;5:2213.

283. Belotti D, Vergani V, Drudis T, et al. The microtubule-affecting drug paclitaxel has antiangiogenic activity. Clin Cancer Res 1996;2:1843.

284. Klauber N, Paragni S, Flynn E, et al. Inhibitor of angiogenesis and breast cancer in mice by the microtuble inhibitors 2-methoxyestradiol and taxol. Cancer Res 1997;57:81.

285. Wang J, Lou P, Lesniewski R. Paclitaxel at ultra low concentrations inhibits angiogenesis without affecting cellular microtubule assembly. Anticancer Drugs 2003;14:13.

286. Roberts JR, Allison DC, Dooley WC, et al. Effects of Taxol on cell cycle traverse: taxol-induced polyploidization as a marker for drug resistance. Cancer Res 2990;50:710.

287. Quillen M, Castello C, Krishan A, et al. Cell surface tubulin in leukemic cells: molecular structure surface binding, turnover, cell cycle expression, and origin. J Cell Biol 1985;101:2345.

288. Ding AH, Porteu F, Sanchez E, et al. Shared actions of endotoxin and Taxol on TNF receptors and TNF release. Science 1990;248:370.

289. Van Bockxmeer FM, Martin CE, Thompson DE, et al. Taxol for the treatment of proliferative vitreoretinopathy. Invest Ophthalmol Vis Sci 1985;26:1140.

290. Sollott SJ, Cheng L, Pauly RR, et al. Taxol inhibits neointimal smooth muscle cell accumulation after angioplasty in the rat. J Clin Invest 1995;95:1869.

291. Laroia ST, Laroia AT. Drug-eluting stents. A review of the current literature. Cardiol Rev 2004;12:37.

292. Roy SN, Horwitz SB. A phosphoglycoprotein with taxol resistance in J774.2 cells. Cancer Res 1985;45:3856.

293. Cole SPC, Sparks KE, Fraser K, et al. Pharmacological characterization of multidrug resistant MRP-transfected human tumor cells. Cancer Res 1994;54:5902.

294. Lorico A, Rappa G, Flavell RA, et al. Double knockout of the MRP gene leads to increased drug sensitivity in vitro. Cancer Res 1996;56:5351.

295. Geney R, Ungureanu M, Li D. Overcoming multidrug resistance in taxane chemotherapy. Clin Chem Lab Med 2002;40:918.

296. Rowinsky EK, Smith L, Chaturvedi P, et al. Pharmacokinetic and toxicologic interactions between the multidrug resistance reversal agent VX-710 and paclitaxel in cancer patients. J Clin Oncol 1998;16:2964.

297. Webster LK, Cosson EJ, Stokes KH, et al. Effect of the paclitaxel vehicle, Cremophor EL, on the pharmacokinetics of doxorubicin and doxorubicinol in mice. Br J Cancer 1996;73:522.

298. Rowinsky EK. Pharmacology and metabolism. In: Marcel Dekker New York. McGuire WG, Rowinsky EK, ed. Paclitaxel in Cancer Treatment. Marcel Dekker New York 1995;91.

299. Patnaik A, Oza AM, Warner E, et al. A phase I dose-finding and pharmacokinetic study of paclitaxel and carboplatin with oral oral valspodar in patients with advanced solid tumors. J ClinOncol 2000;18:3677.

300. Cabral F, Wible L, Brenner S, et al. Taxol-requiring mutants of Chinese hamster ovary cells with impaired mitotic spindle activity. J Cell Biol 1983;97:30.

301. Druckman S, Kavallaris M. Microtubule alterations and resistance to tubulin-binding agents. Int J Oncol 2002;21:621.

302. Haber M, Burkhart CA, Regl DL, et al. Altered expression of Mb2, the class II b-tubulin isotype, in a murine J774.2 cell line with a high level of taxol resistance. J Biol Chem 1995;270:31269.

303. Kavallaris M, Kuo DYS, Burkhart CA, et al. Taxol-resistant ovarian tumors are associated with altered expression of specific beta-tubulin isotypes. J Clin Invest 1997;100:1282.

304. Ranganathan S, Dexter DW, Benetatos CA, et al. Increase of beta(III)- and beta(IVa)- tubulin isotopes in human prostate carcinoma cells as a result of estramustine resistance. Cancer Res 1996;56:2584.

305. Giannakakou P, Sackett DL, Kang YK, et al. Paclitaxel-resistant human ovarian cancer cells have mutant beta-tubulins that exhibit impaired paclitaxel-driven polymerization. J Biol Chem 1997;272:17118.

306. Gonzalez-Garay ML, Chang L, Blade K, et al. A β-tubulin leucine cluster involved in microtubule assembly and paclitaxel resistance. J Biol Chem 1999;274:23875.

307. Dumontet C, Jaffrezou JP, Tsuchiya E, et al. Resistance to microtubule-targeted cytotoxins in a K562 leukemia cell variant

associated with altered tubulin expression and polymerization. Elec J Oncol 1998;2:44.

308. Blade K, Menick DR, Cabral F. Overexpression of class I, II, or IVb beta-tubulin isotypes in CHO cells is insufficient to confer resistance to paclitaxel. J Cell Sci 1999;112:2213.

309. Hari M, Yang H, Zeng C, et al. Expression of class III beta-tubulin reduces microtubule assembly and confers resistance to paclitaxel. Cell Motil Cytoskeleton 2003;56:45.

310. Ranganathan S, Benetatos CA, Colarusso PJ, et al. Altered beta-tubulin isotype expression in paclitaxel-resistant human prostate carcinoma cells. Br J Cancer 1998, 77:562.

311. Kavallaris M, Burkhart CA, Horwitz SB. Antisense oligonucleotides to class III beta-tubulin sensitize drug resistant cells to Taxol. Br J Cancer 1999;80:1020.

312. Monzo M, Rosell R, Sánchez JJ, et al. Paclitaxel resistance in non-small cell lung cancer associated with beta tubulin gene mutations. J Clin Oncol 1999;17:1786.

313. Kelley MJ, Li S, Harpole DH. Genetic analysis of the beta-tubulin gene, TUBB, in non-small cell lung cancer. J Natl Cancer Inst 2001;93:1886.

314. Verrills NM, Flemming CL, Liu M, et al. Microtubule alterations and mutations induced by desoxyepothilone B: implications for drug-target interactions. Chem Biol 2003;10:597.

315. Blade K, Menick DR, Cabral F. Overexpression of class I, II, or Ivb beta-tubulin isotypes in CHO cells is insufficient to confer resistance to paclitaxel. J Cell Sci 1999;112:2213.

316. Rosell R, Fossella F, Milas L. Molecular markers and targeted therapy with novel agents: prospects in the treatment of non-small cell lung cancer. Lung Cancer 2002;38(Suppl 4):43.

317. Gooch JL, Van Den Berg CL, et al. Insulin-like growth factor (IGF)-I rescues breast cancer cells from chemotherapy-induced cell death-proliferative and anti-apoptotic effects. Breast Cancer Res Treat 1999;56:1.

318. Murphy M, Hinmann A, Levine AJ. Wild-type p53 negatively regulates the expression of a microtubule-associated protein. Genes Dev 1996;10:2971.

319. Zhang CC, Yang JM, White E, et al. The role of MAP4 expression in the sensitivity to paclitaxel and resistance to vinca alkaloids in p53 mutant cells. Oncogene 1998;16:1617.

320. Schmidt M, Lu Y, Liu B, et al. Differential modulation of paclitaxel-mediated apoptosis by p21^{Waf1} and p27^{Kip1}. Oncogene 2000; 19:2423.

321. Li W, Fan J, Banerjee D, et al. Overexpression of p21^{waf1} decreases g2-M arrest and apoptosis induced by paclitaxel in human sarcoma cells lacking both p53 and functional rb protein. Mol Pharmacol 1999;55:108.

322. Yu D, Liu B, Jing T, et al. Overexpression of both p185^{c-erB2} and p170^{mdr-1} renders breast cancer cells highly resistant to Taxol. Oncogene 1998;16:2087.

323. Yu D, Liu B, Tan M, et al. Overexpression of c-erbB-2/neu in breast cancer cells confers increased resistance to Taxol via mdr-1-independent mechanisms. Oncogene 1996;13:1359.

324. Slamon DJ, Leyland-Jones B, Shak S, et al. Use of chemotherapy plus a monoclonal antibody against HER2 for metastatic breast cancer that overexpresses HER2. N Engl J Med 2001;344:783.

325. Konecny GE, Thomssen C, Luck HJ, et al. Her-2/neu gene amplification and response to paclitaxel in patients with metastatic breast cancer. J Natl Cancer Inst 2004;96:1141.

326. Hamel E, Lin CM, Johns DG. Tubulin-dependent biochemical assay for the antineoplastic agent Taxol and applications to measurements of the drug in the serum. Cancer Treat Rep 1982;66:1381.

327. Leu J-G, Chen B-X, Schiff PB, et al. Characterization of polyclonal and monoclonal anti-Taxol antibodies and measurement of Taxol in serum. Cancer Res 1993;53:1388.

328. Mortier KA, Verstraete AG, Zhang GF, et al. Enhanced method performance due to a shorter chromatographic run-time in a liquid chromatography-tandem mass spectrometry assay for paclitaxel. J Chromatogr A 2004;1041:235.

329. Gustafson DL, Long ME, Zirrolli JA, et al. Analysis of docetaxel pharmacokinetics in humans with the inclusion of later sampling time-points afforded by the use of a sensitive tandem LCMS assay. Cancer Chemother Pharmacol 2003;52:159.

330. Malingre MM, Beijnen JH, Schellens JHM. Oral delivery of the taxanes. Invest New Drugs 2001;19:155.

331. Huizing MT, Keung ACF, Rosing H, et al. Pharmacokinetics of paclitaxel and metabolites in a randomized comparative study in platinum-pretreated ovarian cancer patients. J Clin Oncol 1993; 11:2127.

332. Gianni L, Kearns C, Gianni A, et al. Nonlinear pharmacokinetics and metabolism of paclitaxel and its pharmacokinetic/pharmacodynamic relationships in humans. J Clin Oncol 1995;13:180.

333. Sonnichsen D, Hurwitz C, Pratt C, et al. Saturable pharmacokinetics and paclitaxel pharmacodynamics in children with solid tumors. J Clin Oncol 1994;12:532.

334. Ohtsu T, Sasaki Y, Tamura T, et al. Clinical pharmacokinetics and pharmacodynamics of paclitaxel: a 3-hour infusion versus a 24-hour infusion. Clin Cancer Res 1995;1:599.

335. Van Tellingen O, Huizing MT, Panday VR, et al. Cremophor EL causes (pseudo) nonlinear pharmacokinetics of paclitaxel in patients. Br J Cancer 1999;81:330.

336. Sparreboom A, van Zuylen L, Brouwer E, et al. Cremophor EL-mediated alterations of paclitaxel distribution in human blood: clinical pharmacokinetic implications. Cancer Res 1999;59: 1454.

337. Gelderblom H, Mross K, ten Tije AJ, et al. Comparative pharmacokinetics of unbound paclitaxel during 1- and 3-hour infusions. J Clin Oncol 2002;20:574.

338. Kumar GN, Walle UK, Bhalla KN, et al. Binding of taxol to human plasma, albumin, and alpha 1-acid glycoprotein. Res Commun Chem Pathol Pharmacol 1993;80:337.

339. Henningsson A, Sparreboom A, Sandstrom M, et al. Population pharmacokinetic modelling of unbound and total plasma concentrations of paclitaxel in cancer patients. Eur J Cancer 2003;39:1105.

340. Lesser G, Grossman SA, Eller S, et al. The neural and extra-neural distribution of systemically administered [3H]paclitaxel in rats: a quantitative autoradiographic study. Cancer Chemother Pharmacol 1995;34:173.

341. Smorenburg CH, Sparreboom A, Bontenbal M, et al. Randomized cross-over evaluation of body-surface area-based dosing versus flat-fixed dosing of paclitaxel. J Clin Oncol 2003;21:197.

342. Glantz MJ, Choy H, Kearns CM, et al. Paclitaxel disposition in plasma and central nervous systems of humans and rats with brain tumors. J Natl Cancer Inst 1995;87:1077.

343. Monsarrat B, Alvinerie P, Dubois J, et al. Hepatic metabolism and biliary clearance of taxol in rats and humans. Monograph Natl Cancer Inst 1993;15:39.

344. Cresteil T, Monsarrat B, Alvinerie P, et al. Taxol metabolism by human liver microsomes: identification of cytochrome P450 isoenzymes involved in its biotransformation. Cancer Res 1994;54:386.

345. Nallani SC, Goodwin B, Maglich JM. Introduction of cytochrome P450 3A by paclitaxel in mice: pivotal role of the nuclear xenobiotic receptor, pregnane X receptor. Drug Metab Dispos 2003;31:681.

346. Harris JW, Rahman A, Kim B-R, et al. Metabolism of taxol by human hepatic microsomes and liver slices: participation of cytochrome P450 3A4 and an unknown P450 enzyme. Cancer Res 1994;15:4026.

347. Kerns CM, Gianni L, Egorin M. Paclitaxel pharmacokinetics and pharmacodynamics. Semin Oncol 1995;22:16.

348. Monsarrat B, Chatelut E, Royer I, et al. Modification of paclitaxel metabolism in a cancer patient by induction of cytochrome P450 3A4. Drug Metab Dispos 1998;26:229.

349. Gianni L, Munzone E, Capri G, et al. Paclitaxel by 3-hour infusion in combination with bolus doxorubicin in women with untreated metastatic breast cancer: high antitumor efficacy and cardiac effects in a dose- finding and sequence- finding study. J Clin Oncol 1995;13:2688.

350. Rowinsky EK, Bonomi P, Jiroutek M, et al. Paclitaxel steady-state plasma concentration as a determinant of disease outcome and toxicity in lung cancer patients treated with paclitaxel and cisplatin. Clin Cancer Res 1999;5:767.

351. Clarke SJ, Rivory LP. Clinical pharmacokinetics of docetaxel. Clin Pharmacokinet 1999;36:99.

352. Bruno R, Hille D, Riva A, et al. Population pharmacokinetic/pharmacodynamics of docetaxel in phase II studies in patients with cancer. J Clin Oncol 1998;16:186.

353. Bruno R, Vivier N, Veyrat-Follet C, et al. Population pharmacokinetics and pharmacokinetic-pharmadynamic relationships for docetaxel. Invest New Drugs 2001;19:163.

354. McLeod HL, Kearns CM, Kuhn JG, et al. Evaluation of the linearity of docetaxel pharmacokinetics. Cancer Chemother Pharmacol 1998;42:155.

355. Marland M, Gaillard C, Sanderink G, et al. Kinetics, distribution, metabolism and excretion of radiolabeled Taxotere (14C-RPR 56976) in mice and dogs. Proc Am Assoc Cancer Res 1993; 34:393.

356. Sparreboom A, Van Tellingen O, Scherrenburg EJ, et al. Isolation, purification and biological activity of major docetaxel metabolites from human feces. Drug Metab Dispos 1996;24:655.

357. Baker SD, Zhao M, Lee CK, et al. Comparative pharmacokinetics of weekly and every-three-weeks docetaxel. Clin Cancer Res 2004;10:1976.

358. Ten Tije AJ, Loos WJ, Zhao M, et al. Limited cerebrospinal fluid penetration of docetaxel. Anticancer Drugs 2004;15:715.

359. Royer I, Bonsarrat B, Sonnier M, et al. Metabolism of docetaxel by human cytochromes P450: interactions with paclitaxel and other antineoplastic agents. Cancer Res 1996;56:58.

360. Shou M, Martinet M, Korzekwa KR, et al. Role of cytochrome P450 3A4 and 3A5 in the metabolism of taxotere and its derivatives: enzyme specificity, interindividual distribution and metabolic contribution in human liver. Pharmacogenetics 1998; 8:8391.

361. Hirth J, Watkins PB, Strawderman M, et al. The effect of an individual's cytochrome CYP3A4 activities on docetaxel clearance. Clin Cancer Res 2000;6:1255.

362. Vigano L, Locatelli A, Grasselli G, et al. Drug interactions of paclitaxel and docetaxel and their relevance for the design of combination therapy. Invest New Drugs 2201;19:197.

363. Rowinsky EK, Gilbert M, McGuire WP, et al. Sequences of taxol and cisplatin: a phase I and pharmacologic study. J Clin Oncol 1991;9:1692.

364. Rowinsky EK, Citardi M, Noe DA, et al. Sequence-dependent cytotoxicity between cisplatin and the antimicrotubule agents taxol and vincristine. J Cancer Res Clin Oncol 1993;119:737.

365. Belani CP, Kearns CM, Zuhowski EG, et al. Phase I trial, including pharmacokinetic and pharmacodynamic correlations, of combination paclitaxel and carboplatin in patients with metastatic non-small-cell lung cancer. J Clin Oncol 1999;17:676.

366. Kearns CM, Egorin MJ. Considerations regarding the less-than-expected thrombocytopenia encountered with combination paclitaxel/carboplatin chemotherapy. Semin Oncol 1997;24 (Suppl 2):S2.

367. Daga H, Isobe T, Miyazaki M, et al. Investigating the relationship between serum thrombopoietin kinetics and the platelet-sparing effect: a clinical pharmacological evaluation of combined paclitaxel and carboplatin in patients with non-small cell lung cancer. Oncol Rep 2004;11:2225.

368. Holmes FA, Madden T, Newman RA, et al. Sequence-dependent alteration of doxorubicin pharmacokinetics by paclitaxel in a phase I study of paclitaxel and doxorubicin in patients with metastatic breast cancer. J Clin Oncol 1996;14: 2713–2721.

369. Gianni L, Vigano L, Locatelli A, et al. Human pharmacokinetic characterization and in vitro study of the interactions between doxorubicin and paclitaxel in patients with breast cancer. J Clin Oncol 1997;15:1906.

370. Perotti A, Cresta S, Grasselli G. Cardiotoxic effects of anthracycline-taxane combinations. Expert Opin Drug Saf 2003;2:59.

371. Gennari A, Salvadori B, Donati S, et al. Cardiotoxicity of epirubicin/paclitaxel-containing regimens: role of cardiac risk factors. J Clin Oncol 1999;11:3596.

372. Kennedy MJ, Zahurak ML, Donehower RC, et al. Phase I and pharmacologic study of sequences of paclitaxel and cyclophosphamide supported by granulocyte colony-stimulating factor in women with previously treated metastatic breast cancer. J Clin Oncol 1995;14:783.

373. Sarvada N, Ishikawa T, Fukase Y, et al. Induction of thymidine phosphorylase activity and enhancement of capecitabine efficacy by taxol/taxotere in human cancer xenografts. Clin Cancer Res 1998;4:1013.

374. Prados MD, Schold SC, Spence AM, et al. Phase II study of paclitaxel in patients with recurrent malignant glioma. J Clin Oncol 1996;14:2316.

375. Monsarrat B, Chatelut E, Royer I, et al. Modification of paclitaxel metabolism in a cancer patient by induction of cytochrome P450 3A4. Drug Metab Dispos 1998;26:229.

376. Desai PB, Duan JZ, Zhu YW, et al. Human liver microsomal metabolism of paclitaxel and drug interactions. Eur J Drug Metab Pharmacokinet 1998;23:417.

377. Bun SS, Ciccolini J, Bun H. Drug interactions of paclitaxel metabolism in human liver microsomes. J Chemother 2003 Jun;15(3):266–74.

378. Wang LZ, Goh BC, Grigg ME, et al. Differences in the induction of cytochrome P450 3A4 by taxane anticancer drugs, docetaxel, and paclitaxel, assessed by employing primary human hepatocytes. Cancer Chemother Pharmacol 2004, 219.

379. Van Veldhuizen PJ, Reed G, et al. Docetaxel and ketoconazole in advanced hormone-refractory prostate carcinoma: a phase I and pharmacokinetic study. Cancer 2003;98:1855.

380. Slichenmyer W, McGuire W, Donehower R, et al. Pretreatment H2 receptor antagonists that differ in P450 modulation activity: comparative effects on paclitaxel clearance rates. Cancer Chemother Pharmacol 1995;36:227.

381. Thompson ME, Highley MS. Interaction between paclitaxel and warfarin. Interaction between paclitaxel and warfarin. Ann Oncol 2003;14:500.

382. James-Dow CA, Klecker RW, Katki AG, et al. Metabolism of Taxol by human and rat liver in vitro. A screen for drug interactions and interspecies differences. Cancer Chemother Pharmacol 1995;36:107.

383. Klecker RW, Jamis-Dow CA, Egorin MJ, et al. Effect of cimetidine, probenecid, and ketoconazole on the distribution, biliary secretion, and metabolism of 3H-Taxol in the Sprague- Dawley rat. Drug Metab Dispos Biol Fate 1994;22:254.

384. Rowinsky EK. The taxanes: dosing and scheduling considerations. Oncology 1997;11(Suppl 2):1.

385. Seidman AD, Berry D, Cirrincione C, et al. CALGB 9840: Phase III study of weekly (W) paclitaxel (P) via 1-hour(h) infusion versus standard (S) 3h infusion every third week in the treatment of metastatic breast cancer (MBC), with trastuzumab (T) for HER2 positive MBC and randomized for T in HER2 normal MBC. Proc Am Soc Clin Oncol 2004;22:14S.

386. Seidman AD, Hochhauser D, Gollub M, et al. Ninety-six-hour paclitaxel infusion after progression during short taxane exposure: a phase II pharmacokinetic and pharmacodynamic study in metastatic breast cancer. J Clin Oncol 1996;14:1877.

387. Seidman AD, Hudis CA, Albanel J, et al. Dose-dense therapy with weekly 1-hour paclitaxel infusions in the treatment of metastatic breast cancer. J Clin Oncol 1998;16:3353.

388. Markman M, Rose PG, Jones E, et al. Ninety-six-hour infusional paclitaxel as salvage therapy of ovarian cancer patients previously failing treatment with 3-hour or 24-hour paclitaxel infusion. J Clin Oncol 1998;16:1849.

389. Holmes FA, Valero V, Buzdar AU, et al. Final results: randomized phase III trial of paclitaxel by 3-hr versus 96-hr infusion in patients with metastatic breast cancer. Proc Am Soc Clin Oncol 1999;18:110a.

390. Wilson WH, Berg S, Bryant G, et al. Paclitaxel in doxorubicin-refractory or mitoxantrone-refractory breast cancer: a phase I/II trial of 96 hour infusion. J Clin Oncol 1994;12:1621.

391. Greco FA, Thomas M, Hainsworth JD. One-hour paclitaxel infusions: review of the safety and efficacy. Cancer Sci Am 1999; 5:179.

392. Hainsworth JD, Burris HA, Greco FA. Weekly administration of docetaxel (Taxotere): summary of clinical data. Semin Oncol 1999;26(Suppl 10):19.

393. Green MC, Buzdar AU, Smith T, et al. Weekly paclitaxel followed by FAC as primary systemic chemotherapy of operable breast cancer improves pathologic complete remission rates when compared to every 3-week paclitaxel therapy followed by FAC-final results of a prospective randomized phase III study. Proc Am Soc Clin Oncol 2002;21:35a.

394. Smith RE, Brown AM, Mamounas EP, et al. Randomized trial of 3-hour versus 24-hour infusion of high-dose paclitaxel in

patients with metastatic or locally advanced breast cancer: National Surgical Adjuvant Breast and Bowel Project Protocol B-26. J Clin Oncol 1999;17:3403.

395. Winer EP, Berry DA, Woolf S, et al. Failure of higher-dose paclitaxel to improve outcome in patients with metastatic breast cancer: cancer and leukemia group B trial 9342. J Clin Oncol 2004;22:2061.

396. Jie C, Tulpule A, Zheng T, et al. Treatment of epidemic AIDS-related Kaposi's sarcoma. Curr Opin Oncol 1997;9:433.

397. Armstrong DK, Bundy BN, Baergen R, et al. Randomized phase III study of intravenous (IV) paclitaxel and cisplatin versus IV paclitaxel, intraperitoneal (IP) cisplatin and IP paclitaxel in optimal stage III epithelial ovarian cancer (OC): a Gynecologic Oncology Group trial (GOG 172). Proc Am Soc Clin Oncol 2002;21:201.

398. Francis P, Rowinsky E, Schneider J, et al. Phase I feasibility and pharmacologic study of intraperitoneal paclitaxel: a Gynecologic Oncology Group study. J Clin Oncol 1995;13:2961.

399. Markman M, Brady MF, Spirtos NM, et al. Phase II trial of intraperitoneal paclitaxel in carcinoma of the ovary, tube, and peritoneum: a Gynecologic Oncology Group study. J Clin Oncol 1998;16:2620.

400. Bookman MA, Kloth DD, Kover PE, et al. Short-course intravenous prophylaxis for paclitaxel-related hypersensitivity reactions. Ann Oncol 1997;8:611.

401. Kloover JS, den Bakker MA, Gelderblom H, et al. Fatal outcome of a hypersensitivity reaction to paclitaxel: a critical review of premedication regimens. Br J Cancer 2004;90:305.

402. Baker SD, Ravdin P, Aylesworth C, et al. A phase I and pharmacokinetic study of docetaxel in cancer patients with liver dysfunction due to malignancies. Proc Am Soc Clin Oncol 1998;17:192.

403. Venock AP, Egorin MJ, Rosner GL, et al. Phase I and pharmacokinetic trial of paclitaxel in patients with hepatic dysfunction. Cancer and leukemia group B 9264. J Clin Oncol 1998;16:1811.

404. Woo MH, Gregornik D, Shearer PD, et al. Pharmacokinetics of paclitaxel in an anephric patient. Cancer Chemother Pharmacol 1999;43:92.

405. Salminen E, Bergman M, Huhtala S, et al. Docetaxel: standard recommended dose of 100 mg/m2 is effective but not feasible for some metastatic breast cancer patients heavily pretreated with chemotherapy—A phase II single-center study. J Clin Oncol 1999;17:1127.

406. Piccart MJ, Klijn J, Paridaens R, et al. Corticosteroids significantly delay the onset of docetaxel-induced fluid retention: final results of a randomized study of the European Organization for Research and Treatment of Cancer, Investigational Drug Branch for Breast Cancer. J Clin Oncol 1997;15.

407. Markman M. Managing taxane toxicities. Support Care Cancer 2003;11:144.

408. Rowinsky EK, Eisenhauer EA, Chaudhry V, et al. Clinical toxicities encountered with taxol. Semin Oncol 1993;20(Suppl 3):1.

409. Eisenhower E, ten Bokkel Huinink W, Swenerton KD, et al. European-Canadian randomized trial of taxol in relapsed ovarian cancer: high vs low dose and long vs. short infusion. J Clin Oncol 1994;12:2654.

410. Weiss R, Donehower RC, Wiernik PH, et al. Hypersensitivity reactions from taxol. J Clin Oncol 1990;8:1263.

411. Peereboom D, Donehower RC, Eisenhauer EA, et al. Successful retreatment with taxol after major hypersensitivity reactions. J Clin Oncol 1993;11:885.

412. Price KS, Castells MC. Taxol reactions. Allergy Asthma Proc 2002;23:205.

413. Olson JK, Sood AK, Sorosky JJ, et al. Taxol hypersensitivity: rapid pretreatment is safe and cost effective. Gynecol Oncol 1996:68:25.

414. Szebeni J, Muggia FM, Alving CR. Complement activation by Cremophor EL as a possible contributor to hypersensitivity to paclitaxel: an in vitro study. J Natl Cancer Inst 1998;90:300.

415. Chaudhry V, Rowinsky EK, Sartorious SE, et al. Peripheral neuropathy from taxol and cisplatin combination chemotherapy: clinical and electrophysiological studies. Ann Neurol 1994;35:490.

416. Rowinsky EK, Chaudhry V, Cornblath DR, et al. The neurotoxicity of taxol. Monogr Natl Cancer Inst 1993;15:107.

417. Gelmon K, Eisenhauer E, Bryce C, et al. Randomized phase II study of high-dose paclitaxel with or without amifostine in patients with metastatic breast cancer. J Clin Oncol 1999; 17:3038.

418. Vahdat L, Papadopoulos K, Lange D, et al. Reduction of paclitaxel-induced per neuropathy with glutamine. Clin Cancer Res 2004;7:1192.

419. Garrison JA, McCune JS, Livingston RB, et al. Myalgias and arthralgias associated with paclitaxel. Oncology 2003;17:271.

420. Capri G, Munzone E, Tarenzi E, et al. Optic nerve disturbances: a new form of paclitaxel neurotoxicity. J Natl Cancer Inst 1994;86:1099.

421. Hofstra LS, de Vries EG, Willemse PH. Ophthalmic toxicity following paclitaxel infusion. Ann Oncol 1997;8:1053.

422. Nieto Y, Cagnoni PJ, Bearman SI, et al. Acute encephalopathy: a new toxicity associated with high-dose paclitaxel. Clin Cancer Res 1999;5:501.

423. Ziske CG, Schottker B, Gorschluter M, et al. Acute transient encephalopathy after paclitaxel infusion: report of three cases. Ann Oncol 2002;13:629.

424. Markman M, Kennedy A, Webser K, et al. Paclitaxel administration to gynecologic cancer patients with major cardiac risk factors. J Clin Oncol 1998;16:3483.

425. Rowinsky EK, McGuire WP, Guarnieri T, et al. Cardiac disturbances during the administration of taxol. J Clin Oncol 1991;9:1704.

426. Arbuck SG, Strauss H, Rowinsky EK, et al. A reassessment of the cardiac toxicity associated with taxol. Monogr Natl Cancer Inst 1993;15:117.

427. Della Torre P, Imondi AR, Bernardi C, et al. Cardioprotection by dexrazoxane in rats treated with doxorubicin and paclitaxel. Cancer Chemother Pharmacol 1999;44:138.

428. Sparano JA, Speyer J, Gradishar WJ, et al. Phase I trial of escalating doses of paclitaxel plus doxorubicin and dexrazoxane in patients with advanced breast cancer. J Clin Oncol 1999;17:880.

429. Jeriah S, Keegan P. Cardiotoxicity associated with paclitaxel/trastuzumab combination chemotherapy. J Clin Oncol 1999; 17:1647.

430. Rowinsky EK, Burke PJ, Karp JE, et al. Phase I and pharmacodynamic study of taxol in refractory adult acute leukemia. Cancer Res 1989;49:4640.

431. Pestalozzi BC, Sotos GA, Choyke PL, et al. Typhlitis resulting from treatment with taxol and doxorubicin in patients with metastatic breast cancer. Cancer 1993;71:1797.

432. Seewaldt VL, Cain JM, Goff BA, et al. A retrospective review of paclitaxel-associated gastrointestinal necrosis in patients with epithelial ovarian cancer. Gynecol Oncol 1997;67:137.

433. Feenstra J, Vermeer RJ, Stricker BH. Fatal hepatic coma attributed to paclitaxel. J Natl Cancer Inst 1997;16:582.

434. Ramanathan RK, Belani CP. Transient pulmonary infiltrates: a hypersensitivity reaction to paclitaxel. Ann Intern Med 1996; 124:278.

435. Ayoub JP, North L, Greer J, et al. Pulmonary changes in patients with lymphoma who receive paclitaxel. J Clin Oncol 1997; 15:2476.

436. Minisini AM, Tosti A, Sobrero AF, et al. Taxane-induced nail changes: incidence, clinical presentation and outcome. Annal Oncol 2003;14:333.

437. Schrijvers D, Wanders J, Dirix L, et al. Coping with toxicities of docetaxel (Taxotere). Ann Oncol 1993;4:610.

438. Bernstein BJ. Docetaxel as an alternative to paclitaxel after acute hypersensitivity reactions. Ann Pharmacother 2000;34:1332.

439. Semb KA, Aamdal S, Oian P. Capillary protein leak syndrome appears to explain fluid retention in cancer patients who receive docetaxel treatment. J Clin Oncol 1998;16:3426–3432.

440. Zimmerman GC, Keeling JH, Barris HA, et al. Acute cutaneous reactions to docetaxel, a new chemotherapeutic agent. Arch Dermatol 1995;131:202.

441. Vukeljia SJ, Baker WJ, Burris HA III, et al. Pyridoxine therapy for palmar-plantar erythrodysesthesia associated with Taxotere. J Natl Cancer Inst 1993;85:1432.

442. Zimmerman GC, Keeling JH, Lowry M, et al. Prevention of docetaxel-induced erythrodysesthesia with local hypothermia. J Natl Cancer Inst 1994;86:557.

443. Wasner G, Hilpert F, Schattschneider J. Docetaxel-induced nail changes-a neurogenic mechanism: a case report. J Neurooncol 2002;58:167.

444. Hilkens PH, Verweij J, Stoter G, et al. Peripheral neurotoxicity induced by docetaxel. Neurology 1996;46:104:2004.

445. Vasey PA. Survival and long-term toxicity results of the SCOTROC study: docetaxel-carboplatin (DC) vs. paclitaxel-carboplatin (PC) in epithelial ovarian cancer. Proc Am Soc Clin Oncol 1992;21:202A.

446. Esamaeli B, Hortobagyi G, Esteva F. Canalicular stenosis secondary to weekly docetaxel: a potentially preventable side effect. Ann Oncol 2002;13:218.

447. Tew KD. The mechanism of action of estramustine. Semin Oncol 1983;10:21.

448. Benson R, Hartley-Asp B. Mechanisms of action and clinical uses of estramustine. Cancer Invest 1990;8:375.

449. Tew KD, Glusker JP, Hartley-Asp B, et al. Preclinical and clinical perspectives on the use of estramustine as an antimitotic drug. Pharmacol Ther 1992;56:323.

450. Fex H, Hogberg B, Konyves I. Estramustine phosphatehistorical overview. Urology 1984;23:4.

451. Forsberg JG, Hoisaeter PA. Effects of hormone-cytostatic complexes on the rat ventral prostate in vivo and in vitro. Vitam Horm 1975;33:137.

452. Lindberg B. Treatment of rapidly progressing prostatic carcinoma with estracyt. J Urol 1972;108:303.

453. Kelly WK, Zhu AX, Scher H, et al. Dose escalation study of intravenous estramustine phosphate in combination with paclitaxel and carboplatin in patients with advanced prostate cancer. Clin Cancer Res 2003;9:2098.

454. Savarese DM, Halabi VH, Akerley WL, et al. Phase II study of docetaxel, estramustine and low-dose hydrocortisone in men with hormone-refractory prostate cancer: a final report of CALGB 9780. J Clin Oncol 2001;19:2509.

455. Hudes G, Haas N, Yeslow G, et al. Phase I clinical and pharmacologic trial of intravenous estramustine phosphate. J Clin Oncol 2002;20:1115.

456. Kanje M, Deinum J, Wallin M, et al. Effect of estramustine phosphate on the assembly of isolated bovine brain microtubules and fast axonal transport in the frog sciatic nerve. Cancer Res 1985;45:2234.

457. Hartley-Asp B. Estramustine-induced mitotic arrest in two human prostatic carcinoma cell lines DU 145 and PC-3. Prostate 1984;5:93.

458. Nilsson T, Muntzing J. Initial clinical studies with estramustine phosphate. Urology 1984;23(6 Suppl):49–50.

459. Stearns ME, Tew KD. Antimicrotubule effects of estramustine, an antiprostatic tumor drug. Cancer Res 1985;45:3891.

460. Stearns ME, Wang M, Tew KD, et al. Estramustine binds a MAP-1-like protein to inhibit microtubule assembly in vitro and disrupt microtubule organization in DU 145 cells. J Cell Biol 1998;107:2647.

461. Dahllof B, Billstrom A, Cabral F, et al. Estramustine depolymerizes microtubules by binding to tubulin. Cancer Res 1993;53:4573.

462. Friden B, Wallin M. Dependency of microtubule-associated proteins (MAPs) for tubulin stability and assembly: use of estramustine phosphate in the study of microtubules. Mol Cell Biol 1991;105:149.

463. Laing N, Dahllof B, Hartley-Asp B, et al. Interaction of estramustine with tubulin isotypes. Biochemistry 1997;36:871.

464. Panda D, Miller HP, Islam K, et al. Stabilization of microtubule dynamics by estramustine by binding to a novel site in tubulin: a possible mechanistic basis for its antitumor action. Proc Natl Acad Sci U S A 1997;94:10560.

465. Eklov S, Mahdy E, Wester K, et al. Estramustine-binding protein (EMBP) content in four different cell lines and its correlation to estramustine induced metaphase arrest. Anticancer Res 1996;16:1819.

466. Walz PH, Bjork P, Gunnarsson PO, et al. Differential uptake of estramustine phosphate metabolites and its correlation with the levels of estramustine binding protein in prostate tumor tissue. Clin Cancer Res 1998;4:2079.

467. Yoshida D, Cornell-Bell A, Piepmeier JM. Selective antimitotic effects of estramustine correlate with its antimicrotubule properties on glioblastoma and astrocytes. Neurosurgery 1994;34:863.

468. Vallbo C, Bergenheim AT, Bergstrom P, et al. Apoptotic tumor cell death induced by estramustine in patients with malignant glioma. Clin Cancer Res 1998;4:87.

469. Johansson M, Bergenheim AT, D'Argy R, et al. Distribution of estramustine in the BT4C rat glioma model. Cancer Chemother Pharmacol 1998;41:317.

470. Bjork P, Borg A, Ferno M, et al. Expression and partial characterization of estramustine-binding protein (EMBP) in human breast cancer and malignant melanoma. Anticancer Res 1991;11:1173.

471. Bergenheim AT, Zackrisson B, Elfverson J, et al. Radiosensitizing effect of estramustine in malignant glioma in vitro and in vivo. J Neurooncol 1995;23:191.

472. Yoshida D, Piepmeier J, Weinstein M. Estramustine sensitizes human glioblastoma cells to irradiation. Cancer Res 1994;54:1415.

473. Stearns ME, Tew KD. Estramustine binds MAP-2 to inhibit microtubule assembly in vitro. J Cell Sci 1988;89:331.

474. Ranganathan S, Dexter DW, Hudes GR. Modulation of endogenous-tubulin isotype expression as a result of human $_{III}$ cDNA transfection into prostate carcinoma cells. Br J Cancer 2001;85:735.

475. Sangrajrang S, Denoulet P, Millot G, et al. Estramustine resistance correlates with tau over-expression in human prostatic carcinoma cells. Int J Cancer 1998;77:625.

476. Speicher LA, Barone LR, Chapman AE, et al. P-glycoprotein binding and modulation of the multidrug-resistant phenotype by estramustine. J Natl Cancer Inst 1994;86:688.

477. Speicher LA, Sheridan VR, Godwin AK, et al. Resistance to the antimitotic drug estramustine is distinct from the multidrug resistant phenotype. Br J Cancer 1991;267.

478. Yang CP, Shen HJ, Horwitz SB. Modulation of the function of P-glycoprotein by estramustine. J Natl Cancer Inst 1994;86:723.

479. Laing NM, Belinsky MG, Kruh GD, et al. Amplification of the ATP-binding cassette 2 transporter gene is functionally linked with enhanced efflux of estramustine in ovarian carcinoma cells. Cancer Res 1998;58:1332.

480. Gunnarsson PO, Andersson SB, Johansson SA, et al. Pharmacokinetics of estramustine phosphate (Estracyt) in prostatic cancer patients. Eur J Clin Pharmacol 1984;26:113.

481. Forshell GP, Muntzing J, Ek A, et al. The absorption, metabolism, and excretion of Estracyt (NSC 89199) in patients with prostatic cancer. Invest Urol 1976;14:128.

482. Dixon R, Brooks M, Gill G. Estramustine phosphate: plasma concentrations of its metabolites following oral administration to man, rat and dog. Res Commun Chem Pathol Pharmacol 1980;27:17.

483. Gunnarsson PO, Forshell GP. Clinical pharmacokinetics of estramustine phosphate. Urology 1984;23:22.

484. Yamazaki H, Shaw DM, Guengerich FP, et al. Roles of cytochromes P450 1A2 and 3A4 in the oxidation of estradiol and estrone in human liver microsomes. Chem Res Toxicol 1998;11:659.

485. Gunnarsson PO, Davidsson T, Andersson SB, et al. Impairment of estramustine phosphate absorption by concurrent intake of milk and food. Eur J Clin Pharmacol 1990;38:189.

486. Von Schoultz B, Carlstrom K, Collste L, et al. Estrogen therapy and liver function-metabolic effects of oral and parenteral administration. Prostate 1989;14:389.

487. Smith PH, Suciu S, Robinson MR, et al. A comparison of the effect of diethylstilbestrol with low dose estramustine phosphate in the treatment of advanced prostatic cancer: final analysis of a phase III trial of the European Organization for Research on Treatment of Cancer. J Urol 1986;136:619.

488. Madison DL, Beer TM. Acute estramustine induced hypocalcemia unmasking severe vitamin D deficiency. Am J Medicine 2002;112:680.

489. Park DS, Vassilopoulou R, Tu S-M. Estramustine-related hypocalcemia in patients with prostate carcinoma and osteoblastic metastases. Urology 2001;58:105.

490. Ferrari AC, Chachoua A, Singh H, et al. A phase I/II study of weekly paclitaxel and 3 days of high dose oral estramustine in patients with hormone-refractory prostate carcinoma. Cancer 2001;91:2039.

491. Sinibaldi VJ, Carducci MA, Moore-Cooper S, et al. Phase II evaluation of docetaxel plus one-day oral estramustine phosphate in

the treatment of patients with androgen independent prostate carcinoma. Cancer 2002;94:1457.

492. Goodin S, Kane MP, Rubin EH. Epothilones: mechanism of action and biologic activity. J Clin Oncol 5-15-2004;22:2015.

493. Stachel SJ, Biswas K, Danishefsky SJ. The epothilones, eleutherobins, and related types of molecules. Curr Pharm Des 2001;7:1277.

494. Bollag DM, McQueney PA, Zhu J, et al. Epothilones, a new class of microtubule-stabilizing agents with a taxol-like mechanism of action. Cancer Res 6-1-1995;55:2325.

495. Verrills NM, Flemming CL, Liu M, et al. Microtubule alterations and mutations induced by desoxyepothilone B: implications for drug-target interactions. Chem Biol 2003;10:597.

496. Mani S, McDaid H, Hamilton A, et al. Phase I clinical and pharmacokinetic study of BMS-247550, a novel derivative of epothilone B, in solid tumors. Clin Cancer Res 2004;10:1289.

497. Rothermel J, Wartmann M, Chen T, et al. EPO906 (epothilone B): a promising novel microtubule stabilizer. Semin Oncol 2003;30:51.

498. Abraham J, Agrawal M, Bakke S, et al. Phase I trial and pharmacokinetic study of BMS-247550, an epothilone B analog, administered intravenously on a daily schedule for five days. J Clin Oncol 2003;21:1866.

499. Chou TC, Zhang XG, Harris CR, et al. Desoxyepothilone B is curative against human tumor xenografts that are refractory to paclitaxel. Proc Natl Acad Sci U S A 1998;95:15798.

500. Dabydeen DA, Florence GJ, Paterson I, et al. A quantitative evaluation of the effects of inhibitors of tubulin assembly on polymerization induced by discodermolide, epothilone B, and paclitaxel. Cancer Chemother Pharmacol 1-22-2004.

501. Hung DT, Chen J, Schreiber SL. (+)-Discodermolide binds to microtubules in stoichiometric ratio to tubulin dimers, blocks taxol binding and results in mitotic arrest. Chem Biol 1996;3:287.

502. Martello LA, LaMarche MJ, He L, et al. The relationship between taxol and (+)-discodermolide: synthetic analogs and modeling studies. Chem Biol 2001;8:843.

503. ter Haar E, Kowalski RJ, Hamel E, et al. Discodermolide, a cytotoxic marine agent that stabilizes microtubules more potently than taxol. Biochemistry 1996;35:243.

504. Honore S, Kamath K, Braguer D, et al. Synergistic suppression of microtubule dynamics by discodermolide and paclitaxel in non-small cell lung carcinoma cells. Cancer Res 7-15-2004;64:4957.

505. Martello LA, McDaid HM, Regl DL, et al. Taxol and discodermolide represent a synergistic drug combination in human carcinoma cell lines. Clin Cancer Res 2000;6:1978.

506. Mita AA, Lockhart C, Chen T-L, et al. A phase I pharmacokinetic (PK) trial of XAA296A (Discodermolide) administered every 3 wks to adult patients with advanced solid malignancies. Proc Am Soc Clin Oncol 2004;23:133.

507. Hamel E, Sackett DL, Vourloumis D, et al. The coral-derived natural products eleutherobin and sarcodictyins A and B: effects on the assembly of purified tubulin with and without microtubule-associated proteins and binding at the polymer taxoid site. Biochemistry 1999;38:5490.

508. Mooberry SL, Tien G, Hernandez AH, et al. Laulimalide and isolaulimalide, new paclitaxel-like microtubule-stabilizing agents. Cancer Res 1999;59:653.

509. Hammond LA, Ruvuna F, Cunningham CC. Phase (Ph) I evaluation of the dolastatin analogue synthadotin (SYN-D;ILX651): Pooled data analysis of three alternate schedules in patients (pts) with advanced solid tumors. Proc Am Soc Clin Oncol 2004;23:212.

510. Bai R, Cichacz ZA, Herald CL, et al. Spongistatin 1, a highly cytotoxic, sponge-derived, marine natural product that inhibits mitosis, microtubule assembly, and the binding of vinblastine to tubulin. Mol Pharmacol 1993;757.

511. Kuznetsov G, Towle MJ, Cheng H, et al. Induction of morphological and biochemical apoptosis following prolonged mitotic blockage by halichondrin B macrocyclic ketone analog E7389. Cancer Res 2004;64:5760.

512. Loganzo F, Discafani CM, Annable T, et al. HTI-286, a synthetic analogue of the tripeptide hemiasterlin, is a potent antimicrotubule agent that circumvents P-glycoprotein-mediated resistance in vitro and in vivo. Cancer Res 2003;1838.

513. Kanthou C, Tozer GM. The tumor vascular targeting agent combretastatin A-4-phosphate induces reorganization of the actin cytoskeleton and early membrane blebbing in human endothelial cells. Blood 2002;99:2060.

514. Davis PD, Dougherty GJ, Blakey DC. ZD6126: a novel vascular-targeting agent that causes selective destruction of tumor vasculature. Cancer Res 2004;62:7247.

515. Goldstein LS, Philip AV. The road less traveled: emerging principles of kinesin motor utilization. Annu Rev Cell Dev Biol 1999;15:141.

516. Vale RD, Milligan RA. The way things move: looking under the hood of molecular motor proteins. Science 2000;288:88.

517. Wood KW, Cornwell WD, Jackson JR. Past and future of the mitotic spindle as an oncology target. Curr Opin Pharmacol 2001;4:370.

518. Blangy A, Lane HA, d'Herin P, et al. Phosphorylation by p34cdc2 regulates spindle association of human Eg5, a kinesin-related motor essential for bipolar spindle formation in vivo. Cell 1995;83:1159.

519. Chu Q, Holen KD, Rowinsky EK, et al. A phase I study to determine the safety and pharmacokinetics of IV administered SB-715992, a novel kinesin spindle protein (KSP) inhibitor, in patients with solid tumors. Proc Am Soc Clin Oncol 2003;22:121.

520. Sakowicz R, Finer JT, Beraud C, et al. Antitumor activity of a kinesin inhibitor. Cancer Res 2004;64:3276.

521. Carmena M, Earnshaw WC. The cellular geography of aurora kinases. Nat Rev Mol Cell Biol 2003;11:842.

522. Harrington EA, Bebbington D, Moore J, et al. VX-680, a potent and selective small-molecule inhibitor of the Aurora kinases, suppresses tumor growth in vivo. Nat Med 2004;10:262.

Clinical and High-Dose Alkylating Agents

12

Kenneth D. Tew   O. Michael Colvin   Roy B. Jones

The alkylating agents are antitumor drugs that act through the covalent binding of alkyl groups to cellular molecules. This binding is mediated by reactive intermediates formed from a more stable parent alkylating compound. Historically, the alkylating agents have played an important role in the development of cancer chemotherapy. The nitrogen mustards mechlorethamine (HN$_2$, "nitrogen mustard") and tris(β-chloroethyl)amine (HN$_3$) were the first non-hormonal agents to show significant antitumor activity in humans.[1-3] The clinical trials of nitrogen mustards in patients with lymphomas evolved from the observation that lymphoid atrophy, in addition to lung and mucous membrane irritation was produced by sulfur mustard during World War I. Antitumor evaluation[4] showed that the related but less reactive nitrogen mustards, the bischloroethylamines (Fig. 12.1), were less toxic and cause regressions of lymphoid tumors in mice. The first clinical studies produced dramatic tumor regressions in some patients with lymphoma, and the antitumor effects were confirmed by an organized multi-institution study.[1-3] This demonstration of efficacy encouraged further efforts to find chemical agents with antitumor activity, leading to the wide variety of antitumor agents in use today. At present, alkylating agents occupy a central position in cancer chemotherapy, both in conventional combination regimens and in high-dose protocols with hematopoietic cell transplantation (HCT). Because of their linear dose-response relationship in cell culture experiments,[5] these drugs have become primary tools used in HCT for a variety of diseases.

CHEMISTRY

Mechanisms of Alkylating Reactions

Traditionally, the pharmacokinetics of alkylating reactions have been described as either a first-order process in which the rate of alkylating agent conversion to reactive intermediate determines the rate of reaction with cellular constituents, or as a second-order process in which tissue constituents must react directly with the intact alkylating agent, resulting in an unstable transition-state molecule (a reactive intermediate composed of the alkylating agent and cellular molecule) that decomposes to form the alkylated cellular constituent. Because alkylating agents are designed to produce reactive intermediates, the parent compounds typically have short elimination half-lives of less than 5 hours.

As a class, the alkylating agents share a common target (DNA) and are cytotoxic, mutagenic, and carcinogenic. The activity of most alkylating agents is enhanced by radiation, hyperthermia, nitroimidazoles, and by glutathione depletion. They differ greatly, however, in their toxicity profiles and antitumor activity. These differences are undoubtedly the result of differences in pharmacokinetic features, lipid solubility, ability to penetrate the central nervous system (CNS), membrane transport properties, detoxification reactions, and specific enzymatic reactions capable of repairing alkylation sites on DNA.[6,7] For example, the nitrosoureas produce a specific site of alkylation on the O-6 position of guanine; resistance to this group of agents is correlated with the presence of a guanine-O^6-alkyl

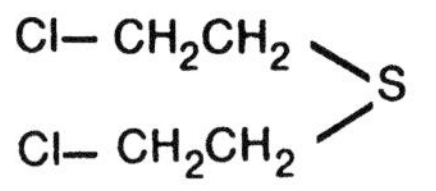

A

Bischloroethylsulfide (sulfur mustard).

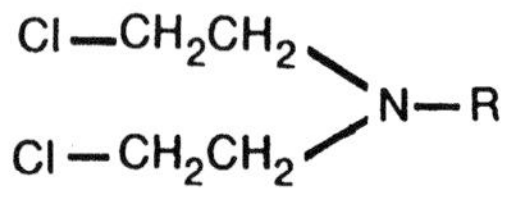

B

Bischloroethylamine (nitrogen mustard general structure). —R = —CH₃ in mechlorethamine. —R = —CH₂CH₂Cl in tris(β-chloroethyl)amine.

Figure 12.1 Structures of bischloroethylsulfide and bischloroethylamine. **A.** Bischloroethylsulfide (sulfur mustard). **B.** Bischloroethylamine (nitrogen mustard general structure).

transferase.[8] Application of techniques such as magnetic resonance imaging and mass spectrometry to the study of the alkylation mechanism and the chemical nature of the intermediates involved are making possible a detailed understanding of these reactions.[9,10] Such approaches, coupled with improved techniques of localizing and studying cellular damage[11,12] and determining sites and mechanisms of detoxification,[13–15] should eventually make it possible to predict the sites of alkylation of an agent and to understand and modify the biologic consequences of such alkylations.

Types of Alkylating Agents Used Clinically

The important pharmacologic properties of the selected clinically useful alkylating agents are summarized in Table 12.1.

Nitrogen Mustards

The prototypic alkylating agents have been the bischloroethylamines or nitrogen mustards. The first nitrogen mustard to be used extensively in the clinic was mechlorethamine (Fig. 12.1), sometimes referred to by its original code name HN₂ or by the term *nitrogen mustard.* The mechanism of alkylation by the nitrogen mustards is shown in Figure 12.2. In the initial step, chlorine is lost and the β-carbon reacts with the nucleophilic nitrogen atom to form the cyclic, positively charged, and very reactive aziridinium moiety. Reaction of the aziridinium ring with a nucleophile (electron-rich atom) yields the initial alkylated product. Formation of a second aziridinium by the remaining chloroethyl group allows for a second alkyla-

tion, which produces a cross-link between the two alkylated nucleophiles.

After introduction of mechlorethamine, a great many analogs were synthesized in which the methyl group was replaced by a variety of chemical groups. Most of these compounds proved to have less antitumor activity than mechlorethamine, but four derivatives seem to have a higher therapeutic index, a broader range of clinical activity, and can be administered both orally and intravenously. These drugs, which for the most part have replaced mechlorethamine in clinical use, are melphalan (L-phenylalanine mustard), chlorambucil, cyclophosphamide, and ifosfamide (Fig. 12.3). The latter two agents are unique in that they require metabolic activation and undergo a complex series of activation and degradation reactions (to be described in detail later in this chapter).

As can be seen from the structures, these derivatives have electron-withdrawing groups substituted on the nitrogen atom. This alteration reduces the nucleophilicity of the nitrogen and renders the molecules less reactive. Melphalan and chlorambucil retain alkylating activity and seem to be more tumor-selective than nitrogen mustard. Cyclophosphamide and ifosfamide, on the other hand, possess no alkylating activity and must be metabolized to produce alkylating compounds. Cyclophosphamide has been the most widely used alkylating agent and has activity against a variety of tumors.[16] In 1972, ifosfamide,[17] an isomeric analog of cyclophosphamide, was introduced into clinical use. It has greater activity against testicular cancer and soft tissue sarcomas.[18,19] Melphalan has been widely used in the treatment of ovarian cancer,[20] multiple myeloma,[21] and carcinoma of the breast.[22] Chlorambucil has been most widely used in the treatment of chronic lymphocytic leukemia,[23,24] lymphomas,[23,25] and ovarian carcinoma[26] but it is unavailable in intravenous form and its use has declined sharply in recent years with the development of more effective treatments for each of the listed diseases. Both intravenous melphalan and cyclophosphamide are now heavily used in high-dose regimens combined with HCT.

Aziridines

The aziridines are analogs of the putative ring-closed intermediates of the nitrogen mustards but are less reactive chemically. Compounds bearing two or more aziridine groups, such as thiotepa (Figure 12.3 [thiotepa, triethylenethiophosphoramide]),[27,28] have shown clinical activity against human tumors. Thiotepa is also used primarily as a component of HCT regimens.

This aziridine compound was originally tested for antitumor activity because the nitrogen mustards alkylate through an aziridine intermediate. Both thiotepa and its primary desulfurated metabolite TEPA (triethylenephosphoramide) have cytotoxic activity in vitro. Although the mechanism of action of these compounds has not been

TABLE 12.1

KEY FEATURES OF SELECTED ALKYLATING AGENTS

	Cyclophosphamide	Ifosfamide	Melphalan	BCNU	Busulfan
Mechanism of action	All agents produce alkylation of DNA through the formation of reactive intermediates that attack nucleophilic sites.				
Mechanisms of resistance	Increased capacity to repair alkylated lesions, e.g., guanine O^6-alkyl transferase (nitrosoureas, busulfan) Increased expression of glutathione-associated enzymes, including γ-glutamyl cysteine synthetase, γ-glutamyl transpeptidase, and glutathione-*S*-transferases Increased aldehyde dehydrogenase (cyclophosphamide) Decreased expression or mutation of p53				
Dose/schedule (mg/m^2):	400–2,000 IV. 100 PO qd	1,000-4,000 IV	8 PO qd × 5 d	200 IV	2–4 mg daily
Oral bioavailability	100%	Unavailable	30% (variable)	Not known	50% or greater
Pharmacokinetics: primary elimination $t_{1/2}$ (h)	3–10 (parent) 1.6 (aldophosphamide) 8.7 (phosphoramide mustard)	7–15 (parent)	1.5 (parent)	0.25 to 0.75[a] (non-linear increase with dose from 170–720 mg/m^2)	
Metabolism	Microsomal hydroxylation Hydrolysis to phosphoramide mustard (active) and acrolein Excretion as inactive oxidation products	Microsomal hydroxylation Hydrolysis to iphosphoramide mustard and acrolein Excretion as inactive oxidation and dechloroethylated products	Chemical decomposition to inert dechlorination products, 20–35% excreted unchanged in urine	Chemical decomposition to active and inert products	Enzymatic conjugation with glutathione
Toxicity					
Myelosuppression	Acute, platelets spared	Acute but mild	Delayed, nadir at 4 weeks	Delayed, nadir 4–6 weeks	Acute and delayed
Alopecia Pulmonary fibrosis Veno-occlusive disease Leukemogenesis Infertility Teratogenesis	Seen with all alkylating agents				
Other	Cystitis; cardiac toxicity; IADH	Encephalopathy	—	Hypotension	Addisonian syndrome, seizures
Precautions	Use MESNA with high-dose therapy	Always coadminister MESNA	Decomposes if administered over <1 hr	—	Monitor AUC with high-dose therapy
Drug interactions	Expect increased cytotoxicity with radiation sensitizers and glutathione depletion		%		Induces phenytoin (Dilantin) metabolism

[a] See reference 276a.
AUC, area under the concentration time curve; BCNU, bischloroethylnitrosourea; IADH, inappropriate antidiuretic hormone syndrome; IV, intravenously; MESNA, 2-mercaptoethane sulfonate; PO, per os; $t_{1/2}$, half-life.

explored thoroughly, they presumably alkylate through opening of the aziridine rings, as shown for the nitrogen mustards. The reactivity of the aziridine groups is increased by protonation and thus is enhanced at the low pH more characteristic of tumors than normal tissues.

Alkyl Alkane Sulfonates

The major clinical representative of the alkyl alkane sulfonates is busulfan (Fig. 12.4), which is widely used in HCT regimens for the treatment of acute and chronic myelogenous leukemia.[29] Its alkylation mechanism is shown in Figure 12.5. Compounds with one to eight methylene units between the sulfonate groups have antitumor activity, but maximal activity is shown by the compound with four methylene units.[30,31]

Busulfan exhibits second-order alkylation kinetics. The compound reacts more extensively with thiol groups of amino acids and proteins[32] than do the nitrogen mustards, and these findings have prompted the suggestion that the alkyl alkane sulfonates may exert their cytotoxic activities

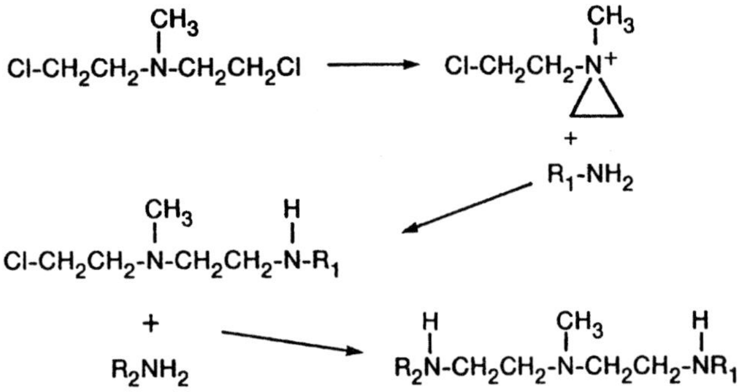

Figure 12.2 Alkylation mechanism of nitrogen mustards. (From Colvin M. Molecular pharmacology of alkylating agents. In: Cooke ST, Prestayko AW. Cancer and Chemotherapy, vol 3. New York: Academic Press, 1981:291.)

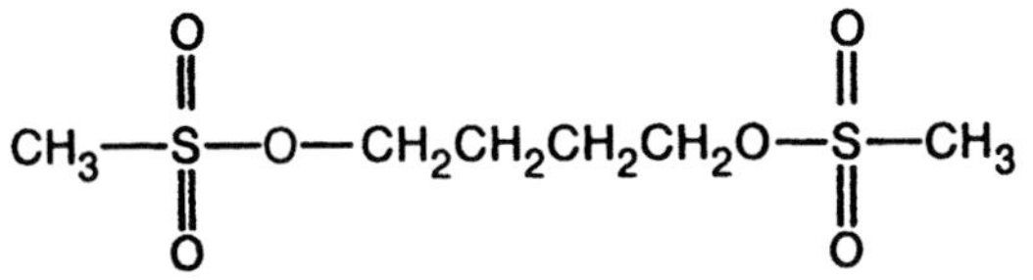

Figure 12.4 Structure of busulfan.

through such thiol reactions along with interactions with DNA.[32,33] Brookes and Lawley[34] were able to demonstrate the reaction of busulfan with the N-7 position of guanine, and Iwanoto et al.[35] have suggested that adenine-to-guanine cross-linking is correlated with the cytotoxic potential of busulfan. Busulfan is markedly cytotoxic to hematopoietic stem cells. This effect is seen clinically in the prolonged aplasia that may follow busulfan administration[36] and can be shown experimentally in stem cell cloning systems.[37] The pharmacologic basis for this property of busulfan is not understood, but has stimulated the use of busulfan in HCT protocols.[38]

Nitrosoureas

The nitrosourea antitumor agents in current use were developed after screening of methylnitrosoguanidine and methylnitrosourea at the Wisconsin Alumni Research Foundation (WARF) and demonstrated modest antitumor activity in experimental animal tumor models.[39] Careful structure-function studies demonstrated that chloroethyl derivatives such as chloroethylnitrosourea and BCNU

(Fig. 12.6) possess greater antitumor activity than methylnitrosourea or other alkyl derivatives, and that the nitrosourea derivatives are more active than the nitrosoguanidines.[39–41] In addition to chloroethyl alkylating activity, the available nitrosoureas can also carbamoylate nucleophiles.[42]

These chloroethylnitrosoureas eradicated intracranially inoculated tumors[41] because of their lipophilic character and ability to cross the blood-brain barrier. In its initial trials, BCNU showed significant activity against brain tumors, colon cancer, and the lymphomas.[43,44] Subsequently, cyclohexylchloroethylnitrosourea (CCNU, lomustine) and methylcyclohexylchloroethylnitrosourea (methyl-CCNU, semustine) (Fig. 12.6) demonstrated greater activity against solid tumors in experimental animals.[45]

The nitrosoureas show partial cross-resistance with other alkylating agents.[41] A number of studies have confirmed that these drugs are indeed alkylating agents, and the mechanism of the alkylation reaction has been established (Fig. 12.7). BCNU is well recognized to cross-link DNA after the formation of monoadducts, particularly at the N7 position of guanine. As shown in Figure 12.7, the diazonium hydroxide intermediate formed during BCNU hydrolysis decomposes to form a 2-chloroethyl carbonium ion (or equivalent) capable of rapid alkylation. In a subsequent step occurring over hours, the chloride is displaced by electron-rich nitrogen on the complementary DNA strand base to form a cross-link. DNA-protein cross-links are also possible.[46,47]

Isocyanates resulting from the spontaneous breakdown of many of the methyl- and chloroethylnitrosoureas are also shown in Figure 12.7. The role of isocyanate-mediated

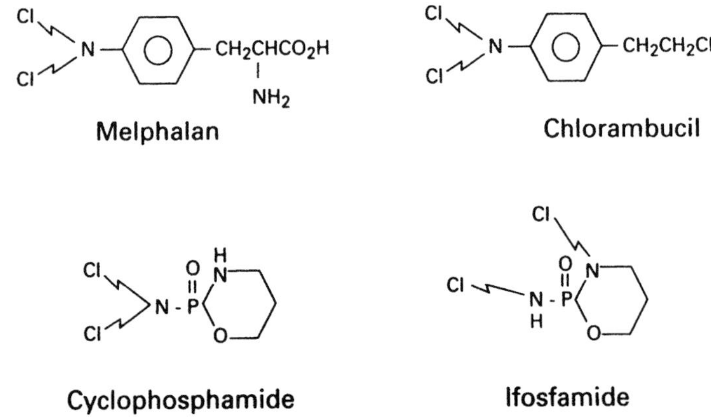

Figure 12.3 Structures of four analogs of mechlorethamine and thiotepa.

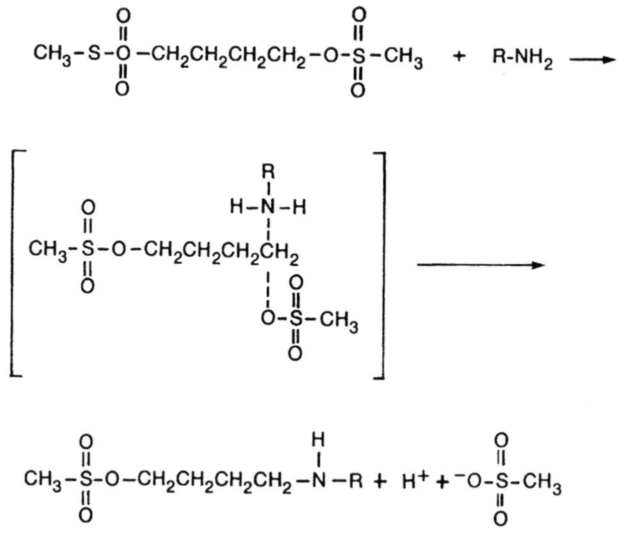

Figure 12.5 Alkylation mechanism of alkane sulfonates. (From Colvin M. Molecular pharmacology of alkylating agents. In: Cooke ST, Prestayko AW. Cancer and Chemotherapy, vol 3. New York: Academic Press, 1981:291.)

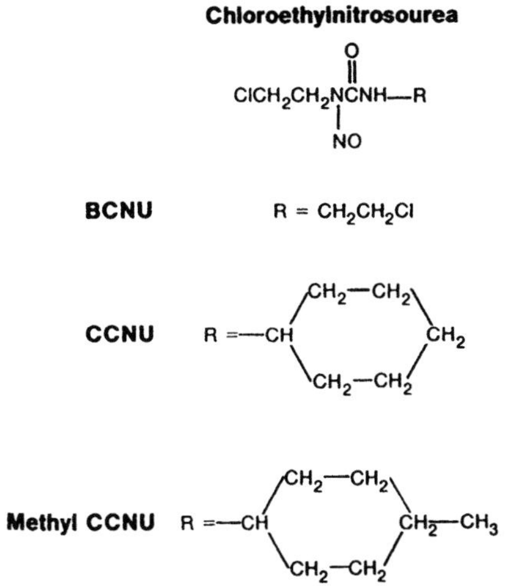

Figure 12.6 Structures of nitrosoureas. BCNU, bischloroethylnitrosourea;CCNU, cyclohexylchloroethylnitrosourea.

carbamoylation in antitumor effects is incompletely understood, but this activity may be responsible for many of the toxicities associated with nitrosourea therapy.[48–50]

Streptozotocin is a unique methylnitrosourea with methylating activity but without carbamoylating activity because the molecule autocarbamoylates through internal cyclization. It is active against islet cell carcinoma.[51,52] The dose-limiting toxicities in humans have been gastrointestinal and renal, and the drug has considerably less hematopoietic toxicity than the other nitrosoureas.

Currently, BCNU is used with HCT regimens for hematopoietic diseases.[53] As predicted from the animal studies, the nitrosoureas have shown significant activity against brain tumors.[54] When used as an adjuvant to radiation therapy, they enhance survival modestly in patients with grade III and IV astrocytomas.[55] The severe hematopoietic depression (especially thrombocytopenia) and pulmonary toxicity produced by these agents are significant limiting factors in their use. BCNU-impregnated wafers implanted directly in brain tumors have been used for regional therapy.

Alkylating Agent–Steroid Conjugates

From the rationale that steroid receptors may serve to localize and concentrate appended drug species in hormone-responsive cancers, a number of synthetic conjugates of mustards and steroids have been developed. Of these drugs, two have made the transition into clinical application. Prednimustine is an ester-linked conjugate of chlorambucil and prednisolone. It appears to function as a prodrug for chlorambucil, releasing the alkylating agent after cleavage by serum esterases.[56,57] Estramustine is a carbamate ester-linked conjugate of nornitrogen mustard and estradiol. Serum esterases are prevalent and readily cleave the ester link of prednimustine with the ultimate release of the hormone and the active alkylating drug.

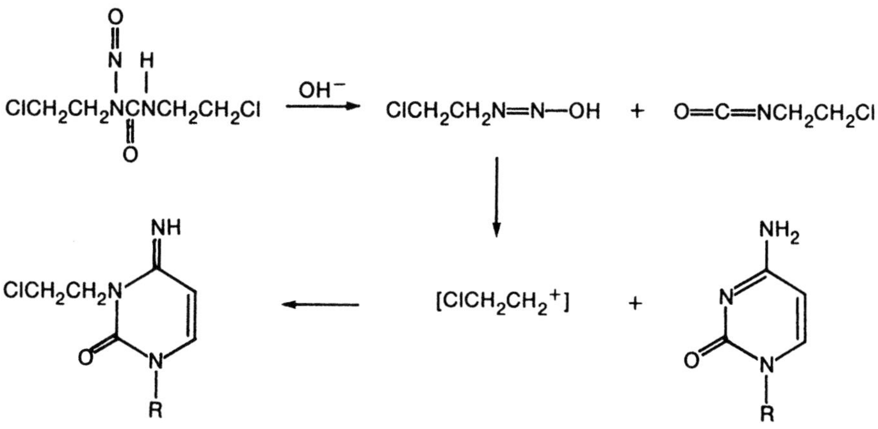

Figure 12.7 Alkylation of nucleoside by bischloroethylnitrosourea (BCNU).

Prednimustine produces altered alkylating agent pharmacokinetics compared with unconjugated chlorambucil because the half-life is prolonged as a consequence of slow hydrolysis of the ester bond.[56] In addition, the elimination phase of chlorambucil in patient plasma is significantly longer after administration of prednimustine than after chlorambucil.[57] Thus, prednimustine acts as a prodrug, delivering alkylating components over a prolonged period.

The pharmacology of estramustine is governed by the presence of the carbamate group in the steroid-mustard linkage. The altered alkylating structure appears to eliminate alkylating activity of the molecule.[58,59] Steroid hormone[60] or other mitotic inhibiting activities[61] may explain the activity of estramustine Neither prednimustine or estramustine is heavily used, but estramustine is being explored for treatment of prostate cancer in conjunction with radiotherapy.

Prodrugs of Alkylating Agents

Therapy with alkylating agents is compromised by their high level of toxicity to normal tissues and their lack of tumor selectivity. Cyclophosphamide and ifosfamide were prodrugs synthesized in the hope that high levels of phosphamidases in epithelial tumors would selectively activate the drugs.[62] A variety of strategies for more selective delivery of alkylating agent to tumor have been explored including cleavable tumor-directed antibody-alkylating agent conjugates,[63,64] alkylating agent-glutathione conjugates, which might be selectively cleaved by glutathione transferase P1 expressed in high levels in tumor cells,[64] or using viral vectors to deliver activating enzymes to tumor cells.[65] The glutathione conjugate is being explored in randomized clinical trials.

CELLULAR PHARMACOLOGY

Sites of Alkylation

Any alkylating agent producing reactive intermediates binds to a variety of cellular constituents[66] including nucleic acids, proteins, amino acids, and nucleotides. As an example, the active alkylating species from a nitrogen mustard demonstrate selectivity for nucleophiles in the following order: (a) oxygens of phosphates, (b) oxygens of bases, (c) amino groups of purines, (d) amino groups of proteins, (e) sulfur atoms of methionine, and (f) thiol groups of cysteinyl residues of glutathione.[67] This ranking, however, assumes there are no steric or hydrophilic/hydrophobic barriers to the tissue nucleophile, and this is seldom the case. In addition, glutathione conjugation is often favored in the presence of glutathione transferases, which offer catalysis. Thus, generalizations about alkylating agent targets are fraught with difficulty.[13-15] In addition, it seems likely that a matrix of biochemical targets of alkylating agents may contribute to cytotoxicity, though DNA is generally favored as the primary target. Proof of this hypothesis may be emerging from three areas of research where cytotoxicity is correlated to: (a) activity of DNA repair enzymes, perhaps best shown for BCNU and repair by alkylguaninealkyltransferase (AGT),[68] (b) changes in a matrix of genetic and epigenetic events measured and analyzed using gene expression arrays,[69] and (c) direct measurement of specific DNA adducts using PCR or mass spectrometric analysis.[70] The stringency of such analyses requires that alternative toxic pathways not involving DNA be excluded, a difficult requirement to meet. For this reason, mechanistic understanding of alkylating agent activity must be considered incomplete.[71-77]

In the DNA molecule, the phosphoryl oxygens of the sugar phosphate backbone are obvious electron-rich targets for alkylation. A number of studies have shown that alkylation of the phosphate groups does occur[78,79] and can result in strand breakage from hydrolysis of the resulting phosphotriesters. Although the biologic significance of the strand breakage caused by phosphate alkylation remains uncertain, the process is so slow that it seems unlikely that it is a major determinant of cytotoxicity, even for monofunctional agents.[80]

Extensive studies with carcinogenic alkylating agents such as methyl methane sulfonate have shown that virtually all the oxygen and nitrogen atoms of the purine and pyrimidine bases of DNA can be alkylated to varying degrees. The relative significance to carcinogenesis or cytotoxicity of alkylation of each of these sites remains uncertain. Various reports have indicated that alkylation of the O-6 atom and of the extracyclic nitrogen of guanine may be of particular importance for carcinogenesis.[81-83]

Studies of the base specificity of alkylation by the chemotherapeutic alkylating agents have been much less extensive. Busulfan and mechlorethamine alkylate the N-7 position of guanine. Guanine cross-links (two guanine molecules abridged at the N-7 position by an alkylating agent) have been isolated from acid hydrolysates of the reaction mixtures.[34]

Reaction of the nitrogen mustard with native DNA, however, produces alkylation of the N-1 position of adenine in addition to N-7–alkylated guanine. The reason for the enhanced alkylation of the N-7 position of guanine is uncertain, but it may be the result of base stacking and charge transfer that enhance the nucleophilic character of the N-7 position.[84] Melphalan preferentially alkylates guanine N-7 or adenine N-3.[70]

Base sequence influences the alkylating reaction. The N-7 position of guanine is most electronegative and, therefore, most vulnerable to attack by the aziridinium cation intermediate of the nitrogen mustards when the base is flanked by guanines on its 3' and 5' sides. The key site of DNA attack for the nitrosoureas as well as nonclassic methylating agents such as procarbazine and dacarbazine seems to be the O-6 methyl group of guanine.[8] Enhanced repair of this site is associated with drug resistance.[85] Thus, the preferred sites for alkylation vary by alkylating agent and chemical environment around the DNA base in question.

DNA Cross-Linking

On the basis of their isolation of the guanines linked at N-7 by alkylating agents, Brookes and Lawley[84,86] postulated that the bifunctional alkylating agents such as the nitrogen mustards produced interstrand and intrastrand DNA-DNA cross- links and that these cross-links were responsible for the inactivation of the DNA and cytotoxicity. On the basis of the Watson-Crick DNA model, these authors suggested that appropriate spatial relationships for cross-linking by nitrogen mustards or sulfur mustard occurred between the N-7 positions of guanine residues in complementary DNA strands (Fig. 12.8).

The importance of cross-linking is supported by the fact that the bifunctional alkylating agents, with few exceptions, are much more effective antitumor agents than the analogous monofunctional agents, as originally described by Loveless and Ross.[87] Furthermore, increasing the number of alkylating units on the molecule beyond two does not usually increase the antitumor activity of the compound.

Direct evidence that DNA cross-linking occurs as the result of treatment of DNA or cells with bifunctional alkylating agents was provided initially by relatively insensitive physical techniques, including sedimentation velocity studies and denaturation-renaturation studies.[46,87-91] These techniques, however, could not detect DNA interstrand cross-linking in mammalian cells exposed to therapeutic levels of alkylating agents in vitro or in tissues after in vivo drug administration. In 1976, a more sensitive assay for DNA interstrand cross-linking in cells, the alkaline elution method,[92] was reported and had the necessary sensitivity to detect DNA cross-linking in cells and tumor-bearing animals exposed to minimal cytotoxic levels of alkylating agents.[11,93,94] These studies, and others using ethidium

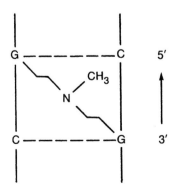

Figure 12.8 Cross-linking of DNA by nitrogen mustard. (Modified and reproduced with permission from Brookes P, Lawley PD. The reaction of mono- and di-functional alkylating agents with nucleic acids. Biochem J 1961;80:486.)

bromide fluorescence to detect cross-links, have shown that DNA cross-linking by bifunctional alkylating agents correlates with cytotoxicity and that DNA in drug-resistant cells has lower levels of cross-linkage.[95,96] The alkaline elution technique also has detected DNA-protein as well as DNA-DNA cross-links,[97] which supports data from previous investigators.[98-100] The work of Ewig and Kohn[97] suggests that DNA-protein cross-links do not play a major role in cytotoxicity.

In addition to these target effect-response studies, inactivation of the AGT promoter in gliomas is correlated with improved antitumor activity and survival in patients treated with BCNU.[101] Becuause AGT repairs guanine alkylation products produced by BCNU, decreased enzyme activity would be expected to increase DNA alkylation, implying that DNA is a critical target for BCNU effects. Thus, evidence increasingly supports the hypothesis that DNA interstrand cross-linking is the major mechanism of alkylating agent cytotoxicity.

Work by Ludlum et al.[47] and Kohn et al.[46] suggests that the chloroethylnitrosoureas cross-link via a unique mechanism. The spontaneous decomposition of the chloroethylnitrosoureas generates a chloroethyldiazonium hydroxide entity[48] that can alkylate DNA bases to produce an alkylating chloroethylamine group on the nucleotide in the DNA strand. This group could then alkylate an adjacent nucleotide on the complementary DNA strand in a slower step, producing an interstrand cross-link. The mechanism of alkylation by thiophosphates such as thiotepa likely begins with protonation of the aziridine N, which leads to ring opening. Cross-linking can proceed by one of several mechanisms, either activation of the free chloroethyl carbon or activation of a second aziridine ring on the original molecule. Although interstrand cross-links are important mediators of the cytotoxic effects of alkylating agents, the monofunctional DNA alkylations exceed cross-links in number and are potentially cytotoxic. This hypothesis is supported by the fact that certain clinically effective agents, such as procarbazine and dacarbazine, are monofunctional alkylating compounds and do not produce cross-links in experimental systems. The basis of the cytotoxic effects of monofunctional alkylation may be single-strand DNA breaks. Although apurinic sites in the DNA lead to spontaneous hydrolysis of an adjacent phosphodiester bond, this process is probably too slow to be of biologic significance.[80] Endonucleases produce single-strand breaks at apurinic sites,[102,103] however, and may be responsible for the toxic and therapeutic effects of the monofunctional agents. The presence of apurinic sites may produce cross-links, but the low frequency of these cross-links makes it unlikely that they are responsible for the antitumor activity of the monofunctional agents.[104]

Limited data suggest that alkylation is nonuniform along the DNA strand and may be concentrated in specific regions. One determinant of regional specificity of DNA alkylations may be chromatin structure[12,105]; areas of active transcription seem to be most vulnerable. The impact of alkylation of specific DNA regions on cytotoxicity requires further study.

In summary, the preponderance of evidence supports the hypothesis that the major factor in the cytotoxicity of most of the clinically effective alkylating agents is interstrand DNA cross-linking, which results in inactivation of the DNA template, cessation of DNA synthesis, and, ultimately cell death. Cell checkpoint proteins, including most prominently p53, are responsible for the recognition of DNA alkylation and strand breaks. Recognition of DNA damage leads to a halt in cell-cycle progression and initiation of programmed cell death. Cells containing mutated p53 have greater resistance to alkylating agents.[106]

An increased knowledge of alkylation mechanisms and targets may make it possible to improve the therapeutic index of these agents. For example, the therapeutic index of alkylating agents should improve if the alkylation of tumor cells were increased without a simultaneous increase in normal tissue alkylation. This might be accomplished by coadministration of the relatively tumor-specific inhibitors of GST P1 which are now under study.[107] As previously noted, GST inhibition increases the antitumor effectiveness of alkylating agents.

Cellular Uptake

The uptake of alkylating agents into cells is a critical determinant of cellular specificity. The cellular uptake of only a few alkylating agents has been examined, however. Wolpert and Ruddon[108] and Goldenberg and Vanstone[109] demonstrated that the uptake of mechlorethamine by Ehrlich ascites tumor cells and by L5178Y lymphoblasts is by active transport systems. Melphalan is transported into several cell types by at least two active transport systems, which also carry leucine and other neutral amino acids across the cell membrane.[110–112] High levels of leucine in the medium protect cells from the cytotoxic effects of melphalan by competing with melphalan for transport into the target cells.[113] In contrast to mechlorethamine and melphalan, which are carried by active transport systems, the highly lipid-soluble nitrosoureas BCNU and CCNU enter cells by passive diffusion.[114]

Studies of cellular uptake of alkylating agents that require metabolic activation (such as cyclophosphamide or ifosfamide) are hampered by uncertainty about whether parent drug, metabolites, or a combination of both are the most critical moiety for transport.

Tumor Resistance

The emergence of alkylating agent–resistant tumor cells is a major problem that limits the clinical effectiveness of these drugs. One mechanism for drug resistance is that of decreased drug entry into the cell. Numerous studies have shown that L5178Y lymphoblast cells resistant to mechlorethamine may have decreased uptake of the drug.[100,108,115] The extracellular domain of the leucine-melphalan transporter expresses CD98.[116] Reduced expression of CD98 on human myeloma cells is associated with melphalan resistance,[117] suggesting that transport alteration may be an important resistance mechanism.

Among other mechanisms of resistance to alkylating agents, changes in sulfhydryl content have been implicated in experimental tumors. For example, the increased nonprotein sulfhydryl content of Yoshida sarcoma cells appears to be responsible for resistance to mechlorethamine.[118] Calcutt and Connors[119] found that tumor cells resistant to alkylating agents often possessed a higher ratio of protein-free to protein-bound thiol compounds and suggested that the increased thiol content might function with and inactivate the alkylating agent intracellularly. Glutathione (GSH) is the major intracellular nonprotein sulfhydryl compound. Increased GSH content of melphalan-resistant ovarian carcinoma cells has been reported,[120] which has led to the experimental use of buthionine sulfoximine, an inhibitor of glutathione synthesis, to reverse resistance to cyclophosphamide, melphalan, and the nitrosoureas in experimental tumors.[121] This reversing agent has been studied clinically but may have limited usefulness as it depletes glutathione from both tumors and normal tissues. Although increased intracellular glutathione content may be found in resistant cells, additional enzymatic detoxification mechanisms that conjugate alkylating intermediates or metabolize them to inactive derivatives at an increased rate have been identified in drug-resistant mutants. Examples of such mechanisms include elevated glutathione transferase levels in mechlorethamine-resistant cells[122] and increased aldehyde dehydrogenase activity, which converts aldophosphamide to its inactive carboxyphosphamide, in cells resistant to cyclophosphamide.[123–125]

Another potential mechanism to explain resistance of cells to alkylating agents is the enhanced repair of the lesions generated by alkylation. Because DNA appears to be the most critical target for the alkylating agents, the repair of DNA has been a major focus of study.[11] Enhanced excision of alkylated nucleotides from DNA appears responsible for the resistance of bacteria to alkylating agents.[46,89,90] Mammalian cells are capable of such excision repair of sulfur mustard–alkylated nucleotides.[126]

Repair of DNA alkylation products and cross-links often involves complex systems involving multiple enzymes. AGT (guanine-O^6-alkyl transferase) repairs single-strand BCNU methylation products in nitrosourea-resistant cells and is an unusual example of a single enzyme repair process. Nucleotide excision repair (NER) is a primary mechanism for excising single-strand alkylation products and may involve up to 25 factors and steps.[127] Interstrand cross-link repair is even more complex and involves some elements of the NER pathway, a variety of less well-understood activities to cleave the second strand, insertion of new bases, and homologous recombination. The complexity of these pathways has limited adequate analysis in this area. In addition, exposure to alkylating agents leads to induction of a series of complementary defensive responses, including decrease in drug-activating enzymes (the P-450 system), increase in glutathione transferase, and increase in DNA repair capacity. This pattern of changes has been most clearly demonstrated in preneoplastic liver nodules after exposure to alkylating carcinogens.[128]

As mentioned previously, apoptotic cell death after DNA damage is mediated through p53, which blocks cell-cycle progression, initiates attempts to repair damage, and ultimately activates apoptotic pathways. Defects in damage recognition or apoptotic signaling may lead to relative resistance.[129] Multiple mechanisms of cellular resistance often occur in a given tumor cell population and are responsible for the drug resistance seen clinically. Goldenberg[130] found that L5178Y lymphoma cells resistant to mechlorethamine are 18.5-fold more resistant to mechlorethamine than the wild-type sensitive cells but are uniformly only twofold to threefold resistant to a variety of other alkylating agents. On this basis, Goldenberg suggested that specific resistance to mechlorethamine occurred because of decreased transport into the cell, whereas the general cross-resistance was the result of other mechanisms, such as enhanced repair capacity. This hypothesis is consistent with the observation of Schabel et al.[131] in experimental animal tumors and with clinical experience. In both situations, varying degrees of cross-resistance between alkylating agents are seen, but a tumor that is resistant to one alkylating agent may remain significantly responsive to another. This finding forms the rational basis for the use of combinations of alkylating agents in high-dose chemotherapy regimens with HCT.[132]

Reversal of Resistance

Drug Modulation

Because of the pivotal importance of GSH to alkylating agent detoxification, four separate approaches to modulation have been adopted: (a) precursors of GSH have been given to replete GSH in normal tissues, thus reducing the host toxicity; (b) specific inhibitors of GSH biosynthetic enzymes have been administered to decrease intracellular GSH; (c) inhibitors of detoxifying enzymes such as GSTs have been given to decrease the tumor cell's ability to protect itself against alkylating metabolites; and (d) other precursor thiols have been administered to protect normal tissues.

Because GSH cannot readily cross cell membranes, early efforts to increase intracellular GSH relied on administration of the constituent amino acids, especially cysteine. More recently, a number of monoesters of GSH have been synthesized that are able to traverse the cell membrane and enhance intracellular GSH.[133] In animal studies,

the GSH-monoethyl ester successfully modulated anticancer drugs such as BCNU, cyclophosphamide, and mitomycin C.[134] Primarily, the ester protected liver, lungs, and spleen. At least in the murine system, it afforded no protection to marrow progenitor cells.

The obverse approach to repletion is depletion of GSH, in an attempt to gain a therapeutic advantage through specific effects in tumor cells. A number of agents, including diethylmaleate, phorone, and dimethylfumarate, have been used and, although successful in achieving tumor cell GSH depletion, have proved to be too toxic to use clinically. The toxicities and complications associated with the use of nonspecific depletors of GSH were circumvented by the design and synthesis of agents that acted as inhibitors of certain enzymes involved in the synthesis of GSH. Direct interference with GSH synthetase results in the buildup of 5-oxoproline, and this has the consequence of marked acidosis in patients.[135] By far the most effective approach to reducing the GSH biosynthetic capacity of a cell has been achieved by administering amino acid sulfoximines,[136,137] which inhibit γ-glutamylcysteine synthetase. The lead compound to emerge from these studies was L-buthionine (SR)-sulfoximine (BSO), the R-stereoisomer of which is the active inhibitor of γ-glutamylcysteine synthetase.[138] A large number of reports now describe low levels of GSH in unperturbed tumor cells adding to the rationale for BSO use to improve the therapeutic index of alkylating agents. Although BSO caused differential sensitization of tumors in animal models,[139] trials in humans failed to clearly demonstrate therapeutic index improvement[140,141] and enthusiasm for clinical use of BSO has waned.

An alternative approach to decreasing GSH effects is to inhibit the enzymes that use GSH as a cofactor. Because GST over-expression was determined to be at least one contributing mechanism to the alkylating agent–resistant phenotype, a rationale was established for the use of GST inhibitors as modulating agents. Because GST P1 often dominates in tumors whereas other subtypes often dominate in normal tissues, inhibitors specific to GST P1 might offer a therapeutic index advantage. Initial studies employed a relatively nonspecific inhibitor of GSTs, ethacrynic acid, a Food and Drug Administration (FDA)-approved diuretic. Preclinical studies were promising,[139,142] but dose escalation was inhibited by diuretic complications. Poor specificity for tumor-associated GST has deterred further development. Specific inhibitors of GST P1 have now been developed and are being studied clinically.[143] In a novel attempt to exploit the association between GST P1 and tumors, a unique drug that is activated by GST P1 to produce an alkylating agent in situ is also undergoing study[144] and a Phase 3 trial in ovarian cancer is underway.

A very different approach to modulation of alkylator toxicity was suggested in studies by the United States Army, which examined over 4,000 synthetic thiol derivatives as radioprotectors.[145] One of these compounds, WR2721,

5-2-(3-aminopropylamino)-has been shown to dephosphorylate selectively in normal tissues through catalysis by alkaline phosphatase.[146] In most tumors, the relatively more acidic microenvironment is believed to inhibit WR2721 activation.[147] WR2721 enhances the dose-modifying factor of cisplatin, melphalan, cyclophosphamide, nitrogen mustard, BCNU, and 5-fluorouracil in preclinical tumor models.[184] In clinical trials WR2721, given as a single dose at 740 mg/m^2 before 1,500 mg/m^2 of cyclophosphamide, does afford protection from granulocytopenia, decreasing the duration and increasing the nadir granulocyte count.[148] More recent studies suggest that WR2721 decreases myelosuppression, neurotoxicity, and nephrotoxicity of the cisplatin-cyclophosphamide combination without compromising the antitumor effect. Hospers et al.[149] have reviewed the recent clinical trials with WR2721 and alkylating agents. Additional studies suggest that coadministration of WR-2721 with high-dose melphalan and HCT may allow delivery of increased doses of melphalan to be delivered with no increase in toxicity.[150]

Nitrosourea Modulation

A modulatory approach specific for nitrosoureas has resulted from studies of DNA repair. Alkyl guanine alkyl transferase (AGT) binds irreversibly to O^6-guanine alkyl adducts and removes them from DNA, inactivating itself in the process. Because an O^6-guanine chloroethyl adduct is produced by BCNU and can lead in a subsequent slow step to DNA cross-linking, AGT inhibitors have been explored in combination with BCNU in cultured human leukemic cells. O^6-benzylguanine was ultimately selected for further study based on a variety of structure-activity and binding studies. The enhancement ratios reported for O^6-benzylguanine were equivalent or superior to those found for other modulating agents. Clinical evidence that response to nitrosoureas and methylating agents is inversely related to the tumor level of AGT supported further development.[151] Unfortunately, a Phase 2 trial of O^6-benzylguanine failed to demonstrate significant activity in patients with nitrosourea-resistant glioma.[152]

Ultimately, studies have shown that alkyl guanine alkyl transferase (AGT) inhibition by DNA methylation of its promoter improves the therapeutic activity of BCNU for brain tumors,[101] and further studies of this promising combination are warranted. Recent supporting data indicates that methylation (silencing) of DNA coding for AGT is correlated with improved sensitivity of human gliomas for BCNU.[153]

CLINICAL PHARMACOLOGY

The primary characteristics of the clinical pharmacokinetics of standard alkylating agents are given in Table 12.1. Although some agents are too reactive chemically to provide more than momentary exposure of tumor cells to parent drug (the best examples are mechlorethamine and BCNU), others are stable in their parent form and require metabolic activation, as in the case of cyclophosphamide and ifosfamide. The clinician must possess a working knowledge of the chemical and metabolic fate of individual alkylating agents to adjust doses for organ dysfunction and to plan rational treatment regimens.

Activation, Decomposition, and Metabolism

Decomposition Versus Metabolism

A principal route of degradation of most of the reactive alkylating agents is spontaneous hydrolysis of the alkylating entity (i.e., alkylation by water).[154-164] For example, mechlorethamine rapidly undergoes reaction to produce 2-hydroxyethyl-2-chloroethylmethylamine and bis-2-hydroxyethylmethylamine (Fig. 12.9).[154] Likewise, both melphalan and chlorambucil undergo similar hydrolysis to form the monohydroxyethyl and bishydroxyethyl products, although less rapidly than the aliphatic nitrogen mustards.[155,156] The hydroxylated products are less active than their chloroalkyl precursors.

Most alkylating agents also undergo some degree of enzymatic metabolism. For example, if mechlorethamine radiolabeled in the methyl group is administered to mice, approximately 15% of the radioactivity can be recovered as exhaled carbon dioxide, which indicates that enzymatic demethylation is occurring.

Cyclophosphamide and Ifosfamide

The widely used drugs cyclophosphamide and ifosfamide are activated to alkylating and cytotoxic metabolites by cytachrome P-450s, particularly the P-450 3A4 subtype.[165] The complex metabolic transformations that cyclophosphamide undergoes are illustrated in Figure 12.10.[164,166] The initial metabolic step is the oxidation of the ring carbon adjacent to the ring nitrogen to produce 4-hydroxycyclophosphamide, which spontaneously ring-opens and establishes equilibrium with aldophosphamide.

The 4-hydroxycyclophosphamide and aldophosphamide may be oxidized by soluble enzymes to produce 4-ketocyclophosphamide and carboxyphosphamide, respectively. These compounds have little cytotoxic activity and represent inactivated urinary excretion products. They account, between them, for approximately 80% of a dose of administered cyclophosphamide.[167,168]

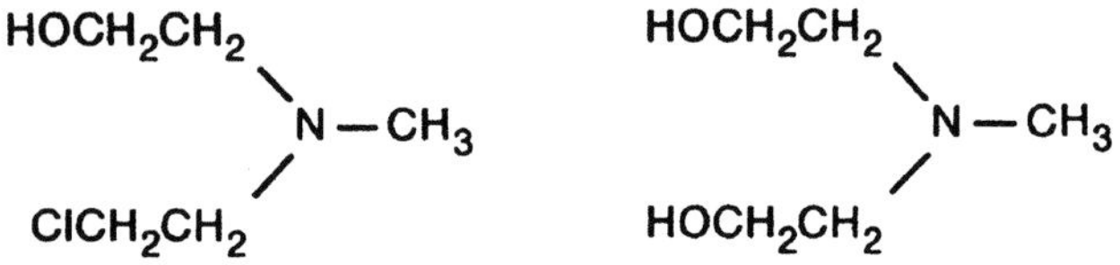

Figure 12.9 Hydrolysis products of mechlorethamine.

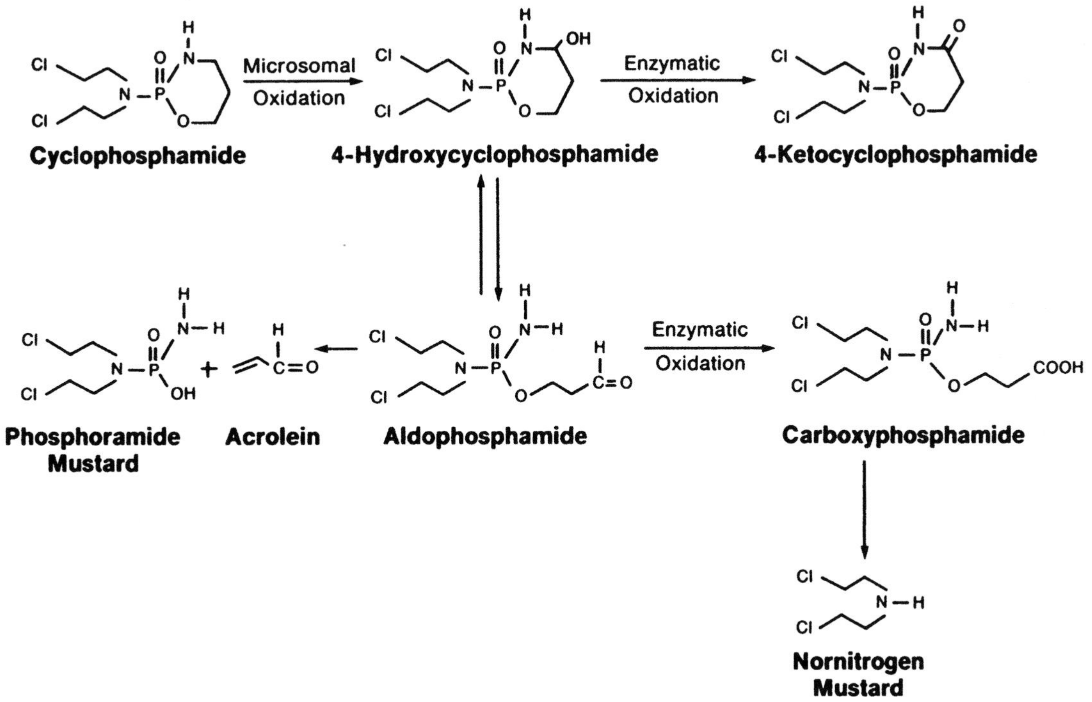

Figure 12.10 Metabolism of cyclophosphamide.

The 4-hydroxycyclophosphamide/aldophosphamide that has escaped enzymatic oxidation by aldehyde dehydrogenase can eliminate acrolein to produce phosphoramide mustard,[169] an active alkylating agent that appears to be responsible for the biologic effects of cyclophosphamide.[170,171] The concentration of aldehyde dehydrogenase in a variety of cell types appears inversely proportional to cytotoxicity, supporting the pivotal role of aldehyde dehydrogenase in determining the cytotoxic specificity of cyclophosphamide.[125] The high enzyme concentration in hematopoietic progenitor cells is suggested to explain the ability of cyclophosphamide to produce major myelosuppression without myeloablation in patients receiving high doses without transplantation.[172] The 4-hydroxycyclophosphamide/aldophosphamide serves as a transport form to deliver the highly polar phosphoramide mustard efficiently into cells.

A related oxazaphosphorine, ifosfamide (Fig. 12.3), also requires P-450 for activation to its active intermediates, which are found in plasma and urine.[173] As with cyclophosphamide, it undergoes hepatic activation to an aldehyde form that decomposes in plasma and peripheral tissues to yield acrolein and its alkylating metabolite.[174] Hydroxylation proceeds at a slower rate for ifosfamide than for cyclophosphamide, which results in a longer plasma half-life for the parent compound. Dechloroethylation of ifosfamide produces inactive metabolites and competes with the activation step as a major pathway of elimination.[175] Both cyclophosphamide (above doses of 4 g/m^2) and ifosfamide (above doses of 5 g/m^2) exhibit dose-dependent

nonlinear pharmacokinetics, with significant delays in elimination at higher doses.[176] Interestingly, both drugs also induce their own metabolism, resulting in significant shortening of the elimination half-life for the parent compound when the drugs are administered on multiple consecutive days.[177]

Nitrosoureas

The decomposition of nitrosoureas to generate the alkylating chloroethyldiazonium hydroxide entity[48] has been mentioned, and the products generated by this decomposition in aqueous solution are illustrated in Figure 12.11. The nitrosoureas also undergo metabolic transformation. Hill et al.[178] demonstrated that BCNU is enzymatically denitrosated by P-450, a finding of possible clinical significance.[179] Enhancement of P-450 activity in vivo by phenobarbital abolished the therapeutic effect of BCNU against the 9L intracerebral rat tumor and decreased the therapeutic activity of CCNU and BCNU against this tumor. The phenobarbital-treated rats had increased plasma clearance of BCNU, with lower plasma levels and lower area under the concentration × time curve (AUC) plasma values of BCNU. The plasma clearance of parent BCNU decreases and the plasma half-life increases as doses escalate from standard-dose (150 to 200 mg/^{2}) to high-dose regimens (600 mg/m^2) (Table 12.1). CCNU and methyl-CCNU undergo hydroxylation of their cyclohexyl ring to produce a series of metabolites that represent the major circulating species after treatment with these drugs.[180,181] These

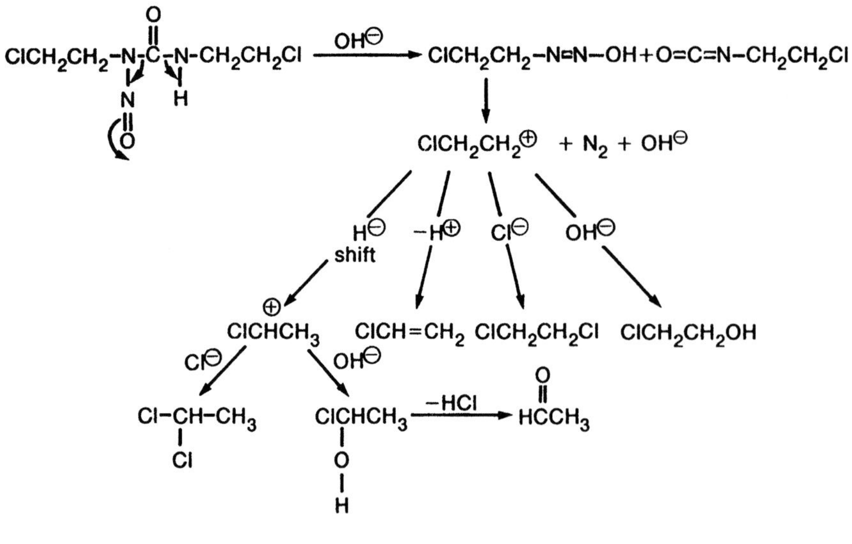

Figure 12.11 Decomposition of bischloroethylnitrosourea (BCNU) in buffered aqueous solution.

metabolites have increased alkylating activity but diminished carbamoylating effects.[182,183]

Clinical Pharmacokinetics

Because of the lack of definitive techniques for measuring certain specific drug and metabolite molecules, the data on the clinical pharmacology of the alkylating agents have been relatively limited. Recently, however, gas chromatography–mass spectrometry and high-pressure liquid chromatography (HPLC) have generated more definitive pharmacokinetic information (Table 12.1).

Melphalan

Several groups have examined the clinical pharmacology of melphalan. Alberts and colleagues[184] studied the pharmacokinetics of melphalan in patients who received 0.6 mg/kg of the drug intravenously. The peak levels of melphalan, as measured by HPLC, were 4.5 to 13 μmol/L (1.4 to 4.1 μg/mL), and the mean terminal-phase half-life ($t_{1/2}\beta$) of the drug in the plasma was 1.8 hours. The 24-hour urinary excretion of the parent drug averaged 13% of the administered dose. Inactive monohydroxy and dihydroxy metabolites appear in plasma within minutes of drug administration. Because renal excretion of drug is an unimportant pathway for drug elimination, full doses of drug are routinely given with hematopoietic cell transplantation in patients with complete renal failure.[185] As renal insufficiency often occurs in patients with myeloma, this flexibility allows a standard transplant regimen to be given to these patients.

Other studies have demonstrated low and variable systemic availability of the drug after oral dosing.[156,186] Food slows its absorption. After oral administration of melphalan, 0.6 mg/kg, much lower peak levels of drug of approximately 1 μmol/L (0.3 μg/mL) were seen. The time to

achieve peak plasma levels varied considerably and occurred as late as 6 hours after dosing. The low bioavailability was caused by incomplete absorption of the drug from the gastrointestinal tract, because 20 to 50% of an oral dose could be recovered in the feces.[186] No drug or drug products were found in the feces after intravenous administration. Not only does oral melphalan show unpredictable bioavailability, but its AUC is reduced one-third by concomitant administration of cimetidine.[187] Use of orally administered melphalan has declined steeply because of these bioavailability issues and because more effective therapies have been developed for breast and ovarian carcinomas and myeloma.

Regional administration of melphalan is possible by both intracavitary[188] and limb perfusion methods.[189]

Chlorambucil

After the oral administration of 0.6 mg/kg of chlorambucil,[156,157] peak levels of 2.0 to 6.3 μmol/L (0.6 to 1.9 μg/mL) occurred within 1 hour. Peak plasma levels of phenylacetic acid mustard, an alkylating metabolite of uncertain but potential importance, ranged from 1.8 to 4.3 μmol/L (0.5 to 1.18 μg/mL), and the peak levels of this metabolite were achieved 2 to 4 hours after dosing. The terminal-phase half-lives for chlorambucil and phenylacetic acid mustard were 92 and 145 minutes, respectively. Less than 1% of the administered dose of chlorambucil was excreted in the urine as either chlorambucil (0.54%) or as phenylacetic acid mustard (0.25%). Approximately 50% of the radioactivity from carbon 14–labeled chlorambucil administered orally was excreted in the urine in 24 hours. Of this material, over 90% appeared to be the monohydroxy and dihydroxy hydrolysis products of chlorambucil and phenylacetic acid mustard. Thus, orally administered chlorambucil is absorbed more completely and more rapidly than melphalan and has a similar terminal-phase half-life.

Cyclophosphamide

The study of the clinical pharmacology of cyclophosphamide has been complicated by the inactivity of the parent compound and by the complex array of metabolites. These metabolites have proved difficult to isolate and measure, and their properties are not yet completely established. The pharmacokinetics and bioavailability of the parent compound have been well established by a number of studies[177,190–196] (Table 12.2).

Cyclophosphamide seems to be reasonably well absorbed after oral administration to humans. D'Incalci et al.[177] found the systemic availability of the unchanged drug after oral administration of 100-mg doses (1 to 2 mg/kg) to be 97% of that after intravenous injection of the same dose. Juma and colleagues[190] found the systemic availability of the drug to be somewhat less and more variable (mean, 74%; range, 34 to 90%) after oral administration of larger doses of 300 mg (3 to 6 mg/kg). A more recent comparison of oral versus intravenous cyclophosphamide in the same patient revealed no difference in the AUC for the primary cytotoxic metabolites, hydroxycyclophosphamide and phosphoramide mustard, after drug administration by the two different routes.[196] After intravenous administration, the peak plasma levels of the parent compound are dose-dependent, with peak levels of 4, 50, and 500 nmol/mL reported after the administration of 1 to 2,[177] 6 to 15,[190] and 60 mg/kg,[191] respectively. The terminal-phase half-life of cyclophosphamide varies considerably among patients, with a range of 3 to 10 hours reported by a number of authors. In patients >19 years of age, the primary half-life for cyclophosphamide is 1.5 hours.[195] Several investigators have reported increased clearance of cyclophosphamide on successive days of high-dose infusion,[193] but this effect can be variable,[197] suggesting that strategies of dose-adjustment aimed at providing uniform exposure of drug or metabolites

may be difficult to achieve. Less than 15% of the parent drug is eliminated in the urine; the major site of clearance is the liver. The pharmacokinetics of the metabolites have been clarified in recent years. Initial measurements of total plasma alkylating activity showed considerable variation across patients, but similar ranges of alkylating activity of the equivalent of 10 to 80 nmol of nitrogen mustard per milliliter after doses of 40 to 60 mg of cyclophosphamide per kilogram have been found by several investigators.[190,198,199] Peak alkylating levels are achieved 2 to 3 hours after drug administration, and Juma et al.[190] found the terminal half-life of plasma alkylating activity to be 7.7 hours. All investigators have noted a plateau-like level of plasma alkylating activity maintained for at least 6 hours.

The predominant metabolites found in plasma are nornitrogen mustard and phosphoramide mustard, with lesser concentrations of the putative transport forms aldophosphamide and 4-hydroxycyclophosphamide (Table 12.2). Of some significance is the fact that reports[200] have questioned the reliability and applicability of earlier gas chromatography methods[191,201] for measuring levels of phosphoramide mustard and nornitrogen mustard in patient plasma. Because of these concerns, the actual quantitation of these metabolites and their half-lives (Table 12.2) remain approximate.

Fenselau et al.[202] identified aldophosphamide as the cyanohydrin derivative in the plasma of patients receiving cyclophosphamide, and Wagner et al.[203] identified a mercaptan derivative of 4-hydroxycyclophosphamide in the plasma of cyclophosphamide-treated patients. Because the two primary metabolites are in equilibrium, the formation of either derivative should allow the measurement of the total of the two metabolites. Wagner et al.[204] used the mercaptan derivatization technique to estimate that peak plasma levels of 1.4 and 2.6 nmol of total 4-hydroxycyclophosphamide/

TABLE 12.2

CLINICAL PHARMACOKINETICS OF CYCLOPHOSPHAMIDE AND METABOLITES

Subject of Study	Cyclophosphamide Dose (mg/kg)	Peak Plasma Concentration, (μmol/L)	Plasma $t_{1/2}$ (hr)	References
Cyclophosphamide	1–2	4	—	236
	6–15	50	3–10	237
	60	500	—	238
Total alkylating activity	40–60	10–80	7.7	237, 244, 245
Phosphoramide mustard	60–75	50–100	—	238
	4–12	3–18	8.7	247
Nornitrogen mustard	60–75	200–500	—	238, 247
	4–9	4–15	3.31	—
Aldophosphamide/4-hydroxycyclophosphamide	10	1.4	15	242, 243, 248, 250, 251
	20	2.6		

$t_{1/2}$, half-life.

aldophosphamide per mL are achieved in humans after injection of doses of 10 and 20 mg of radiolabeled cyclophosphamide per kilogram, respectively. Subsequent studies have determined that 4-hydroxycyclophosphamide/aldophosphamide has a half-life of approximately 1.5 hours in children[195] and 1 to 5 hours in adults receiving conventional[196] or high-dose[205] cyclophosphamide. The AUC for 4-hydroxycyclophosphamide and aldophosphamide at conventional doses of drug ranged from 3 to 19 nmol/mL × hours and seems to be independent of either peak plasma levels or the plasma half-life of the parent drug or hydroxycyclophosphamide.

Because the initial metabolism of cyclophosphamide is hepatic, modulation of the activity of P-450 in vivo might be expected to alter the pharmacokinetics of the drug. Pretreatment with phenobarbital, a known P-450 inducer, reduces the plasma half-life of the parent compound in both humans and experimental animals.[206,207] Also, with repeated doses of cyclophosphamide, the plasma half-life can be shown to become progressively shorter,[177,192] which indicates that cyclophosphamide can induce the P-450 enzymes responsible for its metabolism. The wide variation in the plasma half-life of cyclophosphamide seen in patients can be partly caused by differing previous drug exposure and the consequent differences in hepatic microsomal activity. For example, Egorin et al.[208] found consistently short plasma half-lives of cyclophosphamide (<2 hours) in a group of patients with brain tumors who had had long-term phenobarbital exposure. The net effect of P-450 induction on alkylating metabolite AUC's appears to be variable, however,[209,210] so the use of P-450 inducer pretreatment as a method to improve the therapeutic index of cyclophosphamide would require careful study.

Two authors have reported increased and prolonged plasma levels of cyclophosphamide metabolites in patients with renal failure, and on this basis, a reduction in dosage has been recommended for such patients.[199,211] Because the use of cyclophosphamide in patients with severe renal failure has been incompletely studied, and both parent drug and active metabolites are known to be renally excreted, caution should be used when cyclophosphamide is administered to such patients.[212]

Ifosfamide

The clinical pharmacology of ifosfamide has been studied by Creaven et al.[213] and their colleagues[199,214,215] and has been summarized by Brade et al.[216] and Bagley et al.[199] After single doses of 3.8 to 5.0 g/m^2, the terminal half-life of ifosfamide was 15 hours, considerably longer than the previously cited values of 3 to 10 hours for cyclophosphamide. At ifosfamide doses of 1.6 to 2.4 g/m^2, however, the half-life of the drug was similar to that of cyclophosphamide. Creaven et al.[213] found similar values for alkylating activity in plasma after the administration of 3.8 g/m^2 ifosfamide and 1.1 g/m^2 cyclophosphamide. Also, the alkylating activity excreted in the urine was similar for these doses of the two analogs and ranged from 6 to 15% for ifosfamide, although urinary excretion may approach 50% at high single doses.[216] These findings are consistent with the previous results of Allen and Creaven,[173] which indicate that P-450 activation of ifosfamide to alkylating metabolites proceeds more slowly than the activation of cyclophosphamide and that high doses of ifosfamide seem to saturate the activation mechanism. As with cyclophosphamide, ifosfamide clearance increases during continuous infusion or with multiple daily doses, reaching a steady state 2 to 3 days after drug administration is begun.[217] Norpoth[218] reported that cleavage of the chloroethyl group from the side chain and ring nitrogen is a quantitatively more significant pathway for ifosfamide metabolism than for cyclophosphamide metabolism in humans. Whereas less than 10% of an administered dose of cyclophosphamide is dechlorethylated,[168] as much as 50% of a dose of ifosfamide may be excreted in the urine as dechlorethylated products. These findings suggest that the less rapid oxidative activation at C-4 of ifosfamide allows the chloroethyl group cleavage to become a significantly competing pathway in the in vivo metabolism of the drug. Although oxidation at C-4 of both cyclophosphamide and ifosfamide leads to ring opening and creation of compounds with alkylating activity, the products of side-chain cleavage have little alkylating activity. Thus, at doses below 3.8 g/m^2, the rates of metabolism of cyclophosphamide and ifosfamide are similar, but a lower proportion of the ifosfamide is converted into alkylating and biologically active metabolites.

Because the slower activation rate of ifosfamide results in more prolonged exposure to the bladder-toxic metabolite acrolein, the glutathione analog MESNA is routinely administered in association with ifosfamide.

Thiotepa

Studies using gas chromatographic analysis specific for thiotepa have revealed that it is rapidly desulfurated to TEPA and other alkylating species.[219–224] The conversion of thiotepa to TEPA is mediated by P-450 as confirmed in vitro by incubation of thiotepa with hepatic microsomes. P-450-inducing agents increase thiotepa clearance, but the pharmacodynamic effects of this are unclear. Both thiotepa and TEPA have cytotoxic activity. Aside from individual variability, the plasma terminal half-life of intact thiotepa is a relatively consistent 1.2 to 2 hours. TEPA appears in plasma within 5 minutes of thiotepa administration. In 120 minutes its plasma concentration reaches that of thiotepa, but it persists longer, with a half-life of 3 to 21 hours, so that after 24 hours, TEPA concentration × time exceeds that of the parent drug. In 24 hours, only 1.5% of the administered thiotepa is excreted in the urine unchanged, together with 4.2% as TEPA and 23.5% as other alkylating species.[219] The pharmacokinetics in children resembles that in adults.[220,223]

Nitrosoureas

Levin et al.[225] studied the pharmacokinetics of BCNU in humans and found that after short-term infusion (15 to 75 minutes) of 60 to 170 mg/m², initial peak levels of up to 5 µmol/L of BCNU were achieved. The plasma concentration decay curves were biexponential, with a distribution-phase half-life of 6 minutes and a second-phase half-life of 68 minutes. With high-dose BCNU, longer elimination half-lives of 22 to 45 minutes have been reported.[226,227]

Busulfan

The pharmacokinetics of busulfan have been studied using a variety of sensitive methods.[228–232] The parent compound can be measured by gas chromatography after derivatization[230] or by HPLC using mass spectroscopic detection.[233] Busulfan is routinely administered over 3 to 4 consecutive days, often with dosing every 6 hours. The drug bioavailability is often variable between patients.[234] Because of this difficulty, when busulfan is used in high doses with hematopoietic cell transplantation either therapeutic drug monitoring, a recently approved parenteral busulfan formulation, or both are frequently used to assure uniform drug exposure.[235] The drug exhibits circadian rhythmicity in its pharmacokinetics, particularly in children, with higher drug levels and slower elimination in the evening. The primary elimination half-life is approximately 2.5 hours in both children and adults, although interpatient variability is considerable at both low and high doses.

The relationship between intravenous dose and AUC within the same patient appears to be predictable over multiple days of administration. Because of variable bioavailability, there is less consistency when the oral formulation is used.[236] Clearance declines with age, which leads to underdosing of children in high-dose regimens.[237] Busulfan clearance for patients older than 18 years averages 2.64 to 2.9 mL/minute per kilogrAM, whereas for children aged 2 to 14 clearance averages 4.4 to 4.5 Ml/minute per kilogram, and for children age 3 or younger it is 6.8 to 8.4 mL/-minute per kilogram.[232] Thus, larger doses must be used in the younger age groups to achieve the desired cytotoxic exposure. Although data are incomplete, young children with hepatic disease (e.g., lysosomal storage disease) have a more prolonged half-life (4.9 hours) than their counterparts with normal liver function (2.3 hours).[232] Because of its high lipid solubility and low level of protein binding, busulfan penetrates readily into the brain and cerebrospinal fluid. The ratio of drug concentration in cerebrospinal fluid to plasma approximates 1.[238] Positron-labeled busulfan has been used to track uptake into the brain, revealing that approximately 20% of a standard dose rapidly enters the CNS.[239] This access to the brain may enhance the activity of this drug against leukemia and lymphoma cells in the CNS, but it also may explain its propensity to cause seizures. Prophylaxis with anticonvulsants is required in patients receiving high-dose busulfan. Busulfan enhances the clearance of phenytoin (dilantin) and, in some patients, lowers the drug's plasma concentration below the therapeutic range, which increases the risk of seizures.[240] Phenytoin levels should be monitored in the setting of busulfan therapy or an alternative, non–P-450 metabolized anticonvulsant should be used.

Pharmacokinetic studies have provided insight into both toxic and therapeutic effects of busulfan when used in high doses with hematopoietic cell transplantation. In this setting, busulfan produces hepatic veno-occlusive disease (VOD), which can be fatal. Grochow and colleagues[231] have shown that excessive busulfan exposure increases VOD risk, and Andersson et al.[241] have suggested that excessive exposure also increases the risk of graft-versus-host disease during allotransplantation. Alternatively, inadequate exposures may increase the risk of both leukemia relapse[242] or allotransplant rejection.[243] These data, taken together, highlight the importance of appropriate busulfan exposure during transplantation and the utility of therapeutic drug monitoring in this setting. The impact of PK-directed dosing of other alkylating agents may merit further study.

TOXICITY

Hematopoietic Suppression

The usual dose-limiting toxicity of the alkylating agents is suppression of hematopoiesis. Characteristically, this suppression involves all formed elements of the blood: leukocytes, platelets, and red cells. However, the degree, time course, and cellular pattern of the hematopoietic suppression produced by the various alkylating agents differ. Clinically significant depression of the platelets may be seen when the dose of cyclophosphamide exceeds 30 mg/kg, but a relative platelet sparing is very characteristic of the drug.

Even at the very high doses (200 mg/kg or greater) of cyclophosphamide used in preparation for bone marrow transplantation, recovery of endogenous hematopoietic elements occurs within 21 to 28 days and has allowed these high doses to be used without transplantation in patients with aplastic anemia.[172] This stem cell-sparing property of cyclophosphamide is further reflected by the fact that cumulative damage to the bone marrow is uncommonly seen when cyclophosphamide is given as a single agent, and repeated high doses of the drug can be given without progressive lowering of leukocyte and platelet counts. In contrast to cyclophosphamide, busulfan seems to be especially damaging to bone marrow stem cells,[37,244] and prolonged or permanent hypoplasia of the bone marrow may be seen after busulfan administration. Melphalan seems to be more damaging to hematopoietic stem cells than cyclophosphamide, in that a longer recovery period for hematopoietic cells is seen both in animals[245] and in humans, and a cumulative bone marrow depression may occur with repeated doses of melphalan.

The hematopoietic depression produced by the nitrosoureas is characteristically delayed. The onset of leukocyte and platelet depression occurs 3 to 4 weeks after drug administration and may last an additional 2 to 3 weeks.[43] Thrombocytopenia appears earlier and usually is more severe than leukopenia. Even if the nitrosourea is given at 6-week intervals, hematopoietic recovery may not occur between courses, and the drug dose often must be decreased when repeated courses are used.

The biochemical basis for the stem cell-sparing effect of cyclophosphamide is now known to be the presence of a high level of the enzyme aldehyde dehydrogenase in the early bone marrow progenitor cells.[246] This enzyme metabolizes the reactive intermediate aldophosphamide. The mechanistic and biochemical bases for the profound effect of busulfan and the nitrosoureas on marrow stem cells remain unknown.

Nausea and Vomiting

Although nausea and vomiting are not usually life-threatening toxic reactions, they are a frequent side effect of alkylating agent therapy and usually require potent antiemetics to control. The effectiveness of the newer centrally acting antiemetics suggests that the emetic effect of these drugs is at most only partially mediated by direct gastrointestinal effects .

Interstitial Pneumonitis, Lung Injury, and Fibrosis

Both BCNU[247] and busulfan[248,249] have been observed to produce pulmonary fibrosis when administered in lower doses over prolonged periods. Busulfan is less frequently used in this dosing pattern in recent times, but BCNU is still used in this manner to treat brain tumors. Both drugs are being increasingly used in high dose over 1 to 4 days with hematopoietic cell transplantation. With this dosing pattern, busulfan produces much less lung toxicity. A dose-dependent pattern of acute lung injury from BCNU with HCT is well recognized, varying from a frequency of 5 to 60% ,depending on the regimen and dose of BCNU administered.[250] This acute injury is manifested by cough, dypnea, occasional fever, and frequently minimal radiographic findings.[251] Although these problems can become life-threatening or progress to fibrosis, the acute injury is entirely reversible and treatable with prednisone if diagnosed early. Virtually all other alkylating agents have been associated with similar patterns of acute lung injury or fibrosis, though much less frequently than with BCNU or busulfan.

Renal and Bladder Toxicity

A toxicity that is relatively unique to the oxazaphosphorines (cyclophosphamide and ifosfamide) is hemorrhagic cystitis, which may range from a mild cystitis to severe bladder damage with massive hemorrhage.[252-254] This toxicity is caused by the excretion of acrolein, a metabolite of both cyclophosphamide and ifosfamide in the urine, with subsequent direct irritation of the bladder mucosa.[252,255] This toxicity is usually seen within weeks of the administration of high-dose cyclophosphamide, but can be seen at any time after repeated doses of ifosfamide or lower-dose cyclophosphamide. In HCT-treated patients, bladder hemorrhage occurring later than 4 to 6 weeks after cyclophosphamide treatment is more likely the result of viral cystitis[256] or coagulopathy. The most effective agent for preventing oxazaphosphorine-induced cystitis is 2-mercaptoethane sulfonate (MESNA), which dimerizes to an inactive metabolite in plasma but hydrolyzes in urine to yield the active parent that conjugates with alkylating species and prevents cystitis. MESNA should be administered routinely to all patients receiving ifosfamide and to any patient who has a history of drug-induced cystitis.[257] MESNA is usually given in divided doses every 4 hours in dosages of 60% of those of the alkylating agent. Experiments in animals and clinical evaluation indicate that the systemic administration of sulfhydryl compounds does not impair the antitumor or immunosuppressive effect of cyclophosphamide.[258,259]

Hemorrhagic cystitis is often a devastating, life-threatening, or extremely debilitating treatment complication, so great emphasis should always be placed on prevention. Chronic cystitis caused by cyclophosphamide has been associated with the later development of malignant transitional cell tumors of the bladder.[260]

At high doses of ifosfamide, severe renal tubular damage with elevation of serum urea and creatinine has been seen, and a Fanconi-like syndrome has been described after ifosfamide therapy.[261,262] High-dose cyclophosphamide can also produce the syndrome of inappropriate antidiuretic hormone excretion, resulting in transient water retention.[263] Chronic administration of nitrosoureas can also infrequently produce renal damage.[264-266] High-dose melphalan has also been associated with renal tubular injury and proteinuria.[267]

Alopecia and Allergic Reactions

Alopecia and allergic reactions have been associated with all alkylating agents. Alopecia is almost universal when alkylating agents are used in high doses with hematopoietic cell transplantation.

Gonadal Atrophy

Alkylating agents have profound toxic effects on reproductive tissue; these are discussed in greater detail in Chapter 4. A depletion of testicular germ cells but preservation of Sertoli's cells was described by Spitz[268] in the first extensive review of the histologic effects of mechlorethamine in patients. This toxic effect and its functional counterpart of aspermia have subsequently been well documented in both animals[269] and humans.[270,271] The probability of aspermia increases with increasing dose and cumulative dose of alkylating agents. Because of the widespread availability of sperm banking, patients who will undergo treatment with alkylating agents and who wish to father children should be counseled to be evaluated for sperm banking prior to treatment. Oligospermia or aspermia are also associated with advanced malignancy. There are isolated reports of return of sperm and sperm function after complete aspermia induced by either conventional or high-dose alkylating agents.[272,273] Amenorrhea as a complication of busulfan therapy was reported by Galton et al.[274] Several reports subsequently documented the high incidence of amenorrhea and ovarian atrophy associated with cyclophosphamide therapy.[275–278] A high incidence of amenorrhea after melphalan therapy also has been established. Pathologic examination of the ovaries after alkylating agent-induced amenorrhea reveals the absence of mature or primordial follicles. Endocrinologic studies demonstrate the decreased estrogen and progesterone levels and elevated serum follicle-stimulating hormone and luteinizing hormone levels typical of menopause. The risk of amenorrhea and infertility after alkylating agents increases with increasing age, as well as dose and cumulative dose of alkylating agents used. Preliminary data suggest that hormonal suppression of menses during alkylating agent treatment can increase the probability of later return of menstrual function, and further study is needed.

Teratogenesis

All alkylating agents are teratogenic.[279–281] Studies have been carried out in a number of systems, both in vivo and in embryo culture in vitro.[282–285] The teratogenic action seems to be the result of direct cytotoxicity to the developing embryo by the same mechanisms operative in tumor cells.[286,287]

Because of the demonstrated teratogenicity of the alkylating agents in animals, appropriate concern has existed about the potential effects of their administration to patients during pregnancy. In 1968, Nicholson[288] reviewed literature reports of women treated with cytotoxic agents during pregnancy. In the 25 instances in which the alkylating agents were given during the first trimester of pregnancy and the status of the fetus was recorded, 4 cases of fetal malformation occurred. No instances of malformed fetuses were reported when alkylating agents or other cytotoxic drugs were administered during the second or third trimester. Thus, administration of alkylating agents during the first trimester presents a definite risk of a malformed viable infant, but the administration of such drugs during the second and third trimesters may not increase the risk of fetal malformation above normal. Other reports confirm the risk of malformation in children born to mothers who had received chlorambucil,[289] cyclophosphamide,[290] or nitrogen mustard and procarbazine[291] during the first trimester and the birth of normal infants to mothers receiving alkylating agents during the second or third trimester.[292,293]

Carcinogenesis

Carcinogenesis as a complication of cancer chemotherapy is covered in detail in Chapter 5. Case reports began appearing during the early 1970s of development of an aggressive acute myeloid leukemia in patients treated with alkylating agents. These leukemias are often characterized by a preceding phase of myelodysplasia, alteration of chromosome 5, 7 or 11, and a poor response to treatment. They usually occur between 1 and 5 years following alkylating agent treatment. Cases described have been in patients treated with melphalan,[294,295] cyclophosphamide,[296–298] chlorambucil,[299,300] and the nitrosoureas.[301] The frequency of so-called "secondary leukemia" varies with alkylating agent regimen, use of other carcinogenic treatments such as radiation, and the dose and schedule of the treatments. Less common use of chronic, low-dose alkylating agent therapy for myeloma and ovarian cancer may alter the incidence of secondary leukemia in these diseases.[302] The routine use of sequential chemotherapy and radiation for treatment of Hodgkin's disease is being reduced because of concern for the increased level of secondary leukemia that these regimens produce.[303] Other malignancies, including solid tumors, also have been reported to develop in patients treated with alkylating agents.[303,304] High-dose alkylating agent therapy with HCT produces an increased risk for a variety of solid tumors including lung, skin, and breast cancer, which frequently occur between 10 and 20 years following treatment. This observation reflects both the carcinogenic and curative potential of alkylating agents used in these regimens.

Organ Toxicity in High-Dose Chemotherapy

Alkylating agents have become a logical tool, either alone or in combination, for high-dose chemotherapy regimens.[305–308] Their use is often associated with nonoverlapping tumor resistance and log-linear increases in tumor killing with dose. In this high-dose setting, toxicities that affect the gut, lung, liver, and CNS become dose-limiting and life threatening. A list of the dose-limiting extramedullary toxicities of the alkylating agents is given in Table 12.3. Melphalan produces severe gastrointestinal toxicity.[309] A number of alkylating agents, including the nitrosoureas, busulfan, thiotepa, and carboplatin produce venoocclusive disease of the liver.[235,310]

The highly lipid-soluble alkylators, especially, busulfan, the nitrosoureas, and thiotepa, cause CNS dysfunction, including seizures, altered mental status, cerebellar dysfunction, cranial nerve palsies, and coma.[311–313] High-dose ifosfamide produces neurotoxicity at least partly because of a metabolite chloracetaldehyde[314] (Fig. 12.12)

TABLE 12.3

ALKYLATING AGENTS IN HIGH-DOSE CHEMOTHERAPY

Dose-Limiting Extramedullary Toxicities of Single Agents

Drug	MTD[a] (mg/m²)	Fold Increase Over Standard Dose	Major Organ Toxicities
Cyclophosphamide	7,000	7.0	Cardiac
Ifosfamide	16,000	2.7	Renal, CNS
Thiotepa	1,000	18.0	GI, CNS
Melphalan	180	5.6	GI
Busulfan	640	9.0	GI, hepatic
BCNU	1,050	5.3	Lung, hepatic
Cisplatin	200	2.0	PN, renal
Carboplatin	2,000	5.0	Renal, PN, hepatic
Etoposide	3,000	6.0	GI

Combination High-Dose Chemotherapy Regimens

Regimen	Dose	Major Toxicities	Regimen MTD[b]	References
Cyclophosphamide	6,000			
BCNU	300	Lung, GI	0.47	445
Busulfan	640	Lung, GI, hepatic	1.0	446
Cyclophosphamide	8,000			
Ifosfamide	16,000			
Carboplatin	1,800	Renal, hepatic, GI	0.8	447
Cyclophosphamide	5,250			
Cisplatin	180			
Cyclophosphamide	6,000			
Thiotepa	500	GI, cardiac	0.59	449
Carboplatin	800			
Cyclophosphamide	5,625			
BCNU	600	Lung, hepatic, renal	0.57	450
Cisplatin	165			

[a] See references 91, 438, 444.
[b] See Eder et al.[449] for calculation of regimen MTD.
BCNU, bischloroethylnitrosourea; CNS, central nervous system; GI, gastrointestinal; MTD, maximum tolerated dose; PN, peripheral neuropathy.

Patients with hypoalbuminemia, renal insufficiency, and those treated with higher doses of ifosfamide are at increased risk for neurotoxicity.[315] Concomitant use of aggressive intravenous fluids appears to increase the renal excretion of CNS-toxic metabolites and reduce the risk of CNS injury.

The dose-limiting toxicity of cyclophosphamide is cardiac toxicity.[316–318] This toxicity has been reported at doses of over 100 mg/kg administered during a 48-hour period, and has been noted most often in patients receiving total doses of more than 200 mg/kg with HCT.[318] High-dose cyclophosphamide produces an acute myopericardial injury within days of administration,[319] and life-threatening effects are often produced by pericardial tamponade. Unlike the cumulative and irreversible injury produced by anthracyclines, cyclophosphamide cardiac toxicity is largely reversible if the patient survives for days following the acute toxic episode. No evidence exists for cumulative damage to the heart after repeated moderate or low doses of cyclophosphamide. BCNU and melphalan are also capable of producing reversible cardiac injury in this setting.

Immunosuppression

Numerous reports have detailed that alkylating agents suppress both humoral and cellular immunity in a variety of experimental systems. Cyclophosphamide is a particularly potent immunosuppressive alkylating agent and has been extensively studied.[320–324] Selective effects of cyclophosphamide on different components of the lymphoid system have been described. In vivo, it has been reported to cause selective suppression of B-lymphocyte function and to deplete B lymphocytes.[325,326] Cyclophosphamide, however, can suppress lymphocyte functions that are mediated by T cells, such as the graft-versus-host response and delayed hypersensitivity.[323,327] Appropriate doses of cyclophosphamide in vivo[328] or of activated cyclophosphamide in vitro[329] also have been established to enhance immunologic responses by selective inhibition of the function of

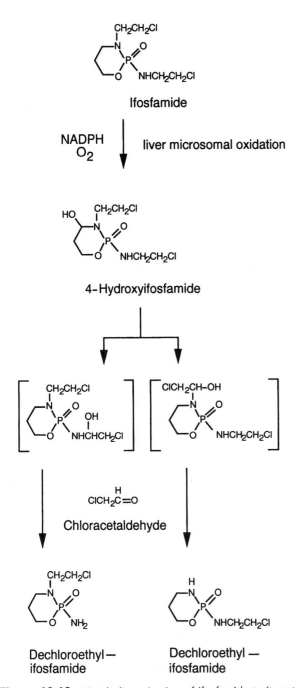

Figure 12.12 Metabolic activation of ifosfamide to its active form, 4-hydroxyifosfamide, and further metabolic transformation to chloracetaldehyde and other end products. NADPH, reduced form of nicotinamide-adenine dinucleotide phosphate.

analog of cyclophosphamide, blocks the differentiation of suppressor T-cell precursors at drug levels that are not cytotoxic and do not produce demonstrable DNA cross-linking in drug- sensitive cell lines.[331]

The clinical significance of the immunosuppression produced by alkylating agents (and other drugs) in the setting of cancer therapy is variable. The major concerns are the danger of increased susceptibility to infection in the immunosuppressed host and the potential interference with a host immune response to the tumor. There is further uncertainty in this area because the immunologic measurements most appropriate to estimate the risks are not certain. Mullins et al.[332] studied the immune responses of patients with solid tumors treated with high-dose cyclophosphamide, 120 mg/kg over a 2-day period. Six of the 12 patients studied became transiently anergic (for 1 to 2 weeks) to skin test antigens to which they had previously been responsive, but the response to these antigens recovered in all patients by 4 weeks after the cyclophosphamide therapy. Nine of the 12 patients showed an adequate antibody response to an antigenic challenge given 24 hours after the cyclophosphamide therapy, despite severe hematopoietic depression. Because most antitumor regimens would not be expected to be as immunosuppressive as the dose of cyclophosphamide used in this study, the results suggest that most intermittent antitumor regimens do not uniformly produce profound immunosuppression and that recovery of the immune response is usually prompt. Continuous drug therapy with cytotoxic agents or high-dose therapy followed by delayed marrow reconstitution are more likely to lead to severe lymphocyte depletion and profound immunosuppression and to be associated with an increased frequency of opportunistic infections.[333]

The immunosuppressive activity of alkylating agents, and of cyclophosphamide in particular, has been used for two types of clinical application. The first use has been for the suppression of the recipient immune response before allogeneic transplantation. Since the demonstration by Santos and colleagues[334] that matched sibling bone marrow can be successfully transplanted into recipients who have been pretreated with large doses of cyclophosphamide, this drug has been one of several agents used for immunosuppressive effect during bone marrow transplantation; the other drugs are methotrexate and calcineurin inhibitors (cyclosporin A, tacrolimus). Cyclophosphamide also has been shown to be effective in controlling kidney graft rejection[335] but has been less widely used for this application than the antimetabolite immunosuppressive agents.

The other use of alkylating agents in patients with non-malignant disease has been in the treatment of immunologic disorders. Osborne et al.,[336] in 1947, reported the successful treatment of a patient with systemic lupus erythematosus using nitrogen mustard. Subsequently, the alkylating agents have been tried in a wide variety of diseases thought to be autoimmune in nature, with variable

suppressor T cells. Several lines of evidence suggest that at least some of the immunosuppressive effects of cyclophosphamide may involve mechanisms other than lethal damage to lymphocytes. Shand and Howard[330] reported that induction of tolerance in B cells by cyclophosphamide in vivo or by activated cyclophosphamide in vitro occurs, is reversible, and is associated with failure of the cyclophosphamide-treated B cell to regenerate a surface immunoglobulin receptor after capping with anti-immunoglobulin serum. Also, 4-hydroperoxycyclophosphamide, an activated results. Cyclophosphamide has been shown to be an effective agent in the treatment of Wegener's granulomatosis,[337] rheumatoid arthritis,[338,339] idiopathic thrombocytopenic purpura,[340] and membranous glomerulonephritis.[341,342] Because of the severe side effects, however, including carcinogenesis, the role of alkylating agents in the treatment of nonmalignant disease must be considered carefully. High-dose cyclophosphamide without HCT has been used to treat aplastic anemia, a disease with a possible autoimmune basis.[172]

REFERENCES

1. Rhoads CP. Nitrogen mustards in treatment of neoplastic disease. JAMA 1946;131:656.
2. Jacobson LP, Spurr CL, Barron ESQ, et al. Studies on the effect of methyl-bis (beta-chloroethyl) amine hydrochloride on neoplastic diseases and allied disorders of the hemapoietic system. JAMA 1946;132:263.
3. Goodman LS, Wintrobe MM, Dameschek W, et al. Use of methyl-bis (beta-chloroethyl) amine hydrochloride for Hodgkin's disease, lymphosarcoma, leukemia. JAMA 1946;132:126.
4. Adair CPJ, Bagg HJ. Experimental and clinical studies on the treatment of cancer by dichloroethylsuphide (mustard gas). Ann Surg 464;93:190.
5. Skipper HE, Schabel FM, Wilcox WS. Experimental evaluation of potential anti-cancer agents XXI. On the criteria and kinetics associated with "curability" of experimental leukemia. Cancer Chemother Rep 1964;35;1.
6. Harris al. DNA repair and resistance to chemotherapy. Cancer Surv 1985;4:601.
7. Russo JE, Hilton J, Colvin OM. The role of aldehydehydrogenase iso-enzymes in cellular resistance to the alkylating agent cyclophosphamide. In: Weiner H, Flynn TG, eds. Enzymology and Molecular Biology of Carbonyl Metabolism. New York: Alan R Liss, 1989:65.
8. Brent TP, Houghton PJ, Houghton JA. O^6-Alkylguanine- DNA alkyltransferase activity correlates with the therapeutic response of human rhabdomyosarcoma xenografts to 1-(2-chloroethyl)-3-(trans-4-methylcyclohexyl)-1-nitrosourea. Proc Natl Acad Sci U S A 1985;82(2987).
9. Colvin M, Brundett RB, Kan MN, et al. Alkylating Properties of phosphoramide mustard. Cancer Res 1976;36:1121.
10. Brundett RB, Cowens JW, Colvin M. Chemistry of nitrosoureas: decomposition of deuterated 1,3 bis(2-chloroethyl)-1-nitrosoureas. J Med Chem 1976;19:958.
11. Ewig RAG, Kohn KW. DNA damage and repair in mouse leukemia L1210 cells treated with nitrogen mustard, 1,3- bis (2-chloroethyl)-1-nitrosourea, and other nitrosoureas. Cancer Res 1977;37:2114.
12. Sudhaker S, Tew KD, Schein PS, et al. Nitrosourea interaction with chromatin and effect on poly (adenosine diphosphate ribose) polymerase activity. Cancer Res 1979;39:1411.
13. Ciaccio PJ, Tew KD, LaCreta FP. The spontaneous and glutathione-S-transferase-mediated reaction of chlorambucil with glutathione. Cancer Commun 1990;2:279.
14. Ciaccio PJ, Tew KD, LaCreta FP. The enzymatic conjugation of chlorambucil with glutathione is catalyzed by human glutathione-S-transferase enzymes and inhibition by ethacrynic acid. Biochem Pharmacol 1991;42:2410.
15. Bolton MG, Colvin OM, Hilton J. Specificity of isozymes of murine glutathione-S-transferase for the conjugation of glutathione with l-phenylalanine mustard. Cancer Res 1991;51:2410.
16. Friedman OM, Myles A, Colvin M. Cyclophosphamide and certain structurally related phosphoramide mustards. Rosowsky A, ed. Advances in Cancer Chemotherapy, vol 1. New York: Marcel Dekker, 1979:179.
17. Drings P, Fritsch H. Erfahrungen mit Iphosphamide in hoher Einzeldosis bei metastasierten soliden Tumoren. Verh Dtsch Ges Inn Med 1972;78:166.
18. Brade W, Seeber S, Herdrich K. Comparative activity of ifosfamide and cyclophosphamide. Cancer Chemother Pharmacol 1986;18(Suppl 2):1.
19. Wiltshaw E, Westbury G, Harmer C, et al. Ifosfamide plus MESNA with and without Adriamycin in soft tissue sarcoma. Cancer Chemother Pharmacol 1986;18(Suppl 2):10.
20. Frick JC, Tretter P, Tretter W, et al. Disseminated carcinoma of the ovary treated by l-phenylalanine mustard. Cancer 1968;21:508.
21. Costa G, Engle RL Jr, Schilling A, et al. Melphalan and prednisone: an effective combination for the treatment of multiple myeloma. Am J Med 1973;54:549.
22. Fisher B, Sherman B, Rockette H, et al. l-Phenylalanine mustard (l-PAM) in the management of premenopausal patients with primary breast cancer. Cancer 1979;44:847.
23. Goldin D, Israels L, Nabarro J, et al. Clinical trials of p-(di- 2-chloroethylamino)-phenylbutyric acid (CB 1348) in malignant lymphoma. BMJ 1955;2:172.
24. Rundles RW, Striggle J, Bell W, et al. Comparison of chlorambucil and Myleran in chronic lymphocytic and granulocytic leukemia. Am J Med 1959;27:424.
25. Zdink E, Stutzman L. Chlorambucil therapy for lymphomas and chronic lymphocytic leukemia. JAMA 1965;191:444.
26. Wiltshaw E. Chlorambucil in the treatment of primary adenocarcinoma of the ovary. J Obstet Gynaecol Br Commonw 1964;72:586.
27. Bateman JC. Chemotherapy of solid tumors with triethylene thiophosphoramide. N Engl J Med 1955;252:879.
28. Ultmann JE, Hyman GA, Crandall C, et al. Methylene thiophosphoramide thio-TEPA in the treatment of neoplastic disease. Cancer 1957;10:902.
29. Santos GW, Tutschka PJ, Brookmeyer R, et al. Marrow transplantation for acute nonlymphocytic leukemia after treatment with busulfan and cyclophosphamide. N Engl Med 1983;309:1347–1353.
30. Haddow A, Timmis GM. Myleran in chronic myeloid leukaemia—chemical constitution and biological action. Lancet 1953;1:207.
31. Timmis GM, Hudson RF. Part I: chemistry of alkylating agents: discussion. Ann N Y Acad Sci 1958;68:727.
32. Roberts JJ, Warwick GP. Mode of action of alkylating agents: formation of S-ethylcysteine from ethyl methanesulphonate in vivo. Nature 1957;179:1181.
33. Roberts JJ, Warwick GP. Metabolic and chemical studies of "Myleran": formation of 3-hydroxytetrahydrothiophene-1,1-dioxide in vivo, and reactions with thiols in vitro. Nature 1959;184:1288.
34. Brookes P, Lawley PD. The alkylation of guanosine and guanylic acid. J Chem Soc 1961;1961:3923.
35. Iwanoto T, Hiraku Y, Oikawa S, et al. DNA intrastrand cross-link at the 5′-GA-3′ sequence formed by busulfan and its role in the cytotoxic effect. Cancer Sci 2004;95: 454–458.
36. Petersen FB, Sanders JE, Storb R, Bensinger WI, Clift RA, Buckner CD. Inadvertent administration of a greater-than-usual pre-marrow transplant dose of busulfan—report of a case. Transplantation 1988;45(4):821–822.
37. Fried W, Kede A, Barone J. Effects of cyclophosphamide and busulfan on spleen-colony-forming units and on hematopoietic stroma. Cancer Res 1977;37:1205.
38. Tutschka PJ, Copelan EA, Klein JP. Bone marrow transplantation for leukemia following a new busulfan and cyclophosphamide regimen. Blood 1987;70:1382.
39. Skinner WA, Gram HF, Greene MO, et al. Potential anticancer agents—XXXI. The relationship of chemical structure to antileukemic activity with analogues. J Med Pharmaceut Chem 1960;2:299.
40. Hyde KA, Acton E, Skinner WA, et al. Potential anticancer agents— LXII. The relationship of chemical structure to antileukemia activity with analogues of 1-methyl-3-nitro-1- nitrosoguanidine (NSC-9369), part II. J Med Pharmaceut Chem 1962;5:1.
41. Schabel FM Jr, Johnston TP, McCaleb GS, et al. Experimental evaluation of potential anticancer agents: VIII. Effects of certain

nitrosoureas on intracerebral L1210 leukemia. Cancer Res 1963; 23:226.

42. Carter SK, Newman JW. Nitrosoureas: 1,3-bis(2-chloroethyl)-1-nitrosourea (NSC-409962;BCNU) and 1-(2-chloroethyl)-3-cyclohexyl-1-nitrosourea (NSC-70937;CCNU)—clinical brochure. Cancer Chemother Rep 3 1968;1:115.

43. DeVita VT, Carbone PP, Owens AH Jr, et al. Clinical trials with 1,3-bis(2-chloroethyl)-1-nitrosourea, NSC-409962. Cancer Res 1965;25:1876.

44. Nissen NI, Pajak TF, Glidewell O, et al. A comparative study of a BCNU containing 4-drug program versus MOPP versus 3-drug combination in advanced Hodgkin's disease. Cancer 1979;43:31.

45. Schabel FM Jr. Nitrosoureas: a review of experimental antitumor activity. Cancer Treat Rep 1976;60:665.

46. Kohn KW, Spears CL, Doty P. Intra-strand crosslink of DNA by nitrogen mustard. J Mol Biol 1966;19:266.

47. Ludlum DB, Kramer BS, Wang J, et al . Reaction of 1,3- bis (2-chloroethyl)-1-nitrosourea with synthetic polynucleotides. Biochemistry 1975;14:5480.

48. Colvin M, Brundrett RB, Cowens JW, et al. A chemical basis for the antitumor activity of chloroethylnitrosoureas. Biochem Pharmacol 1976;25:695–699.

49. Bowdon BJ, Grimsley J, Lloyd HH. Interrelationships of some chemical , physicochemical, and biological activities of several 1-(2-haloethyl)-1-nitrosoureas. Cancer Res 1974;34:194.

50. Panasci LC, Green G, Nagourney R, et al. A structure-activity analysis of chemical and biological parameters of chloroethylnitrosoureas in mice. Cancer Res 1977;37:2615–2618.

51. Broder LE , Carter SK . Pancreatic islet cell carcinoma. Ann Intern Med 1973;79:108.

52. Moertel CG , Hanley JA , Johnson LA . treptozocin alone compared with streptozocin plus fluorouracil in the treatment of advanced islet-cell carcinoma. N Engl J Med 1980;303:1189.

53. Phillips GL, Wolff SN, Fay JW, et al. Intensive 1,3-bis (2-chloroethyl)-1-nitrosourea (BCNU) monochemotherapy and autologous marrow transplantation for malignant glioma. J Clin Oncol 1986;4:639-645.

54. Levin VA, Wilson CB. Nitrosourea pharmacodynamics in relation to the central nervous system. Cancer Treat Rep 1976; 60:725.

55. Eyre HJ, Eltingham JR, Gehan EA, et al. Randomized comparisons of radiotherapy and carmustine versus procarbazine versus decarbazine for the treatment of malignant gliomas following surgery: a Southwest Oncology Group Study. Cancer Treat Rep 1986;70:1085.

56. Hartley-Asp B, Gunnarsson PO, Liljekvist J. Cytotoxicity and metabolism of prednimustine, chlorambucil and prednisolone in a Chinese hamster cell line. Cancer Chemother Pharmacol 1986;16:85.

57. Bastholt L, Johansson C-J, Pfeiffer P, et al. A pharmacokinetic study of prednimustine as compared with prednisolone plus chlorambucil in cancer patients. Cancer Chemother Pharmacol 1991;28:205.

58. Tew KD. The mechanism of action of estramustine. Semin Oncol 1983;10:21.

59. Punzi J, Duax W, Strong P, et al. Molecular conformation of estramustine and two analogues. Mol Pharmacol 1992;41:569.

60. Edman K, Svensson L, Eriksson B, et al. Determination of estramustine phosphate and its metabolites estromustine, estramustine, estrone and estradiol in human plasma by liquid chromatography with florescence detection and gas chromatography with nitrogen-phosphorus and mass spectrometric detection. J Chromatogr B Biomed Sci Appl 2000;738(2):267.

61. Tew KD, Glusker JP, Hartley-Asp B, et al. Preclinical and clinical perspectives on the use of estramustine as an antimitotic drug. Pharmacol Ther 1993;56:323.

62. Gomori G. Histochemical demonstration of sites of phosphamidase activity. Proceedings of the Society for Experimental Biology & Medicine 1948;69;407–409.

63. Deonarain MP, Epenetos AA. Targeting enzymes for cancer therapy: old enzymes in new roles. Br J Cancer 1994;70:786.

64. Niculescu-Duvaz D, Niculescu-Duvaz I, Friedlow F, et al. Self-immolative nitrogen mustard prodrugs for suicide gene therapy. J Med Chem 1998;41:5297.

65. Chase M, Chung RY, Chiocca EA. An oncolytic viral mutant that delivers the CYP2B1 transgene and augments cyclophosphamide chemotherapy. Nat Biotechnol 1998;16:444.

66. Skipper HE, Bennett LL, Langham WH. Overall tracer studies with C^{14}-labeled nitrogen mustard in normal and leukemic mice. Cancer 1951;4:1025.

67. Coles B. Effects of modifying structure on electrophilic reactions with biological nucleophiles. Drug Metab Rev 1985;15:1307.

68. Magull-Seltenreich A, Zeller WJ. Inhibition of O6-alkylguanine-DNA alkyltransferase in animal and human ovarian tumor cell lines by O6-benzylguanine and sensitization to BCNU. Cancer Chemother Pharmacol 1995;35:262–266.

69. Shipp MA, Ross KN, Tamayo P, et al. Diffuse large B-cell lymphoma outcome prediction by gene-expression profiling and supervised machine learning.[comment]. Nature Medicine 2002; 8(1):68–74.

70. Osborne MR, Lawley PD. Alkylation of DNA by melphalan with special reference to adenine derivatives and adenine-guanine cross-linking. Chemicobiol Interact 1993;89:49–60.

71. Drysdale RB, Hopkins A, Thompson RY, et al. Some effects of nitrogen and sulphur mustards on the metabolism of nucleic acids in mammalian cells. Br J Cancer 1958;12:137.

72. Wheeler GP. Studies related to the mechanism of action of cytotoxic alkylating agents: a review. Cancer Res 1962;22:651.

73. Tomisek AJ, Simpson BT. Effect of in vivo cyclophosphamide treatment on the DNA-primary ability of DNA from Fortner plasmacytoma. Proc Am Assoc Cancer Res 1966;7:71.

74. Ruddon RW, Johnson JM. The effect of nitrogen mustard on DNA template activity in purified DNA and RNA polymerase systems. Mol Pharmacol 1968;4:258.

75. Wheeler GP, Alexander JA. Effects of nitrogen mustard and cyclophosphamide upon the synthesis of DNA in vivo and in cell-free preparation. Cancer Res 1969;29:98.

76. Roberts JJ, Brent TP, Crathorn AR. Evidence for the inactivation and repair of the mammalian DNA template after alkylation by mustard gas and half mustard gas. Eur J Cancer 1971;7:515.

77. Goldstein NO, Rutman RJ. The effect of alkylation on the in vitro thymidine-incorporating system of Lettré-Ehrlich cells. Cancer Res 1964;24:1363.

78. Bannon P, Verly W. Alkylation of phosphates and stability of phosphate triesters in DNA. Eur J Biochem 1972;31:103.

79. Lawley PD. Reaction of N-methyl-N-nitrosourea (MNUA) with P-labelled DNA: evidence for formation of phosphotriesters. Chem Biol Interact 1973;7:127.

80. Verly WG. Monofunctional alkylating agents and apurinic sites in DNA. Biochem Pharmacol 1974;23:3.

81. Loveless A. Possible relevance of O-6 alkylating of deoxyguanosine to the mutagenicity and carcinogenicity of nitrosamines and nitrosamides. Nature 1969;233:206.

82. Gerchman LL, Ludlum DB. The properties of O^6-methylguanine in templates for RNA polymerase. Biochim Biophys Acta 1973; 308:310.

83. Weinstein IB, Jeffrey AM, Jennette KW, et al. Benzo[a]pyrene diol epoxides as intermediates in nucleic acid binding in vitro and in vivo. Science 1976;195:592.

84. Brookes P, Lawley PD. The reaction of mono- and difunctional alkylating agents with nucleic acids. Biochem J 1961;80:486.

85. Silber JR, Blank A, Bobola MS, et al. O-6-methylguanine- DNA methyltransferase-deficient phenotype in human gliomas: frequency and time to tumor progression after alkylating agent-based chemotherapy. Clin Cancer Res 1999;5:807.

86. Brookes P, Lawley PD. The action of alkylating agents on deoxyribonucleic acid in relation to biological effects of the alkylating agents. Exp Cell Res 1963;9(Suppl):512.

87. Loveless A, Ross WCJ. Chromosome alteration and tumour inhibition by nitrogen mustards: the hypothesis of cross- linking alkylation. Nature 1950;166:113.

88. Geiduschek EP. "Reversible" DNA. Proc Natl Acad Sci U S A 1961; 47:950.

89. Kohn KW, Steigbiel NH, Spears CL. Cross-linking and repair of DNA in sensitive and resistant strains of E. coli treated with nitrogen mustard. Proc Natl Acad Sci U S A 1965;53:1154.

90. Lawley PD, Brookes P. Cytotoxicity of alkylating agents towards sensitive and resistant strains of *Escherichia coli* in relation to

extent and mode of alkylation of cellular macromolecules and repair of alkylation lesions in deoxyribonucleic acid. Biochem J 1968;109:433.

91. Venitt S. Interstrand cross-links in the DNA of *Escherichia coli* B/r and Bs-1 and their removal by the resistant strain. Biochem Biophys Res Commun 1968;31:355.

92. Kohn KW, Erickson LC, Ewig RAG, et al. Fractionation of DNA from mammalian cells by alkaline elution. Biochemistry 1976; 15:4629.

93. Ross WE, Ewig RAG, Kohn KW. Differences between melphalan and nitrogen mustard in the formation and removal of DNA cross-links. Cancer Res 1978;38:1502.

94. Thomas CB, Osieka R, Kohn KW. DNA cross-linking by in vivo treatment with 1-(2-chloroethyl)-3-(4-methylcyclohexyl)-1-nitrosourea of sensitive and resistant human colon carcinoma xenografts in nude mice. Cancer Res 1978;38:2448.

95. Erickson LC, Bradley MO, Ducore JM, et al. DNA cross-linking and cytotoxicity in normal and transformed human cells treated with antitumor nitrosourea. Proc Natl Acad Sci U S A 1980;77:467.

96. Garcia ST, McQuillan A, Panasci I. Correlation between the cytotoxicity of melphalan and DNA crosslink as detected by the ethidium bromide fluorescence assay in the F$_1$ variant of B16 melanoma cells. Biochem Pharmacol 1988;37:3189.

97. Ewig RAG, Kohn KW. DNA-protein crosslink and DNA interstrand crosslink by haloethylnitrosourea in L1210 cells. Cancer Res 1978;38:3197.

98. Rutman RJ, Steele WJ, Price CC. Experimental chemotherapy studies: I. Chemical and metabolic investigations of chloroquine mustard. Cancer Res 1961;21:1124.

99. Berenbaum MC. Histochemical evidence for crosslink of DNA by alkylating agents in vivo. Biochem Pharmacol 1962;11:1035.

100. Klatt P, Stehlin JS Jr, McBride C, et al. The effect of nitrogen mustard treatment on the DNA of sensitive and resistant Ehrlich tumor cells. Cancer Res 1969;29:286.

101. Esteller M, Garcia-Foncillas J, Andion E, et al. Inactivation of the DNA-repair gene MGMT and the clinical response of gliomas to alkylating agents.[comment][erratum appears in N Engl J Med 2000;343(23):1740]. N Engl J Med 2000;343(19):1350–1354.

102. Verly WG, Paquette Y. An endonuclease for depurinated DNA in *Escherichia coli* B. Cancer J Biochem 1972;50:217.

103. Hadi SM, Goldthwait DA. Endonuclease II of *Escherichia coli*: degradation of partially depurinated DNA. Biochemistry 1971; 10:4986.

104. Burnotte J, Verly WG. Crosslink of methylated DNA by moderate heating at neutral pH. Biochim Biophys Acta 1972;262:449.

105. Tew KD, Sudhakar S, Schein PS, et al. Binding of chlorozotocin and 1-(2-chloroethyl)-3-cyclohexyl-1-nitrosourea to chromatin and nucleosomal fractions of HeLa cells. Cancer Res 1978; 38:3371.

106. Lowe SW, Ruley HE, Jacks T, et al. P53-dependent apoptosis modulates the cytotoxicity of anticancer agents. Cell 1993; 74:957.

107. Morgan AS, Ciaccio PJ, Tew KD, Kauvar LM. Isozyme-specific glutathione S-transferase inhibitors potentiate drug sensitivity in cultured human tumor cell lines. Cancer Chemotherapy & Pharmacology 1996;37(4):363-370.

108. Wolpert MK, Ruddon RW. A study on the mechanisms of resistance to nitrogen mustard (HN2) in Ehrlich ascites tumor cells: comparison of uptake of HN$_2$.^{14}C into sensitive and resistant cells. Cancer Res 1969;29:873.

109. Goldenberg GJ, Vanstone CL. Transport carrier for nitrogen mustard in HN2-sensitive and -resistant L5178Y lymphoblasts. Clin Res 1969;17:665.

110. Goldenberg GJ, Lee M, Lam H-YP, et al. Evidence for carrier-mediated transport of melphalan by L5178Y lymphoblasts in vitro. Cancer Res 1977;37:755.

111. Vistica DT, Rabon A, Rabinowitz M. Effect of l-alpha-amino-gamma-guanidinobutyric acid on melphalan therapy of the L1210 murine leukemia. Cancer Lett 1979;6(6):345.

112. Begleiter A, Lam H-YP, Grover J, et al. Evidence for active transport of melphalan by two amino acid carriers in L5178Y lymphoblasts in vitro. Cancer Res 1979;39:353.

113. Vistica DT, Toal JN, Rabinowitz M. Amino acid conferred protection against melphalan: characterization of melphalan transport

114. Begleiter A, Lam H-YP, Goldenberg GJ, et al. Mechanism of uptake of nitrosourea by L5178Y lymphoblasts in vitro. Cancer Res 1977;37:1022.

115. Goldenberg GJ, Vanstone CL, Israels LG, et al. Evidence for a transport carrier of nitrogen mustard in nitrogen mustard-sensitive and -resistant L5178Y lymphoblasts. Cancer Res 1970; 30:2285.

116. Deves R, Boyd CA. Surface antigen CD98(4F2): not a single membrane protein, but a family of proteins with multiple functions [review]. J Membrane Biol 2000;173(3):165-177.

117. Harada N, Nagasaki A, Hata H, et al. Down-regulation of CD98 in melphalan-resistant myeloma cells with reduced drug uptake. Acta Haematol 2000;103(3):144–151.

118. Hirono I. Non-protein sulphydryl group in the original strain and subline of the ascites tumour resistant to alkylating reagents. Nature 1960;186:1059.

119. Calcutt G, Connors TA. Tumour sulphydryl levels and sensitivity to the nitrogen mustard Merophan. Biochem Pharmacol 1963; 12:839.

120. Hamilton TC, Winker MA, Lovie KG, et al. Augmentation of Adriamycin, melphalan and cisplatin cytotoxicity in drug-resistant and -sensitive human ovarian carcinoma cell lines by buthionine sulfoximine mediated glutathione depletion. Biochem Pharmacol 1985;34:2583.

121. Somfai-Relle S, Suzukake K, Vistica BP, et al. Reduction in cellular glutathione by buthionine sulfoximine and sensitization of murine tumor cells resistant to l-phenylalanine mustard. Biochem Pharmacol 1984;33:485.

122. Robson CN, Lewis AD, Wolf CR, et al. Reduced levels of drug-induced DNA crosslink in nitrogen mustard- resistant Chinese hamster ovary cells expressing elevated glutathione S-transferase activity. Cancer Res 1987;47:6022.

123. Sladek NE. Bioassay and relative cytotoxic potency of cyclophosphamide metabolites generated in vitro and in vivo. Cancer Res 1973;33:1150.

124. Connors TA, Cox PJ, Farmer PB, et al. Some studies of the active intermediate formed in the microsomal metabolism of cyclophosphamide and isophosphamide. Biochem Pharmacol 1974; 23:115.

125. Hilton J. Role of aldehyde dehydrogenase in cyclophosphamide-resistant L1210 leukemia. Cancer Res 1984;44:5156.

126. Crathorne AR, Roberts JJ. Mechanism of the cytotoxic action of alkylating agents in mammalian cells and evidence for the removal of alkylated groups from deoxyribonucleic acid. Nature 1966;211:150.

127. Petit C, Sancar A. Nucleotide excision repair: from e.coli to man. Biochimie 1999;81:15–25.

128. Cowan K, Batist G, Tulpule A, et al. Similar biochemical changes associated with multidrug resistance in human breast cancer cells and carcinogen-induced resistance in xenobiotics in rats. Proc Natl Acad Sci U S A 1986;83:9328.

129. Kirsch D, Kastan M. Tumor-suppressor p53: implications for tumor development and prognosis. J Clin Oncol 1998;16:3158.

130. Goldenberg GJ. The role of drug transport in resistance to nitrogen mustard and other alkylating agents in L5178Y lymphoblasts. Cancer Res 1975;35:687.

131. Schabel FM Jr, Trader MW, Laster WR Jr, et al. Patterns of resistance and therapeutic synergism among alkylating agents. Antibiot Chemother 1978;23:200.

132. Antman K, Eder JP, Elias A, et al. High-dose combination alkylating agent preparative regimen with autologous bone marrow support: the Dana-Farber Cancer Institute/Beth Israel Hospital experience. Cancer Treat Rep 1987;71:19.

133. Puri RN, Meister A. Transport of glutathione as γ-glutamylcysteinylglycyl ester, into liver and kidney. Proc Natl Acad Sci U S A 1983;80:5258.

134. Teicher BA, Crawford JM, Holden SA, et al. Glutathione monoethylester can selectively protect liver from high-dose BCNU or cyclophosphamide. Cancer 1988;62:1275.

135. Meister A. Glutathione deficiency produced by inhibition of its synthesis, and its reversal: applications in research and therapy. Pharmacol Ther 1991;51:155.

136. Sekura R, Meister A. Covalent interaction of l-2-amino-4- oxo-5-chlorpentanoate at the glutamate binding site of γ-glutamylcystein synthetase. J Biol Chem 1977;252:2600.

137. Griffith WO, Meister A. Differential inhibition of glutamine and γ-glutamylcysteine synthetase by alpha alkyl analogues of methionine sulfoximine that induce convulsions. J Biol Chem 1978;253:2333.

138. Campbell EB, Hayward ML, Griffith OW. Analytical and preparative separation of the diastereomers of l-buthionine (SR)-sulfoximine, a potent inhibitor of glutathione biosynthesis. Anal Biochem 1991;194:268.

139. Tew KD, Bomber AM, Hoffman SJ. Ethacrynic acid and piriprost as enhancers of cytotoxicity in drug-resistant and -sensitive cell lines. Cancer Res 1988;48:3622.

140. Bailey HH, Mulcahy RT, Tutsch KD, et al. Phase I clinical trial of intravenous L-buthionine sulfoximine and melphalan: an attempt at modulation of glutathione. J Clin Oncol 1994; 12:194–205.

141. O'Dwyer PJ, Hamilton TC, LaCreta FP, et al. Phase I trial of buthionine sulfoximine in combination with melphalan in patients with cancer. J Clin Oncol 1996;14:249–256.

142. Clapper ML, Hoffman SJ, Tew KD. Sensitization of human colon tumor xenografts to l-phenylalanine mustard using ethacrynic acid. J Cell Pharmacol 1990;1:71.

143. Johansson AS, Ridderstrom M, Mannervik B. The human glutathione transferase P1-1 specific inhibitor TER 117 designed for overcoming cytostatic-drug resistance is also a strong inhibitor of glyoxalase I. Molecular Pharmacology 2000;57(3): 619–624.

144. Morgan AS, Sanderson PE, Borch RF, et al. Tumor efficacy and bone marrow sparing properties of TER286, a cytotoxin activated by glutathione transferase. Cancer Res 1998;58:2568–2575.

145. Yuhas JM, Spellman JM, Culo F. The role of WR-2721 in radiotherapy and/or chemotherapy. Cancer Clin Trials 1980;3:211.

146. Capizzi RL, Scheffler BJ, Schein PS. Amifostine-mediated protection of normal bone marrow from cytotoxic chemotherapy [review]. Cancer 1993;72(11 Suppl):3495–3501.

147. Capizzi RL. The preclinical basis for broad-spectrum selective cytoprotection of normal tissues from cytotoxic therapies by amifostine [review]. Semin Oncol 1999;26(2 Suppl 7):3–21.

148. Glover D, Glick JH, Weiler C. WR2821 protects against the hematologic toxicity of cyclophosphamide: a controlled phase II trial. J Clin Oncol 1986;4:584.

149. Hospers GA, Eisenhauer EA, de Vries EG. The sulfhydryl containing compounds WR-2721 and glutathione as radio- and chemoprotective agents. A review, indications for use and prospects. Br J Cancer 1999;80:629.

150. Phillips GL. The potential of amifostine in high-dose chemotherapy and autologous hematopoietic stem cell transplantation [review]. Semin Oncol 2002;29(6 Suppl 19):53–56.

151. Dolan ME, Pegg AE. O6-Benzylguanine and its role in chemotherapy Clin Cancer Res 1997;8:837.

152. Quinn JA, Pluda J, Dolan ME, et al. Phase II trial of carmustine plus O6-benzylguanine for patients with nitrosourea-resistant, recurrent, or progressive malignant glioma. J Clin Oncol 2002; 20:2277–2283.

153. Esteller M, Herman JG. Generating mutations but providing chemosensitivity: the role of O6-methylguanine DNA methyltransferase in human cancer. Oncogene 2004;23:1–8.

154. Bartlett PD, Ross SD, Swain CG. Kinetics and mechanisms of the reactions of tertiary β-chloroethylamines in solution: III. β-Chloroethyldiethylamine and tris-β-chloroethylamine. J Am Chem Soc 1949;71:1415.

155. Chang SY, Alberts DS, Farquhar D, et al. Hydrolysis and protein binding of melphalan. J Pharm Sci 1978;67:682.

156. Alberts DS, Chang SY, Chen H-SG, et al. Comparative pharmacokinetics of chlorambucil and melphalan in man. Recent Results Cancer Res 1980;74:124.

157. Alberts DS, Chang SY, Chen H-SG, et al. Pharmacokinetics and metabolism of chlorambucil in man: a preliminary report. Cancer Treat Rev 1979;6 (Suppl):9.

158. McLean A, Woods RC, Catovsky D, et al. Pharmacokinetics and metabolism of chlorambucil in patients with malignant disease. Cancer Treat Rev 1979;6 (Suppl):33.

159. Everett JL, Roberts JJ, Ross WCJ. Aryl-2-halogenoalkylamines: XII. Some carboxylic derivatives of N, N-di-2-chloroethylaniline. J Chem Soc 1953;2386.

160. Arnold H, Bourseaux F, Brock N. Neuartige Krebs-Chemotherapeutika aus der Gruppe der zyklischen N-Lost-Phosphamidester. Naturwissenschaften 1958;45:64.

161. Foley GE, Friedman OM, Drolet BP. Studies on the mechanism of action of Cytoxan: I. Evidence of activation in vivo. Proc Am Assoc Cancer Res 1960;3:111.

162. Brock N, Hohorst H-J. Uber die Aktivierung von Cyclophosphamid in vivo und in vitro. Arzneimittelforschung 1963;13:1021.

163. Cohen JL, Jao JY. Enzymatic basis of cyclophosphamide activation by hepatic microsomes of the rat. J Pharmacol Exp Ther 1970;174–206.

164. Friedman OM, Myles A, Colvin M. Cyclophosphamide and related phosphoramide mustards: current status and future prospects. In: Rosowsky A, ed. Advances in Cancer Chemotherapy. New York: Marcel Dekker, 1979:159.

165. Chang TKH, Weber GF, Crespi CL, et al. Differential activation of cyclophosphamide and ifosfamide by cytochromes P450 2B and 3A in human liver microsomes. Cancer Res 1993;53:5629–5637.

166. Colvin M. A review of the pharmacology and clinical use of cyclophosphamide. In: Pinedo HM, ed. Clinical Pharmacology of Antineoplastic Drugs. Amsterdam: Elsevier, 1978:245.

167. Struck RF, Kirk MC, Mellett LB, et al. Urinary metabolites of the antitumor agent cyclophosphamide. Mol Pharmacol 1971;7:519.

168. Bakke JE, Feil WJ, Fjelstul CE, et al. Metabolism of cyclophosphamide by sheep. J Agric Food Chem 1972;20:384.

169. Colvin M, Padgett CA, Fenselau C. A biologically active metabolite of cyclophosphamide. Cancer Res 1973;33:915.

170. Maddock CL, Handler AH, Friedman OM, et al. Primary evaluation of alkylating agent cyclohexylamine salt of N, N- bis (2-chloroethyl)phosphorodiamidic acid (NSC-69945;OMF-59) in experimental antitumor assay systems. Cancer Chemother Rep 1966;50:629.

171. Hohorst H-J, Draeger A, Peter G, et al. The problem of oncostatic specificity of cyclophosphamide (NSC-27271): studies on reactions that control the alkylating and cytotoxic activity. Cancer Treat Rep 1976;60:309.

172. Brodsky RA, Sensenbrenner LL, Jones RJ. Complete remission in severe aplastic anemia after high-dose cyclophosphamide without bone marrow transplantation. Blood 1996;87(2):491–494.

173. Allen LM, Creaven PJ. In vitro activation of isophosphorine (NSC 109724), a new oxazaphosphorine, by rat-liver microsomes. Cancer Chemother Rep 1972;56:603.

174. Low JE, Borch RF, Sladek NE. Further studies on the conversion of 4-hydroxyoxaphosphorines to reactive mustards and acrolein in inorganic buffers. Cancer Res 1983;43:5815.

175. Colvin M. The comparative pharmacology of cyclophosphamide and ifosfamide. Semin Oncol 1982;9(Suppl 1):2.

176. Chen TL, Kennedy MG, Karaly SB, et al. Nonlinear pharmacokinetics of cyclophosphamide and 4-hydroxycyclophosphamide aldophosphamide in patients with metastatic breast cancer receiving high dose chemotherapy followed by autologous bone marrow transplantation. Drug Metab Dispos 1997;25:544.

177. D'Incalci M, Bolis G, Facchinetti T, et al. Decreased half- life of cyclophosphamide in patients under continual treatment. Eur J Cancer 1979;19:7.

178. Hill DL, Kirk MC, Struck RF. Microsomal metabolism of nitrosoureas. Cancer Res 1975;35:296.

179. Levin VA, Stearns J, Byrd A, et al. The effect of phenobarbital pretreatment on the antitumor activity of 1,3-bis (2-chloroethyl)-1-nitrosourea (BCNU), 1-(2-chloroethyl)-3-cyclohexyl-1-nitrosourea (CCNU) and 1-(2-chloroethyl)-3-(2,6-dioxo)-3-piperidyl-1-nitrosourea (PCNU), and on the plasma pharmacokinetics and biotransformation of BCNU. J Pharmacol Exp Ther 1979; 208:1.

180. May HE, Boose R, Reed DJ. Hydroxylation of the carcinostatic 1-(2-chloroethyl)-3-cyclohexyl-1-nitrosourea (CCNU) by rat liver microsomes. Biochem Biophys Res Commun 1974;57:426.

181. Hilton J, Walker MD. Hydroxylation of 1-(2-chloroethyl)-3- cyclohexyl-1-nitrosourea. Biochem Pharmacol 1975;24:2153.

182. Wheeler GP, Johnston TP, Bowdon BJ, et al. Comparison of the properties of metabolites of CCNU. Biochem Pharmacol 1977;26:2331.

183. Reed DJ, May HE. Cytochrome P-450 interactions with the 2-chloroethylnitrosoureas and procarbazine. Biochimie 1978;60:989.

184. Alberts DS, Chang SY, Chen H-SG, et al. Kinetics of intravenous melphalan. Clin Pharmacol Ther 1979;26:73.

185. Tricot G, Alberts DS, Johnson C, et al. Safety of autotransplants with high-dose melphalan in renal failure: a pharmacokinetic and toxicity study. Clin Cancer Res 1996;2:947-952.

186. Tattersall MHN, Weinberg A. Pharmacokinetics of melphalan following oral or intravenous administration in patients with malignant disease. Eur J Cancer 1978;14:507.

187. Sviland L, Robinson A, Proctor SJ, et al. Interaction of cimetidine with oral melphalan. A pharmacokinetic study. Cancer Chemother Pharmacol 1987;20:173.

188. Markman M. Melphalan and cytarabine administered intraperitoneally as single agents and combination intraperitoneal chemotherapy with cisplatin and cytarabine. Semin Oncol 1985;12:33–37.

189. Roberts MS, Wu ZY, Siebert GA, Anissimov YG, Thompson JF, Smithers BM. Pharmacokinetics and pharmacodynamics of melphalan in isolated limb infusion for recurrent localized limb malignancy. Melanoma Research 2001;11(4):423–431.

190. Juma FD, Rogers HJ, Trounce JR. Pharmacokinetics of cyclophosphamide and alkylating activity in man after intravenous and oral administration. Br J Clin Pharmacol 1979;8:209.

191. Jardine I, Fenselau C, Appler M, et al. Quantitation by gas chromatography–chemical ionization mass spectrometry of cyclophosphamide, phosphoramide mustard, and nornitrogen mustard in the plasma and urine of patients receiving cyclophosphamide therapy. Cancer Res 1978;38:408.

192. Erlichman C, Soldin SJ, Hardy RW, et al. Disposition of cyclophosphamide on two consecutive cycles of treatment in patients with ovarian carcinoma. Arzneimittelforschung 1988;38:839.

193. Moore MJ, Hardy RW, Thiessen JJ, et al. Rapid development of enhanced clearance after high-dose cyclophosphamide. Clin Pharmacol Ther 1988;44:622.

194. Egorin MJ, Forrest A, Belani CP, et al. A limited sampling strategy for cyclophosphamide pharmacokinetics. Cancer Res 1989;49:3129.

195. Sladak NE, Doeden D, Powers JF, et al. Plasma concentrations of 4-hydroxycyclophosphamide and phosphoramide mustard in patients repeatedly given high doses of cyclophosphamide in preparation for bone marrow transplantation. Cancer Treat Rep 1984;68:1247.

196. Struck RF, Alberts DS, Horne K, et al. Plasma pharmacokinetics of cyclophosphamide and its cytotoxic metabolites after intravenous versus oral administration in a randomized, crossover trial. Cancer Res 1987;47:2723.

197. Nieto Y, Xu X, Cagnoni PJ, et al. Nonpredictable pharmacokinetic behavior of high-dose cyclophosphamide in combination with cisplatin and 1,3-bis(2-chloroethyl)-1-nitrosourea.[see comment]. Clin Cancer Res 1999;5(4):747–751.

198. Brock N, Gross R, Hohorst H-J, et al. Activation of cyclophosphamide in man and animals. Cancer 1971;27:1512.

199. Bagley CM Jr, Bostick FW, DeVita VT Jr. Clinical pharmacology of cyclophosphamide. Cancer Res 1973;33:226.

200. Phillipou G, Seaborn CJ, Raniolo E. Reproducibility of methods relating to cyclophosphamide metabolic structures. J Natl Cancer Inst 1993;85:1249.

201. Juma FD, Rogers HJ, Trounce JR. The pharmacokinetics of cyclophosphamide, phosphoramide mustard and nor-nitrogen mustard studied by gas chromatography in patients receiving cyclophosphamide therapy. Br J Clin Pharmacol 1980;10:327.

202. Fenselau C, Kan M-NN, Subba Rao S, et al. Identification of aldophosphamide as a metabolite of cyclophosphamide in vitro and in vivo in humans. Cancer Res 1977;37:2538.

203. Wagner T, Peter G, Voelcker G, et al. Characterization and quantitative estimation of activated cyclophosphamide in blood and urine. Cancer Res 1977;37:2592.

204. Wagner T, Heydrich D, Voelcker G, et al. Characterization and quantitative estimation of activated cyclophosphamide in blood and urine. Cancer Res Clin Oncol 1980;96:79.

205. Graham MI, Shaw IC, Souhami RL, et al. Decreased plasma half-life of cyclophosphamide during repeated high-dose administration. Cancer Chemother Pharmacol 1983;10:192.

206. Field RB, Gang M, Kline I, et al. The effect of phenobarbital or 2-diethylaminoethyl-2,2-diphenylvalerate on the activation of cyclophosphamide in vivo. J Pharmacol Exp Ther 1972;180:475.

207. Jao JY, Jusko WJ, Cohen JL. Phenobarbital effects on cyclophosphamide pharmacokinetics in man. Cancer Res 1972;32:2761.

208. Egorin M, Kaplan R, Salcman M, et al. Plasma and cerebrospinal fluid (CSF) pharmacokinetics of cyclophosphamide (CYC) in patients treated with and without dimethyl sulfoxide (DMSO). Proc Am Assoc Cancer Res 1981;22:210.

209. Alberts DS, van Daalen Wetters T. The effects of phenobarbital on cyclophosphamide antitumor activity. Cancer Res 1976;36:2785.

210. Sladek N. Therapeutic efficacy of cyclophosphamide as a function of its metabolism. Cancer Res 1972;32:535.

211. Mouridsen HT, Jacobson E. Pharmacokinetics of cyclophosphamide in renal failure. Acta Pharmacol Toxicol 1975;36:409.

212. Haubitz M, Bohnenstengel F, Brunkhorst R, et al. Cyclophosphamide pharmacokinetics and dose requirements in patients with renal insufficiency. Kidney Int 2002;61(4):1495-1501.

213. Creaven PJ, Allen LM, Alford DA, et al. Clinical pharmacology of isophosphamide. Clin Pharmacol Ther 1974;16:77.

214. Allen LM, Creaven PJ. Pharmacokinetics of ifosfamide. Clin Pharmacol Ther 1975;17:492.

215. Nelson RL, Allen LM, Creaven PJ. Pharmacokinetics of divided-dose ifosfamide. Clin Pharmacol Ther 1976;19:365.

216. Brade WP, Herdrich K, Varini M. Ifosfamide—pharmacology, safety and therapeutic potential. Cancer Treat Rev 1985;12:1.

217. Boddy AV, Cole M, Pearson ADJ, et al. The kinetics of the auto-induction of ifosfamide metabolism during continuous infusion. Cancer Chemother Pharmacol 1995;36:53.

218. Norpoth K. Studies on the metabolism of isophosphamide (NSC-109724) in man. Cancer Treat Rep 1976;60:437.

219. Cohen BE, Egorin ME, Kohlhepp EA, et al. Human plasma pharmacokinetics and urinary excretion of thiotepa and its metabolites. Cancer Treat Rep 1986;70:859.

220. Heideman RL, Cole DE, Balis F, et al. Phase I and pharmacokinetic evaluation of thiotepa in the cerebrospinal fluid and plasma of pediatric patients: evidence for dose-dependent plasma clearance of thiotepa. Cancer Res 1989;49:736.

221. Hogan B. Pharmacokinetics of thiotepa and tepa in the conventional dose-range and its correlation to myelosuppressive effects. Cancer Chemother Pharmacol 1991;27:373.

222. O'Dwyer PJ, LaCreta F, Engstrom PF, et al. Phase I/pharmacokinetic reevaluation of thiotepa. Cancer Res 1991;51:3171.

223. Kletzel M, Kearns GL, Thompson HC Jr. Pharmacokinetics of high-dose thiotepa in children undergoing autologous bone marrow transplantation. Bone Marrow Transplant 1992;10:171.

224. O'Dwyer PJ, LaCreta F, Schilder R, et al. Phase I trial of thiotepa in combination with recombinant human granulocyte-macrophage colony-stimulating factor. J Clin Oncol 1992;10:1352.

225. Levin VA, Hoffman W, Weinkam RJ. Pharmacokinetics of BCNU in man: a preliminary study of 20 patients. Cancer Treat Rep 1978;62:1305.

226. Henner WD, Peters WP, Eder JP, et al. Pharmacokinetics and immediate effects of high-dose carmustine in man. Cancer Treat Rep 1986;70:877.

227. Jones RB, et al. Nitrosoureas. In: Grochow LB, Ames MM, ed. A Clinician's Guide To Chemotherapy Pharmacokinetics and Pharmacodynamics. Baltimore: Williams & Wilkins, 1998:331.

228. Hassan M, Ehrsson H. Urinary metabolites of busulfan in the rat. Drug Metab Dispos 1987;15:399.

229. Hassan M, Öberg G, Ehrsson H, et al. Pharmacokinetic and metabolic studies of high-dose busulphan in adults. Eur J Clin Pharmacol 1989;36:525.

230. Chen T-L, Grochow LB, Hurowitz LA, et al. Determination of busulfan in human plasma by gas chromatography with electron-capture detection. J Chromatogr 1988;425:303.

231. Grochow LB, Jones RJ, Brundrett RB, et al. Pharmacokinetics of busulfan: correlation with veno-occlusive disease in patients

undergoing bone marrow transplantation. Cancer Chemother Pharmacol 1989;25:55.

232. Vassal G, Fischer A, Challine D, et al. Busulfan disposition below the age of three: alteration in children with lysosomal storage disease. Blood 1993;82:1030.

233. Andersson BS, Madden T, Tran HT, et al. Acute safety and pharmacokinetics of intravenous busulfan when used with oral busulfan and cyclophosphamide as pretransplantation conditioning therapy: a phase I study. Biol Blood Marrow Transplant 2000;6(5A):548-554.

234. Peters WP, Henner WD, Grochow LB, et al. Clinical and pharmacologic effects of high-dose single-agent busulfan with autologous bone marrow support in the treatment of solid tumors. Cancer Res 1987;47:6402.

235. Grochow LB, Piantadosi S, Santos G, et al. Busulfan dose adjustment decreases the risk of venooclusive disease in patients undergoing bone marrow transplantation. Proc Am Assoc Cancer Res 1992;33:200.

236. Kashyap A, Wingard J, Cagnoni P, et al. Intravenous versus oral busulfan as part of a busulfan/cyclophosphamide preparative regimen for allogeneic hematopoietic stem cell transplantation: decreased incidence of hepatic venoocclusive disease (HVOD), HVOD-related mortality, and overall 100-day mortality [comment]. Biol Blood Marrow Transplant 2002;8(9):493-500.

237. Grochow LB, Krivit W, Whitley CB, et al. Busulfan disposition in children. Blood 1990;75:1723.

238. Hassan M, Ehrsson H, Smedmyr B, et al. Cerebrospinal fluid and plasma concentrations of busulfan during high-dose therapy. Bone Marrow Transplant 1989;4:113.

239. Hassan M, Thorell J-O, Warne N, et al. ^{11}C-labeling of busulphan. Appl Radiat Isot 1991;42:1055.

240. Grigg AP, Shepherd JD, Phillips GL. Busulphan and phenytoin. Ann Intern Med 1989;111:1049.

241. Andersson BS, Thall PF, Madden T, et al. Busulfan systemic exposure relative to regimen-related toxicity and acute graft-versus-host disease: defining a therapeutic window for i.v. BuCy2 in chronic myelogenous leukemia [comment]. Biol Blood Marrow Transplant 2002;8(9):477-485.

242. Slattery JT, Clift RA, Buckner CD, et al. Marrow transplantation for chronic myeloid leukemia: the influence of plasma busulfan levels on the outcome of transplantation. Blood 1997;89:3055-3060.

243. Slattery JT, Sanders JE, Buckner CD, et al. Graft-rejection and toxicity following bone marrow transplantation in relation to busulfan pharmacokinetics [published erratum appears in Bone Marrow Transplant 1995;16:31-42.

244. Elson LA, Elson LA. Hematological effects of the alkylating agents. Ann N Y Acad Sci 1958;68:826.

245. Botnick LE, Hannon EC, Hellman S. Multisystem stem cell failure after apparent recovery from alkylating agents. Cancer Res 1978;38:1942.

246. Scrobohaci ML, Drouet L, Monem-Mansi A, et al. Liver venoocclusive disease after bone marrow transplantation changes in coagulation parameters and endothelial markers [see comments]. Thromb Res 1991;63(5):509–519.

247. Aronin PA, Mahaley MSJ, Rudnick SA, et al. Prediction of BCNU pulmonary toxicity in patients with malignant gliomas: an assessment of risk factors. N Engl J Med 1980;303:183–188.

248. Burn WA, McFarland W, Matthews MJ. Busulfan-induced pulmonary disease. Am Rev Respir Dis 1970;101:408.

249. Willson JKV. Pulmonary toxicity of antineoplastic drugs. Cancer Treat Rep 1978;62:2003.

250. Cao T.M., Negrin R.S., Stockerl-Goldstein K., et al. Pulmonary toxicity syndrome in breast cancer patients undergoing BCNU-containing high-dose chemotherapy and autologous hematopoietic cell transplantation. Biol Blood Marrow Transplant 2000; 6:387–394.

251. Jones RB, Matthes S, Shpall EJ, et al. BCNU plasma exposure (AUC) correlates with the risk of non- infectious pulmonary injury following cyclophosphamide, cisplatin and BCNU with autologous marrow support. Proc Am Soc Clin Oncol 1992; 11:349.

252. Philips FS, Sternberg SS, Cronin AP, et al. Cyclophosphamide and urinary bladder toxicity. Cancer Res 1961;21:1577.

253. Forni AM, Koss LG, Geller W. Cytological study of the effect of cyclophosphamide on the epithelium of the urinary bladder in man. Cancer 1964;17:1348.

254. Rubin JS, Rubin RT. Cyclophosphamide hemorrhagic cystitis. J Urol 1966;96:313.

255. Bellin HJ, Cherry JM, Koss LG. Effects of a single dose of cyclophosphamide: V. Protection effect of diversion of the urinary stream on dog bladder. Lab Invest 1974;30:43.

256. Arthur RR, Shah KV, Baust SJ, et al. Association of BK viruria with hemorrhagic cystitis in recipients of bone marrow transplants. New Engl J Med 196;315:230–234.

257. Andriole GL, Sandlund JT, Miser JS, et al. The efficacy of Mesna (2-mercaptoethane sodium sulfonate) as a uroprotectant in patients with hemorrhagic cystitis receiving further oxazaphosphorine chemotherapy. J Clin Oncol 1987;5:799.

258. Botta JA Jr, Nelson LW, Weikel JN Jr. Acetylcysteine in the prevention of cyclophosphamide-induced cystitis in rats. J Natl Cancer Inst 1973;51:1051.

259. Kline I, Gang M, Venditti JM. Protection with N-acetylcysteine (NAC) against isophosphamide (ISOPH, NSC- 10924) host toxicity and enhancement of therapy in early murine leukemia L1210. Proc Am Assoc Cancer Res 1972;13:29.

260. Manohoran A. Carcinoma of the urinary bladder in patients receiving cyclophosphamide. Aust N Z J Med 1984;14:507.

261. DeFronzo RA, Abeloff M, Braine H, et al. Renal dysfunction after treatment with isophosphamide (NSC-109724). Cancer Chemother Rep 1974;58(3):375.

262. Moncrieff M, Foot A. Fanconi syndrome after ifosfamide. Cancer Chemother Pharmacol 1989;23:121.

263. DeFronzo RA, Braine HG, Colvin M, et al. Water intoxication in man after cyclophosphamide therapy. Ann Intern Med 1973; 78:861.

264. Silver HKB, Morton DL. CCNU nephrotoxicity following sustained remission in oat cell carcinoma. Cancer Treat Rep 1979;63:226.

265. Schacht RG, Baldwin DS. Chronic interstitial nephritis and renal failure due to nitrosourea (NU) therapy. Kidney Int 1978;14:661.

266. Harmon WE, Cohen HJ, Schneeberger EE, et al. Chronic renal failure in children treated with methyl CCNU. N Engl J Med 1979;300:1200.

267. Peters WP, Stuart A, Klotman M, et al. High dose combination cyclophosphamide, cisplatin and melphalan with autologous bone marrow support: a clinical and pharmacologic study. Cancer Chemo Pharmacol 1989;23:377–383.

268. Spitz S. The histological effects of nitrogen mustards on human tumors and tissues. Cancer 1948;1:383.

269. DeRooij DG, Kramer MR. The effects of three alkylating agents on the seminiferous epithelium of rodents. Virchows Arch (Zellpathol) 1969;4:267.

270. Richter P, Calamera JC, Morgenfeld MC, et al. Effect of chlorambucil on spermatogenesis in the human with malignant lymphoma. Cancer 1970;25:1026.

271. Miller DG. Alkylating agents and human spermatogenesis. JAMA 1971;217:1662.

272. Hinkes E, Plotkin D. Reversible drug-induced sterility in a patient with acute leukemia. JAMA 1973;223:1490.

273. Blake DA, Heller RH, Hsu SH, et al. Return of fertility in a patient with cyclophosphamide-induced azoospermia. Johns Hopkins Med J 1976;139:20.

274. Galton DAG, Till M, Wiltshaw E. Busulfan (1,4-dimethylsulfonoxy-butane, Myleran): summary of clinical results. Ann N Y Acad Sci 1958;68:967.

275. Kumar R, Biggart JD, McEvoy J, et al. Cyclophosphamide and reproductive function. Lancet 1972;1:1212.

276. Sherins RJ, DeVita VT. Effect of drug treatment for lymphoma on male reproductive capacity. Ann Intern Med 1973;79:216.

277. Miller JJ, Williams GF, Leissring JC. Multiple late complications of therapy with cyclophosphamide, including ovarian destruction. Am J Med 1971;50:530.

278. Fosdick WM, Parson JL, Hill DF. Long-term cyclophosphamide therapy in rheumatoid arthritis. Arthritis Rheum 1968;11:151.

279. Haskin D. Some effects of nitrogen mustard on the development of external body form in the fetal rat. Anat Rec 1948;102:493.

280. Bodenstein D. The effects of nitrogen mustard on embryonic amphibian development. J Exp Zool 1948;108:93.

281. Bodenstein D, Goldin A. A comparison of the effects of various nitrogen mustard compounds on embryonic cells. J Exp Zool 1948;108:75.

282. Murphy ML, Karnofsky DA. Effect of azaserine and other growth-inhibiting agents on fetal development of the rat. Cancer 1956; 9:955.

283. Murphy ML, Del Moro A, Lacon C. The comparative effects of five poly-functional alkylating agents on the rat fetus, with additional notes. Ann N Y Acad Sci 1958;68:762.

284. Klein NW, Vogler MA, Chatot CL, et al. The use of cultured rat embryos to evaluate the teratogenic activity of serum: cadmium and cyclophosphamide. Teratology 1958;21:199.

285. Gibson JE, Becker BA. Teratogenicity of structural truncates of cyclophosphamide in mice. Teratology 1971;4:141.

286. Sadler TW, Kochhar DM. Chlorambucil-induced cell death in embryonic mouse limb buds. Toxicol Appl Pharmacol 1976; 37:237.

287. Brummett ES, Johnson EM. Morphological alterations in the developing fetal rat limb due to maternal injection of chlorambucil. Teratology 1979;20:279.

288. Nicholson HO. Cytotoxic drugs in pregnancy. J Obstet Gynaecol Br Commonw 1968;75:307.

289. Steege JF, Caldwell DS. Renal agenesis after first trimester exposure to chlorambucil. South Med J 1980;73:1414.

290. Toledo TM, Harper RC, Moser RH. Fetal effects during cyclophosphamide and irradiation therapy. Ann Intern Med 1971;74:87.

291. Garrett MJ. Teratogenic effects of combination chemotherapy. Ann Intern Med 1974;80:667.

292. Ortega J. Multiple agent chemotherapy including bleomycin of non-Hodgkin's lymphoma during pregnancy. Cancer 1977;40: 2829.

293. Lergier JE, Jiminez E, Maldonado N, et al. Normal pregnancy in multiple myeloma treated with cyclophosphamide. Cancer 1974;34:1018.

294. Rosner F, Grunwald H. Multiple myeloma terminating in acute leukemia. Am J Med 1974;57:927.

295. Einhorn N. Acute leukemia after chemotherapy (melphalan). Cancer 1978;41:444.

296. Rosner F, Grunwald H. Hodgkin's disease and acute leukemia. Am J Med 1975;58:339.

297. Seiidenfeld AM, Smythe HA, Ogryzlo MA, et al. Acute leukemia in rheumatoid arthritis treated with cytotoxic agents. J Rheumatol 1976;3:295.

298. Hochberg MC, Shulman LE. Acute leukemia following cyclophosphamide therapy for Sjögren's syndrome. Johns Hopkins Med J 1978;142:211.

299. Steigbigel RT, Kim H, Potolsky A, et al. Acute myeloproliferative disorder following long-term chlorambucil therapy. Arch Intern Med 1974;134:728.

300. Cardamone JM, Kimmerle RI, Marshall EY. Development of acute erythroleukemia in B-cell immunoproliferative disorders after prolonged therapy with alkylating drugs. Am J Med 1974; 57:837.

301. Cohen RJ, Wiernik PH, Walker MD. Acute nonlymphocytic leukemia associated with nitrosourea chemotherapy: report of two cases. Cancer Treat Rep 1976;60:1257.

302. Reimer RR, Hoover R, Fraumeni JF Jr, et al. Acute leukemia after alkylating-agent therapy of ovarian cancer. N Engl J Med 1977; 297:177.

303. Tucker MA, Coleman CN, Cox RS, et al. Risk of second cancers after treatment for Hodgkin's disease. N Engl J Med 1988;318:76.

304. Penn I. Second malignant neoplasms associated with immunosuppressive medications. Cancer 1976;37:1024.

305. Lazarus HM, Herzig RH, Graham-Pole J, et al. Intensive melphalan chemotherapy and cryopreserved autologous bone marrow transplantation for the treatment of refractory cancer. J Clin Oncol 1983;1:359.

306. Leff RS, Thompson JM, Mosley KR, et al. Phase II trial of high-dose melphalan and autologous bone marrow transplantation for metastatic colon carcinoma. J Clin Oncol 1986;4:1586.

307. Takvorian T, Canellos GP, Ritz J, et al. Prolonged disease-free survival after autologous bone marrow transplantation in patients with non-Hodgkin's lymphoma with a poor prognosis. N Engl J Med 1987;316:1499.

308. Morgan M, Dodds A, Atkinson K, et al. The toxicity of busulfan and cyclophosphamide as the preparative regimen for bone marrow transplantation. Br J Haematol 1990;77:529.

309. McElwain TJ, Hedley DW, Gordon MY, et al. High dose melphalan and non-cryopressed autologous bone marrow treatment of malignant melanoma and neuroblastoma. Exp Hematol 1979;7 (Suppl 5):360.

310. Rollins BJ. Hepatic venoocclusive disease. Am J Med 1988; 81:297.

311. Phillips GL, Fay JW, Wolff SN, et al. 1,3-Bis (2-chloroethyl)-1-nitrosourea (BCNU) and autologous bone marrow transplantation (BMTX) for refractory malignancy. Proc Am Assoc Cancer Res 1980;21:180.

312. Takvorian T, Parker LM, Hochberg FH, et al. Single high dose of BCNU with autologous bone marrow (ABM). Proc Am Soc Clin Oncol 1980;21:341.

313. Steinberg SS, Philips FS, Scholler J. Pharmacological and pathological effects of alkylating agents. Ann N Y Acad Sci 1958;68:811.

314. Goren MP, Right RK, Pratt CB, et al. Dechlorethylation of ifosfamide and neurotoxicity. Lancet 1986;2:1219.

315. Thigpen T. Ifosfamide-induced central nervous system toxicity [editorial]. Gynecol Oncol 1991;42:191.

316. Colvin M, Santos GW. High dose cyclophosphamide administration in man. Proc Am Assoc Cancer Res 1970;11:17.

317. Buckner CD, Rudolph RJ, Fefer A, et al. High dose cyclophosphamide therapy for malignant disease. Cancer 1972;29:357.

318. Steinherz LJ, Steinherz PG. Cyclophosphamide cardiotoxicity. Cancer Bull 1985;37:231.

319. Slavin RE, Millan JC, Mullins GM. Pathology of high dose intermittent cyclophosphamide therapy. Hum Pathol 1975;6:693.

320. Makinodan T, Santos GW, Quinn RP. Immunosuppressive drugs. Pharmacol Rev 1970;22:189.

321. Berenbaum CC, Brown IN. Dose-response relationships for agents inhibiting the immune response. Immunology 1964; 7:65.

322. Santos GW, Owens AH Jr. 19S and 7S antibody production in the cyclophosphamide- or methotrexate-treated rat. Nature 1966; 209:622.

323. Owens AH Jr, Santos GW. The effect of cytotoxic drugs on graft-versus-host disease in mice. Transplantation 1971;11:378.

324. Many A, Schwartz RS. On the mechanisms of immunological tolerance in cyclophosphamide-treated mice. Clin Exp Immunol 1970;6:87.

325. Larman SP, Weidanz WO. The effect of cyclophosphamide on the ontogeny of the humoral immune response in chickens. J Immunol 1970;105:614.

326. Turk JL, Paulter LW. Selective depletion of lymphoid tissue by cyclophosphamide. Clin Exp Immunol 1972;10:285.

327. Turk JL. Studies on the mechanism of action of methotrexate and cyclophosphamide on contact sensitivity in the guinea pig. Int Arch Allergy 1964;24:191.

328. Maguire HC, Ettore VL. Enhancement of dinitrochlorobenzene (DNCB) contact sensitization by cyclophosphamide in the guinea pig. J Invest Dermatol 1967;48:39.

329. Stevenson HC, Fauci AS. XII. Differential effects of in vitro cyclophosphamide on human lymphocyte subpopulations involved in B-cell activation. Immunology 1980;39:391.

330. Shand FL, Howard JG. Cyclophosphamide inhibited B-cell receptor regeneration as a basis for drug-induced tolerance. Nature 1978;271:255.

331. Ozer H, Cowens JW, Nussbaum A, et al. Human immunoregulatory T subset function defined in vitro by cyclophosphamide metabolites. Fed Proc 1981;40:1075.

332. Mullins GM, Anderson PN, Santos GW. High dose cyclophosphamide therapy in solid tumors. Cancer 1975;36:1950.

333. Santos GW. Immunological toxicity of cancer chemotherapy. Recent Results Cancer Res 1974;49:20.

334. Santos GW, Sensenbrenner LL, Anderson PN, et al. HL-A- identical marrow transplants in aplastic anemia, acute leukemia, and lymphosarcoma employing cyclophosphamide. Transplant Proc 1976;8:607.

335. Starzl TE, Groth CG, Putman CW, et al. Cyclophosphamide for clinical renal and hepatic transplantation. Transplant Proc 1973; 5:511.

336. Osborne EO, Jordon JW, Hoak FC, et al. Nitrogen mustard therapy in cutaneous blastomatous disease. JAMA 1947;135:1123.
337. Reza MJ, Dornfield L, Goldberg LS, et al. Long-term follow-up of patients treated with cyclophosphamide. Arthritis Rheum 1975;18:501.
338. Cooperating Clinics Committee of the American Rheumatism Association. A controlled trial of cyclophosphamide in rheumatoid arthritis. N Engl J Med 1970;283:883.
339. Townes AS, Sowa JM, Schulman LE, et al. Controlled trial of cyclophosphamide in rheumatoid arthritis (RA): an 11-month double-blind crossover study. Arthritis Rheum 1972;15:129.
340. Laros RK Jr, Penner JA. "Refractory" thrombocytopenic purpura treated successfully with cyclophosphamide. JAMA 1971;215:445.
341. Weinerman B, Maxwell I, Hryniuk W. Intermittent cyclophosphamide treatment of autoimmune thrombocytopenia. Can Med Assoc J 1974;111:1100.
342. Barratt TM, Soothill JF. Controlled trial of cyclophosphamide in steroid-sensitive relapsing nephrotic syndrome of childhood. Lancet 1970;2:279.

Nonclassic Agents

13

Henry S. Friedman   Steven D. Averbuch
Joanne Kurtzberg

Classic alkylating agents, such as the prototype nitrogen-mustard compounds, typically contain a chloroethyl group, and their biologic activity results from polyfunctional alkylation of biologic macromolecules (see Chapter 12, "Clinical and High-Dose Alkylating Agents"). Compounds with diverse chemical structures are also capable of covalent binding to biologic macromolecules, and they also have important clinical activity. These compounds, referred to as the *nonclassic alkylating agents*, include procarbazine (PCB), dacarbazine (DTIC), and temozolomide (TMZ).

Although these agents lack bifunctionality, as Newell and coworkers[1] point out, they share a common structural feature, an *N*-methyl group, which is important for activity. These agents are essentially prodrugs and must undergo complex metabolic transformation to active intermediates; their precise cellular mechanisms of action and clinical pharmacology are not completely understood, but they are clinically useful, and indeed, PCB and DTIC are part of curative regimens for lymphomas. Additionally, TMZ was recently approved for treatment of patients with recurrent anaplastic astrocytoma in 1999, the first new agent approved for malignant gliomas in more than 30 years.

PROCARBAZINE

PCB was synthesized as part of an effort to develop new monoamine-oxidase inhibitors at the Hoffman-LaRoche Laboratories,[2] and it was found to have antitumor activity in rodent preclinical testing.[3,4] Early clinical trials demonstrated significant efficacy for PCB in the treatment of Hodgkin's disease and lymphomas, with little activity against solid tumors.[5–9] PCB has been used widely in combination with other agents in the treatment of Hodgkin's and non-Hodgkin's lymphomas,[10–13] and, to a lesser extent, in small cell lung carcinoma[14–16] and melanoma.[17,18] Building on earlier experience with the treatment of brain

tumors,[19–21] trials have demonstrated considerable activity against high-grade glioma.[22–24] Nevertheless, there is still little known about PCB's cellular mechanism of action, and information regarding its clinical pharmacology is incomplete.

Mechanism of Action and Cellular Pharmacology

PCB, a prodrug, must undergo metabolism to active species. It enters cells by passive diffusion and thereafter is rapidly converted to cytotoxic metabolites by several possible routes.[25–39] Although selected tumor cells may contain cytosolic enzymes capable of activating PCB,[29] the parent drug is weakly cytotoxic for most tumor cell lines in culture, and its activity is markedly enhanced by allowing chemical decomposition of the drug[25] or cocultivation of tumor cells with rat hepatocytes.[31] However, it is not clear that the cytotoxic species generated by in vitro incubation with hepatic microsomes or intact hepatocytes is the same as that produced in humans.

As indicated in Figure 13.1, potential pathways of activation include chemical decomposition (I) as well as microsomal oxidation (II–V). The active end products have not been identified with certainty; they may be diazonium ions (R—N$^+$ N), methyl or *N*-isopropylbenzamide free radicals, or other species capable of covalently binding to DNA.[40–43] Although most evidence favors a cytotoxic pathway involving the production of methyl or benzylazoxy intermediates by liver cytochrome P-450, with release of these metabolites into plasma and their subsequent uptake and further decomposition to diazonium ions in situ, free-radical species (either a methyl radical or an isopropylbenzylamide radical) can be generated by pathways II and V in the presence of rat liver cytochrome P-450.[44] Thus, it is not clear which of the several putative and positively identified metabolites are responsible for cytotoxicity. The metabolic pathways will be

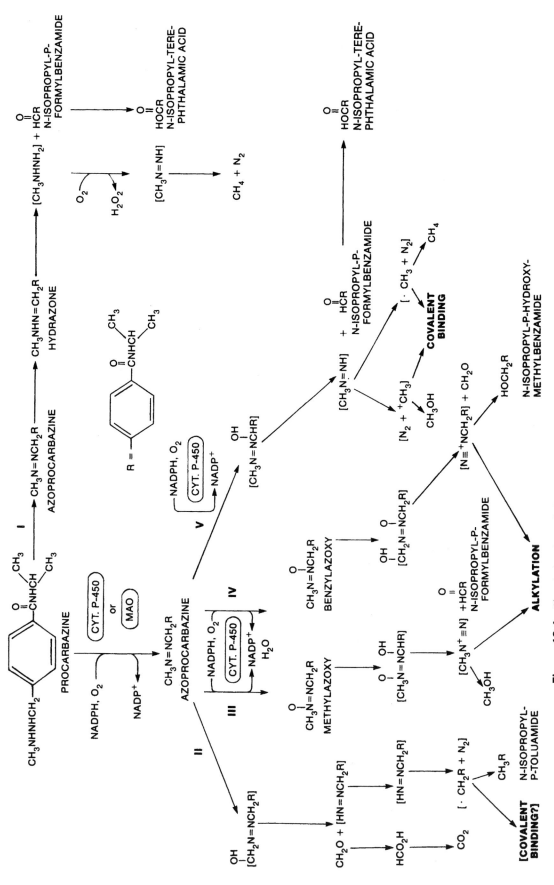

Figure 13.1 Chemical and metabolic reactions of procarbazine, leading to the generation of reactive intermediates. I, Chemical breakdown of procarbazine in aqueous solution; II, III, IV, and V, proposed metabolic activation pathways in vivo. Intermediates not identified in vivo or in vitro are indicated by brackets. See text for detailed description. CYT, cytochrome; MAO, monoamine oxidase; NADP, nicotinamide adenine dinucleotide; NADPH, nicotinamide adenine dinucleotide phosphate.

considered again with respect to PCB pharmacokinetics in humans in a later section, "Clinical Pharmacology."

Several additional cellular effects of PCB and its metabolites have been demonstrated, although it is unclear whether these contribute directly to cytotoxicity. Hydrogen peroxide and formaldehyde are two potentially toxic products generated from PCB and are thought to cause cytotoxicity by interaction with DNA.[45] However, the data demonstrating azo-PCB activity in the absence of hydrogen peroxide generation strongly argue against a role for this toxic byproduct in the cytotoxic activity of PCB.[25,46] Earlier reports and more recent studies using alkaline elution techniques have demonstrated that PCB and its metabolites are capable of causing chromatid and single-strand DNA breaks in murine tumor cells in vitro.[29,47–49] The number of breaks depends on the dosage and time elapsed after treatment, and it has been suggested that the breaks occur during, or soon after, DNA synthesis.[50] Because the percentage of cells undergoing mitosis is also diminished as a function of dosage and time after PCB,[48] it is likely that the most susceptible phase in the cell cycle may be the premitotic G_2 phase. However, this has not been confirmed using current technology, such as cell sorting by flow cytometry. In addition, a G_2 block may simply indicate the physiologic response of cells to DNA injury. Chromatid translocations (sister chromatid exchange) are also observed in murine tumor cells in vivo after PCB treatment, although this effect is not observed in vitro after PCB.[47,48] Again, this result suggests that differences exist in the toxic metabolites generated in vitro versus in vivo. A recent report suggests that procarbazine causes DNA damage through nonenzymatic formation of a Cu(I)-hydroperoxy complex and methyl radicals.[51]

In addition to these effects on nuclear DNA, PCB can inhibit DNA, RNA, and protein synthesis in vitro and in vivo.[26,47,52] Single doses of PCB administered to mice bearing transplanted tumors inhibited DNA incorporation of thymidine by 35 to 70%.[26,47] Maximal inhibition occurred within several hours, and complete recovery was achieved by 8 to 24 hours. De novo purine synthesis and pyrimidine-nucleotide synthesis are inhibited, but there is no effect on nucleoside or nucleotide kinases. PCB produces a similar time course and degree of inhibition for the RNA (uracil) incorporation of orotic acid and for nuclear RNA synthesis. Protein synthesis inhibition cuased by PCB is relatively delayed, reaching a maximum at 12 to 16 hours, and this effect is believed to be a result of the inhibition of nucleic acid synthesis.[26,47,52,53] PCB seems to inhibit normal transfer RNA (tRNA) methylation, and the resulting altered tRNA synthesis and function may well account for some of the effects on nucleic acid and protein synthesis.[43,54]

The most compelling evidence to date suggests that the cytotoxicity of PCB is mediated by its role as a methylating agent. Adult Fisher rats treated with radiolabeled PCB developed large amounts of O^6-[^{14}C]methylguanine compared with 7-[^{14}C]methylguanine.[55] O^6-methylguanine is a known

mutagenic and carcinogenic adduct[56–58] also thought to contribute to cytotoxicity.[59] Accordingly, the observation that administration of PCB to athymic nude mice bearing xenografts derived from human malignant gliomas and medulloblastoma resulted in greater growth delays in those tumors lacking O^6-alkylguanine-DNA alkyl transferase (AGT),[60] the enzyme mediating repair of O^6-methylguanine,[61] is particularly convincing. Four of five tumor lines with AGT levels had growth delays of less than 20 days after PCB, whereas all five lines with undetectable AGT levels had growth delays of more than 30 days. Furthermore, O^6-methylguanine was found in significantly higher levels in two sensitive lines with low-AGT levels as compared with O^6-methylguanine levels in a resistant line with a high-AGT level.

Mechanisms of Resistance

Recent studies have shed light on the cellular mechanism(s) of resistance to PCB. Resistance develops rapidly in tumor cells[3] after exposure to PCB, and one study suggested a direct correlation between the rate of DNA synthesis and the rapidity of resistance development.[26] Resistant cells also were found to contain additional chromosomes.[62] The previously mentioned inverse correlation between central nervous system (CNS) xenograft response to PCB and AGT activity suggests that resistance to this methylating agent is secondary to AGT-mediated repair of O^6-methylguanine, similar to nitrosourea resistance mediated by this enzyme.[61] However, an alternative method of resistance has been defined. Friedman et al.[63] established a methylator- resistant human glioblastoma multiforme xenograft, D-245 MG (PR), in athymic nude mice by serially treating the parent xenograft, D-245 MG, with PCB. D-245 MG xenografts were sensitive to PCB, TMZ, N-methyl-N-nitrosourea, 1,3-bis(2-chloroethyl)-1-nitrosourea, 9-aminocamptothecin, topotecan, CPT-11, cyclophosphamide, and busulfan. D-245 MG (PR) xenografts were resistant to PCB, TMZ, N-methyl-N-nitrosourea, and busulfan, but they were sensitive to the other agents. D-245 MG and D-245 MG (PR) xenografts displayed no AGT alkyl transferase activity, and their levels of glutathione and glutathione-S-transferase were similar. D-245 MG xenografts expressed the human mismatch-repair proteins hMSH2 and hMLH1, whereas D-245 MG (PR) expressed hMLH1 but not hMSH2.

These results indicate that this resistance to PCB and other methylators was secondary to an in vivo-acquired mismatch repair deficiency. This observation is consistent with other reports demonstrating methylator resistance in human tumor cells resulting from mismatch repair deficiency.[64,65]

Drug Interactions

Because PCB undergoes extensive hepatic microsomal metabolism and because it inhibits monoamine oxidase, which is widespread in tissues and plasma, there are many potential drug-drug and drug-food interactions. The activity of other drugs that are inactivated by microsomal metabolism may be enhanced in the presence of PCB, as shown by a prolonged pentobarbital-induced sleep time in animals.[66-69] Therefore, patients taking barbiturates, phenothiazines, narcotics, and other hypnotics or sedatives may experience potentiated effects of these agents. Conversely, these drugs and others, such as cimetidine, that affect hepatic metabolism may increase or decrease PCB metabolism and thereby alter PCB activity and toxicity.[45,70,71] Pretreatment of rats with phenobarbital before PCB administration resulted in increased PCB clearance and a slight decrease in concentrations of the azometabolite. Inasmuch as phenobarbital or phenytoin pretreatment increased the survival of tumor-bearing mice treated with PCB (Table 13.1), it may be presumed that microsomal enzyme induction resulted in increased production of active PCB metabolites.[46] It is not known whether this drug interaction may be useful clinically to achieve therapeutic advantage through biochemical modulation of PCB activity.

Monoamine oxidase inhibition[72] and pyridoxal phosphate depletion[73] by PCB cause CNS depression. This also may potentiate the sedative effects of other CNS depressants. This inhibition of monoamine oxidase also predisposes patients to acute hypertensive reactions after concomitant therapy with tricyclic antidepressants and sympathomimetic drugs, as well as after ingestion of tyramine-rich foods, such as red wine, bananas, ripe cheese, and yogurt. Finally, a disulfiram-like reaction manifested by sweating, facial flushing, and headache may occur in patients who ingest alcohol while taking PCB.

Clinical Pharmacology

PCB hydrochloride is supplied in capsules containing the equivalent of 50 mg of the base for oral administration. As a single agent, the usual dose is 100 to 200 mg/m^2 of body surface area, given daily until myelosuppression occurs. As part of the mechlorethamine, vincristine, PCB, and prednisone (MOPP) combination regimen for Hodgkin's disease, the daily dose of PCB is 100 mg/m^2 of body surface area daily for 14 days.[10]

TABLE 13.1
KEY FEATURES OF PROCARBAZINE (PCB)
[N-ISOPROPYL-α-(2-METHYLHYDRAZINO)-P-TOLUAMIDE, IBENZMETHYZIN, NATULAN, MATULANE, NSC 77213]

Factor	Result
Mechanism of action	Metabolic activation required: methylation of nucleic acids; inhibition of DNA, RNA, and protein synthesis.
Metabolism	Converted to azo-PCB by erythrocyte and liver microsomes
	Subsequent metabolism to N-isopropyl-p-formylbenzamide, N-isopropyl-p-hydroxymethyl benzamide, N-isopropyl-p-toluamide, N-isopropyl-N-isopropylterephthalamic acid (inactive), methane, and carbon dioxide
	Possible formation of methyldiazene free radical "active intermediate"
Pharmacokinetics:	Half-life = 7 min
	Approximately 100% bioavailability from oral route, peak plasma concentration reached within 60 min
	Equilibration between plasma and cerebrospinal fluid in 15–30 min
Elimination	Renal elimination of ≥75% in 24 hr
Drug and food interactions	PCB may inhibit hepatic microsomal drug metabolism and therefore potentiate activity of barbiturates, antihistamines, narcotics, and phenothiazines
	Alcohol use may cause "disulfiram-like" reaction
	Sympathomimetics, tricyclic antidepressants, or tyramine-rich foods may cause severe hypertension from PCB inhibition of monoamine oxidase
Toxicity	Myelosuppression
	Gastrointestinal (nausea and vomiting); rare, hepatic dysfunction
	Neurotoxicity (drowsiness, depression, agitation, paresthesias)
	Cutaneous or pulmonary hypersensitivity (rare)
	Azoospermia; anovulation
	Carcinogenesis (associated with secondary malignancy in treated patients)
	Teratogenesis
Precautions	Dose modification may be necessary in hepatic and/or renal dysfunction
	Avoid alcohol
	Avoid tyramine-rich foods, sympathomimetics, tricyclic antidepressants, hypnotics, antihistamines, narcotics, phenothiazines

The pharmacokinetics and metabolism of PCB have been studied mostly in laboratory animals, and information regarding pharmacokinetics in humans is incomplete.[62,74-77] After oral administration, the drug is rapidly and completely absorbed from the gastrointestinal tract. The biodistribution of PCB is not well known; however, earlier studies using drug that was isotopically labeled at different sites on the molecule showed high levels of radioactivity in the liver, kidney, intestine, and skin at 30 and 60 minutes after drug administration.[76] There is also rapid equilibration of [14C]PCB (labeled in the benzyl ring) between plasma and cerebrospinal fluid (CSF) in dogs and humans.[66] After the intravenous administration of 150 mg [14C]PCB, the plasma half-life ($t_{1/2}$) of parent drug was approximately 7 minutes in humans, whereas studies in dogs and rats demonstrated $t_{1/2}$ of 12 and 24 minutes, respectively.[74] Because single-bolus intravenous dosages of PCB produce a spectrum of toxicity, primarily neurotoxicity,[78] distinct from the myelosuppression seen after oral administration, it is likely that a first-pass effect of orally administered drug through the portal circulation significantly influences drug metabolism and pharmacokinetics. This is supported by the observation of almost complete conversion of PCB to the azometabolite in isolated liver perfusion studies.[35,75] After the intraperitoneal injection of 150 mg PCB in rats, the azometabolite appears in plasma within minutes, peaking at 10 to 20 minutes and then decreasing slowly over several hours concomitant with the appearance of the methyl and benzylazoxy isomers[28] (Fig. 13.2A). Preliminary data in humans show that the methylazoxy isomer is the major plasma metabolite after a single 250 mg/kg oral dose of PCB. This compound peaks at approximately 90 minutes and seems to have an initial plasma half-life of approximately 60 minutes. Azo-PCB and the benzylazoxy isomer are present in relatively equal but lesser concentrations compared to the methylazoxy isomer. Interestingly, PCB treatment seems to alter its own metabolism, a change that may, in turn, influence its activity.[28,46,67] The total and relative plasma concentrations of PCB metabolites are markedly changed after the administration of a fourteenth daily oral dose of PCB[28] (Fig. 13.2B). Of note was the significant increase in azo-PCB concentration, suggesting that prior PCB exposure induces this metabolite's production or delays its clearance. Shiba and Weinkam[46] also observed that prior treatment with PCB enhances PCB antitumor activity in rats.

In all species examined, the major urinary metabolite of PCB is the biologically inactive N-isopropylterephthalamic acid.[66,70,74-76] Approximately 70% of radioactivity administered in the form of [14C]PCB was recovered, primarily as the acid, in the urine during the first 24 hours. There is minimal fecal excretion (4 to 12% over 96 hours), and approximately 30% of radioactivity labeled in the N-methyl group appears as respiratory $^{14}CO_2$.[76,79]

The complex pharmacokinetic and excretion characteristics of PCB reflect the rapid and extensive enzymatic metabolism of this compound, which is necessary for antitumor activity and presumably is responsible for host organ toxic reactions. The proposed metabolic routes for PCB were discussed in detail in the previous edition of this text[80] and were reviewed in detail by Prough and Tweedie[29] (Fig. 13.1). The understanding of PCB metabolism is improving as a result of improved experimental techniques and analytical methods, including high-pressure liquid chromatography (HPLC) and mass spectroscopy.[27,28,33-37,81,82] Again, most of the information in this area is derived from studies in animals in vivo and in vitro. There do not seem to be any major discrepancies in these results in animals as compared with the literature describing human metabolism.[46,66,74,76,83] Nonetheless, the information is not

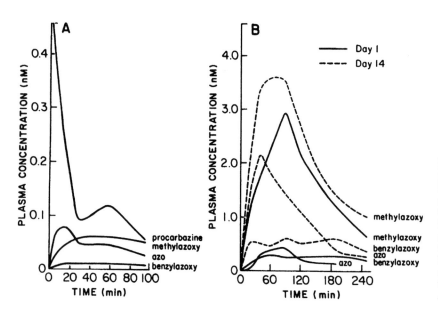

Figure 13.2 A. Procarbazine (PCB) disappearance and azo and azoxy metabolite kinetics in rat plasma after administration of PCB, 150 mg/kg, intraperitoneally. **B.** Plasma concentrations of azo and azoxyprocarbasine metabolites in a patient after the administration of PCB, 250 mg/kg per day, orally, on days 1 and 14 of a 14-day treatment schedule. (From Shiba DA, Weinkam RJ. Quantitative analysis of PCB, PCB metabolites and chemical degradation products with application to pharmacokinetic studies. J Chromatogr 1982; 229:397.)

sufficient to allow assignment of quantitative importance to the several possible alternate routes of metabolism (Fig. 13.1). However, a recent report detailing an improved assay for procarbazine in human plasma by liquid chromatography with electrospray ionization mass spectrometry may facilitate these needed analyses.[84]

PCB is not stable in aqueous solution, decomposing by rapid metal-catalyzed oxidation to azo-PCB with the production of hydrogen peroxide.[29,33,45,66,81] In the presence of light, isomerization to the biologically inactive hydrazone (N-isopropyl-p-formylbenzamide methylhydrazine) occurs slowly. This is followed by hydrolysis to yield the aldehyde, N-isopropyl-p-formylbenzamide, and methylhydrazine. The former compound is further oxidized to N-isopropyl-terephthalamic acid. Earlier studies suggested that this route of chemical decomposition was responsible for the biologic activity of PCB,[45,66,74] but subsequent investigations have shown that the chemical decomposition products are relatively stable under physiologic conditions and that they account for a small proportion of the compounds formed in vitro and in vivo as compared with cytochrome P-450–mediated metabolism.[25,26,29,33-38] Because of PCB's chemical degradation to potentially toxic compounds under common conditions, such as aqueous solvent, trace metal contamination, and air and light exposure, extreme care must be taken in the formulation and storage of PCB solutions intended for parenteral administration. These considerations also apply when evaluating the results of PCB studies in vitro and in vivo.

In biologic systems, the oxidation of PCB to azo-PCB occurs by microsomal cytochrome P-450 oxidoreductase or by mitochondrial monoamine oxidase enzymatic conversion[32,34,75,85,86] (Fig. 13.1). Isolated rat liver perfusion studies, as well as incubation of drug with rat liver microsomes, disclose extensive metabolism of the drug and suggest that the liver is the predominant site of the initial metabolism of PCB.[29,34-38] The subsequent metabolism of azo-PCB may occur by several different routes. Isozymic cytochrome P-450–mediated N-oxidation results in the formation of methyl and benzylazoxy isomers[27,34,87,88] (Fig. 13.1, pathways III and IV). The former is produced in higher quantitative yield during in vitro reactions and is the predominant metabolite of azo-PCB in rat and human plasma.[28,29] It has been proposed that hydroxylation of either carbon atom adjacent to the azoxy function results in unstable compounds that react to produce the reactive alkylating alkyldiazonium ion [R—N$^+$N]. Further microsomal metabolism of the azoxy compounds results in formation of N-isopropyl-p-formylbenzamide or N-isopropyl-p-hydroxymethylbenzamide. These compounds are then oxidized to the major urinary metabolite, N-isopropyl-terephthalamic acid.[27-29,66,74] Alternatively, Moloney and associates[40] recently demonstrated a pathway of metabolic activation of the terminal N-methyl group of azo-PCB that does not involve azoxy formation (Fig. 13.1, pathway V). This pathway involves a P-450–mediated oxidation of the benzyl carbon atom adjacent to the azo function with subsequent formation of N-isopropyl-p-formylbenzamide and a putative unstable methyldiazene intermediate. The proposed intermediate could form either a methyl radical or a carbonium ion, both of which are covalent binding species. If, instead, hydrogen abstraction occurs, as in the presence of reduced glutathione, then methane is formed as a final metabolic product.[38,77] Another pathway that would produce a free-radical intermediate and not involve azoxy formation is the oxidation of the methyl carbon adjacent to the azo function (Fig. 13.1, pathway II). This metabolic route would ultimately lead to formation of CO_2 and N-isopropyl-p-toluamide, a metabolite identified in rat plasma and brain after the administration of PCB.[33,75-77,79,80] Because the azoxy metabolites are the predominant products found in plasma, however, it is likely that pathways III and IV predominate in humans.

Toxicity

After oral administration, PCB causes anorexia and mild nausea and vomiting, which is probably of central origin and often abates with continued use.[89] In some patients, it is often helpful to escalate the dosage in a stepwise fashion over the first several days of drug administration to minimize these gastrointestinal side effects. Mild-to-moderate myelosuppression in the form of reversible leukopenia and thrombocytopenia is the most common dose-limiting toxicity of PCB given orally. Depression of peripheral leukocyte and platelet counts becomes apparent after 1 week of therapy and may persist for 2 weeks or longer after discontinuation of the drug.[90] PCB also may cause hemolysis in patients with glucose-6-phosphate dehydrogenase deficiency.[91] PCB generally does not cause mucosal injury to the rapidly proliferating gastrointestinal epithelium.

Patients receiving PCB orally may occasionally experience neurotoxicity manifest by drowsiness, depression, agitation, paresthesias of the extremities,[92] and reversible orthostatic hypotension.[8] These effects are probably a result of central monoamine oxidase inhibition and may be related to drug-induced depletion of pyridoxal phosphate.[72,73,93] When PCB is administered intravenously, neurotoxic effects become more pronounced and are dose-limiting. After a single high-dose intravenous bolus (2 g/m^2) or a 5-day continuous infusion of PCB, patients experienced severe nausea and vomiting, confusion, and even coma lasting several days.[78,93] Myelosuppression does not occur when PCB is administered in this way. However, there is also a parallel lack of clinical antitumor effect, which emphasizes the importance of first-pass hepatic metabolism for activation of PCB to antiproliferative intermediates. The pattern of toxicity after small, intermittent intravenous doses is more like that seen after oral administration,[1,6] although it is unlikely that this schedule offers any clinical benefit over that of conventional oral dosing.

PCB also may cause hypersensitivity reactions, including maculopapular skin rash, eosinophilia, pulmonary infiltrates, or, rarely, transient hepatic dysfunction.[5,7,94–98] The skin rash usually responds to concomitant glucocorticosteroid treatment, and the PCB may be continued without exacerbation of rash or further sequelae. In contrast, PCB-induced interstitial pneumonitis usually necessitates discontinuation of the drug.

PCB has potent immunosuppressive properties that may contribute to the infectious complications.[99] These immunosuppressive properties have been used to therapeutic advantage for the treatment of lupus erythematosus and in the suppression of graft-versus-host disease after bone marrow transplantation.[100] With the use of newer agents developed for these indications and with the increasing concern over serious late toxic reactions to PCB, this drug should probably not be used for non-neoplastic diseases.

The successful use of PCB-containing chemotherapy combinations resulting in curative and long-term disease-free survival has directed increasing attention and concern to the chronic and late toxicities of this agent. PCB has profound azoospermic,[101,102] teratogenic,[103] mutagenic,[104,105] and carcinogenic[106,107] properties in experimental animals, and most of these effects have been associated with PCB use in humans.

PCB is highly toxic to reproductive organs, causing azoospermia and anovulation.[108–112] More than 90% of men receiving PCB in combination with classic alkylating agents, such as in MOPP combination chemotherapy for Hodgkin's disease, have irreversible azoospermia. Approximately 50% of women thus treated have permanent drug-induced ovarian failure. In pregnant animals, administration of PCB causes congenital skeletal and CNS abnormalities.[103,113] Although evidence for direct causation of lethal and nonlethal mutations in human fetuses is lacking, women of childbearing potential should be advised against pregnancy during chemotherapy. In women treated with MOPP chemotherapy and who regain normal ovarian function, there seems to be no impairment of fertility nor any increased birth defects in offspring.[111,112,114,115]

Mutagenesis and carcinogenesis resulting from PCB have been demonstrated experimentally in vitro and in vivo.[104–107] Nonlymphocytic leukemias and adenocarcinomas developed in rodents and nonhuman primates after PCB administration, and, accordingly, the finite increased incidence of secondary leukemias and solid malignancies in patients after treatment with MOPP combination chemotherapy pointed to PCB as the responsible carcinogen.[116–118] Because this regimen also contains an alkylating agent with carcinogenic properties, it is difficult to assign a direct cause of secondary malignancies to PCB alone.[118] Indeed, studies in experimental systems suggest that additive or interactive effects of classic alkylating agents with PCB may account for the observed mutagenesis.[119]

The mechanisms of PCB gonadal toxicity and somatic genotoxicity are mostly thought to be the same as for its antitumor activity. As for the latter, metabolic conversion of PCB is necessary for its toxic and carcinogenic effects on normal tissue, although it is not clear which metabolic pathways are mechanistically important, nor is it known whether there may be separate mechanisms for anticancer activity and for normal organ toxicity. Yost et al.[120] and Horstman et al.[121] proposed separate mechanisms for PCB spermatotoxicity and anticancer activity based on different activating metabolic pathways. Furthermore, these authors exploited this difference by using antioxidants that protected against PCB spermatotoxicity but did not compromise its antileukemic activity in mice (Table 13.2). These studies, as well as those of Prough and Tweedie[29] and Shiba and Weinkam,[46] which show improved therapeutic benefit from phenobarbital induction of PCB metabolism, suggest that anticancer and toxic effects of PCB may be separable and, therefore, susceptible to modulation for therapeutic advantage. Further investigations of PCB's metabolism and molecular mechanisms of action are necessary to develop clinically useful approaches to lessen toxicity successfully and improve efficacy.

TABLE 13.2

EXPERIMENTAL BIOCHEMICAL MODULATION OF PROCARBAZINE (PCB) EFFICACY AND TOXICITY IN MICE BEARING L1210 LEUKEMIA, INTRAPERITONEALLY

Treatment	Modulation	Life Span Increase (%)[a]	Sperm Count (%)[b]	Reference
PCB 200 mg/kg, IP, daily × 3	None	122		43
PCB 200 mg/kg, IP, daily × 3	Phenytoin 60 mg/kg, PO, for 7 d	146[c]		43
PCB 200 mg/kg, IP, daily × 3	Phenobarbital 48 mg/kg, PO, for 7 d	140[c]		43
PCB 400 mg/kg, IP	None	125	45	108
PCB 400 mg/kg, IP	N-Acetylcysteine 189.9 mg/kg, IP	128	85	108
PCB 400 mg/kg, IP	Sodium ascorbate 307.4 mg/kg, IP	125	90	108

[a] % mean treated/control.
[b] Mean expressed as a percentage of control mice given 0.9% NaCl.
[c] Significant at the 95% confidence limit compared with mice treated with PCB alone.
IP, intraperitoneally; PO, per os.

DACARBAZINE

History

DTIC was chemically synthesized as a result of a rational attempt to develop agents capable of interfering with the synthesis of purines. As reviewed by Montgomery,[122] a series of compounds designed as analogs of aminoimidazole carboxamide (AIC), an intermediate in purine ring synthesis, was synthesized in the late 1950s and had significant antitumor activity in experimental testing. The addition of nitrous acid to form a 5-diazoimidazole derivative seemed to confer this antitumor activity, and the further addition of a third nitrogen group to form the 5-triazene resulted in a light-sensitive compound that spontaneously converted back to the diazo analog. Dimethyl substitution of the triazine resulted in a more stable but still light-sensitive derivative, DTIC, which was highly active and was developed for clinical use.[123]

DTIC is an active single agent in the treatment of metastatic malignant melanoma, producing remissions in 16 to 31% of patients with this disease,[124] and it is also active as a single agent in Hodgkin's disease.[125] Thus, in the United States, DTIC is approved for use in these two diseases. It is frequently used alone or in combination with agents such as nitrosoureas, bleomycin, and vinca alkaloids in melanoma,[126–129] and it is most commonly used as part of the doxorubicin, bleomycin, vinblastine, and DTIC (ABVD) and actinomycin D, bleomycin, and vincristine regimens for Hodgkin's disease.[130,131] In addition, DTIC has demonstrated activity in the treatment of sarcomas,[132–134] childhood neuroblastoma,[135,136] and primary brain tumors.[137] It may be the most active agent alone or in combination for the treatment of malignant amine precursor uptake and decarboxylation and other neuroendocrine tumors.[138–140] The key features of DTIC are summarized in Table 13.3.

General Mechanism of Action and Cellular Pharmacology

The exact mechanism underlying DTIC's antitumor activity remains an enigma. Although DTIC was developed as a purine antimetabolite, there is abundant evidence that its antitumor activity does not result from interference with purine synthesis. The drug is active against several cell lines resistant to the purine analogs 6-thioguanine and 6-mercaptopurine, and it does not demonstrate cell-cycle schedule dependence observed with other antimetabolites.[122] Second, the AIC portion of the molecule is not necessary for antitumor activity.[141,142]

There is mounting evidence to suggest that, similar to PCB, the production of O^6-methylguanine is the primary cytotoxic event after administration of DTIC. Xenografts, or

---

TABLE 13.3

KEY FEATURES OF DACARBAZINE [5-(3,3-DIMETHYL-1-TRIAZENO) IMIDAZOLE-4-CARBOXAMIDE, DTIC, DIC, NSC-45388]

Factor	Result
Mechanism of action	Metabolic activation probably required; methylation of nucleic acids; direct DNA damage; inhibition of purine synthesis.
Metabolism	Oxidative N-methylation to 5-aminoimidazole-4-carboxamide via formation of 5(3-hydroxymethyl-3-methyltriazen-1-yl) imidazole-4-carboxamide and 5-(3-methyltriazen-2-yl) imidazole-4-carboxamide.
	$t_{1/2}\alpha = 3$ min; $t_{1/2}\beta = 41$ min
	$V_d = 0.6$ L/kg; $Cl = 15$ mL/kg/min
	20% protein bound
	Variable oral absorption.
	Poor CSF penetration (plasma/CSF ratio = 7:1 at equilibrium).
Elimination	Renal excretion: 50% as unchanged dacarbazine and 9–18% as 5-aminoimidazole-4-carboxamide.
	Minor hepatobiliary and pulmonary excretion.
Drug and food interactions	*Corynebacterium parvum* may prolong $t_{1/2}$.
Toxicity	Myelosuppression.
	Gastrointestinal (nausea and vomiting).
	Influenza-like syndrome (fever, myalgia, and malaise).
	Infrequent alopecia, cutaneous hypersensitivity, or photosensitivity.
	Rare hepatic vein thrombosis and hepatic necrosis.
	Possible carcinogenesis and teratogenesis.
Precautions	Dose modification may be necessary in hepatic and/or renal dysfunction.

Cl, clearance; CSF, cerebrospinal fluid; $t_{1/2}$, half-life; V_d, apparent volume of distribution.

cell lines with negligible levels of AGT, are more sensitive to DTIC than are xenografts or cell lines with high levels of AGT.[143-149] Furthermore, DTIC depletes AGT levels in human colon cancer HT 29 xenografts in athymic mice[150] and in human peripheral blood cells in patients treated for metastatic melanoma.[151]

The previously mentioned work[143-149] supporting O^6-methylguanine as the major cytotoxic lesion produced by DTIC strongly suggests that elevated levels of AGT may be responsible for resistance to this agent. The inverse relationship between AGT levels and response to DTIC in human xenografts also may be operational in clinical tumor resistance to DTIC.[143-149] Furthermore, resistance to all methylators, including DTIC, is seen in the setting of a deficiency of DNA mismatch repair.[63-65] Finally, Lev et al.[152] have reported DTIC resistance mediated by up-regulation of interleukin 8 and vascular endothelial growth factor in melanoma cells.

Drug Interactions

At present, there are no known drug or food interactions with DTIC that are of clinical importance. Because DTIC has been used in conjunction with immune adjuvants in the treatment of malignant melanoma, there has been some interest in the influence of these agents on DTIC pharmacology. Farquhar and coworkers[153] described an inhibition of DTIC N-demethylase in rats pretreated with bacillus Calmette-Guérin (BCG), suggesting that patients receiving both agents may be less able to activate DTIC. In four patients with melanoma, BCG did not seem to influence DTIC pharmacokinetics, although altered metabolism per se was not examined.[154] In contrast, patients receiving *Corynebacterium parvum* adjuvant immunotherapy did show a prolongation of DTIC serum half-life[155] consistent with the ability of *C. parvum* to depress hepatic microsomal N-demethylation of a variety of drugs.[156] Although the initial step for metabolic activation of DTIC is catalyzed by microsomal cytochrome P-450, the interaction of phenobarbital, or other commonly used cytochrome P-450–inducing agents, with DTIC has not been reported.

DTIC activity against L1210 murine leukemia is potentiated by alkylating agents, such as melphalan, and by doxorubicin.[122] Activity is also enhanced when DTIC is combined with the nitrosoureas bischloromethyl- nitrosourea (BCNU) and chloroethylcyclo-hexylnitrosourea (CCNU). The mechanism(s) for the potentiation observed using these combinations may be related to the ability of nitrosoureas to deplete AGT and thereby sensitize cells to methylating agents.

Clinical Pharmacology

DTIC is supplied in sterile vials containing 100 or 200 mg DTIC for intravenous administration. As a single agent, a dose of up to 1,500 mg/m^2 of body surface area may be given as a single bolus as opposed to the more frequently used schedule of 250 mg/m^2 daily for 5 days every 3 to 4 weeks.[126,128,134,157] The latter schedule was developed in an attempt to minimize the gastrointestinal toxicity from DTIC, which tends to lessen with repeated administration. Most studies, however, fail to show any significant schedule dependency with respect to antitumor efficacy or toxicity.[126,128] DTIC also has been used by intra-arterial infusion for the regional treatment of malignant melanoma involving liver, pelvis, the maxillofacial region, and extremities with high response rates in uncontrolled series.[158-161] It is not known whether in situ melanoma cells in humans are capable of metabolizing DTIC[162]; otherwise, these results are difficult to interpret because DTIC requires metabolic activation for its antitumor activity.

Initial studies of DTIC pharmacokinetics and metabolism in rodents, dogs, and humans used radiochemical[163,164] and colorimetric methods.[165-167] More recently, improved experimental methods, such as HPLC[154,155,168] and mass spectroscopy,[169] have been used to study triazine pharmacology. Because of the scarcity of clinical studies using adequately sensitive and specific techniques, knowledge of DTIC pharmacology in humans remains incomplete. After oral administration, the drug is absorbed slowly and variably[166,167]; therefore, intravenous administration is the preferred route. Intravenous boluses of 2.65 to 6.85 mg/kg (approximately 120 to 300 mg/m^2) produced peak plasma concentrations of nearly 10 to over 30 µg/mL, respectively.[154] After intravenous administration of DTIC, Breithaupt and coworkers[154] found a biphasic plasma disappearance of the parent drug consistent with a two-compartment model with an initial half-life of 3 minutes and a terminal half-life of 41 minutes (Fig. 13.3). This is in contrast to a terminal half-life of 3.2 hours found in an earlier study using HPLC[155] analysis. Approximately 20% of DTIC is loosely bound to plasma protein.[166] In humans, the mean volume of distribution for DTIC was 0.6 L/kg, and the total-body clearance was 15.4 mL/kg per minute.[154] In one study, approximately 50% of an intravenous dose of DTIC was recovered in the urine as parent drug, and the renal clearance was calculated to be between 5 and 10 mL/kg per minute,[154] confirming earlier reports[166,167] that tubular secretion may be involved in the renal excretion of DTIC. Altered schedules of intravenous drug administration did not change the area under the curve (concentration × time), confirming a lack of schedule dependence for DTIC pharmacokinetics.[154]

In dogs[166] and humans,[126] DTIC penetrates poorly into the CSF. At equilibrium, the ratio between plasma and spinal fluid was 7:1. This finding may explain the lack of DTIC activity against intracranial L1210 leukemia.[122] It fails to explain, however, the observations that DTIC has activity against transplantable murine ependymoblastoma[170] and against primary and metastatic brain tumors in humans.[124,127,137]

The major metabolite of DTIC found in plasma and urine is AIC (Fig. 13.3),[154,163,164,166] with cumulative excretion in

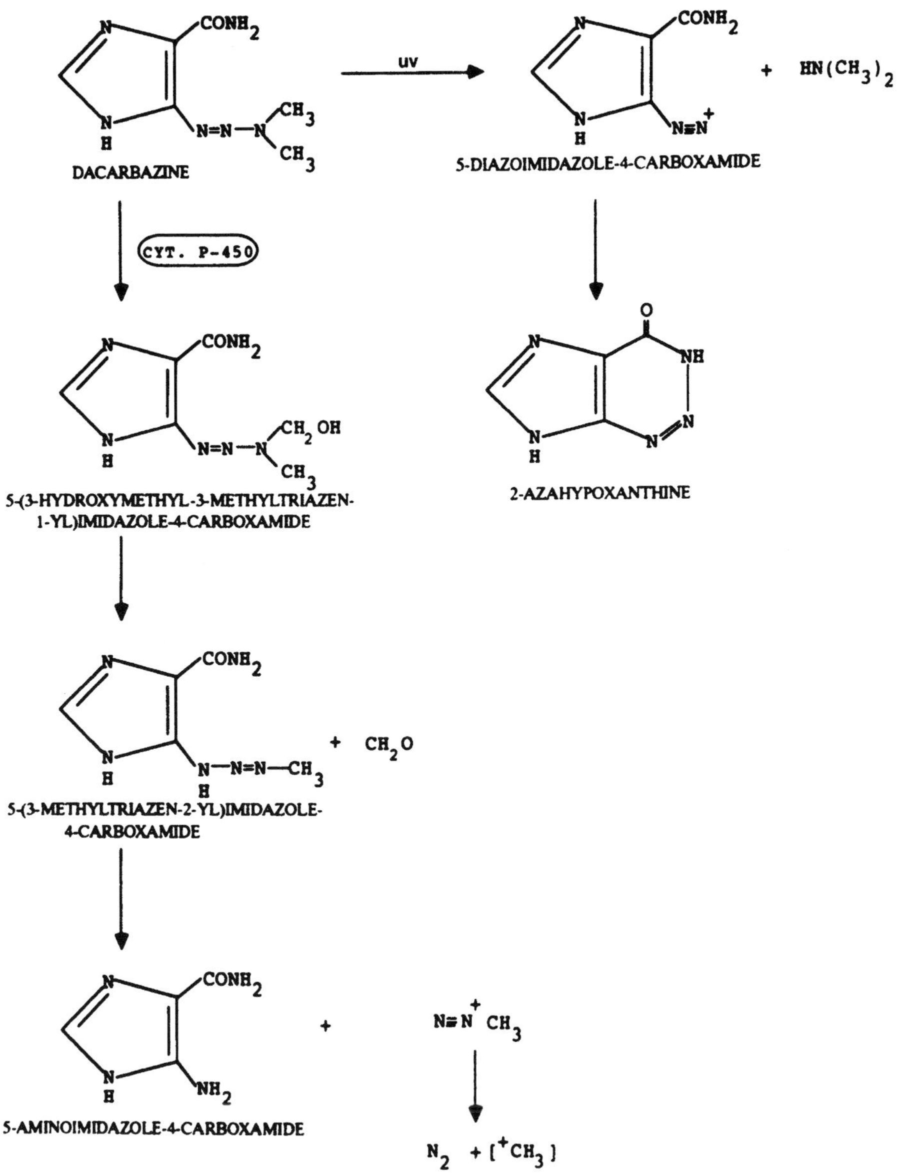

DACARBAZINE

5-DIAZOIMIDAZOLE-4-CARBOXAMIDE

$+ \; HN(CH_3)_2$

CYT. P-450

5-(3-HYDROXYMETHYL-3-METHYLTRIAZEN-1-YL)IMIDAZOLE-4-CARBOXAMIDE

2-AZAHYPOXANTHINE

5-(3-METHYLTRIAZEN-2-YL)IMIDAZOLE-4-CARBOXAMIDE

$+ \; CH_2O$

5-AMINOIMIDAZOLE-4-CARBOXAMIDE

$N \equiv N^+ \; CH_3$

$N_2 \; + \; [^+CH_3]$

Figure 13.3 Plasma concentrations of dacarbazine (DTIC) and 5-aminoimidazole-4-carboxamide (AIC) in a patient after administration of dacarbazine, 6.34 mg/kg, intravenously. (From Breithaupt H, Dammann A, Aigner K. Pharmacokinetics of dacarbazine [DTIC] and its metabolite 5-aminoimidazole-4-carboxamide [AIC] following different dose schedules. Cancer Chemother Pharmacol 1982;9:103.)

the urine accounting for 9 to 20% of parent compound in several patients studied.[154,164] AIC is also formed from DTIC in the presence of liver microsomes[171] and by some tumor cells.[172] After the intraperitoneal administration of [^{14}CO-methyl]DTIC to rats or mice, 4% of the dose is recovered as respiratory $^{14}CO_2$ in 6 hours, and 9% of the dose is recovered as $^{14}CO_2$ in 24 hours.[173,174] Presumably, the expired radiolabeled $^{14}CO_2$ is derived from the formaldehyde produced after N-demethylation of DTIC. These findings, as well as the identification of 5-(3-hydroxymethyl-3-methyltriazen-1-yl) imidazole-4-carboxamide (HMTIC) as a urinary metabolite of DTIC in rats,[175-177] are consistent with a metabolic pathway for DTIC, as shown in Figure 13.4, in which MTIC is the primary active metabolite, responsible for transferring its methyl group to DNA.

Toxicity

The most frequent toxic reaction to DTIC treatment is moderately severe nausea and vomiting, which occurs in 90% of patients.[134,179] These symptoms appear soon after infusion and may persist for up to 12 hours. The severity of gastrointestinal toxicity decreases with successive doses when the drug is given on a 5-day schedule and if the initial dose is decreased.[179] Above 1,200 mg/m^2 as a rapid intravenous bolus, DTIC frequently causes severe, but short-lived, watery diarrhea.[126,157] After rapid infusion of a high dose (>1,380 mg/m^2) of DTIC, hypotension may occur.[157]

Myelosuppression is a common dose-related toxicity of DTIC, although the degree of leukopenia and thrombocytopenia is variably mild to moderate. Significant

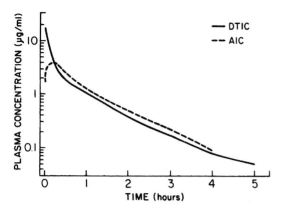

Figure 13.4 Light-activated and metabolic reactions of dacarbazine leading to the generation of reactive intermediates. CYT, cytochrome; uv, ultraviolet.

myelosuppression occurs when more than 1,380 mg/m^2 is given as a single intravenous bolus,[157] whereas studies using a 5-day administration schedule reported increasing frequency of myelosuppression above a total of 1,000 mg/m^2.[126,134] In the latter, nadir leukopenia and thrombocytopenia occurred on day 25, with complete recovery by day 40. This delayed bone marrow recovery is not common, however, and usually there is sufficient recovery so that DTIC may be administered every 21 to 28 days.

Less frequent toxic reactions include a flulike syndrome of fever up to 39°C, myalgias, and malaise lasting several days after DTIC treatment. Headache, facial flushing, facial paresthesias, pain along the injection vein, alopecia, and abnormal hepatic and renal function tests rarely occur. Photosensitivity to DTIC has been reported in several patients, especially after high-dose therapy.[157-180] Therefore, patients should be advised to avoid sunlight exposure for several days after DTIC therapy. Cases of hepatic vein occlusion associated with fever, eosinophilia, and hepatic necrosis and resulting in death have been attributed to DTIC as a distinct clinical pathologic syndrome.[181-185] The mechanism for this toxicity is unknown, but an allergic etiology has been suggested.[184,185]

DTIC causes a number of immunologic effects in vitro and in vivo. The drug markedly depresses antibody responses and allograft rejection in mice for up to 60 days after a single injection.[186] This is probably a specific effect of DTIC because structure activity studies showed different patterns of immunodepression depending on which phenyltriazene analog was tested.[187] DTIC apparently does not directly suppress natural killer cell activity in mice.[188] After DTIC treatment, L1210 or L5178 lymphomas were found to be highly immunogenic, such that large inocula of the DTIC-resistant tumors were rejected by immunocompetent animals. DTIC-treated cells were actually less susceptible to natural killer cell cytolysis in vitro.[189]

DTIC has mutagenic, carcinogenic, and teratogenic properties in experimental systems.[190,191] In rodents, DTIC causes lymphoma and tumors of the thymus, lung, uterus, or mammary glands when given orally or by single or multiple injections.[142,192-194] MTIC treatment also caused similar tumors but in a lower frequency compared with DTIC.[193] It is not firmly established whether DTIC is carcinogenic for humans. In a retrospective analysis of patients receiving either MOPP or ABVD (plus or minus radiation therapy) for Hodgkin's disease, Valagussa et al.[195] reported no treatment-associated secondary malignancies in patients receiving ABVD. Subsequently, isolated cases of acute leukemia occurring after DTIC therapy have been reported,[196-197] but these remain rare. Finally, DTIC causes dose-dependent fetal malformations and fetal resorptions when administered to pregnant rats and rabbits.[198,199] Teratogenic effects were observed in the urogenital system, skeleton, eye, and cardiovascular system.

TEMOZOLOMIDE

History

Several series of 1,2,4-triazines and 1,2,4-triazinones were synthesized in England in the 1960s and 1970s, and selected compounds proved to have activity against murine tumors.[200-204] The most promising was mitozolomide, which was active against a broad spectrum of murine tumors,[203] but it produced severe and unpredictable thrombocytopenia in clinical trials and was abandoned as a clinical candidate.[204]

Selection of the next generation of imidazotetrazinones focused on TMZ, the 3-methyl derivative of mitozolomide (Fig. 13.5). This compound, with a different spectrum of activity against murine tumors,[205] was less active and considerably less toxic than mitozolomide and displayed superb delivery to all body tissues, including the brain.[206,207] TMZ was rationally advanced to clinical trial, partly based on the realization that under physiologic conditions the ring opens with resulting generation of the monomethyl triazine MTIC, the same metabolite formed by metabolic dealkylation of DTIC.[208] The inefficient demethylation of DTIC in humans (despite rapid demethylation in mice) coupled with the conversion of TMZ to MTIC without need for this metabolic step suggested a potential benefit for the use of TMZ. Table 13.4 lists the key features of TMZ.

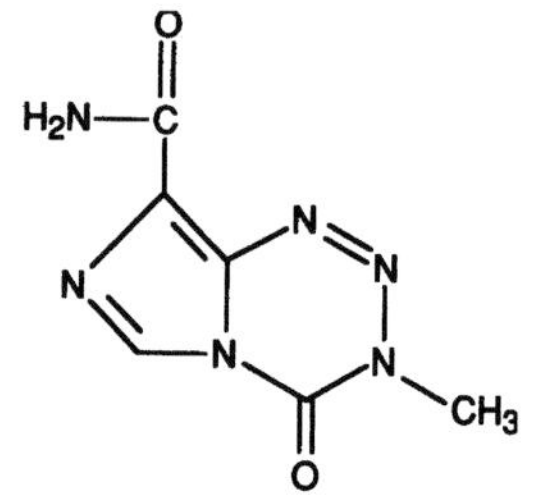

Figure 13.5 Structure of temozolomide.

TABLE 13.4
KEY FEATURES OF TEMOZOLOMIDE {8-CARBAMOYL-3-METHYLIMIDAZO [5,1-D]-1,2,3,5-TETRAZIN-4(3H)-one}

Factor	Result
Mechanism of action	Methylation of nucleic acids
Metabolism	Chemical conversion of 5 (3-methyltria-zeno) imidazole-4-carboxamide
Pharmacokinetics (IV or PO)	Volume of distribution: 28.3 L
	Elimination half-life: 1.8 hr
	Distribution half-life: 0.26 hr
	Clearance: 11.76 L/hr[253]
Drug and food inter-actions	Unknown
Toxicity	Myelosuppression
	Nausea and vomiting
	Elevated hepatic transaminases

IV, intravenously; PO, per os.

Phase 1 trials of intravenous and subsequently oral TMZ began in 1987 with a single-dose schedule and demonstrated the dose-limiting toxicity to be myelosuppression with trivial clinical benefits observed.[209] However, based on preclinical data supporting a multiple-dose regimen, another phase 1 trial using a 5-day schedule was conducted, with myelosuppression again the dose-limiting toxicity. Greater clinical activity was noted with four responses (two partial and two complete) in 23 patients with metastatic melanoma and two partial responses in four patients with high-grade glioma.[209]

Further evaluation in 28 patients with primary brain tumors revealed five radiographic responses in 10 patients with recurrent astrocytoma (the majority of which were high-grade type). Similarly, four radiographic responses were seen in seven patients with newly diagnosed high-grade glioma.[210] It should be noted that radiographic criteria for response were not the conventionally accepted partial or complete response criteria. Nevertheless, these results are provocative and justified further studies in patients with CNS tumors, particularly gliomas.

This study of O'Reilly et al.[210] was extended to 75 patients (48 with recurrent disease and 27 with new diagnoses).[211] Improvements on computed tomography (CT) were seen in 12 (25%) of the patients with recurrent disease and in eight (30%) of the patients with new diagnoses. Twenty-two percent of patients with recurrences and 43% of those with newly diagnosed tumors survived to 1 year.

The Cancer Research Campaign (CRC) conducted a multicenter phase 2 study in which TMZ demonstrated activity in patients with recurrent and progressive high-grade glioma.[212] Objective responses, measured by improvement in neurologic status, were seen in 11 of 103 patients (11%) who received TMZ; five of these patients had improvement on CT or magnetic resonance imaging

(MRI) scans.[212] Objective responses were observed in patients in whom anaplastic astrocytoma, glioblastoma multiforme (grade IV), and unclassified high-grade astrocytoma (grades III–IV) were diagnosed.

The Schering-Plough Research Institute conducted a randomized, multicenter, open-label phase 2 study of TMZ and PCB in 225 patients with glioblastoma multiforme (GBM) at first relapse.[213] The primary objectives were to compare the progression-free survival at 6 months and safety of TMZ and PCB in adult patients with GBM who had failed conventional treatment. The 6-month progression-free survival rate was significantly higher for patients who received TMZ (21%) than for those who received PCB (8%) ($P = .008$). Median progression-free survival for TMZ patients (12.4 weeks) was significantly longer than for PCB patients (8.32 weeks; $P = .0063$). The 6-month overall survival rate for TMZ patients was 60% versus 44% for PCB patients ($P = .019$).

The Schering-Plough Research Institute also conducted an open-label, multicenter phase 2 trial comprising 162 patients with malignant astrocytoma at first relapse.[214] The primary protocol end point, progression-free survival at 6 months, was 46% [95% confidence limit (CL), 38 to 54%]. The median progression-free survival was 5.4 months, and 24% of patients remained progression-free at 12 months based on Kaplan-Meier estimates.

Duke University participated in a Schering-Plough Research Institute multicenter phase II trial evaluating the activity of TMZ *before* radiation therapy in the treatment of newly diagnosed high-grade glioma.[215] Eligibility criteria included residual enhancing disease on postoperative MRI and a Karnofsky performance score (KPS) ≥70%. Thirty-three patients with GBM evaluated for tumor response revealed 3 with complete response, 14 with partial response, 4 with stable disease, and 12 with progressive disease. Five patients with anaplastic astrocytoma evaluated for response revealed one with partial response, two with stable disease, and two with progressive disease. These results with patients with glioblastoma multiforme have been extended to phase 3 trials, confirming an increase in survival when TMZ is used in an adjuvant setting.[216,217] Furthermore, TMZ has been shown to be active in the treatment of other primary brain tumors, including low-grade glioma,[218] oligodendroglioma,[219] and meningioma.[220]

The efficacy of TMZ has also been evaluated in a study of patients with advanced metastatic melanoma, including patients with brain metastases.[221] Among 56 patients (49 with evaluable lesions), complete responses occurred in 3, all with lung metastases only, and partial responses occurred in 9, yielding a response rate of 21%. Stable disease was observed in an additional eight patients.

General Mechanism of Action and Cellular Pharmacology

The spontaneous conversion of TMZ is initiated by the effect of water at the highly electropositive C^4 position of

TMZ. This activity opens the ring, releases CO_2, and generates the reactive methylating agent MTIC. The initial proposal was that this effect of water was catalyzed in the close environment of the major groove of DNA,[222,223] but confirming this mechanism has been difficult, and it is known that TMZ converts readily to MTIC in free solution in the absence of DNA.[224] MTIC degrades to the methyldiazonium cation, which transfers the methyl group to DNA and to the final degradation product AIC, which is excreted via the kidneys.[225,226] The methylation of DNA appears to be the principal mechanism responsible for the cytotoxicity of TMZ to malignant cells (see following discussion). The methyldiazonium cation can also react with RNA and with soluble and cellular protein.[227] However, the methylation of RNA and the methylation or carbamoylation of protein do not appear to have any known significant role in the antitumor activity of TMZ.[227] Further studies are required to clarify the role of these targets in the biochemical mechanism of action of TMZ.

The spontaneous conversion of TMZ and MTIC depends on pH. Under acidic conditions, TMZ is stable; however, its chemical stability decreases at a pH of >7.0 and is converted rapidly to MTIC in that environment.[226] In contrast, MTIC is more stable under basic conditions and rapidly degrades to the methyldiazonium cation and AIC at a pH of <7.0.[226] A comparison of the half-life of TMZ in phosphate buffer (pH, 7.4; $t_{1/2} = 1.83$ hours)[209,226] indicates that the conversion of TMZ to MTIC is a chemically controlled reaction with little or no enzymatic component. The spontaneous conversion of TMZ may contribute to its highly reproducible pharmacokinetics in comparison with other alkylating agents such as DTIC and PCB, which must undergo metabolic conversion in the liver and are thus subject to interpatient variation in metabolic rates of conversion.[223,226]

Among the lesions produced in DNA after treatment of cells with TMZ, the most common is methylation at the N^7 position of guanine, followed by methylation at the O^3 position of adenine and the O^6 position of guanine.[226] Although the N^7-methylguanine and O^3-methyladenine adducts probably contribute to the antitumor activity of TMZ in some, if not all, sensitive cells, their role is controversial.[228] The critical role of the O^6-methylguanine adduct, which accounts for 5% of the total adducts formed by TMZ,[226] in the agent's antitumor activity is supported by the correlation between the sensitivity of tumor cell lines to TMZ and the activity of the DNA repair protein AGT, which specifically removes alkyl groups at the O^6 position of guanine. Cell lines that have low levels of AGT are sensitive to the cytotoxicity of TMZ, whereas cell lines that have high levels of this repair protein are much more resistant to it.[229-232] This correlation also has been observed in human glioblastoma xenograft models.[233-235] The preferential alkylation of guanine and adenine and the correlation of sensitivity to the drug with the ability to repair the O^6-alkylguanine lesion also have been seen with triazine, DTIC, and the nitrosourea alkylating agents BCNU and CCNU.[232,236,237]

The cytotoxic mechanism of TMZ appears to be related to the failure of the DNA mismatch repair system to find a complementary base for methylated guanine. This system involves the formation of a complex of proteins that recognize, bind to, and remove methylated guanine.[238-240] The proposed hypothesis is that when this repair process is targeted to the DNA strand opposite the O^6-methylguanine, it cannot find a correct partner, thus resulting in long-lived nicks in the DNA.[241] These nicks accumulate and persist into the subsequent cell cycle, where they ultimately inhibit initiation of replication in the daughter cells, blocking the cell cycle at the G_2M boundary.[241-245] In murine[242] and human[246] leukemia cells, sensitivity to TMZ correlates with increased fragmentation of DNA and apoptotic cell death. More recent work has shown that TMZ induces G_2-M arrest through activation of Chk1 kinase with subsequent phosphorylation of Ccd 25 phosphatase and cdc2.[247,248] This has been shown to be p53-independent, although p53 status impacts on G_2-M arrest duration and outcome. Specifically, p53 wild-type cells undergo prolonged G_2-M arrest and senescence, whereas p53-deficient cells bypass cell cycle arrest and die by mitotic catastrophe. Since p53-proficient cells were less sensitive than p53-deficient cells to TMZ, it is possible that targeting the G_2 checkpoint might enhance TMZ-induced antitumor activity.[247,248] Additionally, O^6-methylguanine induced apoptosis is executed by the mitochondrial damage pathway, requires DNA replication, and is mediated by p53 and Fas/CD95/Apo-1.[249] Nevertheless, studies confirming that base excision repair mediates TMZ resistance have not yet been conclusively demonstrated.

DNA adducts formed by TMZ and the subsequent DNA damage or alteration of specific genes may cause cell death or reduce the metastatic potential of tumor cells. For example, mutations caused by adduct formation may result in altered surface antigens on tumor cells that contribute enhanced immunogenicity in the host.[250,251] The effects of enhanced immunologic response range from complete tumor rejection to reduced growth rates and reduced metastatic potential.[252] Additional evidence suggests that TMZ can reduce the metastatic potential of Lewis lung carcinoma cells[253] and induce differentiation in the K562 erythroleukemia cell line.[254] It has been postulated that TMZ- induced DNA damage and subsequent cell-cycle arrest may reduce the metastatic properties of some tumor cells.[254]

Mechanism of Resistance

AGT DNA Repair Protein

Several studies have shown that AGT is the primary mechanism of resistance to TMZ and other alkylating agents.[147,257] AGT functions as the first line of defense against TMZ by removing the alkyl groups from the O^6 position of guanine, in effect reversing the cytotoxic lesion of TMZ.[258] AGT levels can be correlated with the sensitivity of tumor cell lines to TMZ and the alkylating agents BCNU and DTIC.[237,246,259–262] The role of AGT in resistance to TMZ is also evidenced by the ability of the virally transfected human AGT gene to confer a high level of resistance to TMZ and other methylating and chloroethylating agents on cells that are devoid of endogenous AGT activity.[263]

AGT levels in human tumor tissues and normal tissue specimens derived from brain, lung, and ovary vary widely over a 100-fold range, with some human tumors having no detectable activity.[264–267] Some specimens from all tumor types examined in these studies have demonstrated a complete absence of AGT activity: as many as 22% of primary brain tumor specimens have no detectable AGT activity.[264] Similar findings with respect to AGT levels in brain tumor cells have been observed in in vitro models.[268] AGT activity has been localized to both the cytoplasm and the nucleus of the cell, although the function of cytoplasmic AGT and its mechanism of transport to the nucleus are unknown.[265] AGT transfers the methyl group to an internal cysteine residue, acting as methyltransferase and methyl acceptor protein. In the process, AGT becomes irreversibly inactivated, and new AGT must be synthesized to restore AGT activity.[61] Therefore, the number of O^6-methylguanine adducts that can be repaired is limited by the number of AGT molecules of the protein available.[61] Recent work has confirmed that elevated AGT levels in newly diagnosed glioblastoma multiforme are directly correlated with lack of response to TMZ[215] or survival following adjuvant therapy with this methylator.[269]

Deficiency in Mismatch Repair Pathway

Although AGT is clearly important in the resistance of cells to TMZ, some cell lines that express low levels of AGT are nevertheless resistant, indicating that other resistance mechanisms may be involved.[270,271] A deficiency in the mismatch repair pathway as a result of mutations in any one of the four proteins that recognize and repair DNA (i.e., GTBP, hMSH2, hPMS2, and hMLH1) can render cells tolerant to methylation and to the cytotoxic effects of TMZ. This deficiency in the mismatch repair pathway results in a failure to recognize and repair the O^6-methylguanine adducts produced by TMZ and other methylating agents.[63,230,272] The DNA damage that results from failure to repair the O^6-methylguanine adducts produces a particular type of genomic instability, microsatellite instability, that is associated with some familial and sporadic cancers, such as hereditary nonpolyposis colorectal cancer.[273,274] The high level of resistance in tumor cells that are deficient in mismatch repair is unrelated to the level of AGT and is, therefore, unaffected by AGT inhibitors.

Base Excision Repair

A series of studies have shown that two Temodar-initiated adducts, N^7-methylguanine and N^3-methyladenine, are not susceptible to AGT and produce cytotoxicity (particularly N^3-methyladenine), independently of DNA mismatch repair activity.[228,275–277] These lesions are promptly repaired by a series of enzymatic steps including N-methylpurine-DNA glycosylase, AP endonuclease, poly (ADP-ribose) polymerase (PARP) DNA polymerase β, x-ray repair cross complementing 1, and ligase III. Sensitization of tumor cells resistant to Temodar because of DNA mismatch repair deficiency have been rendered susceptible to this methylator by inhibition of base excision repair. Strategies have included inhibition of PARP[275–283] and use of methoxyamine.[228] Intriguingly, moderate enhancement of Temodar activity following base excision repair disruption was also seen in DNA mismatch repair proficient cells.[228,275–277] Nevertheless, conclusive evidence confirming that base excision repair mediates TMZ resistance has not yet been published.

Drug Interactions

There are no known adverse reactions with other drugs. It is expected that compounds that deplete AGT will increase TMZ toxicity.

Clinical Pharmacology and Toxicity

TMZ is supplied in capsules containing 5, 25, 100, or 250 mg for oral use. In the initial phase 1 trial in the United Kingdom, TMZ was administered as a single intravenous dose at doses of 50 to 200 mg/m^2 and subsequently was given orally to fasted patients as a single dose, up to a total dose of 200 to 1,200 mg/m^2. Additionally, oral doses of 750 to 1,200 mg/m^2 were divided into five equal doses and administered daily for 5 days at 4-week intervals.

The pharmacokinetics of TMZ were evaluated in the United Kingdom phase 1 trials.[209] After intravenous administration, plasma TMZ concentrations declined biexponentially consistent with a two-compartment open model and a terminal elimination half-life of 1.8 hours. After oral administration, plasma TMZ concentrations were consistent with a one-compartment oral model, with rapid absorption and maximum plasma concentrations occurring 0.7 hour after treatment. The clearance of TMZ was 11.8 L/hr, and the pharmacokinetics were independent of the dosage (with a linear relationship between dose and area under the time × concentration curve). Oral bioavailability was considered to be complete.

In 1993, Schering-Plough began the worldwide development of TMZ using machine-filled capsules that were prepared according to good manufacturing practices, which differed from the hand-filled capsules used in the initial study. Several phase 1 studies have evaluated the safety and tolerability of that new TMZ formulation (Temodar). Data from these studies have confirmed the safety, tolerability, and pharmacokinetics of TMZ reported in the CRC phase 1 study (Table 13.3).[284–292]

Phase 1 studies of TMZ also were expanded to include pediatric cancer patients. A phase 1 study was conducted to define the multiple-dose pharmacokinetics of TMZ in this population. In this study, 19 patients between 3 and 17 years old were given TMZ over a dosage range of 100 to 240 mg/m^2 per day. TMZ was absorbed rapidly, had an AUC that increased in a dosage-related manner, and showed no evidence of accumulation. The plasma half-life, whole-body clearance, and volume of distribution were independent of dosage (Table 13.4).[284] Compared with adult patients treated with 200 mg/m^2 per day, children appeared to have a higher AUC (48.7 versus 34.5 mg/hr per milliliter), most likely because children have a larger ratio of body surface area to volume. Despite higher concentrations at dosages equivalent to those used in adult patients, the bone marrow function in pediatric patients appears to allow greater exposure to the drug before dose-limiting bone marrow toxicity develops.[284]

The effects of food and gastric pH on the pharmacokinetics and bioavailability of orally administered TMZ also have been evaluated. Administration of TMZ after ingestion of food resulted in a small decrease in its oral bioavailability.[289] When TMZ was taken after a meal, a slight (9%), but statistically significant, reduction occurred in the rate and extent of its absorption (Table 13.5). Because AUC confidence levels were within the bioequivalence guidelines of 80 to 125%, it is unlikely that the slight reduction observed in the oral bioavailability of TMZ in the presence of a meal has any clinical effect on the antitumor activity of TMZ.

The oral bioavailability, maximum plasma concentration, and half-life of TMZ were not affected by an increase in gastric pH of 1 to 2 units, resulting from the administration of ranitidine every 12 hours on either the first 2 or the last 2 days of the 5-day TMZ dosing schedule.[291]

Subsequent phase 1 trials sponsored by Schering-Plough in adult[286-291] and pediatric patients[284,293] with advanced cancer also have confirmed that hematologic toxicity, specifically thrombocytopenia and neutropenia, is dose-limiting. Neutropenia or thrombocytopenia appeared 21 to 28 days after the first dose of each cycle and recovered to grade 1 myelosuppression within 7 to 14 days. Grade 4 toxicity occurred at cumulative oral dosages of more than 1,000 mg/m^2 over 5 days, but little other toxicity was seen.[287] Grade 3 or 4 myelosuppression occurred in less than 10% of patients studied.

The effect of prior treatment with chemotherapy, radiation, or both, on the maximum tolerated dose (MTD) of TMZ has been evaluated.[286,290] In one of these studies,[290] 24 patients stratified according to prior exposure to chemotherapy and radiation were given a dosage of 100 mg/m^2 per day of TMZ for 5 days, which was escalated to 150 and 200 mg/m^2 per day in the absence of myelosuppression. The MTD for TMZ was established as 150 mg/m^2 per day.[290] The other similar phase 1 study, reported by the National Cancer Institute, evaluated the safety of TMZ in patients who were stratified on the basis of prior exposure to nitrosourea.[286] The MTD for patients with prior exposure to nitrosourea was 150 mg/m^2 per day, and the MTD for patients without such prior exposure was 250 mg/m^2 per day. An evaluation of the pharmacokinetics of TMZ showed that its clearance from the plasma was significantly less in patients with prior exposure to nitrosourea than it was in patients without such prior exposure.[286] This may have contributed to the lower dose of TMZ that was tolerated by these patients and had a notable effect on the dosing recommendation for these patients.[286]

The results of these studies indicated that a dosage of 200 mg/m^2 of TMZ given on a 5-day schedule and repeated

---

TABLE 13.5

KEY FEATURES OF TEMOZOLOMIDE (8-CARBAMOYL-3-METHYLIMIDAZO [5,1-D]-1,2,3,5-TETRAZIN-4(3H)-ONE)

Mechanism of action:	Methylation of nucleic acids
Metabolism:	Chemical conversion of 5(3-methyltriazeno) imidazole-4-carboxamide
Pharmacokinetic Volume of distribution:	28.3 L
s (i.v. or p.o.):	Elimination half-life: 1.8 h
	Distribution half-life: 0.26 h
	Clearance: 11.76 L/h[253]
Drug and food interactions:	Unknown
Toxicity:	Myelosuppression
	Nausea and vomiting
	Elevated hepatic transaminases

every 28 days is appropriate for patients who are not pre-treated with radiation, chemotherapy, or both. Patients who are pretreated with chemotherapy receive a lower starting dose of TMZ (i.e., 150 mg/m^2), which can be escalated to 200 mg/m^2 in subsequent courses in the absence of grade 3 or 4 myelosuppression.[290]

REFERENCES

1. Newell D, Gescher A, Harland S, et al. N-Methyl antitumor agents: a distinct class of anticancer drugs? Cancer Chemother Pharmacol 1987;19:91.
2. Zeller P, Gutmann H, Hegedus B, et al. Methylhydrazine derivatives, a new class of cytotoxic agents. Experientia 1963;19:129.
3. Bollag W, Grunberg E. Tumour inhibitory effects of a new class of cytotoxic agents: methylhydrazine derivatives. Experientia 1963;19:130.
4. Bollag W. The tumor-inhibitory effects of the methylhydrazine derivative Ro 4-6467/1 (NSC-77213). Cancer Chemother Rep 1963;33:1.
5. Martz G, D'Allessandri A, Keel HJ, et al. Preliminary clinical results with a new anti-tumor agent Ro 4-6467 (NSC- 77213). Cancer Chemother Rep 1963;33:5.
6. Mathe G, Schweisguth O, Schneider M, et al. Methyl hydrazine in the treatment of Hodgkin's disease. Lancet 1963;2:1077.
7. Brunner KW, Young CW. A methylhydrazine derivative in Hodgkin's disease and other malignant neoplasms: therapeutic and toxic effects studies in 51 patients. Ann Intern Med 1965;63:69.
8. Samuels ML, Leary WV, Alexanian R, et al. Clinical trials with N-isopropyl-(2-methylhydrazino)-p-toluamide hydrochloride in malignant lymphoma and other disseminated neoplasia. Cancer 1967;20:1187.
9. Spivack SD. PCB. Ann Intern Med 1974;81:795.
10. DeVita VT, Serpick AA, Carbone PP. Combination chemotherapy in the treatment of advanced Hodgkin's disease. Ann Intern Med 1970;73:881.
11. Stolinsky DC, Solomon J, Pugh R, et al. Clinical experience with PCB in Hodgkin's disease, reticulum cell sarcoma, and lymphosarcoma. Cancer 1970;26:984.
12. DeVita VT, Canellos GP, Chabner B, et al. Advanced diffuse histiocytic lymphoma, a potentially curable disease. Lancet 1975;1:248.
13. DeVita VT, Hubbard SM, Longo DL. The chemotherapy of lymphomas: looking back, moving forward—the Richard and Hinda Rosenthal Foundation award lecture. Cancer Res 1987;47:5810.
14. Samuels ML, Leary WV, Howe CD. PCB (NSC-77213) in treatment of advanced bronchogenic carcinoma. Cancer Chemother Rep 1969;53:135.
15. Gersel Pedersen A, Sorenson S, Aabo K, et al. Phase II study of PCB in small cell carcinoma of the lung. Cancer Treat Rep 1982;66:273.
16. Daniels JR, Chak LY, Sikic BI, et al. Chemotherapy of small cell carcinoma of lung: a randomized comparison of alternating and sequential combination chemotherapy programs. J Clin Oncol 1984;2:1192.
17. Luce JK. Chemotherapy of malignant melanoma. Cancer 1972;30:1604.
18. Carmo-Pereira J, Costa FO, Henriques E. Combination cytotoxic chemotherapy with PCB, vincristine, and lomustine in disseminated malignant melanoma: 8 years follow-up. Cancer Treat Rep 1984;68:1211.
19. Kumar AR, Renaudin J, Wilson CB, et al. PCB hydrochloride in the treatment of brain tumors. J Neurosurg 1974;40:365.
20. Gutin PH, Wilson CB, Kumar AR, et al. Phase II study of PCB, CCNU, and vincristine combination chemotherapy in the treatment of brain tumors. Cancer 1975;35:1398.
21. Levin VA, Rodriguez LA, Edwards MSB, et al. Treatment of medulloblastoma with PCB, hydroxyurea, and reduced radiation dose to whole brain and spine. J Neurosurg 1988;68:383.
22. Rodriguez LA, Prados M, Silver P, et al. Reevaluation of PCB for the treatment of recurrent malignant central nervous system tumors. Cancer 1989;64:2420.
23. Newton HB, Junck L, Bromberg J, et al. PCB chemotherapy in the treatment of recurrent malignant astrocytomas after radiation and nitrosourea. Neurology 1990;40:1743.
24. Newton HB, Bromberg J, Junck L, et al. Comparison between BCNU and PCB chemotherapy for treatment of gliomas. J Neurooncol 1993;15:157.
25. Gale GR, Simpson JG, Smith AB. Studies of the mode of action of N-isopropyl-alpha-(2-methylhydrazino)-p-toluamide. Cancer Res 1967;27:1186.
26. Gutterman J, Huang AT, Hochstein P. Studies on the mode of action of N-isopropyl-alpha-(2-methylhydrazine)-p-toluamide. Proc Soc Exp Biol Med 1969;130:797.
27. Cummings SW, Guengerich FP, Prough RA. The characterisation of N-isopropyl-p-hydroxymethylbenzamide formed during the oxidative metabolism of azoPCB. Drug Metab Dispos 1982;10:459.
28. Shiba DA, Weinkam RJ. Quantitative analysis of PCB, PCB metabolites and chemical degradation products with application to pharmacokinetic studies. J Chromatogr 1982;229:397.
29. Prough RA, Tweedie DJ. PCB. In: Powis G, Prough RA, eds. Metabolism and Action of Anti-Cancer Drugs. London: Taylor & Francis, 1987:29.
30. Lee IP, Dixon RL. Effects of PCB on spermatogenesis determined by velocity sedimentation cell separation. J Pharmacol Exp Ther 1972;181:219.
31. Alley MC, Powis G, Appel PL, et al. Activation and inactivation of cancer chemotherapeutic agents by rat hepatocytes cocultured with human tumor cell lines. Cancer Res 1984; 44:549.
32. Prough RA, Coomes ML, Dunn DL. The microsomal metabolism of carcinogenic and/or therapeutic hydrazines. In: Ullrich V, Roots I, Hildebrandt A, et al., eds. Microsomes and Drug Oxidations. Oxford: Pergamon Press, 1977:500.
33. Weinkam RJ, Shiba DA. Metabolic activation of PCB. Life Sci 1978;22:937.
34. Dunn DL, Lubet RA, Prough RA. Oxidative metabolism of N-isopropyl-alpha-(2-methylhydrazino)-p-toluamide hydrochloride (PCB) by rat liver microsomes. Cancer Res 1979; 39:4555.
35. Prough RA, Wittkop JA, Reed DJ. Evidence for the hepatic metabolism of some monoalkylhydrazines. Arch Biochem Biophys 1969;131:369.
36. Baggiolini M, Dewald B, Aebi H. Oxidation of p-N1-methylhydrazinomethyl)-N-isopropylbenzamide to the methylazo derivative and oxidative cleavage of the N^2-C bond in the isolated perfused rat liver. Biochem Pharmacol 1969;18:2187.
37. Kuttab SH, Tanglerpaibul S, Vouros P. Studies on the metabolism of PCB by mass spectroscopy. Biomed Mass Spectrom 1982;9:78.
38. Molony SJ, Prough RA. Studies on the pathway of methane formation from PCB, a 2-methylbenzyl hydrazine derivative, by rat liver microsomes. Arch Biochem Biophys 1983;221:577.
39. Lam H, Begleiter A, Stein W, et al. On the mechanism of uptake of PCB by L5178Y lymphoblasts in vivo. Biochem Pharmacol 1978;27:1883.
40. Moloney SJ, Wiebkin P, Cummings SW, et al. Metabolic activation of the terminal N-methyl group of N-isopropyl- alpha-(2-methylhydrazino)-p-toluamide hydrochloride (PCB). Carcinogenesis 1985;6:397.
41. Kreis W, Yen Y. An antineoplastic C^{14}-labeled methylhydrazine derivative in P815 mouse leukemia: a metabolic study. Experientia 1965;21:284.
42. Matsumoto H, Higa HH. Studies on methylazoxymethanol, the aglycone of cycasin: methylation of nucleic acids in vitro. Biochem J 1966;98:20C.
43. Kreis W. Metabolism of an antineoplastic methylhydrazine derivative in a P815 mouse neoplasm. Cancer Res 1970; 30:82.
44. Sinha BK. Metabolic activation of PCB: evidence for carbon-centered free radical intermediates. Biochem Pharmacol 1984; 33:2777.
45. Berneis K, Kofler M, Bollag W, et al. The degradation of deoxyribonucleic acid by new tumor inhibiting compounds: the intermediate formation of hydrogen peroxide. Experientia 1963;19:132.

46. Shiba DA, Weinkam RJ. The in vivo cytotoxic activity of PCB and PCB metabolites against L1210 ascites leukemia cells in CDF$_1$ mice and the effects of pretreatment with PCB, phenobarbital, diphenylhydantoin, and methylprednisolone upon in vivo PCB activity. Cancer Chemother Pharmacol 1983;11:124.

47. Therman E. Chromosome breakage by 1-methyl-2-benzylhydrazine in mouse cancer cells. Cancer Res 1972;32:1133.

48. Rutishauser A, Bollag W. Cytological investigations with a new class of cytotoxic agent: methylhydrazine derivatives. Experientia 1963;19:131.

49. Erikson JM, Ducore JM, Prough RA. Genotoxic and cytotoxic effect of PCB (N-isopropyl-alpha-(2-methylhydrazino)-p-toluamide) and its metabolites in L1210 cells. Proc Am Assoc Cancer Res 1987;28:3.

50. Blijleven WG, Vogel E. The mutational spectrum of PCB on *Drosophila melanogaster*. Mutat Res 1977;45:47.

51. Ogawa K, Hiraku Y, Oikawa S, et al. Molecular mechanisms of DNA damage induced by procarbazine in the presence of Cu(II). Mutat Res 2003;539:145.

52. Sartorelli AC, Tsunamura S. Studies on the biochemical mode of action of a cytotoxic methylhydrazine derivative, N-isopropyl-alpha-(2-methylhydrazino)-p-toluamide. Mol Pharmacol 1966;2:275.

53. Koblet H, Diggelmann H. The action of ibenzmethyzin on protein synthesis in the rat liver. Eur J Cancer 1968;4:45.

54. Revel M, Littauer U. The coding properties of methyldeficient phenylalanine transfer RNA from *Escherichia coli*. J Mol Biol 1966;15:389.

55. Meer L, Schold SC, Kleihues P. Inhibition of the hepatic O^6-alkylguanine-DNA alkyltransferase in vivo by pretreatment with antineoplastic agents. Biochem Pharmacol 1989;38:929.

56. Rossi SC, Conrad M, Voigt JM, et al. Excision repair of O^6-methylguanine synthesised at the rat H-rasN-methyl-N- nitrosourea activation site and introduced in *Escherichia coli*. Carcinogenesis (Lond) 1989;10:373.

57. Swenberg JA, Bedell MA, Billings KC, et al. Cell-specific differences in O^6-alkylguanine DNA repair activity during continuous exposure to carcinogen. Proc Natl Acad Sci U S A 1982;79:5499.

58. Bedell MA, Lewis JG, Billings KC, et al. Cell specificity in hepatocarcinogenesis: O^6-methylguanine preferentially accumulates in target cell DNA during continuous exposure of rats to 1,2-dimethylhydrazine. Cancer Res 1982;42:3079.

59. Hall J, Kataoka H, Stephenson C, et al. O^6-Methylguanine and methylphosphotriesters to the cytotoxicity of alkylating agents in mammalian cells. Carcinogenesis (Lond) 1988;9:1587.

60. Schold SC Jr, Brent TP, von Hofe E, et al. O^6-Alkylguanine-DNA alkyltransferase and sensitivity to PCB in human brain tumor xenografts. J Neurosurg 1989;70:573.

61. Pegg AE. Mammalian O^6-alkylguanine-DNA alkyltransferase: regulation and importance in response to alkylating carcinogenic and therapeutic agents. Cancer Res 1990; 50:6119.

62. Huang A, Gutterman J, Hochstein P. Cytogenetic changes induced by PCB in Ehrlich ascites tumor cells. Experientia 1969; 25:203.

63. Friedman HS, Johnson SP, Dong Q, et al. Methylator resistance mediated by mismatch repair deficiency in a glioblastoma multiforme xenograft. Cancer Res 1997;57:2933.

64. Kat A, Thilly WG, Fang WH, et al. An alkylation-tolerant mutator human cell line is deficient in strand specific mismatch repair. Proc Natl Acad Sci U S A 1993;90:6424.

65. Koi M, Umar A, Chauhan DP, et al. Human chromosome 3 corrects mismatch repair deficiency and microsatellite instability and reduces N-methyl-N'-nitro-N-nitrosoguanidine tolerance in colon tumor cells with homozygous hMLH1 mutation. Cancer Res 1994;54:4308.

66. Oliverio VT, Denham C, DeVita VT, et al. Some pharmacologic properties of a new antitumor agent, N-isopropylalpha-(2-methylhydrazino)-p-toluamide hydrochloride (NSC-77213). Cancer Chemother Rep 1964;42:1.

67. Eade N, MacLeod S, Renton K. Inhibition of hepatic microsomal drug metabolism by the hydrazines Ro4-4602, MK486, and PCB hydrochloride. Can J Physiol Pharmacol 1972;50:721.

68. Lee IP, Lucier GW. The potentiation of barbiturate-induced narcosis by PCB. J Pharmacol Exp Ther 1976;196:586.

69. Reed D. Effects in vivo of lymphoma ascites tumors and PCB, alone and in combination, upon hepatic drug-metabolizing enzymes of mice. Biochem Pharmacol 1976;25:153.

70. Schwartz DE. Comparative metabolic studies with natulan, methylhydrazine, and methylamine in rats. Experientia 1966;22:212.

71. Hande KR, Noone RM. Cimetidine prolongs the half-life of PCB and hexamethylmelamine. Proc Am Assoc Cancer Res 1983;24:287.

72. DeVita V, Hahn M, Oliverio V. Monoamine oxidase inhibition by a new carcinostatic agent, PCB. Proc Soc Exp Biol Med 1965;120:561.

73. Chabner BA, DeVita VT, Considine N, et al. Plasma pyridoxal phosphate depletion by the carcinostatic PCB. Proc Soc Exp Biol Med 1969;132:1119.

74. Raaflaub J, Schwartz DE. Uber den Metabolismus eines cytostatisch wirksamen methylhydrazin-derivates (Natulan). Experientia 1965;21:44.

75. Baggliolini M, Bickel HM, Messiha FS. Demethylation in vivo of Natulan, a tumor-inhibiting methylhydrazine derivative. Experientia 1965;21:334.

76. Schwartz DE, Bollag W, Obrecht P. Distribution and excretion studies of PCB in animals and man. Arzneimittel-Forsch 1967;17:1389.

77. Dost FN, Reed DJ. Methane formation in vivo from N-isopropyl-alpha-(2-methylhydrazino)-p-toluamide hydrochloride, a tumor-inhibiting methylhydrazine derivative. Biochem Pharmacol 1967;16:1741.

78. Chabner BA, Sponzo R, Hubbard S, et al. High dose intermittent intravenous infusion of PCB (NSC-77213). Cancer Chemother Rep 1973;57:361.

79. Gescher A, Raymont C. Studies of the metabolism of N- methyl containing antitumor agents: $^{14}CO_2$ breath analysis after administration of ^{14}C-labelled N-methyl drugs, formaldehyde and formate in mice. Biochem Pharmacol 1981;30:1245.

80. Weinkam RJ, Shiba DA. Nonclassical alkylating agents: PCB. In: Chabner BA, ed. Pharmacologic Principles of Cancer Treatment. Philadelphia: Saunders, 1982:340.

81. Gorsen RM, Weiss AJ, Manthei RW. Analysis of PCB and metabolites by gas chromatography-mass spectrometry. J Chromatogr 1980;221:309.

82. Rucki RJ, Ross A, Moros SA. Application of an electrochemical detector to the determination of PCB hydrochloride by high-performance liquid chromatography. J Chromatogr 1980;190:359.

83. Wolff T, Dislerath LM, Worthington MT, et al. Substrate specificity of human liver cytochrome P-450 debrisoquine hydroxylase probed using immunochemical inhibition and chemical modeling. Cancer Res 1985;45:2116.

84. He X, Batchelor TT, Grossman S, Supko JG, and New Approaches to Brain Tumor Therapy (NABTT) CNS Consortium. Determination of procarbazine in human plasma: by liquid chromatography with electrospray ionization mass spectrometry. J Chromatogr B Analyt Technol Biomed Life 2004;799:281.

85. Wittkop JA, Prough RA, Reed DJ. Oxidative demethylation of N-methylhydrazines by rat liver microsomes. Arch Biochem Biophys 1969;134:308.

86. Coomes MW, Prough RA. The mitochondrial metabolism of 1,2-disubstituted hydrazines, PCB and 1,2-dimethylhydrazine. Drug Metab Dispos 1983;11:550.

87. Wiebkin P, Prough RA. Oxidative metabolism of N-isopropyl-alpha-(2-methylazo)-p-toluamide (azoPCB) by rodent liver microsomes. Cancer Res 1980;40:3524.

88. Prough RA, Brown MI, Dannan GA, et al. Major isozymes of rat liver microsomal cytochrome P-450 involved in the N-oxidation of N-isopropyl-alpha-(2-methylazo)-p-toluamide, the azo derivative of PCB. Cancer Res 1984;44:543.

89. DeVita V, Serpick A, Carbone P. Preliminary clinical studies with ibenz-methyzin. Clin Pharmacol Ther 1966;7:542.

90. Hoagland HC. Hematologic complications of cancer chemotherapy. Semin Oncol 1982;9:95.

91. Sponzo RW, Arseneau J, Canellos GP. PCB-induced oxidative haemolysis: relationship to in vivored cell survival. Br J Haematol 1974;27:587.

92. Weiss HD, Walker MD, Wiernik PH. Neurotoxicity of commonly used antineoplastic agents. N Engl J Med 1974;291:75.

93. Casimir A, Kavanagh J, Liu F, et al. Phase I trial of intravenous PCB administered as a 5 day continuous infusion: correlation with plasma levels of pyridoxal phosphate. Proc Am Assoc Cancer Res 1983;24:144.

94. Lokich JJ, Moloney WC. Allergic reaction to PCB. Clin Pharmacol Ther 1972;13:573.

95. Jones SE, Moore M, Blank N, et al. Hypersensitivity of PCB (Matulane) manifested by fever and pleuro pulmonary reaction. Cancer 1972;29:498.

96. Weiss RB. Hypersensitivity reactions to cancer chemotherapy. Semin Oncol 1982;9:5.

97. Dunagin WG. Clinical toxicity of chemotherapeutic agents: dermatologic toxicity. Semin Oncol 1982;9:14.

98. Garbes ID, Henderson ES, Gomez GA, et al. PCB-induced interstitial pneumonitis with a normal chest x-ray: a case report. Med Pediatr Oncol 1986;14:238.

99. Liske R. A comparative study of the action of cyclophosphamide and PCB on the antibody production in mice. Clin Exp Immunol 1973;15:271.

100. Sullivan KM, Shulman HM, Storb R, et al. Chronic graft- versus-host disease in 52 patients: adverse natural course and successful treatment with combination immunosuppression. Blood 1981; 57:26.

101. Parvinen L. Early effects of PCB (N-isopropyl-L-(2-methylhydrazino)-p-toluamide hydrochloride) on rat spermatogenesis. Exp Mol Pathol 1979;30:1.

102. Chryssanthou CP, Wallach RC, Atchison M. Meiotic chromosomal changes and sterility produced by nitrogen mustard and PCB in mice. Fertil Steril 1983;39:97.

103. Chaube S, Murphy M. Fetal malformations produced in rats by PCB. Teratology 1969;2:23.

104. Pueyo C. Natulan induces forward mutations to L-arabinose–resistance in Salmonella typhimurium. Mutat Res 1979;67:189.

105. Gatehouse DG, Paes DJ. A demonstration of the in vitro bacterial mutagenicity of PCB, using the microtitre fluctuation test and large concentrations of S9 fraction. Carcinogenesis 1983; 4:347.

106. Kelly MG, O'Gara RW, Yancey ST, et al. Comparative carcinogenicity of N-isopropyl-alpha-(2-methylhydrazino)-p- toluamide HCl (PCB hydrochloride), its degradation products, other hydrazines, and isonicotinic acid hydrazide. J Natl Cancer Inst 1969;42:337.

107. Sieber SM, Correa P, Dalgard DW, et al. Carcinogenic and other adverse effects of PCB in nonhuman primates. Cancer Res 1978; 38:2125.

108. Schilsky RL, Lewis BJ, Sherins RJ, et al. Gonadal dysfunction in patients receiving chemotherapy for cancer. Ann Intern Med 1980;93:109.

109. Chapman RM. Effect of cytotoxic therapy on sexuality and gonadal function. Semin Oncol 1982;9:84.

110. Waxman JH, Terry YA, Wrigley PF, et al. Gonadal function in Hodgkin's disease: long-term follow up of chemotherapy. Br Med J 1982;285:1612.

111. Schilsky RL, Sherins RJ, Hubbard SM, et al. Long-term follow up of ovarian function in women treated with MOPP chemotherapy for Hodgkin's disease. Am J Med 1981; 71:552.

112. Horning SJ, Hoppe RT, Kaplan HS, et al. Female reproductive potential after treatment for Hodgkin's disease. N Engl J Med 1981;304:1377.

113. Johnson JM, Thompson DJ, Haggerty GC, et al. The effect of prenatal PCB treatment on brain development in the rat. Teratology 1985;32:203.

114. Andrieu JM, Ochoa-Molina ME. Menstrual cycle, pregnancies and offspring before and after MOPP therapy for Hodgkin's disease. Cancer 1983;52:435.

115. Lacher MJ, Toner K. Pregnancies and menstrual function before and after combined radiation and chemotherapy for Hodgkin's disease. Cancer Invest 1986;4:93.

116. Glicksman AS, Pajak TF, Gottlieb A, et al. Second malignant neoplasms in patients successfully treated for Hodgkin's disease: a Cancer and Leukemia Group B study. Cancer Treat Rep 1982; 66:1035.

117. Grunwald HW, Rosner F. Acute myeloid leukemia following treatment of Hodgkin's disease. Cancer 1982;50:676.

118. Henry-Amar M. Quantitative risk of second cancer in patients in first complete remission from early stages of Hodgkin's disease. Natl Cancer Inst Monogr 1988;6:65.

119. Goldstein LS. Dominant lethal mutations induced in mouse spermatogonia by mechlorethamine, PCB, and vincristine administered in 2-drug and 3-drug combinations. Mutat Res 1987;191:171.

120. Yost GS, Horstman MG, El Walily AF, et al. PCB spermatogenesis toxicity: Deuterium isotope effects point to regioselective metabolism in mice. Toxicol Appl Pharmacol 1985; 80:316.

121. Horstman MG, Meadows GG, Yost GS. Separate mechanisms for PCB spermatotoxicity and anticancer activity. Cancer Res 1987;47:1547.

122. Montgomery JA. Experimental studies at Southern Research Institute with DTIC (NSC-45388). Cancer Treat Rep 1976;60: 125.

123. Shealy YF, Montgomery JA, Laster WR Jr. Antitumor activity of triazenoimidazoles. Biochem Pharmacol 1962;11:674.

124. Comis RL. DTIC (NSC 45388) in malignant melanoma: a perspective. Cancer Treat Rep 1976;60:165.

125. Frei E, Luce JK, Talley RW, et al. 5-(3,3-Dimethyl-1-triazeno) imidazole-4-carboxamide (NSC-45388) in the treatment of lymphoma. Cancer Chemother Rep 1972;56:667.

126. Cowan DH, Bergsagel DE. Intermittent treatment of metastatic malignant melanoma with high dose 5-(3,3-dimethyl- 1-triazeno)-imidazole-4-carboxamide (NSC-45388). Cancer Chemother Rep 1971;55:175.

127. Einhorn LH, Furnas B. Combination chemotherapy for disseminated melanoma with DTIC, vincristine, and methyl-CCNU. Cancer Treat Rep 1977;61:881.

128. Pritchard KI, Quirt IC, Cowan DH, et al. DTIC therapy in metastatic melanoma: a simplified dose schedule. Cancer Treat Rep 1980;64:1123.

129. Carey RW, Anderson JR, Green M, et al. Treatment of metastatic malignant melanoma with vinblastine, dacarbazine, and cisplatin: a report from the cancer and leukemia group B. Cancer Treat Rep 1986;70:329.

130. Bonadonna G, Zucali R, Monfardini S, et al. Combination chemotherapy of Hodgkin's disease with adriamycin, bleomycin, vinblastine and imidazole carboxamide versus MOPP. Cancer 36:252, 1975.

131. Bonadonna G, Valagussa P, Santoro A. Alternating non-cross-resistant combination chemotherapy or MOPP in stage IV Hodgkin's disease: a report of 8-year results. Ann Intern Med 1986;104:739.

132. Gottlieb JA, Benjamin RS, Baker LH, et al. Role of DTIC (NSC-45388) in the chemotherapy of sarcoma. Cancer Treat Rep 1976; 60:199.

133. Vogel CL, Primack A, Owor R, et al. Effective treatment of Kaposi's sarcoma with 5-(3,3-dimethyl-1-triazeno) imidazole-4-carboxamide (NSC-45388). Cancer Chemother Rep 1973;57: 65.

134. Luce JK, Thurman WG, Isascs BL, et al. Clinical trials with the anti-tumor agent 5-(3,3-dimethyl-1-triazeno)imidazole-4-carboxamide (NSC-45388). Cancer Chemother Rep 1970;54:119.

135. Finklestein JZ, Albo V, Ertel I, et al. 5-(3,3-Dimethyl-1-triazeno)imidazole-4-carboxamide (NSC-45388) in the treatment of solid tumors in children. Cancer Chemother Rep 1975;59:351.

136. Finklestein JZ, Klemperer MR, Evans A, et al. Multiagent chemotherapy for children with metastatic neuroblastoma: a report from Children's Cancer Study Group. Med Pediatr Oncol 1979;6:179.

137. Eyre HJ, Eltringham JR, Gehan EA, et al. Randomized comparisons of radiotherapy and carmustine versus PCB versus dacarbazine for the treatment of malignant gliomas following surgery: a Southwest Oncology Group Study. Cancer Treat Rep 1986;70: 1085.

138. Kessinger A, Foley JF, Lemon HM. Therapy of malignant APUD cell tumors: effectiveness of DTIC. Cancer 1983; 51:790.

139. Averbuch SD, Steakley CS, Young RC, et al. Malignant pheochromocytoma: effective treatment with a combination of cyclophosphamide, vincristine, and dacarbazine. Ann Intern Med 1988; 109:267.

140. Altimari AF, Badrinath K, Reisel HJ, et al. DTIC therapy in patients with malignant intra-abdominal neuroendocrine tumors. Surgery 1987;102:1009.

141. Clarke DA, Barcley RK, Stock CC, et al. Triazenes as inhibitors of mouse sarcoma 180. Proc Soc Exp Biol Med 1955; 90:484.

142. Schmid FA, Hutchison DJ. Chemotherapeutic, carcinogenic, and cell-regulatory effects of triazenes. Cancer Res 1974;34:1671.

143. Hayward IP, Parsons PG. Comparison of virus reactivation, DNA base damage, and cell cycle effects in autologous melanoma cells resistant to methylating agents. Cancer Res 1984;44:55.

144. Gibson NW, Hartley JA, LaFrance RJ, et al. Differential cytotoxicity and DNA-damaging effects produced in human cells of the Mer+ and Mer– phenotypes by a series of alkyltriazenylimidazoles. Carcinogenesis (Lond) 1986;7:259.

145. Lunn JM, Harris AL, Brown PM, et al. Potential of the cytotoxic action of DTIC: involvement of O^6-methylguanine–DNA-methyltransferase. Br J Cancer 1986;54:186.

146. Catapano CV, Broggini M, Erba E, et al. In vitro and in vivo methazolostone-induced DNA damage and repair in L1210 leukemia sensitive and resistant to chlorethylnitrosoureas. Cancer Res 1987;47:4884.

147. D'Incalci M, Citti L, Taverna P, et al. Importance of DNA repair enzyme O^6-alkyltransferase (AT) in cancer chemotherapy. Cancer Treat Rev 1988;15:279.

148. Lunn JM, Harris AL. Cytotoxicity of 5-(3-methyl-1-triazeno) imidazole-4-carboxamide (MTIC) on Mer+, Mer+, Rem- and Mer- cells: differential potentiation by 3-acetamidobenzamide. Br J Cancer 1988;57:54.

149. Foster BJ, Newell DR, Lunn JM, et al. Correlation of dacarbazine and CB10-277 activity against human melanoma xenografts with O^6-alkyltransferase. Proc Am Assoc Cancer Res 1990;31: 401.

150. Mitchell RB, Dolan ME. Effect of temozolomide and dacarbazine on O^6-alkylguanine–DNA alkyltransferase activity and sensitivity of human tumor cells and xenografts to 1,3- bis(2-chloroethyl)-1-nitrosourea. Cancer Chemother Pharmacol 1993;32:59.

151. Lee SM, Thatcher N, Dougal M, et al. Dosage and cycle effects of dacarbazine (DTIC) and fotemustine on O^6-alkylguanine–DNA alkyltransferase in human peripheral blood mononuclear cells. Br J Cancer 1993;67:216.

152. Lev DC, Ruiz M, Mills L, et al. Dacarbazine causes transcriptional up-regulation of interleukin 8 and vascular endothelial growth factor in melanoma cells: a possible escape mechanism from chemotherapy. Mol Cancer Ther 2003;2:753.

153. Farquhar D, Loo TL, Gutterman JU, et al. Inhibition of drug metabolizing enzymes in the rat after bacillus Calmette-Guérin treatment. Biochem Pharmacol 1976;25:1529.

154. Breithaupt H, Dammann A, Aigner K. Pharmacokinetics of dacarbazine (DTIC) and its metabolite 5-aminoimidazole- 4-carboxamide (AIC) following different dose schedules. Cancer Chemother Pharmacol 1982;9:103.

155. Benvenuto JA, Hall SW, Farquhar D, et al. High-pressure liquid chromatography in pharmacological studies of anticancer drugs. Chromatogr Sci 1979;10:377.

156. Lipton A, Hepner GW, White DS, et al. Decreased hepatic drug demethylation in patients receiving chemo-immunotherapy. Cancer 1978;41:1680.

157. Buesa JM, Gracia M, Valle M, et al. Phase I trial of intermittent high-dose dacarbazine. Cancer Treat Rep 1984;68:499.

158. Savlov ED, Hall TC, Oberfield RA. Intra-arterial therapy of melanoma with dimethyl triazeno imidazole carboxamide (NSC-45388). Cancer 1971;28:1161.

159. Einhorn LH, McBride CM, Luke JK, et al. Intra-arterial infusion therapy with 5-(3,3-dimethyl-1-triazeno)imidazole-4-carboxamide (NSC-45388) for malignant melanoma. Cancer 1973;32:749.

160. Jortay AM, Lejeune FJ, Kenis Y. Regional chemotherapy of maxillofacial malignant melanoma with intracarotid artery infusion of DTIC. Tumori 1977;63:299.

161. Aigner K, Hild P, Henneking K, et al. Regional perfusion with cisplatinum and dacarbazine. Rec Res Cancer Res 1983;86:239.

162. Mizuno NS, Humphrey EW. Metabolism of 5-(3,3-dimethyl-1-triazeno)imidazole-4-carboxamide (NSC 45388) in human and animal tumor tissue. Cancer Chemother Rep 1972; 56:465.

163. Householder GE, Loo TL. Disposition of 5-(3,3-dimethyl- 1-triazeno)imidazole-4-carboxamide, a new antitumor agent. J Pharmacol Exp Ther 1971;179:386.

164. Skibba JL, Ramirez G, Beal DD, et al. Metabolism of 4(5)-(3,3-dimethyl-1-triazeno)imidazole-5(4)-carboxamide to 4(5)-amino-imidazole-5(4)-carboxamide in man. Biochem Pharmacol 1970;19:2043.

165. Loo TL, Stasswender EA. Colorimetric determination of dialkyltriazenoimidazoles. J Pharm Sci 1967;56:1016.

166. Loo TL, Luce JK, Jardine H, et al. Pharmacologic studies of the antitumor agent 5-(dimethyl-triazeno)imidazole-4-carboxamide. Cancer Res 1968;28:2448.

167. Skibba JL, Ramirez G, Beal DD, et al. Preliminary clinical trial and the physiologic disposition of 4(5)-(3,3-dimethyl- 1-triazeno)imidazole-5(4)-carboxamide in man. Cancer Res 1969; 29:1944.

168. Fiore D, Jackson AJ, Didolkar MS, et al. Simultaneous determination of dacarbazine, its photolytic degradation product, 2-azahypoxanthine, and the metabolite 5-aminoimidazole-4-carboxamide in plasma and urine by high- pressure liquid chromatography. Antimicrob Agents Chemother 1985;27:977.

169. Farina P, Benfenati BR, Torti L, et al. Metabolism of the anticancer agent 1-(4-acetylphenyl)-3,3-dimethyltriazene. Biomed Mass Spectrom 1983;10:485.

170. Venditti JM. Antitumor activity of DTIC (NSC-45388) in animals. Cancer Treat Rep 1976;60:135.

171. Hill DL. Microsomal metabolism of triazenylimidazoles. Cancer Res 1975;35:3106.

172. Shealy YF, Krauth CA, Holum B, et al. Synthesis and properties of the antileukemic agent 5(or4)-3,3-bis(2-chloroethyl)1-triazenoimidazole-4(or 5)carboxamide. J Pharm Sci 1969;57:83.

173. Sava G, Giraldi T, Lassiani L, et al. Metabolism and mechanism of the antileukemic action of isomeric aryldimethyltriazenes. Cancer Treat Rep 1982;66:1751.

174. Ray SK, Basak SC, Raychaudhury C, et al. The utility of information content, hydrophobicity, and van der Waals volume in the design of barbiturates and tumor inhibitory triazenes: a comparative study. Arzheim Forsch 1983;33:352.

175. Steven MFG. DTIC: a springboard to new antitumour agents. In: Reinhoudt DW, Connors TA, Pinedo HM, et al., eds. Structure-Activity Relationships of Antitumour Agents. The Hague: Martinus Nijhoff, 1983:183.

176. Wilman DEV, Cox PJ, Goddard PM, et al. Tumor inhibitory triazenes: 3. Dealkylation within an homologous series and its relation to antitumor activity. J Med Chem 1984;27:870.

177. Vaughan K, Tang Y, Llanos G, et al. Studies of the mode of action of antitumor triazenes and triazines: 6. 1-Aryl-3- (hydroxymethyl)-3-methyltriazenes: synthesis, chemistry and antitumor properties. J Med Chem 1984;27:357.

178. Shealy YF. Synthesis and biological activity of 5-amino imidazoles and 5-triazenoimidazoles. J Pharm Sci 1970; 59:1533.

179. Moore GE, Meiselbaugh D. DTIC (NSC-45388) toxicity. Cancer Treat Rep 1976;60:219.

180. Beck TM, Hart NE, Smith CE. Photosensitivity reaction following DTIC administration: report of two cases. Cancer Treat Rep 1980;64:725.

181. Fosch PJ, Cazarnetzki BM, Macher E, et al. Hepatic failure in a patient treated with DTIC for malignant melanoma. J Cancer Res Clin Oncol 1979;95:281.

182. Greenstone MA, Dowd PM, Mikhailidis DP, et al. Hepatic vascular lesions associated with dacarbazine treatment. Br Med J 1981;282:1744.

183. Feaux de Lacroix W, Runne U, Hauk H, et al. Acute liver dystrophy with thrombosis of hepatic veins: a fatal complication of dacarbazine treatment. Cancer Treat Rep 1983; 67:779.

184. McClay E, Lusch CJ, Mastrangelo MJ. Allergy-induced hepatic toxicity associated with dacarbazine. Cancer Treat Rep 1987; 71:219.

185. Ceci G, Bella M, Melissari M, et al. Fatal hepatic vascular toxicity of DTIC: is it really a rare event? Cancer 1988;61:1988.

186. Puccetti P, Giampietri A, Fioretti MC. Long-term depression of two primary immune responses induced by a single dose of 5-(3,3-dimethyl-1-triazeno)-imidazole-4-carboxamide (DTIC). Experientia 34:799, 1978.

187. Nardelli B, Puccetti P, Romani L, et al. Chemical xenogenication of murine lymphoma cells with triazine derivatives: immunotoxicological studies. Cancer Immunol Immunother 17:213, 1984.

188. Mantovani A, Luini W, Peri G, et al. Effect of chemotherapeutic agents on natural cell-mediated cytotoxicity in mice. J Natl Cancer Inst 61:1255, 1978.

189. Romani L, Migliorati G, Bonmassar E, et al. Susceptibility of murine lymphoma cells treated with 5-(3,3- dimethyl-1-triazenyl)-1*H* imidazole-4-carboxamide to NK-mediated cytotoxicity in vitro. Int J Immunopharmacol 1985;5:299.

190. Tamaro M, Dolzani L, Monti-Bragadin C, et al. Mutagenic activity of the dacarbazine analogue *p*-(3,3-dimethyl-1-triazeno) benzoic acid potassium salt in bacterial cells. Pharmacol Res Commun 1986;18:491.

191. Singh B, Gupta RS. Mutagenic responses of thirteen anticancer drugs on mutation at multiple genetic loci and on sister chromatid exchanges in Chinese hamster ovary cells. Cancer Res 1983;43:577.

192. Skibba JL, Erturk E, Bryan GT. Induction of thymic lymphosarcomas and mammary adenocarcinomas in rats by oral administration of the antitumor agent 4(5)-(3,3-dimethyl-1- triazeno)-imidazole-5(4)-carboxamide. Cancer 1970;26:1000.

193. Beal DD, Skibba JL, Croft WA, et al. Carcinogenicity of the antineoplastic agent, 5-(3,3-dimethyl-1-triazeno)-imidazole-4-carboxamide, and its metabolites in rats. J Natl Cancer Inst 1975;54:951.

194. Weisburger JH, Griswold DP, Prejean JD, et al. I: Tumor induction by cytostatics? The carcinogenic properties of some of the principal drugs used in clinical cancer chemotherapy. Rec Res Cancer Res 1975;52:1.

195. Valagussa P, Santoro A, Fossati Bellani F, et al. Absence of treatment-induced second neoplasms after ABVD in Hodgkin's disease. Blood 1982;59:488.

196. Brusamolino E, Papa G, Valagussa P, et al. Treatment- related leukemia in Hodgkin's disease: a multi-institution study on 75 cases. Hematol Oncol 1987;5:83.

197. Carey RW, Kunz VS. Acute nonlymphocytic leukemia (ANLL) following treatment with dacarbazine for malignant melanoma. Am J Hematol 1987;25:119.

198. Chaube S, Swinyard CA. Urogenital anomalies in fetal rats produced by the anticancer agent 4(5)-(3,3-dimethyl-1-triazeno)-imidazole-4-carboxamide. Anat Rec 1976;186:461.

199. Thompson DJ, Molello JA, Sterbing RJ, et al. Reproduction and teratology studies with oncolytic agents in the rat and rabbits: II. 5-(3,3-Dimethyl-1-triazeno)-imidazole-4- carboxamide (DTIC). Toxicol Appl Pharmacol 1975;33:281.

200. Baldwin RW, Partridge MW, Stevens MFG. Pyrazolotriazines: a new class of tumour-inhibitory agents. J Pharm Pharmacol 1966;18S:1S.

201. Harrap KA, Connors TA, Stevens MFG. Second-generation azolotetrazinones. In: New Avenues in Developmental Cancer Chemotherapy. London: Academic Press, 1987:335.

202. Stevens MFG, Hickman JA, Stone R, et al. Antitumor imidazotetrazines: 1. Synthesis and chemistry of 8-carbamoyl- 3(2-chloroethyl)imidazo[5,2-D]-1,2,3,5-tetrazin-4(3*H*)-one, a novel broad-spectrum antitumor agent. J Med Chem 1984;27:196.

203. Hickman JA, Stevens MFG, Gibson NW, et al. Experimental antitumor activity against murine tumor model systems of 8-carbamoyl-3(2-chloroethyl)imidazo[5,1-D]-1,2,3,5-tetrazin-4(3*H*)-one (mitozolomide), a novel broad-spectrum agent. Cancer Res 1985;45:3008.

204. Newlands ES, Backledge G, Slack JA, et al. Phase I clinical trial of mitozolomide. Cancer Treat Rep 1985;69:801.

205. Horspool KR, Stevens MFG, Newton CG, et al. Antitumor imidazotetrazines: 20. Preparation of the 8-acid derivative of mitozolomide and its utility in the preparation of active antitumor agents. J Med Chem 1990;30:1393.

206. Stevens MFG, Hickman JA, Langdon SP, et al. Antitumor activity and pharmacokinetics in mice of 8-carbamoyl- 3(2-chloroethyl) imidazo[5,1-D]-1,2,3,5-tetrazin-4(3*H*)-one (CCRG81045; MB39831), a novel drug with potential as an alternative to dacarbazine. Cancer Res 1987;47:5846.

207. Stevens MFG, Newlands ES. From triazines and triazenes to temozolomide. Eur J Cancer 1993;29A:1045.

208. Tsang LL, Quarterman CP, Gescher A, et al. Comparison of the cytotoxicity in vitro of temozolomide and dacarbazine, prodrugs of 3-methyl-(trizen-1-yl) imidazole-4 carboxamide. Cancer Chemother Pharmacol 1991;27:342.

209. Newlands ES, Blackledge GP, Slack JA, et al. Phase I trial of temozolomide (CCRG81045: MB39831: NSC-362856). Br J Cancer 1992;65:287.

210. O'Reilly SM, Newlands ES, Glaser MG, et al. Temozolomide: a new oral cytotoxic chemotherapeutic agent with promising activity against primary brain tumours. Eur J Cancer 1993;29A:940.

211. Newlands ES, O'Reilly SM, Glaser MG, et al. The Charing Cross Hospital experience with temozolomide in patients with gliomas. Eur J Cancer 1996;32A:2236.

212. Bower M, Newlands ES, Bleehen NM, et al. Multicentre CRC phase II trial of temozolomide in recurrent or progressive high-grade glioma. Cancer Chemother Pharmacol 1997;40:484.

213. Yung A, Levin VA, Brada M, et al. Randomized, multicenter, open-label, Phase II, comparative study of temozolomide and procarbazine in the treatment of patients with glioblastoma multiforme at first relapse. Br J Cancer 2000;83:588–593.

214. Yung A, Prados M, Poisson M, for the Temodal Brain Tumor Group. Multicenter Phase II trial of temozolomide in patients with malignant astrocytoma at first relapse. J Clin Oncol 1999;17:2762–2769.

215. Friedman HS, McLendon RE, Kerby T, et al. DNA mismatch repair and O^6-alkylguanine-DNA alkyltransferase analysis and response to Temodal in newly diagnosed malignant glioma. J Clin Oncol 1998;6:3851.

216. Stupp R, Dietrich P-Y, Ostermann K, et al. Promising survival for patients with newly diagnosed glioblastoma multiforme treated with concomitant radiation plus temozolomide followed by adjuvant temozolomide. J Clin Oncol 20:1375-1382, 2002.

217. Stupp R, Mason WP, Van Den Bent MJ, et al. Concomitant and adjuvant temozolomide and radiotherapy for newly diagnosed glioblastoma multiforme. Conclusive results of a randomized phase III trial by the EORTC Brain and RT Groups and NCIC Clinical Trials Group. Proc Am Soc Clin Oncol 23:1, 2004.

218. Quinn JA, Reardon DA, Friedman AH, et al. Phase II trial of temozolomide in patients with progressive low grade glioma. J Clin Oncol 2003;21:646.

219. van den Bent MJ, Taphoorn MJ, Brandes AA, et al.; European Organization for Research and Treatment of Cancer Brain Tumor Group. Phase II study of first-line chemotherapy with temozolomide in recurrent oligodendroglial tumors: the European Organization for Research and Treatment of Cancer Brain Tumor Group Study 26971. J Clin Oncol 2003;21:2525.

220. Chamberlain MC, Tsao-Wei DD, Groshen S. Temozolomide for treatment-resistant recurrent meningioma. Neurology 2004; 62:1210.

221. Blehen NM, Newlands ES, Lee SM, et al. Cancer Research Campaign phase II trial of temozolomide in metastatic melanoma. J Clin Oncol 1995;13:910.

222. Clark AS, Stevens MFG, Sansom CE, et al. Anti-tumor imidazotetrazines. Part XXI. Mitozolomide and temozolomide: probes for the major groove of DNA. Anti-Cancer Drug Design 1990;5:63.

223. Lowe PR, Sansom CE, Schwalbe CH, et al. Antitumour imidazotetrazines. 25. Crystal structure of 8-carbamoyl-3-methylimidazo[5,1-*d*]-1,2,3,4-tetrazin-4(3*H*)-one (temozolomide) and structural comparisons with the related drugs mitozolomide and DTIC. J Med Chem 1992;35:3377.

224. Clark AS, Deans B, Stevens MGF, et al. Antitumor imidazotetrazines. 32. Synthesis of novel imidazotetrazinones and related bicyclic heterocyles to probe the mode of action of the antitumor drug temozolomide. J Med Chem 1995; 38:1493.

225. Spassova MK, Golovinsky EV. Pharmacobiochemistry of arylalkyltriazenes and their application in cancer chemotherapy. Pharmacol Ther 1985;27:333.

226. Denny BJ, Wheelhouse RT, Stevens MFG, et al. NMR and molecular modeling investigation of the mechanism of activation of the antitumor drug temozolomide and its interaction with DNA. Biochem 1994;33:9045.

227. Bull VL, Tisdale MJ. Antitumor imidazotetrazines—XVI. Macromolecular alkylation by 3-substituted imidazotetrazinones. Biochem Pharmacol 1987;36:3215.

228. Liu L, Taverna P, Whitacre CM, et al. Pharmacologic disruption of base excision repair sensitizes mismatch repair-deficient and –proficient colon cancer cells to methylating agents. Clin Cancer Res 1999;5:2908.

229. D'Atri S, Bonmassar E, Franchi A, et al. Repair of DNA methyl adducts and sensitivity to temozolomide of acute myelogenous leukemia (AML) cells. Exp Hematol 1991; 19:530 (abst 276).

230. Wedge SR, Porteous JK, Newlands ES. 3-Aminobenzamide and/or O^6-benzylguanine evaluated as an adjunct to temozolomide or BCNU treatment in cells of variable mismatch repair status and O^6-alkylguanine-DNA alkyltransferase activity. Br J Cancer 1996;1030.

231. Wedge SR, Porteous JK, May BL, et al. Potentiation of temozolomide and BCNU cytotoxicity by O^6-benzylguanine: a comparative study *in vitro*. Br J Cancer 1996;73:482.

232. Dolan ME, Mitchell RB, Mummert C, et al. Effect of O^6- benzylguanine analogues on sensitivity of human tumor cells to the cytotoxic effects of alkylating agents. Cancer Res 1991;51:3367.

233. Friedman HS, Dolan ME, Pegg AE, et al. Activity of temozolomide in the treatment of central nervous system tumor xenografts. Cancer Res 1995;55:2853.

234. Plowman J, Waud WR, Koutsoukos AD, et al. Preclinical antitumor activity of temozolomide in mice: efficacy against human brain tumor xenografts and synergism with 1,3-bis (2-chloroethyl)-1-nitrosourea. Cancer Res 1994;54:3793.

235. Wedge SR, Porteous JK, Newlands ES. Effect of single and multiple administration of an O^6-benzylguanine/temozolomide combination: an evaluation in a human melanoma xenograft model. Cancer Chemother Pharmacol 1997;40:266.

236. Dolan ME, Moschel RC, Pegg AE. Depletion of mammalian O^6-alkylguanine-DNA alkyltransferase activity by O^6- benzylguanine provides a means to evaluate the role of this protein in protection against carcinogenic and therapeutic alkylating agents. Proc Natl Acad Sci U S A 1990;87:5368.

237. D'Atri S, Piccioni D, Castellano A, et al. Chemosensitivity to triazine compounds and O^6-alkylguanine-DNA alkyltransferase levels: studies with blasts of leukaemic patients. Ann Oncol 1995;6:389.

238. Drummond JT, Li G-M, Longley MJ, et al. Isolation of an hMSH2-p160 heterodimer that restores DNA mismatch repair to tumor cells. Science 1995;268:1909.

239. Palombo F, Gallinari P, Iaccarino I, et al. GTBP, a 160-kilodalton protein essential for mismatch-binding activity in human cells. Science 1995;268:1912.

240. Li G-M, Modrich P. Restoration of mismatch repair to nuclear extracts of H6 colorectal tumor cells by a heterodimer of human MutL homologs. Proc Natl Acad Sci U S A 1995;92:1950.

241. Karran P, Macpherson P, Ceccotti S, et al. O^6-methylguanine residues elicit DNA repair synthesis by human cell extracts. J Biol Chem 1993;268:15878.

242. Taverna P, Catapano CV, Citti L, et al. Influence of O^6- methylguanine on DNA damage and cytotoxicity of temozolomide in L1210 mouse leukemia sensitive and resistant to chloroethylnitrosoureas. Anticancer Drugs 1992;3:401.

243. Karran P, Hampson R. Genomic instability and tolerance to alkylating agents. Cancer Surv 1996;28:69.

244. Karran P, Bignami M. Self-destruction and tolerance in resistance of mammalian cells to alkylation damage. Nucleic Acids Res 1992;20:2933.

245. Ceccotti S, Dogliottie E, Gannon J, et al. O^6-methylguanine in DNA inhibits replication in vitro by human cell extracts. Biochem 1993;32:13664.

246. Tentori L, Graziani G, Gilberti S, et al. Triazine compounds induce apoptosis in O^6alkylguanine-DNA alkyltransferase deficient leukemia cell lines. Leukemia 1995;9:1888.

247. Hirose Y, Berger MS, Pieper RO: Abrogation of the Chk1-mediated G_2 checkpoint pathway potentiates temozolomide-induced toxicity in a p53-independent manner in human glioblastoma cells. Cancer Res 2001;61:5843.

248. Hirose Y, Berger MS, Pieper RO: p53 effects both the duration of G_2/M arrest and the fate of temozolomide-treated human glioblastoma cells. Cancer Res 2001;61:1957.

249. Roos W, Baumgartner M, Kaina B. Apoptosis triggered by DNA damage O6-methylguanine in human lymphocytes requires DNA replication and is mediated by p53 and FAS/CD95/Apo-1. Oncogene 2004;23:359.

250. Puccetti P, Romani L, Fioretti MC. Chemical xenogenization of experimental tumors. Cancer Metastasis Rev 1987; 6:93.

251. Bianchi R, Citti L, Beghetti R, et al. O^6-methylguanine- DNA methyltransferase activity and induction of novel immunogenicity in murine tumor cells treated with methylating agents. Cancer Chemother Pharmacol 1992;29:277.

252. Allegrucci M, Fuschiotti P, Puccetti P, et al. Changes in the tumorigenic and metastatic properties of murine melanoma cells treated with a triazine derivative. Clin Exp Metastasis 1989;7:329.

253. Tentori L, Leonetti C, Aquino A. Temozolomide reduces the metastatic potential of Lewis lung carcinoma (3LL) in mice: role of alpha-6 integrin phosphorylation. Eur J Cancer 1995;31A:746.

254. Tisdale MJ. Antitumor imidazotetrazines-X. Effect of 8-carbamoyl-3-methylimidazo[5,1-*d*]-1,2,3,5-tetrazine-4-(3H)-one (CCRG 81045; M&B 39831; NSC 362856) on DNA methylation during induction of haemoglobin synthesis in human leukaemia cell line K562. Biochem Pharmacol 1986;35:311.

255. Tisdale MJ. Antitumor imidazotetrazines and gene expression. Acta Oncol 1988;27:511.

256. Tisdale MJ. Antitumor imidazotetrazines-XVIII. Modification of the level of 5-methylcytosine in DNA by 3-substituted imidazotetrazinones. Biochem Pharmacol 1989;38:1097.

257. Pegg AE, Dolan ME, Moschel RC. Structure, function, and inhibition of O^6-alkylguanine-DNA alkyltransferase. Prog Nucleic Acid Res Mol Biol 1995;51:167.

258. Pegg AE. Alkylation and subsequent repair of DNA after exposure of dimethylnitrosamine and related carcinogens. Rev Biochem Toxicol 1983;5:83.

259. Tisdale MJ. Antitumor imidazotetrazines-XV. Role of guanine O^6 alkylation in the mechanism of cytotoxicity of imidazotetrazinones. Biochem Pharmacol 1987;36:457.

260. Baer JC, Freeman AA, Newlands ES, et al. Depletion of O^6- alkylguanine-DNA alkyltransferase correlates with potentiation of temozolomide and CCNU toxicity in human tumor cells. Br J Cancer 1993;67:1299.

261. Redmond SMS, Joncourt F, Buser K, et al. Assessment of P- glycoprotein, glutathione-based detoxifying enzymes and O^6-alkylguanine-DNA alkyltransferase as potential indicators of constitutive drug resistance in human colorectal tumors. Cancer Res 1991; 51:2092.

262. Franchi A, Papa G, D'Atri S, et al. Cytotoxic effects of dacarbazine in patients with acute myelogenous leukemia: a pilot study. Haematologica 1992;77:146.

263. Wang G, Weiss, Sheng P, et al. Retrovirus-mediated transfer of the human O^6-methylguanine-DNA-methyltransferase gene into a murine hematopoietic stem cell line and resistance to the toxic effects of certain alkylating agents. Biochem Pharmacol 1996;51:1221.

264. Citron M, Decker R, Chen S, et al. O^6-methylguanine- DNA methyltransferase in human normal and tumor tissue from brain, lung and ovary. Cancer Res 1991;51:4131.

265. Belanich M, Randall T, Pastor MA, et al. Intracellular localization and intracellular heterogeneity of the human DNA repair protein O^6-methylguanine-DNA methyltransferase. Cancer Chemother Pharmacol 1996;37:547.

266. Wiestler O, Kleihues P, Pegg A. O^6-alkylguanine-DNA alkyltransferase activity in human brain and brain tumors. Carcinogenesis 1984;5:121.

267. Frosina G, Rossi O, Arena G, et al. O^6-alkylguanine-DNA alkyltransferase activity in human brain tumors. Cancer Lett 1990; 55:153.

268. Yarosh D. The role of O^6-methylguanine-DNA methyltransferase in cell survival, mutagenesis and carcinogenesis. Mutat Res 1985;145:1.

269. Hegi Hegi ME, Diserens AC, Godard S, et al. Clinical trial substantiates the predictive value of O-6-methylguanine-DNA methyltransferase promoter methylation in glioblastoma patients treated with temozolomide. Clin Cancer Res 2004;10:1871.

270. Walker MC, Masters JRW, Margison GP. O^6-alkylguanine- DNA alkyltransferase activity in nitrosourea sensitivity in human cancer cell lines. Br J Cancer 1990;66:840.

271. Bobola MS, Tseng SH, Blank A, et al. Role of O^6-methylguanine-DNA methyltransferase in resistance of human brain tumor cell lines to the clinically relevant methylating agents temozolomide and streptozotocin. Clin Cancer Res 1996;2:735.

272. Liu L, Markowitz S, Gerson SL. Mismatch repair mutations override alkyltransferase in conferring resistance to temozolomide but not to 1,3-Bis(2-chloroethyl) nitrosourea. Cancer Res 1996; 56:5375.

273. Ionov Y, Peinado MA, Malkhosyan S, et al. Ubiquitous somatic mutations in simple repeated sequences reveal a new mechanism for colonic carcinogenesis. Nature 1993;363:558.

274. Aaltonen LA, Peltomaki P, Leach FS, et al. Clues to the pathogenesis of familial colorectal cancer. Science 1993; 260:812.

275. Tentori L, Leonetti C, Scarsella M, et al. Combined treatment with temozolomide and poly(ADP-ribose) polymerase inhibitor enhances survival of mice bearing hematologic malignancy at the central nervous system site. Blood 2002;99:2241.

276. Tentori L, Portarena I, Torino F, et al. Poly(ADP-Ribose) polymerase inhibitor increases growth inhibition and reduces G_2/M cell accumulation induced by temozolomide in malignant glioma cells. GLIA 2002;40:44.

277. Tentori L, Leonetti C, Scarsella M, et al. Systemic administration of the PARP inhibitor GPI 15427 increases the anti-tumor activity of temozolomide in melanoma, glioma and lymphoma preclinical models in vivo. Proc Am Assoc Cancer Res 2003;44:1253.

278. Boulton S, Pemberton LC, Porteous JK, et al. Potentiation of temozolomide-induced cytotoxicity: a comparative study of the biological effects of poly(ADP-ribose)polymerase inhibitors. Br J Cancer 1995;72:849.

279. Bowman KJ, White A, Golding BT, et al. Potentiation of anti-cancer agent cytotoxicity by the potent poly(ADP-ribose)polymerase inhibitors NU1025 and NU1064. Br J Cancer 1998;78:1269.

280. Tentori L, Turriziani T, Franco D, et al. Treatment with temozolomide and poly(ADP-ribose) polymerase inhibitors induces early apoptosis and increases base excision repair gene transcripts in leukemic cells resistant to triazene compounds. Leukemia 1999;13:901.

281. Calabrese CR, Batey MA, Thomas HD, et al. Identification of potent nontoxic poly(ADP-ribose) polymerase-1 inhibitors: chemopotentiation and pharmacological studies. Clin Cancer Res 2003;9:2711.

282. Miknyoczki SJ, Jones-Bolin S, Pritchard S, et al. Chemopotentiation of temozolomide, irinotecan, and cisplatin activity by CEP-6800, a Poly(ADP-Ribose) polymerase inhibitor. Mol Cancer Ther 2003;2:371.

283. Curtin NJ, Wang LZ, Yiakouvaki A, et al. Novel poly(ADP-ribose) polymerase-1 inhibitor, AG14361, restores sensitivity to temozolomide in mismatch repair-deficient cells. Clin Cancer Res 2004;10:881.

284. Estlin EJ, Lashford L, Ablett S, et al. Phase I study of temozolomide in paediatric patients with advanced cancer. Br J Cancer 1988;78:652.

285. Baker SD, Wirth P, Statkevich P, et al. Absorption, metabolism and exretion of ^{14}C-temozolomide in patients with advanced cancer. Proc Am Soc Clin Oncol 1997;16:214a (abst 749).

286. Dhodapkar JR, Rubin J, Reid JM, et al. Phase I trial of temozolomide (NSC 362856) in patients with advanced cancer. Clin Cancer Res 1997;3:1093.

287. Eckardt JR, Weiss GR, Burris HA, et al. Phase I and pharmacokinetic trial of SCH52365 (temozolomide) given orally daily $\times$ 5 days. Proc Am Soc Clin Oncol 1995;14:484 (abst 1579).

288. Brada M, Moore S, Judson I, et al. A phase I study of SCH 52365 (temozolomide) in adult patients with advanced cancer [abstract 1521] Proc Am Soc Clin Oncol 1995;14:470.

289. Reidenberg P, Willalona M, Eckhardt G, et al. Phase I clinical and pharmacokinetic study of temozolomide in advanced cancer patients stratified by extent of prior therapy [abstract 344]. Ann Oncol 1996;7:99.

290. Reidenberg P, Statkevich P, Judson I, et al. Effect of food on the oral bioavailability of temozolomide, a new chemotherapeutic agent [abstract PIII- 44]. Clin Pharmacol Ther 1996;59:70.

291. Statkevich P, Judson I, Batra V, et al. Effect of ranitidine (R) on the pharmacokinetics (PK) of temozolomide (T) [abstract PI-39]. Clin Pharmacol Ther 1997;61:72.

292. Baker SD, Statkevich P, Rowinsky E, et al. Pharmacokinetics (PK) and pharmacodynamics (PD) of temozolomide (TEM) administered as a single oral dose [abstract PPDM 8378]. Pharm Res 1996;13S:487.

293. Nicholson HS, Krailo M, Ames MM, et al. Phase I study of temozolomide in children and adolescents with recurrent solid tumors: a report from the Children's Cancer Group (CCG). J Clin Oncol 1998;16:3037.

Cisplatin, Carboplatin, and Oxaliplatin

14

Eddie Reed

Rosenberg and colleagues[1,2] in a set of experiments involving *Escherichia coli*, discovered the dramatic inhibitory effects of platinum compounds on cellular replication. Following those seminal studies, a rapid series of basic, preclinical, and clinical studies resulted in Food and Drug Administration (FDA) approval for the treatment of testicular cancer. Within 15 years, cisplatin's effectiveness in ovarian cancer, lung cancer, head and neck cancer, bladder cancer, and other malignancies led to its becoming the most widely used anticancer drug in North America and in Europe.

Because of the particularly troublesome toxicities of renal damage, nausea and vomiting, deafness, and peripheral neuropathy, efforts were made to develop analogs of the drug that would have equivalent clinical effectiveness, but without the toxicities of the parent compound. The first cisplatin analog to meet with widespread clinical use was carboplatin (Figure 14.1). Well-performed clinical studies have shown that carboplatin is equally effective as cisplatin in ovarian cancer, lung cancer, and several other malignancies. However, for unclear reasons, carboplatin is less effective than cisplatin in the treatment of germ cell malignancy. Carboplatin is less neurotoxic, emetogenic, and nephrotoxic than cisplatin. However, carboplatin is not toxicity-free, as will be discussed.

A number of additional platinum analogs have been synthesized for potential clinical use. Of these, only oxaliplatin (Figure 14.1) has reached the stage of FDA approval, as of this writing. For unclear reasons, oxaliplatin is particularly effective in colon cancer, in combination with other agents. Colon cancer is a disease for which neither cisplatin nor carboplatin show meaningful levels of effectiveness. Understanding the molecular basis for these peculiarities for these three compounds could potentially unlock a treasure trove of new insights as to how cancer cells fight off the effects of DNA-damaging agents.

SUBCELLULAR PHARMACOLOGY

The cellular effects of platinum compounds (and the effects of the cell on platinum compounds) have been extensively studied using cisplatin, carboplatin, and oxaliplatin as the experimental tools. Cisplatin is able to cross cellular barriers because of its simple chemistry, although there have been a number of reports of specific transmembrane transport systems that promote efflux of the drug,[3–5] such as the copper efflux transporter described by Kruh.[3] At physiologic pH of 7.4, the chemistry of the molecule is such that dissociation of the chlorides (along with replacement of these chlorides by -OH molecules) results in cisplatin having a neutral charge (Figure 14.2). This makes it possible for ready diffusion across the cellular membrane, flowing with the cisplatin gradient from a high concentration outside the cell to a lower concentration inside the cell. Several important aspects of platinum chemistry are summarized in Table 14.1.

Once inside the cell, three different fates await the compound.[3,5] One fate is to be exported from the cell by one of several specific active transport systems that have been described. A second fate is to be chemically neutralized by proteins that have active sulfhydryl groups, such as glutathione or metallothioneins. A third fate is to react in a relatively nonspecific way with a number of intracellular molecules, which include a range of proteins, RNAs, and DNA (cellular and mitochondrial).

Through this relatively nonspecific interaction of this highly reactive platinum moiety with a range of subcellular

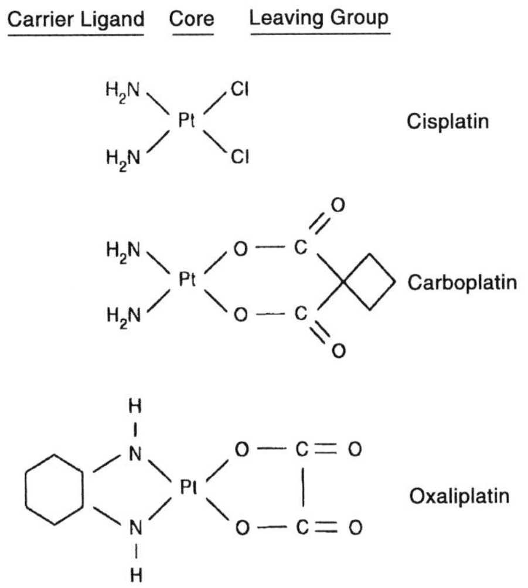

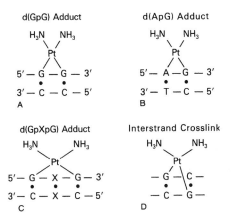

Figure 14.1 Two-dimensional structures are shown for cisplatin, carboplatin, and oxaliplatin. The core structures are the same based on the *cis* configuration of Pt(II). The leaving groups are different for the three compounds. The carrier ligand is different for oxaliplatin

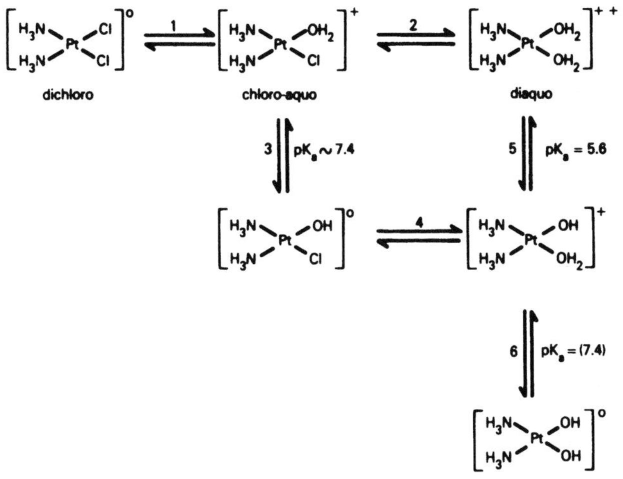

Figure 14.2 Aquation and hydrolysis equilibria of cisplatin (pka values are from ref. 187). Note that reactions 3 and 6 are favored at physiologic pH and yield products that have a neutral charge and that theoretically could readily cross cell membranes.

molecules, cisplatin exerts its effects on the cell. In terms of affinity for these different classes of reactive subcellular moieties, the measured affinity for RNA is greater than that for DNA, which, in turn, is greater than that for proteins. Because of time of transit from cellular membrane into the nucleus, the sum total of reactions with DNA is lower than that with intracellular protein on a molar basis.

It is widely accepted that in most circumstances, the reactions with cellular DNA determine the bulk of cisplatin-related cellular effects. One exception was noted with a Burkitt's lymphoma cell line, in which protein binding was reported to effect cell death in a time frame that could

not be explained by DNA damage.[3] This is presumed to be the exception, rather than the rule.

In early studies comparing cisplatin with transplatin (utilizing a technique called alkaline elution), it was demonstrated that the DNA-damaging effects of cisplatin were responsible for its cell-killing effects.[3] Further, it was found necessary for reactive groups to be in the *cis* configuration to generate effective cell killing. In subsequent, more detailed studies, it was shown by several different groups that the intrastrand N7-d(GpG) and the N7-d (ApG) intrastrand adducts were probably responsible for cell killing of the drug (Figure 14.3).[5] The relative contribution of these adducts to cell killing, as well as other specific DNA lesions such as interstrand cross-links, have never been completely

TABLE 14.1
IMPORTANT ISSUES REGARDING PLATINUM CHEMISTRY

1. Analogs in the *cis* configuration are clinically active. Analogs in the *trans* configuration are not.
2. The bond angles for the platinum core of these drugs are fixed; therefore, DNA bends to accommodate the structure of the drug.
3. The leaving group is important in platinum pharmacology and the specific carrier ligand is important as well.
4. The aquation chemistry of the cisplatin compound suggests movement of the drug across cellular membranes against a concentration gradient. No need exists for active transport into the cell.
5. The aquation chemistry for oxaliplatin is similar to that of cisplatin. For carboplatin, esterase activity for the carboxylato leaving group is necessary to generate the reactive species of the compound.
6. All clinically active platinum compounds that have been studied form bifunctional intrastrand DNA adducts. which appear to be responsible for the cell-killing effect of these analogs.

Figure 14.3 Bifunctional adducts of cisplatin with DNA. Lesions indicated in panels A, B, and C represent different intrastrand adducts, which together account for more than 90% of total platinum binding to DNA. The lesion indicated in panel D is the interstrand cross-link measured by alkaline elution and accounts for less than 5% of total platinum binding to DNA. See text for discussion.

worked out. But it is clear that the intrastrand adducts are more highly correlated with drug-induced cell killing.

The N7-d(GpG) and the N7-d(ApG) adducts account for more than 80% of total platinum-DNA damage that forms after an exposure of cisplatin to isolated DNA;[1,6] or to cells in tissue culture;[7,8] or to cells from patients in clinical settings.[9-11] These two adducts are associated with severe kinking of the DNA double helix.[12] This kinking is recognized and repaired by the nucleotide excision repair pathway, which involves the genes ERCC1, XPA, and others.[13-15] Table 14.2 summarizes the relative proportions of the DNA lesions formed after exposure to cisplatin, carboplatin, or oxaliplatin.

Kinking of the DNA is caused by the fact that the bond angles within the cisplatin molecule are relatively rigid as compared with the DNA double-helix.[12] The DNA double-helix thereby bends to conform to the structure of the platinum molecule. This is in contrast to most bifunctional alkylating agents within which the pivotal carbon molecule has bond angles that "breathe" and allow for the drug to bend to accommodate the structure of the DNA. In addition to the fixed angle bending of the DNA helix, there is evidence for local denaturation of the DNA strand at the site of intrastrand adduct binding.

In addition to cisplatin, carboplatin and oxaliplatin are FDA-approved for the treatment of one or more human malignancies. Carboplatin is similar to cisplatin in most respects. The major subcellular differences between these two drugs include the need for an esterase activity to release the carboxylato moiety of the carboplatin molecule, and thereby to expose the reactive arms for covalent binding to target sites, and a delayed time frame for the formation of the specific DNA lesions such as the N7-d (GpG) and N7-d(GpG) adducts, as compared with cisplatin.[16] Differences in clinical pharmacology and in clinical toxicity are discussed in this chapter. For almost all matters, the subcellular behaviors of cisplatin and carboplatin appear to be practically the same.

Oxaliplatin is FDA-approved for the treatment of colorectal cancer. The major subcellular differences between cisplatin and oxaliplatin include the carrier ligand effects involving the nonreactive moiety of the oxaliplatin compound,[17,18] and differences in the rates of formation and repair of oxaliplatin-DNA damage, as compared with cisplatin.[17,19,20] Differences in clinical pharmacology and in clinical toxicity are also discussed in this chapter.

MECHANISM(S) OF ACTION

The consensus is that cisplatin and its analogs exert their cytotoxic effects by covalently binding to purine DNA bases and disrupting the normal functions of cellular DNA. Platinum analogs that have therapeutic activity form a preponderance of DNA intrastrand adducts as opposed to DNA interstrand cross-links or DNA–platinum-protein cross-links.[3,5] Cisplatin binding to mitochondrial DNA has been described,[21-24] but is of unclear biologic significance. Binding to cellular proteins has been suggested as being of primary importance in one Burkitt's lymphoma cell line in which cell death occurred shortly after cellular exposure and appeared to result from loss of cell membrane integrity.

Early studies of cisplatin and transplatin compared the relative importance of DNA damage versus protein binding in terms of causing tumor cell kill in tissue culture.[3] Some laboratories have sought to correlate tumor cell kill with one or more of the different intrastrand lesions, the N7-d(GpG) adduct or the N7-d(ApG) adduct or the N7-d (GpXpG) adduct.[5] There are conflicting reports over which lesion(s) may be more associated with the cytotoxic effects of these drugs and which lesion(s) may be more associated with the mutagenic effects of these drugs. These studies have not been definitive because of the complexity of the mix of DNA adducts after cisplatin exposure, as shown in Table 14.2. When platinum agents are allowed to react with isolated DNA or cells, or are given to animals, the proportions of the various DNA adducts are relatively constant, which is also listed in Table 14.2.

Cell death may occur through apoptotic or nonapototic pathways. The apoptotic pathways may be mediated through mismatch repair genes,[25-28] p53,[29] or bcl2/bax.[30,31] Overwhelming DNA damage is associated with acute, nonapoptotic cell death. Reports going back more than 3 decades show that cisplatin exerts a positive effect on immune-mediated killing of tumor cells.[3-5] These effects have been reported in vitro in animal models and in human clinical trials. Detailed discussion of these considerations is given in this chapter.

TABLE 14.2
TYPES OF DNA LESIONS CAUSED BY CISPLATIN, CARBOPLATIN, AND OXALIPLATIN

DNA Lesion	% of Total DNA Damage	(Comment)
N7-d(GpG)-intrastrand adduct	~60	Possibly lethal to cells
N7-d(ApG)-intrastrand adduct	~30	Possibly lethal to cells
N7-d(GpXpG)-intrastrand adduct	~10	Potential lethality unclear
N7-d(X)-d(X)-interstrand cross-link	<2	Biologic importance unclear
		Levels correlate with cellular toxicity

With the advent of oxaliplatin, the nature of effects of different carrier ligands on platinum's ability to induce cellular damage, and evade DNA repair processes, have been of particular interest. Saris and colleagues[19] were the first to demonstrate that a ligand bound to the platinum core, when opposite the *cis* configuration of the reactive bonds, can exert tremendous influence on subcellular pharmacology of the drug. The carrier ligand has effects on DNA repair efficiency and on cell-killing efficiency.[17–20,27] It is not clear why oxaliplatin should be particularly active in cases of colon cancer when cisplatin and carboplatin have very limited activity in this disease. One possible explanation has to do with the relative inability to perform replicative bypass over an oxaliplatin-DNA lesion as compared with a cisplatin-carboplatin–DNA lesion. The carrier ligand of oxaliplatin makes replicative bypass of this DNA lesion much more difficult. Thus, cells that depend on replicative bypass as a major mechanism of platinum resistance may be comparatively more sensitive to oxaliplatin than the other platinum compounds. Others have shown that the carrier ligand has substantial effects on the clinical pharmacology of platinum analogs, as will be discussed later.

Platinum agents give additive or synergistic activity with a range of other anticancer agents. Cisplatin is thought to be relatively non–cell cycle-specific in terms of its cell-killing effects. However, it tends to synergize with agents that reduce the intracellular levels of precursors that are needed for DNA replication or repair. This includes antimetabolites such as 5-fluorouracil[32,33] and gemcitabine.[34] Platinums also synergize with agents that alter mitosis, such as paclitaxel, DNA repair activity,[35] and with ERCC1 inhibitors.[36–39] Positive interactions with topoisomerase inhibitors have been described,[40] as well as with agents from other drug classes.[3,5]

In summary, the primary mechanism of cell killing for this class of compounds is covalent binding to purine bases of cellular DNA. This covalent binding leads to bending of the DNA helix at a fixed angle, with local denaturing of the DNA strand. This DNA damage is detected by components of the repair complex and is converted into a strand break. Adducts are removed and breaks are repaired by the nucleotide-excision repair process. When not effectively repaired, cell killing may occur through apoptotic or nonapoptotic pathways. The possible contribution of drug-induced, immune-mediated cell killing, which may occur in the intact host, is discussed later.

IMMUNE EFFECTS OF PLATINUM AGENTS

The first human clinical studies of positive immune modulation by cisplatin were done in a group of 34 patients by Kleinerman and colleagues.[41] They showed that, after receiving cisplatin-based therapy, patients' monocyte function improved by sixfold; this was particularly striking in

patients with epithelial ovarian cancer.[41] In subsequent studies, they showed that cisplatin directly stimulated monocytes and did not stimulate other subsets of immune cells.[42] Follow-up in vitro studies showed that cisplatin and adriamycin had similar monocyte-stimulating effects, but that this effect was not seen with irradiation, L-phenylalanine mustard, mAMSA, or actinomycin D.[43] Similar studies have been reported in murine systems and other preclinical models.[3,5]

Recently, Merritt and colleagues[44] attempted to dissect out the possible mechanism for the observations of Kleinerman and colleagues.[41] In there studies, gene knockout mice were used in a Lewis lung cancer model. The mice were either Fas-negative or Fas-positive. In these studies, the ability of intraperitoneal cisplatin to effect tumor cell kill depended on the presence of Fas. It was concluded that cisplatin-induced cell killing, in this model, depended on the presence of Fas ligand in the tumor cells.

Li and colleagues[45,46] have shown that Jun/JunK is up-regulated after exposure to cisplatin. Several recent studies have shown that up-regulation of Jun/JunK may lead to up-regulation of Fas in Fas-competent cells.[47–49] Collectively, the data suggest a flow in which up-regulation of Jun/JunK may lead in either of three general directions in terms of downstream molecular pathways. In some cells, up-regulation of Jun/JunK may activate DNA repair processes; in some cells, Fas ligand-mediated immunogenicity may dominate; and in other cells, global stress response processes may be activated. In cells where up-regulation of Fas is a major element of the Jun/JunK response, this could lead to greater immunogenicity and greater immune-mediated cell killing after cisplatin treatment. Among the tumor cell types that demonstrate greater immune-mediated cell killing after cisplatin exposure are esophageal cancer,[50] mesothelioma,[51] gastric cancer,[52] melanoma,[53] colorectal cancer,[54] and cervical cancer.[55]

MECHANISMS OF RESISTANCE

The mechanisms of resistance to platinum agents have been studied most extensively for cisplatin. There are four generic pathways through which cells become resistant, or are intrinsically resistant, to platinum compounds: altered cellular accumulation of drug, cytosolic inactivation of drug, increased DNA repair, or an altered apoptotic process that results in increased tolerance to DNA damage.

Eastman and colleagues[6,7] studied the relative contributions of the first three of these processes in L1210 murine leukemia cells. Johnson et al.[56] and Ferry et al.[57] studied the relative contributions of these first three processes in human ovarian cancer cells. In both systems, the observations were very similar. At all levels of cisplatin resistance (up to 100-fold over baseline), all three components of resistance (DNA repair, cytosolic inactivaton, and cellular accumulation of drug) appeared to contribute somewhat to the overall pattern of resistance. However, there were differences regarding the relative contribution of a particular mechanism in the two model systems.

At low levels of cisplatin resistance (about 10- to 15-fold over baseline), the primary determinant of cellular resistance was DNA repair. At intermediate levels of resistance (up to 40- to 50-fold over baseline), the primary determinant of cellular resistance was reduced cellular accumulation of drug. At very high levels of resistance, cytosolic inactivation of drug became the primary determinant of resistance. Each item will be briefly reviewed in turn, moving from the cell membrane in toward the nucleus.

Altered Cellular Accumulaton

Chemically, the pH of the blood compartment is such that the redox state of cisplatin in the blood stream favors the uptake of a neutral species of drug, from the blood into the cell. This uptake is mediated by the drug concentration gradient, from high levels in the blood to the lower levels within the cells.[5] There are no reports of an active uptake process for cisplatin or any of its analogs.

Active efflux of cisplatin has been described in vitro, particularly as medicated by Cu^{II} transporters, ATP7A and ATP7B,[4] and other less well-definied systems.[5] Reduced drug accumulation appears to be a consistent observation in cisplatin-resistant tumor cell lines.

Cytosolic Inactivation of Drug

Proteins or peptides with increased levels of sulfhydryl groups may confer cellular resistance to cisplatin through covalent binding to the active moieties of the compound. Such molecules include glutathione[58,59] and metallothionein.[60,61] Up-regulation of either results in inactivation of the drug before it can reach the nucleus and leads to decreased DNA damage levels after a given level of drug exposure.

DNA Repair

Platinum compounds form bulky lesions with cellular DNA, which are repaired by nucleotide-excision repair (NER).[15,34] This is the same pathway that repairs DNA damage from polycyclic aromatic hydrocarbons and from ultraviolet light. There are 16 proteins involved in the DNA repairosome that repairs cisplatin-DNA adduct. They include ERCC1, XPA, XPF, XPB, XPD, and others.[15] In sequence, the platinum-DNA lesion is recognized by the repairosome, the 3' cut into the DNA strand is made 15 to 23 bases from the site of the lesion, the helicase function is implemented, and then the 5' cut is made.[13,15] The 5' cut is implemented by the ERCC1-XPF heterodimer, which is the last substep in the excision of cisplatin-DNA damage. Gap-filling and ligase activity follows.

Platinum-DNA adduct repair temporally occurs in two phases in vitro.[62,63] The first phase occurs over the first 6 to

8 hours after the drug exposure, during which 60 to 80% of all DNA damage is removed from the cells. The second phase occurs more slowly and may last for many hours. It is not complete after 24 hours. A similar pattern was observed in a study of the in vitro removal of platinum from the DNA of peripheral blood cells,[9] indicating that what happens in vitro parallels what happens in human patients.

Zehn and colleagues[64] and Jones and colleagues[65] showed that the first phase of cisplatin-DNA adduct repair is predominated by transcription-coupled, or gene-specific, repair. In this process, transcriptionally active genes are repaired first, before the rest of the genome. The quiescent parts of cellular DNA are repaired in a more leisurely fashion by the cell, taking many hours. This is a function of the three-dimensional state of DNA structure in which transcriptionally active genes are more open and can be readily accessed by the DNA repair protein machinery. The gene-specific repair of cisplatin-DNA damage occurs over the first 6 to 8 hours after the cisplatin exposure and is most prominent in cisplatin-resistant cells.

Altered Apoptosis/Increased Tolerance To DNA Damage

Apoptosis in response to cisplatin is mediated through the mismatch repair (MMR)[25-28] and other genes as previously discussed. Data exist to suggest that sensitivity to drug-induced apoptosis may be altered in cells that have one or more of several defined defects in MMR. This altered sensitivity to apoptosis results in enhanced tumor cell survival and, therefore, greater resistance to chemotherapy. It has been reported that in each cell line in which this alteration in MMR exists, there is a concurrent enhancement of the activity of NER, thus clouding the issue of which is more important, MMR or NER.

Enhanced replicative bypass of platinum-DNA lesions has been suggested to be a mechanism of tumor cell resistance to platinum compounds. Although demonstrated elegantly in the laboratory, it is not yet clear whether this is important in human tissues. The central considerations related to platinum drug resistance are summarized in Table 14.3.

COMMON END ORGAN TOXICITIES

Kidney Toxicity

Renal toxicity is common with all clinically utilized platinum analogs, and particularly so with cisplatin.[66-68] Kidney damage from carboplatin and from oxaliplatin tend to be less severe, and may be subclinical in many cases. Preclinical models suggest that the proximal renal tubule is less sensitive to platinum damage than the distal tubule, although both are affected by platinum exposures.

Renal clearance may be substantially reduced after several cycles of therapy with cisplatin or carboplatin, even in

TABLE 14.3

MECHANISMS OF CELLULAR RESISTANCE TO PLATINUM COMPOUNDS

Alterations in transmembrane cellular accumulation of drug

No specific transmembrane carrier for cisplatin has ever been identified. The Cu^{++} carrier may play a role.

Altered cellular accumulation has been associated with inhibition of a variety of membrane proteins, including Na, K-adenosine triphosphatase.

Facile transmembrane transit of drug can be explained by the aquation of cisplatin in water.

Cytosolic inactivation of drug

Glutathione conjugation of activated platinum occurs with possible active transport out of the cell for drug conjugated to reduced glutathione by the multidrug resistance protein class of adenosine triphosphate-dependent transporters.

Metallothioneins glutathione and inactivate platinum.

Other sulfhydryl-containing groups, such as proteins, inactivatedrug.

DNA repair

Nucleotide excision repair increases (NER; this pathway is responsible for the repair of cisplatin-DNA damage).

Clinical data show enhanced mRNA expression in platinum-resistant tumors.

Increased NER is associated with high levels of resistance (more than 10-fold over baseline) in cultured cells.

Defective MMR may be responsible for failure to recognize platinum-DNA adducts and for the failure to link unrepaired DNA damage to apoptotic pathways.

Clinical data show enrichment of MMR-defective cells in tumors after platinum therapy.

Defective MMR is associated with low levels of resistance (twofold to threefold over baseline) in cultured cells.

Translesional DNA synthesis is observed to occur preferentially in cisplatin-resistant cells.

In many cell lines, increased NER and defective MMR occur in tandem.

Resistance to apoptosis

Resistance may be mediated through defective MMR proteins, *p53*, *bcl/bax*, or other mechanisms.

Apoptotic response may be *p53*-dependent or *p53*-independent, and caspase-dependent or caspase-independent.

the face of a normal serum creatinine. Alternatively stated, the serum creatinine may remain normal in a patient who has had several cycles of platinum therapy, and the concurrent renal clearance may remain dramatically reduced. This phenomenon has been observed with a number of heavy metals, such as lead. This is important because drugs of other classes (such as antibiotics) may be needed by cancer patients and require adequate renal clearance. Cation loss in the urine is a common component of platinum-related renal toxicity and may include Mg^{2+}, Ca^{2+}, and other heavy metals. The treating physician should consider regular replacement of these cations during the course of treatment, along with over-the-counter supplements such as zinc and selenium. Symptomatic hypomagnesemia and hypocalcemia may result.

Methods used to minimize this toxicity include vigorous intravenous hydration before and after administering cis-

platin, and in cases where renal compromise has been discovered or is suspected, using this same approach with carboplatin and oxaliplatin. The use of mannitol to enhance urine flow may be beneficial, but the use of furosemide may be counterproductive in many patients. Furosemide tends to decrease total body water, which would increase tissue-drug exposure per dose and thereby enhance toxicity. Dosing based on area under the curve (AUC) is particularly important for carboplatin, which is eliminated primarily by renal clearance.

Nausea and Vomiting

Cisplatin is clearly the more emetogenic of the platinum analogs, although severe nausea may be seen with carboplatin and with oxaliplatin.[5,69–71] It is not clear whether this emetogenic effect is mediated primarily through the CNS or through peripheral mechanisms. However, for cisplatin in particular, the most aggressive antiemetic regimens are necessary to ensure patient comfort and patient compliance with future treatment. For cisplatin-containing regimens, it is best to premedicate the patient with dexamethasone, an HT3 antagonist and a substance P antagonist. This approach will address immediate and delayed nausea and vomiting caused by the platinum drugs. Premedication for this side effect should be aggressive and focused on preventing the development of symptoms. Some centers will use H1 and H2 antagonists as well. A less aggressive approach can be used for carboplatin and for oxaliplatin, but the strategy of a preventive approach should be maintained.

Neurotoxicity

Neurotoxicity is a major side effect of cisplatin, and is a frequent problem with carboplatin and oxaliplatin.[5,69,72–74] This can be ameliorated in some cases by amifostine (adisulfide activated in normal cells preferentially). Neurotoxicity can be manifested as peripheral sensory or, less commonly, meta neuropathy, auditory impairment, visual disturbances and, less commonly, cortical blindness, seizures, papilledema, and retrobulbarneuritis. Auditory impairment is discussed later.

The toxicity profile from single-agent oxaliplatin is dominated by peripheral neuropathy with little nephrotoxicity and minimal ototoxicity or hematologic toxicity. This neurotoxicity is manifested in either of two ways. An acute neurotoxicity that appears to be related to dose and duration of drug infusion presents as paresthesias or dysesthesias, commonly triggered by exposure to cold and occurring in the extremities and perioral region. This may also be associated with laryngopharyngeal dysesthesias, which cause difficulty breathing or swallowing. These toxicities are usually associated with the maximal drug doses.

Oxaliplatin generates a chronic neurotoxicity that is associated with cumulative platinum dose. This side effect is virtually identical to cisplatin-related neurotoxicity, with the exception that oxaliplatin-induced neurotoxicity is usually fully reversible over 3 to 4 months after stopping the drug. For cisplatin, peripheral neuropathy can persist for several years after stopping the medication.

Cisplatin-related peripheral neuropathy has been treated by a number of maneuvers over time, all with less-than-desired results. No approach is clearly satisfactory with respect to preventing this toxicity, or treating it once it occurs. This is usually managed by cisplatin dose reductions and/or dose delays. One study assessed the effect of vitamin B6 on preventing peripheral neuropathy in patients with ovarian cancer who received platinum-based combination chemotherapy.[75] The group randomized to received vitamin B6 had significantly less toxicity than the similarly treated group that did not receive vitamin B6. However, the group receiving vitamin B6 also had a significantly reduced response rate and a significantly reduced survival.

Myelosuppression

Trilineage cumulative myelosuppression is commonly seen with cisplatin and with carboplatin, but less so with oxaliplatin. With cisplatin in particular, thrombocytopenia is prominent. Leukopenia can be ameliorated by granulocyte colony-stimulating factor, and anemia responds to erythropoietin. Platinum-based therapy of ovarian cancer is associated with a fourfold increase in the risk of developing acute myelogenous leukemia.[76]

Ototoxicity

Auditory impairment can be overt, with clinically dramatic reductions in auditory acuity after several cycles of cisplatin-based therapy, or they can be more subtle. Some patients may complain of the loss of the ability to filter out extraneous noises during a conversation, for example, in a restaurant. High-frequency tones (4,000 to 8,000 Hz) are most affected.

The chinchilla is thought to be a good model for cisplatin-based hearing loss in humans.[77,78] Studies in this animal model suggest that the mechanism of ototoxicity for platinum compounds is loss of hair cells in the cochlea. At low doses of platinum compounds (50 mg/kg intraperitoneally in the chinchilla), loss of inner hair cells in the cochlea is readily seen. At low doses, observers reported a one-third reduction in the amplitude of conduction within nerve fibers of the eighth nerve. This reduction in amplitude was not accompanied by changes in conduction threshold or in the latency of conduction. At doses fivefold higher, loss of outer hair cells were observed, along with reductions in all three parameters measured in these nerve fibers.

Acute Hypersensitivity

Acute hypersensitivity reactions, including anaphylaxis, can occur with platinum compounds. When this occurs, it is usually after the seventh or eighth exposure to the drug. The frequency of this occurrence is directly related to the number of cycles of platinum therapy a patient has received, beyond six. If treatment with platinum-based therapy is of crucial importance, three are several desensitization regimens published in the older literature. Rarely, hemolytic anemia can be seen with drugs in this class. Acute laryngopharngeal dysesthesias can be seen with oxaliplatin, resulting in difficulty swallowing or breathing. This side effect, when it occurs, is usually completely reversible.

CLINICAL PHARMACOLOGY

The clinical pharmacology profiles of cisplatin, carboplatin, and oxaliplatin are summarized in Tables 14.4, 14.5, and 14.6. The detailed pharmacology of cisplatin and carboplatin has been described in previous chapters of this book and elsewhere.[3–5,69] For oxaliplatin, the volume of distribution is 50-fold greater than for cisplatin. Oxaliplatin undergoes extensive nonenzymatic conversion to reactive species, as does cisplatin and carboplatin. Oxaliplatin is excreted mainly by the kidneys (>50% of excreted drug), and less than 2% is excreted in the feces. About 40% of administered oxaliplatin is sequestered in red blood cells, and this fraction appears to have no clinical significance. Studies in patients with varying levels of renal dysfunction show that for single-agent oxaliplatin, dose reduction is not necessary if the patient has a creatinine clearance of >20 mL/minute.

Drug Infusion Issues

The specifics of the intravenous infusion of cisplatin or carboplatin are not well standardized from institution to institution. However, several matters are clear. Platinum agents should be administered using normal saline, which stabilizes the parent compound; the infusion should specifically exclude Mg^{2+}, aluminum needles, and other reactive species that might chemically neutralize the compound. Vigorous intravenous hydration should be given immediately before and during each infusion.

For all three platinum analogs, shorter infusions (less than 1 hour) appear to be associated with greater acute toxicities. Continuous intravenous infusions for long periods of time (24 hours or more) are associated with dramatic reductions in efficacy. For these reasons, the infusion times for all three of these agents tend to range from 1 hour to approximately 4 hours. There are no prospective randomized trials that show that one specific duration of infusion, between 1 and 4 hours, provides the best therapeutic index for cisplatin or carboplatin. Two-hour infusions appear best for oxaliplatin.

At my institution, cisplatin or carboplatin is administered as a 1-hour intravenous infusion in 250 mL of normal saline. Prehydration and posthydration are essential for cisplatin, and probably should be used for carboplatin as well because 50% reductions in renal clearance

TABLE 14.4
KEY FEATURES OF CISPLATIN

Dosage:	50–75 mg/m^2 IV every 3–4 weeks.
	Other dosing regimens may be used in selected situations.
	Usually administered in normal saline with vigorous IV prehydration (at least 0.5 L of saline with 125 mg of mannitol).
Mechanism of action:	Covalently binds to DNA bases and disrupts DNA function.
	Toxicity may be related to DNA damage and/or protein damage.
Metabolism:	Inactivated intracellularly and in the bloodstream by conjugation to sulfhydryl groups.
	Drug covalently binds to glutathione, metallothionein, and sulfhydryls on proteins.
Pharmaco-kinetics:	After IV bolus, $t_{1/2\alpha}$ = 20–30 min; $t_{1/2\beta}$ = approximately 60 min; $t_{1/2\gamma}$ = approximately 24 hr.
Elimination:	Approximately 25% of an IV dose is excreted from the body during the first 24 hr.
	Of that portion eliminated, excretion is renal > 90%, and bile < 10%.
	Extensive long-term protein binding has been observed in many tissues.
Drug interactions:	Thiosulfates administered IV may inactivate drug systemically.
	Amifostine (WR2721) may also act to inactivate drug, but preferentially in healthy tissues.
	May show enhanced efficacy, and increased toxicity, with a range of other cytotoxic agents.
Toxicity:	Renal insufficiency with cation wasting.
	Nausea and vomiting.
	Peripheral neuropathy.
	Auditory impairment (high tone loss).
	Myelosuppression (thrombocytopenia > WBC > RBC).
	Visual impairment (rare).
	Hypersensitivity (rare).
	Seizures (rare).
	Leukemia.
Precautions:	Use with caution in the presence of other nephrotoxic drugs (such as aminoglycosides).
	Monitor serum electrolytes and cations (especially Mg^{2+} and Ca^{2+}), and creatinine.
	Maintain high urine flow during cisplatin administration.
	Aggressive premedication with antiemetics is recommended.
	Caution should be used if the 24-hr creatinine clearance is <60 mL/min. Consideration should be given to using alternative agents in this setting, although cisplatin can be safely administered if extensive precautions are used.

RBC, red blood cell count; $t_{1/2}$, half-life; WBC, white blood cell count.

may occur in the absence of preinfusion and postinfusion hydration. Platinum-induced reductions in renal function are characteristically nonoliguric and the extent of damage may not be fully reflected by changes in serum creatinine.

The acute neurotoxicity of oxaliplatin is directly related to dose and to the duration of drug infusion. The more severe toxicities are seen at higher doses and with shorter infusion times. Therefore, oxaliplatin doses should never exceed 85 mg/m^2 every 2 weeks, or 130 mg/m^2 every 3 weeks. The oxaliplatin infusion should always be at least over 2 hours in duration.

Platinum-Dosing Strategies

Carboplatin is now most commonly dosed by the AUC for the drug. The most common AUCs for dosing are 5 or 6. The AUC dose is calculated using the Calvert formula, which is: carboplatin dose = target AUC (GFR + 25).[77] An older approach, though currently a less well-accepted alternative, is to use 300 mg/m^2 per dose when the drug is given in combination with a taxane, or 400 mg/m^2 per dose as a single agent. This is based on the clinical observation that, in terms of antitumor efficacy, 1 mg of cisplatin appears to be equivalent to 4 mg of carboplatin; that is, a 75-mg dose of cisplatin is therapeutically equivalent to 300 mg of carboplatin.

Whether one bases dose on AUC or the milligrams per square meter method, the calculated total milligram dosage for any individual tends to be similar if the creatinine clearance is nearly normal. The carboplatin dose should be administered every 21 or 28 days, depending on blood count recovery. In a percentage of patients, cumulative thrombocytopenia will result in dose reductions, or dosing delays, by the fourth or fifth cycle of therapy.

For cisplatin, the dosage should be 50, 60, or 70 mg/m^2 per dose, given every 21 or 28 days depending on blood count recovery. Whereas many institutions give cisplatin over 30 minutes, some data suggest that this shorter infusion may be associated with a higher rate of severe side effects. This author recommends a 1-hour infusion time. Prehydration and posthydration with a total of at least 1 L of normal saline are essential. The preventive approach should be taken with respect to immediate and delayed nausea and vomiting. Such therapy should consist of the combination of a steroid, a HT3 inhibitor, and a substance P inhibitor. Once nausea and vomiting develop from cisplatin, they are very difficult to manage.

Oxaliplatin dosing guidelines are provided in Table 14.6. When given in combination with other agents, as in the treatment of colorectal cancer, these doses should never be exceeded. A number of oxaliplatin-based combination therapy regimens are under investigation in a range of diseases.

CLINICAL CONCEPTS OF PLATINUM RESISTANCE

In the treatment of gynecologic malignancies, specifically in ovarian cancer, the disease may be clinically platinum-sensitive or clinically platinum-resistant.[79,80] Data show that if a patient with ovarian cancer is more than 2 years out from the most recent dose of platinum (having responded to that therapy), there is a >70% likelihood

TABLE 14.5
KEY FEATURES OF CARBOPLATIN

Dosage:	Generally dosed by AUC, in mg/m^2 × min. Usual dosing range is 4–6 mg/m^2 × min.
	Calvert formula is generally used for calculating the AUC. A measured creatinine clearance is recommended.
	Calvert formula is: AUC (carboplatin) = dose/(creatinine clearance + 25).
	The older dosing method is 1 mg cisplatin = 4 mg carboplatin. This approach is not recommended. AUC dosing is associated with greater patient safety, particularly with respect to myelosuppression.
Mechanism of of action:	Covalent binding to DNA.
Metabolism:	Conversion to a DNA-reactive species occurs more quickly in cells than in IV solutions, which suggests the activity of esterases in cleavage of the dicarboxylate side group.
Pharmacokinetics:	After IV bolus, $t_{1/2\alpha}$ = 12–24 min; $t_{1/2\beta}$ = 1.3–1.7 hr; $t_{1/2\gamma}$ = 22–40 hr.
Elimination:	Approximately 90% is excreted in the urine in 24 hr.
Drug interactions:	See cisplatin (Table 14-5).
Toxicity:	Myelosuppression is more prominent than with cisplatin.
	Nausea and vomiting may occur, but are much less prominent than with cisplatin.
	Nephrotoxicity can occur, particularly at higher dosages and in patients with prior renal dysfunction.
Precautions:	AUC dosing is very important in the setting of preexistent renal dysfunction.

AUC, area under the concentration × time curve; $t_{1/2}$, half-life.

that the disease will respond to retreatment with cisplatin- or carboplatin-based therapy.[79] The percentage of patients who will respond decreases with the shortening of the disease-free period. Persons who have disease recurrence within the first 6 months after the most recent dose of platinum have a low likelihood of response to retreatment with cisplatin or carboplatin and are considered to have platinum-resistant disease. This concept is firmly established for cases of epithelial ovarian cancer. The applicability of this concept to other diseases commonly treated with platinum-based therapy is less well established.

Platinum-DNA Adduct and NER Gene Expression Studies

Several groups have conducted a number of studies to assess the possible relationships between platinum-DNA adduct levels in tissues from cancer patients and clinical end points in those patients.[9,10,81–88] In some studies, adduct was measured with the use of an enzyme-linked immunosorbent assay that measured only a fraction of the total amount of DNA damage. In other studies, including this author's laboratory adduct was measured by atomic absorbance spectrometry with Zeeman background correction, which measures total DNA-bound platinum.[81,82]

Generally, platinum-DNA adduct levels in peripheral blood cell DNA appeared to parallel the adduct levels formed in tumor tissues taken from the same patients. Consistent with this observation, platinum-DNA adduct levels in peripheral blood cell DNA correlated well with

independent assessments of tumor response or the duration of progression free survival: the higher the adduct level, the greater the likelihood of response. The correlation between platinum-DNA adduct levels and disease response was consistently seen using treatment programs that were totally or predominantly platinum-based. In treatment regimens that merely contained a platinum agent as one of several clinically active drugs, this relationship did not clearly suggest that the molecular contributions of the non–DNA-damaging agent(s) was critically important to the success of the treatment regimen.

As previously discussed, NER is responsible for the repair of cisplatin-DNA adduct and ERCC1 is an essential gene in the NER pathway. The mRNA expression of ERCC1 in tumor tissues directly correlates with clinical resistance to platinum therapy in ovarian cancer,[89,90] gastric cancer,[91] colorectal cancer,[92] and lung cancer.[93,94] Up-regulation of ERCC1 and other genes in the NER process suggests increased levels of DNA repair activity, which has been clearly demonstrated in vitro,[95,96] and loss of NER proficiency is associated with cisplatin sensitivity of ovarian cancer cells in vitro.[97]

Several studies show that other genes critical to the NER process, such as XPA, XPD, and others, show up-regulation of mRNA expression concurrent with clinical resistance to platinum-based therapy.[88,89] These studies are fully consistent with a large number of in vitro studies showing a similar direct relationship between ERCC1 mRNA expression and cellular resistance to platinum, which has been reviewed in other reports.[15,36]

TABLE 14.6

KEY FEATURES OF OXALIPLATIN

Dosage:	Up to 85 mg/m^2 q2weeks; or up to 130 mg/m^2 q3weeks.
	Given as a 2-, 4-, or 6-hr infusion; 6-hr infusions are used most commonly.
	Administer in a 5% dextrose IV solution.
Mechanism of action:	DNA damage. May have unique properties based on unique carrier ligand. 1,2-diaminocyclohexane carrier ligand is the nonleaving group.
Metabolism:	Not fully characterized. Drug accumulates in red blood cells of humans and rats but does not accumulate in plasma (cisplatin accumulates in plasma with repeated dosing).
Pharmacokinetics:	With a 4-hr infusion:
	Free platinum levels decrease in a triphasic fashion.
	Terminal $t_{1/2}$ = 27.3 hr.
	Volume of distribution = 349 L.
	Total clearance = 222 mL/min; renal clearance = 121 mL/min.
Elimination:	Renal elimination is important. Characterization in humans is not complete.
Drug interactions:	Most effective in gastrointestinal malignancies, given in combination with fluorouracil analogs.
	Synergizes with antimetabolites; additional studies warranted.
Toxicity:	When given with 5-fluorouracil, major toxicities include:
	Myelosuppression (neutropenia primarily).
	Diarrhea ± stomatitis.
	Peripheral neuropathy (sensory much greater than motor).
	Nausea and vomiting, mild to moderate.
	Rare toxicities: anaphylaxis, hemolytic anemia, laryngopharyngeal dysesthesias.
Precautions:	Similar to those for cisplatin and carboplatin (Tables 14-5 and 14-6).

$t_{1/2}$, half-life.

COMMON CLINICAL USES

The platinum compounds constitute the mainstay of therapy for a wide range of malignancies. This includes potentially curative therapies for advanced-stage testicular and ovarian germ cell tumors, epithelial ovarian cancer, and small-cell lung cancer. Effective platinum-based therapies also are in place for advanced stages of non-small cell lung cancer, bladder cancer, colorectal cancer, esophageal cancer, gastric cancer, and head and neck malignancies. Cisplatin, in conjunction with radiation, is curative for early-stage head and neck malignancies and cervical cancer. A better understanding of the molecular processes that underlie the clinical differences between cisplatin, carboplatin, and oxaliplatin may open the door for the development of future agents in this class, with an even better therapeutic index and broader efficacy.

REFERENCES

1. Rosenberg B, Van Camp L, Krigas T. Inhibition of cell division in Escherichia coli by electrolysis products from a platinum electrode. Nature 1965;205:698.
2. Rosenberg B, Van Camp L, Trosko JE, et al. Platinum compounds: a new class of potent antitumor agents. Nature 1969;222:385–386.
3. Kruh GD. Lustrous insights into cisplatin accumulation: copper transporters. Clin Cancer Res 2003;9:5807–5809.
4. Reed E, Dabholkar M, Chabner BA. Platinum analogues. In: Chabner BA, Longo DL, eds. Cancer Chemotherapy. 2nd ed. Philadelphia: Lippincott-Raven Publishers, 1996:357–378.
5. Reed E. Cisplatin and analogs. In: Chabner B A, Longo D L, eds. Cancer Chemotherapy and Biotherapy: Principles and Practice. 3rd ed. Philadelphia: Lippincott Williams & Wilkins, 2001:447–465.
6. Eastman A. Reevaluation of interaction of cis-dichloro (ethylenediammine)platinum(II) with DNA. Biochemistry 1986;25:3912–3915.
7. Eastman A, Schulte N, Sheibani N, et al. Mechanisms of resistance to platinum drugs. In: Nicolini M, ed. Platinum and Other Metal Coordination Compounds in Cancer Chemotherapy. Boston: Martinus Nijhoff, 1988:178–196.
8. Fichtinger-Schepman AM, van der Veer JL, den Hartog JH, et al. Adducts of the antitumor drug cis-diamminedichloroplatinum (II), with DNA: formation, identification and quantitation. Biochemistry 1985;24:707–713.
9. Fichtinger-Schepman AMJ, van Oosterom AT, Lohman PHM, et al. Cis-diamminedichloroplatinum(II)-induced adducts in peripheral leukocytes from seven cancer patients: quantitative immunochemical detection of the adduct induction and removal after a single dose of cis-diamminedichloroplatinum(II). Cancer Res 1987;47:3000–3004.
10. Fichtinger-Schepman AMJ, van Oosterom AT, Lohman PHM, et al. Interindividual human variation in cisplatinum sensitivity, predictable in an in vitro assay? Mutat Res 1987;190:59–62.
11. Fichtinger-Schepman AM, van Dijk-Knijnenburg HC, van der Velde-Visser SD, et al. Cisplatin and carboplatin DNA adducts: is PT-AG the cytotoxic lesion? Carcinogenesis 1995;16:2447–2453.
12. Gelasco A, Lippard SJ. NMR solution structure of a DNA dodecamer duplex containing a cis-diammineplatinum(II) d(GpG)

intrastrand cross-link, the major adduct of the anti-cancer drug cisplatin. Biochemistry 1998;37:9230–9239.

13. Sancar A. Mechanisms of DNA excision repair. Science 1994;266:1954–1956.

14. De Laat WL, Jaspers NG, Hoeijmakers JH. Molecular mechanism of nucleotide excision repair. Genes Dev 1999;13:768–785.

15. Reed E. Platinum-DNA adduct, nucleotide excision repair, and platinum based anti-cancer chemotherapy. Cancer Treat Rev 1998;24:331–344.

16. Micetich Ke, Barnes D, Etickson LC. A comparative study of the cytotoxicity and DNA-damaging effects of cis-diammino(1,1 cyclobutanedicarboxylato)-platinum(II) and cisdiamminedichloroplatinum (II) on LI210 cells. Cancer Res 1985;45:4043–4047.

17. Reardon JT, Vaisman A, Chaney SG, et al. Efficient nucleotide excision repair of cisplatin, oxaliplatin, and bis-aceto-amminedichloro-cyclohexylamine-platinum(IV) (JM216) platinum intrastrand DNA diadducts. Cancer Res 1999;59:3968–3971.

18. Luo FR, Wyrick SD, Chaney SG. Cytotoxicity, cellular uptake, and cellular biotransformations of oxaliplatin in human colon carcinoma cells. Oncol Res 1998;10:595–603.

19. Saris Cp, van de Vaart PJ, Rietbrock RC, et al. In vitro formation of DNA adducts by cisplatin, lobaplatin and oxaliplatin in calf thymus DNA in solution and in cultured human cells. Carcinogenesis 1996;17:2763–2769.

20. Raymond E, Faivre S, Chaney SG, et al. Cellular and molecular pharmacology of oxaliplatin. Mol Cancer Ther 2002;1:227–235.

21. Olivero OA, Semino C, Kassim A, et al. Preferential binding of cisplatin to mitochondrial DNA of Chinese hamster ovary cells. Mutat Res 1995;346:221–230.

22. Olivero OA, Chang PK, Lopez-Larraza DM, et al. Preferential formation and decreased removal of cisplatin-DNA adducts in Chinese hamster ovary cell mitochondrial DNA as compared to nuclear DNA. Mutat Res 1997;391:79–86.

23. Giurgiovich AJ, Diwan BA, Olivero OA, et al. Elevated mitochondrial cisplatin-DNA adduct levels in rat tissues after transplacental cisplatin exposure. Carcinogenesis 1997;18:93–96.

24. Giurgiovich AJ, Diwan BA, Lee KB, et al. Cisplatin-DNA adduct formation in maternal and fetal rat tissues after transplacental cisplatin exposure. Carcinogenesis 1996;17:1665–1669.

25. Aebi S, Fink D, Gordon R, et al. Resistance to cytotoxic drugs in DNA mismatch repair-deficient cells. Clin Cancer Res 1997;3:1763–1767.

26. Drummond JT, Anthoney A, Brown R, et al. Cisplatin and adriamycin resistance are associated with MutL-alpha and mismatch repair deficiency in an ovarian tumor cell line. J Biol Chem 1996;271:19645–19648.

27. Nehma A, Baskaran R, Nebel S, et al. Induction of JNK and c-Abl signalling by cisplatin and oxaliplatin in mismatch repair proficient and -deficient cells. Br J Cancer 1999;79:1104–1110.

28. Vaisman A, Varchenko M, Umar A, et al. The role of hMLH1, hMSH3, and hMSH6 defects in cisplatin and oxaliplatin resistance: correlation with replicative bypass of platinum-DNA adducts. Cancer Res 1998;58:3579–3585.

29. Siemer S, Ornskov D, Guerra B, et al. Determination of mRNA and protein levels of p53, MDM2, and protein kinase CK2 subunits in F9 cells after treatment with the apoptosis-inducing drugs cisplatin and carboplatin. Int J Biochem Cell Biol 1999;31:661–670.

30. Arriola EL, Rodriguez-Lopez AM, Hickman JA, et al. Bcl-2 overexpression results in reciprocal downregulation of Bcl-X(L) and sensitizes human testicular germ cell tumors to chemotherapy-induced apoptosis. Oncogene 1999;18(7):1457–1464.

31. Henkels KM, Turchi JJ. Cisplatin-induced apoptosis proceeds by caspase-3-dependent and -independent pathways in cisplatin-resistant and -sensitive human ovarian cancer cell lines. Cancer Res 1999;59:3077–3083.

32. deBraud F, Munzone E, Nole F, et al. Synergistic activity of oxaliplatin and 5-fluorouracil in patients with metastatic colorectal cancer with progressive disease while on or after 5-fluorouracil. Am J Clin Oncol 1998;21:279–283.

33. Rothenberg ML, Oza AM, Bigelow RH, et al. Superiority of oxaliplatin and fluorouracil-leucovorin compared with either therapy alone in patients with progressive colorectal cancer after irinotecan and fluorouracil-leucovorin: interim results of a phase III trial. J Clin Oncol 2003;21:2059–2069.

34. Villella J, Marchetti D, Odunsi K, et al. Response of combination platinum and gemcitabine chemotherapy for recurrent epithelial ovarian carcinoma. Gynecol Oncol 2004;95:539–545.

35. Altaha R, Liang X, Yu JJ. Reed Excision repair cross complementing-group-1: gene expression and platinum resistance. Int J Mol Med 2004;14:959–970.

36. Li Q, Bostick-Bruton F, Reed. E. Modulation of ERCC-1 mRNA expression by pharmacological agents in human ovarian cancer cells. Biochem Pharmacol 1999;57:347–353.

37. Li Q, Bostick-Bruton F, Reed E. Effect of interleukin-1 and tumor necrosis factor on cisplatin-induced ERCC1 mRNA expression in a human ovarian carcinoma cell line. Anticancer Res 1998;18:2283–2287.

38. Mimnaugh EG, Yunmbam MK, Li Q, et al. Proteasome inhibitors prevent cisplatin-DNA adduct repair and potentiate cisplatin-induced apoptosis in ovarian carcinoma cells. Biochem Pharmacol 2000;60:1343–1354.

39. Bonovich M, Olive M, Reed E, et al. Adenoviral delivery of A FOS, an AP-1 dominant negative, selectively inhibits drug resistance in two human cancer cell lines. Cancer Gene Ther 2002;9:62–70.

40. Von Knethen A, Lotero A, Brune B. Etoposide and cisplatin induced apoptosis in activated RAW 264.7 macrophages is attenuated by cAMP-induced gene expression. Oncogene 1998;17:387–394.

41. Kleinerman ES, Zwelling L A, Howser D, et al. Defective monocyte killing in patients with malignancies and restoration of function during chemotherapy. Lancet 1980;2(8204):1102–1105.

42. Kleinerman ES, Zwelling LA, Muchmore AV. Enhancement of naturally occurring human spontaneous monocyte mediated cytotoxicity by cis-diamminedichloroplatinum(II). Cancer Res 1980;40:3099–3102.

43. Kleinerman ES, Zwelling LA, Schwartz R. Effect of L-phenylalanine mustard, adriamycin, actinomycin D, and4′(acridinylamino) methanesulfo-m-anisidide on naturally occurring human spontaneous monocyte mediated cytotoxicity. Cancer Res 1982;42:1692–1695.

44. Merritt RE, Mahtabifard A, Yamada RE, et al. Cisplatin augments cytotoxic T lymphocyte mediated antitumor immunity in poorly immunogenic murine lung cancer. J Thorac Cardiovasc Surg 2003;126:1609–1617.

45. Li Q, Gardner K, Zhang L, et al. Cisplatin induction of ERCC1 mRNA expression in A2780/CP70 human ovarian cancer cells. J Biol Chem 1998;273:23419–23425.

46. Li Q, Tsang B, Gardner K, et al. Phorbol ester exposure activates an AP-1 associated increase in ERCC1 mRNA expression in human ovarian cancer cells. Cell Mol Life Sci 1999;55:456–466.

47. Gupta S, Natarajan R, Payne SG, et al. Deoxycholic acid activates the c-Jun N-terminal kinase pathway via Fas receptor activation in primary hepatocytes. Role of acidic sphingomyelinase-mediated ceramide generation in Fas receptor activation. J Biol Chem 2004;279:5821–5828.

48. Schwabe RF, Uchinami H, Qian T, et al Differential requirement for c-Jun NH2-terminal kinase in TNF alpha-Fas-mediated apoptosis in hepatocytes. FASEB J 2004;18:720–722.

49. Shangary S, Lerner EC, Zhan Q, et al. Lyn regulates the cell death response to ultraviolet radiation through c-Jun N terminal kinase-dependent Fas ligand activation. Exp Cell Res 2003;289:67–76.

50. Toh U, Sudo T, Kido K, et al. Intraarterial cellular immunotherapy for patients with inoperable liver metastases of esophageal cancer. Gan To Kagaku Ryoho 2002;29:2152–2156.

51. Berghmans T, Paesmans M, Lalami Y, et al. Activity of chemotherapy and immunotherapy on malignant mesothelioma; a systematic review of the literature with meta-analysis. Lung Cancer 2002;38:111–121.

52. Yoshikawa T, Tsuburaya A, Kobayashi O, et al. A combination immunochemotherapy of 5-fluorouracil, cisplatin, leucovorin, and OK-432 for advanced and recurrent gastric carcinoma. Hepatogastroenterology 2003;50:2259–2263.

53. Lens MB, Eisen TG. Systemic chemotherapy in the treatment of malignant melanoma. Expert Opin Pharmacother 2003;4:2205–2211.

54. Ohtsukasa S, Okabe S, Yamashita H, et al. Increased expression of ECA and MHC class I in colorectal cancer cells exposed to chemotherapy drugs. J Cancer Res Clin Oncol 2003;129:719–726.

55. Wilailak S, Dangprasert S, Srisupundit S. Phase I clinical trial of chemoimmunotherapy in combination with radiotherapy in stage IIIB cervical cancer patients. Int J Gynecol Cancer 2003; 13:652–656.

56. Johnson S, Perez R, Godwin A, et al. Role of platinum-DNA adduct formation and removal in cisplatin resistance in human ovarian cancer cell lines. Biochem Pharmacol 1994;47: 689–697.

57. Ferry K, Hamilton T, Johnson S. Increased nucleotide excision repair in cisplatin-resistant ovarian cancer cells: role for ERCC1-XPF. Biochem Pharmacol 2000;60:1305–1313.

58. Godwin A, Meister A, O'Dwyer P, et al. High resistance to cisplatin in human ovarian cacer cell lines is associated with marked increase in glutathione systhesis. Proc Natl Acad Sci U S A 1992; 89:3070–3074.

59. Hosking LK, Whelan RDH, Shellard SA, et al. An evaluation of the role of glutathione and its associated enzymes in the expression of differential sensitivities to antitumor agents shown by a range of human tumour cell lines. Biochem Pharmacol 1990;40:1833–1842.

60. Pattaniak A, Bachowski G, Laib J, et al. Properties of the reaction of cis-dichlorodiammineplatinum(II) with metallothionein. J Biol Chem 1992;267:16121–

61. Kelley S, Basu A, Teicher B, et al. Overexpression of metallothionein confers resistance to anticancer drugs. Science 1988; 241:1813–1815.

62. Lee KB, Parker RJ, Bohr VA, et al. Cisplatin sensitivity/resistance in UV-repair deficient Chinese hamster ovary cells of complementation groups 1 and 3. Carcinogenesis 1993;14:2177–2180.

63. Parker RJ, Eastman A, Bostick-Bruton F, et al. Acquired cisplatin resistance in human ovarian cancer cells is associated with enhanced repair of cisplatin-DNA lesions and reduced drug accumulation. J Clin Invest 1991;87:772–777.

64. Zhen W, Link CJ Jr, O'Connor PM, et al. Increased genespecific repair of cisplatin interstrand crosslinks in cisplatin resistant human ovarian cancer cells. Mol Cell Biol 1992;12:3689–3698.

65. Jones JC, Zhen W, Reed E, et al. Preferential DNA repair of cisplatinum lesions in active genes in CHO cells. J Biol Chem 1991;266: 7101–7107.

66. Cornelison TL, Reed E. Nephrotoxicity and hydration management for cisplatin, carboplatin, and ormaplatin: a review. Gynecol Oncol 50:147–158, 1993.

67. Reed E, Jacob J. Carboplatin and renal dysfunction. Ann Intern Med 1989;110:409.

68. Reed E, Jacob J, Brawley O. Measures of renal function in cisplatin-related chronic renal disease. J Natl Med Assoc 1991;83: 522–526.

69. Reed E. Anticancer drugs. Sect 7, platinum analogs. In: DeVita VT, Hellman S, Rosenberg SA, eds. Cancer Principles and Practice of Oncology. Philadelphia: JB Lippincott, 1993:390–400.

70. Reed E. The chemotherapy of ovarian cancer. PPO Updates 1996; 10(7):1–12.

71. Diaz-Rubio E, SastreJ, Zaniboni A. Oxaliplatin as a single agent in previously untreated colorectal carcinoma patients: a phase II multicentric study. Ann Oncol 1998;9:105–108.

72. Takimoto CH, Remick SC, Sharma S, et al. Administration of oxaliplatin to patients with renal dysfunction: a preliminary report of the National Cancer Institute Organ Dysfunction Working Group. Semin Oncol 2003;30(Suppl 15):20–25.

73. Extra J M, Espie M, Calvo F, et al. Phase I study of oxaliplatin in patients with advanced cancer. Cancer Chemother Pharmacol 1990;25(Suppl 5):299–303.

74. Becouarn Y, Roughier P. Clinical efficacy of oxaliplatin monotherapy: phase II trials in advanced colorectal cancer. Semin Oncol 1998;25(Suppl 5):23–31.

75. Wiernik PH, Yeap B, Vogl SE, et al. Hexamethylmelamine and low or moderate dose cisplatin with or without pyridoxine for treatment of advanced ovarian carcinoma: a study of the Eastern Cooperative Oncology Group. Cancer Invest 1992;10:1–9.

76. Travis LB, Holowaty EJ, Bergfeldt K, et al. Risk of leukemia after platinum-based chemotherapy for ovarian cancer. N Engl J Med 1999;340:351–357.

77. Burkard R, Trautwein P, Salvi R. The effects of click level, click rate, and level of background masking noise on the inferior caliculus potential (ICP) in the normal and carboplatintreated chinchilla. J Acoust Soc Am 1997;102(6):3620–3627.

78. Hofstetter P, Ding D, Salvi R. Magnitude and pattern of inner and outer hair cell loss in chinchilla as a function of carboplatin dose. Audiology 1997;36(6):301–311.

79. Markman M, Rothman R, Hakes T, et al. Second line platinum therapy in patients with ovarian cancer previously treated with cisplatin. J Clin Oncol 1991;9:389–393.

80. Reed E, Jacob J, Ozols RF, et al. 5-Fluouracil and leucovorin in platinum-refractory advanced stage ovarian cancer. Gynecol Oncol, 1992;46:326–329.

81. Reed E, Ozols RF, Tarone R, et al. Platinum-DNA adducts in leukocyte DNA correlate with disease response in ovarian cancer patients receiving platinum-based chemotherapy. Proc Natl Acad Sci U S A 1987;84:5024–5028.

82. Reed E, Yuspa SH, Zwelling LA, et al. Quantitation of cisplatin-DNA intrastrand adducts in testicular and ovarian cancer patients receiving cisplatin chemotherapy. J Clin Invest 1986;77:545–550.

83. Reed E, Ostchega Y, Steinberg S, et al. An evaluation of platinum-DNA adduct levels relative to known prognostic variables in a cohort of ovarian cancer patients. Cancer Res 1990;50:2256–2260.

84. Perera FB, Tang D, Reed E, et al. Multiple biologic markers in testicular cancer patients treated with platinum-based chemotherapy. Cancer Res 1992;52:3558–3565.

85. Parker RJ, Gill I, Tarone R, et al. Platinum-DNA damage in leukocyte DNA of patients receiving carboplatin and cisplatin chemotherapy, measured by atomic absorption spectrometry. Carcinogenesis 1991;12:1253–1258.

86. Reed E, Parker RJ, Gill I, et al. Platinum-DNA adduct in leukocyte DNA of a cohort of 49 patients with 24 different types of malignancy. Cancer Res 1993;53:3694–3699.

87. Schellens JH, Ma J, Planting AS, et al. Relationship between the exposure to cisplatin, DNA-adduct formation in leucocytes and tumor response in patients with solid tumors. Br J Cancer 1996;73:1569–1575.

88. Peng B, Tilby MJ, English MW, et al. Platinum-DNA adduct formation in leucocytes of children in relation to pharmacokinetics after cisplatin and carboplatin therapy. Br J Cancer 1997;76:1466–1473.

89. Dabholkar M, Bostick-Bruton F, Weber C, et al. ERCCI and ERCC2 expression in malignant tissues from ovarian cancer patients. J Natl Cancer Inst 1992;84:1512–1517.

90. Dabholkar M, Vionnet JA, Bostick-Bruton F, et al. mRNA Levels of XPAC and ERCC1 in ovarian tumor tissue correlates with response to platinum containing chemotherapy. J Clin Invest 1994;94:703–708.

91. Metzger R, Leichman CG, Danenberg KD, et al. ERCC1 mRNA levels complement thymidylate synthase mRNA levels in predicting response and survival for gastric cancer patients receiving combination cisplatin and fluorouracil chemotherapy. J Clin Oncol 1998;16:309–316.

92. Shirota Y, Stoehlmacher J, Brabender J, et al. ERCC1 and thymidylate synthase mRNA levels predict survival for colorectal cancer patients receiving combination oxaliplatin and fluorouracil chemotherapy. J Clin Oncol 2001;19:4298–4304.

93. Lord RV, Brabender J, Gandara D, et al. Low ERCC1 expression correlates with prolonges survival after cisplatin plus gemcitabine chemotherapy in non-small cell lung cancer. Clin Cancer Res 2002;8:2286–2291.

94. Rosell R, Taron M, Barnadas A, et al. Nucleotide excision repair pathways involved in cisplatin resistance in non-small-cell lung cancer. Cancer Control 2003;10:297–305.

95. Li Q, Yu JJ, Mu C, et al. Association between the level of ERCC1 expression and the repair of cisplatin-induced DNA damage in human ovarian cancer cells. Anticancer Res 2000;20(2A):645–652.

96. Wang G, Reed E, Li QQ. Molecular basis of cellular response to cisplatin chemotherapy in non-small cell lung cancer. Oncol Rep 2004;12:955–965.

97. Taniguchi T, Tischkowitz M, Ameziane N, et al. Disruption of the Fanconi anemia–BRCA pathway in cisplatin-sensitive ovarian tumors. Nat Med 2003;9:568–574.

Bleomycin

15

John S. Lazo   Bruce A. Chabner

In a search for new antimicrobial and antineoplastic agents, Umezawa and colleagues[1] isolated a number of small glycopeptides from culture broths of the fungus *Streptomyces verticillus*. The most active antitumor agent found was, in fact, a mixture of peptides now known in clinical usage as *bleomycin*, a drug that has important activity against Hodgkin's disease, testicular cancer, malignant pleural effusions, cancers of the cervix and penis, and head and neck cancer. Bleomycin used in combination with vinblastine sulfate or etoposide and *cis*-diamminedichloroplatinum has produced a high rate of cure in patients with germinal neoplasms of the testis.[2] The drug has attracted great interest because of its unique biochemical action, its virtual lack of toxicity for normal hematopoietic tissue, and its ability to cause pulmonary fibrosis. Its primary pharmacologic and pharmacokinetic features are shown in Table 15.1.

STRUCTURE AND MECHANISM OF ACTION

The bleomycins are a family of peptides with a molecular weight of approximately 1,500 (Fig. 15.1). All contain a unique structural component, bleomycinic acid, and differ only in their terminal alkylamine group. Because of their unusual structure, catalytic properties, and important antitumor activity, the bleomycin antibiotics have been the subject of intensive basic and clinical investigation. Bleomycin A_2, the predominant peptide, has been prepared by total chemical synthesis, as has a series of analogs.[3] More than 100 additional bleomycin-like antitumor antibiotics have been isolated or synthesized, but none has yet emerged as superior in clinical activity.

The clinical mixture of bleomycin peptides is formulated as a sulfate salt, and its potency is measured in units (U) of antimicrobial activity. Each unit contains between 1.2 and 1.7 mg of polypeptide protein. The powdered clinical mixture is stable for at least 1 year at room temperature and for 4 weeks after reconstitution in aqueous solution if stored at 4°C.

The multiple glycopeptides found in the clinical preparation of bleomycin have been separated and purified by paper, conventional column, and high-performance liquid chromatography (HPLC).[4,5] The predominant active component, comprising approximately 70% of the commercial preparation, is the A_2 peptide shown in Figure 15.1. The remaining bleomycins differ in the terminal amine. The native compound isolated from *S. verticillus* is a blue-colored Cu(II) coordinated complex. Bleomycin complexes in vitro 1:1 with several endogenous and exogenous metals, including Cu(I), C(II), Fe(II), Fe(III), Co(II), Co(III), Zn(II), Mn(II), and Mn(III). The Co(III) complexes are essentially inert with respect to biologic activity and the exchangeability of their bound metal and thus have been candidates for tumor localization, especially with cobalt 57 (^{57}Co). Unfortunately, the half-life of ^{57}Co is 270 days rather than the desired several hours or days common for clinically useful diagnostic agents. Among endogenous metals, bleomycin has the highest affinity for Cu(II); bleomycin has a fourfold greater affinity for reduced Cu(I) than for Fe(II).[6] In initial clinical trials with Cu(II)·bleomycin, patients experienced profound phlebitis, and the white apobleomycin was soon adopted for clinical use. Nevertheless, after systemic administration, bleomycin appears to speciate rapidly with Cu(II) removed from plasma proteins.[7] The Cu(II)·bleomycin complex is internalized through a poorly described endocytotic system that may include discrete plasma membrane proteins of 250 kd.[8,9] Most investigators believe that the Cu·bleomycin is a prodrug and that cleavage-competent bleomycin is Fe(II)-speciated. Considerable chemical evidence regarding DNA damage produced by Fe(II)·bleomycin exists to support this hypothesis.[6] The primary model was first outlined by Umezawa's group[7] and is schematically represented in Figure 15.2. Cu(II) associated

TABLE 15.1

KEY FEATURES OF BLEOMYCIN PHARMACOLOGY

Mechanism of action	Oxidative cleavage of DNA initiated by hydrogen abstraction
Metabolism	Activated by microsomal reduction
	Degraded by hydrolase found in multiple tissues
Pharmacokinetics	$t_{1/2}\alpha$: 24 min; $t_{1/2}\beta$: 2–4 hr
Elimination	Renal: 45–70% in first 24 hr
Drug interactions	None clearly established at a biochemical level
	Oxygen enhances pulmonary toxicity
	cis-Platinum induces renal failure and increases risk of pulmonary toxicity
Toxicity	Pulmonary interstitial infiltrates and fibrosis
	Desquamation, especially of fingers, elbows
	Raynaud's phenomenon
	Hypersensitivity reactions (fever, anaphylaxis, eosinophilic pulmonary infiltrates)
Precautions	Pulmonary toxicity increased in patients with:
	Underlying pulmonary disease
	Age >70 yr
	Renal insufficiency
	Prior chest irradiation
	O_2 during surgery
	Reduce dose if creatinine clearance <80 mL/min

$t_{1/2}$, half-life.

with intracellular Cu(II)·bleomycin is reduced, possibly by intracellular cysteine-rich proteins, to Cu(I), which is released, and the apobleomycin quickly complexes with Fe(II).[10] Nuclear translocation of the Fe(II)·bleomycin complex proceeds with subsequent chromatin damage. The metal coordination chemistry of bleomycin has been the subject of considerable attention, and primarily on the basis of studies using electron paramagnetic resonance (EPR),[11] crystallography,[12] and Fe(II) surrogate metals such as Cu(II), a square-pyramidal complex, as indicated in Figure 15.1, is most favored.[6,7] Six distinct moieties are required for this metal coordination complex, and the N-1 of the pyrimidine, the N of the imidazole, and the secondary amine are undisputed participants.[6] Debate still exists about the arrangement of the remaining ligands, and this presumably will be resolved with further structural analyses. Although many aspects of the cellular scheme found in Figure 15.2 are biologically and chemically appealing, several questions remain unanswered, including the identity of the sulfhydryl-rich reductant for Cu(II), the recipient and fate of the Cu(I), the intracellular source of Fe(II), the mode by which the metal-bound bleomycin translocates the plasma membrane, and the nucleus. Therefore, others[13,14] have developed a rival hypothesis to explain the antitumor activity and fate of bleomycin. Even though Cu(II)·bleomycin is not highly cytotoxic,[15,16] persuasive arguments for a potential functional role of Cu(I)·bleomycin in the biologic actions of

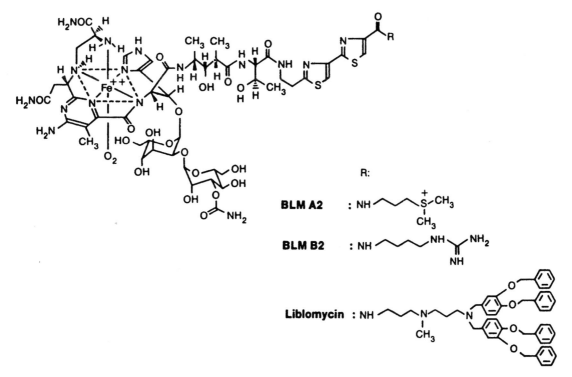

Figure 15.1 Structure of bleomycin·Fe(II) complex. The various substitutions on the amino-terminal end of the molecule are shown for bleomycin A_2 (BLM A2), for bleomycin B_2 (BLM B2; also a component of the clinical preparation), and for one congener, liblomycin.

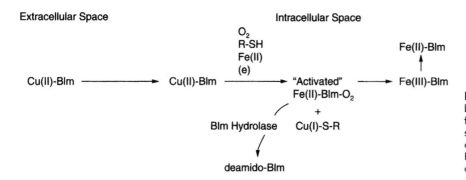

Figure 15.2 Schematic representation of bleomycin (Blm) transformation as it moves from the extracellular to the intracellular space. The Cu(II)·Blm complex in the extracellular space is converted to a cytotoxic Fe(II)·Blm·O₂ complex in the cell. Inactivation of Blm by Blm hydrolase is also shown.

this antineoplastic agent have been presented.[6,14] Thus the widely embraced concept that Fe(II)-complexed bleomycin is the only biologically relevant species may require revision.

MECHANISM OF ACTION

Early mechanistic studies identified a concentration-dependent loss in DNA integrity with loss of cell viability in the absence of marked decreases in either RNA or protein composition. After considering several potential therapeutic targets, including RNA and DNA polymerases and nucleases and DNA ligases, most investigators accepted direct DNA damage as the most attractive candidate for the cytotoxicity and, consequently, the antitumor activity of bleomycin.[6,7] Single- and double-strand DNA damage is readily observed in cultured cells and isolated DNA incubated with bleomycin in solution. This breakage is reflected in the chromosomal gaps, deletions, and fragments seen in cytogenetic studies of whole cells incubated with the drug. Nevertheless, as with many antineoplastic agents, reports exist dissociating DNA damage from cell death.[17] Although this may simply reflect rapid DNA repair, other biochemical targets continue to be examined. For example, bleomycin mediates lipid peroxidation, which certainly has been associated with the lethality of other small redox-active molecules. The fact that bleomycin can participate in the oxidative degradation of the three major classes of RNA—transfer RNA, messenger RNA, and

ribosomal RNA—in a substrate-specific and ternary-structure–dependent manner is also interesting.[18] The cleavage of RNA occurs by H abstraction from the oligoribonucleotides[19] in the presence of DNA and at pharmacologically relevant bleomycin concentrations.[20] This has rekindled interest in the possibility that RNA damage may have therapeutic relevance. Nevertheless, the primacy of DNA damage as the major mechanism of bleomycin cytotoxicity remains.[21]

CHEMISTRY OF BLEOMYCIN-MEDIATED DNA CLEAVAGE

The mechanism by which Fe(II)·bleomycin cleaves DNA has been examined using viral, bacterial, mammalian, and synthetic DNAs. Bleomycin is unlike most DNA-damaging agents because it attacks neither the nucleic bases nor the phosphate linkage. In this multistep process, initially an "activated" Fe(II)·bleomycin·O₂ complex is formed that is kinetically competent to cleave DNA. The binding of dioxygen to Fe(II)·bleomycin proceeds most rapidly in the presence of DNA, which stabilizes the complex.[22] The proposed sequence of events responsible for the production of an activated bleomycin has been deduced from in vitro studies and is briefly outlined in Figure 15.3. Fe(II) combines with apobleomycin, producing an EPR-silent, high-spin Fe(II)·bleomycin complex. With dioxygen, this is rapidly converted to a ternary Fe(II)·bleomycin·O₂ species,

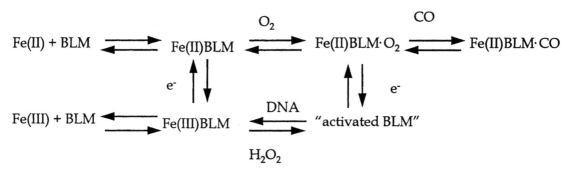

Figure 15.3 Model for the activation of cleavage-competent bleomycin (BLM).

which can be trapped with isocyanide, CO, or NO or can be activated by a $1e^-$ reduction. The e^- can be supplied by a second Fe(II)·bleomycin·O_2 molecule,[8,16] by H_2O_2,[8] by microsomal enzymes and nicotinamide-adenine dinucleotide phosphate (reduced form) (NADPH) organic reductant,[23] or by nuclei and nicotinamide-adenine dinucleotide (reduced form) (NADH).[24] Mossbauer studies[23] suggest that the activated bleomycin has a half-life of a few minutes at 0°C, so it is likely to be reasonably long-lived even at 37°C. In the absence of DNA, the activated species will self-destruct. The association constant of Fe(II)·bleomycin for duplex DNA, however, is approximately 10^5 per M.[25] Thus the second step in the DNA cleavage process readily occurs. The interaction of bleomycin with DNA shows nucleotide sequence selectivity[26] and most likely occurs at the minor groove where the primary DNA target, H4', is located.[21] At saturating concentrations of bleomycin, one molecule of drug associates with four or five base pairs of DNA. The binding between bleomycin and DNA appears to be through electrostatic interactions and partial intercalation (insertion between base pairs) of the amino-terminal tripeptide of bleomycin (called the *S tripeptide*)[27,28] (Fig. 15.4). The bithiazole of the S tripeptide bonds to guanine groups in the favored sequence of GpC and GpT.[26,27] The terminal dimethylsulfonium of bleomycin A_2 and the positively charged terminal amines of other bleomycins also participate in DNA binding, as indicated by broadening of the proton magnetic resonance of the sulfonium moiety in the presence of DNA.[26] If either bleomycin or its S tripeptide is mixed with DNA, linear DNA is lengthened or supercoiled circular DNA is relaxed. Both these effects are indicative of unwinding of the double-helical structure as the result of intercalation[28] and can be produced by bithiazole alone or by bleomycin and bleomycin analogs. Fe(II)·bleomycin exhibits a strong preference for the B-form of DNA rather than for the Z-form,[29] consistent with interactions with the minor groove of DNA.

The third step in the action of bleomycin is the generation of single- and double-strand DNA breaks. During the DNA cleavage process, Fe(II)·bleomycin functions catalytically as a ferrous oxidase[30] with the oxidation of Fe(II) to Fe(III); regeneration of the active Fe(II) requires endogenous reductants, including cytochrome P-450 reductase and NADPH,[31] an enzyme found in the nucleus and nuclear membrane. Under very controlled in vitro conditions, the short-lived oxygenated iron-bleomycin species[32] participates in almost four cleavage events per bleomycin molecule. Others have estimated the reduction of dioxygen by bleomycin, as monitored by measurement of oxygen consumption, with a maximum velocity of 27 mol oxygen consumed per minute per mole of bleomycin.[30] The K_m (binding affinity) of this reaction for Fe(II) is 1.8 mmol/L.[30]

The mechanism of DNA cleavage has been defined by the DNA fragments produced after incubation of the substrate with activated bleomycin.[21,33–36] Incubation of DNA with bleomycin in an aerobic environment results in the scission of the C-3'—C-4' ribose bond via a Criegee-type rearrangement, which produces three types of product, including a 5'-oligonucleotide terminating at its 3' end with a phosphoglycolic acid moiety, a 3'-oligonucleotide containing a 5'-phosphate, and a 3'-(thymin-9'-yl)propenal.[8,16] Exposure to Fe(II)·bleomycin produces the release of all four bases (thymine, cytosine, adenine, and guanine)[34] (Fig. 15.5, pathway A). Under anaerobic conditions, the free-base release is accompanied by production of an oxidatively damaged sugar in the intact DNA strand, which yields DNA cleavage only in basic conditions, namely, pH 12 (Fig. 15.5, pathway B). No base propenal is released. Which of these pathways predominates in intact cells is not known, although both free bases and base propenal adducts are detected in most cells. The base propenal compounds have intrinsic cytotoxicity and may contribute to the damage to cells.[37]

Bleomycin produces both single- and double-strand DNA breaks in a ratio of approximately 10:1. The unexpectedly high frequency of double-strand breaks has been addressed in elegant studies of the effect of bleomycin on hairpin-shaped oligonucleotides that have single-strand gaps corresponding to those produced by bleomycin.[38] The highly electronegative 3'-phosphoglycolate and 5'-phosphate groups remaining at the site of DNA single-strand cleavage

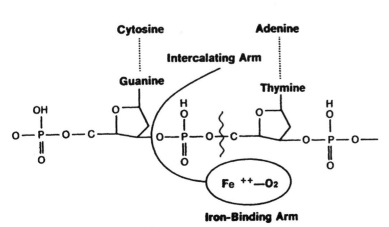

Figure 15.4 Intercalation of the bithiazole groups between DNA base pairs, at least one of which contains the GpT of GpC sequence. Also shown is the apposition of the Fe(II)-binding portion of bleomycin to the deoxyribose group, which is cleaved via hydrogen abstraction at the C-4' of the deoxyribose.

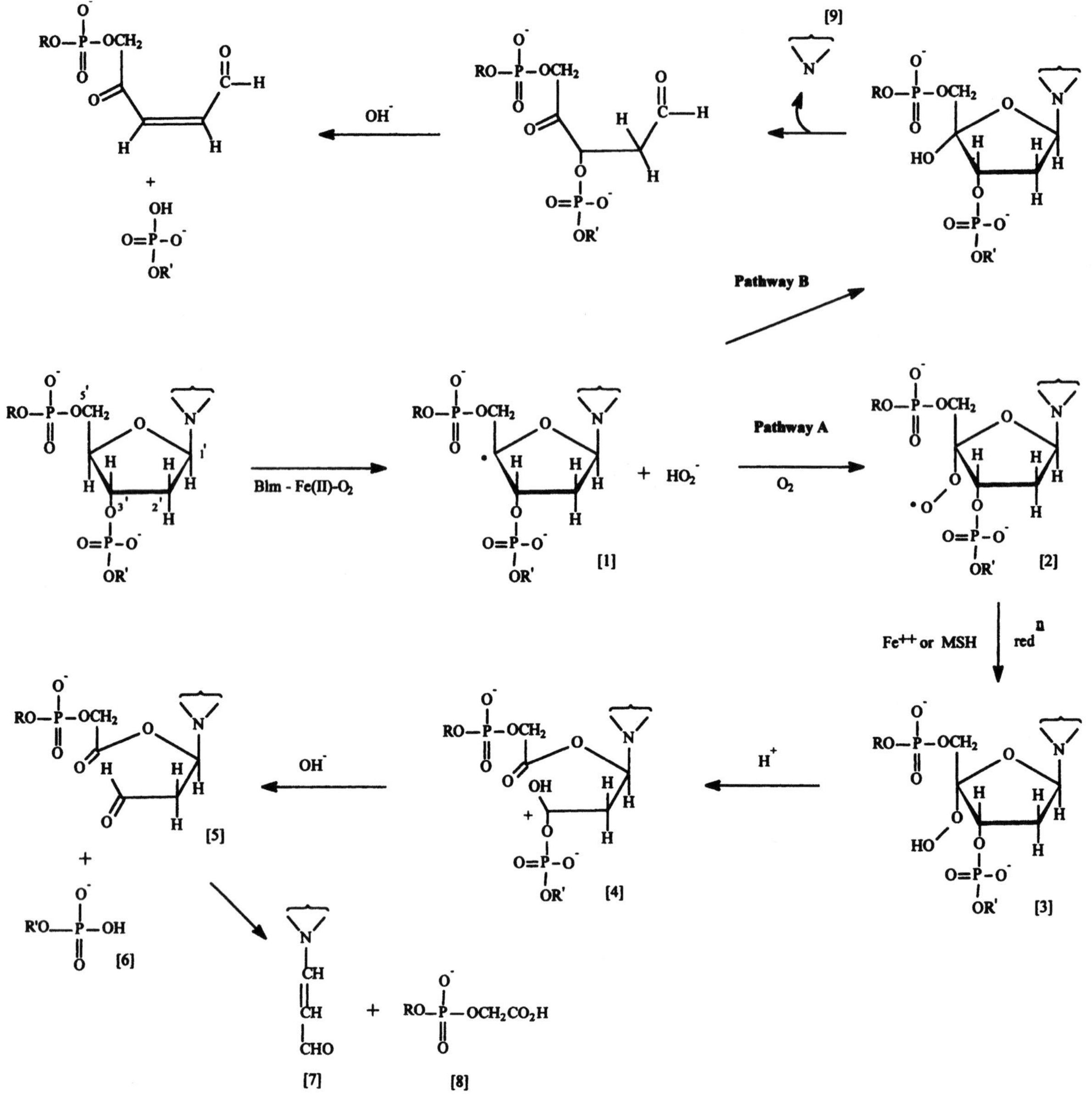

Figure 15.5 Scheme for the cleavage of the 3'—4' deoxyribose bond by the activated bleomycin·Fe(II)·O_2 complex. The activated drug complex initially abstracts a hydrogen radical from the 4' position to produce the unstable intermediate [1] that decomposes in the presence of oxygen (pathway A) to produce the free base propenal [7], leaving a 3'-phosphoglycolate ester [8] and a 5'-phosphate [6] at the free ends of the broken DNA strand. Under conditions of limited oxygen, a free base [9] is released, and DNA strand scission occurs only in the presence of alkali (pH 12).

may promote access of a second bleomycin molecule to the opposing strand, resulting in a double-strand break.

Analysis of the products of DNA cleavage, using either viral or mammalian DNA, has consistently shown a preferential release of thymine or thymine-propenal, with lesser amounts of the other three bases or their propenal adducts.[21,39] The propensity for attack at thymine bases probably results from the previously mentioned preference for partial intercalation of bleomycin between base pairs in which at least one strand contains the sequence 5'-GpT-3'. The specificity for cleavage of DNA at a residue located at

the 3' side of G seems to be absolute.[40] A schematic representation of the intercalation and cleavage processes as conceived by Grollman and Takeshita[41] is given in Figure 15.4 and summarizes the structural and sequence specificities discussed in this chapter.

CELLULAR PHARMACOLOGY

The cellular uptake of bleomycin is slow, and large concentration gradients are maintained between extracellular and intracellular spaces.[42] ^{14}C-bleomycin accumulates at the cell membrane of murine tumor cells, with gradual appearance of labeling at the nuclear membrane only after 4 hours of exposure.[43] The importance of the plasma membrane as a barrier for the highly cationic bleomycins, which also have a significant size, has been clearly documented by studies using electrical permeabilization techniques,[44] which increases intracellular drug and cytotoxicity. A bleomycin-binding membrane protein has been identified with a molecular mass of 250 kd and becomes half-maximally saturated with a bleomycin concentration of 5 μmol/L.[9] This protein may be responsible for the internalization of bleomycin, but additional characterization is necessary to affirm its role in the cytotoxic action of bleomycin. Using a fluorescent mimic of bleomycin or agents that disrupt vacuoles, Mistry et al.[45] and Lazo et al.[8] concluded that the internalized bleomycin is sequestered in cytoplasmic organelles. The process by which the entrapped bleomycin is released from the vesicles is not known.

Once bleomycin is internalized, it either translocates to the nucleus to effect DNA damage or can be degraded by bleomycin hydrolase, which has been characterized and cloned from several species.[46–49] This homomultimeric enzyme metabolizes and inactivates a broad spectrum of bleomycin analogs. The enzyme cleaves the carboxamide amine from the β-aminoalaninamide, yielding a weakly cytotoxic (less than 1/100) deaminobleomycin.[46] Both the primary amino acid sequence and higher-order structure determined by x-ray crystallography reveal that bleomycin hydrolase is a founding member of what is a growing class of self-compartmentalizing or sequestered intracellular proteases.[50,51] Both yeast and human enzymes are homohexamers with a ring or barrel-like structure that have the papain-like active sites situated within a central channel in a manner resembling the organization of the active sites in the 20S proteosome.[50,51] The central channel, which has a strong positive electrostatic potential in the yeast protein, is slightly negative in human bleomycin hydrolase.[51] The yeast enzyme binds to DNA and RNA, but human bleomycin hydrolase lacks this attribute.[48,51,52] The C-terminus requires autoprocessing of the terminal amino acid, and the processed enzyme has both aminopeptidase and peptide ligase activity.[52,53] The kinetic properties of bleomycin hydrolase, such as its pH optimum and salt requirements, are distinct from those of other cysteine proteinases, although the substrate specificity of bleomycin hydrolase is similar to that of cathepsin H.[47] Human bleomycin hydrolase is located on chromosome band 17q11.2 and has one polymorphic site encoding either a valine or isoleucine.[54,55] Bleomycin hydrolase is found in both normal and malignant cells.[48,56] That this is the only enzyme responsible for metabolizing bleomycin was documented with bleomycin hydrolase–null or "knockout" mice.[57] This inactivating enzyme is present in relatively low concentrations in lung and skin, the two normal tissues most susceptible to bleomycin damage.[46,56] Interestingly,

pulmonary bleomycin hydrolase levels are highest in animal species or strains resistant to the pulmonary toxicity of bleomycin.[46] Mice that lack the functional gene are more sensitive to the toxic effects of bleomycin.[57] The enzyme is cytoplasmic but also may be localized to distinct subcellular organelles,[58] although the functional significance of this regionalization requires more investigation. A polymorphism, A[1450]G, in the coding region of the gene may affect catalytic activity and thus sensitivity to bleomycin, but it requires further characterization.[59]

Cells exposed to bleomycin in culture seem to be most susceptible in mitosis or in the G_2, or intermitotic, phase of the cell cycle[60]; in addition, progression of cells through G_2 into mitosis is blocked by the drug.[61] In mouse L cells, S phase is also lengthened before G_2 blockade.[62] Barlogie et al.[63] observed that cell death also occurred in cells exposed during G_1, although cell killing was maximal in G_2.

DNA is more sensitive to DNA cleavage at the G_2-M and G_1 phases of the cell cycle than at S phase, which may reflect differences in chromatin structure.[64] The degree of chromatin compactness dramatically influences bleomycin-induced DNA damage.[65]

Despite the apparent increased toxicity for cells in G_2, no agreement exists regarding preferential kill of logarithmically growing cells as compared with plateau-phase cells; indeed, some workers have observed greater fractional cell kill for plateau-phase cells.[66] The possibility of enhancing cell kill by exposure during G_2 has led to the clinical use of bleomycin by continuous infusion to maximize the chances of tumor cell exposure during the most sensitive phase of the cell cycle. The results of these trials have not been convincing with respect to increasing activity.

The intracellular lesions caused by bleomycin include chromosomal breaks and deletions and both single-strand and (less frequently) double-strand breaks. In nonmitotic cells, DNA is organized into nucleosomes, or small beads, which are joined by long strands, or linker regions. The primary point of attack seems to be in the linker regions of DNA, between nucleosomes.[67] Interestingly, the resulting 180– to 200–base-pair fragments are similar in size to those formed by endonucleases activated during apoptosis.[44] The technique of alkaline elution has been used by Iqbal and coworkers,[68] who observed a biphasic survival curve for cell survival or for DNA single-strand breaks versus dose. The reason for the biphasic characteristics of these curves is unclear, but it may be related to the differing susceptibility of DNA to cleavage by bleomycin during different phases of the cell cycle or the production of small internucleosomal DNA breaks from either direct DNA damage or an apoptotic endonuclease. Clearly, however, cell kill and DNA strand breakage increase in proportion to the duration of drug exposure for at least 6 hours; this finding again implies a greater effectiveness for bleomycin given by prolonged infusion than by intravenous bolus.

Cells are able to repair bleomycin-induced DNA breaks via a complex array of enzymes and pathways specific for both single-strand and double-strand breaks.[59] A delay in plating cells after bleomycin exposure increases plating efficiency, presumably by allowing time for repair of potentially lethal damage.[69] Inhibitors of DNA repair, such as caffeine and 3'-aminobenzamide,[70] accentuate DNA strand breakage and cell kill by bleomycin. Indirect evidence suggests that repair processes similar to those required for repair of lesions induced by *ionizing radiation* play a role in limiting damage due to bleomycin,[71,72] whereas cells deficient in repair mechanisms for *ultraviolet radiation* damage have no increased sensitivity to bleomycin. Cells from patients with ataxia-telangiectasia, which arises from an inherited defect in DNA repair, have increased sensitivity to bleomycin,[73] as do cells deficient in BRCA1, a component of pathways that sense DNA damage and repair double-strand breaks.[74,75]

RESISTANCE

Several intracellular factors have been identified as contributors to bleomycin tumor resistance: increased drug inactivation, decreased drug accumulation, and increased repair of DNA damage, particularly double-strand breaks.[74,75] Early studies[76] demonstrated increased rates of bleomycin inactivation in two bleomycin-resistant rat hepatoma cell lines. Morris et al.[77] raised a neutralizing polyclonal antibody to bleomycin hydrolase and demonstrated an increased level of this enzyme in cultured human head and neck carcinoma cells with acquired resistance to bleomycin. Metabolic inactivation of bleomycin also can contribute to intrinsic bleomycin resistance in human colon carcinoma cells.[78] Treatment of tumor-bearing mice with E-64 before treatment with bleomycin inhibited bleomycin metabolism and increased the antitumor activity of bleomycin without increasing pulmonary toxicity.[78] This provides a potentially novel approach to increase the therapeutic activity of bleomycin.

Increased bleomycin hydrolase activity is not the only mechanism of bleomycin resistance.[79] Some cells selected in culture for bleomycin resistance display enhanced DNA repair capacity.[80] A decrease in drug content is also seen in human tumor cells with acquired resistance to bleomycin.[17] Because Fe(III)·bleomycin requires reduction to Fe(II)·bleomycin, sulfhydryl groups on proteins and peptides are potential factors in drug resistance. Tumor lines with elevated levels of glutathione, selected for resistance to doxorubicin, are collaterally sensitive to bleomycin.[81] The evidence for glutathione enhancement of bleomycin activity is not entirely clear; others have found that buthionine sulfoxamine, a glutathione-depleting agent, enhances tumor sensitivity to bleomycin.[82] Increasing the major protein thiol metallothionein produces a small increase in bleomycin sensitivity, consistent with the proposal that this cysteine-rich protein may assist in the removal of Cu(I) from bleomycin.[10] Bleomycin is not affected by P-glycoprotein, the product of the mul-

tidrug resistance gene, in contrast to many other natural products.

CLINICAL PHARMACOKINETICS

A number of techniques have been developed for assay of bleomycin in biologic fluids, including microbiologic methods,[83] HPLC,[84] biochemical techniques (degradation of DNA),[85] and radioimmunoassay methods.[86] The most rapid and simplest for clinical studies is the radioimmunoassay, which, using bleomycin labeled with iodine-125 or ^{57}Co, has provided insight into the disposition of bleomycin in humans and has superseded the less sensitive and less specific microbiologic assay techniques. The antibodies described by Broughton and Strong[86] react quantitatively with the component peptides of the clinically used bleomycin formulation. The primary component peptides A_2 and B_2 give 75 to 100% reactivity compared with the mixture in standard curve determinations. HPLC, using the ion-pairing technique, allows resolution of the component peptides but is more time-consuming.

The hallmark of bleomycin pharmacokinetics in patients with normal serum creatinine is a rapid two-phase drug disappearance from plasma; 45%[87] to 70%[88] of the dose is excreted in the urine within 24 hours. For intravenous bolus doses, the half-lives for plasma disappearance have varied somewhat among the published studies. Alberts et al.[89] reported α and β half-lives of 24 minutes and 4 hours, respectively, whereas Crooke et al.[90] estimated the β half-life to be approximately 2 hours. Peak plasma concentrations reach 1 to 10 mU/mL for intravenous bolus doses of 15 U/m^2.

For patients receiving bleomycin by continuous intravenous infusion, the postinfusion half-life is approximately 3 hours. Intramuscular injection of bleomycin (2 to 10 U/m^2) gave peak plasma levels of 0.13 to 0.6 mU/mL, or approximately one-tenth the peak level achieved by the intravenous bolus doses.[91] The mean half-life after intramuscular injection was 2.5 hours, or approximately the same as that after intravenous injection. Peak serum concentrations were reached approximately 1 hour after injection (Fig. 15.6). Bleomycin pharmacokinetics also have been studied in patients receiving intrapleural or intraperitoneal injections. These routes have proved effective in controlling malignant effusions due to breast, lung, and ovarian cancer.[92] Intracavitary bleomycin, in doses of 60 U/m^2, gives peak plasma levels of 0.4 to 5.0 mU/mL, with a plasma half-life of 3.4 hours after intrapleural doses and 5.3 hours after intraperitoneal injection.[93] Corresponding intracavitary levels are 10- to 22-fold higher than simultaneous plasma concentrations.[94] Approximately 45% of an intracavitary dose is absorbed into the systemic circulation, and 30% is excreted in the urine as immunoreactive material.

As might be expected, bleomycin pharmacokinetics is markedly altered in patients with abnormal renal function, particularly those with creatinine clearance of less than

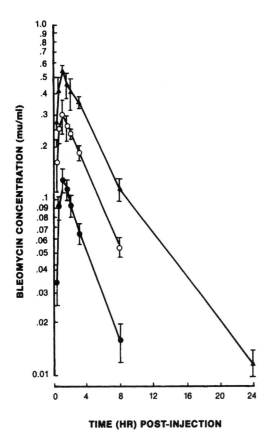

Figure 15.6 Pharmacokinetics of bleomycin after intramuscular administration of 2 (●), 5 (m), and 10 (▲) mg of bleomycin per m². (From Oken MM, Crooke ST, Elson MK, et al. Pharmacokinetics of bleomycin after IM administration in man. Cancer Treat Rep 1981; 65:485.)

35 mL/minute. Alberts et al.[89] noted a terminal half-life of approximately 10 hours in a patient with a slightly elevated creatinine clearance of 1.5 mg/dL, and Crooke et al.[87] reported a patient who showed a creatinine clearance of 10.7 mL/minute and a β half-life of 21 hours. Others have reported a high frequency of pulmonary toxicity in patients with renal dysfunction secondary to cisplatin treatment.[88,95] One report described fatal pulmonary fibrosis that occurred after three doses of 20 U each given to a patient with chronic renal insufficiency (blood urea nitrogen, 48 mg/dL; creatinine, 4.8 mg/dL).[96] The available data are too limited to provide accurate guidelines for dosage adjustment in patients with renal failure. One retrospective study identified a glomerular filtration rate of less than 80 mL/minute as conferring an increased risk of pulmonary toxicity.[97] The prudent course is to decrease dosages by 50% for patients with clearances below 80 mL/minute or to give an alternative regimen such as vinblastine, ifosfamide and cisplatin.[98]

CLINICAL TOXICITY AND SIDE EFFECTS

The most important toxic actions of bleomycin affect the lungs and skin; usually little evidence of myelosuppression is apparent except in patients with severely compromised bone marrow function due to extensive previous chemotherapy.[99] In such patients, myelosuppression is usually mild and is seen primarily with high-dose therapy. Fever occurs during the 48 hours after drug administration in one-quarter of patients.[100] Some investigators advocate using a 1-U test dose of bleomycin in patients receiving their initial dose of drug,[101] because rare instances of fatal acute allergic reactions have been reported.

Pulmonary Toxicity

Pulmonary toxicity is manifest as a subacute or chronic interstitial pneumonitis complicated in its later stages by progressive interstitial fibrosis, hypoxia, and death.[102] Pulmonary toxicity, usually manifested with cough, dyspnea, and bibasilar pulmonary infiltrates on chest radiographs, occurs in 3% to 5% of patients receiving a total dose of less than 450 U bleomycin; it increases significantly to a 10% incidence in those treated with greater cumulative doses.[100] Toxicity is also more frequent in patients older than age 70, in those with underlying emphysema, and in patients receiving single doses greater than 25 U/m².[103] The use of bleomycin in single doses of more than 30 U is to be discouraged, because instances of rapid onset of fatal pulmonary fibrosis 7 to 8 weeks after high-dose bleomycin have been reported.[104] Evidence also exists that previous radiotherapy to the chest predisposes to bleomycin-induced pulmonary toxicity.[105] Although the risk of lung toxicity increases with cumulative doses greater than 450 U, severe pulmonary sequelae have been observed at total doses below 100 U. In the standard regimen for treating testicular cancer, bleomycin is given in doses of 30 U/week for 12 doses, and the incidence of fatal pulmonary toxicity in this low-risk population of young male patients is less than 2%.[2,106]

Pathogenesis of Pulmonary Toxicity

The potential for bleomycin A_2, A_5, A_6, or B_2 to cause pulmonary toxicity is easily demonstrated by intravenous infusion or by direct instillation of the parent molecule into the trachea of a rodent, where it induces an acute inflammatory response, epithelial apoptosis, an alveolar fibrinoid exudate, and, over a period of 1 to 2 weeks, progressive deposition of collagen.[107,108] The terminal amines of these bleomycins are sufficient, by themselves, to cause the toxicity in rodents, and the toxic potency of the bleomycins is directly correlated with the potency of their individual terminal amines, with the A_2 aminopropyl-dimethylsulfonium and the A_5 spermidine having greater effect than the B_2 agmatine.[109] These findings raise the possibility that modification of the terminal amine might allow selection of a less toxic analog for clinical use. Several such analogs have been tested, but clinical superiority has not been demonstrated.

The pathogenesis of bleomycin pulmonary toxicity in rodents serves as a model for understanding pulmonary fibrosis, an end result of a broad range of human diseases induced by drugs, autoimmunity, and infection.[107] The primary model has been the intratracheal instillation of bleomycin in mice or hamsters,[110] although one should note that in clinical drug use the agent is administered parenterally. The drug has direct toxicity to alveolar epithelial cells, causing induction of epithelial apoptosis, intraalveolar inflammation, cytokine release by alveolar macrophages, fibroblast proliferation, and collagen deposition,[110-112] as well as endothelial cell damage in small pulmonary vessels.[113] As changes progress from acute inflammation to interstitial fibrosis, pulmonary function deteriorates, as indicated by a decrease in lung compliance, a decrease in carbon monoxide diffusion capacity, and terminal hypoxia.[114,115] Hydroxyproline deposition parallels the increase in collagen and serves as a quantitative measure of the progression of fibrosis in animal models.[114]

A broad array of cytokines, produced by alveolar macrophages and by endothelial cells in response to bleomycin, have been implicated in the molecular pathogenesis of pulmonary fibrosis. These include transforming growth factor β (TGF-β),[115-117] tumor necrosis factor α (TNF-α),[118-120] interleukin 1β,[120] interleukins 2, 3, 4, 5, and 6,[121,122] and various chemokines. Bleomycin and TGF-β both stimulate the promoter that controls transcription of a collagen precursor.[117] Interleukin 1 augments TGF-β secretion stimulated by bleomycin, whereas TNF-α enhances prostaglandin secretion and fibroblast proliferation.[120]

Genetic experiments have provided further insight into factors that influence susceptibility to fibrosis[120-124] and into the central role of cytokines in bleomycin lung toxicity. They illustrate the importance of drug inactivation, fibrin deposition, and cytokine action in mediating lung injury. Travis and colleagues have shown that strains of mice with greatly increased susceptibility to bleomycin toxicity (and simultaneously to radiation toxicity) can be inbred, although the specific genetic defect is still unclear.[123,124] Other experiments have shown that specific genetic lesions do predispose to pulmonary fibrosis. Bleomycin hydrolase–knockout mice have significantly greater lung and epidermal toxicity than normal controls.[125] Mice lacking plasminogen activator inhibitor 1, a protein that blocks the activation of the major fibrinolytic protease in plasma and in the alveolar space, have decreased susceptibility to bleomycin pulmonary fibrosis,[126] as do mice lacking matrilysin, a matrix metalloproteinase.[127]

Perhaps the most compelling genetic experiments implicate the central role of TGF-β, which is secreted by alveolar macrophages in response to bleomycin.[128] TGF-β is secreted in a complex with a latency-associated peptide and is activated by binding of the complex to αvβ6 integrin found on alveolar epithelial cells and keratinocytes. This binding of the TGF-β complex to its integrin exposes cytokine-binding domains that allow interaction of TGF-β with its receptor(s) and stimulates the production of procollagen by fibroblasts.[129] Mice in which αvβ6 integrin has been knocked out develop an inflammatory alveolar response to bleomycin but do not develop progressive fibrosis.

The stimulus for cytokine and chemokine release is uncertain, although apoptosis of epithelial cells, alveolar macrophages, or lymphocytes may play an important role.[130,131] In mice, genetic deletion of either Fas, which is expressed on pulmonary epithelial cells, or Fas ligand, as expressed on T lymphocytes, does not prevent inflammation but does protect against pulmonary fibrosis.[131] Soluble Fas antigen or anti-Fas ligand antibody also provides protection against fibrosis, presumably by preventing Fas-mediated epithelial apoptosis. CXCL12, a potent chemokine, is secreted by inflammatory cells in response to lung injury and attracts bone marrow–derived stem cells that establish as fibrocytes in the damaged lung.[130] Anti-CXCL12 antibodies protect against bleomycin-induced pulmonary fibrosis.

In addition to providing remarkable insights regarding the pathogenesis of pulmonary fibrosis, these experiments suggest a number of new approaches to the prevention of bleomycin toxicity. Thus, in various animal models, protection is provided by Fas antigen and anti-Fas ligand antibodies[131]; TNF-α–soluble receptor[132]; TGF-β antibodies[133]; granulocyte-macrophage colony–stimulating factor antibodies[134]; pirfenidone, an inhibitor of platelet-derived growth factor function and procollagen transcription[135,136]; the antioxidant amifostine[137]; relaxin, a collagen matrix–degrading protein that increases collagenase secretion and decreases procollagen synthesis[138]; transgenic expression of *Sh ble*, a yeast protein that binds the iron-bleomycin complex and protects against its toxicity[139]; dehydroproline, an inhibitor of procollagen synthesis[140,141]; indomethacin[142]; and anti-CXCL12 antibodies.[130] These findings may be applicable to the general problem of preventing drug-induced or idiopathic pulmonary fibrosis in humans,[143] although none of these agents has yet been shown to be efficacious in a clinical trial.

In general, in animal toxicology experiments, single high doses of bleomycin produce greater pulmonary inflammation and fibrosis than do smaller daily doses or continuous drug infusion,[144,145] but these findings have never been confirmed in humans.

Clinical Syndrome of Pulmonary Toxicity

Clinical symptoms of bleomycin pulmonary injury include a nonproductive cough, dyspnea, and occasionally fever and pleuritic pain. Physical examination usually reveals minimal auscultatory evidence of pulmonary alveolar infiltrates, and initial chest films are often negative or may reveal an increase in interstitial markings, especially in the lower lobes, with a predilection for subpleural areas. Chest radiographs, when positive, reveal patchy reticulonodular

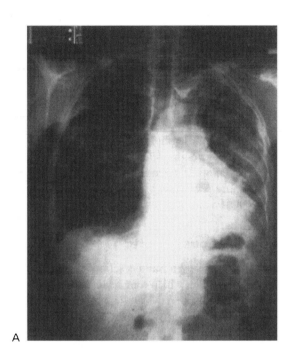
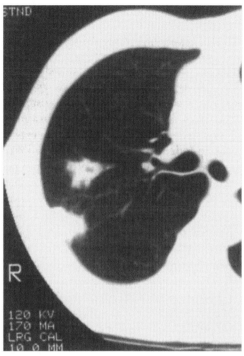

Figure 15.7 **A:** Typical interstitial pulmonary infiltrates, most obvious in left lung, observed during treatment of a patient with testicular carcinoma. **B:** Nodular variant of bleomycin pulmonary toxicity in a patient undergoing treatment for testicular cancer. Computed tomographic scan of chest showing a nodular density with central cavitation. On biopsy, the lesion was found to be composed of granulomas with associated interstitial pneumonitis. Appropriate stains and cultures did not reveal infectious agents. (From Talcott JA, Garnick MB, Stomper PC, et al. Cavitary lung nodules associated with combination chemotherapy containing bleomycin. J Urol 1987;138:619.)

infiltrates, which in later stages may coalesce to form areas of apparent consolidation. In occasional patients, the initial radiographic changes may be discrete nodules indistinguishable from metastatic tumor; central cavitation of nodules may be present[146,147] (Fig. 15.7). Gallium-67 lung scans or computed tomographic scans (Fig. 15.8) may show the presence of a diffuse lung lesion at a time of minimal abnormality on plain films of the chest; computed tomographic scans are much more sensitive than posteroanterior chest films in revealing the extent of pulmonary

fibrosis. Radiologic findings do not differentiate bleomycin lung toxicity from other forms of interstitial lung disease,[148] however, particularly *Pneumocystis carinii* pneumonia. Arterial oxygen desaturation and an abnormal carbon monoxide diffusion capacity are present in symptomatic patients with bleomycin toxicity as well as in patients with other forms of interstitial pulmonary disease. Thus, open lung biopsy is usually required to distinguish between the primary differential diagnostic alternatives, specifically a drug-induced pulmonary lesion, an infectious interstitial

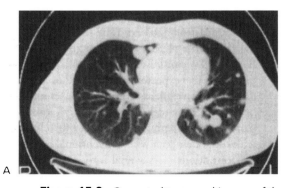
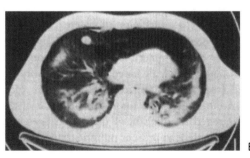

Figure 15.8 Computed tomographic scans of the chest before **(A)** and after **(B)** treatment for testicular cancer. The multiple metastatic pulmonary nodules partially regressed with therapy, but the posttreatment film shows dense bilateral pulmonary fibrosis as well as a large left pneumothorax and pneumomediastinum. The patient died of bleomycin pulmonary toxicity shortly afterward.

pneumonitis, and neoplastic pulmonary infiltration. The findings on histologic examination of human lung after bleomycin treatment closely resemble those previously described in the experimental animal and include necrosis of Type I alveolar cells, an acute inflammatory infiltrate in the alveoli, interstitial and intraalveolar edema, pulmonary hyaline membrane formation, and intraalveolar and, later in the course, interstitial fibrosis. In addition, squamous metaplasia of Type II alveolar lining cells has been described as a characteristic finding.[149] In rare cases, a true hypersensitivity pneumonitis may develop, characterized by underlying eosinophilic pulmonary infiltrates and a prompt clinical response to corticosteroids.[150]

Pulmonary function tests, particularly a rapid fall in the carbon monoxide–diffusing capacity, are of possible value in predicting a high risk of pulmonary toxicity. Most patients treated with bleomycin, however, show a progressive (10 to 15%) fall in diffusion capacity with increasing total dose and a more marked increase in changes above a 270-unit total dose. Whether or not the diffusion capacity test can be used to predict which patients will subsequently develop clinically significant pulmonary toxicity is not clear.[151] Some investigators suggest that bleomycin should be halted if the diffusion capacity for carbon dioxide (DCCO) falls below 40% of the initial value, even in the absence of symptoms. As mentioned earlier, at advanced stages in the evolution of bleomycin pulmonary toxicity, the diffusion capacity as well as arterial oxygen saturation and total lung capacity become markedly abnormal. Long-term assessment of pulmonary function in patients treated with bleomycin for testicular cancer has revealed a return to baseline normal values at a median of 4 years after treatment.[152]

Patients who have received bleomycin seem to be at greater risk of respiratory failure during the postoperative recovery period after surgery,[153] although more recent studies have questioned the association of perioperative oxygen and pulmonary toxicity.[154] In one study, five of five patients treated with 200 U/m² bleomycin (cumulative dose) for testicular cancer died of postoperative respiratory failure; a reduction in inspired oxygen to an inspired oxygen fraction of 0.24 and a decrease in the volume of fluids administered during surgery prevented mortality in subsequent patients.[153] The sensitivity of bleomycin-treated patients to high concentrations of inspired oxygen is intriguing in view of the molecular action of bleomycin, which is dependent on and mediated by the formation of oxygen-derived free radicals. Current safeguards for anesthesia of bleomycin-treated patients include the use of the minimum tolerated concentration of inspired oxygen and modest fluid replacement to prevent pulmonary edema.

No specific therapy is available for patients with bleomycin-induced lung toxicity. Discontinuation of the drug may be followed by a period of continued progression of the pulmonary findings, with partial reversal of the abnormalities in pulmonary function only after several months. The inflammatory component of the pathologic process does resolve in experimental models,[115] and interstitial infiltrates regress clinically, but the reversibility of pulmonary fibrosis has not been documented. The value of corticosteroids in promoting recovery from bleomycin-induced lung toxicity remains controversial; beneficial effects have been described in isolated case studies.[155,156] Long-term follow-up of patients with clinical and radiographic evidence of bleomycin-induced pneumonitis suggests a complete resolution of radiographic, clinical, and pulmonary function abnormalities in a small series of eight patients 2 years after completion of treatment for testicular cancer.[157] However, in more severe cases pulmonary fibrosis may be only partially reversible.

Cutaneous Toxicity

A more common but less serious toxicity of bleomycin is its effect on skin, which may relate to bleomycin hydrolase levels.[56] Approximately 50% of patients treated with conventional once-daily or twice-daily doses of this agent develop erythema, induration, and hyperkeratosis and peeling of skin that may progress to frank ulceration.[100] These changes predominantly affect digits, hands, joints, and areas of previous irradiation. Hyperpigmentation, alopecia, and nail changes also occur during bleomycin therapy. These cutaneous side effects do not necessitate discontinuation of therapy, particularly if clear benefit is being derived from the drug. Rarely, patients may develop Raynaud's phenomenon while receiving bleomycin.[158] Other toxic reactions to bleomycin include hypersensitivity reactions characterized by urticaria, periorbital edema, and bronchospasm.[100]

SCHEDULES OF ADMINISTRATION

Bleomycin has been administered using a number of different schedules and routes of administration. The most common route and schedule is bolus intravenous injection. Because of the greater effect of bleomycin on cells in the mitotic and G_2 phases of the cell cycle, the drug has been given by continuous infusion to produce prolonged exposure to toxic concentrations, but a high incidence of pulmonary toxicity has sometimes resulted. For example, continuous infusion of 25 U/day for 5 days produced the expected rapid onset of pulmonary toxicity, particularly in patients with previous chest irradiation,[105,159] but in addition caused hypertensive episodes in 17% of patients and hyperbilirubinemia in 30%.[103] These latter toxicities are rarely seen with conventional bolus doses.

Continuous intraarterial infusion also has been used for patients with carcinoma of the cervix[160] and of the head and neck.[161] One study[160] noted a disappointing 12% response rate to infusion of 20 U/m² per week for courses of up to 3 weeks. Pulmonary toxicity was observed in 20% of patients.

Bleomycin also has been applied topically as a 3.5% ointment in a xipamide (Aquaphor) base. Two-week courses of treatment produced complete regression of Paget's disease of the vulva in four of seven patients,[162] with no serious local toxicity.

As described previously in the discussion of pharmacokinetics, bleomycin can be used to sclerose the pleural space in patients with malignant effusions. After thorough evacuation of fluid from the pleural space, 40 U/m^2 is dissolved in 100 mL normal saline and instilled through a thoracostomy tube, which is clamped for 8 hours and then returned to suction. In approximately one-third of patients thus treated, the effusion clears completely; this is about the same response rate as obtained with tetracycline instillation.[163,164] The only toxic reactions are fever and pleuritis, both of which resolve in 24 to 48 hours. The intraperitoneal instillation of bleomycin has been used in patients with ovarian cancer, mesothelioma, and other malignancy confined to the peritoneum[93] but with rare responses. Sixty milligrams of bleomycin per m^2 was dissolved in 2 L of saline, and the solution was placed in the peritoneal cavity for a 4- to 8-hour dwell time. Side effects included abdominal pain, fever, rash, and mucositis. A limited pharmacokinetic advantage was observed (the peritoneal area under the concentration × time curve was sevenfold greater than the plasma area under the curve), which provides little justification for this route of administration.

Bleomycin has been instilled into the urinary bladder in doses of 60 U in 30 mL of sterile water.[165] Seven of 26 patients with superficial transitional cell carcinomas had complete disappearance of disease after 7 to 8 weekly treatments, but all had relatively small lesions. The primary toxic reaction was cystitis. Plasma drug level monitoring revealed little evidence of systemic absorption.

RADIATION AND DRUG INTERACTION

Bleomycin is used frequently in combination therapy regimens for treatment of lymphomas and less commonly for squamous carcinomas of the esophagus and head and neck, primarily because of its lack of myelosuppressive toxicity. The pharmacologic basis of synergism between bleomycin and various agents has received considerable attention[166,167] but is only poorly understood. Administration of bleomycin within 3 hours of irradiation, either before or after, produces greater than additive effects,[168] possibly owing to the production of free-radical damage to DNA by both agents. This interaction has been tested in a randomized clinical trial of radiation therapy plus or minus bleomycin, 5 mg twice weekly, in patients with head and neck cancer.[169] In this study, the group receiving bleomycin had a significantly higher complete response rate and a better 3-year disease-free survival rate. As mentioned earlier, synergistic pulmonary toxicity has been reported in patients receiving bleomycin after previous chest irradiation.

REFERENCES

1. Umezawa H, Maeda K, Takeuchi T, et al. New antibiotics, bleomycin A and B. J Antibiot (Tokyo) 1966;19:200.
2. Levi JA, Raghavan D, Harvey V, et al. The importance of bleomycin in combination chemotherapy for good-prognosis germ cell carcinoma. J Clin Oncol 1993;11:1300.
3. Takita T, Umezawa Y, Saito S, et al. Total synthesis of bleomycin A$_2$. Tetrahedron Lett 1982;23:521.
4. Umezawa H, Suhara Y, Takita T, et al. Purification of bleomycin. J Antibiot (Tokyo) 1966;19:210.
5. Mistry JS, Sebti SM, Lazo JS. Separation of bleomycins and their deamido metabolites by high-performance cation-exchange chromatography. J Chromatogr 1990;514:86.
6. Stubbe J, Kozarich JW. Mechanisms of bleomycin-induced DNA degradation. Chem Rev 1987;87:1107.
7. Umezawa H. Advances in bleomycin studies. In: Hecht SM, ed. Bleomycin: Chemical, Biochemical, and Biological Aspects. New York: Springer-Verlag, 1979:24.
8. Lazo JS, Schisselbauer JC, Herring GM, et al. Involvement of the cellular vacuolar system with the cytotoxicity of bleomycin-like agents. Cancer Commun 1990;2:81.
9. Pron G, Belehradek J Jr, Mir LM. Identification of a plasma membrane protein that specifically binds bleomycin. Biochem Biophys Res Commun 1993;194:333.
10. Takahashi K, Takita T, Umezawa H. The nature of thiol compounds which trap cuprous ion reductively liberated from bleomycin-Cu(II) in cells. J Antibiot (Tokyo) 1987;40:348.
11. Dabrowiak JC, Greenaway FT, Santillo FS, et al. The iron complexes of bleomycin and tallysomycin. Biochem Biophys Res Commun 1979;91:721.
12. Takita T, Muraoka Y, Nakatani T, et al. Chemistry of bleomycin, XXI: metal-complex and its implication for the mechanism of bleomycin action. J Antibiot (Tokyo) 1978;31:1073.
13. Ehrenberg GM, Shipley JB, Heimbrook DC, et al. Copper dependent cleavage of bleomycin. Biochemistry 1987;26:931.
14. Hecht SM. The chemistry of activated bleomycin. Acc Chem Res 1986;19:383.
15. Sausville EA, Peisach J, Horwitz SB. Effects of chelating agents and metal ions on the degradation of DNA by bleomycin. Biochemistry 1978;17:2740.
16. Sausville EA, Peisach J, Horwitz SB. A role for ferrous ion and oxygen in the degradation of DNA by bleomycin. Biochem Biophys Res Commun 1976;73:814.
17. Lazo JS, Schisselbauer JC, Meandzija B, et al. Initial single strand DNA damage and cellular pharmacokinetics of bleomycin A$_2$. Biochem Pharmacol 1989;38:2207.
18. Holes CE, Carter BJ, Hecht SM. Characterization of iron (II)·bleomycin–mediated RNA strand scission. Biochemistry 1993;32:4293.
19. Holmes CE, Duff RJ, von der Marvel GA, et al. On the chemistry of DNA degradation by Fe·bleomycin. Bioorganic Med Chem 1997;5:1235.
20. Morgan MA, Hecht SM. Iron (II)·bleomycin–mediated degradation of a DNA-RNA heteroduplex. Biochemistry 1994;33:10286.
21. Burger RM. Cleavage of nucleic acids by bleomycin. *Chem Rev* 1998;98:1153.
22. Fulmer P, Pettering DH. Reaction of DNA-bound ferrous bleomycin with dioxygen: activation versus stabilization of dioxygen. Biochemistry 1994;33:5319.
23. Ciriolo MR, Magliozzo RS, Peisach J. Microsome-stimulated activation of ferrous bleomycin in the presence of DNA. J Biol Chem 1987;262:6290.
24. Mahmutoglu I, Kappus H. Redox cycling of bleomycin-Fe(III) by an NADH-dependent enzyme, and DNA damage in isolated rat liver nuclei. Biochem Pharmacol 1987;36:3677.
25. Burger RM, Kent TA, Horwitz SB, et al. Mossbauer study of iron bleomycin and its activation intermediates. J Biol Chem 1983;258:1559.
26. Kasai H, Naganawa H, Takita T, et al. Chemistry of bleomycin, XXII: interaction of bleomycin with nucleic acids, preferential binding to guanine base and electrostatic effect of the terminal amine. J Antibiot (Tokyo) 1978;31:1316.

27. Umezawa H, Takita T, Sugiura Y, et al. DNA-bleomycin interaction: nucleotide sequence–specific binding and cleavage of DNA by bleomycin. Tetrahedron 1984;40:501.

28. Povirk LF, Hogan M, Dattagupta N. Binding of bleomycin to DNA: intercalation of the bithiazole rings. Biochemistry 1979;18:96.

29. Hertzberg RP, Caranfa MJ, Hecht SM. Degradation of structurally modified DNAs by bleomycin group antibiotics. Biochemistry 1988;27:3164.

30. Caspary WJ, Niziak C, Lanzo DA, et al. Bleomycin A_2: a ferrous oxidase. Mol Pharmacol 1979;16:256.

31. Kilkuskie RE, Macdonald TL, Hecht SM. Bleomycin may be activated for DNA cleavage by NADPH–cytochrome P450 reductase. Biochemistry 1984;23:6165.

32. Burger RM, Horwitz SB, Peisach J, et al. Oxygenated iron bleomycin: a short-lived intermediate in the reaction of ferrous bleomycin with O_2. J Biol Chem 1979;254:12299.

33. Sugiura Y, Kikuchi TK. Formation of superoxide and hydroxy radicals by bleomycin and iron (II). J Antibiot (Tokyo) 1978; 1:1310.

34. Sausville E, Stein R, Peisach J, et al. Properties and products of the degradation of DNA by bleomycin. Biochemistry 1978;17: 2746.

35. Burger RM, Projan SJ, Horwitz SB, et al. The DNA cleavage mechanism of iron-bleomycin. J Biol Chem 1986;261:15955.

36. Rabow L, Stubbe J, Kozarich JW, et al. Identification of the alkalilabile product accompanying cytosine release during bleomycin-mediated degradation of d(CGCGCG). J Am Chem Soc 1986; 108:7130.

37. Grollman AP, Takeshita M, Pillai KM, et al. Origin and cytotoxic properties of base propenals derived from DNA. Cancer Res 1985;45:1127.

38. Keller TJ, Oppenheimer NJ. Enhanced bleomycin-mediated damage of DNA opposite charged nicks: a model for bleomycin-directed double strand scission of DNA. J Biol Chem 1987; 262:15144.

39. Burger RM, Berkowitz AR, Peisach J, et al. Origin of malondialdehyde from DNA degraded by Fe(II)-bleomycin. J Biol Chem 1980;255:11832.

40. Takeshita M, Grollman AP, Ohtsubo E, et al. Interaction of bleomycin with DNA. Proc Natl Acad Sci USA 1978;75:5983.

41. Grollman AP, Takeshita M. Interactions of bleomycin with DNA. In: Weber G, ed. Advances in Enzyme Regulation. Vol 18. Oxford: Pergamon Press, 1980:67.

42. Roy SN, Horwitz SB. Characterization of the association of radiolabeled bleomycin A_2 with HeLa cells. Cancer Res 1984; 44:1541.

43. Fugimito J, Higashi H, Kosaki G. Intracellular distribution of [^{14}C]bleomycin and the cytokinetic effects of bleomycin in the mouse tumor. Cancer Res 1976;36:2248.

44. Touchekti O, Pron G, Belehradek J Jr, et al. Bleomycin, an apoptosis mimetic drug that induces two types of cell death depending on the number of molecules internalized. Cancer Res 1993;53:5462.

45. Mistry JS, Jani JP, Morris G, et al. Synthesis and evaluation of fluoromycin: a novel fluorescence-labeled derivative of talisomycin S_{10b}. Cancer Res 1992;52:709.

46. Lazo JS, Humphreys CJ. Lack of metabolism as the biochemical basis of bleomycin-induced pulmonary toxicity. Proc Natl Acad Sci USA 1983;80:3064.

47. Sebti SM, Mignano JE, Jani JP, et al. Bleomycin hydrolase: molecular cloning, sequencing and biochemical studies reveal membership in the cysteine proteinase family. Biochemistry 1989;28: 6544.

48. Brömme D, Rossi AB, Smeekens SP, et al. Human bleomycin hydrolase: molecular cloning, sequencing, functional expression, and enzymatic characterization. Biochemistry 1996;35: 6706.

49. Enekel C, Wolf DH. BLH1 codes for a yeast thiol aminopeptidase, the equivalent of mammalian bleomycin hydrolase. J Biol Chem 1993;268:7036.

50. Joshua-Tor L, Xu HE, Johnston SA, et al. Crystal structure of a conserved protease that binds DNA: the bleomycin hydrolase, Gal6. Science 1995;269:945.

51. Farrell PA, Gonzalez F, Zheng W, et al. Crystal structure of human bleomycin hydrolase, a self-compartmentalizing cysteine protease. Structure 1999;7:619.

52. Koldamova RP, Lefterov IM, Gadjeva VG, et al. Essential binding and functional domains of human bleomycin hydrolase. Biochemistry 1998;37:2282.

53. Zheng W, Johnston SA, Joshua-Tor L. The unusual active site of Gal6/bleomycin hydrolase can act as a carboxypeptidase, aminopeptidase, and peptide ligase. - 1998;93:103.

54. Montoya SE, Ferrell RE, Lazo JS. Genomic structure and genetic mapping of the human neutral cysteine protease bleomycin hydrolase. Cancer Res 1997;57:4191.

55. Ferrando A, Pendas A, Elena L, et al. Gene characterization, promoter analysis, and chromosomal localization of human bleomycin hydrolase. J Biol Chem 1997;272:33298.

56. Takeda A, Nonaka M, Ishikawa A, et al. Immunohistochemical localization of the neutral cysteine protease bleomycin hydrolase in human skin. Arch Dermatol Res 1999;291:238.

57. Schwartz DR, Homanics GE, Hoyt DG. The neutral cysteine protease bleomycin hydrolase is essential for epidermal integrity and bleomycin resistance. Proc Natl Acad Sci USA 1999;96:4680.

58. Koldamova RP, Lefterov LM, DiSabella MT, et al. An evolutionarily conserved cysteine protease, human bleomycin hydrolase, binds to the human homologue of ubiquitin-conjugating enzyme 9. Mol Pharmacol 1998;54:954.

59. Tuimala J, Szekely G, Gundy S, et al. Genetic polymorphisms of DNA repair and xenobiotic-metabolizing enzymes: role in mutagen sensitivity. Carcinogenesis 2002;23:1003–1008.

60. Barranco SC, Humphrey RM. The effects of bleomycin on survival and cell progression in Chinese hamster cells in vitro. Cancer Res 1971;31:1218.

61. Tobey RA. Arrest of Chinese hamster cells in G_2 following treatment with the antitumor drug bleomycin. J Cell Physiol 1972; 79:259.

62. Wanatabe M, Takabe Y, Katsumata T, et al. Effects of bleomycin on progression through the cell cycle of mouse L cells. Cancer Res 1974;34:2726.

63. Barlogie B, Drewinko B, Schumann J, et al. Pulse cytophotometric analysis of cell cycle perturbation with bleomycin in vitro. Cancer Res 1976;36:1182.

64. Olive PL, Banath JP. Detection of DNA double-strand breaks through the cell cycle after exposure to x-rays, bleomycin, etoposide and ^{125}IdUrd. Int J Radiat Biol 1993;64:349.

65. Lopez-Larraza DM, Bianchi NO. DNA response to bleomycin in mammalian cells with variable degrees of chromatin condensation. Environ Mol Mutagen 1993;21:258.

66. Twentyman PR. Bleomycin: mode of action with particular reference to the cell cycle. Pharmacol Ther 1983;23:417.

67. Kuo MT, Hsu TC. Bleomycin causes release of nucleosomes from chromatin and chromosomes. Nature 1978;271:83.

68. Iqbal ZM, Kohn KW, Ewig RAG, et al. Single-strand scission and repair of DNA in mammalian cells by bleomycin. Cancer Res 1976;36:3834.

69. Barranco SC, Novak JK, Humphrey RM. Studies on recovery from chemically induced damage in mammalian cells. Cancer Res 1975;35:1194.

70. Nakatsugawa S, Dewey WC. The role in cancer therapy of inhibiting recovery from PLD induced by radiation or bleomycin. Int J Radiat Oncol Biol Phys 1984;10:1425.

71. Onishi T, Shimada K, Takagi Y. Effects of bleomycin on *Escherichia coli* strains with various sensitivities to radiation. Biochem Biophys Acta 1973;312:248.

72. Cramer P, Painter RB. Bleomycin-resistant DNA synthesis in ataxia telangiectasia cells. Nature 1981;291:671.

73. Taylor AMR, Rosney CM, Campbell JB. Unusual sensitivity of ataxia telangiectasia cells to bleomycin. Cancer Res 1979;39: 1046.

74. Quinn JE, Kennedy RD, Mullan PB, et al. BRCA1 functions as a differential modulator of chemotherapy-induced apoptosis. Cancer Res 2003;63:6221.

75. Li HR, Shagisultanova EI, Yamashita K, et al. Hypersensitivity of tumor cell lines with microsatellite instability to DNA double strand break producing chemotherapeutic agent bleomycin. Cancer Res 2004;64:4760.

76. Mayaki M, Ono T, Hori S, et al. Binding of bleomycin to DNA in bleomycin-sensitive and resistant rat ascites hepatoma cells. Cancer Res 1975;35:2015.

77. Morris G, Mistry JS, Jani JP, et al. Neutralization of bleomycin hydrolase by an epitope-specific antibody. Mol Pharmacol 1992;42:57.

78. Jani JP, Mistry JS, Morris G, et al. In vivo circumvention of human colon carcinoma resistance to bleomycin. Cancer Res 1992;52:2931.

79. Brabbs S, Warr JR. Isolation and characterization of bleomycin-resistant clones of OHO cells. Genet Res 1979;34:269.

80. Zuckerman JE, Raffin TA, Brown JM, et al. In vitro selection and characterization of a bleomycin-resistant subline of B16 melanoma. Cancer Res 1986;46:1748.

81. Tsuruo T, Hamilton TC, Louie KG, et al. Collateral susceptibility of Adriamycin-, melphalan- and cisplatin-resistant human ovarian tumor cells to bleomycin. Jpn J Cancer Res 1986;77:941.

82. Russo A, Mitchell JB, McPherson S, et al. Alteration of bleomycin cytotoxicity by glutathione depletion or elevation. Int J Radiat Oncol Biol Phys 1984;10:1675.

83. Umezawa H, Takeuchi T, Hori S, et al. Studies on the mechanism of antitumor effect of bleomycin on squamous cell carcinoma. J Antibiot (Tokyo) 1972;25:409.

84. Shiu GK, Goehl TJ. High-performance liquid chromatographic determination of bleomycin A_2 in urine. J Chromatogr 1980;181:127.

85. Galvan L, Strong JE, Crooke ST. Use of PM-2 DNA degradation as a pharmacokinetic assay for bleomycin. Cancer Res 1979;39:3948.

86. Broughton A, Strong JE. Radioimmunoassay of bleomycin. Cancer Res 1976;36:1418.

87. Crooke ST, Luft F, Broughton A, et al. Bleomycin serum pharmacokinetics as determined by a radioimmunoassay and a microbiologic assay in a patient with compromised renal function. Cancer 1977;39:1430.

88. Bennett WM, Pastore L, Houghton DC. Fatal pulmonary bleomycin toxicity in cisplatin-induced acute renal failure. Cancer Treat Rep 1980;64:921.

89. Alberts DS, Chen HSG, Liu R, et al. Bleomycin pharmacokinetics in man, I: intravenous administration. Cancer Chemother Pharmacol 1978;1:177.

90. Crooke ST, Comis RL, Einhorn LH, et al. Effects of variations in renal function on the clinical pharmacology of bleomycin administered as an IV bolus. Cancer Treat Rep 1977;61:1631.

91. Oken MM, Crooke ST, Elson MK, et al. Pharmacokinetics of bleomycin after IM administration in man. Cancer Treat Rep 1981;65:485.

92. Paladine W, Cunningham TJ, Sponzo R, et al. Intracavitary bleomycin in the management of malignant effusions. Cancer 1976;38:1903.

93. Alberts DS, Chen HSG, Mayersohn M, et al. Bleomycin pharmacokinetics in man, II: intracavitary administration. Cancer Chemother Pharmacol 1979;2:127.

94. Howell SB, Schiefer M, Andrews PA, et al. The pharmacology of intraperitoneally administered bleomycin. J Clin Oncol 1987;5:2009.

95. Dalgleish AG, Woods RL, Levi JA. Bleomycin pulmonary toxicity: its relationship to renal dysfunction. Med Pediatr Oncol 1984;12:313.

96. McLeod BF, Lawrence HJ, Smith DW, et al. Fatal bleomycin toxicity from a low cumulative dose in a patient with renal insufficiency. Cancer 1987;60:2617.

97. O'Sullivan JM, Huddart RA, Norman AR, et al. Predicting the risk of bleomycin lung toxicity in patients with germ-cell tumors. Ann Oncology 2003;14:91.

98. Hinton S, Catalano PJ, Einhorn LH, et al. Cisplatin, etoposide and either bleomycin or ifosfamide in the treatment of disseminated germ cell tumors. Cancer 2003;97:1869.

99. Hubbard SP, Chabner BA, Canellos GP, et al. High-dose intravenous bleomycin in treatment of advanced lymphomas. Eur J Cancer 1975;11:623.

100. Blum RH, Carter SK, Agre K. A clinical review of bleomycin—a new antineoplastic agent. Cancer 1973;31:903.

101. Levy RL, Chiarillo S. Hyperpyrexia, allergic-type response, and death occurring with bleomycin administration. Oncology 1980;37:316.

102. Comis RL. Bleomycin pulmonary toxicity: current status and future directions. Semin Oncol 1992;19(Suppl 5):64.

103. Parvinen LM, Kikku P, Maekinen E, et al. Factors affecting the pulmonary toxicity of bleomycin. Acta Radiol Oncol 1983;22:417.

104. Dee GJ, Austin JH, Mutter GL. Bleomycin-associated pulmonary fibrosis: rapidly fatal progression without chest radiotherapy. J Surg Oncol 1987;35:135.

105. Samuels ML, Johnson DE, Holoye PH, et al. Large-dose bleomycin therapy and pulmonary toxicity: a possible role of prior radiotherapy. JAMA 1976;235:1117.

106. Williams SD, Birch R, Einhorn LA, et al. Treatment of disseminated germ cell tumors with cisplatin, bleomycin, and either vinblastine or etoposide. N Engl J Med 1987;316:1435.

107. Harrison JH Jr, Lazo JS. High dose continuous infusion of bleomycin in mice: a new model for drug-induced pulmonary fibrosis. J Pharmacol Exp Ther 1987;243:1185.

108. Hay J, Shahzeidi S, Laurent G. Mechanisms of bleomycin-induced lung damage. Arch Toxicol 1991;65:81.

109. Raisfeld IH. Role of terminal substituents in the pulmonary toxicity of bleomycins. Toxicol Appl Pharmacol 1981;57:355.

110. Huff RA, Bevan DR. Application of alkaline unwinding to analysis of breaks induced by bleomycin in hamster lung DNA in vivo. J Appl Toxicol 1991;11:359.

111. Phan SH, Varani J, Smith D. Rat lung fibroblast collagen metabolism in bleomycin-induced pulmonary fibrosis. J Clin Invest 1985;76:241.

112. Conley NS, Yarbro JW, Ferrari HA, et al. Bleomycin increases superoxide anion generation by pig peripheral alveolar macrophages. Mol Pharmacol 1986;30:48.

113. Adamson IY, Bowden DH. The pathogenesis of bleomycin-induced pulmonary fibrosis in mice. Am J Pathol 1974;77:185.

114. Sikic BI, Young DM, Mimnaugh EG, et al. Quantification of bleomycin pulmonary toxicity in mice by changes in lung hydroxyproline content and morphometric histopathology. Cancer Res 1978;38:787.

115. Phan S, Gharaee-Kermani M, McGarry B, et al. Regulation of rat pulmonary artery endothelial cell transforming growth factor-beta production by Il-1beta and tumor necrosis factor-alpha. J Immunol 1992;149:103.

116. Hoyt DG, Lazo JS. Alterations in pulmonary mRNA encoding procollagens, fibronectin and transforming growth factor-β precede bleomycin-induced pulmonary fibrosis in mice. J Pharmacol Exp Ther 1988;246:765.

117. King SL, Lichter AC, Rowe SW, et al. Bleomycin stimulates pro-alpha (I) collagen promoter through transforming growth factor beta response element by intracellular and extracellular signaling. J Biol Chem 1994;269:13156.

118. Everson MP, Chandler DB. Changes in distribution, morphology, and tumor necrosis factor-alpha secretion of alveolar macrophage subpopulations during the development of bleomycin-induced pulmonary fibrosis. Am J Pathol 1992;140:503.

119. Khalil N, Whitman C, Zuo L, et al. Regulation of alveolar macrophage transforming growth factor-beta secretion by corticosteroids in bleomycin-induced pulmonary inflammation in the rat. J Clin Invest 1993;92:1812.

120. Piguet PF, Collart MA, Grau GE, et al. Tumor necrosis factor/cachectin plays a key role in bleomycin induced pneumopathy and fibrosis. J Exp Med 1989;170:655.

121. Scheule RK, Perkins RC, Hamilton R, et al. Bleomycin stimulation of cytokine secretion by the human alveolar macrophage. Am J Physiol 1992;262:L386.

122. Baecher AC, Barth RK. PCR analysis of cytokine induction profiles associated with mouse strain variation in susceptibility to pulmonary fibrosis. Reg Immunol 1993;5:207.

123. Haston CK, Amos CI, King TM, et al. Inheritance of susceptibility to bleomycin-induced pulmonary fibrosis in the mouse. Cancer Res 1996;56:2596.

124. Haston CK, Travis EL. Murine susceptibility to radiation-induced pulmonary fibrosis is influenced by a genetic factor implicated in susceptibility to bleomycin-induced pulmonary fibrosis. Cancer Res 1997;57:5286.

125. Schwartz DR, Homanics GE, Hoyt DG, et al. The neutral cysteine protease bleomycin hydrolase is essential for epidermal

integrity and bleomycin resistance. Proc Natl Acad Sci USA 1999;96:4680.

126. Eitzman DT, McCoy RD, Zheng X, et al. Bleomycin-induced pulmonary fibrosis in transgenic mice that either lack or overexpress the murine plasminogen activator inhibitor-1 gene. J Clin Invest 1996;97:232.

127. Zuo F, Kaminski N, Eugui E, et al. Gene expression analysis reveals matrilysin as a key regulator of pulmonary fibrosis in mice and humans. PNAS 2002;99:6292.

128. Munger JS, Huang X, Kawakatsu H, et al. The integrin αvβ6 binds and activates latent TGFβ1: a mechanism for regulating pulmonary inflammation and fibrosis. Cell 1999;96:319.

129. Coker RK, Laurent GJ, Shahzeidi S, et al. Transforming growth factors-β1, -β2, and -β3 stimulate fibroblast procollagen production in vitro but are differentially expressed during bleomycin-induced lung fibrosis. Am J Pathol 1997;150:981.

130. Phillips RJ, Burdick MD, Hing K, et al. Circulating fibrocytes traffic to the lungs in response to CXL12 and mediate fibrosis. J Clin Invest 2004;114:438.

131. Kuwano K, Hagimoto N, Kawasaki M, et al. Essential roles of the fas-fas ligand pathway in the development of pulmonary fibrosis. J Clin Invest 1999;104:13.

132. Piguet PK, Besin C. Treatment by human recombinant soluble TNF receptor of pulmonary fibrosis induced by bleomycin or silica in mice. Eur Respir J 1994;7:515.

133. Giri SN, Hyde DM, Hollinger MA. Effect of antibody to transforming growth factor beta on bleomycin-induced accumulation of lung collagen in mice. Thorax 1993;48:959.

134. Piguet PF, Grau GE, deKossodo S. Role of granulocyte-macrophage colony stimulating factor in pulmonary fibrosis induced in mice by bleomycin. Exp Lung Res 1993;19:579.

135. Gurujeyalakshmi G, Hollinger MA, Giri SN. Pirfenidone inhibits PDGF isoforms in bleomycin hamster model of lung fibrosis at the translational level. Am J Physiol 1999;276:L311.

136. Iyer SN, Gurujeyalakshmi G, Giri SN. Effects of pirfenidone on procollagen gene expression at the transcriptional level in bleomycin hamster model of lung fibrosis. J Pharmacol Exp Ther 1999;289:211.

137. Nici L, Santos-Moore A, Kuhn C, et al. Modulation of bleomycin-induced pulmonary toxicity in the hamster by the antioxidant amifostine. Cancer 1998;83:2008.

138. Unemori EN, Pickford LB, Salles AL, et al. Relaxin induces an extracellular matrix-degrading phenotype in human lung fibroblasts in vitro and inhibits lung fibrosis in a murine model in vivo. J Clin Invest 1996;98:2739.

139. Weinbach J, Camus A, Barra J, et al. Transgenic mice expressing the Sh ble bleomycin resistance gene are protected against bleomycin-induced pulmonary fibrosis. Cancer Res 1996;56:5659.

140. Phan SH, Thrall RS, Ward PA. Bleomycin-induced pulmonary fibrosis in rats: biochemical demonstration of increased rates of collagen synthesis. Am Rev Respir Dis 1980;121:501.

141. Kelley J, Newman RA, Evans JN. Bleomycin-induced pulmonary fibrosis in the rat: prevention with an inhibitor of collagen synthesis. J Lab Clin Med 1980;96:954.

142. Thrau RS, McCormick JR, Jack RM, et al. Bleomycin-induced pulmonary fibrosis in the rat: inhibition by indomethacin. Am J Pathol 1979;95:117.

143. Witschi H. Exploitable biochemical approaches for the evaluation of toxic lung damage. Essays Toxicol 1975;6:125.

144. Sikic BI, Collins JM, Mimnaugh EG, et al. Improved therapeutic index of bleomycin when administered by continuous infusion in mice. Cancer Treat Rep 1978;62:2011.

145. Samuels ML, Johnson DE, Holoye PY. Continuous intravenous bleomycin (NSC-125066) therapy with vinblastine (NSC-49842) in stage III testicular neoplasia. Cancer Chemother Rep 1975;59:563.

146. Zucker PK, Khouri NF, Rosenshein NB. Bleomycin-induced pulmonary nodules: a variant of bleomycin pulmonary toxicity. Gynecol Oncol 1987;28:284.

147. Talcott JA, Garnick MB, Stomper PC, et al. Cavitary lung nodules associated with combination chemotherapy containing bleomycin. J Urol 1987;138:619.

148. Richman SD, Levenson SM, Bunn PA, et al. ^{67}Ga-Accumulation in pulmonary lesions associated with bleomycin toxicity. Cancer 1975;36:1966.

149. Burkhardt A, Gebbers JO, Holtje WJ. Die Bleomycin-Lunge. Dtsch Med Wochenschr 1977;102:281.

150. Holoye PY, Luna MA, MacKay B, et al. Bleomycin hypersensitivity pneumonitis. Ann Intern Med 1978;88:47.

151. Comis RL, Kuppinger MS, Ginsberg SJ, et al. Role of single-breath carbon monoxide–diffusing capacity in monitoring the pulmonary effects of bleomycin in germ-free tumor patients. Cancer Res 1979;39:5076.

152. Osanto S, Bukman A, Van Hoek F, et al. Long-term effects of chemotherapy in patients with testicular cancer. J Clin Oncol 1992;10:574.

153. Goldiner PL, Carlon GC, Critkovic E, et al. Factors influencing post-operative morbidity and mortality in patients treated with bleomycin. Br Med J 1978;1:1664.

154. Donat SM, Levy DA. Bleomycin associated pulmonary toxicity: is pre-operative oxygen restriction necessary? J Urology 1998;160:1397.

155. Yagoda A, Etwbanas E, Tan CTC. Bleomycin, an antitumor antibiotic: clinical experience in 274 patients. Ann Intern Med 1972;77:861.

156. Maher J, Daley PA. Severe bleomycin lung toxicity: reversal with high dose corticosteroids. Thorax 1993; 48:92.

157. Van Barneveld PW, Sleijfer DT, van der Mark TW, et al. Natural course of bleomycin-induced pneumonitis: a follow-up study. Am Rev Respir Dis 1987;135:48.

158. Letters to the editor. Cancer Treat Rep 1978;62:569.

159. Einhorn L, Krause M, Hornbach N, et al. Enhanced pulmonary toxicity with bleomycin and radiotherapy in oat cell lung cancer. Cancer 1976;37:2414.

160. Morrow CP, DiSaia PJ, Mangan CF, et al. Continuous pelvic arterial infusion with bleomycin for squamous carcinoma of the cervix recurrent after irradiation therapy. Cancer Treat Rep 1977;61:1403.

161. Bitter K. Pharmacokinetic behaviour of bleomycin–cobalt-57 with special regard to intra-arterial perfusion of the maxillofacial region. J Maxillofac Surg 1976;4:226.

162. Watring WG, Roberts JA, Lagasse LD, et al. Treatment of recurrent Paget's disease of the vulva with topical bleomycin. Cancer 1978;41:10.

163. Kessinger A, Wigton RS. Intracavitary bleomycin and tetracycline in the management of malignant pleural effusions: a randomized study. J Surg Oncol 1987;36:81.

164. Maiche AG, Virkkunen P, Kantkanen T, et al. Bleomycin and mitoxantrone in the treatment of malignant pleural effusions. Am J Clin Oncol 1992;16:50.

165. Bracken RB, Johnson DE, Rodriquez L, et al. Treatment of multiple superficial tumors of bladder with intravesical bleomycin. Urology 1977;9:161.

166. Crooke ST, Bradner WT. Bleomycin: a review. J Med 1976;7:333.

167. Blehan NM, Gillies NE, Twentyman PR. The effect of bleomycin and radiation in combination on bacteria and mammalian cells in culture. Br J Radiol 1974;47:346.

168. Takabe Y, Miyamoto T, Watanabe M, et al. Synergism of x-ray and bleomycin on Ehrlich ascites tumour cells. Br J Cancer 1977;36:391.

169. Fu K, Phillips TL, Silverberg IJ, et al. Combined radiotherapy and chemotherapy with bleomycin and methotrexate for advanced inoperable head and neck cancer: update of a Northern California Oncology Group randomized trial. J Clin Oncol 1987;5:1410.

Antitumor Antibiotics 16

Edwin W. Willems   Kees Nooter   Jaap Verweij

INTRODUCTION

Over several decades, microbial fermentation has yielded many valuable compounds, such as the anthracyclines, the bleomycins, and various unusual nucleosides, which are discussed in separate chapters. In this chapter we review two relatively long-standing antibiotics of diverse structure as well as one of the marine-originated ecteinascidins, namely ecteinascidin-743 (ET-743). Dactinomycin (actinomycin D; DACT) is still one of the most valuable drugs in pediatric oncology, whereas mitomycin C (MMC), although largely replaced by newer classes of agents, is still occasionally used in treating tumors of the gastrointestinal and respiratory tracts and for intravesicular treatment of bladder cancer. ET-743 is a promising anticancer agent with unique mechanisms of action.

DACTINOMYCIN

DACT, a product of the *Streptomyces* yeast species, was discovered in 1940[1] and has since been identified as an active anticancer antibiotic for gestational choriocarcinoma, Wilms tumor, neuroblastoma, childhood rhabdomyosarcoma, and Ewing's sarcoma.[2,3] Numerous analogs have been isolated from various sources, but none has demonstrated superiority over DACT. Its key pharmacological features are given in Table 16.1.

MECHANISM OF ACTION AND CELLULAR PHARMACOLOGY

The structure of DACT[4] is shown in Figure 16.1. It is a chromopeptide consisting of a phenoxazinone planar chromophore with two pentapeptide rings attached.[3] Naturally occurring actinomycins differ in the peptide chains but not in the phenoxazone ring. DACT is known to be a strong DNA-binding drug and a potent inhibitor of RNA and protein synthesis. Actual binding to DNA was shown to be intercalative: the chromophore inserts in between the DNA guanine-cytidine base pairs, while the two chains of the pentapeptide rest in the minor groove.[3] DACT can bind to both non-GpC and GpC-containing sequences. Interaction between GpC sequences leads to formation of two hydrogen bonds between each guanine and a pentapeptide.[3] Besides binding to double-strand DNA, DACT is also known to bind to single-strand DNA (ssDNA).[5] The overall association rate between DACT and DNA does not depend on polynucleotide sequence or length but probably reflects the summation of multiple sites of interaction with DNA.[6] When bound to the ssDNA in the open complex formed by the polymerase, DACT prevents reannealing of ssDNA. Results suggest that stabilization of unusual ssDNA hairpins by DACT may be an important aspect of its potent transcription inhibition activity.[7,8]

Since DACT is taken up in tissues by passive diffusion, its cytotoxic response depends on the ability of the cell to accumulate and retain the drug.[9] It may be noted that increased temperature or alterations in the membrane lipid bilayer markedly enhance transport of DACT in different cells. DACT likely causes cell death by apoptosis, as demonstrated in a variety of cells both in vitro and in vivo.[10] Although high doses of DACT inhibited growth in a human embryonal rhabdomyosarcoma cell line and induced cytotoxicity, at low doses the drug induced morphologic and phenotypic differentiation.[8] Apparently, low-dose DACT releases these cells from their differentiation blockade, allowing them to recover normal myogenic development. This suggests a potential role for differentiation therapy in the treatment of rhabdomyosarcomas.

MECHANISM OF RESISTANCE

Resistance to DACT is related to increased efflux.[11] For example, Chinese hamster ovary cells were found to be

TABLE 16.1
KEY FEATURES OF DACTINOMYCIN

Mechanism of action	Inhibition of RNA and protein synthesis
Metabolism	Unknown
Pharmacokinetics	$t_{1/2}$: 36 hr
Elimination	Renal: 6–30%, Bile: 5–11%
Drug interactions	None
Toxicity	Myelosuppression
	Nausea and vomiting
	Mucositis
	Diarrhea
	Necrosis at extravasation
	Radiation sensitization and recall reactions
Precautions	Avoid extravasation

$t_{1/2}$, half-life.

cross-resistant to DACT and to other drugs such as vinca alkaloids, anthracyclines, and epipodophyllotoxins.[12,13] In several instances, drug resistance could be overcome with verapamil hydrochloride.[14] Human tumor cell lines made resistant to DACT in vitro were found to amplify the P-glycoprotein–encoding MDR gene.[15] Resistance is reversed by drugs that inhibit P-glycoprotein function.[16]

DRUG INTERACTIONS

No pharmacokinetic interactions between DACT and other drugs are known.

CLINICAL PHARMACOLOGY

The pharmacokinetics of DACT have been studied in rat, monkey, and dog.[17] In these species, serum levels of DACT declined rapidly after administration, with concomitant accumulation of drug in the tissues. The mean drug half-life in tissues was 47 hours, and metabolites have not been identified. Urinary excretion varies from 6 to 31%, and bile excretion varies from 5 to 11%. A very limited study in humans yielded similar results,[18] with a very short half-life of distribution and a long plasma elimination half-life (36 hours). Urinary excretion and fecal excretion were 20% and 14%, respectively, and only 3.3% of the urinary excretion consisted of metabolites. Clearly, more extensive and detailed pharmacokinetic studies are required in humans.

By adsorbing DACT onto polybutylcyanoacrylate nanoparticles,[19] one can achieve a significant increase of drug concentration in muscle, spleen, and liver in Wistar rats, whereas urinary excretion is diminished.[20] Similar results were obtained by liposome entrapment of DACT; however, a slow-release system has not yet resulted in a

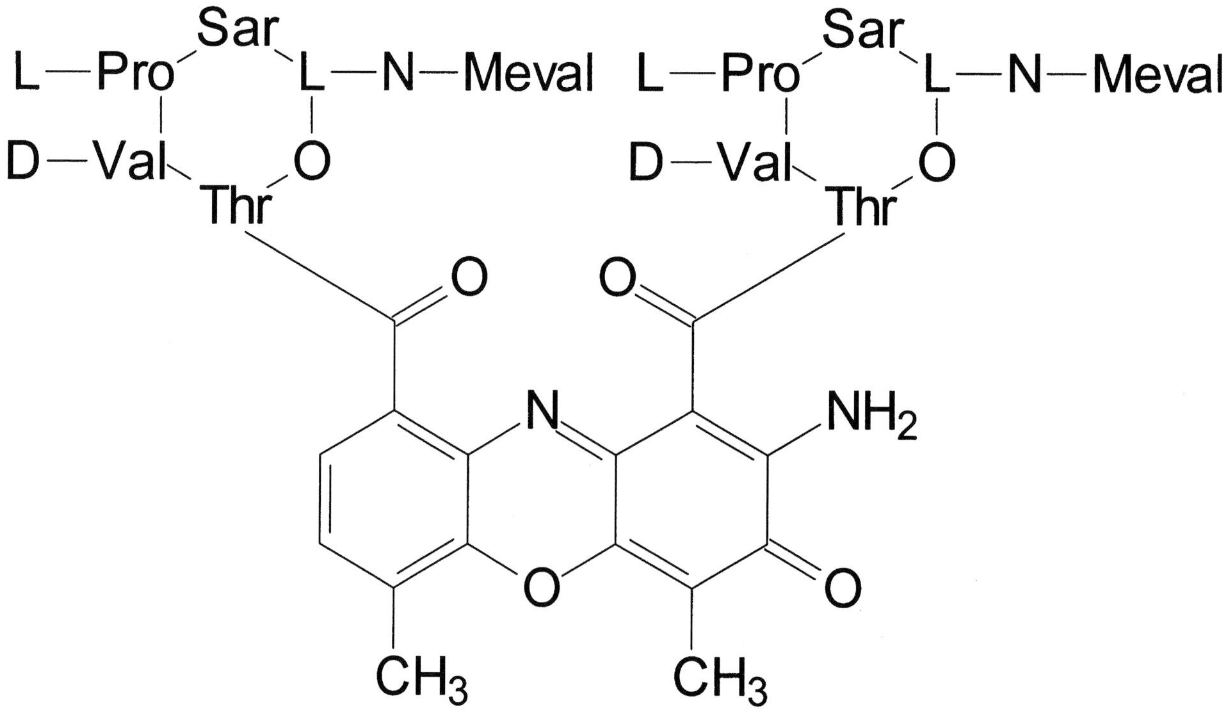

Figure 16.1   Structure of dactinomycin. D-Val, d-valine; L-N-Meval, methylvaline; L-Thr, l-threonine; L-Pro, l-proline; Sar, sarcosine.

higher efficacy.[19] It has been demonstrated in humans that single-dose intermittent schedules or daily administration of DACT for 5 days produce similar antitumor activity without increased toxicity.[21–23]

TOXICITY

At the usual clinical dosages of 10 to 15 mg/kg per day for 5 days, DACT causes nausea, vomiting, diarrhea, mucositis, and hair loss. The major and dose-limiting side effect is myelosuppression, with a white blood cell and platelet nadir occurring 8 to 14 days after drug administration.[23] Drug extravasation results in soft tissue necrosis.[23] In rare cases, DACT treatment leads to severe hepatotoxicity with features of veno-occlusive disease, as in children treated for Wilms tumor.[24] DACT can act as a radiosensitizer and may cause radiation recall phenomena, in which patients receiving DACT experience inflammatory reactions in previously irradiated sites.[25] The clinical consequences of such reactions may be serious, especially with the involvement of lung. Corticosteroids may ameliorate these reactions.

MITOMYCIN C

Mitomycin C (Mutamycin; MMC) was isolated from *Streptomyces caespitosus* in 1958.[26] The initial clinical studies used daily low-dose schedules, which resulted in unacceptably severe, cumulative myelosuppression. Later, an intermittent dosing schedule was introduced, using bolus injections every 4 to 8 weeks, which resulted in more manageable hematological toxicity. With the latter schedule, MMC was found to be active against a wide variety of solid tumors, including breast cancer, non–small cell lung cancer, gastric cancer, pancreatic cancer, gallbladder cancer, colorectal cancer, cervical cancer, prostatic cancer, and superficial bladder cancer. In addition, MMC is used as a radiosensitizer for the treatment of epidermoid anal cancer.[27] Its key pharmacological features are given in Table 16.2.

MECHANISM OF ACTION AND CELLULAR PHARMACOLOGY

MMC (Figure 16.2) and other mitomycins have unique chemical structures in which quinone, aziridine, and carbamate functions are arranged around a pyrrolo [l,2-a]indole nucleus.[28] They are the only known naturally occurring compounds containing an aziridine ring. MMC is soluble in both aqueous and organic solvents. However, because of its chemical instability in solution, the clinical formulation of MMC is a lyophilized form containing mannitol (Mutamycin) or sodium chloride (Mitomycin Kyowa) as excipients. After dissolution in water, MMC is administered intravenously. The stability of

TABLE 16.2
KEY FEATURES OF MITOMYCIN C

Mechanism of action	Alkylation of DNA
Metabolism	Hepatic
Pharmacokinetics	$t_{1/2}\,\alpha$: 2–10 min
	$t_{1/2}\,\beta$: 25–90 min
Elimination	Renal: 1–20%
Drug interaction	None
Toxicity	Myelosuppression
	Necrosis at extravasation
	Hemolytic uremic syndrome
	Interstitial pneumonitis
	Cardiomyopathy
Precautions	Avoid extravasation.

$t_{1/2}$, half-life.

the reconstituted solutions is limited. Storage of MMC at room temperature in unbuffered solutions (pH 7.0) for 5 days seems justified.[29]

Formation of DNA Adducts

MMC cross-links complementary strands of DNA but also induces monofunctional alkylation, with attachment to a single DNA strand.[30] It primarily acts as a DNA replication inhibitor, and although monofunctional alkylation is by far the most frequently observed interaction, DNA interstrand cross-linking is considered to be the most lethal type. DNA cross-linking and alkylation require chemical or enzymatic reduction of the quinone function. The primary mechanism of this process involves the C-1 aziridine and the C-10 carbamate groups, although several additional reactive electrophiles, such as a quinone methide and the oxidized forms of aziridinomitosene and leuco-aziridinomitosene, may alkylate DNA as well.[31,32] Several MMC-induced DNA cross-links have been identified,[33] including 2,7-diaminomitosene, which specifically alkylates guanines in $(G)_n$ tracts of DNA. Selective removal of the aziridine function of MMC results in a switch from minor to major groove alkylation of DNA.[34] Acidic activation of MMC is the second mechanism by which DNA alkylation can be produced.

Reductive Alkylation

MMC is considered the prototypical bioreductive alkylating agent. Two mechanisms exist through which reductive metabolism mediates the cytotoxic effects of MMC.[34–37] First, under anaerobic conditions, one- or two-electron reduction followed by spontaneous loss of methanol leads to the formation of reactive unstable intermediates.

The suggested mechanism included initial formation of a hydroquinone and its rearrangement to yield a

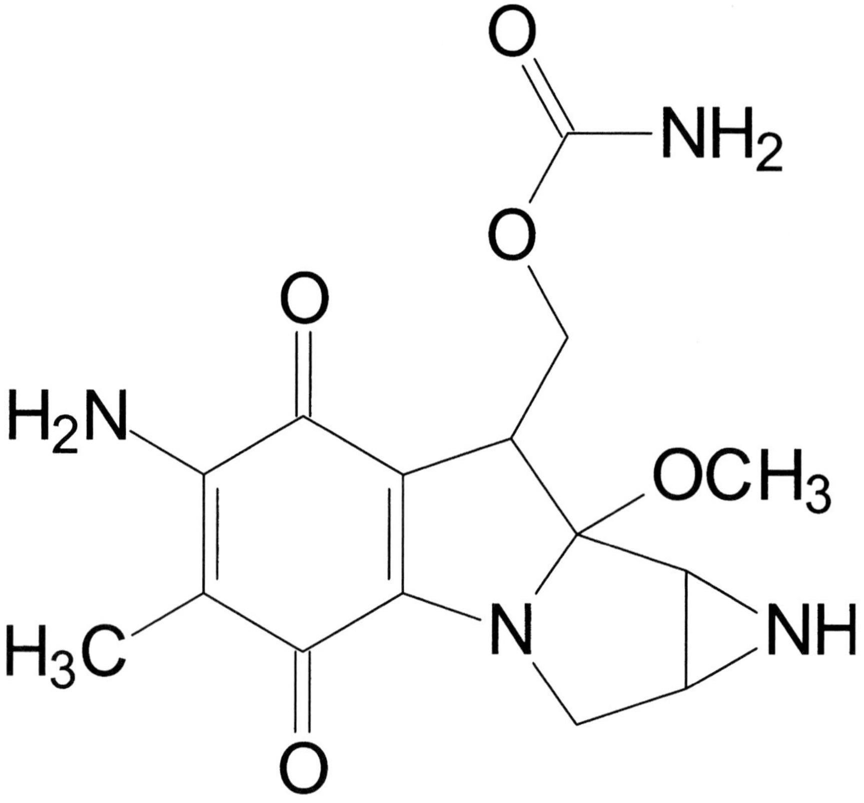

Figure 16.2 Structure of mitomycin C.

quinone-methide followed by a nucleophilic attack of DNA leading to a monoalkylated product. Intramolecular displacement of the carbamate group would then result in a second reactive site that produces a cross-linked adduct. Although the cross-linking of MMC to DNA in viable cells and cell extracts. In vitro reactions depend on the reduced form of nicotinamide adenine dinucleotide phosphate (NADPH) that are capable of activating MMC have been prepared, reproducing the process in models in vitro has been difficult. Although MMC reduction can be easily accomplished, covalent binding to DNA has been difficult to reproduce in cell-free systems. The addition of a reducing agent increases the binding to DNA by creating conditions favorable for the maintenance of the semiquinone radical, the intermediate that is formed by the first electron uptake of MMC. For this reason the semiquinone is believed to bind initially to DNA. It appears that one-electron reduction is sufficient to activate both the C-1 and C-10 electrophilic centers.[38]

Aerobic Activation

Under aerobic conditions a second mechanism comes into play through which MMC develops its cytotoxic effect. Reductive metabolism again leads to the formation of reduced MMC; however, its aerobic fate is different. Molecular oxygen reacts with either the short-lived semiquinone radical or the hydroquinone form to generate the superoxide radical anion, hydroxyl radicals, or hydrogen

peroxide.[39] Formation of these highly reactive species may lead to cytotoxic effects such as lipid peroxidation or nucleic acid damage and can be prevented by free radical scavengers such as mannitol as well as by protective enzymes such as superoxide dismutase or catalase. Whether the reactive intermediate of MMC is formed through the radical semiquinone or the dianion (hydroquinone form) depends on the half-life of the radical anion. In an aprotic environment, the radical anion may have a considerable lifetime; in protic media, however, it exists only a few milliseconds, with rapid uptake of a second electron. Furthermore, oxygen definitely plays an important role, as it is a specific inhibitor of the two-electron pathway because of interaction with and inactivation of the semiquinone species by oxygen.

Several enzyme systems capable of activating MMC include NADPH-cytochrome P-450 reductase, xanthine oxidase, and xanthine dehydrogenase.[35,39] However, a controversial aspect of the bioreductive activation of MMC concerns the role of an enzyme called DT-diaphorase (DTD).[31,34–37] DTD is an obligate two-electron reductase that is characterized by its ability to use both the reduced form of nicotinamide adenine dinucleotide (NADH) and NADPH as electron donors and by its inhibition by dicumarol.[39] Both MMC-induced cytotoxicity and induction of DNA interstrand cross-links were found to be DTD-dependent and could be inhibited by pretreatment of HT-29 colon carcinoma cell lines with dicumarol.[40] The ability of DTD to metabolize MMC to a reactive cytotoxic species suggests that the level of DTD may be an important determinant of the antitumor activity of MMC.

The NADPH–cytochrome P-450 reductase is a flavoprotein containing 1 mole each of flavin mononucleotide and flavin adenine dinucleotide, and its function is to transfer electrons from NADPH to the various forms of cytochrome P-450. The enzyme was shown to be involved in MMC activation to toxic species, with greater cytotoxicity occurring under hypoxic conditions.[41,42] However, similar effects were also shown to occur independent of NADPH–cytochrome P-450.[43] These and other data may suggest that the enzymes involved in the reduction of MMC under hypoxic conditions may not be the same as those observed under aerobic conditions or that the products of reduction, and hence those responsible for alkylation, may differ.

Analysis of DNA Adducts

Several studies have been published on covalent interactions between MMC and DNA or DNA fragments.[33,44] The actual binding site of MMC in DNA is the N-6 position of adenine residues or either the N-2 or N-7 position of guanine residues. Acid-activated MMC was found to alkylate preferentially the guanine N-7 position, in contrast to reductively activated MMC, which preferentially alkylates the guanine N-2 position, possibly because of the different electronic structures of acid-activated and reduction-activated MMC. The activation mechanism of MMC can presumably now be evaluated from analysis of the DNA adducts formed in vivo.

Induction of Apoptosis

Most anticancer drugs kill cells by apoptosis. The intrinsic threshold of a particular cell for induction of apoptosis may determine its sensitivity to the killing effects of drugs and may constitute an alternative mechanism of drug resistance. A number of (proto) oncogenes and tumor suppressor genes influence the apoptotic pathway, including most prominently p53 and its downstream effector p21.[45]

Mutagenesis

Most anticancer drugs are mutagenic, and the alkylating agents in particular have been subject to research on mutagenicity. Although the majority of DNA damage is repaired by the different cellular DNA repair systems, persisting DNA lesions may lead to enhanced mutagenesis owing to the occurrence of errors on replication of a damaged template. Monofunctionally activated MMC has been shown to cause a substantial increase in the mutation frequency in human Ad293 cells transfected with a shuttle vector plasmid pSP189.[46] The observed bias of mutations of G:C and the formation of guanine monoadducts suggest that monoadducts may be responsible for the mutations. In *Saccharomyces cerevisiae* strains, increased mutagenic activity

of MMC in terms of frequencies of reversion of mitotic gene conversion and reversion was observed at applied elevated cytochrome P-450 and glutathione contents,[47] which confirmed the relevance of metabolizing enzymes and mitochondrial function in MMC's mechanism of action.[34][IS1]

MECHANISM OF RESISTANCE

The mechanisms of resistance to MMC are incompletely understood but probably involve changes in drug accumulation, bioactivation, inactivation of the alkylating species, and DNA excision repair. In a series of Chinese hamster ovary cell mutants selected for MMC resistance, a progressive loss of MMC activation capacity and increased capacity for excision repair of DNA was found as cells became more drug resistant.[48] The specific bioactivation enzyme system deficient in the resistant cells was not identified in these studies, although the primary activation mechanism in the sensitive parent was sensitive to dicumarol and, therefore, probably DTD. In some resistant cell lines, MMC shares in the MDR phenotype that encompasses doxorubicin, vincristine, and other natural products and that is mediated by overexpression of the drug efflux protein P-170.[49] On the other hand, several drugs known to reverse MDR induced by other drugs were not capable of reversing MMC-induced MDR, which suggests other pathways contributing to the process.[50] One subline of the HCT 116 human colon carcinoma cell line resistant to MMC had an increased expression of a 148,000–molecular-weight membrane protein, the level of which correlated with the degree of MMC resistance.[51] The investigators observed no in vitro cross-resistance to other natural product–type cytotoxic agents. The increased expression of this cell surface protein in drug-resistant phenotypes may be a useful marker for MMC resistance.

CLINICAL PHARMACOLOGY

MMC has a biexponential decline of the plasma concentration time curves, which corresponds to a two-compartment model with linear pharmacokinetics up to doses as high as 60 mg/m^2.[52,53] After a rapid distribution half-life (2 to 10 minutes), the elimination half-life is 25 to 90 minutes (mean, 54 minutes). A remarkable observation in two studies was an unexplained increase in total-body clearance and a decrease in the area under the plasma concentration time curve of MMC after combination chemotherapy that included 5-fluorouracil and doxorubicin.[52,54] No correlations have been found between pharmacokinetic data for MMC and a wide variety of clinical parameters. Most important, impaired liver or renal function does not seem to change the pharmacokinetic behavior of MMC, and therefore neither impairment requires dosage reduction. Urinary recovery after intravenous administration ranged from 1 to 20%, which cannot explain the rapid plasma clearance. Therefore, the suggestion has been made that MMC is rapidly cleared from plasma by metabolism. The liver is thought to be the major organ of biotransformation,[55] but the spleen, kidney, brain, and heart may also be involved in this process. The presence of oxygen markedly reduced the rate of metabolism of MMC in liver homogenates, compared with metabolism in a similar but anaerobic system. As biotransformation is required for activity, this supports the theory of a more pronounced metabolic activation under anaerobic conditions.

MMC is erratically absorbed after oral administration. Intravesical MMC therapy to treat superficial bladder cancer results in extremely low plasma levels, with virtually no systemic side effects and a significant exposure at the target site (bladder).[56,57] MMC uptake in bladder tissues is linearly related to drug concentration in urine.[58] MMC administered intraperitoneally is rapidly absorbed through the serosal surface into plasma, and hence effective control of local lesions through attainment of high drug levels in the peritoneal cavity is infeasible.[59]

TOXICITY

The most significant and frequent side effect of MMC is a delayed myelosuppression, which seems to be directly related to schedule and total dose.[60] Below a total dose of 50 mg/m^2, hematological toxicity is rare. At higher doses thrombocytopenia is more frequent than leukocytopenia and anemia. Other toxic reactions usually include mild and infrequent anorexia, nausea, vomiting, and diarrhea. Alopecia, stomatitis, and rashes also occur infrequently. Extravasation results in tissue necrosis, with very disabling ulcers that may require plastic surgery. High doses of MMC may result in lethal veno-occlusive liver disease.[61] Other more frequent and potentially lethal side effects include hemolytic uremic syndrome (HUS), interstitial pneumonitis, and cardiac failure. The incidence of MMC-induced HUS seems to be less than 10% and is dose dependent, mainly occurring at cumulative doses >50 mg/m^2.[62,63] No consistently effective treatment for this syndrome is available. It may be noted that red blood cell transfusion should be avoided.

Pulmonary toxicity of MMC consists of an interstitial pneumonitis.[63] Discontinuation of MMC administration may occasionally lead to recovery, and corticosteroid treatment may be helpful in preventing progression of pulmonary dysfunction. The incidence of pulmonary toxicity is approximately 7% of the treated population. Cardiac failure secondary to MMC occurs in a similar percentage, and the incidence rises with cumulative doses >30 mg/m^2.[64]

ECTEINASCINEDIN-743

In the late 1960s, extracts of the Caribbean marine tunicate *Ecteinascidia turbinata* were found to be active as inhibitors of cell proliferation. However, it was not until the last decade that the active compound, ecteinascinedin-743 (ET-743; Yondelis, trabectedin; NSC648766) was isolated, purified, and synthesized;[65-67] see Figure 16.3 for its chemical structure. ET-743 belongs to the class of the tetrahydroisoquinoline compounds, which also comprise antibiotic agents such as saframycins, safracins, and naphthyridinomycins. Most likely, ET-743 is produced by the marine tunicate as a defense mechanism to survive in its natural environment.[65,68]

ET-743 produces 50% cell death at low picomolar or nanomolar concentrations in a wide variety of in vitro models.[65,67,69] ET-743 also displayed in vivo activity in preclinical tumor models of human ovarian, breast, non–small cell lung, melanoma, sarcoma, and renal cancer.[67,69,70] Antitumor effects of ET-743 were observed in clinical phase I trials.[67,71] Currently, phase II/III clinical trials with ET-743 are ongoing, and these suggest activity in soft tissue sarcomas, ovarian and breast cancer, and osteosarcoma.[66,72,73] Its key pharmacological features are given in Table 16.3.

MECHANISMS OF ACTION AND CELLULAR PHARMACOLOGY

The exact mechanism by which ET-743 exerts its antitumor activity is not completely understood, but DNA appears to be the primary target.

DNA Minor Groove Binding

It seems quite clear that the cytotoxic effects of ET-743 result from the selective alkylation (i.e., causing DNA adducts) of the N2 amino group of guanine in GC-rich regions of the minor groove of DNA (5′-PuGC-3′ or 5′-PyrGG-3′), similar to what was previously reported for the structurally related antitumor antibiotics saframycin, quinocarmycin, and naphthyridinomycin.[69,74,75] This type of alkylation depends on dehydration of the carbinolamine functional group of ET-743 leading to the formation of an iminium intermediate that subsequently reacts with and causes binding to DNA.[75] However, the DNA sequence selectivity of ET-743 differs from other alkylating agents, such as CC1065 or tallimustine (FCE 24517), that covalently bind to N3 of adenine in AT-rich regions.[76-78] Two subunits of ET-743 (A and B) are responsible for DNA recognition and bonding, while the third subunit (C) does not have contact with DNA and protrudes out of the minor groove;[75,78,79] the C-unit may directly interact with transcription factors.[78] Differences in DNA alkylating sequence selectivity and DNA bending direction, as well as the fact that the DNA bond is reversible upon denaturation, also distinguish ET-743 from other DNA alkylating agents;[66,72] these differences may partly explain the observed differences in antitumor activity and toxicity. Moreover, the reported

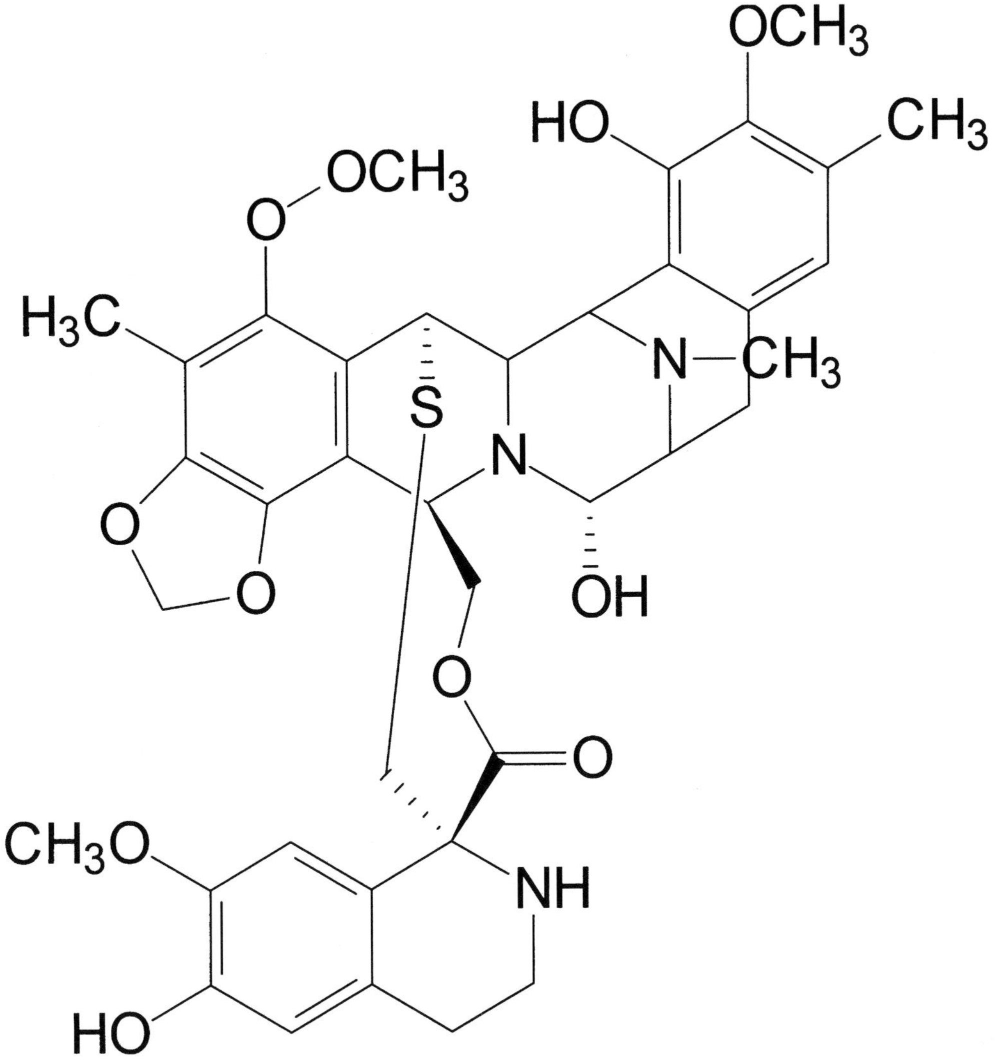

Figure 16.3 Structure of ET-743.

TABLE 16.3
KEY FEATURES OF ET-743

Mechanism of action	Alkylation of DNA, as well as synthesis inhibition of RNA, DNA, and protein
Metabolism	Desmethylation and CYP3A4-mediated oxidation
Pharmacokinetics	Terminal $t_{1/2}$: 55 hr
Elimination	Primarily via bile (<2% in urine)
Drug interactions	None
Toxicity	Neutropenia
	Thrombocytopenia
	Hepatic toxicity
	Nausea and vomiting
	Fatigue
Precautions	Co-medication with CYP3A4 substrates
	Care should be taken in case of bilirubin increase.

$t_{1/2}$, half-life.

structural changes induced by ET-743 could be important in affecting the recognition and binding of transcription factors or DNA-binding proteins.

Recognition of Transcription Factors and DNA-Binding Proteins

Many DNA-binding drugs interfere with important cellular functions, such as DNA repair, replication, and transcription.[68,80] Therefore, an altered transcription of genes that mediate drug action and apoptosis can negatively impact on therapeutic intervention, including in cancer. As a consequence, impairment of the complex interactions between activators (i.e., promoters and enhancer elements) and their DNA targets (i.e., gene-specific DNA-binding proteins, generally transcription factors) could alter the pattern of gene expression.

Several studies have elucidated the inhibitory effect of ET-743 on DNA binding of transcription factors, such as oncogene products (e.g., MYC, c-MYB, and Maf), transcriptional activators regulated during the cell cycle (E2F and SRF), and general transcription factors (e.g., Sp1, TATA-binding protein (TBP), and NF-Y).[65,75] Inhibition of DNA binding for TBP, E2F, SRF, and NF-Y (and SCR, an important activator of the c-fos gene) was observed at higher ET-743 concentrations (>50 μM) than those required for cytotoxicity (<10 nM). This finding is interesting since NF-Y activates the CCAAT element that is present in 25% of eukaryotic promoters,[68] including promoters that regulate genes in the cell cycle.[68,75] In addition, activation of the multidrug resistance gene (MDR1) and heat shock protein 70 (HSP70) promoters, both of which contain the CCAAT box, were significantly inhibited by ET-743, while leaving constitutive gene expression relatively unaffected.[81,82] Therefore, ET-743 is the first pharmacological agent that prevents the activation of MDR1 transcription by multiple stress inducers targeting induced NF-Y-mediated and HSP70-mediated transcription and is distinct from other DNA-interacting anticancer drugs.[82] Interestingly, Martinez and colleagues (2001) have shown that nanomolar concentrations of ET-743 and its synthetic analog phthalascidin (Pt-650) both up-regulate and down-regulate the expression of a variety of genes, including those involved in DNA damage response, transcription, and signal transduction (e.g., protein tyrosine phosphatase, CCAAT displacement protein, and p21/waf1/cip1) in intestinal carcinoma HCT116 and breast MDA-MB-435 cell lines.[82]

The orphan nuclear receptor (SXR) regulates drug metabolism through induction of transcription of the gene for metabolizing cytochrome P-450 enzymes (e.g., CYP2C8 and CYP3A4) and the MDR1 gene that encodes P-glycoprotein (P-gp); P-gp regulates the efflux of a wide range of compounds, including anticancer drugs. ET-743 was found to inhibit SXR and, subsequently, suppress MDR1 gene expression.[65,83] These observations may be relevant in relation to the reported cytotoxicity of ET-743, either alone or in combination with other drugs (see below), since ET-743 could modulate the activity of other anticancer drugs. For example, ET-743 has been shown to inhibit paclitaxel-induced SXR activation and to repress MDR1 transcription through inhibition of SXR at concentrations similar to those required for the above-mentioned inhibition of trichostatin-induced MDR1 transcription.[65]

Interference with DNA Repair Pathways

The cytotoxicity of ET-743 has been investigated in cell lines with specific defects in DNA repair mechanisms.[75,76,84-86] Cells deficient in DNA mismatch repair were as sensitive to ET-743 (but resistant to cisplatin) as proficient (control) cells. Thus, the loss of mismatch repair does not affect the cytotoxicity of ET-743. DNA-dependent protein kinase (DNA-PK) is involved in the DNA double-strand–break repair pathway, which is activated by ionizing radiation and alkylating drugs (chlorambucil). Cells lacking functional

DNA-PK (or inhibited by wortmannin) were severalfold more sensitive to ET-743, although double-strand breaks could not be observed in these cells. Thus, loss of DNA-PK activity enhances ET-743's toxicity.[86] Nucleotide excision repair (NER) represents a major DNA repair system able to handle a broad variety of DNA damages, such as ultraviolet lesions and bulky chemical adducts (as seen with cisplatin and mitomycin treatments). NER-deficient cells are less sensitive to ET-743 than NER-proficient (control) cells, in contrast to the reported sensitivities of several other DNA alkylators.[85] This result was totally unexpected, since it was thought that NER-deficient cells would be unable to recognize and process ET-743-induced DNA damage and would therefore be unable to survive. NER-deficient cells became sensitive to ET-743 when the mutant repair protein (and any one of the several potential mutations) was restored by transfection. Thus, an intact transcription-coupled NER pathway is essential to ET-743 activity and defects in that it confers resistance to ET-743, as shown for cisplatin in mismatch repair–deficient cells.[76,87] In fact, cisplatin-resistant ovarian carcinoma cells (with increased NER) are sensitive to ET-743.[66,72] The unusual pattern of ET-743's sensitivity in NER-deficient cells emphasizes that ET-743 represents a new class of anticancer agents able to interact with DNA in a different way than other alkylating agents, which may explain its remarkable activity against tumors that are not sensitive to other DNA-interacting anticancer agents.

Cell Cycle Perturbation, Topoisomerase I, and the Microtubule Network

ET-743 causes perturbation of the cell cycle at specific phases. In vitro studies have demonstrated that ET-743 decreases the rate of progression of tumor cells through the S phase and causes prolonged p53-independent blockade in G_2/M phase,[77] giving rise to a strong apoptotic response. Interestingly, cells in G1 are more sensitive to ET-743 than cells in S phase or G_2/M phase.[65,70,85] ET-743 does not seem to mediate topoisomerase I–related effects, and its effect on tubulin is not likely related to an antitumor effect.[65,75]

MECHANISMS OF RESISTANCE

Multidrug resistance (MDR) is a phenomenon displayed by many tumors and is characterized by various molecular adaptations in cancer cells to allow increasingly high doses of cytotoxic drugs.[88] Although studies addressing mechanistic aspects of MDR and aberrant apoptosis in cancer cells have yielded valuable insights, only limited knowledge is available about underlying mechanisms involved in the resistance to ET-743. The relationship between ET-743 and MDR1 seems inconclusive.[65,83] ET-743 inhibits activation of expression of MDR1 (by trichostatin) in tumor cells but not activation of constitutive expression in normal cells. In some tumor cell lines, resistance was mediated through MDR, in others it was not.[65] Defects in transcription-coupled NER confer resistance to ET-743, whereas the drug resistance by these cells could be reversed by transfection of the appropriate repair enzyme. In addition, so far, limited evidence is available that ET-743 is a substrate for any of the known ABC transporters (P-gp, MRP1, and BCRP). Moreover, ET-743 shows low or no cross-resistance with several standard chemotherapeutic agents.[73]

DRUG INTERACTIONS

Since it has been demonstrated that ET-743, at least in vitro, is a substrate for CYP3A4 enzymes (see below), it might be expected that the well-known CYP3A4 enzyme inducer dexamethasone increases ET-743's metabolism. However, a combination of both compounds in B16 tumor cells and osteosarcoma xenografts showed increased activity compared to ET-743 alone.[65] This finding may be explained by ET-743–reduced CYP3A4 enzyme expression, repressed CYP3A4 SXR activation, or the presence of cytotoxic metabolites of ET-743 (e.g., N-desmethylyondelis; ET-729). Interestingly, Donald and colleagues (2003) demonstrated the protective effects of single high-dose dexamethasone on ET-743–induced hepatotoxicity in female rats[89]; this protective effect of dexamethasone could, however, not be mimicked in in vitro experiments using liver cells in culture.[90]

CLINICAL PHARMACOLOGY

Due to its limited aqueous solubility, ET-743 has been formulated as a lyophilized pharmaceutical product containing 250 μg ET-743 per dosage unit, 250 mg mannitol (bulking agent), and 0.05 M phosphate buffer (pH 4.0) for stabilization.[65] This formulation is light sensitive and stable at room temperature only for a few hours.

ET-743 is administered to cancer patients in μg/m^2 dosages, resulting in relatively low plasma levels (pg/mL to ng/mL). Several quantitative bioanalytic methods have been developed that are accurate and sensitive, with the lower limit of quantitation in the therapeutic range, including high-performance liquid chromatography (HPLC) and HPLC combined with mass spectrometry.[69,91,92]

Even though metabolism is the most important route for ET-743's elimination (<2% is excreted in the urine as unchanged drug),[69] information on the metabolism of ET-743 is yet sparse and inconclusive. One possible explanation for this apparent discrepancy is that, owing to its relative high potency, metabolite concentrations in vivo are too low to detect with currently available bioanalytic assays. Even though data supporting the role of CYP3A4 enzymes in the disposition and/or antitumor activity of ET-743 in vivo are still lacking, in vitro studies have demonstrated that ET-743 is a substrate for CYP3A4 enzymes. When incubated with human or rat microsomes that express

CYP3A4, ET-743 is metabolized into three species, N-desmethylyondelis (ET-729) and two oxidative degradation products. Rat and human microsomal metabolism of ET-743 was reduced in the presence of chemical CYP3A4 inhibitors or antirat CYP3A2 antiserum and to a much lower extent by CYP2E and CYP2A inhibitors.[93] In human liver panel studies, ET-743 disappearance was highly correlated with CYP3A4 activities. Glucuronidation does not seem to be an important detoxification route for ET-743.[94]

Preclinical studies have demonstrated that exposure time represents an important parameter for the chemosensitivity of cancer cells to ET-743. The drug proved to have a more favorable in vitro therapeutic index when the duration of exposure was extended from 1 hour to periods ranging from 24 hours to 3 days. Many clinical phase I studies with ET-743 have been performed with different infusion schemes: 1-hour, 3-hour, 24-hour, daily times 5, and 72-hour infusion.[65,95] In phase I studies, common pharmacokinetic (PK) parameters, such as clearance, terminal elimination constant (half-life; $t_{1/2}$), area under the concentration time curve (AUC), maximal concentration (C_{max}), and apparent volume of distribution at steady state (V_{ss}), range from 21 to 86 L/h, 26 to 89 h^{-1}, 36 to 55 h·ng/mL, 0.32 to 17 ng/mL, and 808 to 3900 L, respectively. It may be noted from these values that ET-743 is extensively distributed in the body (high V_{ss}), which is reflected by a slow redistribution and elimination (long $t_{1/2}$), although high interpatient variability was observed. Primary dose-limiting toxicity included thrombocytopenia and neutropenia, hepatic toxicity (with 72-hour infusion), and fatigue. Hematological toxicity, which was reversible and dose-dependent, seems to be related to ET-743's C_{max}, while the AUC may be related to the hepatic toxicity observed with longer ET-743 infusions (e.g., 72-hour infusion). No correlations were observed[87] between the grades of nausea, vomiting, or fatigue with either AUC or C_{max}. Except for an observed decrease in clearance with increasing dose (1-hour infusion) and a disproportionate increase of AUC beyond a dose of 1050 μg/m^2 (72-hour infusion), all phase I studies have shown dose-independent kinetics. Preliminary population PK modeling of the phase II study data (24-hour infusion) showed that ET-743's PK profile was best described by a three-compartment model, with an comparable clearance (44 L/hour) as observed in phase I studies. In addition, a correlation between total plasma clearance and age was suggested. A dose of 1,500 μg/m^2 was evaluated in different clinical phase II studies, and activity has been reported for soft tissue sarcoma, ovarian cancer, and breast cancer. Combination studies and phase III studies are currently ongoing.

TOXICITY

With short ET-743 infusions, dose-limiting toxicity was hematological (e.g., thrombocytopenia, neutropenia), but with longer infusions, hepatic toxicity became dose-limiting. The latter consists of acute and reversible transaminitis and cholangitis, which is characterized by elevation of alkaline phosphatases, aspartate aminotransferase, and bilirubin (with peak levels on day 3) and a decrease of hepatic cytochrome P-450 (CYP) enzymes (CYP3A2, CYP1A1/2, and CYP2E1). Pharmacokinetic-pharmacodynamic analyses from clinical studies showed that increasing levels of alkaline phosphatases and aspartate aminotransferase correlated with increasing ET-743 doses and AUC, while neutropenia correlated with C_{max} and AUC.[96] Liver toxicity was also a consistent feature in studies with mice, rats, and monkeys.[70] Donald et al. (2002, 2003) demonstrated that a high dose of dexamethasone protects against ET-743–induced hepatic toxicity in the female rat.[25,90,97] Clinical studies carefully evaluating this finding in cancer patients are ongoing.

REFERENCES

1. Waksman SA, Woodruff HB. Bacteriostatic and bactericidal substances produced by soil *Actinomyces*. Proc Soc Biol Med 1940; 45:609–614.
2. Shannon A, Smith H, Nagel K, et al. Selective thrombocytopenia in children with Wilm tumor: An immune-mediated effect of dactinomycin? Med Pediatric Oncol 2003;41:483–485.
3. Chen FM, Sha F, Chin K, et al. The nature of actinomycin C binding to d(AACCAXYG) sequence motifs. Nucleic Acids Res 2004;32:271–277.
4. Brockmann H. Structural differences of the actinomycins and their derivatives. Ann NY Acad Sci 1960;89:323–335.
5. Yoo H, Rill RL. Actinomycin D binding to unsaturated, single-stranded DNA. J Mol Recognit 2001;14:145–150.
6. Brown SC, Shafer RH. Kinetic studies of actinomycin D binding to mono-, oligo- and polynucleotides. Biochemistry 1987;26: 277–281.
7. Wadkins RM, Vlady B, Tung CS. Actinomycin D binds to metastable hairpins in single-stranded DNA. Biochemistry 1998;37:11915–11923.
8. Marchal JA, Prados J, Melguizo C. Actinomycin D treatment leads to differentiation and inhibits proliferation in rhabdomyosarcoma cells. J Lab Clin Med 1997;130:42–50.
9. Kessel D, Wodinsky I. Uptake in vivo and in vitro of actinomycin D by mouse leukemias as factors in survival. Biochem Pharmacol 1968;17:161–164.
10. Kleeff J, Kornmann M, Sawhney H, et al. Actinomycin C induces apoptosis and inhibits growth of pancreatic cancer cells. Int J Cancer 2000;86:399–407.
11. Goldberg, IH, Beerman TA, Poor R. Antibiotics: nucleic acids as targets in chemotherapy. In: Cancer, Becker FF, ed. New York: Plenum Press,1978.
12. Gupta RS. Podophyllotoxin-resistant mutants of Chinese hamster ovary cells: cross-resistance studies with various microtubule inhibitors and podophyllotoxic analogues. Cancer Res 1983;43: 505–512.
13. Gupta RS. Cross-resistance of vinblastine- and taxol-resistant mutants of Chinese hamster ovary cells to other anticancer drugs. Cancer Treat Rep 1985;69:515–521.
14. Gupta RS. Cross resistance pattern towards anticancer drugs of a human carcinoma multidrug-resistant cell line. Br J Cancer 1988; 58:441–447.
15. Prados J, Melguizo C, Marchal JA, et al. Therapeutic differentiation in a human rhabdomyosarcoma cell line selected for resistance to actinomycin D. Int J Cancer 1998;75:379–383.
16. Hofsli E, Nissen-Meyer J. Reversal of multidrug resistance by lipophilic drugs. Cancer Res 1990;50:3997–4002.
17. Galbraith WM, Mellet LB. Tissue disposition of 3H-actinomycin C (NSC-3053) in the rat, monkey and dog. Cancer Chemother Rep 1975;59:1061–1069.
18. Tattersall MHM, Sodergen JE, Dengupta SL, et al. Pharmacokinetics of actinomycin D in patients with malignant melanoma. Clin Pharmacol Ther 1975;17:701–708.
19. Kedar A, Mayhew EG, Moore RH, et al. Failure of actinomycin D entrapped in liposomes to prolong survival in renal cell adenocarcinoma–bearing mice. Oncology 1981;38:311–314.
20. Kante B, Couvreur P, Speiser P, et al. Tissue distribution of [3H]actinomycin D adsorbed on polybutylcyanoacrylate nanaparticles. Int J Pharm 1980;7:45–53.
21. Blatt J, Trigg ME, Pizzo PA, et al. Single dose actinomycin D in childhood solid tumors. Cancer Treat Rep 1981;65:145–147.
22. Benjamin RS, Hall SW, Burgess MA. A pharmacokinetically based phase I-II study of single dose actinomycin D (NSC-8053). Cancer Treat Rep 1976;60:289–291.
23. Frei E. The clinical use of actinomycin. Cancer Chemother Rep 1974;58:49–54.
24. Hazar V, Kutluk T, Akyuz C, et al. Veno-occlusive disease-like hepatotoxicity in two children receiving chemotherapy for Wilms' tumor and clear sarcoma of kidney. Pediatr Hematol Oncol 1998;15:85–89.
25. D'Angio GJ, Farber S, Maddock CI. Potentiation of x-ray effects by actinomycin D. Radiology 1959;73:175–177.
26. Wakaki S, Marumo H, Tomioka K. Isolations of new fractions of antitumor mitomycins. Antibiot Chemother 1958;8:228–240.
27. Cummings BJ. Anal cancer. Int J Radiat Oncol Biol Phys 1990;19: 1309–1315.
28. Stevens CL, Taylor KG, Munk KE, et al. Chemistry and structure of mitomycin C. J Med Chem 1964;8:1–10.
29. Beijnen JH, Rosing H, Underberg WJM. Stability of mitomycins in infusion fluids. Acta Pharm Chem Sci Ed 1985;13:58–66.
30. Tomasz M, Palom Y. The mitomycin bioreductive antitumor agents: cross-linking and alkylation of DNA as the molecular basis of their activity. Pharmacol Ter 1997;76:73–87.
31. Cummings JS, Spanswick VJ, Smyth JF. Re-evaluation of the molecular pharmacology of mitomycin C. Eur J Cancer 1995;31A: 1918–1933.
32. Suresh Kumar G, Lipman R, Cummings J, et al. Mitomycin C-DNA adducts generated by DT-diaphorase: revised mechanism of the enzymatic reductive activation of mitomycin C. Biochemistry 1997;36:14128–14136.
33. Tomasz M, Lipman R, Chowdary D, et al. Isolation and structure of a covalent cross-link adduct between mitomycin C and DNA. Science 1987;235:1204–1208.
34. Nishiyama M. Suzuki K, Kumazaki T, et al. Molecular targeting of mitomycin C chemotherapy. Int J Cancer 1997;72:649–656.
35. Cummings J, Spanswich VJ, Tomasz M, et al. Enzymology of mitomycin C metabolic activation in tumour tissue. Biochem Pharmacol 1998;56:405–414.
36. Spanswick VJ, Cummings J, Ritchie AA, et al. Pharmacological determinants of the antitumour activity of mitomycin C. Biochem Pharmacol 1998;56:1497–1503.
37. Spanswick VJ, Cummings J, Smyth J. Current issues in the enzymology of mitomycin C metabolic activation. Gen Pharmacol 1998;4:539–544.
38. Kohn H. Mechanistic studies on the mode of reaction of mitomycin C under catalytic and electrochemical reductive conditions. J Am Chem Soc 987;109:1833–1840.
39. Rooseboom M, Commandeur JN, Vermeulen NP. Enzyme-catalyzed activation of anticancer prodrugs. Pharmacol Rev 2004; 56:53–102.
40. Siegel D, Gibson NW, Preusch PC, et sal. Metabolism of mitomycin C by DT-diaphorase: role of mitomycin C-induced DNA damage and cytotoxicity in human colon carcinoma cells. Cancer Res 1990;50:7483–7489.
41. Belcourt MF, Hodnick WF, Rockwell S, et al. Differential toxicity of mitomycin C and porfiromycin to aerobic and hypoxic Chinese hamster ovary cells overexpressing human NADPH:cytochrome c (P-450) reductase. Proc Natl Acad Sci USA 1996;93:456–460.
42. Sawamura AO, Aoyama T, Tamakoshi K, et al. Transfection of human cytochrome P-450 reductase cDNA and its effects on the sensitivities to toxins. Oncology 1996;53:406–411.

43. Hoban PR, Walton MI, Robson CN, et al. Decreased NADPH: cytochrome P-450 reductase activity and impaired drug activation in a mammalian cell line resistant to mitomycin C under aerobic but not hypoxic conditions. Cancer Res 1990;50:4692–4697.

44. Tomasz M, Chowdary D, Lipman R, et al. Reaction with DNA with chemically or enzymatically activated DNA: isolation and structure of the major covalent adducts. Proc Natl Acad Sci USA 1986;83:6702–6706.

45. Beard SE, Capaldi SR, Gee P. Stress responses to DNA damaging agents in the human colon carcinoma cell line, RKO. Mutat Res 1996;371:1–13.

46. Maccubbin AE, Mudipalli A, Nadadur SS, et al. Mutations in a shuttle vector plasmid exposed to monofunctionally activated mitomycin C. Environ Mol Mutagen 1997;29:143–151.

47. Rossi C, Poli P, Candi A, et al. Modulation of mitomycin C mutagenicity on Saccharomyces cerevisiae by glutathion, cytochrome P-450, and mitochondria interactions. Mutat Res 1997;390:113–120.

48. Dulhanty AM, Li M, Whitmore GF. Isolation of Chinese hamster ovary cell mutants deficient in excision repair and mitomycin C bioactivation. Cancer Res 1989;49:117–122.

49. Giavazzi R, Kartner N, Hart IR. Expression of cell surface p-glycoprotein by an adriamycin-resistant murine fibrosarcoma. Cancer Res 1983;43:145–147.

50. Dorr RT, Liddil JD. Modulation of mitomycin C–induced multidrug resistance in vitro. Cancer Chemother Pharmacol 1991;27:290–294.

51. Wilson JK, Lng BH, Marks ME, et al. Mitomycin C resistance in a human colon carcinoma cell line associated with cell surface protein alternations. Cancer Res 1984;44:5880–5885.

52. Den Hartigh J, McVie JG, van Oort WJ, et al. Pharmacokinetics of mitomycin C in humans. Cancer Res 1983;43:5017–5021.

53. Dorr RT. New findings in the pharmacokinetics, metabolic, and drug-resistance aspects of mitomycin C. Semin Oncol 1988;15: 32–41.

54. Verweij J, Stuurman M, de Vries J, et al. The difference in pharmacokinetics of mitomycin C, given either as a single agent or as part of combination chemotherapy. J Cancer Res Clin Oncol 1986; 112:282–284.

55. Fujita H. Comparative studies on the blood level, tissue distribution, excretion and inactivation of anticancer drugs. Jpn J Clin Oncol 1971;12:335–342.

56. Dalton JT, Wientjes MG, Pfeffer M. Studies on mitomycin C absorption after intravesical treatment of superficial bladder tumors. J Urol 1991;132:30–33.

57. Wientjes MG, Badalment RA, Wang RC. Penetration of mitomycin C in human bladder. Cancer Res 1993;53:3314–3320.

58. Gao X, Au JL, Gadalament RA. Bladder tissue uptake of mitomycin C during intravesical therapy is linear with drug concentration in urine. Clin Cancer Res 1998;4:139–143.

59. Colombo R, Da Pozzo JF, Lev A. Neoadjuvant combined microwave-induced local HT and topical chemotherapy versus chemotherapy alone for superficial bladder cancer. J Urol 1996; 155:1227–1232.

60. Crooke ST, Bradner WT. Mitomycin C: a review. Cancer Treat Res 1976;3:121–139.

61. Lazarus HM, Gottfried MR, Herzig RH. Veno-occlusive disease of the liver after high dose mitomycin C therapy and autologous bone marrow transplantation. Cancer 1982;49:1789–1795.

62. Verweij J, de Vries J, Pinedo HM. Mitomycin C–induced renal toxicity, a dose-dependent side effect? Eur J Cancer Clin Oncol 1987; 23:195–199.

63. Verweij J, Van der Burg MEL, Pinedo HM. Mitomycin C induced hemolytic uremic syndrome: sic case reports and review of the literature on renal, pulmonary and cardiac side effect of the drug. Radiother Oncol 1987;8:33–41.

64. Verweij J, van Zanten T, Souren T. Prospective study of the dose relationship of mitomycin C–induced interstitial pneumonitis. Cancer 1987;60:756–761.

65. van Kesteren C, de Vooght MM, Lopez-Lazaro L, et al. Yondelis (trabectedin, ET-743): the development of an anticancer agent of marine origin. Anticancer Drugs 2003;14:487–502.

66 Takebayashi Y, Pourquier P, Zimonjic DB, et al. Antiproliferative activity of ecteinascidin 743 is dependent upon transcription-coupled nucleotide-excision repair. Nat Med 2001;7:961–966.

67. Rinehart KL. Antitumor compounds from tunicates. Med Res Rev 2000;20:1–27.

68. Minuzzo M, Marchini S, Broggini M, et al. Interference of transcriptional activation by the antineoplastic drug ecteinascidin-743. Proc Natl Acad Sci USA 2000;97:6780–6784.

69. Ryan DP, Supko JG, Eder JP, et al. Phase I and pharmacokinetic study of ecteinascidin 743 administered as a 72-hour continuous intravenous infusion in patients with solid malignancies. Clin Cancer Res 2001;7:231–242.

70. Twelves C, Hoekman K, Bowman A, et al. Phase I and pharmacokinetic study of Yondelis (Ecteinascidin-743; ET-743) administered as an infusion over 1 h or 3 h every 21 days in patients with solid tumours. Eur J Cancer 2003;39:1842–1851.

71. Jin S, Gorfajn B, Faricloth G, et al. Ecteinascidin 743, a transcription-targeted chemotherapeutic that inhibits MDR1 activation. Proc Natl Acad Sci USA 2000;97:6775–6779.

72. Takebayashi Y, Goldwasser F, Urasaki, Y. Ecteinascidin 743 induces protein-linked DNA breaks in human colon carcinoma HCT116 cells and is cytotoxic independently of topoisomerase I expression. Clin Cancer Res 2001;7:185–191.

73. Yovine A, Raymond E, Kaci MO, et al. Phase II study of ecteinascidin-743 in advanced pretreated soft tissue sarcoma patients. J Clin Oncol 2004;22:890–899.

74. Sakai R, Rinehart KL, Guan Y, et al. Additional antitumor ecteinascidins from a Caribbean tunicate: crystal structures and activities in vivo. Proc Natl Acad Sci USA 1992;89:11456–11460.

75. D'lncalci M, Erba E, Damia G, et al. Unique features of the mode of action of ET-743. Oncologist 2002;7:210–216.

76. Damia G, Guidi G, D'Incalci M. Expression of genes involved in nucleotide excision repair and sensitivity to cisplatin and melphalan in human cancer cell lines. Eur J Cancer 1998;34:1783–1788.

77. Ryan DP, Puchlaski T, Supko JG, et al. A phase II and pharmacokinetic study of ecteinascidin 743 in patients with gastrointestinal stromal tumors. Oncologist 2002;7:531–538.

78. Pommier Y, Kohlhagen G, Bailly C, et al. DNA sequence- and structure-selective alkylation of guanine N2 in the DNA minor groove by ecteinascidin 743, a potent antitumor compound from the Caribbean tunicate Ecteinascidia turbinata. Biochemistry 1996;35:13303–13309.

79. Zewail-Foote M, Hurley LH. Ecteinascidin 743: a minor groove alkylator that bends DNA toward the major groove. J Med Chem 1999;42:2493–2497.

80. Latchman DS. Transcription factors: an overview. Int J Biochem Cell Biol 1997;29:1305–1312.

81. Friedman D, Hu Z, Kolb EA, et al. Ecteinascidin-743 inhibits activated but not constitutive transcription. Cancer Res 2002;62: 3377–3381.

82. Martinez EJ, Corey EJ, Owa T. Antitumor activity– and gene expression–based profiling of ecteinascidin Et 743 and phthalascidin Pt 650. Chem Biol 2001;8:1151–1160.

83. Jin W, Metobo S, Williams RM. Synthetic studies on ecteinascidin-743: constructing a versatile pentacyclic intermediate for the synthesis of ecteinascidins and safracmycins. Org Lett 2003;5:2095–2098.

84. Damia G, Silvestri S, Carrassa L, et al. Unique pattern of ET-743 activity in different cellular systems with defined deficiencies in DNA-repair pathways. Int J Cancer 2001;92:583–588.

85. Erba E, Bergamaschi D, Bassano L, et al. Ecteinascidin-743 (ET-743), a natural marine compound, with a unique mechanism of action. Eur J Cancer 2001;37:97–105.

86. Scotto KW. ET-743: more than an innovative mechanism of action. Anticancer Drugs 2002;13(Suppl 1):S3–6.

87. Chabner BA. Cytotoxic agents in the era of molecular targets and genomics. Oncologist 2002;7(Suppl 3):34–41.

88. Shao L, Kasanov J, Hornicek FJ, et al. Ecteinascidin-743 drug resistance in sarcoma cells: transcriptional and cellular alterations. Biochem Pharmacol 2003;66:2381–2395.

89. Donald S, Verschoyle RD, Edwards R, et al. Hepatobiliary damage and changes in hepatic gene expression caused by the antitumor drug ecteinascidin-743 (ET-743) in the female rat. Cancer Res 2002;62:4256–4262.

90. Donald S, Verschoyle RD, Edwards R, et al. Complete protection by high-dose dexamethasone against the hepatotoxicity of the novel antitumor drug Yondelis (ET-743) in the rat. Cancer Res 2003;63:5902–5908.

91. Rosing H, Hildebrand MJ, Jimeno J, et al. Quantitative determination of ecteinascidin 743 in human plasma by miniaturized high-performance liquid chromatography coupled with electrospray ionization tandem mass spectrometry. J Mass Spectrom 1998;33:1134–1140.
92. Rosing H, Hildebrand MJ, Jimeno J, et al. Analysis of ecteinascidin 743, a new potent marine-derived anticancer drug, in human plasma by high-performance liquid chromatography in combination with solid-phase extraction. J Chromatogr B Biomed Sci Appl 1998;710(1-2):183–189.
93. Reid JM, Kuffel MJ, Ruben SL, et al. Rat and human liver cytochrome P-450 isoform metabolism of ecteinascidin 743 does not predict gender-dependent toxicity in humans. Clin Cancer Res 2002;8:2952–2962.
94. Sparidans RW, Rosing H, Hildebrand MJ, et al. Search for metabolites of ecteinascidin 743, a novel, marine-derived, anti-cancer agent, in man. Anticancer Drugs 2001;12:653–666.
95. Held-Warmkessel J. Ecteinascidin-743. Clin J Oncol Nurs 2003;7: 313–319.
96. Taamma A, Misset JL, Riofrio M, et al. Phase I and pharmacokinetic study of ecteinascidin-743, a new marine compound, administered as a 24-hour continuous infusion in patients with solid tumors. J Clin Oncol 2001;19:1256–1265.
97. Donald S, Verschoyle RD, Greaves P, et al. Comparison of four modulators of drug metabolism as protectants against the hepatotoxicity of the novel antitumor drug Yondelis (ET-743) in the female rat and in hepatocytes in vitro. Cancer Chemother Pharmacol 2004;53:305–312.

Topoisomerase I–Targeting Drugs

Alex Sparreboom   William C. Zamboni

Topoisomerase I–targeting agents, such as the camptothecin analogs, belong to a class of anticancer drugs that target the DNA-relaxing enzyme topoisomerase I. The first identified compound in this class, camptothecin, is a naturally occurring alkaloid found in the bark and wood of the Chinese tree *Camptotheca acuminata*. The camptothecins have generated broad interest, both as a research tool for studying the molecular function and activity of DNA topoisomerase I and as therapeutic agents with proven activity in the treatment of various human malignancies.

HISTORY

As early as the 1950s, a National Cancer Institute screening program discovered that extracts derived from the *Camptotheca* tree were cytotoxic to cancer cells. Not until 1966, however, did Wall and colleagues identify camptothecin as the active agent.[1] Biochemical studies performed in the early 1970s of the pharmacology of camptothecin showed that it could damage DNA,[2] ultimately inhibiting both DNA and RNA synthesis[3–10]; the mechanisms underlying these drug actions remained obscure. Because of promising preclinical activity, the drug entered clinical trials in the early 1970s under National Cancer Institute sponsorship. Because of its insolubility in aqueous solutions, camptothecin was formulated as its sodium salt (NSC-1000880). In early clinical studies, a few responses were observed in patients with colorectal, stomach, small-bowel, and non–small cell lung cancers (NSCLC) and melanoma. Unfortunately, severe toxicities, including hemorrhagic cystitis, nausea, vomiting, diarrhea, and dose-limiting myelosuppression, were also observed.[11–13] When limited phase II testing failed to demonstrate meaningful

antitumor activity in gastrointestinal cancers[14] and malignant melanoma,[15] further clinical development was halted.

Important advances in the 1980s led to a resurgence of interest in the camptothecins. First was the discovery that camptothecin had a unique molecular target, DNA topoisomerase I, a key nuclear enzyme responsible for relaxing torsionally strained DNA.[16,17] Currently, the camptothecins remain the best-characterized inhibitors of topoisomerase I. Corporate interest in this field led to the synthesis of more soluble and less toxic camptothecin analogs with even greater preclinical anticancer activity, such as irinotecan (CPT-11) and topotecan.[18,19] In 1996, topotecan hydrochloride (Hycamtin) was approved in the United States for use as second-line chemotherapy for patients with advanced ovarian cancer, and in that same year, irinotecan hydrochloride (Camptosar) was approved for use in patients with 5-fluorouracil (5-FU)–refractory advanced colorectal cancer. Additional camptothecin analogs currently in clinical testing include 9-nitrocamptothecin (9-NC), lurtotecan (GG211, GI47211), exatecan mesylate (DX8951f), diflomotecan (BN80915), karenitecin (BNP1350), and gimatecan (ST1481). Several noncamptothecin agents that also interact with topoisomerase I have entered clinical trials, including NB-506, intoplicine (RP60475), TAS 101, and (*N*-[2-(dimethylamino) ethyl] acridine-4-carboxamide. The development of these new agents may further increase the importance of topoisomerase I as a target for cancer chemotherapy.[20]

MECHANISM OF ACTION

DNA topoisomerases are essential enzymes found in all nucleated cells. These enzymes are involved in the regulation of DNA topology and are necessary for the preservation of the integrity of the genetic material during DNA metabolism, including RNA transcription, DNA replication, recombination, chromatin remodeling, chromatin condensation, and repair during cell division.[21,22] Based on their different reaction mechanism and cellular function, there are two types of DNA topoisomerases (type I and type II). Their characteristics are summarized in Table 17.1.

Human topoisomerase I is a monomeric ~91 kd polypeptide of 765 amino acids encoded by an active copy gene located on chromosome 20q12-13.2 and two pseudogenes on chromosomes 1q23-24 and 22q11.2-13.1.[23–25] The coding sequence of the gene is split into 21 exons spread over at least 85 kilobase pairs of human genomic DNA. The human topoisomerase I gene promotor is influenced by positively and negatively acting transcription factors, as described elsewhere.[26]

This protein is comprised of four major domains: a highly charged NH_2-terminal domain, a conserved core domain, a positively charged linker domain, and a highly conserved COOH-terminal domain containing the active site tyrosine, that is, the nucleophilic Tyr^{723} amino acid residue.[25,27] The relaxation of torsionally strained (supercoiled) duplex DNA by human topoisomerase I, with subsequent transcription and replication, is independent of charge (positively or negatively).[25] A transesterification

TABLE 17.1
DIFFERENTIATION OF HUMAN DNA TOPOISOMERASES TYPE I AND II

Type I topoisomerase
  Monomeric protein, molecular weight ~91 kd
  Single-copy gene located on chromosome 20q12–13.2
  Transiently breaks one strand of duplex DNA and forms a
    3′-phospho-tyrosine covalent intermediate
  Single-step changes in the linking number of circular DNAs
  Its expression is continuous during the cell cycle and in
    quiescent cells
  Mainly involved in relaxation of supercoiled DNA during RNA
    transcription
  ATP independent

Type II topoisomerase
  Homodimeric protein, molecular weight 170 kd (isoenzyme IIα)
    and 180 kd (isoenzyme IIβ)
  Single-copy gene located on chromosome 17q21–22 (isoenzyme
    IIα) and chromosome 3p24 (isoenzyme IIβ)
  Breaks both strands of duplex DNA and forms a pair of 5′-
    phosphotyrosine covalent intermediates
  Generates a gate through which another region of DNA can be
    passed
  Double-step changes in the linking number of circular DNAs
  Its expression increases during S phase of the cell cycle
    (especially isoenzyme IIα) and is almost absent in quiescent
    cells (primarily expression of isoenzyme IIβ)
  Involved in DNA replication, recombination, RNA transcription
    and repair
  ATP dependent

reaction takes place by which topoisomerase I cleaves one strand of the double-helix structure of DNA, attacking the C_4-oxygen atom of the active site tyrosine (Tyr^{723}) residue. The enzyme forms a transient, covalent phosphotyrosyl intermediate with the 3′-end of the nicked DNA strand, the so-called cleavable complex.[28] Afterwards, the energy of this covalent attachment is recycled for the reverse transesterification reaction that reseals the DNA strands (religation) and liberates the enzyme. Consequently, for these intertwining processes neither energy cofactors nor metal cations are required by human topoisomerase I.[29] Recent studies have provided more detailed insights into the three-dimensional structure of human topoisomerase I and its interactive function with the DNA molecule.[30,31] In Table 17.2, the principal structural characteristics of human topoisomerase I are summarized.

The mechanism of DNA relaxation after formation of the covalent complex and before religation is still not completely elucidated.[30] So far, two mechanisms are supposed, viz. the strand passage model and the free rotation model. Both models represent the two extremes of a continuum in the conceptual framework for how topoisomerase I might effect changes in linking number.[30,31] In the strand passage (or enzyme-bridging) model, it is hypothesized that the intact DNA strand is passed through an enzyme-bridged gate, which is made by the covalent linkage of the 3′ end and by noncovalent binding to the 5′ end of the broken strand. On the other hand, in the free rotation model, relaxation of torsionally strained duplex DNA is possible due to the releasing of the 5′ end of the broken strand from the active site and its consequent ability to rotate freely about the complementary unbroken strand.[25,31] X-ray crystallographic studies with complexes of human topoisomerase I and DNA led to the proposal that the relaxation of supercoiled DNA proceeds by a controlled rotation mechanism.[30,31]

In the controlled rotation model, the DNA structure is allowed to rotate completely free at 30° intervals downstream of the cleavage site round the intact DNA strand modulated by the interaction of the nose-cone helices of subdomain I and II in a positively charged cavity formed by the cap of the enzyme and the linker domain.[25] In vitro studies with reconstituted human topoisomerase I have revealed the more precise function of the linker region. During the normal relaxation of supercoiled DNA, it acts to slow the relegation.[27] From these studies, it is also hypothesized that the inhibition of DNA relaxation caused by camptothecin—by stabilizing the cleavable complex—depends on a direct effect of the cytotoxic agent on DNA rotation that is mediated by electrostatic interactions between the linker domain and DNA.[27]

When the attachment of camptothecin is modeled in the three-dimensional structure of human topoisomerase I, it is believed that the DNA duplex is extended in such a way that carbon positions 7 and 9 of the camptothecin structure are facing out into open space. These carbon positions are

TABLE 17.2
STRUCTURAL CHARACTERISTICS OF HUMAN DNA TOPOISOMERASE TYPE I

Two domains with essential functions for catalytic activity and relaxation function

I. Core domain (MW 56 kd)
   Amino acid residues 215 to 635 (Ile^{215}–Arg^{635})
   Subdomain I
      Amino acid residues 215 to 232 and 320 to 433
      Two α helices and nine β strands
   Subdomain II
      Amino acid residues 233 to 319
      Five α helices and two β strands
   Subdomain III
      Amino acid residues 434 to 635
      Ten α helices and five β strands
      Contains all active-site residues except the Tyr^{723}
      Extends from the top half of the molecule downward through 2 long α helices that function like a hinge that opens and closes the enzyme around the DNA
   Subdomains I and II are folded tightly together and form the "cap" (top lobe) region of the enzyme
   Subdomains I and II have two long "nose-cone" helices (α5 and β6) that make a ~90° angle with each other and come together in a V-figure at a point 25 Å away from the body of the molecule and enclose a triangular-shaped empty space between them
   Subdomain III forms the bottom lobe of the enzyme
   Subdomains I and III interact via 2 short "lips" opposite from the long-hinge helices
II. COOH-terminal domain (MW 6 kd)
   Amino acids residues 713 to 765 (Gln^{713}–Phe^{765})
   Contains the active site (catalytic) tyrosine Tyr^{723}

Two domains without essential functions for catalytic activity and relaxation function

III. NH$_2$-terminal domain (MW 24 kd)
   Amino acid residues 1 to 214 (Met^1–Gly^{214})
   Is highly charged, has very few hydrophobic amino acids, is largely disordered, and contains several nuclear-targeting signals
   Involved in nucleolar localization through interactions with nucleolin
IV. Linker domain (MW 7 kd)
   Amino acids residues 636 to 712 (Pro^{636}–Lys^{712})
   Coiled-coil structure that is positively charged
   Reaches 50 Å away from the body of the enzyme

very accessible to chemical modifications. Consequently, this gives the opportunity to expand the potency of modified camptothecin analogs by auspicious interactions of these derivatives with distant proteins or DNA atoms at the binding site.[31]

Stabilization of the cleavable complex by camptothecins is not sufficient in itself for the induction of cell death because the complex can reverse spontaneously. The lethal effects of these drugs are caused by the interaction between a moving replication fork (or transcription process) and the drug-stabilized cleavable complex, resulting in irreversible arrest of DNA replication and the formation of a double-strand break located at the fork. This so-called fork

collision model leads to the arrest of the cell cycle in the S/G$_2$ phase and finally to apoptosis.[32] As cells in the S phase division are up to 1,000-fold more sensitive to topoisomerase I inhibitors than cells in the G$_1$ or G$_2$/M phases after exposure, the cytotoxicity of these agents is considered S-phase specific.[33–35]

The time of persistence of the drug-stabilized cleavable complex depends on the production and/or repair of replication or transcription lesions. In general, transcription lesions require longer persistence, that is, greater stability of the cleavable complex, than do replication lesions.[36] Unfortunately, the fraction of replicating cells in tumor tissues is underrepresented. This means that cell kill results predominantly from the transcription lesion mechanism. For this reason, the potency of different camptothecin analogs to stabilize the cleavable complex is of paramount importance for efficacious therapeutic use.[36] Of relevance for all topoisomerase I inhibitors are the data from in vitro experiments that revealed that the cytotoxicity increases with the duration of exposure. Short-time exposures to high concentrations are less effective than long-term exposures to low concentrations.[37,38]

Due to their mechanism of action, topoisomerase I inhibitors are potential mutagens, although their clinical mutagenicity and oncogenicity have not been established.[39–41] Furthermore, the tendency to administer topoisomerase I inhibitors using protracted schedules or prolonged exposure regimens could hypothetically lead to an increased risk of mutagenicity.[42,43]

The stabilization of the cleavable complexes by topoisomerase I inhibitors disrupts the DNA integrity and interferes with the normal processes of DNA topology, including replication, transcription, DNA repair, chromosome condensation, and chromosome separation.[39] The formation of these drug-induced cleavable complexes is essential but is not sufficient in itself to cause cytotoxicity. This implies that cells need to undergo DNA synthesis to yield maximum toxicity.[44–46] Experimental studies showed that in the presence of topoisomerase II inhibitors chromosomal aberrations arise during replication, which seems a more important cause of cytotoxicity.[47] Furthermore, it was postulated that recombination processes must be initiated to bypass the replication block created by topoisomerase II inhibitor–stabilized complexes and that some of these events cause aberrant, illegitimate, or nonhomologous recombination, which may lead to cytotoxicity and/or mutations. Nonhomologous recombination that causes deletions of an essential gene, partially or completely, resulted in the loss of gene products and finally to cell death. In contrast, aberrant recombination or rearrangement causing deletion of a suppressor gene or activation of a proto-oncogene have the potential to induce secondary cancers.[39] Topoisomerase II inhibitors cause an increased risk of acute myeloid leukemia[48] characterized by balanced chromosomal translocations involving either the MLL (ALL-1, HRX) gene[49] at 11q23 or the AML1 gene[50] at 21q22.

In principal, topoisomerase I inhibitors could produce similar molecular alterations as those caused by topoisomerase II inhibitors. Direct comparative in vitro studies have shown that, on a molar basis, the topoisomerase I inhibitors were more mutagenic than the topoisomerase II inhibitor etoposide.[39] Topotecan was found to be less mutagenic than the parent compound camptothecin. So far, the clinical use of topoisomerase I inhibitors has not been linked to secondary malignancies. However, the relative survival time of patients treated with irinotecan or topotecan as compared with those treated with anthracyclines and epipodophyllotoxins (e.g., for lymphomas, testicular cancer, or hematological malignancies) possibly indicates a less clinically apparent mutagenic risk associated with topoisomerase I inhibitors.

MECHANISMS OF RESISTANCE

Based on preclinical studies, it is likely that clinical resistance to the camptothecins might be the result of three main mechanisms: (a) alterations in the target (topoisomerase I), (b) inadequate accumulation of drug in the tumor, and/or (c) alterations in the cellular response to the topoisomerase I–camptothecin interaction.[51,52]

Alterations in Topoisomerase I

Various point mutations of topoisomerase I in different camptothecin-resistant cell lines have been associated with camptothecin resistance.[53-61] The different point mutations in human topoisomerase I in several camptothecin-resistant cell lines are summarized in Table 17.3. These point mutations result in decreased topoisomerase I catalytic activity or impaired binding of camptothecin to topoisomerase I.[53,62] In some models, single amino acid changes resulted in partial resistance, while double mutation induced a synergistic resistance.

TABLE 17.3

DIFFERENT POINT MUTATIONS OF HUMAN TOPOISOMERASE I

CPT-Resistant Cell Line	Point Mutation	Reference
CPT^R-2000 cell line	Gly^{717} to Val and Thr^{729} to Ile	53
CPT-K5 cell line	Asp^{533} to Gly^a and Asp^{583} to Gly	56
PC-7/CPT cell line	Thr^{729} to Ala	57
By in vitro mutagenesis	Gly^{363} to Cys	58
CHO DC3F/C-10	Gly^{505} to Ser	60
U-937/CR cell line	Phe^{361} to Ser	61

^{a}Only Asp^{533} to Gly leads to resistance.

In a small clinical study involving eight NSCLC patients treated with irinotecan, two point mutations were identified that were located near a site in topoisomerase I that was previously identified[62] as a position of a mutation in the camptothecin-resistant human lung cancer cell line PC7/CPT. Although this is the first prospective clinical study demonstrating that point mutations in topoisomerase I occur after chemotherapy with irinotecan, further clinical studies will be needed to verify if the incidence of topoisomerase I gene mutations relates to the occurrence of clinical resistance to topoisomerase I inhibitors.

Altered Cellular Accumulation and Transport of Camptothecins

The role of the P-glycoprotein (ABCB1)–associated multidrug resistance (MDR) phenotype in camptothecin resistance has still not been clearly defined. Irinotecan and SN-38 do not appear to interact significantly with P-glycoprotein,[63] and cross-resistance to irinotecan is not seen in P388 leukemia cells expressing pleiotropic drug resistance to vincristine and doxorubicin.[64] In comparative studies, MDR-expressing sublines were nine-fold more resistant to topotecan than were parental wild-type cells.[65] Although other investigators have confirmed these findings for topotecan, this degree of MDR-associated resistance is much less than the 200-fold change in sensitivity typically described for classic MDR substrates, such as doxorubicin or etoposide.[66-68]

Several camptothecin analogs, including SN-38, topotecan, and 9-aminocamtothecin, are also substrates for other transport systems in addition to P-glycoprotein, such as the MDR-associated protein-1 (MRP1, ABCC1)[69] and the breast cancer resistance protein (BCRP, ABCG2),[70,71] and preliminary evidence for the clinical relevance of this observation to in vivo resistance has been provided.[72] In human colon cancer xenografts that highly express MDR, irinotecan was still quite effective, even against a cell line resistant to topotecan.[73] Thus, different mechanisms of camptothecin resistance may be specific for certain camptothecin analogs. Further characterization of these specific mechanisms of resistance is urgently required.

In addition to active transport, cellular metabolism may be particularly important for irinotecan, which is converted to SN-38 by carboxylesterases.[74] Indeed, increased levels of these esterases is associated with increased sensitivity to irinotecan.[75,76] In addition, there is large interindividual variation in expression of carboxylesterases in colon tumors that may contribute to variation in the therapeutic outcome of irinotecan therapy.[77,78] SN-38 is also conjugated and detoxified by UDP-glucuronosyltransferase (UGT) to yield an SN-38-glucuronide.[79] Furthermore, glucuronidation of SN-38 is associated with increased efflux of the drug from colon cancer cells,[80] and glucuronidation of camptothecins has been associated with altered chemosensitivity of breast cancer and lung cancer cells.[81] It is of interest to note that reactivation of SN-38 in tumor specimens by β-glucuronidases might also take place and may represent an important route of tumor drug activation.[82]

Alternative Mechanisms

Other potential mechanisms of decreased sensitivity to camptothecins include a reduction in the number of cells in the S phase[83] and increased expression of metallothionein.[84] Furthermore, double-stranded DNA break repair activity may also modulate camptothecin-induced cytotoxicity. For example, yeast mutants defective in the RAD52 double-stranded DNA break repair gene are hypersensitive to camptothecin.[85,86]

The key biochemical or molecular determinants of tumor response to clinical camptothecin therapy have not yet been identified. Because of the complex, stepwise pattern of drug-induced perturbations in cellular metabolism, no single parameter may be able to identify sensitive or resistant tumors completely. Although the overall topoisomerase I activity may be important,[87,88] other factors might also be relevant, including topoisomerase I enzyme mutations, the amount of cleavable complexes formed, and the extent of ongoing DNA synthesis. Total topoisomerase I protein levels in tissues as measured by Western immunoblotting correlate poorly with sensitivity to camptothecins in experimental studies.[89] Likewise, total topoisomerase I mRNA does not predict drug sensitivity when different cell lines are compared.[90] This poor correlation between total topoisomerase I expression and drug effects may be due either to posttranslational regulation of the enzyme, to subcellular localization of topoisomerase I away from DNA, or to other as yet unidentified factors. Preliminary studies suggest that camptothecin sensitivity may be predicted by changes in topoisomerase I immunofluorescence patterns indicative of translocation of the protein from the nucleus to the cytoplasm. This change occurs during drug treatment.[91–93] Newer methods of purifying topoisomerase I from human tumor tissues have been developed[94] and may help to further define our understanding of the important determinants of clinical response to topoisomerase I poisons.

Although DNA cleavable complex formation is necessary but not sufficient for drug toxicity, measurement of these lesions as a predictor of drug effects is an attractive approach.[89] The cleavable complex is the specific lesion in the DNA that accumulates within the cell during drug exposure. Clinical measurement of the amount of cleavable complexes formed has been hampered, however, by the lack of sufficiently sensitive tests that can be easily applied to patient tissues.[95–97] One potentially promising approach is the use of ligase-mediated polymerase chain reaction, which does not require radioactive prelabeling of cells to monitor cleavable complex formation.[98]

Also important, but even less well understood, is the role of events downstream from the formation of cleavable

complexes, such as DNA damage repair,[99] the triggering of apoptosis,[100–102] and alterations in the integrity of the G_2 cell-cycle checkpoint.[103,104] For example, two different colon cancer cell lines with different sensitivity to camptothecin were found to differ in their cell-cycle response.[105] In one experiment, the more resistant cells arrested in the G_2 phase of the cell cycle after camptothecin exposure, whereas the more sensitive cells passed through the G_2 checkpoint after experiencing camptothecin-induced damage. The more sensitive cells also showed a greater capacity to arrest in the S phase, and they failed to down-regulate cyclin B–cdc kinase activity after camptothecin exposure. Thus, cell-cycle checkpoint integrity may also be an important determinant of camptothecin sensitivity. Despite the extensive ongoing research in this complex area, however, no single method or molecular marker can as yet reliably predict tumor responsiveness to camptothecins.

CAMPTOTHECIN STRUCTURE-ACTIVITY RELATIONSHIPS

Most of the currently known camptothecin analogs share a basic 5-ring structure with a chiral center located at C20 in the terminal E ring (Fig. 17.1). Structure-activity studies have also shown a close correlation between the ability to inhibit topoisomerase I and overall cytotoxic potency.[106] Some important general relationships have emerged from attempts to synthesize improved analogs.[107,108] While these relationships will clearly be refined in the years to come, current knowledge is potentially adequate for the design of improved analogs of camptothecin. This current knowledge is here summarized rather than described exhaustively. For the purpose of this overview, a number of regions in the camptothecin structure are particularly relevant:

1. It has been shown that the topoisomerase I inhibitory activity of these agents is stereospecific, with the naturally occurring (S)-isomer being manyfold more potent that the (R)-isomer.[16,109]

2. In general, substitutions at C7, C9, and C10 tend to increase topoisomerase I inhibition and sometimes increase water solubility, whereas substitutions at C12 decrease antitumor activity.[110]

3. Similarly, additional ring structures (e.g., between C7-C9 or C10-C11) may increase activity.[111–114]

4. One of the principal chemical features of this class of agents is the presence of a lactone functionality in the E ring, which is not only essential for antitumor activity but also confers a degree of instability to these agents in aqueous solutions.[115] Most camptothecins can undergo a pH-dependent reversible interconversion between this lactone form and a ring-opened carboxylate (or hydroxy acid) form (Fig. 17.1), of which only the lactone form is able to diffuse across cell membranes and exert the characteristic topoisomerase I inhibitory activity. At neutral

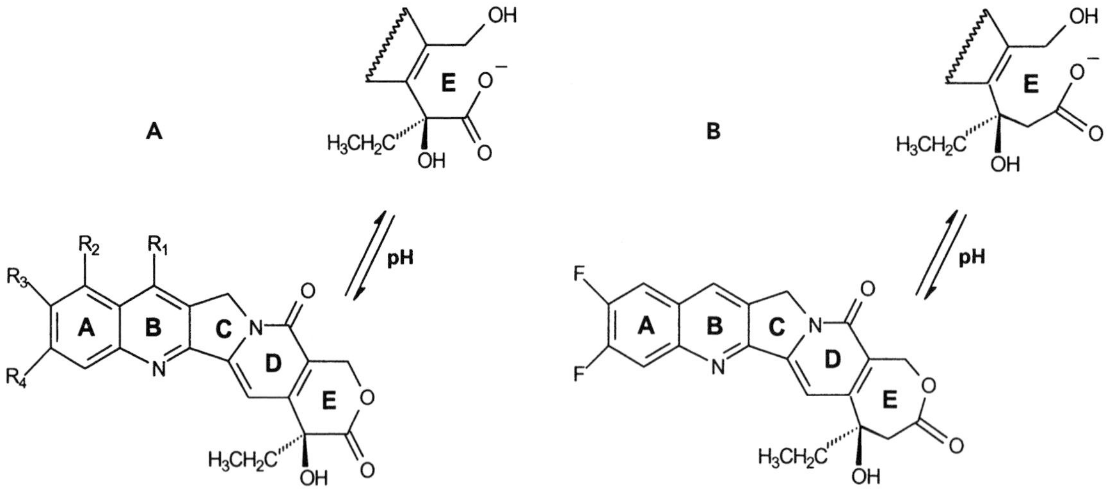

Figure 17.1 Structure of camptothecin analogs (modified from reference 532).

FIGURE A	R_1	R_2	R_3	R_4
Camptothecin	H	H	H	H
9-NC	H	NO_2	H	H
9-AC	H	NH_2	H	H
Topotecan	H	$CH_2N\begin{smallmatrix}CH_3\\CH_3\end{smallmatrix}$	H	H
Irinotecan	CH_2CH_3	H	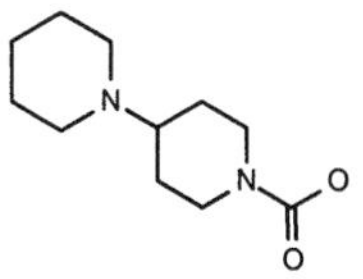 piperidino-piperidine carbonyloxy	H
SN-38	CH_2CH_3	H	OH	H
Lurtotecan	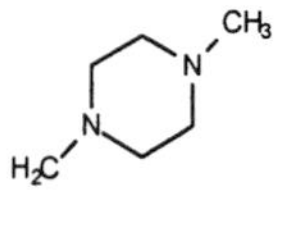 methylpiperazinyl-methyl	H	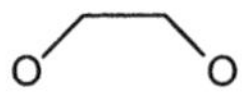 $-O-CH_2-O-$	
Exatecan	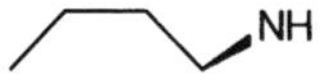 aminopropyl		CH_3	F

or physiologic pH, the equilibrium between the two species favors the carboxylate form for all the camptothecins. As outlined, an understanding of this hydrolysis reaction helps to explain several observations in the early development of these agents. The equilibrium between the lactone moiety ring and the carboxylate form of the camptothecins is not solely dependent on the pH, but also on the presence of specific binding proteins in the biological matrix, most notably human serum albumin (HSA). Following establishment of equilibration at 37°C in phosphate buffered saline, equal amounts of the various camptothecin analogs are present in the pharmacologically active lactone form, with values of 17%, 19%, 15%, 13%, and 15% for camptothecin,

9-amino camptothecin (9-AC), topotecan, irinotecan, and SN-38, respectively.[116] Addition of 40 mg/mL HSA shifts the equilibrium for camptothecin and 9-AC toward the carboxylate form, with approximately 1% present in the lactone form at equilibrium.[117] In contrast to HSA, addition of murine serum albumin to 9-AC leads to approximately 35% existing in the lactone form at equilibrium.[117] As opposed to camptothecin and 9-AC, HSA actually stabilizes the lactone moiety of irinotecan and SN-38, with 30% and 39%, respectively, present in the lactone form at equilibrium, while almost no effect was seen for topotecan.[116,118] It has been proposed that the differences in the percentages present in the lactone form at equilibrium are related to sterical considerations of the various substituents at the R_1 and R_2 positions (Fig. 17.1, panel A). For some of the more recently developed analogs, the substituents cause sterical hindrance and prevent binding of the carboxylate forms to HSA, thus driving the equilibrium towards the lactone species.

TOPOTECAN

Topotecan is a water-soluble camptothecin derivative containing a stable basic side chain at position 9 of the A ring of 10-hydroxycamptothecin (Fig. 17.1). Clinical trials of topotecan were initiated in 1989. In 1996, topotecan was approved in the United States for use as second-line chemotherapy in patients with advanced ovarian cancer, and in 1998 it was approved for the treatment of small cell lung cancer (SCLC) after failure of initial or subsequent chemotherapy. Key features of topotecan are listed in Table 17.4.

Dosages and Routes of Administration

The most common dose and schedule of topotecan administration is a 30-minute intravenous (i.v.) infusion of 1.5 mg/m^2 daily for 5 days every 3 weeks.[119,120] This regimen has undergone the most widespread clinical testing, and it is currently the dosage of topotecan approved by the US Food and Drug Administration (FDA) for treating ovarian and lung cancer patients. Five-day continuous infusions of topotecan at 2.0 mg/m^2 per day have been tested in patients with hematologic malignancies, although in these studies gastrointestinal toxicities such as mucositis and diarrhea became more problematic.[121] Based on a promising theoretical rationale,[35] prolonged 21-day infusion schedules at 0.5 to 0.6 mg/m^2 per day[122] have been disappointing in phase II studies.[123–125] Other schedules tested in phase I or

---

TABLE 17.4
KEY FEATURES OF TOPOTECAN

Mechanism of action	Topoisomerase I poison. Stabilizes the cleavable complex in which topoisomerase I is covalently bound to DNA at a single-stranded break site. Conversion into lethal DNA damage follows when a DNA replication fork encounters these cleavable complexes ("fork collision model").
Metabolism	Nonenzymatic hydrolysis of the lactone ring generates the less active open-ring hydroxy carboxylic acid. *N*-desmethyl metabolite recently characterized in plasma, urine, and feces.
Elimination	About 26% to 41% excreted unchanged in urine over 24 h. Concentrated in the bile at levels that are 1.5 times higher than the simultaneous plasma levels.
Pharmacokinetics	Approximate terminal half-life of topotecan lactone is 2.9 hr (range, 1.6–5.5 h); approximate clearance of 62 L/h/m^2 (range, 14–155 L/h/m^2) reported for 30-min topotecan infusions.
Toxicity	Myelosuppression, predominantly noncumulative neutropenia, with thrombocytopenia and anemia less common Nausea and vomiting (mild) Diarrhea (mild) Fatigue Alopecia Skin rash Elevated liver function test results Mucositis
Modifications for organ dysfunction	In minimally pretreated patients, no dosage adjustments appear to be necessary for patients with mild renal impairment (creatinine clearance 40–60 mL/min), but dosage adjustment to 0.75 mg/m^2/d is recommended for patients with moderate renal impairment (20–39 mL/min). Further dosage adjustments may be necessary for patients with extensive prior chemotherapy or radiation therapy. Studies of small numbers of patients suggest that dosage adjustments are not required for hyperbilirubinemia up to 10 mg/dL.
Precautions	For febrile or severe grade 4 neutropenia lasting >3 d, the dosage for subsequent courses should be reduced by 0.25 mg/m^2/d. Monitoring of blood counts is essential.

phase II studies include a single 30-minute infusion,[126] 24-hour infusions,[127–129] and 3-day,[130,131] 5-day,[130,132] and 14-day continuous infusions.[133] Oral administration has also been tested clinically[134–139] and has been compared with i.v. administration in two randomized studies.[140,141] Finally, intraperitoneal (i.p.),[142,143] intrathecal,[144,145] and individual adaptive, pharmacokinetically guided topotecan studies have been completed.[146,147]

Clinical Pharmacology

Analytic Methodology

Most analytic assays for topotecan in biologic matrices use reversed-phase high-performance liquid chromatography (HPLC) with fluorescence detection (reviewed in reference 148). Deproteinization by rapid precipitation of samples with cold methanol ($-30°C$) can stabilize the topotecan lactone for later analysis.[149] The lactone concentration can then be determined by direct HPLC injection to separate the lactone from the carboxylate forms. In addition, preinjection acidification of plasma samples allows for total plasma topotecan (carboxylate and lactone) to be determined by the same methodology. The plasma carboxylate concentrations are then calculated by subtracting the lactone concentrations from the total drug measurement. A newer validated method for simultaneously measuring both the lactone and carboxylate forms of topotecan in plasma as a single HPLC injection has also been developed,[150] and assays for measuring topotecan in other human matrices, including saliva,[151] urine, feces,[152] whole blood, and erythrocytes have been reported.[153]

General Pharmacokinetics

After i.v. topotecan administration, the lactone ring undergoes rapid hydrolysis to generate the carboxylate species.[154] Less than 1 hour after the start of an infusion, the majority of the circulating drug in plasma is in the carboxylate form, and this species predominates for the duration of the monitoring period.[154] In most studies, the ratio of the lactone to total topotecan area under the concentration versus time curve (AUC) ranged from 20% to 35%.[155] Interindividual variation in the AUC and the total-body clearance was quite large for both lactone and total topotecan (lactone plus carboxylate).[155] In general, plasma concentrations and AUC levels tended to increase with increasing dose levels, consistent with linear pharmacokinetics, although in some studies, nonlinearity in drug clearance at higher dose levels was seen.[126,156]

The kinetics of topotecan were analyzed using a linear, two-compartment, open model in most studies.[155] For topotecan lactone, the terminal half-life ranged from 2.0 to 3.5 hours, which is relatively short compared with that of other camptothecin analogs. Consequently, no accumulation of drug was observed when it was administered daily

for 5 consecutive days.[154] The total-body clearance of topotecan lactone after a 30-minute infusion ranged from 25.7 to 155 L/h/m², and the volume of distribution at steady state ranged from 23 to 25 L/m². No evidence exists that topotecan kinetics changes with repeated dosing cycles.[154] Limited sampling models for topotecan pharmacokinetics have been developed[157,158] and applied to clinical pharmacodynamic studies of topotecan in patients in phase II studies.[159] The pharmacokinetics of topotecan has also been studied in pediatric populations, and no substantial difference from kinetics in adults has been observed.[128,131,160,161] Finally, population pharmacokinetic studies in patients treated with i.v. or orally administered topotecan revealed that patient characteristics (i.e., gender, height, weight) and laboratory values (i.e., serum creatinine concentration) give a moderate ability to predict the clearance of topotecan in an individual patient.[162–167] Although a significant correlation between the clearance of topotecan and patient age has not been established, pharmacokinetic results of a larger number of elderly patients are warranted in order to make more definite conclusions on this specific issue.

Absorption

The most common route for topotecan administration has been i.v.; however, oral formulations using prolonged administration schedules have undergone preclinical[168] and clinical testing.[138,169,170] Animal studies demonstrated an oral bioavailability of approximately 28% and antitumor efficacy equivalent to that with parenteral treatment in four of the five murine models studied.[168] In humans, the reported oral bioavailability ranged from 30 to 42%.[134,136] Plasma concentrations peaked within one hour after oral ingestion, and no difference in the lactone-carboxylate ratio was observed when oral dosing was compared with i.v. administration. Coadministration of food slightly deceased the rate of absorption, but it did not affect the amount of drug absorbed.[134]

The oral bioavailability of topotecan is influenced by many different factors. First, the relatively high pH in the small bowel leads to conversion to the carboxylate form, which is poorly absorbed by the intestinal walls.[171] Second, the bioavailability is reduced by protein-mediated, outward-directed transport of topotecan by ABCG2.[172] Third, the bioavailability is partly influenced by the binding of topotecan to food, proteins, and intestinal fluids and/or by decomposition in the gastrointestinal fluid.

From a clinical point of view, as long as equivalent safety and efficacy can be ensured, the majority of patients prefer oral instead of i.v. administration of chemotherapy,[173] predominantly due to the convenience of administration outside a clinical setting and avoidance of vascular complications related to i.v. access, including catheter-associated infections or potential thrombosis.[170]

From a pharmacological point a view, the oral route of topotecan administration has some disadvantages.

Absorption of topotecan from the gastrointestinal (GI) tract is a prerequisite for its activity, but this process can be influenced by several factors. Delays or losses of the drug during absorption may contribute to variability in drug response or may even result in failure of the treatment.[170] Both anatomical and physiological factors affect the overall rate and extent of absorption from the GI tract, and they influence the precise quantitative prediction. Ideally, a cytostatic drug should have little interpatient variability in absorption and AUC and, even more important, little intrapatient variability with successive doses.[174] As an inverse relationship is demonstrated between decreasing absolute bioavailability of drugs and the interindividual variation in bioavailability, it is recommended that caution be taken in prescribing oral drugs with low oral bioavailability, as the therapeutic index is narrow, and thus either toxic or subtherapeutic dosing may easily occur. For instance, given the relatively low bioavailability of orally administered topotecan and the relatively high variability in the AUC both between patients and within the same patient, this issue of a narrow therapeutic index is clearly demonstrated for the oral administration of topotecan at its maximum tolerated dose (MTD).

The variability of pharmacokinetics of orally administered topotecan can be explained in part by the affinity for drug-transporting proteins expressed in the intestinal epithelium and directed toward the gut lumen. Currently, two major classes of drug pumps, including P-glycoprotein (ABCB1) and ABCG2, have been characterized that may play a role in mediating transmembrane transport of topotecan.[172] These proteins belong to the large superfamily of ATP-binding cassette transporters found in almost all prokaryotic and eukaryotic cells. The characteristic tissue distribution of these drug transporters strengthens the indication that they play an important role in detoxification and protection against xenobiotic substances. In vivo studies with genetic knockout of murine Abcb1 and Abcg2 genes revealed that the intestinal absorption of topotecan was increased in the absence of the transporters.[172] These experimental studies led to the development of clinical trials of anticancer drugs modulated by coadministration of inhibitors of P-glycoprotein and ABCG2. Recently, a proof-of-concept study in 16 patients with solid tumors was reported in which topotecan was administered in the presence and absence of GF120918, a potent inhibitor of ABCG2 and P-glycoprotein.[175] This study showed that the coadministration of the inhibitor of the drug transporters significantly increased the systemic exposure of oral topotecan, with the mean AUC of total topotecan increasing from 32.4 ± 9.6 µg·h/L without coadministration of GF120918 to 78.7 ± 20.6 µg·h/L with coadministration of GF120918 ($P = .008$). Furthermore, the apparent oral bioavailability increased significantly from 40 to 97.1% ($P = .008$).

Other routes of topotecan administration have been tested in preclinical or clinical models. The pharmacokinetics

of intrathecally administered topotecan was studied in nonhuman primates and pediatric patients.[128,176] Intraventricularly administered topotecan showed a 450-fold relative pharmacologic advantage compared with systemic administration. No clinically significant acute or chronic neurologic toxicities were associated with intrathecal drug administration, which suggests that this may be a promising means of delivering this agent to patients with CNS tumors. I.p. topotecan administration was studied in nude mice bearing peritoneally implanted human ovarian cancer xenografts.[177] Excellent antitumor efficacy and modest systemic toxicity were observed, but pharmacokinetic monitoring was not performed, so a rigorous assessment of the relative pharmacokinetic advantage for this regional drug delivery approach could not be made. A phase I study on the i.p. administration of topotecan revealed that the MTD was 20 mg/m^2 once every 3 weeks delivered by the i.p. route, achieving cytotoxic plasma levels of topotecan, with acceptable toxicity and avoidance of myelotoxicity.[143] I.p. total topotecan was cleared from the peritoneal cavity at 0.4 ± 0.3 L/h/m^2 with a half-life of 2.7 ± 1.7 hours. The mean peritoneal to plasma AUC ratio for total topotecan was $54 \pm 34\%$.[143] These data were in good agreement with those from a phase I study using a topotecan 24-hour continuous i.p. infusion.[142] The terminal half-life for peritoneal topotecan and for plasma total topotecan were similar for both studies. These data suggest that it would be possible to combine the i.p. administration of topotecan with other active chemotherapeutic agents. Further efficacy testing of regional topotecan delivery for patients with ovarian cancer was recommended.

Distribution

In experiments in rhesus monkeys, cerebrospinal fluid (CSF) topotecan lactone concentrations were approximately 32% of simultaneous plasma levels, and these concentrations tended to decline in parallel over time.[178,179] A physiologic pharmacokinetic model based on these primate experiments was developed and may help guide future investigations of topotecan's activity against CNS tumors.[179] The pharmacokinetic findings were confirmed in children who received topotecan by 24- or 72-hour continuous i.v. infusions.[180] The median CNS penetration of topotecan lactone and total drug was 29% (range, 10 to 59%) and 50% (range, 11 to 97%), respectively. Due to its hydrophilic properties, topotecan showed a moderate steady-state apparent volume of distribution, approximately only 2 times the body weight for the lactone species and total drug. In comparison with other camptothecin analogs, the fraction of topotecan bound to plasma proteins is much lower. Possibly, this property accounts for the more efficacious penetration of topotecan in cerebrospinal fluid,[181,182] pleural fluid, and ascites[183] than occurs with other camptothecin derivates. Furthermore, the plasma pharmacokinetics of topotecan did not change due to the presence

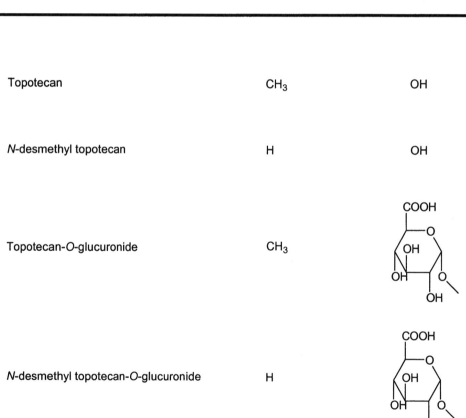

Compound	R1	R2
Topotecan	CH₃	OH
N-desmethyl topotecan	H	OH
Topotecan-O-glucuronide	CH₃	(glucuronide)
N-desmethyl topotecan-O-glucuronide	H	(glucuronide)

Figure 17.2 Structures of topotecan metabolites.

of third spaces (i.e., ascites and/or pleural effusion).[183] The ratio between the exposure to topotecan in the third space and in the plasma compartment was 55%. Consequently, topotecan can be safely administered to patients with malignant ascites and pleural effusion, and it might contribute to local tumor effects due to its substantial penetration in the third space.[183]

Metabolism

Recently, an N-desmethyl metabolite of topotecan was characterized[184] and found to be present at relatively low concentrations in human plasma, urine, and feces after i.v. administration of topotecan (Fig. 17.2).[152] Although a specific interaction with drug metabolism enzymes has not been established, preliminary clinical data suggest enhanced topotecan clearance in pediatric patients simultaneously receiving treatment with agents that induce hepatic cytochrome P-450 enzymes, such as dexamethasone, phenobarbital, and phenytoin.[185] Furthermore, a very low topotecan clearance was described in another patient who was taking terfenadine simultaneously.[161] These observations are consistent with a potential drug interaction at the level of CYP3A; however, additional studies on the metabolism and excretion of topotecan and its potential for drug interactions are clearly warranted.[186]

Topotecan and its main metabolite can also undergo further metabolism into a UGT-mediated glucuronide product (i.e., topotecan-O-glucuronide and N-desmethyl topotecan-O-glucuronide).[187] This is a reversible transformation because β-glucuronidase is able to reform topotecan and N-desmethyl topotecan. Because topotecan is metabolized in the liver only to a minor extent, it is not surprising that the pharmacokinetics in patients with impaired liver function did not significantly differ from those in patients with normal hepatic function.[188] In contrast, patients with moderately impaired renal function had significantly reduced plasma clearance.[189] As a consequence, dose modifications are recommended for patients with impaired renal function and are not required for patients with liver dysfunction.

Excretion

Elimination of the lactone form is thought to result mainly from the rapid hydrolysis to the carboxylate species followed by renal excretion of the open-ring metabolite.[154] Overall, 25 to 49% of the dose administered is excreted as total drug (lactone plus carboxylate) in the urine over a 24-hour period,[155] with a few studies performed in pediatric patients reporting recovery of over 90% of the administered drug during more prolonged urinary collection periods.[190,191] Furthermore, approximately 18% and 33% of the i.v. and oral dose of topotecan, respectively, was excreted unchanged in the feces. As mentioned earlier, in patients with impaired renal function, the clearance of total topotecan is reduced—there is a 33% decrease in patients with a creatinine clearance (CrCl) ranging from 40 to 59 mL/minute and a 75% decrease in patients with a CrCl ranging from 20 to 39 mL/minute—compared with patients with normal renal function (i.e., CrCl ≥ 60 mL/minute).[189] In patients with reduced renal clearance of topotecan, a second plasma peak was seen after the end of infusion due to increased bile excretion, which, in turn, leads to enterohepatic recycling.[192] Nevertheless, this is likely not of clinical relevance. Because altered clearance of topotecan has been observed in patients with impaired renal function,[189] dosage adjustments for this special population have been recommended (see earlier section). Topotecan was concentrated in the bile at levels 1.5 times higher than simultaneous plasma concentrations in one patient with an external biliary drainage catheter, which

suggests that excretion through this route may also be important.[126] As expected, no change in topotecan kinetics was observed in a clinical study of patients with moderately impaired hepatic function.[188]

Pharmacodynamics

Pharmacodynamic correlations between parameters of systemic drug exposure and topotecan drug effects have been observed inconsistently.[19,193,194] In a pediatric study, the topotecan total (lactone plus carboxylate) AUC and lactone plasma AUC correlated with the percentage change in the platelet count and the granulocyte count after a 72-hour drug infusion.[161] Similar correlations between leukocyte or granulocyte counts and total topotecan AUC or topotecan dose have been reported after a 30-minute infusion of topotecan given daily for 5 days,[154] after 20-minute infusions every 3 weeks,[126] and after 24-hour continuous infusions.[156] In each case, measurement of the total topotecan plasma concentration was as informative about drug effects as the lactone drug levels. Thus, the need to measure lactone drug concentrations has been questioned by some investigators.[119] Finally, although interpatient variability in topotecan plasma concentrations is high, the total variability in hematologic toxicity in patients is relatively low when the drug is administered according to standard dosing guidelines.[155] Thus, therapeutic drug monitoring is not useful for this agent. In a clinical study examining sequences of topotecan and cisplatin, the prior administration of cisplatin resulted in substantially greater hematologic toxicity.[195] A pharmacokinetic interaction causing a transient reduction in topotecan clearance when this agent was administered after i.v. cisplatin was thought to be related to subclinical renal tubular toxicity induced by the platinum analog,[195] although this could not be confirmed in subsequent studies.[196,197] More recently, it has been suggested that the administration of topotecan on days 1 to 4 and docetaxel on day 4 resulted in an approximately 50% decrease in docetaxel clearance and was associated with increased neutropenia.[198]

Toxicity

The dosage regimen of topotecan approved for clinical use is 1.5 mg/m^2 per day given as a 30-minute i.v. infusion daily for 5 days every 3 weeks. Dose-related, reversible, and noncumulative myelosuppression is the most important side effect of topotecan.[199] Neutropenia—the nadir is usually approximately 9 days after the start of the treatment, and the median duration is approximately 7 to 10 days— occurred more frequently and is often more severe than thrombocytopenia. Also, neutropenia was more severe in heavily pretreated patients than in minimally pretreated patients.[199] Besides myelosuppression, stomatitis (24 to 28% of patients) and late-onset diarrhea (40%) were noted at higher doses.[19] Other nonhematological toxicities reported included alopecia (76 to 82% of patients), nausea

(75 to 78%), vomiting (53 to 64%), fatigue (30 to 41%), and asthenia (21 to 22%) (reviewed in reference 199).

Numerous phase I clinical trials with topotecan using different schedules of drug administration have been performed.[155] Based on the in vitro data on long-term exposure and the fact that efficacy of the drug has been demonstrated to be dependent on the schedules of administration, two schedules have been selected for phase II studies. First, a 30-minute i.v. infusion daily for 5 consecutive days every 3 weeks at a dose of 1.5 mg/m^2 per day has been used. In this schedule, the dose-limiting toxicity is short-lasting, non-cumulative myelosuppression.[119,120,200] Nonhematological toxicities are usually mild and reversible and include nausea, vomiting, fatigue, alopecia, and sometimes diarrhea. Phase II studies with the drug administered in this schedule revealed response rates ranging from 9.5 to 25% in pre-treated patients with ovarian cancer and response rates of 10 to 39% in patients with SCLC.[201–203] In addition, a comparative, randomized, multicenter trial in which patients with recurrent ovarian cancer were treated showed that topotecan was at least as effective as paclitaxel in terms of response rate (20% vs. 13%), median duration of response, and median time to progression.[204–210] In other tumor types, topotecan was much less active[124,211–231] (see below). A summary of the safety profiles and clinically observed toxicities is provided in Tables 17.5 and 17.4, respectively.[232,233]

Second, as mentioned previously, various schedules focusing on the continuous infusion of topotecan have been studied, including a 24-hour infusion weekly and every 3 weeks; a 72-hour infusion administered weekly, every 14 days, and every 21 days; a 120-hour infusion every 3 to 4 weeks; and 21-day low-dose continuous infusion every 4 weeks. In addition to the dose-limiting toxicity of leukocytopenia, the longest infusion schedules also induce thrombocytopenia.

With the continuous i.v. administration for 21 days every 28 days, the MTD was 0.53 mg/m^2 per day.[122] The steady-state lactone topotecan was only approximately 4 ng/mL. No consistent relationship between drug level and hematological toxicity was found. Of interest, the phase I study showed several partial tumor responses in tumor types that were initially chemotherapy-resistant.[122] In a phase II study with this regimen in patients with progressive and platinum refractory ovarian cancer, the response rate was 37%.[234]

In order to mimic a prolonged exposure regimen and based on the relatively short half-life of the drug (average 2.4 hours), a twice daily oral administration schedule for 21 days every 28 weeks was studied.[135] The dose-limiting side effect was diarrhea, at a dose of 0.6 mg/m^2 twice daily. It occurred in 55% of patients, with day 15 as the median day of onset (range, 12 to 20) and mean period of resolution of 8 days (range, 7 to 16). Administration of high-dose loperamide did not limit the diarrhea.[135] The hematological toxicity was mild and consisted mainly of neutropenia (35%).

TABLE 17.5

SAFETY GUIDELINES FOR THE USE OF TOPOTECAN

Proper patient selection according to known risk factors

For severe neutropenia: renal impairment, prior myelosuppressive chemotherapy (both platinum analogues and alkylating agents), prior bone marrow transplantation, prior wide-field radiotherapy

For severe thrombocytopenia: renal impairment, prior myelosuppressive chemotherapy (especially carboplatin)

Proper training of the treating medical oncologist and his staff and extensive information to the patient

Should include patient information leaflet about the management of toxicities

Dose reduction in case of

Grade 4[a] neutropenia > 2 weeks (with G-CSF[b])

Grade 3[a] neutropenia concomitant with fever and/or infection

Complicated grade 3 or 4 thrombocytopenia

Renal impairment; creatinine clearance < 60 mL/min and extensive prior therapy; creatinine clearance < 40 mL/min and minimal prior therapy

Treatment delay > 2 weeks

Elevated bilirubin in combination with poor performance status and comorbidities

Contraindication for use in patients with

WHO[c] performance status > 2

Predictable poor compliance

Creatinine clearance < 20 mL/min

Baseline serum bilirubin > 1.5 × UNL[d]

Treatment only with caution and close survey between cycles in patient with

WHO performance status = 2

Creatinine clearance < 60 mL/min

Prior myelosuppressive chemotherapy (carboplatin)

Prior abdominopelvic radiation therapy

---

[a]Grade 3 and 4 according to NCI common toxicity criteria (version 2.0).
[b]G-CSF, granulocyte colony–stimulating factor.
[c]WHO, World Health Organization.
[d]UNL, upper normal limit.

Because of this diarrhea occurring beyond day 15, and in view of the emerging insights that topoisomerase I inhibition might be no longer optimal after 14 days of continuous drug administration, a shorter schedule was investigated.[234,235] Patients were treated once daily or twice daily for 10 days every 21 days.[235] In the once daily regimen, dose-limiting thrombocytopenia and diarrhea was seen at a dose of 1.6 mg/m^2 per day. The dose-limiting toxicities (DLTs) were similar, occurring at a dose of 0.8 mg/m^2 twice a day.

Because of the persistence of diarrhea as a side effect in the 10-day schedule, a 5-day schedule was studied.[236] The DLT was neutropenia, similar to the i.v. drug use, with a nadir between day 8 and 15 and a median duration of 6 days (range, 2 to 12). Nonhematological toxicities were mild to moderate. Moderate to severe diarrhea (grade 2 or above) was observed in 21% of the patients, and this event was self-limiting. The recommended dose was 2.3 mg/m^2 per day. Assuming an average body surface area in patients of 1.75 m^2, the recommended dose of 2.3 mg/m^2 per day equals a fixed dose of 4 mg per day. Pharmacokinetics and toxicity were studied at this fixed dose in order to ascertain whether dosing based on per square meter offered any advantage over flat dosing, but such an advantage was not found.[165,236,237]

In summary, hematologic toxicity is more pronounced with the shorter oral regimens but is still mostly mild and noncumulative, whereas diarrhea is a severe and intractable side effect of more prolonged daily administration.[238] An analysis of the pharmacokinetic-pharmacodynamic relationships revealed that the total AUC per course did not differ between the various regimens, and in an analysis of the time over the threshold concentration of 1 ng/mL, it appeared that the daily times 5 schedule provided the best systemic exposure and toxicity profile.[239]

In acute leukemia, the MTD of a daily 30-minute i.v. infusion for 5 consecutive days every 3 weeks was 4.5 mg/m^2 per day.[240] The DLT at higher dose levels was a complex of symptoms, consisting of high fever, rigors, precipitous anemia, and hyperbilirubinemia. Although the precise etiology of these adverse effects was not known, it was believed that high doses of topotecan had induced an acute hemolytic reaction.

Antitumor Activity

The antitumor activity of topotecan, given as a single agent using various schedules of administration, was established in a variety of phase II studies, including ovarian cancer (overall response rate [OR], 14 to 38%), small-cell lung cancer (OR, ~39%; reviewed in references 241 and 242), NSCLC (OR, ~13%; reviewed in reference 243), breast cancer (OR, ~10%),[222] myelodysplastic syndrome (complete response rate [CR], ~37%),[244] and chronic myelomonocytic leukemia (CR, ~27%[245]; reviewed in 246). Marginal activity was seen in head and neck cancer,[219,247] prostate cancer,[248] pancreatic cancer,[224,231] gastric cancer,[225,226] esophageal carcinoma,[217] hepatocellular carcinoma,[227] and recurrent malignant glioma[191,215] and when topcotecan was used as consolidation treatment after first-line standard chemotherapy for ovarian cancer.[249]

In a phase III study, the daily times 5 i.v. topotecan regimen was compared with paclitaxel (3-hour infusion of 175 mg/m^2 per day every 3 weeks) in ovarian cancer. In this disease, topotecan and paclitaxel where equally effective with regard to response rates, progression-free survival, and overall survival.[204,250] The median duration of response was 26 weeks (range, 7 to 84 weeks) for topotecan and 22 weeks (range, 9 to 67 weeks) for paclitaxel. The respective median times to progression were 19 weeks (range, <1 week to 93 weeks) and 15 weeks (range, <1 week to 77 weeks), while the median survival was 63 weeks (range, <1 week to 122 weeks) versus 53 weeks (range, <1 week to 130 weeks).[125]

In an open-label, multicenter study comparing the activity and tolerability of oral versus i.v. topotecan, 266 patients with relapsed epithelial ovarian cancer after failure of one platinum-based regimen, which could have included a taxane, were randomized to both arms.[141] Oral versus i.v. doses of topotecan were administered as 2.3 mg/m^2 per day and as 1.5 mg/m^2 per day, respectively, for 5 consecutive days every 3 weeks. The principal toxicity was noncumulative myelosuppression, although moderate to severe neutropenia was less frequently seen in patients treated with oral topotecan. Furthermore, grade 3 and 4 gastrointestinal toxicity was slightly higher in the oral treatment arm. No difference in response rates between the two treatment arms was reported. Although a small, statistically significant difference in survival favored the i.v. formulation (58 weeks) over the oral formulation (51 weeks) (P = .033), in the context of second-line palliative treatment for ovarian cancer, this outcome has only limited clinical significance.[141] For this reason, oral topotecan could be an alternative treatment modality in this setting because of its convenience and good tolerability. Its definite place has to be clarified in further studies.

Another phase III study compared single agent topotecan with combination chemotherapy consisting of cyclophosphamide, doxorubicin, and vincristine (CAV) in 211 patients with SCLC relapsing after first-line platinum-based chemotherapy.[251] Although the response rate, time to disease progression, and overall survival were similar, the palliation of disease-related symptoms was better with topotecan.[251] In a randomized trial performed by the Eastern Cooperative Oncology Group (ECOG), topotecan was compared with best support of care in patients with extensive SCLC. In this trial, topotecan was administered as consolidation therapy after response induction with cisplatin and etoposide.[201] Although topotecan induced a moderate increase in the time to disease progression, it did not improve survival.[201] Finally, similar to the study of ovarian cancer, oral topotecan was compared to i.v. administration of topotecan in patients with relapsed and chemosensitive SCLC. The oral formulation was found to be similar in efficacy, result in less severe neutropenia, and possess superior drug administration convenience.[140] Based on these data, topotecan has been approved by the FDA for the treatment of recurrent SCLC in the US.[252]

Although topotecan has shown some activity against hematological malignancies, its use for this specific indication needs to be further explored in research.[253] As indicated, the complete remission rate is interesting in myelodysplastic syndromes (MDSs) (37%) and in chronic myelomonocytic leukemia (CMML) (27%).[121,254] Of note, the presence of a mutation of the *ras*-oncogene seems to predict insensitivity to topotecan treatment in CMML. In relapsed or resistant multiple myeloma, the overall response rate was 16% (95% CI, 7 to 31%). Responses have lasted 70 to more than 477 days, with a median progression-free survival of 13 months and a median survival time of 28 months.[228,229]

IRINOTECAN

Irinotecan (7-ethyl-10-[4-(1-piperidino)-1-piperidino]carbonyloxycamptothecin, CPT-11) (Fig.17.1) was the first camptothecin derivative with increased aqueous solubility to enter clinical trials. These began in the 1980s in Japan, where the drug was developed by the Daiichi Pharmaceutical and Yakult Honsha companies. Irinotecan hydrochloride became commercially available in Japan for treatment of lung cancer (SCLC and NSCLC), cervical cancer, and ovarian cancer in 1994. In 1996 irinotecan was approved in the US for use in patients with advanced colorectal cancer refractory to 5-FU, and in 2000 it was approved as a component of first-line therapy in combination with 5-FU/LV for the treatment of metastatic colorectal cancer or for patients who have progressed following initial 5-FU-based therapy. Irinotecan is unique in that it must first be converted by a carboxylesterase-converting enzyme to the active metabolite SN-38 (Fig.17.3).[255,256] SN-38 is the major metabolite believed to be responsible for irinotecan's biologic effects. Key features of irinotecan are listed in Table 17.6.

Dosages and Routes of Administration

The most commonly used schedules of irinotecan administration are a 30- or 90-minute i.v. infusion of 125 mg/m² given weekly for 4 of every 6 weeks or 350 mg/m² given every 3 weeks. In Japan, regimens of 100 mg/m² every week or 150 mg/m² every other week also have been used. The weekly times 4 schedule is more popular in North America, and the every-3-week schedule was developed predominantly in Europe. None of these regimens shows clear superiority with regard to antitumor efficacy in comparative clinical studies.[257,258] Other short infusion schedules tested clinically include daily infusions for 3 days[259] and infusions every 2 weeks.[260]

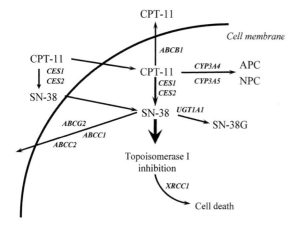

Figure 17.3   Genes involved in irinotecan (CPT-11) activation (modified from reference 337).

Because of the schedule-dependent activity of irinotecan seen in preclinical studies, protracted or repeated irinotecan dosing schedules have been tested in phase I trials. These included short 1-hour infusions of 20 mg/m² per day daily for 5 days[261] and a continuous infusion over 4 days,[262] over 7 days,[263] or over 14 days.[264] The dose-limiting toxicity for all of these protracted administration schedules is diarrhea, with myelosuppression being less common than with the weekly or every-3-weeks short infusion schedules. Despite the somewhat low recommended dosages associated with these protracted administration schedules, the conversion of irinotecan to the active metabolite SN-38 is relatively more efficient. The AUC proportions of SN-38 relative to irinotecan range from 16 to 28%; these values are much greater than the 3 to 4% proportional AUC values of SN-38 to irinotecan seen during weekly or every-3- weeks short infusion schedules, and they are consistent with an increased efficiency of irinotecan enzymatic activation.[257] I.p. dosing, [265,266] intraarterial dosing,[267] and oral dosing of irinotecan[266,268–272] are also under investigation and represent potential strategies for the more convenient delivery of protracted low doses of irinotecan to patients.

Clinical Pharmacology

Analytic Methodology

Both irinotecan and its active metabolite SN-38 circulate in plasma after drug administration. Like all camptothecins, irinotecan and SN-38 both contain a terminal α-hydroxy lactone ring that is unstable in aqueous solutions and undergoes rapid nonenzymatic hydrolysis to the open-ring carboxylate (Fig.17.1). The early pharmacokinetic studies of irinotecan used assays that measured only total (lactone and carboxylate) concentrations of irinotecan and SN-38; however, more recent assays have been validated that can separate both lactone and carboxylate forms (reviewed in reference 148). Virtually all of these assays use reversed-phase HPLC with fluorescence detection. Rapid precipitation of plasma samples with ice cold methanol or acetonitrile (or both) is used to trap the camptothecins in their relative lactone and carboxylate forms, which are later resolved on a reversed-phase HPLC column.[148] Careful attention to sample storage conditions is important for preventing interconversion of the lactone and carboxylate drug species. Newer assays have also been developed for the determination of more recently recognized irinotecan metabolites, including 10-O-glucuronyl-SN-38 (SN-38G),[273,274] 7-ethyl-10-[4-N-(5-aminopentanoic acid)-1-piperidino]-carbonyloxycamptothecin (APC), and 7-ethyl-10-(4-amino-1-piperidino)-carbonyloxycamptothecin (NPC) (Fig. 17.3).[275] Recently, assays for measuring irinotecan and SN-38 in saliva[276] and erythrocytes have also been reported.[277]

TABLE 17.6
KEY FEATURES OF IRINOTECAN

Mechanism of action	After metabolic activation to 7-ethyl-10-hydroxycamptothecin (SN-38), the mechanism of action is the same as for topotecan.
Metabolism	Irinotecan is a prodrug that requires enzymatic cleavage of the C-10 side chain by an irinotecan carboxylesterase–converting enzyme to generate the biologically active metabolite SN-38. Both irinotecan and SN-38 can undergo nonenzymatic hydrolysis of the lactone ring to the open-ring carboxylate species. Irinotecan can also undergo hepatic oxidation of its dipiperidino side chain to form the inactive metabolite 7-ethyl-10-[4-N-(5-aminopentanoic acid)-1-piperidino]carbonyloxycamptothecin (APC).
Elimination	Elimination of irinotecan occurs by urinary excretion, biliary excretion, and hepatic metabolism. About 16.1% (range, 11.1–20.9%) of an administered dose of irinotecan is excreted unchanged in the urine. SN-38 is glucuronidated, and both the conjugated and unconjugated forms are excreted in the bile. SN-38 glucuronide can also be detected in plasma.
Pharmacokinetics	Approximate terminal half-life of irinotecan lactone is 6.8 h (range, 5.0–9.6 h) and approximate clearance is 46.9 L/h/m^2 (range, 39.0–53.5 L/h/m^2). Approximate terminal half-life of SN-38 lactone is 11.05 h (range, 9.1–13.0 h).
Toxicity	Early-onset diarrhea within hours or during the infusion associated with cramping, vomiting, flushing, and diaphoresis. Consider atropine 0.25–1.0 mg s.c. or i.v. in patients experiencing cholinergic symptoms. Late-onset diarrhea can occur later than 12 h after drug administration. Myelosuppression, predominantly neutropenia and less commonly thrombocytopenia. Alopecia Nausea and vomiting Mucositis Fatigue Elevated hepatic transaminases Pulmonary toxicity (uncommon) associated with a reticulonodular infiltrate, fever, dyspnea, and eosinophilia
Modifications for organ dysfunction	No definite recommendations are available for patients with impaired renal or hepatic dysfunction. Extreme caution is warranted in patients with liver dysfunction or Gilbert's disease.
Precautions	Severe delayed-onset diarrhea may be controlled by high-dose loperamide given in an initial oral dose of 4 mg followed by 2 mg every 2 h during the day and 4 mg every 4 h during the night. High-dose loperamide should be started at the first sign of any loose stool and continued until no bowel movements occur for a 12-hr period. Particular caution is also warranted in monitoring and managing toxicities in elderly patients (>64 yr) or those who have previously received pelvic/abdominal irradiation.

General Pharmacokinetics

After short i.v. infusions of irinotecan, both the parent drug and SN-38 are measurable in plasma as the lactone and open-ring carboxylate species (Fig. 17.3). After approximately 1 hour, however, the levels of SN-38 tend to be 50 to 100 times lower than the irinotecan plasma levels, and the overall AUC proportion of SN-38 relative to irinotecan is only approximately 4%.[257] In most[259,278–281] but not all[282] reports, irinotecan and SN-38 plasma concentrations and AUC increased proportionally with increasing dose, which suggests linear pharmacokinetics. Peak plasma levels of irinotecan occurred immediately after the end of the infusion period, whereas SN-38 peak levels tended to occur approximately 2.2 ± 0.1 hours later (range, 1.6 to 2.8 hours).[280] Extremely high interpatient variability in the plasma concentrations of irinotecan and SN-38 is common, although the reasons for this are only partially defined and appear unrelated to body-size measures.[283,284]

The kinetics of irinotecan and SN-38 have been fitted to a biexponential or triexponential model in most studies.[257] For short i.v. infusions, the mean terminal elimination half-life for irinotecan lactone was approximately 6.8 hours (range, 5.0 to 9.6 hours). The plasma half-life of the active metabolite, SN-38 lactone, however, was relatively long compared with that of the other camptothecins; the terminal half-life was approximately 10.4 hours (range, 9.1 to 11.5 hours) for SN-38 lactone. The prolonged duration of exposure to SN-38 is probably a function of its sustained

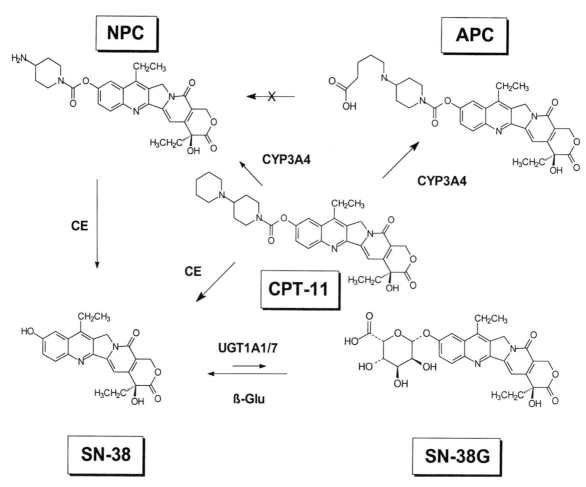

Figure 17.4   Metabolic pathways of irinotecan (CPT-11) (modified from reference 257).

production from irinotecan in tissues, because direct injection of SN-38 into rats resulted in extremely rapid plasma clearance, with a half-life of only 7 minutes.[285,286]

Race, gender, and renal function do not appear to alter the clinical pharmacology of irinotecan.[287,288] However, decreased total irinotecan clearance has been modestly correlated with abnormalities in liver function such as increased serum bilirubin and γ-glutamyl transpeptidase levels in population pharmacokinetic studies.[287,289] These same hepatic abnormalities also correlated with an increased ratio of SN-38 to irinotecan AUC (metabolic ratio), an observation that can be explained by increased conversion of irinotecan to SN-38 or decreased clearance of the SN-38 metabolite, or both.

Several groups have attempted to use population pharmacokinetic analysis using nonlinear mixed effect modeling and Bayesian approaches to predict irinotecan pharmacokinetic profiles.[287,290–292] Limited sampling strategies have also been developed; most have recommended two[293–295] or three[296–298] sampling times to reliably estimate irinotecan, SN-38, or SN-38G AUC values. All have attempted to estimate total irinotecan and SN-38 pharmacokinetic parameters, and none have distinguished between the lactone and carboxylate drug species. A few of these limited sampling methods have been applied to clinical studies of the pharmacokinetics of irinotecan in larger patient populations.[299]

Compared with topotecan, relatively large amounts of both irinotecan and SN-38 in plasma are present in the lactone form. The irinotecan lactone AUC ranged from 33 to 44% of the total irinotecan AUC, and for SN-38 the lactone percentage was even greater, ranging from 30 to 74% in most studies.[257] Thus, compared with other camptothecins, relatively large amounts of the SN-38 circulate in plasma as the biologically active lactone, which may be relevant to irinotecan's clinical activity.

One potential explanation for variation in the lactone to carboxylate ratios for different camptothecins is their differential protein binding. It has been shown that the equilibrium ratio in plasma between the carboxylate and lactone forms of different camptothecin derivatives was greatly affected by their relative degree of albumin binding.[118] For drugs such as camptothecin or 9-AC, the albumin-binding affinity of the open-ring carboxylate was over 200 times greater than the lactone affinity.[118] The overall plasma protein binding for SN-38 is higher than that for irinotecan, with 92 to 96% of total SN-38 being protein-bound in laboratory plasma incubation experiments, compared with 30 to 43% for irinotecan.[300] Serum albumin was the major protein to which both SN-38 and irinotecan were bound.

Thus, several factors in the clinical pharmacology of irinotecan may contribute to its greater antitumor activity relative to other camptothecin derivatives. One is the longer half-life of the active metabolite SN-38.[301] As discussed earlier, this may be due to the slow conversion of irinotecan to SN-38 and enterohepatic recirculation. The second factor is the relatively large amount of circulating SN-38 that is present as the active lactone form. Finally, as discussed previously, the topoisomerase I–DNA cleavable complexes induced by SN-38 are extremely stable compared with those of other camptothecin analogs.[110] All of these factors probably contribute to the clinical antitumor activity of irinotecan.

Because of the greater difficulty in analytic determination of the unstable lactone species in plasma, several investigators have questioned the value of measuring lactone versus total (lactone plus carboxylate) plasma concentrations for pharmacokinetic studies.[302] In any individual, the ratio of lactone to total drug is relatively constant; however, variation between different individuals may be quite high. Nonetheless, pharmacodynamic studies performed to date have not shown a superiority for lactone compared to total plasma drug measurements in predicting clinical drug effects.[257]

Absorption

Although the most common route of irinotecan administration is i.v., oral formulations have been tested in preclinical[268] and clinical studies (reviewed in reference 238). In nude mice, oral administration of irinotecan is active and well tolerated,[266,268,303,304] although the bioavailability in animals is only 12 to 21%.[269] The amount of SN-38 generated from oral administration of irinotecan, however, was threefold higher than that from i.v. administration when the molar AUC ratios of SN-38 to irinotecan were compared.[269] Extensive first-pass metabolism of irinotecan to SN-38 in the intestine and liver was proposed as a potential explanation. In a clinical phase I study, oral irinotecan at 20 to 100 mg/m^2 per day for 5 days every 3 weeks was well tolerated.[271] Because of the occurrence of dose-limiting age-related delayed diarrhea, the recommended phase II oral dosage was 66 mg/m^2 per day for patients younger than 65 years and 50 mg/m^2 per day for older patients. As seen in earlier animal studies, higher molar AUC ratios of SN-38 to irinotecan were generated by the oral route, consistent with greater metabolic conversion of irinotecan to SN-38. I.p. administration has also been examined, and there is evidence that it may result in more efficient activation of irinotecan to SN-38 than i.v. routes of administration.[265,266,305,306]

Distribution

Little is known about the tissue penetration and distribution of irinotecan, although the volume of distribution at steady state is large, with mean values ranging from 76 to 157 L/m^2 for total irinotecan. In rhesus monkeys, the CSF penetration of irinotecan was only $14 \pm 3\%$ of the plasma exposure, which is less than observed for topotecan,[182] and SN-38 was not detectable in the CSF. In nude mice, repeated daily i.p. administration of irinotecan resulted in high prolonged irinotecan and SN-38 concentrations in the intestine[307]; however, penetration into other tissue compartments was not measured. Interestingly, when SN-38 instead of irinotecan was directly administered i.v. to rats, very little tissue accumulation was observed, which suggests that peripheral tissue conversion of irinotecan to the active metabolite may be potentially important for generating its clinical activity.[285]

In a phase II clinical study, i.v. irinotecan at 60 mg/m^2 combined with cisplatin was given to patients with malignant pleural mesothelioma, and pleural fluid pharmacokinetics were monitored in three patients.[308] Irinotecan was detectable in pleural fluid as early as 1 hour after an i.v. infusion, with peak levels occurring after 6 hours. The active metabolite SN-38 was also detected within 1 hour after the end of an infusion; by 6 hours the SN-38 pleural fluid concentrations mirrored plasma concentrations and continued to do so for the remainder of the monitoring period, which lasted 24 to 48 hours. The maximal pleural concentrations of irinotecan and SN-38 were 37% and 76% of the plasma concentrations of drug, respectively. Thus, excellent penetration into the pleural fluid compartment was observed in this study. Dosing guidelines for patients with large third-space fluid collections such as pleural effusions and ascites are not available; however, no clinical reports have been published of excessive irinotecan toxicity in these patients.[308]

Metabolism

Irinotecan is extensively metabolized to a number of active and inactive metabolites (Fig.17.3). This creates the potential for clinically important variability in the kinetics of this agent. Irinotecan carboxylesterase–converting enzyme metabolizes irinotecan to SN-38, which, in turn, is conjugated by liver UDP glucuronosyl transferases (UGTs) to form an inactive β-glucuronic acid derivative, SN-38G. The total amount of SN-38 generated in individual patients is highly variable,[257] which suggests that variations in carboxylesterase-converting enzyme activity may be important in determining irinotecan response and toxicity. The relative AUC value of the active metabolite SN-38 to irinotecan varied from 0.9 to 11% in a pharmacokinetic study of different dosages of irinotecan (dose range, 115 to 600 mg/m^2).[309] Furthermore, this ratio was highest at the lowest doses of irinotecan examined (115 mg/m^2), which suggests that less efficient conversion of irinotecan to SN-38 occurred at higher drug concentrations. Alternatively, variations in the clearance of SN-38 via the UGT pathway provide another potential mechanism for variability in irinotecan pharmacokinetics. Irinotecan is also a substrate for metabolism by the cytochrome P-450 system, which creates an additional potential for drug interactions. Collectively, these studies demonstrate that the metabolic pharmacokinetics of irinotecan is complex and may be mediated by several different families of enzymes, including carboxylesterases, cytochrome P-450 enzymes, and glucuronosyl transferases.

Carboxylesterase-Mediated Metabolism

In rodents, an irinotecan carboxylesterase–converting enzyme that can hydrolyze irinotecan to SN-38 has been purified from rat serum, and high activity is also found in rat and mouse liver, intestinal mucosa, and other tissues.[310] However, carboxylesterase-converting enzyme–specific activity is much lower in human serum[311–313] and in comparable human tissues.[314] The main carboxylesterase responsible for the clinical activation of irinotecan in humans has been proposed to be CES2.[315,316] Human liver carboxylesterase activity is found in hepatic microsomal fractions, and this enzyme has been cloned and characterized.[317] The high interindividual variation observed in human liver and intestinal microsomal carboxylesterase activity could potentially cause clinically important differences in drug metabolism.[318,319] In human and animal studies, no evidence exists that irinotecan induces hepatic or serum carboxylesterase activity.[320]

Carboxylesterase activity and irinotecan metabolism have been studied in detail in human liver microsomes.[257] Rate-limiting deacylation kinetics were observed, with an initial fast "burst" rate of SN-38 release occurring during the first 10 to 15 minutes of incubation, followed by slower steady-state production of SN-38. The overall activity of irinotecan carboxylesterase–converting enzyme was lower in human liver than in rats, with an apparent K_m in humans of 52.9 μmol/L and a V_{max} (maximum reaction velocity) of 0.145 nmol/L per hour. A slight inhibition of irinotecan activation by loperamide suggested that a potential drug interaction could occur when this drug was given concomitantly; however, this finding has not been evaluated further in clinical studies.

The difference between irinotecan lactone and carboxylate forms as substrates for carboxylesterase activation was studied further in human liver microsomes.[321] Irinotecan lactone was more rapidly metabolized than the carboxylate by approximately twofold, with observed K_m values of 23.3 ± 5.3 μmol/L and 48.9 ± 5.5 μmol/L for irinotecan lactone and carboxylate, respectively. Additional studies using the enzyme inhibitor phenylmethyl sulfonyl fluoride suggested that the liver carboxylesterase responsible for SN-38 formation was a serine-dependent hydrolase. Although irinotecan carboxylesterase activity correlated with the

carboxylesterase-mediated hydrolysis of *para*-nitrophenol acetate, this later reaction was over 1 million times more efficient. Thus, irinotecan is a relatively poor substrate for human liver carboxylesterase. High interindividual variability in carboxylesterase-specific activity was seen in 12 different human liver microsomal preparations, with a 5- to 45-fold range of activity depending on the carboxylesterase substrate used.[318] This finding suggests that interindividual variation in this enzyme activity may be an important source of pharmacokinetic and pharmacodynamic variability.

An unresolved issue is whether actual irinotecan carboxylesterase-converting enzyme activity within the tumor itself is an important determinant of irinotecan sensitivity. In general, human irinotecan carboxylesterase-activating activity is difficult to measure in human tissues and in plasma because of its low overall level.[322] In a study of irinotecan carboxylesterase-converting enzyme activity in 53 human colon tumors, the enzyme-specific activity varied 146- fold.[323] Some[324,325] but not all[87,303] studies have found a modest correlation between tumor carboxylesterase-converting enzyme activity and sensitivity to irinotecan. Despite this uncertainty, studies of the use of the mammalian liver carboxylesterase gene to sensitize tumors to irinotecan are under investigation in laboratory model systems.[326–328]

CYP3A-Mediated Metabolism

Under normal circumstances, only a relatively small amount of the total irinotecan metabolized is converted into SN-38. Recently, several additional metabolites of irinotecan have been identified and characterized in human matrices.[329] Oxidation of the terminal piperidino ring by hepatic cytochrome P-450 enzymes, in particular CYP3A4, is thought to be responsible for the formation of APC (Fig.17.3).[330] Overall, the APC metabolite was at least 100-fold less active than SN-38 as an inhibitor of topoisomerase I,[331] and it was found to a poor substrate for conversion to SN-38 by human liver carboxylesterases. In cytotoxicity experiments, APC was also a poor inhibitor of human nasopharyngeal KB cell growth; the concentration showing 50% growth inhibition was comparable to that of irinotecan.[331] Although the APC metabolite does not appear to be responsible for any of irinotecan's clinical toxicities or antitumor effects, its formation may represent an important metabolic pathway for irinotecan clearance.

Another piperidino ring metabolite of irinotecan is NPC, which was characterized in the plasma and urine of patients on irinotecan therapy (Fig.17.3).[332] Like APC, this derivative is a poor inducer of topoisomerase I–cleavable complexes, but unlike APC, this new metabolite is a weak substrate for CES2 and can be enzymatically converted into SN-38.[316,333] Thus, NPC may contribute to the clinical activity of irinotecan. In plasma, the concentration of NPC is less than that of irinotecan or APC. Additional hepatic metabolites of irinotecan were also found in an analysis of human bile obtained from a patient undergoing irinotecan therapy. At least 16 different irinotecan metabolites were partially identified using highly sensitive liquid chromatography/mass spectroscopy and liquid chromatography/tandem mass spectroscopy techniques.[334] These included irinotecan oxidation products involving the C-10 bipiperidine side chain and a decarboxylated camptothecin derivative that lacked the terminal carboxylate group. Alkylated and N-oxidized species were also detected. The exact chemical structure of most of these metabolites and their clinical importance are not yet known, although several metabolites seem to be the result of CYP3A5-mediated conversion.[335]

Because of the genetic diversity in the genes encoding these proteins,[336] it has been suggested that genotyping for CYP3A4 and CYP3A5 variants may be useful for prediction of total hepatic CYP3A activity as well as the pharmacokinetic profile of substrate drugs. However, such studies have demonstrated that genotyping for CYP3A4 and CYP3A5 does not lead to significant correlations with irinotecan pharmacokinetics.[337] This may be due to the low allele frequency of most CYP3A variant genotypes in the Caucasian population (e.g., CYP3A4*17, CYP3A4*18, and CYP3A5*1) or may reflect the absence of a clinically important effect on enzyme activity in vivo (e.g., CYP3A4*1B).[336] Taking into account that CYP3A is a very complex enzyme system and that it is easily influenced by environmental (i.e., comedication, herbal preparations, and/or food substances) and physiologic factors (i.e., aging, disease state, and altered liver and renal function), the role of CYP3A4/5 genotyping in improving treatment with irinotecan remains doubtful.

Because human hepatic CYP3A appears to be important in the metabolism of irinotecan, the potential exists for serious drug-drug interactions. This enzyme is principally responsible for the metabolism of a large number of commonly prescribed drugs. A number of studies evaluating irinotecan in malignant glioma patients revealed that the clearance of irinotecan was significantly faster in patients who required cotreatment with anticonvulsants and glucocorticoids—inducers of CYP3A4—than in patients who did not receive such concomitant treatment.[338–348] A recent investigation also indicates that a significant interaction occurs between irinotecan and the herbal product St. John's wort, likely because of CYP3A4 induction, resulting in 42% decreased circulating concentrations of SN-38.[349] In contrast, inhibition of CYP3A4 activity by agents like ketoconazole[350] or cyclosporin A[351] has been shown to lead to substantially increased exposure to SN-38. It has also been suggested that both irinotecan and SN-38 are mechanism-based inactivators of CYP3A4,[352] although the clinical relevance of this finding is unknown.

UGT-Mediated Metabolism of SN-38

The major metabolite of SN-38 is the glucuronidated derivative SN-38G,[285] which is present in the plasma and bile of patients receiving irinotecan chemotherapy (Fig. 17.3).[353] In pharmacokinetic studies, the peak SN-38G concentrations were seen 10 to 20 minutes after the end of a 90-minute irinotecan infusion.[354] The amount of SN-38G increased from time zero up to 1 hour postinfusion; this was followed by a gradual decline so that by 5 to 6 hours postinfusion the ratio of SN-38G to SN-38 stabilized at 4:1 or 5:1. The decrease in plasma concentrations of SN-38G tended to parallel the decrease in SN-38 over time.[301] These data are consistent with the view that UGT is the rate-limiting step responsible for the elimination of the SN-38 active metabolite.[353]

UGT may also represent a potentially exploitable target for modulating SN-38 pharmacokinetics. In mice, coadministration of irinotecan with valproic acid, an inhibitor of glucuronidation, markedly decreased the amount of SN-38G formed, and it increased the systemic exposure to SN-38 2.7-fold.[355] In contrast, coadministration with phenobarbital, which enhances hepatic glucuronidation, increased the plasma AUC for SN-38G and decreased that for SN-38.[355] If these same drug interactions occur in humans as well as in mice, then a potential strategy for using such agents is suggested, such as administering phenobarbital to decrease gastrointestinal toxicity by increasing SN-38 detoxification.

The UGT isoforms UGT1A1, UGT1A3, UGT1A6, UGT1A7, and UGT1A9 have all been implicated in the glucuronidation of SN-38 in in vitro studies using hepatic liver microsomes.[79] It has been suggested that patients with Gilbert's syndrome, who are genetically deficient in UGT1A1 and have impaired bilirubin conjugating activity, may be at risk for severe irinotecan-induced diarrhea because of an inability to conjugate and detoxify SN-38. The genetic defect in Gilbert's syndrome, which can occur in up to 15% of the population and may be clinically silent, most commonly results from the presence of an additional TA repeat [(TA)₇TAA] (UGT1A1*28) in the promoter region of UGT1A1.[356,357] In a retrospective case control study of 26 Japanese patients who experienced greater toxicity following irinotecan treatment, multivariate analysis suggested that a heterozygous or homozygous genotype for UGT1A1*28 would be a significant risk factor for severe toxicity by this drug.[358] Shortly thereafter, a prospective clinical pharmacogenetic study of 20 patients being treated with irinotecan for solid tumors found that one seventh of heterozygotes experienced grade 4 diarrhea, one fourth of the homozygote variant demonstrated grade 3 neutropenia, while another homozygote demonstrated both grade 3 diarrhea and grade 4 neutropenia.[359] The findings have been independently confirmed by several investigators[337,360–364] and have been propagated as a rationale for performing pretreatment genetic testing on patients receiving irinotecan.

Collectively, the data suggest that much of the variability in irinotecan pharmacokinetics is related to variations in its enzymatic metabolism. The existence of multiple polymorphic metabolic pathways for irinotecan and its metabolites makes this a complex area to study, but ongoing research may provide a better understanding of the clinical impact of these pathways in irinotecan chemotherapy.

Deconjugation of SN-38G

Because hepatic glucuronidation followed by biliary excretion of SN-38G is a major route of drug elimination, the presence of bacterial β-glucuronidase in the intestinal lumen can potentially contribute to irinotecan's gastrointestinal toxicity. Hydrolysis of the inactive glucuronidated SN-38G by bacterial enzymes can release unconjugated SN-38, which results in prolonged exposure of the gastrointestinal mucosa to the active metabolite. This process can also enhance reabsorption of the unconjugated SN-38 from the intestinal lumen via enterohepatic circulation. Inhibition of bacterial β-glucuronidase, however, might prevent deconjugation of SN-38G and promote fecal elimination of drug, thereby lessening gastrointestinal toxicity. Consistent with this hypothesis was the finding that the Chinese herbal medicine Kampo, which contains baicalin, a β-glucuronidase inhibitor, substantially reduced the severity of irinotecan-induced diarrhea in rats.[365] In animal studies, antibiotic administration also protected against drug-associated diarrhea, presumably by altering the gut microbial flora and decreasing intestinal β-glucuronidase activity.[366,367] Coadministration of penicillin and streptomycin sulfate with irinotecan to rats markedly reduced drug-induced diarrhea and cecal damage. Pharmacodynamic studies in these rats receiving both irinotecan and antibiotics showed no difference in blood pharmacokinetics but demonstrated an 85% reduction in SN-38 concentrations within the large intestine.[366,367] A similar approach in humans treated with the antibiotic neomycin has been shown to safely alleviate irinotecan-associated diarrhea without diminishing clinical efficacy.[368]

Excretion

In addition to hepatic metabolism, elimination of irinotecan and its metabolites also occurs by urinary and fecal excretion. Fourteen percent to 37% of the administered irinotecan dose was excreted unchanged in the urine over 48 hours after a short 90-minute infusion.[278,280] Only approximately 0.26% of the administered dose, however, was excreted as SN-38.[278,280] Biliary secretion of irinotecan, SN-38, and SN-38G also appears to be a substantial mechanism of drug elimination. Biliary drug concentrations were measured in two patients; the total irinotecan concentration was 10 to 113 times higher and the SN-38 biliary concentration was 2 to 40 times higher than the simultaneous plasma drug.[278,354] For two other patients, quantitative collection of bile from percutaneous catheters was performed for up to 48 hours after a single dose of irinotecan.[354] The percentage of the total dose

administered that was excreted into the bile as either irinotecan, SN-38, or SN-38G ranged from 24 to 50%.

Biliary transport of irinotecan and its metabolites by the canalicular multispecific organic anion transporter (cMOAT, ABCC2) has been extensively studied using isolated canalicular membrane vesicles obtained from rat liver.[369,370] The ABCC2 system is believed to be responsible for the biliary secretion of irinotecan carboxylate, SN-38 carboxylate, and the carboxylate and lactone forms of SN-38G, but other transport systems in the bile canaliculi may also exist, including ABCG2[371,372] but not ABCB1.[373]

Theoretically, another way of reducing gastrointestinal toxicity is to reduce the amount of free SN-38 in bile by blocking biliary excretion of SN-38 and SN-38G.[374] Cyclosporin A can reduce bile flow and inhibit bile canalicular active transport, and thus it is a potential modulator of SN-38–induced toxicity. Coadministration of cyclosporin A with irinotecan in rats was found to increase the AUCs of irinotecan, SN-38, and SN-38G by 3.4-fold, 3.6-fold, and 1.9-fold, respectively.[375] Overall, nonrenal clearance of irinotecan decreased by 81%, with no change in the calculated volume of distribution, and the terminal half-life of SN-38 increased by approximately twofold. The AUC ratio of SN-38 to irinotecan in plasma was not altered, but the AUC ratio of SN-38 to SN-38G did increase. All of these observations are consistent with cyclosporin-induced inhibition of biliary canalicular transport of irinotecan, SN-38, and SN-38G; however, the precise transport systems affected by this modulation have not been fully characterized. Nonetheless, these observations suggest another possible strategy for reducing the gastrointestinal toxicities of irinotecan.

Fecal loss also contributes to the elimination of irinotecan and its metabolites from the body. In one study, which included 10 patients, the total excretion of irinotecan, SN-38, SN-38G, APC, and NPC in urine accounted for 28.1 ± 10.6% of the administered dose, whereas recovery from feces accounted for 24.4 ± 13.3%.[376] Thus, the total mass balance of known metabolites accounted for only approximately 50% of the total administered dose, which indicates the likely existence of other as yet unidentified metabolites of irinotecan, although a better drug yield was obtained in a small study in which radiolabeled irinotecan was administered.[377]

Pharmacodynamics

The major clinical toxicity of irinotecan is delayed diarrhea, which is believed to result from direct effects of the active metabolite SN-38 on the intestinal epithelium. As previously described, glucuronidation of SN-38 may prevent this toxicity by decreasing the relative amount of biologically active unconjugated SN-38 in the bile and small intestine. In an attempt to identify patients at risk for severe delayed diarrhea during irinotecan therapy, a biliary index was developed to estimate the relative amount of free and unconjugated SN-38 in the biliary system using measured plasma drug concentrations.[374] The biliary index was defined as the product of the AUC of irinotecan and the ratio of the AUC of SN-38 to that of SN-38G. In the original study, nine patients with grade 3 to 4 diarrhea had higher biliary indices (which indicated relatively more unconjugated SN-38 in the bile) than 12 patients with grade 0 to 2 diarrhea.[374] Estimation of the biliary index initially required substantial numbers of pharmacokinetic blood samples to determine the AUCs of irinotecan, SN-38, and SN-38G. However, a limited sampling strategy for estimating the biliary index was recently developed that requires only two blood samples obtained at 3.5 and 7.5 hours after a 90-minute infusion of irinotecan.[288,378] Thus, the biliary index may be able to be estimated during week 1 of therapy, and if it is highly elevated, immediate dosage adjustments can be instituted to decrease the incidence of severe diarrhea. Nevertheless, other studies using a variety of different schedules of administration have not confirmed the utility of the biliary index in predicting clinically significant diarrhea.[299,379,380]

Other pharmacodynamic studies have attempted to correlate the AUC of irinotecan or SN-38 with clinical drug toxicities, with varying results. In early studies of irinotecan in Japan, no correlation between irinotecan or SN-38 AUCs and myelosuppression or diarrhea was noted.[282] In later studies, a strong correlation between the degree of leukopenia and the AUC of irinotecan was reported, whereas the severity of diarrhea correlated better with SN-38 kinetics.[311] Other studies have also found pharmacodynamic correlations between the irinotecan AUC and myelosuppression[279,287,299,381] and/or between the SN-38 AUC and myelosuppression.[279,280,287,299,379,381] For severe diarrhea, inconsistent associations with the irinotecan AUC[259,279,281,381] and with the SN-38 AUC[278,279] or SN-38G AUC[380] have also been reported. Similarly, tumor response does not correlate with plasma pharmacokinetic parameters. Finally, although SN-38 lactone is believed to the biologically active species, measurement of SN-38 lactone kinetics has not been superior to total drug (lactone and carboxylate) measurements in predicting pharmacodynamic end points.[302]

Dosage Adjustments for Abnormal Organ Function

When grade 3 neutropenia or delayed diarrhea occurs, the dose of irinotecan should be reduced by 25 mg/m^2 on the weekly schedule or by 50 mg/m^2 on the every-3-weeks schedule. If grade 4 neutropenia or diarrhea occurred during the previous cycle, the dose of irinotecan should be reduced by 50 mg/m^2 on either schedule. A new course of therapy should not be initiated until any prior neutropenia or diarrhea has resolved. Patients at increased risk for severe diarrhea include those who have had prior pelvic radiation, have poor performance status, are age 65 years or older, or have Gilbert's syndrome.[382]

In pharmacokinetic studies, modest changes in renal function do not appear to affect irinotecan plasma concentrations.[383] In contrast, various studies suggest that elevated bilirubin levels are associated with a decrease in irinotecan clearance and an elevated AUC ratio of SN-38 to irinotecan.[289,291,301,383,384] Therefore, extreme caution is warranted in administering irinotecan to patients with impaired hepatic function and hyperbilirubinemia, and a 1.75-fold (43%) reduction in irinotecan dose has been recommended in patients with bilirubin values 1.51 to 3.0 times the upper limit of normal.[383,384]

Toxicity

Phase I studies were performed first in Japan, later in the US and Europe. The recommended regimen of irinotecan in the US is 125 mg/m^2 administered as a 90-minute i.v. infusion once weekly for 4 or 6 weeks.[278] In Europe, the approved administration schedule of irinotecan is 350 mg/m^2 given as an i.v. infusion over 60 to 90 minutes once every 3 weeks,[280] while a recent reevaluation indicated a MTD of 320 mg/m^2, or 290 mg/m^2 in patients with prior abdominal/pelvic radiation therapy.[385] Finally, in Japan the administration schedule of irinotecan was developed as 100 mg/m^2 every week or 150 mg/m^2 every other week.[282] Remarkably, the dose intensity of all applied dosage regimens of irinotecan is approximately 100 mg/m^2 per week, which suggests a schedule independency. This phenomenon might be explained by the long half-life of SN-38, which is achieved after a single dosage of irinotecan.[301] Although the half-life of SN-38 does not fully support this approach, in an effort to further explore the possible therapeutic advantage of prolonged exposure to camptothecins, protracted or repeated dosing regimens of irinotecan have been studied (see above).

In the US phase I clinical trials, the maximum dose-intensity of irinotecan was achieved with short-time i.v. infusion once every 2 or 3 weeks (mean dose-intensity [DI], 125 mg/m^2 per week; range, 80 to 167 mg/m^2 per week), whereas the lowest dose-intensity was achieved with continuous i.v. infusion (DI, range 27 and 47 mg/m^2 per week).[386] In the weekly times 4 schedule and the daily i.v. infusion over 3 or 5 consecutive days, the mean calculated dose-intensity was 83 mg/m^2 per week (range, 73 to 100 mg/m^2 per week). Thus, the maximum dose-intensity achieved with prolonged exposure schedules of irinotecan is 2 to 3 times lower than that achieved with short-infusion administration. But as indicated previously, irinotecan is more effectively converted to SN-38 during protracted i.v. infusion.

The principal DLT for all schedules used was delayed diarrhea, with or without neutropenia.[257] The frequency of severe diarrhea (grade 3 or 4) was reported as 35% in the phase I studies. The incidence of this toxicity can be reduced by more than 50% if an intensive treatment with loperamide is used, as described in the safety guidelines in Table 17.7. Neutropenia is typically dose-related, is generally of brief duration and noncumulative, and occurred in 14 to 47% of patients treated once every 3 weeks and less frequently using the weekly schedule (12 to 19%).[387–390] In approximately 3% of patients, the neutropenia was associated with fever. In one phase I study, where irinotecan was given as a 96-hour continuous infusion for 2 weeks every 3 weeks, thrombocytopenia was also dose-limiting.[262] Due to inhibition of acetylcholinesterase activity by irinotecan within the first 24 hours after dosing of the drug, an acute cholinergic reaction can be observed. The symptomatology of this syndrome, as well as the other nonhematologic toxicities of irinotecan, is summarized in Table 17.8.

Antitumor Activity

Phase II studies consistently revealed response rates of 10 to 35% to single-agent irinotecan in advanced or metastatic colorectal cancer (reviewed in reference 391) independent of the applied schedules. There was no apparent difference between the applied schedules with respect to the median remission duration and median survival time, respectively 6 to 8 months and 8 to 13 months.[391–393]

In a randomized phase III study comparing treatment with irinotecan given as a 300 to 350 mg/m^2 i.v. infusion every 3 weeks to best supportive care in patients refractory to previous treatment with 5-FU–based chemotherapy, the one-year survival rate was significantly greater for the irinotecan-treated group than for the control group, 36% and 14% ($P <.01$), respectively.[387] Another randomized phase III study, comparing treatment with irinotecan to three different continuous i.v. infusion schedules of 5-FU in patients with previously treated advanced colorectal cancer, revealed a survival advantage for the irinotecan-treated group in comparison to the 5-FU–treated group.[388] The one-year survival rates were 45% and 32%, respectively ($P <.05$). Apart from colorectal cancer antitumor activity,

---

TABLE 17.7
SAFETY GUIDELINES FOR THE USE OF IRINOTECAN

Proper patient selection according to known risk factors
For severe neutropenia: Performance status; serum bilirubin level
For severe diarrhea: Performance status; prior abdominopelvic radiation therapy, hyperleukocytosis
Proper training of the treating medical oncologist and staff and extensive information to the patient
Should include patient information leaflet about management of toxicities
Early use of high-dose loperamide as soon as the first loose stool occurs
Recommendation: 4 mg loperamide for the first intake and then 2 mg every 2 hours at least 12 hours after the last loose stool for a maximum of 48 hours
Early use of oral broad-spectrum antibiotics (e.g., fluoroquinolone) in case of
Any grade 4[a] diarrhea
Febrile diarrhea
Diarrhea with concomitant grade 3[a] or 4 neutropenia
Failure of 48-hour high-dose loperamide therapy
Dose reduction in case of
Grade 4 neutropenia (even asymptomatic)
Grade 3 neutropenia concomitant with fever and/or infection
Severe diarrhea
Contraindication for use in patients with
WHO[b] performance status > 2
Predictable poor compliance
Baseline serum bilirubin > 1.5 × UNL[c]
Treatment only with caution and close survey between cycles in patients with
WHO performance status = 2
Baseline serum bilirubin between 1 and 1.5 × UNL
Prior abdominopelvic radiation therapy
Baseline hyperleukocytosis

---

[a]Grade 3 and 4 according to NCI common toxicity criteria (version 2.0).
[b]WHO, World Health Organization.
[c]UNL, upper normal limit.

TABLE 17.8
MAIN TOXICITIES OF IRINOTECAN

Hematological
Grade 3[a] and 4[a] neutropenia
Dose-dependent and schedule-dependent
Lowest frequencies in protracted dose regimens
Reversible, noncumulative, and of short duration
Febrile neutropenia occurred in about 3% of patients.
Nonhematological
Acute cholinergic-like syndrome (±9% of patients)
Caused by rapid and reversible inhibition of acetylcholinesterase by lactone form of irinotecan and can be induced by coadministration of oxaliplatin.
Symptoms may occur shortly or within several hours after drug administration, and are short lasting, never life threatening.
Symptoms: diarrhea, gastrointestinal cramps, nausea, vomiting, anorexia, asthenia, diaphoresis, chills, malaise, dizziness, visual accommodation disturbances, salivation, lacrimation, and asymptomatic bradycardia
Responsive to and preventable by subcutaneous administration of 0.25 to 1.0 mg atropine.
Delayed-onset diarrhea
Could be severe and unpredictable at all dose levels, with increased intensity and frequency at higher dose levels (±34% of patients grade 3 or 4 after use of loperamide) and occurrence later than 24 hours after drug administration, with peak incidence at day 5 or 6.
Nausea and vomiting (±86% of patients, but ±19% grade ≥ 3)
Manageable with 5-HT3 antagonists.
Other common toxicities
Fatigue (±17%), mucositis (±12%), skin toxicity (±5%), asthenia, alopecia, and elevated liver transaminases
Less common toxicities
Pulmotoxicity (pneumonitis), cardiotoxicity (bradycardia), microscopic hematuria, cystitis, dysarthria, and immune thrombocytopenia

---

[a]Grade 3 and 4 according to NCI common toxicity criteria (version 2.0).

single-agent irinotecan was also moderately active in phase II studies in several other solid malignancies, including breast cancer,[212] relapsed or refractory non-Hodgkin's lymphomas,[394] and SCLC[395] (reviewed in reference 396).

Based on the activity data in colorectal cancer derived from phase I/II studies on the combination of irinotecan with 5-FU/LV, two randomized phase III studies were performed comparing this combination to single agent 5-FU/LV in the first-line treatment of metastatic colorectal cancer.[108,109] Saltz et al. randomized 683 patients to receive either a weekly times 4 regimen of a 90-minute i.v. infusion of irinotecan at a dose of 125 mg/m^2 and a 15-minute i.v. infusion of LV at a dose of 20 mg/m^2, followed by 5-FU i.v. bolus at a dose of 500 mg/m^2 (arm A, $n = 231$); conventional low-dose 5-FU/LV (arm B, $n = 226$); or irinotecan at a dose of 125 mg/m^2 for 4 consecutive weeks every 6 weeks (arm C, $n = 226$).[397] An intention-to-treat analysis showed that the combination of irinotecan and 5-FU/LV (arm A) yielded a significantly higher remission rate ($P < .001$), significantly longer progression-free survival ($P = .004$), and significantly longer median survival ($P = .04$) than single-agent 5-FU/LV (arm B). There was no difference between single-agent irinotecan (arm C) and 5-FU/LV (arm B) in terms of overall response rate, median time to disease progression, and median overall survival time.[397]

Severe diarrhea (grade 3 or 4) (arm A, 23%; arm B, 13%; arm C, 31%) and grade 4 neutropenia (arm A, 42%; arm B, 24%; arm C, 12%) were the most prominent toxicities in this study, but these side effects did not preclude the administration of approximately 75% of the prescribed doses of irinotecan and 5-FU.[397] The reverse side of the study was the bias of unreported toxic deaths in the combination treatment arm (arm A).

Douillard et al. randomized 385 patients to the combination of irinotecan and an infusional schedule of 5-FU.[398,399] The regimens were once weekly, irinotecan 80 mg/m^2 with 5-FU 2,300 mg/m^2 by 24-hour infusion and leucovorin (LV) 500 mg/m^2 (arm A1), or every 2 weeks, irinotecan 180 mg/m^2 on day 1 with 5-FU 400 mg/m^2 bolus and 600 mg/m^2 by 22-hour infusion, and LV 200 mg/m^2 on day 1 and 2 (arm A2).[398] For the control arm (arm B), the regimens were once weekly, 5-FU 2600 mg/m^2 by 24-hour infusion and LV 500 mg/m^2 (arm B1), or every 2 weeks, 5-FU and LV at the same doses and administration as in arm A2.[398] Although there was a good balance between both treatment arms for known risk factors, the number of primary rectal cancers in arm A was slightly higher. Compared with the study by Saltz et al., in this study proportionally more patients had received prior adjuvant 5-FU–based chemotherapy (10% and 25%, respectively). An objective response rate of 41% was reported in treatment arm A (combination irinotecan with 5-FU and LV), compared with 23% in the schedule of 5-FU and LV alone (arm B) ($P < .001$). Also, the median time to disease progression ($P < .001$) and median survival time ($P < .028$) were statistically significant in favor of the combination treatment arm (arm A) compared with the control arm (arm B). The overall treatment response rates were 51% for arm A1 and 38% for arm A2. For the weekly single-agent 5-FU and LV (arm B1) and biweekly 5-FU/LV (arm B2), the overall response rates were 29% and 21%, respectively. More severe neutropenia (29% vs. 21%, $P < .01$) and more severe diarrhea (24% vs. 11%) were seen in the combination arm (arm A) than in the control arm (arm B). The neutropenia was not significantly associated with fever or infection.

In a multiregression Cox model analysis, the influence of baseline characteristics of patients on the efficacy of the cytotoxic therapy in terms of time to progression and survival was determined. This analysis revealed that excellent performance status (WHO 0 vs. 1 or more), extent of organ involvement (1 vs. 2 or more sites), and normal values for lactate dehydrogenase (LDH), bilirubin, and leucocytes were the major prognostic factors for longer overall survival.[391] A significant prolongation of time to progression adjusted for normal values of LDH and disease extent (only one organ site) ($P = .0001$) was established for the combination irinotecan and 5-FU/LV compared with single-agent 5-FU/LV in both studies.[391]

Combined analysis of both studies confirmed that the addition of irinotecan to 5-FU/LV significantly increases response rate, median time to disease progression, and median time of survival, and thus patients with excellent prognostic characteristics will have received a survival benefit from this combination therapy.[391] The above-mentioned treatment schedules used in both studies are approved by the FDA as first-line chemotherapy for patients with metastatic colorectal cancer.[391] Yet randomized trials to evaluate the merits of this combination in the adjuvant setting are ongoing.[399] Furthermore, clinical trials evaluating the antitumor efficacy of irinotecan in combination with the oral fluoropyrimidine capecitabine, which may replace infusional 5-FU, are currently in progress, as are studies evaluating the addition of monoclonal antibodies like bevacizumab to irinotecan-based regimens for metastatic colorectal cancer.[400] Oxaliplatin (see Chapter 14) was approved for use in combination with FU/LCV in 2004 and may replace irinotecan as the preferred partner in colon cancer treatment.

Other Combination Chemotherapy Trials

The combination of irinotecan and raltitrexed was evaluated in two phase I studies, and asthenia was found to be the dose-limiting toxicity in both studies. The recommended doses were irinotecan 350 mg/m^2 and raltitrexed 3 mg/m^2 once every 3 weeks.[401,402] All phase I studies on the combination of irinotecan and cisplatin, except for one, focused on fractioned dose schedules for both agents (reviewed in reference 403). Neutropenia (grade 4 in 35% of the patients) and diarrhea were the dose-limiting toxicities. In only 4% of all patients was neutropenia complicated by fever. A 33% and 65% increase in the dose intensity of irinotecan could be achieved by adding G-CSF to schedules, with neutropenia as the dose-limiting toxicity.[404,405] Only one phase I study involved the 3 weekly administration and studied the relevance of sequence of drug administration.[406] Patients were randomized to receive irinotecan immediately followed by cisplatin in the first course, and the reversed sequence in the second course, or vice versa. Significant differences in toxicity between the treatment schedules were not observed. Neither could a pharmacokinetic interaction be discerned. In addition, irinotecan had no influence on the platinum DNA-adduct formation in peripheral leukocytes in either sequence.[406] Apparently there is no administration sequence that should clearly be favored for this particular topoisomerase I inhibitor.

Phase II studies of this combination indicate high levels of activity in various tumors, but none of these studies were randomized, so their interpretation is difficult.[252] A Phase III study using this combination as first-line chemotherapy for patients with extensive SCLC showed a significant improvement in the 1-year survival rate (60%) in comparison with conventional treatment with etoposide and cisplatin (40%) ($P = .005$).[407]

The combination of irinotecan and oxaliplatin was evaluated in several studies using a once-every-2-weeks schedule and a once-every-3-weeks schedule, with neutropenia and a combination of diarrhea and neutropenia as dose-limiting side effects, respectively.[408–412] Remarkably, the interaction of both drugs showed acute cholinergic toxicities, whose severity is potentiated by oxaliplatin.[413] The recommended dose of oxaliplatin is 85 mg/m^2 for both schedules. The recommended dose of irinotecan is 175 mg/m^2 for the once-every-2-weeks schedule and 200 mg/m^2 for the once-every-3-weeks. In a phase II study in patients with advanced colorectal cancer, this combination was compared with raltitrexed as first-line treatment. The combination showed an acceptable toxicity profile after dose-reduction of irinotecan to 150 mg/m^2 once every 3 weeks.[410]

In phase I and/or II studies, irinotecan has also been combined with numerous other cytotoxic and noncytotoxic agents, including etoposide,[414,415] carboplatin,[416–418] docetaxel,[419–423] paclitaxel,[424,425] gemcitabine,[426] and mitomycin-C,[427,428] and in a triplet combination with carboplatin and docetaxel.[429,430] The various combination treatment regimens with irinotecan have previously been reviewed extensively.[252]

9-NITROCAMPTOTHECIN

The compound 9-NC (RFS2000, rubitecan, Orathecin) is a camptothecin analog (Fig. 17.1, Table 17.9) that has a nitro group in the C-9 position and is highly insoluble in water. 9-NC is partially metabolized in vivo to an active metabolite, 9-AC.[431,432] Since nearly all human cells are able to convert 9-NC to 9-AC, including tumor cells, it has

been difficult to identify whether the 9-NC–mediated antitumor activity is directly associated with the parent drug alone, 9-AC alone, or the combination of both. Most likely the antitumor activity is associated with both 9-NC and 9-AC. However, because in patients most of the drug remains in the 9-NC form, the antitumor activity may be predominantly due to 9-NC.

In preclinical studies, 9-NC has shown excellent anticancer activity in nude mice bearing human tumor xenografts, including breast cancer,[433,434] ovarian cancer,[435] and melanoma.[436,437] It is predominantly being developed clinically as an oral agent to mimic the protracted schedule and maximize patient convenience,[438] in spite of extensive inter- and intrapatient variability in bioavailability.[439] The recommended dose of 9-NC orally is 1.5 mg/m^2 per day for 5 days each week for 8 weeks. This regimen has been used in phase I[440–442] and phase II studies in patients with solid tumors and leukemia[443–448] and in phase III studies in patients with newly diagnosed and refractory pancreatic cancer.[449] Administration of aerosolized liposomal 9-NC in the treatment of advanced pulmonary malignancies is also being evaluated.[450–455]

In a phase II trial of 9-NC at a dosage of 1.5 mg per m^2 per day daily for 5 days each week, a response rate of 32% (95% CI, 20 to 45%) was seen in 60 evaluable patients with advanced pancreatic cancer.[456] Phase III studies of 9-NC administered orally daily for 5 days per week in patients with newly diagnosed and refractory pancreatic cancer have also been completed, although only the results of the randomized phase III study of 9-NC versus best choice in patients with refractory pancreatic cancer have been reported.[449] In patients with measurable disease (59%), there were 12 independently verified (i.e., blinded radiology reviewed) responders of 9-NC (2 CR and 10 PR), for an overall response rate of 11%, compared with one responder (<1%, 1 CR) for patients treated on the best alternative chemotherapy arm ($P < 0.001$). The median progression-free survival (PFS) was significantly longer for the 9-NC arm (58 days) than for the best alternative chemotherapy (48 days) ($P = 0.003$). 9-NC was well tolerated as < 5% of patients discontinued treatment due to toxicity. The results of this study support the notion that 9-NC has an acceptable risk-benefit ratio, is convenient to use, and can achieve tumor growth control in a disease with few treatment options.

Phase II studies of single-agent 9-NC have been performed in patients with various solid tumors. 9-NC has achieved antitumor activity in patients with refractory ovarian cancer[443] and refractory gastric cancer.[457] However, 9-NC has been shown to be inactive against metastatic colorectal cancer,[458] advanced glioblastoma multiforme,[459] soft-tissue sarcoma,[446] urothelial tract cancers,[447] and SCLC.[448] 9-NC has also been evaluated in patients with chronic myeloid leukemia, chronic myelomonocytic leukemia (CML), and myelodysplastic syndromes.[460] Although the response rate in Ph-positive CML is low, one

TABLE 17.9

KEY FEATURES OF SYNTHETIC DERIVATIVES OF CAMPTOTHECIN

a. 9-Nitrocamptothecin

Metabolism	Partial metabolism to the active metabolite 9-aminocamptothecin by an unidentified enzyme. Various oxidation products likely involving multiple CYP isoforms have been identified in bile and urine.
Elimination	About 15% excreted unchanged in urine over 24 h.
Pharmacokinetics	Approximate terminal half-life is 20 hr; measures of exposure increase linearly with an increase in dose; oral bioavailability is highly variable.
Toxicity	Myelosuppression, predominantly noncumulative neutropenia, with thrombocytopenia and anemia less common
	Nausea and vomiting (mild)
	Diarrhea (mild)
	Fatigue
	Alopecia
	Hemorrhagic cystitis (incidence 14% in early trials)
Precautions	Concomitant use of enzyme-inducing anticonvulsants is contraindicated.

b. 9-Aminocamptothecin

Metabolism	Unknown
Elimination	About 30% excreted unchanged in urine over 24 h.
Pharmacokinetics	Approximate terminal half-life is 10–14 h; measures of exposure increase linearly with an increase in dose; oral bioavailability (~50%) is highly variable. Systemic clearance is approximately 24 L/h/m^2. Lactone–total drug ratio is very low (~10%).
Toxicity	Myelosuppression, predominantly noncumulative neutropenia, with thrombocytopenia and anemia less common
	Nausea and vomiting (mild)
	Diarrhea (mild)
	Fatigue
	Alopecia
Precautions	Concomitant use of enzyme-inducing anticonvulsants is contraindicated.

c. Exatecan mesylate (DX-8951f)

Metabolism	Extensive metabolism by the CYP3A4 and CYP1A2 isozymes to inactive metabolites.
Elimination	About 30% excreted unchanged in urine over 24 h.
Pharmacokinetics	Approximate terminal half-life is 8 hr; measures of exposure increase linearly with an increase in dose. Systemic clearance is approximately 1–2 L/h/m^2.
Toxicity	Myelosuppression, predominantly noncumulative neutropenia, with thrombocytopenia and anemia less common
	Nausea and vomiting (mild)
	Diarrhea (mild)
	Fatigue
	Alopecia
Precautions	None identified

d. Lurtotecan (GI147211)

Metabolism	Unknown
Elimination	About 11% excreted unchanged in urine over 24 h.
Pharmacokinetics	Approximate terminal half-life is 4–7 h; measures of exposure increase linearly with an increase in dose. Oral bioavailability is approximately 1.3%. Systemic clearance is approximately 35 L/h/m^2.
Toxicity	Myelosuppression, predominantly noncumulative neutropenia, with thrombocytopenia and anemia less common
	Nausea and vomiting (mild)
	Diarrhea (mild)
	Fatigue
	Alopecia
Precautions	None identified

e. Gimatecan (ST1481)

Metabolism	Unknown
Elimination	Unknown
Pharmacokinetics	Approximate terminal half-life is 100 hr; measures of exposure increase linearly with an increase in dose.
Toxicity	Myelosuppression, predominantly noncumulative neutropenia, with thrombocytopenia and anemia less common
	Nausea and vomiting (mild)
	Alopecia
Precautions	Concomitant use of enzyme-inducing anticonvulsants is contraindicated.

f. Diflomotecan (BN80915)

Metabolism	Unknown

(continued)

TABLE 17.9

KEY FEATURES OF SYNTHETIC DERIVATIVES OF CAMPTOTHECIN (*continued*)

Elimination	About 5% excreted unchanged in urine over 24 h.
Pharmacokinetics	Approximate terminal half-life is 4 h; measures of exposure increase linearly with an increase in dose. Oral bioavailability is approximately 60–75%.
Toxicity	Myelosuppression, predominantly noncumulative neutropenia, with thrombocytopenia and anemia less common
	Nausea and vomiting (mild)
	Diarrhea (mild)
Precautions	None identified

cytogenetic response was noted. Further studies are needed to better define the dose and schedule of 9-NC for the treatment of CML and MDS.[460] An evaluation of the feasibility of combining 9-NC with other cytotoxic agents, including gemcitabine[461] and capecitabine[441] in patients with solid tumors, is currently ongoing.

9-AMINOCAMPTOTHECIN

9-AC is a camptothecin derivative (Fig. 17.1, Table 17.9) with impressive preclinical activity in human xenograft models of colon cancer,[109,462] malignant melanoma,[436] prostate cancer,[463] breast cancer,[433] ovarian cancer,[435] acute leukemia,[464] bladder cancer,[465] and CNS metastatic tumors.[462] In three human colon cancer xenografts, 9-AC was highly active, exhibited minimal systemic toxicity, and produced a better antitumor response than a panel of nine anticancer agents, including 5-FU, doxorubicin, melphalan, methotrexate, vincristine, vinblastine, and several nitrosourea compounds.[109]

Clinical testing of 9-AC began in 1993 with initial phase I trials of the drug administered as a 72-hour infusion every 2 weeks[466] or 3 weeks.[467,468] This schedule was selected because of the preclinical studies demonstrating that prolonged drug exposures were needed to see any biologic effect and that short i.v. infusions had no activity in animal models.[469] More recently, other schedules of 9-AC administration have been developed, including a prolonged 120-hour infusion weekly,[470] a 24-hour infusion weekly for 4 of 5 weeks,[471] and a short i.v. infusion daily for 5 days every 3 weeks.[472] On all of these schedules, the major dose-limiting toxicities are neutropenia and, to a lesser extent, thrombocytopenia. Other common toxicities included anemia, fatigue, nausea and vomiting, diarrhea, alopecia, and mucositis. The compound 9-AC is not associated with pulmonary toxicity or hemorrhagic cystitis, and the diarrhea is much less severe than that seen with irinotecan. Phase I trials involving pediatric patients[473] and acute leukemia patients[474] have also been completed. Oral administration[475,476] and i.p. schedules for 9-AC have also been studied.[477]

In pharmacokinetic studies, the amount of 9-AC that is present in plasma relative to the total drug level (lactone plus carboxylate) is quite low, with most reported values below 10%.[117] This observation is consistent with earlier studies demonstrating that 9-AC lactone exhibits greater instability in human plasma than do other camptothecin derivatives such as topotecan or irinotecan.[478] Most of the reported terminal elimination half-lives for total 9-AC in plasma have been in the range of 7 to 10 hours.[479] Reports suggest that patients receiving anticonvulsant medications may have increased clearance and lower plasma drug levels of 9-AC.[480] In pharmacodynamic studies, 9-AC steady-state plasma concentrations[481,482] and AUC[471,472,483] correlated with the dose-limiting toxicity of neutropenia.

In phase II studies of 72-hour infusions of 9-AC administered at 50 to 59 μg/m^2 per hour every 2 weeks to 16 previously treated patients with metastatic colorectal cancer, no responses were observed, and the myelosuppressive toxicity was substantial.[484] Grade 4 neutropenia occurred in 56% of patients, and febrile neutropenia occurred in 31%. In another trial in which 17 previously untreated patients with this disease were given a lower dose of 35 μg/m^2 per hour for 72 hours every 2 weeks, no responses were observed.[485] In heavily pretreated patients with relapsed or refractory lymphoma administered 9-AC at 40 μg/m^2 per hour over 72 hours every 3 weeks with G-CSF support,[486] the response rate was 25% (95% CI, 13 to 41%), with 10 partial responses seen in 40 evaluable patients. The median duration of response was 5 months (range, 1 to 10 months), and the median survival time was 12.5 months. In 58 untreated patients with advanced NSCLC treated with 46 to 59 μg/m^2 per hour over 72 hours every 2 weeks, the overall response rate was 8.6% (95% CI, 2.9 to 19%),[487] and the median survival was 5.4 months. Again, myelosuppressive toxicity was substantial, with grade 4 neutropenia seen in 31% of patients overall. Using similar treatment schedules, 9-AC was found to have minimal activity in refractory breast cancer[488] and metastatic colorectal cancer.[489] Thus, in phase II trials, the antitumor activity of 9-AC on the 72-hour infusion schedule has been disappointing. Efforts to improve its activity include the development of longer infusion schedules.[470] Seventeen previously untreated patients with metastatic colorectal cancer were given 9-AC as a 120-hour infusion at 20 μg/m^2 per hour for 120 hours every week for 3 of 4 weeks; however, no responses occurred.[490]

Thus, despite its impressive preclinical activity in human colon cancer xenograft models, 9-AC has not shown effective antitumor activity in the clinical studies completed to date. One potential explanation for this discrepancy may be the inability to achieve the necessary plasma drug concentrations needed for antitumor efficacy.[491] Because human bone marrow stem cells are more sensitive to 9-AC than is murine bone marrow, dose-limiting myelosuppression made it impossible to achieve the same plasma drug concentrations in humans that were associated with optimal antitumor efficacy in the preclinical animal models.[492]

EXATECAN MESYLATE (DX-8951F)

The hexacyclic camptothecin analog exatecan mesylate (DX-8951f) ([1S,9S]-1-amino-9-ethyl-5-fluoro-1,2,3,9,12, 15-hexahydro-9-hydroxy-4-methyl-10 H,13H-benzo[de]-pyrano[3′,4′:6,7]-indolizino[1,2-b]quinoline-10,13-dione monomethane sulfonate, dihydrate) is a synthetic derivative with an amino group at C-1 and a fluorine atom at C-5 (Table 17.9). The compound has increased aqueous solubility in comparison with other camptothecin analogs. As exatecan does not require enzymatic activation, inter-individual variability in efficacy and side effects might be reduced as compared to some prodrug analogs.[493] The anhydrous free-base form of the drug is referred to as DX-8951. The lactone form of DX-8951 is hydrolyzed into an open-ring hydroxy-acid form, comparable with most other camptothecins. Similarly, the lactone and hydroxy-acid form coexist in solution according to a reversible pH-dependent equilibrium.[494,495]

Exatecan showed superior and a broader spectrum of antitumor activity in vitro and in vivo in comparison with some other camptothecin analogs tested.[496–502] Comparable with other camptothecin derivatives, exatecan is metabolized by CYP3A4 and CYP1A2, resulting in the formation of at least two hydroxylated metabolites referred to as UM-1 and UM-2.[503] The antitumor activity of these metabolites is much less potent than the parent compound itself.[494,504]

Phase I clinical studies included DX-8951f administered as a 30-min i.v. infusion once every week[505] or every 3 weeks,[506,507] as a 30-min i.v. infusion daily for 5 days[508] or 7 days every 3 weeks,[509] as a 24-hour continuous i.v. infusion every week[510] or every 3 weeks,[511] and as a protracted 5- to 21-day infusion.[512]

Reversible, noncumulative, and dose-related neutropenia was the DLT in all schedules.[505–512] With the prolonged continuous infusion schedules, thrombocytopenia was an added DLT, especially in heavily pretreated patients.[511,512] Neutrophil and platelet count nadirs occurred between days 10 – 15, with recovery by day 22. Non-hematological toxicities included mild to moderate gastrointestinal toxicity (nausea, vomiting, stomatitis, diarrhea), fatigue, asthenia and alopecia.[505–508,510–512] Transient and reversible liver dysfunction was also observed and in a Japanese study this event was dose-limiting at the dose of 6.65 mg/m^2.[506,508] In

advanced leukemia, stomatitis was dose limiting.[509] Remarkably, the MTD in leukemia (0.9 mg/m^2/daily for 5 days) is almost double of that observed in solid tumors.[509]

For phase II clinical trials, the 30-min infusion regimen with daily administration for 5 consecutive days every 3 weeks was selected because this schedule in phase I studies showed the most prominent signs of antitumor activity. However, at this dose and schedule, DX-8951f appears to lack significant activity in metastatic breast cancer,[513] NSCLC,[514] advanced ovarian cancer,[515] and colorectal cancer.[516]

LURTOTECAN

Like exatecan, lurtotecan (GI147211, GG211) is a hexacyclic camptothecin analog currently under clinical investigation as an anticancer drug (Table 17.9). Lurtotecan is a water-soluble, totally synthetic derivative with a dioxalane moiety between C-10 and C-11.[517] Because of the agent's low oral bioavailability,[518] lurtotecan has been evaluated clinically in various phase I trials using a 30-minute i.v. infusion given daily for 5 consecutive days[519,520] or a 72-hour[521] or 21-day[522] continuous i.v. infusion. The dose-limiting toxicity in all schedules was myelosuppression, including severe neutropenia and thrombocytopenia. Nonhematological toxicities were various and only mild to moderate. In phase II trials, lurtotecan has shown only modest activity in breast cancer, colorectal cancer, NSCLC,[523] and SCLC.[524] Overall, the data suggest that the hematological toxicity profile, antitumor activity, and pharmacokinetic profiles closely resemble those observed with topotecan.[525]

GIMATECAN

Gimatecan (ST1481) is an orally administered camptothecin with a relatively long plasma half-life (>80 hours; Table 17.9).[526] Gimatecan lacks schedule-dependency and has a favorable in vivo therapeutic index in several human tumor xenografts.[527,528] Thus, several schedules of orally administered gimatecan have been evaluated in phase I studies. Gianni and colleagues evaluated gimatecan administered orally daily for 5 days for 1 week (schedule A), 2 weeks (schedule B), or 3 weeks (schedule C), repeated every 4 weeks.[529] The qualitative toxicity pattern was similar in all schedules, and late onset thrombocytopenia followed by neutropenia was dose limiting in all schedules. The MTD on schedule A was 5.6 mg/m^2 per cycle, and on schedule B and C it was 7.2 mg/m^2 per cycle. Partial responses were documented in patients with NSCLC, breast cancer, and rhabdomyosarcoma.

A phase I/II study of gimatecan administered orally once a day for 5 consecutive days repeated every 28 days was performed in patients with recurrent malignant glioma where the dose was independently escalated based on concurrent use of enzyme-inducing anticonvulsants

(EIAEDs).[530] The mean ± SD terminal half-lives in the EIAED and non-EIAED groups were 6.3 ± 4.7 hours and 71 ± 28 hours, respectively. In addition, the AUC of day 5 in the EIAED group was 81% lower than in the non-EIAED group. Thus, the apparent clearance of gimatecan is markedly increased in patients coadministered EIAEDs. In addition, the authors concluded that the drug is well tolerated and shows initial promise in the treatment of patients with malignant glioma.

Due to the long plasma half-life, Zhu and colleagues performed a phase I trial of gimatecan administered orally once a week for 3 of 4 weeks at doses from 0.26 to 1.32 mg/m^2 per week, without significant toxicity.[531] Gimatecan was rapidly absorbed and slowly eliminated, with a mean apparent half-life of 108 ± 40 hours. The authors concluded that administration of gimatecan orally once a week at doses that are well tolerated provides continuous exposure to potentially effective plasma concentrations of the drug.

HOMOCAMPTOTHECINS

Diflomotecan (BN80915) belongs to the class of fluorinated homocamptothecins (Table 17.9). Homocamptothecins are synthetic, water-insoluble camptothecin analogs with a stabilized lactone ring due to modification of the naturally occurring 6-membered ring into a 7-membered ring by insertion of a methylene spacer between the alcohol and the carboxyl moiety.[532] The inductive effect from the electronegative oxygen of the adjacent hydroxyl group causes higher reactivity of the carboxyl group of camptothecins. By inserting a methylene spacer between the carboxylic and alcoholic functions of the E ring, it was believed that the electronic influence of the hydroxyl group was removed.[533] The alcohol moiety was seen as an important structure for stabilizing the cleavable complex, because neither deshydroxy-camptothecin nor the nonnatural enantiomer of camptothecin is biologically active.[533] Since a one-carbon ring expansion is chemically termed a homologation, these new lactone- or E-ring modified compounds were named homocamptothecins.

In comparison with most other camptothecins, which show rapid hydrolysis of the lactone moiety until a pH and protein–dependent equilibrium has been reached, homocamptothecins display a slow and irreversible hydrolytic lactone-ring opening.[534] This key feature, irreversibility of the E-ring opening, may lead to reduced toxicity.

Diflomotecan has entered phase I clinical testing. Oral diflomotecan administered once daily for 5 days every 3 weeks, was limited by dose-dependent myelosuppression.[535] Other toxicities observed were gastrointestinal (i.e., mild nausea and vomiting, alopecia, and fatigue). The recommended dose for phase II studies is 0.27 mg given once daily for 5 days every 3 weeks.

Oral diflomotecan exerts an apparent linear, dose-independent pharmacokinetic profile over a large dose range studied, with high inter- and intrapatient variability. It was also reported that flat dosing of oral diflomotecan resulted in the same variation in AUC as dosing per square meter would have done, as already established for many other cytotoxic agents.[237] The oral bioavailability (F) of diflomotecan at the recommended dose was 67.1%, which is much better than for other oral topoisomerase I inhibitors such as topotecan (F = 30 to 44%)[134,136] and 9-AC (F = 48.6%).[536] Preliminary pharmacogenetic analysis has indicated that the ABCG2 421C>A genotype significantly affects the systemic disposition of diflomotecan.[537] This suggests that, in the future, population pharmacokinetic studies incorporating this pharmacogenetic information might enable a reduction in interindividual pharmacokinetic variability.

SILATECANS AND HOMOSILATECANS

Since the closed, active lactone ring is a structural requirement for effective biologic activity of the camptothecins,[115] many researchers have investigated various modifications of the camptothecins in an effort to promote lactone stability yet retain antitumor efficacy. One approach to synthesize a more stable topoisomerase I inhibitor has included structural modifications that eliminate the highly preferential binding of the carboxylate form to HSA and thus reduce the rate of hydrolysis. In addition, the discovery of lactone stabilization through lipid bilayer partitioning has led to the design of more lipophilic analogs in order to promote partitioning of these agents into the lipid bilayers of erythrocytes and protect the active lactone form from hydrolysis.[538]

The synthesis of 7-silycamptothecins by adding a silyl group at position 7 with various substitutions at position 10 has demonstrated increased stability of the lactone ring.[539,540] The addition of a silyl group may limit drug inactivation by both protein binding and hydrolysis of the lactone ring and may also enhance lipophilicity, which would increase in vivo activity while possibly limiting toxicity.[541] The majority of these new compounds demonstrate potencies comparable to or better than other camptothecin derivatives. Two of the leading members of this class, DB-67 and karenitecin (BNP1350), are in preclinical and phase II development, respectively. Preclinical nonhuman primate and phase I clinical studies of karenitecin indicated the percent lactone was 104% and 87 ± 11%, respectively.[542,543] DB-67 was found to have antitumor activity more potent than that of topotecan and at least comparable to that of SN-38 against a panel of five high-grade glioma cell lines.[541] Although the results of this study are promising for the future treatment of human gliomas, it is unclear if the increased stability of the lactone ring in human blood and its potentially increased lipophilicity will translate into increased activity in humans. One potential problem is that silatecans have low penetration into the CSF.[542]

Homocamptothecins have been further modified to form homosilatecans.[544] In addition to the expanded β-hydroxylactone E ring, each of the homosilatecans also contains a silylalkyl functionality at the 7-position. As with the silatecans, this functionality group increases the lipophilicity while reducing the strength of carboxylate interactions with HSA. Two homosilatecans, DB-90 and DB-91, contain amino and hydroxyl groups at the 10-position, respectively, to further reduce binding of the carboxylate form to HSA. Homosilatecans display improved lipophilicity and stability in human whole blood compared with camptothecin and topotecan. Interestingly, homosilatecans display similar stability in human and mouse blood, which contrasts with the interspecies variations in blood stability observed for camptothecins.[544] Thus, preclinical animal modeling and efficacy studies with the homosilatecans may be predictive of their use in a clinical setting.

ALTERNATIVE FORMULATIONS AND PRODRUGS

Several different liposomal formulations of camptothecin analogs, including camptothecin,[545] topotecan,[546] irinotecan,[547] SN-38,[548] lurtotecan,[549] and 9-NC,[451] have been designed. The main goals of these strategies were to overcome the limited water solubility of camptothecins, increase the lactone stability, prolong the duration of exposure in plasma and tumor, and improve the therapeutic index by increasing tumor delivery of the active drug and reducing toxicity. In addition, since camptothecin analogs are topoisomerase inhibitors that exhibit cell cycle–dependent antitumor activity, the prolonged exposures may increase cytotoxic effects.[35]

Liposomal Lurtotecan

Because the oral bioavailability of lurtotecan was previously shown to be highly variable and as low as 10%,[518] alternative methods of drug administration are currently being developed, including a new liposomal formulation (OSI-211; also known as NX 211). Preclinical data have been generated demonstrating that this unilamellar liposomal formulation of lurtotecan has a significant therapeutic advantage over the free drug, showing increased antitumor activity in xenograft models, which is consistent with increased systemic exposure and enhanced tumor-specific delivery of the drug.[550] Based on these exciting data, phase I clinical trials have been performed, with OSI-211 given to cancer patients as a 30-minute infusion either once[551] or daily for 3 days every 3 weeks.[552–554] As expected, the dose-limiting toxicities in these trials were neutropenia and thrombocytopenia, and pharmacological findings seem to agree with the preclinical profile of this agent. Indeed, the clearance of total lurtotecan following administration of

OSI-211 was approximately 25-fold slower than that of the free drug,[551] which might prove to be beneficial for the pharmacodynamic outcome of treatment. A phase II study in which OSI-211 was delivered at a dose of 2.4 mg/m^2 on days 1 and 8 of a 3-week schedule lacked significant activity in patients with topotecan-resistant ovarian cancer.[555] Clinical evaluation of this agent in other patient populations and/or with alternative schedules is currently ongoing.

Liposomal SN-38

SN-38, the active metabolite of irinotecan, thus far has not been used as an anticancer drug due to poor solubility in any pharmaceutically acceptable solvent as well as its rapid elimination.[285] An alternative i.v. formulation involving liposomal encapsulation of SN-38 has been recently presented.[548] The liposomal formulation of SN-38 overcomes the need for administration of the prodrug, irinotecan, and the variability associated with irinotecan administration and subsequent formation of SN-38 by CES2. SN-38 has low affinity to lipid membranes, and it tends to precipitate in aqueous phase, resulting in very low drug-to-liposome entrapment. A novel liposomal formulation of SN-38 has been developed to overcome these issues.[548] In this liposomal formulation, SN-38 drug partitions into the bilayer of the liposome. As a result, SN-38 in biological solutions (e.g., blood or plasma) may be immediately released from the liposome. Thus, SN-38 is likely to predominantly exist in the circulation as released, nonencapsulated SN-38. In view of the important role of UGT1A1*28 in SN-38 elimination, pharmacogenetic analyses of UGT1A1*28 have been implemented prospectively as part of a phase I study of liposomal encapsulated SN-38 in patients with advanced cancer.[556]

Stealth-Liposomal CKD602

Pegylation of liposomes (Stealth$^{(R)}$) was initially developed to avoid uptake of liposomes by the mononuclear phagocyte system (MPS), thus allowing liposomes to remain in the circulation for longer periods of time than nonpegylated liposomes.[557–559] Stealth liposomal CKD602 (S-CKD602) is a liposomal formulation similar to Stealth liposomal doxorubicin (Doxil)[560]: the drug is contained in the core of the liposome, and the outer layer of the liposomal bilayer contains a phospholipid covalently bound to methoxypolyethylene glycol (MPEG). The purpose of the encapsulating CKD602 in a Stealth liposome is to maintain the lactone stability, prolong the elimination half-life in plasma, increase the drug exposure in the tumor, and potentially improve antitumor efficacy. In preclinical studies, S-CKD602 produced significantly enhanced antitumor efficacy over that of nonliposomal CKD602 in human xenograft models of ovarian, melanoma, colon, and SCLC carcinomas.[561,562] S-CKD602 is currently being evaluated in a phase I study.

Polyethylene Glycol-Conjugated Prodrugs

An alternative strategy to optimize the therapeutic indices and feasibility of administering camptothecin involves conjugating camptothecin to a chemically modified polyethylene glycol (PEG) macromolecule.[563-565] The highly water soluble and stable prodrug pegylated camptothecin (PEG-CPT, EZ-246, Prothecin) undergoes enzymatic hydrolysis that releases camptothecin in tissues and biological fluids. An advantage of this approach is that the acylated camptothecin prodrug maintains the E ring in its desired active lactone form.[564] Selective tumor distribution may also occur as a result of the high molecular and specific physiochemical properties of PEG-camptothecin, which potentially results in enhanced vascular permeation and intratumoral retention. Furthermore, PEG-camptothecin has demonstrated an impressive and broad spectrum of antitumor activity in xenograft models.[564]

In a phase I study in patients with advanced solid tumors, the recommended dose of PEG- camptothecin was 7,000 mg/m^2 as a 1-hour infusion every 3 weeks.[566] The primary toxicity was myelosuppression; cystitis, nausea, vomiting, and diarrhea were also observed but were rarely severe. The plasma dispositions of PEG-camptothecin and released camptothecin are complex, reflecting the interplay between both forms. The elimination half-life (77 $\pm$ 37 hour) of PEG- camptothecin is significantly longer than that reported for most other camptothecin analogs.[566] In addition, released camptothecin accumulated slowly in plasma. A phase II study of PEG-camptothecin in patients with adenocarcinoma of the stomach and gastroesophageal junction reported responses in 4 of 15 patients.[567] The regimen was well tolerated, with a low incidence of grade 3 and 4 toxicities. Two subjects developed grade 2 cystitis and also reported dehydration.

CONCLUSION

Over the past several years, the camptothecins have evolved from an experimental class of antitumor agents into established agents with documented clinical utility in the treatment of human malignancies. Despite our growing understanding of the pharmacology of the topoisomerase I inhibitors, several important issues must still be resolved. One is to determine the optimal method of combining these agents with other active drugs or treatment modalities such as radiation and biologic agents. Current laboratory and clinical investigations of camptothecin drug combinations may help guide further clinical development in this area. A more difficult question is why marked differences exist in the clinical activity of different camptothecin derivatives. Agents such as camptothecin and 9-AC are potent inhibitors of topoisomerase I at the molecular level, yet their clinical utility appears to be much less than that of topotecan or irinotecan. Some of this variation may be related to the clinical pharmacology of these agents, but pharmacologic differences do not fully explain the differences in clinical efficacy. Further studies of their molecular pharmacology and a clearer understanding of the relevant molecular determinants of response to the topoisomerase I poisons may help to clarify these issues and aid development of even more effective topoisomerase I poisons.

Almost 40 years after they first showed promising anticancer activity in a National Cancer Institute screening program, the camptothecins are established agents for the treatment of human cancer. Nonetheless, we are still learning how to optimally incorporate these agents into effective cancer treatments. The development of the camptothecins has also helped to elucidate the basic function of the topoisomerase I protein at the molecular level, and these agents have provided investigators with a valuable research tool for studying this important enzyme. The documented clinical activity of the camptothecins has highlighted topoisomerase I as a key target for cancer chemotherapy and has thereby allowed the development of completely new pharmacologic strategies for the treatment of human cancer.

REFERENCES

1. Wall ME, Wani MC, Cook CE, et al. Plant antitumor agents, I: the isolation and structure of camptothecin, a novel alkaloidal leukemia and tumor inhibitor from *Camptotheca acuminata*. J Am Chem Soc 1966;88:3888–3890.
2. Horwitz SB, Horwitz MS. Effects of camptothecin on the breakage and repair of DNA during the cell cycle. Cancer Res 1973; 33:2834–2836.
3. Bosmann HB. Camptothecin inhibits macromolecular synthesis in mammalian cells but not in isolated mitochondria of *E. coli*. Biochem Biophys Res Commun 1970;41:1412–1420.
4. Horwitz SB, Chang CK, Grollman AP. Studies on camptothecin, I: effects of nucleic acid and protein synthesis. Mol Pharmacol 1971;7:632–644.
5. Wu RS, Kumar A, Warner JR. Ribosome formation is blocked by camptothecin, a reversible inhibitor of RNA synthesis. Proc Natl Acad Sci USA 1971;68:3009–3014.
6. Gallo RC, Whang-Peng J, Adamson RH. Studies on the antitumor activity, mechanism of action, and cell cycle effects of camptothecin. J Natl Cancer Inst 1971;46:789–795.
7. Kessel D. Effects of camptothecin on RNA synthesis in leukemia L1210 cells. Biochim Biophys Acta 1971;246:225–232.
8. Kessel D, Bosmann HB, Lohr K. Camptothecin effects on DNA synthesis in murine leukemia cells. Biochim Biophys Acta 1972; 269:210–216.
9. Kessel D, Dysard R. Effects of camptothecin on RNA synthesis in L-1210 cells. Biochim Biophys Acta 1973;312:716–721.
10. Abelson HT, Penman S. Selective interruption of high molecular weight RNA synthesis in HeLa cells by camptothecin. Nat New Biol 1972;237:144–146.
11. Gottlieb JA, Guarino AM, Call JB, et al. Preliminary pharmacologic and clinical evaluation of camptothecin sodium (NSC-100880). Cancer Chemother Rep 1970;54:461–470.
12. Creaven PJ, Allen LM, Muggia FM. Plasma camptothecin (NSC-100880) levels during a 5-day course of treatment: relation to dose and toxicity. Cancer Chemother Rep 1972;56:573–578.
13. Muggia FM, Creaven PJ, Hansen HH, et al. Phase I clinical trial of weekly and daily treatment with camptothecin (NSC-100880): correlation with preclinical studies. Cancer Chemother Rep 1972;56:515–521.

14. Moertel CG, Schutt AJ, Reitemeier RJ, et al. Phase II study of camptothecin (NSC-100880) in the treatment of advanced gastrointestinal cancer. Cancer Chemother Rep 1972;56:95–101.

15. Gottlieb JA, Luce JK. Treatment of malignant melanoma with camptothecin (NSC-10080). Cancer Treat Rep 1972;56:103–105.

16. Hsiang YH, Hertzberg R, Hecht S, et al. Camptothecin induces protein-linked DNA breaks via mammalian DNA topoisomerase I. J Biol Chem 1985;260:14873–14878.

17. Hsiang YH, Liu LF. Identification of mammalian DNA topoisomerase I as an intracellular target of the anticancer drug camptothecin. Cancer Res 1988;48:1722–1726.

18. Iyer L, Ratain MJ. Clinical pharmacology of camptothecins. Cancer Chemother Pharmacol 1998;42(Suppl):S31–43.

19. Mathijssen RH, Loos WJ, Verweij J, et al. Pharmacology of topoisomerase I inhibitors irinotecan (CPT-11) and topotecan. Curr Cancer Drug Targets 2002;2:103–123.

20. Pizzolato JF, Saltz LB. The camptothecins. Lancet 2003;361:2235–2242.

21. Wang JC. DNA topoisomerases. Annu Rev Biochem 1985;54:665–697.

22. Vosberg HP. DNA topoisomerases: enzymes that control DNA conformation. Curr Top Microbiol Immunol 1985;114:19–102.

23. Juan CC, Hwang JL, Liu AA, et al. Human DNA topoisomerase I is encoded by a single-copy gene that maps to chromosome region 20q12-13.2. Proc Natl Acad Sci USA 1988;85:8910–8913.

24. Kunze N, Yang GC, Jiang ZY, et al. Localization of the active type I DNA topoisomerase gene on human chromosome 20q11.2-13.1, and two pseudogenes on chromosomes 1q23-24 and 22q11. 2-13.1. Hum Genet 1989;84:6–10.

25. Redinbo MR, Champoux JJ, Hol WG. Structural insights into the function of type IB topoisomerases. Curr Opin Struct Biol 1999;9:29–36.

26. Heiland S, Knippers R, Kunze N. The promoter region of the human type-I-DNA-topoisomerase gene: protein-binding sites and sequences involved in transcriptional regulation. Eur J Biochem 1993;217:813–822.

27. Stewart L, Ireton GC, Champoux JJ. A functional linker in human topoisomerase I is required for maximum sensitivity to camptothecin in a DNA relaxation assay. J Biol Chem 1999;274:32950–32960.

28. Keck JL, Berger JM. Enzymes that push DNA around. Nat Struct Biol 1999;6:900–902.

29. Stewart L, Ireton GC, Champoux JJ. The domain organization of human topoisomerase I. J Biol Chem 1996;271:7602–7608.

30. Stewart L, Redinbo MR, Qiu X, et al. A model for the mechanism of human topoisomerase I. Science 1998;279:1534–1541.

31. Redinbo MR, Stewart L, Kuhn P, et al. Crystal structures of human topoisomerase I in covalent and noncovalent complexes with DNA. Science 1998;279:1504–1513.

32. Hsiang YH, Lihou MG, Liu LF. Arrest of replication forks by drug-stabilized topoisomerase I-DNA cleavable complexes as a mechanism of cell killing by camptothecin. Cancer Res 1989;49:5077–5082.

33. Drewinko B, Freireich EJ, Gottlieb JA. Lethal activity of camptothecin sodium on human lymphoma cells. Cancer Res 1974;34:747–750.

34. D'Arpa P, Beardmore C, Liu LF. Involvement of nucleic acid synthesis in cell killing mechanisms of topoisomerase poisons. Cancer Res 1990;50:6919–6924.

35. Gerrits CJ, de Jonge MJ, Schellens JH, et al. Topoisomerase I inhibitors: the relevance of prolonged exposure for present clinical development. Br J Cancer 1997;76:952–962.

36. Kohn KW, Pommier Y. Molecular and biological determinants of the cytotoxic actions of camptothecins: perspective for the development of new topoisomerase I inhibitors. Ann NY Acad Sci 2000;922:11–26.

37. Burris HA 3rd, Hanauske AR, Johnson RK, et al. Activity of topotecan, a new topoisomerase I inhibitor, against human tumor colony-forming units in vitro. J Natl Cancer Inst 1992;84:1816–1820.

38. Verweij J, Schellens JH. Topoisomerase I inhibition: a new target or new missiles? Ann Oncol 1995;6:102–104.

39. Hashimoto H, Chatterjee S, Berger NA. Mutagenic activity of topoisomerase I inhibitors. Clin Cancer Res 1995;1:369–376.

40. Anderson RD, Berger NA. International Commission for Protection against Environmental Mutagens and Carcinogens: mutagenicity and carcinogenicity of topoisomerase-interactive agents. Mutat Res 1994;309:109–142.

41. Baguley BC, Ferguson LR. Mutagenic properties of topoisomerase-targeted drugs. Biochim Biophys Acta 1998;1400:213–222.

42. Cosentino L, Heddle JA. A comparison of the effects of diverse mutagens at the lacZ transgene and Dlb-1 locus in vivo. Mutagenesis 1999;14:113–119.

43. Shaver-Walker PM, Urlando C, Tao KS, et al. Enhanced somatic mutation rates induced in stem cells of mice by low chronic exposure to ethylnitrosourea. Proc Natl Acad Sci USA 1995 92:11470–11474.

44. Chatterjee S, Trivedi D, Petzold SJ, et al. Mechanism of epipodophyllotoxin-induced cell death in poly(adenosine diphosphate-ribose) synthesis-deficient V79 Chinese hamster cell lines. Cancer Res 1990;50:2713–2718.

45. Holm C, Covey JM, Kerrigan D, et al. Differential requirement of DNA replication for the cytotoxicity of DNA topoisomerase I and II inhibitors in Chinese hamster DC3F cells. Cancer Res 1989;49:6365–6368.

46. Chow KC, Ross WE. Topoisomerase-specific drug sensitivity in relation to cell cycle progression. Mol Cell Biol 1987;7:3119–3123.

47. Berger NA, Chatterjee S, Schmotzer JA, et al. Etoposide (VP-16-213)–induced gene alterations: potential contribution to cell death. Proc Natl Acad Sci USA 1991;88:8740–8743.

48. Pui CH, Relling MV, Rivera GK, et al. Epipodophyllotoxin-related acute myeloid leukemia: a study of 35 cases. Leukemia 1995;9:1990–1996.

49. Broeker PL, Super HG, Thirman MJ, et al. Distribution of 11q23 breakpoints within the MLL breakpoint cluster region in de novo acute leukemia and in treatment-related acute myeloid leukemia: correlation with scaffold attachment regions and topoisomerase II consensus binding sites. Blood 1996;87:1912–1922.

50. Stanulla M, Wang J, Chervinsky DS, et al. Topoisomerase II inhibitors induce DNA double-strand breaks at a specific site within the AML1 locus. Leukemia 1997;11:490–496.

51. Rasheed ZA, Rubin EH. Mechanisms of resistance to topoisomerase I–targeting drugs. Oncogene 2003;22:7296–7304.

52. Chrencik JE, Staker BL, Burgin AB, et al. Mechanisms of camptothecin resistance by human topoisomerase I mutations. J Mol Biol 2004;339:773–784.

53. Wang LF, Ting CY, Lo CK, et al. Identification of mutations at DNA topoisomerase I responsible for camptothecin resistance. Cancer Res 1997;57:1516–1522.

54. Andoh T, Ishii K, Suzuki Y, et al. Characterization of a mammalian mutant with a camptothecin-resistant DNA topoisomerase I. Proc Natl Acad Sci USA 1987;84:5565–5569.

55. Sugimoto Y, Tsukahara S, Oh-hara T, et al. Decreased expression of DNA topoisomerase I in camptothecin-resistant tumor cell lines as determined by a monoclonal antibody. Cancer Res 1990;50:6925–6930.

56. Tamura H, Kohchi C, Yamada R, et al. Molecular cloning of a cDNA of a camptothecin-resistant human DNA topoisomerase I and identification of mutation sites. Nucleic Acids Res 1991;19:69–75.

57. Kubota N, Kanzawa F, Nishio K, et al. Detection of topoisomerase I gene point mutation in CPT-11 resistant lung cancer cell line. Biochem Biophys Res Commun 1992;188:571–577.

58. Benedetti P, Fiorani P, Capuani L, et al. Camptothecin resistance from a single mutation changing glycine 363 of human DNA topoisomerase I to cysteine. Cancer Res 1993;53:4343–4348.

59. Knab AM, Fertala J, Bjornsti MA. Mechanisms of camptothecin resistance in yeast DNA topoisomerase I mutants. J Biol Chem 1993;268:22322–22330.

60. Tanizawa A, Beitrand R, Kohlhagen G, et al. Cloning of Chinese hamster DNA topoisomerase I cDNA and identification of a single point mutation responsible for camptothecin resistance. J Biol Chem 1993;268:25463–25468.

61. Rubin E, Pantazis P, Bharti A, et al. Identification of a mutant human topoisomerase I with intact catalytic activity and resistance to 9-nitro-camptothecin. J Biol Chem 1994;269:2433–2439.

62. Tsurutani J, Nitta T, Hirashima T, et al. Point mutations in the topoisomerase I gene in patients with non-small cell lung cancer treated with irinotecan. Lung Cancer 2002;35:299–304.

63. Jansen WJ, Hulscher TM, van Ark-Otte J, et al. CPT-11 sensitivity in relation to the expression of P170-glycoprotein and multidrug resistance–associated protein. Br J Cancer 1998;77:359–365.

64. Tsuruo T, Matsuzaki T, Matsushita M, et al. Antitumor effect of CPT-11, a new derivative of camptothecin, against pleiotropic drug–resistant tumors in vitro and in vivo. Cancer Chemother Pharmacol 1988;21:71–74.

65. Chen AY, Yu C, Potmesil M, et al. Camptothecin overcomes MDR1-mediated resistance in human KB carcinoma cells. Cancer Res 1991;51:6039–6044.

66. Hendricks CB, Rowinsky EK, Grochow LB, et al. Effect of P-glycoprotein expression on the accumulation and cytotoxicity of topotecan (SK&F 104864), a new camptothecin analogue. Cancer Res 1992;52:2268–2278.

67. Mattern MR, Hofmann GA, Polsky RM, et al. In vitro and in vivo effects of clinically important camptothecin analogues on multidrug-resistant cells. Oncol Res 1993;5:467–474.

68. Hoki Y, Fujimori A, Pommier Y. Differential cytotoxicity of clinically important camptothecin derivatives in P-glycoprotein–overexpressing cell lines. Cancer Chemother Pharmacol 1997; 40:433–438.

69. Jonsson E, Fridborg H, Csoka K, et al. Cytotoxic activity of topotecan in human tumour cell lines and primary cultures of human tumour cells from patients. Br J Cancer 1997;76:211–219.

70. Doyle LA, Yang W, Abruzzo LV, et al. A multidrug resistance transporter from human MCF-7 breast cancer cells. Proc Natl Acad Sci USA 1998;95:15665–15670.

71. Miyake K, Mickley L, Litman T, et al. Molecular cloning of cDNAs which are highly overexpressed in mitoxantrone-resistant cells: demonstration of homology to ABC transport genes. Cancer Res 1999;59:8–13.

72. Candeil L, Gourdier I, Peyron D, et al. ABCG2 overexpression in colon cancer cells resistant to SN38 and in irinotecan-treated metastases. Int J Cancer 2004;109:848–854.

73. Houghton PJ, Cheshire PJ, Hallman JC, et al. Therapeutic efficacy of the topoisomerase I inhibitor 7-ethyl-10-(4-[1-piperidino]-1-piperidino)-carbonyloxy-camptothecin against human tumor xenografts: lack of cross-resistance in vivo in tumors with acquired resistance to the topoisomerase I inhibitor 9-dimethylaminomethyl-10-hydroxycamptothecin. Cancer Res 1993;53:2823–2829.

74. Danks MK, Potter PM. Enzyme-prodrug systems: carboxylesterase/CPT-11. Methods Mol Med 2004;90:247–262.

75. Danks MK, Morton CL, Pawlik CA, et al. Overexpression of a rabbit liver carboxylesterase sensitizes human tumor cells to CPT-11. Cancer Res 1998;58:20–22.

76. Wierdl M, Wall A, Morton CL, et al. Carboxylesterase-mediated sensitization of human tumor cells to CPT-11 cannot override ABCG2-mediated drug resistance. Mol Pharmacol 2003;64: 279–288.

77. Sanghani SP, Quinney SK, Fredenburg TB, et al. Carboxylesterases expressed in human colon tumor tissue and their role in CPT-11 hydrolysis. Clin Cancer Res 2003;9:4983–4991.

78. Xu G, Zhang W, Ma MK, et al. Human carboxylesterase 2 is commonly expressed in tumor tissue and is correlated with activation of irinotecan. Clin Cancer Res 2002;8:2605–2611.

79. Hanioka N, Ozawa S, Jinno H, et al. Human liver UDP-glucuronosyltransferase isoforms involved in the glucuronidation of 7-ethyl-10-hydroxycamptothecin. Xenobiotica 2001;31:687–699.

80. Cummings J, Boyd G, Ethell BT, et al. Enhanced clearance of topoisomerase I inhibitors from human colon cancer cells by glucuronidation. Biochem Pharmacol 2002;63:607–613.

81. Jinno H, Tanaka-Kagawa T, Hanioka N, et al. Glucuronidation of 7-ethyl-10-hydroxycamptothecin (SN-38), an active metabolite of irinotecan (CPT-11), by human UGT1A1 variants, G71R, P229Q, and Y486D. Drug Metab Dispos 2003;31:108–113.

82. Dodds HM, Tobin PJ, Stewart CF, et al. The importance of tumor glucuronidase in the activation of irinotecan in a mouse xenograft model. J Pharmacol Exp Ther 2002;303:649–655.

83. Chen AY, Liu LF. DNA topoisomerases: essential enzymes and lethal targets. Annu Rev Pharmacol Toxicol 1994;34:191–218.

84. Chun JH, Kim HK, Kim E, et al. Increased expression of metallothionein is associated with irinotecan resistance in gastric cancer. Cancer Res 2004;64:4703–4706.

85. Eng WK, Faucette L, Johnson RK, et al. Evidence that DNA topoisomerase I is necessary for the cytotoxic effects of camptothecin. Mol Pharmacol 1988;34:755–760.

86. Nitiss J, Wang JC. DNA topoisomerase–targeting antitumor drugs can be studied in yeast. Proc Natl Acad Sci USA 1988; 85:7501–7505.

87. Jansen WJ, Zwart B, Hulscher ST, et al. CPT-11 in human colon-cancer cell lines and xenografts: characterization of cellular sensitivity determinants. Int J Cancer 1997;70:335–340.

88. Matsumoto Y, Fujiwara T, Honjo Y, et al. Quantitative analysis of DNA topoisomerase I activity in human and rat glioma: characterization and mechanism of resistance to antitopoisomerase chemical, camptothecin-11. J Surg Oncol 1993;53:97–103.

89. Goldwasser F, Bae I, Valenti M, et al. Topoisomerase I–related parameters and camptothecin activity in the colon carcinoma cell lines from the National Cancer Institute anticancer screen. Cancer Res 1995;55:2116–2121.

90. Perego P, Capranico G, Supino R, et al. Topoisomerase I gene expression and cell sensitivity to camptothecin in human cell lines of different tumor types. Anticancer Drugs 1994;5:645–649.

91. Buckwalter CA, Lin AH, Tanizawa A, et al. RNA synthesis inhibitors alter the subnuclear distribution of DNA topoisomerase I. Cancer Res 1996;56:1674–1681.

92. Baker SD, Wadkins RM, Stewart CF, et al. Cell cycle analysis of amount and distribution of nuclear DNA topoisomerase I as determined by fluorescence digital imaging microscopy. Cytometry 1995;19:134–145.

93. Danks MK, Garrett KE, Marion RC, et al. Subcellular redistribution of DNA topoisomerase I in anaplastic astrocytoma cells treated with topotecan. Cancer Res 1996;56:1664–1673.

94. Florell SR, Martinchick JF, Holden JA. Purification of DNA topoisomerase I from the spleen of a patient with non-Hodgkin's lymphoma. Anticancer Res 1996;16:3467–3474.

95. Subramanian D, Kraut E, Staubus A, et al. Analysis of topoisomerase I/DNA complexes in patients administered topotecan. Cancer Res 1995;55:2097–2103.

96. Kaufmann SH, Svingen PA, Gore SD, et al. Altered formation of topotecan-stabilized topoisomerase I–DNA adducts in human leukemia cells. Blood 1997;89:2098–2104.

97. Boege F. Analysis of eukaryotic DNA topoisomerases and topoisomerase-directed drug effects. Eur J Clin Chem Clin Biochem 1996;34:873–888.

98. Pondarre C, Strumberg D, Fujimori A, et al. In vivo sequencing of camptothecin-induced topoisomerase I cleavage sites in human colon carcinoma cells. Nucleic Acids Res 1997;25:4111–4116.

99. Fujimori A, Gupta M, Hoki Y, et al. Acquired camptothecin resistance of human breast cancer MCF-7/C4 cells with normal topoisomerase I and elevated DNA repair. Mol Pharmacol 1996;50:1472–1478.

100. Adjei PN, Kaufmann SH, Leung WY, et al. Selective induction of apoptosis in Hep 3B cells by topoisomerase I inhibitors: evidence for a protease-dependent pathway that does not activate cysteine protease P32. J Clin Invest 1996;98:2588–2596.

101. Shimizu T, Pommier Y. DNA fragmentation induced by protease activation in p53-null human leukemia HL60 cells undergoing apoptosis following treatment with the topoisomerase I inhibitor camptothecin: cell-free system studies. Exp Cell Res 1996;226:292–301.

102. Gupta M, Fan S, Zhan Q, et al. Inactivation of p53 increases the cytotoxicity of camptothecin in human colon HCT116 and breast MCF-7 cancer cells. Clin Cancer Res 1997;3:1653–1660.

103. Dubrez L, Goldwasser F, Genne P, et al. The role of cell cycle regulation and apoptosis triggering in determining the sensitivity of leukemic cells to topoisomerase I and II inhibitors. Leukemia 1995;9:1013–1024.

104. Gradzka I, Szumiel I. Discrepancy between the initial DNA damage and cell survival after camptothecin treatment in two murine lymphoma L5178Y sublines. Cell Biochem Funct 1996;14: 163–171.

105. Goldwasser F, Shimizu T, Jackman J, et al. Correlations between S and G2 arrest and the cytotoxicity of camptothecin in human colon carcinoma cells. Cancer Res 1996;56:4430–4437.

106. Takimoto CH, Wright J, Arbuck SG. Clinical applications of the camptothecins. Biochim Biophys Acta 1998;1400:107–119.

107. Chourpa I, Beljebbar A, Sockalingum GD, et al. Structure-activity relation in camptothecin antidrug drugs: why a detailed molecular characterisation of their lactone and carboxylate forms by Raman and SERS spectroscopies? Biochim Biophys Acta 1997; 1334:349–360.

108. Thomas CJ, Rahier NJ, Hecht SM. Camptothecin: current perspectives. Bioorg Med Chem 2004;12:1585–1604.

109. Giovanella BC, Stehlin JS, Wall ME, et al. DNA topoisomerase I–targeted chemotherapy of human colon cancer in xenografts. Science 1989;246:1046–1048.

110. Tanizawa A, Fujimori A, Fujimori Y, et al. Comparison of topoisomerase I inhibition, DNA damage, and cytotoxicity of camptothecin derivatives presently in clinical trials. J Natl Cancer Inst 1994;86:836–842.

111. Sugimori M, Ejima A, Ohsuki S, et al. Synthesis and antitumor activity of ring A- and F-modified hexacyclic camptothecin analogues. J Med Chem 1998;41:2308–2318.

112. Luzzio MJ, Besterman JM, Emerson DL, et al. Synthesis and antitumor activity of novel water soluble derivatives of camptothecin as specific inhibitors of topoisomerase I. J Med Chem 1995; 38:395–401.

113. Uehling DE, Nanthakumar SS, Croom D, et al. Synthesis, topoisomerase I inhibitory activity, and in vivo evaluation of 11-aza-camptothecin analogs. J Med Chem 1995;38:1106–1118.

114. Vladu B, Woynarowski JM, Manikumar G, et al. Seven- and 10-substituted camptothecins: dependence of topoisomerase I–DNA cleavable complex formation and stability on the 7- and 10-substituents. Mol Pharmacol 2000;57:243–251.

115. Chourpa I, Riou JF, Millot JM, et al. Modulation in kinetics of lactone ring hydrolysis of camptothecins upon interaction with topoisomerase I cleavage sites on DNA. Biochemistry1998; 37:7284–7291.

116. Burke TG, Munshi CB, Mi Z, et al. The important role of albumin in determining the relative human blood stabilities of the camptothecin anticancer drugs. J Pharm Sci 1995;84:518–519.

117. Loos WJ, Verweij J, Gelderblom HJ, et al. Role of erythrocytes and serum proteins in the kinetic profile of total 9-amino-20(S)-camptothecin in humans. Anticancer Drugs 1999;10:705–710.

118. Burke TG, Mi Z. The structural basis of camptothecin interactions with human serum albumin: impact on drug stability. J Med Chem 1994;37:40–46.

119. Saltz L, Sirott M, Young C, et al. Phase I clinical and pharmacology study of topotecan given daily for 5 consecutive days to patients with advanced solid tumors, with attempt at dose intensification using recombinant granulocyte colony-stimulating factor. J Natl Cancer Inst 1993;85:1499–1507.

120. Verweij J, Lund B, Beijnen J, et al. Phase I and pharmacokinetics study of topotecan, a new topoisomerase I inhibitor. Ann Oncol 1993;4:673–678.

121. Beran M, Kantarjian H. Topotecan in the treatment of hematologic malignancies. Semin Hematol 1998;35:26–31.

122. Hochster H, Liebes L, Speyer J, et al. Phase I trial of low-dose continuous topotecan infusion in patients with cancer: an active and well-tolerated regimen. J Clin Oncol 1994;12:553–559.

123. Mainwaring PN, Nicolson MC, Hickish T, et al.Continuous infusional topotecan in advanced breast and non–small-cell lung cancer: no evidence of increased efficacy. Br J Cancer 1997;76:1636–1639.

124. Kindler HL, Kris MG, Smith IE, et al. Phase II trial of topotecan administered as a 21-day continuous infusion in previously untreated patients with stage IIIB and IV non-small-cell lung cancer. Am J Clin Oncol 1998;21:438–441.

125. Gore M, Rustin G, Schuller J, et al. Topotecan given as a 21-day infusion in the treatment of advanced ovarian cancer. Br J Cancer 2001;84:1043–1046.

126. Wall JG, Burris HA 3rd, Von Hoff DD, et al. A phase I clinical and pharmacokinetic study of the topoisomerase I inhibitor topotecan (SK&F 104864) given as an intravenous bolus every 21 days. Anticancer Drugs 1992;3:337–345.

127. Haas NB, LaCreta FP, Walczak J, et al. Phase I/pharmacokinetic study of topotecan by 24-hour continuous infusion weekly. Cancer Res 1994;54:1220–1226.

128. Blaney SM, Balis FM, Cole DE, et al. Pediatric phase I trial and pharmacokinetic study of topotecan administered as a 24-hour continuous infusion. Cancer Res 1993;53:1032–1036.

129. Abbruzzese JL, Madden T, Sugarman SM, et al. Phase I clinical and plasma and cellular pharmacological study of topotecan without and with granulocyte colony-stimulating factor. Clin Cancer Res 1996;2:1489–1497.

130. Burris HA 3rd, Awada A, Kuhn JG, et al. Phase I and pharmacokinetic studies of topotecan administered as a 72 or 120 h continuous infusion. Anticancer Drugs 1994;5:394–402.

131. Pratt CB, Stewart C, Santana VM, et al. Phase I study of topotecan for pediatric patients with malignant solid tumors. J Clin Oncol 1994;12:539–543.

132. Rowinsky EK, Adjei A, Donehower RC, et al. Phase I and pharmacodynamic study of the topoisomerase I-inhibitor topotecan in patients with refractory acute leukemia. J Clin Oncol 1994; 12:2193–2203.

133. Denschlag D, Watermann D, Horig K, et al. Topotecan as a continuous infusion over 14 days in recurrent ovarian cancer patients. Anticancer Res 2004;24:1267–1269.

134. Herben VM, Rosing H, ten Bokkel Huinink WW, et al. Oral topotecan: bioavailability and effect of food co-administration. Br J Cancer 1999;80:1380–1386.

135. Creemers GJ, Gerrits CJ, Eckardt JR, et al. Phase I and pharmacologic study of oral topotecan administered twice daily for 21 days to adult patients with solid tumors. J Clin Oncol 1997;15:1087–1093.

136. Schellens JH, Creemers GJ, Beijnen JH, et al. Bioavailability and pharmacokinetics of oral topotecan: a new topoisomerase I inhibitor. Br J Cancer 1996;73:1268–1271.

137. Beran M, O'Brien S, Thomas DA, et al. Phase I study of oral topotecan in hematological malignancies. Clin Cancer Res 2003; 9:4084–4091.

138. Daw NC, Santana VM, Iacono LC, et al. Phase I and pharmacokinetic study of topotecan administered orally once daily for 5 days for 2 consecutive weeks to pediatric patients with refractory solid tumors. J Clin Oncol 2004;22:829–837.

139. Clarke-Pearson DL, Van Le L, Iveson T, et al. Oral topotecan as single-agent second-line chemotherapy in patients with advanced ovarian cancer. J Clin Oncol 2001;19:3967–3975.

140. von Pawel J, Gatzemeier U, Pujol JL, et al. Phase II comparator study of oral versus intravenous topotecan in patients with chemosensitive small-cell lung cancer. J Clin Oncol 2001;19: 1743–1749.

141. Gore M, Oza A, Rustin G, et al. A randomised trial of oral versus intravenous topotecan in patients with relapsed epithelial ovarian cancer. Eur J Cancer 2002;38:57–63.

142. Plaxe SC, Christen RD, O'Quigley J, et al. Phase I and pharmacokinetic study of intraperitoneal topotecan. Invest New Drugs 1998;16:147–153.

143. Hofstra LS, Bos AM, de Vries EG, et al. A phase I and pharmacokinetic study of intraperitoneal topotecan. Br J Cancer 2001; 85:1627–1633.

144. Blaney SM, Cole DE, Godwin K, et al. Intrathecal administration of topotecan in nonhuman primates. Cancer Chemother Pharmacol 1995;36:121–124.

145. Blaney SM, Heideman R, Berg S, et al. Phase I clinical trial of intrathecal topotecan in patients with neoplastic meningitis. J Clin Oncol 2003;21:143–147.

146. Montazeri A, Culine S, Laguerre B, et al. Individual adaptive dosing of topotecan in ovarian cancer. Clin Cancer Res 2002;8: 394–399.

147. Santana VM, Zamboni WC, Kirstein MN, et al. A pilot study of protracted topotecan dosing using a pharmacokinetically guided dosing approach in children with solid tumors. Clin Cancer Res 2003;9:633–640.

148. Loos WJ, de Bruijn P, Verweij J, et al. Determination of camptothecin analogs in biological matrices by high-performance liquid chromatography. Anticancer Drugs 2000;11:315–324.

149. Beijnen JH, Smith BR, Keijer WJ, et al. High-performance liquid chromatographic analysis of the new antitumour drug SK&F 104864-A (NSC 609699) in plasma. J Pharm Biomed Anal 1990; 8:789–794.

150. Loos WJ, Stoter G, Verweij J, et al. Sensitive high-performance liquid chromatographic fluorescence assay for the quantitation of topotecan (SKF 104864-A) and its lactone ring–opened product (hydroxy acid) in human plasma and urine. J Chromatogr B Biomed Appl 1996;678:309–315.

151. Boucaud M, Pinguet F, Poujol S, et al. Salivary and plasma pharmacokinetics of topotecan in patients with metastatic epithelial ovarian cancer. Eur J Cancer 2001;37:2357–2364.

152. Rosing H, van Zomeren DM, Doyle E, et al. Quantification of topotecan and its metabolite N-desmethyltopotecan in human plasma, urine and faeces by high-performance liquid chromatographic methods. J Chromatogr B Biomed Sci Appl 1999;727: 191–203.

153. Loos WJ, van Zomeren DM, Gelderblom H, et al. Determination of topotecan in human whole blood and unwashed erythrocytes by high-performance liquid chromatography. J Chromatogr B Analyt Technol Biomed Life Sci 2002;766:99–105.

154. Grochow LB, Rowinsky EK, Johnson R, et al. Pharmacokinetics and pharmacodynamics of topotecan in patients with advanced cancer. Drug Metab Dispos 1992;20:706–713.

155. Herben VM, ten Bokkel Huinink WW, Beijnen JH. Clinical pharmacokinetics of topotecan. Clin Pharmacokinet 1996;31:85–102.

156. van Warmerdam LJ, ten Bokkel Huinink WW, Rodenhuis S, et al. Phase I clinical and pharmacokinetic study of topotecan administered by a 24-hour continuous infusion. J Clin Oncol 1995; 13:1768–1776.

157. van Warmerdam LJ, Verweij J, Rosing H, et al. Limited sampling models for topotecan pharmacokinetics. Ann Oncol 1994;5: 259–264.

158. Minami H, Beijnen JH, Verweij J, et al. Limited sampling model for area under the concentration time curve of total topotecan. Clin Cancer Res 1996;2:43–46.

159. van Warmerdam LJ, Creemers GJ, Rodenhuis S, et al. Pharmacokinetics and pharmacodynamics of topotecan given on a daily-times-five schedule in phase II clinical trials using a limited-sampling procedure. Cancer Chemother Pharmacol 1996; 38:254–260.

160. Tubergen DG, Stewart CF, Pratt CB, et al. Phase I trial and pharmacokinetic (PK) and pharmacodynamics (PD) study of topotecan using a five-day course in children with refractory solid tumors: a pediatric oncology group study. J Pediatr Hematol Oncol 1996;18:352–361.

161. Stewart CF, Baker SD, Heideman RL, et al. Clinical pharmacodynamics of continuous infusion topotecan in children: systemic exposure predicts hematologic toxicity. J Clin Oncol 1994;12: 1946–1954.

162. Gallo JM, Laub PB, Rowinsky EK, et al. Population pharmacokinetic model for topotecan derived from phase I clinical trials. J Clin Oncol 2000;18:2459–2467.

163. Montazeri A, Boucaud M, Lokiec F, et al. Population pharmacokinetics of topotecan: intraindividual variability in total drug. Cancer Chemother Pharmacol 2000;46:375–381.

164. Loos WJ, Gelderblom HJ, Verweij J, et al. Gender-dependent pharmacokinetics of topotecan in adult patients. Anticancer Drugs 2000;11:673–680.

165. Loos WJ, Gelderblom H, Sparreboom A, et al. Inter- and intrapatient variability in oral topotecan pharmacokinetics: implications for body-surface area dosage regimens. Clin Cancer Res 2000;6:2685–2689.

166. Mould DR, Holford NH, Schellens JH, et al. Population pharmacokinetic and adverse event analysis of topotecan in patients with solid tumors. Clin Pharmacol Ther 2002;71:334–348.

167. Leger F, Loos WJ, Fourcade J, et al. Factors affecting pharmacokinetic variability of oral topotecan: a population analysis. Br J Cancer 2004;90:343–347.

168. McCabe FL, Johnson RK. Comparative activity of oral and parenteral topotecan in murine tumor models: efficacy of oral topotecan. Cancer Invest 1994;12:308–313.

169. Wagner S, Erdlenbruch B, Langler A, et al. Oral topotecan in children with recurrent or progressive high-grade glioma: a Phase I/II study by the German Society for Pediatric Oncology and Hematology. Cancer 2004;100:1750–1757.

170. Sparreboom A, de Jonge MJ, Verweij J. The use of oral cytotoxic and cytostatic drugs in cancer treatment. Eur J Cancer 2002;38:18–22.

171. Davies BE, Minthorn EA, Dennis MJ, et al. The pharmacokinetics of topotecan and its carboxylate form following separate intravenous administration to the dog. Pharm Res 1997;14:1461–1465.

172. Jonker JW, Smit JW, Brinkhuis RF, et al. Role of breast cancer resistance protein in the bioavailability and fetal penetration of topotecan. J Natl Cancer Inst 2000;92:1651–1656.

173. Liu G, Franssen E, Fitch MI, et al. Patient preferences for oral versus intravenous palliative chemotherapy. J Clin Oncol 1997; 15:110–115.

174. DeMario MD, Ratain MJ. Oral chemotherapy: rationale and future directions. J Clin Oncol 1998;16:2557–2567.

175. Kruijtzer CM, Beijnen JH, Rosing H, et al. Increased oral bioavailability of topotecan in combination with the breast cancer resistance protein and P-glycoprotein inhibitor GF120918. J Clin Oncol 2002;20:2943–2950.

176. Blaney S, Berg SL, Pratt C, et al. A phase I study of irinotecan in pediatric patients: a pediatric oncology group study. Clin Cancer Res 2001;7:32–37.

177. Pratesi G, Tortoreto M, Corti C, et al. Successful local regional therapy with topotecan of intraperitoneally growing human ovarian carcinoma xenografts. Br J Cancer 1995;71:525–528.

178. Blaney SM, Cole DE, Balis FM, et al. Plasma and cerebrospinal fluid pharmacokinetic study of topotecan in nonhuman primates. Cancer Res 1993;53:725–727.

179. Sung C, Blaney SM, Cole DE, et al. A pharmacokinetic model of topotecan clearance from plasma and cerebrospinal fluid. Cancer Res 1994;54:5118–5122.

180. Baker SD, Heideman RL, Crom WR, et al. Cerebrospinal fluid pharmacokinetics and penetration of continuous infusion topotecan in children with central nervous system tumors. Cancer Chemother Pharmacol 1996;37:195–202.

181. Zamboni WC, Luftner DI, Egorin MJ, et al. The effect of increasing topotecan infusion from 30 minutes to 4 hours on the duration of exposure in cerebrospinal fluid. Ann Oncol 2001;12:119–122.

182. Blaney SM, Takimoto C, Murry DJ, et al. Plasma and cerebrospinal fluid pharmacokinetics of 9-aminocamptothecin (9-AC), irinotecan (CPT-11), and SN-38 in nonhuman primates. Cancer Chemother Pharmacol 1998;41:464–468.

183. Gelderblom H, Loos WJ, Verweij J, et al. Topotecan lacks third space sequestration. Clin Cancer Res 2000;6:1288–1292.

184. Rosing H, Herben VM, van Gortel-van Zomeren DM, et al. Isolation and structural confirmation of N-desmethyl topotecan, a metabolite of topotecan. Cancer Chemother Pharmacol 1997;39:498–504.

185. Zamboni WC, Gajjar AJ, Heideman RL, et al. Phenytoin alters the disposition of topotecan and N-desmethyl topotecan in a patient with medulloblastoma. Clin Cancer Res 1998;4:783–789.

186. Zamboni WC, Houghton PJ, Johnson RK, et al. Probenecid alters topotecan systemic and renal disposition by inhibiting renal tubular secretion. J Pharmacol Exp Ther 1998;284:89–94.

187. Rosing H, van Zomeren DM, Doyle E, et al. O-glucuronidation, a newly identified metabolic pathway for topotecan and N-desmethyl topotecan. Anticancer Drugs 1998;9:587–592.

188. O'Reilly S, Rowinsky E, Slichenmyer W, et al. Phase I and pharmacologic studies of topotecan in patients with impaired hepatic function. J Natl Cancer Inst 1996;88:817–824.

189. O'Reilly S, Rowinsky EK, Slichenmyer W, et al. Phase I and pharmacologic study of topotecan in patients with impaired renal function. J Clin Oncol 1996;14:3062–3073.

190. Furman WL, Baker SD, Pratt CB, et al. Escalating systemic exposure of continuous infusion topotecan in children with recurrent acute leukemia. J Clin Oncol 1996;14:1504–1511.

191. Blaney SM, Phillips PC, Packer RJ, et al. Phase II evaluation of topotecan for pediatric central nervous system tumors. Cancer 1996;78:527–531.

192. Herben VM, Schoemaker E, Rosing H, et al. Urinary and fecal excretion of topotecan in patients with malignant solid tumours. Cancer Chemother Pharmacol 2002;50:59–64.

193. Zamboni WC, D'Argenio DZ, Stewart CF, et al. Pharmacodynamic model of topotecan-induced time course of neutropenia. Clin Cancer Res 2001;7:2301–2308.

194. Zamboni WC, Houghton PJ, Hulstein JL, et al. Relationship between tumor extracellular fluid exposure to topotecan and tumor response in human neuroblastoma xenograft and cell lines. Cancer Chemother Pharmacol 1999;43:269–276.

195. Rowinsky EK, Kaufmann SH, Baker SD, et al. Sequences of topotecan and cisplatin: phase I, pharmacologic, and in vitro studies to examine sequence dependence. J Clin Oncol 1996; 14:3074–3084.

196. de Jonge MJ, Loos WJ, Gelderblom H, et al. Phase I pharmacologic study of oral topotecan and intravenous cisplatin: sequence-

dependent hematologic side effects. J Clin Oncol 2000;18: 2104–2115.

197. Gelderblom H, Loos WJ, Sparreboom A, et al. Influence of the cisplatin hydration schedule on topotecan pharmacokinetics. Eur J Cancer 2003;39:1542–1546.

198. Zamboni WC, Egorin MJ, Van Echo DA, et al. Pharmacokinetic and pharmacodynamic study of the combination of docetaxel and topotecan in patients with solid tumors. J Clin Oncol 2000; 18:3288–3294.

199. Brogden RN, Wiseman LR. Topotecan. A review of its potential in advanced ovarian cancer. Drugs 1998;56:709–723.

200. Rowinsky EK, Grochow LB, Hendricks CB, et al. Phase I and pharmacologic study of topotecan: a novel topoisomerase I inhibitor. J Clin Oncol 1992;10:647–656.

201. Schiller JH, Kim K, Hutson P, et al. Phase II study of topotecan in patients with extensive-stage small-cell carcinoma of the lung: an Eastern Cooperative Oncology Group Trial. J Clin Oncol 1996;14:2345–2352.

202. Ardizzoni A, Hansen H, Dombernowsky P, et al. Topotecan, a new active drug in the second-line treatment of small-cell lung cancer: a phase II study in patients with refractory and sensitive disease. The European Organization for Research and Treatment of Cancer Early Clinical Studies Group and New Drug Development Office, and the Lung Cancer Cooperative Group. J Clin Oncol 1997;15:2090–2096.

203. Ardizzoni A, Manegold C, Debruyne C, et al. European Organization for Research and Treatment of Cancer (EORTC) 08957 phase II study of topotecan in combination with cisplatin as second-line treatment of refractory and sensitive small cell lung cancer. Clin Cancer Res 2003;9:143–150.

204. ten Bokkel Huinink W, Gore M, Carmichael J, et al. Topotecan versus paclitaxel for the treatment of recurrent epithelial ovarian cancer. J Clin Oncol 1997;15:2183–2193.

205. ten Bokkel Huinink W, Carmichael J, Armstrong D, et al. Efficacy and safety of topotecan in the treatment of advanced ovarian carcinoma. Semin Oncol 1997;24:S5-19–S15-25.

206. Creemers GJ, Gerrits CJ, Schellens JH, et al. Phase II and pharmacologic study of topotecan administered as a 21-day continuous infusion to patients with colorectal cancer. J Clin Oncol 1996;14:2540–2545.

207. Kudelka AP, Tresukosol D, Edwards CL, et al. Phase II study of intravenous topotecan as a 5-day infusion for refractory epithelial ovarian carcinoma. J Clin Oncol 1996;14:1552–1557.

208. Rose PG, Gordon NH, Fusco N, et al. A phase II and pharmacokinetic study of weekly 72-h topotecan infusion in patients with platinum-resistant and paclitaxel-resistant ovarian carcinoma. Gynecol Oncol 2000;78:228–234.

209. Markman M, Blessing JA, DeGeest K, et al. Lack of efficacy of 24-h infusional topotecan in platinum-refractory ovarian cancer: a Gynecologic Oncology Group trial. Gynecol Oncol 1999;75: 444–446.

210. Markman M, Blessing JA, Alvarez RD, et al. Phase II evaluation of 24-h continuous infusion topotecan in recurrent, potentially platinum-sensitive ovarian cancer: a Gynecologic Oncology Group study. Gynecol Oncol 2000;77:112–115.

211. Lynch TJ Jr, Kalish L, Strauss G, et al. Phase II study of topotecan in metastatic non-small-cell lung cancer. J Clin Oncol 1994;12: 347–352.

212. Perez EA, Hillman DW, Mailliard JA, et al. Randomized phase II study of two irinotecan schedules for patients with metastatic breast cancer refractory to an anthracycline, a taxane, or both. J Clin Oncol 2004;22:2849–2855.

213. Perez-Soler R, Fossella FV, Glisson BS, et al. Phase II study of topotecan in patients with advanced non-small-cell lung cancer previously untreated with chemotherapy. J Clin Oncol 1996;14: 503–513.

214. Creemers GJ, Wanders J, Gamucci T, et al. Topotecan in colorectal cancer: a phase II study of the EORTC Early Clinical Trials Group. Ann Oncol 1995;6:844–846.

215. Macdonald D, Cairncross G, Stewart D, et al. Phase II study of topotecan in patients with recurrent malignant glioma. National Clinical Institute of Canada Clinical Trials Group. Ann Oncol 1996;7:205–207.

216. Macdonald JS, Benedetti JK, Modiano M, et al. Phase II evaluation of topotecan in patients with advanced colorectal cancer: a

Southwest Oncology Group trial (SWOG 9241). Invest New Drugs 1997;15:357–359.

217. Macdonald JS, Jacobson JL, Ketchel SJ, et al. A phase II trial of topotecan in esophageal carcinoma: a Southwest Oncology Group study (SWOG 9339). Invest New Drugs 2000;18:199–202.

218. Maksymiuk AW, Marschke RF Jr, Tazelaar HD, et al. Phase II trial of topotecan for the treatment of mesothelioma. Am J Clin Oncol 1998;21:610–613.

219. Murphy BA, Leong T, Burkey B, et al. Lack of efficacy of topotecan in the treatment of metastatic or recurrent squamous carcinoma of the head and neck: an Eastern Cooperative Oncology Group trial (E3393). Am J Clin Oncol 2001;24:64–66.

220. Miller DS, Blessing JA, Kilgore LC, et al. Phase II trial of topotecan in patients with advanced, persistent, or recurrent uterine leiomyosarcomas: a Gynecologic Oncology Group study. Am J Clin Oncol 2000;23:355–357.

221. Weitz JJ, Marschke RF Jr, Sloan JA, et al. A randomized phase II trial of two schedules of topotecan for the treatment of advanced stage non-small cell lung cancer. Lung Cancer 2000; 28:157–162.

222. Levine EG, Cirrincione CT, Szatrowski TP, et al. Phase II trial of topotecan in advanced breast cancer: a Cancer and Leukemia Group B study. Am J Clin Oncol 1999;22:218–222.

223. Witte RS, Manola J, Burch PA, et al. Topotecan in previously treated advanced urothelial carcinoma: an ECOG phase II trial. Invest New Drugs 1998;16:191–195.

224. Stevenson JP, Scher RM, Kosierowski R, et al. Phase II trial of topotecan as a 21-day continuous infusion in patients with advanced or metastatic adenocarcinoma of the pancreas. Eur J Cancer 1998;34:1358–1362.

225. Saltz LB, Schwartz GK, Ilson DH, et al. A phase II study of topotecan administered five times daily in patients with advanced gastric cancer. Am J Clin Oncol 1997;20:621–625.

226. Benedetti JK, Burris HA 3rd, Balcerzak SP, et al. Phase II trial of topotecan in advanced gastric cancer: a Southwest Oncology Group study. Invest New Drugs 1997;15:261–264.

227. Wall JG, Benedetti JK, O'Rourke MA, et al. Phase II trial of topotecan in hepatocellular carcinoma: a Southwest Oncology Group study. Invest New Drugs 1997;15:257–260.

228. Kraut EH, Walker MJ, Staubus A, et al. Phase II trial of topotecan in malignant melanoma. Cancer Invest 1997;15:318–320.

229. Kraut EH, Crowley JJ, Wade JL, et al. Evaluation of topotecan in resistant and relapsing multiple myeloma: a Southwest Oncology Group study. J Clin Oncol 1998;16:589–592.

230. O'Reilly S, Donehower RC, Rowinsky EK, et al. A phase II trial of topotecan in patients with previously untreated pancreatic cancer. Anticancer Drugs 1996;7:410–414.

231. Scher RM, Kosierowski R, Lusch C, et al. Phase II trial of topotecan in advanced or metastatic adenocarcinoma of the pancreas. Invest New Drugs 1996;13:347–354.

232. Armstrong D, O'Reilly S. Clinical guidelines for managing topotecan-related hematologic toxicity. Oncologist 1998;3:4–10.

233. Heron JF. Topotecan: an oncologist's view. Oncologist 1998;3: 390–402.

234. Hochster H, Liebes L, Speyer J, et al. Effect of prolonged topotecan infusion on topoisomerase 1 levels: a phase I and pharmacodynamic study. Clin Cancer Res 1997;3:1245–1252.

235. Gerrits CJ, Burris H, Schellens JH, et al. Oral topotecan given once or twice daily for ten days: a phase I pharmacology study in adult patients with solid tumors. Clin Cancer Res 1998;4:1153–1158.

236. Gerrits CJ, Burris H, Schellens JH, et al. Five days of oral topotecan (Hycamtin), a phase I and pharmacological study in adult patients with solid tumours. Eur J Cancer 1998;34:1030–1035.

237. Baker SD, Verweij J, Rowinsky EK, et al. Role of body surface area in dosing of investigational anticancer agents in adults, 1991–2001. J Natl Cancer Inst 2002;94:1883–1888.

238. Gelderblom HA, de Jonge MJ, Sparreboom A, et al. Oral topoisomerase 1 inhibitors in adult patients: present and future. Invest New Drugs 1999;17:401–415.

239. Gerrits CJ, Schellens JH, Burris H, et al. A comparison of clinical pharmacodynamics of different administration schedules of oral topotecan (Hycamtin). Clin Cancer Res 1999;5:69–75.

240. Rowinsky EK, Grochow LB, Sartorius SE, et al. Phase I and pharmacologic study of high doses of the topoisomerase I inhibitor

topotecan with granulocyte colony-stimulating factor in patients with solid tumors. J Clin Oncol 1996;14:1224–1235.

241. Greco FA. Topotecan as first-line therapy for small cell lung cancer. Lung Cancer 2003;41(Suppl 4):S9–16.

242. Greco FA, Hainsworth JD. Emerging role of topotecan in first-line therapy of small-cell lung cancer. Clin Lung Cancer 2003; 4:279–287.

243. Eckardt J. Single-agent chemotherapy for non-small cell lung cancer. Lung Cancer 2003;41(Suppl 4):S17–22.

244. Kollmannsberger C, Mross K, Jakob A, et al. Topotecan: a novel topoisomerase I inhibitor: pharmacology and clinical experience. Oncology 1999;56:1–12.

245. Gore SD, Rowinsky EK, Miller CB, et al. A phase II "window" study of topotecan in untreated patients with high risk adult acute lymphoblastic leukemia. Clin Cancer Res 1998;4:2677–2689.

246. Takimoto CH, Arbuck SG. Topoisomerase I inhibitors. In: Chabner BA, Longo DL, eds., Cancer Chemotherapy and Biotherapy: Principles and Practice, 3rd ed. Philadelphia: Lippincott Williams & Wilkins, 2001:579–646.

247. Robert F, Soong SJ, Wheeler RH. A phase II study of topotecan in patients with recurrent head and neck cancer: identification of an active new agent. Am J Clin Oncol 1997;20:298–302.

248. Hudes GR, Kosierowski R, Greenberg R, et al. Phase II study of topotecan in metastatic hormone-refractory prostate cancer. Invest New Drugs 1995;13:235–240.

249. De Placido S, Scambia G, Di Vagno G, et al. Topotecan compared with no therapy after response to surgery and carboplatin/paclitaxel in patients with ovarian cancer: Multicenter Italian Trials in Ovarian Cancer (MITO-1) randomized study. J Clin Oncol 2004;22:2635–2642.

250. ten Bokkel Huinink W, Lane SR, Ross GA. Long-term survival in a phase III, randomised study of topotecan versus paclitaxel in advanced epithelial ovarian carcinoma. Ann Oncol 2004;15: 100–103.

251. von Pawel J, Schiller JH, Shepherd FA, et al. Topotecan versus cyclophosphamide, doxorubicin, and vincristine for the treatment of recurrent small-cell lung cancer. J Clin Oncol 1999; 17:658–667.

252. Garcia-Carbonero R, Supko JG. Current perspectives on the clinical experience, pharmacology, and continued development of the camptothecins. Clin Cancer Res 2002;8:641–661.

253. Kantarjian H. New advances in the treatment of hematologic malignancies: focus on topoisomerase I inhibitors: introduction. Semin Hematol 1998;35:1–2.

254. Beran M, Kantarjian H, O'Brien S, et al. Topotecan, a topoisomerase I inhibitor, is active in the treatment of myelodysplastic syndrome and chronic myelomonocytic leukemia. Blood 1996; 88:2473–2479.

255. Kaneda N, Nagata H, Furuta T, et al. Metabolism and pharmacokinetics of the camptothecin analogue CPT-11 in the mouse. Cancer Res 1990;50:1715–1720.

256. Kawato Y, Aonuma M, Hirota Y, et al. Intracellular roles of SN-38, a metabolite of the camptothecin derivative CPT-11, in the antitumor effect of CPT-11. Cancer Res 1991;51:4187–4191.

257. Mathijssen RH, van Alphen RJ, Verweij J, et al. Clinical pharmacokinetics and metabolism of irinotecan (CPT-11). Clin Cancer Res 2001;7:2182–2194.

258. Fuchs CS, Moore MR, Harker G, et al. Phase III comparison of two irinotecan dosing regimens in second-line therapy of metastatic colorectal cancer. J Clin Oncol 2003;21:807–814.

259. Catimel G, Chabot GG, Guastalla JP, et al. Phase I and pharmacokinetic study of irinotecan (CPT-11) administered daily for three consecutive days every three weeks in patients with advanced solid tumors. Ann Oncol 1995;6:133–140.

260. Rothenberg ML, Kuhn JG, Schaaf LJ, et al. Alternative dosing schedules for irinotecan. Oncology (Huntingt) 1998;12:68–71.

261. Furman WL, Stewart CF, Poquette CA, et al. Direct translation of a protracted irinotecan schedule from a xenograft model to a phase I trial in children. J Clin Oncol 1999;17:1815-1824.

262. Takimoto CH, Morrison G, Harold N, et al. Phase I and pharmacologic study of irinotecan administered as a 96-hour infusion weekly to adult cancer patients. J Clin Oncol 2000;18:659–667.

263. Masi G, Falcone A, Di Paolo A, et al. A phase I and pharmacokinetic study of irinotecan given as a 7-day continuous infusion in

metastatic colorectal cancer patients pretreated with 5-fluorouracil or raltitrexed. Clin Cancer Res 2004;10:1657–1663.

264. Herben VM, Schellens JH, Swart M, et al. Phase I and pharmacokinetic study of irinotecan administered as a low-dose, continuous intravenous infusion over 14 days in patients with malignant solid tumors. J Clin Oncol 1999;17:1897–1905.

265. Guichard S, Chatelut E, Lochon I, et al. Comparison of the pharmacokinetics and efficacy of irinotecan after administration by the intravenous versus intraperitoneal route in mice. Cancer Chemother Pharmacol 1998;42:165–170.

266. Choi SH, Tsuchida Y, Yang HW. Oral versus intraperitoneal administration of irinotecan in the treatment of human neuroblastoma in nude mice. Cancer Lett 1998;124:15–21.

267. van Riel JM, van Groeningen CJ, Kedde MA, et al. Continuous administration of irinotecan by hepatic arterial infusion: a phase I and pharmacokinetic study. Clin Cancer Res 2002;8:405–412.

268. Thompson J, Zamboni WC, Cheshire PJ, et al. Efficacy of oral irinotecan against neuroblastoma xenografts. Anticancer Drugs 1997;8:313–322.

269. Stewart CF, Zamboni WC, Crom WR, et al. Disposition of irinotecan and SN-38 following oral and intravenous irinotecan dosing in mice. Cancer Chemother Pharmacol 1997;40:259–265.

270. Zamboni WC, Houghton PJ, Thompson J, et al. Altered irinotecan and SN-38 disposition after intravenous and oral administration of irinotecan in mice bearing human neuroblastoma xenografts. Clin Cancer Res 1998;4:455–462.

271. Drengler RL, Kuhn JG, Schaaf LJ, et al. Phase I and pharmacokinetic trial of oral irinotecan administered daily for 5 days every 3 weeks in patients with solid tumors. J Clin Oncol 1999;17:685–696.

272. Gupta E, Vyas V, Ahmed F, et al. Pharmacokinetics of orally administered camptothecins. Ann NY Acad Sci 2000;922:195–204.

273. Hanioka N, Jinno H, Nishimura T, et al. High-performance liquid chromatographic assay for glucuronidation activity of 7-ethyl-10-hydroxycamptothecin (SN-38), the active metabolite of irinotecan (CPT-11), in human liver microsomes. Biomed Chromatogr 2001;15:328–333.

274. Sparreboom A, de Bruijn P, de Jonge MJ, et al. Liquid chromatographic determination of irinotecan and three major metabolites in human plasma, urine and feces. J Chromatogr B Biomed Sci App 1998;712:225–235.

275. Owens TS, Dodds H, Fricke K, et al. High-performance liquid chromatographic assay with fluorescence detection for the simultaneous measurement of carboxylate and lactone forms of irinotecan and three metabolites in human plasma. J Chromatogr B Analyt Technol Biomed Life Sci 2003;788:65–74.

276. Poujol S, Pinguet F, Malosse F, et al. Sensitive HPLC-fluorescence method for irinotecan and four major metabolites in human plasma and saliva: application to pharmacokinetic studies. Clin Chem 2003;49:1900–1908.

277. de Jong FA, Mathijssen RH, de Bruijn P, et al. Determination of irinotecan (CPT-11) and SN-38 in human whole blood and red blood cells by liquid chromatography with fluorescence detection. J Chromatogr B Analyt Technol Biomed Life Sci 2003;795: 383–388.

278. Rothenberg ML, Kuhn JG, Burris HA 3rd, et al. Phase I and pharmacokinetic trial of weekly CPT-11. J Clin Oncol 1993;11:2194–2204.

279. Abigerges D, Chabot GG, Armand JP, et al. Phase I and pharmacologic studies of the camptothecin analog irinotecan administered every 3 weeks in cancer patients. J Clin Oncol 1995;13:210–221.

280. Rowinsky EK, Grochow LB, Ettinger DS, et al. Phase I and pharmacological study of the novel topoisomerase I inhibitor 7-ethyl-10-[4-(1-piperidino)-1-piperidino]carbonyloxycamptothecin (CPT-11) administered as a ninety-minute infusion every 3 weeks. Cancer Res 1994;54:427–436.

281. Ohe Y, Sasaki Y, Shinkai T, et al. Phase I study and pharmacokinetics of CPT-11 with 5-day continuous infusion. J Natl Cancer Inst 1992;84:972–974.

282. Negoro S, Fukuoka M, Masuda N, et al. Phase I study of weekly intravenous infusions of CPT-11, a new derivative of camptothecin, in the treatment of advanced non-small-cell lung cancer. J Natl Cancer Inst 1991;83:1164–1168.

283. Mathijssen RH, Verweij J, de Jonge MJ, et al. Impact of body-size measures on irinotecan clearance: alternative dosing recommendations. J Clin Oncol 2002;20:81–87.

284. de Jong FA, Mathijssen RH, Xie R, et al. Flat-fixed dosing of irinotecan: influence on pharmacokinetic and pharmacodynamic variability. Clin Cancer Res 2004;10:4068–4071.

285. Atsumi R, Okazaki O, Hakusui H. Pharmacokinetics of SN-38 [(+)-(4S)-4,11-diethyl-4,9-dihydroxy-1H-pyrano[3′,4′:6,7]-indolizino[1,2-b]quinoline-3,14(4H,12H)-dione], an active metabolite of irinotecan, after a single intravenous dosing of 14C-SN-38 to rats. Biol Pharm Bull 1995;18:1114–1119.

286. Kaneda N, Hosokawa Y, Yokokura T, et al. Plasma pharmacokinetics of 7-ethyl-10-hydroxycamptothecin (SN-38) after intravenous administration of SN-38 and irinotecan (CPT-11) to rats. Biol Pharm Bull 1997;20:992–996.

287. Chabot GG, Abigerges D, Catimel G, et al. Population pharmacokinetics and pharmacodynamics of irinotecan (CPT-11) and active metabolite SN-38 during phase I trials. Ann Oncol 1995;6:141–151.

288. Gupta E, Mick R, Ramirez J, et al. Pharmacokinetic and pharmacodynamic evaluation of the topoisomerase inhibitor irinotecan in cancer patients. J Clin Oncol 1997;15:1502–1510.

289. Meyerhardt JA, Kwok A, Ratain MJ, et al. Relationship of baseline serum bilirubin to efficacy and toxicity of single-agent irinotecan in patients with metastatic colorectal cancer. J Clin Oncol 2004;22:1439–1446.

290. Xie R, Mathijssen RH, Sparreboom A, et al. Clinical pharmacokinetics of irinotecan and its metabolites: a population analysis. J Clin Oncol 2002;20:3293–3301.

291. Klein CE, Gupta E, Reid JM, et al. Population pharmacokinetic model for irinotecan and two of its metabolites, SN-38 and SN-38 glucuronide. Clin Pharmacol Ther 2002;72:638–647.

292. Yamamoto N, Tamura T, Karato A, et al. CPT-11: population pharmacokinetic model and estimation of pharmacokinetics using the Bayesian method in patients with lung cancer. Jpn J Cancer Res 1994;85:972–977.

293. Yamamoto N, Tamura T, Nishiwaki Y, et al. Limited sampling model for the area under the concentration versus time curve of irinotecan and its application to a multicentric phase II trial. Clin Cancer Res 1997;3:1087–1092.

294. Nakashima H, Lieberman R, Karato A, et al. Efficient sampling strategies for forecasting pharmacokinetic parameters of irinotecan (CPT-11): implication for area under the concentration-time curve monitoring. Ther Drug Monit 1995;17:221–229.

295. Sasaki Y, Mizuno S, Fujii H, et al. A limited sampling model for estimating pharmacokinetics of CPT-11 and its metabolite SN-38. Jpn J Cancer Res 1995;86:117–123.

296. Chabot GG. Limited sampling models for simultaneous estimation of the pharmacokinetics of irinotecan and its active metabolite SN-38. Cancer Chemother Pharmacol 1995;36:463–472.

297. Mathijssen RH, van Alphen RJ, de Jonge MJ, et al. Sparse-data set analysis for irinotecan and SN-38 pharmacokinetics in cancer patients co-treated with cisplatin. Anticancer Drugs 1999;10:9–16.

298. Sloan JA, Atherton P, Reid J, et al. Limited sampling models for CPT-11, SN-38, and SN-38 glucuronide. Cancer Chemother Pharmacol 2001;48:241–249.

299. Canal P, Gay C, Dezeuze A, et al. Pharmacokinetics and pharmacodynamics of irinotecan during a phase II clinical trial in colorectal cancer. Pharmacology and Molecular Mechanisms Group of the European Organization for Research and Treatment of Cancer. J Clin Oncol 1996;14:2688–2695.

300. Combes O, Barre J, Duche JC, et al. In vitro binding and partitioning of irinotecan (CPT-11) and its metabolite, SN-38, in human blood. Invest New Drugs 2000;18:1–5.

301. Kehrer DF, Yamamoto W, Verweij J, et al. Factors involved in prolongation of the terminal disposition phase of SN-38: clinical and experimental studies. Clin Cancer Res 2000;6:3451–3458.

302. Sasaki Y, Yoshida Y, Sudoh K, et al. Pharmacological correlation between total drug concentration and lactones of CPT-11 and SN-38 in patients treated with CPT-11. Jpn J Cancer Res 1995;86:111–116.

303. Kawato Y, Furuta T, Aonuma M, et al. Antitumor activity of a camptothecin derivative, CPT-11, against human tumor xenografts in nude mice. Cancer Chemother Pharmacol 1991;28:192–198.

304. Kunimoto T, Nitta K, Tanaka T, et al. Antitumor activity of 7-ethyl-10-[4-(1-piperidino)-1-piperidino]carbonyloxy-camptothecin, a novel water-soluble derivative of camptothecin, against murine tumors. Cancer Res 1987;47:5944–5947.

305. Verschraegen CF, Jaeckle K, Giovanella B, et al. Alternative administration of camptothecin analogues. Ann NY Acad Sci 2000;922:237–246.

306. Matsui A, Okuda M, Tsujitsuka K, et al. Pharmacology of intraperitoneal CPT-11. Surg Oncol Clin N Am 2003;12:795–811, xv.

307. Araki E, Ishikawa M, Iigo M, et al. Relationship between development of diarrhea and the concentration of SN-38, an active metabolite of CPT-11, in the intestine and the blood plasma of athymic mice following intraperitoneal administration of CPT-11. Jpn J Cancer Res 1993;84:697–702.

308. Nakano T, Chahinian AP, Shinjo M, et al. Cisplatin in combination with irinotecan in the treatment of patients with malignant pleural mesothelioma: a pilot phase II clinical trial and pharmacokinetic profile. Cancer 1999;85:2375–2384.

309. Rivory LP, Haaz MC, Canal P, et al. Pharmacokinetic interrelationships of irinotecan (CPT-11) and its three major plasma metabolites in patients enrolled in phase I/II trials. Clin Cancer Res 1997;3:1261–1266.

310. Tsuji T, Kaneda N, Kado K, et al. CPT-11 converting enzyme from rat serum: purification and some properties. J Pharmacobiodyn 1991;14:341–349.

311. Sasaki Y, Hakusui H, Mizuno S, et al. A pharmacokinetic and pharmacodynamic analysis of CPT-11 and its active metabolite SN-38. Jpn J Cancer Res 1995;86:101–110.

312. Guemei AA, Cottrell J, Band R, et al. Human plasma carboxylesterase and butyrylcholinesterase enzyme activity: correlations with SN-38 pharmacokinetics during a prolonged infusion of irinotecan. Cancer Chemother Pharmacol 2001;47:283–290.

313. Shingyoji M, Takiguchi Y, Watanabe-Uruma R, et al. In vitro conversion of irinotecan to SN-38 in human plasma. Cancer Sci 2004;95:537–540.

314. Satoh T, Hosokawa M, Atsumi R, et al. Metabolic activation of CPT-11, 7-ethyl-10-[4-(1-piperidino)-1- piperidino]carbonyloxy-camptothecin, a novel antitumor agent, by carboxylesterase. Biol Pharm Bull 1994;17:662–664.

315. Bencharit S, Morton CL, Howard-Williams EL, et al. Structural insights into CPT-11 activation by mammalian carboxylesterases. Nat Struct Biol 2002;9:337–342.

316. Sanghani SP, Quinney SK, Fredenburg TB, et al. Hydrolysis of irinotecan and its oxidative metabolites, 7-ethyl-10-[4-N-(5-aminopentanoic acid)-1-piperidino] carbonyloxycamptothecin and 7-ethyl-10-[4-(1-piperidino)-1-amino]-carbonyloxycamptothecin, by human carboxylesterases CES1A1, CES2, and a newly expressed carboxylesterase isoenzyme, CES3. Drug Metab Dispos 2004;32:505–511.

317. Danks MK, Morton CL, Krull EJ, et al. Comparison of activation of CPT-11 by rabbit and human carboxylesterases for use in enzyme/prodrug therapy. Clin Cancer Res 1999;5:917–924.

318. Hosokawa M, Endo T, Fujisawa M, et al. Interindividual variation in carboxylesterase levels in human liver microsomes. Drug Metab Dispos 1995;23:1022–1027.

319. Khanna R, Morton CL, Danks MK, et al. Proficient metabolism of irinotecan by a human intestinal carboxylesterase. Cancer Res 2000;60:4725–4728.

320. Kaneda N, Kurita A, Hosokawa Y, et al. Intravenous administration of irinotecan elevates the blood beta-glucuronidase activity in rats. Cancer Res 1997;57:5305–5308.

321. Haaz MC, Rivory LP, Riche C, et al. The transformation of irinotecan (CPT-11) to its active metabolite SN-38 by human liver microsomes: differential hydrolysis for the lactone and carboxylate forms. Naunyn Schmiedebergs Arch Pharmacol 1997;356:257–262.

322. Atsumi R, Okazaki O, Hakusui H. Metabolism of irinotecan to SN-38 in a tissue-isolated tumor model. Biol Pharm Bull 1995;18:1024–1026.

323. Guichard S, Terret C, Hennebelle I, et al. CPT-11 converting carboxylesterase and topoisomerase activities in tumour and normal colon and liver tissues. Br J Cancer 1999;80:364–370.

324. Ogasawara H, Nishio K, Kanzawa F, et al. Intracellular carboxyl esterase activity is a determinant of cellular sensitivity to the antineoplastic agent KW-2189 in cell lines resistant to cisplatin and CPT-11. Jpn J Cancer Res 1995;86:124–129.

325. van Ark-Otte J, Kedde MA, van der Vijgh WJ, et al. Determinants of CPT-11 and SN-38 activities in human lung cancer cells. Br J Cancer 1998;77:2171–2176.

326. Meck MM, Wierdl M, Wagner LM, et al. A virus-directed enzyme prodrug therapy approach to purging neuroblastoma cells from hematopoietic cells using adenovirus encoding rabbit carboxylesterase and CPT-11. Cancer Res 2001;61:5083–5089.

327. Wierdl M, Morton CL, Weeks JK, et al. Sensitization of human tumor cells to CPT-11 via adenoviral-mediated delivery of a rabbit liver carboxylesterase. Cancer Res 2001;61:5078–5082.

328. Stubdal H, Perin N, Lemmon M, et al. A prodrug strategy using ONYX-015-based replicating adenoviruses to deliver rabbit carboxylesterase to tumor cells for conversion of CPT-11 to SN-38. Cancer Res 2003;63:6900–6908.

329. Sai K, Kaniwa N, Ozawa S, et al. A new metabolite of irinotecan in which formation is mediated by human hepatic cytochrome P-450 3A4. Drug Metab Dispos 2001;29:1505–1513.

330. Haaz MC, Rivory L, Riche C, et al. Metabolism of irinotecan (CPT-11) by human hepatic microsomes: participation of cytochrome P-450 3A and drug interactions. Cancer Res 1998; 58:468–472.

331. Rivory LP, Riou JF, Haaz MC, et al. Identification and properties of a major plasma metabolite of irinotecan (CPT-11) isolated from the plasma of patients. Cancer Res 1996;56:3689–3694.

332. Dodds HM, Haaz MC, Riou JF, et al. Identification of a new metabolite of CPT-11 (irinotecan): pharmacological properties and activation to SN-38. J Pharmacol Exp Ther 1998;286: 578–583.

333. Haaz MC, Riche C, Rivory LP, et al. Biosynthesis of an aminopiperidino metabolite of irinotecan [7-ethyl-10-[4-(1-piperidino)-1-piperidino]carbonyloxycamptothecine] by human hepatic microsomes. Drug Metab Dispos 1998;26:769–774.

334. Lokiec F, du Sorbier BM, Sanderink GJ. Irinotecan (CPT-11) metabolites in human bile and urine. Clin Cancer Res 1996;2: 1943–1949.

335. Santos A, Zanetta S, Cresteil T, et al. Metabolism of irinotecan (CPT-11) by CYP3A4 and CYP3A5 in humans. Clin Cancer Res 2000;6:2012–2020.

336. Xie HG, Wood AJ, Kim RB, et al. Genetic variability in CYP3A5 and its possible consequences. Pharmacogenomics 2004;5: 243–272.

337. Mathijssen RH, Marsh S, Karlsson MO, et al. Irinotecan pathway genotype analysis to predict pharmacokinetics. Clin Cancer Res 2003;9:3246–3253.

338. Friedman HS, Petros WP, Friedman AH, et al. Irinotecan therapy in adults with recurrent or progressive malignant glioma. J Clin Oncol 1999;17:1516–1525.

339. Crews KR, Stewart CF, Jones-Wallace D, et al. Altered irinotecan pharmacokinetics in pediatric high-grade glioma patients receiving enzyme-inducing anticonvulsant therapy. Clin Cancer Res 2002;8:2202–2209.

340. Kuhn JG. Influence of anticonvulsants on the metabolism and elimination of irinotecan: a North American Brain Tumor Consortium preliminary report. Oncology (Huntingt) 2002;16: 33–40.

341. Mathijssen RH, Sparreboom A, Dumez H, et al. Altered irinotecan metabolism in a patient receiving phenytoin. Anticancer Drugs 2002;13:139–140.

342. Murry DJ, Cherrick I, Salama V, et al. Influence of phenytoin on the disposition of irinotecan: a case report. J Pediatr Hematol Oncol 2002;24:130–133.

343. Buckner JC, Reid JM, Wright K, et al. Irinotecan in the treatment of glioma patients: current and future studies of the North Central Cancer Treatment Group. Cancer 2003;97:2352–2358.

344. Cloughesy TF, Filka E, Kuhn J, et al. Two studies evaluating irinotecan treatment for recurrent malignant glioma using an every-3-week regimen. Cancer 2003;97:2381–2386.

345. Gajjar A, Chintagumpala MM, Bowers DC, et al. Effect of intrapatient dosage escalation of irinotecan on its pharmacokinetics in pediatric patients who have high-grade gliomas and receive enzyme-inducing anticonvulsant therapy. Cancer 2003; 97:2374–2380.

346. Gilbert MR, Supko JG, Batchelor T, et al. Phase I clinical and pharmacokinetic study of irinotecan in adults with recurrent malignant glioma. Clin Cancer Res 2003;9:2940–2949.

347. Cloughesy TF, Filka E, Nelson G, et al. Irinotecan treatment for recurrent malignant glioma using an every-3-week regimen. Am J Clin Oncol 2002;25:204–208.

348. Raymond E, Fabbro M, Boige V, et al. Multicentre phase II study and pharmacokinetic analysis of irinotecan in chemotherapy-naive patients with glioblastoma. Ann Oncol 2003;14:603–614.

349. Mathijssen RH, Verweij J, de Bruijn P, et al. Effects of St. John's wort on irinotecan metabolism. J Natl Cancer Inst 2002;94: 1247–1249.

350. Kehrer DF, Mathijssen RH, Verweij J, et al. Modulation of irinotecan metabolism by ketoconazole. J Clin Oncol 2002;20: 3122–3129.

351. Chester JD, Joel SP, Cheeseman SL, et al. Phase I and pharmacokinetic study of intravenous irinotecan plus oral ciclosporin in patients with fluorouracil-refractory metastatic colon cancer. J Clin Oncol 2003;21:1125–1132.

352. Hanioka N, Ozawa S, Jinno H, et al. Interaction of irinotecan (CPT-11) and its active metabolite 7-ethyl-10-hydroxycamptothecin (SN-38) with human cytochrome P450 enzymes. Drug Metab Dispos 2002;30:391–396.

353. Rivory LP, Robert J. Identification and kinetics of a beta-glucuronide metabolite of SN-38 in human plasma after administration of the camptothecin derivative irinotecan. Cancer Chemother Pharmacol 1995;36:176–179.

354. Lokiec F, Canal P, Gay C, et al. Pharmacokinetics of irinotecan and its metabolites in human blood, bile, and urine. Cancer Chemother Pharmacol 1995;36:79–82.

355. Gupta E, Wang X, Ramirez J, et al. Modulation of glucuronidation of SN-38, the active metabolite of irinotecan, by valproic acid and phenobarbital. Cancer Chemother Pharmacol 1997;39: 440–444.

356. Iyer L, King CD, Whitington PF, et al. Genetic predisposition to the metabolism of irinotecan (CPT-11): role of uridine diphosphate glucuronosyltransferase isoform 1A1 in the glucuronidation of its active metabolite (SN-38) in human liver microsomes. J Clin Invest 1998;101:847–854.

357. Iyer L, Hall D, Das S, et al. Phenotype-genotype correlation in vitro SN-38 (active metabolite of irinotecan) and bilirubin glucuronidation in human liver tissue with UGT1A1 promoter polymorphism. Clin Pharmacol Ther 1999;65:576–582.

358. Ando Y, Saka H, Ando M, et al. Polymorphisms of UDP-glucuronosyltransferase gene and irinotecan toxicity: a pharmacogenetic analysis. Cancer Res 2000;60:6921–6926.

359. Iyer L, Das S, Janisch L, et al. UGT1A1*28 polymorphism as a determinant of irinotecan disposition and toxicity. Pharmacogenomics J 2002;2:43–47.

360. Ando Y, Ueoka H, Sugiyama T, et al. Polymorphisms of UDP-glucuronosyltransferase and pharmacokinetics of irinotecan. Ther Drug Monit 2002;24:111–116.

361. Gagne JF, Montminy V, Belanger P, et al. Common human UGT1A polymorphisms and the altered metabolism of irinotecan active metabolite 7-ethyl-10-hydroxycamptothecin (SN-38). Mol Pharmacol 2002;62:608–617.

362. Toffoli G, Cecchin E, Corona G, et al. Pharmacogenetics of irinotecan. Curr Med Chem Anti-Canc Agents 2003;3:225–237.

363. Innocenti F, Undevia SD, Iyer L, et al. Genetic variants in the UDP-glucuronosyltransferase 1A1 gene predict the risk of severe neutropenia of irinotecan. J Clin Oncol 2004;22:1382–1388.

364. Sai K, Saeki M, Saito Y, et al. UGT1A1 haplotypes associated with reduced glucuronidation and increased serum bilirubin in irinotecan-administered Japanese patients with cancer. Clin Pharmacol Ther 2004;75:501–515.

365. Takasuna K, Kasai Y, Kitano Y, et al. Protective effects of kampo medicines and baicalin against intestinal toxicity of a new anticancer camptothecin derivative, irinotecan hydrochloride (CPT-11), in rats. Jpn J Cancer Res 1995;86:978–984.

366. Takasuna K, Hagiwara T, Hirohashi M, et al. Involvement of beta-glucuronidase in intestinal microflora in the intestinal toxicity of the antitumor camptothecin derivative irinotecan hydrochloride (CPT-11) in rats. Cancer Res 1996;56:3752–3757.

367. Takasuna K, Hagiwara T, Hirohashi M, et al. Inhibition of intestinal microflora beta-glucuronidase modifies the distribution of the active metabolite of the antitumor agent irinotecan hydrochloride (CPT-11) in rats. Cancer Chemother Pharmacol 1998;42: 280–286.

368. Kehrer DF, Sparreboom A, Verweij J, et al. Modulation of irinotecan-induced diarrhea by cotreatment with neomycin in cancer patients. Clin Cancer Res 2001;7:1136–1141.

369. Chu XY, Kato Y, Niinuma K, et al. Multispecific organic anion transporter is responsible for the biliary excretion of the camptothecin derivative irinotecan and its metabolites in rats. J Pharmacol Exp Ther 1997;281:304–314.

370. Chu XY, Kato Y, Sugiyama Y. Multiplicity of biliary excretion mechanisms for irinotecan, CPT-11, and its metabolites in rats. Cancer Res 1997;57:1934–1938.

371. Nakatomi K, Yoshikawa M, Oka M, et al. Transport of 7-ethyl-10-hydroxycamptothecin (SN-38) by breast cancer resistance protein ABCG2 in human lung cancer cells. Biochem Biophys Res Commun 2001;288:827–832.

372. Bates SE, Medina-Perez WY, Kohlhagen G, et al. ABCG2 mediates differential resistance to SN-38 (7-ethyl-10-hydroxycamptothecin) and homocamptothecins. J Pharmacol Exp Ther 2004;310:836–842.

373. Iyer L, Ramirez J, Shepard DR, et al. Biliary transport of irinotecan and metabolites in normal and P-glycoprotein-deficient mice. Cancer Chemother Pharmacol 2002;49:336–341.

374. Gupta E, Lestingi TM, Mick R, et al. Metabolic fate of irinotecan in humans: correlation of glucuronidation with diarrhea. Cancer Res 1994;54:3723–3725.

375. Gupta E, Safa AR, Wang X, et al. Pharmacokinetic modulation of irinotecan and metabolites by cyclosporin A. Cancer Res 1996;56:1309–1314.

376. Sparreboom A, de Jonge MJ, de Bruijn P, et al. Irinotecan (CPT-11) metabolism and disposition in cancer patients. Clin Cancer Res 1998;4:2747–2754.

377. Slatter JG, Schaaf LJ, Sams JP, et al. Pharmacokinetics, metabolism, and excretion of irinotecan (CPT-11) following i.v. infusion of [(14)C]CPT-11 in cancer patients. Drug Metab Dispos 2000;28:423–433.

378. Mick R, Gupta E, Vokes EE, et al. Limited-sampling models for irinotecan pharmacokinetics-pharmacodynamics: prediction of biliary index and intestinal toxicity. J Clin Oncol 1996;14:2012–2019.

379. de Jonge MJ, Verweij J, de Bruijn P, et al. Pharmacokinetic, metabolic, and pharmacodynamic profiles in a dose-escalating study of irinotecan and cisplatin. J Clin Oncol 2000;18:195–203.

380. Xie R, Mathijssen RH, Sparreboom A, et al. Clinical pharmacokinetics of irinotecan and its metabolites in relation with diarrhea. Clin Pharmacol Ther 2002;72:265–275.

381. de Forni M, Bugat R, Chabot GG, et al. Phase I and pharmacokinetic study of the camptothecin derivative irinotecan, administered on a weekly schedule in cancer patients. Cancer Res 1994;54:4347–4354.

382. Rougier P, Bugat R. CPT-11 in the treatment of colorectal cancer: clinical efficacy and safety profile. Semin Oncol 1996;23:34–41.

383. Venook AP, Enders Klein C, Fleming G, et al. A phase I and pharmacokinetic study of irinotecan in patients with hepatic or renal dysfunction or with prior pelvic radiation: CALGB 9863. Ann Oncol 2003;14:1783–1790.

384. Raymond E, Boige V, Faivre S, et al. Dosage adjustment and pharmacokinetic profile of irinotecan in cancer patients with hepatic dysfunction. J Clin Oncol 2002;20:4303–4312.

385. Pitot HC, Goldberg RM, Reid JM, et al. Phase I dose-finding and pharmacokinetic trial of irinotecan hydrochloride (CPT-11) using a once-every-three-week dosing schedule for patients with advanced solid tumor malignancy. Clin Cancer Res 2000;6:2236–2244.

386. Rothenberg ML. The current status of irinotecan (CPT-11) in the United States. Ann NY Acad Sci 1996;803:272–281.

387. Cunningham D, Glimelius B. A phase III study of irinotecan (CPT-11) versus best supportive care in patients with metastatic colorectal cancer who have failed 5-fluorouracil therapy. V301 Study Group. Semin Oncol 1999;26:6–12.

388. Rougier P, Van Cutsem E, Bajetta E, et al. Randomised trial of irinotecan versus fluorouracil by continuous infusion after fluorouracil failure in patients with metastatic colorectal cancer. Lancet 1998;352:1407–1412.

389. Rougier P, Bugat R, Douillard JY, et al. Phase II study of irinotecan in the treatment of advanced colorectal cancer in chemotherapy-naive patients and patients pretreated with fluorouracil-based chemotherapy. J Clin Oncol 1997;15:251–260.

390. Rothenberg ML, Cox JV, DeVore RF, et al. A multicenter, phase II trial of weekly irinotecan (CPT-11) in patients with previously treated colorectal carcinoma. Cancer 1999;85:786–795.

391. Vanhoefer U, Harstrick A, Achterrath W, et al. Irinotecan in the treatment of colorectal cancer: clinical overview. J Clin Oncol 2001;19:1501–1518.

392. Goldberg RM. Current approaches to first-line treatment of advanced colorectal cancer. Clin Colorectal Cancer 2004;4 (Suppl 1):S9–15.

393. Rothenberg ML. Current status of second-line therapy for metastatic colorectal cancer. Clin Colorectal Cancer 2004;4 (Suppl 1):S16-21.

394. Ribrag V, Koscielny S, Vantelon JM, et al. Phase II trial of irinotecan (CPT-11) in relapsed or refractory non-Hodgkin's lymphomas. Leuk Lymphoma 2003;44:1529–1533.

395. Meert AP, Berghmans T, Branle F, et al. Phase II and III studies with new drugs for non-small cell lung cancer: a systematic review of the literature with a methodology quality assessment. Anticancer Res 1999;19:4379–4390.

396. Rosen LS. Irinotecan in lymphoma, leukemia, and breast, pancreatic, ovarian, and small-cell lung cancers. Oncology (Huntingt) 1998;12:103–109.

397. Saltz L. Irinotecan-based combinations for the adjuvant treatment of stage III colon cancer. Oncology (Huntingt) 2000;14:47–50.

398. Douillard JY. Irinotecan and high-dose fluorouracil/leucovorin for metastatic colorectal cancer. Oncology (Huntingt) 2000;14:51–55.

399. Douillard JY, Barbarot V, Bennouna J. Update on European adjuvant trials with irinotecan for colorectal cancer. Oncology (Huntingt) 2002;16:13–15.

400. Hurwitz H, Fehrenbacher L, Novotny W, et al. Bevacizumab plus irinotecan, fluorouracil, and leucovorin for metastatic colorectal cancer. N Engl J Med 2004;350:2335–2342.

401. Stevenson JP, Redlinger M, Kluijtmans LA, et al. Phase I clinical and pharmacogenetic trial of irinotecan and raltitrexed administered every 21 days to patients with cancer. J Clin Oncol 2001;19:4081–4087.

402. Ford HE, Cunningham D, Ross PJ, et al. Phase I study of irinotecan and raltitrexed in patients with advanced gastrointestinal tract adenocarcinoma. Br J Cancer 2000;83:146–152.

403. de Jonge MJ, Sparreboom A, Verweij J. The development of combination therapy involving camptothecins: a review of preclinical and early clinical studies. Cancer Treat Rev 1998;24:205–220.

404. Masuda N, Fukuoka M, Kudoh S, et al. Phase I study of irinotecan and cisplatin with granulocyte colony-stimulating factor support for advanced non-small-cell lung cancer. J Clin Oncol 1994;12:90–96.

405. Mori K, Hirose T, Machida S, et al. A phase I study of irinotecan and infusional cisplatin with recombinant human granulocyte colony-stimulating factor support in the treatment of advanced non-small cell lung cancer. Eur J Cancer 1997;33:503–505.

406. de Jonge MJ, Verweij J, Planting AS, et al. Drug-administration sequence does not change pharmacodynamics and kinetics of irinotecan and cisplatin. Clin Cancer Res 1999;5:2012–2017.

407. Noda K, Nishiwaki Y, Kawahara M, et al. Irinotecan plus cisplatin compared with etoposide plus cisplatin for extensive small-cell lung cancer. N Engl J Med 2002;346:85–91.

408. Goldwasser F, Gross-Goupil M, Tigaud JM, et al. Dose escalation of CPT-11 in combination with oxaliplatin using an every two weeks schedule: a phase I study in advanced gastrointestinal cancer patients. Ann Oncol 2000;11:1463–1470.

409. Wasserman E, Cuvier C, Lokiec F, et al. Combination of oxaliplatin plus irinotecan in patients with gastrointestinal tumors: results of two independent phase I studies with pharmacokinetics. J Clin Oncol 1999;17:1751–1759.

410. Scheithauer W, Kornek GV, Raderer M, et al. Randomized multicenter phase II trial of oxaliplatin plus irinotecan versus raltitrexed as first-line treatment in advanced colorectal cancer. J Clin Oncol 2002;20:165–172.

411. Goldberg RM, Sargent DJ, Morton RF, et al. A randomized controlled trial of fluorouracil plus leucovorin, irinotecan, and

oxaliplatin combinations in patients with previously untreated metastatic colorectal cancer. J Clin Oncol 2004;22:23–30.

412. Tournigand C, Andre T, Achille E, et al. FOLFIRI followed by FOLFOX6 or the reverse sequence in advanced colorectal cancer: a randomized GERCOR study. J Clin Oncol 2004;22: 229–237.

413. Valencak J, Raderer M, Kornek GV, et al. Irinotecan-related cholinergic syndrome induced by coadministration of oxaliplatin. J Natl Cancer Inst 1998;90:160.

414. Karato A, Sasaki Y, Shinkai T, et al. Phase I study of CPT-11 and etoposide in patients with refractory solid tumors. J Clin Oncol 1993;11:2030–2035.

415. Masuda N, Fukuoka M, Kudoh S, et al. Phase I and pharmacologic study of irinotecan and etoposide with recombinant human granulocyte colony-stimulating factor support for advanced lung cancer. J Clin Oncol 1994;12:1833–1841.

416. Fukuda M, Oka M, Soda H, et al. Phase I study of irinotecan combined with carboplatin in previously untreated solid cancers. Clin Cancer Res 1999;5:3963–3969.

417. Naka N, Kawahara M, Okishio K, et al. Phase II study of weekly irinotecan and carboplatin for refractory or relapsed small-cell lung cancer. Lung Cancer 2002;37:319–323.

418. Yamada M, Kudoh S, Fukuda H, et al. Dose-escalation study of weekly irinotecan and daily carboplatin with concurrent thoracic radiotherapy for unresectable stage III non-small cell lung cancer. Br J Cancer 2002;87:258–263.

419. Fisher MD. Phase II and phase III trials: docetaxel/irinotecan versus docetaxel/cisplatin in advanced non-small-cell lung cancer (WJTOG 9803). Clin Lung Cancer 2001;2:178–179.

420. Masuda N, Negoro S, Kudoh S, et al. Phase I and pharmacologic study of docetaxel and irinotecan in advanced non-small-cell lung cancer. J Clin Oncol 2000;18:2996–3003.

421. Couteau C, Risse ML, Ducreux M, et al. Phase I and pharmacokinetic study of docetaxel and irinotecan in patients with advanced solid tumors. J Clin Oncol 2000;18:3545–3552.

422. Adjei AA, Klein CE, Kastrissios H, et al. Phase I and pharmacokinetic study of irinotecan and docetaxel in patients with advanced solid tumors: preliminary evidence of clinical activity. J Clin Oncol 2000;18:1116–1123.

423. Font A, Sanchez JM, Rosell R, et al. Phase I study of weekly CPT-11 (irinotecan)/docetaxel in patients with advanced solid tumors. Lung Cancer 2002;37:213–218.

424. Hotta K, Ueoka H, Kiura K, et al. A phase I study and pharmacokinetics of irinotecan (CPT-11) and paclitaxel in patients with advanced non-small cell lung cancer. Lung Cancer 2004;45: 77–84.

425. Kasai T, Oka M, Soda H, et al. Phase I and pharmacokinetic study of paclitaxel and irinotecan for patients with advanced non-small cell lung cancer. Eur J Cancer 2002;38:1871–1878.

426. Freitas JR, Rocha-Lima CM. Therapy of advanced non-small-cell lung cancer with irinotecan and gemcitabine in combination. Clin Lung Cancer 2002;4(Suppl 1):S26–29.

427. Yamao T, Shirao K, Matsumura Y, et al. Phase I-II study of irinotecan combined with mitomycin-C in patients with advanced gastric cancer. Ann Oncol 2001;12:1729–1735.

428. Scheithauer W, Kornek GV, Brugger S, et al. Randomized phase II study of irinotecan plus mitomycin C vs. oxaliplatin plus mitomycin C in patients with advanced fluoropyrimidine/leucovorin-pretreated colorectal cancer. Cancer Invest 2002;20:60–68.

429. Fujita A, Ohkubo T, Hoshino H, et al. Phase I study of carboplatin, irinotecan and docetaxel on a divided schedule with recombinant human granulocyte colony stimulating factor support in patients with stage IIIB or IV non-small cell lung cancer. Anticancer Drugs 2002;13:505–509.

430. Pectasides D, Visvikis A, Kouloubinis A, et al. Weekly chemotherapy with carboplatin, docetaxel and irinotecan in advanced non-small-cell lung cancer: a phase II study. Eur J Cancer 2002;38:1194–1200.

431. Pantazis P, Harris N, Mendoza J, et al. Conversion of 9-nitro-camptothecin to 9-amino-camptothecin by human blood cells in vitro. Eur J Haematol 1994;53:246–248.

432. Pantazis P, Harris N, Mendoza J, et al. The role of pH and serum albumin in the metabolic conversion of 9-nitrocamptothecin to 9-aminocamptothecin by human hematopoietic and other cells. Eur J Haematol 1995;55:211–213.

433. Pantazis P, Kozielski AJ, Vardeman DM, et al. Efficacy of camptothecin congeners in the treatment of human breast carcinoma xenografts. Oncol Res 1993;5:273–281.

434. Pantazis P, Early JA, Kozielski AJ, et al. Regression of human breast carcinoma tumors in immunodeficient mice treated with 9-nitrocamptothecin: differential response of nontumorigenic and tumorigenic human breast cells in vitro. Cancer Res 1993; 53:1577–1582.

435. Pantazis P, Kozielski AJ, Mendoza JT, et al. Camptothecin derivatives induce regression of human ovarian carcinomas grown in nude mice and distinguish between non-tumorigenic and tumorigenic cells in vitro. Int J Cancer 1993;53:863–871.

436. Pantazis P, Hinz HR, Mendoza JT, et al. Complete inhibition of growth followed by death of human malignant melanoma cells in vitro and regression of human melanoma xenografts in immunodeficient mice induced by camptothecins. Cancer Res 1992;52:3980–3987.

437. Pantazis P, Early JA, Mendoza JT, et al. Cytotoxic efficacy of 9-nitrocamptothecin in the treatment of human malignant melanoma cells in vitro. Cancer Res 1994;54:771–776.

438. Zamboni WC, Hamburger DR, Jung LL, et al. Relationship between systemic exposure of 9-nitrocamptothecin (9NC, Rubitecan, RFS2000) and its 9-aminocamptothecin (9AC) metabolite and response in human colon cancer xenografts [abstract]. Proc AACR-NCI-EORTC 2001:400.

439. Zamboni WC, Bowman LC, Tan M, et al. Interpatient variability in bioavailability of the intravenous formulation of topotecan given orally to children with recurrent solid tumors. Cancer Chemother Pharmacol 1999;43:454–460.

440. Verschraegen CF, Natelson EA, Giovanella BC, et al. A phase I clinical and pharmacological study of oral 9-nitrocamptothecin, a novel water-insoluble topoisomerase I inhibitor. Anticancer Drugs 1998;9:36–44.

441. Michaelson MD, Ryan DP, Fuchs CS, et al. A phase I study of 9-nitrocamptothecin given concurrently with capecitabine in patients with refractory, metastatic solid tumors. Cancer 2003; 97:148–154.

442. Zamboni WC, Jung LL, Egorin MJ, et al. Phase I and pharmacologic studies of intermittently administered 9-nitrocamptothecin in patients with advanced solid tumors. Clin Cancer Res 2004; 10:5058–5064.

443. Verschraegen CF, Gupta E, Loyer E, et al. A phase II clinical and pharmacological study of oral 9-nitrocamptothecin in patients with refractory epithelial ovarian, tubal or peritoneal cancer. Anticancer Drugs 1999;10:375–383.

444. Konstadoulakis MM, Antonakis PT, Tsibloulis BG, et al. A phase II study of 9-nitrocamptothecin in patients with advanced pancreatic adenocarcinoma. Cancer Chemother Pharmacol 2001; 48:417–420.

445. Ellerhorst JA, Bedikian AY, Smith TM, et al. Phase II trial of 9-nitrocamptothecin (RFS 2000) for patients with metastatic cutaneous or uveal melanoma. Anticancer Drugs 2002;13:169–172.

446. Patel SR, Beach J, Papadopoulos N, et al. Results of a 2-arm phase II study of 9-nitrocamptothecin in patients with advanced soft-tissue sarcomas. Cancer 2003;97:2848–2852.

447. de Jonge MJ, Droz JP, Paz-Ares L, et al. Phase II study of 9-nitro-camptothecin (RFS 2000) in patients with advanced or metastatic urothelial tract tumors. Invest New Drugs 2004;22:329–333.

448. Punt CJ, de Jonge MJ, Monfardini S, et al. RFS2000 (9-nitro-camptothecin) in advanced small cell lung cancer, a phase II study of the EORTC New Drug Development Group. Eur J Cancer 2004;40:1332–1334.

449. Jacobs AD, Burris HA, Rivkin S, et al. A randomized phase III study of rubitecan (ORA) vs. best choice (BC) in 409 patients with refractory pancreatic cancer: report from a North-American multi-center study [abstract]. Proc Am Soc Clin Oncol 2004; 23:315.

450. Verschraegen CF, Gilbert BE, Loyer E, et al. Clinical evaluation of the delivery and safety of aerosolized liposomal 9-nitro-20(s)-camptothecin in patients with advanced pulmonary malignancies. Clin Cancer Res 2004;10:2319–2326.

451. Knight V, Koshkina NV, Waldrep JC, et al. Anticancer effect of 9-nitrocamptothecin liposome aerosol on human cancer xenografts in nude mice. Cancer Chemother Pharmacol 1999;44:177–186.

452. Knight V, Kleinerman ES, Waldrep JC, et al. 9-Nitrocamptothecin liposome aerosol treatment of human cancer subcutaneous xenografts and pulmonary cancer metastases in mice. Ann NY Acad Sci 2000;922:151–163.

453. Knight V, Koshkina N, Waldrep C, et al. Anti-cancer activity of 9-nitrocamptothecin liposome aerosol in mice. Trans Am Clin Climatol Assoc 2000;111:135–145.

454. Koshkina NV, Kleinerman ES, Waidrep C, et al. 9-Nitrocamptothecin liposome aerosol treatment of melanoma and osteosarcoma lung metastases in mice. Clin Cancer Res 2000;6:2876–2880.

455. Lawson KA, Anderson K, Snyder RM, et al. Novel vitamin E analogue and 9-nitrocamptothecin administered as liposome aerosols decrease syngeneic mouse mammary tumor burden and inhibit metastasis. Cancer Chemother Pharmacol 2004;54:421–431.

456. Stehlin JS, Giovanella BC, Natelson EA, et al. A study of 9-nitrocamptothecin (RFS-2000) in patients with advanced pancreatic cancer. Int J Oncol 1999;14:821–831.

457. Ebrahimi B, Phan A, Yao J, et al. Phase II clinical trial of rubitecan against advanced gastric adenocarcinoma [abstract]. Proc Am Soc Clin Oncol 2002;596a.

458. Schoffski P, Herr A, Vermorken JB, et al. Clinical phase II study and pharmacological evaluation of rubitecan in non-pretreated patients with metastatic colorectal cancer: significant effect of food intake on the bioavailability of the oral camptothecin analogue. Eur J Cancer 2002;38:807–813.

459. Raymond E, Campone M, Stupp R, et al. Multicentre phase II and pharmacokinetic study of RFS2000 (9-nitro-camptothecin) administered orally 5 days a week in patients with glioblastoma multiforme. Eur J Cancer 2002;38:1348–1350.

460. Cortes J, O'Brien S, Giles F, et al. 9-Nitro-20-(S)-camptothecin (9-NC, RFS2000) in chronic myeloid leukemia (CML), chronic myelomonocytic leukemia (CMML) and myelodysplastic syndromes (MDS) [abstract]. Proc Am Soc Clin Oncol 2000;19:7.

461. Fracasso PM, Rader JS, Govindan R, et al. Phase I study of rubitecan and gemcitabine in patients with advanced malignancies. Ann Oncol 2002;13:1819–1825.

462. Potmesil M, Vardeman D, Kozielski AJ, et al. Growth inhibition of human cancer metastases by camptothecins in newly developed xenograft models. Cancer Res 1995;55:5637–5641.

463. de Souza PL, Cooper MR, Imondi AR, et al. 9-Aminocamptothecin: a topoisomerase I inhibitor with preclinical activity in prostate cancer. Clin Cancer Res 1997;3:287–294.

464. Jeha S, Kantarjian H, O'Brien S, et al. Activity of oral and intravenous 9-aminocamptothecin in SCID mice engrafted with human leukemia. Leuk Lymphoma 1998;32:159–164.

465. Keane TE, El-Galley RE, Sun C, et al. Camptothecin analogues/cisplatin: an effective treatment of advanced bladder cancer in a preclinical in vivo model system. J Urol 1998;160:252–256.

466. Dahut W, Harold N, Takimoto C, et al. Phase I and pharmacologic study of 9-aminocamptothecin given by 72-hour infusion in adult cancer patients. J Clin Oncol 1996;14:1236–1244.

467. Rubin E, Wood V, Bharti A, et al. A phase I and pharmacokinetic study of a new camptothecin derivative, 9-aminocamptothecin. Clin Cancer Res 1995;1:269–276.

468. Eder JP Jr, Supko JG, Lynch T, et al. Phase I trial of the colloidal dispersion formulation of 9-amino-20(S)-camptothecin administered as a 72-hour continuous intravenous infusion. Clin Cancer Res 1998;4:317–324.

469. Giovanella BC, Stehlin JS, Hinz HR, et al. Preclinical evaluation of the anticancer activity and toxicity of 9-nitro-20(S)-camptothecin (rubitecan). Int J Oncol 2002;20:81–88.

470. Thomas RR, Dahut W, Harold N, et al. A phase I and pharmacologic study of 9-aminocamptothecin administered as a 120-h infusion weekly to adult cancer patients. Cancer Chemother Pharmacol 2001;48:215–222.

471. Siu LL, Oza AM, Eisenhauer EA, et al. Phase I and pharmacologic study of 9-aminocamptothecin colloidal dispersion formulation given as a 24-hour continuous infusion weekly times four every 5 weeks. J Clin Oncol 1998;16:1122–1130.

472. Herben VM, van Gijn R, Schellens JH, et al. Phase I and pharmacokinetic study of a daily times 5 short intravenous infusion schedule of 9-aminocamptothecin in a colloidal dispersion formulation in patients with advanced solid tumors. J Clin Oncol 1999;17:1906–1914.

473. Langevin AM, Casto DT, Thomas PJ, et al. Phase I trial of 9-aminocamptothecin in children with refractory solid tumors: a Pediatric Oncology Group study. J Clin Oncol 1998;16:2494–2499.

474. Vey N, Kantarjian H, Tran H, et al. Phase I and pharmacologic study of 9-aminocamptothecin colloidal dispersion formulation in patients with refractory or relapsed acute leukemia. Ann Oncol 1999;10:577–583.

475. Mani S, Iyer L, Janisch L, et al. Phase I clinical and pharmacokinetic study of oral 9-aminocamptothecin (NSC-603071). Cancer Chemother Pharmacol 1998;42:84–87.

476. de Jonge MJ, Punt CJ, Gelderblom AH, et al. Phase I and pharmacologic study of oral (PEG-1000) 9-aminocamptothecin in adult patients with solid tumors. J Clin Oncol 1999;17:2219–2226.

477. Muggia FM, Liebes L, Hazarika M, et al. Phase I and pharmacologic study of i.p. 9-aminocamptothecin given as six fractions over 14 days. Anticancer Drugs 2002;13:819–825.

478. Mi Z, Malak H, Burke TG. Reduced albumin binding promotes the stability and activity of topotecan in human blood. Biochemistry 1995;34:13722–13728.

479. Takimoto CH, Dahut W, Harold N, et al.Clinical pharmacology of 9-aminocamptothecin. Ann NY Acad Sci 1996;803:324–326.

480. Grossman SA, Hochberg F, Fisher J, et al. Increased 9-aminocamptothecin dose requirements in patients on anticonvulsants. NABTT CNS Consortium. The New Approaches to Brain Tumor Therapy. Cancer Chemother Pharmacol 1998;42:118–126.

481. Takimoto CH, Dahut W, Marino MT, et al. Pharmacodynamics and pharmacokinetics of a 72-hour infusion of 9-aminocamptothecin in adult cancer patients. J Clin Oncol 1997;15:1492–1501.

482. Minami H, Lad TE, Nicholas MK, et al. Pharmacokinetics and pharmacodynamics of 9-aminocamptothecin infused over 72 hours in phase II studies. Clin Cancer Res 1999;5:1325–1330.

483. de Jonge MJ, Verweij J, Loos WJ, et al. Clinical pharmacokinetics of encapsulated oral 9-aminocamptothecin in plasma and saliva. Clin Pharmacol Ther 1999;65:491–499.

484. Saltz LB, Kemeny NE, Tong W, et al. 9-Aminocamptothecin by 72-hour continuous intravenous infusion is inactive in the treatment of patients with 5-fluorouracil-refractory colorectal carcinoma. Cancer 1997;80:1727–1732.

485. Pazdur R, Diaz-Canton E, Ballard WP, et al. Phase II trial of 9-aminocamptothecin administered as a 72-hour continuous infusion in metastatic colorectal carcinoma. J Clin Oncol 1997;15:2905–2909.

486. Wilson WH, Little R, Pearson D, et al. Phase II and dose-escalation with or without granulocyte colony-stimulating factor study of 9-aminocamptothecin in relapsed and refractory lymphomas. J Clin Oncol 1998;16:2345–2351.

487. Vokes EE, Ansari RH, Masters GA, et al. A phase II study of 9-aminocamptothecin in advanced non-small-cell lung cancer. Ann Oncol 1998;9:1085–1090.

488. Kraut EH, Balcerzak SP, Young D, et al. A phase II study of 9-aminocamptothecin in patients with refractory breast cancer. Cancer Invest 2000;18:28–31.

489. Pitot HC, Knost JA, Mahoney MR, et al. A North Central Cancer Treatment Group phase II trial of 9-aminocamptothecin in previously untreated patients with measurable metastatic colorectal carcinoma. Cancer 2000;89:1699–1705.

490. Pazdur R, Medgyesy DC, Winn RJ, et al. Phase II trial of 9-aminocamptothecin (NSC 603071) administered as a 120-hr continuous infusion weekly for three weeks in metastatic colorectal carcinoma. Invest New Drugs 1998;16:341–346.

491. Kirstein MN, Houghton PJ, Cheshire PJ, et al. Relation between 9-aminocamptothecin systemic exposure and tumor response in human solid tumor xenografts. Clin Cancer Res 2001;7:358–366.

492. Erickson-Miller CL, May RD, Tomaszewski J, et al. Differential toxicity of camptothecin, topotecan and 9-aminocamptothecin to human, canine, and murine myeloid progenitors (CFU-GM) in vitro. Cancer Chemother Pharmacol 1997;39:467–472.

493. Mitsui I, Kumazawa E, Hirota Y, et al. A new water-soluble camptothecin derivative, DX-8951f, exhibits potent antitumor activity against human tumors in vitro and in vivo. Jpn J Cancer Res 1995;86:776–782.

494. Oguma T, Yamada M, Konno T, et al. High-performance liquid chromatographic analysis of lactone and hydroxy acid of new

antitumor drug, DX-8951 (exatecan), in mouse plasma. Biol Pharm Bull 2001;24:176–180.

495. De Jager R, Cheverton P, Tamanoi K, et al. DX-8951f: summary of phase I clinical trials. Ann NY Acad Sci 2000;922:260–273.

496. Lawrence RA, Izbicka E, De Jager RL, et al. Comparison of DX-8951f and topotecan effects on tumor colony formation from freshly explanted adult and pediatric human tumor cells. Anticancer Drugs 1999;10:655–661.

497. Vey N, Giles FJ, Kantarjian H, et al. The topoisomerase I inhibitor DX-8951f is active in a severe combined immunodeficient mouse model of human acute myelogenous leukemia. Clin Cancer Res 2000;6:731–736.

498. Kumazawa E, Jimbo T, Ochi Y, et al. Potent and broad antitumor effects of DX-8951f, a water-soluble camptothecin derivative, against various human tumors xenografted in nude mice. Cancer Chemother Pharmacol 1998;42:210–220.

499. Takiguchi S, Kumazawa E, Shimazoe T, et al. Antitumor effect of DX-8951, a novel camptothecin analog, on human pancreatic tumor cells and their CPT-11-resistant variants cultured in vitro and xenografted into nude mice. Jpn J Cancer Res 1997;88:760–769.

500. Nomoto T, Nishio K, Ishida T, et al. Characterization of a human small-cell lung cancer cell line resistant to a new water-soluble camptothecin derivative, DX-8951f. Jpn J Cancer Res 1998;89:1179–1186.

501. Ishii M, Iwahana M, Mitsui I, et al. Growth inhibitory effect of a new camptothecin analog, DX-8951f, on various drug-resistant sublines including BCRP-mediated camptothecin derivative-resistant variants derived from the human lung cancer cell line PC-6. Anticancer Drugs 2000;11:353–362.

502. Sun FX, Tohgo A, Bouvet M, et al. Efficacy of camptothecin analog DX-8951f (exatecan mesylate) on human pancreatic cancer in an orthotopic metastatic model. Cancer Res 2003;63:80–85.

503. Atsumi R, Oguma T, Yoshioka N, et al. Urinary metabolites of DX-8951, a novel camptothecin analog, in rats and humans. Arzneimittelforschung 2001;51:253–257.

504. Oguma T, Konno T, Inaba A, et al. Validation study of assay method for DX-8951 and its metabolite in human plasma and urine by high-performance liquid chromatography/atmospheric pressure chemical ionization tandem mass spectrometry. Biomed Chromatogr 2001;15:108–115.

505. Braybrooke JP, Boven E, Bates NP, et al. Phase I and pharmacokinetic study of the topoisomerase I inhibitor, exatecan mesylate (DX-8951f), using a weekly 30-minute intravenous infusion, in patients with advanced solid malignancies. Ann Oncol 2003;14:913–921.

506. Minami H, Fujii H, Igarashi T, et al. Phase I and pharmacological study of a new camptothecin derivative, exatecan mesylate (DX-8951f), infused over 30 minutes every three weeks. Clin Cancer Res 2001;7:3056–3064.

507. Boige V, Raymond E, Faivre S, et al. Phase I and pharmacokinetic study of the camptothecin analog DX-8951f administered as a 30-minute infusion every 3 weeks in patients with advanced cancer. J Clin Oncol 2000;18:3986–3992.

508. Rowinsky EK, Johnson TR, Geyer CE Jr, et al. DX-8951f, a hexacyclic camptothecin analog, on a daily-times-five schedule: a phase I and pharmacokinetic study in patients with advanced solid malignancies. J Clin Oncol 2000;18:3151–3163.

509. Giles FJ, Cortes JE, Thomas DA, et al. Phase I and pharmacokinetic study of DX-8951f (exatecan mesylate), a hexacyclic camptothecin, on a daily-times-five schedule in patients with advanced leukemia. Clin Cancer Res 2002;8:2134–2141.

510. Sharma S, Kemeny N, Schwartz GK, et al. Phase I study of topoisomerase I inhibitor exatecan mesylate (DX-8951f) given as weekly 24-hour infusions three of every four weeks. Clin Cancer Res 2001;7:3963–3970.

511. Royce ME, Hoff PM, Dumas P, et al. Phase I and pharmacokinetic study of exatecan mesylate (DX-8951f): a novel camptothecin analog. J Clin Oncol 2001;19:1493–1500.

512. Garrison MA, Hammond LA, Geyer CE Jr, et al. A phase I and pharmocokinetic study of exatecan mesylate administered as a protracted 21-day infusion in patients with advanced solid malignancies. Clin Cancer Res 2003;9:2527–2537.

513. Esteva FJ, Rivera E, Cristofanilli M, et al. A phase II study of intravenous exatecan mesylate (DX-8951f) administered daily for 5 days every 3 weeks to patients with metastatic breast carcinoma. Cancer 2003;98:900–907.

514. Braybrooke JP, Ranson M, Manegold C, et al. Phase II study of exatecan mesylate (DX-8951f) as first line therapy for advanced non-small cell lung cancer. Lung Cancer 2003;41:215–219.

515. Verschraegen CF, Kudelka AP, Hu W, et al. A phase II study of intravenous exatecan mesylate (DX-8951f) administered daily for 5 days every 3 weeks to patients with advanced ovarian, tubal or peritoneal cancer resistant to platinum, taxane and topotecan. Cancer Chemother Pharmacol 2004;53:1–7.

516. Royce ME, Rowinsky EK, Hoff PM, et al. A phase II study of intravenous exatecan mesylate (DX-8951f) administered daily for five days every three weeks to patients with metastatic adenocarcinoma of the colon or rectum. Invest New Drugs 2004;22:53–61.

517. Emerson DL, Besterman JM, Brown HR, et al. In vivo antitumor activity of two new seven-substituted water-soluble camptothecin analogues. Cancer Res 1995;55:603–609.

518. Gerrits CJ, Schellens JH, Creemers GJ, et al. The bioavailability of oral GI147211 (GG211), a new topoisomerase I inhibitor. Br J Cancer 1997;76:946–951.

519. Gerrits CJ, Creemers GJ, Schellens JH, et al. Phase I and pharmacological study of the new topoisomerase I inhibitor GI147211, using a daily × 5 intravenous administration. Br J Cancer 1996;73:744–750.

520. Eckhardt SG, Baker SD, Eckardt JR, et al. Phase I and pharmacokinetic study of GI147211, a water-soluble camptothecin analogue, administered for five consecutive days every three weeks. Clin Cancer Res 1998;4:595–604.

521. Paz-Ares L, Kunka R, DeMaria D, et al. A phase I clinical and pharmacokinetic study of the new topoisomerase inhibitor GI147211 given as a 72-h continuous infusion. Br J Cancer 1998;78:1329–1336.

522. Stevenson JP, DeMaria D, Sludden J, et al. Phase I/pharmacokinetic study of the topoisomerase I inhibitor GG211 administered as a 21-day continuous infusion. Ann Oncol 1999;10:339–344.

523. Gamucci T, Paridaens R, Heinrich B, et al. Activity and toxicity of GI147211 in breast, colorectal and non-small-cell lung cancer patients: an EORTC-ECSG phase II clinical study. Ann Oncol 2000;11:793–797.

524. Sessa C, Wanders J, Roelvink M, et al. Second-line treatment of small-cell lung cancer with the camptothecin-derivative GI147211: a study of the EORTC Early Clinical Studies Group (ECSG). Ann Oncol 2000;11:207–210.

525. Schellens JH, Heinrich B, Lehnert M, et al. Population pharmacokinetic and dynamic analysis of the topoisomerase I inhibitor lurtotecan in phase II studies. Invest New Drugs 2002;20:83–93.

526. Supko JG, Alderson L, Wen P, et al. Pharmacokinetics of gimatecan, an orally administered camptothecin analogue, in patients with malignant gliomas [abstract]. Proc Am Soc Clin Oncol 2004;23:136.

527. Petrangolini G, Pratesi G, De Cesare M, et al. Antiangiogenic effects of the novel camptothecin ST1481 (gimatecan) in human tumor xenografts. Mol Cancer Res 2003;1:863–870.

528. Pratesi G, Beretta GL, Zunino F. Gimatecan, a novel camptothecin with a promising preclinical profile. Anticancer Drugs 2004;15:545–552.

529. Gianni L, Hess D, Baselga J, et al. A phase I study of the oral camptothecin gimatecan with a design of concerted dose escalation in three schedules of different dosing-duration [abstract]. Proc Am Soc Clin Oncol 2003;22:138.

530. Alderson L, Supko J, Maestri X, et al. Phase I/II trial of gimatecan in patients with recurrent malignant glioma [abstract]. Proc Am Soc Clin Oncol 2003;22:104.

531. Zhu AX, Ready NE, Clark JW, et al. Phase I trial of gimatecan given orally once a week for 3 of 4 weeks in patients with advanced solid tumors [abstract]. Proc Am Soc Clin Oncol 2003;22:138.

532. Kehrer DF, Soepenberg O, Loos WJ, et al. Modulation of camptothecin analogs in the treatment of cancer: a review. Anticancer Drugs 2001;12:89–105.

533. Lavergne O, Demarquay D, Bailly C, et al. Topoisomerase I-mediated antiproliferative activity of enantiomerically pure fluorinated homocamptothecins. J Med Chem 2000;43:2285–2289.

534. Lesueur-Ginot L, Demarquay D, Kiss R, et al. Homocamptothecin, an E-ring modified camptothecin with enhanced lactone stability,

retains topoisomerase I-targeted activity and antitumor properties. Cancer Res 1999;59:2939–2943.

535. Gelderblom H, Salazar R, Verweij J, et al. Phase I pharmacological and bioavailability study of oral diflomotecan (BN80915), a novel E-ring-modified camptothecin analogue in adults with solid tumors. Clin Cancer Res 2003;9:4101–4107.

536. Sparreboom A, de Jonge MJ, Punt CJ, et al. Pharmacokinetics and bioavailability of oral 9-aminocamptothecin capsules in adult patients with solid tumors. Clin Cancer Res 1998;4:1915–1919.

537. Sparreboom A, Gelderblom H, Marsh S, et al. Diflomotecan pharmacokinetics in relation to ABCG2 421C>A genotype. Clin Pharmacol Ther 2004;76:38–44.

538. Burke TG, Mishra AK, Wani MC, et al. Lipid bilayer partitioning and stability of camptothecin drugs. Biochemistry 1993;32:5352–5364.

539. Bom D, Curran DP, Kruszewski S, et al. The novel silatecan 7-tert-butyldimethylsilyl-10-hydroxycamptothecin displays high lipophilicity, improved human blood stability, and potent anticancer activity. J Med Chem 2000;43:3970–3980.

540. Josien H, Bom D, Curran DP. 7-Silylcamptothecins (silatecans): a new family of camptothecin antitumor agents. Bioorg Med Chem Lett 1997;7:3189–3194.

541. Pollack IF, Erff M, Bom D, et al. Potent topoisomerase I inhibition by novel silatecans eliminates glioma proliferation in vitro and in vivo. Cancer Res 1999;59:4898–4905.

542. Thompson PA, Berg SL, Aleksic A, et al. Plasma and cerebrospinal fluid pharmacokinetic study of BNP1350 in nonhuman primates. Cancer Chemother Pharmacol 2004;53:527–532.

543. Schilsky RL, Hausheer FH, Bertucci D, et al. Phase I trial of karenitecin administered intravenously daily for five consecutive days in patients with advanced solid tumors using accelerated dose titration [abstract]. Proc Am Soc Clin Oncol 2000;19:195a.

544. Curran DP, Josien H, Bom D, et al. The cascade radical annulation approach to new analogues of camptothecins. combinatorial synthesis of silatecans and homosilatecans. Ann NY Acad Sci 2000;922:112–121.

545. Koshkina NV, Gilbert BE, Waldrep JC, et al. Distribution of camptothecin after delivery as a liposome aerosol or following intramuscular injection in mice. Cancer Chemother Pharmacol 1999;44:187–192.

546. Subramanian D, Muller MT. Liposomal encapsulation increases the activity of the topoisomerase I inhibitor topotecan. Oncol Res 1995;7:461–469.

547. Sadzuka Y, Hirotsu S, Hirota S. Effective irinotecan (CPT-11)-containing liposomes: intraliposomal conversion to the active metabolite SN-38. Jpn J Cancer Res 1999;90:226–232.

548. Zhang JA, Xuan T, Parmar M, et al. Development and characterization of a novel liposome-based formulation of SN-38. Int J Pharm 2004;270:93–107.

549. Colbern GT, Dykes DJ, Engbers C, et al. Encapsulation of the topoisomerase I inhibitor GL147211C in pegylated (STEALTH) liposomes: pharmacokinetics and antitumor activity in HT29 colon tumor xenografts. Clin Cancer Res 1998;4:3077–3082.

550. Emerson DL, Bendele R, Brown E, et al. Antitumor efficacy, pharmacokinetics, and biodistribution of NX 211: a low-clearance liposomal formulation of lurtotecan. Clin Cancer Res 2000;6:2903–2912.

551. Kehrer DF, Bos AM, Verweij J, et al. Phase I and pharmacologic study of liposomal lurtotecan, NX 211: urinary excretion predicts hematologic toxicity. J Clin Oncol 2002;20:1222–1231.

552. Gelmon K, Hirte H, Fisher B, et al. A phase 1 study of OSI-211 given as an intravenous infusion days 1, 2, and 3 every three weeks in patients with solid cancers. Invest New Drugs 2004;22:263–275.

553. Giles FJ, Tallman MS, Garcia-Manero G, et al. Phase I and pharmacokinetic study of a low-clearance, unilamellar liposomal formulation of lurtotecan, a topoisomerase 1 inhibitor, in patients with advanced leukemia. Cancer 2004;100:1449–1458.

554. MacKenzie MJ, Hirte HW, Siu LL, et al. A phase I study of OSI-211 and cisplatin as intravenous infusions given on days 1, 2 and 3 every 3 weeks in patients with solid cancers. Ann Oncol 2004;15:665–670.

555. Seiden MV, Muggia F, Astrow A, et al. A phase II study of liposomal lurtotecan (OSI-211) in patients with topotecan resistant ovarian cancer. Gynecol Oncol 2004;93:229–232.

556. Kraut EH, Fishman MN, LoRusso PM, et al. Pharmacogenomic and pharmacokinetic assessment of liposome encapsulated SN38 (LE-SN38) in advanced cancer patients [abstract]. Proc Am Soc Clin Oncol 2004;23:163.

557. Drummond DC, Meyer O, Hong K, et al. Optimizing liposomes for delivery of chemotherapeutic agents to solid tumors. Pharmacol Rev 1999;51:691–743.

558. Papahadjopoulos D, Allen TM, Gabizon A, et al. Sterically stabilized liposomes: improvements in pharmacokinetics and antitumor therapeutic efficacy. Proc Natl Acad Sci USA 1991;88:11460–11464.

559. Allen TM, Hansen C. Pharmacokinetics of stealth versus conventional liposomes: effect of dose. Biochim Biophys Acta 1991;1068:133–141.

560. Cheung TW, Remick SC, Azarnia N, et al. AIDS-related Kaposi's sarcoma: a phase II study of liposomal doxorubicin. The TLC D-99 Study Group. Clin Cancer Res 1999;5:3432–3437.

561. Stewart BE, Engbers CM, Modi NB, et al. Safety evaluation of STEALTH liposomal CKD-602 [abstract]. Proc Soc Toxicol 2004;78:139.

562. Yu N, Conway C, Nicol F. STEALTH liposome formulation enhances antitumor efficacy of CKD-602, a topoisomerase I inhibitor, in human tumor xenograft models [abstract]. Proc Am Assoc Cancer Res 2004;45:710.

563. Greenwald RB, Choe YH, McGuire J, et al. Effective drug delivery by PEGylated drug conjugates. Adv Drug Deliv Rev 2003;55:217–250.

564. Conover CD, Greenwald RB, Pendri A, et al. Camptothecin delivery systems: enhanced efficacy and tumor accumulation of camptothecin following its conjugation to polyethylene glycol via a glycine linker. Cancer Chemother Pharmacol 1998;42:407–414.

565. Conover CD, Greenwald RB, Pendri A, et al. Camptothecin delivery systems: the utility of amino acid spacers for the conjugation of camptothecin with polyethylene glycol to create prodrugs. Anticancer Drug Des 1999;14:499–506.

566. Rowinsky EK, Rizzo J, Ochoa L, et al. A phase I and pharmacokinetic study of pegylated camptothecin as a 1-hour infusion every 3 weeks in patients with advanced solid malignancies. J Clin Oncol 2003;21:148–157.

567. Scott LC, Evans T, Yao JC, et al. Pegamotecan (EZ-246), a novel PEGylated camptothecin conjugate, for treatment of adenocarcinomas of the stomach and gastrointestinal (GE) junction: preliminary results of a single agent phase 2 study [abstract]. Proc Am Soc Clin Oncol 2004;23:320.

Anthracyclines and Anthracenediones

18

James H. Doroshow

DAUNORUBICIN (DAUNOMYCIN) AND DOXORUBICIN

The anthracycline antibiotics doxorubicin and daunorubicin, initially discovered over 40 years ago,[1,2] are among the most widely used antineoplastic agents in current clinical practice; their antineoplastic spectrum of action compares favorably with the alkylating agents and the taxanes. Doxorubicin and daunorubicin are especially active against the hematopoietic malignancies such as acute lymphocytic and acute myelogenous leukemia, Hodgkin's and non-Hodgkin's lymphoma, and multiple myeloma, as well as carcinomas of the breast, lung, ovary, stomach, and thyroid, sarcomas of bone and soft tissue origin, and various childhood malignancies. The key features of the two most commonly used anthracyclines, daunorubicin and doxorubicin, are summarized in Table 18.1, and the structures of the anthracyclines now in use are shown in Figure 18.1. Doxorubicin is currently used principally for the treatment of solid tumors, especially breast cancer and lymphoma, while daunorubicin is routinely utilized as part of chemotherapeutic induction programs for acute myelogenous leukemia (AML) and acute lymphocytic leukemia (ALL). The doxorubicin analog epirubicin is similar to the parent compound with respect to its acute toxicity profile and spectrum of antitumor efficacy but is significantly less potent and only slightly less cardiotoxic. The modestly decreased cardiac toxicity of epirubicin is only a marginal advantage, since other means are currently available to lessen the risk of anthracycline-induced heart damage. Idarubicin, a daunorubicin analog, has significant activity in the treatment of AML but is less active against solid tumors, and thus it is an appropriate alternate anthracycline only in the setting of acute leukemia.

In the clinic, the anthracyclines doxorubicin and daunorubicin have no known antagonistic interactions with any of the other commonly used anticancer agents. Furthermore, these drugs are active over a wide range of doses and in a variety of administration schedules; essentially equivalent antitumor activity is observed whether the anthracycline is given as a single large bolus dose once a month, as a weekly intravenous bolus, or as a prolonged infusion.[3,4] However, changes in drug scheduling do change the pattern of normal tissue injury. The combination of broad antitumor activity, lack of antagonism with other antitumor agents, and flexibility in dose and schedule make doxorubicin and daunorubicin very useful in the design of drug combinations. As a result, anthracycline-containing combination chemotherapy protocols have become standard therapy for cancers of the breast and thyroid; bone and soft tissue sarcomas; essentially all hematologic malignancies; and many childhood solid tumors. Although the acute toxicities associated with anthracycline administration, such as myelosuppression, mucositis, and alopecia, are important in clinical practice, the toxic reaction that causes the greatest concern is the unique cumulative cardiac injury produced by these drugs. Elucidation of the biochemical mechanisms of this cardiac toxicity resulted in the identification of an iron-chelating agent with its own modest antineoplastic activity, dexrazoxane (ICRF-187), which can block the cardiac toxicity of the anthracycline antibiotics in a wide range of animal models. Prospective, randomized clinical trials have shown that this agent is highly effective in reducing the cardiac toxicity of doxorubicin. This development, as well as the demonstration of a steep dose-response curve for doxorubicin in the treatment of solid tumors[5] and the feasibility of utilizing colony-stimulating factors with or without peripheral

TABLE 18.1
KEY FEATURES OF DAUNORUBICIN AND DOXORUBICIN

Mechanism of action	Pleiotropic effects including (1) activation of signal transduction pathways, (2) generation of reactive oxygen intermediates, (3) stimulation of apoptosis, and (4) inhibition of DNA topoisomerase II catalytic activity
Metabolism	1. Reduction of side-chain carbonyl to alcohol, resulting in some loss of cytotoxicity 2. One-electron reduction to semiquinone free-radical intermediate by flavoproteins, leading to aerobic production of superoxide anion, hydrogen peroxide, and hydroxyl radical 3. Two-electron reduction, resulting in formation of aglycone species that can be conjugated for export in bile
Pharmacokinetics	*Doxorubicin:* V_d = 25 liters; protein binding = 60–70%; CSF/plasma ratio, very low; $t_{1/2\alpha}$ = 10 min; $t_{1/2\beta}$ = 1–3 hr; $t_{1/2\gamma}$ = 30 hr. Circulates predominantly as parent drug; doxorubicinol is most common metabolite, although a substantial fraction of patients form doxorubicin 7-deoxyaglycone and doxorubicinol 7-deoxyaglycone; substantial interpatient variation in biotransformation; no apparent dose-related change in clearance; clearance in men > women. *Daunomycin:* V_d, protein binding, and CSF/plasma ratio similar to doxorubicin; $t_{1/2\alpha}$ = 40 min; $t_{1/2\beta}$ = 20–50 hr. Metabolism to daunomycinol faster than for equivalent doxorubicin metabolism, although interpatient variation remains high.
Elimination	Only 50 to 60% of parent drug accounted for by known routes of elimination, which include reduction of the side-chain carbonyl by hepatic aldoketoreductases, aglycone formation, and excretion of biliary conjugates and metabolites. A substantial fraction of the parent compound is bound to DNA and cardiolipin in tissues and is slowly dissociated, contributing to prolonged disappearance. While changes in anthracycline pharmacokinetics may be difficult to demonstrate in patients with mild alterations in liver function, drug clearance is definitely decreased in the presence of significant hyperbilirubinemia or patients with a marked burden of metastatic tumor in liver.
Drug interactions	Heparin binds to doxorubicin, causing aggregation; coadministration of both drugs leads to increased doxorubicin clearance. In rodents, phenobarbital has been shown to increase, and morphine decrease, doxorubicin disappearance; drugs that diminish hepatic reduced glutathione pools (acetaminophen and BCNU) sensitize the liver to anthracycline toxicity.
Toxicity	1. Myelosuppression 2. Mucositis 3. Alopecia 4. Cardiac toxicity 5. Severe local tissue damage after drug extravasation
Precautions	1. Acute and chronic cardiac decompensation can occur. Most common is cumulative dose-related congestive cardiomyopathy, which is more frequent in patients with underlying hypertensive heart disease or those who have received mediastinal radiation with a cardiac dose > 2000 cGy. 2. Radiation sensitization of normal tissues, including chest wall and esophagus, is common and may occur many years after radiation exposure. 3. Extravasation damage to extremities has resulted in loss of limb function.

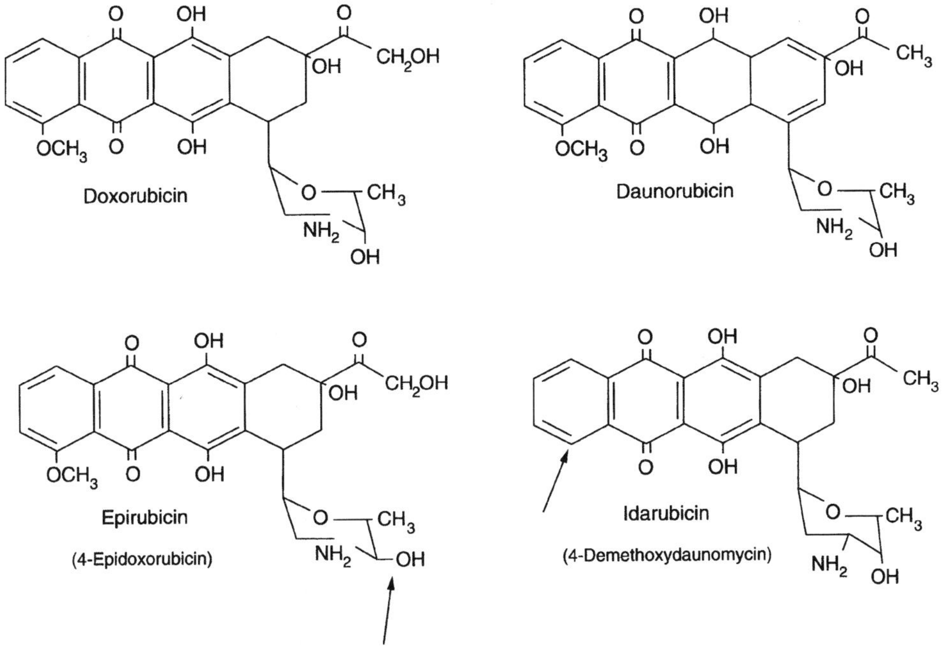

Figure 18.1 Structures of the four anthracyclines in current clinical use. For epirubicin and idarubicin, arrows point to the sites where these new drugs differ from doxorubicin and daunomycin, respectively.

blood progenitor support to ameliorate the bone marrow toxicity of the anthracyclines, has permitted a significant increase in the dose intensity, dose density, and duration of anthracycline therapy and may further increase the clinical utility of this family of drugs.[6–9]

General Mechanism of Action and Cellular and Molecular Pharmacology

Transmembrane Transport

The initial studies of anthracycline cellular pharmacokinetics reported the existence of a carrier-mediated transport system. This was based on the apparent saturation kinetics for uptake, and the K_m and V_{max} for this carrier were calculated. However, the physical properties of doxorubicin vary over the concentration range at which these studies were done; both doxorubicin and daunorubicin self-associate like other planar molecules by ring stacking, forming polymers.[10] This results in progressively less of the added drug being available for uptake into the cell.[11] It now seems clear that for doxorubicin and daunorubicin, transmembrane movement is by free diffusion of the un-ionized drug.[12] Furthermore, the uptake of the less polar daunorubicin is substantially faster than that of doxorubicin, which is itself substantially faster than the uptake of its polar alcohol metabolite.[13]

The daunosamine sugar can become protonated within the physiologic pH range with a pKa of 7.6.[14,15] For this reason, both extracellular and intracellular pH can have a significant impact on anthracycline uptake and cytotoxicity.[16–18] For example, intracellular acidosis would result in enhanced drug accumulation because un-ionized drug would enter, would become protonated, and would be unable to diffuse out of the cell. Conversely, relative acidification of the extracellular fluid would result in a shift of drug out of the cell. In this regard, it should be pointed out that tumor masses as small as 1 cm can exhibit extracellular pHs as low as 6 to 6.5.[19] More recent in vivo measurements utilizing ^{31}P magnetic resonance spectroscopy have demonstrated that the intracellular pH of tumor cells in xenograft models is most frequently neutral to alkaline while the extracelluar pH is acidic.[15] Thus, it is not surprising that simultaneous alkalinization of intra- and extracellular pH has been demonstrated to enhance the uptake and cytotoxicity of doxorubicin in cell culture and in SCID mice carrying the human MCF-7 breast carcinoma.[15,17] Furthermore, the acidification of intracellular organelles, including lysosomes, the Golgi network, and endosomes, in doxorubicin-resistant tumor cells significantly increases drug sequestration in these sites away from targets critical for tumor cell killing; blockade of sodium-proton exchange in acidic organelles produces a redistribution of doxorubicin into the cytoplasm and nucleus that can partially restore doxorubicin sensitivity in cells expressing the multidrug-resistance phenotype.[20,21]

The cellular pharmacology of the anthracyclines is also characterized by the ability of essentially all nucleated cells to accumulate these drugs to an extraordinary degree.[22] Ratios between the intracellular and extracellular concentration of daunorubicin and doxorubicin are routinely on the order of 30- to 1000-fold both at the end of a short-term in vitro incubation and in leukemic blasts at the end of an anthracycline infusion.[23] The accumulation of the anthracyclines is due to DNA binding, rapid association with cell membranes, and storage in several different intracellular compartments; furthermore, there are significant differences in the degree of accumulation based on cell and tissue type.[22] This phenomenon is important both for understanding the pharmacokinetics of these drugs and for the therapeutic efficacy of prolonged intravenous infusions.

Recent studies have demonstrated that once the anthracyclines diffuse through the plasma membrane, a substantial portion of the drug is bound to the 20S fraction of the proteasome.[24,25] Following proteasomal binding, anthracyclines are actively transported to the nucleus in an ATP-requiring, nuclear pore–dependent process that utilizes nuclear localization signals found in the 20S proteasomal subunits. The anthracyclines then dissociate from the proteasome due to the higher binding affinity of DNA. This process may facilitate the induction of cellular death programs by the anthracyclines and could provide a rationale for the combination of the anthracyclines with other agents that target proteasomal function.[26,27]

In addition to the diffusion of the anthracyclines across the cell membrane, active drug efflux occurs in some cells. The initial demonstration of ATP-dependent drug efflux resulted from the elucidation of the role of the multidrug resistance transporter in acquired anthracycline resistance.[28–31] Cells expressing the *MDR1* gene product efflux anthracyclines utilizing the P170 glycoprotein, a membrane protein capable of pumping a wide range of natural products, including the anthracyclines, out of cells. The P170 glycoprotein has adenosine triphosphate binding sites, and drug efflux is dependent on the presence of adequate intracellular ATP pools. Recently, other ATP-dependent drug efflux mechanisms capable of transporting anthracyclines against a concentration gradient have been discovered and may contribute to tumor cell drug resistance and to transport of the anthracycline antibiotics in normal host tissues, including the liver. These efflux mechanisms transport unmodified and/or glutathione-conjugated drug molecules.[32–40]

It is apparent from the studies reviewed above that while the general processes by which anthracyclines cross cell membranes have been examined in outline form, the kinetics of this process have not been established definitively, as is the case for methotrexate. The major barrier to such studies is the tendency for these drugs to bind to many intracellular proteins, DNA, phospholipids, and, perhaps, glycosaminoglycans. Because only free drug is presumably available for transport, efflux should be examined as a function of free, not total or bound, drug. However, this has rarely been done in studies of drug efflux utilizing anthracycline-resistant cell lines. Furthermore, the elucidation of several different energy-dependent efflux proteins in both tumor cells and normal tissues complicates the interpretation of prior studies while at the same time providing continuing opportunities for additional evaluations of cellular pharmacokinetic processes.

DNA Intercalation, Topoisomerase II Interactions, and Other Effects on DNA

DNA Intercalation

There remains considerable controversy over the mechanism of action of the anthracyclines and thus over the importance of various intracellular targets. However, there is no disagreement with the observation that the bulk of intracellular drug is in the nucleus and that a portion of the anthracycline in the nucleus is intercalated into the DNA double helix (Fig. 18.2). Detailed studies of daunorubicin affinity for DNA have identified a preference for dGdC-rich regions that are flanked by A:T base pairs.[41] In short

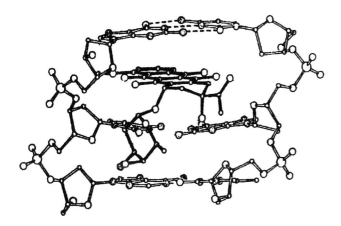

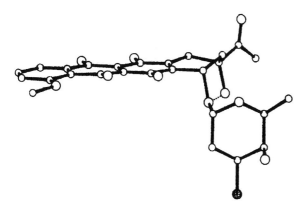

Figure 18.2 Three-dimensional view of daunomycin free and intercalated into DNA. This view shows the planar nature of the drug chromophore and how this is critical to DNA intercalation.

defined DNA sequences prepared by PCR, daunorubicin binds preferentially to either 5'(A or T)GC or 5'(A or T)CG triplets.[42] The consensus sequence for highest doxorubicin affinity is 5'-TCA.[43] With respect to DNA interactions, the anthracycline molecule (Fig. 18.1) can be separated by function into three domains: the planar ring, which actually intercalates into DNA; the side chain (and its associated D ring), which provides an important hydrogen-bonding function; and the daunosamine sugar, which binds to the minor groove and plays a critical role in base recognition and sequence specificity.[42]

It has generally been assumed that all of the drug within the nucleus is intercalated. When tumor cells exposed to doxorubicin or daunorubicin are examined by fluorescence microscopy, an intense nuclear fluorescence is observed, and many investigators have assumed that the intensity of this fluorescence is a measure of drug intercalated into DNA. However, anthracycline fluorescence is quenched significantly upon intercalation, and in fact, this quenching has been used to measure intercalation.[44] Thus, the nuclear fluorescence of the anthracyclines is likely to be due to binding of the drug to components of the nucleus by a non-intercalative mechanism. In fact, stable, covalently bound doxorubicin-DNA adducts (containing the daunosamine sugar) have recently been produced under conditions favored by the iron-dependent redox chemistry in which doxorubicin participates.[45]

Because the anthracyclines concentrate in the nucleus and are good DNA intercalators, DNA intercalation was presumed initially to play an important role in their mechanism of action. Several proposals were advanced to describe how DNA intercalation might lead to tumor cell kill, the best documented of which were studies demonstrating inhibition of RNA and DNA polymerases by the anthracyclines.[46,47] Unfortunately, the drug concentrations required for inhibition of these enzymes are far in excess of that which can be achieved in vivo, which probably explains the lack of correlation between inhibition of RNA and DNA synthesis and the cytotoxicity of doxorubicin.[48]

Topoisomerase II Interactions

An important advance in our understanding of anthracycline-DNA interactions occurred with the demonstration that anthracyclines cause protein-associated DNA breaks measured by filter elution, which in some cell lines are correlated with cytotoxicity.[49–51] Subsequent investigations have shown that the formation of protein-associated DNA breaks is caused by the formation of a ternary drug-DNA-enzyme "cleavable complex" involving the anthracycline antibiotic and DNA topoisomerase II, an enzyme associated with the nuclear matrix that plays a critical role in releasing torsional strain in DNA as well as in chromosome condensation.[52] Anthracyclines inhibit topoisomerase II by trapping DNA strand passage intermediates that can be detected as protein-associated DNA single- and double-strand breaks linked to the enzyme.[53,54] It had previously been presumed that through intercalation the anthracyclines altered the three-dimensional conformation of DNA, which arrested the cycle of topoisomerase II action at the point of DNA cleavage. However, topoisomerase II–associated DNA cleavage can be demonstrated at doxorubicin concentrations (10^{-8} M) well below the dissociation constant for DNA intercalation,[55] as well as with anthracycline analogs that do not intercalate into DNA.[56] Thus it is possible that anthracyclines may stimulate topoisomerase II–mediated DNA cleavage by a nonintercalative mechanism. Studies evaluating the interaction of the anthracyclines with topoisomerase II have demonstrated that doxorubicinone actively inhibits the purified enzyme, suggesting that the anthracycline sugar is not required for enzyme inhibition. Since the daunosamine sugar plays an important role in DNA binding, it may be possible to dissociate DNA intercalation further as a mechanism of action.[54] It has been demonstrated that the anthracyclines produce topoisomerase-related DNA cleavage in specific regions of the DNA (with an adenine at the 3′ end of one break site); this may provide a clue to gene-specific effects of these drugs, including specific sites of cleavage by anthracycline analogs.[57,58] It is also now clear, as will be described subsequently, that anthracycline resistance may be associated with alterations in the level or function of topoisomerase II, indicating a potentially important role for this enzyme in anthracycline action.[59–61]

Recent molecular studies performed both in human cell lines and in yeast model systems have more clearly defined the role of the alpha isoform of topoisomerase II in the production of protein-associated DNA cleavage after doxorubicin exposure.[62,63] Overexpression of the antisense construct of topoisomerase IIα in human U937 monocytic leukemia cells down-regulates topoisomerase IIα mRNA levels by >70%, with a concomitant reduction in the cytotoxicity of daunorubicin. Furthermore, a detailed reexamination of doxorubicin-related single-strand cleavage and topoisomerase-DNA complex formation has confirmed this process to be ATP-dependent and specific for topoisomerase II (not I),[64] an observation originally described more than a decade earlier.[65]

Although anthracycline interactions with DNA topoisomerase II clearly occur in many mammalian cell lines, it is likely that the formation of cleavable complexes alone is only potentially lethal and is not in itself sufficient for tumor cell killing. Although the initial correlations of protein-associated single-strand cleavage and cytotoxicity in L1210 cells, which were performed at clinically relevant drug concentrations, suggested a direct relationship between topoisomerase II–mediated DNA damage and cytotoxicity for doxorubicin,[49,66] subsequent investigations have demonstrated a dissociation between tumor cell killing and the kinetics of DNA break formation and disappearance for doxorubicin and its analogs.[67] In some cell lines, only DNA double-strand cleavage can be associated with cytotoxicity,[68] and in others, DNA single-strand cleavage is modest

and double-strand cleavage essentially undetectable at even supralethal drug concentrations.[69,70] Furthermore, recent evidence from several different model systems does not provide uniform support for a causal relationship between the level of topoisomerase II and the sensitivity of human cell lines to doxorubicin in vitro.[71,72] Finally, correlations between topoisomerase IIα content or activity in primary tumors and clinical outcome for breast cancer patients treated with anthracyclines have not been demonstrable.[73,74]

It has been appreciated for some time that in addition to stabilization of the cleavable complex, the anthracyclines and a number of other antineoplastic compounds can inhibit the catalytic activity of the enzyme without trapping the complex.[53,75] This observation, important for the development of new anthracyclines as well as combination regimens, underlies the recent demonstration that certain anthracycline analogs (not doxorubicin) antagonize the cytotoxicity and DNA cleavage of etoposide through inhibition of cleavable complex formation.[76–78] Furthermore, certain anthracycline analogs have recently been found that inhibit both topoisomerase I and II, which may explain their nonoverlapping resistance profiles and altered spectrum of action.[79–81] Doxorubicin is also known to exhibit more cytotoxicity than expected per DNA break. This might mean either that doxorubicin-associated breaks are qualitatively different from those produced by other topoisomerase II–active drugs or that other mechanisms of action might be operating in parallel. Thus, questions remain regarding the precise role of cleavable complex formation in the cytotoxicity of the anthracycline antibiotics.

Other Effects on DNA

In addition to the physicochemical effects of the anthracyclines on DNA and their interactions with topoisomerase II, doxorubicin produces other effects on DNA. Among the most important of these is that doxorubicin and daunorubicin form DNA-anthracycline complexes that significantly modify the ability of a specific class of nuclear enzymes, the helicases, to dissociate duplex DNA into DNA single strands in an ATP-dependent fashion; the entire process of strand separation is thus hindered, limiting replication.[82] This effect occurs at clinically relevant drug concentrations (<1 μM) and parallels, at least in part, the cytotoxic spectrum of several anthracycline analogs.[83] The mechanism of helicase inhibition involves the formation of an irreversible ternary complex between anthracyclines that possess an unblocked daunosamine sugar, DNA, and the helicase.[84] Given the diversity of human DNA helicases, differential effects of the anthracyclines could be related to their interactions with this class of nuclear enzymes. It has also been shown that in the absence of significant DNA double-strand cleavage, doxorubicin interferes with DNA unwinding and produces nonoligosomal fragmentation of nascent DNA during continuous exposure to very low drug concentrations.[70,85] This DNA effect is associated with tumor cell differentiation and suppression of *c-myc* oncogene expression by both doxorubicin and certain of its analogs and suggests yet another potential growth inhibitory pathway for the anthracyclines.[86,87]

As will be reviewed subsequently, it has also been demonstrated that doxorubicin can undergo cycles of reduction and oxidation in essentially all intracellular compartments, including the nucleus and the mitochondrion, leading to the formation of reactive oxygen species.[88] Doxorubicin redox cycling has been shown to oxidize DNA bases in human chromatin and in intact tumor cells, which may provide a cytotoxic mechanism unrelated to strand cleavage.[89-91] Mitochondrial DNA is also susceptible to oxidative stress in vitro and in the rat after doxorubicin administration where the production of 8-hydroxyguanosine, a byproduct of hydroxyl radical attack on DNA, is significantly increased in cardiac and liver mitochondria above the level observed in nuclear DNA from these two organs.[92-94]

Evidence of DNA base oxidation has also recently been demonstrated in patients treated with anthracycline antibiotics. Urinary hydroxymethyluracil (an oxidative by-product of thymine) has been observed within 24 hours of drug treatment in patients receiving combination chemotherapy that included an anthracycline.[95,96] Following bolus therapy with the anthracycline analog epirubicin, a wide variety of oxidized DNA bases can be found in chromatin isolated from patient lymphocytes using gas chromatography/mass spectroscopy (GC/MS).[97] In patients receiving a 96-hour infusion of doxorubicin, producing steady-state drug levels of 0.1 μM, a 2- to 5-fold increase in 13 different oxidized DNA bases, including thymine glycol, 5-OH-hydantoin, 5-OH-uracil, 4,6-diamino-5-formamindo-pyrimidine, and 5,6-di-OH-uracil, was observed by GC/MS in peripheral blood mononuclear cells beginning 72 hours after the initiation of treatment.[98] These data are important because this spectrum of DNA base damage is the same as that produced by ionizing radiation, which is known to be produced by the hydroxyl radical.[99,100] Thus, these studies provide unequivocal evidence of the oxidative metabolism of doxorubicin and its analogs under clinical conditions.

It is important to remember that doxorubicin and daunorubicin are both mutagens and carcinogens;[101] only recently have investigators begun to map the base substitutions and deletions produced by doxorubicin that appear to occur adjacent to preferential doxorubicin DNA binding sequences. Furthermore, it is now well established that therapy with doxorubicin (or epirubicin), when used in combination with cyclophosphamide, is associated with a dramatically increased risk of a second malignancy, specifically acute mono- or myelomonocytic leukemia.[102-104]

Because of the inhibitory effects of oxidized DNA bases on the action of DNA polymerases and other DNA repair mechanisms, as well as their own intrinsic mutagenic properties, the clinical investigations that demonstrate the production of oxidized DNA bases in hematopoietic cells after treatment with doxorubicin indicate a potential mechanism for anthracycline-related mutagenicity and carcinogenicity, as well as provide insights into the mechanism of tumor cell killing by the anthracyclines and their potentially adverse consequences for the synthesis of genes comprising the mitochondrial respiratory chain.[105-108]

In addition to the production of oxidized DNA bases, the intracellular reactive oxygen metabolism of the anthracyclines leads to the iron-dependent production of formaldehyde from a variety of intracellular carbon sources, which can subsequently react to produce a drug-formaldehyde conjugate containing two anthracycline molecules.[109-111] Such conjugates have a unique ability to form novel covalent DNA cross-links that markedly enhance the therapeutic activity of the anthracycline. They also provide the opportunity to produce targeted anthracycline prodrugs that possess a unique spectrum of anticancer activity.[112,113]

Drug Activation by One- and Two-Electron Reduction

During DNA intercalation and binding to topoisomerase II, the anthracyclines act as chemically inert compounds that owe their activity to their ability to bind to key macromolecules and distort the three-dimensional geometry of these targets. However, the anthracyclines are chemically reactive and possess an extraordinarily rich chemistry that even now has not been fully documented.[114,115]

One-Electron Reduction

The one-electron reduction of the anthracyclines was initially described in hepatic microsomal systems[116-118] but was later shown to play a central role in the cardiac toxicity of this class of drugs[119-121] and may be involved in antitumor activity as well.[122-124] All of the clinically active anthracyclines are anthraquinones. As is true of quinones in general,[125,126] the anthracyclines are able to undergo one- and two-electron reduction to reactive compounds that cause widespread damage to intracellular macromolecules, including lipid membranes, DNA bases, and thiol-containing transport proteins (Fig. 18.3).[127-130] As outlined in Figure 18.4, the one-electron reduction of doxorubicin or daunorubicin may occur in essentially all intracellular compartments, including the nuclear membrane, and is catalyzed by flavin-centered dehydrogenases or reductases, including cytochrome P-450 reductase, NADH dehydrogenase (complex I of the mitochondrial electron transport chain), xanthine oxidase, and cytochrome b_5 reductase.[131-133] In addition, recent studies demonstrate that all three isoforms of nitric oxide synthase (at their flavoprotein domains) are capable of catalyzing the one-electron reduction of doxorubicin, with the subsequent production of superoxide and a decrease in nitric oxide.[134,135] Furthermore, doxorubicin can directly inhibit nitric oxide synthase activity,[135,136] which could produce significant alterations in vascular tone both in the heart and in tumors.[137,138] It can

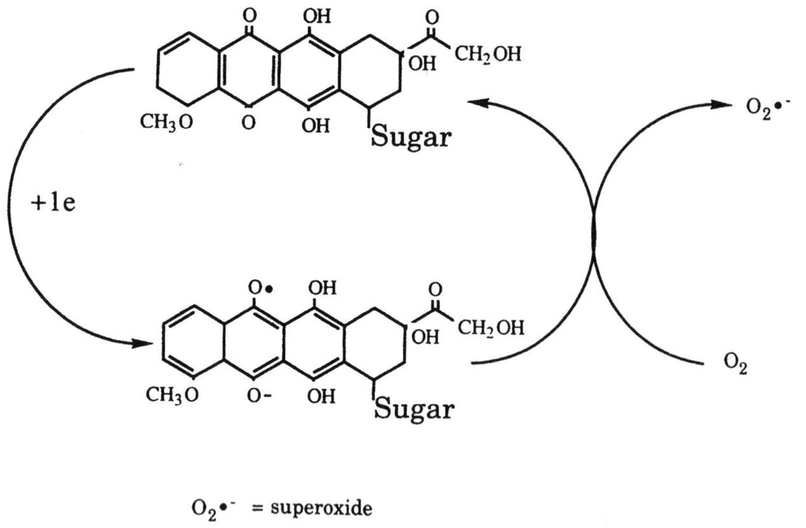

Figure 18.3 One-electron reduction of doxorubicin. This reduction occurs at the quinone oxygens of the chromophore. The semiquinones react rapidly with oxygen, when it is available, to yield the one-electron reduction product of oxygen, superoxide.

also be metabolized by lactoperoxidase and nitrite.[139] All of these flavoenzymes are widely distributed in mammalian tissues, and anthracycline-mediated free-radical formation has been demonstrated in a wide range of organs and tumor cell lines. In addition to flavoproteins, doxorubicin can be reduced in the heart by oxymyoglobin, leading to the production of strong oxidant species.[140]

One-electron reduction of the anthracyclines leads to the formation of the corresponding semiquinone free radical. In the presence of oxygen, this free radical rapidly donates its electron to oxygen to generate superoxide anion ($O_2^{\bullet-}$). Although not highly toxic itself, the dismutation of superoxide yields hydrogen peroxide (H_2O_2). Under biological conditions, the anthracycline semiquinone or reduced metal ions such as iron reductively cleave hydrogen peroxide to produce the hydroxyl radical ($OH^{\bullet}$) or a higher oxidation state metal with the chemical characteristics of the hydroxyl radical, one of the most reactive and destructive chemical species known.[141,142] It is now commonly accepted that reduced metals are critical components in the formation of toxic free-radical intermediates and may well contribute to the cytotoxicity of the anthracyclines.[143] However, it remains an area of active investigation how reduced metal species, including iron, become available for these free-radical reactions.

Because oxygen radical formation occurs as a result of normal metabolic processes (including mitochondrial respiration) and is a common mechanism of action for several naturally occurring toxins, most mammalian cells have elaborate defenses against oxygen radical toxicity.[144] Superoxide dismutase, catalase, and glutathione peroxidase act in concert to reduce superoxide, hydrogen peroxide, and lipid hydroperoxides to water or nontoxic lipid alcohols without the formation of the hydroxyl or peroxyl radicals (Fig. 18.4). Glutathione, a sulfur-containing tripeptide, can react with many radicals as well as function as part of the glutathione peroxidase cycle to reduce peroxides to

less reactive compounds. There are also specific DNA repair systems to handle oxidative damage to DNA.[145-147] However, antioxidant defenses are not equally distributed in various tissues in the body. For example, glutathione concentration is higher in the liver than in most other tissues and tumors. Catalase activity is lower in the heart than in the liver.[120,148] Likewise, the activity of several flavoproteins capable of activating the anthracyclines differs from tissue to tissue. These variations in drug activation and antioxidant defense provide ample opportunity for tissue specificity in terms of toxicity and antitumor activity. For example, the unique cardiac toxicity of the anthracyclines may result, in part, from the low level of cardiac catalase coupled with the extraordinary cardiac content of mitochondria and myoglobin, which enhance drug activation, as well as the sensitivity of cardiac glutathione peroxidase to free-radical attack,[120,149] which destroys the activity of this critical enzyme at the same time that anthracycline administration stimulates cardiac hydrogen peroxide formation.[150] In contrast, while anthracyclines can easily be activated to reactive intermediates by hepatic enzymes, the liver has a more active free-radical defense system and is able to actively efflux anthracyclines and anthracycline metabolites. The importance of hepatic antioxidant systems is shown by the fact that pretreatment in rodents with agents that significantly diminish the level of reduced glutathione, such as carmustine (BCNU) or acetaminophen, dramatically sensitizes hepatocytes to doxorubicin-induced free-radical injury.[151,152]

The role of oxygen radical formation in tumor cell killing rather than cardiac toxicity continues to be defined.[153-156] However, several lines of evidence support this hypothesis. First, doxorubicin resistance in tumor cell lines can frequently be reversed by agents that decrease glutathione concentration.[157-162] This observation cannot be explained by DNA or topoisomerase interactions. Second, anthracycline-enhanced free-radical formation has been

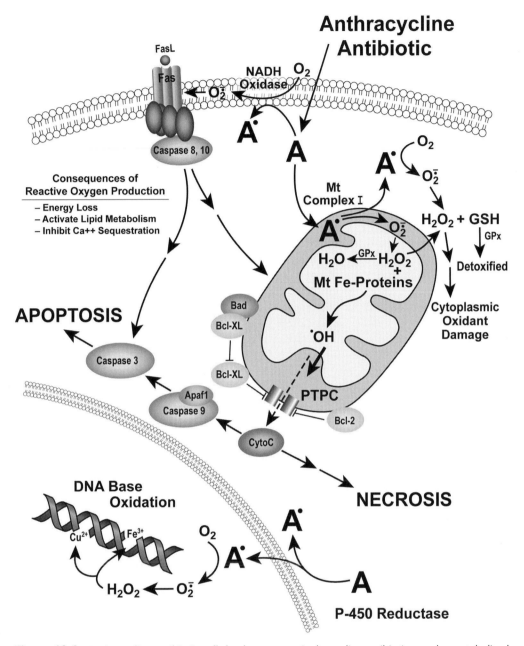

Figure 18.4 Anthracycline antibiotic cell death program. Anthracycline antibiotics can be metabolized at the cell surface, at complex I of the mitochondrial electron transport chain, in the cytosol, or at the nuclear envelop by flavin-containing dehydrogenases, leading to the production of reactive oxygen species with the potential to alter intracellular iron stores at multiple intracellular sites. This free-radical cascade can initiate both apoptotic and necrotic death programs associated with mitochondrial membrane injury, DNA base oxidation, altered calcium sequestration, energy loss, and altered proliferative potential. The effects of anthracycline-enhanced reactive oxygen production are modulated by intracellular antioxidant enzymes (glutathione peroxidase, catalase) and antiapoptotic proteins. (Please see color insert.)

detected in a range of tumor cell lines,[122,163,164] the best studied of which are human breast cancer cell lines where both intra- and extracellular reactive oxygen species were demonstrated.[123,165] Extracellular as well as intracellular antioxidants have also been demonstrated to decrease the cytotoxicity of the anthracyclines in a wide variety of cells, including human tumor cell lines.[123,124,143,166–170] In addition, some anthracycline-resistant cancer cell lines exhibit

increases in various aspects of the oxygen free-radical defense system, including increases in glutathione and the selenoprotein glutathione peroxidase.[161,171–174] Alterations in glutathione peroxidase activity produced by manipulation of selenium status significantly affect tumor cell killing by doxorubicin.[175,176] Transfection of the human cytosolic glutathione peroxidase in the sense orientation produces doxorubicin resistance[177] while antisense expression sensitizes cells to doxorubicin cytotoxicity.[178] Finally, 4-fold overexpression of the manganese superoxide dismutase in CHO cells produces 2.5-fold resistance to doxorubicin,[179] while inhibition of the copper-zinc superoxide dismutase with 1,25-dihydroxyvitamin D_3 significantly enhances doxorubicin-related cytotoxicity.[180]

Reservations about the role of oxygen radical formation in tumor cell killing arise from several observations. First, most of the studies demonstrating anthracycline-enhanced hydroxyl radical formation have utilized drug concentrations in excess of that which would be clinically relevant. This limitation is in part technical in that it is not possible at present to detect hydroxyl radicals at concentrations much below 10^{-7}. However, recent studies using fluorescent probes to detect hydrogen peroxide production by flow cytometry after doxorubicin exposure in human colon carcinoma cells successfully demonstrated peroxide formation after treatment with 0.4 μM of doxorubicin,[164] and enhanced oxidative respiration and reactive oxygen production have been observed in human breast cancer cells using chemiluminescent probes at doxorubicin levels between 0.05 and 0.1 μM.[181] Second, many tumors for which doxorubicin has great clinical utility, such as breast cancer, are clearly hypoxic, and thus the applicability of the chemistry outlined in Figures 18.3 and 18.4 might be questioned. However, under low partial pressures of oxygen, iron-mediated lipid peroxidation and DNA damage from the doxorubicin semiquinone are actually enhanced.[182] Third, there is no question that glutathione depletion does not sensitize all tumor cell lines to the cytotoxic effect of doxorubicin[183] and that many doxorubicin-resistant cells have no alteration in antioxidant defense enzymes.[184] Fourth, it has frequently been presumed that oxygen radical–mediated effects on DNA were unlikely because intercalated drug could not be reduced. However, doxorubicin covalently bound to oligonucleotides can still be activated by cytochrome P-450 reductase,[185] and daunorubicin intercalated into calf thymus DNA can be reduced by a superoxide-generating system; under these circumstances the semiquinone is accessible to hydrogen peroxide for reaction, and the disproportionation of the semiquinone to the 7-deoxyaglycone may occur by intramolecular electron transfer, with migration of electrons over several base pairs.[186–188] Finally, as outlined previously, recent studies have demonstrated the presence of oxidized DNA bases, by-products of anthracycline redox cycling, in both the urine[96] and peripheral blood mononuclear cells of patients receiving anthracycline therapy.[97,189] These reports provide the first, albeit indirect, evidence demonstrating the products of redox cycling in human tissues after anthracycline administration using standard treatment schedules.

Role of Iron

Although free-radical formation was originally proposed as the basis for anthracycline cardiac toxicity in 1977 and various animal model studies suggested that hydroxyl radical

scavengers could blunt doxorubicin-related heart damage, free-radical scavengers were initially unsuccessful cardioprotective agents in humans.[190] These results suggested that some additional variable was involved. This variable proved to be the interaction of anthracyclines with iron. Because of its reactivity, free-iron concentrations in the body are in the range of approximately 10^{-13} M, whereas total iron concentrations are between 10^{-4} and 10^{-5} M. Most of the iron in tissues is stored in ferritin. Doxorubicin has been found to release iron from ferritin in two ways. The drug can slowly abstract iron from the ferritin shell directly;[191] a much more rapid release of iron follows conversion of the anthracycline to its semiquinone, which can release iron under hypoxic conditions or through the reducing power of the superoxide anion in air.[192,193] Doxorubicin can also release nonheme, nonferritin iron from microsomes.[194–197] In addition, doxorubicin can increase the uptake of iron by a transferrin receptor–mediated process, enhancing intracellular iron availability.[198] The hydroxyquinone structure of doxorubicin and daunorubicin represents a powerful site for chelation of metal ions, especially ferric iron. Iron anthracycline complexes have been shown to possess a wide range in interesting biochemical properties in vitro.[199,200] These complexes can bind DNA by a mechanism distinct from intercalation, cause oxidative destruction of membranes, and oxidize critical sulfhydryl groups. It remains unclear, however, whether these tight-binding iron-anthracycline complexes are stable and produce toxic effects intracellularly[201,202] or whether the "delocalization" of catalytic amounts of protein-bound iron by anthracycline-stimulated free-radical formation is responsible for hydroxyl radical formation in tissues.

These investigations suggested that the most effective way to interfere with the generation of highly reactive oxidants after anthracycline exposure would be to pretreat with a chelating agent that might withdraw iron from free-radical reactions. This hypothesis has been confirmed, and an iron chelator, dexrazoxane (ICRF-187), has been shown to prevent doxorubicin-induced lipid peroxidation[203] and cardiac toxicity in a wide range of animal models.[204,205] Randomized, controlled clinical trials in humans have confirmed the ability of this agent to diminish markedly the cardiac toxicity of doxorubicin.[206,207] Dexrazoxane is a highly effective iron chelator in vivo; during phase I studies, it caused a 10-fold increase in urinary iron clearance.[208,209] Dexrazoxane is itself a prodrug in that it must undergo hydrolysis to become an effective iron chelator (Fig. 18.5). This hydrolysis to ICRF-198, the major iron-binding metabolite of dexrazoxane, can occur spontaneously at physiologic pH but is markedly enhanced after uptake into cardiac myocytes, with conversion of the parent drug to ICRF-198 in less than 60 seconds.[210] The parent drug is very lipid soluble and enters cells by passive diffusion. ICRF-198 has been demonstrated to efflux iron from iron-loaded myocytes; these studies suggest that the same

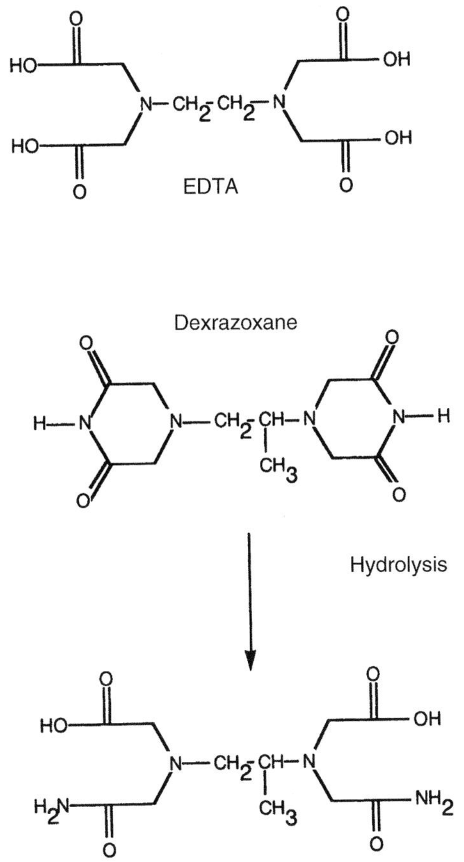

Figure 18.5 Dexrazoxane and its analogy to EDTA (ethylenediaminetetraacetic acid). Dexrazoxane is much more nonpolar because the carboxylic acid groups have been fused into amide rings. This allows ready entry into the cell. Dexrazoxane can undergo hydrolysis to yield a carboxylamine able to bind iron.

chelating ability may be available to remove iron that has been released from cardiac iron-storage proteins.[210]

Important additional studies have further amplified our understanding of the role of iron in anthracycline biochemistry and in the mechanism of drug-induced cardiac toxicity.[211–214] The alcohol metabolite of doxorubicin, doxorubicinol, which is produced by the two-electron reduction of the C-13 side chain carbonyl group, has been demonstrated to cause the delocalization of low-molecular-weight Fe(II) species from the iron-sulfur center of aconitase in a redox-dependent fashion. The formation of a doxorubicin-iron complex with aconitase interferes with critical interconversions of cytosolic aconitase with iron regulatory protein-1(IRP-1); IRP-1 plays an essential role in iron homeostasis and, hence, in the regulation of critical intracellular metabolic processes (such as the action of mitochondrial electron transport proteins, myoglobin, and various cytochromes). These effects of doxorubicin metabolites suggest that iron-dependent reactions occur that may not be directly related to the formation of reactive oxygen species. This could help to explain the utility of dexrazoxane, compared to free-radical scavengers that do

not chelate iron, in the prevention of both acute and chronic anthracycline cardiotoxicity.[197]

Doxorubicin is a powerful chelator of other metal ions, including Cu^{2+} and Al^{3+}. The chelation of aluminum by doxorubicin is effective enough that a doxorubicin solution left in contact with aluminum foil for only 1 hour will change from the orange-red of doxorubicin to the bright cherry red of the aluminum complex. A similar reaction occurs with iron-containing alloys; doxorubicin left within a syringe needle for any significant period of time will also change color by virtue of chelation of metal from the needle. For this reason, every effort should be made in the clinic to keep anthracyclines from prolonged contact with any metal surface.

Two-Electron Reduction of the Anthracyclines

Two-electron reduction of doxorubicin (which may occur by sequential one-electron reductions or directly when strong reducing agents are applied) results in the formation of an unstable quinone methide, which rapidly undergoes a series of reactions leading to the formation of the corresponding deoxyaglycone (Fig. 18.6).[114] It is now established that deoxyaglycones are formed in vivo.[215,216] Because the deoxyaglycones exhibit far less cytotoxicity than the parent drug, the current consensus is that this is a pathway for drug inactivation. It is likely that in the absence of oxygen the one-electron reduction product, the semiquinone, reacts with itself to yield parent drug and the two-electron reduction product. The quinone methide intermediate in this pathway has been proposed as a potential monofunctional alkylating agent; however, there is little evidence that this intermediate plays an important cytotoxic role in tumor cells. Finally, two-electron reduction of the anthracyclines using powerful reducing agents to convert doxorubicin to its inactive deoxyaglycone metabolite has been advocated as a means to reduce local tissue injury after anthracycline extravasation.[217] Direct enzymatic two-electron reduction is unlikely to occur under physiologic conditions.[218]

Signal Transduction, Membrane-Related Actions of the Anthracyclines, Apoptosis, and Cellular Senescence

Membrane Perturbations

It has been appreciated for more than a decade that the anthracycline antibiotics are membrane-active compounds that produce myriad effects at the cell surface.[219] It is only in the more recent past that events occurring at the cell surface have been related more clearly to anthracycline cytotoxicity and DNA damage. Doxorubicin alters the fluidity of both tumor cell plasma membranes[220,221] and cardiac mitochondria;[127] it binds avidly to phospholipids, including cardiolipin,[222,223] causes an up-regulation of epidermal growth factor receptor (but not p185[HER-2/neu]),[224,225] inhibits

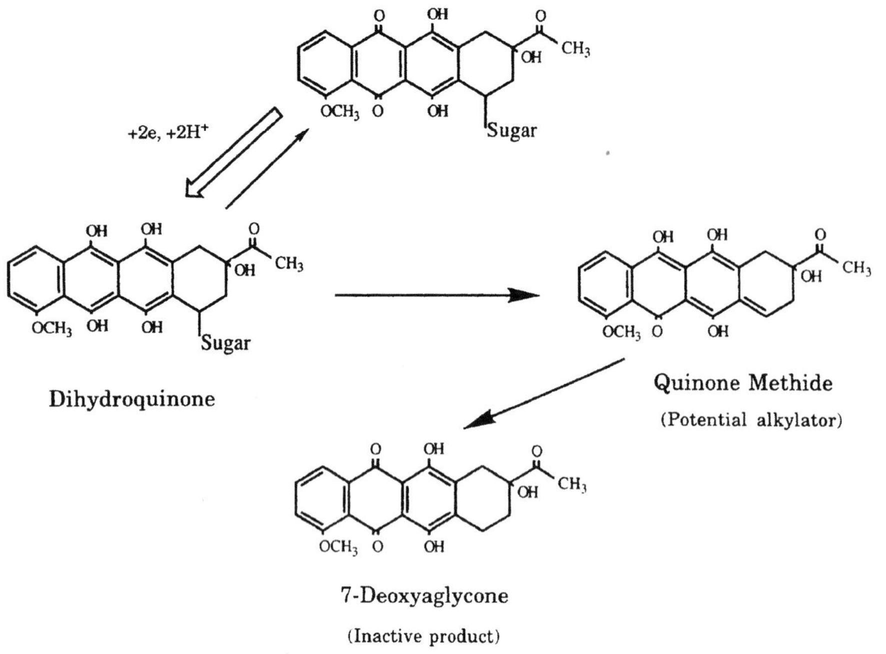

Figure 18.6 Two-electron reduction of anthraquinones. The immediate product is the dihydroquinone, which is not stable. This undergoes rearrangement with loss of the sugar to yield the quinone methide. This structure has activity as an alkylator in pure chemical systems. The most likely fate, however, is progression, via a second arrangement, to yield the 7- deoxyaglycone. This final product is much less active than the parent drug.

the transferrin reductase of the plasma membrane,[226] induces iron-dependent protein oxidation in erythrocyte plasma membranes in vivo[227], and can be actively cytotoxic without entering the cell.[228,229] Furthermore, recent studies suggest that the presence of extracellular doxorubicin is of critical importance for membrane interactions that are intimately related to the evolution of tumor cell kill[230] and that doxorubicin cytotoxicity can be manipulated by membrane phospholipid alterations [231-233] that increase drug uptake but not intracellular distribution. The confluence of these studies suggests that plasma membrane–associated events, modulated by lipid metabolism, could be involved in the mechanism of action of the anthracyclines.

Signal Transduction and Anthracyclines

Communication between the cell surface and the nucleus plays a crucial role in growth control; several important signal transduction pathways for mitogenic stimuli can be initiated at the plasma membrane.[234-238] If membrane interactions by the anthracyclines are important for their mechanism of action, it should be possible to show that these compounds interact significantly with known signal transduction programs.[239]

Several laboratories have provided essential pieces of evidence linking anthracycline action to effects on specific signal transduction pathways, including the protein kinase C system. Although at high concentrations (>100 μM), anthracyclines can inhibit protein kinase C,[240,241] the doxorubicin-iron complex is more active as an inhibitor of diacylglycerol at 10-fold lower concentrations.[242] At clinically relevant levels, doxorubicin increases the turnover of phosphoinositides and phosphatidylcholine in sarcoma

180 cells, which leads to the accumulation of diacylglycerol and inositol phosphates and a twofold increase in cytosolic protein kinase C activity.[243] Furthermore, activation of the protein kinase C pathway by phorbol esters enhances doxorubicin cytotoxicity and drug-related DNA-protein cross-links, whereas down-regulation of protein kinase C partially prevents cell kill.[244] Since protein kinase C can phosphorylate topoisomerase II,[245] it is possible that the initiation of membrane signalling by doxorubicin could be involved in the regulation of anthracycline-mediated DNA damage.

The importance of the sphingomyelin pathway in signal transduction has become increasingly clear during the past five years.[234] In addition to participating in protein kinase C–related signal transduction, sphingolipid metabolites are involved in transducing signals from a wide variety of cell surface molecules, including interferon-γ, TNF-α, and Fas/APO-1. Recent data suggest that the activation of sphingomyelinases by a variety of cellular stresses, including exposure to the anthracyclines, leads to the release of the critical signalling intermediate ceramide from membrane sphingomyelin.[246-248] Intracellular ceramide accumulation can produce profound effects on cell cycle progression as well as on the effector arm of the cell death program.[249-251] Expression of glucosylceramide synthase (the enzyme that converts ceramide to glucosylceramide) in human MCF-7 cells blocks doxorubicin-induced increases in ceramide after drug exposure, leading to an 11-fold increase in IC_{50} concentration.[252]

Signal transduction pathways involving protein kinase C and ceramide also appear to be involved in the regulation of the function of the P170 glycoprotein and the enhanced export of anthracyclines in drug-resistant cells;[253-255]

inhibition of protein kinase C has been shown to down-regulate P170 glycoprotein function and enhance the sensitivity of myeloid leukemia cells to daunorubicin, providing a novel strategy for overcoming multidrug resistance.[256] Furthermore, certain agents that reverse multidrug resistance, such as cyclosporin A and verapamil, may in part be active through an inhibition of ceramide glycosylation.[257]

Anthracyclines and Apoptosis

The explosive growth of our understanding of apoptosis (programmed cell death)[258–260] has provided crucial links between many of the pleiotropic effects of the anthracyclines that have been described previously, including anthracycline-related alterations in membrane biochemistry, signal transduction, mitochondrial metabolism, DNA damage, and free-radical formation.

Doxorubicin or daunorubicin exposure can produce the morphological changes associated with apoptosis, such as chromatin condensation, internucleosomal DNA fragmentation, reduced cell volume, and cytoplasmic blebbing in a wide variety of cell lines, including HeLa cells,[261] P388 murine leukemia cells,[262] M1 myeloid leukemia cells,[263] murine small intestinal crypt epithelium,[264] thymocytes,[265,266] and others.[156,267] In general, the degree of anthracycline-related apoptosis varies considerably between experimental model systems; in cell culture, the full expression of apoptotic morphology is often not observed until 48 to 120 hours after drug treatment. This variability is due, in part, to wide variation in the expression of both proapoptotic and antiapoptotic molecules in cultured tumor cells, a degree of variability that has also been observed in human tumor samples.[38,268–270]

Intensive investigative efforts have begun to determine the molecular mechanisms of anthracycline-related apoptosis. The picture that is starting to emerge is of a series of biochemical interactions by the anthracycline antibiotics with a wide variety of different initiating death signals ultimately utilizing common effector molecules to produce apoptosis and/or necrotic cell kill. One of the best-described death stimuli is the interaction of the CD95 (APO-1/Fas) surface receptor with its natural ligand CD95L or structurally related antibodies to form a signalling complex that activates proteases of the caspase family to effect the ultimate biochemical reactions resulting in apoptotic morphology. This pathway, which plays a critical role in the regulation of lymphoid cell growth, has been shown to be active in some solid tumors and leukemias. Recent experiments initially suggested that doxorubicin produced apoptosis by inducing CD95L and CD95 receptor formation and that CEM cells, Jurkat T cells, and neuroblastoma cells resistant to anti-CD95 antibody were resistant to doxorubicin-induced apoptosis.[271–273] Although doxorubicin clearly appears to up-regulate CD95L expression after doxorubicin exposure in HeLa cells transfected with a CD95L reporter construct,[274] a series of recent studies in different cell lines have determined that acquired resistance to CD95 by clonal selection or by treatment with other anti-CD95 antibodies that inhibit CD95-mediated apoptosis does not concomitantly engender resistance to doxorubicin-related apoptosis,[275,276] that CD95 and CD95L are frequently not up-regulated following doxorubicin exposure,[277] and that anthracycline-mediated activation of caspase 8, previously supposed to modulate CD95-induced apoptosis specifically, occurs in the absence of signalling through the CD95/CD95L pathway.[278] All of these experiments support the hypothesis that doxorubicin and CD95 utilize common downstream effectors of apoptosis but that the initiating death stimulus for either of these molecules may vary.

Apoptosis due to the anthracyclines has also been clearly related to ceramide generation,[246,279] which links the plasma membrane biochemistry of doxorubicin with the induction of the cell death cascade. Only recently, however, has the molecular ordering of anthracycline-induced apoptosis begun to be examined. In these studies, ceramide generation following sphingomyelinase activation leads to important effects on mitochondrial permeability, the activation of proapoptotic caspases, and serine-threonine protein phosphatases.[234,249,280] Yet it remains to be determined whether ceramide production after anthracycline exposure is associated principally with the activation of cell death signals to the mitochondria or with the effector phase of apoptosis.[281]

One of the critical steps in translating a wide variety of apoptotic stimuli into either apoptotic or necrotic cell death is the induction of cytochrome c release from the space between the inner and outer mitochondrial membrane.[258,282,283] Cytochrome c release can lead to caspase activation or to altered mitochondrial electron transport, with subsequent apoptosis or necrosis. Anthracyclines are fully capable of inducing cytochrome c release independent of DNA damage.[284,285] In light of the previously described extensive binding and metabolism of the anthracyclines by complex I of the mitochondrial electron transport chain,[132] it is likely that reactive oxygen species, produced by anthracycline-treated mitochondria, can damage mitochondrial membrane integrity and may play an important initiating role in doxorubicin-related apoptosis. Recent studies indicate that various free-radical scavengers inhibit programmed cell death following anthracycline exposure.[90,156,168,169,286] Furthermore, cytokine-mediated induction of ceramide production has been found to be redox-sensitive, and overexpression of antioxidant genes in human tumor cells prevents ceramide production and partially blocks apoptosis.[287,288] These recent observations link many of the known but pleiotropic biochemical effects of the anthracyclines; further studies are likely to define the order of anthracycline-related death signals at the molecular level and the relationship of these signals to intracellular anthracycline metabolism.

Two major endogenous modulators of programmed cell death, Bcl-2 and p53, as well as their associated downstream effectors, play critical roles in regulating anthracycline-related apoptosis. The Bcl-2 protein functions in the outer membranes of mitochondria, nuclei, and the endoplasmic reticulum as an inhibitor of cell death; it has been clearly shown to block apoptosis following anthracycline exposure in many experimental systems.[289,290] Furthermore, in acute myelogenous leukemic blasts and HL-60 cells, the cytotoxicity of daunorubicin is increased by exposure to *bcl-2* antisense oligonucleotides.[291] The biochemical mechanisms through which Bcl-2 inhibits cell death continue to be elucidated; however, it is currently appreciated that Bcl-2 represses cytochrome *c* release from mitochondria, interferes with caspase activation, blocks the apoptotic effects of reactive oxygen species, and binds to transcription factors involved in doxorubicin-mediated apoptosis, such as nuclear factor-κB.[292–297] Bcl-2 has also been demonstrated to suppress p53-mediated transcriptional activation of several genes involved in the apoptotic process after doxorubicin exposure in MCF-7 cells.[292]

It appears that programmed cell death resulting from doxorubicin exposure is modulated by the interplay between the expression of *bcl-2* and the *p53* tumor suppressor gene.[298] P53 functions as a transcription factor that causes cell cycle arrest or apoptosis after DNA damage; among the genes activated by p53 are the cyclin-dependent kinase inhibitor *p21*, *cyclin G*, and the apoptosis-inducing gene *bax*. Exposure to anthracyclines leads to elevated steady-state levels of p53 in cells expressing the wild-type gene,[267,299] which produces cell cycle arrest or apoptosis depending on the cell type studied. G_1 arrest is due to the induction of p21 in both p53-dependent and p53-independent contexts, which leads to apoptosis or cellular senescence.[299–302] Studies also suggest that p53 induction after doxorubicin treatment produces up-regulation of cyclin G expression, with a consequent increase in the accumulation of cells in the G_2/M as well as G_1 phase of the cell cycle.[303] Finally, mutations in *p53*, found in almost half of human tumors, lead to diminished apoptosis and doxorubicin resistance in many different tumor cell types.[304–306]

Anthracyclines and Cellular Senescence

Recent studies have demonstrated that in addition to necrotic or apoptotic death phenotypes, exposure of mammalian cells to the anthracycline antibiotics may produce prolonged growth arrest that in morphologic and enzymatic terms resembles replicative senescence.[307] This response may occur whether or not p53 mutations are present and is characterized by the inability of cells undergoing terminal differentiation to form colonies, while at the same time remaining metabolically active but nonproliferative; furthermore, although not required for the initiation of cellular senescence, both p53 and p21 are positive regulators of the senescence phenotype.[308–310] cDNA microarray analysis has demonstrated that doxorubicin-related senescence is associated with the inhibition of genes associated with cell proliferation and the up-regulation of tumor suppressors.[311] The discovery of this novel antiproliferative pathway induced by the anthracycline antibiotics provides

additional insight into the pleiotropic nature of their antineoplastic mechanism of action as well as possible new approaches to enhancing their use in oncologic practice.[312]

Mechanisms of Resistance

Enhanced Drug Efflux

P170 Glycoprotein–Mediated Anthracycline Efflux

A majority of the doxorubicin-resistant cell lines developed in the laboratory exhibit increased expression of the P170 glycoprotein. At present, the role of this protein in enhancing drug efflux and as a mechanism of experimental drug resistance has been conclusively established.[28,313,314] The evidence supporting this role includes (a) a good correlation between the presence of this protein and a pattern of broad-spectrum drug resistance that includes the anthracyclines, vinca alkaloids, actinomycin D, and the epipodophyllotoxins[315]; (b) transfer of the cloned *MDR1* gene for this protein that demonstrates the full phenotype of multidrug resistance, including resistance to doxorubicin[316]; and (c) the reversal of anthracycline resistance by a range of compounds, such as verapamil, cyclosporine A, calmodulin inhibitors, and tamoxifen, that block P170-mediated drug efflux by binding to this protein.[317–322] The genetic mechanism behind this increased expression in selected lines in vitro is variable. In some cell lines demonstrating very high levels of anthracycline resistance, the notable finding has been gene amplification, either present in double minutes or integrated within the chromosome as homogeneous staining regions; other lines show only increased messenger RNA coding for the P170 glycoprotein.[323,324] The nature of the resistance that develops after a single prolonged exposure to doxorubicin in a human sarcoma cell line was evaluated using classic fluctuation analysis; induction of *MDR1* expression was not demonstrated, but rather resistance to doxorubicin arose from a spontaneous mutation with an apparent rate of approximately 2×10^{-6} per cell generation.[325] It is also clear that the expression of the *MDR1* gene may, under some circumstances, be transcriptionally modulated by doxorubicin itself as well as inhibitors of protein kinase C and calmodulin.[254,326,327] For resistance that develops in vivo, the situation is more complex, with most tumors and many normal tissues exhibiting increased expression of a single gene copy.[315]

Although the physiologic role for this protein has not been established unequivocally, its expression has been documented in a range of normal tissues. Elevated expression is seen in colon mucosa, kidney, adrenal medulla, adrenal cortex, the blood-brain barrier, and many normal bone marrow elements.[328–330] In addition, expression in liver is increased after both partial hepatectomy and exposure to carcinogens such as 2-acetylaminofluorene.[331] The combination of partial hepatectomy and carcinogen exposure is synergistic, resulting in over a 100-fold increase in expression. Based on this information, it has been postulated that the P170 glycoprotein is part of an integrated system for protecting cells against toxic xenobiotics.[332,333] Other components of this system include the mixed-function oxidases, glutathione transferases, glucuronyl transferases, glutathione, and glutathione peroxidase.

A wide range of human tumors has been examined before and after treatment with anthracyclines and other drugs that participate in the multidrug-resistance phenotype. Increased expression of the P170 glycoprotein is found before treatment in renal, colon, and adrenal carcinomas, some neuroblastomas and soft tissue sarcomas, and occasionally in tumors of lymphoid or myeloid origin. For patients with acute lymphocytic and myelocytic leukemias, expression of P170 glycoprotein carries an adverse prognosis.[334,335] P170 glycoprotein expression is rarely found at significant levels either before or after therapy in small cell carcinoma of the lung, but expression is clearly increased posttreatment in some patients failing primary therapy for leukemia, lymphoma, or myeloma.[336,337] Expression in breast cancer is variable.[338,339] Clinical trials evaluating the effect of multidrug-reversal agents on the efficacy of anthracycline-containing chemotherapeutic programs have begun to be available.[340–342] In general, the initial studies of this approach demonstrate that clinical strategies to overcome P170 glycoprotein–mediated drug resistance are most likely to be effective for patients with hematologic malignancies, that better reversing agents able to be administered at the appropriate dose with an acceptable toxicity profile are urgently needed, and that, not unexpectedly, the pharmacokinetics of the anthracyclines may be significantly altered by drugs such as cyclosporine A, which markedly decreases the clearance of doxorubicin and doxorubicinol.[343] Despite these difficulties, a recent large randomized trial for patients with AML demonstrated significantly improved relapse-free and overall survival when cyclosporine A was added to daunorubicin as part of a standard cytosine arabinoside and daunorubicin induction regimen.[344] It remains to be determined whether these results reflect reversal of P-glycoprotein–mediated acquired resistance or are due to the increased levels of daunorubicin and its alcohol metabolite found in patients treated with cyclosporine A.

Multidrug Resistance Protein and Other ATP-Dependent Efflux Mechanisms

In some doxorubicin-resistant cell lines that exhibit decreased drug accumulation, P170 glycoprotein is not overexpressed, and verapamil produces quite variable alterations in resistance.[345,346] These results are explained by a unique, ATP-dependent efflux protein that was discovered in the doxorubicin-selected human small cell cancer line H69/AR. Its mRNA encodes a 190-kd protein that is a member of the ATP-binding cassette transmembrane transporter superfamily.[32] The encoded glycoprotein has also been found in doxorubicin-resistant HL-60 leukemia cells

and the doxorubicin-resistant HT1080/DR4 human sarcoma line, both of which lack P170 glycoprotein expression.[33,347] A wide variety of other experimental tumor cell systems have also been demonstrated to overexpress the multidrug resistance protein (MRP).[348–350] The overexpression of MRP in drug-sensitive HeLa cells has been shown to produce resistance to doxorubicin, etoposide, and vincristine but not to cisplatin or traditional alkylating agents; thus, MRP expression alone, in the absence of alterations in MDR1 expression or levels of topoisomerase II, can produce anthracycline resistance. Furthermore, doxorubicin export by the *MRP* gene product is as efficient as that by the P-glycoprotein.[351] In contrast to human sarcoma cells, doxorubicin selection of leukemic cells in vitro leads first to the overexpression of MRP at low drug concentrations, with the subsequent expression of the P170 glycoprotein.[352] Furthermore, MRP may function coordinately with MDR1 to produce anthracycline resistance in patients with acute leukemia, suggesting that MRP may play an important role in the clinic.[353,354] These studies also suggest that critical tissue specificities may be involved in the evolution of the overexpression of different transport proteins.

MRP expression occurs widely in normal tissues except the liver and small intestine, where expression is limited.[355] Studies utilizing *MRP* knockout models[356] have suggested a variety of physiological functions for the multidrug resistance protein. These include transport of heavy metals; modulation of ion channels; transport of glutathione conjugates, including leukotriene C_4; and the cotransport of GSH with and without other xenobiotics such as the anthracyclines.[35,37] Although transport of chemically prepared conjugates of doxorubicin or daunorubicin with glutathione by membrane vesicles from cells overexpressing MRP has been documented,[37] the occurrence of such conjugates in vivo has not yet been observed. It is more likely that MRP plays a critical role in the cotransport of GSH with the anthracyclines as part of a series of related gene products rather than as a single GS-X pump.[357]

When additional multidrug-resistant tumor cell lines were discovered that relied on enhanced drug efflux but lacked either the P170 glycoprotein or overexpression of MRP, studies revealed a novel ATP-binding cassette transporter, initially in breast cancer cells resistant to the combination of doxorubicin and verapamil.[358,359] This transporter was initially named the breast cancer resistance protein (BCRP) because it was cloned from MCF-7 breast cancer cells. Doxorubicin can, at variable levels, be transported by BCRP; however, this depends on the presence of a specific mutation in BCRP at arginine 482 that increases drug efflux.[360] BCRP more effectively transports mitoxantrone, camptothecin-related topoisomerase I inhibitors, and quinazoline *ErbB1* inhibitors. The role of BCRP expression in the development of anthracycline resistance for patients with acute leukemia is under active investigation.[361,362]

Other ATP-dependent doxorubicin efflux pumps have also been characterized.[34] Furthermore, a 110-kd lung resistance-related protein has been identified as the major vault protein, a critical component of certain subcellular organelles[39]; this protein has been associated with an adverse prognosis in patients with AML treated with anthracycline-containing chemotherapy.[38,40]

These more recent discoveries, taken together with the finding of an entire family of genes encoding multidrug resistence associated proteins (MRPs),[357] suggest the possibility that several distinct efflux mechanisms exist for the anthracyclines. This is entirely consistent with the redundant mechanisms present in mammalian cells to resist the toxicity of xenobiotics.

Altered Topoisomerase II Activity

Altered topoisomerase II activity has been implicated as a cause of resistance involving the anthracyclines. The resistance pattern of cells selected for topoisomerase II–mediated drug insensitivity may differ from the classic profile of *MDR1* substrates. Nonetheless, it is clear that doxorubicin resistance in P388 and L1210 cells, MCF-7 breast cancer cells, and human small cell lung cancer and melanoma lines can be associated with reduced DNA topoisomerase II activity and drug-induced DNA cleavage.[60,363–368] When tumor cells are selected for anthracycline resistance in the presence of the cyclosporine A analog PSC-833, which binds the P-glycoprotein, doxorubicin resistance develops in the context of significant reductions in topoisomerase IIα mRNA and protein as well as diminished catalytic activity without overexpression of MDR1, MRP, or the lung resistance-associated protein.[369] It is relatively common for tumor cells selected with an anthracycline alone to exhibit both altered topoisomerase II activity and expression of the P170 glycoprotein or MRP.[364,368,370] The mechanisms of decreased topoisomerase activity that have been described from in vitro studies include the presence of mutations in the topoisomerase IIα gene,[63] decreased topoisomerase IIα gene copy number,[61] and transcriptional downregulation of topoisomerase gene expression.[371] Perhaps the most persuasive evidence that changes in topoisomerase II activity are causally related to doxorubicin resistance has been provided by studies that demonstrate reversal of resistance after transfer of a fully functional topoisomerase II gene into resistant cells.[372] The importance of these observations for our understanding of anthracycline resistance at the clinical level remains to be elucidated. However, in a related clinical study, the activity of topoisomerase II in acute myelogenous leukemia cells varied over a more than 20-fold range, with significant cell-to-cell heterogeneity; there was no relationship between enzyme levels and drug sensitivity.[373]

Altered Free Radical Biochemistry, Sensitivity to Apoptosis, and Other Mechanisms of Anthracycline Resistance

The relationship between changes in intracellular free-radical detoxifying species and doxorubicin resistance has been reviewed above. It is sufficient here to emphasize that there are considerable, and probably tissue-specific, variations in the ability of cells to respond to a drug-induced free-radical challenge through enhanced antioxidant defense.[374,375]

In addition to changes in drug export, topoisomerase II activity, or defenses against free radicals, it has recently been appreciated that other resistance mechanisms are at work to prevent doxorubicin-related cell death. Clearly, overexpression of *bcl-2* can significantly diminish the toxicity of doxorubicin, as can mutations in *p53*.[289,304,306] However, as described above, the varied downstream effectors of anthracycline-mediated programmed cell death may individually play critical roles in drug sensitivity beyond that produced by *bcl-2* or p53 per se.[257,376–378] Furthermore, in light of the broad importance of these mediators of tumor cell killing for essentially all classes of antineoplastic agents,[379] it is also likely that alterations in components of the cell death cascade play an important role in resistance to the anthracyclines acquired in the clinic prior to anthracycline administration.

Potent nuclear DNA repair systems also contribute substantially to the ability of tumor cells to withstand the cytotoxic effects of doxorubicin.[380] Attention has focused on the loss of DNA mismatch repair genes, such as *MLH1*, in the production of the doxorubicin-resistant phenotype, although the pathways to cell death that are interfered with remain unclear at present.[381–384] Mutations producing decreased levels of poly(ADP-ribose)polymerase in V79 cells also dramatically decrease the efficacy of doxorubicin.[385] Since ADP-ribosylation is a well-known posttranslational modification of topoisomerase II and plays an important role in NAD$^+$ utilization, these results suggest that critical aspects of intermediary metabolism may modify the relationship between DNA cleavage reactions and tumor cell killing.[386–388] Inhibitors of this enzyme are also capable of producing doxorubicin resistance in human tumor cells.[389,390] However, resistance patterns apparently mediated by alterations in ADP-ribosylation may, in fact, represent partial blockade of certain downstream effectors of the apoptotic cascade, since poly(ADP-ribose)polymerase is a critical substrate for the caspases.[258]

Additional mechanisms of DNA repair of relevance to the pharmacology of the anthracycline antibiotics are the activities of the hereditary breast cancer susceptibility genes *BRCA1* and *2* that participate in a common DNA damage response pathway.[391] *BRCA1* and *2* are initially upregulated, then depleted by exposure to doxorubicin in p53-competent cells.[392,393] It has been suggested that a deficiency in *BRCA1* may sensitize cells to killing by doxorubicin; however, this has not been universally observed.[394,395] The level of *BRCA1* mRNA expression may also provide predictive information regarding overall therapeutic efficacy in women treated with an anthracycline-containing chemotherapeutic program.[396]

Drug Interactions

Very few drug interactions have been documented for the anthracyclines. Heparin, a large polyanion, binds to the aminosugar of doxorubicin and daunorubicin, creating insoluble aggregates. Coadministration of heparin and doxorubicin can lead to an increase in the rate of doxorubicin clearance. In rodents, phenobarbital has been shown to increase, and morphine decrease, doxorubicin disappearance.[397,398]

Doxorubicin and daunorubicin can cause radiosensitization of normal tissues and subsequent radiation recall. The most significant aspect of this problem occurs with the heart. A cardiac radiation exposure of 2,000 cGy given in conventional 200-cGy per day fractionation results in a doubling of the rate at which cardiac toxicity develops so that a cumulative doxorubicin dose of 250 mg/m² is equivalent to a dose of 500 mg/m² in the absence of radiation. This is not an uncommon problem, in that doxorubicin is used for first-line therapy of breast cancer and Hodgkin's disease, for which mediastinal or chest wall radiation therapy is also often used. Recent radiation techniques have reduced the cardiac radiation dose that occurs during treatment following breast-conserving surgery, which lessens this risk somewhat.

Recently, the disposition of doxorubicin was found to be significantly altered when it was administered immediately after a short i.v. infusion of paclitaxel.[399] This is due to the presence of high levels of Cremophor EL, the diluent in which paclitaxel is prepared, in the plasma after paclitaxel administration. Cremophor EL is a substrate for the P-glycoprotein and can significantly affect the biliary excretion of doxorubicin.[400] This interaction is not observed if paclitaxel is given over 24 hours (which lowers the concentration of the diluent in plasma) or if docetaxel, rather than paclitaxel, is combined with doxorubicin, since the former taxane is not prepared in Cremophor EL.

Clinical Pharmacology

Dose and Schedule of Administration

Doxorubicin has been successfully administered using a wide range of schedules, and at present there is little evidence that changes in schedule make any significant difference in antitumor activity. As mentioned earlier, the antitumor activity of doxorubicin is proportional to the area under the curve (AUC), not to peak drug levels. Thus, a dose of 60 mg/m² is approximately equally effective administered as a bolus or infused over 1, 2, or 4 days. Myelosuppression is also proportional to AUC and changes very little over this broad range of schedules. The most common schedule has been 45 to 60 mg/m² every 18 to 21 days. Because of evidence that peak level correlates with cardiac toxicity, weekly dosing at 20 to 30 mg/m² has also been evaluated and seems to be both less cardiotoxic

and approximately as effective as bolus dosing. This trend has been extended to the administration of a 96-hour infusion that is convincingly less cardiotoxic while preserving antitumor activity.[401] As an added benefit, prolonged infusions dramatically lessen the nausea and vomiting associated with bolus administration of doxorubicin. The only major negative aspect of infusional doxorubicin is a tendency for mucositis to increase in intensity as the infusion is prolonged. Daunorubicin is usually administered as a brief intravenous infusion in doses of 30 to 45 mg/m² daily for 3 days as induction therapy for AML.

Pharmacokinetics and Metabolism

The basic pharmacokinetic constants for doxorubicin and daunorubicin are listed in Table 18.1. The pharmacokinetics of these drugs are dominated by tissue binding. During the early distributive phase, drug levels fall rapidly as the drug gains ready access to all tissues of the body except the brain. During this phase, the bulk of the drug binds to DNA throughout the body, and in general tissue levels of the drug are proportional to their DNA content.[402] In addition, plasma protein binding accounts for approximately 75% of the drug in the plasma.[403] In spite of this plasma protein binding, tissue-plasma ratios range from 10:1 to 500:1 by virtue of the higher affinity of the drugs for DNA than for plasma. Tumor levels have rarely been measured in humans, but multiple myeloma patients were studied during a 96-hour infusion of doxorubicin. Doxorubicin levels of about 10 μM were documented in myeloma cells by the end of the infusion.[404] However, with the extensive binding of these drugs to DNA and proteins, the free-drug pool probably represents a very small fraction of the drug concentrations measured in both plasma and cells. Unfortunately, there have been no detailed studies of the pharmacokinetics of this free-drug pool.

After bolus administration, or after the conclusion of a constant i.v. infusion, an initial doxorubicin half-life of 10 minutes is followed by a secondary half-life of 1 to 3 hours. The terminal half-life of 30 to 50 hours accounts for over 70% of the total drug AUC for doxorubicin. As a result of this prolonged terminal phase, plasma levels of drug remain above 10 nM for the greater part of a week after a single dose of 60 mg/m² of doxorubicin.[403] In tissue culture, levels as low as 1 to 5 nM are cytotoxic for sensitive tumor cells after extended exposures. Even accounting for the difference in protein content between tissue culture media and plasma, these results suggest that drug levels sufficient for tumor cell kill may persist for prolonged periods. Doxorubicinol is the primary metabolite of doxorubicin in human plasma but is present in concentrations far smaller than those of the parent compound. Approximately 50% of the drug is excreted in the bile, both as parent drug and as various metabolites, including glucuronides and sulfates. Less than 10% of the administered drug appears in the urine; however, this is sufficient to cause a reddish-orange discoloration of the urine in many patients. When administered at higher than standard dose levels (>100 mg/m^2), peak plasma levels of doxorubicin may reach 6-7 μM. When administered as a continuous i.v. infusion at high dose (150 to 165 mg/m^2), steady state doxorubicin concentrations are approximately 0.1 μM.[405] The relationship of AUC to dose appears to be linear up to a doxorubicin dose level of 165 mg/m^2 whether the drug is administered as a bolus or as a continuous infusion.[405,406]

Pharmacokinetic studies of gender and body surface area[407,408] revealed, unexpectedly, that men with normal hepatic function were found to have approximately twice the clearance of doxorubicin (administered as an i.v. bolus) as compared with women; higher drug clearance was associated with an increased conversion rate of doxorubicin to its major alcohol metabolite. The pharmacodynamic implications of these findings are uncertain. The pharmacokinetics of the anthracycline analog epirubicin is independent of body surface area; normalization of epirubicin dose based on surface area has no effect on the drug's observed AUC. Although neutropenia correlated well with epirubicin AUC when the drug was administered as a single agent, the absence of an effect of body surface area normalization on systemic exposure suggests that this procedure neither reduces interpatient variability in anthracycline pharmacokinetics nor variability in hematopoietic toxicity following epirubicin treatment. Drug administration at fixed milligram increments for this drug would appear to be rational, safe, and more efficient than current standard practice.

For daunorubicin, metabolism to daunorubicinol is a major determinant of its plasma pharmacology. The parent drug is cleared rapidly from plasma, with a primary half-life of 40 minutes; the loss of parent drug from plasma correlates with the rapid appearance of C^4-O-demethyl daunorubicin, daunorubicinol, their aglycones, and various sulfate and glucuronide metabolites in bile. Within hours after a bolus dose of daunorubicin, the predominant circulating form of the drug is the alcohol metabolite,[409] which has a longer half-life (23 to 40 hours) than its parent. The opposite is the case for doxorubicin, where doxorubicinol is typically a minor part of the total AUC.[410] The formation of either doxorubicinol or daunorubicinol is a function of the enzymatic conversion of the side-chain carbonyl to an alcohol by one or more enzymes in the hepatic aldoketoreductase family.[411–415]

Over the years, there has been considerable controversy as to the importance of the aglycone metabolites of the anthracyclines. There are two families of aglycones to be considered, the 7-deoxy and 7-hydroxy aglycones. As mentioned earlier, the 7-deoxyaglycones are the result of a two-electron reduction of the parent drug to a quinone methide, with subsequent elimination of the sugar. It is important to emphasize that the full two-electron reduction of the anthracyclines to the 7-deoxyaglycone stage occurs stepwise, after initial one-electron reduction by microsomal or mitochondrial flavin-containing enzymes. Thus, the demonstration of 7-deoxy by-products has been argued to be de facto evidence of an anthracycline redox cycle. The 7-hydroxyaglycones result from hydrolysis of the sugar-anthraquinone bond. The latter can arise artifactually during the processing and analysis of the drug. This has especially been a problem with older techniques that depend upon thin-layer chromatography. In the past, many investigators seem to have been confused about the distinction between these two aglycone families, and thus the importance of the 7-deoxyaglycones was dismissed by some. It is now clear that the 7-deoxyaglycones are indeed circulating metabolites of both daunorubicin and doxorubicin. In addition, the formation of the 7-deoxyaglycones exhibits large patient-to-patient variability. 7-Deoxydoxorubicin can range from 1 to 5% of the total drug. In contrast, 7-deoxydoxorubicinol aglycone can range from 0 to 20%.[215]

Doxorubicinol and daunorubicinol are cytotoxic metabolites but are considerably less active than the parent compound.[416] As mentioned earlier, deoxyaglycones are much less active than the corresponding parent drug and are currently viewed as a pathway of drug inactivation. In one study, aglycone levels in patients with acute myelogenous leukemia were statistically significantly higher in nonresponders than in responders.[417]

Although the bulk of doxorubicin elimination occurs by hepatic metabolism and biliary excretion, the evidence that doses of doxorubicin or daunorubicin must be reduced in patients with compromised hepatic function is somewhat difficult to interpret.[418–421] Altered patterns of metabolism have been observed in individual patients, with prolonged terminal half-life of parent drug, and decreased clearance of doxorubicinol. Patients with abnormal liver function also have a diminished capacity to clear doxorubicin when it is administered as an infusion or a bolus.[421,422] However, no consistent pattern of increased toxicity has emerged in patients with mildly decreased drug clearance. Moderate to severe alterations in hepatic function, however, increase AUC significantly.[423] Physicians are advised to reduce doses routinely in patients with moderate or severe hepatic dysfunction or when marked replacement of the liver by tumor is present, in which case all forms of chemotherapy carry increased risk.

Toxicity

Table 18.1 provides a summary of the common toxicities of the anthracyclines.

Bone Marrow Suppression and Mucositis

Bone marrow suppression and mucositis are common to other anticancer drugs, and there is nothing unusual about these toxic reactions after anthracycline administration. Both myelosuppression and mucositis follow an acute course, with maximal toxicity within 7 to 10 days of drug administration and rapid recovery thereafter. For daunorubicin, bone marrow suppression is more common than mucositis and is the usual dose-limiting toxicity. Doxorubicin causes these two reactions in more equal severity after bolus dose administration. With weekly dosing or continuous infusion, mucositis frequently becomes the dose-limiting toxicity.

Extravasation Injury

Extravasation of most anthracyclines leads to severe local injury that can continue to progress over weeks to months. The drug has been shown to bind locally to tissues and can still be detected at high levels at the base of a drug-induced ulcer in the soft tissues of the hand or forearm months later.[424–426] These lesions are very difficult to treat. Skin grafting is usually not successful unless preceded by extensive excision of the involved tissue. However, debridement of dead tissue should be undertaken with extreme caution during the initial phases of extravasation injury, and local wound care to prevent infection is most important.[427] A wide range of treatments have been used immediately after extravasation in an attempt to lessen the injury. These have included ice, steroids, vitamin E, DMSO, and bicarbonate.[428,429] More recently, the cardioprotectant dexrazoxane has been used to treat acute anthracycline extravasations in combination with subcutaneous granulocyte-macrophage colony-stimulating factor to promote wound healing.[430]

Cardiac Toxicity

The cardiac toxicity exhibited by doxorubicin and the other anthracyclines is unique in its pathology and mechanism.[431,432] Although the major limiting factors in the clinical use of anthracyclines in adults are bone marrow suppression, mucositis, and drug resistance on the part of the tumor, for individual patients, most commonly with the use of doxorubicin in breast cancer, cardiac toxicity can develop while the patient's tumor is still responsive to the drug. This is a problem not only for the use of the anthracyclines alone or in combination with other chemotherapeutic agents but also with the monoclonal antibody trastuzumab. Trials have demonstrated synergistic cardiac toxicity for the combination of doxorubicin and trastuzumab,[433] an antibody directed against the *HER2/neu* oncoprotein, which is itself active in the treatment of advanced breast cancer.[434] The observed potentiation of anthracycline-induced heart damage by trastuzumab has eliminated its concurrent use with doxorubicin in the population of patients whose tumors exhibit high levels of *HER2/neu* expression, a group that could benefit most from this combination.[435] Finally, children seem to be more sensitive to the cardiac toxicity of this drug, and this has become a significant problem in the use of doxorubicin in pediatric oncology.[436–439] Advances in our understanding of the impact of schedule on the cardiac toxicity

of these drugs and the development of successful antidotal agents may reduce the importance of this problem in the future.

Clinical Presentation and Management

The anthracyclines manifest both acute and chronic cardiac toxicity. Acute toxicity is detected most commonly as a range of arrhythmias, including heart block. In its more extreme form, this acute injury can include a pericarditis-myocarditis syndrome with onset of fever, pericarditis, and congestive heart failure.[440] This syndrome can occur at low cumulative doses of doxorubicin and can have a fatal outcome. In animal models, doxorubicin administration causes significant increases in circulating catecholamines and histamine, and coadministration of α- and β-adrenergic antagonists along with H_1 and H_2 blockers has lessened acute and subacute doxorubicin toxicity.[441] Clinical trials have not been conducted to see if such treatment might be effective in the management of the acute toxicity of doxorubicin in humans, perhaps because this syndrome is relatively uncommon and idiosyncratic. There has been no clear correlation between the manifestation of arrhythmias and the development of the chronic cardiomyopathy. There is essentially no experience with re-treating patients who have survived the pericarditis-myocarditis syndrome with doxorubicin or daunorubicin.

Cardiac toxicity has been best documented for doxorubicin administered as a bolus dose of 45 to 60 mg/m^2 every 21 to 28 days. With this schedule, cardiac toxicity develops as a result of cumulative injury to the myocardium. The pathology of this toxicity, determined after endomyocardial biopsy, has been described in detail; a useful grading system correlates well with the risk of clinical cardiac toxicity[442,443] (Table 18.2). These studies have shown that with each dose of doxorubicin there is progressive injury to the myocardium so that the grade increases steadily with total dose of drug administered. The major changes observed in myocytes are dilation of the sarcoplasmic reticulum and disruption of myofibrils. Early in the development of this toxicity, these changes appear focally in scattered myocytes

TABLE 18.2

CRITERIA FOR GRADING ANTHRACYCLINE CARDIOMYOPATHY

Grade	Criteria
0	No change from normal
1	Scanty cells with early myofibrillar loss and/or distended sarcoplasmic reticulum
2	Groups of cells with marked myofibrillar loss and/or cytoplasmic vacuolization
3	Diffuse cell damage with total loss of contractile elements, loss of organelles and mitochondria, and nuclear degeneration

surrounded by normal-appearing cells. As the toxicity progresses, the frequency of these altered cells increases until a significant proportion of the myocardium is involved. Late in the development of this toxicity, the picture is complicated by the development of diffuse myocardial fibrosis. This pathology is unique to the anthracyclines and allows the pathologist definitely to distinguish this cardiac toxicity from other processes such as viral cardiomyopathy or ischemic heart injury. In addition, Billingham's grading system has allowed correlation of the findings among studies done at a range of institutions and has made possible the advances that have now significantly lessened the risk of this problem.

The clinical risk of congestive heart failure is low at total doses below 250 to 300 mg/m² of doxorubicin or 600 to 700 mg/m² of daunorubicin,[444,445] although cases of fatal congestive cardiomyopathy have been observed after a single dose of doxorubicin. Above these doses, the risk steadily accelerates. The total dose limit at which the risk becomes unacceptable is largely arbitrary, and as discussed above, the risk may in part be dependent on the treatment schedule used. For doxorubicin, the most commonly used total dose limit applied in the past has been 450 to 500 mg/m², at which the risk of clinically evident cardiac toxicity has generally been believed to be 1 to 10% (Figure 18.7). The corresponding limit applied for daunorubicin has been 900 to 1,000 mg/m². However, recent large trials that have prospectively evaluated heart function with radionuclide-gated cardiac blood pool scans strongly suggest that subclinical, but not inconsequential, reductions in ejection fraction can be detected routinely after 250 to 300 mg/m² of doxorubicin.[446–448] Furthermore, changes in ejection fraction may or may not predict the development of heart failure in a specific patient. As mentioned below, certain patients, especially those with breast cancer, may approach

this total dose limit with a tumor that is still responsive to doxorubicin when there are few other therapeutic options. It has been established that changing from bolus to 96-hour infusion or the addition of dexrazoxane after a cumulative doxorubicin dose level of 300 mg/m² will allow a substantial duration of additional anthracycline therapy with a significantly reduced risk of severe cardiac toxicity.[3,449,450]

It has often been said that doxorubicin-induced cardiac toxicity is difficult to treat and is associated with a high mortality.[451] While doxorubicin-induced congestive heart failure may have a fatal outcome, it is eminently treatable with standard measures, and many patients (probably well over half) recover or stabilize at a lower, but clinically acceptable, level of cardiac function.[451,452] It is important to point out, however, that congestive heart failure may occur many months after the discontinuation of doxorubicin and that patients who have been stabilized with adequate medical management are at increased risk during subsequent intercurrent illnesses.[451,453] Children are clearly at risk for developing congestive heart failure many years after discontinuing doxorubicin even if treated long term with an angiotensin-converting enzyme inhibitor.[454]

There are now a number of techniques available to detect the cardiac toxicity early (Table 18.3). Endomyocardial biopsy provides a definitive assessment of risk. However, this may not be available to the clinician. Ejection fraction measurement by electrocardiogram (ECG)–gated radioisotopic cardiac blood pool scan has been shown to provide an accurate measure of cardiac contractility.[455,456] A significant drop in contractility by this technique is usually seen before the onset of congestive heart failure, but this may not be the case in an individual patient.[457] Because of these techniques, clinically significant cardiac toxicity is now detected much earlier, and this has done much to lessen the mortality of this complication. Medical management centers around afterload reduction. With conservative treatment, many patients experience gradual improvement in function, and a few patients can have a rather dramatic return of exercise tolerance. This improvement can, however, take more than 1 year.

Lessening the Risk of Cardiac Toxicity

Fortunately, much can now be done to lessen the risk of cardiac toxicity. First, patient characteristics associated with increased risk have been identified. Hypertension and pre-existing cardiac disease predisposing to diastolic dysfunction significantly increase the risk that a patient will develop clinically apparent cardiac abnormalities at a lower cumulative drug dose. Cardiac radiation exposure clearly increases the sensitivity of the heart to anthracyclines; at a radiation dose of 2,000 cGy, the slope of the cardiac biopsy score versus the cumulative doxorubicin dose doubles so that a dose of 250 mg/m² becomes equal to a dose of 500 mg/m² in the absence of radiation.[458] Modern advances in computer-based radiation treatment

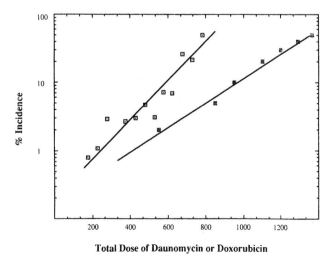

Figure 18.7   Incidence of congestive heart failure as a function of cumulative dose (in mg/m²) of either daunomycin (■) or doxorubicin (□). Daunomycin is a much less potent cardiotoxin than doxorubicin. (Redrawn from data presented in references 400 and 401.)

TABLE 18.3

PHYSIOLOGIC TESTS OF CARDIAC FUNCTION

Test Used	Pertinent Measurement	Value Considered to Indicate Cardiomyopathy	Advantages	Disadvantages
Systolic time intervals	PEP/LVET	1. Greater than 0.42–0.45 2. Increase of > 0.07 from control	Simple to perform; inexpensive	Large standard error; strongly affected by load factors
Echocardiography	Fractional shortening; ejection fraction	Less than 30%; < 45%	Equipment widely available; personnel trained to perform tests widely available; moderate cost	Limited interpretability in significant proportion of adults; assumes uniformity of function and normal left ventricular geometry; measurements subject to error
ECG	QRS voltage	Decrease in precardial leads of ≥ 30%	Simple to perform; inexpensive	Large standard error of lead position; lacks adequate sensitivity; detects abnormalities associated with cardiomyopathy rather than predicting changes
Cardiac catheterization	Ejection fraction; cardiac output; pressure measurement	Below 45%; resting cardiac index of < 2.5 L/min; exercise increase < 5; pulmonary wedge pressure > 12 mmHg; resting right ventricular end-diastolic pressure >12 mmHg	Allows comprehensive assessment of cardiac function and endomyocardial biopsy if desired	Invasive, with the risks that this entails; expensive and difficult to perform repeated measurements
Radionuclide cardiography	Ejection fraction; dV/dt during diastole and systole	Decrease of > 15% from pretreatment ejection fraction; or decrease to < 45%; failure to increase EF by > 5% with exercise	Accurate measure of ventricular volumes; essentially noninvasive; easy to obtain values under varying conditions	Some operator-dependent variability in interpretation; moderately expensive

planning should be used to minimize cardiac radiation exposure in patients with breast cancer and lymphoma who will receive an anthracycline.

It is now clear that the risk of cardiac toxicity from doxorubicin is a function of peak drug level, not AUC.[401] In contrast, both in vitro and in patients, the antitumor activity of doxorubicin is a function of AUC, not peak drug level. Thus, shifting from bolus drug administration to weekly dosing or prolonged infusion results in a significant reduction in the incidence of cardiac toxicity.[459] In clinical settings where cardiac toxicity has proved to be a serious problem, such as in breast cancer or in the pediatric malignancies, where the incidence of cardiac dysfunction is higher and the late consequences more profound,[460] consideration should be given to the use of prolonged intravenous infusions or the cardioprotective agent dexrazoxane. However, in the pediatric cancer patient population, the use of dexrazoxane appears to be more effective than 48-hour doxorubicin infusions in lessening anthracycline cardiotoxicity.[461,462]

Dexrazoxane is the first agent that has shown consistent ability to block the development of anthracycline-induced cardiac toxicity in a wide range of animal models. Randomized, controlled clinical trials have proven that this agent dramatically reduces the incidence of cardiac toxicity in patients with breast cancer without significantly altering the antitumor activity of anthracycline-containing combinations.[206,449,450,463,464] In the first such study, 92 patients with advanced breast cancer received either 5-fluorouracil, doxorubicin, and cyclophosphamide or the same regimen plus dexrazoxane. The latter was given in doses of 1,000 mg/m² by intravenous infusion 30 minutes before the chemotherapeutic drugs. Patients receiving dexrazoxane had an equivalent response rate and duration of time to disease progression as those not receiving dexrazoxane. However, the dexrazoxane-treated patients had significantly smaller decreases in left ventricular ejection fraction at each dose level of doxorubicin, their cardiac biopsies reflected less histologic change, and 11 patients treated with dexrazoxane tolerated doxorubicin doses above

600 mg/m^2 while only 1 patient not receiving dexrazoxane remained on study above this dose level. The only negative aspect of this trial was a modest increase in myelosuppression in the arm receiving dexrazoxane. These results have been confirmed in larger trials with both doxorubicin and its analog epirubicin and have led to the approval of dexrazoxane by the US Food and Drug Administration as a cardioprotectant in patients receiving >300 mg/m^2 of doxorubicin. This approach also appears to be applicable to pediatric patients with sarcomas receiving doxorubicin.[438,461] To maintain its cardioprotective properties while reducing drug-related granulocytopenia, the currently recommended dose of dexrazoxane is 10 times the doxorubicin dose on a milligram per milligram basis administered no more than 30 minutes before the anthracycline infusion is initiated.

Putative Biochemical Mechanisms of Anthracycline Cardiac Toxicity

In addition to the pathologic picture outlined above, any hypothesis that seeks to explain the cardiac toxicity of the anthracyclines must also account for the alterations in cardiac biochemistry that occur after doxorubicin exposure. The consistent changes observed involve marked alterations in calcium handling in the heart muscle and include loss of high-affinity calcium-binding sites, elevation of cardiac calcium content, and mitochondrial accumulation of calcium.[465–469] The other alteration frequently described is a diminished capacity for ATP generation. In terms of muscle physiology, these changes are critical. Calcium plays a central role in linking electrical excitation with contraction; each cycle of muscle contraction is triggered by a rapid rise in free intracellular calcium, and relaxation is dependent on a rapid drop in free calcium. In addition, calcium has been shown to play a major role in regulating the beat-to-beat force of cardiac muscle contraction. The two major sites for the beat-to-beat regulation of calcium are the sarcoplasmic reticulum and mitochondria. Sarcoplasmic reticulum avidly binds calcium that is rapidly released when a wave of electrical depolarization sweeps through the sarcoplasmic membrane. Because extensions of the sarcoplasmic reticulum are in intimate contact with the contractile fibers, sarcoplasmic depolarization leads to rapid onset of muscle contraction. The cardiac mitochondria will accumulate calcium if it is available in preference to making ATP. In general, no mechanism has been offered for a direct interaction of doxorubicin with calcium. Since anthracyclines are good metal chelators, one possibility is that the drugs chelate calcium and as a result alter the distribution of this metal ion. However, doxorubicin does not chelate calcium within the physiologic concentration range for calcium. The pathology of anthracycline cardiac toxicity suggests another, more reasonable hypothesis: the major site of anatomical damage after drug exposure is the sarcoplasmic reticulum, a major site of calcium regulation. Doxorubicin injury to the sarcoplasmic reticulum leads to calcium release.[470] Calcium is then taken up by the mitochondria, which do that in preference to ATP generation. This sequence would account for the lower ATP levels and the accumulation of calcium within the mitochondria.

How do the anthracyclines trigger damage to the sarcoplasmic reticulum? The hypothesis that best explains the above phenomenon is that the cardiac toxicity of the anthracyclines results from drug-induced free-radical formation (Table 18.4). Within the heart muscle there are several sites where enzyme activity is capable of reducing doxorubicin to the corresponding semiquinone; doxorubicin-stimulated oxygen radical formation by cardiac sarcoplasmic reticulum, cytosol, and mitochondria has been conclusively demonstrated.[471,472] The non-redox-active anthracycline 5-iminodaunorubicin does not generate reactive oxygen species in the sarcoplasmic reticulum or mitochondria and is markedly less cardiotoxic than its parent molecule.[473] Doxorubicin can also induce peroxidation of the sarcoplasmic reticulum lipid and oxidant-related sulfhydryl loss; progression of this oxidative damage to the membrane is associated with a drop in both high-affinity calcium binding and the force of contraction.[129,465] Recent

TABLE 18.4

MECHANISMS OF ANTHRACYCLINE CARDIAC TOXICITY

Oxidative Mechanisms	Nonoxidative Mechanisms
Inhibition of calcium sequestration by sarcoplasmic reticulum; 10- to 20-fold decrease in IC$_{50}$ by enzymatic drug activation	Inhibition of mitochondrial cytochrome oxidase; >0.5 mmol/L drug required
Inhibition of NADH dehydrogenase between its flavin and iron-sulfur center; requires low micromolar drug concentrations	Direct oxidation of ryanodine receptor sulfhydryls
Lipid membrane peroxidation	Down-regulation of cardiac β-adrenergic receptors
Oxidation of oxymyoglobin; potential for the production of "ferryl" myoglobin, a strong oxidant	Inhibition of specific cardiac mRNAs for α-actin, troponin I
Iron "delocalization"	

IC^{50}, concentration that inhibits 50%; mRNA, messenger RNA; NADH, nicotinamide adenine dinucleotide (reduced form).
Summarized in reference 189.

studies demonstrate, furthermore, that redox cycling of the doxorubicin quinone selectively inhibits critical hyperreactive sulfhydryl groups on the ryanodine-sensitive calcium channel of the sarcoplasmic reticulum, resulting in enhanced channel activation and subsequent alterations in calcium homeostasis.[474] These observations show that doxorubicin is reduced to a semiquinone at the sarcoplasmic reticulum and that this leads to oxidative damage to the sarcoplasmic membrane, with subsequent loss of the capacity of this membrane to bind calcium, thus disrupting the linkage between electrical excitation and contraction. To confirm that oxygen radicals are indeed formed in the heart after doxorubicin exposure, isolated perfused beating rat hearts have been exposed to doxorubicin, and electron spin resonance has been used to detect hydroxyl radicals. In this setting, hydroxyl radicals could easily be detected after exposure of the heart to drug levels (1 μM) attained following bolus dosing at 60 mg/m^2 but not at concentrations obtained during a 96-hour infusion (0.04 to 0.1 μM).[150] Thus, it seems clear that doxorubicin can trigger the formation of reactive oxygen species in vivo and that this occurs at concentrations that are associated with the development of cardiac toxicity.

As outlined in Table 18.4, the anthracyclines can produce a wide variety of toxic effects in the heart, some of which may contribute to their clinical cardiac toxicity.[475,476] Unfortunately, many of the effects described occur at unrealistically high drug concentrations and do not help to explain the specificity of anthracycline cardiac damage. These considerations do not apply to studies that demonstrate specific down-regulation of cardiac α-actin and troponin I mRNAs[477] in a fashion that is not inhibited by free-radical scavengers.[478] Taken together with studies that have examined the effect of doxorubicin on the activation of other cardiac-specific genes and regulatory pathways,[479,480] it seems likely that the pathogenesis of anthracycline cardiac toxicity and its morphological expression may be understood more clearly in the future at the transcriptional level.

Why is the heart, and not other tissues, a target for this free-radical damage? Several factors are probably involved. First, cardiac tissue has very low levels of catalase activity; overexpression of catalase in the hearts of transgenic mice reduces the cardiac toxicity of doxorubicin.[148] This leaves glutathione peroxidase as the only known pathway for hydrogen peroxide detoxification in the heart. However, doxorubicin administration can produce a rapid drop in glutathione peroxidase activity. Thus, at a time when doxorubicin is stimulating the formation of hydrogen and lipid peroxides, it is also eliminating the major pathway for peroxide removal. This observation suggests that limitations in the ability of the heart enzymatically to detoxify oxygen radicals provide an important basis for it sensitivity to doxorubicin.[481] This hypothesis has received support from an unusual experiment. Prolonged exercise causes a marked increase in the activities of superoxide dismutase and glutathione peroxidase in rodents; these mice are then

more resistant to the cardiac toxicity of doxorubicin.[482] It is also highly likely that the robust affinity of the anthracyclines for mitochondrial lipids[483] enhances drug binding in a site-specific manner that markedly increases drug-related cardiac mitochondrial reactive oxygen production.[484–486] Furthermore, the heart is extraordinarily rich in iron proteins that are capable of donating their metal to catalyze strong oxidant formation.

In summary, the free-radical hypothesis has been very effective in accounting for the various characteristics of anthracycline cardiomyopathy. In addition, this hypothesis has led to the identification of an agent that is successful at dramatically reducing the cardiac toxicity of doxorubicin in humans without compromising the antitumor efficacy of this valuable anticancer agent.

DOXORUBICIN ANALOGS

A large number of doxorubicin analogs have been brought to clinical trial in the hope of finding a compound with less cardiac toxicity and a broader spectrum of antitumor action.[487,488] The most promising of these analogs are (a) idarubicin, an agent with marked activity in acute nonlymphocytic leukemia and acute lymphocytic leukemia, and (b) epirubicin, which has activity in breast cancer. The important features of these two agents, with relevant references, are given in Table 18.5.[80,127,346,489–506]

MITOXANTRONE

In the search for analogs of the anthracyclines, a variety of multiringed planar structures with the potential for DNA intercalation have been evaluated for antitumor activity. A promising related class of compounds, the anthracenediones, were synthesized by chemists at American Cyanamid Laboratories[507] in the late 1970s and were found to have potent antitumor activity against the P388 and L1210 leukemias. The most active of this series tested was mitoxantrone (dihydroanthracenedione), a planar tetracyclic compound having two symmetrical aminoalkyl side arms but no glycosidic substituent as found in the active anthracyclines (Fig. 18.8). Against P388, it is one of the most active agents tested, yielding a 500% increase in life span and a high percentage of cures.[508] Subsequent preclinical and clinical evaluation has demonstrated significant differences between this agent and the anthracyclines in terms of mechanism of action, the lesser cardiac toxicity of the anthracenediones, and their diminished potential for extravasation injury and for causing nausea and vomiting or alopecia. Their narrow spectrum of antitumor activity, confined to breast and prostate cancer and the leukemias and lymphomas, has limited the opportunity to replace doxorubicin with mitoxantrone in clinical practice. However, because of the favorable toxicity profile of mitoxantrone,

TABLE 18.5

KEY FEATURES OF ANTHRACYCLINE ANALOGS

	Idarubicin	Epirubicin
Mechanism of action	DNA strand breakage mediated by topoisomerase II; free radical–induced injury; induction of apoptosis	Same
Mechanism of resistance	1. Multidrug resistance mediated by MDR1 or MRP 2. Topoisomerase II mutations 3. Altered apoptotic response	Same
Dose/schedule (mg/m²)	10–15 IV q3wk 10 IV × 3 d (leukemia) 45 PO q3wk	90–110 IV q3wk
Pharmacokinetics 　Elimination half-life 　　Parent compound 　13-ol metabolite 　Other metabolite 　Oral bioavailability	 11.3 hr 40-60 hr 30%	 18.3 hr 21.1 hr 12.1 hr (epiglucuronide)
Metabolism	Primary metabolite, 13-epirubicinol, is cytotoxic and exceeds level of parent compound in plasma	Primary metabolites are glucuronides of parent and 13-ol
Excretion	80% excreted in urine as 13-ol	Primarily parent compound, 13-ol, and glucuronides
Toxicity	1. Leukopenia 2. Thrombocytopenia 3. Cardiotoxicity (less than doxorubicin)	1. Leukopenia 2. Thrombocytopenia 3. Cardiotoxicity equal to doxorubicin
Drug interactions	None established	None established
Precautions	None established	Possible dose reduction in hepatic dysfunction

it is an appropriate agent for use in an elderly patient population, such as men with hormone-refractory prostate cancer, where treatment can provide significant palliative benefit.[509,510]

Mechanism of Action

Like the anthracyclines, mitoxantrone binds avidly to nucleic acids and inhibits DNA and RNA synthesis. Its mode of binding to DNA includes intercalation between opposing DNA strands, with preference for GC base pairs.[511] Careful studies of the stoichiometry of binding and electron microscopic evaluation of the distortions produced in vitro in plasmid DNA indicate an additional type of binding that produces a compaction of chromatin[512] and, with plasmid DNA, lacelike intertwining of the DNA strands. These effects are dependent on the presence of the highly positively charged aminoalkyl side chains and probably represent electrostatic cross-linking of DNA strands. Also found are single- and double-strand breaks in DNA.[513]

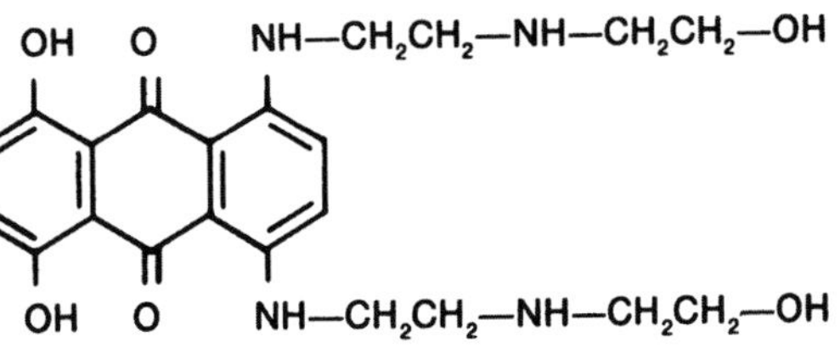

Because the drug has the basic quinone structure found in the anthracyclines, its ability to generate free radicals in a manner similar to that of doxorubicin has been examined. These studies revealed that the drug has a much reduced potential to undergo one-electron reduction, compared to doxorubicin,[514,515] and is less readily reduced enzymatically.[516] Since some of the single-strand breaks are protein-associated, it appears that these breaks result from the formation of a cleavable complex with topoisomerase II, which occurs in mitoxantrone-treated cells.[517] This possibility is heightened by the finding that there is little evidence of lipid peroxidation in cardiac tissue, modest stimulation of oxygen consumption in vitro, and, indeed, inhibition of doxorubicin-induced lipid peroxidation by mitoxantrone;[518] all of these findings argue against a free-radical mechanism of tissue injury by mitoxantrone and favor enzyme-mediated DNA cleavage. The reduced potential for free-radical formation may also explain the lesser cardiotoxicity of mitoxantrone, although this drug is able to oxidize critical sulfhydryl groups on the ryanodine receptor of the sarcoplasmic reticulum.[475,476,519] As is the case for the anthracyclines, mitoxantrone can also readily stimulate apoptosis in a variety of cell lines.[520,521] Ceramide-dependent pathways have been implicated as part of the molecular ordering of mitoxantrone-induced programmed cell death.[248]

OH　O　NH—CH₂CH₂—NH—CH₂CH₂—OH

OH　O　NH—CH₂CH₂—NH—CH₂CH₂—OH

Figure 18.8 Structure of mitoxantrone.

Mechanisms of Drug Resistance

As a planar anthraquinone analog, it is not surprising that mitoxantrone shares cross-resistance with many of the natural products, including the vinca alkaloids and doxorubicin.[522-524] This resistance may be mediated by amplification of the P170 glycoprotein (classic MDR1); however, in some cell lines, decreased intracellular drug accumulation is related to the overexpression of the multidrug resistance protein (MRP).[525,526] Alterations in topoisomerase II function have also been well described as a mechanism of mitoxantrone resistance.[527] In fact, there are now clear examples in which tumor cells develop pleiotropic resistance based both on enhanced efflux and altered topoisomerase function.[528] Recent studies have also clarified a series of prior observations suggesting that mitoxantrone resistance in vitro could occur in the absence of alterations in topoisomerase II or enhanced expression of MDR1 or MRP.[359,523,529,530] These investigations have identified a novel member of the ATP-binding cassette superfamily of transporters that encodes a 655–amino acid protein (termed the breast cancer resistance protein) that is capable of enhancing the efflux of mitoxantrone and the anthracyclines from mitoxantrone-selected tumor cell lines. Additional mechanisms of mitoxantrone resistance have been related to altered intracellular pH in tumor cells[531] and to modifications in the cellular apoptotic program.

Drug Interactions

Mitoxantrone is frequently used in combination with arabinosylcytosine in the treatment of acute nonlymphocytic leukemia, and there is evidence for biochemical synergy of the two agents. In studies of leukemic cells taken from patients during therapy, coadministration of mitoxantrone and arabinosylcytosine enhanced the accumulation of araCTP in leukemic blast cells.[532] In the same study, mitoxantrone alone produced no detectable single-strand breaks but in combination with arabinosylcytosine induced easily detectable single-strand breaks as determined by alkaline elution of blast cell DNA. The molecular basis for these favorable interactions is not understood. Like doxorubicin, mitoxantrone sensitizes cells to both hyperthermia and ionizing radiation.[533]

Dosage

The recommended dosage for bolus intravenous administration of mitoxantrone is 12 mg/m^2 per day for 3 days for treatment of AML and 12 to 14 mg/m^2 per day once every 3 weeks for patients with solid tumors. The drug has definitely established activity against breast cancer,[534] ovarian cancer,[535] non-Hodgkin's lymphoma,[536] and prostate cancer[509] as well as against acute leukemia.[537] The drug is administered as a 30-minute infusion and rarely causes extravasation injury if infiltrated. Mitoxantrone should not be administered in solutions containing heparin.

Pharmacokinetics

Mitoxantrone can be measured in plasma and urine by HPLC.[538,539] The plasma disappearance of mitoxantrone is characterized by a rapid preliminary phase of clearance, with half-lives of approximately 10 minutes($t_{1/2\alpha}$) and 1.1 to 1.6 hours ($t_{1/2\beta}$)[538,539] followed by a long terminal half-life of 23 to 42 hours. During this final phase of drug disappearance, the drug concentration in plasma approximates 1 ng/mL (or 2 nM), a level at the margin of cytotoxicity. The pharmacokinetics of mitoxantrone are linear over the dose range from 8 to 14 mg/m^2 administered as a short infusion.[540] Less than 30% of the drug can be accounted for by the fraction of drug that appears in the urine (less than 10%) or the stool (less than 20%). Like doxorubicin, the drug distributes in high concentrations into tissues (liver > bone marrow > heart > lung > kidney) and remains in these sites for weeks after therapy.[538] Although specific guidelines are not available for dose adjustment in patients with hepatic dysfunction, several authors have noted a prolongation of the terminal half-life to >60 hours in patients with liver impairment.[539,541]

The specific metabolites of mitoxantrone have not been well characterized.[542] The side chains undergo oxidation, yielding the mono- and dicarboxylic acids of anthracenedione, and both have been recovered from urine.[543] Neither has antitumor activity.

As an alternative to intravenous infusion, mitoxantrone has been administered by hepatic intra-arterial infusion[544] and by intraperitoneal instillation.[545,546] These trials were based on the observation that mitoxantrone has a steep dose-response curve in vitro and that optimal concentrations of drug (1 to 10 μg/mL) are achieved only briefly during standard intravenous therapy. Local concentrations much higher than those realized in systemic administration can be achieved by either the intra-arterial or intraperitoneal routes. During intraperitoneal trials, patients with ovarian or colon cancer received 12 to 38 mg/m^2 as a single dose every 4 weeks in 2 liters of dialysate. A 1,400-fold advantage was found for intraperitoneal drug concentrations over simultaneous plasma levels. The terminal half-life for disappearance of drug from the intraperitoneal space was 9 hours. Toxicity was primarily leukopenia at the highest doses of drug. Abdominal discomfort and tenderness, as well as catheter dysfunction due to the formation of a fibrous sheath reflecting serositis, are not uncommon with intraperitoneal mitoxantrone.

Toxicity

The primary advantages of mitoxantrone in comparison with doxorubicin are its much reduced incidence of cardiac toxicity, the mild nausea and vomiting that follows intravenous administration, and the minimal alopecia. Early trials of mitoxantrone revealed occasional episodes of cardiac failure,[547] primarily in patients who had not been helped by prior doxorubicin. There is no doubt that patients will develop congestive heart failure after treatment with mitoxantrone in the absence of prior anthracycline exposure, although the incidence is less than 5%.[533,548,549] Our appreciation for the cumulative cardiac toxicity of mitoxantrone has recently been enhanced by reports of heart damage occurring in patients with multiple sclerosis (for which mitoxantrone has been approved by the US Food and Drug Administration).[550,551] In this setting, 5% of patients who receive over 100 mg/m^2 of mitoxantrone develop an asymptomatic decrease in left ventricular ejection fraction. The incidence of cardiac toxicity is greatest in patients who have received prior anthracyclines or chest irradiation[552] and in those with underlying cardiac disease.[533,549,552]

Other toxicities include a reversible leukopenia, with recovery within 14 days of drug administration; mild thrombocytopenia; nausea and vomiting; and, rarely, abnormal liver enzymes in patients receiving dose levels appropriate for solid tumors.[553] One minor, and at times alarming, side effect of mitoxantrone is a bluish discoloration of the sclera, fingernails, and urine.[554]

In summary, mitoxantrone has not replaced doxorubicin in solid tumor chemotherapy, primarily because of its lesser activity against breast cancer. However, because of its advantageous toxicity profile, it is useful in the palliative therapy of hormone-resistant prostate cancer and is effective in combination therapy for the lymphomas and leukemias.

REFERENCES

1. Di Marco A, Gaetani M, Orezzi P, et al. "Daunomycin," a new antibiotic of the rhodomycin group. Nature 1964;201:706–707.
2. Arcamone F, Cassinelli G, Fantini G, et al. Adriamycin, 14-hydroxy-daunomycin, a new antitumor antibiotic from *S. peucetius* var. *caesius*. Biotechnol Bioeng 1969;11:1101–1110.
3. Legha SS, Benjamin RS, Mackay B, et al. Adriamycin therapy by continuous intravenous infusion in patients with metastatic breast cancer. Cancer 1982;49:1762–1766.
4. Legha SS, Benjamin RS, Mackay B, et al. Role of adriamycin in breast cancer and sarcomas. In: Muggia FM, Young CW, Carter SK, eds. Anthracycline Antibiotics in Cancer Therapy. The Hague: Martinus Nijhoff, 1982:432–444.
5. Jones RB, Holland JF, Bhardwaj S, et al. A phase I-II study of intensive-dose adriamycin for advanced breast cancer. J Clin Oncol 1987;5:172–177.
6. Bronchud MH, Howell A, Crowther D, et al. The use of granulocyte colony-stimulating factor to increase the intensity of treatment with doxorubicin in patients with advanced breast and ovarian cancer. Br J Cancer 1989;60:121–125.
7. Somlo G, Doroshow JH, Forman SJ, et al. High-dose doxorubicin, etoposide, and cyclophosphamide with autologous stem cell reinfusion in patients with responsive metastatic or high-risk primary breast cancer. Cancer 1994;73:1678–1685.
8. Morgan RJ Jr, Doroshow JH, Venkataraman K, et al. High-dose infusional doxorubicin and cyclophosphamide: feasibility study of tandem high-dose chemotherapy cycles without stem cell support. Clin Cancer Res 1997;3:2337–2345.
9. Citron ML, Berry DA, Cirrincione C, et al. Randomized trial of dose-dense versus conventionally scheduled and sequential versus concurrent combination chemotherapy as postoperative adjuvant treatment of node-positive primary breast cancer: first report of Intergroup Trial C9741/Cancer and Leukemia Group B Trial 9741. J Clin Oncol 2003;21:1431–1439.
10. Dalmark M, Johansen P. Molecular association between doxorubicin (Adriamycin) and DNA-derived bases, nucleosides, nucleotides, other aromatic compounds, and proteins in aqueous solution. Mol Pharmacol 1982;22:158–165.
11. Dalmark M, Strom HH. A Fickian diffusion transport process with features of transport catalysis: doxorubicin transport in human red blood cells. J Gen Physiol 1981;78:349–364.
12. Peterson C, Trouet A. Transport and storage of daunorubicin and doxorubicin in cultured fibroblasts. Cancer Res 1978;38:4645–4649.
13. Bachur NR, Steele M, Meriwether WD, et al. Cellular pharmacodynamics of several anthracycline antibiotics. J Med Chem 1976;19:651–654.
14. Gianni L, Corden B, Myers C. The biochemical basis of anthracycline toxicity and antitumor action. Rev Biochem Toxicol 1983;5:1–82.
15. Raghunand N, He X, van Sluis R, et al. Enhancement of chemotherapy by manipulation of tumour pH. Br J Cancer 1999;80:1005–1011.
16. Peterson C, Baurain R, Trouet A. The mechanism for cellular uptake, storage, and release of daunorubicin: studies on fibroblasts in culture. Biochem Pharmacol 1980;29:1687–1692.
17. Gerweck LE, Kozin SV, Stocks SJ. The pH partition theory predicts the accumulation and toxicity of doxorubicin in normal and low-pH-adapted cells. Br J Cancer 1999;79:838–842.
18. Schindler M, Grabski S, Hoff E, et al. Defective pH regulation of acidic compartments in human breast cancer cells (MCF-7) is normalized in adriamycin-resistant cells (MCF-7adr). Biochemistry 1996;35:2811–2817.
19. Vaupel PW, Frinak S, Bicher HI. Heterogeneous oxygen partial pressure and pH distribution in C3H mouse mammary adenocarcinoma. Cancer Res 1981;41:2008–2013.
20. Altan N, Chen Y, Schindler M, et al. Defective acidification in human breast tumor cells and implications for chemotherapy. J Exp Med 1998;187:1583–1598.
21. Simon SM, Schindler M. Cell biological mechanisms of multidrug resistance in tumors. Proc Natl Acad Sci USA 1994;91:3497–3504.
22. Johnson BA, Cheang MS, Goldenberg GJ. Comparison of adriamycin uptake in chick embryo heart and liver cells and murine L5178Y lymphoblasts in vitro: role of drug uptake in cardiotoxicity. Cancer Res 1986;46:218–223.
23. Peterson C, Paul C, Gahrton G. Studies on the cellular pharmacology of daunorubicin and doxorubicin in experimental systems and human leukemia. In: Mathe G, Maral R, De Jager R, eds. Anthracyclines: Current Status and Future Developments. New York: Masson Publishing USA, 1983:85–89.
24. Kiyomiya K, Matsuo S, Kurebe M. Proteasome is a carrier to translocate doxorubicin from cytoplasm into nucleus. Life Sci 1998;62:1853–1860.
25. Kiyomiya K, Matsuo S, Kurebe M. Mechanism of specific nuclear transport of adriamycin: the mode of nuclear translocation of adriamycin-proteasome complex. Cancer Res 2001;61:2467–2471.
26. Kiyomiya K, Kurebe M, Nakagawa H, et al. The role of the proteasome in apoptosis induced by anthracycline anticancer agents. Int J Oncol 2002;20:1205–1209.
27. Cusack JC. Rationale for the treatment of solid tumors with the proteasome inhibitor bortezomib. Cancer Treat Rev 2003;29 (Suppl 1):21–31.
28. Kartner N, Riordan JR, Ling V. Cell-surface P-glycoprotein associated with multidrug resistance in mammalian cell lines. Science 1983;221:1285–1288.
29. Ueda K, Cardarelli C, Gottesman MM, et al. Expression of a full-length cDNA for the human "MDR1" gene confers resistance to colchine, doxorubicin, and vinblastine. Proc Natl Acad Sci USA 1987;84:3004–3008.
30. Pastan I, Gottesman MM. Multidrug resistance. Annu Rev Med 1991;42:277–286.
31. Horio M, Chin KV, Currier SJ, et al. Transepithelial transport of drugs by the multidrug transporter in cultured Madin-Darby canine kidney cell epithelia. J Biol Chem 1989;264:14880–14884.
32. Cole SPC, Bhardwaj G, Gerlach JH, et al. Overexpression of a transporter gene in a multidrug-resistant human lung cancer cell line. Science 1992;258:1650–1654.
33. Slovak ML, Ho JP, Bhardwaj G, et al. Localization of a novel multidrug resistance-associated gene in the HT1080/DR4 and H69AR human tumor cell lines. Cancer Res 1993;53:3221–3225.
34. Awasthi S, Singhal SS, Srivastava SK, et al. Adenosine triphosphate-dependent transport of doxorubicin, daunomycin, and

vinblastine in human tissues by a mechanism distinct from the P-glycoprotein. J Clin Invest 1994;93:958–965.

35. Jedlitschky G, Leier I, Buchholz U, et al. ATP-dependent transport of glutathione S-conjugates by the multidrug resistance-associated protein. Cancer Res 1994;54:4833–4836.

36. Yi J-R, Lu S, Fernandez-Checa J, et al. Expression cloning of a rat hepatic reduced glutathione transporter with canalicular characteristics. J Clin Invest 1994;93:1841–1845.

37. Priebe W, Krawczyk M, Kuo MT, et al. Doxorubicin- and daunorubicin-glutathione conjugates, but not unconjugated drugs, competitively inhibit leukotriene C4 transport mediated by MRP/GS-X pump. Biochem Biophys Res Commun 1998;247:859–863.

38. Borg AG, Burgess R, Green LM, et al. Overexpression of lung-resistance protein and increased P-glycoprotein function in acute myeloid leukaemia cells predict a poor response to chemotherapy and reduced patient survival. Br J Haematol 1998;103:1083–1091.

39. Schroeijers AB, Scheffer GL, Flens MJ, et al. Immunohistochemical detection of the human major vault protein LRP with two monoclonal antibodies in formalin-fixed, paraffin-embedded tissues. Am J Pathol 1998;152:373–378.

40. Michieli M, Damiani D, Ermacora A, et al. P-glycoprotein, lung resistance-related protein and multidrug resistance associated protein in de novo acute non-lymphocytic leukaemias: biological and clinical implications. Br J Haematol 1999;104:328–335.

41. Chaires JB, Fox KR, Herrera JE, et al. Site and sequence specificity of the daunomycin-DNA interaction. Biochemistry 1987;26:8227–8236.

42. Bailly C, Suh D, Waring MJ, et al. Binding of daunomycin to diaminopurine- and/or inosine-substituted DNA. Biochemistry 1998;37:1033–1045.

43. Trist H, Phillips DR. In vitro transcription analysis of the role of flanking sequence on the DNA sequence specificity of adriamycin. Nucl Acids Res 1989;17:3673–3688.

44. Calendi E, Marco A, Reggiani M, et al. On physicochemical interactions between daunomycin and nucleic acids. Biochem Biophys Acta 1965;103:25–54.

45. Zeman SM, Phillips DR, Crothers DM. Characterization of covalent adriamycin-DNA adducts. Proc Natl Acad Sci USA 1998;95:11561–11565.

46. Zunino F, Ganbetta R, DiMarco A, et al. A comparison of the effects of daunomycin and adriamycin on various DNA polymerases. Cancer Res 1975;35:754–760.

47. Zunino F, Gambetta R, DiMarco A. The inhibition in vitro of DNA polymerase and RNA polymerase by daunomycin and adriamycin. Biochem Pharmacol 1975;24:309–311.

48. Siegfried JM, Sartorelli AC, Tritton TR. Evidence for the lack of relationship between inhibition of nucleic acid synthesis and cytotoxicity of adriamycin. Cancer Biochem Biophys 1983;6:137–142.

49. Ross WA, Glaubiger DL, Kohn KW. Protein-associated DNA breaks in cells treated with adriamycin and ellipticine. Biochim Biophys Acta 1978;519:23–30.

50. Zwelling LA, Michaels S, Erickson LC, et al. Protein-associated deoxyribonucleic acid strand breaks in L1210 cells treated with the deoxyribonucleic acid intercalating agents 4'-(9- acridinylamino) methanesulfon-m-anisidide and adriamycin. Biochemistry 1981;20:6553–6563.

51. Kohn KW. Beyond DNA cross-linking: history and prospects of DNA-targeted cancer treatment. Fifteenth Bruce F. Cain Memorial Award Lecture. Cancer Res 1996;56:5533–5546.

52. Liu LF. DNA topoisomerase poisons as antitumor drugs. Annu Rev Biochem 1989;58:351–375.

53. Tewey KM, Chen GI, Nelson EM, et al. Intercalative antitumor drugs interfere with the breakage-reunion reaction of mammalian DNA topoisomerase. J Biol Chem 1984;259:9182–9187.

54. Pommier Y. DNA topoisomerase I and II in cancer chemotherapy: update and perspectives. Cancer Chemother Pharmacol 1993;32:103–108.

55. Potmesil M, Kirschenbaum S, Israel M, et al. Relationship of adriamycin concentrations to the DNA lesions induced in hypoxic and euoxic L1210 cells. Cancer Res 1983;43:3629–3633.

56. Levin M, Silber R, Israel M, et al. Protein-associated DNA breaks and DNA-protein cross-links caused by DNA nonbinding derivatives of adriamycin in L1210 cells. Cancer Res 1981;41:1006–1010.

57. Capranico G, Kohn KW, Pommier Y. Local sequence requirements for DNA cleavage by mammalian topoisomerase II in the presence of doxorubicin. Nucl Acids Res 1990;18:6611–6619.

58. Binaschi M, Farinosi R, Borgnetto ME, et al. In vivo site specificity and human isoenzyme selectivity of two topoisomerase II-poisoning anthracyclines. Cancer Res 2000;60:3770–3776.

59. Glisson B, Gupta R, Hodges P, et al. Cross-resistance to intercalating agents in an epipodophyllotoxin-resistant Chinese hamster ovary cell line: evidence for a common intracellular target. Cancer Res 1986;46:1939–1942.

60. Sinha BK, Haim N, Dusre L, et al. DNA strand breaks produced by etoposide (VP-16,213) in sensitive and resistant human breast tumor cells: implications for the mechanism of action. Cancer Res 1988;48:5096–5100.

61. Withoff S, Keith WN, Knol AJ, et al. Selection of a subpopulation with fewer DNA topoisomerase II alpha gene copies in a doxorubicin-resistant cell line panel. Br J Cancer 1996;74:502–507.

62. Towatari M, Adachi K, Marunouchi T, et al. Evidence for a critical role of DNA topoisomerase IIalpha in drug sensitivity revealed by inducible antisense RNA in a human leukaemia cell line. Br J Haematol 1998;101:548–551.

63. Patel S, Sprung AU, Keller BA, et al. Identification of yeast DNA topoisomerase II mutants resistant to the antitumor drug doxorubicin: implications for the mechanisms of doxorubicin action and cytotoxicity. Mol Pharmacol 1997;52:658–666.

64. Sorensen M, Sehested M, Jensen PB. Effect of cellular ATP depletion on topoisomerase II poisons: abrogation of cleavable-complex formation by etoposide but not by amsacrine. Mol Pharmacol 1999;55:424–431.

65. Kupfer G, Bodley AL, Liu LF. Involvement of intracellular ATP in cytotoxicity of topoisomerase II-targeting antitumor drugs. NCI Monogr 1987;4:37–40.

66. Ross WE, Zwelling LA, Kohn KW. Relationship between cytotoxicity and DNA strand breakage produced by adriamycin and other intercalating agents. Int J Radiat Oncol Biol Phys 1979;5:1221–1224.

67. Zwelling LA, Kerrigan D, Michaels S. Cytotoxicity and DNA strand breaks by 5-iminodaunorubicin in mouse leukemia L1210 cells: comparison with adriamycin and 4'-(9- acridinylamino)methanesulfon-m-anisidide. Cancer Res 1982;42:2687–2691.

68. Goldenberg GJ, Wang H, Blair GW. Resistance to adriamycin: relationship of cytotoxicity to drug uptake and DNA single- and double-strand breakage in cloned cell lines of adriamycin-sensitive and -resistant P388 leukemia. Cancer Res 1986;46:2978–2983.

69. Munger C, Ellis A, Woods K, et al. Evidence for inhibition of growth related to compromised DNA synthesis in the interaction of daunorubicin with H-35 rat hepatoma. Cancer Res 1988;48:2404–2411.

70. Fornari FA, Randolph JK, Yalowich JC, et al. Interference by doxorubicin with DNA unwinding in MCF-7 breast tumor cells. Mol Pharmacol 1994;45:649–656.

71. Binaschi M, Farinosi R, Austin CA, et al. Human DNA topoisomerase IIalpha-dependent DNA cleavage and yeast cell killing by anthracycline analogues. Cancer Res 1998;58:1886–1892.

72. Yamazaki K, Isobe H, Hanada T, et al. Topoisomerase II alpha content and topoisomerase II catalytic activity cannot explain drug sensitivities to topoisomerase II inhibitors in lung cancer cell lines. Cancer Chemother Pharmacol 1997;39:192–198.

73. Sandri MI, Hochhauser D, Ayton P, et al. Differential expression of the topoisomerase II alpha and beta genes in human breast cancers. Br J Cancer 1996;73:1518–1524.

74. Jarvinen TA, Holli K, Kuukasjarvi T, et al. Predictive value of topoisomerase IIalpha and other prognostic factors for epirubicin chemotherapy in advanced breast cancer. Br J Cancer 1998;77:2267–2273.

75. Pommier Y, Leteurtre F, Fesen MR, et al. Cellular determinants of sensitivity and resistance to DNA topoisomerase inhibitors. Cancer Invest 1994;12:530–542.

76. Jensen PB, Sorensen BS, Demant EJ, et al. Antagonistic effect of aclarubicin on the cytotoxicity of etoposide and 4'-(9-acridinylamino)methanesulfon-m-anisidide in human small cell lung

cancer cell lines and on topoisomerase II-mediated DNA cleavage. Cancer Res 1990;50:3311–3316.

77. Sorensen BS, Sinding J, Andersen AH, et al. Mode of action of topoisomerase II-targeting agents at a specific DNA sequence: uncoupling the DNA binding, cleavage and religation events. J Mol Biol 1992;228:778–786.

78. Jensen PB, Sorensen BS, Sehested M, et al. Different modes of anthracycline interaction with topoisomerase II: separate structures critical for DNA-cleavage, and for overcoming topoisomerase II-related drug resistance. Biochem Pharmacol 1993; 45:2025–2035.

79. Nitiss JL, Pourquier P, Pommier Y. Aclacinomycin A stabilizes topoisomerase I covalent complexes. Cancer Res 1997;57:4564–4569.

80. Fukushima T, Inoue H, Takemura H, et al. Idarubicin and idarubicinol are less affected by topoisomerase II-related multidrug resistance than is daunorubicin. Leuk Res 1998;22:625–629.

81. Guano F, Pourquier P, Tinelli S, et al. Topoisomerase poisoning activity of novel disaccharide anthracyclines. Mol Pharmacol 1999;56:77–84.

82. Bachur NR, Yu F, Johnson R, et al. Helicase inhibition by anthracycline anticancer agents. Mol Pharmacol 1992;41:993–998.

83. Bachur NR, Johnson R, Yu F, et al. Anthracycline antihelicase action: new mechanism with implications for guanosine-cytidine intercalation specificity. In: Priebe W, ed. Anthracycline Antibiotics: New Analogues, Methods of Delivery, and Mechanisms of Action. Washington, DC: American Chemical Society, 1995: 204–221.

84. Bachur NR, Lun L, Sun PM, et al. Anthracycline antibiotic blockade of SV40 T antigen helicase action. Biochem Pharmacol 1998;55:1025–1034.

85. Fornari FA Jr, Jarvis WD, Grant S, et al. Induction of differentiation and growth arrest associated with nascent (nonoligosomal) DNA fragmentation and reduced c-myc expression in MCF-7 human breast tumor cells after continuous exposure to a sublethal concentration of doxorubicin. Cell Growth Different 1994; 5:723–733.

86. Fornari FAJ, Jarvis DW, Grant S, et al. Growth arrest and non-apoptotic cell death associated with the suppression of c-myc expression in MCF-7 breast tumor cells following acute exposure to doxorubicin. Biochem Pharmacol 1996;51:931–940.

87. Gewirtz DA, Randolph JK, Chawla J, et al. Induction of DNA damage, inhibition of DNA synthesis and suppression of c-myc expression by the anthracycline analog, idarubicin (4-demethoxy-daunorubicin) in the MCF-7 breast tumor cell line. Cancer Chemother Pharmacol 1998;41:361–369.

88. Bachur NR, Gee MV, Friedman RD. Nuclear catalyzed antibiotic free radical formation. Cancer Res 1982;42:1078–1081.

89. Akman SA, Doroshow JH, Burke TG, et al. DNA base modifications induced in isolated human chromatin by NADH dehydrogenase-catalyzed reduction of doxorubicin. Biochemistry 1992; 31:3500–3506.

90. Muller I, Jenner A, Bruchelt G, et al. Effect of concentration on the cytotoxic mechanism of doxorubicin: apoptosis and oxidative DNA damage. Biochem Biophys Res Commun 1997;230: 254–257.

91. Gajewski E, Synold TW, Akman SA, et al. Doxorubicin-induced oxidative DNA base modification and apoptosis in human MCF-10A breast cancer cells at clinically achievable drug concentrations. Proc Amer Assoc Cancer Res 1999;40:646.

92. Lin SW, Akman SA, Chen V, et al. Comparison of doxorubicin and H_2O_2-mediated oxidative DNA damage and repair in mitochondrial and nuclear DNA of human fibroblasts by quantitative extra long PCR. Proc Amer Assoc Cancer Res 1999;40:403.

93. Palmeira CM, Serrano J, Kuehl DW, et al. Preferential oxidation of cardiac mitochondrial DNA following acute intoxication with doxorubicin. Biochim Biophys Acta 1997;1321:101–106.

94. Serrano J, Palmeira CM, Kuehl DW, et al. Cardioselective and cumulative oxidation of mitochondrial DNA following subchronic doxorubicin administration. Biochim Biophys Acta 1999;1411:201–205.

95. Faure H, Coudray C, Mousseau M, et al. 5-Hydroxymethyluracil excretion, plasma TBARS and plasma antioxidant vitamins in adriamycin-treated patients. Free Radic Biol Med 1996;20:979–983.

96. Faure H, Mousseau M, Cadet J, et al. Urine 8-oxo-7,8-dihydro-2-deoxyguanosine vs. 5-(hydroxymethyl) uracil as DNA oxidation marker in adriamycin-treated patients. Free Radic Res 1998;28: 377–382.

97. Olinski R, Jaruga P, Foksinski M, et al. Epirubicin-induced oxidative DNA damage and evidence for its repair in lymphocytes of cancer patients who are undergoing chemotherapy. Mol Pharmacol 1997;52:882–885.

98. Doroshow JH, Synold TW, Somlo G, et al. Oxidative DNA base modifications in peripheral blood mononuclear cells of patients treated with high-dose infusional doxorubicin. Blood 2001;97: 2839–2845.

99. Senturker S, Dizdaroglu M. The effect of experimental conditions on the levels of oxidatively modified bases in DNA as measured by gas chromatography-mass spectrometry: how many modified bases are involved? prepurification or not? Free Radic Biol Med 1999;27:370–380.

100. Nackerdien Z, Olinski R, Dizdaroglu M. DNA base damage in chromatin of gamma-irradiated cultured human cells. Free Radic Res Commun 1992;16:259–273.

101. Westendorf J, Marquardt Hi, Marquardt H. Structure-activity relationship of anthracycline-induced genotoxicity in vitro. Cancer Res 1984;44:5599–5604.

102. Bjergaard-Pedersen J, Sigsgaard TC, Nielsen D, et al. Acute monocytic or myelomonocytic leukemia with balanced chromosome translocations to band 11q23 after therapy with 4-epi-doxorubicin and cisplatin or cyclophosphamide for breast cancer. J Clin Oncol 1992;10:1444–1451.

103. Diamandidou E, Buzdar AU, Smith TL, et al. Treatment-related leukemia in breast cancer patients treated with fluorouracil-doxorubicin-cyclophosphamide combination adjuvant chemotherapy: the University of Texas M.D. Anderson Cancer Center experience. J Clin Oncol 1996;14:2722–2730.

104. Hoffmann L, Moller P, Pedersen-Bjergaard J, et al. Therapy-related acute promyelocytic leukemia with t(15;17) (q22;q12) following chemotherapy with drugs targeting DNA topoisomerase II: a report of two cases and a review of the literature. Ann Oncol 1995;6:781–788.

105. Breimer LH. Molecular mechanisms of oxygen radical carcinogenesis and mutagenesis: the role of DNA base damage. Mol Carcinogenesis 1990;3:188–197.

106. Hsie AW, Recio L, Katz DS, et al. Evidence for reactive oxygen species inducing mutations in mammalian cells. Proc Natl Acad Sci USA 1986;83:9616–9620.

107. Jaruga P, Dizdaroglu M. Repair of products of oxidative DNA base damage in human cells. Nucleic Acids Res 1996;24:1389–1394.

108. Melov S, Coskun P, Patel M, et al. Mitochondrial disease in superoxide dismutase 2 mutant mice. Proc Natl Acad Sci USA 1999;96:846–851.

109. Taatjes DJ, Gaudiano G, Koch TH. Production of formaldehyde and DNA-adriamycin or DNA-daunomycin adducts, initiated through redox chemistry of dithiothreitol/iron, xanthine oxidase/NADH/iron, or glutathione/iron. Chem Res Toxicol 1997; 10:953–961.

110. Taatjes DJ, Fenick DJ, Koch TH. Nuclear targeting and nuclear retention of anthracycline-formaldehyde conjugates implicates DNA covalent bonding in the cytotoxic mechanism of anthracyclines. Chem Res Toxicol 1999;12:588–596.

111. Burke PJ, Koch TH. Doxorubicin-formaldehyde conjugate, doxoform: induction of apoptosis relative to doxorubicin. Anticancer Res 2001;21:2753–2760.

112. Burke PJ, Koch TH. Design, synthesis, and biological evaluation of doxorubicin-formaldehyde conjugates targeted to breast cancer cells. J Med Chem 2004;47:1193–1206.

113. Dernell WS, Powers BE, Taatjes DJ, et al. Evaluation of the epi-doxorubicin-formaldehyde conjugate, epidoxoform, in a mouse mammary carcinoma model. Cancer Invest 2002;20:713–724.

114. Abdella BRJ, Fisher J. A chemical perspective on the anthracycline antitumor antibiotics. Environ Health Perspect 1985; 64:3–18.

115. Fisher J, Ramakrishnan K, Becvar JE. Direct enzyme-catalyzed reduction of anthracyclines by reduced nicotinamide adenine dinucleotide. Biochemistry 1983;22:1347–1355.

116. Handa K, Sato S. Generation of free radicals of quinone group-containing anti-cancer chemicals in NADPH-microsome system as evidenced by initiation of sulfite oxidation. Gann 1975;66:43–47.

117. Goodman J, Hochstein P. Generation of free radicals and lipid peroxidation by redox cycling of adriamycin and daunomycin. Biochem Biophys Res Commun 1977;77:797–803.

118. Bachur NR, Gordon SL, Gee MV. A general mechanism for microsomal activation of quinone anticancer agents to free radicals. Cancer Res 1977;38:1745–1752.

119. Myers CE, McGuire WP, Liss RH, et al. Adriamycin: the role of lipid peroxidation in cardiac toxicity and tumor response. Science 1977;197:165–167.

120. Doroshow JH, Locker GY, Myers CE. Enzymatic defenses of the mouse heart against reactive oxygen metabolites: alterations produced by doxorubicin. J Clin Invest 1980;65:128–135.

121. Doroshow JH, Locker GY, Ifrim I, et al. Prevention of doxorubicin cardiac toxicity in the mouse by N-acetylcysteine. J Clin Invest 1981;68:1053–1064.

122. Doroshow JH. Role of hydrogen peroxide and hydroxyl radical formation in the killing of Ehrlich tumor cells by anticancer quinones. Proc Natl Acad Sci USA 1986;83:4514–4518.

123. Sinha BK, Katki AG, Batist G, et al. Differential formation of hydroxyl radical by adriamycin in sensitive and resistant MCF-7 human breast tumor cells: implications for the mechanism of action. Biochemistry 1987;26:3776–3781.

124. Doroshow JH. Glutathione peroxidase and oxidative stress. Toxicol Lett 1995;82/83:395–398.

125. Doroshow JH, Hochstein P. Redox cycling and the mechanism of action of antibiotics in neoplastic diseases. In: Autor AP, ed. Pathology of Oxygen. New York: Academic Press, 1982:245–259.

126. O'Brien PJ. Molecular mechanisms of quinone cytotoxicity. Chem Biol Interact 1991;80:1–41.

127. Praet M, Laghmiche M, Pollakis G, et al. In vivo and in vitro modifications of the mitochondrial membrane induced by 4' epi-adriamycin. Biochem Pharmacol 1986;35:2923–2928.

128. Carmichael AJ, Riesz P. Photoinduced reactions of anthraquinone antitumor agents with peptides and nucleic acid bases: an electron spin resonance and spin trapping study. Arch Biochem Biophys 1985;237:433–444.

129. Harris RN, Doroshow JH. Effect of doxorubicin-enhanced hydrogen peroxide and hydroxyl radical formation on calcium sequestration by cardiac sarcoplasmic reticulum. Biochem Biophys Res Commun 1985;130:739–745.

130. Vile G, Winterbourn C. Thiol oxidation and inhibition of Ca-ATPase by adriamycin in rabbit heart microsomes. Biochem Pharmacol 1990;39:769–774.

131. Pan SS, Pedersen L, Bachur NR. Comparative flavoprotein catalysis of anthracycline antibiotic reductive cleavage and oxygen consumption. Mol Pharmacol 1981;19:184–186.

132. Doroshow JH, Davies KJ. Redox cycling of anthracyclines by cardiac mitochondria, II: formation of superoxide anion, hydrogen peroxide, and hydroxyl radical. J Biol Chem 1986;261:3068–3074.

133. Thornally PJ, Bannister WH, Bannister JV. Reduction of oxygen by NADH/NADH dehydrogenase in the presence of adriamycin. Free Radic Res Commun 1986;2:163–171.

134. Vasquez-Vivar J, Martasek P, Hogg N, et al. Endothelial nitric oxide synthase-dependent superoxide generation from adriamycin. Biochemistry 1997;36:11293–11297.

135. Garner AP, Paine MJ, Rodriguez-Crespo I, et al. Nitric oxide synthases catalyze the activation of redox cycling and bioreductive anticancer agents. Cancer Res 1999;59:1929–1934.

136. Luo D, Vincent SR. Inhibition of nitric oxide synthase by antineoplastic anthracyclines. Biochem Pharmacol 1994;47:2111–2112.

137. Ursell PC, Mayes M. Anatomic distribution of nitric oxide synthase in the heart. Int J Cardiol 1995;50:217–223.

138. Thomsen LL, Miles DW. Role of nitric oxide in tumour progression: lessons from human tumours. Cancer Metastasis Rev 1998;17:107–118.

139. Reszka KJ, McCormick ML, Britigan BE. Peroxidase- and nitrite-dependent metabolism of the anthracycline anticancer agents daunorubicin and doxorubicin. Biochemistry 2001;40:15349–15361.

140. Doroshow JH. Anthracycline-enhanced cardiac oxygen radical metabolism. In: Singal PK, ed. Free Radicals in the Pathophysiology of Heart Disease. Boston: Martinus Nijhoff, 1988:31–40.

141. Kalyanaraman B, Sealy RC, Sinha BK. An electron spin resonance study of the reduction of peroxides by anthracycline semiquinones. Biochim Biophys Acta 1984;799:270–275.

142. Kalyanaraman B, Morehouse KM, Mason RP. An electron paramagnetic resonance study of the interactions between the adriamycin semiquinone, hydrogen peroxide, iron- chelators, and radical scavengers. Arch Biochem Biophys 1991;286:164–170.

143. Doroshow JH. Prevention of doxorubicin-induced killing of MCF-7 human breast cancer cells by oxygen radical scavengers and iron chelating agents. Biochem Biophys Res Commun 1986;135:330–335.

144. Doroshow JH, Esworthy RS. The role of antioxidant defenses in the cardiotoxicity of anthracycline. In: Muggia FM, Green MD, Speyer JL, eds. Cancer Treatment and the Heart. Baltimore: The Johns Hopkins University Press, 1992:47–58.

145. Breimer LH. Repair of DNA damage induced by reactive oxygen species. Free Radic Res Commun 1991;14:159–171.

146. Sancar A. DNA repair in humans. Annu Rev Genet 1995;29:69–105.

147. Taffe BG, Larminat F, Laval J, et al. Gene-specific nuclear and mitochondrial repair of formamidopyrimidine DNA glycosylase-sensitive sites in Chinese hamster ovary cells. Mutat Res 1996;364:183–192.

148. Kang YJ, Chen Y, Epstein PN. Suppression of doxorubicin cardiotoxicity by overexpression of catalase in the heart of transgenic mice. J Biol Chem 1996;271:12610–12616.

149. Tabatabaie T, Floyd RA. Susceptibility of glutathione peroxidase and glutathione reductase to oxidative damage and the protective effect of spin trapping agents. Arch Biochem Biophys 1994;314:112–119.

150. Rajagopalan S, Politi PM, Sinha BK, et al. Adriamycin-induced free radical formation in the perfused rat heart: implications for cardiotoxicity. Cancer Res 1988;48:4766–4769.

151. Babson JR, Abell NS, Reed DJ. Protective role of the glutathione redox cycle against adriamycin-mediated toxicity in isolated hepatocytes. Biochem Pharmacol 1981;30:2299–2304.

152. Reed DJ. Regulation of reductive processes by glutathione. Biochem Pharmacol 1986;35:7–13.

153. Keizer HG, Pinedo HM, Schuurhuis GJ, et al. Doxorubicin (adriamycin): a critical review of free radical-dependent mechanisms of cytotoxicity. Pharmacol Ther 1990;47:219–231.

154. Cervantes A, Pinedo HM, Lankelma J, et al. The role of oxygen-derived free radicals in the cytotoxicity of doxorubicin in multidrug resistant and sensitive human ovarian cancer cells. Cancer Lett 1988;41:169–177.

155. Gewirtz DA. A critical evaluation of the mechanisms of action proposed for the antitumor effects of the anthracycline antibiotics adriamycin and daunorubicin. Biochem Pharmacol 1999;57:727–741.

156. Simizu S, Takada M, Umezawa K, et al. Requirement of caspase-3(-like) protease-mediated hydrogen peroxide production for apoptosis induced by various anticancer drugs. J Biol Chem 1998;273:26900–26907.

157. Hamilton TC, Winker MA, Louie KG, et al. Augmentation of adriamycin, melphalan, and cisplatin cytotoxicity in drug-resistant and -sensitive human ovarian carcinoma cell lines by buthionine sulfoximine mediated glutathione depletion. Biochem Pharmacol 1985;34:2583–2586.

158. Kramer RA, Zahker J, King G. Role of glutathione redox cycle in acquired and de novo multidrug resistance. Science 1988;241:694–697.

159. Dusre L, Mimnaugh EG, Myers CE, et al. Potentiation of adriamycin cytotoxicity by buthione sulfoximine in multidrug resistant breast tumor cells. Cancer Res 1989;49:8–15.

160. Lee FY, Siemann DW, Sutherland RM. Changes in cellular glutathione content during adriamycin treatment in human ovarian cancer: a possible indicator of chemosensitivity. Br J Cancer 1989;60:291–298.

161. Samuels BL, Murray JL, Cohen MB, et al. Increased glutathione peroxidase activity in a human sarcoma cells line with inherent doxorubicin resistance. Cancer Res 1991;51:521–527.

162. Nair S, Singh SV, Samy TS, et al. Anthracycline resistance in murine leukemic P388 cells: role of drug efflux and glutathione related enzymes. Biochem Pharmacol 1990;39:723–728.
163. Benchekroun MN, Sinha BK, Robert J. Doxorubicin-induced oxygen free radical formation in sensitive and doxorubicin-resistant variants of rat glioblastoma cell lines. FEBS Lett 1993;326:302–305.
164. Ubezio P, Civoli F. Flow cytometric detection of hydrogen peroxide production induced by doxorubicin in cancer cells. Free Radic Biol Med 1994;16:509–516.
165. Alegria AE, Samuni A, Mitchell JB, et al. Free radicals induced by adriamycin-sensitive and adriamycin-resistant cells: a spin-trapping study. Biochemistry 1989;28:8653–8658.
166. Bredehorst R, Panneerselvam M, Vogel C-W. Doxorubicin enhances complement susceptibility of human melanoma cells by extracellular oxygen radical formation. J Biol Chem 1987; 262:2034–2041.
167. Kule C, Ondrejickova O, Verner K. Doxorubicin, daunorubicin, and mitoxantrone cytotoxicity in yeast [published erratum appears in Mol Pharmacol 1995;47:882]. Mol Pharmacol 1994;46:1234–1240.
168. Quillet-Mary A, Mansat V, Duchayne E, et al. Daunorubicin-induced internucleosomal DNA fragmentation in acute myeloid cell lines. Leukemia 1996;10:417–425.
169. Ikeda K, Kajiwara K, Tanabe E, et al. Involvement of hydrogen peroxide and hydroxyl radical in chemically induced apoptosis of HL-60 cells. Biochem Pharmacol 1999;57:1361–1365.
170. Mallery SR, Clark YM, Ness GM, et al. Thiol redox modulation of doxorubicin mediated cytotoxicity in cultured AIDS-related Kaposi's sarcoma cells. J Cell Biochem 1999;73:259–277.
171. Hosking LK, Whelan RD, Shellard SA, et al. An evaluation of the role of glutathione and its associated enzymes in the expression of differential sensitivities to antitumor agents shown by a range of human tumour cell lines. Biochem Pharmacol 1990;40: 1833–1842.
172. Benchekroun MN, Pourquier P, Schott B, et al. Doxorubicin-induced lipid peroxidation and glutathione peroxidase activity in tumor cell lines selected for resistance to doxorubicin. Eur J Biochem 1993;211:141–146.
173. Sinha BK, Mimnaugh EG, Rajagopalan S, et al. Adriamycin activation and oxygen free radical formation in human breast tumor cells: protective role of glutathione peroxidase in adriamycin resistance. Cancer Res 1989;49:3844–3848.
174. Benchekroun MN, Catroux P, Montaudon D, et al. Development of mechanisms of protection against oxidative stress in doxorubicin-resistant rat tumoral cells in culture. Free Radic Res Commun 1990;11:137–144.
175. Doroshow JH. Redox cycling and the antitumor activity of the anthracyclines. In: Davies KJA, Ursini F, eds. The Oxygen Paradox. Padua: CLEUP University Press, 1995:469–477.
176. Vanella A, Campisi A, di Giacomo C, et al. Enhanced resistance of adriamycin-treated MCR-5 lung fibroblasts by increased intracellular glutathione peroxidase and extracellular antioxidants. Biochem Mol Med 1997;62:36–41.
177. Doroshow JH, Esworthy RS, Chu FF, et al. Glutathione peroxidase and resistance to oxidative stress. In: Tew KD, Pickett CB, Mantle TJ, et al., eds. Structure and Function of Glutathione Transferases. Boca Raton: CRC Press, 1993:269–277.
178. Taylor SD, Davenport LD, Speranza MJ, et al. Glutathione peroxidase protects cultured mammalian cells from the toxicity of adriamycin and paraquat. Arch Biochem Biophys 1993;305:600–605.
179. Hirose K, Longo DL, Oppenheim JJ, et al. Overexpression of mitochondrial manganese superoxide dismutase promotes the survival of tumor cells exposed to interleukin-1, tumor necrosis factor, selected anticancer drugs, and ionizing radiation. FASEB J 1993;7:361–368.
180. Ravid A, Rocker D, Machlenkin A, et al. 1,25-Dihydroxyvitamin D3 enhances the susceptibility of breast cancer cells to doxorubicin-induced oxidative damage. Cancer Res 1999;59:862–867.
181. Bustamante J, Galleano M, Medrano EE, et al. Adriamycin effects on hydroperoxide metabolism and growth of human breast tumor cells. Breast Cancer Res Treat 1990;17:145–153.
182. Winterbourn CC, Gutteridge JM, Halliwell B. Doxorubicin-dependent lipid peroxidation at low partial pressures of O$_2$. J Free Radic Biol Med 1985;1:43–49.
183. Bellamy WT, Dalton WS, Meltzer P, et al. Role of glutathione and its associated enzymes in multidrug-resistant human myeloma cells. Biochem Pharmacol 1989;38:787–793.
184. Crescimanno M, D'Alessandro N, Armata M-G, et al. Modulation of the antioxidant activities in dox-sensitive and -resistant Friend leukemia cells: effect of doxorubicin. Anticancer Res 1991;11: 901–904.
185. Dikalov SI, Rumyantseva GV, Weiner LM, et al. Hydroxyl radical generation by oligonucleotide derivatives of anthracycline antibiotic and synthetic quinone. Chem Biol Interact 1991;77: 325–339.
186. Rouscilles A, Houee-Levin C, Gardes-Albert M, et al. t-Radiolysis study of the reduction by COO$^-$ free radicals of daunorubicin intercalated in DNA. Free Radic Biol Med 1989;6:37–43.
187. Houee-Levin C, Gardes-Albert KB, Rouscilles A, et al. One-electron reduction of daunorubicin intercalated in DNA or in protein: a gamma radiolysis study. Free Radic Res Commun 1990;11:127–136.
188. Houee-Levin C, Gardes-Albert M, Rouscilles A, et al. Intramolecular semiquinone disproportionation in DNA: pulse radiolysis study of the one-electron reduction of daunorubicin intercalated in DNA. Biochemistry 1991;30:8216–8222.
189. Gajewski E, Synold TW, Akman SA, et al. Oxidative DNA base modification in patients (pts) treated with high dose infusional doxorubicin (DOX). Proc Amer Assoc Cancer Res 1998;39:489.
190. Myers CE, Bonow R, Palmeri S, et al. Prevention of doxorubicin cardiomyopathy by N-acetylcysteine. Semin Oncol 1983;10:53–55.
191. Demant EJ. Transfer of ferritin-bound iron to adriamycin. FEBS Lett 1984;176:97–100.
192. Thomas CE, Aust SD. Release of iron from ferritin by cardiotoxic anthracycline antibiotics. Arch Biochem Biophys 1986;248: 684–689.
193. Monteiro HP, Vile GF, Winterbourn CC. Release of iron from ferritin by semiquinone, anthracycline, bipyridyl, and nitroaromatic radicals. Free Radical Biol Med 1989;6:587–591.
194. Minotti G. Adriamycin-dependent release of iron from microsomal membranes. Arch Biochem Biophys 1989;268:398–403.
195. Minotti G. Reactions of adriamycin with microsomal iron and lipids. Free Radic Res Commun 1989;7:143–148.
196. Minotti G. NADPH- and adriamycin-dependent microsomal release of iron and lipid peroxidation. Arch Biochem Biophys 1990;277:268–276.
197. Minotti G, Menna P, Salvatorelli E, et al. Anthracyclines: molecular advances and pharmacologic developments in antitumor activity and cardiotoxicity. Pharmacol Rev 2004;56:185–229.
198. Kotamraju S, Chitambar CR, Kalivendi SV, et al. Transferrin receptor-dependent iron uptake is responsible for doxorubicin-mediated apoptosis in endothelial cells: role of oxidant-induced iron signaling in apoptosis. J Biol Chem 2002;277:17179–17187.
199. Myers CE, Gianni L, Zweier J, et al. The role of iron in adriamycin biochemistry. Fed Proc 1986;45:2792–2797.
200. Zweier JL, Gianni L, Muindi J, et al. Differences in O$_2$ reduction by the iron complexes of adriamycin and daunomycin: the importance of the sidechain hydroxyl group. Biochim Biophys Acta 1986;884:326–336.
201. Gelvan D, Samuni A. Reappraisal of the association between adriamycin and iron. Cancer Res 1988;48:5645–5649.
202. Gelvan D, Berg E, Saltman P, et al. Time-dependent modifications of ferric-adriamycin. Biochem Pharmacol 1990;39:1289–1295.
203. Vile GF, Winterbourn CC. dl-N,N'-dicarboxamidomethyl-N,N'-dicarboxymethyl-1,2-diaminopropane (ICRF-198) and d-1,2-bis(3,5-dioxopiperazine-1-yl)propane (ICRF-187) inhibition of Fe^{3+} reduction, lipid peroxidation, and CaATPase inactivation in heart microsomes exposed to adriamycin. Cancer Res 1990; 50:2307–2310.
204. Herman EH, Ferrans VJ, Young RS, et al. Effect of pretreatment with ICRF-187 on the total cumulative dose of doxorubicin tolerated by beagle dogs. Cancer Res 1988;48:6918–6925.
205. Herman EH, Ferrans VJ. Examination of the potential long-lasting protective effect of ICRF-187 against anthracycline-induced chronic cardiomyopathy. Cancer Treat Rev 1990;17:155–160.
206. Speyer JL, Green MD, Kramer E, et al. Protective effect of the bispiperazinedione ICRF-187 against doxorubicin-induced cardiac

toxicity in women with advanced breast cancer. N Engl J Med 1988;319:745–752.
207. Speyer JL, Green MD, Zeleniuch-Jacquotte A, et al. ICRF-187 permits longer treatment with doxorubicin in women with breast cancer. J Clin Oncol 1992;10:117–127.
208. Von Hoff DD, Howser D, Lewis BJ, et al. Phase I study of ICRF-187 using a daily for 3 days schedule. Cancer Treat Rep 1981;65:249–252.
209. Tetef ML, Synold TW, Chow W, et al. Phase I trial of 96-hour continuous infusion of dexrazoxane in patients with advanced malignancies. Clin Cancer Res 2001;7:1569–1576.
210. Doroshow JH. Role of reactive-oxygen metabolism in cardiac toxicity of anthracycline antibiotics. In: Priebe W, ed. Anthracycline Antibiotics: New Analogues, Methods of Delivery, and Mechanisms of Action. Washington, DC: American Chemical Society, 1995:259–267.
211. Minotti G, Cairo G, Monti E. Role of iron in anthracycline cardiotoxicity: new tunes for an old song? FASEB J 1999;13:199–212.
212. Minotti G, Cavaliere AF, Mordente A, et al. Secondary alcohol metabolites mediate iron delocalization in cytosolic fractions of myocardial biopsies exposed to anticancer anthracyclines: novel linkage between anthracycline metabolism and iron-induced cardiotoxicity. J Clin Invest 1995;95:1595–1605.
213. Minotti G, Mancuso C, Frustaci A, et al. Paradoxical inhibition of cardiac lipid peroxidation in cancer patients treated with doxorubicin: pharmacologic and molecular reappraisal of anthracycline cardiotoxicity. J Clin Invest 1996;98:650–661.
214. Minotti G, Recalcati S, Mordente A, et al. The secondary alcohol metabolite of doxorubicin irreversibly inactivates aconitase/iron regulatory protein-1 in cytosolic fractions from human myocardium. FASEB J 1998;12:541–552.
215. Cummings J, Milstead R, Cunningham D, et al. Marked interpatient variation in adriamycin biotransformation to 7-deoxyaglycones: evidence from metabolites identified in serum. Eur J Cancer Clin Oncol 1986;22:991–1001.
216. Cummings J, Smyth JF. Pharmacology of adriamycin: the message to the clinician. Eur J Cancer Clin Oncol 1988;24:579–582.
217. Averbuch SD, Boldt M, Gaudiano G, et al. Experimental chemotherapy-induced skin necrosis in swine: mechanistic studies of anthracycline antibiotic toxicity and protection with a radical dimer compound. J Clin Invest 1988;81:142–148.
218. Powis G, Gasdaska PY, Gallegos A, et al. Over-expression of DT-diaphorase in transfected NIH 3T3 cells does not lead to increased anticancer quinone drug sensitivity: a questionable role for the enzyme as a target for bioreductively activated anticancer drugs. Anticancer Res 1995;15:1141–1145.
219. Tritton TR. Cell surface actions of adriamycin. Pharmacol Ther 1991;49:293–309.
220. Siegfried JA, Kennedy KA, Sartorelli AC, et al. The role of membranes in the mechanism of action of the antineoplastic agent adriamycin: spin-labelling studies with chronically hypoxic and drug-resistant tumor cells. J Biol Chem 1983;258:339–343.
221. Sugiyama M, Sakanashi T, Okamoto K, et al. Membrane fluidity in Ehrlich ascites tumor cells treated with adriamycin. Biotechnol Appl Biochem 1986;8:217–221.
222. Goormaghtigh E, Brasseur R, Huart P, et al. Study of the adriamycin-cardiolipin complex structure using attenuated total reflection infrared spectroscopy. Biochemistry 1987;26:1789–1794.
223. Heywang C, Saint-Pierre CM, Masson CM, et al. Orientation of anthracyclines in lipid monolayers and planar asymmetrical bilayers: a surface-enhanced resonance Raman scattering study. Biophys J 1998;75:2368–2381.
224. Zuckier G, Tritton TR. Adriamycin causes up regulation of epidermal growth factor receptors in actively growing cells. Exp Cell Res 1983;148:155–161.
225. Pegram M, Hsu S, Lewis G, et al. Inhibitory effects of combinations of HER-2/neu antibody and chemotherapeutic agents used for treatment of human breast cancers. Oncogene 1999;18:2241–2251.
226. Sun IL, Navas P, Crane FL, et al. Diferric transferrin reductase in the plasma membrane is inhibited by adriamycin. Biochem Int 1987;14:119–127.
227. DeAtley SM, Aksenov MY, Aksenova MV, et al. Adriamycin induces protein oxidation in erythrocyte membranes. Pharmacol Toxicol 1998;83:62–68.
228. Tritton TR, Yee G. The anticancer agent adriamycin can be actively cytotoxic without entering cells. Science 1982;217:248–250.
229. Rogers KE, Carr BI, Tokes ZA. Cell surface-mediated cytotoxicity of polymer-bound adriamycin against drug-resistant hepatocytes. Cancer Res 1983;43:2741–2748.
230. Vichi P, Tritton TR. Adriamycin: protection from cell death by removal of extracellular drug. Cancer Res 1992;52:4135–4138.
231. Burns CP, Spector AA. Membrane fatty acid modification in tumor cells: a potential therapeutic adjunct. Lipids 1987;22:178–184.
232. Spector AA, Burns CP. Biological and therapeutic potential of membrane lipid modifications in tumors. Cancer Res 1987;47:4529–4537.
233. Burns CP, North JA, Petersen ES, et al. Subcellular distribution of doxorubicin: comparison of fatty acid-modified and unmodified cells. Proc Soc Exp Biol Med 1988;188:455–460.
234. Hannun YA. Functions of ceramide in coordinating cellular responses to stress. Science 1996;274:1855–1859.
235. Leevers SJ, Vanhaesebroeck B, Waterfield MD. Signalling through phosphoinositide 3-kinases: the lipids take centre stage. Curr Opin Cell Biol 1999;11:219–225.
236. Haimovitz-Friedman A. Radiation-induced signal transduction and stress response. Radiat Res 1998;150:S102–108.
237. Bredel M, Pollack IF. The p21-Ras signal transduction pathway and growth regulation in human high-grade gliomas. Brain Res Brain Res Rev 1999;29:232–249.
238. Kyriakis JM. Making the connection: coupling of stress-activated ERK/MAPK (extracellular-signal-regulated kinase/mitogen-activated protein kinase) core signalling modules to extracellular stimuli and biological responses. Biochem Soc Symp 1999;64:29–48.
239. Tritton TR, Hickman JA. How to kill cancer cells: membranes and cell signaling as targets in cancer chemotherapy. Cancer Cells 1990;2:95–105.
240. Palayoor ST, Stein JM, Hait WN. Inhibition of protein kinase C by antineoplastic agents: implications for drug resistance. Biochem Biophys Res Commun 1987;148:718–725.
241. Donella-Deana A, Monti E, Pinna LA. Inhibition of tyrosine protein kinases by the antineoplastic agent adriamycin. Biochem Biophys Res Commun 1989;160:1309–1315.
242. Hannun YA, Foglesong RJ, Bell RM. The adriamycin-iron(III) complex is a potent inhibitor of protein kinase C. J Biol Chem 1989;264:9960–9966.
243. Posada J, Vichi P, Tritton TR. Protein kinase C in adriamycin action and resistance in mouse sarcoma 180 cells. Cancer Res 1989;49:6634–6639.
244. Tritton TR. Cell death in cancer chemotherapy: the case of adriamycin. In: Tomei LD, Cope FO, eds. Apoptosis: The Molecular Basis of Cell Death. Cold Spring Harbor, NY: Cold Spring Harbor Laboratory Press, 1991:121–137.
245. Sahyoun N, Wolf M, Besterman J, et al. Protein kinase C phosphorylates topoisomerase II: topoisomerase activation and its possible role in phorbol ester-induced differentiation of HL-60 cells. Proc Natl Acad Sci USA 1986;83:1603–1607.
246. Jaffrezou JP, Levade T, Bettaieb A, et al. Daunorubicin-induced apoptosis: triggering of ceramide generation through sphingomyelin hydrolysis. EMBO J 1996;15:2417–2424.
247. Bose R, Verheij M, Haimovitz-Friedman A, et al. Ceramide synthase mediates daunorubicin-induced apoptosis: an alternative mechanism for generating death signals. Cell 1995;82:405–414.
248. Bettaieb A, Plo I, Mansat-De M, et al. Daunorubicin- and mitoxantrone-triggered phosphatidylcholine hydrolysis: implication in drug-induced ceramide generation and apoptosis. Mol Pharmacol 1999;55:118–125.
249. Tepper AD, de Vries E, van Blitterswijz WJ, et al. Ordering of ceramide formation, caspase activation, and mitochondrial changes during CD95- and DNA damage-induced apoptosis. J Clin Invest 1999;103:971–978.
250. Mansat V, Bettaieb A, Levade T, et al. Serine protease inhibitors block neutral sphingomyelinase activation, ceramide generation, and apoptosis triggered by daunorubicin. FASEB J 1997;11:695–702.
251. Allouche M, Bettaieb A, Vindis C, et al. Influence of Bcl-2 overexpression on the ceramide pathway in daunorubicin-induced apoptosis of leukemic cells. Oncogene 1997;14:1837–1845.

252. Liu YY, Han TY, Giuliano AE, et al. Expression of glucosylceramide synthase, converting ceramide to glucosylceramide, confers adriamycin resistance in human breast cancer cells. J Biol Chem 1999;274:1140–1146.

253. Fine RL, Patel J, Chabner BA. Phorbol esters induce multidrug resistance in human breast cancer cells. Proc Natl Acad Sci USA 1988;85:582–586.

254. Yu G, Ahmad S, Aquino A, et al. Transfection with protein kinase Ca confers increased multidrug resistance to MCF-7 cells expressing P-glycoprotein. Cancer Commun 1991;3:181–189.

255. Budworth J, Gant TW, Gescher A. Co-ordinate loss of protein kinase C and multidrug resistance gene expression in revertant MCF-7/Adr breast carcinoma cells. Br J Cancer 1997;75:1330–1335.

256. Laredo J, Huynh A, Muller C, et al. Effect of the protein kinase C inhibitor staurosporine on chemosensitivity to daunorubicin of normal and leukemic fresh myeloid cells. Blood 1994;84:229–237.

257. Lavie Y, Cao H, Volner A, et al. Agents that reverse multidrug resistance, tamoxifen, verapamil, and cyclosporin A, block glycosphingolipid metabolism by inhibiting ceramide glycosylation in human cancer cells. J Biol Chem 1997;272:1682–1687.

258. Reed JC. Dysregulation of apoptosis in cancer. J Clin Oncol 1999;17:2941–2953.

259. Wickremasinghe RG, Hoffbrand AV. Biochemical and genetic control of apoptosis: relevance to normal hematopoiesis and hematological malignancies. Blood 1999;93:3587–3600.

260. Hannun YA. Apoptosis and the dilemma of cancer chemotherapy. Blood 1997;89:1845–1853.

261. Skladanowski A, Konopa J. Adriamycin and daunomycin induce programmed cell death (apoptosis) in tumour cells. Biochem Pharmacol 1993;46:375–382.

262. Ling Y-H, Priebe W, Perez-Soler R. Apoptosis induced by anthracycline antibiotics in P388 parent and multidrug-resistant cells. Cancer Res 1993;53:1845–1852.

263. Lotem J, Sachs L. Hematopoietic cytokines inhibit apoptosis induced by transforming growth factor beta 1 and cancer chemotherapy compounds in myeloid leukemic cells. Blood 1992;80:1750–1757.

264. Thakkar NS, Potten CS. Inhibition of doxorubicin-induced apoptosis in vivo by 2-deoxy-d-glucose. Cancer Res 1993;53:2057–2060.

265. Onishi Y, Azuma Y, Sato Y, et al. Topoisomerase inhibitors induce apoptosis in thymocytes. Biochim Biophys Acta 1993;1175:147–154.

266. Zaleskis G, Berleth E, Verstovsek S, et al. Doxorubicin-induced DNA degradation in murine thymocytes. Mol Pharmacol 1994;46:901–908.

267. Chernov MV, Stark GR. The p53 activation and apoptosis induced by DNA damage are reversibly inhibited by salicylate. Oncogene 1997;14:2503–2510.

268. Teixeira C, Reed JC, Pratt MAC. Estrogen promotes chemotherapeutic drug resistance by a mechanism involving bcl-2 proto-oncogene expression in human breast cancer cells. Cancer Res 1995;55:3902–3907.

269. Strobel T, Swanson L, Korsmeyer S, et al. BAX enhances paclitaxel-induced apoptosis through a p53-independent pathway. Proc Natl Acad Sci USA 1996;93:14094–14099.

270. Makris A, Powles TJ, Dowsett M, et al. Prediction of response to neoadjuvant chemoendocrine therapy in primary breast carcinomas. Clin Cancer Res 1997;3:593–600.

271. Friesen C, Herr I, Krammer PH, et al. Involvement of the CD95 (APO-1/FAS) receptor/ligand system in drug-induced apoptosis in leukemia cells. Nat Med 1996;2:574–577.

272. Fulda S, Sieverts H, Friesen C, et al. The CD95 (APO-1/Fas) system mediates drug-induced apoptosis in neuroblastoma cells. Cancer Res 1997;57:3823–3829.

273. Fulda S, Susin SA, Kroemer G, et al. Molecular ordering of apoptosis induced by anticancer drugs in neuroblastoma cells. Cancer Res 1998;58:4453–4460.

274. Mo YY, Beck WT. DNA damage signals induction of Fas ligand in tumor cells. Mol Pharmacol 1999;55:216–222.

275. Eischen CM, Kottke TJ, Martins LM, et al. Comparison of apoptosis in wild-type and Fas-resistant cells: chemotherapy-induced apoptosis is not dependent on Fas/Fas ligand interactions. Blood 1997;90:935–943.

276. Landowski TH, Shain KH, Oshiro MM, et al. Myeloma cells selected for resistance to CD95-mediated apoptosis are not cross-resistant to cytotoxic drugs: evidence for independent mechanisms of caspase activation. Blood 1999;94:265–274.

277. McGahon AJ, Costa PA, Daly L, et al. Chemotherapeutic drug-induced apoptosis in human leukaemic cells is independent of the Fas (APO-1/CD95) receptor/ligand system. Br J Haematol 1998;101:539–547.

278. Wesselborg S, Engels IH, Rossmann E, et al. Anticancer drugs induce caspase-8/FLICE activation and apoptosis in the absence of CD95 receptor/ligand interaction. Blood 1999;93:3053–3063.

279. Come MG, Bettaieb A, Skladanowski A, et al. Alteration of the daunorubicin-triggered sphingomyelin-ceramide pathway and apoptosis in MDR cells: influence of drug transport abnormalities. Int J Cancer 1999;81:580–587.

280. Herr I, Wilhelm D, Bohler T, et al. Activation of CD95 (APO-1/Fas) signaling by ceramide mediates cancer therapy-induced apoptosis. EMBO J 1997;16:6200–6208.

281. Laurent G, Jaffrezou JP. Signaling pathways activated by daunorubicin. Blood 2001;98:913–924.

282. Garland JM, Rudin C. Cytochrome c induces caspase-dependent apoptosis in intact hematopoietic cells and overrides apoptosis suppression mediated by bcl-2, growth factor signaling, MAP-kinase-kinase, and malignant change. Blood 1999;92:1235–1246.

283. Kroemer G, Zamzami N, Susin SA. Mitochondrial control of apoptosis. Immunol Today 1997;18:44–51.

284. Green PS, Leeuwenburgh C. Mitochondrial dysfunction is an early indicator of doxorubicin-induced apoptosis. Biochim Biophys Acta 2002;1588:94–101.

285. Clementi ME, Giardina B, Di Stasio E, et al. Doxorubicin-derived metabolites induce release of cytochrome c and inhibition of respiration on cardiac isolated mitochondria. Anticancer Res 2003;23:2445–2450.

286. Doroshow JH, Matsumoto L, van Balgooy J. Modulation of doxorubicin-induced, oxygen radical mediated apoptosis by glutathione peroxidase and free radical scavengers in human breast cancer cells. Proc Amer Assoc Cancer Res 1999;40:16.

287. Singh I, Pahan K, Khan M, et al. Cytokine-mediated induction of ceramide production is redox-sensitive: implications to proinflammatory cytokine-mediated apoptosis in demyelinating diseases. J Biol Chem 1998;273:20354–20362.

288. Gouaze V, Mirault ME, Carpentier S, et al. Glutathione peroxidase-1 overexpression prevents ceramide production and partially inhibits apoptosis in doxorubicin-treated human breast carcinoma cells. Mol Pharmacol 2001;60:488–496.

289. Ohmori T, Podack ER, Nishio K, et al. Apoptosis of lung cancer cells caused by some anti-cancer agents (MMC, CPT-11, ADM) is inhibited by BCL-2. Biochem Biophys Res Commun 1993;192:30–36.

290. Reed JC. Bcl-2 and the regulation of programmed cell death. J Cell Biol 1994;124:1–6.

291. Campos L, Sabido O, Rouault J-P, et al. Effects of BCL-2 antisense oligodeoxynucleotides on in vitro proliferation and survival of normal marrow progenitors and leukemic cells. Blood 1994;84:595–600.

292. Froesch BA, Aime-Sempe C, Leber B, et al. Inhibition of p53 transcriptional activity by Bcl-2 requires its membrane-anchoring domain. J Biol Chem 1999;274:6469–6475.

293. Hockenbery DM, Oltvai ZN, Yin X-M, et al. Bcl-2 functions in an antioxidant pathway to prevent apoptosis. Cell 1993;75:241–251.

294. Decaudin D, Geley S, Hirsch T, et al. Bcl-2 and Bcl-XL antagonize the mitochondrial dysfunction preceding nuclear apoptosis induced by chemotherapeutic agents. Cancer Res 1997;57:62–67.

295. Boland MP, Foster SJ, O'Neill LA. Daunorubicin activates NFkappaB and induces kappaB-dependent gene expression in HL-60 promyelocytic and Jurkat T lymphoma cells. J Biol Chem 1997;272:12952–12960.

296. Wang CY, Mayo MW, Baldwin AS Jr. TNF- and cancer therapy-induced apoptosis: potentiation by inhibition of NF-kappaB. Science 1996;274:784–787.

297. Jeremias I, Kupatt C, Baumann B, et al. Inhibition of nuclear factor kappaB activation attenuates apoptosis resistance in lymphoid cells. Blood 1998;91:4624–4631.

298. Haldar S, Negrini M, Monne M, et al. Down-regulation of *bcl-2* by *p53* in breast cancer cells. Cancer Res 1994;54:2095–2097.

299. Bacus SS, Yarden Y, Oren M, et al. Neu differentiation factor (heregulin) activates a p53-dependent pathway in cancer cells. Oncogene 1996;12:2535–2547.

300. Gartenhaus RB, Wang P, Hoffmann P. Induction of the WAF1/CIP1 protein and apoptosis in human T-cell leukemia virus type I-transformed lymphocytes after treatment with adriamycin by using a p53-independent pathway. Proc Natl Acad Sci USA 1996;93:265–268.

301. Michieli P, Chedid M, Lin D, et al. Induction of WAF1/CIP1 by a p53-independent pathway. Cancer Res 1994;54:3391–3395.

302. Wang Y, Blandino G, Givol D. Induced p21waf expression in H1299 cell line promotes cell senescence and protects against cytotoxic effect of radiation and doxorubicin. Oncogene 1999;18:2643–2649.

303. Shimizu A, Nishida J, Ueoka Y, et al. CyclinG contributes to G2/M arrest of cells in response to DNA damage. Biochem Biophys Res Commun 1998;242:529–533.

304. Lowe SW, Ruley HE, Jacks T, et al. p53-dependent apoptosis modulates the cytotoxicity of anticancer agents. Cell 1993;74:957–967.

305. Lowe SW, Bodis S, McClatchey A, et al. p53 status and the efficacy of cancer therapy in vivo. Science 1994;266:807–810.

306. Aas T, Borresen AL, Geisler S, et al. Specific p53 mutations are associated with de novo resistance to doxorubicin in breast cancer patients. Nat Med 1996;2:811–814.

307. Chang BD, Broude EV, Dokmanovic M, et al. A senescence-like phenotype distinguishes tumor cells that undergo terminal proliferation arrest after exposure to anticancer agents. Cancer Res 1999;59:3761–3767.

308. Chang BD, Broude EV, Fang J, et al. p21Waf1/Cip1/Sdi1-induced growth arrest is associated with depletion of mitosis-control proteins and leads to abnormal mitosis and endoreduplication in recovering cells. Oncogene 2000;19:2165–2170.

309. Chang BD, Watanabe K, Broude EV, et al. Effects of p21Waf1/Cip1/Sdi1 on cellular gene expression: implications for carcinogenesis, senescence, and age-related diseases. Proc Natl Acad Sci USA 2000;97:4291–4296.

310. Chang BD, Xuan Y, Broude EV, et al. Role of p53 and p21Waf1/Cip1 in senescence-like terminal proliferation arrest induced in human tumor cells by chemotherapeutic drugs. Oncogene 1999;18:4808–4818.

311. Chang BD, Swift ME, Shen M, et al. Molecular determinants of terminal growth arrest induced in tumor cells by a chemotherapeutic agent. Proc Natl Acad Sci USA 2002;99:389–394.

312. Berns A. Senescence: a companion in chemotherapy? Cancer Cell 2002;1:309–311.

313. Gros P, Croop J, Housman D. Mammalian multidrug resistance gene: complete cDNA sequence indicates strong homology to bacterial transport proteins. Cell 1986;47:371–380.

314. Gros P, BenNeriah Y, Croop J, et al. Isolation and expression of a complementary DNA that confers multidrug resistance. Nature 1986;332:728–731.

315. Endicott JA, Ling V. The biochemistry of P-glycoprotein-mediated multidrug resistance. Annu Rev Biochem 1989;58:137–171.

316. Sugimoto Y, Tsuruo T. DNA-mediated transfer and cloning of a human multidrug-resistant gene of adriamycin-resistant myelogenous leukemia K562. Cancer Res 1987;47:2620–2625.

317. Hamada H, Hagiwara T, Nakajma T, et al. Phosphorylation of Mr 170,000 to 180,000 glycoprotein species specific to multidrug-resistant tumor cells: effects of verapamil, trifluoperazine and phorbol esters. Cancer Res 1987;47:2860–2865.

318. Chambers SK, Hait WN, Kacinski BM, et al. Enhancement of anthracycline growth inhibition in parent and multidrug-resistant Chinese hamster ovary cells by cyclosporin A and its analogues. Cancer Res 1989;49:6275–6279.

319. Coley HM, Twentyman PR, Workman P. The efflux of anthracyclines in multidrug-resistant cell lines. Biochem Pharmacol 1993;46:1317–1326.

320. Kang Y, Perry RR. Modulatory effects of tamoxifen and recombinant human a-interferon on doxorubicin resistance. Cancer Res 1993;53:3040–3045.

321. Merlin J-L, Guerci A, Marchal S, et al. Comparative evaluation of S9788, verapamil, and cyclosporine A in K562 human leukemia cell lines and in P-glycoprotein-expressing samples from patients with hematologic malignancies. Blood 1994;84:262–269.

322. Alvarez M, Pauli K, Monks A, et al. Generation of a drug resistance profile by quantitation of *mdr*-1/P-glycoprotein in the cell lines of the national cancer institute anticancer drug screen. J Clin Invest 1995;95:2205–2214.

323. Lemontt JF, Azzaria M, Gross P. Increased *mdr* gene expression and decreased drug accumulation in multidrug-resistant human melanoma cells. Cancer Res 1988;48:6348–6353.

324. Noonan KE, Beck C, Holzmayer TA, et al. Quantitative analysis of *MDR1* (multidrug resistance) gene expression in human tumors by polymerase chain reaction. Proc Natl Acad Sci USA 1990;87:7160–7164.

325. Chen G, Jaffrezou J-P, Fleming WH, et al. Prevalence of multidrug resistance related to activation of the *mdr1* gene in human sarcoma mutants derived by single-step doxorubicin selection. Cancer Res 1994;54:4980–4987.

326. Morton KA, Jones BJ, Sohn MH, et al. Enrichment for metallothionein does not confer resistance to cisplatin in transfected NIH/3T3 cells. J Pharmacol Exp Ther 1993;267:697–702.

327. Chaudhary PM, Roninson IB. Induction of multidrug resistance in human cells by transient exposure to different chemotherapeutic drugs. J Natl Cancer Inst 1993;85:632–639.

328. Fojo AT, Ueda K, Siamon DJ, et al. Expression of a multidrug resistance gene in human tumors and tissues. Proc Natl Acad Sci USA 1987;84:265–269.

329. Sparreboom A, van Asperen J, Mayer U, et al. Limited oral bioavailability and active epithelial excretion of paclitaxel (Taxol) caused by P-glycoprotein in the intestine. Proc Natl Acad Sci USA 1997;94:2031–2035.

330. Egashira M, Kawamata N, Sugimoto K, et al. P-glycoprotein expression on normal and abnormally expanded natural killer cells and inhibition of P-glycoprotein function by cyclosporin A and its analogue PSC833. Blood 1999;93:599–606.

331. Fairchild CR, Ivy SP, Rushmore T, et al. Carcinogen-induced *mdr* overexpression is associated with xenobiotic resistance in rat preneoplastic liver nodules and hepatocellular carcinomas. Proc Natl Acad Sci USA 1987;84:7701–7705.

332. Myers CE, Cowan K, Sinha BK, et al. The phenomenon of pleiotropic drug resistance. In: De Vita VT Jr, Hellman S, Rosenberg SA, eds. Important Advances in Oncology. Philadelphia: JB Lippincott, 1987:27–38.

333. Yeh GC, Lopaczynska J, Poore CM, et al. A new functional role for P-glycoprotein: efflux pump for benzo(a)pyrene in human breast cancer MCF-7 cells. Cancer Res 1992;52:6692–6695.

334. Marie J-P, Zittoun R, Sikic BI. Multidrug resistance (*mdr*1) gene expression in adult acute leukemias: correlations with treatment outcome and in vitro drug sensitivity. Blood 1991;78:586–592.

335. Goasguen JE, Dossot J-M, Fardel O, et al. Expression of the multidrug resistance-associated P-glycoprotein (P-170) in 59 cases of de novo acute lymphoblastic leukemia: prognostic implications. Blood 1993;81:2394–2398.

336. Chabner BA, Fojo A. Multidrug resistance: P-glycoprotein and its allies—the elusive foes. J Natl Cancer Inst 1989;81:910–913.

337. Grogan TM, Spier CM, Salmon SE, et al. P-glycoprotein expression in human plasma cell myeloma: correlation with prior chemotherapy. Blood 1993;81:490–495.

338. Keith WN, Stallard S, Brown R. Expression of mdr1 and GST-p in human breast tumors: comparison to in vitro chemosensitivity. Br J Cancer 1990;61:712–716.

339. Verrelle P, Meissonnier F, Fonck Y, et al. Clinical relevance of immunohistochemical detection of multidrug resistance P-glycoprotein in breast carcinoma. J Natl Cancer Inst 1991;83:111–116.

340. Miller TP, Grogan TM, Dalton WS, et al. P-glycoprotein expression in malignant lymphoma and reversal of clinical drug resistance with chemotherapy plus high-dose verapamil. J Clin Oncol 1991;9:17–24.

341. Wishart GC, Bissett D, Paul J, et al. Quinidine as a resistance modulator of epirubicin in advanced breast cancer: mature results of a placebo-controlled randomized trial. J Clin Oncol 1994;12:1771–1777.

342. Lum BL, Fisher GA, Brophy NA, et al. Clinical trials of modulation of multidrug resistance: pharmacokinetic and pharmacodynamic considerations. Cancer 1993;72:3502–3514.

343. Bartlett NL, Lum BL, Fisher GA, et al. Phase I trial of doxorubicin with cyclosporine as a modulator of multidrug resistance. J Clin Oncol 1994;12:835–842.

344. List AF, Kopecky KJ, Willman CL, et al. Benefit of cyclosporine (Csa) modulation of anthracycline resistance in high-risk AML: a Southwest Oncology Group (SWOG) study. Blood 1998;92 (Suppl. 1):312a.

345. Slovak ML, Hoeltge GA, Dalton WS, et al. Pharmacological and biological evidence for differing mechanisms of doxorubicin resistance in two human tumor cell lines. Cancer Res 1988; 48:2793–2797.

346. Mirski SE, Gerlach JH, Cole SP. Multidrug resistance in a human small cell line selected in adriamycin. Cancer Res 1987;47:2594–2598.

347. Krishnamachary N, Center MS. The MRP gene associated with a non-P-glycoprotein multidrug resistance encodes a 190-kDa membrane bound glycoprotein. Cancer Res 1993;53:3658–3661.

348. Eijdems EW, Zaman GJ, de Haas M, et al. Altered MRP is associated with multidrug resistance and reduced drug accumulation in human SW-1573 cells. Br J Cancer 1995;72:298–306.

349. Welters MJ, Fichtinger-Schepman AM, Baan RA, et al. Role of glutathione, glutathione S-transferases and multidrug resistance-related proteins in cisplatin sensitivity of head and neck cancer cell lines. Br J Cancer 1998;77:556–561.

350. Moran E, Cleary I, Larkin AM, et al. Co-expression of MDR-associated markers, including P-170, MRP and LRP and cytoskeletal proteins, in three resistant variants of the human ovarian carcinoma cell line, OAW42. Eur J Cancer 1997;33:652–660.

351. Marbeuf-Gueye C, Broxterman HJ, Dubru F, et al. Kinetics of anthracycline efflux from multidrug resistance protein-expressing cancer cells compared with P-glycoprotein-expressing cancer cells. Mol Pharmacol 1998;53:141–147.

352. Slapak CA, Mizunuma N, Kufe DW. Expression of the multidrug resistance associated protein and p-glycoprotein in doxorubicin-selected human myeloid leukemia cells. Blood 1994;84:3113–3121.

353. Schneider E, Cowan KH, Bader H, et al. Increased expression of the multidrug resistance-associated protein gene in relapsed acute leukemia. Blood 1995;85:186–193.

354. Legrand O, Simonin G, Beauchamp-Nicoud A, et al. Simultaneous activity of MRP1 and Pgp is correlated with in vitro resistance to daunorubicin and with in vivo resistance in adult acute myeloid leukemia. Blood 1999;94:1046–1056.

355. Rappa G, Finch RA, Sartorelli AC, et al. New insights into the biology and pharmacology of the multidrug resistance protein (MRP) from gene knockout models. Biochem Pharmacol 1999; 58:557–562.

356. Lorico A, Rappa G, Flavell RA, et al. Double knockout of the MRP gene leads to increased drug sensitivity in vitro. Cancer Res 1996;56:5351–5355.

357. Kool M, de Haas M, Scheffer GL, et al. Analysis of expression of cMoat (MRP2), MRP3, MRP4, and MRP5, homologues of the multidrug resistance-associated protein (MRP1), in human cancer cell lines. Cancer Res 1997;57:3537–3547.

358. Doyle LA, Ross DD. Multidrug resistance mediated by the breast cancer resistance protein BCRP (ABCG2). Oncogene 2003;22:7340–7358.

359. Doyle LA, Yang W, Abruzzo LV, et al. A multidrug resistance transporter from human MCF-7 breast cancer cells. Proc Natl Acad Sci USA 1998;95:15665–15670.

360. Allen JD, Jackson SC, Schinkel AH. A mutation hot spot in the Bcrp1 (Abcg2) multidrug transporter in mouse cell lines selected for doxorubicin resistance. Cancer Res 2002;62:2294–2299.

361. Plasschaert SL, Van Der Kolk DM, De Bont ES, et al. The role of breast cancer resistance protein in acute lymphoblastic leukemia. Clin Cancer Res 2003;9:5171–5177.

362. Sargent JM, Williamson CJ, Maliepaard M, et al. Breast cancer resistance protein expression and resistance to daunorubicin in blast cells from patients with acute myeloid leukaemia. Br J Haematol 2001;115:257–262.

363. Deffie AM, Batra JK, Goldenberg GG. Direct correlation between DNA topoisomerase II activity and cytotoxicity in adriamycin-sensitive and -resistant P388 leukemia cell lines. Cancer Res 1989;49:58–62.

364. Ganapathi R, Grabowski D, Ford J, et al. Progressive resistance to doxorubicin in mouse leukemia L1210 cells with multidrug resistance phenotype: reductions in drug-induced topoisomerase II-mediated DNA cleavage. Cancer Commun 1989;1:217–224.

365. de Jong S, Zijlstra JG, de Vries EGE, et al. Reduced DNA topoisomerase II activity and drug-induced DNA cleavage activity in an adriamycin-resistant human small cell lung carcinoma cell line. Cancer Res 1990;50:304–309.

366. Ramachandran C, Samy TS, Huang XL, et al. Doxorubicin-induced DNA breaks, topoisomerase II activity and gene expression in human melanoma cells. Biochem Pharmacol 1993;45:1367–1371.

367. Son YS, Suh JM, Ahn SH, et al. Reduced activity of topoisomerase II in an adriamycin-resistant human stomach-adenocarcinoma cell line. Cancer Chemother Pharmacol 1998;41:353–360.

368. Wyler B, Shao Y, Schneider E, et al. Intermittent exposure to doxorubicin in vitro selects for multifactorial non-P-glycoprotein-associated multidrug resistance in RPMI 8226 human myeloma cells. Br J Haematol 1997;97:65–75.

369. Beketic-Oreskovic L, Duran GE, Chen G, et al. Decreased mutation rate for cellular resistance to doxorubicin and suppression of mdr1 gene activation by the cyclosporin PSC 833 [see comments]. J Natl Cancer Inst 1995;87:1593–1602.

370. Friche E, Danks MK, Schmidt CA, et al. Decreased DNA topoisomerase II in daunorubicin-resistant Ehrlich ascites tumor cells. Cancer Res 1991;51:4213–4218.

371. Wang H, Jiang Z, Wong YW, et al. Decreased CP-1 (NF-Y) activity results in transcriptional down-regulation of topoisomerase IIalpha in a doxorubicin-resistant variant of human multiple myeloma RPMI 8226. Biochem Biophys Res Commun 1997; 237:217–224.

372. McPherson JP, Deffie AM, Jones NR, et al. Selective sensitization of adriamycin-resistant P388 murine leukemia cells to antineoplastic agents following transfection with human DNA topoisomerase II alpha. Anticancer Res 1997;17:4243–4252.

373. Kaufman SH, Karp JE, Jones RJ, et al. Topoisomerase II levels and drug sensitivity in adult acute myelogenous leukemia. Blood 1994;83:517–530.

374. Lee FY, Vessey AR, Siemann DW. Glutathione as a determinant of cellular response to doxorubicin. NCI Monogr 1988;6:211–215.

375. Capranico G, Babudri N, Casciarri G, et al. Lack of effect of glutathione depletion on cytotoxicity, mutagenicity and DNA damage produced by doxorubicin in cultured cells. Chem Biol Interact 1986;57:189–201.

376. Yamamoto M, Maehara Y, Oda S, et al.. The p53 tumor suppressor gene in anticancer agent-induced apoptosis and chemosensitivity of human gastrointestinal cancer cell lines. Cancer Chemother Pharmacol 1999;43:43–49.

377. Meng RD, Phillips P, el-Deiry WS. p53-independent increase in E2F-1 expression enhances the cytotoxic effects of etoposide and of adriamycin. Int J Oncol 1999;14:5–14.

378. Kuhl JS, Krajewski S, Duran GE, et al. Spontaneous overexpression of the long form of the Bcl-X protein in a highly resistant P388 leukaemia. Br J Cancer 1997;75:268–274.

379. Reed JC. Bcl-2 and the regulation of programmed cell death. J Cell Biol 1994;124:1–6.

380. Nielsen D, Maare C, Skovsgaard T. Cellular resistance to anthracyclines. Gen Pharmacol 1996;27:251–255.

381. Brown R, Hirst GL, Gallagher WM, et al. hMLH1 expression and cellular responses of ovarian tumour cells to treatment with cytotoxic anticancer agents. Oncogene 1997;15:45–52.

382. Durant ST, Morris MM, Illand M, et al. Dependence on RAD52 and RAD1 for anticancer drug resistance mediated by inactivation of mismatch repair genes. Curr Biol 1999;9:51–54.

383. Belloni M, Uberti D, Rizzini C, et al. Induction of two DNA mismatch repair proteins, MSH2 and MSH6, in differentiated human neuroblastoma SH-SY5Y cells exposed to doxorubicin. J Neurochem 1999;72:974–979.

384. Fink D, Aebi S, Howell SB. The role of DNA mismatch repair in drug resistance. Clin Cancer Res 1998;4:1–6.

385. Chatterjee S, Cheng MF, Berger NA. Hypersensitivity to clinically useful alkylating agents and radiation in poly(ADP-ribose) polymerase-deficient cell lines. Cancer Commun 1990;2:401–407.

386. Darby MK, Schmitt B, Jongstra-Bilen J, et al. Inhibition of calf thymus type II DNA topoisomerase by poly(ADP-ribosylation). EMBO Journal 1985;4:2129–2134.

387. Berger NA. Poly(ADP-ribose) in the cellular response to DNA damage. Radiat Res 1985;101:4–15.

388. Yamamoto K, Tsukidate K, Farber JL. Differing effects of the inhibition of poly(ADP-ribose) polymerase on the course of oxidative cell injury in hepatocytes and fibroblasts. Biochem Pharmacol 1993;46:483–491.

389. Tanizawa A, Kubota M, Takimoto T, et al. Prevention of adriamycin-induced interphase death by 3-aminobenzamide and nicotinamide in a human promyelocytic leukemia cell line. Biochem Biophys Res Commun 1987;144:1031–1036.

390. Doroshow JH, Van Balgooy C, Akman SA. Effect of poly (ADP-ribose) polymerase inhibition on protein-associated DNA single-strand cleavage and cytotoxicity by anthracycline antibiotics. Proc Amer Assoc Cancer Res 1995;36:444.

391. Chen JJ, Silver D, Cantor S, et al. BRCA1, BRCA2, and Rad51 operate in a common DNA damage response pathway. Cancer Res 1999;59:1752s–1756s.

392. MacLachlan TK, Dash BC, Dicker DT, et al. Repression of BRCA1 through a feedback loop involving p53. J Biol Chem 2000;275:31869–31875.

393. Su J, Ciftci K. Changes in BRCA1 and BRCA2 expression produced by chemotherapeutic agents in human breast cancer cells. Int J Biochem Cell Biol 2002;34:950–957.

394. Fedier A, Steiner RA, Schwarz VA, et al. The effect of loss of Brca1 on the sensitivity to anticancer agents in p53-deficient cells. Int J Oncol 2003;22:1169–1173.

395. Tassone P, Tagliaferri P, Perricelli A, et al. BRCA1 expression modulates chemosensitivity of BRCA1-defective HCC1937 human breast cancer cells. Br J Cancer 2003;88:1285–1291.

396. Egawa C, Motomura K, Miyoshi Y, et al. Increased expression of BRCA1 mRNA predicts favorable response to anthracycline-containing chemotherapy in breast cancers. Breast Cancer Res Treat 2003;78:45–50.

397. Reich SD, Bachur NR. Alterations in adriamycin efficacy by phenobarbital. Cancer Res 1976;36:3803–3806.

398. Innis JD, Meyer M, Hurwitz A. A novel acute toxicity resulting from the administration of morphine and adriamycin to mice. Toxicol Appl Pharmacol 1987;90:445–453.

399. Holmes FA, Madden T, Newman RA, et al. Sequence-dependent alteration of doxorubicin pharmacokinetics by paclitaxel in a phase I study of paclitaxel and doxorubicin in patients with metastatic breast cancer. J Clin Oncol 1996;14:2713–2721.

400. Sparreboom A, van Tellingen O, Nooijen WJ, et al. Nonlinear pharmacokinetics of paclitaxel in mice results from the pharmaceutical vehicle Cremophor EL. Cancer Res 1996;56:2112–2115.

401. Legha SS, Benjamin RS, Mackay B, et al. Reduction of doxorubicin cardiotoxicity by prolonged continuous intravenous infusion. Ann Intern Med 1982;96:133–139.

402. Terasaki T, Iga T, Sugiyama Y, et al. Experimental evidence of characteristic tissue distribution of adriamycin: tissue DNA concentration as a determinant. Pharmacol Rev 1989;53:496–501.

403. Greene R, Collins J, Jenkins J, et al. Plasma pharmacokinetics of adriamycin and adriamycinol: implications for the design of in vitro experiments and treatment protocols. Cancer Res 1983;43:3417–3422.

404. Speth PAJ, Linssen PCM, Holdrinet RSG, et al. Plasma and cellular adriamycin concentrations in patients with myeloma treated with 96-hour continuous infusion. Clin Pharmacol Ther 1987;41:661–665.

405. Synold T, Doroshow JH. Anthracycline dose intensity: clinical pharmacology and pharmacokinetics of high-dose doxorubicin administered as a 96-hour continuous intravenous infusion. J Infus Chemother 1996;6:69–73.

406. Bronchud MH, Margison JM, Howell A, et al. Comparative pharmacokinetics of escalating doses of doxorubicin in patients with metastatic breast cancer. Cancer Chemother Pharmacol 1990;25:435–439.

407. Dobbs NA, Twelves CJ, Gillies H, et al. Gender affects doxorubicin pharmacokinetics in patients with normal liver biochemistry. Cancer Chemother Pharmacol 1995;36:473–476.

408. Dobbs NA, Twelves CJ. What is the effect of adjusting epirubicin doses for body surface area? Br J Cancer 1998;78:662–666.

409. Huffman DH, Bachur NR. Daunorubicin metabolism in acute myelocytic leukemia. Blood 1972;39:637–643.

410. Gill P, Favre R, Durand A, et al. Time dependency of adriamycin and adriamycinol kinetics. Cancer Chemother Pharmacol 1983;10:120–124.

411. Lovless H, Arena E, Felsted RL, et al. Comparative mammalian metabolism of adriamycin and daunorubicin. Cancer Res 1978;38:593–598.

412. Felsted RL, Gee M, Bachur NR. Rat liver daunorubicin reductase: an aldo-keto reductase. J Biol Chem 1974;249:3672–3679.

413. Felsted RL, Richter DR, Bachur NR. Rat liver aldehyde reductase. Biochem Pharmacol 1977;26:1117–1124.

414. Felsted RL, Bachur NR. Mammalian carbonyl reductases. Drug Metab Rev 1980;11:1–60.

415. Forrest GL, Akman S, Doroshow J, et al.. Genomic sequence and expression of a cloned human carbonyl reductase gene with daunorubicin reductase activity. Mol Pharmacol 1991;40:502–507.

416. Ozols RF, Willson JKV, Weltz MD, et al. Inhibition of human ovarian cancer colony formation by adriamycin and its major metabolites. Cancer Res 1980;40:4109–4112.

417. Gessner T, Preisler HD, Azarnia N, et al. Plasma levels of daunomycin metabolites and the outcome of ANLL therapy. Med Oncol Tumor Pharmacother 1987;4:23–31.

418. Benjamin RS. A practical approach to adriamycin (NSC-123127) toxicology. Cancer Chemother Rep 1975;6:191–194.

419. Brenner DE, Wiernik PH, Wesley M, et al. Acute doxorubicin toxicity: relationship to pretreatment liver function, response and pharmacokinetics in patients with acute nonlymphocytic leukemia. Cancer 1984;53:1042–1048.

420. Chan KK, Chlebowski RT, Tong M, et al. Clinical pharmacokinetics of adriamycin in hepatoma patients with cirrhosis. Cancer Res 1980;40:1263–1268.

421. Ackland SP, Ratain MJ, Vogelzang NJ, et al. Pharmacokinetics and pharmacodynamics of long-term continuous-infusion doxorubicin. Clin Pharmacol Ther 1989;45:340–347.

422. Twelves CJ, Dobbs NA, Gillies HC, et al. Doxorubicin pharmacokinetics: the effect of abnormal liver biochemistry tests. Cancer Chemother Pharmacol 1998;42:229–234.

423. Doroshow J, Chan K. Relationship between doxorubicin clearance and indocyanine green dye pharmacokinetics in patients with hepatic dysfunction. Proc Amer Soc Clin Oncol 1982;1:11.

424. Sonneveld P, Wassenaar HA, Nooter K. Long persistence of doxorubicin in human skin after extravasation. Cancer Treat Rep 1984;68:895–896.

425. Dorr RT, Dordal MS, Koenig LM, et al. High levels of doxorubicin in the tissues of a patient experiencing extravasation during a 4-day infusion. Cancer 1989;64:2462–2464.

426. Andersson AP, Dahlstrom KK, Dahlstrom KK. Clinical results after doxorubicin extravasation treated with excision guided by fluorescence microscopy. Eur J Cancer 1993;29A:1712–1714.

427. Heitmann C, Durmus C, Ingianni G. Surgical management after doxorubicin and epirubicin extravasation. J Hand Surg [Br] 1998;23:666–668.

428. Bertelli G, Gozza A, Forno GB, et al. Topical dimethylsulfoxide for the prevention of soft tissue injury after extravasation of vesicant cytotoxic drugs: a prospective clinical study. J Clin Oncol 1995;13:2851–2855.

429. Disa JJ, Chang RR, Mucci SJ, et al. Prevention of adriamycin-induced full-thickness skin loss using hyaluronidase infiltration. Plast Reconstr Surg 1998;101:370–374.

430. El Saghir N, Otrock Z, Mufarrij A, et al. Dexrazoxane for anthracycline extravasation and GM-CSF for skin ulceration and wound healing. Lancet Oncol 2004;5:320–321.

431. Doroshow JH. Doxorubicin-induced cardiac toxicity. N Engl J Med 1991;324:843–845.

432. Singal PK, Iliskovic N. Doxorubicin-induced cardiomyopathy. N Engl J Med 1998;339:900–905.

433. Slamon D, Leyland-Jones B, Shak S, et al. Addition of Herceptin[tm] (humanized anti-HER2 antibody) to first line chemotherapy for HER2 overexpressing metastatic breast cancer (HER2+/MBC) markedly increases anticancer activity: a randomized, multinational controlled phase III trial. Proc Amer Soc Clin Oncol 1998;17:98a.

434. Cobleigh MA, Vogel CL, Tripathy D, et al. Efficacy and safety of Herceptin™ (humanized anti-HER2 antibody) as a single agent in 222 women with HER2 overexpression who relapsed following chemotherapy for metastatic breast cancer. Proc Amer Soc Clin Oncol 1998;17:97a.

435. Paik S, Bryant J, Park C, et al. erbB-2 and response to doxorubicin in patients with axillary lymph node-positive, hormone receptor-negative breast cancer [see comments]. J Natl Cancer Inst 1998;90:1361–1370.

436. Lipshultz SE, Colan SD, Gelber RD, et al. Late cardiac effects of doxorubicin (adriamycin) therapy for childhood acute lymphoblastic leukemia. N Engl J Med 1991;324:808–915.

437. Schwartz CL, Hobbie WL, Truesdell S, et al. Corrected QT interval prolongation in anthracycline-treated survivors of childhood cancer. J Clin Oncol 1993;11:1906–1910.

438. Wexler LH, Andrich MP, Venzon D, et al. Randomized trial of the cardioprotective agent ICRF-187 in pediatric sarcoma patients treated with doxorubicin. J Clin Oncol 1996;14:362–372.

439. Kremer LC, Caron HN. Anthracycline cardiotoxicity in children. N Engl J Med 2004;351:120–121.

440. Bristow MR, Thompson PD, Martin RP, et al. Early anthracycline cardiotoxicity. Am J Med 1978;65:823–832.

441. Bristow MR, Minobe WA, Billingham ME, et al. Anthracycline-associated cardiac and renal damage in rabbits. Lab Invest 1981;45:157–168.

442. Billingham ME, Mason JW, Bristow MR, et al. Anthracycline cardiomyopathy monitored by morphologic changes. Cancer Treat Rep 1978;62:865–872.

443. Bristow MR, Mason JW, Billingham ME, et al. Doxorubicin cardiomyopathy: evaluation by phonocardiography, endomyocardial biopsy, and cardiac catheterization. Ann Intern Med 1978;88:168–175.

444. Von Hoff DD, Rozencweig M, Layard M, et al. Daunomycin-induced cardiotoxicity in children and adults: a review of 110 cases. Am J Med 1977;62:200–208.

445. Von Hoff DD, Layard MW, Basa P, et al. Risk factors for doxorubicin-induced congestive heart failure. Ann Intern Med 1979;91:710–717.

446. Swain SM. Adult multicenter trials using dexrazoxane to protect against cardiac toxicity. Semin Oncol 1998;25:43–47.

447. Cottin Y, Touzery C, Dalloz F, et al. Comparison of epirubicin and doxorubicin cardiotoxicity induced by low doses: evolution of the diastolic and systolic parameters studied by radionuclide angiography. Clin Cardiol 1998;21:665–670.

448. Perez EA, Suman VJ, Davidson NE, et al. Effect of doxorubicin plus cyclophosphamide on left ventricular ejection fraction in patients with breast cancer in the North Central Cancer Treatment Group N9831 Intergroup Adjuvant Trial. J Clin Oncol 2004;22:3700–3704.

449. Swain SM, Whaley FS, Gerber MC, et al. Delayed administration of dexrazoxane provides cardioprotection for patients with advanced breast cancer treated with doxorubicin-containing therapy [see comments]. J Clin Oncol 1997;15:1333–1340.

450. Swain SM, Whaley FS, Gerber MC, et al. Cardioprotection with dexrazoxane for doxorubicin-containing therapy in advanced breast cancer. J Clin Oncol 1997;15:1318–1332.

451. Moreb JS, Oblon DJ. Outcome of clinical congestive heart failure induced by anthracycline chemotherapy. Cancer 1992;70:2637–2641.

452. Haq MM, Legha SS, Choksi J, et al. Doxorubicin-induced congestive heart failure in adults. Cancer 1985;56:1361–1365.

453. Buzdar AU, Marcus C, Smith TL, et al. Early and delayed clinical cardiotoxicity of doxorubicin. Cancer 1985;55:2761–2765.

454. Lipshultz SE, Lipsitz SR, Sallan SE, et al. Long-term enalapril therapy for left ventricular dysfunction in doxorubicin-treated survivors of childhood cancer. J Clin Oncol 2002;20:4517–4522.

455. Alexander J, Dainiak N, Berger HJ, et al. Serial assessment of doxorubicin cardiotoxicity with quantitative radionuclide angiocardiography. N Engl J Med 1979;300:278–283.

456. Dresdale A, Bonow RO, Wesley R, et al. Prospective evaluation of doxorubicin-induced cardiomyopathy resulting from postsurgical adjuvant treatment of patients with soft tissue sarcomas. Cancer 1983;52:51–60.

457. Swain SM, Whaley FS, Ewer MS. Congestive heart failure in patients treated with doxorubicin: a retrospective analysis of three trials. Cancer 2003;97:2869–2879.

458. Billingham ME, Bristow MR, Glatstein E, et al. Adriamycin cardiotoxicity: endomyocardial biopsy evidence of enhancement by irradiation. Am J Surg Pathol 1977;1:17–23.

459. Torti FM, Bristow MR, Howes AE, et al. Reduced cardiotoxicity of doxorubicin delivered on a weekly schedule: assessment by endomyocardial biopsy. Ann Intern Med 1983;99:745–749.

460. Goorin AM, Chauvenet AR, Perez-Atayde AR, et al. Initial congestive heart failure, six to ten years after doxorubicin chemotherapy for childhood cancer. J Pediatr 1990;116:144–147.

461. Lipshultz SE, Rifai N, Dalton VM, et al. The effect of dexrazoxane on myocardial injury in doxorubicin-treated children with acute lymphoblastic leukemia. N Engl J Med 2004;351:145–153.

462. Lipshultz SE, Giantris AL, Lipsitz SR, et al. Doxorubicin administration by continuous infusion is not cardioprotective: the Dana-Farber 91-01 acute lymphoblastic leukemia protocol. J Clin Oncol 2002;20:1677–1682.

463. Lopez M, Vici P, Di Lauro K, et al. Randomized prospective clinical trial of high-dose epirubicin and dexrazoxane in patients with advanced breast cancer and soft tissue sarcomas. J Clin Oncol 1998;16:86–92.

464. Venturini M, Michelotti A, Del Mastro L, et al. Multicenter randomized controlled clinical trial to evaluate cardioprotection of dexrazoxane versus no cardioprotection in women receiving epirubicin chemotherapy for advanced breast cancer. J Clin Oncol 1996;14:3112–3120.

465. Singal PK, Pierce GN. Adriamycin stimulates low-affinity Ca^{2+} binding and lipid peroxidation but depresses myocardial function. Am J Physiol 1986;250:H419–425.

466. Singal PK, Deally CMR, Weinberg LE. Subcellular effects of adriamycin in the heart: a concise review. J Mol Cell Cardiol 1987;19:817–828.

467. Singal PK, Forbes MS, Sperelakis N. Occurrence of intramitochondrial Ca^{2+} granules in a hypertrophied heart exposed to adriamycin. Can J Physiol Pharmacol 1984;62:1239–1244.

468. Villani F, Piccinini F, Merelli P, et al. Influence of adriamycin on calcium exchangeability in cardiac muscle and its modification by ouabain. Biochem Pharmacol 1978;27:985–987.

469. Milei J, Boveris A, Llesuy S, et al. Amelioration of adriamycin-induced cardiotoxicity in rabbits by prenylamine and vitamins A and E. Am Heart J 1986;111:95–102.

470. Keung EC, Toll L, Ellis M, et al. L-type cardiac calcium channels in doxorubicin cardiomyopathy in rats: morphological, biochemical, and functional correlations. J Clin Invest 1991;87:2108–2113.

471. Doroshow JH. Effect of anthracycline antibiotics on oxygen radical formation in rat heart. Cancer Res 1983;43:460–472.

472. Davies KJ, Doroshow JH, Hochstein P. Mitochondrial NADH dehydrogenase-catalyzed oxygen radical production by adriamycin, and the relative inactivity of 5-iminodaunorubicin. FEBS Lett 1983;153:227–230.

473. Jensen RA, Acton EM, Peters JH. Electrocardiographic and transmembrane potential effects of 5-iminodaunorubicin in the rat. Cancer Res 1984;44:4030–4039.

474. Feng W, Liu G, Xia R, et al. Site-selective modification of hyperreactive cysteines of ryanodine receptor complex by quinones. Mol Pharmacol 1999;55:821–831.

475. Abramson JJ, Salama G. Critical sulfhydryls regulate calcium release from sarcoplasmic reticulum. J Bioenerg Biomembr 1989;21:283–294.

476. Pessah IN, Durie EL, Schiedt MJ, et al. Anthraquinone-sensitized $Ca2+$ release channel from rat cardiac sarcoplasmic reticulum: possible receptor-mediated mechanism of doxorubicin cardiomyopathy. Mol Pharmacol 1990;37:503–514.

477. Papoian T, Lewis W. Adriamycin cardiotoxicity in vivo: selective alterations in rat cardiac mRNAs. Am J Pathol 1990;136:1201–1207.

478. Torti SV, Akimoto H, Lin K, et al. Selective inhibition of muscle gene expression by oxidative stress in cardiac cells. J Mol Cell Cardiol 1998;30:1173–1180.

479. Kurabayashi M, Dutta S, Jeyaseelan R, et al. Doxorubicin-induced Id2A gene transcription is targeted at an activating transcription

factor/cyclic AMP response element motif through novel mechanisms involving protein kinases distinct from protein kinase C and protein kinase A. Mol Cell Biol 1995;15:6386–6397.

480. Jeyaseelan R, Poizat C, Baker RK, et al. A novel cardiac-restricted target for doxorubicin. CARP, a nuclear modulator of gene expression in cardiac progenitor cells and cardiomyocytes. J Biol Chem 1997;272:22800–22808.

481. Nakano E, Takeshige K, Toshima Y, et al. Oxidative damage in selenium deficient hearts on perfusion with adriamycin: protective role of glutathione peroxidase system. Cardiovasc Res 1989; 23:498–504.

482. Kanter MM, Hamlin RL, Unverferth DV, et al. Effect of exercise training on antioxidant enzymes and cardiotoxicity of doxorubicin. J Appl Physiol 1985;59:1298–1303.

483. Nicolay K, Fok JJ, Voorhout W, et al. Cytofluorescence detection of adriamycin-mitochondria interactions in isolated, perfused rat heart. Biochim Biophys Acta 1986;887:35–41.

484. Nohl H. Identification of the site of adriamycin-activation in the heart cell. Biochem Pharmacol 1988;37:2633–2637.

485. Goormaghtigh E, Pollakis G, Ruysschaert JM. Mitochondrial membrane modifications induced by adriamycin-mediated electron transport. Biochem Pharmacol 1983;32:889–893.

486. Nohl H, Gille L, Staniek K. The exogenous NADH dehydrogenase of heart mitochondria is the key enzyme responsible for selective cardiotoxicity of anthracyclines. Z Naturforsch [C] 1998;53:279–285.

487. Weiss RB. The anthracyclines: will we ever find a better doxorubicin? Semin Oncol 1992;19:670–686.

488. Lown JW. Anthracycline and anthraquinone anticancer agents: current status and recent developments. Pharmacol Ther 1993; 60:185–214.

489. LeBot MA, Begue JM, Kernaleguen D, et al. Different cytotoxicity and metabolism of doxorubicin, daunorubicin, epirubicin, esorubicin and idarubicin in cultured human and rat hepatocytes. Biochem Pharmacol 1988;37:3877–3887.

490. Bertelli G, Amoroso D, Pronzato P, et al. Idarubicin: an evaluation of cardiac toxicity in 77 patients with solid tumors. Anticancer Res 1988;8:645–646.

491. Dodion P, Sanders C, Rombaut W, et al. Effect of daunorubicin, carminomycin, idarubicin, and 4-demethoxydaunorubicinol against normal myeloid stem cells and human malignant cells in vitro. Eur J Cancer Clin Oncol 1987;23:1909–1914.

492. Tamassia V, Pacciarini MA, Moro E, et al. Pharmacokinetic study of intravenous and oral idarubicin in cancer patients. Int J Clin Pharmacol Res 1987;7:419–426.

493. Capranico G, Riva A, Tinelli S, et al. Markedly reduced levels of anthracycline-induced strand breaks in resistant P388 leukemia cells and isolated nuclei. Cancer Res 1987;47:3752–3756.

494. Tan CT, Hancock C, Steinherz P, et al. Phase I and clinical pharmacological study of 4- demethoxydaunorubicin (idarubicin) in children with advanced cancer. Cancer Res 1987;47:2990–2995.

495. Gillies HC, Herriott D, Liang R, et al. Pharmacokinetics of idarubicin (4-demethoxydaunorubicin; IMI-30; NSC 256439) following intravenous and oral administration in patients with advanced cancer. Br J Clin Pharmacol 1987;23:303–310.

496. Zwelling LA, Bales E, Altschuler E, et al. Circumvention of resistance by doxorubicin, but not by idarubicin, in a human leukemia cell line containing an intercalator-resistant form of topoisomerase II: evidence for a non-topoisomerase II-mediated mechanism of doxorubicin cytotoxicity. Biochem Pharmacol 1993;45:516–520.

497. Maessen PA, Mross KB, Pinedo HM, et al. Improved method for the determination of 4'-epidoxorubicin and seven metabolites in plasma by high-performance liquid chromatography. J Chromatogr 1987;417:339–346.

498. Hortobagyi GN, Yap HY, Kau SW, et al. A comparative study of doxorubicin and epirubicin in patients with metastatic breast cancer. Am J Clin Oncol 1989;12:57–62.

499. Havsteen H, Brynjolf I, Svahn T, et al. Prospective evaluation of chronic cardiotoxicity due to high-dose epirubicin or combination chemotherapy with cyclophosphamide, methotrexate, and 5-fluorouracil. Cancer Chemother Pharmacol 1989;23:101–104.

500. Robert J, Vrignaud P, Nguyen-Ngoc T, et al. Comparative pharmacokinetics and metabolism of doxorubicin and epirubicin in

patients with metastatic breast cancer. Cancer Treat Rep 1985; 69:633–640.

501. Camaggi CM, Strocchi E, Tamassia V, et al. Pharmacokinetic studies of 4'-epidoxorubicin in cancer patients with normal and impaired renal function and with hepatic metastases. Cancer Treat Rep 1982;66:1819–1824.

502. Vile GF, Winterbourn CC. Microsomal lipid peroxidation induced by adriamycin, epirubicin, daunorubicin and mitoxantrone: a comparative study. Cancer Chemother Pharmacol 1989;24:105–108.

503. Fukushima T, Yamashita T, Yoshio N, et al. Effect of PSC 833 on the cytotoxicity of idarubicin and idarubicinol in multidrug-resistant K562 cells. Leuk Res 1999;23:37–42.

504. Chan EM, Thomas MJ, Bandy B, et al. Effects of doxorubicin, 4'-epirubicin, and antioxidant enzymes on the contractility of isolated cardiomyocytes. Can J Physiol Pharmacol 1996;74:904–910.

505. Bontenbal M, Andersson M, Wildiers J, et al. Doxorubicin vs epirubicin: report of a second-line randomized phase II/III study in advanced breast cancer. EORTC Breast Cancer Cooperative Group. Br J Cancer 1998;77:2257–2263.

506. Ryberg M, Nielsen D, Skovsgaard T, et al. Epirubicin cardiotoxicity: an analysis of 469 patients with metastatic breast cancer. J Clin Oncol 1998;16:3502–3508.

507. Murdock KC, Wallace RE, Durr FE, et al. Antitumor agents, I: 1,4-Bis((aminoalkyl)amino)-9,10- anthracenediones. J Med Chem 1979;22:1024–1030.

508. Johnson RK, Zee-Cheng RKY, Lee WW, et al. Experimental antitumor activity of aminoanthraquinones. Cancer Treat Rep 1979; 63:425–439.

509. Moore MJ, Osoba D, Murphy K, et al. Use of palliative end points to evaluate the effects of mitoxantrone and low-dose prednisone in patients with hormonally resistant prostate cancer. J Clin Oncol 1994;12:689–694.

510. Bloomfield DJ, Krahn MD, Neogi T, et al. Economic evaluation of chemotherapy with mitoxantrone plus prednisone for symptomatic hormone-resistant prostate cancer: based on a Canadian randomized trial with palliative end points. J Clin Oncol 1998; 16:2272–2279.

511. Foye WD, Vajrargupta D, Sengupta SK. DNA binding specificity and RNA polymerase inhibitory activity of bis(aminoalkyl) anthraquinones and bis(methylthio)vinyl quinolinium iodides. J Pharm Sci 1982;71:253–257.

512. Lown JW, Hanstock CC, Bradley RD, et al. Interactions of the antitumor agents, mitoxantrone and bisantrene, with deoxyribonucleic acids studied by electron microscopy. Mol Pharmacol 1984;25:178–184.

513. Bowden GT, Roberts R, Alberts DS, et al. Comparative molecular pharmacology in leukemic L1210 cells of the anthracene anticancer drugs mitoxantrone and bisantrene. Cancer Res 1985;45: 4915–4920.

514. Butler J, Hoey BM. Are reduced quinones necessarily involved in the antitumor activity of quinone drugs. Br J Cancer 1987;55 (Suppl 8):53–59.

515. Nguyen B, Gutierrez PL. Mechanism(s) for the metabolism of mitoxantrone: electron spin resonance and electrochemical studies. Chem Biol Interact 1990;74:139–162.

516. Doroshow JH, Davies KJ. Comparative cardiac oxygen radical metabolism by anthracycline antibiotics, mitoxantrone, bisantrene, 4'-(9-acridinylamino)-methanesulfon-m-anisidide, and neocarzinostatin. Biochem Pharmacol 1983;32:2935–2939.

517. Crespi MO, Ivanier SE, Genovese J, et al. Mitoxantrone affects topoisomerase activities in human breast cancer cells. Biochem Biophys Res Commun 1986;136:521–528.

518. Kharasch ED, Novak RF. Inhibition of adriamycin-stimulated microsomal lipid peroxidation by mitoxantrone and ametantrone. Biochem Biophys Res Commun 1982;108:1346–1352.

519. Abramson JJ, Buck E, Salama G, et al. Mechanism of anthraquinone-induced calcium release from skeletal muscle sarcoplasmic reticulum. J Biol Chem 1988;263:18750–18758.

520. Bhalla K, Ibrado AM, Tourkina E, et al. High-dose mitoxantrone induces programmed cell death or apoptosis in human myeloid leukemia cells. Blood 1993;82:3133–3140.

521. Bellosillo B, Colomer D, Pons G, et al. Mitoxantrone, a topoisomerase II inhibitor, induces apoptosis of B-chronic lymphocytic leukaemia cells. Br J Haematol 1998;100:142–146.

522. Inaba M, Nagashima K, Sakurai Y. Cross-resistance of vincristine-resistant sublines of P388 leukemia to mitoxantrone with special emphasis on the relationship between in vitro and in vivo cross-resistance. Gann 1984;75:625–630.

523. Dalton WS, Cress AE, Alberts DS, et al. Cytogenetic and phenotypic analysis of a human colon carcinoma cell line resistant to mitoxantrone. Cancer Res 1988;48:1882–1888.

524. Bhalla K, Hindenburg A, Taub RN, et al. Isolation and characterization of an anthracycline-resistant human leukemic cell line. Cancer Res 1985;45:3657–3662.

525. Nakagawa M, Schneider E, Dixon KH, et al. Reduced intracellular drug accumulation in the absence of P-glycoprotein (mdr1) overexpression in mitoxantrone-resistant human MCF-7 breast cancer cells. Cancer Res 1992;52:6175–6181.

526. Satake S, Sugawara I, Watanabe M, et al. Lack of a point mutation of human DNA topoisomerase II in multidrug-resistant anaplastic thyroid carcinoma cell lines. Cancer Lett 1997;116:33–39.

527. Schneider E, Horton JK, Yang CH, et al. Multidrug resistance-associated protein gene overexpression and reduced drug sensitivity of topoisomerase II in a human breast carcinoma MCF7 cell line selected for etoposide resistance. Cancer Res 1994;54:152–158.

528. Hazlehurst LA, Foley NE, Gleason-Guzman MC, et al. Multiple mechanisms confer drug resistance to mitoxantrone in the human 8226 myeloma cell line. Cancer Res 1999;59:1021–1028.

529. Miyake K, Mickley L, Litman T, et al. Molecular cloning of cDNAs which are highly overexpressed in mitoxantrone-resistant cells: demonstration of homology to ABC transport genes. Cancer Res 1999;59:8–13.

530. Ross DD, Yang W, Abruzzo LV, et al. Atypical multidrug resistance: breast cancer resistance protein messenger RNA expression in mitoxantrone-selected cell lines. J Natl Cancer Inst 1999;91:429–433.

531. Kozin SV, Gerweck LE. Cytotoxicity of weak electrolytes after the adaptation of cells to low pH: role of the transmembrane pH gradient. Br J Cancer 1998;77:1580–1585.

532. Heinemann V, Murray D, Walters R, et al. Mitoxantrone-induced DNA damage in leukemia cells is enhanced by treatment with high-dose arabinosylcytosine. Cancer Chemother Pharmacol 1988;22:205–210.

533. Shenkenberg TD, VonHoff DD. Mitoxantrone: a new anticancer drug with significant clinical activity. Ann Intern Med 1986;105:67–81.

534. Neidhart JA, Gochnour D, Roach R, et al. A comparison of mitoxantrone and doxorubicin in breast cancer. J Clin Oncol 1986;4:672–677.

535. Lawton F, Blackledge G, Mould J, et al. Phase II study of mitoxantrone in epithelial ovarian cancer. Cancer Treat Rep 1987;71:627–629.

536. Coltman CAJ, McDaniel TM, Balcerzak SP, et al. Mitoxantrone hydrochloride (NSC-310739) in lymphoma. Invest New Drugs 1983;1:65–70.

537. Birot-Babapalle F, Catovsky D, Slocumbe G, et al. Phase II study of mitoxantrone and cytarabine in acute myeloid leukemia. Cancer Treat Rep 1987;71:161–163.

538. Alberts DS, Peng YM, Leigh S, et al. Disposition of mitoxantrone in cancer patients. Cancer Res 1985;45:1879–1884.

539. Smyth JF, Macpherson JS, Warrington PS, et al. The clinical pharmacology of mitoxantrone. Cancer Chemother Pharmacol 1986;17:149–152.

540. Repetto L, Vannozzi MO, Balleari E, et al. Mitoxantrone in elderly patients with advanced breast cancer: pharmacokinetics, marrow and peripheral hematopoietic progenitor cells. Anticancer Res 1999;19:879–884.

541. Savaraj N, Lu K, Manuel V, et al. Pharmacology of mitoxantrone in cancer patients. Cancer Chemother Pharmacol 1982;8:113–117.

542. Wolf CR, Macpherson JS, Smyth JF. Evidence for the metabolism of mitozantrone by microsomal glutathione transferases and 3-methylcholanthrene-inducible glucuronosyl transferases. Biochem Pharmacol 1986;35:1577–1581.

543. Chiccarelli FS, Morrison JA, Cosulich DB, et al. Identification of human urinary mitoxantrone metabolites. Cancer Res 1986;46:4858–4861.

544. Shepherd FA, Evans WK, Blackstein ME, et al. Hepatic arterial infusion of mitoxantrone in the treatment of primary hepatocellular carcinoma. J Clin Oncol 1987;5:635–640.

545. Alberts DS, Surwit EA, Peng YM, et al. Phase I clinical and pharmacokinetic study of mitoxantrone given to patients by intraperitoneal administration. Cancer Res 1988;48:5874–5877.

546. Husain A, Sabbatini P, Spriggs D, et al. Phase II trial of intraperitoneal cisplatin and mitoxantrone in patients with persistent ovarian cancer. Gynecol Oncol 1999;73:96–101.

547. Yap HY, Blumenschein GR, Schell FC, et al. Dihydroanthracenedione: a promising new drug in the treatment of metastatic breast cancer. Ann Intern Med 1981;95:694–697.

548. Underferth DV, Underferth BJ, Balcerzak SP, et al. Cardiac evaluation of mitoxantrone. Cancer Treat Rep 1983;67:343–350.

549. Benjamin RS, Chawla SP, Ewer MS, et al. Evaluation of mitoxantrone cardiac toxicity by nuclear angiography and endomyocardial biopsy: an update. Invest New Drugs 1985;3:117–121.

550. Ghalie RG, Edan G, Laurent M, et al. Cardiac adverse effects associated with mitoxantrone (Novantrone) therapy in patients with MS. Neurology 2002;59:909–913.

551. Gonsette RE. Mitoxantrone in progressive multiple sclerosis: when and how to treat? J Neurol Sci 2003;206:203–208.

552. Prai GR, Reed NS, Ruddell NST. A case of mitoxantrone-associated cardiomyopathy without prior anthracycline therapy. Br J Radiol 1987;60:1125–1126.

553. Arlin ZA, Silver R, Cassileth P. Phase I-II trial of mitoxantrone in acute leukemia. Cancer Treat Rep 1985;69:61–64.

554. Speechly-Dick ME, Owen ERTC. Mitoxantrone-induced onycholysis. Lancet 1988;1:113.

Topoisomerase II Inhibitors: The Epipodophyllotoxins, Acridines, and Ellipticines

19

Yves Pommier   *François Goldwasser*

INTRODUCTION

DNA topoisomerase II (Top2) inhibitors have been the subject of considerable biochemical, pharmacological, and clinical investigation. In addition to the epipodophyllotoxins, acridines, ellipticines, and bisdioxopiperazines considered in this chapter, other drugs interact with Top2, including anthracyclines, mitoxantrone, and anthrapyrazoles. However, these other drugs exhibit other mechanisms of action and are described separately (see chater 18).

The inhibition of cellular topoisomerase by antitumor agents such as adriamycin and ellipticine was first hypothesized by Kohn and coworkers in the late 1970s before eukaryotic topoisomerase II (Top2) had been identified.[1] This hypothesis was based on the observations that the DNA breaks induced by adriamycin and ellipticine had unique characteristics in DNA alkaline elution assays: (a) they were only detectable after full deproteinization and therefore were called *protein-associated* (or *protein-linked*) *strand breaks,* and (b) they were associated with an equal frequency of DNA-protein cross-links. The demonstration that the drug-induced protein-associated strand breaks were mediated through inhibition of Top2 took a few more years. This discovery was facilitated by cellular pharmacology studies of amsacrine, a far more potent inducer of protein-linked DNA breaks than anthracyclines or ellipticines.[2,3] Liu and coworkers, who had isolated mammalian Top2, showed that a number of inducers of protein-linked DNA breaks were acting through Top2.[4] Independently, Kohn and coworkers demonstrated that the protein linked to DNA upon m-AMSA treatment is Top2.[5] The term *cleavage* (or *cleavable*) *complex* is commonly used to define the enzyme-DNA complex, because cleavage is only detectable after strong protein denaturation by sodium dodecylsulfate (SDS). Our knowledge regarding both the Top2 enzyme and the mechanisms of action of and resistance to Top2 poisons has considerably increased. We better understand the wide variability in the spectrum of antitumoral activity of Top2 poisons as well as some of their specific toxic effects. Interference of these agents with Top2 has led to a model of *MLL* gene translocations and leukemia in which Top2-mediated chromosomal breakage occasionally is resolved by translocation.[6]

Extracts from the mayapple or mandrake plant have long been used in folk medicine. The active principle in this plant, podophyllotoxin, acts as an antimitotic agent that binds to tubulin at a site distinct from that occupied by the vinca alkaloids. A number of semisynthetic derivatives of podophyllotoxin have been made. Two glycosidic

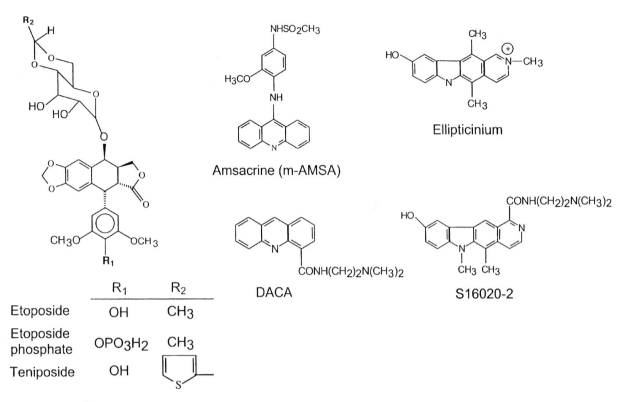

Figure 19.1   Chemical structures of the epipodophyllotoxins (VP-16 and VM-26), the acridines (m-AMSA and DACA), and the ellipticines and olivacines (ellipticinium and S16020-2).

derivatives, teniposide (VM-26) and etoposide (VP-16) (Fig.19.1), are active against a number of human malignancies. Etoposide was approved by the US Food and Drug Administration (FDA) for marketing by Bristol Laboratories under the trade name VePesid in early 1984. Teniposide (Vumon) has been used in Europe for several years and was approved by the FDA in 1992 for refractory childhood leukemia. More recently, etoposide phosphate (Etopofos; Fig.19.1) was designed as a prodrug of etoposide in order to obtain a water-soluble compound activated specifically with antibody alkaline phosphatase conjugates at the tumor site.[7,8] In fact, etoposide phosphate is almost immediately converted to etoposide in the patient plasma by host endogenous phosphatase. Thus, etoposide phosphate simplifies the formulation of etoposide by being water-soluble and readily converted to etoposide.

It is now well established that etoposide and teniposide exert their antineoplastic effect by inhibiting Top2 and that, in contrast to the parent compound (podophyllotoxin), they are inactive against tubulin. Etoposide and teniposide are very active against malignancies with a high proliferation rate. Etoposide is a key agent in germ-cell malignancies,[9,10] small cell lung cancer, poorly differentiated carcinomas, and poorly differentiated endocrine tumors and is given as first-line therapy in combination with cisplatin. Etoposide is also used in second-line regi-

mens or salvage therapies in non-Hodgkin's lymphomas (NHLs), including HIV-associated NHLs[11]; high-risk metastatic gestational trophoblastic tumors[12]; Kaposi's sarcomas; osteosarcomas; Ewing's sarcomas; neuroblastomas; and leukemias. It is also one of the important agents used in preparatory regimens for bone marrow transplantation.[13]

Teniposide (VM-26) is mainly used in pediatry and neuro-oncology. Teniposide is active in combination in pediatric tumors such as retinoblastoma, neuroblastoma,[14] and acute myelocytic leukemias,[15–17] as salvage therapy for initial induction failures in childhood acute lymphoblastic leukemia (ALL), and for non-Hodgkin's lymphoma.[18] Teniposide is active against recurrent oligodendroglioma[19] and is also incorporated in chemotherapy regimens in primary central nervous system lymphoma.[20] Teniposide is known as active in small cell lung cancer and in bladder cancer (by both intravenous and intravesical routes)[21,22] but is infrequently used in these diseases.

Amsacrine, or 4'(9-acridinylamino)-methanesulfon-m-aniside (m-AMSA; Fig. 19.1), is the first rationally synthesized aminoacridine anticancer agent to undergo full clinical development. Amsacrine has substantial efficacy in acute myeloblastic leukemia (AML) and ALL[23,24] but has largely been replaced by newer agents. The acridine derivative, N-[2-(dimethylamino)ethyl]acridine-4-carboxamide

(DACA; Fig. 19.1), displays high activity against solid tumors in mice[23] and exhibits a dual mode of cytotoxic action involving topoisomerases I and II.[24,25] It has not proven effective in trials thus far.

Representing a third structural class of Top2 inhibitors, ellipticine is an alkaloid derived from the Apocynaceae family, including *Ochrosia, Bleekeria vitensis,* and *Aspidosperma subincanum.*[26] Despite its promising preclinical activity, severe toxic effects observed in animal studies hampered the progress of ellipticine toward clinical trials. The semi-synthetic derivative 2-*N*-methyl-9-hydroxyellipticinium acetate (NMHE = ellipticinium; Fig.19.1) was briefly tested in breast cancer trials. The drug S16020-2 is a new olivacine derivative structurally related to ellipticinium[27] (Fig.19.1). S16020-2 is highly cytotoxic in vitro[28] and displays outstanding antitumor activity against various experimental tumors, especially some solid tumor models.[29–31] Its activity is notably higher than that of ellipticinium and comparable to that of doxorubicin HCl, although with a different tumor specificity. S16020-2 is being tested in clinical trials.[32]

Catalytic inhibitors of Top2 have also been identified (see Table 19.2). One of them, dexrazoxane, a bisdioxopiperazine derivative, has been approved as a cardioprotective agent in association with anthracyclines.[33–35] Among the bis(*N*-acyloxymethyl) dioxopiperazine derivatives, sobuzoxane (MST-16) has antitumoral activity in non-Hodgkin's lymphoma and T-cell leukemia patients[36,37] and has obtained official approval in Japan.

MOLECULAR AND CELLULAR PHARMACOLOGY

DNA Topoisomerase II

Enzymology and Functions

The length of eukaryotic DNA and its anchorage to nuclear matrix attachment regions limit the free rotation of one strand around the other as the two strands of the DNA double helix are separated for DNA metabolism (transcription, replication, recombination, and repair). DNA topoisomerases catalyze the unlinking of the DNA strands by making transient DNA strand breaks and allowing the DNA to rotate around or traverse through these breaks.[38] Three families of topoisomerases are known in humans: topoisomerase I (Top1), topoisomerase II (Top2), and topoisomerase III (Top3)[38] (Table 19.1). DNA gyrase and topoisomerase IV (topo IV) are the bacterial equivalents of eukaryotic Top2. Quinolones (nalidixic acid, ciprofloxacin, norfloxacin, and derivatives), which are widely used antibiotics, act by inhibiting DNA gyrase and topo IV but have no or very limited effect on the host human Top2.[39,40]

Topoisomerase-mediated DNA breaks occur through transesterification reactions in which a DNA phospho-ester bond is transferred to a specific enzyme tyrosine residue while the enzyme generates a break in the DNA phosphodiester backbone. Type 1 enzymes (Top1 and Top3) make DNA single-strand breaks, whereas the type 2 enzymes (Top2α and Top2β) make DNA double-strand

TABLE 19.1
MAMMALIAN DNA TOPOISOMERASES

	Topoisomerases I	Topoisomerase IIα	Topoisomerase IIβ	Topoisomerases III
Size of monomer	100 kd (Top1 nuclear) 72 kd (Top1 mt) Acting as monomer	170 kd Acting as dimer	180 kd Acting as dimer	110 kd
Size of mRNA	4.2 kb (Top1 nuclear) 1.8 kb (Top1 mt)	6.2 kb	6.5 kb	3.8 kb (main transcript; ref. 260)
Chromosome location	20q12–13.2 (Top1 nuclear) 8q24.3 (Top1 mt)	17q21–22	3p24	17p11.2–12 (Top3α) 22q11–12 (Top3β)
Catalytic intermediate	DNA SSB Covalent linkage to 3' DNA terminus	DNA DSB Covalent linkage to 5' DNA termini	DNA DSB Covalent linkage to 5' DNA termini	DNA SSB Covalent linkage to 5' DNA termini
ATP dependence	No	Yes	Yes	No
Cell cycle expression	Throughout	G$_2$/M	Throughout	
Specific inhibitors indolocarbazoles	Camptothecins, indeno-isoquinolines, (reviewed in ref. 261)	Top2 poisons and catalytic inhibitors, intercalators (see Table 19.2)	Same as topoisomerase IIα (preference for amsacrine, mitoxantrone; see ref. 262)	Unknown

SSB, single-strand breaks; DSB, double-strand breaks.
Top1mt: mitochondrial Top1 is the most recently discovered human Top1 gene (ref. 263).

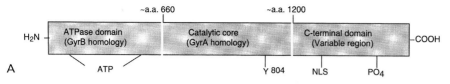

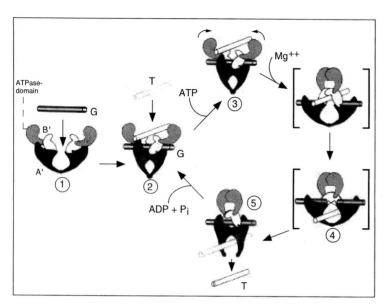

Figure 19.2 A: Domain structure of Top2. The three major domains of eukaryotic are illustrated, as well as the site of ATP binding (ATP), the active-site tyrosine (Y805 for Top 2α and Y826 for Top 2β), the nuclear localization sequence(s) (NLS), and the sites of phosphorylation (PO$_4$). The N-terminal domain (homologous to the gyrase B subunit) extends from amino acid 1 to about 660. The catalytic core domain (homologous to the A subunit of gyrase) extends from about residue 660 to 1,200, and the C-terminal domain (no corresponding homology with gyrase) extends from about residue 1,200 to the C-terminus of the enzyme. **B:** Model for the catalytic cycle of type II topoisomerases (according to reference 41). The unliganded enzyme binds to duplex DNA (labeled G) across the A′ domains (step 1). A second duplex DNA strand (labeled T) and ATP bind to the enzyme (steps 2 and 3). Nucleotide binding promotes dimerization of the ATPase domains and closure of the clamp (curved arrows, step 3). Cleavage of the G-strand allows the passage of the T-strand through the cleaved G-strand (step 4 is diagrammed in brackets to indicate that the cleavage complex is a short-lived intermediate in the proposed transportation event). Following G-strand religation, the T-strand is released through the dimer interface in the A′ region (step 5). ATP hydrolysis completes the enzyme catalytic cycle.

breaks. In the case of Top1, the enzyme catalytic tyrosine becomes linked to the 3′-terminus of the cleaved DNA, while in the case of Top3 the linkage is to the 5′-DNA terminus of the break. In Top2-mediated reactions, each enzyme molecule of a homodimer becomes linked to the 5′-terminus of each of the cleaved DNA strands (Table 19.1, Fig. 19.4).

Both Top1 and Top2 can remove DNA supercoiling by catalyzing DNA relaxation. They can complement each other in this function, at least in yeast, where the absence of Top1 can be compensated for by the presence of the other topoisomerase. However, yeast strains deficient in Top2 are not viable and die at mitosis because Top2 is essential for chromosome condensation and for the proper segregation of mitotic and meiotic chromosomes.[38] The reason is that, in addition to its DNA-relaxing activity, Top2 can separate two linked circles of duplex DNA (decatenation). Top2 also catalyzes the reverse reaction (catenation) by allowing one duplex to pass through a double-stranded gap created in the other duplex (strand passage reaction; see next section and Fig. 19.2). Decatenation is essential at the end of DNA replication for the separation of daughter DNA molecules and the segregation of newly replicated chromosomes. The accumulation of Top2 at the end of the S phase and during G$_2$ and its concentration in the chromosome scaffold are consistent with the enzyme's role in separating chromatin loops and condensing DNA at mitosis (see Table 19.1).

Mammalian cells have two Top2 isoenzymes, termed *Top2α* and *Top2β* (Table 19.1). They differ in molecular mass, enzymatic properties, chromosome localization, sequence, cell cycle regulation, and cellular and tissue distribution. Although the cellular concentration of Top2β is relatively constant throughout the cell cycle, the Top2α level is tightly linked to the proliferative state of the cell. The concentration of the α isoform increases two- to three-fold during G$_2$/M and is, order of magnitude, higher in rapidly proliferating cells than in quiescent populations.

DNA Topoisomerase II Catalytic Cycle

A description of the Top2 catalytic cycle is essential for understanding how Top2 poisons stabilize the cleavage complex of the DNA strand passage reaction (see Fig. 19.2; for more details, see references 41, 42). In contrast to Top1, Top2 enzymes function as a homodimers. Their catalytic activity requires the presence of magnesium as well as ATP as an exogenous energy source. Hence Top2 enzymes act as DNA-dependent ATPases. Recent structural and mechanistic studies reveal a remarkable dynamic behavior of the enzyme structure during its catalytic cycle.[41,42] Top2 catalyzes DNA strand passage according to the two-gate model shown in Figure 19.2.[41,42] The enzyme forms a dimer and initiates its catalytic cycle by binding to its DNA substrate with a preference for DNA crossover regions. Hence, Top2 interactions with DNA are determined both by DNA superstructure (DNA crossovers, bends, etc.) and local DNA sequence. Although Top2 enzymes interact with preferred sequences, they do not have the sequence specificity of restriction endonucleases. This lack of stringency probably allows the enzyme to act at multiple sites of the genome in order to perform its vital functions.

Top2 assumes at least two alternative conformations, open or closed clamp forms in the absence or presence of ATP, respectively.[41,42] The enzyme binds two segments of duplex DNA, referred to as the G and T segments. The G (for *gate*) segment is the one cleaved by the enzyme in order to pass the T (for *transported*) segment through the enzyme-DNA complex (Fig. 19.2). Upon ATP binding, Top2 undergoes a conformational change from an open to a closed clamp form (step 3). In the presence of a divalent cation (under physiological conditions Mg^{++}), the tyrosine active residue of each Top2 monomer (tyrosine 805 for human Top2α) attacks a DNA phosphodiester bond four bases apart on the G duplex and becomes covalently linked to the 5′ ends of the broken DNA while the 3′-ends are 3′-hydroxyls. The T segment can then pass through the gap produced in the G segment (step 4). Cleavage of the G duplex is reversible in nature, and under normal conditions the cleavage complex is a short-lived intermediate. After strand passage the T segment is released from the clamp, and the broken ends of the G segment are religated by Top2 (step 5). Upon hydrolysis of ATP by the intrinsic ATPase activity of the enzyme, the Top2-DNA complex is converted back to the open clamp form with release of the G segment. Thus closing and opening of the Top2 clamp are coupled with ATP binding and hydrolysis, respectively. Through its ability to open both strands of a DNA duplex and to catalyze strand passage in concerted reactions, Top2 can perform a variety of DNA topoisomerization reactions. Whereas DNA relaxation is common to Top1, conversion of circular DNA to knotted forms and removal of preexisting knots are specific to Top2. These biochemical reactions are commonly used to assay topoisomerase activities in vitro: relaxation of supercoiled plasmid DNA in the absence of ATP and Mg $^{++}$ in the case of Top1 and decatenation of kinetoplast DNA (kDNA) and unknotting of P4 DNA in the case of Top2.[43]

DNA Topoisomerase II Poisons

Mechanisms of Top2 Inhibition by Anticancer Drugs

The antitumor Top2 inhibitors poison the enzyme by stabilizing the DNA cleavage complexes (step 4 in Fig. 19.2) rather than preventing enzyme catalytic activity. The production of DNA cleavage complexes is due to an inhibition of DNA religation in the case of VP-16, VM-26, and m-AMSA.[44–46] On the other hand, compounds such as quinolones act by inducing the formation of cleavage complexes rather than by inhibiting religation.[47] The cleavage

complexes can be detected in cells as protein-linked DNA breaks by alkaline elution or by SDS-KCl precipitation assays (for review, see references 1, 43). Cellular topoisomerase-DNA complexes can also be detected using the ICE bioassay (immunocomplex topo assay).[48] Inhibition of Top2 catalytic activity without the trapping of cleavage complexes (Table 19.2; Fig. 19.3) was first demonstrated for strong DNA intercalating agents at drug concentrations that saturate the DNA. It is attributed to DNA structural alterations that prevent the enzyme from binding to DNA (steps 1 and 2 in Fig. 19.2) or prevent initiation of the cleavage complex.[49,50] Other DNA binders such as merbarone and the bisdioxopiperazines (ICRF-159, ICRF-187 [= dexrazoxane], and ICRF-193) produce the "closed clamp" type of inhibition, for example, inhibition of Top2 catalytic activity without the trapping of cleavage complexes[51,52] (see Table 19.2). Hence three types of curves that relate drug concentrations to cleavage complexes can be observed for Top2 inhibitors (Fig. 19.3): (a) a monotonal increase of cleavage complexes with drug concentration in the case of non-DNA or weak DNA binders (VP-16, VM-26, m-AMSA, quinolones), (b) a bell-shaped curve (with initial increase in cleavage complexes with increasing drug concentrations, followed by a decrease in cleavage complexes at higher concentrations) in the case of DNA intercalators (ellipticines, anthracyclines, mitoxantrone, anthrapyrazoles), and (c) a monotonal decrease of cleavage complexes in the case of some bulky intercalators (ethidium bromide, ditercalinium, aclarubicin) or non-DNA binders (bisdioxopiperazines) (see Table 19.2) that inhibit catalytic activity without trapping cleavage complexes.

At the biochemical level, Top2 inhibitors exhibit different effects (Table 19.3). The kinetics of cleavage complex formation and reversal in drug-treated cells vary from slow in the case of doxorubicin[2] and ellipticine[53] to very rapid in the case of VP-16, m-AMSA, and ellipticinium.[2,54] The higher cytotoxicity of doxorubicin versus VP-16 may be explained by the importance of persistent cleavage complexes for cytotoxicity. Most drugs induce not only Top2-mediated DNA double-strand breaks but also Top2-mediated single-strand breaks, the ratio of which varies widely among drugs. Ellipticines produce almost exclusively DNA double-strand breaks, while VP-16 and amsacrine produce 10 to 20 single-strand breaks per double-strand break.[2,44,54] Anthracyclines produce a mixture of single-strand and double-strand breaks.[2] Hence the higher cytotoxicity of anthracyclines compared with amsacrine or VP-16 may be due to the higher frequency of DNA double-strand breaks, which may be more cytotoxic than single-strand breaks.[44] Finally, the DNA sequence and genomic localization of Top2 cleavage complexes vary among drugs.[55] Drugs that are chemically and structurally related frequently produce closely related patterns of Top2 cleavage, whereas compounds structurally and electronically unrelated produce different patterns both in purified DNA and in drug-treated cells.[44,55,56]

TABLE 19.2

TOPOISOMERASE II INHIBITORS

	Poisons	Refs.	Suppressors	Refs.
Intercalators and DNA binders	Doxorubicin		Doxorubicin (high conc.)	
	Daunorubicin		Daunorubicin (high conc.)	
	Epirubicin		Epirubicin (high conc.)	
	Idarubicin	See 44, 45, 58	Idarubicin (high conc.)	See 45, 46
	Amsacrine		Amsacrine (high conc.)	
	Mitoxantrone		Mitoxantrone (high conc.)	
	Elliptinium		Elliptinium (high conc.)	
	Actinomycin D*		Actinomycin D* (high conc.)	
	Anthrapyrazoles	264	Anthrapyrazoles (high conc.)	264
	Menogaril	265	Menogaril (high conc.)	265
	Intoplicine*	266	Intoplicine* (high conc.)	266
	Saintopin*	267	Saintopin* (high conc.)	267
	Amonafide	268	Amonafide (high conc.)	268
	Streptonigrin	269, 270	Bulgarein	271
	Makaluvamines	272	Ethidium bromide	273
	Alkylating anthraquinones	274	Ditercalinium	275, 276
	Olivacines	27		
	Bisantrenes	277		
Nonintercalators	VP-16, VM-26	278–280	Distamycin, Hoechst 33258	281
	Aza IQD*	282	Merbarone	283
	Flavones-flavonones	284	Bisdioxopiperazines	51
	Isoflavones (genistein)	285	Suramin	286
	Nitroimidazole (Ro 15-0216)	287	Novobiocin	288
	Terpenoids	289	Chloroquine	290
	Naphthoquinones	291	Fostriecin	292
	Withangulatin	293	Aclarubicin (aklavin, oxaunomycin, β-rhodomycinone)	294
	Polyaromatic quinones	295	Quinobenoxazines	296
	Quinolones (CP-115,953)	297		
	Azatoxins	298		

*Dual Top1 and Top2 inhibitor.
See Fig. 19.3 and text for definition of poisons and suppressors.

Base-Sequence Preference of Top2 Inhibitors and Drug-Binding Model

The DNA sequencing of drug-induced cleavage sites shows that each class of inhibitor tends to act at Top2 cleavage sites with different base sequence preferences at the 3'- and/or 5'-terminus of the Top2-mediated DNA double-strand break[57-60] (Fig.19.4). These drug-specific preferences for certain bases immediately flanking the cleavage sites suggest that the drugs interact directly with these bases. Since all Top2 inhibitors, whether intercalator or not, have a planar aromatic portion that in some cases mimics a base pair (see Fig.19.1), the simplest explanation is that the drugs stack inside the cleavage sites at the enzyme-DNA interface. Depending on the drug structure, preferential base stacking would take place either at the 3'- or the 5'-terminus. This hypothesis implies that topoisomerases first cleave the DNA at many sites and that the drugs bind specifically to some sites and prevent DNA religation.[61]

The base sequence analysis data suggest that stacking at one cleavage site is sufficient for the creation of a DNA double-strand break, a theory consistent with the concerted action of both enzyme monomers during catalysis.[57,61-63] This type of inhibition, which we refer to as "interfacial inhibition," is one of nature's paradigms for noncompetitive protein inhibition.[64]

Determinants of Sensitivity and Resistance to Top2 Inhibitors

Figure 19.5 summarizes the multiple factors that determine the cytotoxicity of Top2 inhibitors. Before topoisomerase inhibitors reach their nuclear target, they have to be taken up by the cells and transported to the nucleus. Reduced drug accumulation and/or altered intracellular drug distribution is a dominant feature of many drug-resistant cell lines. Most clinical antitumor Top2 inhibitors are substrates for the 170-kd transmembrane glycoprotein Pgp, which is a product of the *MDR1* gene and responsible

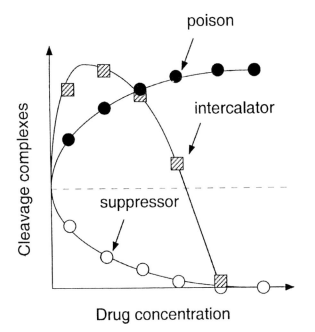

Figure 19.3 Different modes of drug inhibition of Top2. Top2 poisons such as the epipodophyllotoxins (VP-16 and VM-26) and the azatoxins (solid circles) only trap the Top2 cleavage complexes with increasing efficiency as their dose increases. Top2 suppressors such as the bis-dioxopiperazines (open circles) are pure catalytic inhibitors that only inhibit the formation of cleavage complexes. The hatched squares correspond to biphasic inhibitors such as DNA intercalators (anthracyclines, ellipticines, acridines; see Table 19.2), which enhance Top2 cleavage complexes at low concentrations and suppress cleavage complexes at higher concentrations.

TABLE 19.3	
DIFFERENCES AMONG TOPOISOMERASE II INHIBITORS	
Other targets besides Top2	Free radicals: anthracyclines, mitoxantrone
	DNA intercalation (e.g., anthracyclines, mitoxantrone, ellipticines)
Different effects on Top2	Base sequence preferences and location of DNA cleavage sites (see Fig. 18-3)
	Ratio of DNA double- to single-strand breaks: ellipticine > anthracyclines > amsacrine/epipodophyllotoxins
	Kinetics of trapping Top2 cleavage complexes (slow for anthracyclines; fast for epipodophyllotoxins/amsacrine)
	Inhibition of cleavage complexes at higher concentration (intercalators)
	Pure Top2 poisons (epipodophyllotoxins)
Mechanisms of resistance	Substrates for transmembrane transporters: anthracyclines and epipodophyllotoxins more than mitoxantrone, amsacrine, and ellipticines
	Specific Top2 mutations affect drug binding differentially (refs. 299–307)

See text for references.

for the classical MDR (multidrug-resistance) phenotype.[65] MDR-sensitive drugs include doxorubicin and analogs, mitoxantrone, anthrapyrazones, ellipticines, VP-16, and to a lesser extent m-AMSA analogs. Hence, cells overexpressing Pgp are generally resistant to Top2 inhibitors because the drugs are actively extruded from the cells. The amino group on the daunosamine sugar of anthracyclines is probably involved in the drug recognition by Pgp. This is probably why the deamino derivative hydroxyrubicin is less subject to drug resistance while retaining Top2 inhibitory activity.[66]

Although drug metabolism is not necessary for activity of the Top2 inhibitors described in this chapter, some drugs undergo metabolic modifications that may affect the way they interact with Top2 or/and DNA. Anthracyclines participate in redox reactions that lead to the formation of free radicals that damage cellular lipids or DNA (see chapter 18). Some adriamycin-resistant and mitoxantrone-resistant cell lines show increased levels of cellular glutathione (GSH) or GSH-conjugating enzymes, which may be a result of GSH-mediated drug inactivation with or without subsequent drug efflux mediated by the putative ATP-dependent glutathione S-conjugate export pump.[67] The VP-16 metabolites demethylated on the podophyllotoxin phenyl ring and without the sugar are at least as active as VP-16 against purified Top2 (Fig.19.6).[68] These

metabolites are more susceptible to oxidation-reduction reactions and may exhibit a shorter half-life and higher reactivity toward other macromolecules than Top2.[69] In the case of the ellipticines, similar oxidation-reduction reactions and free-radical formation have been identified and may be responsible for lesions that contribute to the drugs' cytotoxic effects.[70,71]

The intracellular distribution of Top2 inhibitors has been well characterized for the anthracyclines. Drug-resistant cells tend to exclude doxorubicin from their nuclei. These observations suggest that a nuclear transporter may exist. In the case of m-AMSA, cellular uptake studies suggest that the drug may be retained in some slowly exchangeable intracellular compartment.[72] An altered intracellular drug distribution with drug sequestration in cytoplasmic organelles has been described.[73]

In contrast to other chemotherapeutic agents such as antifolates, the degree of cellular sensitivity to Top2 inhibitors correlates with the abundance of the target enzyme. Indeed, the higher the levels of Top2, the more sensitive is the cell, because more cleavage complexes are formed and more consecutive genotoxic and cytotoxic lesions accumulate (see Fig. 19.5). Cancer cells often have a higher level of Top2α, and the Top2 content in cancer cells is less regulated by growth conditions.[74,75] Top2β appears to be also up-regulated in neoplastic cells compared to normal, quiescent tissues.[76] Coamplification of the *erbB2*, *Top2α*, and retinoid acid receptor α genes, all localized on chromosome 17q, has been observed in breast cancer cells.[77] Top2α expression can also be stimulated by Top1 inhibitors (see "Therapeutic Interaction"

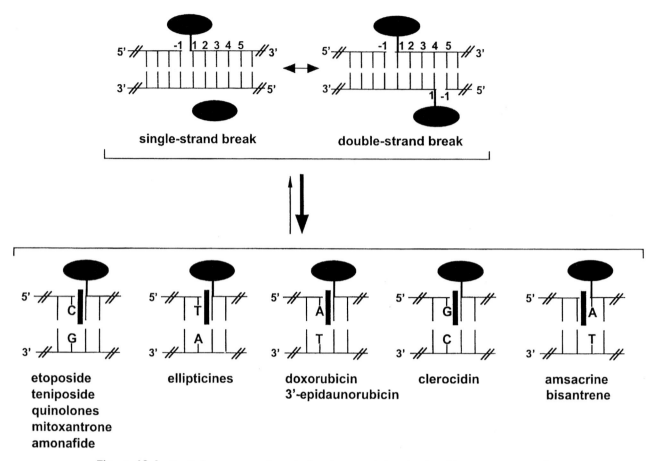

Figure 19.4 Top2 cleavage complexes in the absence of drug (top) and base sequence preferences for Top2 inhibitors. Top2 is shown as filled circles.

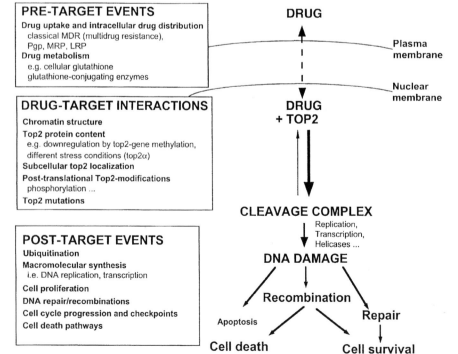

Figure 19.5 Determinants of sensitivity and resistance to Top2 inhibitors. (LRP, lung resistance–related protein; MRP, multidrug resistance protein; Pgp, P-glycoprotein.)

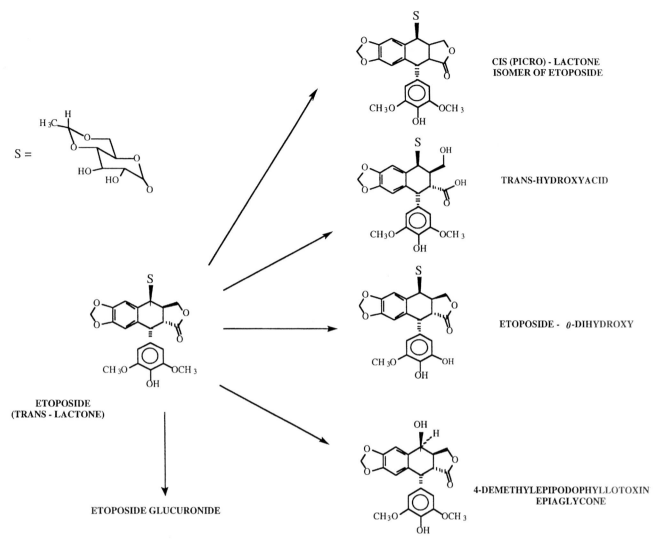

Figure 19.6 Metabolism of etoposide. Both etoposide-o-dihydroxy and 4-demethylepipodophyllotoxin aglycone are active against Top2.

below). Treatment of AML patients with topotecan leads on average to a threefold increase in Top2α expression.[78] Furthermore, a permanent twofold increase of both Top2α and β was reported for topotecan-resistant human cell lines.[79]

Many cell lines resistant to Top2 inhibitors show decreased Top2 protein levels. The two main mechanisms for decreased Top2 transcription are likely to involve DNA modifications (promoter mutations, gene rearrangements, CpG methylation) and transcription factor alterations. Methylation of the Top2 gene has been reported in association with decreased transcription.[80] Different stress conditions can decrease Top2α expression. For instance, p53, which itself is activated by DNA damage, down-regulates Top2α.[81,82] Glucose-regulated stress, such as hypoxia and nutrient deprivation, also lead to decreased expression of Top2α protein with associated resistance to VP–16.[83,84] These findings may be relevant for poorly vascularized human tumors. It seems that it is mostly Top2α that is altered in cell lines selected with VP-16 or teniposide.[85,86] Although Top2α is also affected in cell lines selected with DNA intercalators such as mitoxantrone, doxorubicin, and the ellipticines, the most dramatic changes seem to concern the β-isoform, which is strongly down-regulated or even missing.[87,88]

Another way of diminishing drug-induced cleavage complexes is by a shift in enzyme localization from the nucleus toward the cytoplasm, as observed for several cell lines resistant to Top2 inhibitors.[86,87,89] In such cases, the cytoplasmic Top2α is still catalytically active and able to carry out its normal functions during mitosis when the nuclear membrane is disassembled.

Top2 mutations have been observed in cell lines selected in vitro. The Top2 mutations are clustered in two regions, one located near the ATP binding site and the other around the catalytic tyrosine (Fig. 19.2). The presence of mutations near the catalytic tyrosine is consistent with the drug-stacking model at the interface of the enzyme-DNA complex.[64] The existence of the second mutation cluster near the putative ATP-binding site suggests that Top2 folding brings this second region near the catalytic domain and that Top2 inhibitors bind at the interface of these two Top2 regions.[61,90,91] The differential resistance to epipodophyllotoxins, m-AMSA, and quinolones of some of the drug-resistant mutants is consistent with preferential interactions of each class of drugs with certain Top2 amino acids and with the preferred DNA bases around the Top2 cleavage sites.

Changes in Top2 phosphorylation may also contribute to Top2-mediated drug resistance. However, in resistant cell lines, reduced cleavage complexes have been associated with both hyperphosphorylation and hypophosphorylation of Top2. Decreased Top2α protein levels were associated with hyperphosphorylation of the enzyme in VP-16-resistant cell lines.[92] Hypophosphorylated Top2α has been reported for VP-16-resistant erythroleukemia[93] and HL-60 cells[94] and for teniposide-resistant leukemia cell lines.[95] Top2 phosphorylation increases in parallel with the cellular need for the enzyme: during the S phase of the cell cycle, with a peak at the G_2 phase.[96] Casein kinase II is probably the main kinase responsible for Top2 phosphorylation in cells.[97–99] Drug-induced cleavage complexes are reduced to approximately 50% after in vitro phosphorylation of Top2α by casein kinase II and protein kinase C.[100] This finding is in contrast with Top1 phosphorylation, which increases camptothecin activity.[101]

Since both normal and cancer cells express Top2, it is likely that drug-induced cleavage complexes are not sufficient for selective killing of cancer cells. DNA synthesis inhibition provides only partial protection against VP-16.[102] The interaction of transcription with cleavage complexes may play a prominent role in the activity of Top2 inhibitors, since VP-16 cytotoxicity is decreased by RNA synthesis inhibitors.[103,104] The dependence of Top1 and Top2 inhibitor cytotoxicity on ongoing replication and transcription probably explains why simultaneous treatment with camptothecin and VP-16 has been found to be antagonistic.[103–105] VP-16 may suppress camptothecin effects by inhibiting replication, and camptothecin may suppress the effects of VP-16 by inhibiting transcription.

Poly(adenosine diphosphoribose) synthesis also may be important for cell killing, since poly(adenosine diphosphoribose polymerase)-deficient Chinese hamster cells are resistant to VP-16 and hypersensitive to camptothecin.[106] These observations indicate that events downstream from the cleavage complexes are critical to cytotoxicity. Such events may involve the accumulation of genetic alterations, such as sister chromatid exchanges (SCE),[107] illegitimate recombinations,[108,109] and apoptosis.[110]

DNA repair must intervene to correct drug-induced and topoisomerase-mediated DNA damage. Yeast cells are usually resistant to topoisomerase inhibitors unless they are RAD52 mutants, for example, deficient in DNA double-strand break repair.[111] The ubiquitin proteolysis pathway has been reported to be responsible for ubiquitination and degradation of Top1 and Top2 cleavage complexes.[112] Abnormal cell cycle control (checkpoints) has recently emerged as a key element in possibly explaining the differential responses of normal versus neoplastic cells to DNA damage. Therefore, alterations of cell cycle control may play a critical role in the cytotoxicity of topoisomerase inhibitors. Lack of arrest in G1, as in cells with mutated or absent p53 genes, may not provide the cell with the time required to repair damage and may lead to an accumulation of further damage. Hence deregulation of cyclins, cell cycle–regulated kinases and phosphatases, and p53 mutations may sensitize cells to topoisomerase inhibitors.[113–116] Furthermore, pharmacological abrogation of drug induced S-phase and G_2-phase checkpoints may provide a novel effective strategy for enhancing the chemotherapeutic activity of topoisomerase inhibitors.[117]

Another determinant of sensitivity to topoisomerase inhibitors is the predisposition of the cell to undergo apoptosis.[110] Some cells, such as human leukemia HL-60 cells, are known to be hypersensitive to a variety of injuries, including DNA damage by topoisomerase inhibitors. The underlying mechanism for this hypersensitivity may be the facile induction of apoptosis.[118] Overexpression of the c-myc proto-oncogene and down-regulation of the bcl-2 gene have been involved in committing the cells to an apoptosis-prone phenotype. p53 could play a key role in the case of VP-16 and mediate apoptosis in response to DNA damage without regulating apoptosis induced by glucocorticoids. Apoptosis also may play a role in drug-induced side effects such as hematopoietic or intestinal toxicity. Indeed, hematopoietic progenitors may be prone to apoptosis. Hence studies on the pharmacologic regulation of apoptosis may prove useful. Several classes of agents can suppress topoisomerase inhibitor–induced apoptosis,[118] and bcl-2 overexpression renders cells resistant to VP-16.[119]

In summary, cellular response to Top2 inhibitors is complex, and several mechanisms are commonly associated in laboratory cell lines: Pgp and/or MRP overexpression, reduction of Top2 protein levels, changes in subcellular localization, Top2 phosphorylation, and Top2 mutations. This multifactorial resistance is likely to be applicable to human cancers, which underlines the importance of a multiparametric approach for the evaluation of clinical response to Top2 inhibitors.

CLINICAL PHARMACOLOGY

Epipodophyllotoxins

Two epipodophyllotoxins derivatives are presently used in cancer chemotherapy, etoposide (VP-16) and teniposide (VM-26). Etoposide phosphate is an improved formulation of etoposide. Etoposide remains one of the most active anticancer agents, and it is used as a key component for chemotherapy, especially for testicular cancers; as an adjuvant (EP protocols)[9]; for first-line metastatic (BEP regimen) and second-line salvage therapies (VIP regimen); and in intensification regimens. Teniposide is a more potent Top2 inhibitor (about 10-fold with purified Top2), and it is mainly used in pediatric tumors and in neuro-oncology.

Drug Assays

Quantitation of epipodophyllotoxins and their metabolites involves either HPLC or immuno-based assays. Two immuno-based assays have been developed more recently: radioimmunoassays (RIAs) and ELISA methods. An ELISA method with a sensitivity of 0.5 ng/mL and with no cross-reactivity with the aglycone metabolite has been developed.[120]

Pharmacokinetics

Intravenous Etoposide

For both epipodophyllotoxins, there is significant interpatient variability in pharmacokinetic parameters.[121,122] Following an i.v. dose, etoposide decay in plasma follows a two-compartment pharmacokinetic model with a terminal half-life of 6 to 8 hours in patients with normal renal function (Table 19.4). Interpatient and intrapatient variability in pharmacokinetic parameters following i.v. administration is substantial and can exceed 35%.[123,124] The volume of distribution[123] averages 4 to 10 L/m². The peak plasma concentration and the area under the curve (AUC) are proportional to the administered dose[125,126] up to doses of 800 mg/m², and the elimination half-life is independent of dose. However, protein binding averages 96% but is nonlinear and influenced by the individual concentration of drug and albumin,[127,128] resulting in elevated free-drug concentrations in patients with low serum albumin. Other conditions, including elevated serum bilirubin concentrations, that compete for albumin binding also increase the concentration of the free, or biologically active, drug, resulting in greater toxicity.[129,130] Thus, the toxicity of etoposide correlates best with the pharmacokinetics of the unbound fraction of the drug. Etoposide penetrates the CSF poorly, with CSF concentrations less than 5% of simultaneously measured plasma levels.[121,123,131] Pleural fluid penetration and ascitic fluid penetration of etoposide are poor.[121,131]

Etoposide is eliminated by both renal and nonrenal mechanisms.[132] Approximately 40% of administered etoposide is cleared through the kidney unchanged.[123,124,126,129,133] Etoposide dosage should be reduced in proportion to reductions in creatinine clearance.[129,130] Hemodialysis membranes are not permeable to etoposide, and the pharmacokinetics of etoposide are not affected by the interval between chemotherapy and hemodialysis.[134]

Several metabolites of etoposide have been identified in humans[121,130,135] (Figure 19.6). The main metabolite is etoposide-glucuronide, which is eliminated in the urine. A catechol metabolite with significant cytotoxic activity is formed following etoposide O-demethylation in the liver.[136] Cytochrome P450 3A metabolizes etoposide to a catechol metabolite, which is further oxidized to a quinone. The etoposide-o-dihydroxy also can be converted to the o-quinone derivative. Both of these, as well as the 4-demethylepipodophyllotoxin, remain active against Top2. Ortho-quinone and semi-quinone free radicals of etoposide may covalently bind to DNA and induce DNA strand breakage.[137,138] Biliary excretion is a minor route of elimination. Minor alterations in liver function, such as transaminase elevations, do not require dose reduction if renal function remains normal,[139] but elevated bilirubin may decrease the clearance of unbound etoposide[127] and increases the unbound fraction of drug, leading to a greater hematologic toxicity. Therefore, etoposide dose should be reduced by 50% in patients with total bilirubin levels of 1.5 to 3.0 mg/dL. No etoposide should be given in patients with more than 5.0 mg/dL bilirubin.[140] Age-related reduction in etoposide clearance has been suggested.[141]

Dose-Escalation Strategies with Etoposide

High-dose etoposide (VP-16) with bone marrow transplantation. Etoposide has been used in most high-dose protocols because its nonhematologic toxicity is only moderate.[142] At very high doses up to 1,500 mg/m², bone marrow rescue is necessary, and the dose-limiting toxicities becomes mucositis and

TABLE 19.4
KEY FEATURES OF EPIPODOPHYLLOTOXIN DERIVATIVES

	Etoposide (VP-16)	Teniposide (VM-26)
Mechanism of action	Inhibition of Top2, Nonintercalator	Same but ≈ 10-fold more potent
Pharmacokinetics	Terminal half-life = 6–8 hr	Terminal half-life = 9.5–21 hr
Elimination	Hepatic metabolism, Renal excretion 35–40%	Probable hepatic metabolism
Toxicities	Neutropenia, Thrombocytopenia, (mild) Alopecia, Hypersensitivity, Mucositis (high doses)	Same as etoposide
Precautions	Reduced dose proportionate to creatinine clearance	Possible increased toxicity in hepatic failure

hepatotoxicity. The maximal tolerated dose (MTD) of etoposide administered as a single agent is up to 2.5 g/m². Between 2.5 and 3.5 g/m², the CSF concentration of etoposide becomes significant.

- **Loco-regional infusions of etoposide.** Based on the previous demonstration of a high peritoneal-plasma ratio of drug exposure for intraperitoneal etoposide, intraperitoneal administrations of etoposide have been done in ovarian cancer patients with peritoneal carcinomatosis.[143-145] The doses of etoposide[143,144,146,147] ranged from 100 to 600 mg/m². The calculated peritoneal-plasma ratio of unbound etoposide was 35. Etoposide can be combined intraperitoneally with cisplatin.[147]

The administration of intrapleural etoposide has been proposed as a way to prevent the recurrence of neoplastic pleural effusions.[148] Incomplete and slow systemic absorption from intrapleurally administered drug has been documented.[149] The intraventricular administration of etoposide is feasible.[150] CSF peak levels exceed more than 100-fold those achieved with intravenous infusion. The half-life in CSF based on the pharmacokinetic data analysis of four patients was 7.4 ± 1.2 hours. Intrathecal injections of etoposide have been reported using a 0.5-mg dose daily for 5 days, followed by a second course with two injections per day of the same dose.[151] No toxic effect was reported. The intra-arterial route (using carotid or vertebral arteries) has been used to increase etoposide uptake in brain tumors.[152] Intra-arterial infusion of etoposide has been used also for the treatment of liver metastases of testicular tumors.[153]

Oral Etoposide

Prolonged administration of etoposide aims for extended Top2 inhibition, thus preventing tumor cells from repairing DNA breaks. Oral administration of etoposide represents the most feasible and economic strategy to maintain effective concentrations of drug for extended times. Nevertheless, the efficacy of oral etoposide therapy is contingent on circumventing pharmacokinetic limitations, mainly low and variable bioavailability.[154] Inhibition of small-bowel and hepatic metabolism of etoposide with specific cytochrome P450 inhibitors or inhibition of the intestinal P-glycoprotein efflux pump has been attempted to increase the bioavailability of oral etoposide, but the best results were obtained with daily oral administration of low etoposide doses (50 to 100 mg/day for 14 to 21 days). Saturable absorption of etoposide was reported for doses greater than 200 mg/day, whereas lower doses were associated with increased bioavailability, although they were characterized by high interpatient and intrapatient variability. Pharmacokinetic parameters such as plasma trough concentration between two oral administrations [C(24,trough)], drug exposure time above a threshold value, and area under the plasma concentration-time curve have been correlated with the pharmacodynamic

effect of oral etoposide. Pharmacokinetic-pharmacodynamic relationships indicate that severe toxicity is avoided when peak plasma concentrations do not exceed 3 to 5 mg/L and C(24,trough) is under the threshold limit of 0.3 mg/L.

Oral etoposide is formulated in a hydrophilic gelatin capsule. Peak plasma levels are obtained 0.5 to 4 hours after administration.[155] The mean bioavailability is 50%,[126,155-159] with substantial interpatient and intrapatient variability (range, 19 to 100%).[123,126,160-162] The bioavailability of doses lower than 100 mg (50 mg/m²) approaches 75%,[159] whereas the bioavailability of doses above 100 mg/m² decreases below 50%. Etoposide has been given orally over a prolonged 21-day schedule at a dose of 50 mg/m² per day with dose-limiting myelosuppression. The 50 mg/m² dose has a higher bioavailability (91% to 96%) than that generally reported for higher doses of etoposide, and many patients maintained plasma concentrations of 1 µg/mL or greater for the entire period of treatment. Bioavailability is not linear and decreases with doses greater than 200 mg,[161] possibly implying a saturable absorptive mechanism in the gastrointestinal (GI) tract. In addition to saturation of uptake, the very low aqueous solubility and the low stability at acid pH likely contribute to the erratic etoposide bioavailability.[157,161,163] The intestinal P-glycoprotein mediates the efflux of etoposide, and the use of P-glycoprotein–inhibiting agents such as quinidine might increase the intestinal absorption of etoposide.[164] Oral bioavailability of etoposide is not affected by food or by concurrent i.v. chemotherapy.[160] A pharmacodynamic model was prospectively tested for the therapeutic monitoring of 21-day oral etoposide[165] (see below).

Oral etoposide is well tolerated in the elderly[166] and active in NHL and AL patients. However, a study compared the effects of oral etoposide and intravenous etoposide in advanced small cell lung cancer patients on survival and quality of life[167] and indicated that the oral route had a lower antitumoral activity and should not be used as first-line treatment for this disease.[167]

In conclusion, the development of oral etoposide was emphasized both because it might allow prolonged exposure to active concentrations of etoposide and because it appeared as an interesting alternative to improve quality of life in patients treated with palliative chemotherapy. However, both the high interindividual variation in bioavailability and the results of the only study that compared oral and intravenous etoposide suggest restrictions for its use as first-line therapy.

Etoposide Phosphate (Etopophos)

Etoposide phosphate (Etopophos) is an improved formulation of etoposide. It is a water-soluble prodrug of etoposide that is rapidly and completely converted to etoposide after intravenous dosing, regardless of the duration of administration, the dose used, or the treatment schedule.[168-170] Therefore, etoposide phosphate does not expose the bloodstream to detergents or oils, as does the formulation of the lipid-soluble etoposide and teniposide. Etoposide can be administered as an i.v. infusion in saline solution over 5 minutes without signs of hypotension or acute effects.[168] Since it is not formulated with polyethylene glycol, polysorbate 80, or ethanol, etoposide phosphate does not cause acidosis, even when given at high doses. When given as a continuous infusion, etoposide phosphate was stable in pumps for at least 7 days.

The molecular weights of etoposide and etoposide phosphate are 558.57 and 568.55, respectively. To avoid confusion, doses of etoposide phosphate may be expressed as molar equivalent doses of etoposide. The toxicity of etoposide and etoposide phosphate are similar.[171] The MTD was 100 mg/m^2 per day of etoposide equivalent for 5 days or 150 mg/m^2 per day for dosing on days 1, 3, and 5. Etoposide phosphate may exhibit better intestinal absorption than etoposide, with a mean bioavailability of 68%. Etoposide phosphate was proposed as a means to overcome the intersubject and intrasubject variability in absorption observed with oral etoposide.[172] However, the same large interindividual variability of etoposide phosphate and etoposide AUC was observed, with 42.3% and 48.4%, as the coefficients of variation.[173]

In conclusion, etoposide phosphate is an improved formulation of etoposide and is better suited for bolus administration, high-dose treatment, and continuous infusions, provided equivalent antitumor activity is demonstrated.

Teniposide (VM-26)

Like etoposide, teniposide demonstrates biexponential disposition following intravenous administration. Only 10 to 20% of administered teniposide is found in the urine as metabolites. The large volume of distribution is consistent with the high degree of protein binding (>99%). Its non-renal clearance is similar to that of etoposide, as is the volume of distribution. An inverse relationship between serum γ-glutamyl-transpeptidase and teniposide plasma clearance has been reported, suggesting an important hepatic component to clearance. A linear relationship exists between dose and AUC.

In mice, teniposide's highest concentrations are in the liver, kidneys, and small intestine. The lowest concentrations are found in the brain. In humans, CSF levels of teniposide are barely detectable, although teniposide is considered clinically more effective than etoposide in the treatment of malignant gliomas. Teniposide slowly diffuses into and is then slowly eliminated from third-space compartments such as ascites.

Teniposide is available only for intravenous administration, but the i.v. formulation of teniposide can be used orally. The bioavailability of oral teniposide appears similar to that of oral etoposide in that absorption is decreased at higher doses and is increased with smaller consecutive daily doses. The mean bioavailability is 41%.[162] The MTD for oral teniposide given over 21

days is 100 mg/day, and the dose-limiting toxicity is myelosupression.[162,174]

Pharmacodynamics

Etoposide activity shows marked schedule dependency[123] and is both concentration-dependent and time-dependent.[123] Etoposide clearance is not correlated with body surface area.[175] Dosing according to body surface area is a poor predictor of the peak or steady-state etoposide concentration or AUC.[176] Hematologic toxicity correlates better to the AUC of unbound etoposide than to the AUC of total etoposide.[177] Steady-state etoposide plasma levels of more than 1 μg/mL are tumoricidal but are associated with severe myelosuppression when the etoposide plasma levels are continuously higher than 3 μg/mL. The maintenance of a minimum plasma concentration between 2 and 3 μg/mL appears critical for efficacy. Intrapatient pharmacokinetic variability is small (12 to 15%).[176] In the absence of measured plasma concentrations, simplifying VP-16 dosing to a fixed dose independent of body surface area—260 mg instead of 150 mg/m^2—has been suggested.[176] However, several studies indicated that patients with impaired renal or liver function or elderly patients are at risk for increased hematological toxicity, and hence it was proposed that the etoposide dose be reduced and individualized in these patients.[178]

Various limited-sampling methods have been proposed to estimate etoposide AUC from one or two plasma concentration measurements.[179,180]

In patients receiving 21-day oral VP-16, etoposide plasma concentrations are correlated with the neutrophil count at the nadir.[165]

Toxicity

Hematotoxicity

Myelosupression is the dose-limiting toxicity of etoposide. Although the single MTD is 300 mg/m^2, doses of 150 mg/m^2 for 3 days and 45 mg/m^2 for 7 days have been studied. Bone marrow toxicity is not cumulative. When given orally over 21 days, etoposide is generally well tolerated at a MTD of 50 mg/m^2 per day. Myelosuppression is the dose-limiting toxicity, with leukocyte nadirs occurring between days 22 and 29.

Nonhematological Toxicities

Common nonhematological toxicities include nausea and vomiting in 10 to 20% of patients and alopecia in 10 to 30% of patients, depending on dose and schedule. Rare cases of anaphylaxis and chemical phlebitis have been reported. Hypotension, fever, bronchospasm, diarrhea, and mucositis are uncommon.[181] Hypotension has been noted in 5 to 8% of patients receiving etoposide but is rare when the drug is given over 1 hour and is probably related to the vehicle (polysorbate 80 plus polyethylene glycol).[181]

Etoposide-Induced Secondary Leukemia

The increased frequency of illegitimate recombination events induced by Top2-reactive agents may account for their leukemogenicity.[107]. Etoposide was demonstrated to be mutagenic in patients.[182] Acute myelogenous leukemia (AML) cases related to prior treatment with epipodophyllotoxins (etoposide and teniposide) have been identified.[6,183–188] In contrast to alkylating agent–associated secondary AML, epipodophyllotoxin-associated AML exhibits a shorter latency period, with a median of 24 to 30 months.[6,186,189] The epipodophyllotoxin phenotype is most often monocytic (FAB M4 or M5). Acute promyelocytic leukemia following treatment with epipodophyllotoxin occurs infrequently.[187,188] Secondary myelodysplastic syndrome and chronic myelogenous leukemia have been described.[6] Therapy-related leukemia and myelodysplasia were also reported following prolonged administration of oral etoposide in breast cancer patients and NHL patients.[190,191] In one review of 37 patients, 21 of 30 patients had M-4 or M-5 AML, with 14 of 28 patients having an 11q23 abnormality. The mean latency period was 33 months. Other studies suggest a shorter latency of 2 years.[6,185,186] Weekly or biweekly schedules of etoposide might be associated with increased risk of secondary leukemia.[6] The administration of L-asparaginase prior to etoposide might also increase the risk of leukemia.[6,192]

The follow-up by the National Cancer Institute Cancer Therapy Evaluation Program of patients treated with epipodophyllotoxins did not show evidence of significant variations in the incidence of secondary leukemias in patients who had received low (.1.5 g/m^2), moderate (1.5 to 2.99 g/m^2), or high cumulative doses (>3 g/m^2).[186] The calculated 6-year rate for development of leukemia was between 0.7% and 3.2%, and the highest rate was observed in the group of patients who received the lowest doses.[186] Most other studies found a correlation between the cumulative dose of etoposide and the risk of secondary leukemias. In the Indiana University experience, among the patients with germ cell malignancies treated with cisplatinum, etoposide, and bleomycin (PEB) at conventional doses, 2 of 538 patients developed AML after 22 months to 3 years.[193] The median follow-up was 4.9 years. The etoposide dose was an important factor for the occurrence of AML following etoposide and cisplatin combination chemotherapy for advanced non–small cell lung cancer.[194] The median etoposide dose was 6.8 g/m^2 in 4 out of 114 patients who developed AML after 13, 19, 28, and 35 months after the beginning of the treatment, compared with a median etoposide dose of 3.0 g/m^2 in the nonleukemic patients. In another report of 212 patients treated with PEB for germ cell tumors, 5 patients developed acute nonlymphocytic leukemia (ANLL) for a mean cumulative risk of 4.7%.[195] All these patients had cumulative etoposide doses

above 2,000 mg/m^2, whereas none of the 130 patients with cumulative dose below 2,000 mg/m^2 developed leukemia. In a series of 734 children treated with epipodophyllotoxins, 21 developed secondary AML. The overall risk of developing a secondary leukemia was 3.8%. Subgroup analysis revealed that the risk was substantially greater when the drug was given on a weekly or biweekly schedule (12%). The cumulative risk was substantially less (1.6%) in the children not treated with etoposide or treated with etoposide only during remission induction or every 2 weeks during continuation treatment.[186,196] In a case-control study of the French Society of Pediatric Oncology, 61 patients with secondary leukemia were matched with 196 controls. In multivariate analysis, the risk of leukemia correlated with the type of primary tumor (excess risk in case of Hodgkin's disease and osteosarcoma) and with the cumulative dose of etoposide.[197] The risk of leukemia in patients who received more than 6g/m² was 200-fold higher. The risk of leukemia was not increased by exposure to alkylating agents or radiotherapy. Not only etoposide but also its catechol and quinone metabolites can induce in vitro Top2 cleavage complexes near the translocation breakpoints and are likely to also play a role in the creation of Top2-mediated chromosomal breakage.[198]

These leukemias frequently involved the long arm of chromosome 11, with translocation of the *MLL* (myeloid-lymphoid leukemia or mixed-lineage leukemia) gene, which resides at chromosome band 11q23, but other less common abnormalities involved chromosomes 3, 8, 15, 16, 17, 21, or 22.[100,199–202] Most of the breakpoints in the *MLL* gene occur in a 9-kilobase region that includes exons 5 to 11. This genomic region includes DNA sequences potentially involved in illegitimate recombinations, such as Alu sequences, VDJ recombinase recognition sites, and Top2 consensus-binding sequences. The *MLL* gene appears to play a role in the regulation of the differentiation of hematopoietic stem cells. Its overall sequence composition is AT-rich. AT-rich sequences often correspond to nuclear matrix attachment regions (MARs), where Top2 cleavage complexes are preferentially formed.[203] More than 20 different translocations involving chromosome 11q23 have been described. DNA topoisomerase II cleavage assays have shown a correspondence between Top2 cleavage sites and the translocation breakpoints. The mechanism of the translocation might be a chromosomal breakage by Top2 followed by the recombination of DNA free ends during DNA repair.

Clinical Resistance

Several studies have found an association between Top2α expression and tumor cell proliferation.[204,205] Consistently higher Top2α mRNA levels were observed in high- grade than in low-grade non-Hodgkin's lymphomas[206] and in small cell than in non–small cell lung cancer.[207] Increased Top2α was correlated with a poor prognosis in breast cancer patients.[208] In contrast to Top2α,Top2β is expressed in both proliferating and quiescent cells.[76] Several studies have investigated the relationship between Top2 levels in leukemia cells and the response to Top2 inhibitor–containing chemotherapy. No correlation was seen between Top2α or Top2β expression, as assessed by Western blot, and the response to Top2 poisons in adult acute leukemias.[209,210] Both negative estrogen receptor status and c-erbB2 overexpression are associated with high Top2α expression in breast cancer.[211] The overexpression of Top2α does not correlate with the antitumoral effect of anthracyclines.[212] However, the clinical response to etoposide phosphate infusion and cisplatin in heavily pretreated metastatic breast cancer patients correlated with tumor Top2α expression.[213]

Acridines

Amsacrine Pharmacokinetics

The key pharmacologic features of amsacrine are given in Table 19.5.

Amsacrine is metabolized via two major routes (Fig. 19.7), both of which result in the formation of conjugated thiols. The major route of metabolism and elimination of amsacrine in the mouse and the rat is cytochrome P-450–dependent. In the liver, the major metabolite is the amsacrine-glutathion-5'-conjugate. Amsacrine and to a greater degree its metabolites are also excreted in urine. The cellular pharmacokinetics suggest that the cellular uptake occurs by a rapid and passive diffusion. Neither amsacrine nor its metabolites penetrate the blood-brain barrier, and amsacrine does not achieve appreciable levels in the CSF.[214]

TABLE 19.5
KEY FEATURES OF AMSACRINE

Mechanism of action	Inhibition of DNA topoisomerase II, with possible selectivity for Top2β Weak intercalator
Pharmacokinetics	Plasma disappearance: Initial half-life = 30 min Terminal half-life = 7–9 hr Protein binding: 50% after 2 hr
Metabolism	Conjugation with glutathione
Elimination	Biliary route (65%, as metabolites) Urinary route (35–50%, as metabolites and parent drug)
Toxicities	Myelosuppression Mucositis Vomiting Hepatotoxicity Ventricular arrhythmias
Precautions	Increased toxicity if renal or liver failure; reduce dose by 30%. Monitoring of serum electrolytes; avoid hypokalemia.

Toxicity of Amsacrine

Hematotoxicity of Amsacrine

A number of single-dose and multiple-dose schedules have been tested in phase I trials in adult patients.[215] The oral route is not used because of large and unpredictable interindividual variability in absorption. The optimal schedule appears to be 150 mg/m² per day for 5 days for adult patients with leukemia. Myelosuppression is the most important and dose-limiting toxicity.

Nonhematological Toxicities of Amsacrine

Amsacrine causes phlebitis. Consequently, it is recommended to dilute amsacrine in 500 mL of 5% dextrose and to use a central line for continuous infusion or repeated treatments to avoid reactions at the injection site. Hearing loss and allergic reactions (anaphylaxis, urticaria and rashes, allergic edema) are relatively rare.

Nausea and vomiting are common with amsacrine.[216] Diarrhea is less common and occurs in 5 to 17% of patients. In a trial incorporating dose escalation, the stomatitis was dose-related and relatively infrequent at doses under 120 mg/m². Stomatitis becomes dose limiting for treatments with very high doses in association with bone marrow rescue.[217]

The incidence of hepatotoxicity may reach 35%.[218] Elevation of bilirubin, the most frequent abnormality,[219] is usually dose-related and reversible.[216] Increased liver transaminases are also dose-dependent and reversible.[220] Increased alkaline phosphatases are rare.[221] However, two cases of fatal hepatotoxicity have been reported, both in heavily pretreated patients.[218,220] Since amsacrine is conjugated in the liver and is excreted in large part via the biliary system, at least 30% dose reduction is generally recommended in patients with impaired hepatic function (elevated bilirubin).

Cardiotoxicity has been reported in children and adults with both high- and low-dose treatments. Although its incidence is low (<5% in most large series), patients may develop arrhythmia, conducting disturbances, congestive heart failure during and after amsacrine administration, and sudden death.[216,222–224] More commonly, the heart rate is decreased by about 10%.[225] Because hypokalemia may exacerbate arrhythmias, it has been recommended that serum potassium levels be maintained at or above 4 mEq/L at the time of drug administration.[226] Normally, this value can be obtained readily with an infusion of potassium chloride at a rate of 10 mEq/hour administered over 10 hours before amsacrine treatment. In most patients, amsacrine produces a significant prolongation (0.05 to 0.064 seconds) of the corrected QT (QTc) interval.[222,227] The amsacrine-associated QTc prolongation may persist for up to 90 minutes. Tachyarrhythmias in the setting of QTc prolongation usually arise by triggered automaticity and may be precipitated by adrenergic hyperactivity. A prospective study suggested that this effect was present in most

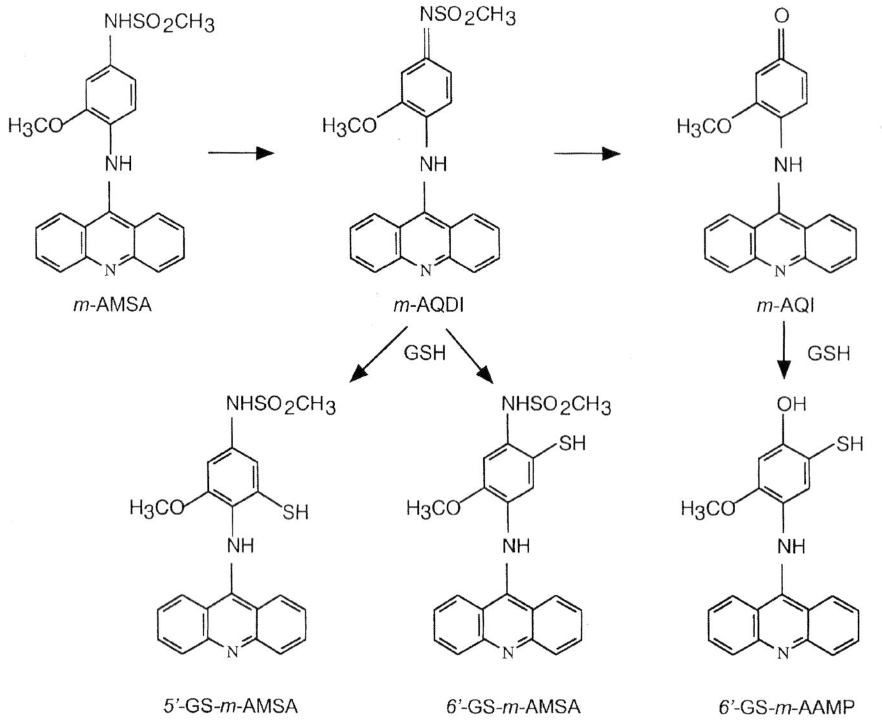

Figure 19.7 Metabolism of amsacrine (m-AMSA).

patients and occurred with each dose. Amsacrine also may reduce significantly the serum sodium and magnesium concentrations 20 minutes after the start of the infusion. The effect is transient and reverses by 24 hours after the infusion.[228] The decrease in magnesium levels may contribute to the amsacrine-induced cardiac arrhythmias.[225,229] Nevertheless, amsacrine has been administered safely to patients with myocardial dysfunction.[226]

The impact of amsacrine treatments on fertility has been reported by Da Cunha and coworkers,[230] who found that amsacrine has temporary and reversible effects on sperm count and motility.[230]

In summary, the optimal schedule of administration for amsacrine appears to be a single daily dose. It seems that little advantage is gained by continuous infusion schedules. Patients with normal hepatic function or mild liver dysfunction should tolerate full drug doses. Patients with significant liver dysfunction manifested by serum bilirubin greater than 2 mg/dL should have an initial 30% dose reduction. Subsequent dose escalation may be possible based on clinical tolerance. Patients with moderate renal dysfunction (serum creatinine in the range of 1.2 to 2 mg/dL) should receive full-dose therapy; however, oliguric patients or those with more serious renal disease (serum creatinine greater than 2 mg/dL) should have an initial 30% dose reduction.

DACA

The acridinecarboxamide N-[2-(dimethylamino)ethyl] acridine-4-carboxamide (DACA; Fig. 19.1) is a lipophilic mono-intercalator that entered phase I and II clinical trials on the basis of its mixed inhibition of both topoisomerases I and II[24,25] and its activity in experimental solid tumors.[23] However, 120-hour continuous infusions failed to produce clinical antitumoral activity in patients with ovarian cancer[231] or non–small cell lung cancer.[232]

Ellipticine and Olivacine Derivatives

Ellipticines and olivacines have in common the absence of dose-limiting myelosuppression and the absence of alopecia. Elliptinium is presently only available in Europe, and its use is severely limited by its propensity to cause severe intravascular hemolysis and by its modest antitumor activity. One olivacine derivative (S16020-S; Fig. 19.1) is presently in phase I-II clinical trials.

Therapeutic Interactions with the Top2 Inhibitors

Platinum Derivatives and Radiotherapy

Therapeutic synergy between etoposide and cis-platinum has been demonstrated, and this combination is very effective in the treatment of germ cell tumors and small cell lung cancers.[233] The synergism between etoposide and platinum derivatives has also been found in experimental systems[234] but its mechanisms remain poorly understood. Top2 inhibition might interfere with the repair of the platinum cross-links or produce complex DNA damage that might be inefficiently repaired in tumor cells. In a model of SCLC xenografts, the combination of ifosfamide and etoposide tended to be more potentiating than the standard combination of cisplatin and etoposide.[235]

In a randomized crossover study, the potential interaction between the platinum agents cisplatin and carboplatin and the metabolism of etoposide was explored.[236] Etoposide was given over three days. At first cycle, etoposide was administered with a platinum drug on day 2, and the alternate platinum was administered on the second course. Neither cisplatin nor carboplatin coadministration affected the pharmacokinetics of etoposide during cycle 1. The AUC of etoposide was increased (28%) on day 3 of cycle 2 when cisplatin was given on day 2. These results are consistent with a previous report of reduction of the total clearance of etoposide during concomitant treatment with cisplatin.[237] However, given the pharmacokinetic variability seen with etoposide, the clinical impact of these variations is small at conventional doses. The clearance of etoposide is substantially lower in patients receiving concomitant high doses of carboplatin prior to undergoing autologous bone marrow transplantation.[238]

Etoposide is an excellent radiosensitizer and is widely used in therapeutic protocols combining chemotherapy and concurrent radiotherapy, especially in lung cancer patients.[239]

Topoisomerase I Inhibitors: The Camptothecins

The interactions between inhibitors of Top1 and Top2 are complex. Tumor heterogeneity might contribute to the efficacy of concurrent administrations of Top2 and Top1 inhibitors. S-phase cells might be most sensitive to camptothecins, while the cytotoxicity of Top2 inhibitors is less cell cycle–dependent. Local pharmacokinetics might also a contributing factor. In cell culture experiments, simultaneous exposure to etoposide and to the topoisomerase I inhibitor camptothecin is antagonistic unless the two drugs are administered with a 4- to 6-hour interval.[105] This in vitro antagonism has been confirmed in mouse xenograft systems in vivo for the association of etoposide with either of the two camptothecin derivatives CPT-11 (irinotecan)[240] or topotecan.[241] Cell cycle responses probably play a key role in the antagonism observed in these simultaneous exposure schedules. Top2 inhibitors deplete the S-phase cells by producing a G_2 arrest, whereas Top1 inhibitors are most cytotoxic in S-phase because of a requirement of active replication for the generation of irreversible DNA lesions.[105,242] In the sequential schedules, compensatory enzyme changes might contribute to the enhanced activity. The combination of a Top1 inhibitor with a Top2 inhibitor is associated with a depletion of the target topoisomerase mRNA and protein and with reciprocal increases in the alternate topoisomerase mRNA and, to a lesser extent, protein.[240] For these reasons, considerable clinical research has focused on the sequential administration of Top1 and Top2 poisons. A compensatory increase in Top2α and increased sensitivity to etoposide have been reported following treatment with topotecan.[241] The Top2α

levels declined 5 days after the last dose of topotecan and resulted in restoration of the original response of xenografts to etoposide.[241] Hence, schedule dependency plays a crucial role in optimizing the effectiveness of combination chemotherapy with Top1 and Top2 inhibitors.

Clinical trials to date have explored the following:

Simultaneous administration of either CPT-11 (irinotecan) or topotecan with etoposide. A phase I combination study was conducted starting with 30 mg/m^2 per day of CPT-11 and 40 mg/m^2 per day of VP-16 given simultaneously from day 1 to 3. Cytolysis and hyperbilirubinemia were observed as dose-limiting toxicities resulting from this first dose level. The SN-38 enterohepatic circulation and drug-drug interactions have been suggested as playing a role.[243] Another phase I combination study tested 60 to 90 mg/m^2 per day of CPT-11 on days 1, 8, and 15 with 80 mg/m^2 per day of VP-16 on days 1 to 3 every 3 weeks, with G-CSF support.[244] Dose-limiting toxicities were diarrhea and leukopenia.[244] The concurrent administration of CPT-11 and etoposide for 3 days has also been evaluated.[245] The main dose-limiting toxicity was diarrhea. Granulocytopenia was also severe. The recommended doses were 60 mg/m^2 per day in combination with 60 mg/m^2 per day of CPT-11, and these doses required prophylactic administration of G-CSF.[245] The concurrent administration of 5-day etoposide and CPT-11 led to granulocytopenia as a dose-limiting toxicity.[246] Several phase II clinical trials have combined etoposide with either CPT-11[247] or topotecan.[248]

Sequential administration of topotecan (72 hours continuous infusion on days 1 to 3) and etoposide (75 or 100 mg/m^2 per day as a 2-hour infusion on days 8 to 10) has been studied in patients with solid tumors.[249] In two of the six patients, Top1 levels in their tumors were successively measured and showed either modest or substantial decrements following topotecan treatment, while in one of these six patients, tumor Top2 levels increased.[249] Sequential administration of intravenous topotecan and oral etoposide was also evaluated but not at optimum intervals.[250]

The pharmacologically guided addition of etoposide to weekly chemotherapy consisting of cisplatin and irinotecan has been investigated.[251] The Top2 poison was given 2 days after each dose of irinotecan. The dose-limiting toxicities included diarrhea and neutropenia. The quantitation of Top2α protein in peripheral blood mononuclear cells revealed an increase of Top2α at the time of etoposide administration in two patients. Evidence of antitumoral activity was seen in previously treated patients with mesothelioma and gastric, breast, and ovarian cancer.[252]

Alternatively, sequential administration starting with the Top2 poison has also been tested using the combination of doxorubicin and topotecan.[253] The MTD was 25 mg/m^2 of doxorubicin followed 2 days later by 1.75 mg/m^2 per day of topotecan for 3 days. The treatment appeared feasible and active, encouraging phase II trials.

Another phase I-II study evaluated two sequences—Top1 inhibition followed by Top2 inhibition, or the reverse—using infusions of topotecan and oral etoposide in patients with small cell lung cancer. The dose-limiting toxicity was neutropenia. The combination was feasible and effective.[254].

These studies support the continued development of sequential Top1 and Top2 targeting in the treatment of solid tumors.

Association of Topoisomerase II Inhibitors

Topoisomerase II inhibitors may be combined together. Etoposide is commonly given with adriamycin in various combination protocols for the treatment of Hodgkin's lymphomas. Mitoxantrone and VP-16 or amsacrine and VP-16 have been combined in the treatment of acute myelogenous leukemia.[255] Such associations may be justified because anthracyclines and mitoxantrone exhibit marked differences in the genomic location of cleavage complexes and therefore may selectively target different portions of the genome[55] (see "Base-Sequence Preference of Top2 Inhibitors and Drug-Binding Model" discussed earlier in the chapter).

The pharmacokinetics of etoposide were found unaffected by the dexrazoxane rescue used to reduce the extracerebral toxicity of high-dose etoposide.[256]

Other Agents

The human colony-stimulating factors (CSFs) accelerate hematopoietic recovery from etoposide-induced myelosuppression. In addition, CSFs may limit etoposide-induced myelosuppression by inhibiting apoptosis in the normal bone marrow cells. CSFs can also modulate the growth and drug response of tumor cells with functional receptors for these cytokines. Granulocyte colony-stimulating factor (G-CSF) enhances etoposide-containing standard chemotherapy when given until 48 hours before the next chemotherapy course.[257]

Anticonvulsivant therapy, when used concomitantly with etoposide, may induce hepatic enzyme induction, resulting in a higher etoposide clearance.[238,258]

Warfarin. Etoposide might displace warfarin from its protein-binding sites, resulting in early elevation in prothrombin time.[259] A close monitoring of the INR is recommended to adjust the dosage of warfarin.

REFERENCES

1. Kohn KW. Beyond DNA cross-linking: history and prospects of DNA-targeted cancer treatment. Fifteenth Bruce F. Cain Memorial Award Lecture. Cancer Res 1996;56:5533–5546.

2. Zwelling LA, Michaels S, Erickson LC, et al. Protein-associated deoxyribonucleic acid strand breaks in L1210 cells treated with the deoxyribonucleic acid intercalating agents 4'-(9- acridinylamino) methanesulfon-m-anisidide and adriamycin. Biochemistry 1981; 20:6553–6563.

3. Pommier Y, Kerrigan D, Schwartz R, et al. The formation and resealing of intercalator-induced DNA strand breaks in isolated L1210 cell nuclei. Biochem Biophys Res Commun 1982;107: 576–583.

4. Nelson EM, Tewey KM, Liu LF. Mechanism of antitumor drug action: poisoning of mammalian DNA topoisomerase II on DNA by 4'-(9-acridinylamino)-methanesulfon-m- anisidide. Proc Natl Acad Sci USA 1984;81:1361–1365.

5. Minford J, Pommier Y, Filipski J, et al. Isolation of intercalator-dependent protein-linked DNA strand cleavage activity from cell nuclei and identification as topoisomerase II. Biochemistry 1986;25:9–16.

6. Felix CA. Secondary leukemias induced by topoisomerase-targeted drugs. Biochim Biophys Acta 1998;1400:233–235.

7. Senter PD, Saulnier MG, Schreiber GJ, et al. Anti-tumor effects of antibody-alkaline phosphatase conjugates in combination with etoposide phosphate. Proc Natl Acad Sci USA 1988;85: 4842–4846.

8. Haisma HJ, Boven E, van Muijen M, et al. Analysis of a conjugate between anti-carcinoembryonic antigen monoclonal antibody and alkaline phosphatase for specific activation of the prodrug etoposide phosphate. Cancer Immunol Immunother 1992;34: 343–348.

9. Kondagunta GV, Sheinfeld J, Mazumdar M, et al. Relapse-free and overall survival in patients with pathologic stage II nonseminomatous germ cell cancer treated with etoposide and cisplatin adjuvant chemotherapy. J Clin Oncol 2004;22:464–467.

10. Kellie SJ, Boyce H, Dunkel IJ, et al. Primary chemotherapy for intracranial nongerminomatous germ cell tumors: results of the second international CNS germ cell study group protocol. J Clin Oncol 2004;22:846–853.

11. Sparano JA, Lee S, Chen MG, et al. Phase II trial of infusional cyclophosphamide, doxorubicin, and etoposide in patients with HIV-associated non-Hodgkin's lymphoma: an Eastern Cooperative Oncology Group trial (E1494). J Clin Oncol 2004;22:1491–1500.

12. Escobar PF, Lurain JR, Singh DK, et al. Treatment of high-risk gestational trophoblastic neoplasia with etoposide, methotrexate, actinomycin D, cyclophosphamide, and vincristine chemotherapy. Gynecol Oncol 2003;91:552–557.

13. Mollee P, Gupta V, Song K, et al. Long-term outcome after intensive therapy with etoposide, melphalan, total body irradiation and autotransplant for acute myeloid leukemia. Bone Marrow Transplant 2004;33:1201–1208.

14. Bowman LC, Castleberry RP, Cantor A, et al. Genetic staging of unresectable or metastatic neuroblastoma in infants: a Pediatric Oncology Group study. J Natl Cancer Inst 1997;89:373–380.

15. Bjorkholm M. Etoposide and teniposide in the treatment of acute leukemia. Med Oncol Tumor Phar 1990;7:3–10.

16. Amylon MD, Shuster J, Pullen J, et al. Intensive high-dose asparaginase consolidation improves survival for pediatric patients with T cell acute lymphoblastic leukemia and advanced stage lymphoblastic lymphoma: a Pediatric Oncology Group study. Leukemia 1999;13:335–342.

17. Campbell M, Salgado C, Quintana J, et al. Improved outcome for acute lymphoblastic leukemia in children of a developing country: results of the Chilean trial PINDA 87. Med Pediatr Oncol 1999;33:88–94.

18. Solal-Celigny P, Lepage E, Brousse N, et al. Doxorubicin-containing regimen with or without interferon alfa-2b for advanced follicular lymphomas: final analysis of survival and toxicity in the Groupe d'Etude des Lymphomes Folliculaires 86 trial. J Clin Oncol 1998;16:2332–2338.

19. Brandes AA, Basso U, Vastola F, et al. Carboplatin and teniposide as third-line chemotherapy in patients with recurrent oligodendroglioma or oligoastrocytoma: a phase II study. Ann Oncol 2003;14:1727–1731.

20. Poortmans PM, Kluin-Nelemans HC, Haaxma-Reiche H, et al. High-dose methotrexate-based chemotherapy followed by consolidating radiotherapy in non-AIDS-related primary central nervous system lymphoma: European Organization for Research

and Treatment of Cancer Lymphoma Group Phase II Trial 20962. J Clin Oncol 2003;21:4483–4488.

21. Oishi N, Berenberg J, Blumenstein BA, et al. Teniposide in metastatic renal and bladder cancer: a Southwest Oncology Group study. Cancer Treat Rep 1987;71:1307–1308.

22. Lum BL, Torti FM. Adjuvant intravesicular pharmacotherapy for superficial bladder cancer. J Natl Cancer Inst 1991;83:682–694.

23. Baguley BC, Zhuang L, Marshall E. Experimental solid tumour activity of N-[2-(dimethylamino)ethyl]acridine-4-carboxamide. Cancer Chemother Pharmacol 1995;36:244–248.

24. Bridewell DJA, Finlay GJ, Baguley BC. Mechanism of cytotoxicity of N-[2-(dimethylamino)ethyl]acridine-4-carboxamide and of its 7-chloro derivative: the roles of topoisomerases I and II. Cancer Chemother Pharmacol 1999;43:302–308.

25. Gamage SA, Spicer JA, Atwell GJ, et al. Structure-activity relationships for substituted Bis(acridine-4-carboxamides): a new class of anticancer agents. J Med Chem 1999;42:2383–2393.

26. Cragg G, Suffness M. Metabolism of plant-derived anticancer agents. Pharmacol Ther 1988;37:425–461.

27. Le Mee S, Pierre A, Markovits J, et al. S16020-2, a new highly cytotoxic antitumor olivacine derivative: DNA interaction and DNA topoisomerase II inhibition. Mol Pharmacol 1998;53:213–220.

28. Leonce S, Perez V, Casabianca Pignede MR, et al. In vitro cytotoxicity of S 16020-2, a new olivacine derivative. Invest New Drugs 1996;14:169–180.

29. Guilbaud N, Kraus-Berthier L, Saint-Dizier D, et al. In vivo antitumor activity of S16020-2, a new olivacine derivative. Cancer Chemother Pharmacol 1996;38:513–521.

30. Guilbaud N, Kraus-Berthier L, Saint-Dizier D, et al. Antitumor activity of S16020-2 in two orthotopic models of lung cancer. Anticancer Drugs 1997;8:276–282.

31. Kraus-Berthier L, Guilbaud N, Jan M, et al. Experimental antitumour activity of S16020-2 in a panel of human tumours. Eur J Cancer 1997;33:1881–1887.

32. Awada A, Giacchetti S, Gerard B, et al. Clinical phase I and pharmacokinetic study of S 16020, a new olivacine derivative: report on three infusion schedules. Ann Oncol 2002;13:1925–1932.

33. Earhart RH, Tutsch KD, Koeller JM, et al. Pharmacokinetics of (+)-1,2-di(3,5-dioxopiperazin-1-yl)propane intravenous infusions in adult cancer patients. Cancer Res 1982;42:5255–5261.

34. Speyer JL, Green MD, Kramer E, et al. Protective effect of the bispiperazinedione ICRF-187 against doxorubicin induced cardiac toxicity in women with advanced breast cancer. N Engl J Med 1988;319:745–752.

35. Speyer JL, Green MD, Zeleniuch-Jacquotte A, et al. ICRF-187 permits longer treatment with doxorubicin in women with breast cancer. J Clin Oncol 1992;10:117–127.

36. Ohno R, Yamada K, Hirano M, et al. The Tokai Blood Cancer Study Group: phase II study: treatment of non-Hodgkin's lymphoma with an oral antitumor derivative of bis(2,6-dioxopiperazine). J Natl Cancer Inst 1992;84:435–438.

37. Ohno R, Masaoka T, Shirakawa S, et al. Treatment of adult T-cell leukemia/lymphoma with MST-16, a new oral antitumor drug and a derivative of bis(2,6-dioxopiperazine). Cancer 1993;71:2217–2221.

38. Wang JC. Cellular roles of DNA topoisomerases: a molecular perspective. Nat Rev Mol Cell Biol 2002;3:430–440.

39. Levine C, Hiasa H, Marians KJ. DNA gyrase and topoisomerase IV: biochemical activities, physiological roles during chromosome replication, and drug sensitivities. Biochim Biophys Acta 1998;1400:29–43.

40. Hooper DC. Clinical applications of quinolones. Biochim Biophys Acta 1998;1400:45–61.

41. Berger JM. Type II DNA topoisomerases. Curr Opin Struct Biol 1998;8:26–32.

42. Wang JC. Moving one DNA double helix through another by a type II DNA topoisomerase: the story of a simple molecular machine. Q Rev Biophys 1998;31:107–144.

43. Pourquier P, Kohlhagen G, Ueng L-M, et al. Topoisomerase I and II activity assays. In: Brown R, Böger-Brown U, eds. Methods in Molecular Medicine: Cytotoxic Drug Resistance Mechanisms. Vol. 28. Totowa, NJ: Humana Press, 1999:95–110.

44. Pommier Y. DNA topoisomerase II inhibitors. In: Teicher BA, ed. Cancer Therapeutics: Experimental and Clinical Agents. Totowa, NJ: Humana Press, 1997:153–174.

45. Liu L. DNA Topoisomerases: Topoisomerase-Targeting Drugs. New York: Academic Press, 1994.

46. Burden DA, Osheroff N. Mechanism of action of eukaryotic topoisomerase II and drugs targeted to the enzyme. Biochim Biophys Acta 1998;1400:139–154.

47. Corbett AH, Osheroff N. When good enzymes go bad: conversion of topoisomerase II to a cellular toxin by antineoplastic drugs. Chem Res Toxicol 1993;6:585–597.

48. Subramanian D, Kraut E, Staubus A, et al. Analysis of topoisomerase I/DNA complexes in patients administered topotecan. Cancer Res 1995;55:2007–2103.

49. Pommier Y, Schwartz RE, Zwelling LA, et al. Effects of DNA intercalating agents on topoisomerase II induced DNA strand cleavage in isolated mammalian cell nuclei. Biochemistry 1985;24:6406–6410.

50. Tewey KM, Chen GL, Nelson EM, et al. Intercalative antitumor drugs interfere with the breakage-reunion reaction of mammalian DNA topoisomerase II. J Biol Chem 1984;259:9182–9187.

51. Andoh T. Bis(2,6-dioxopiperazines), catalytic inhibitors of DNA topoisomerase II, as molecular probes, cardioprotectors and antitumor drugs. Biochimie 1998;80:235–246.

52. Classen S, Olland S, Berger JM. Structure of the topoisomerase II ATPase region and its mechanism of inhibition by the chemotherapeutic agent ICRF-187. Proc Natl Acad Sci USA 2003;100:10629–10634.

53. Zwelling LA, Michaels S, Kerrigan D, et al. Protein-associated deoxyribonucleic acid strand breaks produced in mouse leukemia L1210 cells by ellipticine and 2-methyl-9- hydroxyellipticinium. Biochem Pharmacol 1982;31:3261–3267.

54. Long BH, Musial ST, Brattain MG. Single- and double-strand DNA breakage and repair in human lung adenocarcinoma cells exposed to etoposide and teniposide. Cancer Res 1985;45:3106–3112.

55. Pommier Y, Orr A, Kohn KW, et al. Differential effects of amsacrine and epipodophyllotoxins on topoisomerase II cleavage in the human c-myc protooncogene. Cancer Res 1992;52:3125–3130.

56. Capranico G, Zunino F, Kohn KW, et al. Sequence-selective topoisomerase II inhibition by anthracycline derivatives in SV40 DNA: relationship with DNA binding affinity and cytotoxicity. Biochemistry 1990;29:562–569.

57. Capranico G, Kohn KW, Pommier Y. Local sequence requirements for DNA cleavage by mammalian topoisomerase II in the presence of doxorubicin. Nucleic Acids Res 1990;18:6611–6619.

58. Capranico G, Binaschi M. DNA sequence selectivity of topoisomerases and topoisomerase poisons. Biochim Biophys Acta 1998;1400:185–194.

59. Pommier Y, Capranico G, Orr A, et al. Local base sequence preferences for DNA cleavage by mammalian topoisomerase II in the presence of amsacrine or teniposide [published erratum appears in Nucleic Acids Res 1991;19:7003]. Nucleic Acids Res 1991;19:5973–5980.

60. Pommier Y, Kohn KW, Capranico G, et al. Base sequence selectivity of topoisomerase inhibitors suggests a common model for drug action. In: Andoh T, Ikeda H, Oguro M, eds. Molecular Biology of DNA Topoisomerases and Its Application to Chemotherapy. Boca Raton, FL: CRC Press, 1993:215–229.

61. Strumberg D, Nitiss JL, Dong J, et al. Importance of the fourth alpha-helix within the CAP homology domain of type II topoisomerase for DNA cleavage site recognition and quinolone action. Antimicrob Agents Chemother 2002;46:2735–2746.

62. Bromberg KD, Burgin AB, Osheroff N. A two-drug model for etoposide action against human topoisomerase IIalpha. J Biol Chem 2003;278:7406–7412.

63. Khan QA, Kohlhagen G, Marshall R, et al. Position-specific trapping of topoisomerase II by benzo[a]pyrene diol epoxide adducts: implications for interactions with intercalating anticancer agents. Proc Natl Acad Sci USA 2003;100:12498–12503.

64. Pommier Y, Cherfils J. Interfacial protein inhibition: a nature's paradigm for drug discovery. Trends Pharmacol Sci. 2005;28:136–145.

65. Gottesman MM, Fojo T, Bates SE. Multidrug resistance in cancer: role of ATP-dependent transporters. Nat Rev Cancer 2002;2:48–58.

66. Solary E, Ling YH, Perez-Soler R, et al. Hydroxyrubicin, a deaminated derivative of doxorubicin, inhibits mammalian DNA topoisomerase II and partially circumvents multidrug resistance. Int J Cancer 1994;58:85–94.

67. Ishikawa T. The ATP-dependent glutathione S-conjugate export pump [see comments]. Trends Biochem Sci 1992;17:463–468.

68. Leteurtre F, Madalengoitia J, Orr A, et al. Rational design and molecular effects of a new topoisomerase II inhibitor, azatoxin [published erratum appears in Cancer Res 1992;52:6136]. Cancer Res 1992;52:4478–4483.

69. Sinha BK, Eliot HM. Etoposide-induced DNA damage in human tumor cells: requirement for cellular activating factors. *Biochim Biophys Acta* 1991;1097:111–116.

70. Auclair C. Multimodal action of antitumor agents on DNA: the ellipticine series. Arch Biochem Biophys 1987;259:1–14.

71. Paoletti C, Le Pecq JB, Dat-Xuong N, et al. Antitumor activity, pharmacology, and toxicity of ellipticines, ellipticinium, and 9-hydroxy derivatives: preliminary clinical trials of 2-methyl-9-hydroxy ellipticinium (NSC 264-137). Recent Results Cancer Res 1980;74:107–123.

72. Zwelling LA, Kerrigan D, Michaels S, et al. Cooperative sequestration of m-AMSA in L1210 cells. Biochem Pharmacol 1982;31:3269–3277.

73. Schuurhuis GJ, Broxterman HJ, Ossenkoppele GJ, et al. Functional multidrug resistance phenotype associated with combined overexpression of Pgp/MDR1 and MRP together with 1-beta-D-arabinofuranosylcytosine sensitivity may predict clinical response in acute myeloid leukemia. Clin Cancer Res 1995;1:81–93.

74. Hsiang YH, Wu HY, Liu LF. Proliferation-dependent regulation of DNA topoisomerase II in cultured human cells. Cancer Res 1988;48:3230–3235.

75. Nelson WG, Cho KR, Hsiang YH, et al. Growth-related elevations of DNA topoisomerase II levels found in Dunning R3327 rat prostatic adenocarcinomas. Cancer Res 1987;47:3246–3250.

76. Turley H, Comley M, Houlbrook S, et al. The distribution and expression of the two isoforms of DNA topoisomerase II in normal and neoplastic human tissues. Br J Cancer 1997;75:1340–1346.

77. Keith WN, Douglas F, Wishart GC, et al. Co-amplification of erbB2, topoisomerase II alpha and retinoic acid receptor alpha genes in breast cancer and allelic loss at topoisomerase I on chromosome 20. Eur J Cancer 1993;10:1469–1475.

78. Nicklee T, Crump M, Hedley DW. Effects of topoisomerase I inhibition on the expression of topoisomerase II alpha measured with fluorescence image cytometry. Cytometry 1996;25:205–210.

79. Sorensen M, Sehested M, Jensen PB. Characterisation of a human small-cell lung cancer cell line resistant to the DNA topoisomerase I-directed drug topotecan. Br J Cancer 1995;72:399–404.

80. Tan KB, Mattern MR, Eng WK, et al. Nonproductive rearrangement of DNA topoisomerase I and II genes: correlation with resistance to topoisomerase inhibitors. J Natl Cancer Inst 1989;81:1732–1735.

81. Sandri MI, Isaacs RJ, Ongkeko WM, et al. p53 regulates the minimal promoter of the human topoisomerase IIalpha gene. Nucleic Acids Res 1996;24:4464–4470.

82. Wang Q, Zambetti GP, Suttle DP. Inhibition of DNA topoisomerase II alpha gene expression by the p53 tumor suppressor. Mol Cell Biol 1997;17:389–397.

83. Yun J, Tomida A, Nagata K, et al. Glucose-regulated stresses confer resistance to VP-16 in human cancer cells through a decreased expression of DNA topoisomerase II. Oncol Res 1995;7:583–590.

84. Teicher BA, Holden SA, Rose CM. Effect of oxygen on the cytotoxicity and antitumor activity of etoposide. J Natl Cancer Inst 1985;75:1129–1133.

85. Hashimoto S, Chatterjee S, Ranjit GB, et al. Drastic reduction of topoisomerase II alpha associated with major acquired resistance to topoisomerase II active agents but minor perturbations of cell growth [published erratum appears in Oncol Res 1995;7:565]. Oncol Res 1995;7:407–416.

86. Feldhoff PW, Mirski SE, Cole SP, et al. Altered subcellular distribution of topoisomerase II alpha in a drug-resistant human small cell lung cancer cell line. Cancer Res 1994;54:756–762.

87. Harker WG, Slade DL, Parr RL, et al. Alterations in the topoisomerase II alpha gene, messenger RNA, and subcellular protein distribution as well as reduced expression of the DNA topoisomerase II beta enzyme in a mitoxantrone-resistant HL-60 human leukemia cell line. Cancer Res 1995;55:1707–1716.

88. Dereuddre S, Frey S, Delaporte C, et al. Cloning and characterization of full-length cDNAs coding for the DNA topoisomerase II beta from Chinese hamster lung cells sensitive and resistant 9-OH-ellipticine. Biochim Biophys Acta 1995;1264:178–182.

89. Wessel I, Jensen PB, Falck J, et al. Loss of amino acids 1490Lys-Ser-Lys1492 in the COOH-terminal region of topoisomerase IIalpha in human small cell lung cancer cells selected for resistance to etoposide results in an extranuclear enzyme localization. Cancer Res 1997;57:4451–4454.

90. Liu Q, Wang JC. Similarity in the catalysis of DNA breakage and rejoining by type IA and IIA DNA topoisomerases. Proc Natl Acad Sci USA 1999;96:881–886.

91. Fass D, Bogden CE, Berger JM. Quaternary changes in topoisomerase II may direct orthogonal movement of two DNA strands. Nat Struct Biol 1999;6:322–326.

92. Matsumoto Y, Takano H, Fojo T. Cellular adaptation to drug exposure: evolution of the drug-resistant phenotype. Cancer Res 1997;57:5086–5092.

93. Ritke MK, Murray NR, Allan WP, et al. Hypophosphorylation of topoisomerase II in etoposide (VP-16)-resistant human leukemia K562 cells associated with reduced levels of beta II protein kinase C. Mol Pharmacol 1995;48:798–805.

94. Ganapathi R, Constantinou A, Kamath N, et al. Resistance to etoposide in human leukemia HL-60 cells: reduction in drug-induced DNA cleavage associated with hypophosphorylation of topoisomerase II phosphopeptides. Mol Pharmacol 1996;50:243–248.

95. Chen M, Beck WT. DNA topoisomerase II expression, stability, and phosphorylation in two VM-26-resistant human leukemic CEM sublines. Oncol Res 1995;7:103–111.

96. Heck MM, Hittelman WN, Earnshaw WC. In vivo phosphorylation of the 170-kDa form of eukaryotic DNA topoisomerase II: cell cycle analysis. J Biol Chem 1989;264:15161–15164.

97. Cardenas ME, Dang Q, Glover CV, et al. Casein kinase II phosphorylates the eukaryote-specific C-terminal domain of topoisomerase II in vivo. EMBO J 1992;11:1785–1796.

98. Ackerman P, Glover CV, Osheroff N. Phosphorylation of DNA topoisomerase II in vivo and in total homogenates of *Drosophila* Kc cells: the role of casein kinase II. J Biol Chem 1988;263:12653–12660.

99. Bojanowski K, Filhol O, Cochet C, et al. DNA topoisomerase II and casein kinase II associate in a molecular complex that is catalytically active. J Biol Chem 1993;268:22920–22926.

100. DeVore RF, Corbett AH, Osheroff N. Phosphorylation of topoisomerase II by casein kinase II and protein kinase C: effects on enzyme-mediated DNA cleavage/religation and sensitivity to the antineoplastic drugs etoposide and 4'-(9- acridinylamino) methane-sulfon-m-anisidide. Cancer Res 1992;52:2156–2161.

101. Pommier Y, Kerrigan D, Hartman KD, et al. Phosphorylation of mammalian DNA topoisomerase I and activation by protein kinase C. J Biol Chem 1990;265:9418–9422.

102. Holm C, Covey JM, Kerrigan D, et al. Differential requirement of DNA replication for the cytotoxicity of DNA topoisomerase I and II inhibitors in Chinese hamster DC3F cells. Cancer Res 1989;49:6365–6368.

103. D'Arpa P, Beardmore C, Liu LF. Involvement of nucleic acid synthesis in cell killing mechanisms of topoisomerase poisons. Cancer Res 1990;50:6919–6924.

104. Kaufmann SH. Antagonism between camptothecin and topoisomerase II-directed chemotherapeutic agents in a human leukemia cell line. Cancer Res 1991;51:1129–1136.

105. Bertrand R, O'Connor PM, Kerrigan D, et al. Sequential administration of camptothecin and etoposide circumvents the antagonistic cytotoxicity of simultaneous drug administration in slowly growing human colon carcinoma HT-29 cells. Eur J Cancer 1992;743–748.

106. Chatterjee S, Cheng MF, Berger NA. Hypersensitivity to clinically useful alkylating agents and radiation in poly(ADP-ribose) polymerase-deficient cell lines. Cancer Commun 1990;2:401–407.

107. Pommier Y, Zwelling LA, Kao-Shan CS, et al. Correlations between intercalator-induced DNA strand breaks and sister

chromatid exchanges, mutations, and cytotoxicity in Chinese hamster cells. Cancer Res 1985;45:3143–3149.

108. Pommier Y, Bertrand R. The mechanism of formation of chromosomal aberrations: role of eukaryotic DNA topoisomerases. In: Kirsch IR, ed. The Causes and Consequences of Chromosomal Aberrations. Boca Raton, FL: CRC Press, 1993:277.

109. Zhu J, Schiestl RH. Topoisomerase I involvement in illegitimate recombination in *Saccharomyces cerevisiae*. Mol Cell Biol 1996; 16:1805–1812.

110. Sordet O, Khan Q, Kohn KW, et al. Apoptosis induced by topoisomerase inhibitors. Curr Med Chem Anticancer Agents 2003;3:271–290.

111. Nitiss J, Wang JC. DNA topoisomerase-targeting antitumor drugs can be studied in yeast. Proc Natl Acad Sci USA 1988;85:7501–7505.

112. Desai SD, Liu LF, Vazquez-Abad D, et al. Ubiquitin-dependent destruction of topoisomerase I is stimulated by the antitumor drug camptothecin. J Biol Chem 1997;272:24159–24164.

113. Goldwasser F, Shimizu T, Jackman J, et al. Correlations between S and G_2 arrest and the cytotoxicity of camptothecin in human colon carcinoma cells. Cancer Res 1996;56:4430–4437.

114. O'Connor PM, Kohn KW. A fundamental role for cell cycle regulation in the chemosensitivity of cancer cells? Semin Cancer Biol 1992;3:409–416.

115. Shao RG, Cao CX, Zhang H, et al. Replication-mediated DNA damage by camptothecin induces phosphorylation of RPA by DNA-dependent protein kinase and dissociates RPA:DNA-PK complexes. EMBO J 1999;18:1397–1406.

116. Gupta M, Fan S, Zhan Q, et al. Inactivation of p53 increases the cytotoxicity of camptothecin in human colon HCT116 and breast MCF-7 cancer cells. Clin Cancer Res 1997;3:1653–1660.

117. Shao RG, Cao CX, Shimizu T, et al. Abrogation of an S-phase checkpoint and potentiation of camptothecin cytotoxicity by 7-hydroxystaurosporine (UCN-01) in human cancer cell lines, possibly influenced by p53 function. Cancer Res 1997;57:4029–4035.

118. Bertrand R, Solary E, Jenkins J, et al. Apoptosis and its modulation in human promyelocytic HL-60 cells treated with DNA topoisomerase I and II inhibitors. Exp Cell Res 1993;207:388–397.

119. Kamesaki S, Kamesaki H, Jorgensen TJ, et al. bcl-2 protein inhibits etoposide-induced apoptosis through its effects on events subsequent to topoisomerase II-induced DNA strand breaks and their repair [published erratum appears in Cancer Res 1994;54:3074]. Cancer Res 1993;53:4251–4256.

120. Henneberry HP, Aherne GW, Marks V. An ELISA for the measurement of VP16 (etoposide) in unextracted plasma. J Immunol Methods 1988;107:205–209.

121. Hande KR, Wedlund PJ, Noone RM, et al. Pharmacokinetics of high-dose etoposide (VP-16-213) administered to cancer patients. Cancer Res 1984;44:379.

122. Rodman JH, Abromowitch M, Sinkule JA, et al. Clinical pharmacodynamics of continuous infusion teniposide: systemic exposure as a determinant of response in a phase I trial. J Clin Oncol 1987;9:1480–1486.

123. D'Incalci M, Farina P, Sessa P, et al. Pharmacokinetics of VP16-213 given by different administration methods. Cancer Chemother Pharmacol 1982;7:141.

124. Henwood J, Brogden R. Etoposide: a review of its pharmacodynamic and pharmacokinetic properties, and therapeutic potential in combination chemotherapy of cancer. Drugs 1990;39:438.

125. Allen L, Creaven P. Comparison of the human pharmacokinetics of VM-26 and VP-16, two antineoplastic epipodophyllotoxin glucopyranoside derivatives. Eur J Cancer 1975;18:697.

126. Smyth RL, Pfeffer M, Scalzo A, et al. Bioavailability and pharmacokinetics of VP-16. Semin Oncol 1985;12:48–51.

127. Stewart CF, Arbuck SG, Fleming RA, et al. Changes in the clearance of total and unbound etoposide in patients with liver dysfunction. J Clin Oncol 1990;8:1874–1879.

128. Stewart CF, Fleming RA, Arbuck SG, et al. Prospective evaluation of a model for predicting etoposide plasma protein binding in cancer patients. Cancer Res 1990;50:6854–6856.

129. Arbuck SG, Douglass HO, Crom WR, et al. Etoposide pharmacokinetics in patients with normal and abnormal organ function. J Clin Oncol 1986;4:1690.

130. D'Incalci M, Rossi C, Zucchetti M, et al. Pharmacokinetics of etoposide in patients with abnormal renal and hepatic function. Cancer Res 1986;46:2566–2571.

131. Holthuis JJ, Postmus PE, Van Oort WJ, et al. Pharmacokinetics of high dose etoposide (VP16-213). Eur J Cancer Clin Oncol 1986;22:1149–1155.

132. Steward DJ, Richard MT, Hugenholtz H, et al. Penetration of VP-16 (etoposide) into human intracerebral and extracerebral tumours. J Neurooncol 1984;2:133.

133. Clark PI, Slevin ML. The clinical pharmacology of etoposide and teniposide. Clin Pharmacokinet 1987;12:223–252.

134. Suzuki S, Koide M, Sakamoto S, et al. Pharmacokinetics of carboplatin and etoposide in a haemodialysis patient with Merckel-cell carcinoma. Nephrol Dial Transplant 1997;12:137–140.

135. Hande KR, Anthony LB, Wolff SN, et al. Etoposide clearance in patients with hepatic dysfunction. Clin Pharmacol Ther 1987;41:161.

136. Stremetzne S, Jaehde U, Schunack W. Determination of the cytotoxic catechol metabolite of etoposide (3'O-demethyletoposide) in human plasma by high-performance liquid chromatography. J Chromatogr B Biomed Sci Appl 1997;703:209–215.

137. Mans DR, Lafleur MV, Westmijze EJ, et al. Formation of different reaction products with single- and double-strand DNA by the *ortho*-quinone and the semi-quinone free radicals of etoposide (VP-16-213). Biochem Pharmacol 1991;43:2131–2139.

138. Mans DR, Lafleur MV, Westmijze EJ, et al. Reactions of glutathione with the catechol, the *ortho*-quinone and the semi-quinone free radical of etoposide: consequences for DNA inactivation. Biochem Pharmacol 1992;43:1761–1768.

139. Hande KR, Wolff SN, Greco A, et al. Etoposide kinetics in patients with obstructive jaundice. J Clin Oncol 1990;8:1101–1107.

140. Perry MC. Hepatotoxicity of chemotherapeutic agents. Semin Oncol 1982;9:65–74.

141. Sekine I, Fukuda H, Kunitoh H, et al. Cancer chemotherapy in the elderly. Jpn J Clin Oncol 1998;28:463–473.

142. Beyer J, Kramar A, Mandanas R, et al. High-dose chemotherapy as salvage treatment in germ cell tumors: a multivariate analysis of prognostic variables. J Clin Oncol 1996;14:2638–2645.

143. Reichman B, Markman M, Hakes T, et al. Intraperitoneal cisplatin and etoposide in the treatment of refractory/recurrent ovarian carcinoma. J Clin Oncol 1988;7:1327–1332.

144. Howell SB, Kirmani S, Lucas WE, et al. A phase II trial of intraperitoneal cisplatin and etoposide for primary treatment of ovarian epithelial cancer. J Clin Oncol 1990;8:137–145.

145. Barakat RR, Almadrones L, Venkatraman ES, et al. A phase II trial of intraperitoneal cisplatin and etoposide as consolidation therapy in patients with stage II–IV epithelial ovarian cancer following negative surgical assessment. Gynecol Oncol 1998;69:17–22.

146. O'Dwyer PJ, LaCreta FP, Daugherty JP, et al. Phase I pharmacokinetic study of intraperitoneal etoposide. Cancer Res 1991;51:2041–2046.

147. O'Dwyer PJ, LaCreta FP, Hogan M, et al. Pharmacologic study of etoposide and cisplatin by the intraperitoneal route. J Clin Pharmacol 1991;31:253–258.

148. Holoye PY, Jeffries DG, Dhingra HM, et al. Intrapleural etoposide for malignant effusion. Cancer Chemother Pharmacol 1990;26:147–150.

149. Jones J, Olman E, Egorin M, et al. A case report and description of the pharmacokinetic behavior of intrapleurally instilled etoposide. Cancer Chemother Pharmacol 1985;14:172–174.

150. Fleischhack G, Reif S, Hasan C, et al. Feasibility of intraventricular administration of etoposide in patients with metastatic brain tumours. Br J Cancer 2001;84:1453–1459.

151. Gaast AV, Sonneveld P, Mans DR, et al. Intrathecal administration of etoposide in the treatment of malignant meningitis: feasibility and pharmacokinetic data. Cancer Chemother Pharmacol 1992;29:335–337.

152. Savaraj N, Feun LG, Lu K, et al. Clinical pharmacology of intracarotid etoposide. Cancer Chemother Pharmacol 1986;16:292–294.

153. Tanase K, Tawada M, Moriyama N, et al. Intra-arterial infusion chemotherapy for liver metastases of testicular tumors: report of two cases. Hinyokika Kiyo 2000;46:823–827.

154. Toffoli G, Corona G, Basso B, et al. Pharmacokinetic optimisation of treatment with oral etoposide. Clin Pharmacokinet 2004; 43:441–466.

155. Steward DJ, Nundy D, Maroun JA, et al. Bioavailability, pharmacokinetics, and clinical effects of an oral preparation of etoposide. Cancer Treat Rep 1985;69:269–273.

156. Brunner KW, Sonntag RW, Ryssel HJ, et al. Comparison of the biologic activity of VP16-213 given IV and orally in capsules or drink ampoules. Cancer Treat Rep 1976;60:1377.

157. Slevin ML, Joel SP, Whomsley R, et al. The effect of dose on the bioavailability of oral etoposide: confirmation of a clinically relevant observation. Cancer Chemother Pharmacol 1989;24:329–331.

158. van der Gast A, Vlastuin M, Kok T, et al. What is the optimal dose and duration of treatment with etoposide? II: comparative pharmacokinetic study of three schedules: 1×100 mg, 2×50 mg, and 4×25 mg of oral etoposide daily for 21 days. Semin Oncol 1992; 19:8–12.

159. Hande KR, Krozely MG, Greco A, et al. Bioavailability of low-dose oral etoposide. J Clin Oncol 1993;11:374–377.

160. Harvey VJ, Slevin ML, Joel SP, et al. The effect of food and concurrent chemotherapy on the bioavailability of oral etoposide. Br J Cancer 1985;52:363–367.

161. Harvey VJ, Slevin ML, Joel SP, et al. The effect of dose on the bioavailability of oral etoposide. Cancer Chemother Pharmacol 1986;16:178–181.

162. Splinter TAW, Holthuis JJM, Kok TC, et al. Absolute bioavailability and pharmacokinetics of oral teniposide. Semin Oncol 1992;19:28–34.

163. Stahelin HF, von Wartburg A. The chemical and biological route from podophyllotoxin glucoside to etoposide: Ninth Cain Memorial Award. Cancer Res 1991;51:5–15.

164. Huang JD, Leu BL, Lai MD. Induction and inhibition of intestinal P-glycoprotein and effects on etoposide. Proc Am Assoc Cancer Res 1994;35:353.

165. Miller AA, Tolley EA, Niell HB. Therapeutic drug monitoring of 21-day oral etoposide in patients with advanced non-small cell lung cancer. Clin Cancer Res 1998;4:1705–1710.

166. Westeel V, Murray N, Gelmon K, et al. New combination of the old drugs for elderly patients with small-cell lung cancer: a phase II study of the PAVE regimen. J Clin Oncol 1998;16:1940–1947.

167. Souhami RL, Spiro SG, Rudd RM, et al. Five-day oral etoposide treatment for advanced small-cell lung cancer: randomized comparison with intravenous chemotherapy. J Natl Cancer Inst 1997;89:577–580.

168. Budman DR, Igwemezie LN, Kaul S, et al. Phase I evaluation of a water-soluble etoposide prodrug, etoposide phosphate, given as a 5-minute infusion on days 1, 3, and 5 in patients with solid tumors. J Clin Oncol 1994;12:1902–1909.

169. Fields SZ, Igwemezie LN, Kaul S, et al. Phase I study of etoposide phosphate (Etopophos) as a 30-minute infusion on days 1, 3, and 5. Clin Cancer Res 1995;1:105–111.

170. Millward MJ, Newell DR, Mummaneni V, et al. Phase I and pharmacokinetic study of a water-soluble etoposide prodrug, etoposide phosphate (BMY-40481). Eur J Cancer 1995;31A:2409–2411.

171. Kaul S, Igwemezie LN, Steward DJ, et al. Pharmacokinetics and bioequivalence of etoposide following intravenous administration of etoposide phosphate and etoposide in patients with solid tumors. J Clin Oncol 1995;13:2835–2841.

172. Sessa C, Zucchetti M, Cerny T, et al. Phase I clinical and pharmacokinetic study of oral etoposide phosphate. J Clin Oncol 1995; 13:200–209.

173. de Jong RS, Mulder NH, Uges DR, et al. Randomized comparison of etoposide pharmacokinetics after oral etoposide phosphate and oral etoposide. Br J Cancer 1997;75:1660–1666.

174. Smit EF, Splinter TAW, Kok TC. A phase I study of daily oral teniposide for 20 days. Semin Oncol 1992;19:40–42.

175. Mick R, Rarain MJ. Modeling interpatient pharmacodynamic variability of etoposide. J Natl Cancer Inst 1991;83:1560–1564.

176. Ratain MJ, Mick R, Schilsky RL, et al. Pharmacologically based dosing of etoposide: a means of safely increasing dose intensity. J Clin Oncol 1991;9:1480–1486.

177. Stewart CF, Arbuck SG, Fleming RA, et al. Relation of systemic exposure to unbound etoposide and hematologic toxicity. Clin Pharmacol Ther 1991;50:385–393.

178. Pfuger K-H, Hahn M, Holz J-B, et al. Pharmacokinetics of etoposide: correlation of pharmacokinetic parameters with clinical conditions. Cancer Chemother Pharmacol 1993;31:350–356.

179. Gentili D, Zucchetti M, Torri V, et al. A limited-sampling model for the pharmacokinetics of etoposide given orally. Cancer Chemother Pharmacol 1993;32:482–486.

180. Lum BL, Lane KJ, Synold TW, et al. Validation of a limited sampling model to determine etoposide area under the curve. Pharmacotherapy 1997;17:887–890.

181. O'Dwyer P, Weiss R. Hypersensitivity reactions induced by etoposide. Cancer Treat Rep 1984;68:959–961.

182. Karnaoukhova L, Moffat J, Martins H, et al. Mutation frequency and spectrum in lymphocytes of small cell lung cancer patients receiving etoposide chemotherapy. Cancer Res 1997;57: 4393–4407.

183. Smith MA, Rubinstein L, Cazenave L, et al. Report of the cancer-therapy evaluation program monitoring plan for secondary acute myeloid-leukemia following treatment with epipodophyllotoxins. J Natl Cancer Inst 1993;85:554–558.

184. Smith MA, Rubinstein L, Ungerleider RS. Therapy-related acute myeloid leukemia following treatment with epipodophyllotoxins: estimating the risks. Med Pediatr Oncol 1994;23:86–98.

185. Smith MA, McCaffrey RP, Karp JE. The secondary leukemias: challenges and research directions. J Natl Cancer Inst 1996; 88:407–418.

186. Smith MA, Rubinstein L, Anderson JR, et al. Secondary leukemia or myelodysplastic syndrome after treatment with epipodophyllotoxins. J Clin Oncol 1999;17:569–577.

187. Detourmignies L, Castaigne S, Stoppa AM, et al. Therapy-related acute promyelocytic leukemia: a report on 16 cases. J Clin Oncol 1992;10:1430–1435.

188. Fenaux P, Lucidarme D, Lai J-L, et al. Favorable cytogenetic abnormalities in secondary leukemia. Cancer 1989;63:2505–2508.

189. Kapoor G, Kadam PR, Chougule A, et al. Secondary ANLL with t(11;19)(q23;p13) following etoposide and cisplatin for ovarian germ cell tumor. Indian J Cancer 1997;34:84–87.

190. Takeda K, Shinohara K, Kameda N, et al. A case of therapy-related acute myeloblastic leukemia with t(16;21)(q24;q22) after chemotherapy with DNA-topoisomerase II inhibitors, etoposide and mitoxantrone, and the alkylating agent, cyclophosphamide. Int J Hematol 1998;67:179–186.

191. Yagita M, Ieki Y, Onishi R, et al. Therapy-related leukemia and myelodysplasia following oral administration of etoposide for recurrent breast cancer. Int J Oncol 1998;13:91–96.

192. Pui CH, Relling MV, Behm FG, et al. L-asparaginase may potentiate the leukemogenic effect of the epipodophyllotoxins. Leukemia 1995;9:1680–1684.

193. Nichols CR, Breeden ES, Loehrer PJ, et al. Secondary leukemia associated with a conventional dose of etoposide: review of serial germ-cell tumor protocols. J Natl Cancer Inst 1993;85:36–40.

194. Ratain MJ, Kaminer LS, Bitran JD, et al. Acute nonlymphocytic leukemia following etoposide and cisplatin combination chemotherapy for advanced non-small-cell carcinoma of the lung. Blood 1987;70:1412–1417.

195. Pedersen-Bjergaard J, Daugaard G, Hansen SW, et al. Increased risk of myelodysplasia and leukaemia after etoposide, cisplatin, and bleomycin for germ-cell tumours. Lancet 1991;338:359–363.

196. Pui CH, Ribeiro RC, Hancock ML, et al. Acute myeloid leukemia in children treated with epipodophyllotoxins for acute lymphoblastic leukemia. N Engl J Med 1991;325:1682–1687.

197. Le Deley MC, Leblanc T, Shamsaldin A, et al. Risk of secondary leukemia after a solid tumor in childhood according to the dose of epipodophyllotoxins and anthracyclines: a case-control study by the Societe Francaise d'Oncologie Pediatrique. J Clin Oncol 2003;21:1074–1081.

198. Lovett BD, Blair IA, Pang S, et al. Etoposide metabolites enhance DNA topoisomerase II cleavage proximal to leukemia-associated *MLL* translocation breakpoints [abstract]. Proc Am Assoc Cancer Res 1999;40. Abstract 4506.

199. Pedersen-Bjergaard J, Sigsgaard TC, Nielsen D, et al. Acute monocytic or myelomonocytic leukemia with balanced chromosome translocations to band 11q23 after therapy with 4-epi-doxorubicin and cisplatin or cyclophosphamide for breast cancer. J Clin Oncol 1992;10:1444–1451.

200. Pedersen-Bjergaard J, Rowley JD. The balanced and unbalanced chromosome aberrations of acute myeloid leukemia may develop in different ways and may contribute differently to malignant transformation. Blood 1994;83:2780–2786.

201. Pedersen-Bjergaard J, Pedersen M, Roulston D, et al. Different genetic pathways in leukemogenesis for patients presenting with therapy-related myelodysplasia and therapy-related acute myeloid leukemia. Blood 1995;86:3542–3552.

202. Nasr F, Macintyre E, Venuat A-M, et al. Translocation t(4;11) (q21;q23) and *MLL* gene rearrangement in acute lymphoblastic leukemia secondary to anti topoisomerase II anticancer agents. Leuk Lymphoma 1997;25:399–401.

203. Pommier Y, Cockerill PN, Kohn KW, et al. Identification within the simian virus 40 genome of a chromosomal loop attachment site that contains topoisomerase II cleavage sites. J Virol 1990;64: 419–423.

204. D'Andrea MR, Farber PA, Foglesong PD. Immunohistochemical detection of DNA topoisomerases IIa and IIb compared with detection of Ki-67, a marker of cellular proliferation in human tumors. Appl Immunohistochem 1994;2:177–185.

205. Kreipe H, Alm P, Olsson H, et al. Prognostic significance of a formalin-resistant nuclear proliferation antigen in mammary carcinomas as determined by the monoclonal antibody Ki-S1. Am J Pathol 1993;142:651–657.

206. Holden JA, Perkins SL, Snow GW, et al. Immunohistochemical staining for DNA topoisomerase II in non-Hodgkin's lymphomas. Am J Clin Pathol 1995;104:54–59.

207. Guinee DG, Holden JA, Benfield JR, et al. Comparison of DNA topoisomerase IIa expression in small cell and nonsmall cell carcinoma of the lung: in search of a mechanism of chemotherapeutic response. Cancer 1996;78:729–735.

208. Sandri MI, Hochhauser D, Ayton RC, et al. Differential expression of the topoisomerase IIalpha and beta genes in human breast cancers. Br J Cancer 1996;73:1518–1524.

209. Kaufmann SH, Karp JE, Jones RJ, et al. Topoisomerase II levels and drug sensitivity in adult acute myelogeneous leukemia. Blood 1994;83:517–530.

210. Kaufmann SH, Karp JE, Burke PJ, et al. Addition of etoposide to initial therapy of adult acute lymphoblastic leukemia: a combined clinical and laboratory study. Leuk Lymphoma 1996;23: 71–83.

211. Jarvinen TA, Holli K, Kuukasjarvi T, et al. Predictive value of topoisomerase IIalpha and other prognostic factors for epirubicin chemotherapy in advanced breast cancer. Br J Cancer 1998;77:2267–2273.

212. Petit T, Wilt M, Velten M, et al. Comparative value of tumour grade, hormonal receptors, Ki-67, HER-2 and topoisomerase II alpha status as predictive markers in breast cancer patients treated with neoadjuvant anthracycline-based chemotherapy. Eur J Cancer 2004;40:205–211.

213. Braybrooke JP, Levitt NC, Joel S, et al. Pharmacokinetic study of cisplatin and infusional etoposide phosphate in advanced breast cancer with correlation of response to topoisomerase IIalpha expression. Clin Cancer Res 2003;9:4682–4688.

214. Hall SW, Friedman J, Legha S, et al. Human pharmacokinetics of a new acridine derivative, 4'-(9-acridinylamino)methanesulfon-*m*-anisidide (NSC 249992). Cancer Res 1983;43:3422.

215. Cassileth PA, Gale RP. Amsacrine: a review. Leuk Res 1986; 10:1257–1265.

216. Legha SS, Keating MJ, McCredie KB, et al. Evaluation of AMSA in previously treated patients with acute leukemia: results of therapy in 109 adults. Blood 1982;60:484–490.

217. Meloni G, De Fabritis P, Petti MC. BAVC regimen and autologous bone marrow transplantation in patients with acute myelogenous leukemia in second remission. Blood 1990;75:2282–2285.

218. Berman E, Arlin ZA, Gaynor J, et al. Comparative trial of cytarabine and thioguanine in combination with amsacrine or daunorubicin in patients with untreated acute nonlymphocytic leukemia: results of the L-16M protocol. Leukemia 1989;3:115–121.

219. Arlin ZA, Sklaroff RB, Gee TS, et al. Phase I and II trial of 4'-(9-acridinylamino)-methanesulfon-*m*-anisidide in patients with acute leukemia. Cancer Res 1980;40:3304–3306.

220. Applebaum F, Schulman H. Fatal hepatotoxicity associated with AMSA therapy. Cancer Treat Rep 1982;66:1863.

221. Louie AC, Issel BF. Amsacrine (AMSA): a clinical review. J Clin Oncol 1985;3:562–592.

222. Weiss RB, Moquin D, Adams JD, et al. Electrocardiogram abnormalities induced by amsacrine. Cancer Chemother Pharmacol 1983;10:133–134.

223. Weiss RB, Grillo-Lopez AJ, Marsoni S, et al. Amsacrine-associated cardiotoxicity: an analysis of 82 cases. J Clin Oncol 1986;4:918–928.

224. Weiss RB. Hypersensitivity reactions. Semin Oncol 1992;19: 458–477.

225. Seymour JF. Induction of hypomagnesemia during amsacrine treatment. Am J Hematol 1993;42:262–267.

226. Arlin ZA, Feldman EJ, Mittelman A, et al. Amsacrine is safe and effective therapy for patients with myocardial dysfunction and acute leukemia. Cancer 1991;68:1198–1200.

227. Schwartz C, Bender K, Burke P, et al. QT interval prolongation and cardiac dysrhythmia in a patient receiving amsacrine. Cancer Treat Rep 1984;68:1043–1044.

228. Shinar E, Hasin Y. Acute electrocardiographic changes induced by amsacrine. Cancer Treat Rep 1984;68:1169–1172.

229. Tzivoni D, Keren A. Suppression of ventricular arrhythmias by magnesium. Am J Cardiol 1990;65:1397–1399.

230. da Cunha MF, Meistrich MF, Haq MM, et al. Temporary effects of AMSA chemotherapy on spermatogenesis. Cancer 1982;49: 2459–2462.

231. Dittrich C, Dieras V, Kerbrat P, et al. Phase II study of XR5000 (DACA), an inhibitor of topoisomerase I and II, administered as a 120-h infusion in patients with advanced ovarian cancer. Invest New Drugs 2003;21:347–352.

232. Dittrich C, Coudert B, Paz-Ares L, et al. Phase II study of XR 5000 (DACA), an inhibitor of topoisomerase I and II, administered as a 120-h infusion in patients with non-small cell lung cancer. Eur J Cancer 2003;39:330–334.

233. Matsui K, Masuda N, Fukuoka M, et al. Phase II trial of carboplatin plus oral etoposide for elderly patients with small-cell lung cancer. Br J Cancer 1998;77:1961–1965.

234. Eder JP, Teicher BA, Holden SA, et al. Ability of four potential topoisomerase II inhibitors to enhance the cytotoxicity of cis-diaminedichloroplatinum (II) in Chinese hamster ovary cells and in epipodophyllotoxin-resistant subline. Cancer Chemother Pharmacol 1990;26:423–428.

235. Nemati F, Livartowski A, De Cremoux P, et al. Distinctive potentiating effects of cisplatin and/or ifosfamide combined with etoposide in human small cell lung carcinoma xenografts. Clin Cancer Res 2000;6:2075–2086.

236. Thomas HD, Porter DJ, Bartelink I, et al. Randomized cross-over clinical trial to study potential pharmacokinetic interactions between cisplatin or carboplatin and etoposide. Br J Clin Pharmacol 2002;53:83–91.

237. Relling M, McLeod H, Bowman L, et al. Etoposide pharmacokinetics and pharmacodynamics after acute and chronic exposure to cisplatin. Clin Pharmacol Ther 1994;56:503–511.

238. Rodman J, Murry D, Madden T, et al. Altered etoposide pharmacokinetics and time to engraftment in pediatric patients undergoing autologous bone marrow transplantation. J Clin Oncol 1994;12:2390–2397.

239. Edelman MJ, Chansky K, Gaspar LE, et al. Phase II trial of cisplatin/etoposide and concurrent radiotherapy followed by paclitaxel/carboplatin consolidation for limited small-cell lung cancer: Southwest Oncology Group 9713. J Clin Oncol 2004;22:127–132.

240. Eder JP, Chan V, Wong J, et al. Sequence effect of irinotecan (CPT-11) and topoisomerase II inhibitors in vivo. Cancer Chemother Pharmacol 1998;42:327–335.

241. Whitacre CM, Zborowska E, Gordon NH, et al. Topotecan increases topoisomerase IIalpha levels and sensitivity to treatment with etoposide in schedule-dependent process. Cancer Res 1997;57:1425–1428.

242. Pommier Y, Pourquier P, Fan Y, et al. Mechanism of action of eukaryotic DNA topoisomerase I and drugs targeted to the enzyme. Biochim Biophys Acta 1998;1400:83–105.

243. Ohtsu T, Sasaki Y, Igarashi T, et al. Unexpected hepatotoxicities in patients with non-Hodgkin's lymphoma treated with irinotecan (CPT-11) and etoposide. Jpn J Clin Oncol 1998;28:502–506.

244. Masuda N, Fukuoka M, Kudoh S, et al. Phase I and pharmacologic study of irinotecan and etoposide with recombinant

human granulocyte colony-stimulating factor support for advanced lung cancer. J Clin Oncol 1994;9:1833–1841.

245. Karato A, Yatsuma S, Shinkai T, et al. Phase I study of CPT-11 and etoposide in patients with refractory solid tumors. J Clin Oncol 1993;11:2030–2035.

246. Clark PI, Sutton P, Smith DB, et al. A phase I study of a 5 day schedule of intravenous topotecan and etoposide in untreated small cell lung cancer [abstract]. Proc Annu Meet Am Soc Clin Oncol 1999;18. Abstract 1926.

247. Nakamura S, Kudoh S, Komuta K, et al. Phase II study of irinotecan combined with etoposide for previously untreated extensive-disease small-cell lung cancer: a study of the West Japan Lung Cancer Group [abstract]. Proc Annu Meet Am Soc Clin Oncol 1999;18. Abstract 1815.

248. Oshita F, Noda K, Nishiwaki Y, et al. Phase II study of irinotecan and etoposide in patients with metastatic non-small-cell lung cancer. J Clin Oncol 1997;15:304–309.

249. Hammond LA, Eckardt JR, Ganapathi R, et al. A phase I and translational study of sequential administration of the topoisomerase I and II inhibitors topotecan and etoposide. Clin Cancer Res 1998;4:1459–1467.

250. Herben VM, ten Bokkel Huinink WW, Dubbelman AC, et al. Phase I and pharmacological study of sequential intravenous topotecan and oral etoposide. Br J Cancer 1997;76:1500–1508.

251. Aisner J, Musanti R, Beers S, et al. Sequencing topotecan and etoposide plus cisplatin to overcome topoisomerase I and II resistance: a pharmacodynamically based phase I trial. Clin Cancer Res 2003;9:2504–2509.

252. Licitra EJ, Vyas V, Nelson K, et al. Phase I evaluation of sequential topoisomerase targeting with irinotecan/cisplatin followed by etoposide in patients with advanced malignancy. Clin Cancer Res 2003;9:1673–1679.

253. Seiden MV, Ng SW, Supko JG, et al. A phase I clinical trial of sequentially administered doxorubicin and topotecan in refractory solid tumors. Clin Cancer Res 2002;8:691–697.

254. Mok TS, Wong H, Zee B, et al. A Phase I-II study of sequential administration of topotecan and oral etoposide (topoisomerase I and II inhibitors) in the treatment of patients with small cell lung carcinoma. Cancer 2002;95:1511–1519.

255. Wahlin A, Brinch L, Hornsten P, et al. Outcome of a multicenter treatment program including autologous or allogeneic bone marrow transplantation for de novo acute myeloid leukemia. Eur J Haematol 1997;58:233–240.

256. Schroeder PE, Hofland KF, Jensen PB, et al. Pharmacokinetics of etoposide in cancer patients treated with high-dose etoposide and with dexrazoxane (ICRF-187) as a rescue agent. Cancer Chemother Pharmacol 2004;53:91–93.

257. Tjan-Heijnen VC, Biesma B, Festen J, et al. Enhanced myelotoxicity due to granulocyte colony-stimulating factor administration until 48 hours before the next chemotherapy course in patients with small-cell lung carcinoma. J Clin Oncol 1998;16:2708–2714.

258. Vecht CJ, Wagner GL, Wilms EB. Interactions between antiepileptic and chemotherapeutic drugs. Lancet Neurol 2003;2:404–409.

259. Le AT, Hasson NK, Lum BL. Enhancement of warfarin response in a patient receiving etoposide and carboplatin chemotherapy. Ann Pharmacother 1997;31:1006–1008.

260. Kim JC, Yoon JB, Koo HS, et al. Cloning and characterization of the 5′-flanking region for the human topoisomerase III gene [In Process Citation]. J Biol Chem 1998;273:26130–26137.

261. Meng L-H, Liao Z-H, Pommier Y. Non-camptothecin DNA topoisomerase I inhibitors in cancer chemotherapy. Curr Topics Med Chem 2003;3:305–320.

262. Errington F, Willmore E, Tilby MJ, et al. Murine transgenic cells lacking DNA topoisomerase IIbeta are resistant to acridines and mitoxantrone: analysis of cytotoxicity and cleavable complex formation. Mol Pharmacol 1999;56:1309–1316.

263. Zhang H, Barcelo JM, Lee B, et al. Human mitochondrial topoisomerase I. Proc Natl Acad Sci USA 2001;98:10608–10613.

264. Gogas H, Mansi JL. New drugs: the anthrapyrazoles. Cancer Treat Rev 1996;21:541–552.

265. Taguchi T, Ohta K, Hotta T, et al. Menogaril (TUT-7) late phase II study for malignant lymphoma, adult T- cell leukemia and lymphoma (ATLL) [in Japanese]. Gan To Kagaku Ryoho 1997;24:1263–1271.

266. Poddevin B, Riou JF, Lavelle F, et al. Dual topoisomerase I and II inhibition by intoplicine (RP-60475), a new antitumor agent in early clinical trials. Mol Pharmacol 1993;44:767–774.

267. Yamashita Y, Kawada S, Fujii N, et al. Induction of mammalian DNA topoisomerase I and II mediated DNA cleavage by saintopin, a new antitumor agent from fungus. Biochemistry 1991;30:5838–5845.

268. Nitiss JL, Zhou J, Rose A, et al. The bis(naphthalimide) DMP-840 causes cytotoxicity by its action against eukaryotic topoisomerase II. Biochemistry 1998;37:3078–3085.

269. Leteurtre F, Kohlhagen G, Pommier Y. Streptonigrin-induced topoisomerase II sites exhibit base preference in the middle of the enzyme stagger. Biochem Biophys Res Commun 1994;203:1259–1267.

270. Capranico G, Palumbo M, Tinelli S, et al. Unique sequence specificity of topoisomerase II DNA cleavage stimulation and DNA binding mode of streptonigrin. J Biol Chem 1994;40:25004–25009.

271. Fujii N, Yamashita Y, Saitoh Y, et al. Induction of mammalian DNA topoisomerase I-mediated DNA cleavage and DNA winding by bulgarein. J Biol Chem 1993;268:13160–13165.

272. Matsumoto SS, Haughey HM, Schmehl DM, et al. Makaluvamines vary in ability to induce dose-dependent DNA cleavage via topoisomerase II interaction [In Process Citation]. Anticancer Drugs 1999;10:39–45.

273. Rowe T, Kupfer G, Ross W. Inhibition of epipodophyllotoxin cytotoxicity by interference with topoisomerase-mediated DNA cleavage. Biochem Pharmacol 1985;34:2483–2487.

274. Kong XB, Rubin L, Chen LI, et al. Topoisomerase II-mediated DNA cleavage activity and irreversibility of cleavable complex formation induced by DNA intercalator with alkylating capability. Mol Pharmacol 1992;41:237–244.

275. Hernandez L, Cholody WM, Hudson EA, et al. Mechanism of action of bisimidazoacridones, new drugs with potent, selective activity against colon cancer. Cancer Res 1995;55:2338–2345.

276. Markovits J, Pommier Y, Mattern MR, et al. Effects of the bifunctional antitumor intercalator ditercalinium on DNA in mouse leukemia L1210 cells and DNA topoisomerase II. Cancer Res 1986;46:5821–5826.

277. Zagotto G, Oliva A, Guano F, et al. Synthesis, DNA-damaging and cytotoxic properties of novel topoisomerase II-directed bisantrene analogues. Bioorg Med Chem Lett 1998;8:121–126.

278. Long BH, Musial ST, Brattain MG. Comparison of cytotoxicity and DNA breakage activity of congeners of podophyllotoxin including VP16-213 and VM26: a quantitative structure-activity relationship. Biochemistry 1984;23:1183–1188.

279. Kerrigan D, Pommier Y, Kohn KW. Protein-linked DNA strand breaks produced by etoposide and teniposide in mouse L1210 and human VA-13 and HT-29 cell lines: relationship to cytotoxicity. NCI Monogr 1987;4:117–121.

280. Hande KR. Etoposide: four decades of development of a topoisomerase II inhibitor. Eur J Cancer 1998;34:1514–1521.

281. Fesen M, Pommier Y. Mammalian topoisomerase II activity is modulated by the DNA minor groove binder distamycin in simian virus 40 DNA. J Biol Chem 1989;264:11354–11359.

282. Riou JF, Helissey P, Grondard L, et al. Inhibition of eukaryotic DNA topoisomerase I and II activities by indoloquinolinedione derivatives. Mol Pharmacol 1991;40:699–706.

283. Fortune JM, Osheroff N. Merbarone inhibits the catalytic activity of human topoisomerase IIalpha by blocking DNA cleavage. J Biol Chem 1998;273:17643–17650.

284. Constantinou A, Mehta R, Runyan C, et al. Flavonoids as DNA topoisomerase antagonists and poisons: structure-activity relationships. J Nat Prod 1995;58:217–225.

285. McCabe MJ Jr, Orrenius S. Genistein induces apoptosis in immature human thymocytes by inhibiting topoisomerase-II. Biochem Biophys Res Commun 1993;194:944–950.

286. Bojanowski K, Lelievre S, Markovits J, et al. Suramin is an inhibitor of DNA topoisomerase II in vitro and in Chinese hamster fibrosarcoma cells. Proc Natl Acad Sci USA 1992;89:3025–3029.

287. Sorensen BS, Jensen PS, Andersen AH, et al. Stimulation of topoisomerase II mediated DNA cleavage at specific sequence

elements by the 2-nitroimidazole Ro 15-0216. Biochemistry 1990;29:9507–9515.

288. Utsumi H, Shibuya ML, Kosaka T, et al. Abrogation by novo-biocin of cytotoxicity due to the topoisomerase II inhibitor amsacrine in Chinese hamster cells. Cancer Res 1990;50: 2577–2581.

289. Kawada S, Yamashita Y, Fujii N, et al. Induction of a heat-stable topoisomerase II-DNA cleavable complex by nonintercalative terpenoides, terpentecin and clerocidin. Cancer Res 1991;51: 2922–2925.

290. Chen M, Beck WT. Teniposide-resistant CEM cells, which express mutant DNA topoisomerase II alpha, when treated with non-complex-stabilizing inhibitors of the enzyme, display no cross-resistance and reveal aberrant functions of the mutant enzyme. Cancer Res 1993;53:5946–5953.

291. Fujii N, Yamashita Y, Arima Y, et al. Induction of topoisomerase II-mediated DNA cleavage by the plant naphthoquinones plumbagin and shikonin. Antimicrob Agents Chemother 1992; 36:2589–2594.

292. Gedik CM, Collins AR. Comparison of effects of fostriecin, novo-biocin, and camptothecin, inhibitors of DNA topoisomerases, on DNA replication and repair in human cells. Nucleic Acids Res 1990;18:1007–1013.

293. Juang JK, Huang HW, Chen CM, et al. A new compound, with-angulatin A, promotes type II DNA topoisomerase-mediated DNA damage. Biochem Biophys Res Commun 1989;159: 1128–1134.

294. Holm B, Jensen PB, Sehested M, et al. In vivo inhibition of etoposide-mediated apoptosis, toxicity, and antitumor effect by the topoisomerase II-uncoupling anthracycline aclarubicin. Cancer Chemother Pharmacol 1994;34:503–508.

295. Fujii N, Tanaka F, Yamashita Y, et al. UCE6, a new antitumor antibiotic with topoisomerase I-mediated DNA cleavage activity produced by actinomycetes: producing organism, fermentation, isolation and biological activity. J Antibiot (Tokyo) 1997;50: 490–495.

296. Permana PA, Snapka RM, Shen LL, et al. Quinobenoxazines: a class of novel antitumor quinolones and potent mammalian DNA topoisomerase II catalytic inhibitors. Biochemistry 1994; 33:11333–11339.

297. Robinson MJ, Martin BA, Gootz TD, et al. Effects of novel fluoro-quinolones on the catalytic activities of eukaryotic topoisomerase II: influence of the C-8 fluorine group. Antimicrob Agents Chemother 1992;36:751–756.

298. Leteurtre F, Sackett DL, Madalengoitia J, et al. Azatoxin deriva-tives with potent and selective action on topoisomerase II. Biochem Pharmacol 1995;49:1283–1290.

299. Campain JA, Gottesman MM, Pastan I. A novel mutant topoisomerase II alpha present in VP-16-resistant human melanoma cell lines has a deletion of alanine 429. Biochemistry 1994;33: 11327–11332.

300. Bugg BY, Danks MK, Beck WT, et al. Expression of a mutant DNA topoisomerase II in CCRF-CEM human leukemic cells selected for resistance to teniposide. Proc Natl Acad Sci USA 1991;88: 7654–7658.

301. Lee MS, Wang JC, Beran M. Two independent amsacrine-resis-tant human myeloid leukemia cell lines share an identical point mutation in the 170 kDa form of human topoisomerase II. J Mol Biol 1992;223:837–843.

302. Chan VT, Ng SW, Eder JP, et al. Molecular cloning and identifica-tion of a point mutation in the topoisomerase II cDNA from an etoposide-resistant Chinese hamster ovary cell line. J Biol Chem 1993;268:2160–2165.

303. Kubo A, Yoshikawa A, Hirashima T, et al. Point mutations of the topoisomerase IIalpha gene in patients with small cell lung can-cer treated with etoposide. Cancer Res 1996;56:1232–1236.

304. Patel S, Fisher LM. Novel selection and genetic characterisation of an etoposide-resistant human leukaemic CCRF-CEM cell line. Br J Cancer 1993;67:456–463.

305. Danks MK, Warmoth MR, Friche E, et al. Single-strand confor-mational polymorphism analysis of the M(r) 170,000 isozyme of DNA topoisomerase II in human tumor cells. Cancer Res 1993;53:1373–1379.

306. Hashimoto S, Danks MK, Chatterjee S, et al. A novel point muta-tion in the 3′ flanking region of the DNA-binding domain of topoisomerase II alpha associated with acquired resistance to topoisomerase II active agents. Oncol Res 1995;7:21–29.

307. Kohno K, Danks MK, Matsuda T, et al. A novel mutation of DNA topoisomerase II alpha in an etoposide-resistant human cancer cell line. Cellular Pharmacol 1995;2:87–90.

Asparaginase

20

Bruce A. Chabner   *Alison M. Friedmann*

The growth of malignant as well as normal cells depends on the availability of specific nutrients and cofactors used in protein synthesis. Some of these nutrients can be synthesized within the cell, but others such as essential amino acids are required from external sources. Nutritional therapy for cancer has been directed at identifying differences between the host and malignant cells that might be exploited in treatment; these attempts have been largely unsuccessful because of difficulties in producing a deficiency state by dietary means and a lack of clear differences in the nutritional requirements of rapidly proliferating host cells and the tumor. The only exception has been the use of L-asparaginase in the treatment of childhood acute leukemia.

L-Asparagine is a nonessential amino acid synthesized by transamination of L-aspartic acid (Fig. 20.1). The amine group is donated by glutamine, and the reaction is catalyzed by the enzyme L-asparagine synthetase. This enzyme is constitutive in many tissues, which accounts for the modest toxicity of asparagine depletion from the plasma, but the capacity to synthesize asparagine is lacking in certain human malignancies, particularly those of lymphocytic derivation. In tumor cells lacking L-asparagine synthetase, such as L5178Y murine leukemia cells,[1] the amino acid can be obtained only from a culture medium or, in vivo, from plasma.

The enzyme L-ASP (L-asparagine amidohydrolase, EC 3.5.1.1), which catalyzes the hydrolysis of asparagine to aspartic acid and ammonia as end products, is found in many plants and microorganisms and in the plasma of certain animals. General interest in L-ASP as a therapeutic agent was the result of an unexplained observation by Kidd,[2] who in 1953 reported that the growth of transplantable lymphomas in rodents was inhibited by guinea pig serum but not by rabbit, horse, or human serum. Ten years later, Broome[3] demonstrated that the responsible factor was the enzyme L-ASP. Subsequently, highly purified preparations of enzyme from *Escherichia coli*[4] and *Erwinia carotovora* (also known as *Erwinia chrysanthemi*)[5] showed significant activity against childhood acute lymphocytic leukemia (ALL) and have become standard components of remission induction, consolidation, and reinduction therapy in this disease and in adult ALL, contributing to the 80% or greater 5-year disease-free survival in childhood ALL and 35 to the 50% 5-year disease-free survival in adult ALL.[6] A chemically modified enzyme, pegaspargase, having a longer half-life and reduced immunogenicity, is approved for use in patients hypersensitive to the native *E. coli* enzyme. Pegaspargase is being used increasingly in pediatric ALL regimens because it has a significantly lower incidence of allergic reactions and reduces the frequency of painful intramuscular injections for the child. The clinical and biochemical features of L-ASP chemotherapy have been summarized in several comprehensive reviews.[7] The key features of L-ASP pharmacology are listed in Table 20.1.

PROPERTIES AND MECHANISM OF ACTION

L-ASP (L-Asp) purified from *E. coli*[8] has been used most widely in both basic and clinical research, although L-ASP obtained from other sources, including *E. chrysanthemi*, *Serratia marcescens*, guinea pig serum, and the serum of other members of the species *Caviodea*, also possesses antitumor activity. The purified bacterial enzyme has a molecular weight of 133,000 to 141,000 Da and is composed of four subunits, each with one active site.[9] The gene coding for the *E. chrysanthemi*[10] enzyme has been cloned and sequenced and expressed in *E. coli*.[11] Preparations of enzyme from different bacterial strains and by different purification methods show slight differences in enzyme characteristics. For the bacterial enzymes, the specific activity of purified enzyme is usually 300 to 400 μmol of substrate cleaved per minute per milligram of protein; the isoelectric point lies between pH 4.6 and 5.5 for the *E. coli* enzyme

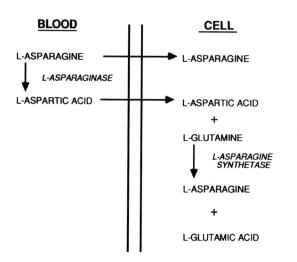

Figure 20.1 Sources of L-asparagine for peripheral tissues. The amino acid may be obtained directly from the circulating blood pool of L-asparagine or may be synthesized by transamination of L-aspartic acid, with L-glutamine acting as the NH_2 donor in a reaction catalyzed by L-asparagine synthetase. The liver is a major source of L-asparagine found in plasma.

and is 8.6 for the *Erwinia* protein; and the K_m (Michaelis-Menten constant) for asparagine is usually 1×10^{-5} mol per liter.[9,12] The *E. coli* enzyme contains 321 amino acids in each subunit (molecular weight 34,080 Da),[13] and the *Erwinia* subunit has a molecular weight of 32,000 Da.[14] (See reference 9 for the amino acid sequence of the *E. coli* enzyme.) The crystal structure of the *E. coli* enzyme has been solved.[13] It has only a 46% homology with the *E. chrysanthemi* enzyme; the two enzymes lack antigenic cross-reactivity and differ in biochemical properties. For example, ammonia activates *E. coli* asparaginase, whereas oxygen represses its synthesis; neither affects the *Erwinia* enzyme.[14]

The *E. coli* and *Erwinia* enzymes are highly specific for L-asparagine as substrates and have less than 10% activity for the D-isomer, for *N*-acylated derivatives, or for L-asparagine in peptide linkage. In contrast, the enzyme from *Saccharomyces cerevisiae* has equal or greater activity with D-asparagine and with *N*-substituted substrates.[15]

The hydrolysis of L-asparagine proceeds according to a reaction mechanism that involves an initial displacement of the amino acid NH_2 group during the formation of an enzyme-aspartyl intermediate, followed by hydrolytic cleavage of the latter bond to generate free L-aspartate and active enzyme. The reaction may be summarized $E + Asn \leftrightarrow NH_3 E \bullet Asp \rightarrow E + Asp + NH_3$, where $E \bullet Asp$ represents the enzyme-aspartyl intermediate.[15] The reaction is irreversibly inhibited by the L-asparagine analog 5-diazo-4-oxo-l-norvaline, which binds covalently to the enzyme's active site.[16]

CELLULAR PHARMACOLOGY AND RESISTANCE

The enzyme L-ASP owes its antitumor effects to the rapid and complete depletion of circulating pools of L-asparagine. In clinical practice, hyperdiploid subtypes of ALL display marked sensitivity to treatment, for unexplained reasons.[17] Similarly, intensive therapy with L-ASP appears to be important in the effective treatment of the less common T cell variety of ALL.[18] Plasma L-asparagine levels (usually in the range of 4×10^{-5} mol/L) are more than sufficient for L-asparagine–requiring tumor cells, which can grow at a normal rate in tissue culture medium containing 1×10^{-6} mol/L asparagine.[19] Because the K_m of the *E. coli* enzyme for L-asparagine is 1×10^{-5} mol/L, the hydrolysis of L-asparagine proceeds at less than maximal velocity once plasma levels fall below this concentration, and considerable excess L-ASP is required in plasma to degrade L-asparagine to sufficiently low concentrations to halt tumor growth. The critical enzyme concentration for maintaining depletion of L-asparagine appears to be at least 0.03 u/mL, but it is possibly 10-fold higher.[20]

The cellular effects of L-ASP result from inhibition of protein synthesis. Cytotoxicity correlates well with inhibition of protein synthesis. Inhibition of nucleic acid synthesis is also observed in sensitive cells but is believed to be secondary to the block in protein synthesis. Cells insensitive to asparagine depletion from growth medium in vitro are also insensitive to L-ASP and show little inhibition of protein synthesis in the presence of the enzyme. These resistant cells have high endogenous activity of asparagine synthetase.[21] The dependence on asparagine exhibited by sensitive cells may be related not only to the requirement for the amino acid itself as a constituent of protein but also to its role as a donor of the NH_2 group in the synthesis of glycine.[22] The mechanism of cell death may be the activation of programmed cell death, or apoptosis, as suggested by both in vitro and in vivo experiments.[23]

Resistance to L-Asparaginase

Resistance emerges rapidly when L-ASP is employed as a single agent, both in animal tumor systems and in humans. Early studies in cell culture[21] and cells taken from resistant leukemia patients[24] demonstrated elevated levels of asparagine synthetase (AspS), indicating the selection of cells that up-regulate the synthesis of asparagine in the presence of the enzyme. Subsequent studies showed that up-regulation was associated with hypomethylation of the AspS gene.[25] However, there is, as yet, no clear correlation of AspS expression and sensitivity to L-ASP in tissue culture studies or prospective clinical trials of human ALL.[26] For example, AspS levels are high in the cells from patients with the (12:21) *TEL/AML1* translocation, a type of ALL that exhibits high sensitivity to L-ASP both in vitro and in patients.[26] Further, there is no evidence for greater AspS

TABLE 20.1

KEY FEATURES OF *ESCHERICHIA COLI* L-ASP PHARMACOLOGY

	L-Asparaginase (*E. Coli*)	Pegaspargase
Mechanism of action	Depletion of the essential amino acid asparagine leads to inhibition of protein synthesis.	Same
Pharmacokinetics	Plasma half-life: 30 hr Blood levels proportional to dose	6 days
Dosage	1,000–25,000 IU/m^2/dose, variable	2,500 IU/m^2 q1–2 weeks
Elimination	Metabolic degradation, immune clearance	Same
Toxicities	Decreased protein synthesis	Same
	Decreased pro-and anticoagulant clotting factors lead to thrombosis and (less commonly) hemorrhage.	Same
	Hypoalbuminemia	
	Hyperglycemia	
	Hypersensitivity reactions	
	Anaphylaxis	
	Serum sickness	
	Cerebral dysfunction	
	Pancreatitis	
	Elevated hepatic enzymes	
Drug interactions	Asparaginase blocks methotrexate action, "rescues" from methotrexate toxicity.	Same
Precautions	Use with caution in patients with hepatic dysfunction or pancreatitis.	If hypersensitive to pegaspargase, switch to *Erwinia* L-asparaginase.
	If history of hypersensitivity to the drug, switch to Pegaspargase or *Erwinia* asparaginase.	

induction after treatment in resistant versus sensitive ALL cells. Definitive studies of the role of AspS are not yet available.[27] Other possible mechanisms of resistance in ALL have been reported, including the development of neutralizing antibodies (referred to as "silent hypersensitivity")[29] and defective induction of apoptosis, a change that confers resistance to glucocorticoids as well.[30] A 35-gene expression profile highly predictive of L-ASP resistance in vitro and in clinical outcomes has been reported but does not include AspS as a contributor.[28]

Chemical Modification

In an attempt to reduce the immunogenicity of L-ASP, to eliminate L-glutaminase activity from the molecule, and to prolong the enzyme's plasma half-life, the *E. coli* asparaginase has been subjected to various modifications. Most bacterial L-ASP preparations contain significant L-glutaminase activity (3 to 5% of the L-ASP activity), activity linked to immunosuppression and cerebral dysfunction. Attempts to eliminate the L-glutaminase activity[31] have met with limited success; the nitrated enzyme has little L-glutaminase but also has reduced L-ASP action.

A second objective has been to reduce immunogenicity. The *E. coli* enzyme, modified by conjugation with 5,000 Da of monomethoxypolyethylene glycol (PEG), displays a

similar decrease in immunogenicity and a 5- to 10-fold increase in plasma half-life and retains 50% of its initial activity.[32] The PEG-asparaginase (pegaspargase) is active and nonimmunogenic in about 70% of patients hypersensitive to the native enzyme. A copolymer of asparaginase with albumin has markedly reduced immunoreactivity and "satisfactory" activity in mice.[33] PEG-asparaginase is an effective alternative for patients hypersensitive to the *E. coli* enzyme and is increasingly employed in primary treatment regimens.[34]

Pharmacologic Considerations

The in vivo clearance rate of the enzyme and its K_m are two important factors that may play roles in determining the efficacy of asparaginase as an antitumor agent. L-ASPs isolated from *Bacillus coagulans*, *Fusarium tricinctum*, and *Candida albicans* are devoid of antitumor activity and are almost completely cleared from the circulation in 30 minutes to 1 hour after intravenous administration into mice. On the other hand, enzymes derived from guinea pig serum and from *E. coli* and *Erwinia* exhibit antitumor activity and have a much longer half-life.[35,36]

The affinity of the enzyme for L-asparagine is another important factor that affects the antitumor activity of L-ASP.[37] Serum concentrations of L-asparagine are 30 to

50 μmol/L, which exceeds the K_m of the bacterial enzymes used in clinical chemotherapy. Thus substrate hydrolysis occurs rapidly under physiologic conditions. As serum levels of the amino acid fall, they approach and then fall below the K_m, which slows the rate of hydrolysis. *E. coli* L-asparaginase and *Erwinia* L-asparaginase, which possess strong antitumor activity, have K_m values of 1 to 1.25×10^{-5} mol/L, whereas lower-affinity L-ASPs from agouti or guinea pig serum[37] or other bacterial sources[38] have only moderate or no antitumor activity.[39]

CLINICAL PHARMACOLOGY

Drug Assay and Pharmacokinetics

L-ASP is easily measured in biologic fluids by assays that detect ammonia release[40] or by a coupled enzymatic assay.[41] The drug is given subcutaneously, intramuscularly, or intravenously; the intramuscular and subcutaneous routes produce peak blood levels 50% lower than the intravenous route but may be less immunogenic. For the *E. coli* enzyme, the usual dosages are a single dose of up to 25,000 IU/m^2 weekly, 5,000 to 10,000 IU/m^2 every other day or every third day for 2 to 4 weeks, or daily doses of 1,000 to 10,000 IU/m^2 for 10 to 20 days. A comparison of the clinical effectiveness of various doses of L-ASP given three times per week demonstrated a higher complete remission rate for doses of 6,000 IU/m^2 or higher than for doses 3,000 IU/m^2 or less[42] (Fig. 20.2). L-ASP activity is detectable in the bloodstream for 2 to 3 weeks after large single doses of the *E. coli* enzyme (25,000 IU/m^2), but depletion of asparagine lasts for only 1 week or less.[42] Thus asparagine levels return toward normal even in the presence of low levels of the enzyme. The threshold at which recovery takes place appears to be 0.03 IU/mL of plasma. However, accurate measurement of serum asparagine levels requires that blood be collected and stored in the presence of an L-ASP inhibitor, such as 5-diazo-4-oxo-l-nor valine.[43] The enzyme distributes primarily within the intravascular space. The cerebrospinal fluid (CSF) concentration of asparagine falls rapidly, however, and an antileukemic effect is exerted in this sanctuary, despite the poor penetration of enzyme into the CSF.[21] The drug can be given directly into the CSF but exits rapidly from this site, and use of this route seems to have no clear therapeutic advantage.

The concentration of L-ASP in plasma is proportional to dose for doses up to 200,000 IU/m^2 and has a primary half-life of 30 hours.[44] The *Erwinia* enzyme, although preserving activity in patients hypersensitive to the *E. coli* preparation, has the disadvantage of a shorter half-life in plasma (16 hours)[44] and does not give equivalent therapeutic results when used with the same dose and schedule as the *E. coli* enzyme (5,000 U/m^2 three times per week). A doubling of the dosage of *Erwinia* enzyme (10,000 U/m^2 per day or 20,000 IU/m^2 3 days per week) is recommended

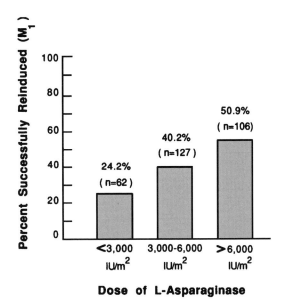

Figure 20.2 Relationship between dose of L-ASP and response in the treatment of acute lymphoblastic leukemia. Patients received the indicated doses every other day, three doses per week, for a maximum of 6 weeks. Successful induction is judged by achievement of an M_1 bone marrow status. (From Ertel IJ, Nesbit ME, Hammond D, et al. Effective dose of L-ASP for induction of remission in previously treated children with acute lymphocytic leukemia: a report from Children's Cancer Study Group. Cancer Res 1979;39:3893.)

to maintain continuous asparagine depletion and equivalent antitumor effects.[45] In patients who develop neutralizing antibodies to the enzyme, plasma clearance is greatly accelerated, and enzyme activity may be undetectable in plasma as soon as 4 hours after administration.[46]

Covalent linkage of L-ASP with PEG has succeeded in markedly reducing the clearance of the enzyme, whereas the volume of distribution remains equivalent to the average plasma volume in humans. In plasma, pegaspargase has a half-life of 6 days, considerably longer than that of the native enzyme; the total clearance is 5.3 ± 3.1 mL/hour per m^2 or 0.13 ± 0.08 mL/hour per kg, and the apparent volume of distribution is 2.1 ± 0.6 L/m^2 or 52.3 ± 16.1 mL/kg.[47] The recommended dosage of pegaspargase is 2,500 U per m^2 every week or every two weeks.[21] This dose results in plasma L-ASP activity of more than 0.1 μmL for at least 7 days. In patients showing hypersensitivity to *E. coli* asparaginase, both native and PEG-linked enzyme may have a shorter half-life, although the PEG enzyme remains active in hypersensitive patients.

Toxicity

The primary toxicities of L-ASP, listed in Table 20.2, fall into two main groups: those related to immunologic sensitization to the foreign protein and those resulting from depletion of asparagine pools and inhibition of protein synthesis. Hypersensitivity reactions to L-ASP are of great

TOXICITY OF L-ASP

Reaction	%
Immediate reaction	70
Nausea, vomiting, fever, chills	
Hypersensitivity reactions	<10
Urticaria	
Bronchospasm	
Hypotension	
Decreased protein synthesis	100
Albumin	
Insulin	
Clotting factors II, V, VII, VIII, IX, X	
Serum lipoproteins	
Antithrombin III	
Cerebral dysfunction	33
Disorientation	
Coma	
Seizures	
Organ toxicities	
Pancreatitis	15
Liver function test abnormalities	100
Azotemia (? increased nitrogen load)	68

From Ohnuma T, Holland JF, Sinks LF. Biochemical and pharmacological studies with L-ASP in man. Cancer Res 1970;30:2297.

concern because they are a common and potentially fatal complication of therapy, particularly when the drug is used as a single agent.[46] Up to 40% of patients receiving single-agent treatment develop some evidence of sensitization.[48] Possibly because of the immunosuppressive effect of corticosteroids, 6-mercaptopurine, and other antileukemic agents, the incidence of hypersensitivity reactions falls to less than 20% in patients receiving combination chemotherapy. Other factors that increase the incidence of reactions include the use of dosages above 6,000 IU/m^2 per day, intravenous as opposed to intramuscular administration, and repeated courses of treatment.[49] Reactions to an initial dose rarely occur; more commonly, hypersensitivity phenomena appear during the second week of treatment or later.[50]

The clinical manifestations of hypersensitivity vary from urticaria (approximately two thirds of reported reactions) to true anaphylactic reactions (hypotension, laryngospasm, cardiac arrest). Rarely, serum sickness–type responses—with arthralgias, proteinuria, and fever—may develop several weeks after an extended course of treatment.[50] Fatal reactions occur in less than 1% of patients treated, but evidence of hypersensitivity should prompt a change in treatment to L-ASP derived from *Erwinia*[5] or to pegaspargase. (The *Erwinia* drug is not sold commercially, but for treatment of ALL it may be available through Ipsen Pharmaceuticals, Ltd, and its US distributor, McKesson BioService Corp; phone 301-315-8460.) Allergic reactions to *Erwinia* L-ASP may occur as an independent phenomenon in

patients who have not previously received *E. coli* enzyme[51] and may ultimately develop in 5 to 20% of patients receiving multiple courses of this enzyme. PEG-asparaginase can also be used in hypersensitive patients, among whom a 30% incidence of allergy to the new drug can be expected.

Because of the frequency and severity of allergic reactions to L-ASP, routine skin testing was recommended for prediction of allergy before the first dose of drug. Allergic reactions may occur in patients with negative skin tests,[52] however, and positive skin tests are not invariably predictive of reactions. Hypersensitive patients usually have both immunoglobulin E and immunoglobulin G antibodies to L-ASP in serum,[53] but more than half the patients with such antibodies do not display an allergic reaction to the drug clinically. Thus the antibody tests have limited value for predicting which patients will have an allergic reaction. Routine skin testing is not recommended for pegaspargase. However, only personnel trained in and prepared for the management of anaphylaxis should administer L-ASP, and patients are generally observed closely for a minimum of 1 hour following its administration.

Other toxic effects result from inhibition of protein synthesis; these include hypoalbuminemia, decrease in clotting factors, decreased serum insulin with hyperglycemia, and decreased serum lipoproteins. Abnormalities in clotting function are regularly observed in association with L-ASP therapy and can lead to thromboembolism in 2 to 11% of ALL patients, most frequently during induction therapy and when glucocorticoids are being administered concurrently.[54–57] Hemorrhagic events occur less frequently and are probably secondary to decreased synthesis of vitamin K–dependent factors, with prolongation of the prothrombin time, partial thromboplastin time, and thrombin time[50,58] and decrease in factors IX and X.[59] Platelets from L-ASP–treated subjects display deficient aggregation in response to collagen but not to adenosine diphosphate, arachidonic acid, or epinephrine.[60] Two instances have been reported of a spontaneous intracranial hemorrhage in a child with marked hypofibrinogenemia.[61]

Inhibition of the synthesis of anticoagulant proteins is likely responsible for thrombotic events. L-ASP decreases the synthesis of antithrombin III, a physiologic anticoagulant and protease inhibitor. Circulating levels of this factor fall to 50% or less compared with levels in controls after single large doses of L-ASP.[50] Also inhibited are the syntheses of vitamin K–dependent inhibitors of clotting, protein C, and its cofactor protein S.

Thrombosis in the central nervous system is a particularly problematic complication of therapy with L-ASP.[62–64] This occurred in 1% of patients receiving 30 weeks of continuous L-ASP therapy in a Dana Farber Cancer Institute pediatric ALL trial.[65] It typically involves the transverse or sagittal sinus circulation of the brain, where it causes seizures, headache, confusion, and stroke symptoms. Subclinical sinus occlusions can be detected by magnetic resonance imaging in patients with modest complaints of headache and undoubtedly occur more frequently than recognized clinically. Catheter-related venous thrombosis may give rise to superior vena cava or internal jugular vein thrombosis.[55]

Interestingly, L-ASP–associated thromboses are thought to occur with increased frequency in patients with underlying inherited disorders of clotting.[54] A survey of 289 children with ALL treated in a German cooperative group (Bonn, Frankfurt, Munster group) trial disclosed events in 32 patients, of whom 27 (85%) had one or more defects predisposing to thrombosis. These defects included the TT677 mutation in methylene tetrahydrofolate reductase (which causes homocysteine elevation in plasma), factor V Leiden, deficiency in protein C or protein S, elevated lipoprotein(a), and the G20210A variant of prothrombin. In this study, 27 of 58 patients (47%) with one or more of these defects experienced a thrombotic event, compared with only 5 of 231 patients (2%) with no prothrombotic defect. The overall incidence of prothrombotic abnormalities in a White population is approximately 20%. Prophylactic anticoagulation for patients at high risk may be effective but requires more extensive study in view of the possibility of hemorrhagic side effects of anticoagulation.[55] A careful family history should be obtained prior to the initiation of L-ASP therapy, with consideration given to obtaining laboratory tests to screen for prothrombotic conditions.

In an attempt to prevent thrombosis, pilot trials have used prophylactic replacement of antithrombin III in children undergoing L-ASP treatment[66] and have observed no thrombotic episodes in the small numbers of children thus treated. A second study of 17 adult patients receiving L-ASP with recombinant antithrombin III (AT) found no posttreatment episodes of thrombosis, as compared to 10 episodes in 54 patients not receiving AT.[67]

Other toxicities are not as easily explained by the drug's mode of action. In 25% of patients, cerebral dysfunction with confusion, stupor, or frank coma may develop. The latter syndrome resembles ammonia toxicity and has, in some cases, been associated with elevated serum ammonia levels.[63] Some of these mental status changes probably represent incompletely evaluated episodes of cortical sinus thrombosis, which is visualized by MRI.[64]

Acute pancreatitis is an infrequent complication that occurs in fewer than 15% of patients, but it may progress to severe hemorrhagic pancreatitis. In most of the affected individuals, a transient increase in serum amylase concentration may coincide with mild nausea, vomiting, and abdominal pain, and these signs of pancreatitis quickly resolve with discontinuation of the drug. L-ASP is frequently the cause of abnormal liver function test results, including increased serum levels of bilirubin, serum glutamic-oxaloacetic transaminase, and alkaline phosphatase. Liver biopsy reveals fatty metamorphosis that is probably due to decreased mobilization of lipids.

Approximately two thirds of patients receiving L-ASP experience nausea, vomiting, and chills as an immediate reaction, but these side effects can be mitigated by administration of antiemetics, antihistamines, or, in extreme cases, corticosteroids. Close attention should be given to any symptoms that may be mediated by allergy, as a local allergic reaction frequently heralds a subsequent life-threatening systemic hypersensitivity reaction. L-ASP has no known toxicity to gastrointestinal mucosa or bone marrow and is thus a favorable agent for use in combination chemotherapy.

The only well-established drug interaction of L-ASP is its ability to terminate the action of methotrexate.[68] The antagonism of L-asparaginase when given before methotrexate is possibly the result of inhibition of protein synthesis, with consequent prevention of cell entry into the vulnerable S phase of the cell cycle. An alternative explanation for antagonism is derived from the inhibition of methotrexate polyglutamylation by L-asparaginase pretreatment,[69] with decreased retention of methotrexate by tumor cells. After a single intravenous dose of L-ASP, inhibition of DNA synthesis lasts for approximately 10 days, a period during which cells are refractory to methotrexate. This interval is followed by a period of increased DNA synthetic activity as cells recover from the block in protein synthesis; during this recovery period, cells are thought to be particularly vulnerable to methotrexate.[70] These considerations form the rationale for clinical trials that use an initial dose of L-ASP, followed in 10 to 14 days by methotrexate, and then a second dose of L-ASP to abbreviate methotrexate toxicity.[71] The results of this approach are inconclusive.

The immunosuppressive properties of L-ASP have been demonstrated in animals and may contribute to high rates of infection with bacteria and fungal organisms, as reported in certain ALL trials in which patients were randomized to receive or not receive high doses of E. coli L-ASP.[72] Hyperglycemia, hypoalbuminemia, and catheter-related thrombosis in patients treated with the drug may also contribute to the risk of infection.

REFERENCES

1. Haley EE, Fischer GA, Welch AD. The requirement for L-asparagine of mouse leukemic cells L5178Y in culture. Cancer Res 1961;21:532.
2. Kidd JG. Regression of transplanted lymphomas induced in vivo by means of normal guinea pig serum, I: course of transplanted cancers of various kinds in mice and rats given guinea pig serum, horse serum, or rabbit serum. J Exp Med 1953;98:565.
3. Broome JD. Evidence that the L-ASP of guinea pig serum is responsible for its antilymphoma effects, I: properties of the L-ASP of guinea pig serum in relation to those of the antilymphoma substance. J Exp Med 1963;118:99.
4. Hill JM, Loeb E, MacLellan A, et al. Response to highly purified L-ASP during therapy of acute leukemia. Cancer Res 1969;29:1574.
5. Ohnuma T, Holland JF, Meyer P. Erwinia carotovora asparaginase in patients with prior anaphylaxis to asparaginase from E. coli. Cancer 1972;30:376.
6. Todeschini G, Tecchio C, Meneghini V, et al. Estimated 6-year event-free survival of 55% in 60 consecutive adult acute lymphoblastic leukemia patients treated with an intensive phase II protocol based on a high induction dose of daunorubicin. Leukemia 1998;12:144.

7. Daenen S, van Imhoff GW, van den Berg E, et al. Improved outcome of adult acute lymphoblastic leukaemia by moderately intensified chemotherapy which includes a pre-induction course for rapid tumour reduction: preliminary results on 66 patients. Br J Haematol 1998;100:273.

8. Braun S, Schlimok G, Heumos I, et al. ErbB2 overexpression on occult metastatic cells in bone marrow predicts poor clinical outcome of stage I-III breast cancer patients. Cancer Res 2001;61:1890.

9. Ho PK, Milikin EB, Bobbitt JL, et al. Crystalline L-ASP from E. coli B: purification and chemical characterization. J Biol Chem 1970; 245:3703.

10. Maita T, Matsuda G. The primary structure of L-ASP from Escherichia coli. Hoppe Seylers Z Physiol Chem 1980;361:105.

11. Gilbert HJ, Blazek R, Bullman HMS, et al. Cloning and expression of the Erwinia chrysanthemi asparaginase gene in Escherichia coli and Erwinia carotovora. J Gen Microbiol 1986;132:151.

12. Minton NP, Bullman HMS, Scawen MD, et al. Nucleotide sequence of the Erwinia chrysanthemi NCPPB 1066 L-asparaginase gene. Gene 1986;46:25.

13. Howard JB, Carpenter FH. L-ASP from Erwinia carotovora: substrate specificity and enzymatic properties. J Biol Chem 1972;247:1020.

14. Swain AL, Jaskolski M, Housset D, et al. Crystal structure of Escherichia coli L-ASP, an enzyme used in cancer therapy. Proc Natl Acad Sci USA 1993;90:1474.

15. Wade HE, Robinson HK, Phillips BW. L-ASP and glutaminase activities of bacteria. J Gen Microbiol 1971;69:249.

16. Dunlop PC, Meyer GM, Roon RJ. Reactions of asparaginase II of Saccharomyces cerevisiae: a mechanistic analysis of hydrolysis and hydroxylaminolysis. J Biol Chem 1980;255:1542.

17. Lachman LB, Handschumacher RE. The active site of L-asparaginase: dimethylsulfoxide effect of 5-diazo-4-oxo-l-norvaline interactions. Biochem Biophys Res Commun 1976;73:1094.

18. Pui CH, Relling MV, Downing JR. Acute lymphoblastic leukemia. N Engl J Med. 2004;350:1535.

19. Amylon MD, Shuster J, Pullen J, et al. Intensive high-dose asparaginase consolidation improves survival for pediatric patients with T cell acute lymphoblastic leukemia and advanced stage lymphoblastic lymphoma: a Pediatric Oncology Group study. Leukemia 1999;13:335.

20. Haley EE, Fischer GA, Welch AD. The requirement for L-asparagine of mouse leukemia cells L5178Y in culture. Cancer Res 1961;21:532.

21. Hawkins DS, Park JR, Thomson BG, et al. Asparaginase pharmacokinetics after intensive polyethylene glycol-conjugated L-asparaginase therapy for children with relapsed acute lymphoblastic leukemia. Clin Cancer Res 2004;10:5335.

22. Horowitz B, Madras BK, Meister A, et al. Asparagine synthetase activity of mouse leukemia. Science 1968;160:533.

23. Keefer JF, Moraga DA, Schuster SM. Comparison of glycine metabolism in mouse lymphoma cells either sensitive or resistant to L-ASP. Biochem Pharmacol 1985;34:559.

24. Story MD, Voehringer DW, Stephens LC, et al. L-ASP kills lymphoma cells by apoptosis. Cancer Chemother Pharmacol 1993;32:129.

25. Haskell CM, Canellos GP. L-ASP resistance in human leukemia-asparagine synthetase. Biochem Pharmacol 1969;18:2578.

26. Worton KS, Kerbel RS, Andrulis IL. Hypomethylation and reactivation of the asparagine synthetase gene induced by L-asparaginase and ethyl methanesulfonate. Cancer Res 1991;51:985.

27. Stams WAG, Den Boer ML, Beverloo HB, et al. Sensitivity to L-asparaginase is not associated with expression levels of asparagine synthetase in t(12;21) pediatric ALL. Blood 2003;101:2743.

28. Irino T, Kitoh T, Koami K, et al. Establishment of real-time polymerase chain reaction method for quantitative analysis of asparagine synthetase expression. J Mol Diagnostics 2004;6:217.

29. Asselin BL. The three asparaginases: comparative pharmacology and optimal use in childhood leukemia. Adv Exp Med Biol 1999;456:621.

30. Holleman A, Den Boer ML, Kazemier KM, et al. Resistance to different classes of drugs is associated with impaired apoptosis in childhood acute lymphoblastic leukemia. Blood 2003; 102:4541.

31. Liu YP, Handschumacher RE. Nitroasparaginase: subunit cross-linkage and altered substrate specificity. J Biol Chem 1972;247:66.

32. Keating MJ, Holmes R, Lerner S, et al. L-ASP and PEG asparaginase: past present and future. Leuk Lymphoma 1993;10(Suppl):153.

33. Yasura T, Kamisaki Y, Wada H, et al. Immunological studies on modified enzymes, I: soluble L-ASP/mouse albumin copolymer with enzyme activity and substantial loss of immunosensitivity. Int Arch Allergy Appl Immunol 1981;64:11.

34. Molino A, Pelosi G, Micciolo R, et al. Bone marrow micrometastases in 109 breast cancer patients: correlations with clinical and pathological features and prognosis. Breast Cancer Res Treat 1997;42:23.

35. Campbell HA, Mashburn LT, Boyse SE, et al. Two L-ASPs from E. coli B: their separation, purification, and antitumor activity. Biochemistry 1967;6:721.

36. Mashburn LT, Landin LM. Some physiochemical aspects of L-ASP therapy. Recent Results Cancer Res 1970;33:48.

37. Broome JD. Factors which may influence the effectiveness of L-ASPs as tumor inhibitors. Br J Cancer 1968;22:595.

38. Yellin TO, Wriston JC Jr. Purification and properties of guinea pig serum asparaginase. Biochemistry 1966;5:1605.

39. Law AS, Wriston JC Jr. Purification and properties of Bacillus coagulans L-ASP. Arch Biochem Biophys 1971;147:744.

40. Roberts J, Holcenberg JS, Dolowy WC. Isolation, crystallization, and properties of Achromobacteraceae glutaminase-asparaginase with antitumor activity. J Biol Chem 1972;247:84.

41. Cooney DA, Capizzi RI, Handschumacher RE. Evaluation of L-asparagine metabolism in animals and man. Cancer Res 1970; 30:929.

42. Ertel IJ, Nesbit ME, Hammond D, et al. Effective dose of L-asparaginase for induction of remission in previously treated children with acute lymphocytic leukemia: a report from Children's Cancer Study Group. Cancer Res 1979;39:3893.

43. Asselin BL, Lorenson MY, Whitin JC, et al. Measurement of serum L-asparagine in the presence of L-ASP requires the presence of an L-ASP inhibitor. Cancer Res 1991;51:6568.

44. Asselin BL, Whitin JC, Coppola DJ, et al. Comparative pharmacokinetic studies of three asparaginase preparations. J Clin Oncol 1993;11:1780.

45. Otten J, Suciu S, Lutz P, et al. The importance of L-ASP (A'ASE) in the treatment of acute lymphoblastic leukemia in children: results of the EORTC 58881 randomized phase trial showing greater efficiency of Escherichia coli as compared to Erwinia A'ASE [abstract]. Blood 1996;88(Suppl 1):669. Abstract 2663.

46. Peterson RC, Handschumacher RF, Mitchell MS. Immunological responses to L-ASP. J Clin Invest 1971;50:1080.

47. Ho DH, Brown NS, Yen A, et al. Clinical pharmacology of polyethylene glycol-L-ASP. Drug Metab Disp 1986;14:349.

48. Clavell LA, Gelber RD, Cohen HJ, et al. Four-agent induction and intensive asparaginase therapy for treatment of childhood acute lymphoblastic leukemia. N Engl J Med 1986;315:657.

49. Jones B, Holland JF, Glidewell O, et al. Optimal use of L-asparaginase (NSC-109229) in acute lymphocytic leukemia. Med Pediatr Oncol 1977;3:387.

50. Rutter DA. Toxicity of asparaginases. Lancet 1975;1:1293.

51. Land VJ, Sutow WW, Fernbach DJ, et al. Toxicity of L-asparaginase in children with advanced leukemia. Cancer 1972;40:339.

52. Khan A, Hill JM. Atopic hypersensitivity to L-ASP. Int Arch Allergy 1971;40:463.

53. Killander D, Dohlwitz A, Engstedt L, et al. Hypersensitive reactions and antibody formation during L-ASP treatment of children and adults with acute leukemia. Cancer 1976;37:220.

54. Nowak-Gottl U, Wermes C, Junker R, et al. Prospective evaluation of the thrombotic risk in children with acute lymphoblastic leukemia carrying the MTHFR TT 677 genotype, the prothrombin G20210A variant, and further prothrombotic risk factors. Blood 1999;93:1595.

55. Sills RH, Nelson DA, Stockman JA III. L-ASP-induced coagulopathy during therapy of acute lymphocytic leukemia. Med Pediatr Oncol 1978;4:311.

56. Sutor AH, Mall V, Thomas KB. Bleeding and thrombosis in children with acute lymphoblastic leukaemia, treated according to the ALL-BFM-90 protocol. Klin Padiatr 1999;211:201.

57. Nowak-Gottl U, Ahlke E, Fleischhack G, et al. Thromboembolic events in children with acute lymphoblastic leukemia (BFM protocols): prednisone versus dexamethasone administration. Blood 2003;101:2529.

58. Gralnick HR, Henderson E. Hypofibrinogenemia and coagulation factor deficiencies with L-ASP treatment. Cancer 1970;27:1313.

59. Ramsay NKC, Coccia PF, Krivit W, et al. The effect of L-asparaginase on plasma coagulation factors in acute lymphoblastic leukemia. Cancer 1977;40:1398.

60. Shapiro RS, Gerrard JM, Ramsay NK, et al. Selective deficiency in collagen-induced platelet aggregation during L-asparaginase therapy. Am J Pediatr Hematol Oncol 1980;2:207.

61. Cairo MS, Lazarus K, Gilmore RL, et al. Intracranial hemorrhage and focal seizures secondary to use of L-ASP during induction therapy of acute lymphocytic leukemia. J Pediatr 1980;97:829.

62. Mitchell L, Hoogendoorn H, Giles AR, et al. Increased endogenous thrombin generation in children with acute lymphoblastic leukemia: risk of thrombotic complications in L-ASP-induced antithrombin III deficiency. Blood 1994;83:386.

63. Leonard JV, Kay JDS. Acute encephalopathy and hyperammonaemia complicating treatment of acute lymphoblastic leukaemia with asparaginase. Lancet 1986;1:162.

64. Bushara KO, Rust RS. Reversible MRI lesions due to pegaspargase treatment of non-Hodgkin's lymphoma. Pediatr Neurol 1997;17:185.

65. Silverman LB, Gelber RD, Dalton VK, et al. Improved outcome for children with acute lymphoblastic leukemia: results of Dana-Farber Consortium Protocol 91-01. Blood 2001;97:1211.

66. Alberts SR, Bretscher M, Wiltsie JC, et al. Thrombosis related to the use of L-ASP in adults with acute lymphoblastic leukemia: a need to consider coagulation monitoring and clotting factor replacement. Leuk Lymphoma 1999;32:489.

67. Elliott MA, Wolf RC, Hook CC, et al. Thromboembolism in adults with acute lymphoblastic leukemia during induction with L-asparaginase-containing multi-agent regimens: incidence, risk factors, and possible role of antithrombin. Leuk Lymphoma 2004;45:1545.

68. Capizzi RL. Schedule-dependent synergism and antagonism between methotrexate and L-ASP. Biochem Pharmacol 1974;23:151.

69. Jolivet J, Cole DE, Holcenberg JS, et al. Prevention of methotrexate polyglutamate formation. Cancer Res 1985;45:217.

70. Lobel JS, O'Brien RT, McIntosh S, et al. Methotrexate and asparaginase combination chemotherapy in refractory acute lymphoblastic leukemia of childhood. Cancer 1979;43:1089.

71. Harris RE, McCallister JA, Provisor DS, et al. Methotrexate/L-ASP combination chemotherapy for patients with acute leukemia in relapse: a study of 36 children. Cancer 1980;46:2004–2008.

72. Liang DC, Hung IJ, Yang CP, et al. Unexpected mortality from the use of *E. coli* L-ASP during remission induction therapy for childhood acute lymphoblastic leukemia: a report from the Taiwan Pediatric Oncology Group. Leukemia 1999;13:155.

Delivering Anticancer Drugs to Brain Tumors

21

Maciej M. Mrugala   *Tracy T. Batchelor*   *Jeffrey G. Supko*

There were an estimated 41,300 new primary brain tumors diagnosed in the United States in 2004.[1] Malignant gliomas (anaplastic astrocytoma and glioblastoma) are the most common malignant primary brain tumors and represent the most frequent indication for cytotoxic chemotherapy in neuro-oncology. The goal of adjuvant chemotherapy for malignant glioma is eradication of the residual macroscopic and microscopic tumor felt to be the reason for surgical and radiation failure. Temozolomide, an orally administered alkylating agent, significantly extends progression-free and overall survival when administered concurrently with radiation in patients with newly diagnosed glioblastoma.[2] In addition, locally delivered chemotherapy in the form of 1,3-bis(2 chloroethyl)-1-nitrosourea (carmustine; BCNU) polymers also extends survival in patients with malignant glioma when applied at the time of the initial debulking procedure.[3] However, the survival benefits of adjuvant chemotherapy for patients with malignant gliomas are modest, as demonstrated by an absolute increase in 1-year survival of 6% in one meta-analysis of 12 randomized clinical trials.[4]

Mechanisms of chemotherapy resistance of brain tumors include factors common to other tumors such as multidrug resistance and increased efficiency of DNA damage-repair systems.[5] In addition, treating malignant brain tumors represents a unique challenge for oncologists due to the presence of the blood-brain barrier (BBB), a physiologic impediment between the circulatory system of the brain and that of the body. The accessibility of many anticancer drugs to brain tumors is at least partially constrained by the BBB. Therefore, difficulty in achieving adequate and sufficiently sustained levels of the cytotoxic moiety at the tumor site is a significant factor contributing to the failure of systemic chemotherapy for malignant

brain tumors.[6,7] Accordingly, the development of treatment strategies for brain tumors has emphasized techniques that are intended to overcome this barrier and improve drug delivery to these tumors. In addition, the use of multiple ancillary agents in the medical management of brain tumor patients, particularly glucocorticoids and enzyme-inducing antiseizure medications, increases the risk for drug interactions that may impact the efficacy or toxicity of chemotherapy. This chapter reviews the current state of approaches for delivering anticancer drugs to brain tumors, the various techniques that are available for assessing drug distribution to brain tumors, and important pharmacologic interactions that may affect both the accessibility of anticancer drugs to the CNS and the systemic pharmacokinetics of the anticancer agent.

BLOOD-BRAIN BARRIER

Three main factors influence the extent to which a systemically administered anticancer agent distributes into the brain and brain tumors: (a) the plasma concentration-time profile of the drug; (b) regional blood flow; and (c) transport of the agent through the BBB and blood-tumor barrier (BTB). The two former considerations are common to all solid tumors, whereas the latter is specific to brain tumors.[6] Erhlich was the first to propose the concept of the BBB at the beginning of the 20th century. On administering the dye trypan blue to rats by intravenous injection, he observed that all body organs were stained except for the brain and spinal cord.[8] The anatomic basis of the BBB was determined three decades ago with the introduction of the electron microscope. It results from a modification of the normal vascular endothelium whereby a sheet of cells is

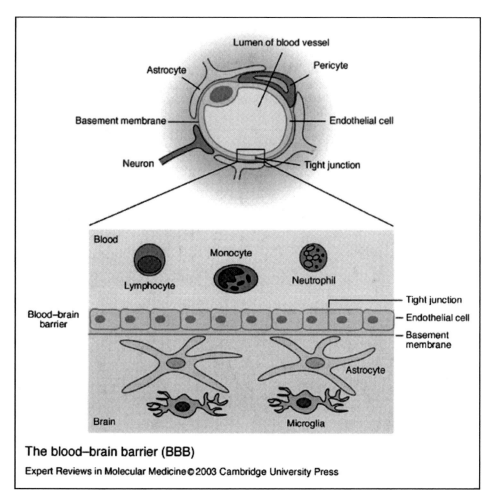

The blood–brain barrier (BBB)

Expert Reviews in Molecular Medicine © 2003 Cambridge University Press

Figure 21.1 Schematic representation of the normal intracerebral capillary. Crucial elements for building the blood-brain barrier (basement membrane and endothelial tight junctions) are visualized. (Reproduced with permission from Karen Francis, Johan van Beek, Cecale Canova, et al. Innate Immunity and Brain Inflammation: the key role of complement. *Expert Reviews in molecular Medicine* pp. 1–19. Cambridge: Cambridge University Press, 2003.)

connected by tight junctions on a basement membrane (Fig.21.1). The area of the exchange surface is 12 m^2, and the physiologic role of the BBB is assumed to include maintenance of a constant biochemical content of the interstitial milieu and protection of the brain from foreign and undesirable molecules.[9] Low hydraulic conductance, low ionic permeability, and high electrical resistance contribute to the very low permeability for hydrophilic non-electrolytes in the absence of a membrane carrier.[10] These properties, together with the lack of intracellular fenestrations and pinocytotic vesicles and the presence of a thicker basal lamina, create a physiologic barrier that is relatively impermeable to many water-soluble compounds.[11,12]

Some drugs use specific transport mechanisms present in the endothelial cell to traverse the BBB.[13] However, most cytotoxic drugs that gain access to the CNS, as exemplified by the chloroethylnitrosourea alkylating agents, cross the BBB by passive diffusion. Aside from pharmacokinetic properties, the main factors that influence the extent to which these compounds distribute into the CNS include lipid solubility, molecular mass, charge, and plasma protein binding. Specifically, small organic compounds with a molecular weight less than 200 that are lipid soluble, neu-

tral at physiologic pH, and are not highly bound to plasma proteins readily cross the BBB.[10]

A second component of the BBB is the expression of P-glycoprotein on the luminal surface of brain capillary endothelial cells.[14] The presence of P-glycoprotein has been implicated in the active efflux of many chemotherapeutic drugs from the brain, including the vinca alkaloids and doxorubicin. Expression of P-glycoprotein has also been reported in malignant gliomas and may serve as another mechanism of chemotherapy resistance.[15,16] Agents that reverse the function of P-glycoprotein, such as verapamil, may increase passage of doxorubicin across the BBB.

The normal physiologic structure of the BBB is disrupted in vasculature within and adjacent to brain tumors. The barrier is usually more permeable in the center of a malignant tumor as opposed to the well-vascularized and infiltrating edge that exhibits variable degrees of BBB integrity.[17] Figure 21.2 contrasts the normal BBB with that disrupted by a brain tumor. Vick and colleagues identified junctional clefts in the endothelial cells of capillaries adjacent to brain tumors.[18] These clefts correlated with the density of infiltrating tumor cells and were present in brain capillaries not in direct contact with the tumor. Evidence

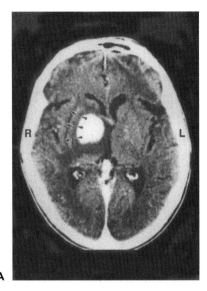
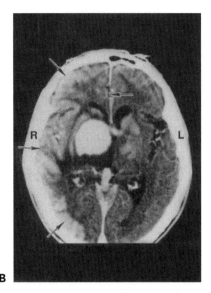
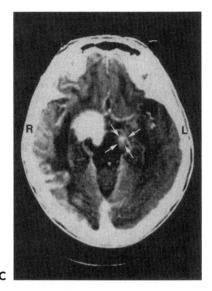

Figure 21.2   Heterogenecity of the blood-brain barrier. Contrast-enhanced CT scans of the basal ganglia of a 61-year-old woman with a primary CNS lymphoma, indicating that the permeability of the blood-tumor barrier is inconsistent for a given patient or even a given tumor nodule. **A.** CT scan demonstrating a bright, uniformly enhancing lesion in the right basal ganglia. The surrounding hypodense signal in the brain tissue around the tumor (arrowheads) should be noted. **B.** CT scan obtained after contrast agent administration. Contrast material was administered immediately after osmotic BBBD and CT scans were obtained 30 minutes after the first BBBD treatment in order to confirm and assess the grade of BBBD. The patient underwent right internal carotid artery disruption in the anterior and middle cerebral artery distributions (arrows). Opening of the brain tissue around the tumor in the area of the peritumoral hypodense signal evident in the CT scan in A should be noted. **C.** CT scan obtained after BBBD in a patient with a right hemiparesis that was unexplained, because the only visible tumor was in the right cerebrum (**A**). BBBD the day after the CT scan in (A) extended into the posterior circulation via the posterior communicating artery. A left-side brainstem lesion not apparent in pre-BBBD imaging studies was noted. The right hemiparesis was thus attributable to a brainstem tumor (arrows) on the left that was not apparent on pre-BBBD MRI scans (intact BBB and no edema). (Reproduced with permission from Neuwelt EA. Mechanisms of disease: the blood-brain barrier Neurosurgery 2004;54:131–140.)

also exists that the microvasculature of these tumors lacks the properties of a normal BBB and has greater permeability as a result. Morphologic studies have demonstrated that the BTB differs anatomically from the normal BBB, with open tight junctions, gap junctions, fenestrations, and numerous intracellular vesicles.[6,19] The increased permeability of these blood vessels forms the basis of contrast enhancement of brain tumors on CT and MRI scans. Iodinated, water-soluble contrast agents do not penetrate areas of the brain with an intact BBB but are able to penetrate brain tumors.[20] These alterations in permeability are highly variable between tumors and within the same tumor.[21] For example, low-grade gliomas and proliferating edges of malignant gliomas seem to have a normally functioning, selective BBB and consequently do not typically show contrast enhancement on CT and MRI studies. A large variation in the enhancement patterns of malignant brain tumors on CT scans is common.[22,23] Approximately 30% of patients with a type of malignant glioma, anaplastic astrocytoma, are reported to have nonenhancing lesions.[22] Finally, positron emission tomography (PET) studies have shown that alterations in permeability usually occur in the central part of large tumors, whereas the periphery is intact.[24] The presence of a selective, normal BBB near the proliferating edge of a brain tumor may result in variable delivery of water-soluble drugs in this region and may contribute significantly to the high local failure rate of conventional anticancer drugs.

The central role hypothesized for the BBB in the resistance of brain tumors to chemotherapy has been questioned by some authorities. It has been suggested that, because the BBB adjacent to tumors and the BTB lack the normal properties of an intact BBB, drug delivery to these areas should not be compromised.[18] Indirect support for this argument comes from the observation that brain tumors occasionally respond to cytotoxic drugs that would not be expected to cross the BBB due to their physicochemical properties. A more consistent observation, however, has been that the most effective classes of antineoplastic drugs against malignant brain tumors are lipid-soluble molecules that can easily penetrate an intact BBB. Moreover, in addition to the existence of normal BBB at the proliferating edge of brain tumors, PET studies have demonstrated that, whereas the BBB and BTB may be abnormal at the time of diagnosis, these structures may become normalized on subsequent treatment.[25] These latter observations support a pivotal role for the BBB and BTB in the resistance of brain tumors to systemically administered chemotherapy.

DRUG DELIVERY METHODS

Following the administration of an anticancer drug by the intravenous or oral routes, the BBB can effectively impede the distribution of drug molecules from systemic circulation into the CNS. Consequently, considerable effort has been expended to develop drug delivery strategies that either entirely circumvent the BBB or modulate the permeability of the barrier to enhance the extent of drug distribution into the brain from systemic circulation. These techniques include intra-arterial administration, BBB disruption with hyperosmolar solutions[26] or biomolecules, high-dose chemotherapy, intrathecal injection, and local delivery by direct intratumoral injection of free drug or implantation of drug embedded in a controlled-release biodegradable delivery system. Even when drugs have crossed the BBB, however, their migration to tumor cells may be hindered by increased intercapillary distances, greater interstitial pressure, lower microvascular pressure, and the sink effect exerted by normal brain tissue.[27]

Intra-arterial Administration

The theoretical advantage for delivering anticancer drugs by the intra-arterial route is related to the ratio of systemic to regional blood flow. In comparison to intravenous injection, a considerably higher local drug concentration can be achieved with intra-arterial injection, thereby increasing the amount of the agent driven across the BBB. This has been confirmed experimentally, including in a report of a two- to threefold increase in tumor concentration of cisplatin and a chloroethylnitrosourea, respectively, in the brains of animals after intra-arterial administration as compared to intravenous administration.[28] With this technique, sufficient local drug concentrations can be achieved with smaller than conventional doses, so that systemic side effects are minimized.[29] The pharmacokinetic advantages of intra-arterial administration occur only during the first passage through the CNS, because the drug then enters venous circulation, and the plasma profile is indistinguishable from that afforded by intravenous administration.

This approach has been clinically evaluated in various settings, including neoadjuvant and adjuvant therapy and recurrent malignant glioma.[30–32] Thus far, clinical trials of intra-arterial chemotherapy for malignant gliomas have not demonstrated improvement in survival over conventional intravenous therapy. A phase III study involving 315 patients with malignant gliomas failed to show any advantages of adjuvant intra-arterial BCNU over intravenous infusion of the same drug.[33] Moreover, subjects in the intra-arterial BCNU arm of this trial experienced significant treatment-related toxicities, with 10% developing leukoencephalopathy and 15% developing ipsilateral blindness. Another randomized clinical trial compared intra-arterial and intravenous ACNU (nimustine). There was no significant difference in the progression-free sur-

vival and overall survival in each treatment arm. However, toxicity associated with intra-arterial ACNU was modest. No cases of leukoencephalopathy and only one case of transient visual impairment were reported.[34]

Potential disadvantages of the intra-arterial route include local complications related to catheterization (thrombosis, bleeding, infection) and neurological sequela, including orbital and cranial pain, retinal toxicity, leukoencephalopathy, or cortical necrosis.[30,33,35] In addition, prodrugs requiring hepatic activation, such as cyclophosphamide, procarbazine, and irinotecan, are not suitable for use by the intra-arterial route One factor that partly explains the unique toxicities associated with intra-arterial administration is the "streaming" effect.[36] Infusion of drug into the high-pressure, rapidly moving arterial bloodstream results in incomplete mixing of the drug and plasma and great variability in the amount of drug reaching different regions of the vascular territory. Depending on the characteristics of the distribution pattern, higher concentrations of drug might be achieved in normal brain, whereas lower amounts reach the tumor. Different strategies have been attempted to minimize the streaming effect, including rapid infusion,[36] superselective cannulation of the feeding artery,[35,37] diastole-phased pulsatile infusion,[38,39] and local blood flow adjusted dosage.[37] All of these techniques were combined in a phase I trial involving 21 brain tumor patients treated with intra-arterial carboplatin. The neurologic side effects were minor, and a twofold escalation of the dose beyond the conventional intra-arterial dose was achieved, with promising results.[37] Despite its serious limitations, there have been a few reports of promising results in patients receiving intra-arterial therapy for primary brain tumors. Intra-arterial carboplatin and etoposide were demonstrated to be safe and useful in the treatment of progressive optic-hypothalamic gliomas in children.[40] The safety and efficacy of intra-arterial chemotherapy with multiple agents in conjunction with osmotic disruption of the BBB were established.[41] It seems that intra-arterial chemotherapy, with all its current limitations, is slowly moving forward and may achieve wider applications. Perfection of the delivery techniques and development of newer, less toxic compounds should increase its efficacy and safety.

Blood-Brain Barrier Disruption

Blood-Brain Barrier (BBB) disruption involves the use of hyperosmolar solutions or biomolecules to increase the permeability of the BBB and improve drug delivery to brain tumors. The specific mechanisms underlying osmotic opening of the BBB and BTB are not entirely understood. Preliminary explanations emphasized endothelial cell shrinkage and resultant separation of tight junctions upon exposure to a hyperosmotic environment.[42] In addition to cellular shrinkage, osmotic stress releases biologically active compounds from endothelial cells, including serine proteases, that could potentially degrade the collagen matrix of the endothelial basement membrane. Finally, cellular shrinkage may also trigger second messenger signals and calcium influx, which could affect the integrity of tight junctions.[9]

Methods for disrupting the BBB involving both intravenous and intra-arterial administration have been developed for use in brain tumor patients.[42] The results of nonrandomized studies have been encouraging for certain brain tumor subtypes, especially primary CNS lymphoma. Potential advantages of this method include increased tumor delivery of drug and lack of systemic toxicity from cytotoxic chemotherapy. Another possible advantage of this technique is avoiding the sink effect seen with other procedures used for delivering chemotherapy to brain tumors. The *sink effect* refers to the selective achievement of higher concentrations of a drug in areas of disrupted BBB in the tumor than in the rest of the brain. As a result of this concentration gradient, the drug rapidly diffuses out of the tumor into the surrounding brain and compromises tumor exposure time. Because BBB disruption theoretically affects the endothelium of both normal brain and brain tumor, a nonselective increase in drug delivery into both areas occurs, and no concentration gradient is established. Despite these potential advantages, the technique of BBB disruption is complex and requires transfemoral angiography and general anesthesia. Moreover, an attendant risk of stroke as well as a high frequency of seizures are associated with this method. These factors have limited the application of this technique.[43,44]

Tumor location and vascular supply determine the arterial circulation that is catheterized and infused. Most commonly, one major artery (left carotid, right carotid, left or right vertebral) is cannulated and treated. Some have advocated that documentation of BBB disruption with iodinated contrast agents be obtained before chemotherapy administration. Given the technical requirements of this procedure, it has not been widely adopted, and no definitive conclusions about the efficacy of the technique can be derived from the results of clinical trials that have been published to date. Other, less invasive techniques of BBB disruption are being investigated. It was recently shown that focused ultrasound exposure, when applied in the presence of preformed gas bubbles, can cause MRI-proven reversible opening of BBB in rabbits.[45] There is also interest in evaluating the use of biological agents to increase permeability of the BBB. Experimental data have demonstrated the effectivness of several such vasoactive compounds, including histamine, leukotriene C4, beta-interferon, tumor necrosis factor-alpha, and bradykinin. The bradykinin analog RMP-7 (Cereport) selectively increases delivery of radiolabeled carboplatin to brain tumor in animal xenograft models and improves survival. However, a recent randomized double-blind, placebo controlled phase II study showed that RMP-7 does not improve efficacy of carboplatin in patients with recurrent malignant glioma.[46]

High-Dose Chemotherapy

Considering that the BBB is a major factor in brain tumor resistance to chemotherapy and that diffusion across this barrier depends on the concentration-time profile of the free fraction of drug (i.e., drug that is not bound to plasma proteins), the assumption has been that increasing the administered dose would drive more drug across the BBB.[6] The rationale for high-dose chemotherapy (HDCT) was derived from the relatively linear in vitro dose-response curve exhibited by the classic alkylating agents and the assumption that intrinsic cellular resistance could be overcome by increasing the dose. In the context of treating brain tumors, the argument has been made that HDCT could overcome the previously mentioned sink effect and provide higher drug concentrations in the tumor for sustained periods. A number of phase I and II studies have been undertaken to evaluate this approach.[47] Despite the theoretical advantages, HDCT for recurrent malignant glioma has not made a significant impact on patient survival, although cases of long-term survival have been observed anecdotally. Among patients with newly diagnosed tumors, the median survival achieved using HDCT with bone marrow or stem cell rescue is comparable to that with conventional-dose chemotherapy (12 to 26 months versus 10 to 12 months, respectively). Treatment-related morbidity and mortality have been high, however, with a mortality rate as great as 27% in one early study. More recently, HDCT with autologous stem cell rescue was successfully used in treatment of medulloblastoma and malignant astrocytic tumors in children.[48] Safety and efficacy of this modality was also addressed by investigators in the treatment of recurrent CNS germinomas and malignant astrocytomas in adults.[49,50] Prolonged tumor control was achieved when HDCT in conjunction with stem cell rescue was used in the treatment of newly diagnosed anaplastic oligodendroglioma.[51] The strategy of HDCT followed by stem cell rescue may become an effective treatment strategy for potentially chemosensitive brain tumors such as anaplastic oligodendroglioma and primary CNS lymphoma.[52]

Intrathecal Administration

Intrathecal chemotherapy involves the direct injection of drug into the CSF and is an obvious way to bypass the BBB. It is accomplished by injecting drug into the lumbar subarachnoid space, the cerebral ventricles, or the basal cisterns, with or without the use of catheters, pumps, or ventricular reservoirs.[53] The rationale is that the cells lining the fluid spaces of the brain are permeable, which results in a free exchange of molecules from extracellular fluid (ECF) to CSF and vice versa. Relatively small doses of a drug given by intrathecal injection can achieve high local concentrations due to the low volume of CSF (approximately 150

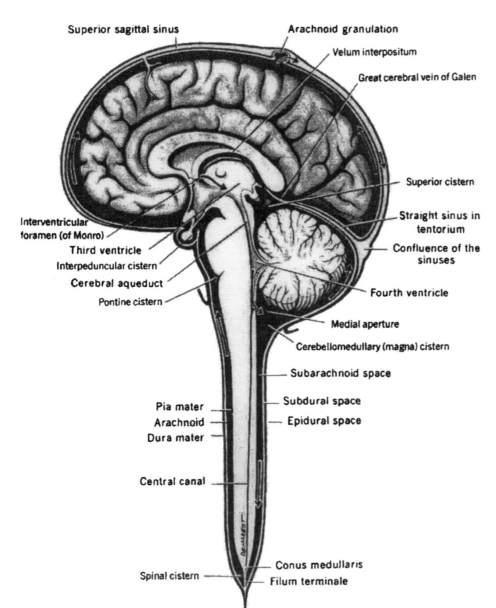

Superior sagittal sinus

Arachnoid granulation

Velum interpositum

Great cerebral vein of Galen

Superior cistern

Straight sinus in tentorium

Confluence of the sinuses

Interventricular foramen (of Monro)

Third ventricle

Interpeduncular cistern

Cerebral aqueduct

Pontine cistern

Fourth ventricle

Medial aperture

Cerebellomedullary (magna) cistern

Subarachnoid space

Subdural space

Pia mater

Arachnoid

Dura mater

Epidural space

Central canal

Conus medullaris

Spinal cistern

Filum terminale

Figure 21.3 The subarachnoid spaces and cisterns of the brain and spinal cord. Schematic representation of cerebrospinal fluid pathways (arrows). (Reprinted with permission from Fix J. High-Yield Neuroanatomy. 2nd ed. Philadelphia: Lippincott Williams & Wilkins, 2000.)

mL), minimizing systemic toxicity. Furthermore, because of the intrinsically low levels of enzymes in the CSF, some potentially useful agents that are subject to rapid metabolism in blood remain in the active form in the CNS for a longer periods of time. The three drugs used most commonly in this manner are methotrexate sodium, cytosine arabinoside (ara-C), and thiotepa (thiotriethylene phosphoramide). These agents have been used mainly for the treatment of leptomeningeal metastases from systemic cancer.[54]

Intrathecal drug administration has several disadvantages, including the necessity to establish access to the CSF compartment. A ventricular access device is usually implanted in the frontal horn of the lateral ventricle to facilitate the administration of drug and minimize patient discomfort. This entails a small surgical risk of hemorrhage

and infection. Moreover, the catheter may malfunction over time and require replacement.[55] Intrathecal drug administration also has numerous pharmacokinetic limitations. Among these, the drug must overcome bulk flow of CSF to penetrate the cisterns and ventricles (Fig. 21.3). In addition, the flow of interstitial fluid produced by brain cells and microvessels from ECF to CSF counteracts the diffusion of drug from CSF to ECF. Estimates are that CSF is completely renewed every 6 to 8 hours; thus, the concentration of a drug injected into the CSF decreases continuously as a consequence of this process, which can only be overcome by a continuous infusion or sustained-release system to maintain a clinically relevant concentration. Development of a liposomal form of ara-C allows sustained release of this drug into CSF and increases the effective half-life of the agent in the CSF by almost 50-fold.[56]

Another pharmacologic disadvantage of the intrathecal route is the fact that production of CSF by the choroid plexus and its elimination into the venous circulation may be altered by the tumor itself, which disturbs bulk flow and modifies drug distribution and diffusion. For example, the clearance of methotrexate from CSF is decreased in the presence of leukemic meningitis.[57,58] Moreover, diffusion in the ventricular space is heterogeneous[59] and may result in uncertain and potentially toxic local concentrations in CSF, even if continuous-infusion devices are used.[53] Finally, and most important, brain tumors are often in locations not adjacent to the ventricular system and may require diffusion of drug from CSF to tumor over a distance of several centimeters, which impairs the ability to achieve cytotoxic concentrations of the drug at the site of the tumor. In the case of methotrexate, the concentration of drug has been calculated to be no more than 0.1% of the CSF concentration 1 cm from the ependymal edge 48 hours after intrathecal administration.[60] However, the relationship is quite complex. Whereas compounds with greater lipophilicity will access the ECF more effectively, they will also be subject to a higher rate of removal by the vascular and cellular compartments, thereby limiting the extent of drug penetration into brain tissue.[61] Therefore, at this point in time, intrathecal chemotherapy is not feasible for brain tumors and is restricted to the treatment and prevention of leptomeningeal metastases.[62]

Intratumoral Administration

The simplest and most direct way to guarantee that a cytotoxic drug reaches its target is to deliver it directly into the tumor or into the cavity left after tumor resection. As with intrathecal injection, this bypasses most of the previously mentioned obstacles pertaining to systemic drug administration for treating brain tumors. Systemic toxicity may also be reduced because substantially lower doses of drug may be given, and only a relatively small amount of drug distributes from the CNS to the bloodstream. A particularly attractive advantage of this strategy is that anticancer drugs that are normally impeded by the BBB may be used. Conceptually, the low permeability of the BBB to such compounds should promote their retention within the CNS by inhibiting distribution into the bloodstream. Due to the high local drug concentrations that can be achieved, better distribution of drug may be provided within the tumor by diffusion and convection driven by the hydrostatic pressure of the tumor. The two techniques that have been most commonly used for directly introducing chemotherapeutic agents into brain tumors are (a) parenteral delivery as either a bolus injection or continuous infusion through a cannula and (b) implantation of drug embedded in a slow-release carrier system.

The feasibility of intratumoral infusion has been demonstrated in a number of clinical trials involving approximately 10 different anticancer agents.[63] These studies, however, have not shown a clear survival advantage or direct evidence of increased drug delivery within the tumor. Furthermore, toxicity has been observed with this technique, including nervous system injury and infection.[63] Even if intratumoral infusion does avoid some obstacles to drug delivery, it does not circumvent the sink effect or problems associated with drug stability. Indeed, drug molecules released into the ECF must penetrate the brain interstitial tissue to reach tumor cells.[27] Before reaching its target, the compound could be inactivated by binding to normal tissue, metabolism, chemical degradation, or elimination by the microvascular circulation.[64] Finally, obstruction of the catheter by tissue debris can occur.[63,64]

Controlled-release methods using polymer, microsphere, and liposomal carriers have been studied extensively in vitro and in vivo.[7] The goal of this strategy is to provide constant delivery of a cytotoxic drug into the tumor using a matrix that also protects the unreleased drug from hydrolysis and metabolism. Use of a solid polymeric matrix to facilitate the delivery of chemotherapeutic agents directly to brain tumors has several potential advantages. Biodegradable carriers have been developed that are unaffected by interstitial pH and provide near zero-order release of drug, with minimal inflammatory response.[65] Potential disadvantages include the fact that drug release cannot be controlled once the device has been implanted without physically removing it. Other potential problems include unpredictable diffusion, stability of the device and drug in the aqueous milieu, and the possibility that the polymer may not release the drug as intended.

A biodegradable polyanhydride solid matrix, poly [bis(*p*-carboxyphenoxy)propane-sebacic acid] or p(CPP-SA), has been developed that releases drug by a combination of diffusion and hydrolytic polymer degradation.[66] Preclinical studies have demonstrated that this system is biocompatible and results in reproducible and sustained continuous release of BCNU. More than 300 patients with recurrent[67,68] and newly diagnosed[3,69,70] malignant gliomas have been treated with the BCNU polymer in phase I–II clinical trials and phase III placebo-controlled studies. A phase III study in patients with recurrent malignant glioma demonstrated that intratumoral implantation of a 3.85% BCNU polymer was safe and resulted in minimal systemic side effects from BCNU. Median survival was significantly longer in subjects with glioblastoma who received the active polymer than in those who did not, even after adjustment for known prognostic factors.[67] A phase III randomized placebo controlled trial examining BCNU polymer application in glioblastoma patients at the time of primary surgical resection also showed survival benefit.[3] A phase I study designed to increase the amount of BCNU in the polymer (up to 20%) demonstrated that at the highest doses BCNU plasma levels were significantly (500-fold) lower than those associated with systemic BCNU toxicity. As a result, no BCNU-related systemic toxicity was seen.[71] However, risk of local neurotoxicity may be increased at higher BCNU concentrations in the polymer. Other studies of this delivery strategy are assessing use of the BCNU polymer in combination with systemic chemotherapy and incorporating other anticancer drugs into the polymer.[72] A clinical trial to evaluate intratumoral implantation of 5-fluorouracil–releasing microspheres has been initiated.[73]

Nonchemotherapeutic approaches involving intratumoral administration are also being investigated. A fusion protein consisting of interleukin 13 (IL-13) linked to a mutated form of *Pseudomonas* exotoxin (IL-13 PE38QQR) that is administered by convection-enhanced delivery (see below) has entered phase I/II trials.[74] In addition, intratumoral administration of chimeric proteins of transforming growth factor (TGF-α) and mutated *Pseudomonas* exotoxin PE-38 (TP-38) directed against the epidermal growth factor (EGFR) is being studied.[73]

Convection-Enhanced Delivery

Experimental evidence has demonstrated that properties of the brain parenchyma may impede delivery of drugs to the site of a brain tumor. Therefore, the BBB may not be the only obstacle that must be overcome for successful delivery of a cytotoxic drug to a brain tumor. Diffusion barriers intrinsic to brain tissue may also be important in limiting drug delivery to tumors. The hydrostatic pressure of brain tissue and the solubility of the drug are important factors that determine the diffusion of drug into surrounding tissue. Convection-enhanced delivery (CED) is a pressure gradient–dependent method developed to overcome these potential barriers; it consists of a direct infusion of drug solution through a catheter surgically implanted in the brain tumor.[75] Experimental studies of CED have demonstrated that drug delivery with this method is dependent on the anatomic site of the catheter. Infusion into gray matter results in spherical distribution of the drug, whereas infusion into white matter results in distribution along white matter fiber pathways. Therefore, the specific anatomic location of the brain tumor may be an important determinant of drug delivery.

Studies of the delivery of ara-C to rat brain after intravenous, intrathecal, and intraventricular administration and CED have been conducted.[76] Using quantitative autoradiographic analysis, it was demonstrated that drug concentration in brain tissue after CED was 4,000-fold higher than after intravenous administration. Moreover, the volume of distribution was 10-fold higher after CED than after intrathecal or intraventricular administration. Experience with the use of CED in the treatment of patients with brain tumors has been limited. In a phase I study involving 18 patients with recurrent malignant

gliomas, a high-flow interstitial microinfusion of a conjugated form of diphtheria toxin was conducted.[77] In 9 of 15 evaluable patients, at least a 50% regression of tumor was apparent on MRI, and two complete responses were observed. The treatment was well tolerated, and no treatment-related deaths or systemic toxicity occurred. The dose-limiting toxicity was local brain injury, which may have been the result of endothelial damage of cerebral capillaries.

ASSESSING DRUG DELIVERY TO THE BRAIN

The clinical effectiveness of chemotherapy ultimately depends upon exposing tumor cells to adequate concentrations of the biologically active form of anticancer drugs for a sufficient duration of time. Distribution of drug from the administration site to the tumor and its subsequent elimination from the body are dependent upon the physicochemical properties of the drug and numerous physiological factors. Penetration of the BBB or BTB is an additional complexity in the use of parenterally or orally adminstered anticancer agents against tumors residing within the CNS, one that is not a consideration in the treatment of hematological malignancies or solid tumors.[6,27,78] Characterizing the exposure of brain tumors to chemotherapeutic agents presents an extremely challenging problem. As is the case with any organ or tissue, the time course of the concentration of a drug or active metabolite within a tumor cannot be discerned from experimental data limited to measurements made in plasma, serum, or whole blood. Although some temporal relationship undoubtedly exists between drug concentrations in plasma and those in tumor, elucidating the tumor concentration-time profile necessarily requires measuring drug levels within the tumor itself.

Determining whether adequate concentrations of the active form of a drug reach the target tissue is extremely important in the context of phase I trials to evaluate the efficacy of new anticancer drugs for treating brain tumors. Because objective antitumor responses occur infrequently in phase I studies, the availability of data regarding the extent to which a chemotherapeutic agent reaches a brain tumor would provide a rational basis for selecting drugs that warrant further clinical evaluation. As described in this section, the principal techniques that are less invasive and potentially more informative than tissue biopsy studies for assessing the pharmacokinetics of anticancer drugs in the CNS and brain tumors include CSF sampling, microdialysis, and noninvasive imaging. Although no single method can be uniformly applied for monitoring drugs in human tissues in vivo, these techniques are nevertheless becoming increasingly important to the clinical development of anticancer drugs for the treatment of brain tumors.

Direct Measurment in Tumor Tissue

The traditional method for evaluating drug distribution to a solid tumor by directly measuring its concentration in tissue has numerous deficiencies. Subjecting brain cancer patients to the risks of an intracranial surgical procedure that may have little or no direct benefit to the treatment of their disease raises ethical concerns. It may be possible to circumvent this problem by obtaining tissue when a biopsy was diagnostically indicated or during a necessary tumor debulking procedure. Nevertheless, measuring the concentration of drug in a single biopsy specimen provides very limited information unless the tissue is obtained while drug is being given in a manner that provides continuous systemic exposure to the agent. Otherwise, the most appropriate time to obtain a single biopsy specimen relative to drug administration is speculative at best, as the presence or absence of a measurable drug concentration has little interpretive value. Acquiring serial tumor specimens from the same patient presents even greater practical constraints than conducting a single biopsy, and the effect of prior procedures on altering the transport of drug to and from the tumor represents a significant confounding factor. Conceivably, as part of a phase II study in which a moderately sized cohort of patients with comparable disease characteristics are treated with the same dose of drug, single biopsies of the tumor and adjacent peritumoral tissue could be performed in different patients over a range of times relative to drug administration, allowing a composite or pooled tissue concentration-time course to be constructed.

Cerebrospinal Fluid

Pharmacologic studies of anticancer agents directed against brain tumors often include the determination of drug or drug metabolite concentrations in the CSF as a surrogate for tumor levels and as a measure of drug delivery beyond the BBB. An understanding of the composition and normal physiology of CSF is important to discern the significance of drug level monitoring in this compartment. The most distinctive difference between CSF and plasma is the substantially lower concentration of proteins in CSF. Because of this, the total concentration of compounds that are poorly soluble in water or that bind avidly to proteins would be expected to be lower in CSF than in plasma or brain tissue, although the free concentration may be increased. In addition, CSF is slightly more acidic than plasma (pH of 7.32 versus 7.40), and this differential could conceivably influence the transport and retention of a drug in CSF, as well as its chemical stability relative to that in plasma, for compounds that have a functional group with a pK_a in the 7 to 8 range.

Fig. 21.3 depicts the normal process involved in CSF formation and flow. The volume of CSF contained within the ventricles, cisterns, and subarachnoid space of a normal adult is approximately 150 mL.[79] Approximately 500 mL of CSF is produced every 24 hours, predominantly by the choroid plexus within the cerebral ventricles; therefore, the entire CSF volume is replenished three times during the course of a day. CSF formed in the lateral ventricles flows into the third ventricle and then into the fourth ventricle. Upon exiting from the fourth ventricle, it passes into the basal cisterns and the cerebral and spinal subarachnoid spaces, descending through the posterior aspect of the spinal cord and returning through the anterior aspect. Ascending CSF passes over the cerebral hemispheres toward the major dural sinuses, where absorption of CSF into the venous system occurs at the arachnoid villi. The presence of a brain tumor can significantly diminish both the formation and flow of CSF.[80]

Concentration gradients between the ventricular and lumbar regions exist for endogenous constituents of CSF as well as for xenobiotics that have gained access to the CSF. The concentration of systemically administered drugs is generally higher in CSF collected from the ventricles than from the lumbar region, as drug distribution in the CNS follows CSF flow.[81] Because drug levels are often determined in CSF acquired by lumbar puncture, it should be recognized that this may significantly underestimate the concentrations in the ventricular region. Similarly, drug administered directly into lumbar CSF is poorly distributed to the ventricles.[59,82] Although patients cannot be subjected to frequently repeated lumbar punctures, ventricular access devices such as the Ommaya reservoir may be used to facilitate the serial acquisition of CSF specimens for drug level monitoring in the brain. Therefore, the specific space from which CSF samples were collected must be taken into account whenever drug concentrations reported in different studies are compared. Furthermore, in the process of collecting CSF specimens, the fluid balance or bulk volume of CSF could be significantly altered, which affects pressure equilibrium and flow between the various CSF compartments as well as the concentration gradients between CSF and plasma.

The presence of drug in the CSF represents a strong, but not definitive, indication that the compound has gained access to brain tissue, inclusive of tumors. Some level of uncertainty exists because the vascular supply to the choroid plexus, hypophysis, and pineal gland is not protected by the BBB. Although comprising a comparably small exchange surface, these do provide a direct pathway for the transport of compounds into the CSF. To further complicate matters, the absence of measurable drug or metabolite levels in the CSF does not absolutely imply that the agent has failed to reach a brain tumor. Conceivably, the majority of a compound reaching brain tissue could be trapped in the intracellular space, extensively bound to tissue protein, subject to chemical or enzymatic conversion to unknown products, or effluxed back into the bloodstream before migrating from interstitial spaces to the CSF. Accordingly, many drugs have been found to achieve higher concentrations in a brain tumor than would have been predicted from plasma and CSF data.[83,84] Despite the limitations of CSF as an indirect measure of drug delivery to a brain tumor, it is an accessible compartment, and CSF sampling remains an important method for screening drug access to the CNS.

Microdialysis

Inadequate transport of drug from systemic circulation to the interstitial space surrounding tumor cells is considered one of the primary reasons for the failure of chemotherapy for malignant gliomas.[27] Microdialysis is a technique that enables the concentration of a compound with appropriate physicochemical characteristics to be continuously measured in ECF within a tumor or normal tissues in a living subject.[85] Commercially available microdialysis catheters consist of a chamber that is less than 1 mm in diameter fitted with a semipermeable membrane that has a molecular weight cutoff ranging from 20 to 100 kd and into which two sections of microcatheter are fused. The device is stereotactically implanted such that the membrane resides within the desired area of the brain or tumor and the microcatheters are externalized. One of the microcatheters is connected to a syringe pump containing an appropriate perfusion fluid, and dialysate is collected from the other microcatheter. A sterile solution that approximates the composition of CSF, typically a Ringer's solution, is used as the perfusion fluid and delivered at flow rates in the microliter-per-minute range. In theory, microdialysis mimics the passive function of a capillary blood vessel.[85–87] Water, inorganic ions, and small hydrophilic organic molecules freely diffuse across the membrane of the probe, which is impermeable to proteins and protein-bound compounds. Lipophilic organic compounds are poorly recovered.

Considerable experience has been gained with the use of microdialysis, in both animal models and human subjects, since the technique was first introduced some 3 decades ago.[88] The greatest advantages of the technique for pharmacodynamic and pharmacokinetic studies is the facilitation of direct, serial sampling of ECF from a highly localized area of intact tissue.[78,89] Microdialysis has been thoroughly evaluated in head injury patients for monitoring lactic acid, glucose, glutamic acid, γ-aminobutyric acid, oxygen partial pressure, and pH, both for diagnostic intent and for assessing the effect of therapeutic interventions.[78,90–92] Insertion and removal of the dialysis probe results in minimal injury to normal brain tissue, alteration of fluid balance, or disruption of the BBB.[78,93,94] Although it can be performed safely, microdialysis is nevertheless an invasive surgical procedure with a small risk of bleeding at the insertion site and of discomfort for the patient.

Due to the low flow rate at which the perfusion solution is delivered, the perfusate must generally be collected over intervals ranging from 5 to 30 minutes in order to obtain a sufficient volume for chemical analysis. Consequently, microdialysis may not be suitable for studying systems in which the concentration of the compound of interest is changing rapidly relative to this time frame. The perfusate obtained by microdialysis can be analyzed directly by methods such as reversed-phase high-performance liquid chromatography, liquid chromatography/mass spectrometry, or capillary electrophoresis without the need for any preliminary sample preparation to remove macromolecules, as is generally required for assays performed on plasma.[78,95,96] Due to the dynamic nature of the system, in which the concentration of compounds in the ECF may be constantly changing while the perfusion fluid within the dialysis probe is continually flowing, steady-state conditions between the sampled fluid and dialysis fluid are not achieved. Nevertheless, it has been conclusively established that the in vivo recovery of an analyte, defined as its concentration in the dialysate relative to that in the sampled fluid, is independent of the concentration in the sampled fluid. Because the drug concentration in the dialysate is generally much lower than in ECF, the diluting effect of the technique demands a very sensitive analytical method to enable the detection of low concentrations of an analyte in very small sample volumes.[78]

The initial preclinical application of the technique to monitor the distribution of an anticancer drug to a brain tumor was described by de Lange, who measured the concentration of methotrexate in a rodent brain tumor model.[97] The results obtained with microdialysis were comparable to those in previous studies of methotrexate distribution to tumors based on the classic methods of autoradiography and tissue excision.[98] Subsequently, the technique has been used to define the concentration-time profile of camptothecin and topotecan in rodent brain tumor models[99,100] as well as of other antineoplastic agents in various preclinical tumor models.[85,86,101,102] Despite the demonstrated potential offered by the technique, there are still no published reports in which microdialysis has been used to study the intratumoral disposition of an anticancer drug in brain cancer patients. Publications documenting the use of the technique in patients with non-CNS solid tumors have solely described the monitoring of carboplatin levels in melanomas[103]and the delivery of 5-fluorouracil to breast tumors.[89] In the latter study, a relationship between the area under the interstitial concentration-time curve of 5-fluorouracil and therapeutic response was established. However, the feasibility of using microdialysis in the reverse application, for intratumoral drug delivery, has been demonstrated in a small cohort of glioma patients.[104]

Noninvasive Imaging

With continual improvements in spatial resolution, temporal resolution, and sensitivity, imaging techniques such as magnetic resonance spectroscopy (MRS) and PET offer the ability to noninvasively monitor the concentration of a drug or its metabolites within brain tumors and surrounding normal tissue. MRS involves the application of a strong magnetic field to the brain, which induces the absorption of energy in the radiofrequency range by atomic nuclei with appropriate spin characteristics. The frequencies of energy required to effect a transition between nuclear spin states are characteristic for each different nucleus and can be readily distinguished by a spectrometer. The isotopes of atoms amenable to detection by MRS that are of greatest interest with regard to drug level monitoring include ^{1}H, ^{2}H (deuterium), ^{11}B, ^{13}C, ^{15}N, ^{19}F, and ^{31}P. These are stable isotopes, although not always the most abundant isotopic form of an atom (e.g., ^{13}C). The spatial location and connectivity of atoms in the immediate vicinity of any given nucleus within a molecule influence the effective magnetic field experienced by the nucleus; this results in small but distinctive shifts in the resonance energy that convey structural information. The physical configuration of the instrumentation used for in vivo MRS results in a very substantial reduction in the resolution that can be achieved with analytical spectrometers. Whereas in vivo MRS can readily distinguish different atomic nuclei, the amount of detail pertaining to the type of molecule or functional group to which similar nuclei are bound is limited.

The intense signals associated with ^{1}H and ^{31}P, which result from the ubiquitous presence of these nuclei in bio-organic molecules, are used advantageously for diagnostic MRI. However, ^{1}H and ^{31}P MRS cannot generally be used to monitor xenobiotics in vivo, due to the intensity of the natural background signals, unless a compound has nuclei with chemical shifts that differ substantially from the resonance frequencies arising from endogenous molecules. Examples of the latter situation include the detection of iproplatin by ^{1}H MRS and ifosfamide by ^{31}P MRS.[105,106] Aside from these considerations, the relatively poor sensitivity of MRS is perhaps the single factor that most severely limits its utilization for in vivo drug level monitoring. A molecule must generally be present at concentrations in the low millimolar range to produce a detectable signal. Relatively few cytotoxic drugs achieve these concentrations in plasma or tissues. Furthermore, the anticancer agents that are currently being advanced into clinical trials tend to be increasingly potent, with MTDs that provide peak plasma concentrations in the nanomolar to low micromolar range in patients. The detection limits of MRS can be improved to some degree by increasing the data acquisition time. This sacrifices temporal resolution, however, which may be extremely important for pharmacokinetic studies. MRS does not permit the determination of the absolute concentration of a drug in vivo, although changes in relative concentration during the course of a single experiment can be readily followed. Another important consideration in using MRS to study the time course of a drug in brain tumors is that the spatial resolution is not particularly good, being approximately 1 cm^2 with current instrumentation.[107]

Despite these limitations, MRS has proven to be extremely valuable for studying the tissue pharmacokinetics of some fluorinated drugs, such as 5-fluorouracil.[107–110] The ^{19}F nucleus represents an ideal object for in vivo MRS studies. Spectra acquired from MRS scans of the human body show no background signals in the region where ^{19}F resonates due to the lack of endogenous fluorinated organic compounds. Moreover, the nuclear spin characteristics of ^{19}F provide an excellent signal.[107] An MRS study involving 103 patients with extraneural malignancies demonstrated that therapeutic response to 5-fluorouracil was significantly correlated with the half-life of the drug within tumors.[107,109,111] Gemcitabine hydrochloride is another fluorinated anticancer agent for which ^{19}F MRS has been successfully used for in vivo pharmacokinetic studies.[112,113] Although the feasibility of the approach has been demonstrated, very little clinical experience has been gained with the use of MRS for studying the distribution of anticancer drugs to brain tumors.

Dynamic PET imaging is an established technique for defining the time course of radiolabeled anticancer drugs within brain tumors and surrounding normal tissue in patients. In comparison with MRS, PET enables radiolabeled compounds to be detected with 10^6 to 10^9 times greater sensitivity and superior temporal resolution due to shorter data acquisition time.[114] Furthermore, whereas MRS is effectively limited to monitoring the relative change in concentration of a compound during the course of a study, PET provides a quantitative measurement of radioactivity. In addition, excellent spatial resolution, on the order of 6 mm or better, can be achieved with the current generation of detectors in whole-body PET scanners.[115]

The ability to use this methodology ultimately depends on developing a suitable procedure to introduce a positron-emitting radionuclide into the drug molecule. The fact that substituting a stable atom with a radioisotope of the same element does not affect the physicochemical, pharmacokinetic, or biologic properties of a drug has been well established. The radionuclides that have been most commonly used for PET pharmacokinetic studies are ^{11}C, ^{18}F, and ^{13}N.[115] Because these radionuclides have very short half-lives, namely 10 minutes for ^{13}N, 20 minutes for ^{11}C, and 110 minutes for ^{18}F, a cyclotron and remote-controlled radiochemical synthesis facility are required for on-site generation of the radionuclide and immediate preparation of the labeled drug.[115,116] As a consequence, the technique is expensive, and relatively few institutions in the United States have assembled the physical facilities required to undertake PET pharmacokinetic studies.

The most informative application of PET to pharmacokinetic studies entails the simultaneous acquisition of two sets of data as follows. A series of tomographic images are acquired for a total period of 1 to 2 hours after bolus intravenous administration of a tracer dose of the radiolabeled drug, which typically ranges from 100 to 1,000 MBq, together with the usual dose of unlabeled drug. The time over which individual images are measured generally increases during the course of the experiment and can range from 5 seconds to 10 minutes, as dictated by the combined rates of radioactive decay of the tracer and elimination of the drug from the body. The time-averaged concentration of radiotracer in discrete regions of interest within the image are used to construct time-activity curves. Arterial blood is also serially collected from the patient throughout the experiment for independent measurement of the radiotracer concentration in whole blood or plasma by liquid scintillation counting. The empirical kinetic model that best relates the time course of radiotracer in tissue to its concentration in plasma is then identified.[117]

In addition to its inherent expense and technical complexities, PET has a number of other distinct limitations when applied to the study of the tissue pharmacokinetics of a drug. The time period over which a radiolabeled drug can be monitored after administration of a tracer dose is effectively limited to three to four times the half-life of radioactive decay. The maximum duration of an experiment is therefore only 90 minutes for a ^{11}C-labeled drug and 6 to 8 hours when ^{18}F is used as the radiotracer. For some drugs, this may not be enough time to adequately define the time course of the uptake or decline of radiotracer in the tumor. Furthermore, expecting patients to remain within the confines of the PET camera for more than 60 to 90 minutes is unreasonable, and demands on the instrument for routine diagnostic use may also represent a significant factor that limits the duration of an experiment.

Another important deficiency is that PET measures total radioactivity without distinguishing alterations in the chemical structure of the labeled molecule. Because PET cannot distinguish the parent drug from metabolites that retain the label, or free from protein-bound drug, it may not be suitable for studying the distribution of drugs that are extensively metabolized or highly protein bound. These factors need to be taken into consideration for each individual agent when analyzing and interpreting kinetic data from PET studies.[117] Nevertheless, PET can provide highly informative insights and answer the critical question of whether radiotracer originating from the drug accumulates within a tumor.

Dynamic PET imaging has been used to study the distribution of the radiolabeled forms of several clinically approved and investigational anticancer agents to human brain tumors, including ^{11}C-BCNU,[118,119] ^{13}N-cisplatin,[120] 5-^{18}F-fluorouracil,[114] and ^{11}C-temozolomide.[117] PET has been used to demonstrate that the initial uptake of radioactivity originating from ^{11}C-temozolomide in plasma was seven times greater in brain tumors than in normal brain tissue, with the kinetic behavior in these two regions becoming almost indistinguishable by 30 minutes after dosing.[117] In consideration of these results, the markedly greater accumulation of radiolabeled agent in the tumor than in normal brain tissue, clearly evident in the PET images, was attributed to increased drug delivery due to a breakdown of the BBB within the tumor. The suggestion that the initial uptake of temozolomide from plasma could be an important determinant of its efficacy against human brain tumors has potential clinical significance.

DRUG INTERACTIONS AFFECTING BRAIN TUMOR THERAPY

Patients with primary or metastatic brain tumors are usually excluded from initial phase I clinical trials of investigational new anticancer drugs because of difficulties in differentiating potential indications of drug-related neurotoxicity from complications associated with the tumor. Furthermore, the additional supporting medications used in the clinical management of patients with brain tumors, especially antiseizure drugs and corticosteroids, could suppress the presentation of symptoms indicative of drug-related neurotoxicity. Until recently, the maximum tolerated dose of an investigational chemotherapeutic agent determined in adult patients with systemic solid tumors was used directly in phase II trials to assess clinical activity against brain tumors, without provisions to further refine the dose. It has become recognized that this practice often resulted in significantly undertreating patients with CNS malignancies as a consequence of pharmacokinetic interactions with concurrent medications that can enhance the elimination of anticancer drugs from systemic circulation as well as impede their access to the CNS.[121,122]

Interactions Affecting the Elimination of Anticancer Agents

As indicated in Chapter 3, metabolism represents a quantitatively significant pathway of elimination for many anticancer chemotherapeutic agents. That certain classes of compounds can induce or suppress the expression of CYP450 enzymes and thereby alter the extent to which other drugs are metabolized by these pathways is well known.[121,122] In addition, competitive inhibition could result from the concurrent administration of two or more drugs that are substrates for the same CYP450 isozyme. These effects may not result in a clinically significant alteration in the pharmacokinetic behavior of most drugs. However, anticancer agents are typically administered at relatively high doses, close to the threshold of tolerability, and thus may utilize a greater capacity of the elimination pathways than drugs given for other indications. Accordingly, the potential for clinically significant pharmacokinetic interactions are greater for chemotherapeutic agents than for other classes of drugs.[123]

Antiseizure drugs such as phenytoin, carbamazepine, and phenobarbital, which are commonly administered on a long-term basis to brain tumor patients, are potent inducers of many of the most important CYP450 enzymes involved in drug metabolism, such as CYP2C8, CYP2C9, and CYP3A4.[124] Patients who are being treated with these medications exhibit increased systemic clearance of epipodophyllotoxins,[125,126] vinca alkaloids,[127] taxanes,[128] and the camptothecins.[129,130] Administering standard doses of these chemotherapeutic agents together with an enzyme-inducing antiseizure drug results in lower plasma concentrations of the anticancer drug and reduced systemic toxicity. In consideration of the potential for pharmacokinetic interactions such as these, phase I studies are now being routinely designed to independently establish the maximum tolerated dose of new chemotherapeutic agents in brain tumor patients stratified according to whether or not they are receiving enzyme-inducing antiseizure drugs. Table 21.1 lists approved anticancer drugs for which pharmacokinetic interactions with enzyme-inducing antiseizure drugs have been evaluated in a clinical study in brain cancer patients and their effect on anticancer drug clearance.

Corticosteroids such as dexamethasone are widely used for the treatment of vasogenic brain edema and increased intracranial pressure in patients with brain tumors. Dexamethasone induces CYP3A4 by a pretranslational mechanism involving a glucocorticoid-responsive sequence in the promoter of the gene encoding the enzyme.[131] In addition, dexamethasone is a potent inducer of CYP2C8 and CYP2C9. Preclinical studies have shown that the pharmacokinetic behavior of cyclophosphamide and ifosfamide were markedly affected by pretreatment with corticosteroids.[132–134] Docetaxel metabolism was shown to be induced by dexamethasone in vitro, and decreased plasma concentrations of the drug have been demonstrated in a rodent model.[135,136] Corticosteroids appear to have little or no effect on the pharmacokinetics of the chloroethylnitrosourea alkylating agents.[137] In addition to interactions originating from the induction of drug-metabolizing enzymes, the potential also exists for diminished elimination of an anticancer agent in brain cancer patients due to competitive inhibition of a major drug-metabolizing enzyme by a supporting medication.

Therapies That Modulate Drug Distribution to the Brain

Corticosteroids have a well-established effect on decreasing the permeability of the BBB and BTB to a wide variety of molecules. Preclinical studies have shown that dexamethasone significantly reduces the transport through the BBB of water,[138] small organic molecules with molecular weights in the 100 to 350 range,[139,140] and macromolecules such as horseradish peroxidase.[141] Treatment with corticosteroids diminishes the permeability of experimental brain tumors, brain tissue immediately adjacent to tumor, and normal brain tissue distant to tumor, but the effect is most pronounced within the tumor itself.[142] These findings have been corroborated in studies of brain tumor patients. A marked reduction in the permeability of tumor and normal brain tissue to ^{82}Rb, as measured by PET imaging, was evident within 6 hours after the administration of dexamethasone by bolus injection to patients, and the effect persisted for at least 24 hours.[143] The magnitude of the decreased uptake of ^{82}Rb ranged from 6 to 48%.[144] Similar results have been observed in other studies using CT scanning[145] and MRI.[146,147] The effect of corticosteroids on the uptake of systemically administered chemotherapeutic agents has been evaluated in nude mice bearing intracranially implanted xenografts of human glioma. Steroid administration decreased the amount of carboplatin,[148] cisplatin,[149] and methotrexate[150] in the tumor and surrounding brain tissue by 20 to 40%. The extent to which the distribution of an anticancer agent to brain tumors is affected by corticosteroids in humans, however, remains to be determined.

TABLE 21.1

INFLUENCE OF ENZYME-INDUCING ANTISEIZURE DRUGS ON THE TOTAL BODY CLEARANCE OF INTRAVENOUSLY ADMINISTERED CHEMOTHERAPEUTIC AGENTS IN CANCER PATIENTS

Anticancer Agent	Infusion Time (h)	Dose (mg/m²) −EIASD	Dose (mg/m²) +EIASD	Total Body Clearance[a] (l/hr/m²) −EIASD	Total Body Clearance[a] (l/hr/m²) +EIASD	Difference (%)	Ref.
Etoposide	6.0	320–500	320–500	0.80	1.42	76.9	126[a]
Irinotecan	1.5	112–125	411	18.8	29.7	58.0	130
Paclitaxel	3.0	240	240	4.76	9.75	104.8	129
Teniposide	4.0	200	200	0.78	1.92	146.2	125
Topotecan	0.5	2.0	2.0	20.8	30.6	47.1	129
Vincristine[b]	0.25	2.0	2.0	34.1	55.5	62.6	127

[a]Mean or median values.
[b]Dose and clearance values are not normalized to body surface area.

The effect of radiotherapy on the integrity of the BBB and consequent penetration of drug into brain tumors remains an open area of investigation. Conflicting observations have been reported and may be attributed to marked differences in radiation treatment protocols, the methods used to assess the impact of the treatments on the function of the BBB, and the time course of changes in vascular physiology.[151] Consideration of the evidence derived from preclinical investigations indicates that the BBB in normal tissue becomes more permeable shortly after delivery of radiation according to the standard regimen of 5 days per week for 6 weeks.[152] This is entirely consistent with the finding that P-glycoprotein labeling decreased by 60% in the endothelial cells of brain vessels in a rodent after irradiation.[153] Slowly progressive alterations in the microvasculature of the irradiated tissue eventually result in decreased permeability.

The optimal schedule for delivering chemotherapy when used in combination with radiotherapy for treating brain tumors has not been conclusively established. The accumulation of methotrexate in a brain tumor model in mice was impaired by delivering radiation either before or concurrently with the systemically administered drug and resulted in shorter survival times; this suggests that chemotherapy should be given before radiation treatments.[154] In contrast, clinical observations indicating that a 30- to 40-Gy dose of radiation increased the permeability of the BBB within the irradiated tumor by 74% but only by 24% in normal surrounding tissue, as assessed by scintigraphy, were the basis for advocating the administration of anticancer drugs after radiotherapy.[155] Another study involving pediatric leukemia patients found no difference in the CSF-to-plasma concentration ratio of chemotherapeutic agents when given before, during, or after radiotherapy.[156] Finally, concurrent administration of temozolomide and radiation in patients with newly diagnosed glioblastoma has been demonstrated to extend progression-free survival and overall survival, suggesting clinical benefit for this strategy.[2] Because clinical trials for many new anticancer agents in brain tumor patients are now conducted in both the preradiation and postradiation periods, comparison of drug distribution into the CNS and brain tumors for these settings may be warranted.

CONCLUSION

Treatment strategies for the most common type of primary brain tumor, malignant glioma, are rapidly expanding. The persistence of normal BBB near the proliferating edge of the tumor, coupled with normalization of other areas of the BBB with treatment, emphasize the importance of strategies aimed at improving drug delivery across the BBB and to the tumor. In addition to the methods discussed in this review, cytotoxic drugs specifically designed for BBB penetration represent an important class of therapies to be assessed in the future. Methods for evaluating the success of these strategies are under development. Pharmacokinetic studies have assumed great importance in the development of antineoplastic therapy for hematologic and solid malignancies. Although application of the same principles to studies of brain tumor therapies is a relatively recent development and represents a unique set of challenges, these correlative studies add valuable information for the assessment of new brain tumor therapies. Moreover, with the emergence of cytostatic therapies for cancer, the traditional radiographic endpoints are insufficient, and these evaluative methods are likely to become surrogate endpoints in future clinical trials of these therapies. Finally, drug interactions have assumed great importance in brain tumor clinical trials owing to the recognition that many common supporting medications used in this patient population affect the metabolism of cytotoxic drugs through induction of the CYP450 enzyme family. The development of noninvasive methods that more readily facilitate evaluation of drug distribution and accumulation in local tissue and tumor is a fundamental challenge for the future. The availability of such techniques will allow efficient assessment of promising agents for the treatment of malignant gliomas.

REFERENCES

1. CBTRUS. Statistical Report: Primary Brain Tumors in the United States, 1997–2001. Central Brain Tumor Registry of the United States, 2004.
2. Stupp R, Mason WP, van den Bent MJ, et al. Radiotherapy plus concomitant and adjuvant temozolomide for glioblastoma. N Engl J Med 2005;352:987.
3. Westphal M, Hilt DC, Bortey E, et al. A phase 3 trial of local chemotherapy with biodegradable carmustine (BCNU) wafers in patients with primary malignant glioma. Neurooncol 2003;5:79.
4. Stewart LA. Chemotherapy in adult high-grade glioma: a systematic review and meta-analysis of individual patient data from 12 randomized trials. Lancet 2002;359:1011.
5. Phillips PC. Antineoplastic drug resistance in brain tumors. Neurol Clin 1991;9:383.
6. Greig NH. Optimizing drug delivery to brain tumors. Cancer Treat Rev 1987;14:1.
7. Sipos EP, Brem H. New delivery systems for brain tumor therapy. Neurol Clin 1995;13:813.
8. Pardridge WM, Oldendorf WH, Cancilla P, et al. Blood-brain barrier: interface between internal medicine and the brain. Ann Intern Med 1986;105:82.
9. Zlokovic BV, Apuzzo ML. Strategies to circumvent vascular barriers of the central nervous system. Neurosurgery 1998;43:877.
10. Crone C. The blood-brain barrier: a modified tight epithelium. In: Suckling AJ, Rumsby MG, Bradbury MWB, eds. The Blood-Brain Barrier in Health and Disease. Chichester, England: Ellis Horwood, 1986:17.
11. Muldoon LL, Pagel MA, Kroll RA, et al. A physiological barrier distal to the anatomic blood-brain barrier in a model of transvascular delivery. Am J Neuroradiol 1999;20:217.
12. Fishman RA. Cerebrospinal Fluid in Diseases of the Nervous System. Philadelphia: WB Saunders, 1992:43.
13. Greig NH, Momma S, Sweeney DJ, et al. Facilitated transport of melphalan at the rat blood-brain barrier by the large neutral amino acid carrier system. Cancer Res 1987;47:1571.
14. Henson JW, Cordon-Cardo C, Posner JB. P-glycoprotein expression in brain tumors. J Neurooncol 1992;14:37.

15. Fenart L, Buee-Scherrer V, Descamps L, et al. Inhibition of P-glycoprotein: rapid assessment of its implication in blood-brain barrier integrity and drug transport to the brain by an in vitro model of the blood-brain barrier. Pharm Res 1998;15:993.

16. Tsuji A. P-glycoprotein–mediated efflux transport of anticancer drugs at the blood-brain barrier. Ther Drug Monit 1998; 20:588.

17. Neuwelt EA. Mechanism of disease: the blood-brain barrier. Neurosurgery 2004;54:131.

18. Vick NA, Khandekar JD, Bigner DD. Chemotherapy of brain tumors: the "blood brain barrier" is not a factor. Arch Neurol 1977;34:523.

19. Waggener JD, Beggs JL. Vasculature of neural neoplasms. Adv Neurol 1976;15:27.

20. Steinhoff H, Grumme T, Kazner E, et al. Axial transverse computerized tomography in 73 glioblastomas. Acta Neurochir 1978; 42:45.

21. Blasberg RG, Groothuis DR. Chemotherapy of brain tumors: physiological and pharmacokinetic considerations. Semin Oncol 1986;13:70.

22. Chamberlain MC, Murovic JA, Levin VA. Absence of contrast enhancement on CT brain scans of patients with supratentorial malignant gliomas. Neurology 1988;38:1371.

23. DeAngelis LM. Cerebral lymphoma presenting as a nonenhancing lesion on computed tomographic/magnetic resonance scan. Ann Neurol 1993;33:308.

24. Brooks DJ, Beaney RP, Thomas DG. The role of positron emission tomography in the study of cerebral tumors. Semin Oncol 1986;13:83.

25. Orr RJ, Brada M, Flower MA, et al. Measurements of blood-brain barrier permeability in patients undergoing radiotherapy and chemotherapy for primary cerebral lymphoma. Eur J Cancer 1991;27:1356.

26. Rapoport SI, Fredericks WR, Ohno K, et al. Quantitative aspects of reversible osmotic opening of the blood-brain barrier. Am J Physiol 1980;238:R421.

27. Jain RK. Transport of molecules in the tumor interstitium: a review. Cancer Res 1987;47:3039.

28. Yamada K, Ushio Y, Hayakawa T, et al. Distribution of radiolabeled 1-(4-amino-2-methyl-5-pyrimidinyl)methyl-3-(2-chloroethyl)-3-nitrosourea hydrochloride in rat brain tumor: intraarterial versus intravenous administration. Cancer Res 1987;47:2123.

29. Bullard DE, Bigner SH, Bigner DD. Comparison of intravenous versus intracarotid therapy with 1,3-bis(2-chloroethyl)-1-nitrosourea in a rat brain tumor model. Cancer Res 1985;45:5240.

30. Fine HA, Dear KB, Loeffler JS, et al. Meta-analysis of radiation therapy with and without adjuvant chemotherapy for malignant gliomas in adults. Cancer 1993;71:2585.

31. Larner JM, Phillips CD, Dion JE, et al. A phase 1-2 trial of superselective carboplatin, low-dose infusional 5-fluorouracil and concurrent radiation for high-grade gliomas. Am J Clin Oncol 1995;18:1.

32. Stewart DJ, Grahovac Z, Hugenholtz H, et al. Combined intraarterial and systemic chemotherapy for intracerebral tumors. Neurosurgery 1987;21:207.

33. Shapiro WR, Green SB, Burger PC, et al. A randomized comparison of intra-arterial versus intravenous BCNU, with or without intravenous 5-fluorouracil, for newly diagnosed patients with malignant glioma. J Neurosurg 1992;76:772.

34. Kochi M, Kitamura I, Goto T, et al. Randomized comparison of intra-arterial versus intravenous infusion of ACNU for newly diagnosed patients with glioblastoma. J Neurooncol 2000;49:63.

35. Tamaki M, Ohno K, Niimi Y, et al. Parenchymal damage in the territory of the anterior choroidal artery following supraophthalmic intracarotid administration of CDDP for treatment of malignant gliomas. J Neurooncol 1997;35:65.

36. Blacklock JB, Wright DC, Dedrick RL, et al. Drug streaming during intra-arterial chemotherapy. J Neurosurg 1986;64:284.

37. Cloughesy TF, Gobin YP, Black KL, et al. Intra-arterial carboplatin chemotherapy for brain tumors: a dose escalation study based on cerebral blood flow. J Neurooncol 1997;35:121.

38. Saris SC, Blasberg RG, Carson RE, et al. Intravascular streaming during carotid artery infusions: demonstration in humans and reduction using diastole-phased pulsatile administration. J Neurosurg 1991;74:763.

39. Gobin PY, Cloughesy TF, Chow KL, et al. Intraarterial chemotherapy for brain tumors by using a spatial dose fractionation algorithm and pulsatile delivery. Radiology 2001;218:724.

40. Osztie E, Varallyay P, Doolittle ND, et al. Combined intraarterial carboplatin, intraarterial etoposide phosphate, and iv cytoxan chemotherapy for progressive optic-hypothalamic gliomas in young children. Am J Neuororadiol 2001;22:818.

41. Doolittle ND, Miner ME, Hall WA, et al. Safety and efficacy of multicenter study using intraarterial chemotherapy in conjunction with osmotic opening of blood-brain barrier for the treatment of patients with malignant brain tumors. Cancer 2000; 88:637.

42. Kroll RA, Neuwelt EA. Outwitting the blood-brain barrier for therapeutic purposes: osmotic opening and other means. Neurosurgery 1998;42:1083.

43. Gumerlock MK, Neuwelt EA. Chemotherapy of brain tumors: innovative approaches. In: Morantz RA, Walsh JW, eds. Brain Tumors. New York: Marcel Dekker, 1994:763.

44. Neuwelt EA, Howieson J, Frenkel EP, et al. Therapeutic efficacy of multiagent chemotherapy with drug delivery enhancement by blood-brain barrier modification in glioblastoma. Neurosurgery 1986;19:573.

45. Sheikov N, McDonnold N, Vykhodsteva N, et al. Cellular mechanisms of blood-brain barrier opening induced by ultrasound in presence of microbubbles. Ultrasound Med Biol 2004; 30:979.

46. Prados MD, Schold SC Jr, Fine HA, et al. A randomized, double-blind, placebo-controlled, phase 2 study of RMP-7 in combination with carboplatin administered intravenously for the treatment of recurrent malignant glioma. Neuro-oncol. 2003; 5:96.

47. Fernandez-Hidalgo OA, Vanaclocha V, Vieitez JM, et al. High-dose BCNU and autologous progenitor cell transplantation given with intra-arterial cisplatinum and simultaneous radiotherapy in the treatment of high-grade gliomas: benefit for selected patients. Bone Marrow Transplant 1996;18:143.

48. Perez Martinez A, Quintero CV, Gonzalez VM, et al. High-dose chemotherapy with autologous stem cell rescue in children with high-risk and recurrent brain tumors. Ann Pediatr 2004;61:8.

49. Modak S, Gardner S, Dunkel IJ, et al. Tiothepa-based high-dose chemotherapy with autologous stem-cell rescue in patients with recurrent or progressive CNS germ cell tumors. J Clin Oncol 2004;22:1934.

50. Chen B, Ahmed T, Mannancheril A, et al. Safety and efficacy of high-dose chemotherapy with autologous stem cell transplantation for patients with malignant astrocytomas. Cancer 2004; 100:2201.

51. Abrey L, Childs BH, Paleologos N, et al. High-dose chemotherapy with stem cell rescue as initial therapy for anaplastic ologodendroglioma. J Neuro-Onc 2003;65:127.

52. Abrey LE, Moskowitz CH, Mason WP, et al. Intensive methotrexate and cytarabine followed by high-dose chemotherapy with autologous stem-cell rescue in patients with newly diagnosed primary CNS lymphoma: an intent-to-treat analysis. J Clin Oncol 2003;21:4151.

53. Bakhshi S, North RB. Implantable pumps for drug delivery to the brain. J Neurooncol 1995;26:133.

54. Pinkel D, Woo S. Prevention and treatment of meningeal leukemia in children. Blood 1994;84:355.

55. Chamberlain MC, Kormanik PA, Barba D. Complications associated with intraventricular chemotherapy in patients with leptomeningeal metastases. J Neurosurg 1997;87:694.

56. Chamberlain MC, Kormanik P, Howell SB, et al. Pharmacokinetics of intralumbar DTC-101 for the treatment of leptomeningeal metastases. Arch Neurol 1995;52:912.

57. Ettinger LJ, Chervinsky DS, Freeman AI, et al. Pharmacokinetics of methotrexate following intravenous and intraventricular administration in acute lymphocytic leukemia and non-Hodgkin's lymphoma. Cancer 1982;50:1676.

58. Bleyer WA, Drake JC, Chabner BA. Neurotoxicity and elevated cerebrospinal-fluid methotrexate concentration in meningeal leukemia. N Engl J Med 1973;289:770.

59. Shapiro WR, Young DF, Mehta BM. Methotrexate: distribution in cerebrospinal fluid after intravenous, ventricular and lumbar injections. N Engl J Med 1975;293:161.
60. Blasberg RG, Patlak C, Fenstermacher JD. Intrathecal chemotherapy: brain tissue profiles after ventriculocisternal perfusion. J Pharmacol Exp Ther 1975;195:73.
61. Blasberg RG. Methotrexate, cytosine arabinoside, and BCNU concentration in brain after ventriculocisternal perfusion. Cancer Treat Rep 1977;61:625.
62. Chamberlain MC. Leptomeningeal metastases: a review of evaluation and treatment. J Neurooncol 1998;37:271.
63. Walter KA, Tamargo RJ, Olivi A, et al. Intratumoral chemotherapy. Neurosurgery 1995;37:1128.
64. Mak M, Fung L, Strasser JF, et al. Distribution of drugs following controlled delivery to the brain interstitium. J Neurooncol 1995;26:91.
65. Wu MP, Tamada JA, Brem H, et al. In vivo versus in vitro degradation of controlled release polymers for intracranial surgical therapy. J Biomed Mater Res 1994;28:387.
66. Leong KW, D'Amore PD, Marletta M, et al. Bioerodible polyanhydrides as drug-carrier matrices, II: biocompatibility and chemical reactivity. J Biomed Mater Res 1986;20:51.
67. Brem H, Piantadosi S, Burger PC, et al. Placebo-controlled trial of safety and efficacy of intraoperative controlled delivery by biodegradable polymers of chemotherapy for recurrent gliomas. The Polymer-Brain Tumor Treatment Group. Lancet 1995;345:1008.
68. Brem H, Mahaley MS Jr, Vick NA, et al. Interstitial chemotherapy with drug polymer implants for the treatment of recurrent gliomas. J Neurosurg 1991;74:441.
69. Brem H, Ewend MG, Piantadosi S, et al. The safety of interstitial chemotherapy with BCNU-loaded polymer followed by radiation therapy in the treatment of newly diagnosed malignant gliomas: phase I trial. J Neurooncol 1995;26:111.
70. Valtonen S, Timonen U, Toivanen P, et al. Interstitial chemotherapy with carmustine-loaded polymers for high-grade gliomas: a randomized double-blind study. Neurosurgery 1997;41:44.
71. Olivi A, Barker F, Tatter S, et al. Toxicities and pharmacokinetics of interstitial BCNU administrated via wafers: results of a phase I study in patients with recurrent malignant glioma. Proc Am Soc Clin Oncol 1999;18:142a.
72. Limentani S, Asher A, Fraser R, et al. A phase I trial of surgery, Gliadel and carboplatin in combination radiation therapy for anaplastic astrocytoma (AA) or glioblastoma multiforme (GBM). Proc Am Soc Clin Oncol 1999;18:151a.
73. Mrugala MM, Kesari S, Ramakrishna N, et al. Therapy for recurrent malignant glioma in adults. Expert Rev Anticancer Ther 2004;4:759.
74. Kunwar S. Convection enhanced delivery of IL13-PE38QQR for treatment of recurrent malignant glioma: presentation of interim findings from ongoing phase 1 studies. Acta Neurochir 2003;88(Suppl):105.
75. Groothius DR. The blood-brain and blood tumor barriers: a review of strategies for increasing drug delivery. Neuro-oncol 2000;2:45.
76. Groothuis DR, Benalcazar H, Allen CV, et al. Comparison of cytosine arabinoside delivery to rat brain by intravenous, intrathecal, intraventricular and intraparenchymal routes of administration. Brain Res 2000;856:281.
77. Laske DW, Youle RJ, Oldfield EH. Tumor regression with regional distribution of the targeted toxin TF-CRM107 in patients with malignant brain tumors. Nat Med 1997;3:1362.
78. De Lange EC, Danhof M, de Boer AG, et al. Methodological considerations of intracerebral microdialysis in pharmacokinetic studies on drug transport across the blood-brain barrier. Brain Res Brain Res Rev 1997;25:27.
79. Cserr HF. Physiology of the choroid plexus. Physiol Rev 1971;51:273.
80. Fishman RA. Cerebrospinal Fluid in Diseases of the Nervous System. Philadelphia: WB Saunders, 1992:23.
81. Zamboni WC, Gajjar AJ, Mandrell TD, et al. A four-hour topotecan infusion achieves cytotoxic exposure throughout the neuraxis in the nonhuman primate model: implications for treatment of children with metastatic medulloblastoma. Clin Cancer Res 1998;4:2537.

82. Blaney SM, Poplack DG, Godwin K, et al. Effect of body position on ventricular CSF methotrexate concentration following intralumbar administration. J Clin Oncol 1995;13:177.
83. Donelli MG, Zucchetti M, D'Incalci M. Do anticancer agents reach the tumor target in the human brain? Cancer Chemother Pharmacol 1992;30:251.
84. Stewart DJ. A critique of the role of the blood-brain barrier in the chemotherapy of human brain tumors. J Neurooncol 1994;20:121.
85. Johansen MJ, Newman RA, Madden T. The use of microdialysis in pharmacokinetics and pharmacodynamics. Pharmacotherapy 1997;17:464.
86. Mary S, Muret P, Makki S, et al. A new technique for study of cutaneous biology, microdialysis. Ann Dermatol Venereol 1999;126:66.
87. Groth L. Cutaneous microdialysis: methodology and validation. Acta Derm Venereol 1996;197(Suppl):1.
88. Ungerstedt U, Pycock C. Functional correlates of dopamine neurotransmission. Bull Schweiz Akad Med Wiss 1974;30:44.
89. Muller M, Mader RM, Steiner B, et al. 5-Fluorouracil kinetics in the interstitial tumor space: clinical response in breast cancer patients. Cancer Res 1997;57:2598.
90. Hamani C, Luer MS, Dujovny M. Microdialysis in the human brain: review of its applications. Neurol Res 1997;19:281.
91. Landolt H, Langemann H. Cerebral microdialysis as a diagnostic tool in acute brain injury. Eur J Anaesthesiol 1996;13:269.
92. Benveniste H, Hansen AJ, Ottosen NS. Determination of brain interstitial concentrations by microdialysis. J Neurochem 1989;52:1741.
93. Major O, Shdanova T, Duffek L, et al. Continuous monitoring of blood-brain barrier opening to Cr51-EDTA by microdialysis following probe injury. Acta Neurochir Suppl (Wien) 1990;51:46.
94. Westergren I, Nystrom B, Hamberger A, et al. Intracerebral dialysis and the blood-brain barrier. J Neurochem 1995;64:229.
95. Hogan BL, Lunte SM, Stobaugh JF, et al. On-line coupling of in vivo microdialysis sampling with capillary electrophoresis. Anal Chem 1994;66:596.
96. Chen A, Lunte CE. Microdialysis sampling coupled on-line to fast microbore liquid chromatography. J Chromatogr A 1995;691:29.
97. De Lange EC, Bouw MR, Mandema JW, et al. Application of intracerebral microdialysis to study regional distribution kinetics of drugs in rat brain. Br J Pharmacol 1995;116:2538.
98. Devineni D, Klein-Szanto A, Gallo JM. In vivo microdialysis to characterize drug transport in brain tumors: analysis of methotrexate uptake in rat glioma-2 (RG-2)-bearing rats. Cancer Chemother Pharmacol 1996;38:499.
99. El-Gizawy SA, Hedaya MA. Comparative brain tissue distribution of camptothecin and topotecan in the rat. Cancer Chemother Pharmacol 1999;43:364.
100. Zamboni WC, Houghton PJ, Hulstein JL, et al. Relationship between tumor extracellular fluid exposure to topotecan and tumor response in human neuroblastoma xenograft and cell lines. Cancer Chemother Pharmacol 1999;43:269.
101. Palsmeier RK, Lunte CE. Microdialysis sampling in tumor and muscle: study of the disposition of 3-amino-1,2,4-benzotriazine-1,4-di-N-oxide (SR 4233). Life Sci 1994;55:815.
102. Ekstrom O, Andersen A, Warren DJ, et al. Evaluation of methotrexate tissue exposure by in situ microdialysis in a rat model. Cancer Chemother Pharmacol 1994;34:297.
103. Blochl-Daum B, Muller M, Meisinger V, et al. Measurement of extracellular fluid carboplatin kinetics in melanoma metastases with microdialysis. Br J Cancer 1996;73:920.
104. Ronquist G, Hugosson R, Sjolander U, et al. Treatment of malignant glioma by a new therapeutic principle. Acta Neurochir 1992;114:8.
105. He Q, Bhujwalla ZM, Maxwell RJ, et al. Proton NMR observation of the antineoplastic agent iproplatin in vivo by selective multiple quantum coherence transfer (Sel-MQC). Magn Reson Med 1995;33:414.
106. Rodrigues LM, Maxwell RJ, McSheehy PM, et al. In vivo detection of ifosfamide by ^{31}P-MRS in rat tumours: increased uptake and cytotoxicity induced by carbogen breathing in GH3 prolactinomas. Br J Cancer 1997;75:62.

107. Wolf W, Waluch V, Presant CA. Non-invasive ^{19}F-NMRS of 5-fluorouracil in pharmacokinetics and pharmacodynamic studies. NMR Biomed 1998;11:380.

108. Findlay MP, Leach MO. In vivo monitoring of fluoropyrimidine metabolites: magnetic resonance spectroscopy in the evaluation of 5-fluorouracil. Anticancer Drugs 1994;5:260.

109. Presant CA, Wolf W, Waluch V, et al. Association of intratumoral pharmacokinetics of fluorouracil with clinical response. Lancet 1994;343:1184.

110. Maxwell RJ. New techniques in the pharmacokinetic analysis of cancer drugs, III: nuclear magnetic resonance. Cancer Surv 1993; 17:415.

111. Presant CA, Wolf W, Albright MJ, et al. Human tumor fluorouracil trapping: clinical correlations of in vivo ^{19}F-nuclear magnetic resonance spectroscopy pharmacokinetics. J Clin Oncol 1990;8:1868.

112. Kristjansen PE, Quistorff B, Spang-Thomsen M, et al. Intratumoral pharmacokinetic analysis by ^{19}F-magnetic resonance spectroscopy and cytostatic in vivo activity of gemcitabine (dFdC) in two small cell lung cancer xenografts. Ann Oncol 1993;4:157.

113. Wolf W, Waluch V, Presant CA, et al. Pharmacokinetic imaging of gemcitabine in human tumors using noninvasive ^{19}F-MRS. Proc Am Assoc Cancer Res 1999;40:384.

114. Kissel J, Brix G, Bellemann ME, et al. Pharmacokinetic analysis of 5-[^{18}F]fluorouracil tissue concentrations measured with positron emission tomography in patients with liver metastases from colorectal adenocarcinoma. Cancer Res 1997;57:3415.

115. Tilsley DW, Harte RJ, Jones T, et al. New techniques in the pharmacokinetic analysis of cancer drugs, IV: positron emission tomography. Cancer Surv 1993;17:425.

116. Rubin RH, Fischman AJ. Positron emission tomography in drug development. Q J Nucl Med 1997;41:171.

117. Meikle SR, Matthews JC, Brock CS, et al. Pharmacokinetic assessment of novel anti-cancer drugs using spectral analysis and positron emission tomography: a feasibility study. Cancer Chemother Pharmacol 1998;42:183.

118. Tyler JL, Yamamoto YL, Diksic M, et al. Pharmacokinetics of superselective intra-arterial and intravenous ^{11}C-BCNU evaluated by PET. J Nucl Med 1986;27:775.

119. Diksic M, Sako K, Feindel W, et al. Pharmacokinetics of positron-labeled 1,3-bis(2-chloroethyl)nitrosourea in human brain tumors using positron emission tomography. Cancer Res 1984; 44:3120.

120. Ginos JZ, Cooper AJ, Dhawan V, et al. [^{13}N]-cisplatin PET to assess pharmacokinetics of intra-arterial versus intravenous chemotherapy for malignant brain tumors. J Nucl Med 1987; 28:1844.

121. Van Meerten E, Verweij J, Schellens JH. Antineoplastic agents: drug interactions of clinical significance. Drug Saf 1995; 12:168.

122. McLeod HL. Clinically relevant drug-drug interactions in oncology. Br J Clin Pharmacol 1998;45:539.

123. Kivisto KT, Kroemer HK, Eichelbaum M. The role of human cytochrome P450 enzymes in the metabolism of anticancer agents: implications for drug interactions. Br J Clin Pharmacol 1995;40:523.

124. Tanaka E. Clinically significant pharmacokinetic drug interactions between antiepileptic drugs. J Clin Pharm Ther 1999;24:87.

125. Baker DK, Relling MV, Pui CH, et al. Increased teniposide clearance with concomitant anticonvulsant therapy. J Clin Oncol 1992;10:311.

126. Rodman JH, Murry DJ, Madden T, et al. Altered etoposide pharmacokinetics and time to engraftment in pediatric patients undergoing autologous bone marrow transplantation. J Clin Oncol 1994;12:2390.

127. Villikka K, Kivisto KT, Maenpaa H, et al. Cytochrome P450-inducing antiepileptics increase the clearance of vincristine in patients with brain tumors. Clin Pharmacol Ther 1999;66:589.

128. Chang SM, Kuhn JG, Rizzo J, et al. Phase I study of paclitaxel in patients with recurrent malignant glioma: a North American Brain Tumor Consortium report. J Clin Oncol 1998;16:2188.

129. Zamboni WC, Gajjar AJ, Heidman RL, et el. Phenytoin alters the disposition of topotecan and N-desmethyltopotecan in a patient with medulloblastoma. Clin Cancer Res 1998;4:783.

130. Gilbert MR, Supko JG, Batchelor T, et al. Phase I clinical trial and pharmacokinetic study of irinotecan in adult patients with recurrent malignant glioma. Clin Cancer Res, 2003;9:2940.

131. Liddle C, Goodwin BJ, George J, et al. Separate and interactive regulation of cytochrome P450 3A4 by triiodothyronine, dexamethasone, and growth hormone in cultured hepatocytes. J Clin Endocrinol Metab 1998;83:2411.

132. Chang TK, Yu L, Maurel P, et al. Enhanced cyclophosphamide and ifosfamide activation in primary human hepatocyte cultures: response to cytochrome P-450 inducers and autoinduction by oxazaphosphorines. Cancer Res 1997;57:1946.

133. Brain EG, Yu LJ, Gustafsson K, et al. Modulation of P450-dependent ifosfamide pharmacokinetics: a better understanding of drug activation in vivo. Br J Cancer 1998;77:1768.

134. Yu LJ, Drewes P, Gustafsson K, et al. In vivo modulation of alternative pathways of P-450-catalyzed cyclophosphamide metabolism: impact on pharmacokinetics and antitumor activity. J Pharmacol Exp Ther 1999;288:928.

135. Marre F, Sanderink GJ, de Sousa G, et al. Hepatic biotransformation of docetaxel (Taxotere) in vitro: involvement of the CYP3A subfamily in humans. Cancer Res 1996;56:1296.

136. Kamataki T, Yokoi T, Fujita K, et al. Preclinical approach for identifying drug interactions. Cancer Chemother Pharmacol 1998; 42:S50.

137. Levin VA, Stearns J, Byrd A, et al. The effect of phenobarbital pretreatment on the antitumor activity of 1,3-bis (2-chloroethyl)-1-nitrosourea (BCNU), 1-(2-chloroethyl)-3-cyclohexyl-1-nitrosourea (CCNU) and 1-(2-chloroethyl)-3-(2,6-dioxo-3-piperidyl)-1-nitrosourea (PCNU), and on the plasma pharmacokinetics and biotransformation of BCNU. J Pharmacol Exp Ther 1979;208:1.

138. Reid AC, Teasdale GM, McCulloch J. The effects of dexamethasone administration and withdrawal on water permeability across the blood-brain barrier. Ann Neurol 1983;13:28.

139. Ziylan YZ, LeFauconnier JM, Bernard G, et al. Effect of dexamethasone on transport of alpha-aminoisobutyric acid and sucrose across the blood-brain barrier. J Neurochem 1988;51: 1338.

140. Ziylan YZ, Lefauconnier JM, Bernard G, et al. Regional alterations in blood-to-brain transfer of alpha-aminoisobutyric acid and sucrose, after chronic administration and withdrawal of dexamethasone. J Neurochem 1989;52:684.

141. Hedley-Whyte ET, Hsu DW. Effect of dexamethasone on blood-brain barrier in the normal mouse. Ann Neurol 1986; 19:373.

142. Shapiro WR, Hiesiger EM, Cooney GA, et al. Temporal effects of dexamethasone on blood-to-brain and blood-to-tumor transport of ^{14}C-alpha-aminoisobutyric acid in rat C6 glioma. J Neurooncol 1990;8:197.

143. Jarden JO, Dhawan V, Moeller JR, et al. The time course of steroid action on blood-to-brain and blood-to-tumor transport of +[82]Rb: a positron emission tomographic study. Ann Neurol 1989;25:239.

144. Jarden JO, Dhawan V, Poltorak A, et al. Positron emission tomographic measurement of blood-to-brain and blood-to-tumor transport of +[82]Rb: the effect of dexamethasone and whole-brain radiation therapy. Ann Neurol 1985;18:636.

145. Yeung WT, Lee TY, Del Maestro RF, et al. Effect of steroids on iopamidol blood-brain transfer constant and plasma volume in brain tumors measured with X-ray computed tomography. J Neurooncol 1994;18:53.

146. Andersen C, Astrup J, Gyldensted C. Quantitation of peritumoural oedema and the effect of steroids using NMR-relaxation time imaging and blood-brain barrier analysis. Acta Neurochir Suppl (Wien) 1994;60:413.

147. Ostergaard L, Hochberg FH, Rabinov JD, et al. Early changes measured by magnetic resonance imaging in cerebral blood flow, blood volume, and blood-brain barrier permeability following dexamethasone treatment in patients with brain tumors. J Neurosurg 1999;90:300.

148. Matsukado K, Nakano S, Bartus RT, et al. Steroids decrease uptake of carboplatin in rat gliomas—uptake improved by intracarotid infusion of bradykinin analog, RMP-7. J Neurooncol 1997;34:131.

149. Straathof CS, van den Bent MJ, Ma J, et al. The effect of dexamethasone on the uptake of cisplatin in 9L glioma and the area of brain around tumor. J Neurooncol 1998;37:1.

150. Neuwelt EA, Barnett PA, Bigner DD, et al. Effects of adrenal cortical steroids and osmotic blood-brain barrier opening on methotrexate delivery to gliomas in the rodent: the factor of the blood-brain barrier. Proc Natl Acad Sci USA 1982;79:4420.

151. Trnovec T, Kallay Z, Bezek S. Effects of ionizing radiation on the blood brain barrier permeability to pharmacologically active substances. Int J Radiat Oncol Biol Phys 1990;19:1581.

152. d'Avella D, Cicciarello R, Angileri FF, et al. Radiation-induced blood-brain barrier changes: pathophysiological mechanisms and clinical implications. Acta Neurochir Suppl (Wien) 1998;71: 282.

153. Mima T, Toyonaga S, Mori K, et al. Early decrease of P-glycoprotein in the endothelium of the rat brain capillaries after moderate dose of irradiation. Neurol Res 1999;21:209.

154. Remsen LG, McCormick CI, Sexton G, et al. Decreased delivery and acute toxicity of cranial irradiation and chemotherapy given with osmotic blood-brain barrier disruption in a rodent model: the issue of sequence. Clin Cancer Res 1995;1:731.

155. Qin DX, Zheng R, Tang J, et al. Influence of radiation on the blood-brain barrier and optimum time of chemotherapy. Int J Radiat Oncol Biol Phys 1990;19:1507.

156. Riccardi R, Riccardi A, Lasorella A, et al. Cranial irradiation and permeability of blood-brain barrier to cytosine arabinoside in children with acute leukemia. Clin Cancer Res 1998;4:69.

Food and Drug Administration Role in Oncology Product Development

22

Thomas G. Roberts Jr.

At present, in the fourth quarter of 2004, there are more than 400 agents in clinical trials for the treatment of cancer, more than the number in any other therapeutic drug class.[1] The sponsor of each of these agents ultimately seeks approval by the US Food and Drug Administration (FDA) to market their product in the United States for at least one indication.[a] However, each year only 2 to 7 new drugs and biologics for the treatment of cancer obtain this goal. FDA approval of the product represents the final hurdle that sponsors must clear in their time-consuming efforts to discover and optimize lead compounds, test new drugs in animals, and conduct clinical studies in humans. Without this license, the effort to develop a new drug, which may have consumed hundreds of millions of dollars and spanned more than a decade of time, is spent in vain.[2,3] Sponsors face considerable odds in their quest to gain FDA approval; the low odds of success are major contributors to the

expense and risk associated with cancer drug development.[4,5] The most recent estimate of the average total cost (i.e., preclinical plus clinical costs) of developing a representative new drug from concept to FDA approval is $802 million,[b] with an average clinical development time of over 6 years.[3,5] Highly active products in a market without competition can generally be developed quickly, but many compounds are not highly active and require time and careful planning to demonstrate their potential.

Making decisions about the safety and efficacy of new drugs for licensure is just one of the roles of the FDA. The agency participates in the regulation of almost every step of clinical development. This regulation includes the oversight of clinical research, the evaluation of marketing claims for drugs seeking approval, and the monitoring of postmarketing activity for safety.[6] Over time, the FDA has evolved its approach to these regulatory activities. During the last 15 years, in particular, decisions by the FDA have become more transparent, and the relationship between the agency and the pharmaceutical industry has become more collaborative. Sponsors now consult with the agency throughout all stages of development, particularly in defining endpoints, selecting indications, and designing clinical trials. The FDA has also shown flexibility with respect to its approval and review policies. This flexibility has been

---

[a] This chapter focuses on the laws and regulations specific to the United States FDA. Thus, the information presented in this chapter may not apply to analogous regulatory agencies, though the United States Food and Drug Administration is a partner to the International Conference on Harmonization.

[b] This figure accounts for the cost of developing other drugs that fail as well as the opportunity cost of capital. When postapproval development costs are added, this number increases to $897 million.

especially evident with respect to drugs intended to treat serious or life-threatening illnesses such as cancer and AIDS. In response to criticism about the pace of drug development and FDA review, programs such as Fast Track Designation, Priority Review, and Accelerated Approval have been introduced to allow patients suffering from cancer and other life-threatening illnesses to receive new medicines at relatively early stages of development. In this chapter, we discuss the role of the FDA and focus in particular on the requirements for achieving marketing approval.

THE AUTHORITY OF THE FDA

The mandate of the FDA has evolved over the 20th century to assume three fundamental assurances: safety, efficacy, and adequate and accurate labeling.[6] Prior to the 20th century, therapeutic products received little regulation, and fraudulent claims of medicines escaped the control of the government. In 1902 the United States became the first country to establish federal control over therapeutic products with the passage of the Biologics Control Act, whose purpose was to define and regulate the safety of biologic products. In 1938, Congress enacted the Federal Food, Drug, and Cosmetic Act, which, for the first time, required drugs to be safe for their intended use. It was not until almost 25 years later, in 1962, that Congress amended the 1938 act by codifying a requirement that therapeutic drugs also demonstrate efficacy in addition to safety. Under the amendments, Congress indicated that the FDA should require "full reports of investigations which have been made to show whether or not such drug is safe for use and whether such drug is effective in use."[7] Over the last 40 years, Congress has enacted subsequent laws governing the FDA, such as the Orphan Drug Act, the Federal Advisory Committee Act, and the Food and Drug Administration Modernization Act of 1997, statutes that are discussed later in the chapter.

In addition to laws originating in the US Congress, the FDA derives its authority and direction from multiple *regulations*. The executive branch develops regulations to provide interpretation of the laws. Regulations do not require congressional action, but they are subjected to a period of public review and scrutiny. When finalized, however, they are binding until revised or withdrawn. They are published in the Code of Federal Regulations. The FDA regulations stipulate, "The purpose of conducting clinical investigations of a drug is to distinguish the effect of a drug from other influences, such as spontaneous change in the course of the disease, placebo effect, or biased observation."[8] The regulations specify further that reports of "adequate and well-controlled investigations" are required to provide the primary basis for determining whether there is "substantial evidence" to support the claims of effectiveness for new drugs.

In addition to the laws and regulations governing the agency, the FDA itself can issue *guidance documents* to reflect its current thinking. These documents are not binding, but they can be helpful to industry in its interpretation of the laws and regulations. Examples of FDA guidance documents include "Guidance on Providing Clinical Evidence of Effectiveness for Human Drug and Biological Products," issued in May 1998, and a series of guidances issued in conjunction with the International Conference on Harmonization on the conduct and analysis of clinical studies. When issues arise that require greater clarification, the Federal Advisory Committee Act provides the FDA authority to consult a panel of outside experts to solicit advice and recommendations on policy.[6] By statute the FDA can only receive advice from chartered advisory committees. There is an Oncologic Drugs Advisory Committee (ODAC) that has a statutorily mandated pediatric oncology subcommittee. The ODAC has a committee chairperson and 12 voting members, who each serve staggered 4-year terms. At least one of the members is a patient representative and another is a statistician. The FDA typically follows the advice of the ODAC in response to questions addressed to the committee. However, the agency does not present all reviews for licensing applications to this committee and renders approval decisions based on the totality of the evidence, of which ODAC opinions represent a part.

INTERACTIONS BETWEEN THE FDA AND SPONSORS

It would be incorrect to think that sponsors and the FDA interact only at the time of FDA review of a licensing application. With increasing frequency, the FDA and drug sponsors communicate formally throughout the drug development process (Fig. 22.1).

Prior to the initiation of clinical testing of an investigational agent, a drug sponsor must file an investigational new drug (IND) application, and the FDA must grant permission to proceed with clinical studies. The IND application must include a copy of the protocol for each proposed study; a description of the physical, chemical, and biological characteristics of the agent; information on absorption, distribution, metabolism, and excretion; and an integrated summary of animal toxicology data.[9] IND filing is also required for the use of approved products that a sponsor wants to study in new populations or in regimens for which the risks are unknown. The IND approval process provides federal oversight of clinical investigations and is designed to protect potentially vulnerable research subjects.

After the FDA grants IND approval, the investigational agent enters into sequential phases of clinical development, with each phase representing a distinct set of goals and challenges. Phase I trials represent the first experience with the agent, regimen, or dosing schedule in humans. The major

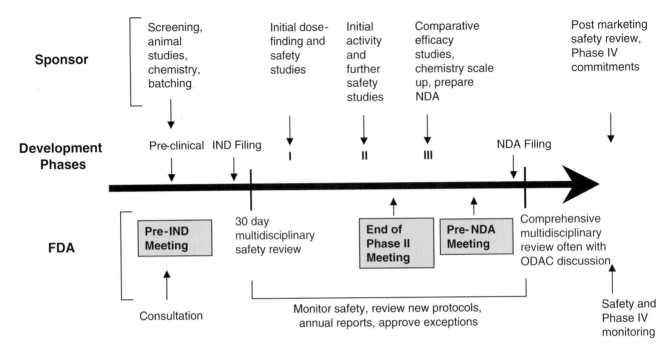

Figure 22.1 Overview of the drug development process. The multiple interactions between drug sponsors and the FDA reflect the convergence of the duties and responsibilities throughout the phases of development. IND, initial new drug application; NDA, new drug application; ODAC, Oncologic Drug Advisory Committee.

objectives of phase I trials are to determine the maximum tolerated dose that is appropriate to use in phase II trials, characterize the toxicity profile, and collect relevant pharmacokinetic data. To meet these objectives, investigators typically treat cohorts of 3 to 6 advanced cancer patients with escalating doses of the investigational agent until a dose-limiting toxicity (DLT) is identified; additional patients are then treated at the dose just below the DLT level to confirm its safety. The purpose of phase II trials is to determine a preliminary assessment of the agent's efficacy and safety in a particular type of cancer. Phase II trials typically do not include a concurrent control group and usually enroll 15 to 50 patients. Phase III trials are large, randomized, multi-institutional, resource-intensive efforts that seek to determine if the investigational treatment shows clinically important benefit over a widely accepted standard of care.[3,10] A sponsor may refer to a phase III trial as a *registration trial* or *pivotal trial* if it plans to use the data generated by the study as the primary basis for marketing approval.

The optimal times for the sponsor to solicit FDA input occur when particular landmarks are reached in the development process. Prior to filing a formal IND application, it can be helpful to the sponsor to request a Pre-IND Meeting to solicit FDA advice regarding requirements for preclinical studies and to discuss clinical development scenarios, particularly for new molecular entities (NMEs).

After the completion of phase I trials, a sponsor may request an End of Phase I Meeting to help in the planning of phase II trials, but such meetings are not universally sought. Once data are available from phase II studies, however, the

sponsor almost always requests a meeting to discuss safety issues and/or approaches that are likely to establish efficacy of its products. In this critical End of Phase II Meeting, the sponsor can discuss clinical trial design and analysis plans for proposed registration studies. The goal of a registration study is to design and complete a trial or group of trials that will produce the relevant data from which a marketing claim may be made. Table 22.1 outlines the many issues that sponsors must consider as they design and execute these pivotal studies. A analysis of NMEs approved from 1987 to 1995 demonstrated that agents that were discussed in Pre-IND and End of Phase II conferences with the FDA had shorter development times than those that were not discussed.[11]

At the conclusion of the End of Phase II Meeting, the sponsor can submit a detailed proposal for their critical phase III trial. This proposal is submitted for *Special Protocol Assessment*, with a legally mandated FDA review time of 45 days. In its assessment of the protocol, the FDA responds to specific questions the sponsor may have and provides general comments. Three types of studies are eligible for Special Protocol Assessment: animal carcinogenicity studies, product stability protocols, and clinical protocols for Phase III studies intended to form the basis for an efficacy claim. If the FDA concurs with the protocol, then a commitment exists to accept the design and size of the study as appropriate for approval, but the agency makes no commitment for ultimate approval, which ultimately depends on the data. Additional meetings are often scheduled before filing for a licensing application (Biologic Licensing Application [BLA] or New Drug Application

TABLE 22.1

KEY QUESTIONS THAT SPONSORS MUST CONSIDER IN THE PLANNING OF REGISTRATION TRIALS

What are the key endpoints?

Is the expectation to prolong life or improve quality of life (or both)?

Is the nature of the anticipated benefit clinically meaningful?

Is the benefit measured directly or through a surrogate? Is the surrogate validated?

Is the data analysis plan stated in advance?

Does the analysis plan address the endpoints appropriately?

Is the comparator for a controlled study reasonable and appropriate?

Is the target patient population representative of people with the disease or condition?

What is the burden of visits and tests?

Is Accelerated Approval (using a surrogate) considered?

If Accelerated Approval is considered, what is the proposed follow-up study?

[NDA]) to address particular chemical and manufacturing concerns (Product Meeting) and to seek input on the organization and format of the licensing application (Pre-BLA or Pre-NDA Meeting) and the product labeling.

FDA PROGRAMS WITH SPECIAL RELEVANCE TO ONCOLOGY

The regulatory review process has undergone significant evolution since 1980, prompted by concerns that patients lacked access to innovative therapies and were impacted negatively by a lengthy review process.[12,13] AIDS advocates lobbying for early access to antiretroviral drugs provided the initial impetus for a series of programs designed to expedite the drug development process, and advocates from the cancer community joined in these efforts shortly thereafter,[14] especially those concerned with breast cancer. The programs initiated in response to the AIDS crisis have also become available to cancer products. Table 22.2 presents some of the reform programs introduced since 1980 with particular relevance to cancer.

Orphan Drugs

In 1983, The US Congress enacted the Orphan Drug Act, allowing the FDA to provide incentives and grants for certain drugs intended to treat diseases with a prevalence of less than 200,000 people in the United States or those that affect more than 200,000 people but for which there is no reasonable expectation that the costs of development would be recovered from sales in the United States. The designation applies to a product used for a specific disease. Because there are more than 200 histological neoplastic subtypes, many cancer indications have the potential to obtain Orphan Drug designation. Orphan Drug designation qualifies the sponsor for a longer period of marketing exclusivity (7 years starting on the approval date, compared with 5 years), a 50% tax credit for money spent on

clinical trials for the orphan indication, exemptions from application filing user fees, and the option to compete for FDA development grants.[15] As of 2004, there have been approximately 40 cancer drugs or biologics that have been approved for marketing with Orphan Drug designation since the inception of the program. Cancer drugs and biologics comprise about 20% of all Orphan Drug approvals over this time period. Examples of approved products with Orphan Drug designation include pemetrexed (Alimta) in the treatment of malignant pleural mesothelioma, bortezomib (Velcade) in the treatment of multiple myeloma, and rituximab (Rituxan) in the treatment of non-Hodgkin's B-cell lymphoma. The Orphan Drug Program has been successful in providing incentives for sponsors to develop agents for rare diseases, but the program was not designed to address the criteria for approval nor to establish new target goals for FDA review times.

The "Fast Track" Programs

Over the period from 1992 to 1997, the US Congress enacted two laws, the Prescription Drug User Fee Act of 1992 (PDUFA) and the FDA Modernization Act of 1997 (FDAMA), which together have had a major impact on the process that the agency uses for reviewing and approving cancer drugs.[16] The legislation in these statutes is far-reaching, but from the perspective of medical oncology, the three programs introduced over this time period with the greatest impact are Fast Track Designation, Priority Review, and Accelerated Approval. Each of these programs exerts its impact at different stages of the drug development process.

Fast Track Designation

The Fast Track mechanism represents a formal structure by which sponsors may interact with the FDA. As described in the FDAMA, Fast Track designation can be granted to the combination of a product and a claim that the product addresses an unmet medical need for a serious or life-

TABLE 22.2		
RECENT FDA POLICY CHANGES RELEVANT TO CANCER		
Year(s)	Action	Result
1980s	Multiple guidance documents	Efficacy is defined as a demonstration of prolongation of life, a better life, or an established surrogate for at least one of these.
1983	Orphan Drug Act	Enables FDA to promote research and marketing of drugs for rare diseases (prevalence less than 200,000 in the United States), providing tax credits for clinical research and allowing 7 years of postapproval marketing exclusivity (compared to 5 years for regular approvals).
1991	Joint FDA/NCI proposal	Disease-free survival is allowed as a valid endpoint in the adjuvant setting if a large proportion of recurrences are symptomatic. Tumor response rates may be taken into consideration along with response duration, drug toxicity, and relief of tumor-related symptoms.
1992	Prescription Drug User Fee Act is enacted and Subpart H is added	*Accelerated Approval* is allowed for serious or life-threatening diseases when the new drug appears to provide benefit over available therapy but when the demonstrated benefit does not meet the standard for regular approval; response rates alone may provide a basis for Accelerated Approval when they are "reasonably likely surrogates" for clinical benefit. *Priority review* is instituted for those products that provide significant improvements in safety or efficacy in treating, diagnosing, or preventing serious disease; the FDA is required to review 90% of priority-related drug applications within 6 months of filing date. Payment of *user fees* by sponsors is tied to a series of FDA performance goals that commit the agency to accelerating the review process.
1997	FDA Modernization Act	Allows the FDA to consider data from "one adequate and well-controlled clinical investigation" with confirmatory evidence if data are sufficient to establish effectiveness. Codifies the *Fast Track Processes* for speeding the development of drugs that address unmet needs.

NCI, National Cancer Institute.

threatening illness. The benefits of Fast Track designation, if granted, include scheduled meetings to seek FDA input into development plans, the option of submitting an NDA in sections rather than all components simultaneously, and the option of requesting evaluation of studies using surrogate endpoints. For the most part, these interactions were already available to sponsors prior to the FDAMA, but the Fast Track mechanism formalized the approach for a subset of drugs. Since its inception, approximately half of the Fast Track designations have gone to drugs for the treatment of cancer or HIV/AIDS. In a survey of industry representatives, respondents indicated that the FDA has been able to approve 75% of the requests for Fast Track designation within 2 months.[16] Initially in 1998, and then updated in 2004, the FDA issued a guidance document describing the Fast Track programs in more detail.[17]

Accelerated Approval

Of the programs that have been designed to expedite the drug development process, none has had more impact or has generated more public commentary than Accelerated Approval. The Accelerated Approval regulations were added in 1992 (under Subpart H for drugs and under Subpart E for biologics). These provisions allow the FDA to approve agents intended to treat serious or life-threatening illnesses before the clinical benefit necessary to meet the standard for Regular Approval has been demonstrated. Using the Accelerated Approval mechanism, the FDA can grant a provisional approval on the basis of a surrogate measure of clinical benefit (e.g., tumor shrinkage) if the treatment is considered superior to available therapy for a serious or life-threatening illness.[18] The FDA grants the approval con-

TABLE 22.3

ACCELERATED APPROVALS IN ONCOLOGY THROUGH AUGUST 2004

Drug or Biologic (Trade Name)	Approval Year	Disease Indication	Response Rate[a]	Postmarketing Status
Liposomal doxorubicin (Doxil)	1995	Kaposi's sarcoma	27–48%	Not yet upgraded
Dexrazoxane (Zinecard)	1995	Reduction of doxorubicin toxicity	NA	Regular approval
Amifostine (Ethyol)	1996	Reduction of cisplatin toxicity	NA	Not yet upgraded
Docetaxel (Taxotere)	1996	Breast cancer	35%	Regular approval
Irinotecan (Camptosar)	1996	Colon cancer	12–15%	Regular approval
Capecitabine (Xeloda)	1998	Breast cancer	26%	Regular approval
Liposomal doxorubicin (Doxil)	1999	Ovarian cancer	0–22%	Not yet upgraded
Temozolomide (Temodar)	1999	Anaplastic astrocytoma	22%	Not yet upgraded
Denileukin diftitox (Ontak)	1999	Cutaneous T-cell lymphoma	23–36%	Not yet upgraded
Liposomal cytarabine (DepoCyt)	1999	Lymphomatous meningitis	41%	Not yet upgraded
Celecoxib (Celebrex)	1999	Reduction of colonic polyps	NA	Not yet upgraded
Gemtuzumab ozogamycin (Mylotarg)	2000	Acute myelogenous leukemia	22–33%	Not yet upgraded
Alemtuzumab (Campath)	2001	Chronic lymphocytic leukemia	21–33%	Not yet upgraded
Imatinib mesylate (Gleevec)	2001	Chronic myelogenous leukemia	31–93%	Regular approval
Imatinib mesylate (Gleevec)	2002	Gastrointestinal stromal tumor	33–43%	Not yet upgraded
Ibritumomab tiuxetan (Zevalin)	2002	Low-grade non-Hodgkin's lymphoma	74–80%	Not yet upgraded
Oxaliplatin (Eloxatin)	2002	Colon cancer	NA	Regular approval
Anastrozole (Arimidex)[b]	2002	Breast cancer	NA	Not yet upgraded
Imatinib mesylate (Gleevec)	2002	Newly diagnosed CML	NA	Not yet upgraded
Gefitinib (Iressa)	2003	Non–small cell lung cancer	10–20%	Phase III trial showed no benefit; marketing was suspended in December 2005
Bortezomib (Velcade)	2003	Multiple myeloma	28%	Recent approval
Tositumomab (Bexxar)	2003	Low-grade non-Hodgkin's lymphoma	63–68%	Recent approval
Cetuximab (Erbitux)	2004	Colon cancer	NA	Recent approval

[a]Response rates are from studies directly supporting approval in the agent's first marketing claim. Response data were obtained either from the FDA website or from the product label. Because the studies were often performed in chemotherapy refractory patients, response rates may be higher when the agents are administered in earlier settings. Agents without response rates noted were approved on the basis of other surrogates for clinical benefit, such as an interim analysis of a Phase III trial in the cases of oxaliplatin and anastrozole.
[b]Anastrozole was approved for the adjuvant treatment of postmenopausal women with hormone receptor positive early breast cancer. All other accelerated approvals have been either for the treatment of advanced cancers or for the reduction of chemotherapy-related toxicity.
NA, not applicable.
Adapted with permission from US Food and Drug Administration. Fast Track Drug Development Programs: Designation, Development, and Application Review. Rockville, MD: US Food and Drug Administration, September 1998.

ditionally and receives the sponsor's agreement to complete confirmatory phase IV trials in a timely manner during the postapproval period. If these trials do not confirm a clinical benefit, the drug can be withdrawn from the market. To date, however, the FDA has requested suspension of marketing of only a single product,[c] despite the fact that as of August 2004 sponsors had completed the phase IV trials required for an upgrade to Regular Approval in only 6 of the 23 oncology-related approvals.[19] Table 22.3 lists oncology agents approved using the Accelerated Approval mechanism through August 2004. The FDA and others in the

medical community have expressed concern over the failure of sponsors to complete confirmatory phase IV studies,[20, 21] prompting a focus on the issue during the March 2003 meeting of the ODAC. The regulatory standard for an Accelerated Approval can be less challenging than the standard for Regular Approval, because Regular Approval is predicated on the demonstration of a clinical benefit (e.g., prolonged survival or an improved quality of life) and not on a surrogate endpoint.

The FDA granted its first oncology-related Accelerated Approvals in 1995 (dexrazoxane for cardiomyopathy and liposomal doxorubicin for the treatment of AIDS-related Kaposi's sarcoma). Since then approximately 30% of the agents approved in medical oncology have utilized this mechanism. A recent review of the Accelerated Approval Program from 1992 through 1997 estimated that access to the program shortened overall development time by as much

[c] The sponsor and FDA jointly agreed to suspend marketing for gifitinib in December of 2004, following analysis of a Phase III trial that failed to show a survival benefit for gefitinib in non small-cell lung cancer. In June of 2005 gifitinib's label was changed to indicate that it is only to be used in patients who have previously taken gifitinib and are benefitting or have benefitted.

as 4 years in some instances.[22] It should be noted that Priority Review designation and eligibility for Accelerated Approval are assessed independently, and therefore the FDA may make discordant decisions in granting these designations. It is possible to receive Accelerated Approval and a Standard Review (10-month target), and it possible to receive Regular Approval with a Priority Review (6-month target).[6]

Priority Review

Whereas Fast Track designation applies throughout the development process, and Accelerated Approval applies following an intermediate stage of development before formal demonstration of clinical benefit, Priority Review is relevant only after a claim has been submitted to the FDA for review. As described in the PDUFA and the FDAMA, the FDA designates reviews for NDAs as either Standard or Priority. A Standard Designation sets the target date for the agency to complete all aspects of a review and to take action on the application (i.e., approve or not approve) at 10 months after the date of NDA filing. In comparison, a Priority Designation sets the target date for the FDA action at 6 months. Similar to the Fast Track program, Priority Review is intended for those products that address unmet medical needs. Fast Track designation does not automatically lead to eligibility for Priority Review, but FDA guidance states that achieving Fast Track Designation means that a product "ordinarily will be eligible for Priority Review."[17] Since 1994, approximately 50 cancer-related marketing claims involving 24 drugs have been granted Priority Review by the FDA, including such drugs as docetaxel (Taxotere) in the treatment of advanced non–small cell lung cancer after failure of prior platinum-based chemotherapy and topotecan (Hycamptin) in the treatment of patients with metastatic carcinoma of the ovary after failure of initial or subsequent chemotherapy. The quickest Priority Reviews to date were the reviews of imatinib mesylate (Gleevec) for the treatment of chronic myelogenous leukemia and of oxaliplatin (Eloxatin) in combination with 5-fluorouracil and leucovorin for the treatment of relapsed or refractory colorectal cancer; the claims for these drug uses received approval after just 10 weeks and 7 weeks of FDA review, respectively.

EVIDENCE REQUIRED FOR APPROVAL

Strategies for Registration

The FDA does not approve a drug but rather approves a claim about the use of a drug.[6] However, it is common after approval for oncologists to use agents for other than the approved claim.[23] A sponsor can take multiple pathways to gain approval for the first marketing claim of its drug or biologic agent. A major decision that the sponsor must make is for what line of treatment it will seek approval. A common approach is to begin therapeutic development with the use of a new single-agent as second- or third-line therapy for relapsed or refractory disease. The assumption is that activity in treatment-experienced patients will translate into clinical benefit for treatment-naïve patients. The phase II trials of gifitinib (Iressa) for the treatment of advanced non–small cell lung cancer after failure of platinum- and docetaxel-based chemotherapies illustrate this approach, since the data from these trials supported an Accelerated Approval for gefitinib in the third-line setting.[24,25] In comparison, first-line approvals tend to be more difficult to achieve, since the new agent must prove at least as good as the best treatment available. In order to show either an outcome difference or establish noninferiority, trials supporting first-line approvals will typically require more patients and longer follow-up than trials in refractory or relapsed populations, unless the new agent is impressively superior to available therapy. First-line approvals are also less likely to earn an Accelerated Approval, because there is at least one first-line regimen established for most cancers, and Accelerated Approval requires a demonstration of superiority if a standard therapy exists.

A common strategy in the first-line setting is to examine whether a new agent adds any benefit (or risk) to an established regimen. The registration trial of bevacizumab (Avastin) provides a recent example of this strategy: previously untreated patients with metastatic colorectal cancer were randomly assigned to receive irinotecan, bolus fluorouracil, and leucovorin (IFL) plus bevacizumab versus IFL alone.[26] Despite the risks associated with seeking a first-line indication, the effort can be worthwhile because a first-line approval will apply to a larger treatment population.

Another decision that sponsors must make is how many registration studies to undertake. In general, the FDA regards the results of a single trial supporting approval as inadequate evidence.[27] However, a single study may be considered adequate for licensing when the study is a large and well designed multicenter study, the implementation is of unquestionable quality, the findings appear clinically important, the results are statistically persuasive, and the confirmation of the results would present ethical or logistical hurdles.

General Approval Considerations

From a regulatory perspective, an intervention is a substance administered to a patient or a procedure performed on a patient with the intention of altering or interfering with the natural history of a disease. If the intervention disrupts or arrests the disease process so that suffering will be relieved or survival will be extended, and if it provides an acceptable risk for further suffering or loss of life, then the intervention can be considered a safe and effective treatment and is therefore eligible for FDA approval. At the most fundamental level, the agency must determine if there are differences between the treatment and control groups and then determine if the differences are due to the intervention under review. Establishing an appropriate control is therefore critical, because it is often difficult to determine efficacy without a control. Controls can either be historical or concurrent, and sponsors using the Accelerated Approval mechanism have usually employed historical controls in their phase II trials that support approval. However, concurrent controls have multiple advantages. Specifically, concurrent controls assure consistency of diagnosis, uniform techniques and frequency of clinical assessments of response and toxicity, a common level of supportive care, and consistency of administration of an intervention. Concurrent controls also allow for the possibility of reducing bias through blinding, although it is often difficult to blind cancer trials because of side effects. The goal of clinical research is to minimize bias and uncertainty, and concurrent controls with effective randomization can minimize both. When registration studies use an active concurrent control, it is usually the best available treatment.

The regulations guide the overall process of FDA approval, but the steps and the sequence of steps that the agency can take in this process are not completely standardized and therefore allow for some flexibility. During a review of a licensing application, the separate disciplines at the FDA review all primary data. The agency determines the nature of the claim, prepares a survey of available therapies that address the same problem (focusing on the nature and duration of the treatment effect of each therapy), and reconstructs what data and analysis would support a new claim. The FDA then identifies the key elements of the submission that provide the data to support the claim. The agency reviews the study protocols (focusing on eligibility, endpoints, measured variables, and planned analysis) and conducts its own analysis with regard to each patient's meeting eligibility, having the requisite measurements, and completing the study. The treatment effect is then determined, and the FDA analysis is compared to the sponsor's planned and submitted analyses.

If the FDA analysis demonstrates that the efficacy of the experimental treatment is either inferior to a control or cannot be distinguished from placebo effect, then there is no need for further analysis, and the application is denied. If the agency determines that the efficacy of the treatment is either superior to or at least not inferior to an active control, and if dropouts and censored patients can be adequately accounted for, the FDA proceeds with a safety analysis for each study to determine an estimate of the risk-benefit ratio (Fig. 22.2). Although a discussion of noninferiority is beyond the scope of this chapter, the factors that are critical in the design and analysis of a noninferiority study are the magnitude and reproducibility of the active control effect; defining the acceptable margin of retaining the active control effect; and describing in detail the analytic plan, including provisions for missing data and censoring. After completing its analysis, the agency compares

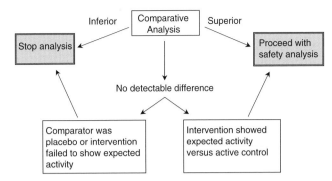

Figure 22.2 Flow diagram of the initial FDA review process. The first step is to determine if the intervention showed its expected activity. If the expected activity is not demonstrated, the analysis is stopped without proceeding to a safety analysis. If the expected activity is demonstrated, the agency proceeds with a safety analysis, and the intervention may be eligible for approval if a favorable risk-benefit ratio is found.

the efficacy data and safety data to the proposed marketing claims and then, if approval can be made, adjusts the claims in alignment with the conclusions supported by the data.

Assessment of Benefit

The assessment of risk is reasonably standard for oncology studies, and the same principles of a graded scale (e.g., NCI Common Toxicity Criteria) are applied to the oncology field as is done in other areas of medicine. The assessment of benefit on the other hand is less standardized (Table 22.4) and is often the subject of considerable dialogue and discussion.

Response Rates

In the early 1970s and 1980s, the FDA approved oncology drugs on the basis of response rate alone, i.e., the fraction of patients experiencing tumor shrinkage. By the mid-1980s

TABLE 22.4

TYPES OF ENDPOINTS USED IN CLINICAL ONCOLOGY

Survival
  Overall
  Disease-free
Progression
  Tumor (usually based on imaging results)
  Onset or worsening of disease-related symptoms
Response
  Tumor (usually based on imaging results)
  Patient benefit (palliation, improvement in symptoms)
Protection against adverse events with no decrease in survival
Reduction in the risk of disease
  From initial onset in a high risk population
  From recurrence in adjuvant setting

the ODAC advised the FDA against using response rate as the sole basis for approval, since the possible benefit of a response may be outweighed by toxicity. Moreover, the correlation between response rate and survival benefit had not been established for most solid tumors.[28] In response to this recommendation, the FDA adopted a new position calling for an improvement in survival or patient symptoms as the standard for Regular Approval.[29] Guidance documents promulgated in the 1980s specified further that the requirement for efficacy should be demonstrated by prolongation of life, a better life (e.g., relief of symptoms), or an established surrogate for at least one of these.[18]

In 1991, the National Cancer Institute and the FDA jointly examined the potential of various endpoints to demonstrate clinical benefit and again considered the issue of whether response rates could be used as a valid endpoint for drug approval. The two agencies concluded that complete responses of reasonable duration, particularly in acute leukemia, could be a potentially valid endpoint, as long as they correlated with clinical benefits such as reduced transfusion requirements. Partial responses were also considered as possibly valid endpoints, but only after considering their duration, the associated toxicity, and the potential to relieve tumor-related symptoms.[30]

A summary of the endpoints used in studies to support licensure for 90 separate claims for a variety of indications between 1985 and 2003 is shown in Table 22.5. The data show that most applications have multiple endpoints, and in most cases the determination of approving a claim for marketing was made on the totality of the evidence and not on a single endpoint. If several endpoints indicate the same trend, the support for considering approval is usually increased. Table 22.6 presents a tabulation of the endpoints from Table 22.5 to indicate their frequency in the aggregate of all 90 approved claims. The data show that few endpoints were used as sole criteria for marketing approval, but response rate was used most frequently, appearing in 60% of all claims and about 75% of Accelerated Approvals. In the hematologic malignancies, complete responses of a predetermined duration can be considered of patient benefit due to absence of disease complications such as bleeding, need for transfusions, or infections. Overall survival was used as a component of 27% of all claims but as a single criterion in only 5% of claims—twice for first-line colorectal cancer, once for first-line glioblastoma multiforme, and once each for second-line non–small cell lung cancer and glioblastoma multiforme. The frequency of use of overall survival and time to disease progression is quite similar. Disease-free survival and recurrence rate have been primarily used in the adjuvant setting.

The difficulty in establishing a coherent policy on the use of response rates to support approval relates to the lack of a documented relationship between tumor response and clinical benefit for most tumors. This relationship has been evaluated adequately in only a few tumor types, often with conflicting results. For example, Buyse et al. performed a meta-analysis of 25 trials in colorectal cancer involving flu-

oropyrimidines and concluded that tumor response was a significant independent predictor of survival.[31] In contrast, Chen et al. did not find a significant correlation of phase II response rates with median survival times in phase III trials of the same regimen in small cell lung cancer.[32] Variations in the definition of response exist and may account for some differences in interpretation. Response rates may provide a reasonable surrogate for survival, but only in certain diseases and with certain drugs. At present, the FDA continues to approve agents on the basis of response rates, but most of these approvals only meet the standard for Accelerated Approvals (Table 22.3) and therefore require confirmatory trials that employ clinical benefit endpoints.

Time to Tumor Progression

Some agents, particularly those with mechanisms of actions that are not cytotoxic, may produce clinical benefit by delaying tumor progression, with relatively low response rates. For these agents, time to tumor progression (TTP) or progression-free survival (PFS) may be a more appropriate surrogate endpoint than response. TTP or PFS is typically defined as the time from enrollment to documented progression of tumor size based on imaging tests (and not on biochemical tumor markers). The difference between TTP and PFS is that, in the latter, death is considered progression. Two major benefits of using progression include the potential need for smaller sample sizes and shorter follow-up times than for overall survival studies. Delayed progression in conjunction with response rates has been considered an adequate surrogate for clinical benefit in evaluating hormonal treatments for breast cancer, supporting Regular Approvals for exemestane, toremifene, anastrozole, letrozole, and fulvestrant in randomized trials comparing each of these with tamoxifen or with another approved hormonal agent.[18]

The ODAC has had difficulty accepting TTP as an endpoint for first-line indications for a number of submissions.[6] Their negative assessments relate to the general limitations of using TTP as an endpoint. First, TTP can only be evaluated reliably in the context of randomized trials, due to the difficulty of comparing results from historical controls in which assessment of tumor status posttherapy is not consistent across trials. In addition, there are few historical control databases that have used TTP as an endpoint. Second, even in randomized trials, TTP outcomes may be influenced by the frequency of obtaining imaging studies. If effective blinding is not performed, investigator bias may influence decisions regarding the timing of imaging studies and the interpretation of clinical data. More recent ODAC discussion of progression as a basis for approval has resulted in a reevaluation of the applicability and definition of this endpoint. The committee expressed a preference for progression-free survival over time to progression because PFS includes deaths from all causes,

TABLE 22.5

ENDPOINTS FOR APPROVALS OF ONCOLOGY DRUG MARKETING APPLICATIONS JANUARY 1, 1985, TO NOVEMBER 1, 2003

Disease Indication	Line(s) of Treatment	Accelerated Approval?	Endpoint(s)	No. of Claims	Percentage of Total Claims
Acute lymphocytic leukemia	First, Second		CR	3	3%
AIDS-related Kaposi's sarcoma	First		RR, TTP	2	2%
AIDS-related Kaposi's sarcoma	Second	YES	RR	1	1%
AIDS-related Kaposi's sarcoma	Second		RR	2	2%
Acute myelogenous leukemia	Second	YES	CR	1	1%
Acute myelogenous leukemia	First, second		CR	8	9%
B-cell chronic lymphocytic leukemia	Second	YES	RR	1	1%
B-cell chronic lymphocytic leukemia	Second		RR	1	1%
Bladder cancer	Second		RR	1	1%
Central nervous system cancer	First		OS	1	1%
Central nervous system cancer	Second		OS	1	1%
Central nervous system cancer	Second	YES	RR	1	1%
Breast cancer	Adjuvant	YES	DFS	1	1%
Breast cancer	Adjuvant		DFS, OS	5	6%
Breast cancer, metastatic	First		RR, TTP, 1-year survival	3	3%
Breast cancer, metastatic	Second	YES	RR	2	2%
Breast cancer, metastatic	Second		RR,TTP	6	7%
Chronic myelogenous leukemia	First	YES	CR	1	1%
Chronic myelogenous leukemia	Second	YES	CR	1	1%
Chronic myelogenous leukemia	Second		CR	1	1%
Colorectal cancer	Adjuvant		Recurrence rate	1	1%
Colorectal cancer, metastatic	First		OS	2	2%
Colorectal cancer, metastatic	Second	YES	RR, TTP	2	2%
Colorectal cancer, metastatic	Second		RR, OS	1	1%
Cutaneous T-cell lymphoma	Second		RR	3	3%
Esophageal cancer	Palliative		Symptom benefit	1	1%
Lymphoma, follicular	Second	YES	RR	1	1%
Lymphoma, follicular	Second		RR	1	1%
Gastrointestinal stromal tumor	First, second	YES	RR	1	1%
Hairy cell leukemia	First		CR, RR, TTP	3	3%
Hairy cell leukemia	Second		CR	1	1%
Lung cancer, non-small cell	First		OS, RR, TTP	4	4%
Lung cancer, non	Second		OS	1	1%
Lung cancer, non	Third	YES	RR	1	1%
Lung cancer, non	Palliative		Symptom benefit	1	1%
Lung cancer, small-cell	First		OS, RR	2	2%
Lung cancer, small-cell	Second		RR, symptom benefit	1	1%
Lymphoma, non-Hodgkin's	Second	YES	RR	2	2%
Lymphomatous meningitis	Second	YES	RR	1	1%
Melanoma	Adjuvant		DFS, OS	1	1%
Multiple myeloma	Third	YES	RR	1	1%
Multiple myeloma	Third		RR	1	1%
Osteosarcoma	First		RR	1	1%
Ovarian cancer	First		OS, RR	2	2%
Ovarian cancer	Second	YES	RR	1	1%
Ovarian cancer	Second		RR, TTP, OS	3	3%
Pancreas cancer	First, second		OS, symptom benefit	1	1%
Pleural effusion, malignant	Palliative		Recurrence rate	2	2%
Prostate cancer	Palliative		Symptom benefit	2	2%
Testicular cancer	Third		RR, DFS	2	2%

CR, complete response rate; RR, overall response rate; TTP, time to tumor progression, DFS, disease-free survival; OS, overall survival.
Data are from the FDA.

TABLE 22.6

TABULATION OF REGISTRATION STUDY ENDPOINTS THAT SUPPORTED MARKETING CLAIMS FROM JANUARY 1, 1985, TO NOVEMBER 1, 2003

Endpoint	Regular Approval	Accelerated Approval	Total[a]
CR	3%	18%	21%
RR	17%	43%	60%
TTP	2%	23%	26%
OS	0%	27%	27%
DFS	1%	9%	10%
1-year survival rate	0%	3%	3%
Recurrence rate	0%	3%	3%
Symptom benefit	0%	7%	7%

CR, complete response rate; RR, overall response rate; TTP, time to tumor progression; OS, overall survival; DFS, disease-free survival.
[a]Totals exceed 100% because most applications included multiple endpoints.
Data are from the FDA.

including disease progression and drug toxicity. The use of PFS in appropriate disease settings is attractive because of the shorter time frame to assess results compared with overall survival and because of the absence of potential confounding of a survival effect by subsequent therapy.

Relief of Tumor-Related Symptoms

Relief of tumor-related symptoms has been used as a primary or supportive basis for licensing in 6 applications for antitumor products between 1985 and 2003 (Table 22.5). Examples of symptom benefit supporting licensure include the approval of mitoxantrone in combination with corticosteroids as initial chemotherapy for the treatment of patients with pain related to advanced hormone-refractory prostate cancer; the pre-defined "clinical benefit response," a composite endpoint of pain, weight gain, and performance status, that provided support for the approval of gemcitabine for the treatment of locally advanced or metastatic pancreatic cancer, even though a small but significant improvement in survival was the primary basis for approval; changes in respiratory symptoms in small cell lung cancer associated with topotecan use; and changes in respiratory symptoms in non–small cell lung cancer associated with the use of porfimer sodium in the photodynamic treatment of endobronchial lesions.

Survival

Of all of the possible endpoints to assess benefit, survival is the least prone to bias and the least controversial in terms of its ability to support an FDA approval. In fact, all other endpoints used to justify approval must not be used to support a treatment that has a negative impact on survival.[6] Survival as an endpoint, however, is not without its limitations. The accurate recording of survival times requires long follow-up and potentially large sample sizes depending upon the mag-

nitude of drug effect. Subsequent treatments after progression can also confound or mitigate the interpretation of survival effect, particularly in crossover study designs. In part due to these limitations, over the last 18 years overall survival has contributed to the basis for approval in only 27% of claims and formed the primary basis for approval in only 8% of claims (Tables 22.5 and 22.6).

The industry and the FDA are keenly interested in the employment of new endpoints to support approvals. Potential endpoints of particular interest include progression-free survival (including symptomatic progression), surrogate biomarkers,[33] and patient-reported outcomes. The FDA is also interested in the use of interim analysis based on endpoints that differ from the endpoints planned for final analysis and in the use of methods to reduce bias such as centralized endpoint assessment committees.[34]

APPROVAL STATISTICS

Over the past 10 to 15 years, a growing number of academic and industry groups have begun to study trends in FDA actions and have monitored statistics such as development and review times. This work reflects the growing importance of cancer drugs and biologics as an industry sector. In 2003, the total worldwide market for oncology-related products was approximately $36.8 billion, and expenditures on oncology-related products have grown to almost 10% of the total $430 billion worldwide market for pharmaceuticals.[35] By 2008, the oncology market is projected to exceed $60 billion.

Review Times

Regulatory review represents only 5 to 10% of total clinical development time for most new oncology products (Fig. 22.3).[6] This percentage has decreased over time, from

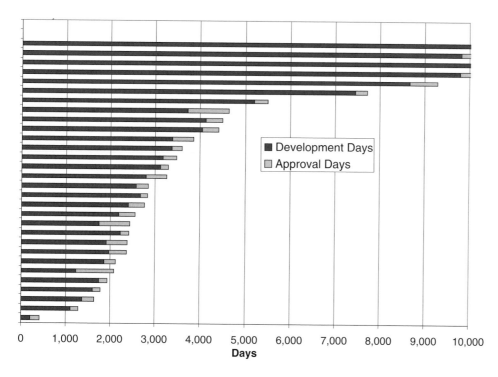

Figure 22.3 Development and approval times for new molecular entities approved 1995–2002. Regulatory review time (approval period) now represents approximately 5 to 10% of total clinical development time for most new oncology products. (The data are from the FDA.)

33% in the 1960s to approximately 25% in the 1980s and to approximately 15% in the early 1990s.[22] This trend is not unique to oncology products. The approval phase of drug development has fallen for drugs across all therapeutic classes. However, the trend toward decreasing review times has been most pronounced in the fields of cancer and AIDS. Of the 50 fastest drug approvals from the period 1963 to 2002, almost half involved agents used to treat cancer, AIDS, or AIDS-related opportunistic infections.[36]

Beginning in 1993, the payment of user fees by drug sponsors became linked to a series of FDA performance goals that committed the agency to incremental shortening of the review process.[22] Under the most recent amendments to these laws in 2002, the FDA is mandated to review and act on 90% of Standard Review original applications within 10 months of receipt, and on 90% of Priority Review original applications within 6 months.[12] There is evidence that the agency is able to meet these targets. At least one recent analysis demonstrated that from 1980 to 2001, the mean time period for approval for antineoplastic products granted Priority Review was 42% shorter than those granted Standard Review.[12]

Development Times

There is also evidence that the Accelerated Approval mechanism is having its intended effect. In a Tufts Center for the Study of Drug Development analysis of new therapeutics approved for marketing in the United States between 1980 and 2001, antineoplastic small molecule drugs that received accelerated approval had clinical development times that were on average 43% shorter than agents that did not utilize this mechanism.[12] Despite

the shortened development times of molecules approved under the Accelerated Approval mechanism, cancer drugs as a class tend to have longer development times than agents in other therapeutic categories. For example, in a Tuft's Center analysis involving a sample of 38 antineoplastic drugs approved from 1980 to 2001, the length of clinical trials was 81.6 months, and the median approval time was 12.8 months (for a total development time of 101 months). In contrast, cardiovascular drugs had a median length of clinical trials of 59.6 months and a median approval time of 26.7 months (for a total of 91.7 months).[12]

Levels of Innovation

The approval of NMEs, defined as medications containing an active substance that has never before been approved for marketing in any form in the United States, or new biopharmaceuticals is often taken as a measure of innovation in the pharmaceutical industry.[37] In general there has been a decline in the number of NMEs or biopharmaceuticals over time across therapeutic classes. In contrast, the number of NMEs approved per year in the oncology field increased substantially from 1991 to 2000, although it has plateaued since 2001 (Fig 22.4). In 2003, the FDA approved seven oncology-related NMEs, the most of any therapeutic class.

FUTURE CHALLENGES

The FDA continues to strive to become more collaborative in its approach to reviewing drugs for approval and to streamline the regulatory and product development processes. In May 2003, the NCI and the FDA (both of which are Health

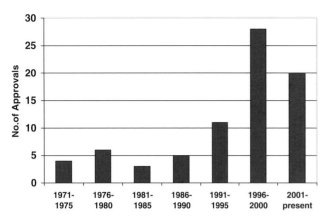

Figure 22.4 Number of approved new molecules for cancer use by the FDA. The number of approvals per 5-year period was relatively constant through 1990 and has increased substantially since then. (Adapted with permission from Rothenberg ML, Carbone DP, Johnson DH. Improving the evaluation of new cancer treatments: challenges and opportunities [opinion]. Nat Rev Cancer 2003;3:303–309. Data are updated through August 2004 and are available from the FDA at: http://www.accessdata.fda.gov/scripts/cder/onctools/statistics.cfm#count.)

and Human Service agencies) agreed to share knowledge and resources to facilitate the development of new cancer drugs. In particular, the agreement focused on developing markers of clinical benefit; creating a cancer bioinformatics infrastructure to improve data collection across all of the sectors involved in the development and delivery of cancer therapies; and encouraging collaborative training, rotations, and joint appointments in the two agencies.[38]

The future will bring many challenges for the FDA in its regulation of cancer-related products. Integrating pharmacogenomic data into the review process represents one such challenge. The expanded use of imaging to answer questions of drug mechanism, distribution, and efficacy in human subjects is another accelerating trend in cancer drug development. To this point, observers in the academic community have recently called upon the agency to mandate sponsors of new targeted anticancer treatments to invest in the research that can define subsets of patients who are likely to have responses to treatment based on the molecular signatures of their tumors.[17] Whether the agency will move toward requiring sponsors to invest in studies to define molecular signatures of response is unclear. Two additional challenges are the need to cooperate with the Center for Medicare and Medicaid Services and the continuing need to balance early access to potentially life saving drugs with the assurances of safety and efficacy. Guiding the FDA in these challenges will be the increasing trends toward more transparency, flexibility, and cooperation.

ACKNOWLEDGMENT

The author would like to thank Steven Hirschfeld of the Food and Drug Administration for his participation in helpful discussions.

ADDITIONAL RESOURCES

The Center for Biologics Evaluation and Research: http://www.fda.gov/cber/
The Center for Drug Evaluation and Research: http://www.fda.gov/cder/
Oncology Tools Website: http://www.fda.gov/cder/cancer
Public discussion of clinical trial endpoints: http://www.fda.gov/cder/drug/cancer_endpoints/default.htm

REFERENCES

1. IMS LifeCycle, R&D focus. In: Parexel's Pharmaceutical R&D Statistical Sourcebook 2003. Waltham, MA: Parexel.
2. Dimasi JA. New drug development in the United States from 1963 to 1999. Clin Pharmacol Ther 2001;69:286–296.
3. Roberts TG Jr, Lynch TJ Jr, Chabner BA. The phase III trial in the era of targeted therapy: unraveling the "go or no go" decision. J Clin Oncol Oct 1 2003;21:3683–3695.
4. Von Hoff DD. There are no bad anticancer agents, only bad clinical trial designs. Twenty-first Richard and Hinda Rosenthal Foundation Award Lecture. Clin Cancer Res 1998;4:1079–1086.
5. DiMasi JA, Hansen RW, Grabowski HG. The price of innovation: new estimates of drug development costs. J Health Econ 2003;22:151–185.
6. Hirschfeld S, Pazdur R. Oncology drug development: United States Food and Drug Administration perspective. Crit Rev Oncol Hematol 2002;42:137–143.
7. Mark B. McClellan, Commissioner, Food and Drug Administration. Speech before the Food and Drug Law Institute, April 1, 2003. Available at http://www.fda.gov/speeches/speechli.htm. Accessed April 28, 2003.
8. CFR Title 21 Part 314, Subpart D, Section 126.
9. US Food and Drug Administration. Content and Format of Investigational New Drug Applications (INDs) for Phase 1 Studies of Drugs, Including Well-Characterized, Therapeutic, Biotechnology-derived Products. Rockville, MD: US Food and Drug Administration, November 1995.
10. Roberts TG Jr, Lynch TJ Jr, Chabner BA. Identifying agents to test in Phase III clinical trials. In: Figg WD, ed. Pharmacokinetics and Pharmacodynamics of Anti-cancer Drugs. Totowa, NJ: Humana Press, 2004.
11. DiMasi JA, Manocchia M. Initiatives to speed new drug development and regulatory review: the impact of FDA-sponsored conferences. Drug Inf J 1997;31:771–788.
12. Reichert JM. Trends in development and approval times for new therapeutics in the United States. Nat Rev Drug Discov 2003;2:695–702
13. Lasagna L. Congress, the FDA, and new drug development: before and after 1962. Perspect Biol Med 1989;32:322–343.
14. Anderson LF. Cancer and AIDS groups push for changes in drug approval process. J Natl Cancer Inst 1989;81:829–831.
15. Milne CP. Orphan products: pain relief for clinical development headaches. Nat Biotechnol 2002;20:780–784.
16. Milne C-P. Fast track designation under the food and drug administration: the industry experience. Drug Inf J 2001;35:71–83.
17. US Food and Drug Administration. Fast Track Drug Development Programs: Designation, Development, and Application Review. Rockville, MD: US Food and Drug Administration, September 1998.
18. Johnson JR, Williams G, Pazdur R. End points and United States Food and Drug Administration approval of oncology drugs. J Clin Oncol 2003;21:1404–1411.
19. Roberts TG Jr, Chabner BA. Beyond fast track for drug approvals. N Engl J Med 2004;351:501–505.
20. Mitka M. Accelerated approval scrutinized: confirmatory phase 4 studies on new drugs languish. JAMA 2003;289:3227–3229.
21. Schilsky RL. Hurry up and wait: is accelerated approval of new cancer drugs in the best interests of cancer patients? J Clin Oncol 2003;21:3718–3720.

22. Shulman SR, Wood-Armany MJ. Accelerating access to cancer drugs. J Biolaw Business 1999;2(2):38–44.
23. Laetz T, Silberman G. Reimbursement policies constrain the practice of oncology. JAMA 1991;266:2996–2999.
24. Kris MG, Natale RB, Herbst RS, et al. Efficacy of gefitinib, an inhibitor of the epidermal growth factor receptor tyrosine kinase, in symptomatic patients with non-small cell lung cancer: a randomized trial. JAMA 2003;290:2149–2158.
25. Fukuoka M, Yano S, Giaccone G, et al. Multi-institutional randomized phase II trial of gefitinib for previously treated patients with advanced non-small-cell lung cancer. J Clin Oncol 2003;21:2237–2246.
26. Hurwitz H, Fehrenbacher L, Novotny W, et al. Bevacizumab plus irinotecan, fluorouracil, and leucovorin for metastatic colorectal cancer. N Engl J Med 2004;350:2335–2342.
27. US Food and Drug Administration. Providing Clinical Evidence of Effectiveness of Human Drugs and Biological Products. Rockville, MD: US Food and Drug Administration, May 1998.
28. Pazdur R. Response rates, survival, and chemotherapy trials. J Natl Cancer Inst 2000;92:1552–1553.
29. Johnson JR, Temple R. Food and Drug Administration requirements for approval of new anticancer drugs. Cancer Treat Rep 1985;69:1155–1159.
30. O'Shaughnessy JA, Wittes RE, Burke G, et al. Commentary concerning demonstration of safety and efficacy of investigational anticancer agents in clinical trials. J Clin Oncol 1991;9: 2225–2232.
31. Buyse M, Thirion P, Carlson RW, et al. Relation between tumour response to first-line chemotherapy and survival in advanced colorectal cancer: a meta-analysis. Meta-Analysis Group in Cancer. Lancet 2000;356:373–378.
32. Chen TT, Chute JP, Feigal E, et al. A model to select chemotherapy regimens for phase III trials for extensive-stage small-cell lung cancer. J Natl Cancer Inst 2000;92:1601–1607.
33. Kelloff GJ, Coffey DS, Chabner BA, et al. Prostate-specific antigen doubling time as a surrogate marker for evaluation of oncologic drugs to treat prostate cancer. Clin Cancer Res 2004;10: 3927–3933.
34. US Food and Drug Administration. On the Establishment and Operation of Clinical Trial Data Monitoring Committees. This is a Draft Guidance by the FDA available at: http://www.fda.gov/ohrms/dockets/98fr/010489gd.pdf Rockville, MD: US Food and Drug Administration, November 2001.
35. Cowen SG. Pharmaceutical therapeutic categories outlook: comprehensive study. 2004. P. 375.
36. A closer look at the FDA's 50 fastest drug approvals, 1963–2001. In: Parexel's Pharmaceutical R&D Statistical Sourcebook 2002. Waltham, MA: Parexel.
37. Frantz S. 2003 approvals: a year of innovation and upward trends. Nat Rev Drug Discov 2004;3:103–105.
38. US Food and Drug Administration. NCI and FDA announce joint program to streamline cancer drug development. May 30, 2003. Available at: http://www.fda.gov/bbs/topics/NEWS/2003/NEW00912.html. Accessed July 12, 2004.
39. Rothenberg ML, Carbone DP, Johnson DH. Improving the evaluation of new cancer treatments: challenges and opportunities [opinion]. Nat Rev Cancer 2003;3:303–309.

Central Venous Catheters: Care and Complications

23

Rachel P. Rosovsky   David J. Kuter

INTRODUCTION

Central venous catheters (CVCs) have become an integral part of treating patients both in and out of the hospital. They allow for easy administration of medications and uncomplicated withdrawal of blood samples. In cancer patients, who often require long-term chemotherapy, these devices have become the standard of care, and their use is increasing steadily every year. Unfortunately, these instruments are also associated with adverse events, most commonly, mechanical, infectious, and thrombotic complications. Recent research has focused on identifying the risk factors for and incidence, prevention, and treatment of these complications. Several studies have shown, for example, that antimicrobial-impregnated catheters can lower the risk of infection and decrease medical costs.[1-3] Unfortunately, only a few randomized or controlled studies involving CVCs and thrombosis exist, and results from these studies are often inconsistent and controversial.[4-10] Additional studies are clearly needed to help guide the optimal management of these complications.

This chapter reviews central venous catheters. We briefly mention the types of instruments available as well as the major indications for their usage. The majority of the review will focus on the complications of CVCs, most notably infectious and thrombotic. We will discuss the risk factors, the strategies for prevention, the current options for treatment, and new developments.

HISTORICAL PERSPECTIVE

The history of the central venous catheter dates back to 1656 when Christopher Wren (1632–1723) administered wine and ale to living dogs via an intravenous cannula. He describes in his writings how the animals became somnolent or vomited after being injected with alcoholic substances, opiates, or purgatives.[11-16] Wren's colleagues performed subsequent experiments with venous catheters involving the transfusion of blood products between animals and humans.[17] Unfortunately, some of these studies resulted in the death of either the animal or human. This outcome halted interest in and further investigation of venous cannulae for a number of centuries.

It was not until 1952, when Aubaniac described cannulating the subclavian vein of a wounded soldier for the purpose of resuscitation, that interest in the clinical uses of CVCs was renewed.[18-20] Fortunately, this attention led to the development of better technology, and over the past 30 years a number of devices for the semipermanent cannulation of the central venous system have been introduced. In 1973, Broviac developed the first long-term CVC for parenteral nutrition.[21] This was followed by the Hickman catheter in 1979, the first permanent venous-access device used for cancer chemotherapy.[22] Totally implantable venous access devices (Fig. 23.1), ones that are placed subcutaneously and contain their own ports attached to a centrally placed catheter, became available in the early 1980s.[23] The most recent advancement has been the peripherally implanted central catheter (PICC).[24]

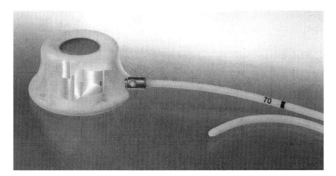

Figure 23.1 Cutaway photo of Port-a-Cath implantable port showing the injection site, reservoir, and attached catheter. (Courtesy of Smith Medical MD, Inc. St. Paul, Minnesota.)

CURRENT DEVICES

A wide variety of CVCs are currently available (Table 23.1). There are a number of short-term devices, including percutaneous lines and peripherally inserted central catheters (PICCs), that are usually employed for less than one month's duration. Alternatively, long-term catheters can remain in place for months to years; these include the surgically tunneled catheters described above (the Broviac and the Hickman, as well as, more recently, the Groshong and the Quinton) and the totally implanted venous access devices that contain their own port (the Mediport, the Infuse-a-Port, and the Port-a-Cath) (Figure 23.1). There are several standard techniques presently practiced for the insertion of a CVC.[25] The choice of catheter and the insertion strategy depend on a number of variables, most importantly the indication for its usage. However, patient characteristics, including any history of failed attempts, previous surgeries, comorbidities, skeletal deformities, and scarring, also need to be accessed.[26]

CURRENT USES

Central venous catheters have become essential for the management of cancer patients. In the United States, more than 5 million CVCs are inserted every year.[27] They not

TABLE 23.1

TYPES OF CENTRAL VENOUS CATHETERS

Short-term devices (1–14 days)
  Percutaneous internal jugular, subclavian, femoral lines
  Peripherally inserted central catheters (PICC)
Long-term devices (months to years)
  Surgically tunneled catheters (Hickman, Broviac, Groshong, Quinton)
  Totally implanted venous access devices (Mediport, Infus-a-Port, Port-a-Cath)

TABLE 23.2

INCIDENCE OF COMPLICATIONS OF CENTRAL VENOUS CATHETERS

Early
  Arrhythmia: 13%
  Arterial puncture: 2.8–3.8%
  Malposition of reservoir: 2%
  Pneumothorax: 1–1.8%
  Wound dehiscence: 1.5%
  Hemorrhage: 1.1–1.2 %
  Failure of insertion: 1.2%
Late
  Infection: 4–38%
  Catheter fracture and embolization: 3%
  Migration of catheter tip: 7.4%
  Thrombosis: ~41% (range 12–74%)
    Asymptomatic: ~29% (range: 5–62%)
    Symptomatic: ~12% (range: 5–41%)
Sequelae of CVC-related thrombosis
  Postphlebitic syndrome: 15–35%
  Pulmonary embolization: ~11% (range: 7–31%)
    Symptomatic: ~6% (range: 3–14%)
    Asymptomatic: ~5% (range: 3–15%)

only allow for intravenous administration of drugs, antibiotics, blood products, fluids, and nutrition but also facilitate easy drawing of blood samples to monitor for potential complications of treatments and disease. Eliminating frequent venipunctures clearly increases a patient's level of comfort. Whether the use of CVCs translates into extending life or improving quality of life is currently being investigated.[28]

COMPLICATIONS

Unfortunately, CVCs are associated with a number of early and late complications (Table 23.2), which can be both harmful to the patient and costly to treat. Most of the mechanical complications occur during the insertion process, although many of the infectious and thrombotic complications occur after the catheter has remained in place for some time. The reported incidence of catheter-related complications varies greatly among different studies, largely due to the different study designs, diagnostic protocols, and patient population.

EARLY COMPLICATIONS

Types of Early Complications

Arrhythmias occur in up to 13% of patients and are one of the most common complications that happen during

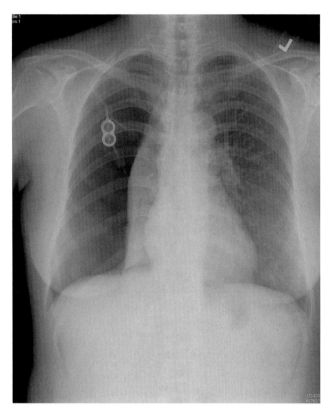

Figure 23.2 Pneumothorax, a potential early complication of CVC. (Courtesy of the Interventional Radiology Department, Brigham and Women's Hospital, Boston, MA.)

or immediately after the insertion process; however, they are usually self-limiting and rarely cause hemodynamic instability. Most of the other early adverse events are mechanical in nature, with an incidence range of 1 to 20%.[17,27] The most commonly reported ones are a venous tear, arterial puncture, or cannulation, which can then cause a hematoma or dissection, or a lung or pleural laceration, which can result in a pneumothorax (Figure 23.2) or hemothorax.[18,26,29] Injury to adjacent nerves or anatomic structures can also occur during the insertion process. Catheter malposition or breakage can occur early or late, as can a rare but potentially lethal complication, an air embolus.[18,25,27] The incidence of failed attempts has been reported to be as high as 5%. Lastly, there are a few case reports of the serious and occasionally fatal complication of cardiac tamponade.[30] Postinsertion care must include a chest x-ray to confirm the correct position of the catheter and the absence of injury to the vessels, lung, and pericardium.

Risks for Early Complications

The risk factors for the early mechanical complications are directly related to the site of CVC insertion as well as patient and catheter-related factors.[18,29] For the percutaneous devices, the frequency of mechanical complica-

tions such as hematoma or infection is higher with a femoral approach than with a subclavian or internal jugular approach.[18,29] However, if one only looks at the serious complications, the femoral and subclavian rates are similar.[27,29]

The type of material used for catheters and the time of their insertion also confer certain risks. Stiff CVCs are easier to insert but have a higher rate of mechanical complications.[18] When the insertion procedure for short-term percutaneous catheters is performed after hours, the complication rate is higher.[29,31] Lastly, thrombocytopenia, altered local anatomy, prior catheterization, recent myocardial infarction, severe obesity, and atherosclerosis are a few of the patient-related factors that can also increase the risk of adverse events.[18]

Prevention of Early Complications

There are a number of strategies one can utilize to reduce the risks of early complications. Perhaps the most important one is to know the patient and to determine the best insertion technique based on that patient's anatomy, comorbidities, and other characteristics. Prior surgeries or radiotherapy in the clavicular region, for example, may cause an alteration in the anatomy or surface landmarks used to locate a vein. Therefore, the contralateral side should be the preferred location in these patients.

Another preventive approach includes the use of ultrasound to aid in localizing the vessel to be cannulated. Ultrasonography decreases the risks associated with an internal jugular vein catheterization but does not clearly benefit the subclavian vein approach.[32] Obviously, the more experienced the physician, the less risk of a complication. One study showed that after three attempts, the incidence of mechanical complications increased to six times the rate after one attempt.[26,33]

As important as these pre-procedure strategies is the ability to recognize and treat complications. For example, an air embolus can usually be prevented by placing the patient in Trendelenburg's position during the insertion process and occluding the catheter hub at all times. However, if an air embolus is suspected or occurs, immediately placing the patient in this position and administering 100% oxygen can facilitate the resorption of air and prevent a potentially fatal outcome.[27]

LATE COMPLICATIONS: GENERAL

Types, Risks, and Prevention of General Late Complications

Infection and thrombosis are the most common late complications associated with CVCs, and they will be discussed separately. The other late complications occur at a rate of 3 to 8%.[17] CVC breakage can develop if defective material is used or if excessive manipulation is applied during the insertion process. CVCs also break due to a phenomenon associated with subclavian catheters termed the "pinch-off syndrome." Because the subclavian catheter is situated between the clavicle and the first rib, over time repeated compression can cause the catheter to fracture, resulting in extravasation of fluids, catheter breakage, and catheter embolization.[18,25] Extravasation of fluid also develops with CVC dislocation, malposition, or damage. Several other late complications also sometimes occur, though infrequently; these include arteriovenous fistulas, cerebrovascular accidents, cardiac aneurysms, and intracardiac abscesses.[18] Lastly, there are additional difficulties associated with CVC removal, but these are beyond the scope of this review.

The strategies to reduce the risks of late complications are similar to the ones presented in the section on early complications. One specific strategy to prevent the pinch-off syndrome is important to mention, however. Utilizing a more lateral approach or an alternative insertion site is recommended, especially in patients with known narrow thoracic inlet syndrome.[25]

LATE COMPLICATIONS: THROMBOSIS

Types of Thrombosis

Fibrin Sheath Formation

Several types of thrombi can occur with CVCs. Fibrin sheaths, or sleeve thrombi, form on the outside of catheters. They are ubiquitous, according to both autopsy and imaging studies, but rarely cause any difficulties unless they occlude the tip of the catheter.[34–37]

Although the time of formation of the fibrin sheath has not been adequately studied, data from several studies suggest that the sheath develops within 24 hours of catheter insertion.[35] Furthermore, electron microscopy and quantitative microbiologic testing of these fibrin sheaths show that they are always colonized by cocci.[38–40]

The presence of a sheath, however, does not predict subsequent deep venous thrombosis (DVT) of the vessel in which the catheter is placed. In one study, only 1 of 16 patients with a fibrin sheath developed thrombosis over a median of 12.5 months.[34] Furthermore, embolization of the fibrin sheath is uncommon and rarely symptomatic because of the small volume of the embolus.[41]

Intraluminal Thrombosis

A very common and underreported event is the development of clotting within the lumen of the catheter.[42–44] This event is often uncovered when the catheter fails to allow blood to be withdrawn or fails to allow infusion through a port. The frequency of catheter clotting varies widely among different studies. Anderson et al. reported 40 of 43 patients (93%) had this complication. In a large study by Schwarz et al, 122 out of 923 patients (13.2%) had this problem, for a frequency of 0.81 events per 1,000 catheter days, a rate comparable to the 0.6 per 1,000 catheter days reported by Ray.[42,44,45] These intraluminal thrombi can be lysed in most situations (80 to 95%) with local infusion of fibrinolytic agents such as urokinase, streptokinase, or tissue plasminogen activator.[46,47]

The inability to withdraw blood ("ball valve effect") does not, however, correlate with the presence of intraluminal thrombosis. In a study by Gould et al., 57% of thrombosed CVCs versus 27% of nonthrombosed CVCs failed to allow withdrawal of blood.[48] When the CVCs that had problems with blood withdrawal were analyzed by venography, 58% were thrombosed but 42% were not,[49] leading to the conclusion that nonthrombotic mechanical problems commonly prevented blood flow.

Central Venous Catheter-Related Blood Vessel Thrombosis (Deep Venous Thrombosis)

Catheter-related DVT is the most challenging thrombotic complication associated with long-term CVCs. These mural thrombi may partially or completely block the blood vessel, and their reported incidence from several prospective and a limited number of retrospective studies ranges from 5 to 75%.[17,50] The wide variability is due, in part, to the variation in the catheter type, the position, the duration of insertion, and the underlying disease. In addition, there is a lack of uniform standards in defining, identifying, and reporting this sort of information.

When diagnostic tests are used to evaluate patients who present with symptoms such as erythema or numbness of the extremity, swelling or pain in the arm, neck, or head, phlegmasia, or venous distension, the reported incidence of CVC-related DVT varies from 5 to 41% (Figure 23.3).[17,50] When surveillance venography or ultrasound are used to evaluate the patient, irrespective of symptoms, the rate of CVC-related DVT ranges from 12 to 75%.[17,50]

The time of onset of CVC-related DVT has been studied longitudinally in only a small number of individuals. In the most extensive study, by De Cicco et al., serial venography was done, on average, 8, 30, and 105 days after insertion of a CVC.[41] Of the DVTs that ultimately developed, 64% occurred by day 8 and 98% by day 30. In another study, 98% of all DVTs occurred in the first 8 days, and in a third study, 68% occurred within the first 30 days.[41,51,52] Further analysis of the time course of thrombus formation is essential for helping to guide future studies addressing the timing and duration of anticoagulation prophylaxis to prevent CVC-related DVT (see "Prevention and Prophylaxis of Central Venous Catheter-Related Deep Venous Thrombosis" later in the chapter).

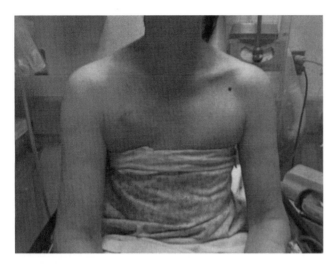

Figure 23.3 Venous distention and swelling of the arm. (Courtesy of Rachel Rosovsky, MD.)

Risk of Central Venous Catheter-Related Thrombosis

Patient-Related Risk Factors

Several observational and prospective studies have tried to elucidate the potential risk factors that may be important in the development of DVTs in CVCs. Both patient-related and catheter-related risks exist. The mere presence of malignancy is perhaps the most important patient-related risk factor, and there is a suggestion that some types of malignancy, such as adenocarcinoma of the lung, have higher rates of catheter-related DVTs than others, such as head and neck cancer.[44] This may be related to the activation of the coagulation system in these different malignancies, tumor-related changes in blood flow in the upper torso, or levels of tissue factor or tissue factor pathway inhibitor. It is probably related to the general increased risk of thrombosis that occurs in oncology patients, as has been discussed elsewhere.[53–56].

The type of chemotherapy also appears to influence the rate of CVC-related thrombosis. Clotting occurred in 6 of 11 catheters (55%) through which sclerosing chemotherapy was infused but in only 9 of 29 (31%) infused with nonsclerosing chemotherapy.[4]

Controversy exists as to whether inherited thrombophilia is a risk factor. One study suggests that low levels of antithrombin III are associated with a greater risk of thrombosis.[57] Another study found that 32% of patients who had CVC-related thrombosis had a diagnosis of a hypercoagulable state; most had an elevated anticardiolipin antibody but no increase in prothrombin 20210A mutation, factor V Leiden, protein C deficiency, or protein S deficiency.[58] Other studies evaluating factor V Leiden have yielded inconsistent results. Although there is a positive correlation of thrombosis with factor V Leiden in pediatric patients who have acute lymphoblas-

tic leukemia, there are conflicting results involving adults.[58–60]

In addition to thrombophilic molecular abnormalities, there are acquired forms of thrombophilia that contribute to the development of clots. Venous stasis caused by an indwelling CVC and vessel damage caused by chemotherapy or by injury during the insertion process are two components of Virchow's triad that are additional contributors to this multifactorial process. The role of an elevated platelet count, however, remains controversial.[4,61]

Catheter-Related Risk Factors

Catheters have undergone major design changes to reduce catheter-related complications. Polyvinylchloride and polyethylene CVCs, for example, have been replaced by the less thrombogenic silicone and polyurethane CVCs.[62] In addition to the catheter material, several other features of CVCs affect their thrombotic risk. Triple-lumen catheters have been shown to carry a higher risk of thrombosis than single- or double-lumen catheters.[62] Catheters inserted on the left side clot more frequently than those inserted in the right.[41] Finally, the position of the catheter tip needs to be at the junction of the superior vena cava (SVC) and the right atrium.[63] Placement of the catheter tip at a distal or high position in the SVC results in a higher rate of thrombosis than placement more centrally or lower in the SVC.[64]

Overall, CVCs are a "stress test" of the coagulation system in cancer patients and can precipitate thrombosis due to multiple mechanisms related to the host and/or to the device itself.

Complications of Central Venous Catheter-Related Deep Venous Thrombosis

A number of sequelae can potentially develop in patients with CVC-related DVT. Catheter dysfunction may be the first sign of a partially or completely occluded vessel and requires either flushing or removal and replacement of the device. This management can be expensive and can cause discomfort and anxiety for the patient. Postphlebitic syndrome occurs in 15 to 35% of patients with CVC-related DVT and can also cause discomfort for the patient in the form of chronic pain, edema, and functional impairment of the limb.[17,65]

The relationship between CVC-related DVT and pulmonary emboli has been examined in a few small studies, and these reveal an incidence of pulmonary emboli in up to 25% of CVC-related DVT (Figure 23.4). These are usually asymptomatic and small and fortunately rarely fatal.[66–68]

Patients with CVC-related DVT are also at risk for infections. This association has been proven in a number of

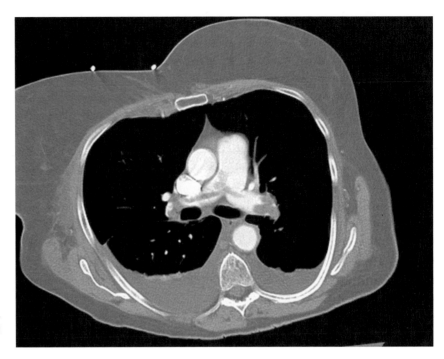

Figure 23.4 Pulmonary embolus. (Courtesy of Samual Goldhaber, MD, Brigham and Women's Hospital, Boston, MA.)

studies and is discussed in "Late Complications: Infection" later in this chapter.

Pathological effects of CVCs on blood vessels have also been identified, largely through autopsy studies. Hemorrhage, thrombosis, calcification, ulceration, and inflammation are found in a greater number of cannulated blood vessels than in those that are not cannulated.[69]

Diagnosis of Central Venous Catheter-Related Deep Venous Thrombosis

Although contrast venography is considered the "gold standard" for diagnosing CVC-related DVT, it is expensive and invasive and requires contrast agents. Consequently, ultrasound with Doppler and color imaging is often used instead. The criteria used to diagnose a DVT by ultrasound include the absence of spontaneous flow or the presence of turbulent flow, abnormal waveforms peripheral to an occluded segment that do not vary with respirations or cardiac pulsations, and visualization of a thrombus or inability to compress the vein.

Studies evaluating the efficacy of ultrasound in the diagnosis of suspected upper-extremity DVTs report sensitivities of 54 to 100% and specificities of 94 to 100%.[70] It is unfortunate that there are only a limited number of studies that directly address the accuracy of ultrasound in diagnosing suspected CVC-related DVT. Koksoy et al. studied 44 patients with CVC-related DVT and found that color Doppler ultrasound had a sensitivity and specificity of 94% and 96%, respectively.[71] Of importance, the sensitivity of duplex ultrasound decreases significantly when used in the asymptomatic patient.

Two factors that influence the sensitivity of ultrasound are the location of the clot and the presence of the catheter. Clots located in the jugular, axillary, or subclavian veins are picked up more frequently than those located in the innominate or superior vena caval veins.[72] In addition, the presence of a catheter can alter not only the venous tone but also the venous flow, making it more difficult to interpret findings visualized on ultrasound.

Newer diagnostic tools currently being investigated include magnetic resonance venography and spiral computed tomography. Preliminary studies show promising results with these newer modalities; however, randomized trials are necessary to compare them with the current standard of venography.[73,74]

In practice, color Doppler ultrasound is the first tool to use in diagnosing suspected CVC-related thrombosis. If a negative result is obtained and the clinical suspicion is high, however, additional testing with serial ultrasounds or venography is warranted. Diagnosing asymptomatic clots remains a challenge and has uncertain importance clinically.

Treatment of Central Venous Catheter-Related Deep Venous Thrombosis

Due to the lack of prospective or comparative studies, there are currently no standard guidelines for the treatment of CVC-related DVT. Consequently, patients with this complication are treated in a manner similar to those patients with lower-extremity DVT. Unfractionated heparin (UFH) or low molecular weight heparin (LMWH) is given for 5 to 7 days, and then patients are continued on Coumadin. Recent studies favor LMWH because it seems to be as effective as UFH and can be given as an outpatient treatment.[75] In addition, cancer patients may derive greater benefit from LMWH than from warfarin.[76] Pentasaccharides and oral direct thrombin inhibitors have not yet been studied in this situation. The optimal duration of anticoagulation is unknown. Most studies show that 6 months is effective; however, patients with active cancer may benefit from indefinite use. Please refer to Table 23.3 for the authors' approach to the treatment of CVC-related thrombosis.

Two other more aggressive options—systemic thrombolysis and thrombectomy—have not been studied in a randomized fashion and, as a result, are not practiced routinely. In addition, the issue of whether to remove a functional but partially clotted catheter has not been extensively studied and remains controversial. Inserting another catheter is costly and associated with increased morbidity.

If a patient has a contraindication to anticoagulation therapy, then a superior caval vein filter can be placed. This filter has the potential to prevent subsequent complications with CVC-related DVT, such as a pulmonary embolus or superior vena cava syndrome.[77] The long-term consequences, however, must be taken into account when considering the use of such devices. The authors believe that their use is rarely indicated.

If the thrombus is located at the tip of the catheter or within its lumen, then local measures are effective. Low-dose thrombolytic therapy—for example, low doses of alteplase, urokinase, or streptokinase given locally as a bolus or infusion—has been shown to restore patency in most patients.[78] Occasionally, patients will need repeated boluses to achieve flow.

The optimal way to treat CVC-related DVT is to try to prevent it from occurring in the first place. Much controversy exists as to the best way to accomplish this, and there are ongoing studies addressing this issue.

Prevention and Prophylaxis of Central Venous Catheter-Related Deep Venous Thrombosis

The complications associated with CVC-related thrombosis may cause significant morbidity and occasional mortality in patients, and as a result there have been major efforts to identify mechanisms to decrease this risk. Not only are biomaterials (polymers and plasticizers) of low thrombogenicity currently being used, but there are ongoing studies to evaluate the benefit of impregnating catheters with antithrombotic substances such as heparin–antithrombin III.[79] Early attempts to impregnate catheters with UFH resulted in rapid leaching from the catheter surface. Recent attempts, however, use a more successful bonding procedure. In addition, catheter designs have been developed to optimize blood flow around the catheter.

The most common procedure used to reduce CVC-related thrombosis is the routine flushing of catheter ports with UFH or other substances. Flushing occurs routinely, from once weekly to thrice weekly. Studies have shown that a 50-unit UFH flush is as effective as a 1,000-unit UFH flush.[80] Surprisingly, recent studies show that a simple saline flush is as effective as a 100-unit UFH flush in preventing thrombi.[81]

The most controversial strategy for decreasing the thrombotic risk associated with CVCs in cancer patients is to use low-dose warfarin, LMWH, or UFH for the purpose of systemic prophylactic anticoagulation. Most of the early studies suggested that low-dose warfarin or LMWH was effective in preventing CVC-related DVTs, whereas the majority of the later studies have suggested the opposite.

Early Prophylactic Anticoagulation Studies

The first study to demonstrate efficacy with low-dose warfarin was a randomized, open-labeled, prospective trial in 1990. Bern et al. compared 1 mg of warfarin given to 42 cancer patients and placebo given to another 40 cancer patients. They evaluated all patients with venography at either 90 days or before if symptoms developed. Total catheter-related DVT rates were 9.5% in patients who received warfarin versus 37.5% in those who received placebo.[4]

The next study to show a benefit from systemic anticoagulation was performed in 1996 by Monreal et al. Similar to the Bern study, it was a randomized, open-label, prospective study of 29 cancer patients and required mandatory venography at 90 days or prior if symptoms developed. The researchers found that only 1 of 16 (6%) of the patients who received dalteparin (2,500 U daily) developed a DVT, as compared with 8 of 13 (62%) of the patients who

---

TABLE 23.3
TREATMENT OF CENTRAL VENOUS CATHETER–RELATED DEEP VENOUS THROMBOSIS

1. If the CVC is nonfunctional, then it is removed and replaced as necessary in another vascular bed. If it is functional, then the CVC is kept in place if still needed.
2. All patients with adequate renal clearance receive dalteparin (150 IU/kg SQ daily) or enoxaparin (1.5 mg/kg SQ daily).
3. In the absence of active malignancy, all are then converted to warfarin (international normalized ratio [INR] 2–3) and treated for 3 to 6 months. In the presence of active malignancy, all are kept on the LMWH for at least 3 to 6 months.
4. Patients with heparin-induced thrombocytopenia are treated with fondaparinux (5 mg SQ daily).
5. Patients with reduced renal function are treated initially with unfractionated heparin, followed by warfarin.

received no treatment.[9] Because of the highly statistically significant difference in outcome ($P = .02$), accrual to this study was closed early.

A third study, performed by Boraks et al., obtained similar results regarding the efficacy of anticoagulation prophylaxis. This nonrandomized study compared 108 patients with hematological malignancies who received 1mg of warfarin prophylactically to a historical control group. Unlike the Bern and Monreal studies, patients were evaluated with venography only if symptoms suspicious for DVT developed. Symptomatic DVTs were discovered in 5% of the treatment group as compared with 13% of the control group. Interestingly, the time to clot development also differed in the two groups. DVTs appeared in the treated group after an average of 72 days versus 16 days in the patients who were not treated.[5]

Subsequently, a number of other studies have been performed to assess the utility of low-dose warfarin prophylaxis. Three have shown a probable benefit but of borderline statistical significance, due to the small number of patients studied. In a prospective, nonrandomized study, 1 mg of warfarin resulted in no CVC-related DVTs in 52 patients (0%), versus 4 of 65 CVC-related DVTs (6%) in patients not receiving warfarin ($P = .06$).[82] In a retrospective, nonrandomized study, symptomatic CVC-related DVTs developed in 4 of 96 patients (4%) treated with 1 mg of warfarin but in 24 out of 209 patients (11%) who received no warfarin ($P = .04$).[83] Of 949 patients with Quinton-type catheters who received 1 mg warfarin per day, the clinical DVT rate was 5.1%, and clinical complications were not apparent.[10]

Old Guidelines and Barriers to Prophylactic Anticoagulation

Based on the earlier positive studies, detailed above, guidelines from the Sixth American College of Chest Physicians (ACCP) Conference on Antithrombotic Therapy in 2000 stated that warfarin (1mg/day) and LMWH (administered once a day) are valid prophylactic options for CVCs.[84–86] Despite these recommendations, less than 10% of patients with CVCs received systemic prophylaxis.[82] There are multiple reasons for this infrequent use of anticoagulation, including a lack of appreciation of the problem among health care providers; the absence of large, randomized, placebo-controlled trials; and concerns regarding the safety of anticoagulation use.

The early studies evaluating the efficacy of systemic prophylaxis suffered from several limitations: they included small numbers of patients studied, they had high dropout rates, most failed to use venographic endpoints, and most were not placebo-controlled.

A genuine concern about the bleeding risk of systemic anticoagulation in potentially thrombocytopenic or anorectic chemotherapy patients was another reason for the lack of routine systemic prophylaxis for CVCs. Ten percent of

the patients in the study by Bern[4] developed a prothrombin time greater than 15 seconds and required holding of their warfarin; 5% of the patients in the study by Boraks[5] developed a prothrombin time greater than 20 seconds and required holding of their warfarin.

The heparins also have some disadvantages that possibly contributed to their low rate of usage. There is the major inconvenience of daily subcutaneous injection of UFH or LMWH, as well as the high cost of the latter. Also in the asthenic or elderly cancer patient with reduced glomerular filtration rate, even low prophylactic doses of LMWH may accumulate and cause bleeding. This adverse effect of LMWH is amplified in patients with reduced renal function due to disease or chemotherapy.

Lastly, concerns regarding the safety of systemic anticoagulation in cancer patients with CVCs likely contribute to the low compliance rate. Considerable recent data, for example, have brought into question the safety of low-dose warfarin in patients receiving 5-flurouracil–based chemotherapy. Magagnoli et al. demonstrated an increased likelihood of an elevated INR (international normalized ratio) and possible bleeding when low-dose warfarin is used in patients with 5-flurouracil–based chemotherapy regimens.[87,88] In patients on full-dose warfarin who then receive 5-flurouracil, the average warfarin dose to maintain a therapeutic INR declines by nearly half and requires careful weekly monitoring.[89] Similar effects have been noted with capecitabine, the prodrug of 5-flurouracil.[90,91]

Recent Prophylactic Anticoagulation Studies

Questions about the design and outcome of the early positive anticoagulation studies prompted a number of confirmatory studies to be performed to assess the utility of prophylactic anticoagulation in patients with CVCs. The majority of these studies have revealed no benefit in preventing or decreasing the rate of CVC-related DVT.

In a nonrandomized study of 160 patients with melanoma or renal cell cancer being treated with interleukin-2, warfarin (1 mg/day) did not reduce the CVC-related DVT rate.[92] In a nonblinded study of patients with hematological malignancies, Heaton et al. randomized 88 patients with double-lumen subclavian Hickman CVCs to warfarin (1 mg/day) or no therapy.[93] After 90 days, there was no difference in the rate of clinically significant thrombi for those treated with warfarin; 8 of 45 patients (18%) treated with warfarin had clinically evident thrombi, versus 5 of 43 patients (12%) not treated.

Similar studies done with LMWH also have failed to show any difference in CVC-related DVT. Pucheu et al. prospectively compared patients given 2,500 anti-Xa units of dalteparin subcutaneously daily with untreated historical controls using ultrasonography at 1, 3, and 12 months to screen for DVT.[94] Documented DVT occurred in only 3 of 46 patients (6.5%) who received dalteparin, and all were without symptoms. In the historical control group, 11 of 72 patients(15%) developed documented DVT, which was not a statistically significant difference. In the largest randomized, blinded, placebo-controlled study ever performed to evaluate CVC prophylaxis in cancer patients, 194 patients received placebo injections and 294 received dalteparin (5,000 IU subcutaneously daily) for 16 weeks.[95] Clinical DVT occurred in 5.3% of placebo and in 5.8% of dalteparin-treated patients, which was not a statistically significant difference. The low rate of DVT in the placebo group was among the lowest seen in any CVC prophylaxis study and may reflect improvements in catheter design and placement, local care, or patient selection. There was no difference in infection rate.

Current Guidelines on Prophylactic Anticoagulation

Many of the recent prophylactic anticoagulation studies, which are both large and placebo-controlled, fail to show any reduction in the rate of CVC-related DVT. These newer studies prompted the American College of Chest Physicians (ACCP) to change their guidelines in 2004. The recently published guidelines from the Seventh ACCP Conference on Antithrombotic Therapy state that the routine use of low-dose warfarin or LMWH to try to prevent thrombosis related to long-term indwelling CVCs in cancer patients is not warranted.[96] In addition to the lack of benefit, concerns regarding the safety of low-dose warfarin in cancer patients are being raised.

Future Possibilities in Thrombosis Prevention

Given the recent data on low-dose warfarin and LMWH in preventing CVC-related DVT, larger, placebo-controlled studies of these drugs could be considered in the future; however, it may be more fruitful, instead, to consider newer antithrombotic agents. The two newest anticoagulants are the direct thrombin inhibitors (DTIs), such as ximelegatran, and the factor Xa inhibitors, such as the pentasaccharides fondaparinux and idraparinux. DTIs have some advantages over warfarin in that they are not affected by diet, antibiotics, or inhibitors of the CYP-450 system, such as 5-flurouracil and capecitabine.[97–100] The factor Xa inhibitors have recently been approved for prophylaxis and treatment of venous thromboembolism and are superior to LMWH in terms of efficacy and bleeding rates.[101–103] Large, randomized, placebo-controlled trials are needed to determine if these newer agents will reduce the DVT rate in cancer patients with CVCs. However, as recent reports suggest, the rates of thrombosis in untreated patients[95] appear to be decreasing and may make even an effective anticoagulant of limited importance in this setting.

LATE COMPLICATIONS: INFECTION

Types of Central Venous Catheter-Related Infection

The incidence and mortality associated with catheter-related infections (CRIs) are difficult to ascertain because of the lack of consensus on definitions. The incidence ranges from 2 to 43%,[26,29] and the mortality, in bacteremic patients, can be as high as 35%.[104]

Several types of vascular CRI exist; these include catheter colonization, phlebitis, exit-site infection, tunnel infection, pocket infection, and bloodstream infection.[105,106] The ability to identify each type has important therapeutic implications. A less serious infection, such as an infection at the exit-site, may require only intravenous antibiotics, whereas a more serious one, such as a tunnel infection, may warrant removal and replacement of the catheter.

The seriousness of an infection and the risks associated with it also depend on the type of organism present. Coagulase-negative *Staphylococcus* species are the most common cause of catheter-related infections and the least virulent. *Staphylococcus aureus*, Gram-negative bacilli, and *Candida* species are the next most common and have the potential to be extremely virulent and cause serious complications.[105,107]

The clinical performance of the patient also has important implications for management decisions and outcome. Immunocompromised or critically ill patients are at significant risk for morbidity and mortality and commonly require removal of their catheter.[105,107]

Risks of Central Venous Catheter-Related Infection

There are many patient- and catheter-related risks factors associated with the development of CRIs. Malignancy, AIDS, and neutropenia are a few of the host factors that predispose patients to an increased risk.[106] As discussed in previous sections, the composition of the catheter and the site of insertion confer certain risks. For percutaneous devices, a subclavian approach is thought to be associated with less risk.[29,108] Occlusive plastic dressings, frequent manipulations, and nonsterile techniques are associated with increased infection risk.

One important identifiable risk factor for CRIs is the presence of thrombosis. This association was first suggested in the early 1980s when a higher rate of bacteremia was discovered in patients with documented CVC thromboses as compared with those without clots.[109] Further studies have confirmed this correlation.[69,92,110] This finding is not surprising given that, as mentioned earlier, almost all catheters develop a fibrin sheath and almost all fibrin sheaths become colonized with cocci.[34–36] To date, none of the anticoagulation studies have shown any reduction in the rate of infection.

Diagnosis of Central Venous Catheter-Related Infection

Techniques for diagnosing CRIs can be divided into those that require catheter removal and those that allow it to remain in place. The "role plate, sonication, and flushing" methods require removal of the catheter, while the newer approach, the "differential time to positivity" (DTP), involves drawing blood cultures from the central line and peripheral veins simultaneously and does not require removal.[106,107] Once a CRI has been identified, it is important to determine if the infection is confined to the catheter or present in the bloodstream. Catheter-related bloodstream infections (CRBIs) often require further workup to detect the seeding of other tissues, along with the possible development of endocarditis, osteomyelitis, or septic thrombophlebitis.[106,107]

Prevention of Central Venous Catheter-Related Infection

The simplest way to prevent infection is to practice meticulous sterile techniques, not only during the insertion process but also during the maintenance period. Aggressive handwashing by medical personnel is an absolute necessity. Using adhesive anchoring devices instead of sutures for catheter securement has dramatically decreased CRBIs. Recognizing the signs and symptoms of localized, systemic, or metastatic infections can help prevent progression. Removing the catheters as soon as they are no longer needed is important because the risk of developing a CRBI increases with time. In addition, poor functioning of a catheter may be a sign of occlusion, and it should be removed if the problem cannot be resolved by simple measures.

Besides the patient's skin, another common source of infection is the catheter hub. Disinfecting the hub each time it is accessed can decrease infection risk. New aseptic hub attachments have recently been developed, but their effectiveness needs to be evaluated in future randomized controlled trials.[27,111,112]

Although the use of combined antimicrobial and antiseptic flushes has been shown to decrease the rate of CRBIs,[110] there is great concern that flushing will promote the development of antibiotic-resistant organisms, such as vancomycin-resistant enterococci and/or fungal species. As a result, the prophylactic use of antibiotic locks or flushes is not currently recommended.[113,114]

The use of antimicrobial-impregnated catheters, however, is a routine and encouraged practice. Over the past few decades, several randomized trials have consistently shown a decrease in catheter colonization and CRBI. Presently, catheters are impregnated with either chlorhexidine and silver sulfadiazine or minocycline and rifampin; both types have been well studied and both show benefit.[2,3,115,116] Although a recent analysis raised questions about the methodology and benefits of these

trials,[117] the Guidelines for the Prevention of Intravascular Catheter-Related Infections recommend their use in catheters expected to remain in place for more than 5 days.[115] Future developments to decrease infection risk include using silver iontophoretic devices, electrically charged catheters, and techniques to limit bacterial adhesion.[18,104]

Treatment of Central Venous Catheter-Related Infection

The most important decision to make when managing CRIs is whether or not to remove the catheter. This assessment depends on the patient, the organism, the extent of the infection, and the type of catheter. Patients who are critically ill, suffer from persistent bacteremia, or have metastatic seeding of their infection should have their catheter removed. Tunnel or port infections warrant catheter removal. In addition, infections caused by difficult- to-treat organisms (e.g., *S. aureus*), virulent Gram-negative infections, and fungal infections carry a high risk of mortality if the catheter is not removed. Prompt recognition of a CRI and administration of antibiotics can help decrease morbidity and mortality, especially in critically ill patients.

CONCLUSION

CVC-related complications are a common clinical problem that may affect nearly half of all cancer patients with CVCs. The mechanical, thrombotic, and infectious complications can result in clinical symptoms, loss of catheter function, postphlebitic syndrome of the upper extremity, pulmonary embolus, increased cost, high morbidity, and even high mortality. Numerous risk factors, both patient- and catheter-related, have been identified and are currently being modified to reduce the rates and types of complications.

Given their common occurrence, further efforts to understand and prevent CVC-related complications are of importance. Efforts should include not only studies of modalities for earlier diagnosis of complications and assessment of anticoagulant and antibiotic efficacies but also studies to determine additional risk factors for CVC-related thrombosis and infection, the timing of onset of these complications, the exploration and implementation of newer preventative agents, the optimal duration and types of treatments, and the natural history of these CVC-related complications.

REFERENCES

1. Darouiche RO, Raad, II, Heard SO, et al. A comparison of two antimicrobial-impregnated central venous catheters. Catheter Study Group. N Engl J Med 1999;340:1–8.

2. Raad I, Darouiche R, Dupuis J, et al. Central venous catheters coated with minocycline and rifampin for the prevention of catheter-related colonization and bloodstream infections: a randomized, double-blind trial. The Texas Medical Center Catheter Study Group. Ann Intern Med 1997;127:267–274.
3. Maki DG, Stolz SM, Wheeler S, et al. Prevention of central venous catheter-related bloodstream infection by use of an antiseptic-impregnated catheter: a randomized, controlled trial. Ann Intern Med 1997;127:257–266.
4. Bern MM, Lokich JJ, Wallach SR, et al. Very low doses of warfarin can prevent thrombosis in central venous catheters: a randomized prospective trial. Ann Intern Med 1990;112:423–428.
5. Boraks P, Seale J, Price J, et al. Prevention of central venous catheter associated thrombosis using minidose warfarin in patients with haematological malignancies. Br J Haematol 1998; 101:483–486.
6. Bozzetti F, Terno G, Bonfanti G, et al. Prevention and treatment of central venous catheter sepsis by exchange via a guidewire: a prospective controlled trial. Ann Surg 1983;198:48–52.
7. Massicotte P, Julian JA, Gent M, et al. An open-label randomized controlled trial of low molecular weight heparin compared to heparin and Coumadin for the treatment of venous thromboembolic events in children: the REVIVE trial. Thromb Res 2003; 109:85–92.
8. Mismetti P, Mille D, Laporte S, et al. Low-molecular-weight heparin (nadroparin) and very low doses of warfarin in the prevention of upper extremity thrombosis in cancer patients with indwelling long-term central venous catheters: a pilot randomized trial. Haematologica 2003;88:67–73.
9. Monreal M, Alastrue A, Rull M, et al. Upper extremity deep venous thrombosis in cancer patients with venous access devices: prophylaxis with a low molecular weight heparin (Fragmin). Thromb Haemost 1996;75:251–253.
10. Nightingale CE, Norman A, Cunningham D, et al. A prospective analysis of 949 long-term central venous access catheters for ambulatory chemotherapy in patients with gastrointestinal malignancy. Eur J Cancer 1997;33:398–403.
11. Bennett JA. A study of Parentalia, with two unpublished letters of Sir Christopher Wren. Ann Sci 1973;30:129–147.
12. Bennett JA. A note on theories of respiration and muscular action in England c. 1660 (Christopher Wren). Med Hist 1976; 20:59–69.
13. Bergman NA. Early intravenous anesthesia: an eyewitness account. Anesthesiology 1990;72:185–186.
14. Buess H. [Christopher Wren and the discovery of intravenous injections]. Z Krankenpfl 1973;66:274–275.
15. Kenney CA. A historical review of the illustrations of the circle of Willis from antiquity to 1664. J Biocommun 1998;25:26–31.
16. Keys TE. Historical vignettes. Sir Christopher Wren. Anesth Analg 1974;53:853.
17. Kuter DJ. Thrombotic complications of central venous catheters in cancer patients. Oncologist 2004;9:207–216.
18. Polderman KH, Girbes AR. Central venous catheter use, II: infectious complications. Intensive Care Med 2002;28:18–28.
19. Aubaniac R. Subclavian intravenous injection: advantages and technic. Presse Med 1952;60:1456.
20. Aubaniac R. Subclavian intravenous transfusion: advantages and technic. Afr Francaise Chir 1952;8:131–135.
21. Broviac JW, Cole JJ, Scribner BH. A silicone rubber atrial catheter for prolonged parenteral alimentation. Surg Gynecol Obstet 1973;136:602–606.
22. Hickman RO, Buckner CD, Clift RA, et al. A modified right atrial catheter for access to the venous system in marrow transplant recipients. Surg Gynecol Obstet 1979;148:871–875.
23. Niederhuber JE, Ensminger W, Gyves JW, et al. Totally implanted venous and arterial access system to replace external catheters in cancer treatment. Surgery 1982;92:706–712.
24. Bregenzer T, Conen D, Sakmann P, et al. Is routine replacement of peripheral intravenous catheters necessary? Arch Intern Med 1998;158:151–156.
25. Galloway S, Bodenham A. Long-term central venous access. Br J Anaesth 2004;92:722–734.
26. Mansfield PF, Hohn DC, Fornage BD, et al. Complications and failures of subclavian-vein catheterization. N Engl J Med 1994; 331:1735–1738.
27. McGee DC, Gould MK. Preventing complications of central venous catheterization. N Engl J Med 2003;348:1123–1133.
28. Cadman A, Lawrance JA, Fitzsimmons L, et al. To clot or not to clot? That is the question in central venous catheters. Clin Radiol 2004;59:349–355.
29. Merrer J, De Jonghe B, Golliot F, et al. Complications of femoral and subclavian venous catheterization in critically ill patients: a randomized controlled trial. JAMA 2001;286: 700–707.
30. Booth SA, Norton B, Mulvey DA. Central venous catheterization and fatal cardiac tamponade. Br J Anaesth 2001;87:298–302.
31. Martin MJ, Husain FA, Piesman M, et al. Is routine ultrasound guidance for central line placement beneficial? A prospective analysis. Curr Surg 2004;61:71–74.
32. Randolph AG, Cook DJ, Gonzales CA, et al. Ultrasound guidance for placement of central venous catheters: a meta-analysis of the literature. Crit Care Med 1996;24:2053–2058.
33. Sznajder JI, Zveibil FR, Bitterman H, et al. Central vein catheterization: failure and complication rates by three percutaneous approaches. Arch Intern Med 1986;146:259–261.
34. Starkhammar H, Bengtsson M, Morales O. Fibrin sleeve formation after long term brachial catheterisation with an implantable port device: a prospective venographic study. Eur J Surg 1992; 158:481–484.
35. Hoshal VL Jr, Ause RG, Hoskins PA. Fibrin sleeve formation on indwelling subclavian central venous catheters. Arch Surg 1971;102:253–258.
36. Bona RD. Thrombotic complications of central venous catheters in cancer patients. Semin Thromb Hemost 1999;25:147–155.
37. Balestreri L, De Cicco M, Matovic M, et al. Central venous catheter-related thrombosis in clinically asymptomatic oncologic patients: a phlebographic study. Eur J Radiol 1995;20: 108–111.
38. Tenney J, Moody M, Newman K, et al. Adherent microorganisms on luminal surfaces of long-term intravenous catheters: importance of *Staphylococcus epidermidis* in patients with cancer. Arch Intern Med 1986;146:1949–1954.
39. Raad I, Costerton W, Sabharwal U, et al. Ultrastructural analysis of indwelling vascular catheters: a quantitative relationship between luminal colonization and duration of placement. J Infect Dis 1993;168:400–407.
40. Raad, II, Hohn DC, Gilbreath BJ, et al. Prevention of central venous catheter-related infections by using maximal sterile barrier precautions during insertion. Infect Control Hosp Epidemiol 1994;15:231–238.
41. De Cicco M, Matovic M, Balestreri L, et al. Central venous thrombosis: an early and frequent complication in cancer patients bearing long-term Silastic catheter: a prospective study. Thromb Res 1997;86:101–113.
42. Ray S, Stacey R, Imrie M, et al. A review of 560 Hickman catheter insertions. Anaesthesia 1996;51:981–985.
43. Schwarz RE, Coit DG, Groeger JS. Transcutaneously tunneled central venous lines in cancer patients: an analysis of device-related morbidity factors based on prospective data collection. Ann Surg Oncol 2000;7:441–449.
44. Anderson AJ, Krasnow SH, Boyer MW, et al. Thrombosis: the major Hickman catheter complication in patients with solid tumor. Chest 1989;95:71–75.
45. Schwarz R, Coit D, Groeger J. Transcutaneously tunneled central venous lines in cancer patients: an analysis of device-related morbidity factors based on prospective data collection. Ann Surg Oncol 2000;7:441–449.
46. Lawson M, Bottino J, Hurtibise M. The use of urokinase to restore patency of occluded central venous catheters. Ann J Intraven Ther Clin Nutr 1982;9:29–32.
47. Hurtibise M, Bottino J, Lawson M. Restoring patency of occluded central venous catheters. Arch Surg 1980;115:212–213.
48. Gould J, Carloss H, Skinner W. Groshong catheter-associated subclavian venous thrombosis. Am J Med 1993;95:419–423.
49. Stephens L, Haire W, Kotulak G. Are clinical signs accurate indicators of the cause of central venous catheter occlusion? JPEN J Parenter Enteral Nutr 1995;19:75–79.
50. Verso M, Agnelli G. Venous thromboembolism associated with long-term use of central venous catheters in cancer patients. J Clin Oncol 2003;21:3665–3675.

51. Curelaru I, Bylock A, Gustavsson B, et al. Dynamics of thrombophlebitis in central venous catheterization via basilic and cephalic veins. Acta Chir Scand 1984;150:285–293.

52. Lokich JJ, Becker B. Subclavian vein thrombosis in patients treated with infusion chemotherapy for advanced malignancy. Cancer 1983;52:1586–1589.

53. Durica SS. Venous thromboembolism in the cancer patient. Curr Opin Hematol 1997;4:306–311.

54. Letai A, Kuter DJ. Cancer, coagulation, and anticoagulation. Oncologist 1999;4:443–449.

55. Prandoni P, Piccioli A, Girolami A. Cancer and venous thromboembolism: an overview. Haematologica 1999;84:437–445.

56. Valente M, Ponte E. Thrombosis and cancer. Minerva Cardioangiol 2000;48:117–127.

57. De Cicco M, Matovic M, Balestreri L, et al. Antithrombin III deficiency as a risk factor for catheter-related central vein thrombosis in cancer patients. Thromb Res 1995;78:127–137.

58. Leebeck F, Stadhouders N, van Stein D, al e. Hypercoagulability states in upper-extremity deep venous thrombosis. Ann J Hematol 2001;67:15–19.

59. Fijnheer R, Paijmans B, Verdonck LF, et al. Factor V Leiden in central venous catheter-associated thrombosis. Br J Haematol 2002;118:267–270.

60. Wermes C, von Depka Prondzinski M, et al. Clinical relevance of genetic risk factors for thrombosis in paediatric oncology patients with central venous catheters. Eur J Pediatr 1999;158 (Suppl 3):S143–146.

61. Haire WD, Lieberman RP, Edney J, et al. Hickman catheter-induced thoracic vein thrombosis: frequency and long-term sequelae in patients receiving high-dose chemotherapy and marrow transplantation. Cancer 1990;66:900–908.

62. Borow M, Crowley JG. Evaluation of central venous catheter thrombogenicity. Acta Anaesthesiol Scand Suppl 1985;81: 59–64.

63. Luciani A, Clement O, Halimi P, et al. Catheter-related upper extremity deep venous thrombosis in cancer patients: a prospective study based on Doppler US. Radiology 2001;220: 655–660.

64. Puel V, Caudry M, Le Metayer P, et al. Superior vena cava thrombosis related to catheter malposition in cancer chemotherapy given through implanted ports. Cancer 1993;72:2248–2252.

65. Prandoni P. Antithrombotic strategies in patients with cancer. Thromb Haemost 1997;78:141–144.

66. Monreal M, Davant E. Thrombotic complications of central venous catheters in cancer patients. Acta Haematol 2001;106: 69–72.

67. Monreal M, Lafoz E, Ruiz J, et al. Upper-extremity deep venous thrombosis and pulmonary embolism: a prospective study. Chest 1991;99:280–283.

68. Monreal M, Raventos A, Lerma R, et al. Pulmonary embolism in patients with upper extremity DVT associated to venous central lines: a prospective study. Thromb Haemost 1994;72: 548–550.

69. Raad, II, Luna M, Khalil SA, et al. The relationship between thrombotic and infectious complications of central venous catheters. JAMA 1994;271:1014–1016.

70. Mustafa B, Rathbun S, Whitsett T, et al. Sensitivity and specificity of ultrasonography in the diagnosis of upper extremity deep vein thrombosis: a systemic review. Arch Intern Med 2002;162: 401–404.

71. Koksoy C, Kuzu A, Kutlay J, et al. The diagnostic value of colour Doppler ultrasound in central venous catheter related thrombosis. Clin Radiol 1995;50:687–689.

72. Chait P, Dinyari M, Massicotte P. The sensitivity and specificity of lineograms and ultrasound compared with venography for the diagnosis of central venous line related thrombosis in symptomatic children: the LUV study. Thromb Haemost 2001;86 (Suppl) abstract p697.

73. Forneris G, Quarello F, Pozzato M, et al. [Spiral x-ray computed tomography in the diagnosis of central venous catheterization complications. Nephrologie 2001;22:495–499.

74. Haire W, Lynch T, Lund G, et al. Limitations of magnetic resonance imaging and ultrasound-directed (duplex) scanning in the diagnosis of subclavian vein thrombosis. J Vasc Surg 1991; 13:391–397.

75. Savage K, Wells P, Schultz V, et al. Outpatient use of low molecular weight heparin (dalteparin) for the treatment of deep vein thrombosis of the upper extremity. Thromb Haemost 1999; 82:1008–1010.

76. Lee A, Levine M, Baker R, et al. Low-molecular weight heparin versus a coumarin for the prevention of recurrent venous thromboembolism in patients with cancer. N Engl J Med 2003; 349: 146–153.

77. Spence L, Gironta M, Malde H, et al. Acute upper extremity deep venous thrombosis: safety and effectiveness of superior vena cava filters. Radiology 1999;210:53–58.

78. Ponec D, Irwin D, Haire W, et al. Recombinant tissue plasminogen activator (alteplase) for restoration of flow in occluded central venous access devices: a double-blind placebo-controlled trial. The Cardiovascular Thrombolytic to Open Occluded Lines (COOL) efficacy trial. J Vasc Interv Radiol 2001;12:951–955.

79. Chan A, Du Y, Berry L, et al. Covalent antithrombin-heparin complex coated catheter prevents thrombosis in a rabbit central venous catheter model. Thromb Haemost 2001;86(Suppl 1):310S.

80. Brown-Smith JK, Stoner MH, Barley ZA. Tunneled catheter thrombosis: factors related to incidence. Oncol Nurs Forum 1990;17:543–549.

81. Stephens L, Haire W, Tarantolo S, et al. Normal saline versus heparin flush for maintaining central venous catheter patency during apheresis collection of peripheral blood stem cells (PBSC). Transfus Sci 1997;18:187–193.

82. Carr KM, Rabinowitz I. Physician compliance with warfarin prophylaxis for central venous catheters in patients with solid tumors. J Clin Oncol 2000;18:3665–3667.

83. Minassian VA, Sood AK, Lowe P, et al. Long-term central venous access in gynecologic cancer patients. J Am Coll Surg 2000;191: 403–409.

84. Geerts WH, Heit JA, Clagett GP, et al. Prevention of venous thromboembolism. Chest 2001;119(Suppl 1):132S–175S.

85. Guyatt G, Schunemann H, Cook D, et al. Grades of recommendation for antithrombotic agents. Chest 2001;119(Suppl 1): 3S–7S.

86. Hirsh J, Dalen J, Guyatt G. The sixth (2000) ACCP guidelines for antithrombotic therapy for prevention and treatment of thrombosis. American College of Chest Physicians. Chest 2001;119 (Suppl 1):1S–2S.

87. Masci G, Magagnoli M, Zucali P, et al. Minidose warfarin prophylaxis for catheter-associated thrombosis in cancer patients: can it be safely associated with fluorouracil-based chemotherapy? J Clin Oncol 2003;21:736–739.

88. Magagnoli M, Masci G, Carnaghi C, et al. Minidose warfarin is associated with a high incidence of international normalized ratio elevation during chemotherapy with FOLFOX regimen. Ann Oncol 2003;14:959–960.

89. Kolesar J, Johnson C, Freeberg B, et al. Warfarin-5-FU interaction: a consecutive case series. Pharmacology 1999;19:1445–1449.

90. Copur M, Ledakis P, Boulton M, et al. An adverse interaction between warfarin and capecitabine: a case report and review of the literature. Clin Colorectal Cancer 2001;1:182–184.

91. Reigner B, Blesch K, Weidekamm E. Clinical pharmacokinetics of capecitabine. Clin Pharmacokinet 2001;40:85–104.

92. Eastman ME, Khorsand M, Maki DG, et al. Central venous device-related infection and thrombosis in patients treated with moderate dose continuous-infusion interleukin-2. Cancer 2001; 91:806–814.

93. Heaton DC, Han DY, Inder A. Minidose (1 mg) warfarin as prophylaxis for central vein catheter thrombosis. Intern Med J 2002;32:84–88.

94. Pucheu A, Leduc B, Sillet-Bach I, et al. Experimental prevention of deep venous thrombosis with low-molecular-weight heparin using implantable infusion devices. Ann Cardiol Angeiol (Paris) 1996;45:59–63.

95. Reichardt P, Kretzschmar A, Biakhov M, et al. A phase III randomized, double-blind, placebo-controlled study evaluating the efficacy and safety of daily low-molecular-weight heparin (dalteparin sodium, Fragmin) in preventing catheter-related complications (CRCs) in cancer patients with central venous catheter (CVCs). Proc ASCO 2002;21:369a.

96. Geerts W, Pineo G, Heit J, et al. Prevention of venous thromboembolism. Chest 2004;126:3385–4005.

97. Colwell CW Jr, Berkowitz SD, Davidson BL, et al. Comparison of ximelagatran, an oral direct thrombin inhibitor, with enoxaparin for the prevention of venous thromboembolism following total hip replacement: a randomized, double-blind study. J Thromb Haemost 2003;1:2119–2130.

98. Gustafsson D. Oral direct thrombin inhibitors in clinical development. J Intern Med 2003;254:322–334.

99. Eriksson H, Wahlander K, Gustafsson D, et al. A randomized, controlled, dose-guiding study of the oral direct thrombin inhibitor ximelagatran compared with standard therapy for the treatment of acute deep vein thrombosis. THRIVE I. J Thromb Haemost 2003;1:41–47.

100. de Moerloose P, Boehlen F. Two new antithrombotic agents (fondaparinux and ximelagatran) and their implications in anesthesia. Can J Anaesth 2002;49(6):S5–10.

101. Bauer KA, Eriksson BI, Lassen MR, et al. Fondaparinux compared with enoxaparin for the prevention of venous thromboembolism after elective major knee surgery. N Engl J Med 2001; 345:1305–1310.

102. Eriksson BI, Lassen MR. Duration of prophylaxis against venous thromboembolism with fondaparinux after hip fracture surgery: a multicenter, randomized, placebo-controlled, double-blind study. Arch Intern Med 2003;163:1337–1342.

103. Turpie AG, Bauer KA, Eriksson BI, et al. Fondaparinux vs enoxaparin for the prevention of venous thromboembolism in major orthopedic surgery: a meta-analysis of 4 randomized double-blind studies. Arch Intern Med 2002;162:1833–1840.

104. Pittet D, Tarara D, Wenzel RP. Nosocomial bloodstream infection in critically ill patients: excess length of stay, extra costs, and attributable mortality. JAMA 1994;271:1598–1601.

105. Hall K, Farr B. Diagnosis and management of long-term central venous catheter infections. J Vasc Interv Radiol 2004;15: 327–334.

106. Fatkenheuer G, Cornely O, Seifert H. Clinical management of catheter-related infections. Clin Microbiol Infect 2002;8: 545–550.

107. Raad, II, Hanna HA. Intravascular catheter-related infections: new horizons and recent advances. Arch Intern Med 2002;162: 871–878.

108. Lam S, Scannell R, Roessler D, et al. Peripherally inserted central catheters in an acute-care hospital. Arch Intern Med 1994;154: 1833–1837.

109. Press O, Ramsey P, Larson E, et al. Hickman catheter infections in patients with malignancies. Medicine 1984;63:189–200.

110. Henrickson KJ, Axtell RA, Hoover SM, et al. Prevention of central venous catheter-related infections and thrombotic events in immunocompromised children by the use of vancomycin/ ciprofloxacin/heparin flush solution: a randomized, multicenter, double-blind trial. J Clin Oncol 2000;18:1269–1278.

111. Sequra M, Alvarez-Lerma F, Tellado J, et al. Advances in surgical technique: a clinical trial on the prevention of catheter-related sepsis using a new hub model. Ann Surg 1996;223:363–369.

112. Luna L, Masdeu G, Perez M, et al. Clinical trial evaluating a new hub device designed to prevent catheter-related sepsis. Eur J Clin Microbiol Infect Dis 2000;19:655–662.

113. O'Grady N, Alexander M, Dellinger P, et al. Guidelines for the prevention of intravascular catheter-related infections. Clin Infect Dis 2002;35:1281–1307.

114. Spafford P, Sinkin R, Cox C, et al. Recommendations for preventing the spread of vancomycin resistance: recommendations of the Hospital Infection Control Practices Advisory Committee (HICPAC). MMWR 1994;44:1–13.

115. O'Grady NP, Alexander M, Dellinger EP, et al. Guidelines for the prevention of intravascular catheter-related infections. The Hospital Infection Control Practices Advisory Committee, Center for Disease Control and Prevention. US Pediatrics 2002;110(5):e51.

116. Brun-Buisson C, Doyon F, Sollet JP, et al. Prevention of intravascular catheter-related infection with newer chlorhexidine-silver sulfadiazine-coated catheters: a randomized controlled trial. Intensive Care Med 2004;30:837–843.

117. McConnell SA, Gubbins PO, Anaissie EJ. Do antimicrobial-impregnated central venous catheters prevent catheter-related bloodstream infection? Clin Infect Dis 2003;37:65–72.

Pharmacogenetics

24

Jeanne Fourie   *Robert B. Diasio*

INTRODUCTION

Interindividual differences in drug efficacy and safety are important barriers to optimal treatment with anticancer chemotherapeutic agents. As a general rule, individual variations in drug effects may stem from variability in the pharmacokinetics and/or pharmacodynamics of the therapeutic compound and may have both genetic and nongenetic causes. Nongenetic causes may include differences in age, organ function, concomitant therapy, and drug interactions as well as variability in exposure to foodstuff, tobacco smoke, and other environmental factors among patients.[1,2] Genetic factors however, have been shown to be integral determinants of drug response and are estimated to account for 20 to 95% of the variability in drug disposition and drug effects.[3] Pharmacogenetics is the study of the hereditary basis of interindividual variability in drug efficacy and safety resulting from the effects of a single gene or a set of candidate genes.[4] Such inherited changes or human genetic variation may include, at a molecular level, single-nucleotide polymorphisms (SNPs) or insertions, deletions, and tandem repeats in candidate genes or genomic regions that can collectively affect the regulation and function of proteins relevant to drug disposition and pharmacodynamic effects. In particular, there is already an extensive list of genes identified through the focused pharmacogenetic approach that encode proteins that alter the pharmacokinetics and pharmacodynamics of drug response through effects on drug-metabolizing enzymes, drug transporters, and drug targets or via genes that influence disease predisposition or progression. In general, the majority of identified genetic polymorphisms have been monogenic with high penetrance; for example, the cytochrome P450 2D6 (CYP2D6) genetic polymorphism has a marked effect on the pharmacokinetic parameters of drugs that are activated or inactivated via oxidative metabolism by this enzyme, and it warrants substantially different doses of these drugs during treatment of poor metabolizers.[5-9]

It is noteworthy that the observed marked variability in drug efficacy and safety in the clinic cannot be fully explained by polymorphisms in any single gene. Most drug effects and treatment outcomes are determined by networks of genes and interactions among these genes, including additional multiple low-penetrance genes, which may be more difficult to identify through large population studies. With the completion of the Human Genome Project and advances in technologies such as high-throughput sequencing, DNA and protein microarrays, and bioinformatics, there is a unique opportunity to investigate all forms of variability in drug response using the rapidly emerging field of pharmacogenomics, which is focused more broadly on elucidation of the polygenic determinants of drug efficacy and safety.[10-12] Pharmacogenomics may be particularly valuable for improvement of the efficacy and safety of cancer chemotherapeutic agents, as these agents in general have very narrow therapeutic windows. Ultimately, pharmacogenetics and pharmacogenomics may further pave the way to individualized drug therapy and the abandonment of anticancer drug therapy based on treatment with a single uniform dose. Such advances may customize in the near future the choice of drug dosages and/or the type of prescription and thereby minimize variability in therapeutic response or unexpected toxicity as well as lead to the design of highly targeted and specific treatment options for particular segments of a population.

Currently, a number of genes implicated in pharmacological traits have been identified, and their molecular mechanisms and clinical impact in cancer chemotherapy have been increasingly elucidated. In this chapter, we provide an overview of the general principles of pharmacogenetics and of specific genetic polymorphisms that are pertinent for the clinical pharmacology of specific cancer chemotherapy agents in current medical use. Furthermore, we discuss the future importance of pharmacogenomics in developing individualized anticancer chemotherapeutic strategies.

IMPACT OF GENETIC VARIATION ON CANCER CHEMOTHERAPY

Human genetic variability is a determinant of anticancer drug efficacy and safety. This variability, which is the basis of the disciplines of pharmacogenetics and pharmacogenomics, encompasses an array of different types of DNA sequence modifications as well as individual differences in gene expression and regulation. In the present overview, we focus on the most common form of variation in genetic sequence, known as single-nucleotide polymorphism. A polymorphism is defined as a "Mendelian or monogenic trait that exists in the population in at least two phenotypes (and presumably at least two genotypes), neither of which is rare—that is, neither of which occurs with a frequency of less than 1 to 2%."[13] Such polymorphisms may include nonsynonymous SNPs, which are within the open reading frame of the gene and may result in significant amino acid substitutions in the encoded protein, affecting protein function or quantity. Other SNPs are characterized as synonymous polymorphisms in the coding region of the DNA, or SNPs in promoter and enhancer regions of a gene that affect transcription and gene regulation, and intronic SNPs, which may lead to, splice variants, mRNA.[14-19] In addition to these SNPs, other sources of variation in DNA sequence include insertions, deletions, and gene duplications, all of which contribute to the complex and multifactorial phenotypes of drug efficacy and safety.

Although virtually all drugs are susceptible to the consequences of genetic variability, the application of pharmacogenetic concepts may be especially important in anticancer chemotherapeutic treatment. Anticancer agents frequently are prodrugs that require enzymatic bioactivation to their cytotoxic active forms, while the active forms of these compounds may also undergo further enzymatic detoxification. In both instances, the involved enzyme systems may exhibit genetic polymorphisms, and therefore small but significant changes in anticancer drug metabolism, distribution, transport, or excretion due to modifications such as decreased production of an altered protein (e.g., an enzyme) or increases in the protein amount can lead to interpatient variability in drug effect. Anticancer agents generally have a relatively narrow therapeutic index. In the current treatment strategy, anticancer agents are administered in "standard" doses to patients. This uniform

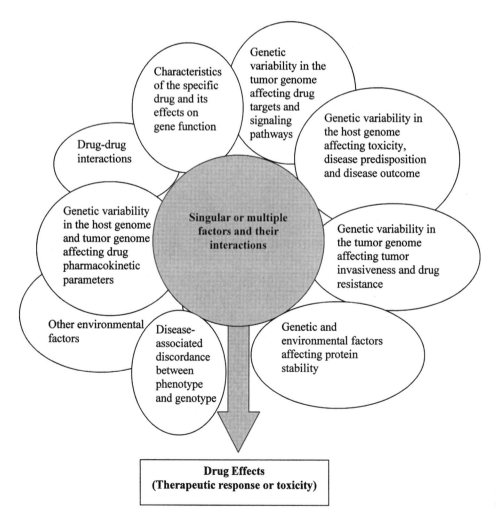

Figure 24.1 Factors influencing drug response.

approach to pharmacotherapy prevents the recognition of interindividual variability in drug metabolism and disposition as part of an individualized drug treatment plan.

Chemotherapeutic drug response is a complex outcome, or phenotype, that is affected by interactions between a network of different genes, including interactions between host and tumor genomes, as most anticancer agents do not selectively target tumor tissue. Genetic polymorphisms in pharmacokinetic pathways may collectively impact drug efficacy and host of tumor toxicity through regulation of drug bioavailability, retention, and efflux and detoxification or metabolism in host or tumor cells. Genetic polymorphisms may further occur in genes that encode drug targets or signal pathways involved in drug response as well as in genes that influence tumor or disease characteristics such as invasiveness and drug resistance. The complexity of variability in human drug response may be additionally affected by differences in the frequencies and types of genetic polymorphisms that are prevalent in ethnically defined populations as well as the specific characteristics of the drugs and disease status, all of which may impact gene function. The various factors that can influence drug response in cancer chemotherapy are presented in Figure 24.1. A major aim of pharmacogenetics and pharmacogenomics is to discern which genetic polymorphisms are important in drug response and how knowledge of this variability can be used in the individualization of drug therapy.

METHODS AND RESEARCH STRATEGIES IN PHARMACOGENETICS

Candidate Gene Approach

The methods used to evaluate pharmacogenetic variability in drug response have evolved over the past several decades to include the candidate gene approach, biochemical or pharmacological pathway approaches, and genomic discovery strategies.[20] Initially, pharmacogenetic studies dating from the 1950s relied on clinical observation for the identification of inherited differences in drug effects.[21-24] Such scientific enquiries are often classified as "from phenotype to genotype" and were driven by reports of unusual drug effects in the form of severe drug toxicity or therapeutic failure. For instance, hemolysis was observed subsequent to the administration of a clinically approved antimalarial drug (primaquine) in African-American soldiers during World War II. This observed sensitivity to a drug was later reported to be produced by a deficiency of glucose-6-phosphate dehydrogenase.[25,26] These early studies were the basis for the development of the "candidate gene approach," wherein the aim is to investigate whether distinct phenotypes observed in pharmacodynamic or pharmacokinetic parameters can be associated with a particular candidate gene and a polymorphic genotype using a hypothesis-based study design. This approach relies on previous knowledge of the pharmacokinetic and/or pharmacodynamic parameters of the drug studied, the disease pathophysiology, and the biochemical roles of proteins encoded by particular genes. This prior knowledge facilitates the rational selection and investigation of the clinical relevance of genetic polymorphisms harbored within a given set of candidate genes that may influence the drug response. To date, this methodology has been useful in the identification of numerous SNPs in mainly high-penetrance genes generally encoding drug-metabolizing enzymes, drug transporters, or drug targets producing distinct and easily recognized polymorphic phenotypes in drug response.[14,16,27,28] SNPs identified through the candidate gene approach have been shown to have a significant effect on drug efficacy and toxicity (e.g., CYP2D6 and TPMT), and in rare cases this information has been used to predict anticancer drug response.[29-31]

The candidate gene approach showed considerable clinical benefit in the identification of monogenic SNPs influencing drug metabolism and bioavailability. Antineoplastic agents characteristically are administered at maximally tolerated doses, and plasma concentrations often correlate with efficacy and/or toxicity. Thus, a wide variation in plasma concentration-time course (pharmacokinetics) between individuals can lead to adverse drug events and unpredictability in drug efficacy. An example of the importance of variability in drug pharmacokinetics affecting drug response is the cyclin-dependent kinase inhibitor flavopiridol: the risk of dose-limiting diarrhea is increased in cancer patients with a poor drug glucuronidation phenotype characterized by a low metabolic ratio of flavopiridol glucuronide to flavopiridol.[32]

A knowledge of the mechanisms governing individual differences in pharmacokinetics may allow dose modification before initiation of pharmacotherapy to achieve optimal drug concentrations and therapeutic effects. Because most human cancers may progress in a relatively short time frame, rapid optimization of drug therapy by genetic or phenotypic tests may be crucial to reduce the long-term morbidity and mortality in treatment of patients with cancer. Genetic polymorphisms in drug-metabolizing enzymes are of particular clinical relevance in explaining pharmacokinetic variability if (1) the polymorphism predicts enzyme activity, (2) the particular enzyme activity predicts drug plasma concentration, and (3) the drug plasma concentration predicts drug efficacy or toxicity.

Pharmacokinetics-Based Individualization of Drug Therapy in the Clinic

The presence of a genetic polymorphism that may affect a particular drug response is often detected by measuring the levels of drug or key metabolite(s) in patients with drug toxicity, treatment failure, or a marked favorable response. However, one may miss excessively elevated drug or metabolite levels if the plasma (serum), urine, or tissue samples are not appropriately timed in relation to the drug administration. A more useful approach for the identification of pharmacogenetic syndromes is to administer a known dose of a drug under controlled testing conditions such that the concentration-time course (pharmacokinetics) of the drug or key metabolite(s) in plasma (serum), urine, or tissue samples, or a combination of the three, can be established. With particular cancer chemotherapeutic agents, where there is a suspect clinically relevant risk of serious toxicity, a test dose may be used prospectively to forecast and lessen the safety risk. Another particularly useful approach is to administer a radioactive tracer dose of a drug to permit accurate quantification of the levels of the drug and various metabolites over time. This method has been used in the identification and characterization of pharmacogenetic syndromes affecting 5-fluorouracil metabolism.[33]

Genotypic or Phenotypic Tests and the Individualization of Drug Therapy

Once a particular pharmacogenetic syndrome has been identified, pharmacokinetic analysis may be of limited clinical feasibility due to its labor-intensiveness. In addition, observation of changes in drug concentration alone may not allow an understanding of the metabolic pathways responsible for drug metabolism. Therefore, genotypic or phenotypic tests can be more beneficial than pharmacokinetic studies in therapeutic drug monitoring and the individualization of drug therapy. Its advantages over pharmacokinetic analysis are summarized below:

- Genotypic and phenotypic tests are less invasive, as they require a single blood, plasma, serum, urine, or tissue sample for assessment of polymorphisms that may affect drug pharmacokinetics and response.
- Genotypic or phenotypic tests can help predict drug response and toxicity. Drug treatment may be altered to prevent potentially lethal toxicity or lack of efficacy due to genetic polymorphisms in genes that influence drug effects.
- The genotypic or phenotypic profile may also be informative in combination treatment with other therapeutic agents.
- The genotypic or phenotypic profile may be applicable to the individual patient's treatment with a drug in the same or a different drug class (e.g., metabolized through the same polymorphic drug-metabolizing enzyme).
- The genotypic or phenotypic test may provide insight into pharmacodynamic variability and the mechanistic basis for variability in drug response or may help in the identification of patients possibly at risk for rapid disease progression or tumor invasiveness.

The choice of a genetic versus a phenotypic test (predictor) of drug effects is usually associated with specific and/or overlapping advantages and disadvantages, summarized in Table 24.1.

Family Studies (Pattern of Inheritance of Drug Effects)

Cancer chemotherapy drugs are too toxic for the family study approach to assessing patterns of inheritance of drug response used for drugs from other therapeutic classes.[34] Other phenotypic tests such as assessment of the activity of a drug-metabolizing enzyme or determination of substrate levels in family members can define the pattern of inheritance.

Once a pharmacokinetic or pharmacodynamic alteration has been defined in an individual patient, studies in the family can provide insight into whether the genetic polymorphism is an autosomal or sex-linked trait and whether the pattern of inheritance is dominant, codominant, or recessive.

With availability of data from the human genome project and the functional assignment of enzyme activity to a particular gene, it is becoming possible to delineate the inheritance of a specific gene. Techniques that can identify a specific DNA sequence or SNP, such as allele-specific polymerase chain reaction-based (PCR-based) methods, should make this technically straightforward.[35]

Population Studies

Population studies are aimed at the assessment of the frequency of the pharmacogenetic syndrome within the general population as well as frequency differences between populations. As with family studies, population studies can use either phenotypic or genotypic tests. The frequency of individuals with particular phenotypic characteristics can be estimated using the Hardy-Weinberg equation.[36] Population studies to assess the specific phenotype or activity of a particular protein may show unimodal or bimodal patterns of distribution. A unimodal distribution in the activity of a particular enzyme, such as a Gaussian or normal distribution pattern, suggests mutations or genetic alterations that lead to a range of activities in the population studied. In contrast, bimodal distributions may indicate mutations that lead to reduced or greater than normal activity in a subset of the population.[37] The evaluation of particular phenotypes in population studies related to chemotherapeutic drug metabolism may require assessments using a safer probe drug that is metabolized through the same potential polymorphic drug-metabolizing enzyme but without posing a risk of toxicity to the healthy individual participating in the study. Results from a population study comparing cancer patients to healthy volunteers indicated that cancer stage may also influence the phenotype of an important drug-metabolizing enzyme CYP2C19, for which genotype normally predicts phenotype in the healthy population.[38,39] In this study, patients with advanced cancer had the extensive metabolizer genotype; however, 25% of the patients displayed a poor metabolizer phenotype. This discordance between phenotype

TABLE 24.1

CHARACTERISTICS OF PHENOTYPIC VERSUS GENOTYPIC PREDICTORS OF DRUG RESPONSE

	Advantages	Disadvantages
Phenotypic test	May use easily accessible biological sample (e.g., plasma, urine, or tissue) to reflect phenotype in poorly accessible tissue. Represents the combined effects of the genes and the environment on the phenotypic measure. Unlike genotypic tests, are able to identify cancer or disease associated changes in phenotype, which may not be reflected in genotype.	Phenotype in normal tissue may not reflect that in tumor tissue. Knowledge of pattern or characteristics of phenotypic variability present in population is required to assess the clinical importance of the specific phenotype in individual patients. Requires feasibility for routine clinical testing. Development requires it to be practical and inexpensive with high diagnostic sensitivity and specificity. Phenotype may change over time under the influence of other gene products or environmental factors. A broad range of variability in the phenotype is required within the population studied in order for the test to be of clinical relevance.
Genotypic test	Genotype may be assessed from a single blood sample without the need for probe drug administration for phenotyping. Allows analysis of the mechanisms of variability in drug effects in patients clinically unsuitable for phenotypic test or for the collection of pooled biological samples necessary for phenotyping. Knowledge of specific genetic alteration causing genetic polymorphism may provide information on the precise molecular mechanism involved.	Must test specific alleles causing the phenotypic changes and thus may require technological proficiency. Population studies required to assess relative importance and variability in specific genotype in particular patient populations or ethnic groups. Particular genotype may produce a widely variable range in phenotype and therefore may be less sensitive or clinically useful than phenotypic tests. May not predict variability in pharmacokinetic or pharmacodynamic parameters if variability is caused by more than one polymorphism in a single gene, interactions between different genes, or interactions between the environment and the genetic polymorphism. Genotype in normal tissue may not be reflective of that found in tumor tissue. Requires ease of interpretation for therapeutic drug optimization in a clinical setting.

and genotype and the decreased activity of CYP2C19 observed in terminally ill cancer patients may influence the clinical efficacy and toxicity of therapeutic agents (e.g. cyclophosphamide) and should be investigated with respect to other drug-metabolizing enzymes.[39] The characterization of genes and related phenotypes involved in anticancer drug pharmacokinetic or pharmacodynamic variability or those involved in cancer predisposition may be limited to investigations using individuals with the particular cancer or those already being treated with a particular chemotherapeutic agent.

Some pharmacogenetic syndromes are associated with multiple alleles (see "Pathway Approach" later in the chapter). Thus, population studies provide the relative frequency of the various alleles associated with a specific pharmacological syndrome.

After an assessment of phenotypic and genotypic markers in the general population, it may be useful to undertake surveys in other populations, including patients affected with specific types of cancer or being treated with a particular chemotherapeutic agent. Such studies may define the frequency of the pharmacogenetic syndrome in the cancer patient population at risk. Other demographic factors, such as race, age, and gender, may influence the risk to specific groups.

The methodologies discussed above have had specific applications in the identification of SNPs in single genes using the candidate gene approach. The genetic polymorphisms in single genes have not thus far explained a large proportion of the individual variability in drug response, mainly because most drug response phenotypes are thought to be determined by the interactions among multiple genes as well as with the environment. Therefore, the candidate gene strategy has limited value for identifying polygenic determinants of variability in drug response. On the other hand, this approach may offer an advantage for testing "specific" biological or pharmacological hypotheses in a given and often limited clinical sample of patients.

Genome-wide studies require larger numbers of subjects to achieve statistical power to identify multiple low-penetrance genes, a requirement seldom fulfilled in small heterogeneous patient samples.

Pathway Approach

The complexity inherent in the genetic determination of drug response warrants the use of methodologies that can evaluate the contribution of polymorphisms in several genes, which may interact in additive, synergistic, or antagonistic ways to influence a single drug response. The biological pathway approach to the analysis of pharmacogenetic variation allows for the investigation of associations between genetic polymorphisms within a particular biological pathway of relevance to the pharmacokinetics or pharmacodynamics of a chemotherapeutic agent and is hypothesis-driven.[20] Similar to the candidate gene approach, this approach requires an understanding of the biochemical pathways and specific molecular and signaling interactions involved in these pathways. Pharmacogenetics, however, not only is concerned with the effects of genes on drug response but also considers the effects of drugs on gene function and the interactions between genes that are caused by drugs (pharmacological pathways). This has led to the elucidation of the targets that drugs act on and also of the signaling pathways and of polymorphisms in key rate-limiting steps within these pathways that may be involved in the mechanism of action of drugs. Through investigations of the effects of drugs *on* genes, one may be able to discern the putative drug targets and the related biological pathways. Polymorphisms in such pathways may in turn influence drug efficacy or resistance to anticancer agents.

Genomics Approach

Pharmacogenomics is the study of variation in drug response utilizing genome-wide approaches. Methodologies include gene expression arrays and proteomics assays, which are designed to assess differences in gene and protein expression profiles.[20] These techniques are being widely applied to define profiles associated with drug response, tumor response, or disease predisposition. Such studies may provide insight into mechanisms for severe toxicity in subsets of patients which, if unexplained, could lead to the termination of development of an agent that might be effective in some patient subsets. These techniques are associated with false-positive and false-negative results. Therefore, subsequent to the identification of a gene or protein potentially implicated in drug response or disease outcome using genomic approaches, a hypothesis-based follow-up research strategy is required (e.g., biochemical functional analysis, large-scale epidemiological studies).

EXAMPLES OF GENETIC VARIATIONS THAT INFLUENCE ANTICANCER CHEMOTHERAPEUTIC DRUG EFFICACY AND SAFETY IN HUMANS

Several pharmacogenetic syndromes are associated with certain cancer chemotherapy agents.[36,40–46] Tables 24.2 and 24.3 list the best-characterized polymorphic enzymes and proteins relevant to cancer chemotherapy.

Thiopurine S-Methyltransferase and 6-Mercaptopurine (6-MP)

The purine antimetabolite 6-mercaptopurine (6-MP) is commonly used in the treatment of childhood acute lymphoblastic leukemia (ALL).[47] This inactive prodrug requires metabolism through an enzymatic pathway involving hypoxanthine phosphoribosyl transferase, leading to the formation of thioguanine nucleotides (TGN), which can be incorporated into DNA to produce antineoplastic activity. Alternatively, 6-MP may be inactivated through oxidation by xanthine oxidase or may produce anticancer activity through its S-methylation by thiopurine S-methyl transferase (TPMT, E.C. 2.1.167).[42,47] Methylation via TPMT results in the formation of 6-methylmercaptopurine nucleotide, which mediates anticancer activity through its inhibition of phosphoribosyl diphosphate amidotransferase, an enzyme involved in de novo purine synthesis.[48] The activation via TPMT has been shown to be the more clinically relevant pathway affecting 6-MP efficacy in the treatment of chronic lymphocytic leukemia; hematological toxicity is due to the negligible detoxifying xanthine oxidase expression in hematological tissues.[11] Genetic polymorphisms in the *TPMT* gene have been associated with considerable variability in both the efficacy and toxicity of 6-MP in childhood ALL.

TABLE 24.2
POLYMORPHISMS IN DRUG-METABOLIZING ENZYMES

Polymorphic Enzyme	Chemotherapeutic Agent
Thiopurine S-methyltransferase	6-MP
Dihydropyrimidine dehydrogenase	5-FU, capecitabine
UDP-glucuronosyltransferase 1A1	Irinotecan, SN-38
Glutathione S-transferase	Chlorambucil, phosphoramide mustard
Sulfotransferase SULT1A1	Tamoxifen
CYP2D6	Tamoxifen
N-acetyltransferases	Amonafide (no longer in clinical development)
Methyltetrahydrofolate reductase	Methotrexate
CYP3A4, CYP3A5, CYP3A7	Etoposide, cyclophosphamide

TABLE 24.3
POLYMORPHISMS IN DRUG TARGETS OR GENES AFFECTING DRUG RESISTANCE

Polymorphic Protein	Chemotherapeutic Agent
Aromatase (CYP19)	Aromatase inhibitors
ERCC1, XPD and XRCC1 DNA repair proteins	Platinum-based compounds
Thymidylate synthase	5-FU
ABCB1 (MDR-1)	Natural product anticancer drugs

TPMT Genetic Polymorphisms

Genetic polymorphisms are the molecular basis of variability in TPMT activity[49,50] in most patients. To date, nine *TPMT* alleles have been associated with decreased TPMT activity,[50] with single nucleotide polymorphisms resulting in amino acid substitutions (*TPMT*2, *TPMT*3A, *TPMT*3B, *TPMT*3C, *TPMT*3D, *TPMT*5, and *TPMT*6), a premature stop codon (*TPMT*3D), and destruction of the splice site between intron 9 and exon 10 (*TPMT*4). In addition to the alleles that confer decreased enzymatic activity, a single nucleotide polymorphism has been identified that leads to increased TPMT activity (*TPMT*1A). Of these identified alleles, three (*TPMT*2, *TPMT*3A, and *TPMT*3C) are responsible for approximately 95% of the intermediate or low enzyme activity observed in patients.[47,51–54] Furthermore, the decrease in enzymatic activity associated with these three alleles is due to characteristic effects of each specific single nucleotide polymorphism on the activity of the expressed protein as well as rapid proteolysis of the variant proteins compared to the wild-type protein.[55,56]

Pattern-of-Inheritance and Population Studies

TPMT genotype is responsible for considerable interindividual and interethnic differences in phenotype. Patients with one wild-type allele and one variant allele have intermediate activity compared to those who are homozygous for the wild-type allele. Patients with two variant alleles lack significant TPMT activity (are TPMT-deficient).[51,52,57] Approximately 10% of the general population have intermediate TPMT activity, and 0.3% have low or insignificant enzyme activity.[51,52] As a result of the multiple variant *TPMT* alleles, each associated with variable TPMT enzyme activity, allele-specific PCR or PCR-RFLP has been utilized to detect alleles associated with variability in enzyme activity in different ethnic groups. In the Caucasian population, *TPMT*3A is the most common variant allele (3.2 to 5.7% of *TPMT* alleles), while *TPMT*3C has an allele frequency of 0.2 to 0.8% and *TPMT*2 a frequency of 0.2 to 0.5%.[47,51] For African and Asian populations however, the *TPMT*3C allele has been the only variant allele identified in published studies to date.[47,58,59]

Clinical Relevance

TPMT genetic polymorphisms are linked to variability in the efficacy and toxicity of 6-MP. This variability is of considerable clinical importance due to the large fraction of the general population that is heterozygous for the mutant *TPMT* alleles (5 to 10%), leading to decreased TPMT enzymatic activity. If the TPMT activity is relatively low, more 6-MP is available. However, pharmacokinetic studies have demonstrated that this may not be reflected in the plasma concentrations of 6-MP.[60] Red blood cell TGN concentrations are a better predictor; when elevated, they predict toxicity. Low TGN concentrations may predict failure to respond and could provide a rationale for increasing the dose of 6-MP to individualize therapy.[61]

Among the subset of ALL patients who were intolerant to 6-MP therapy (i.e., they developed hematopoietic toxicity, hepatotoxicity, mucositis, and/or other toxicities requiring dose reductions or delays in subsequent chemotherapy cycles), sixfold overrepresentation of *TPMT* deficients and heterozygotes was observed.[62] Looking at hematopoietic toxicity alone, this overrepresentation was even more significant; in particular, 71% of patients who experienced hematopoietic toxicity were deficient or heterozygous for the *TPMT* variant alleles, compared to the general population of ALL patients, among whom 8 to 10% are *TPMT* homozygous mutant or heterozygous.[62] It was further indicated that once *TPMT* deficiency or heterozygosity was determined in these ALL patients and an appropriate 6-MP dose reduction was made for subsequent therapy, patients were able to undergo 6-MP treatment without acute dose-limiting toxicity and were able to maintain red blood cell TGN levels similar to or greater than those achieved by full doses in homozygous wild-type patients.[51,62–64] These data provide strong evidence that the diagnosis of *TPMT* deficiency or heterozygosity before initiation of 6-MP treatment may help to increase the efficacy of 6-MP, limit toxicity, and increase the event-free survival of ALL patients.[11]

Dihydropyrimidine Dehydrogenase and 5-Fluorouracil (5-FU)

Fluoropyrimidines constitute an important class of antineoplastic agents, with the prototype agent 5-fluorouracil (5-FU) being one of the most commonly prescribed anticancer drugs.[65,66] This agent is used particularly in the treatment of solid tumors of the breast, head, neck, and gastrointestinal tract.[67–70] The oral fluoropyrimidine prodrug capecitabine is also being widely tested in various types of cancer.[71] The biological activity of 5-FU is mediated through activation or anabolism of the parent prodrug to 5-fluoro-2-deoxyuridine monophosphate (5-FdUMP), which subsequently inhibits thymidylate synthase (TS), an enzyme required for de novo pyrimidine synthesis. On the other hand, 80 to 90% of the administered intravenous

5-FU dose is inactivated through catabolism in the liver, where the rate-limiting enzyme is dihydropyrimidine dehydrogenase (DPD, EC1.3.1.2).[33,72]

Catabolism has been shown to be important in 5-FU response. In particular, DPD exhibits a wide interindividual variation in activity of up to 20-fold, and patients with low or negligible DPD activity are unable to efficiently inactivate 5-FU, leading to decreased catabolism, which can produce severe 5-FdUMP–mediated gastrointestinal, hematopoietic, and neurological toxicities.[46,73–76]

DPD Genetic Polymorphisms

Genetic polymorphisms in the *DPYD* gene lead to complete or partial loss of DPD enzyme activity and thus may be responsible for the considerable patient-to-patient variability in therapeutic efficacy and toxicity.[73,76–78] The syndrome of DPD deficiency, resulting from molecular defects in the gene coding for DPD (*DPYD*), leads to complete or partial loss of DPD enzyme activity.[79]

More than 30 sequence variations in the *DPYD* gene have been identified, producing multiple complex heterozygote genotypes that are inherited in an autosomal codominant fashion.[80] Analyses of the prevalence of the specific variant alleles have shown that the most common inactivating allele (*DPYD*2A*) is characterized by a G to A transition at the invariant GT splice donor site flanking exon 14 of the *DPYD* gene.[73] This mutation leads to truncated mRNA due to skipping of exon 14, which results in a nonfunctional protein.[73,74,81] A second single nucleotide polymorphism associated with DPD deficiency is *DPYD*13*, which is characterized by a T to G transition at a domain important to enzyme activity.[82] Familial studies have indicated that DPD deficiency is inherited in an autosomal codominant fashion and that DPD deficiency most likely results from multiple mutations at a single gene locus. For instance, a profoundly deficient patient with heterozygous mutations for both *DPYD*13* and *DPYD*2A* and a spouse with normal DPD activity had two partially deficient offspring (one child being heterozygous for the *DPYD*2A* variant allele and one child being heterozygous for the *DPYD*13* variant allele).[82] To date, however, the identified *DPYD* variant alleles do not explain all observed cases of DPD deficiency, as many patients with severe 5-FU toxicity have no detected mutations in the *DPYD* gene.[83] Further studies are thus warranted to fully elucidate the complex molecular and genetic mechanisms leading to DPD deficiency and 5-FU toxicity.

Pattern-of-Inheritance and Population Studies

Partial and complete DPD deficiencies occur in approximately 0.1% and 3 to 5% of the general population, respectively.[77] The high prevalence of this syndrome suggests that DPD deficiency may predispose a significant segment of the general population to an increased risk of altered 5-FU pharmacokinetics and toxicity. However, the complexity of this syndrome, along with the multiple heterozygous genotypes observed in population studies, may limit the usefulness of genotyping for a single mutation in this gene.[84] Previous reports of sequence variations in this gene have not consistently predicted DPD enzyme activity and identified patients at risk for 5-FU–mediated toxicity due to DPD deficiency.[83,85,86] This suggests that, in addition to the investigation of variations in the *DPYD* gene, further investigations should explore other markers that may act alone or together with DPD to produce 5-FU toxicity. Measurement of DPD activity may be more beneficial than genotypic tests in screening for DPD deficiency. Several genotypic and phenotypic methods, including high-performance liquid chromatography (semiautomated radioassay), mass spectrometry, thin-layer chromatography, and denaturing high-performance liquid chromatography, have been developed to identify DPD deficiency in cancer patients.[87–90] Unfortunately, all of these methods remain too complicated and time consuming for routine clinical use and are unavailable in most treatment centers. Due to the complexity of DPD deficiency and its suggested importance in a significant portion of patients with unpredictable severe 5-FU toxicity, rapid screening tests are needed to assess DPD activity in cancer patients prior to treatment with fluoropyrimidine chemotherapeutic agents. A simple 2-^{13}C uracil breath test (UraBT) has shown potential for rapidly assessing DPD activity in healthy individuals as well as cancer patients. This test is based on the metabolism of 2-^{13}C uracil by the enzymes of the pyrimidine-catabolic pathway to produce $^{13}CO_2$; the $^{13}CO_2$ profiles of individuals with normal DPD activity and deficient DPD activity are distinct.[91] The clinical utility of this test is still requires further investigation.

Clinical Implications

DPD has been identified as having a pivotal role in the modulation of 5-FU plasma concentrations. Studies with thymine and uracil (both endogenous substrates for DPD) and 5-FU have shown that all three substrates have similar affinities for DPD and that 5-FU degradation is inhibited by both thymine and uracil, leading to altered 5-FU pharmacokinetics and, in turn, increased toxicity.[92,93] Furthermore, the inability to degrade 5-FU in patients with decreased DPD activity is associated with an increased risk for the development of 5-FU–related severe toxicity.[94] Pharmacokinetic studies in patients receiving 5-FU by continuous infusion have demonstrated that plasma 5-FU levels have a circadian variation. This circadian variation was further shown to inversely correlate with the circadian variation in DPD activity from peripheral blood mononuclear cells, suggesting that plasma 5-FU levels are regulated by DPD.[95] The determination of variability in DPD activity could aid in the prediction of altered 5-FU plasma concentrations, which in turn may allow for the development of individualized 5-FU–based pharmacotherapy strategies.

There are marked interindividual differences in response, survival, and toxicity among patients treated with 5-FU. For example, patients with metastatic colorectal cancer have been shown to exhibit an overall response rate of 26% to 5-FU treatment.[96] DPD activity has been related to 5-FU efficacy and toxicity.[33,97,98] Interestingly, DPD also appears to serve a critical role in tumor response to 5-FU, with low intratumor expression of the DPD gene (*DPYD*) shown to predict favorable response to this agent and increased survival time in patients with colorectal cancer.[97]

5-FU toxicity is common; 31 to 34% of patients with colorectal cancer treated with 5-FU displayed dose-limiting grade 3 to grade 4 hematological toxicity.[99] DPD deficiency accounts for 43 to 60% of patients with severe toxicity to 5-FU (in some cases severe enough to result in death).[100,101] The other determinants of 5-FU toxicity are undefined.

UDP-Glucuronosyl-Transferase 1A1 and Irinotecan

Irinotecan (CPT-11), a synthetic analog of camptothecin, is commonly used in the treatment of several solid tumors, including advanced colorectal cancer. This prodrug requires metabolic activation to the active metabolite 7-ethyl-10-hydroxycamptothecin (SN-38) by carboxylesterase 2, with its antineoplastic activity resulting from the inhibition of topoisomerase I.[102] The active metabolite, SN-38, is further glucuronidated via hepatic UDP-glucuronosyl-transferase 1A1 (UGT1A1) to the more polar and inactive metabolite SN-38-glucuronide, which can undergo elimination via the bile and urine.[103] CPT-11 may also undergo phase I oxidative metabolism through CYP3A4 and CYP3A5. This oxidative metabolism predominantly leads to inactive metabolites and decreases the fraction of administered CPT-11 available for activation to SN-38.[104] Optimum treatment with CPT-11 is hindered by severe dose-limiting diarrhea and neutropenia, which are associated with decreased UGT1A1-mediated inactivation of SN-38.[103,105] Accordingly, the main focus of pharmacogenetic studies has been to elucidate the mechanisms of CPT-11–mediated toxicity, including the variability in the metabolism of CPT-11 and genetic polymorphisms associated with UGT1A1-mediated glucuronidation.

UGT1A1 genetic polymorphisms

The polymorphic phase II detoxification enzyme UGT1A1 is responsible for the inactivation through glucuronidation of a variety of endogenous (bilirubin) and exogenous substrates. Over 30 genetic variants have been identified for *UGT1A1*, a large fraction of which influence the expression and function of the enzyme.[106,107] The commonly observed Gilbert's syndrome is characterized by mild unconjugated hyperbilirubinemia and is associated with homozygosity

for the dinucleotide (TA) insertion in the $(TA)_6TAA$ element in the *UGT1A1* promoter region[108] in the Caucasian population. This polymorphism results in the *UGT1A1*28* variant allele, which has seven TA repeats, in contrast to six repeats observed in the wild-type *UGT1A1*1* allele. Functionally, the variant allele leads to a 70% decrease in *UGT1A1* gene expression compared to the *UGT1A1*1* allele.[109-111] The *UGT1A1*28* allele is less frequent in Asian populations than in Caucasian populations. In fact, missense mutations are more frequently observed in the Asian population, including mutations in the first exon (*UGT1A1*6* and *UGT1A1*27*).[112]

Pattern-of-Inheritance and Population Studies

The frequency of the *UGT1A1*28* allele is approximately 35% in Caucasians and African Americans, while it is present at a much lower frequency in Asian populations. This variable prevalence of the *UGT1A1*28* allele based on ethnic origin is in part responsible for the wide range in frequency reported for the homozygous *UGT1A1*28* genotype in different populations (0.5 to 23%).[106,111,113] Interestingly, other missense mutations in the coding region of *UGT1A1* are thought to be responsible for cases of Gilbert's syndrome observed in Asian populations. Particularly, the most common variant present in Asian populations is the *UGT1A1*6* allele, which has an allelic frequency from 13 to 23%.[114,115] This mutation is of functional significance and results in a 30% and 60% decrease in bilirubin-glucuronidation for heterozygotes and homozygotes, respectively. These data suggest that, regardless of mutation type, individuals with Gilbert's syndrome may be at increased risk for CPT-11–mediated toxicity. Further studies are required to assess the clinical importance of these mutations as well as polymorphisms in other genes affecting both the efficacy and safety of CPT-11 in various populations.

Clinical Implications

The suggested cause of CPT-11–induced severe diarrhea is direct enteric injury due to biliary excretion of the active metabolite SN-38 in the absence of adequate glucuronidation.[116] Clinical data have shown an inverse relationship between SN-38 glucuronidation rates and severity of diarrhea in patients treated with escalating doses of CPT-11 (ref.[103]).

Particular genetic polymorphisms in the *UGT1A1* gene have been implicated in the occurrence of CPT-11–induced toxicity. The *UGT1A1*28* mutation was associated with grade 4 leukopenia and grade 3 to grade 4 diarrhea in Japanese cancer patients.[112] The frequency of the *UGT1A1*28* variant was 3.5-fold higher in patients with severe toxicity than in those with no CPT-11–induced toxicity. The *UGT1A1*6* allele frequency was not altered between the two patient groups, while all patients heterozygous for the

UGT1A1*27 allele experienced severe drug-induced toxicity. Interestingly, patients with a UGT1A1*28 mutation in combination with either a UGT1A1*6 or UGT1A1*27 allele also had an increased risk of severe toxicity. In another study, the ratios of SN-38 glucuronide to SN-38 were significantly lower in UGT1A1*28 carriers than in homozygous carries of the UGT1A1*1 allele.[105] As a result of the high prevalence of the UGT1A1*28 polymorphism, especially in African American and Caucasian populations, further studies are required to determine whether dose adjustment based on UGT1A1 genotype would have beneficial or adverse effects on the response to CPT-11.

Glutathione-S-Transferase

Glutathione-dependent detoxification of reactive electrophiles, including cytotoxic chemotherapeutic agents, is catalyzed by the glutathione S-transferase (GST) superfamily of isozymes, which consists of five subclasses (GSTA1, GSTP1, GSTM1, GSTT1, and GSTZ1).[117] Several studies described below have reported associations between GST polymorphisms and the efficacy and/or toxicity of various antineoplastic agents as well as disease outcome.

GST Genetic Polymorphisms

Polymorphisms that occur in the human GST genes may have several effects on protein expression and function; for example, gene duplication can lead to ultrarapid metabolizing phenotypes (e.g., GSTM1*Ax2), and SNPs can result in increased or decreased protein function.[118] One such characterized polymorphism in the coding region of GSTP1, for instance, leads to a protein with decreased catalytic activity. Gene deletions may also result in null phenotypes; for instance, patients homozygous for the GSTM1*0 or GSTT1*0 "null" allele, where the GSTM1 or GSTT1 gene has been deleted, cannot express the corresponding GST protein.[119-122]

Pattern-of-Inheritance and Population Studies

A significant number of genetic polymorphisms in the GST genes have been identified; however, few have been studied extensively. As a result of the homozygous GSTM1*0 genotype, GSTM1 activity is not present in approximately 50 to 60% of Caucasian and Saudi Arabian populations and 22% of a Nigerian population.[123] Similarly, the homozygous GSTT1*0 genotype results in the absence of catalytically active protein.[118] Population studies have revealed 64.4% and 9% frequencies for this GSTT1*0 null phenotype in Chinese and Mexican populations, respectively.[124]

Clinical Significance

GST polymorphisms have been investigated for their contribution as factors affecting chemotherapeutic response, treatment outcome, and survival in patients with various types of cancer. The GSTM1 and GSTT1 null phenotypes (homozygous GSTM1*0 or GSTT1*0) have been associated with an increased risk of aplastic anemia[125] and a number of forms of cancer, including lung, colon, head, neck, and bladder cancer and postmenopausal breast cancer and ovarian cancer.[125,126] Overexpression of GST enzymes is associated with resistance to several cancer chemotherapeutic agents, including chlorambucil, carmustine, nitrogen mustard, melphelan, and the active metabolite of cyclophosphamide (phosphoramide mustard), which are all substrates for GST and are inactivated via GSH conjugation.[118]

GST genetic polymorphisms have not been found to have consistent effects on disease outcome and survival. Ovarian cancer patients with the combination GSTM1 null and GSTT1 null genotypes demonstrated a decreased survival and reduced progression-free interval when compared with patients without these null genotypes.[127] Further, the patients with both null genotypes displayed a lack of response to treatment with cisplatin and alkylating agents, compared with a 54% response rate for patients with alternate genotype combinations.[127] These data are inconsistent with the suggested biological mechanism in which a lack of detoxification by GST would be hypothesized to produce improved response and survival rates compared with those for patients without the null genotypes. Contrary results were shown for breast cancer patients homozygous for both the GSTM1*0 and GSTT1*0 alleles compared with patients without the null genotypes.[128] In this study, patients who had the null genotypes and were treated with cyclophosphamide combination therapy had a smaller risk of recurrence and hazard of death than patients without the null genotypes. Reduced inactivation of cyclophosphamide-generated reactive oxygen species through a lack of GST activity may produce improved antitumor activity and survival rates in breast cancer.[128]

Conflicting results have also been reported for patients with childhood ALL. In one report, patients with at least two of the genotypes associated with decreased or lack of GST activity (GSTM1*0, GSTT1*0, or GSTP1Val105 homozygous genotypes) had a 3.5-fold increased risk of recurrence compared with patients who did not have these genotypes.[129] In contrast to these results, another similar investigation could not demonstrate any effects of the GSTM1*0 and GSTT1*0 alleles on patient survival.[130] Given the complexity and high degree of genetic variability observed in the GST family of enzymes, exact relationships between genotype/phenotype and response to chemotherapy or disease outcome need further clarification. This may be achieved by using rapid, high-throughput methods capable of assessing multiple GST genotypes or by using RNA and GST protein expression techniques. Further, correlative studies investigating plasma pharmacokinetics or GST substrates and GST activity may shed further light on possible clinically relevant applications for the individualization of chemotherapeutic treatment.

Thymidylate Synthase and 5-FU

Like polymorphisms in genes important for drug metabolism, polymorphisms in the genes for drug targets are also important determinants of drug response and disease outcome. Thymidylate synthase (TS) is the main target of 5-FU. The 5-FU metabolite FdUMP produces a stable complex with TS and a methyl cofactor, leading to inhibition of dTMP synthesis and DNA synthesis.[45] Variability in response to 5-FU has been linked to several TS gene (*TYMS*) genetic polymorphisms.[131–133]

TS Genetic Polymorphisms

To date, three polymorphisms in the *TYMS* gene have been identified. A polymorphism within the 5'-promotor enhancer region (*TSER*) of the *TYMS* gene consists of tandem repeats of 28 base pairs ranging from two (*TSER*2) to nine (*TSER*9) copies.[134] The role of most of these alleles in TS expression is currently unknown; however, patients homozygous for the *TSER*3 genotype have increased intratumor TS messenger RNA levels[135] and elevated TS protein levels [136] compared with patients with the homozygous *TSER*2 genotype.[135,137,138] Two additional polymorphisms have been identified. The first is a single nucleotide polymorphism within the second repeat of the *TSER*3 allele (G→C, *3RG* and *3RC* alleles). It has been suggested this polymorphism affects the level of TS expression by abolishing a USF1-binding site.[139] The second polymorphism described is a 6bp deletion located in the 3'UTR, 447 base pairs downstream from the stop codon.[140]

Pattern-of-Inheritance and Population Studies

The polymorphisms in which there is a double (*TSER*2) and triple (*TSER*3) tandem repeat of 28 base pairs are observed most frequently in Caucasian populations, with higher repeats (*TSER*4, *TSER*5, and *TSER*9 alleles) mainly found in African populations.[141] When Asian populations are considered, the homozygous (*TSER*3) genotype is approximately twice as frequent (67%) as in Caucasians (38%). Using RFLP analysis, the frequency of the *3RC* allele in different ethnic populations was determined to be 56%, 47%, 28%, and 37% for non-Hispanic Whites, Hispanic Whites, African Americans, and Singapore Chinese, respectively.[139] Lastly, the 6–base pair deletion polymorphism displayed frequencies of 41%, 26%, 52%, and 76% in non-Hispanic Whites, Hispanic Whites, African-Americans, and Singapore Chinese, respectively.[142,143]

Clinical Significance

Variability in response to 5-FU has been linked to TS, with drug resistance and poor prognosis associated with overexpression of the gene.[144–148] Several studies have linked the double- and triple-repeat allelic variants (*TSER*2 and *TSER*3) with response to 5-FU. Pullarkat and colleagues (2001) demonstrated that patients homozygous for the *TSER*3 allele had a 3.6-fold higher level of TS mRNA than those homozygous for the *TSER*2 allele.[135] These researchers also found that colorectal cancer patients homozygous for the *TSER*2 genotype had a response rate of 50%, compared with 9% for those homozygous for the *TSER*3 genotype.[135] Moreover, patients with the homozygous *TSER*2 genotype had less severe side effects in response to 5-FU than those with the *TSER*3 homozygous genotype. In another study, colorectal cancer patients homozygous or heterozygous (*TSER*2/*TSER*3) for the *TSER*2 allele displayed a higher probability of pathological downstaging (60%) subsequent to neoadjuvant 5-FU–based chemotherapy than patients' homozygotes for the *TSER*3 allele (22%).[137] Currently, however, some ambiguity exists regarding the definitions of "good" and "poor" outcome in these studies, and larger trials are needed to elucidate the importance of *TSER* polymorphisms and other *TYMS* polymorphisms in determining chemotherapeutic outcome.

With respect to the *3RC* variant allele, in a trial with 208 colorectal cancer patients, a 1.3-fold (95% CI, 0.9–1.9) increased risk of colorectal cancer was found in patients with the *3RG* allele compared with controls; however, the specific functional significance of this polymorphism is unclear.[149] Another study reported a decreased response to 5-FU in patients homozygous for the variant 6–base pair deletion located in the 3'UTR (447 base pairs downstream from the stop codon), with an odds ratio of 2.0 for 5-FU–based chemotherapy.[150] Overall, these studies suggest that determination of the *TSER* genotype may be a clinically useful tool in the prediction of response to 5-FU.

Sulfotransferase 1A1 and Tamoxifen

The triphenylethylene antiestrogenic compound tamoxifen is commonly used for the treatment of hormone-responsive breast cancer as well as for the prevention of breast cancer.[151] The parent compound is subject to extensive hepatic metabolism, leading to the major metabolites *N*-desmethyl-tamoxifen, tamoxifen-*N*-oxide, and 4-hydroxy-tamoxifen (4-OH-tam). The therapeutic efficacy of this antiestrogen is attributed to the parent compound (tamoxifen), its cytochrome P450–mediated hydroxylated metabolite (4-OH-tam), and 4hydroxy-*N*-desmethyl-tamoxifen (endoxifen), which is formed through hydroxylation of *N*-desmethyl-tam by CYP2D6. 4-OH-tam has been shown to be significantly more potent than the parent compound, with a 33-fold increased affinity for human breast cancer estrogen receptors.[152] The plasma concentration of endoxifen is dependent on the highly polymorphic *CYP2D6* genotype of the patient.[153,154] This suggests that polymorphisms within the *CYP2D6* gene influencing protein function, as well as the administration of concomitant substrates or inhibitors of CYP2D6, may affect the therapeutic outcome of tamoxifen therapy. However, additional studies are required to characterize the clinical relevance of variability in the CYP2D6 gene as a factor in the response to tamoxifen.

One other important class of enzymes involved in the metabolism of tamoxifen consists of the hepatic phenol sulfotransferases. These enzymes are classified as phase II drug-metabolizing enzymes and are important in the sulfation-mediated metabolism of endogenous substrates (e.g., steroids), the inactivation of xenobiotics, and the activation of procarcinogens. There are six characterized isoforms within the phenol sulfotransferase (SULT) family of enzymes, and among these the SULT1A1 isoform plays a critical role in the trans-selective sulfation of 4-OH-tam.[155] A functionally significant genetic polymorphism in the SULT1A1 gene has been identified, and data suggest an association with breast cancer risk and therapeutic response to tamoxifen.[156]

SULT1A1 Genetic Polymorphism and Pattern of Inheritance

A single nucleotide polymorphism characterized by a G→A transition in codon 213 leading to an Arg to His amino acid substitution (SULT1A1*2) has been described for the SULT1A1 gene.[157–159] Population studies have indicated the presence of the variant SULT1A1*2 allele at frequencies of 0.321% and 0.269% in Caucasian and Nigerian populations, respectively.[160] Functionally, this polymorphism results in a 10-fold decrease in phenol SULT activity in individuals homozygous for the variant allele (SULT1A1*2), compared with those homozygous for the wild-type allele (SULT1A1*1).[159]

Clinical Significance

Considerable interpatient variability is associated with 4-OH-tam plasma and tumor tissue concentrations, ranging from 28 to 69% of those determined for tamoxifen.[161] Additionally, variability in 4-OH-tam concentration and response to tamoxifen may be associated with the reported induction of SULT1A mRNA by 4-OH-tam[156] as well as with prognosis, as the SULT1A1*2 allele leads to a SULT protein with lower catalytic activity than does the SULT1A1*1 allele.[159] With respect to the potential association between the risk of breast cancer and the SULT1A1 genotype, results have been inconsistent. One study in postmenopausal woman reported a significant association between the variant SULT1A1*2 allele and an increased risk for breast cancer.[162] In contrast, another study reported no association between the SULT1A1 genotype and risk for breast cancer.[156]

Nowell and colleagues demonstrated an association between the SULT1A1 polymorphism and breast cancer outcome in women treated with adjuvant tamoxifen. Specifically, women homozygous for the SULT1A1*2 allele

displayed a threefold increased risk of death (hazard rate, 2.9; 95% CI, 1.1–7.6) compared with patients with the heterozygous (SULT1A1*2/SULT1A1*1) genotype or the homozygous SULT1A1*1 genotype. Additionally, in patients not treated with tamoxifen, no association was noted between survival and the SULT1A1 polymorphism.[163]

As the results from current studies do not provide consistent evidence regarding the clinical relevance of the SULT1A1 genotype and its relevance in breast cancer chemotherapeutic treatment, further prospective studies are required to assess the impact of the SULT1A1 genotype on disease outcome and therapeutic outcomes as well as the relevance of other polymorphic enzymes involved in the metabolism of tamoxifen.

Aromatase (CYP19) and Aromatase Inhibitors

Estrogens have an established role in the development of several cancers, including breast carcinogenesis.[164] In postmenopausal women, estrogen is associated with increased breast cancer risk.[165] While estrogen is primarily produced in the ovaries before menopause, most circulating estrogens in postmenopausal women are synthesized from adrenal androgens in adipose tissue, where the final stage of synthesis is catalyzed by the cytochrome P450 hemoprotein-containing enzyme aromatase (CYP19).[166,167] The abnormal expression of this enzyme has been observed in several human cancers, including breast, uterine, testicular, and adrenal tumors.[168–171] Based on these data, the regulation of estrogen synthesis through the inhibition of CYP19 has become a strategy for the prevention or treatment of breast cancer. The first aromatase inhibitor (AI) shown to be beneficial in the treatment of advanced breast cancer was the cytochrome P450 inhibitor aminoglutethimide.[172,173] Unfortunately, this compound lacked specificity, and its unfavorable side-effect profile led to the development of more specific second-generation (e.g., formestane and fadrazole) and third-generation AIs.[174,175] Currently, third-generation clinical agents have more than a 1000-fold increased potency compared with aminoglutethimide[176] and are associated with fewer side effects.[177] They can be classified into two types according to structure. Specifically, exemestane is a steroidal (type I) AI that binds irreversibly to the androgen-binding site of CYP19, while anastrozole, letrozole, and vorozole are nonsteroidal AIs (type II) that bind to the heme moiety of CYP19.[174,178] These agents have increased efficacy over tamoxifen in the treatment of hormone-dependent recurrent or advanced breast cancers[179,180] and are more effective than tamoxifen in adjuvant and neoadjuvant settings as well as breast cancer prevention.[181]

CYP19 Genetic Polymorphisms

Causal genetic variations underlying common complex human diseases such as breast cancer can be studied through haplotype-based genetic association. Such studies are based on dividing the human genome into genomic segments (blocks) that show little evidence of historical recombination and low haplotype diversity.[182] Because of the high degree of linkage disequilibrium observed among SNPs within these blocks, it has been suggested that ancestral disease variants may be identified through evaluation of the underlying haplotypes.[183] Hairman and colleagues (2003) determined that the CYP19 locus contains five blocks of linkage disequilibrium; in addition, one of these blocks covers all of the coding region exons and introns of the CYP19 gene and contains four common haplotypes in the Caucasian population.[183] Importantly, it was shown within this block that the *3'UTR t* allele (rs10046) uniquely tags the most common haplotype.

Clinical Significance

Nine prospective studies have reported that circulating levels of several steroid hormones, including estrogens and androgens, are directly related to the risk of breast cancer in postmenopausal women.[184] Furthermore, the CYP19 *3'UTR t-c* SNP (rs10046) has been shown to be most strongly associated with circulating estradiol levels in postmenopausal women, compared with other investigated SNPs in genes coding for enzymes regulating sex hormones, and the CYP19 *3'UTR t* allele in particular was associated with the highest estradiol levels in this study.[185] Further analysis indicated that homozygotes for the *3'UTR c* allele had significantly smaller mean estradiol-testosterone ratios than homozygotes for the *3'UTR t*[185]; however, CYP19 SNPs only explained a small percentage of the variance in the estradiol-testosterone ratios in these postmenopausal women. Genetic variability in the CYP19 gene may be responsible for only a marginal increase in risk of breast cancer compared with other genetic variants.[185] This conclusion is consistent with the current view that the genetic predisposition to breast cancer is the result of a few high-penetrance genes (e.g., *BRCA1* and *BRCA2*), coupled with multiple as yet unidentified lower penetrance genes.

The presence of a SNP in the 3'UTR of the CYP19 gene may be associated with an improved response to letrozole in the treatment of postmenopausal metastatic breast cancer patients.[186] The significance of these early findings, as well as the possible mechanisms involved, requires further study.

ERCC1, XPD, and XRCC1 in Platinum Chemotherapy

Cisplatin, carboplatin, and oxaliplatin are platinum analogs routinely used in the treatment of non–small cell lung carcinoma and ovarian, breast, gastrointestinal, and testicular cancers.[187] The cytotoxic mechanism of these agents involves the inhibition of DNA replication through the formation of inter- and intrastrand helix-deforming DNA adducts.[188] Enhanced DNA repair is an important mechanism of plat-

inum resistance. The repairosome responsible for nucleotide excision repair (NER) consists of more than 16 gene products, and polymorphisms in particular genes involved in this repair pathway may influence the response to platinum therapy. The relevant genes include the excision repair cross-complementation group 1 gene (*ERCC1*) and the xeroderma pigmentosum group D gene (*XPD*) as well as the x-ray cross-complementing gene (*XRCC1*) involved in the repair of single-strand breaks following base excision repair.[189-192]

ERCC1, XPD and XRCC1 Genetic Polymorphisms and Patterns of Inheritance

Common polymorphisms within the *XPD* gene include the nonsynonymous SNP leading to a single amino acid change from lysine to glutamine at codon 751 of the XPD protein, which is implicated in the response to platinum agents,[193] and the G→A transition at codon 312 leading to an amino acid change from aspartic acid to asparagine.[194] These polymorphisms have a high prevalence in the general population, with allele frequencies of 29% and 42% for the SNP at codon 751 and 312, respectively.[194] Similar associations have been made at codon 118 of *ERCC1* (118C/T), which is located 42 before the start of the helix-turn-helix sites at exon 4. The nonsynonymous SNP localized at this site is characterized by a nucleotide alteration, AAC to AAT, resulting in asparagine, and it has an allele frequency of 46% in the general population. It is associated with diminished *ERCC1* mRNA and protein levels.[194,195] Another common polymorphism in the *ERCC1* gene, C8092A, is located in the 3' untranslated region of the gene, has an allele frequency of 4% in the general population, and may be associated with the risk of adult-onset glioma. The polymorphism affects *ERCC1* mRNA stability.[194,196]

An *XRCC1* gene SNP polymorphism characterized by a G→A transition at codon 399 (Arg399Gln) results in an arginine to glutamine amino acid change, has an allele frequency of 25%, and, like the *XPD* and *ERCC1* polymorphisms, is associated with improved platinum response.[194]

Clinical Significance

Polymorphisms in the *XPD*, *ERCC1*, and *XRCC1* DNA repair genes are related to the therapeutic outcome of platinum-based chemotherapy.[45]

The *Lys751Gln* polymorphism in the *XPD* gene was shown to affect response to fluorouracil/oxaliplatin treatment in a clinical trial with 73 patients diagnosed with metastatic colorectal cancer. Specifically, 24% of patients with the *Lys751/Lys751* genotype responded to this combination treatment but only 10% of patients with the *Lys751/Gln751* genotype and 10% of patients with the *Gln751/Gln751* genotype responded. The median survival for those with the *Lys751/Lys751* genotype was 17.4 months (95% CI, 7.9–26.5), compared with 12.8 months (95% CI, 8.5–25.9) for those with the *Lys751/Gln751* genotype and 3.3 months (95% CI, 1.4–6.5) for patients with the *Gln751/Gln751* genotype.[193] In 31 women with breast cancer, the mechanism for this observed increased response predicted by the *Lys751/Lys751* genotype was shown to be a result of a reduced DNA repair capacity.[197] However, these results were not supported by two subsequent studies that suggested that individuals homozygous for the wild-type allele (*Lys751/Lys751*) had greater repair capacity than patients with at least two of the variant alleles (*Asn312* or *Gln751*).[198,199] Therefore, even though the mechanism for the predictive value of the polymorphism at codon 751 may not be elucidated at present, this genotype may still be useful in the prediction of the therapeutic response to platinum agents.

Variability in the *ERCC1* function has been investigated for its utility in pharmacogenetic approaches aimed at the possible improvement of platinum-based chemotherapeutic response and survival outcomes. High expression of this gene is associated with resistance to platinum-based therapy in human ovarian and gastric tumor specimens.[190,192] In patients with advanced non–small cell lung carcinoma treated with platinum-based chemotherapy, two common *ERCC1* polymorphisms (*118C/T* and *C8092A*) were investigated for their possible association with overall survival.[196] In this study, an increased overall survival time of 22.3 months was noted for patients with the *C8092/C8092* genotype, compared with 13.4 months for those with the *C8092/A8092* or *A8092/A8092* genotypes. These data provide initial evidence suggesting that copies of the *A8092* allele are associated with poor outcome. Interestingly, no significant association was observed between the *118C/T* polymorphism and overall survival; however, further studies with larger sample sizes may be required to assess the influence of this polymorphism.

The *XRCC1* gene involved in DNA repair mechanisms has also been investigated for the potential association between its polymorphic variants and response to platinum analogs. Functionally, patients with genotypes containing the *399Gln* variant allele displayed decreased DNA repair capacity of the *XRCC1* protein compared with individuals homozygous for the wild-type *399Arg* genotype.[200] In 61 advanced colorectal cancer patients treated with 5-FU and oxaliplatin, 18% of the patients responded to treatment, with 66% having stable disease and 16% having progressive disease. Of the responders, the majority of patients (73%) carried the *Arg/Arg* genotype, with 66% of the nonresponders having the *Arg/Gln* or *Gln/Gln* genotypes.[201] These preliminary studies are encouraging; however, the relationship between DNA repair capacity and response to platinum chemotherapy still remains to be defined.

Epidermal Growth Factor Receptor Mutations and Gefitinib

The epidermal growth factor receptor (EGFR, erb-B1) is a member of the tyrosine kinase receptor family and is implicated in tumor growth through several mechanisms, including inhibition of apoptosis, cellular proliferation, and promotion of angiogenesis.[202] The altered expression and deregulation of this receptor led to the rational development of the reversible EGFR inhibitor gefitinib, which is approved as third-line therapy for non–small cell lung carcinoma.[203,204] Results from initial clinical studies indicated tumor response only in a small subset of patients with chemotherapy-refractory advanced non–small cell carcinoma.[205,206] However, the responding subset (~10%) showed a remarkably rapid and significant response.[207] *EGFR* genetic variability was assessed in primary tumors from patients with non–small cell lung cancer who responded to gefitinib, who had no response to gefitinib, and who had not been exposed to gefitinib. Somatic mutations in the tyrosine kinase domain of the *EGFR* gene were observed in eight of the nine patients with gefitinib-responsive cancer. These mutations were absent in patients with no response to gefitinib. Mutated receptors appeared to show increased tyrosine kinase activity in response to EGF and enhanced sensitivity to inhibition by gefitinib compared with wild-type receptors.[208] These findings illustrate the validity of and potential for optimization of targeted therapies through understanding the molecular basis of response.

OTHER GENETIC POLYMORPHISMS OF POTENTIAL IMPORTANCE IN THE RESPONSE TO CHEMOTHERAPY

Over the years a number of additional genes with characterized polymorphisms have been identified and are being evaluated for their potential contribution to variability in response to different chemotherapeutic agents. Among these, the ATP-binding cassette (ABC) transporters have been established as playing a role in the pharmacokinetics of a large number of anticancer agents, including irinotecan, etoposide, and doxorubicin.[209] Preliminary data have also suggested a role for the polymorphic methylenetetrahydrofolate reductase gene (*MTHFR*) in the predisposition to severe myelotoxicity subsequent to treatment of breast cancer patients with methotrexate; however, larger trials are needed to investigate the role of specific polymorphisms in this gene in the response and toxicity of various chemotherapeutic agents.[210] Other polymorphic genes currently considered to influence variability in drug response are various cytochrome P450 enzymes (CYP2D6, CYP2C9, CYP2C19, CYP3A4, CYP3A5, CYP3A7), *N*-acetyltransferases, aldehyde dehydrogenase, O^6-alkyl-guanine alkyl transferase, and NAD(P)H:quinone oxidoreductase.[40,41] A largely ignored area of investigation is the impact of aging on the phenotypes of drug metabolism. It is conceivable that some of the extreme variability in drug tolerance seen in aged cancer patients is related to an accelerated decline in the function of particular allelotypes with age. Despite the known importance of many gene products for pharmacogenetic syndromes associated with drugs from other classes,[34,211,212] limited clinical evidence indicates that polymorphisms of the relevant genes have a significant clinical impact on currently used cancer chemotherapy drugs. To further characterize these genes, as well as future polymorphic genes that may be implicated in the variable response to new and currently used chemotherapeutic agents, prospective clinical trials with the inclusion of phenotypic/genotypic correlative components are essential.

CONCLUSION

Optimum cancer treatment is hindered by the significant interpatient variability in disease outcome and chemotherapeutic efficacy and toxicity. To date, pharmacogenetic studies have mainly involved hypothesis-driven, focused investigations aimed at understanding the genetic basis of this variability through determining the effects of specific polymorphic genes on drug pharmacodynamics and pharmacokinetics and disease outcome. The influence of specific polymorphic genes on drug response is variable, but no single polymorphic change can adequately explain all variations in therapeutic efficacy and safety. With many of these investigations, specific conclusions regarding the clinical relevance of the particular polymorphic gene for drug response require large phase I and II clinical trials, with the assessment of relationships between the specific genotypes and specific clinical outcomes.

Pharmacogenetic and pharmacogenomic approaches may significantly enhance drug efficacy and limit toxicity by leading to an "individualized approach to drug therapy" that theoretically has the potential to allow for the selection of the optimum drug or drug combination and the optimum dosage to maximally benefit a specific population or a specific patient. However, an improved understanding of the genetic basis for interindividual differences in drug response is required. Therapeutic response is a multifaceted entity influenced by the contributions of many genes as well as interactions among genes and the environment. New genomic and proteomic methods have the potential to elucidate mechanisms of variability in drug response and improve cancer diagnosis, predict tumor response to particular drugs, and individualize treatment to increase the efficacy and decrease the toxicity of chemotherapeutic agents.

REFERENCES

1. Zevin S, Benowitz NL. Drug interactions with tobacco smoking: an update. Clin Pharmacokinet 1999;36:425–438.
2. Loebstein R, Yonath H, Peleg D, et al. Interindividual variability in sensitivity to warfarin: nature or nurture? Clin Pharmacol Ther 2001;70:159–164.
3. Kalow W, Tang BK, Endrenyi L. Hypothesis: comparisons of inter- and intra-individual variations can substitute for twin studies in drug research: pharmacogenetics in biological perspective. Pharmacogenetics 1998;8:283–289.
4. Kalow W. Pharmacogenetics in biological perspective. Pharmacol Rev 1997;49:369–379.
5. Flockhart DA, Oesterheld JR. Cytochrome P450-mediated drug interactions. Child Adolesc Psychiatr Clin N Am 2000;9:43–76.
6. Lin KM, Anderson D, Poland RE. Ethnicity and psychopharmacology: bridging the gap. Psychiatr Clin North Am 1995;18:635–647.
7. Alfaro CL, Lam YW, Simpson J, et al. CYP2D6 inhibition by fluoxetine, paroxetine, sertraline, and venlafaxine in a crossover study: intraindividual variability and plasma concentration correlations. J Clin Pharmacol 2000;40:58–66.
8. Ozdemir V, Shear NH, Kalow W. What will be the role of pharmacogenetics in evaluating drug safety and minimising adverse effects? Drug Saf 2001;24:75–85.
9. Alvan G, Bertilsson L, Dahl ML, et al. Moving toward genetic profiling in patient care: the scope and rationale of pharmacogenetic/ecogenetic investigation. Drug Metab Dispos 2001;29(4 Pt 2):580–585.
10. Goldstein DB, Tate SK, Sisodiya SM. Pharmacogenetics goes genomic. Nat Rev Genet 2003;4:937–947.
11. Evans WE. Pharmacogenomics: marshalling the human genome to individualise drug therapy. Gut 2003;52(Suppl 2):10–18.
12. Kalow W. Pharmacogenetics and personalised medicine. Fundam Clin Pharmacol 2002;16:337–342.
13. Vogel FM, Motulsky AG. Human Genetics. Problems and Approaches. Berlin: Springer-Verlag, 1986:498–544.
14. Evans WE, Relling MV. Pharmacogenomics: translating functional genomics into rational therapeutics. Science 1999;286:487–491.
15. Meyer UA, Zanger UM. Molecular mechanisms of genetic polymorphisms of drug metabolism. Annu Rev Pharmacol Toxicol 1997;37:269–296.
16. Evans WE, Johnson JA. Pharmacogenomics: the inherited basis for interindividual differences in drug response. Annu Rev Genomics Hum Genet 2001;2:9–39.
17. Evans WE, McLeod HL. Pharmacogenomics: drug disposition, drug targets, and side effects. N Engl J Med 2003;348:538–549.
18. Weinshilboum R. Inheritance and drug response. N Engl J Med 2003;348:529–537.
19. Weinshilboum R, Wang L. Pharmacogenetics: inherited variation in amino acid sequence and altered protein quantity. Clin Pharmacol Ther 2004;75:253–258.
20. Ulrich CM, Robien K, McLeod HL. Cancer pharmacogenetics: polymorphisms, pathways and beyond. Nat Rev Cancer 2003;3:912–920.
21. Alving AS, Carson PE, Flanagan CL, et al. Enzymatic deficiency in primaquine-sensitive erythrocytes. Science 1956;124:484–485.
22. Hughes HB, Biehl JP, Jones AP, et al. Metabolism of isoniazid in man as related to the occurrence of peripheral neuritis. Am Rev Tuberc 1954;70:266–273.
23. Evans DA, Manley KA, McKusick VA. Genetic control of isoniazid metabolism in man. Br Med J 1960;5197:485–491.
24. Kalow W. Familial incidence of low pseudocholinesterase level. Lancet 1956;ii:576.
25. Motulsky AG. Drug reactions enzymes, and biochemical genetics. J Am Med Assoc 1957;165:835–837.
26. Beutler E. The hemolytic effect of primaquine and related compounds: a review. Blood 1959;14:103–139.
27. McLeod HL, Evans WE. Pharmacogenomics: unlocking the human genome for better drug therapy. Annu Rev Pharmacol Toxicol 2001;41:101–121.
28. Roses AD. Pharmacogenetics. Hum Mol Genet 2001;10:2261–2267.
29. Gonzalez FJ, Skoda RC, Kimura S, et al. Characterization of the common genetic defect in humans deficient in debrisoquine metabolism. Nature 1988;331:442–446.
30. Ingelman-Sundberg M, Oscarson M, McLellan RA. Polymorphic human cytochrome P450 enzymes: an opportunity for individualized drug treatment. Trends Pharmacol Sci 1999;20:342–349.
31. Marshall E. Preventing toxicity with a gene test. Science 2003;302:588–590.
32. Innocenti F, Stadler WM, Iyer L, et al. Flavopiridol metabolism in cancer patients is associated with the occurrence of diarrhea. Clin Cancer Res 2000;6:3400–3405.

33. Heggie GD, Sommadossi JP, Cross DS, et al. Clinical pharmacokinetics of 5-fluorouracil and its metabolites in plasma, urine, and bile. Cancer Res 1987;47:2203–2206.

34. Kalow W. Pharmacoanthropology and the genetics of drug metabolism. In: Kalow W, ed. Pharmacogenetics of Drug Metabolism. New York: Pergamon Press, 1992;865–877

35. Sasvari-Szekely M, Gerstner A, Ronai Z, et al. Rapid genotyping of factor V Leiden mutation using single-tube bidirectional allele-specific amplification and automated ultrathin-layer agarose gel electrophoresis. Electrophoresis 2000;21:816–821.

36. Lu Z, Diasio RB. Polymorphic drug-metabolizing enzymes. In: Schilsky RL, Milano GA, Ratain MJ, eds. Principles of Antineoplastic Drug Development and Pharmacology. New York: Dekker, 1996: 281–385.

37. Relling MV, Dervieux T. Pharmacogenetics and cancer therapy. Nat Rev Cancer 2001;1:99–108.

38. Chang TK, Yu L, Goldstein JA, et al. Identification of the polymorphically expressed CYP2C19 and the wild-type CYP2C9-ILE359 allele as low-Km catalysts of cyclophosphamide and ifosfamide activation. Pharmacogenetics 1997;7:211–221.

39. Williams ML, Bhargava P, Cherrouk I, et al. A discordance of the cytochrome P450 2C19 genotype and phenotype in patients with advanced cancer. Br J Clin Pharmacol 2000;49:485–488.

40. Boddy AV, Ratain MJ. Pharmacogenetics in cancer etiology and chemotherapy. Clin Cancer Res 1997;3:1025–1030.

41. Iyer L, Ratain MJ. Pharmacogenetics and cancer chemotherapy. Eur J Cancer 1998;34:1493–1499.

42. Krynetski EY, Evans WE. Pharmacogenetics of cancer therapy: getting personal. Am J Hum Genet 1998;63:11–16.

43. Iyer L. Inherited variations in drug-metabolizing enzymes: significance in clinical oncology. Mol Diagn 1999;4:327–333.

44. Desai AA, Innocenti F, Ratain MJ. Pharmacogenomics: road to anticancer therapeutics nirvana? Oncogene 2003;22:6621–6628.

45. Watters JW, McLeod HL. Cancer pharmacogenomics: current and future applications. Biochim Biophys Acta 2003;1603:99–111.

46. Innocenti F, Ratain MJ. Update on pharmacogenetics in cancer chemotherapy. Eur J Cancer 2002;38:639–644.

47. McLeod HL, Krynetski EY, Relling MV, et al. Genetic polymorphism of thiopurine methyltransferase and its clinical relevance for childhood acute lymphoblastic leukemia. Leukemia 2000; 14:567–572.

48. Vogt MH, Stet EH, De Abreu RA, et al. The importance of methylthio-IMP for methylmercaptopurine ribonucleoside (Me-MPR) cytotoxicity in Molt F4 human malignant T-lymphoblasts. Biochim Biophys Acta 1993;1181:189–194.

49. Lee D, Szumlanski C, Houtman J, et al. Thiopurine methyltransferase pharmacogenetics: cloning of human liver cDNA and a processed pseudogene on human chromosome 18q21.1. Drug Metab Dispos 1995;23:398–405.

50. Szumlanski C, Otterness D, Her C, et al. Thiopurine methyltransferase pharmacogenetics: human gene cloning and characterization of a common polymorphism. DNA Cell Biol 1996; 15:17–30.

51. Yates CR, Krynetski EY, Loennechen T, et al. Molecular diagnosis of thiopurine S-methyltransferase deficiency: genetic basis for azathioprine and mercaptopurine intolerance. Ann Intern Med 1997;126:608–614.

52. Otterness D, Szumlanski C, Lennard L, et al. Human thiopurine methyltransferase pharmacogenetics: gene sequence polymorphisms. Clin Pharmacol Ther 1997;62:60–73.

53. Krynetski EY, Schuetz JD, Galpin AJ, et al. A single point mutation leading to loss of catalytic activity in human thiopurine S-methyltransferase. Proc Natl Acad Sci USA 1995;92:949–953.

54. Tai HL, Krynetski EY, Yates CR, et al. Thiopurine S-methyltransferase deficiency: two nucleotide transitions define the most prevalent mutant allele associated with loss of catalytic activity in Caucasians. Am J Hum Genet 1996;58:694–702.

55. Tai HL, Krynetski EY, Schuetz EG, et al. Enhanced proteolysis of thiopurine S-methyltransferase (TPMT) encoded by mutant alleles in humans (TPMT*3A, TPMT*2): mechanisms for the genetic polymorphism of TPMT activity. Proc Natl Acad Sci USA 1997;94:6444–6449.

56. Tai HL, Fessing MY, Bonten EJ, et al. Enhanced proteasomal degradation of mutant human thiopurine S-methyltransferase (TPMT) in mammalian cells: mechanism for TPMT protein deficiency inherited by TPMT*2, TPMT*3A, TPMT*3B or TPMT*3C. Pharmacogenetics 1999;9:641–650.

57. Weinshilboum RM, Sladek SL. Mercaptopurine pharmacogenetics: monogenic inheritance of erythrocyte thiopurine methyltransferase activity. Am J Hum Genet 1980;32:651–662.

58. Ameyaw MM, Collie-Duguid ES, Powrie RH, et al. Thiopurine methyltransferase alleles in British and Ghanaian populations. Hum Mol Genet 1999;8:367–370.

59. Kubota T, Chiba K. Frequencies of thiopurine S-methyltransferase mutant alleles (TPMT*2, *3A, *3B and *3C) in 151 healthy Japanese subjects and the inheritance of TPMT*3C in the family of a propositus. Br J Clin Pharmacol 2001;51:475–477.

60. Lennard L, Lilleyman JS. Individualizing therapy with 6-mercaptopurine and 6-thioguanine related to the thiopurine methyltransferase genetic polymorphism. Ther Drug Monit 1996;18: 328–334.

61. Lennard L, Keen D, Lilleyman JS. Oral 6-mercaptopurine in childhood leukemia: parent drug pharmacokinetics and active metabolite concentrations. Clin Pharmacol Ther 1986;40:287–292.

62. Evans WE, Hon YY, Bomgaars L, et al. Preponderance of thiopurine S-methyltransferase deficiency and heterozygosity among patients intolerant to mercaptopurine or azathioprine. J Clin Oncol 2001;19:2293–2301.

63. Relling MV, Hancock ML, Boyett JM, et al. Prognostic importance of 6-mercaptopurine dose intensity in acute lymphoblastic leukemia. Blood 1999;93:2817–2823.

64. Relling MV, Hancock ML, Rivera GK, et al. Mercaptopurine therapy intolerance and heterozygosity at the thiopurine S-methyltransferase gene locus. J Natl Cancer Inst 1999;91:2001–2008.

65. Milano G, Etienne MC. Fluorinated pyrimidines. In: Grochow L, Ames M, eds. A Clinician's Guide to Chemotherapy, Pharmacokinetics and Pharmacodynamics. Baltimore: Williams and Wilkins, 1998:289–300.

66. Allegra CJ, Grem JL. Antimetabolites. In: Devita VT, Rosenberg SA, eds. Cancer Principles and Practice of Oncology. Philadelphia: Lippincott-Raven, 1997:432–451.

67. Nishida M. Pharmacological and clinical properties of Xeloda (capecitabine), a new oral active derivative of fluoropyrimidine. Nippon Yakurigaku Zasshi, 2003;122:549–553.

68. Andre T, Louvet C, de Gramont A. Colon cancer: what is new in 2004? Bull Cancer 2004;91(1):75–80.

69. Argiris A, Haraf DJ, Kies MS, et al. Intensive concurrent chemoradiotherapy for head and neck cancer with 5-fluorouracil- and hydroxyurea-based regimens: reversing a pattern of failure. Oncologist 2003;8:350–360.

70. Diasio RB, Harris BE. Clinical pharmacology of 5-fluorouracil. Clin Pharmacokinet 1989;16:215–237.

71. Meropol NJ. Oral fluoropyrimidines in the treatment of colorectal cancer. Eur J Cancer 1998;34:1509–1513.

72. Daher GC, Harris BE, Diasio RB. Metabolism of pyrimidine analogues and their nucleosides. Pharmacol Ther 1990;48:189–222.

73. Wei X, McLeod HL, McMurrough J, et al. Molecular basis of the human dihydropyrimidine dehydrogenase deficiency and 5-fluorouracil toxicity. J Clin Invest 1996;98:610–615.

74. van Kuilenburg AB, Muller EW, Haasjes J, et al. Lethal outcome of a patient with a complete dihydropyrimidine dehydrogenase (DPD) deficiency after administration of 5-fluorouracil: frequency of the common IVS14+1G>A mutation causing DPD deficiency. Clin Cancer Res 2001;7:1149–1153.

75. Diasio RB. Clinical implications of dihydropyrimidine dehydrogenase on 5-FU pharmacology. Oncology (Huntingt) 2001;15 (1 Suppl 2):21–26; discussion 27.

76. Diasio RB, Beavers TL, Carpenter JT. Familial deficiency of dihydropyrimidine dehydrogenase: biochemical basis for familial pyrimidinemia and severe 5-fluorouracil-induced toxicity. J Clin Invest 1988;81:47–51.

77. Lu Z, Zhang R, Carpenter JT, et al. Decreased dihydropyrimidine dehydrogenase activity in a population of patients with breast cancer: implication for 5-fluorouracil-based chemotherapy. Clin Cancer Res 1998;4:325–329.

78. Etienne MC, Lagrange JL, Dassonville O, et al. Population study of dihydropyrimidine dehydrogenase in cancer patients. J Clin Oncol 1994;12:2248–2253.

79. Lu Z, Zhang R, Diasio RB. Dihydropyrimidine dehydrogenase activity in human peripheral blood mononuclear cells and liver: population characteristics, newly identified deficient patients, and clinical implication in 5-fluorouracil chemotherapy. Cancer Res 1993;53:5433–5438.

80. van Kuilenburg AB. Dihydropyrimidine dehydrogenase and the efficacy and toxicity of 5-fluorouracil. Eur J Cancer 2004;40: 939–950.

81. Johnson MR, Hageboutros A, Wang K, et al. Life-threatening toxicity in a dihydropyrimidine dehydrogenase-deficient patient after treatment with topical 5-fluorouracil. Clin Cancer Res 1999;5:2006–2011.

82. Johnson MR, Wang K, Diasio RB. Profound dihydropyrimidine dehydrogenase deficiency resulting from a novel compound heterozygote genotype. Clin Cancer Res 2002;8:768–774.

83. Collie-Duguid ES, Etienne MC, Milano G, et al. Known variant DPYD alleles do not explain DPD deficiency in cancer patients. Pharmacogenetics 2000;10:217–223.

84. Ezzeldin H, Johnson MR, Okamoto Y, et al. Denaturing high performance liquid chromatography analysis of the DPYD gene in patients with lethal 5-fluorouracil toxicity. Clin Cancer Res 2003;9:3021–3028.

85. Fernandez-Salguero PM, Sapone A, Wei X, et al. Lack of correlation between phenotype and genotype for the polymorphically expressed dihydropyrimidine dehydrogenase in a family of Pakistani origin. Pharmacogenetics 1997;7:161–163.

86. Vreken P, Van Kuilenburg AB, Meinsma R, et al. Dihydropyrimidine dehydrogenase (DPD) deficiency: identification and expression of missense mutations C29R, R886H and R235W. Hum Genet 1997;101:333–338.

87. Fernandez-Salguero P, Gonzalez FJ, Etienne MC, et al. Correlation between catalytic activity and protein content for the polymorphically expressed dihydropyrimidine dehydrogenase in human lymphocytes. Biochem Pharmacol 1995;50:1015–1020.

88. Johnson MR, Yan J, Shao L, et al. Semi-automated radioassay for determination of dihydropyrimidine dehydrogenase (DPD) activity: screening cancer patients for DPD deficiency, a condition associated with 5-fluorouracil toxicity. J Chromatogr B Biomed Sci Appl 1997;696:183–191.

89. Ezzeldin H, Okamoto Y, Johnson MR, et al. A high-throughput denaturing high-performance liquid chromatography method for the identification of variant alleles associated with dihydropyrimidine dehydrogenase deficiency. Anal Biochem 2002; 306:63–73.

90. Kuhara T, Ohdoi C, Ohse M, et al. Rapid gas chromatographic-mass spectrometric diagnosis of dihydropyrimidine dehydrogenase deficiency and dihydropyrimidinase deficiency. J Chromatogr B Analyt Technol Biomed Life Sci 2003;792:107–115.

91. Mattison LK, Ezzeldin H, Carpenter M, et al. Rapid identification of dihydropyrimidine dehydrogenase deficiency by using a novel 2-13C-uracil breath test. Clin Cancer Res 2004;10:2652–2658.

92. Milano G, Fischel JL, Etienne MC, et al. Inhibition of dihydropyrimidine dehydrogenase by alpha-interferon: experimental data on human tumor cell lines. Cancer Chemother Pharmacol 1994;34:147–152.

93. Yan J, Tyring SK, McCrary MM, et al. The effect of sorivudine on dihydropyrimidine dehydrogenase activity in patients with acute herpes zoster. Clin Pharmacol Ther 1997;61:563–573.

94. Maring JG, van Kuilenburg AB, Haasjes J, et al. Reduced 5-FU clearance in a patient with low DPD activity due to heterozygosity for a mutant allele of the DPYD gene. Br J Cancer 2002; 86:1028–1033.

95. Harris BE, Song R, Soong SJ, et al. Relationship between dihydropyrimidine dehydrogenase activity and plasma 5-fluorouracil levels with evidence for circadian variation of enzyme activity and plasma drug levels in cancer patients receiving 5-fluorouracil by protracted continuous infusion. Cancer Res 1990;50:197–201.

96. Leichman CG, Lenz HJ, Leichman L, et al. Quantitation of intratumoral thymidylate synthase expression predicts for disseminated colorectal cancer response and resistance to protracted-infusion fluorouracil and weekly leucovorin. J Clin Oncol 1997;15:3223–3229.

97. Salonga D, Danenberg KD, Johnson M, et al. Colorectal tumors responding to 5-fluorouracil have low gene expression levels of

98. dihydropyrimidine dehydrogenase, thymidylate synthase, and thymidine phosphorylase. Clin Cancer Res 2000;6:1322–1327.

98. Grem JL. 5-Fluoropyrimidines. In: Chabner BA, Longo DL, eds. Cancer Chemotherapy and Biotherapy. 2nd ed. Philadelphia: WB Saunders, 1996:149–212.

99. Toxicity of fluorouracil in patients with advanced colorectal cancer: effect of administration schedule and prognostic factors. Meta-Analysis Group in Cancer. J Clin Oncol 1998;16:3537–3541.

100. Van Kuilenburg AB, Meinsma R, Zoetekouw L, et al. Increased risk of grade IV neutropenia after administration of 5-fluorouracil due to a dihydropyrimidine dehydrogenase deficiency: high prevalence of the IVS14+1g>a mutation. Int J Cancer 2002; 101:253–258.

101. Johnson MR, Diasio RB. Importance of dihydropyrimidine dehydrogenase (DPD) deficiency in patients exhibiting toxicity following treatment with 5-fluorouracil. Adv Enzyme Regul 2001;41:151–157.

102. Rothenberg ML, Kuhn JG, Burris HA 3rd, et al. Phase I and pharmacokinetic trial of weekly CPT-11. J Clin Oncol 1993;11: 2194–2204.

103. Gupta E, Lestingi TM, Mick R, et al. Metabolic fate of irinotecan in humans: correlation of glucuronidation with diarrhea. Cancer Res 1994;54:3723–3725.

104. Santos A, Zanetta S, Cresteil T, et al. Metabolism of irinotecan (CPT-11) by CYP3A4 and CYP3A5 in humans. Clin Cancer Res 2000;6:2012–2020.

105. Iyer L, Das S, Janisch L, et al. UGT1A1*28 polymorphism as a determinant of irinotecan disposition and toxicity. Pharmacogenomics J 2002;2(1):43–47.

106. Burchell B, Hume R. Molecular genetic basis of Gilbert's syndrome. J Gastroenterol Hepatol 1999;14:960–966.

107. Tukey RH, Strassburg CP. Human UDP-glucuronosyltransferases: metabolism, expression, and disease. Annu Rev Pharmacol Toxicol 2000;40:581–616.

108. Sampietro M, Iolascon A. Molecular pathology of Crigler-Najjar type I and II and Gilbert's syndromes. Haematologica 1999;84: 150–157.

109. Bosma PJ, Chowdhury JR, Bakker C, et al. The genetic basis of the reduced expression of bilirubin UDP-glucuronosyltransferase 1 in Gilbert's syndrome. N Engl J Med 1995;333:1171–1175.

110. Monaghan G, Ryan M, Seddon R, et al. Genetic variation in bilirubin UPD-glucuronosyltransferase gene promoter and Gilbert's syndrome. Lancet 1996;347:578–581.

111. Beutler E, Gelbart T, Demina A. Racial variability in the UDP-glucuronosyltransferase 1 (UGT1A1) promoter: a balanced polymorphism for regulation of bilirubin metabolism? Proc Natl Acad Sci USA 1998;95:8170–8174.

112. Ando Y, Saka H, Ando M, et al. Polymorphisms of UDP-glucuronosyltransferase gene and irinotecan toxicity: a pharmacogenetic analysis. Cancer Res 2000;60:6921–6926.

113. Monaghan G, Foster B, Jurima-Romet M, et al. UGT1*1 genotyping in a Canadian Inuit population. Pharmacogenetics 1997;7: 153–156.

114. Sato H, Adachi Y, Koiwai O. The genetic basis of Gilbert's syndrome. Lancet 1996;347:557–558.

115. Akaba K, Kimura T, Sasaki A, et al. Neonatal hyperbilirubinemia and mutation of the bilirubin uridine diphosphate-glucuronosyltransferase gene: a common missense mutation among Japanese, Koreans and Chinese. Biochem Mol Biol Int 1998;46: 21–26.

116. Araki E, Ishikawa M, Iigo M, et al. Relationship between development of diarrhea and the concentration of SN-38, an active metabolite of CPT-11, in the intestine and the blood plasma of athymic mice following intraperitoneal administration of CPT-11. Jpn J Cancer Res 1993;84:697–702.

117. Coles BF, Kadlubar FF. Detoxification of electrophilic compounds by glutathione S-transferase catalysis: determinants of individual response to chemical carcinogens and chemotherapeutic drugs? Biofactors 2003;17:115–130.

118. Townsend D, Tew K. Cancer drugs, genetic variation and the glutathione-S-transferase gene family. Am J Pharmacogenomics 2003;3:157–172.

119. Hayes JD, Pulford DJ. The glutathione S-transferase supergene family: regulation of GST and the contribution of the isoenzymes

to cancer chemoprotection and drug resistance. Crit Rev Biochem Mol Biol 1995;30:445–600.

120. Hayes JD, Strange RC. Glutathione S-transferase polymorphisms and their biological consequences. Pharmacology 2000;61: 154–166.

121. Landi S. Mammalian class theta GST and differential susceptibility to carcinogens: a review. Mutat Res 2000;463:247–283.

122. Rebbeck TR. Molecular epidemiology of the human glutathione S-transferase genotypes GSTM1 and GSTT1 in cancer susceptibility. Cancer Epidemiol Biomarkers Prev 1997;6:733–743.

123. McLellan RA, Oscarson M, Alexandrie AK, et al. Characterization of a human glutathione S-transferase mu cluster containing a duplicated GSTM1 gene that causes ultrarapid enzyme activity. Mol Pharmacol 1997;52:958–965.

124. Nelson HH, Wiencke JK, Christiani DC, et al. Ethnic differences in the prevalence of the homozygous deleted genotype of glutathione S-transferase theta. Carcinogenesis 1995;16: 1243–1245.

125. Lee KA, Kim SH, Woo HY, et al. Increased frequencies of glutathione S-transferase (GSTM1 and GSTT1) gene deletions in Korean patients with acquired aplastic anemia. Blood 2001; 98:3483–3485.

126. Lohmueller KE, Pearce CL, Pike M, et al. Meta-analysis of genetic association studies supports a contribution of common variants to susceptibility to common disease. Nat Genet 2003;33:177–182.

127. Howells RE, Redman CW, Dhar KK, et al. Association of glutathione S-transferase GSTM1 and GSTT1 null genotypes with clinical outcome in epithelial ovarian cancer. Clin Cancer Res 1998;4:2439–2445.

128. Ambrosone CB, Sweeney C, Coles BF, et al. Polymorphisms in glutathione S-transferases (GSTM1 and GSTT1) and survival after treatment for breast cancer. Cancer Res 2001;61:7130–7135.

129. Stanulla M, Schrappe M, Brechlin AM, et al. Polymorphisms within glutathione S-transferase genes (GSTM1, GSTT1, GSTP1) and risk of relapse in childhood B-cell precursor acute lymphoblastic leukemia: a case-control study. Blood 2000;95:1222–1228.

130. Chen CL, Liu Q, Pui CH, et al. Higher frequency of glutathione S-transferase deletions in black children with acute lymphoblastic leukemia. Blood 1997;89:1701–1707.

131. Chu E, Ju J, Schmitz J. Antifolate drugs in cancer therapy. In: Jackman A, ed. Anticancer Drug Development Guide. Totowa, NJ: Humana Press, 1999:397–408.

132. Chu E, Koeller DM, Casey JL, et al. Autoregulation of human thymidylate synthase messenger RNA translation by thymidylate synthase. Proc Natl Acad Sci USA 1991;88:8977–8981.

133. Dolnick BJ. Thymidylate synthase and the cell cycle: what should we believe? Cancer J 2000;6:215–216.

134. Marsh S, McLeod HL. Thymidylate synthase pharmacogenetics in colorectal cancer. Clin Colorectal Cancer 2001;1:175–178; discussion 179–181.

135. Pullarkat ST, Stoehlmacher J, Ghaderi V, et al. Thymidylate synthase gene polymorphism determines response and toxicity of 5-FU chemotherapy. Pharmacogenomics J 2001;1:65–70.

136. Kawakami K, Omura K, Kanehira E, et al. Polymorphic tandem repeats in the thymidylate synthase gene is associated with its protein expression in human gastrointestinal cancers. Anticancer Res 1999;19(4B):3249–3252.

137. Villafranca E, Okruzhnov Y, Dominguez MA, et al. Polymorphisms of the repeated sequences in the enhancer region of the thymidylate synthase gene promoter may predict downstaging after preoperative chemoradiation in rectal cancer. J Clin Oncol 2001; 19:1779–1786.

138. Marsh S, McKay JA, Cassidy J, et al. Polymorphism in the thymidylate synthase promoter enhancer region in colorectal cancer. Int J Oncol 2001;19:383–386.

139. Mandola MV, Stoehlmacher J, Muller-Weeks S, et al. A novel single nucleotide polymorphism within the 5′ tandem repeat polymorphism of the thymidylate synthase gene abolishes USF-1 binding and alters transcriptional activity. Cancer Res 2003;63: 2898–2904.

140. Ulrich CM, Bigler J, Velicer CM, et al. Searching expressed sequence tag databases: discovery and confirmation of a common polymorphism in the thymidylate synthase gene. Cancer Epidemiol Biomarkers Prev 2000;9:1381–1385.

141. Marsh S, Ameyaw MM, Githang'a J, et al. Novel thymidylate synthase enhancer region alleles in African populations. Hum Mutat 2000;16:528.

142. Mandola MV, Stoehlmacher J, Zhang W, et al. A 6 bp polymorphism in the thymidylate synthase gene causes message instability and is associated with decreased intratumoral TS mRNA levels. Pharmacogenetics 2004;14:319–327.

143. Lenz H.-J, Zang W, Zahedy S, et al. A 6 basepair deletion in the 3 UTR of the thymidylate synthase(TS) gene predicts TS mRNA expression in colorectal tumors: a possible candidate gene for colorectal cancer risk. Proc Am Assoc Cancer Res 2002;43:660.

144. Johnston PG, Fisher ER, Rockette HE, et al. The role of thymidylate synthase expression in prognosis and outcome of adjuvant chemotherapy in patients with rectal cancer. J Clin Oncol 1994;12:2640–2647.

145. Pestalozzi BC, McGinn CJ, Kinsella TJ, et al. Increased thymidylate synthase protein levels are principally associated with proliferation but not cell cycle phase in asynchronous human cancer cells. Br J Cancer 1995;71:1151–1157.

146. Lenz HJ, Leichman CG, Danenberg KD, et al. Thymidylate synthase mRNA level in adenocarcinoma of the stomach: a predictor for primary tumor response and overall survival. J Clin Oncol 1996;14:176–182.

147. Kornmann M, Link KH, Lenz HJ, et al. Thymidylate synthase is a predictor for response and resistance in hepatic artery infusion chemotherapy. Cancer Lett 1997;118(1):29–35.

148. Aschele C, Debernardis D, Casazza S, et al. Immunohistochemical quantitation of thymidylate synthase expression in colorectal cancer metastases predicts for clinical outcome to fluorouracil-based chemotherapy. J Clin Oncol 1999;17:1760–1770.

149. Stoehlmacher I, Mandola MV, Yun J, et al. Alterations of the thymidylate synthase (TS) pathway and colorectal cancer risk: the impact of three TS polymorphisms. Proc Am Assoc Cancer Res 2003;44:597.

150. McLeod HL, Sargent DJ, Marsh S, et al. Pharmacogenetic analysis of systemic toxicity and response after 5-fluorouracil (5FU)/CPT-11, 5FU/oxaliplatin (oral), or CPT-11/oxal therapy for advanced colorectal cancer. Proc Am Assoc Clin Oncol 2003;22:252.

151. Fisher B, Costantino JP, Wickerham DL, et al. Tamoxifen for prevention of breast cancer: report of the National Surgical Adjuvant Breast and Bowel Project P-1 study. J Natl Cancer Inst 1998;90: 1371–1388.

152. Fabian C, Tilzer L, Sternson L. Comparative binding affinities of tamoxifen, 4-hydroxytamoxifen, and desmethyltamoxifen for estrogen receptors isolated from human breast carcinoma: correlation with blood levels in patients with metastatic breast cancer. Biopharm Drug Dispos 1981;2:381–390.

153. Johnson MD, Zuo H, Lee KH, et al. Pharmacological characterization of 4-hydroxy-N-desmethyl tamoxifen, a novel active metabolite of tamoxifen. Breast Cancer Res Treat 2004;85:151–159.

154. Stearns V, Johnson MD, Rae JM, et al. Active tamoxifen metabolite plasma concentrations after coadministration of tamoxifen and the selective serotonin reuptake inhibitor paroxetine. J Natl Cancer Inst 2003;95:1758–1764.

155. Nishiyama T, Ogura K, Nakano H, et al. Reverse geometrical selectivity in glucuronidation and sulfation of cis- and trans-4-hydroxytamoxifens by human liver UDP-glucuronosyltransferases and sulfotransferases. Biochem Pharmacol 2002;63:1817–1830.

156. Seth P, Lunetta KL, Bell DW, et al. Phenol sulfotransferases: hormonal regulation, polymorphism, and age of onset of breast cancer. Cancer Res 2000;60:6859–6863.

157. Zhu X, Veronese ME, Bernard CC, et al. Identification of two human brain aryl sulfotransferase cDNAs. Biochem Biophys Res Commun 1993;195:120–127.

158. Jones AL, Hagen M, Coughtrie MW, et al. Human platelet phenol-sulfotransferases: cDNA cloning, stable expression in V79 cells and identification of a novel allelic variant of the phenol-sulfating form. Biochem Biophys Res Commun 1995;208:855–862.

159. Raftogianis RB, Wood TC, Otterness DM, et al. Phenol sulfotransferase pharmacogenetics in humans: association of common SULT1A1 alleles with TS PST phenotype. Biochem Biophys Res Commun 1997;239:298–304.

160. Coughtrie MW, Gilissen RA, Shek B, et al. Phenol sulphotransferase SULT1A1 polymorphism: molecular diagnosis and allele

frequencies in Caucasian and African populations. Biochem J 1999;337(Pt 1):45–49.

161. MacCallum J, Cummings J, Dixon JM, et al. Concentrations of tamoxifen and its major metabolites in hormone responsive and resistant breast tumours. Br J Cancer 2000;82:1629–1635.

162. Zheng W, Xie D, Cerhan JR, et al. Sulfotransferase 1A1 polymorphism, endogenous estrogen exposure, well-done meat intake, and breast cancer risk. Cancer Epidemiol Biomarkers Prev 2001;10:89–94.

163. Nowell S, Sweeney C, Winters M, et al. Association between sulfotransferase 1A1 genotype and survival of breast cancer patients receiving tamoxifen therapy. J Natl Cancer Inst 2002;94: 1635–1640.

164. Henderson BE, Ross RK, Pike MC, et al. Endogenous hormones as a major factor in human cancer. Cancer Res 1982;42:3232–3239.

165. Endogenous sex hormones and breast cancer in postmenopausal women: reanalysis of nine prospective studies. J Natl Cancer Inst 2002;94:606–616.

166. Miller WR, Hawkins RA, Forrest AP. Significance of aromatase activity in human breast cancer. Cancer Res 1982;42(Suppl 8): 3365s–3368s.

167. Steinkampf MP, Mendelson CR, Simpson ER. Regulation by follicle-stimulating hormone of the synthesis of aromatase cytochrome P-450 in human granulosa cells. Mol Endocrinol 1987;1: 465–471.

168. Phornphutkul C, Okubo T, Wu K, et al. Aromatase p450 expression in a feminizing adrenal adenoma presenting as isosexual precocious puberty. J Clin Endocrinol Metab 2001;86:649–652.

169. Sumitani H, Shozu M, Segawa T, et al. In situ estrogen synthesized by aromatase P450 in uterine leiomyoma cells promotes cell growth probably via an autocrine/intracrine mechanism. Endocrinology 2000;141:3852–3861.

170. Inkster S, Yue W, Brodie A. Human testicular aromatase: immunocytochemical and biochemical studies. J Clin Endocrinol Metab 1995;80:1941–1947.

171. Esteban JM, Warsi Z, Haniu M, et al. Detection of intratumoral aromatase in breast carcinomas: an immunohistochemical study with clinicopathologic correlation. Am J Pathol 1992;140: 337–343.

172. Thompson EA Jr, Siiteri PK. Utilization of oxygen and reduced nicotinamide adenine dinucleotide phosphate by human placental microsomes during aromatization of androstenedione. J Biol Chem 1974;249:5364–5372.

173. Santen RJ, Santner S, Davis B, et al. Aminoglutethimide inhibits extraglandular estrogen production in postmenopausal women with breast carcinoma. J Clin Endocrinol Metab 1978;47: 1257–1265.

174. Karaer O, Oruc S, Koyuncu FM. Aromatase inhibitors: possible future applications. Acta Obstet Gynecol Scand 2004;83:699–706.

175. Mokbel K. The evolving role of aromatase inhibitors in breast cancer. Int J Clin Oncol 2002;7:279–283.

176. Yue W, Mor G, Naftolin F, et al. Aromatase inhibitors in breast cancer. In: Robertson JFR, Nicholson RI, Hayes DF, eds. Endocrine Therapy of Breast Cancer. London: Martin Dunitz, 2002: 75–106.

177. Santen RJ. Inhibition of aromatase: insights from recent studies. Steroids 2003;68:559–567.

178. Brodie AM, Njar VC. Aromatase inhibitors and breast cancer. Semin Oncol 1996;23(4 Suppl 9):10–20.

179. Bonneterre J, Buzdar A, Nabholtz JM, et al. Anastrozole is superior to tamoxifen as first-line therapy in hormone receptor positive advanced breast carcinoma. Cancer 2001;92:2247–2258.

180. Mouridsen H, Gershanovich M, Sun Y, et al. Superior efficacy of letrozole versus tamoxifen as first-line therapy for postmenopausal women with advanced breast cancer: results of a phase III study of the International Letrozole Breast Cancer Group. J Clin Oncol 2001;19:2596–2606.

181. Ellis MJ, Coop A, Singh B, et al. Letrozole is more effective neoadjuvant endocrine therapy than tamoxifen for ErbB-1-and/or ErbB-2-positive, estrogen receptor-positive primary breast cancer: evidence from a phase III randomized trial. J Clin Oncol 2001;19:3808–3816.

182. Gabriel SB, Schaffner SF, Nguyen H, et al. The structure of haplotype blocks in the human genome. Science 2002;296:2225–2229.

183. Haiman CA, Stram DO, Pike MC, et al. A comprehensive haplotype analysis of CYP19 and breast cancer risk: the Multiethnic Cohort. Hum Mol Genet 2003;12:2679–2692.

184. Hankinson SE, Willett WC, Manson JE, et al. Plasma sex steroid hormone levels and risk of breast cancer in postmenopausal women. J Natl Cancer Inst 1998;90:1292–1299.

185. Dunning AM, Dowsett M, Healey CS, et al. Polymorphisms associated with circulating sex hormone levels in postmenopausal women. J Natl Cancer Inst 2004;96:936–945.

186. Lloveras B, Monzo M, Colomer R, et al. Letrozole efficacy is related to human aromatase CYP19 single nucleotide polymorphisms (SNPs) in metastatic breast cancer patients. Journal of Clinical Oncology 2004;22:507.

187. Goetz MP, Ames MM, Weinshilboum RM. Primer on medical genomics, Part XII: pharmacogenomics: general principles with cancer as a model. Mayo Clin Proc 2004;79:376–384.

188. Jamieson ER, Lippard SJ. Structure, recognition, and processing of cisplatin-DNA adducts. Chem Rev 1999;99:2467–2498.

189. Furuta T, Ueda T, Aune G, et al. Transcription-coupled nucleotide excision repair as a determinant of cisplatin sensitivity of human cells. Cancer Res 2002;62:4899–4902.

190. Dabholkar M, Vionnet J, Bostick-Bruton F, et al. Messenger RNA levels of XPAC and ERCC1 in ovarian cancer tissue correlate with response to platinum-based chemotherapy. J Clin Invest 1994; 94:703–708.

191. Li Q, Yu JJ, Mu C, et al. Association between the level of ERCC-1 expression and the repair of cisplatin-induced DNA damage in human ovarian cancer cells. Anticancer Res 2000;20(2A):645–652.

192. Metzger R, Leichman CG, Danenberg KD, et al. ERCC1 mRNA levels complement thymidylate synthase mRNA levels in predicting response and survival for gastric cancer patients receiving combination cisplatin and fluorouracil chemotherapy. J Clin Oncol 1998;16:309–316.

193. Park DJ, Stoehlmacher J, Zhang W, et al. A xeroderma pigmentosum group D gene polymorphism predicts clinical outcome to platinum-based chemotherapy in patients with advanced colorectal cancer. Cancer Res 2001;61:8654–8658.

194. Shen MR, Jones IM, Mohrenweiser H. Nonconservative amino acid substitution variants exist at polymorphic frequency in DNA repair genes in healthy humans. Cancer Res 1998;58: 604–608.

195. Yu JJ, Mu C, Lee KB, et al. A nucleotide polymorphism in ERCC1 in human ovarian cancer cell lines and tumor tissues. Mutat Res 1997;382:13–20.

196. Zhou W, Gurubhagavatula S, Liu G, et al. Excision repair cross-complementation group 1 polymorphism predicts overall survival in advanced non-small cell lung cancer patients treated with platinum-based chemotherapy. Clin Cancer Res 2004;10: 4939–4943.

197. Lunn RM, Helzlsouer KJ, Parshad R, et al. XPD polymorphisms: effects on DNA repair proficiency. Carcinogenesis 2000;21: 551–555.

198. Spitz MR, Wu X, Wang Y, et al. Modulation of nucleotide excision repair capacity by XPD polymorphisms in lung cancer patients. Cancer Res 2001;61:1354–1357.

199. Qiao Y, Spitz MR, Shen H, et al. Modulation of repair of ultraviolet damage in the host-cell reactivation assay by polymorphic XPC and XPD/ERCC2 genotypes. Carcinogenesis 2002;23:295–299.

200. Lunn RM, Langlois RG, Hsieh LL, et al. XRCC1 polymorphisms: effects on aflatoxin B1-DNA adducts and glycophorin A variant frequency. Cancer Res 1999;59:2557–2561.

201. Stoehlmacher J, Ghaderi V, Iobal S, et al. A polymorphism of the XRCC1 gene predicts for response to platinum based treatment in advanced colorectal cancer. Anticancer Res 2001;21(4B): 3075–3079.

202. El-Rayes BF, LoRusso PM. Targeting the epidermal growth factor receptor. Br J Cancer 2004;91:418–424.

203. Green MR. Targeting targeted therapy. N Engl J Med 2004; 350:2191–2193.

204. Mendelsohn J, Baselga J. Status of epidermal growth factor receptor antagonists in the biology and treatment of cancer. J Clin Oncol 2003;21:2787–2799.

205. Kris MG, Natale RB, Herbst RS, et al. Efficacy of gefitinib, an inhibitor of the epidermal growth factor receptor tyrosine

kinase, in symptomatic patients with non-small cell lung cancer: a randomized trial. JAMA 2003;290:2149–2158.

206. Fukuoka M, Yano S, Giaccone G, et al. Multi-institutional randomized phase II trial of gefitinib for previously treated patients with advanced non-small-cell lung cancer. J Clin Oncol 2003; 21:2237–2246.

207. Cohen MH, Williams GA, Sridhara R, et al. United States Food and Drug Administration Drug Approval summary: Gefitinib (ZD1839; Iressa) tablets. Clin Cancer Res 2004;10:1212–1218.

208. Lynch TJ, Bell DW, Sordella R, et al. Activating mutations in the epidermal growth factor receptor underlying responsiveness of non-small-cell lung cancer to gefitinib. N Engl J Med 2004; 350:2129–2139.

209. Sparreboom A, Danesi R, Ando Y, et al. Pharmacogenomics of ABC transporters and its role in cancer chemotherapy. Drug Resist Updat 2003;6:71–84.

210. Toffoli G, Veronesi A, Boiocchi M, et al. MTHFR gene polymorphism and severe toxicity during adjuvant treatment of early breast cancer with cyclophosphamide, methotrexate, and fluorouracil (CMF). Ann Oncol 2000;11:373–374.

211. Kalow W. Pharmacogenetics: its biologic roots and the medical challenge. Clin Pharmacol Ther 1993;54:235–241.

212. Meyers U, Skoda RC, Zanger UM, et al. The genetic polymorphism of debrisoquine/sparteine metabolism: molecular mechanisms. In: Kalow W, ed. Pharmacogenetics of Drug Metabolism. New York: Pergamon Press, 1992;609–623.

New Targets for Anticancer Therapeutics

25

A. Dimitrios Colevas   Orit Scharf
Lyudmila A. Vereshchagina   Janet E. Dancey   S. Percy Ivy
Len Neckers   Bennett Kaufman   Richard Swerdlow

This chapter summarizes the molecular basis of oncology interest, preclinical development, and early clinical trials of a selection of investigational agents targeting five cellular processes: the cell cycle via cyclin-dependent kinase inhibition (CDKI), the mitotic apparatus via kinesin spindle protein inhibition (KSPI), cell-cell communication via integrin inhibition, intracellular signal transduction via molecular target of rapamycin (mTOR) inhibition, and posttranslational protein processing via heat shock protein 90 (HSP90) inhibition.

All the molecular targets of the agents discussed here are known to be functional in both normal and cancer cells. The rationale for development is therefore not based on the premise that these targets are uniquely expressed in cancer cells, as was the case, for example, with imatinib in diseases associated with Bcr-Abl expression. Targeting a critical cellular process or molecular pathway at any point in that process or pathway may perturb cells sufficiently to alter their survival or growth. The key, therefore, is to elucidate which process or pathway is uniquely essential to cancer cell growth or differentially sensitive to disruption in cancer cells. Because many cancers harbor abnormalities in the pRb pathway or overexpress cyclins, CDK inhibitors are a logical target in these cancers. Cell division is a sine qua non of cancer, while most somatic cells rest in G_0. Targeting of proteins expressed only during cell division, such as kinesin spindle proteins, might selectively perturb cancer cells. Tissue-specific integrin expression, such as exclusive neo-endothelial expression of the $\alpha_v\beta_3$ heterodimer, as well as overexpression of $\alpha_v\beta_3$ in certain cancers, suggests that an $\alpha_v\beta_3$ integrin inhibitor would have cancer-specific activity.

Both mTOR and Hsp90 inhibition could have cancer-specific activity by virtue of the fact that the targeted pathways in the former and molecular entities in the latter seem to be particularly relevant to growth and/or survival of selected cancers. Therefore, the agents described in this chapter have been chosen for development due to their ability to alter pathways rather than target oncogenic gene products.

The preclinical support for the molecular pathway cancer-specific activity of the above agents is summarized in this chapter. It is important to recognize that these preclinical data are derived from experiments in artificial systems that historically have been poor predictors of clinical efficacy. Therefore, the definitive evaluation of the potential of these agents will depend on the results of the ongoing clinical trials.

CYCLIN-DEPENDENT KINASE INHIBITORS

Introduction

The four phases of the cell cycle (G_1, S, G_2, and M) are characterized by distinct cellular processes that are required for proper cell division.[1] Each phase transition is tightly regulated by cyclin-dependent kinase (CDK) complexes composed of a cyclin and a kinase.[2] Mitogen-dependent accumulation of cyclin D–dependent kinases triggers the phosphorylation of the retinoblastoma (Rb) protein by CDK4 and/or CDK6 (G_1) as well as by CDK2 (G_1/S interphase), and this phosphorylation then enables complexes of the E2F transcription factor to activate transcription of target genes (e.g., enzymes required for DNA synthesis such as thymidine kinase and dihydrofolate reductase), leading to cell division.[3,4] This process is then accelerated by the cyclin E–CDK2 complex, which acts through positive feedback to facilitate progressive rounds of Rb phosphorylation and E2F release. Another regulation point is the G_2/M transition, where specific expression of regulators is essential to control the correct sequence of events; CDK1 cooperates with other kinases and phosphatases to regulate the final phases of the cell cycle.[3] Most human neoplasms are characterized by dysregulation of components of the Rb pathway. This dysregulation leads to aberrant progression into the S phase while ignoring growth-factor and cell-cycle control signals.[5] These observations have stimulated a great interest in development of pharmacological small-molecule CDK inhibitors. Several small-molecule CDK inhibitors that bind at the ATP-binding site of CDKs are being studied in clinical trials (alvocidib or flavopiridol, UCN-01, CYC202 or R-roscovitine, BMS-381032, and E7070 or indisulam) (Table 25.1 and Fig. 25.1).[6,7]

Alvocidib (Flavopiridol)

Alvocidib (NSC 649890, Flavopiridol, L86-8275, HMR 1275; Sanofi-Aventis Pharmaceuticals, Inc., Bridgewater,

NJ; Fig. 25.1) is a synthetic flavone derived from a natural product, rohitukine, isolated from the stem bark of *Dysoxylum binectariferum*, a plant indigenous to India.[24,25] The biology and chemistry of alvocidib and its mechanism of action, pharmacology, preclinical studies, and clinical experience have been the subject of several review articles.[3,6,8,9,26] The antitumor activity of alvocidib has been linked to CDK inhibition, induction of apoptosis, and inhibition of transcription and angiogenesis. Alvocidib disrupts progression of cells through the cell cycle at G_1/S and G_2/M.[24] Alvocidib directly inhibits CDK 1, 2, 4, 6, and 7 in the 30- to 300-nM range.[9] In addition, alvocidib inhibits epidermal growth factor receptor (EGFR) tyrosine kinase, the serine/threonine kinases, PKC and PKA, mitogen-activated protein kinase (MAPK) Erk-1, and src family kinases at concentrations in the micromolar range.[9] The efficacy of alvocidib is not solely based on cell cycle arrest.[27] Alvocidib also inhibits the positive transcription elongation factor (P-TEFb; $IC_{50} < 10$ nM).[10] Alvocidib down-regulates expression of cyclin D1 by reducing cyclin D1 mRNA and inhibiting transcription of cyclin D1 promoter.[11] Alvocidib induces apoptosis in various tumor and normal cells in vitro as well as in tumor xenografts in vivo, particularly those of hematopoietic origin, independent of Bcl-2 and p53 status.[9,28,29] Thus, available data indicate

TABLE 25.1
CDK INHIBITORS IN CLINICAL DEVELOPMENT

Agent	CDK/Cyclin Target*	Prominent In Vitro/In Vivo Preclinical Data	Clinical
Alvocidib (3, 6, 8–12)	**CDK1/cyclin B, CDK2/cyclin A, CDK2/cyclin E, CDK4/cyclin D, CDK6/cyclin D, CDK 7/cyclin H (TFIIH), CDK9/cyclin T (P-TEFb),** cyclin D1 protein↓	Average $IC_{50} = 0.066$ μM; G_1/S, G_2/M arrest; apoptosis (↑); angiogenesis (↓)	Phase I and phase II single-agent and combination studies (+ paclitaxel, cisplatin, carboplatin, docetaxel, irinotecan, gemcitabine, ara-C, bortezomib, trastuzumab, doxorubicin, imatinib, dapsipeptide, SAHA). Promising activity in CLL.
R-roscovitine (CYC202) (13–16)	**CDK2/cyclin A, CDK2/cyclin E, CDK7/cyclin H, CDK5/p35, CDC2/cyclin B,** CDK9/cyclin T, CDK1/cyclin B, cyclin D1 protein↓	Average $IC_{50} = 15.2$ μM; 45–62% tumor growth (↓) in xenograft models; G_1/S, G_2/M arrest; apoptosis (↑)	Phase I single-agent studies: oral BID. Phase II combination studies: + capecitabine in breast cancer; + gemcitabine/cisplatin in NSCLC.
Indisulam (E7070) (17–19)	CDK2/cyclin E activity↓; CDK2, CDK4, CDC2, Cyclin A, B1, H proteins↓	$IC_{50} = 0.1–4.4$ μg/mL; T/C < 42% and 73–85% tumor volume (↓) in xenograft models; G_1/S, G_2/M arrest; apoptosis (↑)	Phase I and phase II single-agent studies: IV d×5, q7d, q21d.
BMS-387032 (20–23)	**CDK2/cyclin E, CDK1/cyclin B, CDK4/cyclin D**	Cellular cytotoxicity $IC_{50} = 0.095$ μM; tumor growth (↓) and 9/16 cured mice in xenograft model experiments; cell cycle arrest; apoptosis (↑)	Phase I single-agent studies: 1-hr IV q7d, q21d; 24-hr CIV q21d.

*****Bold** implies $IC_{50} < 1$ μM.

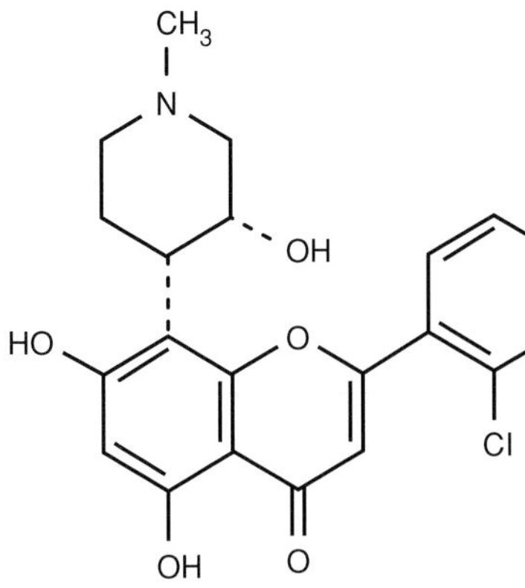

Figure 25.1 Chemical structure of alvocidib.

that alvocidib can target a variety of key regulatory molecules involved in cell cycle progression and apoptosis.

Alvocidib has demonstrated a potent antiproliferative activity in the National Cancer Institute's (NCI) 60–cell line drug screen (average IC$_{50}$ = 66 nM), with no obvious tumor-type selectivity.[8] IC$_{50}$ values ranged from approximately 50 to 200 nM, similar to concentrations required to inhibit CDKs.[24] Alvocidib inhibits growth of human tumor xenografts, including head and neck squamous cell carcinoma (HNSCC) and lung, colon, ovary, gastric, and breast cancer, and causes regression in glioma, leukemia, and lymphoma models.[30–33]

Alvocidib is being clinically developed by Sanofi-Aventis in collaboration with the NCI. Several different schedules of administration have been explored. The initial phase I studies tested multiple-day continuous infusions (CIVs) based on nonclinical data suggesting that prolonged exposure optimized anticancer activity. With a 72-hour CIV on an every-2-week schedule, the maximum tolerated dose (MTD) and recommended phase II dose (RP2D) is 40 to 50 mg/m^2 per day × 3, with secretory diarrhea as the dose-limiting toxicity (DLT).[34,35] Other prominent adverse events include proinflammatory syndrome and thrombosis. The steady-state levels achieved at MTD (300-nM range) are below what is predicted to be active from several nonclinical models. Subsequent studies of 1-, 3-, or 5-consecutive-day 1-hour infusions of alvocidib have yielded MTDs of 62.5, 50, and 37.5 mg/m^2 per day, respectively.[36–38] Neutropenia, fatigue, and hepatotoxicity are the DLTs, and nausea and vomiting have been significant.[36,38] Micromolar plasma concentrations, reached at the MTDs, are short-lived. Hints of activity from these trials included a gastric cancer patient with a complete response (CR) for 48 months and a patient with renal cell cancer (RCC) who achieved a partial response.[34,35] Because minimal anticancer activity has been seen in these single-agent phase II trials on these schedules, additional schedules have been tested, including weekly 1-hour and 24-hour infusions.

Alvocidib on these additional schedules is tolerable at doses tested on the above schedules with similar pharmacokinetics (PKs).[39–41]

Based on the observation that free alvocidib levels in human plasma are significantly lower than in bovine plasma, two groups have pursued a hybrid schedule of bolus followed by infusional alvocidib in order to achieve micromolar steady-state concentrations for several hours. Alvocidib given weekly by 30-minute intravenous (IV) bolus followed by 4-hour IV in patients with fludarabine-refractory chronic lymphocytic leukemia (CLL) has resulted in micromolar concentrations for several hours, tumor lysis syndrome as a DLT at 80 mg/m^2 per dose, and dramatic activity against fludarabine-resistant CLL, including nine sustained partial responses in the first 23 patients treated.[12,42]

Based on nonclinical evidence of synergism, alvocidib has been combined with the following agents in clinical trials: paclitaxel, docetaxel, irinotecan, gemcitabine, cisplatin, carboplatin, imatinib, trastuzumab, 5-fluorouracil (5-FU), bortezomib, suberoylanilide hydroxamic acid (SAHA), and doxorubicin and also with radiation.[43–50] Combinations with multiple agents have included gemcitabine plus irinotecan, oxaliplatin plus 5-FU, irinotecan plus 5-FU, leucovorin plus 5-FU, cytosine arabinoside plus mitoxantrone, fludarabine plus rituximab, paclitaxel plus cisplatin or carboplatin, and irinotecan plus cisplatin.[51–55] Generally, the doses of alvocidib achievable when combined with conventional agents are in the same range or slightly lower than the single-agent MTD as a 1-hour, 24-hour, or 72-hour infusion. One notable exception is the combination of alvocidib with taxanes, where the tolerability of the combinations is sensitive to the schedule and administration of these agents, despite no known PK interaction.[43–45,51,52] The hybrid bolus followed by continuous infusion schedule has yet to be tested in combination with other agents.

Clinical PK data for alvocidib are summarized in Table 25.2. Mean steady-state alvocidib concentrations achieved using 72-hour CIV were not adequate after correction for the conversion from bovine to human plasma environment.[35,56] Preliminary data suggest that levels greater than 1 μm are sustained for more than 5 hours in patients treated using the hybrid infusion.[12] The postinfusional peak concentration (C$_{max}$) of alvocidib appears to be related to enterohepatic recirculation, and nonlinear elimination has been observed at alvocidib doses above 50 mg/m^2 per day, but there is evidence of postinfusional C$_{max}$ with the 1-hour infusion.[26,56] Dose-corrected areas under the curve (AUCs) are similar with the 72- and 1-hour infusions.[26] Alvocidib is highly protein bound, with a mean unbound fraction of 6%.[56] Irinotecan increases the metabolism of alvocidib, but no other PK interactions are known for the above combinations.[50] The systemic glucuronidation of alvocidib is inversely associated with the risk of developing diarrhea in metastatic renal cancer patients.[57]

TABLE 25.2
CLINICAL PK PARAMETERS OF ALVOCIDIB UNDER DIFFERENT SCHEDULES

Schedule	72-hr CIV q2wks	1–hr IV d×5 q3wk	1-hr IV d×5 q3wk	1-hr IV d×3 q3wk	1-hr IV d×1 q3wk	1-hr IV qwk×3	24-hr CIV qwk×4	30-min IV →4-hr IV qwk×4 q6wk
Dose (mg/m^2/d)	50 and 78 (34)	8–56 (35)	12–52.5 (36)	50 and 62.5 (36)	62.5 and 78 (36)	80 mg/m^2 (39)	40–100 mg/m^2 (40)	60 mg/m^2/dose (42)
C_{max} (μM)	C_{ss} 0.271 (50 mg/m^2/d); 0.344 (78 mg/m^2/d) (34)	C_{ss} 0.417 ± 0.099 (MTD = 40 mg/m^2/d) (35)	1.7 (37.5 mg/m^2/d) (36)	3.2 (50 mg/m^2/d) (36)	3.9 (62.5 mg/m^2/d) (36)	5.3 (39)	0.924 (100 mg/m^2) (40)	1.2–5 (42)
$t_{1/2}$ (hr)	$t_{1/2\beta}$ = 11.6 (1.3–29.1) (34)	$t_{1/2\alpha}$ = 1.1; $t_{1/2\beta}$ = 27.3 ± 18.3 (35)		$t_{1/2\beta}$ = 5.2 ± 4.9 (37)				$t_{1/2\beta}$ = 10.1 ± 4.7 (42)
AUC (μM·h)		29 ± 13 (MTD = 40 mg/m^2/d) (35)				28 (39)	22 (100 mg/m^2) (40)	15 ± 8.4 (42)
Cl (L/hr/m^2)	17.23 (11.5–27.3) (34)	10.5 ± 2.6 (MTD = 40 mg/m^2/d) (35)		13.8 ± 4.9 (37)				10.2 ± 4.2 (42)
Vd_{ss} (L/m^2)	131.16 (24.3–516.7) (34)			64.9 ± 43.41 (37)				129.2 (42)

Phase II Trials

Alvocidib has been administered as a 1-hour IV infusion daily for 3 days every 3 weeks in patients with mantle cell lymphoma, metastatic malignant melanoma, and advanced RCC. Responses were seen in 3/31, 0/17, and 2/34 patients, respectively. Four RCC patients remained progression free during treatment for over 1 year.[58–60] In single-agent phase II trials using the 72-hour CIV every-2-week schedule, response rates in patients with advanced colorectal cancer (ACRC), metastatic non–small cell lung cancer (NSCLC), metastatic androgen-independent prostate cancer, metastatic gastric cancer, and metastatic renal cancer were 0/18, 0/20, 0/36, 0/14, and 2/34, respectively.[61–65]

Future Prospects

Because clinically significant antineoplastic activity using alvocidib as a single agent on the 1-hour and 72-hour infusion schedules has not been seen, further efforts are focused on clinical development in four areas. First, the promising activity in CLL on the hybrid schedule will be the subject of follow-up phase II studies. Second, the utility of combining alvocidib with conventional agents continues to be explored. Third, based on promising preclinical synergy data, NCI is sponsoring combinations of alvocidib with other targeted therapies, including histone deacetylase inhibitors, imatinib, and rituxumab. And finally, there are a number of ongoing clinical trials with embedded correlative studies designed to ask whether or not alvocidib in fact inhibits its purported targets in human tumors.

Other CDK inhibitors currently undergoing clinical trials include oral R-roscovitine (CYC202; Cyclacel, Dundee, UK; phase I single-agent and phase II combination studies with capecitabine in breast cancer and with gemcitabine/cisplatin in NSCLC), BMS-387032 (Bristol-Myers Squibb in collaboration with the NCI; phase I trials), and indisulam (E7070; Eisai; phase I and II single-agent studies).[15,16,18,19,21–23]

SB-715992 (KINESIN SPINDLE KINASE INHIBITOR)

The kinesin superfamily of proteins consists of motor proteins that utilize energy released by hydrolysis of ATP to produce directed force along microtubules.[66] Kinesins are divided into two major groups by their function; those involved in vesicle transport and membrane organization and those involved in cell division (mitotic kinesins).[67] Expression of mitotic kinesins is increased in tumor tissues relative to normal adjacent tissues.[68,69] Mitotic kinesins are predominantly expressed during cell division, further suggesting that they may be more specific anti-mitotic targets than tubulin, which is present in all cells during all phases of the cell cycle.[67] The kinesin spindle protein (KSP; also known as Eg5) is a mitotic kinesin required in early mitosis for the establishment of mitotic spindle bipolarity and for cell cycle progression through mitosis.[70,71] SB-715992 (GlaxoSmithKline) is a 2-(aminomethyl) quinazolinone inhibitor of KSP, with broad antiproliferative activity both in vitro and in vivo,[72] and it is the first mitotic KSP inhibitor to enter clinical trials.[73] SB-715992 is 70,000-fold more selective for KSP than other kinesins and disrupts the assembly of functional mitotic spindles, thereby causing cell cycle arrest and subsequent cell death.[73]

Preclinical Studies

In vitro studies have shown that SB-715992 has a Ki of 0.6 nM and cytotoxic activity at less than 10 nM in a spectrum of tumor cell lines.[74] It caused complete tumor regression in two human colon tumor xenografts and tumor growth delay in another. On the other hand, a mammary tumor xenograft was completely refractory to SB-715992. SB-715992 is growth inhibitory in other pancreatic and colon carcinoma xenograft models.[72] Efficacy is dose-related, and in the most sensitive tumor models, regressions were seen at doses as low as one third of the MTD.[74] Equivalent efficacy and toxicity were seen regardless of administration method.[74]

Clinical Trials

GlaxoSmithKline has sponsored two clinical trials with SB-715992. One study administered 1-8 mg/m^2 on days 1, 8, and 15 every 28 days.[75] Twenty-seven patients with solid tumors were treated, and two patients developed a DLT (grade 3 neutropenia) at a dose of 8 mg/m^2. As a result, the 7 mg/m^2 dose was expanded and no grade 3/4 adverse events were observed. Increases in AUC and C_{max} were dose-related. PK parameters measured on days 1 and 15 of the first cycle were as follows: C_{max} = 349 and 218 ng/mL; Cl = 1,596 and 7,546 mL/hour; and volume of distribution at steady state (Vd_{ss}) = 235 and 240 L, respectively. The RP2D for this study was 7 mg/m^2.

In the second study, SB-715992 was administered intravenously at doses of 1 to 21 mg/m^2 every 21 days.[76] Forty-two patients with solid tumors were treated, and two DLTs were observed at 21 mg/m^2, grade 4 neutropenia lasting more than 5 days and grade 4 neutropenic fever (one patient each). The 18 mg/m^2 dose level was expanded, and 12 patients were treated at this dose. Two DLTs have been observed, grade 4 neutropenia in both cases. Non-dose-limiting grade 3/4 neutropenia occurred in seven patients and grade 4 leukopenia occurred in one patient. Common grade 2 drug-related adverse events at doses greater than 6 mg/m^2 included fatigue, leukopenia, and anemia. Stable disease was observed in four patients for 5 to 11 cycles. AUC and C_{max} increased in a dose-dependent manner, and median PK values were as follows: C_{max} = 473 ng/mL; AUC=5,074 ng·h/mL; $t_{1/2}$ = 33 hours, Cl = 6,656 mL/hour;

and Vd_{ss} = 236 L. Monopolar mitotic spindles were observed in a tumor biopsy from a patient with squamous cell carcinoma of the head and neck (SCCHN), at a dose of 16 mg/m^2. The RP2D in this study was 18 mg/m^2 every 21 days.

In addition to these studies, the NCI is sponsoring phase I and II studies of SB-715992 in patients with solid tumors, acute leukemia, RCC, colorectal cancer, hepatocellular carcinoma, prostate cancer, SCCHN, and melanoma.

α_v ANTAGONISTS AS NOVEL ANTICANCER AGENTS

Introduction

Integrins are a widely expressed family of cell adhesion receptors that recognize extracellular matrix proteins and cell-surface molecules through short peptide sequences.[77] The integrins consist of two distinct noncovalently associated subunits; 18 α- and 8 β-subunits combine in a restricted repertoire to form 24 known heterodimers.[78] Several integrins share the α_v subunit and interact strongly with the Arg-Gly-Asp (RGD) peptide sequence found within specific extracellular matrices and cell surface proteins. The $\alpha_v\beta_3$ and $\alpha_v\beta_5$ integrins are overexpressed on endothelial cells during tumor angiogenesis[77–79] and participate in other events promoting tumor progression, such as cell migration and capillary morphogenesis. $\alpha_v\beta_3$ has a limited tissue distribution. It is not typically expressed on epithelial cells and appears at minimal levels on intestinal and vascular cells.[80] In contrast, it is extensively expressed on some tumor cells, including late-stage glioblastoma,[81,82] ovarian carcinoma,[83] melanoma,[84,85] pancreatic carcinoma,[86] and prostate cancer.[87]

The importance of both $\alpha_v\beta_3$ and $\alpha_v\beta_5$ in tumor angiogenesis[88] has generated an interest in antagonists to these integrins. Both blocking antibodies directed against the extracellular domain (LM609) and RGD peptides disrupt blood vessel formation in several in vitro and in vivo models.[80] In tumor models, this inhibition disrupts tumor-associated angiogenesis and in some cases causes tumor regression as well.[89] Humanized LM609, known as MEDI-522 (Vitaxin; MedImmune, Inc.), and the cyclic RGD peptide EMD 121974 (Cilengitide; Merck KgaA/EMD Pharmaceuticals) are both currently being evaluated in clinical trials.

MEDI-522 (Vitaxin)

Preclinical Studies

Antibodies directed against $\alpha_v\beta_3$ integrin cause dose-dependent regression of CAM blood vessels as a result of apoptosis associated with activation of endothelial cell p53 and increased expression of p21$^{waf1/cip1}$.[90,91]

Clinical Trials

MedImmune, Inc. is sponsoring two phase I studies in cancer patients. In one study, MEDI-522 was administered to patients with refractory solid tumors at doses up to 6 mg/kg as a single dose, followed 2 to 5 weeks later by weekly doses for up to 1 year.[92] The majority of MEDI-522-related adverse events were mild to moderate in severity, with the most common being infusion-type reactions. No anti–MEDI-522 antibodies were observed. Preliminary pharmacokinetic (PK) results showed a nonlinear increase in terminal half-life with increasing doses, reaching 130 hours following the 4 mg/kg dose level. At 6 mg/kg per week, mean serum trough levels of MEDI-522 ranged from 24 to 37 μg/mL. In the other phase I study, MEDI-522 was administered to patients with irinotecan-refractory colorectal cancer at dose levels of 4 to 10 mg/kg.[93] MedImmune is currently enrolling patients into two phase II studies (melanoma and prostate cancer), and the NCI is sponsoring two phase I studies in patients with solid tumors. The NCI studies are being conducted in patients with advanced solid tumors utilizing a drug administration schedule similar to that used in the MedImmune-sponsored studies.

EMD 121974 (Cilengitide)

Preclinical Studies

EMD 121974 (Merck KgaA, Germany, and EMD Pharmaceuticals Inc.; Fig. 25.2) is the inner salt of a cyclized pentapeptide containing the RGD sequence and is a potent and selective antagonist of the $\alpha_v\beta_3$ and $\alpha_v\beta_5$ integrins.[94] EMD 121974 has been shown to bind to integrins $\alpha_v\beta_3$ and $\alpha_v\beta_5$, with IC_{50} values of 1 nM and 140 nM, respectively,[95] and it inhibits integrin binding to extracellular matrix proteins.[96] In addition, EMD 121974 inhibits the growth of WM164 melanoma tumor in vivo.[96] EMD 121974 inhibits the M21 melanoma xenograft model at 10 to 15 mg/kg administered once or twice a day or every other day.[95] EMD 121974 inhibits medulloblastoma (DAOY) and glioblastoma (U87MG) orthotopic xenografts

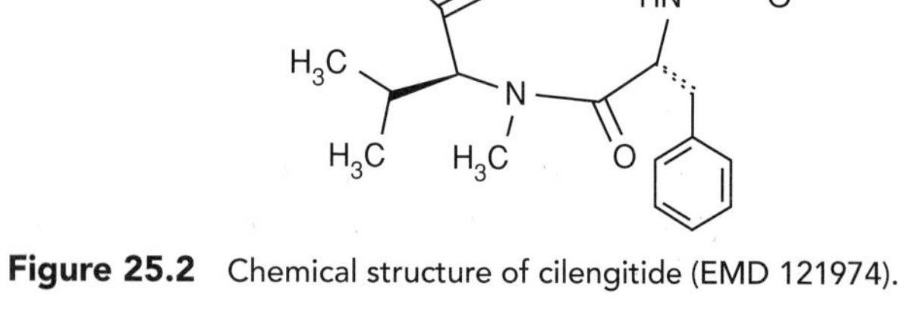

Figure 25.2 Chemical structure of cilengitide (EMD 121974).

at ~5 mg/kg administered intraperitoneally.[97] All treated mice survived without evidence of morbidity, and only residual tumor cells or small clusters could be seen (<1 mm³ in size).

Toxicology

Four weeks of daily IV bolus administration of EMD 121974 to mice resulted in no evidence of treatment-related effects up to the highest dose level of 90 mg/kg.[95] In cynomolgus monkeys, EMD 121974 administered intravenously daily at doses up to 90 mg/kg showed dose-related anemia and reticulocytosis at the end of the study period, with normalization of both parameters after 4 weeks. No bone marrow abnormality was observed at necropsy.[95]

Clinical Studies

Merck KgaA/EMD Pharmaceuticals has sponsored several phase I and II studies with EMD 121974. In a phase I study, EMD 121974 was administered by a 1-hour IV infusion at doses of 30 to 1,600 mg/m² twice weekly to patients with advanced solid tumors.[95] PK parameters were approximately linear, and C_{max} was generally observed at the end of the infusion period. Mean systemic clearance (CL) was 34 to 66 mL/min per m², and Vd_{ss} was 9 to 17 L/m². Systemic exposure to EMD 121974 was dose-dependent. The target plasma concentration of 11 to 13 mg/mL, derived from murine PK models, was attained at a dose of 120 mg/m². Hematologic adverse events consisted of grade 2 anemia. Nonhematologic adverse events were generally mild, never exceeding grade 2, and consisted of nausea, anorexia, vomiting, fatigue, and malaise. No DLT occurred.

The NCI is sponsoring several phase I and II studies with EMD 121974. The New Approaches to Brain Tumor Therapy consortium (NABTT) treated 51 malignant glioma patients with EMD 121974 at a starting dose of 120 mg/m² twice weekly, escalating up to 2,400 mg/m².[98] Two complete responses (at 360 and 2,400 mg/m²) and three partial responses (two at 120 mg/m² and one at 360 mg/m²) have been confirmed. DLTs included grade 4 arthralgia at 480 mg/m²; thrombocytopenia at 600 mg/m²; and anorexia, hypoglycemia, and hyponatremia at 1,800 mg/m². The MTD was not reached. Since no serious adverse events or biologic activity had been observed with lower doses of EMD 121974, patients with solid tumors enrolled in another phase I study were treated at 600, 1,200, and 2,400 mg/m² twice weekly. PK analysis from these two studies demonstrates that the twice-weekly schedule appears to maintain the preclinically effective plasma concentration of 1 μM for less than 24 hours. In a study of children with refractory brain tumors in which EMD 121974 is administered at a starting dose of 120 mg/m² twice weekly for 4 weeks, the study has accrued patients up to the 1,200 mg/m² dose level.

Because responses have occurred in patients receiving low as well as high doses of EMD 121974, and because there seems to be no dose-related toxicity in the dose ranges studied, the NCI is sponsoring several phase II studies to be conducted with two doses: 500 mg and 2,000 mg administered intravenously twice weekly. A phase II study in melanoma patients is currently enrolling patients. In addition, a phase I-II study of EMD 121974 combined with radiation therapy in newly diagnosed glioblastoma multiforme patients has been recently approved. During the phase I portion of this study, patients will be administered EMD 121974 at a starting dose of 500 mg twice weekly, escalating to 2,000 mg concurrently with conventional radiation therapy. In the phase II portion of the study, patients will receive either 500 mg or 2,000 mg of EMD 121974 during radiation. Additional phase II studies with EMD 121974 in patients with carcinoma of the prostate and glioblastoma are planned.

INHIBITORS OF THE MAMMALIAN TARGET OF RAPAMYCIN

Introduction

The mammalian target of rapamycin (mTOR) is a downstream protein kinase of the phosphatidylinositol 3-kinase (PI3K)/Akt signaling pathway. By targeting mTOR, the immunosuppressant and antiproliferative agent rapamycin inhibits signals required for cell cycle progression, cell growth, and proliferation in normal and malignant cells. Currently, mTOR inhibitors rapamycin (sirolimus, Wyeth) and derivatives temsirolimus (CCI-779, Wyeth), everolimus, (RAD001, Novartis Pharma AG), and AP23573 (Ariad Pharmaceuticals) are being evaluated in cancer clinical trials. An additional agent, TAFA-93 (Isotechnika), has recently entered human trials for the prevention of organ rejection after transplantation.

Biochemistry of the PI3K-Akt-mTOR Pathway

The mTOR is a serine-threonine kinase that regulates both cell growth and cell cycle progression by integrating signals from nutrient and growth factor stimuli.[99,100] mTOR functions in a protein complex that integrates signals from a variety of sources, including growth factors, energy stores, and hypoxia, with the protein translation apparatus.[101]

Growth factor receptor-stimulated mTOR regulation proceeds through the PI3K and Akt pathways (Fig. 25.3). In response to extracellular stimuli, PI3K phosphorylates phosphatidylinositol-4, 5- bis-phosphate (PIP_2) to generate phosphatidylinositol-3, 4, 5- triphosphate (PIP_3). The formation of PIP_3 leads to the binding and activation of phosphatidylinositol-dependent kinase-1 (PDK1) and Akt at the plasma membrane.[100] The tumor suppressor phos-

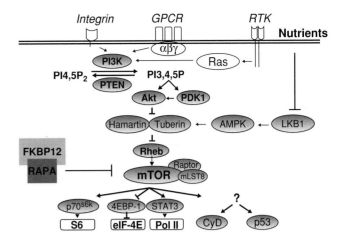

Figure 25.3 Growth factor receptor (GFR, integrin and G-protein coupled receptor [GPCR]) stimulation leads to activation of PI3K, phosphorylation of the 3'-OH of phosphatidylinositol-4, 5-bis-phosphate ($PI4,5,P_2$) to generate phosphatidylinositol-3, 4, 5-triphosphate ($PI3,4,5P_3$). $PI3,4,5P_3$ then recruits phosphatidylinositol-dependent kinase-1 (PDK1) and Akt, to the plasma membrane to be activated. The tumor suppressor phosphatase PTEN (for phosphatase and tensin homolog deleted on chromosome 10) dephosphorylates $PI3,4,5,P_3$ at the D-3 position of the inositol ring. Activated Akt phosphorylates and inhibits the tuberous sclerosis complex (TSC), removing its inhibitory effect on Ras-related small GTPase Rheb (Ras homolog enriched in brain). TSC2 is also inhibited by the presence of amino acids, allowing Rheb to activate mTOR through an unknown mechanism. Activation of mTOR in complex with other proteins such as raptor (regulatory associated protein of mTOR) and mammalian ortholog of LST8 (mLST8) leads to phosphorylation of eukaryotic initiation factor 4E (eIF-4E)–binding protein (4E-BP1) and ribosomal protein S6 kinase 1 (S6K1). This interaction results in an increase in translation rates of a subset of mRNAs, including those encoding proteins required for cell cycle progression such as cyclin D (CyD). Rapamycin (RAPA) in complex with FK506-binding protein of 12 kd (FKBP12) inhibits mTOR. See text for additional details.

phatase PTEN (for phosphatase and tensin homolog deleted on chromosome 10) dephosphorylates PIP_3, reversing the action of PI3K. Activated Akt phosphorylates and inhibits the tuberous sclerosis complex (TSC), which is composed of TSC1 (hamartin) and TSC2 (tuberin) heterodimer that inhibits cell cycle progression and cell proliferation.[102,103] TSC2 acts as a GTPase-activating protein (GAP) toward the Ras-related small GTPase Rheb (Ras-homolog-enriched-in-brain),[104] a positive upstream regulator of mTOR. Activation of TSC2 by the tumor suppressor gene product LKB1, as may occur in a nutrient-deprived state, inhibits Rheb and results in the down-regulation of mTOR. In contrast, inhibition of TSC2, as occurs in the presence of amino acids, with Akt phosphorylation, or through loss of TSC2 function through mutation, as occurs in tuberous sclerosis patients, leads to mTOR activation and phosphorylation of the downstream mTOR targets.[103] The net result of these signaling interactions suggests a model in which growth factor signaling through PI3K-Akt is coordinated with nutrient availability signaling through LKB1-TSC1/2 to Rheb and mTOR.

mTOR functions in a complex with at least two other proteins: regulatory associated protein of mTOR (raptor)[105,106] and mammalian ortholog of LST8.[106,107] Current evidence suggests that activated mTOR, in complex with raptor and possibly other proteins, leads to phosphorylation of two key proteins: eukaryotic initiation factor 4E (eIF-4E) binding protein-1 (4E-BP1) and protein S6 kinase 1 (S6K1)[108,109] (see Fig. 25.3). Activation of mTOR, leads to phosphorylation of 4E-BP1, release of eIF-4E to bind to cap mRNA transcripts and other initiation complex proteins, and the initiation of cap-dependent translation. This effect on translation of certain regulatory mRNAs may be one means by which mTOR regulates cell growth.[110]

A second mTOR target is the phosphorylation and activation of S6K1. Previously, activation of S6K1 had been correlated with increased translation of 5' terminal oligopyrimidine tract (TOP) mRNAs, which encode components of the translational apparatus.[111] However, the translation of TOP mRNAs may occur independent of S6K1 function (for recent reviews, see refs. 110, 112). The recent results lead to the conclusion that regulation of TOP mRNA translation is primarily through the PI3K pathway, with little role for mTOR.[110] S6K1 has been implicated in glucose homeostasis and regulation of eukaryotic elongation factor 2 kinase.[110]

Consistent with the role of mTOR as a controller of cellular growth, mTOR activation leads to the phosphorylation of several additional downstream signaling effectors and transcription factors, which in turn influence cell proliferation, survival, and angiogenesis. Many, though not all, of the protean functions of mTOR appear to be sensitive to inhibition by rapamycin. The many cellular signaling processes in which mTOR participates and the inhibition of some of these processes by rapamycins have contributed to interest in mTOR inhibition as a strategy for therapeutic development.

mTOR in Human Cancer

Although mutations of mTOR have not been reported in human cancers, both aberrant PI3K-dependent signaling and aberrant protein translation have been identified in a wide variety of malignancies and may contribute to oncogenesis and malignant progression. For example, components of the PI3K pathway that are mutated in different human tumors include activation mutations of growth factor receptors, amplification and/or overexpression of PI3K and Akt, as well as loss of PTEN. The resultant aberrant pathway signaling not only leads to a growth advantage during carcinogenesis and stimulates cancer cell proliferation but also contributes to treatment resistance due to a high PI3K-Akt–mediated survival threshold.[100] If such cancer cells are "addicted" to the growth and survival signaling

effects of the PI3K-Akt pathway, it is possible that this dependency will result in cancer cell sensitivity to mTOR inhibition.

In addition to cancer cell dependency on aberrant PI3K signaling for proliferation and survival, endothelial cell proliferation may also be dependent on mTOR signaling. Endothelial cell proliferation is stimulated by vascular endothelial cell growth factor (VEGF) activation of the PI3K-Akt-mTOR pathway. VEGF production may be partly controlled by mTOR signaling through mTOR effects on the expression of hypoxia-inducible factor-α (HIF1α).[113–115]

Rapamycin and Derivatives

Rapamycin (sirolimus, Rapamune, Wyeth; Fig. 25.4) is a macrocyclic lactone produced by *Streptomyces hygroscopicus*, a soil bacterium native to Easter Island (Rapa Nui). Rapamycin is used as an immunosuppressant for the prophylaxis of renal allograft rejection. Rapamycin's immunosuppressant effects are due to its inhibition of the biochemical events required for the progression of interleukin-2 (IL-2) stimulated T cells from the G_1 to the S phase of the cell cycle. However, rapamycin and derivatives also inhibit cellular proliferation in a variety of tumor models and are currently under clinical evaluation as potential cancer therapeutics.

Mechanism of Action

Rapamycin targets the ubiquitously expressed FK506-binding protein of 12 kd (FKBP12). The FKBP12-rapamycin

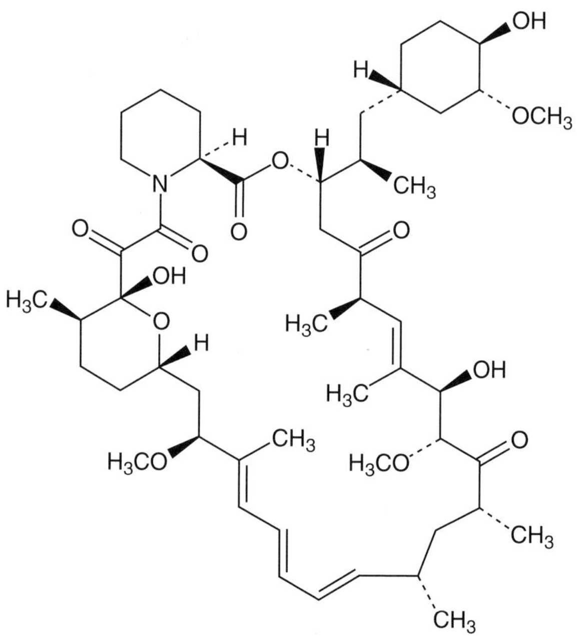

Figure 25.4 Chemical structure of rapamycin. (Reproduced with permission from Huang S, Bjornsti MA, Houghton PJ. Rapamycins: mechanism of action and cellular resistance. Cancer Biol Ther 2003;2:222–232.)

complex binds to the FKBP12-rapamycin–binding (FRB) domain adjacent to the kinase domain of mTOR and may inhibit mTOR by modifying the conformation and/or composition of the multiprotein mTOR complexes. By disrupting these protein complexes, rapamycin may impair either upstream signaling leading to mTOR activation or kinase access to downstream substrates.[116,117] Rapamycin and its derivatives share the following features: inhibition of cellular proliferation by inducing G_1 phase arrest, induction of apoptosis in selected models, and limited normal tissue toxicity.

The rapamycins may inhibit tumor and endothelial cell proliferation in picomolar to nanomolar concentrations and may add to the cytotoxicity of other chemotherapeutic agents and radiation.[118–123] Rapamycins induce reduction of cyclins, particularly cyclin D,[124,125] as well as increase cyclin-dependent kinase inhibitors $p21^{Cip1}$ and $p27^{Kip1}$.[126,127] In most instances, inhibition of TOR by rapamycin leads to an antiproliferative response. However, there are examples in which rapamycin induces apoptosis.[128,129] Rapamycin-induced apoptosis may depend on the functions of p53, $p21^{Cip1}$, and $p27^{Kip}$.[128–130] Rapamycin inhibits endothelial cell proliferation in the presence of hypoxia, inhibits endothelial cell proliferation due to VEGF stimulation through inhibition of mTOR, and decreases VEGF synthesis through enhanced HIF1α degradation.[131–133] Therefore, the expected clinical activity of rapamycin would be delayed tumor progression rather than tumor regression in most patients with sensitive disease; however, tumor regression through rapamycin-induced apoptosis could occur.

Determinants of Sensitivity and Resistance to mTOR Inhibition

Genetic mutations and/or compensatory aberrant signal transduction both upstream and downstream of mTOR influence tumor cells sensitivity to rapamycins.[134,135] Expression and function of the ataxia-telangiectasia gene product ATM and of 14-3-3, p53, PI3K-Akt, and PTEN have been reported to correlate with rapamycin sensitivity (for reviews, see refs. 134, 135). Inhibition of phosphorylation of S6K1, its target ribosomal S6 protein, and 4E-BP1 correlates with rapamycin sensitivity but is not sufficient for in vitro sensitivity in all cases.[135,136]

Rapamycin and related compounds exert selective cytostatic/cytotoxic effects on PTEN -/- tumors in vivo.[137,138] However, the loss of PTEN function does not correlate with rapamycin sensitivity in all models. Aberrant proliferative and prosurriral signaling through the PI3K-Akt pathway may occur not only through loss of the tumor suppressor PTEN, but also through abnormal stimulation of growth factor receptors, PI3K or Akt. These protein kinases may be activated through abnormal paracrine or loops or through activating mutations and/or amplification.

Rapamycin may add to the cytotoxic effects of standard cancer drugs; however, tumor cell responsiveness to these combinations will be determined by the molecular pheno-type of particular cancer cells. Lymphomas expressing Akt but not those expressing bcl-2 were sensitized by rapamycin to chemotherapy-induced apoptosis. Overexpression of the mTOR downstream target eIF-4E renders cells insensitive to concomitant administration of rapamycin and chemotherapy.[139] Cancer cells overexpressing Akt that are exposed to rapamycin may be rendered sensitive to standard cancer drugs and be triggered to undergo apoptosis when exposed to the combination, but tumor cells overexpressing eIF-4E or bcl-2 may be insensitive to rapamycin and remain resistant to standard cancer therapies.

Preclinical Anticancer Activity of mTOR Inhibitors

All the rapamycins under clinical development have antiproliferative activity in a variety of hematological and solid tumor systems as single agents and in combinations with standard cancer therapeutics agents and radiation.[119–121,123,140–148] Rapamycins easily cross the blood-brain barrier.[119] Therefore, rapamycins may have a role as single agents and in combination with standard therapies in a variety of malignancies, including malignancies within the CNS. While the data are limited, the antitumor effects of rapamycin and its derivatives temsirolimus and everolimus appear to be similar.[149–151]

Pharmacology of Rapamycin and Derivatives

Rapamycin and its derivative everolimus are orally administered, and the efficiency of absorption is modulated by p-glycoproteins (reviewed in ref. 152). Rapamycin has a terminal half-life of 62 hours in renal transplant recipients and a bioavailability of approximately 15%.[152] Everolimus has a bioavailability of approximately 30% and a half-life of 30 hours. Both rapamycin and everolimus have been reported to be metabolized by liver and intestinal cytochrome P450 enzyme CYP3A4, and metabolites are mainly excreted through the gastrointestinal tract. Significant interindividual pharmacokinetic variability has been reported and may be explained by interpatient p-glycoprotein and P450 enzyme system variability . The terminal half-life for intravenous temsirolimus is 13 to 22 hours and is associated with significant metabolism to rapamycin.[153] AP23573 has a median half-life of 49 hours and no appreciable conversion to rapamycin.[154,155]

Toxicity of Rapamycin and Derivatives

Although rapamycins induce immunosuppression with chronic oral dosing, prolonged immunosuppression is not a desirable effect for a cancer therapeutic, particularly when combined with myelosuppressive agents. Intermittent dosing models of the rapamycins were effective in inducing tumor growth delay without causing prolonged immunosuppression.[118,156] Rapamycin and everolimus have been associated with thrombocytopenia, leukopenia, and elevated serum lipids and creatinine in organ transplant recipients. In addition, there have been rare reports of pneumonitis associated with these agents.[157,158] Temsirolimus, everolimus, and AP23573 all induce reversible mucositis and myelosuppression in cancer patients. Given the structural similarities between rapamycin and its ester derivatives temsirolimus, everolimus, and AP23573, their activity, metabolism, and toxicity profiles would be expected to overlap.

Temsirolimus (CCI-779)

Temsirolimus (Fig. 25.5) is the only rapamycin derivative for which there are both intravenous and oral formulations. Human T-cell leukemia, prostate cancer, breast cancer, small cell lung carcinoma, glioma, melanoma, and rhabdomyosarcoma cell lines were among the most sensitive to temsirolimus.[118,119,148] Results from three phase I studies in cancer patients evaluating increasing doses of temsirolimus on different schedules have been reported. The first study evaluated pharmacokinetics and biological effects of temsirolimus administered as a 30-minute IV infusion daily for 5 days every 2 weeks in doses ranging from 0.75 to 19.1 mg/m^2 per day.[159,160] Grade 3 toxicities included hypocalcemia, elevation in hepatic transaminases, vomiting, and thrombocytopenia. Other toxicities were mild to moderate and included neutropenia, rash, mucositis, diarrhea, asthenia, fever, and hyperlipidemia. Hypersensitivity reactions were observed. In heavily pre-

treated patients, the RP2D was 15 mg/m^2 per day but has yet to be determined in minimally pretreated patients. In the second study, 24 patients received temsirolimus weekly as a 30-minute infusion over a dose range of 7.5 to 220 mg/m^2 per week.[153] No immunosuppressive effect was reported. At 220 mg/m^2 per week, dose-limiting manic-depressive syndrome, stomatitis, and asthenia seen in two of nine patients prevented further dose escalation. Mucocutaneous reactions were the most frequent drug-related toxicities. Other grade 3 or 4 toxicities included elevations of total cholesterol, triglycerides, and hepatic enzymes, as well as neutropenia, thrombocytopenia, and hypophosphatemia. Of 11 males who had normal baseline testosterone levels, 9 showed reduction of these levels, along with increased follicle-stimulating hormone and/or luteinizing hormone levels. All toxicities were reversible upon treatment discontinuation.

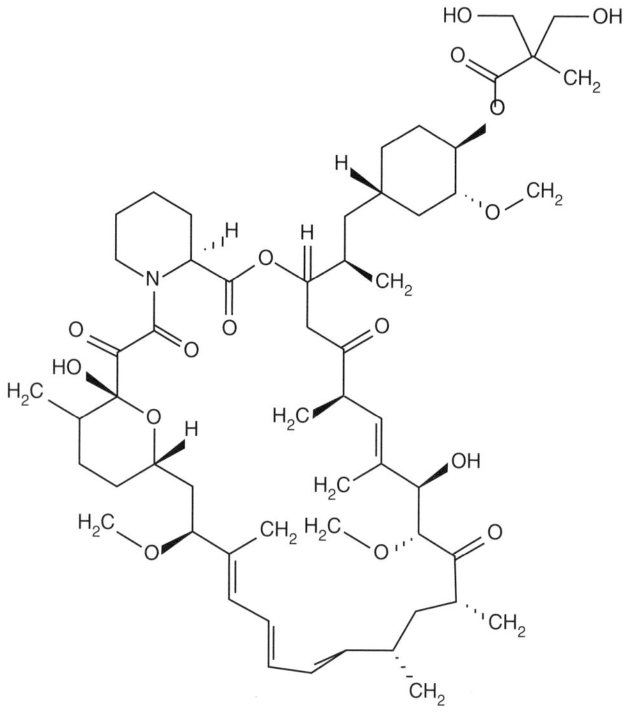

The pharmacokinetics of temsirolimus are complex. Following treatment, temsirolimus blood levels decrease in a polyexponential manner. AUCs increase proportionally with doses up to 150 mg. At doses higher than 300 mg, aberrantly high AUCs and low clearance have been seen in some patients. The mean Vd$_{ss}$ is large, 127 to 384 L. Clearance of temsirolimus increases with increasing dose, ranging from 19 to 51 L/hour. The mean terminal half-life for temsirolimus appears to decrease with increasing dose, from 22 hours following the 34 mg/m^2 dose to 13 hours following the 220 mg/m^2 dose. Significant conversion of temsirolimus to rapamycin occurs, with a mean AUC ratio (rapamycin/temsirolimus) of ~2.5 to 3.5. The mean terminal half-life for rapamycin ranges from 61 to 69 hours.

The pharmacokinetic profile and the MTD of temsirolimus administered intravenously once per week in patients with recurrent malignant gliomas taking enzyme-inducing antiepileptic drugs (EIAEDs) has also been evaluated.[161] The MTD was determined to be 250 mg administered intravenously once per week. The pharmacokinetic profiles were similar to those previously described, but the AUC of rapamycin was 1.6-fold lower for patients on EIAEDs. A phase II study is ongoing to determine the efficacy of this agent at 250 mg administered intravenously once per week in patients taking EIAEDs.

A phase I study evaluating the safety and tolerability of oral temsirolimus, 25 to 100 mg daily for 5 days every 2 weeks, indicated that at the 100-mg dose level two of six patients experienced dose-limiting toxicity consisting of grade 3 stomatitis, grade 3 AST elevation, or grade 3 solar-plantar desquamative rash.[162] The MTD/RP2D was 75-mg daily for 5 days. Preliminary pharmacokinetic data indicate that the oral agent undergoes moderately rapid absorption, that exposure is related to dose, and that rapamycin is a major metabolite. Phase II trials in patients with RCC,[163] breast carcinoma,[164–166] and mantle cell lymphoma (MCL)[167] indicated that temsirolimus may induce objective responses and/or prolong progression-free survival (PFS) compared to historical data.

Figure 25.5 Chemical structure of temsirolimus (CCI-779). (Reproduced with permission from Huang S, Bjornsti MA, Houghton PJ. Rapamycins: mechanism of action and cellular resistance. Cancer Biol Ther 2003;2:222–232.)

In the RCC phase II study, 111 patients were randomly assigned to receive 25, 75, or 250 mg of temsirolimus weekly as a 30-minute IV infusion. The reported objective response rate was 7%, and minor responses were noted in 26% of patients. Median time to tumor progression was 5.8 months, and median survival was 15 months. Neither toxicity nor efficacy was significantly influenced by dose. Eight of the nine patients treated with a single dose of 25, 75, or 250 mg had evidence of S6K activity inhibition in peripheral blood mononuclear cells (PBMCs) that was independent of the administered dose.[168]

A phase II trial of 109 advanced breast cancer patients, the majority having previously been treated with chemotherapy, found no significant difference in efficacy among patients who received 75- or 250-mg weekly doses.[164-166] However, toxicity was higher among patients receiving 250 mg weekly. Among the 98 evaluable patients, the objective response rate was 10% (10/98), and the median response duration was 5.4 months. No patients with HER-2 negative tumors had any significant response. Four patient tumors were negative for PTEN, and three of the patients with these tumors had objective tumor responses. Three specimens had HER-2 gene overexpression as shown by Herceptin test or FISH analysis, and two of the patients with these tumors had objective responses to the drug. These findings suggest that PTEN mutation and/or HER-2 overexpression in breast cancer may predict response to mTOR inhibitors.

The most promising activity has been reported in an abstract from a phase II study in which a 250-mg dose of temsirolimus is administered intravenously once weekly to previously treated patients with MCL. An overall objective response rate of 44% was seen among 18 eligible patients.[167] The 250-mg dose was not well tolerated; therefore, the trial has been modified to evaluate a lower dose (25 mg).

Two studies evaluating temsirolimus with standard agents suggest enhanced toxicity at relatively modest doses of temsirolimus. Temsirolimus given intravenously once weekly over a dose range of 5 to 25 mg with interferon-α given subcutaneously 3 times 6 million units (MU) weekly[169] necessitated dose reductions or delays in 7 of 20 patients because of hyperlipidemia, leukopenia, and hyperglycemia. In the second study, patients were treated with escalating doses of temsirolimus administered intravenously followed by leucovorin (LV), 200 mg/m² administered intravenously over 1 hour, and 5-fluorouracil (5-FU), 2,000 to 2,600 mg/m² via 24-hour IV infusion.[170] Stomatitis was the dose-limiting toxicity for the 75-mg/m² dose, and 2 of 15 patients who received 45 mg/m² temsirolimus with 5-FU and LV died from mucositis with bowel perforation. No pharmacokinetic interaction between temsirolimus and 5-FU was observed. Thus it appears that enhanced toxicity may be seen with combinations of temsirolimus and some standard anticancer agents.

Everolimus (RAD001)

Everolimus is the 42-O-(2-hydroxyethyl) derivative of rapamycin (Fig. 25.6). Preclinical studies have shown dose-dependent inhibition of tumor growth and reduced tumor vascularity.[171-173] Everolimus also potentiated the anticancer activity of a number of agents, including paclitaxel, gemcitabine, and gefitinib.[171-173]

Recently, a phase I study of everolimus administered orally 1 day a week was preliminarily reported.[171] Among patients receiving doses of 5 to 30 mg once weekly, everolimus was well tolerated, with only mild to moderate anorexia, fatigue, rash, mucositis, headache, hyperlipidemia, and gastrointestinal toxicities. Pharmacokinetic results showed that exposure (AUC) increased in proportion to dose. A plateau in peak plasma concentration occurred at doses greater than or equal to 20 mg, and the terminal half-life of the agent was 26 to 38 hours. Although the MTD was not defined, at doses of 20 mg or greater, seven of eight patients exhibited inhibition of S6K1 activity in PBMCs for at least 7 days. The data from the nonclinical and clinical studies suggest that weekly administration of 20 mg everolimus in patients gives plasma concentrations and sustained S6K1 inhibition equivalent to the pharmacokinetic and pharmacodynamic changes that correlate with antitumor effects in rodents treated at an equivalent dose and schedule,[171,172,174] and 20 mg once weekly was identified as the initial dosage for subsequent clinical investigation.[172]

A phase I study evaluating everolimus combined with gemcitabine found that 600 mg/m² gemcitabine plus 20 mg everolimus per week was not tolerated in a majority of

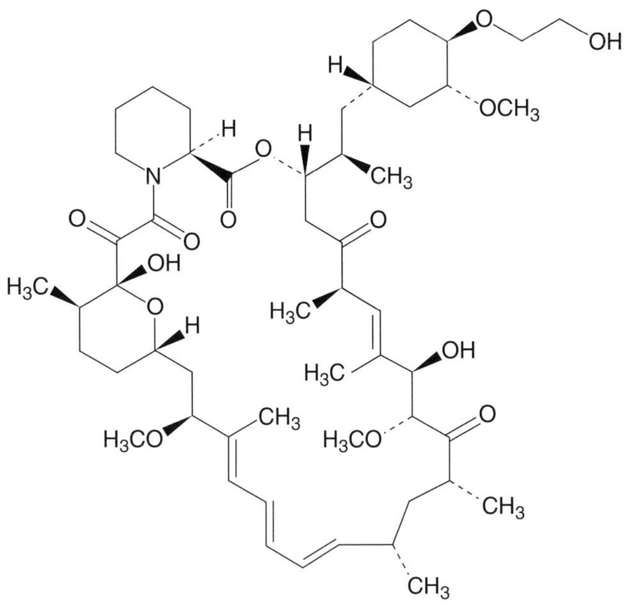

Figure 25.6 Chemical structure of everolimus. (Reproduced with permission from Huang S, Bjornsti MA, Houghton PJ. Rapamycins: mechanism of action and cellular resistance. Cancer Biol Ther 2003;2:222–232.)

patients due to myelosuppression. No apparent pharmacokinetic interaction was observed. The results of this trial are consistent with the experience with temsirolimus in combination with standard anticancer agents and suggest that modifications of dose and possibly schedule of administration of rapamycins may be required to optimize combination regimens.

AP23573

AP23573 was identified among a series of semisynthesized phosphorus-containing, C43-modified rapamycin analogs.[175] AP23573 is not a prodrug for rapamycin.[175] AP23573 potently inhibits human tumor cell line proliferation in vitro and induces partial tumor regressions in several xenograft models.[156] Tumor mTOR signaling, measured by levels of phosphorylated ribosomal S6 protein, was completely abolished for 2 to 3 days after a single administration of 1 mg/kg AP23573. As in the case of other rapamycins, in vitro studies showed that the antitumor activity of AP23573 adds to that of cytotoxic agents such as camptothecin, cisplatin, and 5-FU (ref. 156) as well as docetaxel, doxorubicin, topotecan, and trastuzumab.[176]

Two phase I trials, evaluating single daily IV doses of drug for 5 consecutive days every 14 days[154,155] and single weekly doses,[177,178] are underway. When AP23573 was administered as a 30-minute IV weekly infusion, its side effects were generally mild to moderate and reversible. The DLT was oral mucositis at 100 mg. Other grade 1 to 2 toxicities included anorexia, diarrhea, fatigue, mucositis/stomatitis, rash, and anemia. In the second study, AP23573 was administered as a 30-minute IV infusion daily for 5 days every 2 weeks in 4-week cycles.[154,155] As with the weekly schedule, dose-limiting mucositis (grade 3) occurred in two of four patients at 28 mg (140 mg total dose). Other reported toxicities included grade 3 neutropenia, thrombocytopenia, and rash and grade 1 to 2 fatigue, mucositis/stomatitis, anemia, and leukopenia. The RP2D is 18.75 mg daily for 5 days.

Pharmacokinetic analyses in these studies showed modest interindividual variability and nonproportional increase in AUC and peak concentration with dose. Unlike temsirolimus, no appreciable rapamycin was measurable. Clearance increased with dose, consistent with the saturation of distribution sites. On the weekly schedule, the drug concentration generally remained above in vitro antiproliferation IC_{50} levels until the next weekly dose. The terminal half-life was 50.5 to 65.7 hours for the daily-for-5-days schedule and 39.2 to 52 hours for the weekly schedule.

Pharmacodynamic assessment of target inhibition in PBMCs was determined by measuring phospho-4E-BP1 inhibition. Phospho-4E-BP1 levels were reduced by at least 90% within 1 hour after infusion of AP23573,[179] they remained reduced by more than 70% 48 hours after dosing, and this level of inhibition persisted in some patients for 7 to 10 days. AP23573 levels greater than 10 ng/mL gen-erally correlated with greater than 70% inhibition of phospho-4E-BP1.

Conclusions

mTOR inhibitors appear to be well tolerated, and there has been some evidence of antitumor activity in cancer patients. The most common toxicities seen are skin reactions, stomatitis, and myelosuppression. Hyperlipidemia and hyperglycemia have also been reported. These adverse effects are transient, reversible, and generally mild to moderate in severity. To date, there has been no evidence of clinically significant immunosuppression with intermittent schedules.

For temsirolimus and everolimus, the RP2Ds are below the agents' MTDs; conversely, the RP2Ds of AP23573 are the MTDs. Pharmacodynamic assays assessing inhibition of either S6K1 or 4E-BP1 phosphorylation in PBMC samples from patients treated with temsirolimus, everolimus, or AP23573 demonstrate that inhibition of mTOR kinase targets tracks with blood levels of the agents. Whether the degree and duration of inhibition in human tumors are similar to those observed in PBMCs is currently unknown. The RP2Ds of the agents appear to be within the range that can be expected to induce target inhibition based on preclinical models.

Antitumor activity has been reported among patients with a variety of malignancies with all agents. With the exception of MCL, the response rates have been low. It seems likely that only a subset of patients will have tumors sensitive to single-agent mTOR inhibitors. Limited clinical results describing correlations between objective responses seen in breast cancer patients with tumors that have HER-2 amplification or PTEN mutations suggest that the nonclinical results demonstrating correlations between enhanced signaling through the PI3K-Akt pathway may correlate with activity. Limited experience with temsirolimus or everolimus combined with cytotoxic agents suggests that doses well below the MTDs of mTOR inhibitors may be sufficient to accentuate the toxicity of standard agents. Whether antitumor activity will also be enhanced remains an unanswered question.

17-ALLYLAMINOGELDANAMYCIN (17-AAG) AND 17-(DIMETHYLAMINOETHYLAMINO)-17-DEMETHOXYGELDANAMYCIN (17-DMAG)

Introduction

The benzoquinoid ansamycin antibiotics, first isolated from the actinomycete *Streptomyces hygroscopicus* var. *geldanus* var. *nova*,[180] include geldanamycin and its semisynthetic derivatives 17-allylamino-17-demethoxygeldanamycin (17-AAG) and 17-dimethylaminoethylamino-17-demethoxygeldanamycin (17-DMAG) (see Fig. 25.7 for structure of

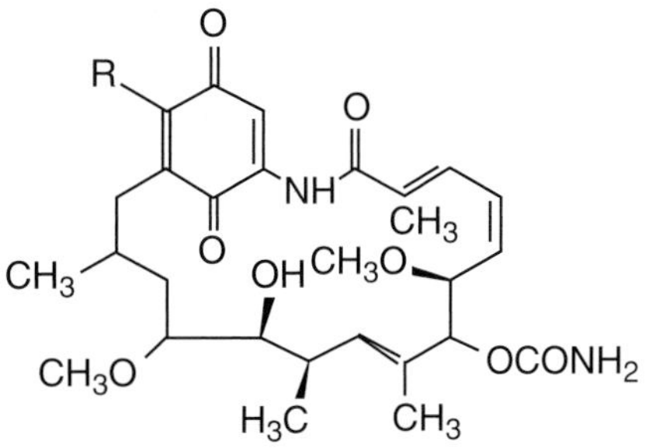

Compound	R Group
17-Allylaminogeldanamycin (17-AAG)	$CH_2=CH-CH_2-OH$
17-Aminogeldanamycin (17-AG)	NH_2
Proposed epoxide metabolite	$\overset{O}{\overset{\triangle}{H_2C-CH-CH_2}}$
Proposed diol metabolite	$\overset{OH}{\underset{OH}{\overset{\mid}{H_2C-CH-CH_2}}}$
Geldanamycin	CH_3O

Figure 25.7 Structure of geldanamycin and its derivatives.

geldanamycin and its derivatives). These small molecules inhibit the chaperone function of the heat shock protein Hsp90[181] and are currently being evaluated in phase I and II clinical trials. The parent compound, geldanamycin, is broadly cytotoxic in the NCI 60-cell line screen[182]; its poor solubility and unacceptable liver toxicity in dogs precluded testing in humans.

Because 17-AAG is less toxic than geldanamycin in rats[183] and caused growth inhibition in breast,[184] melanoma,[185] and ovarian mouse xenograft models, the NCI initiated phase I trials in 1999. Development of 17-DMAG followed soon afterwards.

Background

In the mid-1980s, while searching for compounds to inhibit the activity of malfunctioning oncogenes,[186,187] Uehara and his associates discovered the benzoquinone ansamycin antibiotics. These compounds were able to convert transformed Rous sarcoma virus-infected rat kidney cells to normal morphology. Although initially ascribed to inhibition of protein tyrosine kinase activity, the activity was subsequently shown to be related to binding to the 90-kd heat shock protein Hsp90, resulting in inhibition of src-Hsp90 heteroprotein complex formation.[188]

Heat shock proteins (Hsps, or molecular chaperones) are among the most abundant proteins found in mammalian cells.[189] Hsps are highly conserved proteins necessary for the conformational stability and functional activity of a variety of client proteins that mediate various signal transduction pathways and in some cases possess oncoprotein activity. Hsp90 also activates steroid hormone receptors (e.g., estrogen and androgen). In association with several different co-chaperones, including Hsp70 and p23, Hsp90 forms heteroprotein complexes.[190] The N-terminal domain of Hsp90 contains the binding site for ATP/ADP, is highly conserved, and binds geldanamycin.[191,192] Inhibition of Hsp90 leads to accumulation of misfolded client proteins that are then targeted for polyubiquitination and degradation by the proteasome.[193]

The geldanamycins' affinity for Hsp90's ATP-binding pocket makes them appealing therapeutic agents for treating a variety of oncologic conditions that are driven by or express clients of Hsp90.[194,195] Figure 25.8 (a and b) depicts this process.

To date, more than 100 client proteins of Hsp90 have been identified.[196] Oncologists are particularly interested in the Hsp90 client proteins listed below.[181,184,188,197–200]

- Metastable signaling proteins (e.g., soluble kinases Raf-1, AKT, IKK)
- Mutated signaling proteins (e.g., p53, KIT, FLT3, B-Raf)
- Chimeric signaling proteins (e.g., NPM-ALK, Bcr-Abl)
- Steroid receptors and bHLH/Pas domain transcription factors (e.g., androgen/estrogen/progesterone receptors, HIF-1α)
- Transmembrane tyrosine kinases—immature versus mature (e.g., HER2, EGFR, MET, KIT, IGFR)

Mechanism of Action

The geldanamycins appear to simultaneously inhibit overlapping signaling pathways and tumor cell receptors that depend on these pathways for proliferation and survival signaling. The NCI is exploring single-agent studies in diseases

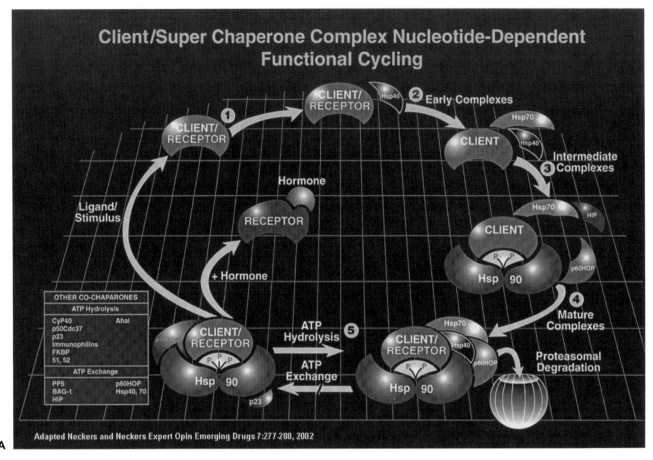

Figure 25.8 A   Hsp90 Chaperone Complex Cycling and Conformational Shuttle. A wide variety of client/receptor proteins, including oncoproteins, require chaperoned folding to achieve an active conformation for signaling and receptor/ligand interactions. 1. The client/receptor protein initially binds to Hsp40. 2. Following the initial binding of Hsp40, additional co-chaperones, such as Hsp70, are recruited for the formation of early complexes. 3. Hsp40 is released and the binding of Hip/Hop defines the formation of the intermediate Hsp90 chaperone complex. 4. The mature Hsp90 complex is formed following the release of Hsp40 and binding of Hip. This event leads to the entry of the complex into a shuttle that is ATP dependent and maintains the client/receptor in an actively-folded conformation. The active conformation then proceeds to signaling or leads to regulated degradation through E3 ligase-mediated ubiquitination. 5. The conformational shuttle is driven by ATP exchange and hydrolysis, and occurs in response to binding of other co-chaperones (Neckers and Neckers, *Expert Opin Emerging Drugs*, 2002;7:277–288.)

known to express clients of Hsp90: melanoma, anaplastic large cell lymphoma, mastocytosis, medullary thyroid carcinoma, renal cell carcinoma, Her-2-positive breast cancer, and hormone-refractory prostate cancer.

In addition, phase I combination studies were undertaken early in development to evaluate 17-AAG's biomodulatory and molecular-targeted effects with current chemotherapy for acute myelogenous leukemia (AML) and chronic lymphocytic leukemia (CLL) and with gemcitabine/cisplatin, imatinib mesylate, bortezomib (PS-341), irinotecan, Raf-1 kinase inhibitor, rituximab, and the taxanes.

Effects of Geldanamycin Derivatives on p53, p185[erbB2], and Raf-1

In vitro experiments with geldanamycin derivatives demonstrated that doses four to five times greater than the cytotoxic IC_{50} values (IC_{50} = 6–600 nM) were required to

achieve maximal effects on mutant p53, p185[erbB2], and Raf-1.[201]

Burger et al. studied melanoma xenografts that were sensitive (MEXF 276 [T/C = 6%]) or resistant (MEXF 514 [T/C = 60%]) to 17-AAG in addition to other derivative cell lines in order to better define the inhibition of Hsp90 chaperone function.[185] Hsp90 was abundantly expressed in 17-AAG–responsive MEXF 276 tumors, but expressed at lower levels in 17-AAG–resistant MEXF 514 tumors and in normal tissues. Hsp90 expression diminished markedly in the sensitive MEXF 276 tissue but not in the resistant MEXF 462 tumors treated with 80 mg/kg 17-AAG.[185] Apoptosis occurred concurrently with diminished Hsp90 expression in MEXF 276 tissues: the apoptotic index rose from 9 to 45% during drug treatment. When cell lines were exposed to concentrations of 17-AAG that cause total growth inhibition, a rapid decline in Hsp90 in the sensitive MEXF 276 cells was accompanied by translocation of Hsp90 from the

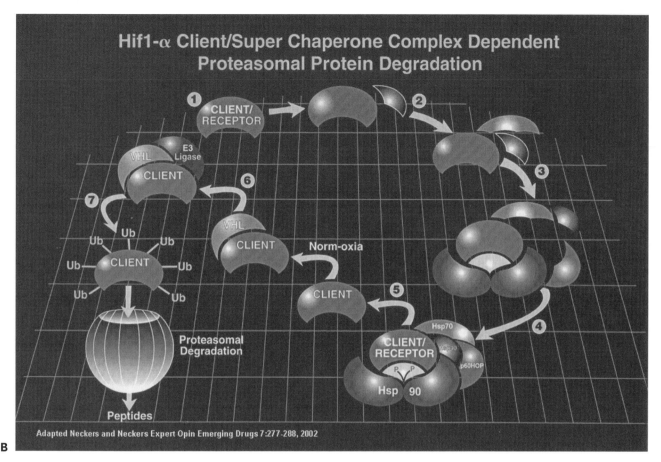

Figure 25.8 B The Hsp90 Chaperone/Client/Receptor Complex and Proteasome-Mediated Degradation The Hsp90 chaperone supercomplex cycles from early to intermediate to mature complex formation after client/receptor binding. Drive by ATP hydrolysis during the binding of co-chaperones including CyP40, p50[cdc37], p23, immunophilins, FKBP51, 52 and Aha, the chaperone supercomplex will release the client in normoxic conditions. VHL binding proceeds E3 ligase binding, by which clients are polyubiquitinated and thereby targeted for proteasomal degradation.

cytoplasm and nucleus to cell membranes. In the resistant MEXF 514, 17-AAG did not alter Hsp90 levels. After 8 hours of exposure to 17-AAG in MEXF 276 cells, Hsp90 depletion and down-regulation of Raf-1 and p185[erbB2] were observed.

Lower single-doses of 17-AAG in the 500 nM range were adequate to produce a reduction in Raf-1 protein levels detected by Western blotting at 24 hours in both HCT116 and HT29 colon adenocarcinoma cell lines.[202] In addition to Raf-1 inhibition, 17-AAG inhibited constitutive MAP kinase phosphorylation detected in HCT116 cells. Raf-1 expression was evaluated in a variety of colon adenocarcinoma cells treated with iso-effective doses of 17-AAG. The minimum effective concentration of 17-AAG was defined as that sufficient to deplete Raf-1 protein at 24 hours. In addition, total and phosphorylated Erk1/2 and c-Akt were also depleted, proliferation was inhibited in a dose-dependent manner, and an increase in floating apoptotic cells was seen.[203] This is the first report of 17-AAG–induced apoptosis mediated by the phosphoinositol-3-kinase/Akt pathway. With one exception, the expression of Bad, Bax, and Bag-1 was similar for all cell lines, and phosphoryla-tion of Bad at serine-136 but not at serine-112 was inhibited by 17-AAG.

Effects of Geldanamycin Derivatives on Other Oncoproteins and Receptors

The Bcr-Abl TK is a client protein that is chaperoned by Hsp90.[204-207] Bhalla et al. studied the apoptotic effects of 17-AAG on Bcr-Abl levels in vitro. Intracellular expression of Bcr-Abl and c-Raf protein levels were decreased following exposure to 17-AAG, as was Akt kinase activity. The binding of Bcr-Abl shifted from Hsp90 to Hsp70 after exposure to 17-AAG and induced the proteasomal degradation of Bcr-Abl, as was previously reported by An et al.[205] Treatment with the proteasome inhibitor bortezomib (PS-341) and 17-AAG resulted in down-regulation of Bcr-Abl levels and inhibition of apoptosis of both the p185- and p210-expressing cell lines. Shiotsu et al. reported that an oxime derivative of radicicol (another Hsp90 inhibitor distinct from 17-AAG), when used as a single agent, induced erythroid differentiation in K562 leukemia cells through destabilization of Bcr-Abl association with

Hsp90.[206] Further, Blagoskonny et al. demonstrated that Hsp90 inhibition with quite low doses of geldanamycin (90 nM), while not apoptotic on its own, selectively sensitized Bcr-Abl–expressing leukemia cells to cytotoxic chemotherapeutic agents such as doxorubicin and paclitaxel.[207] Imatinib mesylate–sensitive and imatinib mesylate–resistant Bcr-Abl–positive acute and chronic myelogenous leukemia cells both exhibit a reduction in Bcr-Abl expression when treated with 17-AAG.[208,209]

Growth inhibition has been observed after treatment with 17-AAG in several breast cancer cell lines with differing levels of oncogene p185[erbB2] expression. Cells with wild-type and mutated Rb appear to induce apoptosis differentially after exposure to 17-AAG.[210–212] Thus, the Rb context of the breast cancer cellular environment seems to dictate response. The breast cell lines with p185[erbB2] amplification were 10- to 100-fold more sensitive to treatment with 17-AAG. Apoptosis occurred earlier and at lower concentrations in cells overexpressing p185[erbB2]. The p185[erbB2] expression was down-regulated to almost undetectable levels 24 hours following treatment with 17-AAG. Down-regulation was associated with a number of cell cycle effects:

- arrest of cells predominantly in G_1
- accumulation of hypophosphorylated Rb
- down-regulation of cyclin D expression
- transient differentiation characterized by flattening and enlarging of the cytoplasm, intracellular lipid accumulation, and induction of milk fat globule proteins with apoptosis[210–212]

17-AAG–mediated inhibition of the Akt kinase–dependent pathway resulted in a posttranscriptional decrease in cyclin D.[210] 17-AAG does not affect PI3 kinase. Although phosphorylated AKT and Akt kinase activities were lost within 30 minutes of treatment with 17-AAG, this preceded the change in Akt protein in cells with high p185[erbB2] Akt protein expression. However, activated Akt decreased gradually over 24 hours in breast cancer cells with low p185[erbB2] expression. Differentiation was not seen in Rb-negative cells, although these cells did undergo apoptosis following drug treatment.[210,211] Transfection of Rb into cells that are not replete with Rb led to G_1 block, differentiation, and apoptosis. These studies suggest that the geldanamycins will be most effective in specific tumors and cellular environments in combination with other drugs.

The 17-AAG (200 nM)–mediated G_1 arrest observed in wild-type Rb-positive non–small cell lung cancer (NSCLC) and small cell lung cancer (SCLC) cell lines resulted in the loss of CDK4, CDK6, and cyclin E expression following a 6-hour exposure, but no changes in the levels of D-type cyclins were observed.[213] Rb-negative lung cancer cell lines did not undergo G_1 arrest when exposed to 17-AAG at concentrations from 200 nM to 5 μM.

Using MCF-7 and T47D human breast cancer cells, Bagatell et al. demonstrated that steroid receptors were destabilized and depleted by 17-AAG, geldanamycin, and KF58333.[214] Estrogen-supplemented, T47D-bearing SCID mice exhibited a marked reduction of progesterone receptor levels in the uterus and tumor following intraperitoneal (IP) administration of 17-AAG (75-mg/kg IP dose per day for 2 days). Three-week growth delay, after treatment with a 50-mg/kg IP dose per day for 5 days, was observed in established hormone-responsive MCF-7 and T47D xenografts. The role of 17-AAG–mediated alterations in steroid hormone receptor levels and clinical activity of 17-AAG will need to be established in future studies.

Nonclinical Rationale for Disease-Specific and Combination Studies

An extensive body of nonclinical work provides the rationale for clinical combination studies of the geldanamycins. The concepts supporting a combination of 17-AAG with imatinib mesylate were reviewed above. Combining the geldanamycins with other agents documented to be active in a specific disease seem rational under the following circumstances:

- the specific disease expresses client proteins.
- the specific disease relies on a client protein in a specific pathway.
- the disease is known to have a molecularly targeted critical pathway.

Preliminary results from colony-forming assays used to investigate the effects of 17-AAG and cytotoxic agents in two ovarian cell lines, A2780 and SKOV3, show that drug interactions with 17-AAG are both drug-specific and cell line–specific.[215] 17-AAG alone caused a G_1 block in A2780 cells and inhibited cell cycle progression in G_1-synchronized SKOV3 cells but did not produce a G_1 block in SKOV3 cells growing asynchronously. In both cell lines, 17-AAG and gemcitabine were generally antagonistic, while doxorubicin and docetaxel were generally additive with 17-AAG. 17-AAG and cisplatin were additive in A2780 cells and mildly synergistic in SKOV3 cells, whereas 17-AAG and etoposide were antagonistic in A2780 cells and moderately synergistic in SKOV3 cells.

17-AAG and cisplatin were additive in the colon adenocarcinoma cell line HCT116 but antagonistic in the colon cell line HT29.[216] 17-AAG and cisplatin were also antagonistic in HCTp5.2 cells, which express dominant negative p53. Induction of c-Jun by cisplatin was unaffected by 17-AAG in HCT116 cells and greatly diminished in HT29 cells. These preliminary results suggest that the combination of 17-AAG and cisplatin is additive in colon cancer cells with normal p53 but antagonistic in p53-deficient lines. Interference with cisplatin-induced apoptosis is a possible reason for 17-AAG's antagonistic action in HT29 cells.

The ability of 17-AAG to sensitize NSCLC cells expressing high levels of p185[erbB2] to paclitaxel-mediated growth arrest and apoptosis was sequence-dependent.[217] Exposure of NSCLC cell lines with low (H460 and H1299) or high (H358, H322, H661, H522) constitutive levels of p185[erbB2] to 17-AAG (20 or 80 nM) for 24 hours resulted in a significant dose-dependent reduction of p185^{erbB2} levels in all lines. Exposure of the NSCLC cells to 17-AAG for 96 hours resulted in a dose-dependent inhibition of NSCLC cell proliferation, with estimated IC$_{50}$ values of 60 to 180 nM. With concurrent exposure to 17-AAG and paclitaxel, the paclitaxel IC$_{50}$ was significantly reduced ($P \leq 0.001$) in cell lines that had high constitutive levels of p185^{erbB2}. The cytotoxic effects were synergistic in cells expressing high levels of p185^{erbB2} but only additive in cells expressing low levels of p185^{erbB2}. However, when cells were pretreated with 17-AAG for 24 hours before concurrent exposure to both agents, the paclitaxel IC$_{50}$ values were increased. Flow-cytometric analysis revealed that 17-AAG induced a G$_1$ phase arrest in NSCLC cells, which may have rendered these cells refractory to the cytotoxic effects of subsequent paclitaxel treatment, since cells are resistant to microtubule damage during the G$_1$ phase.[218]

The tumoricidal and antiangiogenic effects of the paclitaxel–17-AAG combination were evaluated in H358 tumor xenografts (a lung cancer line expressing high levels of p185^{erbB2}) in nude mice.[219,220] VEGF and p185^{erbB2} levels were reduced 2-fold and 3-fold, respectively, in H358 cells exposed to 17-AAG, and sensitivity to paclitaxel was enhanced 3- to 25-fold. Apoptosis induction was significantly increased in cells treated with the combination compared with cells treated with paclitaxel alone (32.6% vs. 9.5%, $P = 0.02$). Combinations of 17-AAG (10 or 25 mg/kg) and paclitaxel (1 mg/kg) were administered intraperitoneally per week for 4 weeks to nude mice bearing H358 tumor xenografts. The survival of animals treated with the combination was significantly longer ($P < 0.01$) than the survival of animals treated with 17-AAG or paclitaxel alone. VEGF expression and a strong reduction of capillary density occurred in tumors treated with either 17-AAG or 17-AAG–paclitaxel; however, a substantial degree of apoptosis was noted only in tumors treated with the combination. The antiproliferative and apoptotic effects induced by paclitaxel or doxorubicin in breast cancer cells with high expression of p185^{erbB2} were enhanced at concentrations of 17-AAG that down-regulated Akt kinase.[210] In cells with intact Rb, pretreatment with 17-AAG decreased paclitaxel-induced apoptosis; however, apoptosis was enhanced when 17-AAG was given after paclitaxel. The schedule dependency was not observed in Rb-negative cells or with doxorubicin.

The Chk1 pathway has emerged as a critical moderator of cellular responses activated by replication stress and various types of DNA damage.[221,222] Chk1, an Hsp90 client, is lost when cells are treated with 17-AAG. When U937 monocytic leukemia cells are treated concurrently with minimally toxic concentrations of 17-AAG (400 nM) and UCN-01 (a Chk1 inhibitor; 75 nM), apoptosis as a result of mitochondrial injury occurred.[223] Arlander et al. showed that the combination of gemcitabine and 17-AAG was markedly more effective at killing ML-1 cells than either drug alone.[224]

Recently, Schrump et al. reported that acetylation is a critical regulator of Hsp90 function.[225] Although histone deacetylase inhibitors (HDACIs) are so named because they induce hyperacetylation of the amino-terminal lysine residues of core nucleosomal histones, causing chromatin remodeling and altered gene expression,[226] HDACIs also promote hyperacetylation of various nonhistone proteins, including Hsp90. For example, Schrump et al. showed that, in NSCLC cells, the depsipeptide HDACI FR901228 induced Hsp90 hyperacetylation, antagonized the binding of ATP to Hsp90, remodeled Hsp90 co-chaperone complexes, and promoted ubiquitin-dependent and proteasome-dependent degradation of several Hsp90 client proteins, including mutated p53, ErbB1, ErbB2, and c-Raf.[225] Bhalla et al. have confirmed and extended these initial observations, demonstrating that, similar to FR901228, the HDACI LAQ824 induced Hsp90 acetylation, inhibited its binding to ATP, and stimulated enhanced degradation of the Hsp90 clients ErbB2, Akt, and c-Raf-1[227] as well as Bcr-Abl.[204,228] 17-AAG has been reported to act synergistically with HDACIs such as suberoylanilide hydroxamic acid (SAHA) to induce mitochondrial damage, caspase activation, and apoptosis in HL-60 human promyelocytic and Jurkat lymphoblastic leukemia cells.[229,230]

Oxygen homeostasis is critical in the cancer cell environment and is tightly regulated in both tumor and normal tissues. Regulation occurs through hypoxia-inducible factor 1 (HIF-1) and the highly homologous HIF-2 proteins. HIF-1 is an Hsp90 client protein.[231] HIF-1 proteins function as nuclear transcription factors and transactivate numerous target genes, many of which are implicated in the promotion of angiogenesis, such as VEGF, and in the adaptation to hypoxia.[232,233] These labile proteins are expressed in low concentrations in normoxic cells; their stability and activation increase severalfold in hypoxic conditions. Von Hipple-Lindau factor (VHL)–mediated protein binding in normoxia accounts for the instability. HIF is not degraded in hypoxic conditions because VHL function is compromised.

Both the geldanamycins and radicicol, another Hsp90 inhibitor, diminish the transcription of HIF-induced downstream effectors like VEGF231.[234-236] Proteasomal degradation of HIF is critical to the modulation of its downstream effectors. Geldanamycin decreases HIF expression by promoting the protein's VHL-independent proteasomal degradation.[235] Geldanamycin has been shown to induce proteosomal degradation of HIF-1α in prostate cancer cells[237] and to block HIF-1 induction, leading to the diminished cellular migration of U78MG, LN229, and U251MG glioma cells.[238]

The c-Met receptor TK and its ligand, hepatocyte growth factor (HGF), play a pivotal role in angiogenesis, cellular motility, differentiation, growth, and invasion in a variety of solid tumors,[239] including colorectal cancer (CRC)[240-243] and SCLC.[244] The geldanamycin analogs have been shown to disrupt the c-Met/HGF axis.[245] Treatment of VoLo human colon cancer cell lines with c-Met antisense oligonucleotides decreased c-Met protein levels, leading to programmed cell death[246]; however, the effectiveness of CRC treatment via inhibition of Hsp90-c-Met interactions by the geldanamycins has not been studied yet. No direct association was seen between Hsp90 and c-Met itself.

Oncogene-producing, dominant, gain-of-function mutations of receptor protein tyrosine kinases (RTKs) can confer uncontrolled proliferation, disordered differentiation, or uncontrolled survival through activation of multiple downstream signaling cascades.[247] These mutated oncogenic RTKs depend on Hsp90 for appropriate folding and activity. One such gain of function mutation involves the RET receptor TK and is associated with human cancer and several human neuroendocrine diseases. Point mutations of RET are responsible for multiple endocrine neoplasia type 2 (MEN2A, MEN2B) and familial medullary thyroid carcinoma (FMTC). Somatic gene rearrangements juxtaposing the TK domain of RET to heterologous gene partners are found in papillary carcinomas of the thyroid (PTC).[247–249]

To study inhibition of RET TK activity using growth inhibition assays in MTC cells, the activities of two TK inhibitors and 17-AAG were tested in the TT MTC cell line.[250] Following treatment with 200 μM genistein, a soy-based inhibitor in the Ras/PI3K pathway, or 6 μM 17-AAG for 48 hours, RET TK activity was inhibited by 87% and 72%, respectively. At the highest drug concentrations tested (100 μM imatinib mesylate, 139 μM genistein, and 3.41 μM 17-AAG), TT cell proliferation at 48 hours was inhibited by 89%, 90%, and 94%, respectively. Thus, 17-AAG, as well as other Hsp90 inhibitors, is an attractive pharmacologic agent for use in systemic therapy in patients with recurrent metastatic MTC for which nonsurgical therapy has been ineffective.

Metabolism

In human or murine hepatic microsome assays, 17-aminogeldanamycin (17-AG), a diol, and an epoxide are the three major metabolites of 17-AAG.[251] The 17-AAG diol was the major metabolite in human hepatic microsomes, followed by 17-AG; in contrast, 17-AG was the most abundant metabolite in murine microsomes. Acrolein, a nephrotoxin, is a potential by-product of the 17-AG metabolite. Finally, the epoxide is probably formed by addition of oxygen across the double bond of the allylamino side chain. CYP3A4 enzymatic metabolism is responsible for 17-AG and epoxide formation. Microsomal epoxide hydrolase catalyzes the conversion of the diol to 17-AG, which does not undergo further microsomal metabolism. 17-AAG metabolites are active and may have clinical significance. The biologically active epoxides and acrolein may induce toxic effects in humans.[251] Pharmacodynamic studies show that the 17-AG metabolite is as active as 17-AAG in decreasing cellular p185[erbB2] in human breast cancer SKBr3 cells in culture.[252] 17-AG

causes growth inhibition in six human colon cancer lines and three ovarian cancer cell lines.[253]

The quinone-metabolizing enzyme DT-diaphorase may alter 17-AAG's antitumor activity and toxicologic properties.[253] 17-AAG growth inhibitory activity was increased 32-fold by transfection of the active DT-diaphorase gene NQO1 into the DT-diaphorase–deficient BE human colon carcinoma cell line, and concomitant depletion of Raf-1 and mutant p53 protein confirmed the Hsp90 inhibition mechanism of action. Increased growth inhibition was not observed with the parent compound, geldanamycin. The increased sensitivity to 17-AAG in cell lines transfected with NQO1 was also seen in xenograft models.

In contrast to 17-AAG, 17-DMAG appears to be only minimally metabolized by CYP3A4.[254] Therefore, intestinal CYP3A4 should not impede 17-DMAG's oral activity. 17-AG does not appear to be a metabolite of 17-DMAG based on the lack of conversion at the 17 position of the compound. The marked metabolic differences between 17-AAG and 17-DMAG suggest that they may have distinct toxicity profiles and therapeutic indices.

In vitro Antitumor Studies

17-AAG exhibited a clear differential pattern of activity in the NCI in vitro cancer screen, with a mean concentration causing 50% growth inhibition (GI_{50}) of 0.19 μM and a mean concentration resulting in total growth inhibition value of 18.7 μM. Overall, the melanoma cell line panel was the most sensitive to 17-AAG, but greater than average sensitivity was demonstrated by individual cell lines in the leukemia, NSCLC, colon, ovarian, breast, prostate, and renal cancer panels.

Banerji et al. describe studies designed to provide the basis for selection of molecular pharmacodynamic markers for a clinical trial of 17-AAG.[255] The CML cell line K562 and normal human peripheral blood lymphocytes/ mononuclear cells (PBMCs) were treated with 17-AAG in vitro, and client proteins were measured by Western blotting. Raf-1 and the src family kinase member Lck were depleted following 24 hours of exposure to ≥500 nM 17-AAG. Hsp70 was also induced in response to 17-AAG. Hsp70, Hsp28, and Hsf1 were induced in K562 cells by geldanamycin, suggesting that the functional inactivation of Hsp90 may stimulate the expression of heat shock proteins in this cell line through activation of Hsf1.[256] When nude mice bearing human ovarian cancer xenografts were treated with a single IP dose of 17-AAG (80 mg/kg), client protein changes were observed at 24 hours in A2780 but not in CH1 tumors.[255]

Four cell lines (H460, H358, H322, and H661) that express varying levels of ErbB1 (EGFR) and ErbB2 (HER2/neu) oncogenes were assayed for expression of these oncogenes, the cell adhesion molecule E-cadherin, secretion of the matrix metalloproteinase 9 (MMP-9), VEGF, and their ability to invade Matrigel after 48-hour exposure to 17-AAG.[257] 17-AAG significantly depleted erbB1 or erbB2 levels in NSCLC cells expressing high levels of these proteins and effectively inhibited their growth, with IC$_{50}$ values ranging from 50 to 90 nM. Drug treatment also enhanced E-cadherin expression in H322 and H358 cells and inhibited secretion of MMP-9 and VEGF secretion by tumor cells. 17-AAG diminished hypoxia-induced up-regulation of VEGF expression as well as growth factor–mediated augmentation of MMP-9 secretion. It profoundly inhibited the ability of H322 and H358 cells to migrate through Matrigel in response to chemoattractant. Thus, 17-AAG's ability to inhibit the metastatic phenotype of lung cancer cells may make it a novel pharmacologic agent for specific molecular intervention in lung cancer.

Recently, Mimnaugh et al. showed that combining a low dose of 17-AAG (50 nM) with a low and clinically achievable dose of the proteasome inhibitor Velcade (PS-341, bortezomib) resulted in a markedly enhanced cytotoxicity that was correlated with a dramatic accumulation of insoluble polyubiquitinated proteins.[258] These investigators also demonstrated that transformed cells were much more sensitive to this drug regimen than were nontransformed cells, suggesting that the combination of an Hsp90 inhibitor and a proteasome inhibitor may prove particularly toxic to cancer cells.

In Vivo Antitumor Studies

Antitumor activity of 17-AAG has been demonstrated in melanoma,[185] breast,[259] ovarian,[255] and colon[253] xenograft models.

Mice with established BT-474 (high-level p185^{erbB2} expression) xenografts were treated with 17-AAG (20, 50, or 75 mg/kg) by daily IP injection for 5 days every 3 weeks.[260,261] Dose-dependent growth inhibition occurred without excess toxicity in the 17-AAG–treated animals. Maximum tumor regression (58%) at the 75 mg/kg–dose level was noted on day 25. 17-AAG cleared rapidly, with no drug detectable in serum by 10 hours. Expression of p185^{erbB2} and phosphorylated AKT decreased 1 hour after a single IP dose of 17-AAG 50 mg/kg, and the loss persisted 24 hours posttreatment. Total AKT protein was not changed.

Mice with established CWR22 prostate cancer xenografts using both the androgen-dependent parental line and androgen-independent sublines have been treated with 5-day cycles of 17-AAG (25 or 50 mg/kg) or vehicle alone.[262] Dose-dependent growth inhibition was noted without excess toxicity in the treated groups using both intermittent and continuous dosing schedules. A 74% loss of p185^{erbB2} and a 58% loss of AR expression were noted 2 hours posttreatment.

The growth of C6 glioma xenografts in nude mice[263] was greatly inhibited when 17-AAG (80 mg/kg) was injected intraperitoneally for 9 days (4 days the first week and 5 days the second week), starting 13 days after C6 cell implantation. The differences in tumor volumes between the 17-AAG group and a vehicle control group were significant ($P = 0.017$) at all time points from day 18 to day 35.

The mean tumor volume of the 17-AAG group on day 35 (the last day tumor volume was measured) was less than one third that of the tumor volume of the vehicle control group.

Combination with Radiation

Exposure of human prostate tumor cells (LNCaP), grown as spheroids, to 17-AAG (100 or 1,000 nM) for 96 hours before or after LET (low linear energy transfer), high dose rate irradiation (2 or 6 Gy) demonstrated supra-additive sequence-dependent responses.[264] Although incubation with 17-AAG or irradiation alone resulted in growth delays, all spheroids, except 6 of 23 exposed to 1,000 nM 17-AAG, regrew to control volumes after the delay. After the sequence consisting of 6 Gy of radiation followed by 100 nM 17-AAG, 5 of 12 spheroids failed to regrow, and after the reverse sequence (100 nM 17-AAG followed by 6 Gy of radiation), 10 of 12 failed to regrow. After the 1,000 nM 17-AAG and 6 Gy sequences, all spheroids failed to regrow. Similarly, Bisht et al. reported that 17-AAG and 17-DMAG are both potent radiosensitizers in vitro and in vivo.[265] These investigators showed that treatment of two human cervical carcinoma cell lines with these Hsp90 inhibitors resulted in an enhanced response to radiation within 6 to 48 hours after drug exposure. In addition, clinically achievable amounts of 17-AAG dramatically sensitized tumor xenografts to single and fractionated courses of irradiation and enhanced programmed and nonprogrammed cell death in the tumors.

Toxicity

Single dose range–finding, multiple dose range–finding, 5-day daily dose, and multiple-dose/DMSA formulation toxicity studies have been conducted in rats. Additionally, single dose range–finding/microdispersed formulation, multiple dose range–finding reconstituted lyophilized formulation, and 5-day daily dose with microdispersed and DMSA-formulated 17-AAG have been conducted. In those studies, the following trends were noted:

- Doses of geldanamycin exceeding 5 mg/kg in rats were generally toxic, leading to death.
- A single dose of microdispersed 17-AAG could be given in doses up to 25 mg/kg in both rats and dogs; the MTD when given daily for 5 days was 25 mg/kg per day for rats and 7.5 mg/kg per day for dogs.
- Lyophilized 17-AAG was tolerated in rats at doses up to 30 mg/kg when given daily or twice daily and in dogs at doses of 10 mg/kg per day.
- Hepatotoxicity, renal failure, and gastrointestinal toxicities (mainly emesis and diarrhea) were the DLTs in both species. Dogs also experienced gallbladder toxicities.

For 17-DMAG, similar studies were conducted, with the following results:

- When given intravenously or intraperitoneally, the maximum daily dose was 12 to 15 mg/m² per day in rats and 8 mg/m² per day in dogs.
- The main DLTs in both species were renal, gastrointestinal, hepatobiliary, and bone marrow effects.

Nonclinical Pharmacokinetics

Plasma pharmacokinetics (PK) of 17-AAG were measured by HPLC following IV administration of 27, 40, or 60 mg/kg to CD2F1 mice.[266] By noncompartmental analysis, AUCs (402, 625, and 1,739 µg/mL·min, respectively) increased proportionally for the lower doses, but a greater than linear increase was observed at the highest dose. Analysis with the trapezoidal function gave more linear AUCs: 375, 624, and 1,373 µg/mL· min, respectively, for the doses used. Total body clearance varied from 34.5 to 66.3 mg/kg per minute. The plasma data were best approximated by a two-compartment, open, linear model. Terminal half-lives ($t_{1/2}$) were 73, 87, and 361 minutes following doses of 27, 40, and 60 mg/kg, respectively. In dogs given 1-hour IV infusions of 2 to 10 mg/kg per day for 5 days, the mean $t_{1/2}$ was dose-independent and ranged from 46 to 73 minutes.[267]

In a preliminary report of studies performed in normal mice and SCID mice bearing MDA-MB-453 xenografts, both 17-AAG and 17-AG levels were below detection in normal tissues 7 hours after a single injection of 40 mg/kg 17-AAG.[259] However, 17-AAG and 17-AG levels were 0.5 to 1 µg/g in tumor tissue for more than 48 hours.

The pharmacokinetic-pharmacodynamic relationships for 17-AAG were investigated in nude mice bearing human ovarian cancer xenografts CH1 and A2780.[268,269] Following a single IP dose of 80 mg/kg, the half-lives in plasma, liver, and tumor were 0.88, 0.86, and 7.5 hours in the A2780-bearing mice and 0.89, 1.73, and 3.86 hours in the CH1-bearing mice, respectively, confirming other reports of differential drug accumulation in tumor.[268] There was no tumor response on the single-dose regimen, and Western blotting showed a minimal induction of Hsp70 at 16 to 24 hours in A2780 xenografts but not in CH1 xenografts. Tumor response was obtained with multiple dosing. The growth delay was greater in A2780 tumors (6.8 days) than in H1 tumors (2 days), and tumor growth resumed 2 to 4 days after dosing ceased. On day 4, expression of Raf-1, Lck, and CDK4 was reduced and expression of Hsp70 was increased in the mouse peripheral blood leukocytes (PBLs).[269] With the exception of Lck, which is not expressed in A2780 tumors, these changes were mirrored in the tumor tissue. These preliminary reports suggest that the use of PBLs to measure pharmacodynamic endpoints may be possible in clinical trials. The same markers are being used to guide the phase I study of 17-AAG at the investigator's institution.

Clinical Pharmacology

Plasma PKs were described in patients entered in a phase I trial of 17-AAG given daily for 5 days every 3 weeks.[270–272]

TABLE 25.3
PHARMACOKINETIC DATA FOR 17-AAG

Schedule	d×5			d×5	qwk×3 q4wk	qwk	
Parameter (units)	10–56 mg/m²	40 mg/m²	56 mg/m²	80 mg/m²	15–112 mg/m²	10–450 mg/m²	450 mg/m²
17-AAG							
Sample size	n = 15	n = 5	n = 7	n = 1	n = 9	n = 22	NA
C_{max} (nM)	530–3170	1860 ± 660	2080	2700 (30 min)			16710
$AUC_{(INF)}$ (nM·h)			6708				
$t_{1/2}$ (hr)	2.5 ± 0.5		3.8	1.5	2.8		
CL	41.0 ± 13.5 L/hr		19.9 L/hr/m²		26.6 (12.5–293.1) L/hr/m²	47.3 L/hr	
Vd_{ss} (L/m²)	86.6 ± 34.6		92			186 L	
72-hr urinary recovery	10.6%						
Reference	(271, 272)	(271)	(272)	(273)	(274, 275)	(276)	(276)
17-AG							
Sample size				n = 1			
C_{max} (nM)			770	607 (60 min)			
$AUC_{(INF)}$ (nM·hr)			5558				
$t_{1/2}$ (hr)			8.6	1.75	4.6		
CL L/hr/m²			30.8				
Vd_{ss}(L/m²)			203				
72-hr urinary recovery	7.8%						
Reference	(272)		(272)	(273)			

NA, not available.

TABLE 25.4

DCTD, NCI–SPONSORED 17-AAG AND COMBINATION PHASE I CLINICAL TRIALS

No. of Patients Planned/ Disease Type	Agent(s)	Dose/Schedule	Toxicities
70/Solid tumor	17-AAG	Dose escalation from 150 mg/m^2 (level 1) to 480 mg/m^2 (level 5) IV twice/wk for 2 wks followed by a 1 wk rest for patients with solid tumors; in adult leukemia patients, the rest is omitted	
36/Solid tumor	17-AAG	Dose escalation from 150 mg/m^2 (level 1) to 480 mg/m^2 (level 5) IV twice/wk for 2 wks followed by a 1 wk rest for patients with solid tumors; in adult leukemia patients, the rest is omitted	
38/Solid tumor	17-AAG	Dose escalations from 40 mg/m^2/day (level 1) to 301 mg/m^2/d (level 7) given on days 1, 4, 15, and 18 of a 4-wk cycle	Gr 2 hepatitis, gr 3 nausea, dypsnea
96/Solid tumor and refractory hematological malignancies	17-AAG	150 mg/m^2 twice/wk for 12 wks and escalated by 40% with each cohort; an MTD is defined independently for each population	Nausea, vomiting secondary to pancreatitis, and gr 3 fatigue
24/Solid tumor	17-AAG	220 mg/m^2/wk for 12 wks, escalating to 700 mg/m^2/wk	Gr 3 reversible hepatitis
130/Solid tumor	17-AAG	Cohort 1: from 10 mg/m^2/dose to 603 mg/m^2/dose on days 1, 8, and 15 in a 28-day cycle Cohort 2: from 10 mg/m^2/dose to 603 mg/m^2/dose on days 1, 4, 8, and 11 in a 21-day cycle	Gr 4 elevated SGOT, dypsnea, hypoxia
66/Solid tumor	17-AAG, gemcitabine and cisplatin	Cohort A: 17-AAG 154 mg/m^2 IV over 1 hr on days 1 and 8, every 21 days; gemcitabine 500 mg/m^2 IV over 30 min on days 1 and 8, every 21 days; cisplatin 30 mg/m^2 IV over 2 hrs on days 1 and 8, every 21 days B, C, D: An MTD of 17-AAG 154 mg/m^2 IV over 1 hr on days 1 and 8, every 21 days; gemcitabine 750 mg/m^2 IV over 30 min on days 1 and 8, every 21 days; cisplatin 40 mg/m^2 IV over 2 hrs on days 1 and 8, every 21 days	
30/Solid tumor	17-AAG and docetaxel	Schedule 1: Docetaxel 55 to 75 mg/m^2 IV over 1 hr on day 1, every 21 days; 17-AAG 80 to 650 mg/m^2 IV over 1 hr on day 1, every 21 days Schedule 2: Docetaxel 35 mg/m^2 IV over 1 hr on days 1, 8, and 15 every 28 days; 17-AAG 160 to 450 mg/m^2 IV over 1 hr on days 1, 8, and 15 every 28 days	
35/Solid tumor	17-AAG and paclitaxel	17-AAG 100 to 225 mg/m^2 IV over 1 hr on days 1, 4, 8, 11, 15, and 18 every 28 days Paclitaxel 80 mg/m^2 IV over 1 hr on days 1, 8, and 15 every 28 days	
18/CML	17-AAG and imatinib	Imatinib 600 mg/day PO once a day started 4–5 days prior to the first 17-AAG treatment; 17-AAG 20 to 60 mg/m^2 days 1 and 4 of wks 1 and 2, each 3 wks	Just opening
36/ALL	17-AAG and cytarabine	Cytarabine 400 mg/m^2/day CIV days 1–5; 17-AAG 100 mg/m^2 to 400 mg/m^2 IV over 60 min on days 3 and 6; repeat 30 $\pm$ 5 days after marrow recovery or hospital discharge	
30/CLL	17-AAG, fludarabine and rituximab	17-AAG 100 to 360 mg/m^2 IV over 60 min on days 1, 4, 8, 11, 15 and 18 of a 28-day cycle; fludarabine 25 mg/m^2 IVPB will be administered on days 1–5; rituximab day 1, cycle 1, 100 mg IVPB over 4 hrs; day 3, cycle 1, 375 mg/m^2 using standard escalation; day 5, cycle 1, 375 mg/m^2 using standard escalation	
74/Hematologic unspecified	17-AGG and bortezomib	17-AAG 100 mg/m^2 to 250 mg/m^2 administered over 1 hr immediately prior to PS-341 0.7 to 1.3 mg/m^2 on days 1, 4, 8, and 11 of each cycle	
42/Solid tumor	17-AAG and bortezomib	17-AAG 100 mg/m^2 to 250 mg/m^2 administered over 1 hr immediately prior to PS-341 0.7 to 1.3 mg/m^2 on days 1, 4, 8, and 11 of each cycle	
27/Solid tumor	17-AAG and BAY 43-9006	BAY 43-9006 400 mg BID starting 2 wks prior to 17-AAG 100 mg/m^2 to 250 mg/m^2 on days 1, 8, and 15 every 28 days	
46/Solid tumor	17-AAG and irinotecan	Irinotecan 85 mg/m^2 to 125 mg/m^2 followed by 17-AAG 220 mg/m^2 to 450 mg/m^2 once/wk for 2 wks in a 21-day cycle	

TABLE 25.5

DCTD, NCI–SPONSORED 17-AAG PHASE II CLINICAL TRIALS

No. of Patients Planned/Disease Type	Dose/Schedule
40/Ovarian epithelial cancer stage IV	17-AAG 220 mg/m^2 IV over 1 hr on days 1, 4, 8, and 11, every 21 days
26/Clear cell carcinoma of the kidney	17 AAG 300 mg/m^2 IV over 1–2 hrs on days 1, 8, 15, every 28 days
36/Malignant mast cell neoplasm	17-AAG 220 mg/m^2 IV over 1 hr on days 1, 4, 8, and 11, every 3 wks
58/Renal cell carcinoma stage IV	17-AAG 220 mg/m^2 IV over 60–90 min twice/wk for 2 wks; cycle = 21 days
50/Malignant melanoma stage IV	17-AAG 450 mg/m^2 IV over 1–2 hr every wk × 6 wks, every 8 wks
72/Medullary thyroid cancer	17-AAG 220 mg/m^2 IV over 1 hr on days 1, 4, 8, and 11, every 21 days
25/Malignant melanoma stage IV	17-AAG 450 mg/m^2 IV over 1 hr once every 7 days, for 12 wks
41/Breast cancer stage IV	17-AAG 220 mg/m^2 IV over 1 hr on days 1, 4, 8, and 11, every 21 days
28/Prostate cancer stage IV	17 AAG 300 mg/m^2 IV over 1–2 hrs on days 1, 8, 15, every 28 days
70/Mantle cell lymphoma	17-AAG 220 mg/m^2 IV over 1 hr on days 1, 4, 8, and 11, every 21 days

One patient each was treated at dose levels of 10, 14, 20, and 28 mg/m^2, eight patients at 40 mg/m^2, and seven patients at 56 mg/m^2. A two-compartment, open model best fit the PK data.[271] Mean values for terminal $t_{1/2}$, clearance, and Vd_{ss} were 2.5 ± 0.5 hours, 41.0 ± 13.5 L/hour, and 86.6 ± 34.6 L/m^2, respectively. Peak plasma concentrations reached $3,170 \pm 1,310$ nM at 56 mg/m^2.[271] Using noncompartmental analysis of data from patients treated with 56 mg/m^2, the average values for 17-AAG and 17-AG, respectively, were as follows: $C_{max} = 2,080$ and 770 nM; AUC = 6,708 and 5,558 nM · hour; terminal $t_{1/2} = 3.8$ and 8.6 hours.[272] Clearances of 17-AAG and 17-AG were 19.9 and 30.8 L/m^2 per hour, and the Vd_{ss} values were 92 and 203 L/m^2, respectively. Over all dose levels, the total amount of drug recovered in urine was 10.6% for 17-AAG and 7.8% for 17-AG. There were no significant differences between day 1 and day 5 PK values. The MTD was

40 mg/m^2, a dose at which Hsp90 inhibition would be expected. Another phase I trial that used the same daily × 5 schedule provided PK data for the 80 mg/m^2 dose.[273] The $t_{1/2}$ was 1.5 hours, and the peak plasma level was 2,700 nM at 30 minutes. Plasma levels at 1, 6, 24, 72, and 96 hours were 1,930, 190, 36, 63, and 57 nM, respectively. For the active metabolite, 17-AG, the $t_{1/2}$ was 1.75 hours, and the peak plasma level was 607 nM at 1 hour. 17-AG plasma levels at 0.5, 6, 24, 72, and 96 hours were 262, 138, 46, 101, and 39 nM, respectively. Thus, concentrations exceeded in vitro and xenograft concentrations of 10 to 500 nM for cell kill.

Preliminary PK and pharmacodynamic data have also been reported from a phase I trial of 17-AAG given once weekly for 3 out of every 4 weeks.[274,275] The median clearance of 17-AAG from plasma samples ($n = 9$) drawn on day 1 was 412 mL/m^2 per minute (range 208 to 4,885). The

---

TABLE 25.6

DCTD, NCI–SPONSORED 17-DMAG PHASE I CLINICAL TRIALS

No. of Patients Planned/Disease Type	Dose/Schedule
30/Solid tumor	17-DMAG 2.5 mg/m^2 to 40 mg/m^2 IV wkly × 3
40/Solid tumor	17-DMAG 1mg/m^2 to 40 mg/m^2 IV over 1 hr on days 1 and 4 each wk; cycle = 4 wks
30/Solid tumor	17-DMAG 1.25 mg/m^2 to 10 mg/m^2 IV over 1 hr each wk; cycle = 4 wks
60/Solid tumor	17-DMAG 1.5 mg/m^2 to 19 mg/m^2 IV over 1 hr daily × 5, every 21 days

C_{max} increased linearly with dose, and the $t_{1/2}$ was 166 ± 115 minutes.[275] The $t_{1/2}$ for 17-AG was 277 minutes (4.6 hours). 17-AAG was a substrate for both the CYP3A4 and CYP3A5 enzyme systems.[275]

Pharmacokinetic data for 17-AAG from NCI-sponsored trials are summarized in Table 25.3.

Clinical Trial Data

A phase I Institute of Cancer Research (UK) trial of 17-AAG in solid tumors used a once weekly administration schedule. The starting dose was 10 mg/m^2 per week administered intravenously once weekly in a cohort of three patients. Doses were doubled in each succeeding cohort.[277] Adverse events included grade 1 to 2 nausea and grade 1 to 2 fatigue in 3 and 9 of the first 15 patients, respectively. One patient experienced grade 3 vomiting at the 80 mg/m^2 per week dose. Grade 3 nausea and vomiting occurred in two of six patients treated at the 320 mg/m^2 per week dose, following which the dose was escalated by 40% to 450 mg/m^2 per week.[276] The DLT at 450 mg/m^2 per week was a grade 3 to 4 elevation of AST/ALT in one of six patients.[278] A total of 28 patients have been treated on this trial. Among the six patients treated in the 320 to 450 mg/m^2 per week dose range, two patients showed stable disease for 27 and 91 weeks, respectively.

PD marker analysis of tumor biopsies done before and 24 hours after treatment in nine patients showed depletion of c-Raf in four of seven samples (where the marker was expressed) and CDK4 depletion and Hsp70 induction in eight of the nine samples.[278] At the highest dose level, PK analysis indicated a $t_{1/2}$ of 5.8 ± 1.9 hours, a Vd$_{ss}$ of 274 ± 108 L, clearance of 35.5 ± 16.6 L/h, and a C_{max} of 16.2 ± 6.3 μM (ref. 278), which is above the levels of 375 nM to 10 μM reported to inhibit Hsp90 in vitro.[279] Although an MTD was not established in this trial, the RP2D is likely to be 450 mg/m^2 per week, as there was evidence of tumor target inhibition at that dose level.[278] Analysis of duration of target inhibition is ongoing.

The NCI, has sponsored 17 phase I studies (7 single agent and 10 combination) to evaluate 17-AAG. An overview of these trials is presented in Tables 25.4 and 25.5. Table 25.6 shows the four trials currently being planned or conducted with 17-DMAG. Of note, dosing was adjusted based on results from early phase I work. In one study, patients with advanced solid tumors were treated with a 60-minute IV infusion for 5 consecutive days every 3 weeks. An MTD of 40 mg/m^2 per dose was established.[271] In a second study, patients with advanced solid tumors who received daily doses for 5 days every 3 weeks reached an MTD of 80 mg/m^2 per dose.[273] Increasing the dosing interval to days 1, 8, and 15 of a 3-week cycle resulted in an MTD of 308 mg/m^2 per dose,[274] and this protocol was amended to alter the dosing to days 1, 4, 8, and 11 based on PK endpoints. Additionally, when patients were dosed once weekly for 4 weeks, dosing could be escalated to 450 mg/m^2 per dose.[276,277] Thus, protocols have been amended to reflect the best dosing schedule.

The Hsp90 inhibitors are a class of agents that affect a diverse group of client proteins involved in oncogenesis. Many of these clients are expressed in a disease-specific fashion. The development of these inhibitors as biomodulators is complex and not necessarily governed by standard approaches. The clinical approach taken with the Hsp90 inhibitors was to proceed simultaneously with single-agent phase II studies as well as disease-specific combinations that would be used to evaluate the biomodulatory effects of the geldanamycins. The ongoing clinical trials outlined in the tables will be used to assess activity of the agents in a disease-specific fashion and to provide a response comparison for the phase I combinations in order to proceed into disease-specific phase II investigations. As these studies mature and reach completion, the role of Hsp90 inhibitors in the treatment of cancer should be better defined with regard to their activity and molecular targeted effects.

REFERENCES

1. Bohnsack BL, Hirschi KK. Nutrient regulation of cell cycle progression. Annu Rev Nutr 2004;24:433–453.
2. Hartwell LH, Kastan MB. Cell cycle control and cancer. Science 1994;266:1821–1828.
3. Senderowicz AM. Small-molecule cyclin-dependent kinase modulators. Oncogene 2003;22:6609–6620.
4. Sherr CJ. Cancer cell cycles. Science 1996;274:1672–1677.
5. Senderowicz AM. Novel direct and indirect cyclin-dependent kinase modulators for the prevention and treatment of human neoplasms. Cancer Chemother Pharmacol 2003;52(Suppl 1):S61–73.
6. Fischer PM, Gianella-Borradori A. CDK inhibitors in clinical development for the treatment of cancer. Expert Opin Investig Drugs 2003;12:955–970.
7. Hardcastle IR, Golding BT, Griffin RJ. Designing inhibitors of cyclin-dependent kinases. Annu Rev Pharmacol Toxicol 2002;42:325–348.
8. Dai Y, Grant S. Small molecule inhibitors targeting cyclin-dependent kinases as anticancer agents. Curr Oncol Rep 2004;6:123–130.
9. Sedlacek HH. Mechanisms of action of flavopiridol. Crit Rev Oncol Hematol 2001;38:139–170.
10. Chao SH, Price DH. Flavopiridol inactivates P-TEFb and blocks most RNA polymerase II transcription in vivo. J Biol Chem 2001;276:31793–31799.
11. Carlson B, Lahusen T, Singh S, et al. Down-regulation of cyclin D1 by transcriptional repression in MCF-7 human breast carcinoma cells induced by flavopiridol. Cancer Res 1999;59:4634–4641.
12. Lin TS, Dalton JT, Wu D, et al. Flavopiridol given as a 30-min intravenous (IV) bolus followed by 4-hr continuous IV infusion (CIVI) results in clinical activity and tumor lysis in refractory chronic lymphocytic leukemia (CLL). Proc ASCO 2004;23:A6564.
13. McClue SJ, Blake D, Clarke R, et al. In vitro and in vivo antitumor properties of the cyclin dependent kinase inhibitor CYC202 (R-roscovitine). Int J Cancer 2002;102:463–468.
14. Whittaker SR, Walton MI, Garrett MD, et al. The cyclin-dependent kinase inhibitor CYC202 (R-roscovitine) inhibits retinoblastoma protein phosphorylation, causes loss of cyclin D1, and activates the mitogen-activated protein kinase pathway. Cancer Res 2004;64:262–272.
15. White JD, Cassidy J, Twelves C, et al. A phase I trial of the oral cyclin dependent kinase inhibitor CYC202 in patients with advanced malignancy. Proc ASCO 2004;23:A3042.
16. Pierga J-Y, Faivre S, Vera K, et al. A phase I and pharmacokinetic (PK) trial of CYC202, a novel oral cyclin-dependent kinase (CDK) inhibitor, in patients (pts) with advanced solid tumors. Proc ASCO 2003;22:A840.
17. Fukuoka K, Usuda J, Iwamoto Y, et al. Mechanisms of action of the novel sulfonamide anticancer agent E7070 on cell cycle

progression in human non-small cell lung cancer cells. Invest New Drugs 2001;19:219–227.

18. Supuran CT. Indisulam: an anticancer sulfonamide in clinical development. Expert Opin Investig Drugs 2003;12:283–287.

19. Van Kesteren C, Beijnen JH, Schellens JH. E7070: a novel synthetic sulfonamide targeting the cell cycle progression for the treatment of cancer. Anticancer Drugs 2002;13:989–997.

20. Misra RN, Xiao HY, Kim KS, et al. N-(cycloalkylamino)acyl-2-aminothiazole inhibitors of cyclin-dependent kinase 2. N-[5-[[[5-(1,1-dimethylethyl)-2-oxazolyl]methyl]thio]-2-thiazolyl]-4-piperidinecarboxamide (BMS-387032), a highly efficacious and selective antitumor agent. J Med Chem 2004;47:1719–1728.

21. McCormick J, Gadgeel SM, Helmke W, et al. Phase I study of BMS-387032, a cyclin dependent kinase (CDK) 2 inhibitor. Proc ASCO 2003;22:A835.

22. Shapiro G, Lewis N, Bai S, et al. A phase I study to determine the safety and pharmacokinetics (PK) of BMS-387032 with a 24-hr infusion given every three weeks in patients with metastatic refractory solid tumors. Proc ASCO 2003;22:A799.

23. Jones SF, Burris HA, Kies M, et al. A phase I study to determine the safety and pharmacokinetics (PK) of BMS-387032 given intravenously every three weeks in patients with metastatic refractory solid tumors. Proc ASCO 2003;22:A798.

24. Kaur G, Stetler-Stevenson M, Sebers S, et al. Growth inhibition with reversible cell cycle arrest of carcinoma cells by flavone L86-8275. J Natl Cancer Inst 1992;84:1736–1740.

25. Naik RG, Dattige SL, Bhat SV, et al. An anti-inflammatory cum immunomodulatory piperidinylbenzopyranone from *Dysoxylum binectariferum*: isolation, structure, and total synthesis. Tetrahedron 1988;44:2081–2086.

26. Zhai S, Senderowicz AM, Sausville EA, et al. Flavopiridol, a novel cyclin-dependent kinase inhibitor, in clinical development. Ann Pharmacother 2002;36:905–911.

27. Bible KC, Kaufmann SH. Flavopiridol: a cytotoxic flavone that induces cell death in noncycling A549 human lung carcinoma cells. Cancer Res 1996;56:4856–4861.

28. Byrd JC, Shinn C, Waselenko JK, et al. Flavopiridol induces apoptosis in chronic lymphocytic leukemia cells via activation of caspase-3 without evidence of bcl-2 modulation or dependence on functional p53. Blood 1998;92:3804–3816.

29. Shapiro GI, Koestner DA, Matranga CB, et al. Flavopiridol induces cell cycle arrest and p53-independent apoptosis in non-small cell lung cancer cell lines. Clin Cancer Res 1999;5: 2925–2938.

30. Czech J, Hoffmann D, Naik R, et al. Antitumoral activity of flavone L86-8275. Int J Cancer 1995;6:31–36.

31. Patel V, Senderowicz AM, Pinto D, Jr, et al. Flavopiridol, a novel cyclin-dependent kinase inhibitor, suppresses the growth of head and neck squamous cell carcinomas by inducing apoptosis. J Clin Invest 1998;102:1674–1681.

32. Newcomb EW, Crisan D, Miller DC, et al. Therapeutic potential of flavopiridol in GL261 mouse glioma model. Proc AACR 2003;44:A714.

33. Arguello F, Alexander M, Sterry JA, et al. Flavopiridol induces apoptosis of normal lymphoid cells, causes immunosuppression, and has potent antitumor activity in vivo against human leukemia and lymphoma xenografts. Blood 1998;91:2482–2490.

34. Senderowicz AM, Headlee D, Stinson SF, et al. Phase I trial of continuous infusion flavopiridol, a novel cyclin-dependent kinase inhibitor, in patients with refractory neoplasms. J Clin Oncol 1998;16:2986–2999.

35. Thomas JP, Tutsch KD, Cleary JF, et al. Phase I clinical and pharmacokinetic trial of the cyclin-dependent kinase inhibitor flavopiridol. Cancer Chemother Pharmacol 2002;50:465–472.

36. Tan AR, Headlee D, Messmann R, et al. Phase I clinical and pharmacokinetic study of flavopiridol administered as a daily 1-hour infusion in patients with advanced neoplasms. J Clin Oncol 2002;20:4074–4082.

37. Zhai S, Sausville EA, Senderowicz AM, et al. Clinical pharmacology and pharmacogenetics of flavopiridol 1-h i.v. infusion in patients with refractory neoplasms. Anticancer Drugs 2003;14:125–135.

38. Senderowicz A, Messmann R, Arbuck S, et al. A phase I trial of 1 hour infusion of flavopiridol (FLA), a novel cyclin-dependent kinase inhibitor, in patients with advanced neoplasms. Proc ASCO 2000;19:A796.

39. Mizunuma N, Nagasaki E, Hatake K, et al. A phase I trial with a weekly one-hour infusion of flavopiridol (HMR1275), a cyclin dependent kinase (CDK) inhibitor. Proc ASCO 2004;23:A3160.

40. Sasaki Y, Sasaki T, Minami H, et al. A phase I pharmacokinetic (PK)- pharmacodynamic (PD) study of flavopiridol by 24 hours continuous infusion (CI) repeating every week. Proc Am Soc Clin Oncol 2002;21:A371.

41. Gries J-M, Bond J, Rodrigues L, et al. Phase I study of flavopiridol 24 hour infusion monotherapy in solid tumors (HMR1275/1002). Proc ASCO 2003;22:A564.

42. Byrd JC. Personal communication. 2004.

43. Kasimis B, Rocha-Lima C, Cogswell J, et al. Phase I study evaluating 1-hour flavopiridol (HMR1275) in combination with docetaxel (D) in previously treated non-small cell lung cancer (NSCLC) patients (pts) (HMR1275B/1008). Proc ASCO2003;22:A2689.

44. Rathkopf D, Fornier M, Shah M, et al. A phase I dose finding study of weekly, sequential docetaxel (Doc) followed by flavopiridol (F) in patients with advanced solid tumors. Proc ASCO 2004;23:A3072.

45. Schwartz GK, O'Reilly E, Ilson D, et al. Phase I study of the cyclin-dependent kinase inhibitor flavopiridol in combination with paclitaxel in patients with advanced solid tumors. J Clin Oncol 2002;20:2157–2170.

46. Bible KC, Lensing JL, Nelson SA, et al. A phase I trial of flavopiridol combined with cisplatin in patients with advanced malignancies. Proc AACR 2002;43:A2749.

47. Shah MA, Kortmansky J, Gonen M, et al. Mature results of a phase I study of irinotecan (CPT) and flavopiridol (F): a clinically and biologically active regimen. Proc ASCO 2003;22:A1051.

48. Patel B, El-Rayes BF, Gadgeel SM, et al. A phase I study of flavopiridol and docetaxel. Proc ASCO 2003;22:A932.

49. Tan AR, Zhai S, Berman AW, et al. Phase I trial of docetaxel followed by infusional flavopiridol over 72 hours in patients with metastatic breast cancer. Proc ASCO 2002;21:A1955.

50. Shah MA, Kortmansky J, Gonen M, et al. A phase I/pharmaceutical study of weekly sequential irinotecan (CPT) and flavopiridol (F). Proc ASCO 2002;21:A373.

51. Shah MA, Kaubisch A, O'Reilly E, et al. A phase IB clinical trial of the sequence dependent combination of paclitaxel (P) and cisplatin with the cyclin dependent kinase (CDK) inhibitor flavopiridol in patients with advanced solid tumors. Proc AACR 2001;42:A2917.

52. Gries JM, Kasimis B, Schwarzenberger P, et al. Phase I study of HMR1275 (flavopiridol) in non-small cell lung cancer (NSCLC) patients after 24 hr IV administration in combination with paclitaxel and carboplatin. Proc ASCO 2002;21:A372.

53. Shah MA, Kortmansky J, Gonen M, et al. A phase I study of weekly irinotecan (CPT), cisplatin (CIS) and flavopiridol (F). Proc ASCO 2004;23:A4027.

54. Bible KC, Lensing JL, Nelson SA, et al. A phase 1 trial of flavopiridol combined with 5-fluorouracil (5-FU) and leucovorin (CF) in patients with advanced malignancies. Proc ASCO 2003;22:A872.

55. Gries J, Kasimis B, Schwarzenberger P, et al. Phase I study of flavopiridol (HMR1275) in combination with paclitaxel and carboplatin in non-small cell lung cancer (NCSLC) patients. Eur J Cancer 2002;38 (Suppl 7):49 (A152).

56. Rudek MA, Bauer KS Jr, Lush RM 3rd, et al. Clinical pharmacology of flavopiridol following a 72-hour continuous infusion. Ann Pharmacother 2003;37:1369–1374.

57. Innocenti F, Stadler WM, Iyer L, et al. Flavopiridol metabolism in cancer patients is associated with the occurrence of diarrhea. Clin Cancer Res 2000;6:3400–3405.

58. Kouroukis CT, Belch A, Crump M, et al. Flavopiridol in untreated or relapsed mantle-cell lymphoma: results of a phase II study of the National Cancer Institute of Canada Clinical Trials Group. J Clin Oncol 2003;21:1740–1745.

59. Burdette-Radoux S, Tozer RG, Lohman R, et al. NCIC CTG phase II study of flavopiridol in patients with previously untreated metastatic malignant melanoma (IND.137). Proc ASCO 2002; 21:A1382.

60. Van Veldhuizen PJ, Faulkner JR, Lara PN, et al. A phase II study of flavopiridol (Flavo) in patients (pts) with advanced renal cell cancer: results of Southwest Oncology Group trial S0109. Proc ASCO 2003;22:A1553.

61. Aklilu M, Kindler HL, Donehower RC, et al. Phase II study of flavopiridol in patients with advanced colorectal cancer. Ann Oncol 2003;14:1270–1273.
62. Shapiro GI, Supko JG, Patterson A, et al. A phase II trial of the cyclin-dependent kinase inhibitor flavopiridol in patients with previously untreated stage IV non-small cell lung cancer. Clin Cancer Res 2001;7:1590–1599.
63. King DM, Lara P, Gandara DR, et al. A phase II trial of flavopiridol in patients with metastatic androgen independent prostate cancer. Proc ASCO 2003;22:A1736.
64. Schwartz GK, Ilson D, Saltz L, et al. Phase II study of the cyclin-dependent kinase inhibitor flavopiridol administered to patients with advanced gastric carcinoma. J Clin Oncol 2001;19:1985–1992.
65. Stadler WM, Vogelzang NJ, Amato R, et al. Flavopiridol, a novel cyclin-dependent kinase inhibitor, in metastatic renal cancer: a University of Chicago Phase II Consortium study. J Clin Oncol 2000;18:371–375.
66. Vale RD, Fletterick RJ. The design plan of kinesin motors. Annu Rev Cell Dev Biol 1997;13:745–777.
67. Funk CJ, Davis AS, Hopkins JA, et al. Development of high-throughput screens for discovery of kinesin adenosine triphosphatase modulators. Anal Biochem 2004;329:68–76.
68. Hegde PS, Cogswell J, Carrick K, et al. Differential gene expression analysis of kinesin spindle protein in human solid tumors. Proc ASCO 2003;39:A535.
69. Mak J, Freedman R, Beraud C. Utilization of gene expression profiles to identify mitotic kinesins. Proc AACR 2002;93:A5375.
70. Yan Y, Sardana V, Xu B, et al. Inhibition of a mitotic motor protein: where, how, and conformational consequences. J Mol Biol 2004;335:547–554.
71. Nigg EA, Blangy A, Lane HA. Dynamic changes in nuclear architecture during mitosis: on the role of protein phosphorylation in spindle assembly and chromosome segregation. Exp Cell Res 1996;229:174–180.
72. Gonzales P, Boehme M, Bienek A, et al. Breadth of anti-tumor activity of CK0238273 (SB-715992), a novel inhibitor of the mitotic kinesin KSP. Proc AACR 2002;95:A1337.
73. Chu Q, Holen KD, Rowinsky EK, et al. A phase I study to determine the safety and pharmacokinetics of IV administered SB-715992, a novel kinesin spindle protein (KSP) inhibitor, in patients (pts) with solid tumors. Proc ASCO 2003;39:A525.
74. Johnson RK, McCabe FL, Caulder E, et al. SB-715992, a potent and selective inhibitor of the mitotic kinesin KSP, demonstrates broad-spectrum activity in advanced murine tumors and human tumor xenografts. Proc AACR 2002;93:A1335.
75. Burris HA, Lorusso P, Jones S, et al. Phase I trial of novel kinesin spindle protein (KSP) inhibitor SB-715992 IV days 1, 8, 15 q 28 days. Proc ASCO 2004;40:A2004.
76. Chu Q, Holen KD, Rowinsky EK, et al. A phase I trial of novel kinesin spindle protein (KSP) inhibitor SB-715992 administered intravenously once every 21 days. Proc ASCO 2004;40:A2078.
77. Kerr JS, Slee AM, Mousa SA. The alpha v integrin antagonists as novel anticancer agents: an update. Expert Opin Investig Drugs 2002;11:1765–1774.
78. Tucker GC. Alpha v integrin inhibitors and cancer therapy. Curr Opin Investig Drugs 2003;4:722–731.
79. Hood JD, Cheresh DA. Role of integrins in cell invasion and migration. Nat Rev Cancer 2002;2:91–100.
80. Eliceiri BP, Cheresh DA. The role of alphav integrins during angiogenesis: insights into potential mechanisms of action and clinical development. J Clin Invest 1999;103:1227–1230.
81. Gladson CL, Cheresh DA. Glioblastoma expression of vitronectin and the alpha v beta 3 integrin: adhesion mechanism for transformed glial cells. J Clin Invest 1991;88:1924–1932.
82. Gladson CL. Expression of integrin alpha v beta 3 in small blood vessels of glioblastoma tumors. J Neuropathol Exp Neurol 1996;55:1143–1149.
83. Liapis H, Adler LM, Wick MR, et al. Expression of alpha(v)beta3 integrin is less frequent in ovarian epithelial tumors of low malignant potential in contrast to ovarian carcinomas. Hum Pathol 1997;28:443–449.
84. Felding-Habermann B, Mueller BM, Romerdahl CA, et al. Involvement of integrin alpha v gene expression in human melanoma tumorigenicity. J Clin Invest 1992;89:2018–2022.
85. Hieken TJ, Farolan M, Ronan SG, et al. Beta3 integrin expression in melanoma predicts subsequent metastasis. J Surg Res 1996;63:169–173.
86. Hosotani R, Kawaguchi M, Masui T, et al. Expression of integrin alphaVbeta3 in pancreatic carcinoma: relation to MMP-2 activation and lymph node metastasis. Pancreas 2002;25:e30–35.
87. Zheng DQ, Woodard AS, Fornaro M, et al. Prostatic carcinoma cell migration via alpha(v)beta3 integrin is modulated by a focal adhesion kinase pathway. Cancer Res 1999;59:1655–1664.
88. Friedlander M, Brooks PC, Shaffer RW, et al. Definition of two angiogenic pathways by distinct alpha v integrins. Science 1995;270:1500–1502.
89. Brooks PC, Montgomery AM, Rosenfield M, et al. Integrin alphavbeta3 antagonists promote tumor regression by inducing apoptosis of angiogenic blood vessels. Cell 1994;79:1157–1164.
90. Brooks PC, Montgomery AM, Rosenfeld M, et al. Integrin alpha v beta 3 antagonists promote tumor regression by inducing apoptosis of angiogenic blood vessels. Cell 1994;79:1157–1164.
91. Stromblad S, Becker JC, Yebra M, et al. Suppression of p53 activity and p21WAF1/CIP1 expression by vascular cell integrin alphaVbeta3 during angiogenesis. J Clin Invest 1996;98:426–433.
92. Faivre SJ, Chieze S, Marty M, et al. Safety profile and pharmacokinetic analysis of Medi-522, a novel humanized monoclonal antibody that targets αvβ3 integrin receptor, in patients with refractory solid tumors. Proc ASCO 2003;39:A832.
93. Pizzolato JF, Sharma S, Maki R, et al. Phase I study of Medi-522, an avb3 integrin inhibitor, in patients (pts) with irinotecan-refractory colorectal cancer (CRC). Proc ASCO 2003;39:A983.
94. Nisato RE, Tille JC, Jonczyk A, et al. alpha v beta 3 and alpha v beta 5 integrin antagonists inhibit angiogenesis in vitro. Angiogenesis 2003;6:105–119.
95. Eskens FA, Dumez H, Hoekstra R, et al. Phase I and pharmacokinetic study of continuous twice weekly intravenous administration of Cilengitide (EMD 121974), a novel inhibitor of the integrins alphavbeta3 and alphavbeta5 in patients with advanced solid tumours. Eur J Cancer 2003;39:917–926.
96. Mitjans F, Meyer T, Fittschen C, et al. In vivo therapy of malignant melanoma by means of antagonists of alphav integrins. Int J Cancer 2000;87:716–723.
97. MacDonald TJ, Taga T, Shimada H, et al. Preferential susceptibility of brain tumors to the antiangiogenic effects of an alpha(v) integrin antagonist. Neurosurgery 2001;48:151–157.
98. Nabors LB, Rosenfeld SS, Mikkelson T, et al. Abstracts from the Ninth Annual Meeting of the Society for Neuro-Oncology, November 18–21: a phase I trial of EMD 121974 for treatment of patients with recurrent malignant gliomas. Neuro-Oncol 2004;6:379(TA-39).
99. Huang S, Houghton PJ. Targeting mTOR signaling for cancer therapy. Curr Opin Pharmacol 2003;3:371–377.
100. Vivanco I, Sawyers CL. The phosphatidylinositol 3-Kinase AKT pathway in human cancer. Nat Rev Cancer 2002;2:489–501.
101. Brugarolas J, Lei K, Hurley RL, et al. Regulation of mTOR function in response to hypoxia by REDD1 and the TSC1/TSC2 tumor suppressor complex. Genes Dev 2004;18:2893–2904.
102. Kwiatkowski DJ. Tuberous sclerosis: from tubers to mTOR. Ann Hum Genet 2003;67:87–96.
103. Kwiatkowski DJ. Rhebbing up mTOR: new insights on TSC1 and TSC2, and the pathogenesis of tuberous sclerosis. Cancer Biol Ther 2003;2:471–476.
104. Manning BD, Cantley LC. Rheb fills a GAP between TSC and TOR. Trends Biochem Sci 2003;28:573–576.
105. Hara K, Maruki Y, Long X, et al. Raptor, a binding partner of target of rapamycin (TOR), mediates TOR action. Cell 2002;110:177–189.
106. Kim DH, Sarbassov DD, Ali SM, et al. mTOR interacts with raptor to form a nutrient-sensitive complex that signals to the cell growth machinery. Cell 2002;110:163–175.
107. Loewith R, Jacinto E, Wullschleger S, et al. Two TOR complexes, only one of which is rapamycin sensitive, have distinct roles in cell growth control. Mol Cell 2002;10:457–468.
108. Gingras AC, Raught B, Sonenberg N. Control of translation by the target of rapamycin proteins. Prog Mol Subcell Biol 2001;27:143–174.

109. Abraham RT. Mammalian target of rapamycin: immunosuppressive drugs uncover a novel pathway of cytokine receptor signaling. Curr Opin Immunol 1998;10:330–336.

110. Bjornsti MA, Houghton PJ. The TOR pathway: a target for cancer therapy. Nat Rev Cancer 2004;4:335–348.

111. Dennis PB, Fumagalli S, Thomas G. Target of rapamycin (TOR): balancing the opposing forces of protein synthesis and degradation. Curr Opin Genet Dev 1999;9:49–54.

112. Holland EC, Sonenberg N, Pandolfi PP, et al. Signaling control of mRNA translation in cancer pathogenesis. Oncogene 2004;23: 3138–3144.

113. Mayerhofer M, Valent P, Sperr WR, et al. BCR/ABL induces expression of vascular endothelial growth factor and its transcriptional activator, hypoxia inducible factor-1alpha, through a pathway involving phosphoinositide 3-kinase and the mammalian target of rapamycin. Blood 2002;100:3767–3775.

114. Humar R, Kiefer FN, Berns H, et al. Hypoxia enhances vascular cell proliferation and angiogenesis in vitro via rapamycin (mTOR)-dependent signaling. FASEB J 2002;16:771–780.

115. Gao N, Zhang Z, Jiang BH, et al. Role of PI3K/AKT/mTOR signaling in the cell cycle progression of human prostate cancer. Biochem Biophys Res Commun 2003;310:1124–1132.

116. Oshiro N, Yoshino K, Hidayat S, et al. Dissociation of raptor from mTOR is a mechanism of rapamycin-induced inhibition of mTOR function. Genes Cells 2004;9:359–366.

117. Yonezawa K, Tokunaga C, Oshiro N, et al. Raptor, a binding partner of target of rapamycin. Biochem Biophys Res Commun 2004;313:437–441.

118. Gibbons JJ, Discafani C, Peterson R, et al. The effect of CCI-779, a novel macrolide anti-tumor agent, on the growth of human tumor cells in vitro and in nude mouse xenografts in vivo. Proc AACR 1999;40:A2000.

119. Geoerger B, Kerr K, Tang CB, et al. Antitumor activity of the rapamycin analog CCI-779 in human primitive neuroectodermal tumor/medulloblastoma models as single agent and in combination chemotherapy. Cancer Res 2001;61:1527–1532.

120. Eshleman JS, Carlson BL, Mladek AC, et al. Inhibition of the mammalian target of rapamycin sensitizes U87 xenografts to fractionated radiation therapy. Cancer Res 2002;62:7291–7297.

121. Grunwald V, DeGraffenried L, Russel D, et al. Inhibitors of mTOR reverse doxorubicin resistance conferred by PTEN status in prostate cancer cells. Cancer Res 2002;62:6141–6145.

122. Shi Y, Gera J, Hu L, et al. Enhanced sensitivity of multiple myeloma cells containing PTEN mutations to CCI-779. Cancer Res 2002;62:5027–5034.

123. Shi Y, Frankel A, Radvanyi LG, et al. Rapamycin enhances apoptosis and increases sensitivity to cisplatin in vitro. Cancer Res 1995;55:1982–1988.

124. Decker T, Hipp S, Ringshausen I, et al. Rapamycin-induced G1 arrest in cycling B-CLL cells is associated with reduced expression of cyclin D3, cyclin E, cyclin A, and survivin. Blood 2003;101: 278–285.

125. Albers MW, Williams RT, Brown EJ, et al. FKBP-rapamycin inhibits a cyclin-dependent kinase activity and a cyclin D1-Cdk association in early G1 of an osteosarcoma cell line. J Biol Chem 1993;268:22825–22829.

126. Luo Y, Marx SO, Kiyokawa H, et al. Rapamycin resistance tied to defective regulation of p27Kip1. Mol Cell Biol 1996;16: 6744–6751.

127. Zezula J, Sexl V, Hutter C, et al. The cyclin-dependent kinase inhibitor p21cip1 mediates the growth inhibitory effect of phorbol esters in human venous endothelial cells. J Biol Chem 1997;272:29967–29974.

128. Huang S, Liu LN, Hosoi H, et al. p53/p21(CIP1) cooperate in enforcing rapamycin-induced G(1) arrest and determine the cellular response to rapamycin. Cancer Res 2001;61:3373–3381.

129. Huang S, Shu L, Easton J, et al. Inhibition of mammalian target of rapamycin activates apoptosis signal-regulating kinase 1 signaling by suppressing protein phosphatase 5 activity. J Biol Chem 2004;279:36490–36496.

130. Huang S, Shu L, Dilling MB, et al. Sustained activation of the JNK cascade and rapamycin-induced apoptosis are suppressed by p53/p21(Cip1). Mol Cell 2003;11:1491–1501.

131. Guba M, von Breitenbuch P, Steinbauer M, et al. Rapamycin inhibits primary and metastatic tumor growth by antiangiogenesis: involvement of vascular endothelial growth factor. Nat Med 2002;8:128–135.

132. Zhong H, Hanrahan C, van der Poel H, et al. Hypoxia-inducible factor 1alpha and 1beta proteins share common signaling pathways in human prostate cancer cells. Biochem Biophys Res Commun 2001;284:352–356.

133. Zhong H, Chiles K, Feldser D, et al. Modulation of hypoxia-inducible factor 1alpha expression by the epidermal growth factor/phosphatidylinositol 3-kinase/PTEN/AKT/FRAP pathway in human prostate cancer cells: implications for tumor angiogenesis and therapeutics. Cancer Res 2000;60:1541–1545.

134. Huang S, Bjornsti MA, Houghton PJ. Rapamycins: mechanism of action and cellular resistance. Cancer Biol Ther 2003;2:222–232.

135. Huang S, Houghton PJ. Mechanisms of resistance to rapamycins. Drug Resist Updat 2001;4:378–391.

136. Noh WC, Mondesire WH, Peng J, et al. Determinants of rapamycin sensitivity in breast cancer cells. Clin Cancer Res 2004;10:1013–1023.

137. Podsypanina K, Lee RT, Politis C, et al. An inhibitor of mTOR reduces neoplasia and normalizes p70/S6 kinase activity in PTEN+/− mice. Proc Natl Acad Sci USA 2001;98:10320–10325.

138. Neshat MS, Mellinghoff IK, Tran C, et al. Enhanced sensitivity of PTEN-deficient tumors to inhibition of FRAP/mTOR. Proc Natl Acad Sci USA 2001;98:10314–10319.

139. Li S, Takasu T, Perlman DM, et al. Translation factor eIF4E rescues cells from Myc-dependent apoptosis by inhibiting cytochrome c release. J Biol Chem 2003;278:3015–3022.

140. Douros J, Suffness M. New antitumor substances of natural origin. Cancer Treat Rev 1981;8:63–87.

141. Eng CP, Sehgal SN, Vezina C. Activity of rapamycin (AY-22,989) against transplanted tumors. J Antibiot (Tokyo) 1984;37: 1231–1237.

142. Muthukkumar S, Ramesh TM, Bondada S. Rapamycin, a potent immunosuppressive drug, causes programmed cell death in B lymphoma cells. Transplantation 1995;60:264–270.

143. Seufferlein T, Rozengurt E. Rapamycin inhibits constitutive p70s6k phosphorylation, cell proliferation, and colony formation in small cell lung cancer cells. Cancer Res 1996;56: 3895–3897.

144. Hosoi H, Dilling MB, Liu LN, et al. Studies on the mechanism of resistance to rapamycin in human cancer cells. Mol Pharmacol 1998;54:815–824.

145. Hosoi H, Dilling MB, Shikata T, et al. Rapamycin causes poorly reversible inhibition of mTOR and induces p53-independent apoptosis in human rhabdomyosarcoma cells. Cancer Res 1999;59:886–894.

146. Grewe M, Gansauge F, Schmid RM, et al. Regulation of cell growth and cyclin D1 expression by the constitutively active FRAP-p70s6K pathway in human pancreatic cancer cells. Cancer Res 1999;59:3581–3587.

147. Majewski M, Korecka M, Kossev P, et al. The immunosuppressive macrolide RAD inhibits growth of human Epstein-Barr virus-transformed B lymphocytes in vitro and in vivo: a potential approach to prevention and treatment of posttransplant lymphoproliferative disorders. Proc Natl Acad Sci USA 2000;97: 4285–4290.

148. Dudkin L, Dilling MB, Cheshire PJ, et al. Biochemical correlates of mTOR inhibition by the rapamycin ester CCI- 779 and tumor growth inhibition. Clin Cancer Res 2001;7:1758–1764.

149. Dancey J, Rapamycin-Sensitive Signal-Transduction Pathways: Protein Translation Control of Cell Proliferation. American Society of Clinical Oncology Educational Book. Alexandria, VA: Lippincott Williams and Wilkins, 2000:68–75.

150. Aguirre D, Boya P, Bellet D, et al. Bcl-2 and CCND1/CDK4 expression levels predict the cellular effects of mTOR inhibitors in human ovarian carcinoma. Apoptosis 2004;9:797–805.

151. deGraffenried LA, Friedrichs WE, Russell DH, et al. Inhibition of mTOR activity restores tamoxifen response in breast cancer cells with aberrant Akt activity. Clin Cancer Res 2004;10:8059–8067.

152. Neuhaus P, Klupp J, Langrehr JM. mTOR inhibitors: an overview. Liver Transpl 2001;7:473–484.

153. Raymond E, Alexandre J, Faivre S, et al. Safety and pharmacokinetics of escalated doses of weekly intravenous infusion of CCI-779, a novel mTOR inhibitor, in patients with cancer. J Clin Oncol 2004;22:2336–2347.

154. Mita MM, Rowinsky EK, Goldston ML, et al. Phase I, pharmacokinetic (PK), and pharmacodynamic (PD) study of AP23573, an mTOR inhibitor, administered IV daily × 5 every other week in patients (pts) with refractory or advanced malignancies. Proc ASCO 2004;23:A3076.

155. Mita MM, Rowinsky EK, Mita AC, et al. Phase I, pharmacokinetic (PK), and pharmacodynamic (PD) study of AP23573, an mTOR Inhibitor, administered IV daily × 5 every other week in patients (pts) with refractory or advanced malignancies. 16th EORTC-NCI-AACR Symposium on Molecular Targets and Cancer Therapeutics. EJC 2004;2(Suppl):A409.

156. Clackson T, Metcalf CA, Rivera VM, et al. Broad anti-tumor activity of AP23573, an mTOR inhibitor in clinical development. Proc ASCO 2003;22:A882.

157. Lennon A, Finan K, FitzGerald MX, et al. Interstitial pneumonitis associated with sirolimus (rapamycin) therapy after liver transplantation. Transplantation 2001;72:1166–1167.

158. Atkins MB, Hidalgo M, Stadler W, et al. A randomized double-blind phase 2 study of intravenous CCI-779 administered weekly to patients with advanced renal cell carcinoma. Proc ASCO 2002;21:A36.

159. Hidalgo M, Rowinsky E, Erlichman C, et al. A phase I and pharmacological study of CCI-779, a rapamycin ester cell cycle inhibitor. Ann Oncol 2000;11:133 (A606O).

160. Hidalgo M, Rowinsky E, Erlichman C, et al. Phase I and pharmacological study of CCI-779, a cell cycle inhibitor. Proceedings of the 11th NCI-EORTC-AACR Symposium on New Drugs in Cancer Therapy. Clin Cancer Res 2000;6(Supp):A413.

161. Chang SM, Kuhn J, Wen P, et al. Phase I/pharmacokinetic study of CCI-779 in patients with recurrent malignant glioma on enzyme-inducing antiepileptic drugs. Invest New Drugs 2004; 22:427–435.

162. Forouzesh B, Buckner J, Adjei A, et al. Phase I, bioavailability, and pharmacokinetic study of oral dosage of CCI-779 administered to patients with advanced solid malignancies. EJC 2002; 38:A168.

163. Atkins MB, Hidalgo M, Stadler WM, et al. Randomized phase II study of multiple dose levels of CCI-779, a novel mammalian target of rapamycin kinase inhibitor, in patients with advanced refractory renal cell carcinoma. J Clin Oncol 2004;22:909–918.

164. Chan S, Johnston S, Scheulen ME, et al. First report: a phase 2 study of the safety and activity of CCI-779 for patients with locally advanced or metastatic breast cancer failing prior chemotherapy. Proc ASCO 2002;21:A175.

165. Chan S, Scheulen ME, Johnston S, et al. Phase 2 study of two dose levels of CCI-779 in locally advanced or metastatic breast cancer (MBC) failing prior anthracycline and/or taxane regimens. Proc ASCO 2003;22:A774.

166. Chan S. Targeting the mammalian target of rapamycin (mTOR): a new approach to treating cancer. Br J Cancer 2004;91: 1420–1424.

167. Witzig TE, Geyer SM, Salim M, et al. A phase II trial of the rapamycin analog CCI-779 in previously treated mantle cell non-Hodgkin's lymphoma: interim analysis of 18 patients. Proc Am Soc Hematol 2003;102:A2374.

168. Peralba JM, DeGraffenried L, Friedrichs W, et al. Pharmacodynamic evaluation of CCI-779, an inhibitor of mTOR, in cancer patients. Clin Cancer Res 2003;9:2887–2892.

169. Dutcher JP, Hudes G, Motzer R, et al. Preliminary report of a phase 1 study of intravenous (IV) CCI-779 given in combination with interferon-α (IFN) to patients with advanced renal cell carcinoma (RCC). Proc ASCO 2003;22:A854.

170. Punt CJ, Boni J, Bruntsch U, et al. Phase I and pharmacokinetic study of CCI-779, a novel cytostatic cell-cycle inhibitor, in combination with 5-fluorouracil and leucovorin in patients with advanced solid tumors. Ann Oncol 2003;14:931–937.

171. O'Donnell A, Faivre S, Judson I, et al. A phase I study of the oral mTOR inhibitor RAD001 as monotherapy to identify the optimal biologically effective dose using toxicity, pharmacokinetic (PK) and pharmacodynamic (PD) endpoints in patients with solid tumours. Proc ASCO 2003;22:A803.

172. Lane H, Tanaka C, Kovarik J, et al. Preclinical and clinical pharmacokinetic/pharmacodynamic (PK/PD) modeling to help define an optimal biological dose for the oral mTOR inhibitor, RAD001, in oncology. Proc ASCO 2003;22:A951.

173. Di Cosimo S, Matar P, Rojo F, et al. The mTOR pathway inhibitor RAD001 induces activation of AKT which is completely abolished by gefitinib, an anti-EGFR tyrosine kinase inhibitor, and combined sequence specific treatment results in greater antitumor activity. Proc AACR 2004;45:A5345.

174. Boulay A, Zumstein-Mecker S, Stephan C, et al. Antitumor efficacy of intermittent treatment schedules with the rapamycin derivative RAD001 correlates with prolonged inactivation of ribosomal protein S6 kinase 1 in peripheral blood mononuclear cells. Cancer Res 2004;64:252–261.

175. Metcalf III CA, Bohacek R, Rozamus LW, et al. Structure-based design of AP23573, a phosphorus-containing analog of rapamycin for anti-tumor therapy. Proc AACR 2004;45:A2476.

176. Rivera VM, Tang H, Metcalf CA III, et al. Anti-proliferative activity of the mTOR inhibitor AP23573 in combination with cytotoxic and targeted agents. Proc AACR 2004;45:A3887.

177. Desai AA, Janisch L, Berk LR, et al. A phase I trial of a novel mTOR inhibitor AP23573 administered weekly (wkly) in patients (pts) with refractory or advanced malignancies: a pharmacokinetic (PK) and pharmacodynamic (PD) analysis. Proc ASCO 2004;23:A3150.

178. Desai AA, Janisch L, Berk LR, et al. A phase 1 trial of weekly (wkly) AP23573, a novel mTOR inhibitor, in patients (pts) with advanced or refractory malignancies: a pharmacokinetic (PK) and pharmacodynamic (PD) analysis. 16th EORTC-NCI-AACR Symposium on Molecular Targets and Cancer Therapeutics. EJC 2004;2(Suppl):A390.

179. Rivera V, Berk L, Mita M, et al. Pharmacodynamic evaluation of the mTOR inhibitor AP23573 in phase 1 clinical trials. 16th EORTC-NCI-AACR Symposium on Molecular Targets and Cancer Therapeutics EJC 2004;2(Suppl):A411.

180. DeBoer C, Meulman PA, Wnuk RJ, et al. Geldanamycin, a new antibiotic. J Antibiot (Tokyo) 1970;23:442–447.

181. Schulte TW, Neckers LM. The benzoquinone ansamycin 17-allylamino-17-demethoxygeldanamycin binds to HSP90 and shares important biologic activities with geldanamycin. Cancer Chemother Pharmacol 1998;42:273–279.

182. Supko JG, Hickman RL, Grever MR, et al. Preclinical pharmacologic evaluation of geldanamycin as an antitumor agent. Cancer Chemother Pharmacol 1995;36:305–315.

183. Page J, Heath J, Fulton R, et al. Comparison of geldanamycin (NSC-122750) and 17-allylaminogeldanamycin (NSC-330507D) toxicity in rats. Proc AACR 1997;38:A2067.

184. Paine-Murrieta G, Cook P, Taylor CW, et al. The anti-tumor activity of 17-allylaminogeldanamycin is associated with modulation of target protein levels in vivo. Proc AACR 1999;40:A119.

185. Burger AM, Fiebig HH, Newman DJ, et al. Antitumor activity of 17-allylaminogeldanamycin (NSC 330507) in melanoma xenografts is associated with decline in Hsp90 protein expression. 10th NCI-EORTC Symposium on New Drugs in Cancer Therapy. 1998:A504.

186. Uehara Y, Hori M, Takeuchi T, et al. Screening of agents which convert "transformed morphology" of Rous sarcoma virus-infected rat kidney cells to "normal morphology": identification of an active agent as herbimycin and its inhibition of intracellular src kinase. Jpn J Cancer Res 1985;76:672–675.

187. Uehara Y, Hori M, Takeuchi T, et al. Phenotypic change from transformed to normal induced by benzoquinonoid ansamycins accompanies inactivation of p60src in rat kidney cells infected with Rous sarcoma virus. Mol Cell Biol 1986;6: 2198–2206.

188. Whitesell L, Mimnaugh EG, De Costa B, et al. Inhibition of heat shock protein HSP90-pp60v-src heteroprotein complex formation by benzoquinone ansamycins: essential role for stress proteins in oncogenic transformation. Proc Natl Acad Sci USA 1994;91:8324–8328.

189. Mosser DD, Morimoto RI. Molecular chaperones and the stress of oncogenesis. Oncogene 2004;23:2907–2918.

190. Scheibel T, Buchner J. The Hsp90 complex: a super-chaperone machine as a novel drug target. Biochem Pharmacol 1998;56: 675–682.

191. Grenert JP, Sullivan WP, Fadden P, et al. The amino-terminal domain of heat shock protein 90 (hsp90) that binds geldanamycin is an ATP/ADP switch domain that regulates hsp90 conformation. J Biol Chem 1997;272:23843–23850.

192. Prodromou C, Roe SM, O'Brien R, et al. Identification and structural characterization of the ATP/ADP-binding site in the Hsp90 molecular chaperone. Cell 1997;90:65–75.

193. Mimnaugh EG, Chavany C, Neckers L. Polyubiquitination and proteasomal degradation of the p185c-erbB-2 receptor protein-tyrosine kinase induced by geldanamycin. J Biol Chem 1996; 271:22796–22801.

194. Neckers L, Ivy SP. Heat shock protein 90. Curr Opin Oncol 2003;15:419–424.

195. Neckers L. Hsp90 inhibitors as novel cancer chemotherapeutic agents. Trends Mol Med 2002;8:S55–61.

196. Picard D. Continuously updated table of Hsp90 interactors. 2004. www.picard.ch/downloads/Hsp90interactors.pdf

197. Chavany C, Mimnaugh E, Miller P, et al. p185erbB2 binds to GRP94 in vivo: dissociation of the p185erbB2/GRP94 heterocomplex by benzoquinone ansamycins precedes depletion of p185erbB2. J Biol Chem 1996;271:4974–4977.

198. Stancato LF, Sakatsume M, David M, et al. Beta interferon and oncostatin M activate Raf-1 and mitogen-activated protein kinase through a JAK1-dependent pathway. Mol Cell Biol 1997;17:3833–3840.

199. Stepanova L, Leng X, Parker SB, et al. Mammalian p50Cdc37 is a protein kinase-targeting subunit of Hsp90 that binds and stabilizes Cdk4. Genes Dev 1996;10:1491–1502.

200. Segnitz B, Gehring U. The function of steroid hormone receptors is inhibited by the hsp90-specific compound geldanamycin. J Biol Chem 1997;272:18694–18701.

201. An WG, Schnur RC, Neckers L, et al. Depletion of p185erbB2, Raf-1 and mutant p53 proteins by geldanamycin derivatives correlates with antiproliferative activity. Cancer Chemother Pharmacol 1997;40:60–64.

202. Clarke PA, Hostein I, Banerji U, et al. Gene expression profiling of human colon cancer cells following inhibition of signal transduction by 17-allylamino-17-demethoxygeldanamycin, an inhibitor of the hsp90 molecular chaperone. Oncogene 2000;19: 4125–4133.

203. Hostein I, Robertson D, DiStefano F, et al. Inhibition of signal transduction by the Hsp90 inhibitor 17-allylamino-17-demethoxygeldanamycin results in cytostasis and apoptosis. Cancer Res 2001;61:4003–4009.

204. Nimmanapalli R, O'Bryan E, Bhalla K. Geldanamycin and its analogue 17-allylamino-17-demethoxygeldanamycin lowers Bcr-Abl levels and induces apoptosis and differentiation of Bcr-Abl-positive human leukemic blasts. Cancer Res 2001;61:1799–1804.

205. An WG, Schulte TW, Neckers LM. The heat shock protein 90 antagonist geldanamycin alters chaperone association with p210bcr-abl and v-src proteins before their degradation by the proteasome. Cell Growth Differ 2000;11:355–360.

206. Shiotsu Y, Neckers LM, Wortman I, et al. Novel oxime derivatives of radicicol induce erythroid differentiation associated with preferential G(1) phase accumulation against chronic myelogenous leukemia cells through destabilization of Bcr-Abl with Hsp90 complex. Blood 2000;96:2284–2291.

207. Blagosklonny MV, Fojo T, Bhalla KN, et al. The Hsp90 inhibitor geldanamycin selectively sensitizes Bcr-Abl-expressing leukemia cells to cytotoxic chemotherapy. Leukemia 2001;15:1537–1543.

208. Bhalla KM, Nimmanapalli R, O'Bryan E. 17-allylamino-17-demethoxygeldanamycin (17-AAG) lowers Bcr-Abl levels and induces differentiation and apoptosis of STI-571 sensitive and resistant Bcr-ABl positive acute leukemia cells. Proc AACR 2001;42:A800.

209. Gorre ME, Ellwood-Yen K, Chiosis G, et al. BCR-ABL point mutants isolated from patients with imatinib mesylate-resistant chronic myeloid leukemia remain sensitive to inhibitors of the BCR-ABL chaperone heat shock protein 90. Blood 2002;100: 3041–3044.

210. Munster PN, Basso A, Solit D, et al. Modulation of Hsp90 function by ansamycins sensitizes breast cancer cells to chemotherapy-induced apoptosis in an RB- and schedule-dependent manner. See Sausville EA. Combining cytotoxics and 17-allylamino, 17-demethoxygeldanamycin: sequence and tumor biology matters. Clin Cancer Res 2001;7:2155–2158, 2228–2236.

211. Munster PN, Srethapakdi M, Moasser MM, et al. Inhibition of heat shock protein 90 function by ansamycins causes the morphological

and functional differentiation of breast cancer cells. Cancer Res 2001;61:2945–2952.

212. Munster PN, Marchion DC, Basso AD, et al. Degradation of HER2 by ansamycins induces growth arrest and apoptosis in cells with HER2 overexpression via a HER3, phosphatidylinositol 3'-kinase-AKT-dependent pathway. Cancer Res 2002;62: 3132–3137.

213. Jiang J, Shapiro GI. 17-AAG induces Rb-dependent G1 arrest in lung cancer cell lines. Proc AACR 2002;43:A332.

214. Bagatell R, Khan O, Paine-Murrieta G, et al. Destabilization of steroid receptors by heat shock protein 90-binding drugs: a ligand-independent approach to hormonal therapy of breast cancer. Clin Cancer Res 2001;7:2076–2084.

215. Wessinger NL, Kane SE. 17-AAG combinations with conventional chemotherapeutic agents in two ovarian cancer cell lines. Proc AACR 2002;43:A4706.

216. Vasilevskaya IA, Rakitina TV, O'Dwyer PJ. Geldanamycin and its 17-allylamino-derivative antagonize the action of cisplatin in human colon cancer cells. Proc AACR 2002;43:A1647.

217. Nguyen DM, Chen A, Mixon A, et al. Sequence-dependent enhancement of paclitaxel toxicity in non-small cell lung cancer by 17-allylamino 17-demethoxygeldanamycin. J Thorac Cardiovasc Surg 1999;118:908–915.

218. Donaldson KL, Goolsby GL, Kiener PA, et al. Activation of p34cdc2 coincident with taxol-induced apoptosis. Cell Growth Differ 1994;5:1041–1050.

219. Nguyen DM, Lorang D, Chen A, et al. Synergistic tumoricidal effect of the paclitaxel and 17 allylamino geldanamycin (17AAG) combination in non small cell lung cancer: in vitro and in vivo analysis. Proc AACR 2002;43:A366.

220. Nguyen DM, Lorang D, Chen GA, et al. Enhancement of paclitaxel-mediated cytotoxicity in lung cancer cells by 17-allylamino geldanamycin: in vitro and in vivo analysis. Ann Thorac Surg 2001; 72:371–378; discussion 378–379.

221. Abraham RT. Cell cycle checkpoint signaling through the ATM and ATR kinases. Genes Dev 2001;15:2177–2196.

222. Zhou BB, Elledge SJ. The DNA damage response: putting checkpoints in perspective. Nature 2000;408:433–439.

223. Jia W, Yu C, Rahmani M, et al. Synergistic antileukemic interactions between 17-AAG and UCN-01 involve interruption of RAF/MEK- and AKT-related pathways. Blood 2003;102: 1824–1832.

224. Arlander SJ, Eapen AK, Vroman BT, et al. Hsp90 inhibition depletes Chk1 and sensitizes tumor cells to replication stress. J Biol Chem 2003;278:52572–52577.

225. Yu X, Guo ZS, Marcu MG, et al. Modulation of p53, ErbB1, ErbB2, and Raf-1 expression in lung cancer cells by depsipeptide FR901228. J Natl Cancer Inst 2002;94:504–513.

226. Rosato RR, Grant S. Histone deacetylase inhibitors in clinical development. Expert Opin Investig Drugs 2004;13:21–38.

227. Fuino L, Bali P, Wittmann S, et al. Histone deacetylase inhibitor LAQ824 down-regulates Her-2 and sensitizes human breast cancer cells to trastuzumab, Taxotere, gemcitabine, and epothilone B. Mol Cancer Ther 2003;2:971–984.

228. Nimmanapalli R, Fuino L, Bali P, et al. Histone deacetylase inhibitor LAQ824 both lowers expression and promotes proteasomal degradation of Bcr-Abl and induces apoptosis of imatinib mesylate-sensitive or -refractory chronic myelogenous leukemia-blast crisis cells. Cancer Res 2003;63:5126–5135.

229. Rahmani M, Yu C, Dai Y, et al. Coadministration of the heat shock protein 90 antagonist 17-allylamino-17-demethoxygeldanamycin with suberoylanilide hydroxamic acid or sodium butyrate synergistically induces apoptosis in human leukemia cells. Cancer Res 2003;63:8420–8427.

230. Rahmani M, Chunrong Y, Dai Y, et al. Co-administration of the heat shock protein 90 antagonist 17-AAG with SAHA or sodium butyrate synergistically induces apoptosis in human leukemia cells. Proc AACR 2004;45:A458.

231. Gradin K, McGuire J, Wenger RH, et al. Functional interference between hypoxia and dioxin signal transduction pathways: competition for recruitment of the Arnt transcription factor. Mol Cell Biol 1996;16:5221–5231.

232. Harris AL. Hypoxia: a key regulatory factor in tumour growth. Nat Rev Cancer 2002;2:38–47.

233. Semenza GL. Targeting HIF-1 for cancer therapy. Nat Rev Cancer 2003;3:721–732.

234. Hur E, Kim HH, Choi SM, et al. Reduction of hypoxia-induced transcription through the repression of hypoxia-inducible factor-1alpha/aryl hydrocarbon receptor nuclear translocator DNA binding by the 90-kDa heat-shock protein inhibitor radicicol. Mol Pharmacol 2002;62:975–982.

235. Isaacs JS, Jung YJ, Mimnaugh EG, et al. Hsp90 regulates a von Hippel Lindau-independent hypoxia-inducible factor-1 alpha-degradative pathway. J Biol Chem 2002;277:29936–29944.

236. Minet E, Mottet D, Michel G, et al. Hypoxia-induced activation of HIF-1: role of HIF-1alpha-Hsp90 interaction. FEBS Lett 1999;460:251–256.

237. Mabjeesh NJ, Post DE, Willard MT, et al. Geldanamycin induces degradation of hypoxia-inducible factor 1alpha protein via the proteosome pathway in prostate cancer cells. Cancer Res 2002;62:2478–2482.

238. Zagzag D, Nomura M, Friedlander DR, et al. Geldanamycin inhibits migration of glioma cells in vitro: a potential role for hypoxia-inducible factor (HIF-1alpha) in glioma cell invasion. J Cell Physiol 2003;196:394–402.

239. To CT, Tsao MS. The roles of hepatocyte growth factor/scatter factor and met receptor in human cancers [review]. Oncol Rep 1998;5:1013–1024.

240. Di Renzo MF, Olivero M, Giacomini A, et al. Overexpression and amplification of the met/HGF receptor gene during the progression of colorectal cancer. Clin Cancer Res 1995;1:147–154.

241. Fujita S, Sugano K. Expression of c-met proto-oncogene in primary colorectal cancer and liver metastases. Jpn J Clin Oncol 1997;27:378–383.

242. Umeki K, Shiota G, Kawasaki H. Clinical significance of c-met oncogene alterations in human colorectal cancer. Oncology 1999;56:314–321.

243. Takeuchi H, Bilchik A, Saha S, et al. c-MET expression level in primary colon cancer: a predictor of tumor invasion and lymph node metastases. Clin Cancer Res 2003;9:1480–1488.

244. Maulik G, Kijima T, Ma PC, et al. Modulation of the c-Met/hepatocyte growth factor pathway in small cell lung cancer. Clin Cancer Res 2002;8:620–627.

245. Webb CP, Hose CD, Koochekpour S, et al. The geldanamycins are potent inhibitors of the hepatocyte growth factor/scatter factor-met-urokinase plasminogen activator-plasmin proteolytic network. Cancer Res 2000;60:342–349.

246. Kitamura S, Kondo S, Shinomura Y, et al. Met/HGF receptor modulates bcl-w expression and inhibits apoptosis in human colorectal cancers. Br J Cancer 2000;83:668–673.

247. Ichihara M, Murakumo Y, Takahashi M. RET and neuroendocrine tumors. Cancer Lett 2004;204:197–211.

248. Santoro M, Melillo RM, Carlomagno F, et al. Molecular mechanisms of RET activation in human cancer. Ann NY Acad Sci 2002;963:116–121.

249. Jhiang SM. The RET proto-oncogene in human cancers. Oncogene 2000;19:5590–5597.

250. Cohen MS, Hussain HB, Moley JF. Inhibition of medullary thyroid carcinoma cell proliferation and RET phosphorylation by tyrosine kinase inhibitors. Surgery 2002;132:960–966; discussion 966–967.

251. Egorin MJ, Rosen DM, Wolff JH, et al. Metabolism of 17-(allylamino)-17-demethoxygeldanamycin (NSC 330507) by murine and human hepatic preparations. Cancer Res 1998;58: 2385–2396.

252. Schnur RC, Corman ML, Gallaschun RJ, et al. erbB-2 oncogene inhibition by geldanamycin derivatives: synthesis, mechanism of action, and structure-activity relationships. J Med Chem 1995;38:3813–3820.

253. Kelland LR, Sharp SY, Rogers PM, et al. DT-diaphorase expression and tumor cell sensitivity to 17-allylamino, 17-demethoxygeldanamycin, an inhibitor of heat shock protein 90. J Natl Cancer Inst 1999;91:1940–1949.

254. Egorin MJ, Lagattuta TF, Hamburger DR, et al. Pharmacokinetics, tissue distribution, and metabolism of 17-(dimethylaminoethylamino)-17-demethoxygeldanamycin (NSC 707545) in CD2F1 mice and Fischer 344 rats. Cancer Chemother Pharmacol 2002;49:7–19.

255. Banerji U, Walton MI, Orr R, et al. Development and validation of pharmacodynamic endpoints in tumor and normal tissue to assess the effect of the Hsp90 molecular chaperone inhibitor 17-allylamino-17-demethoxy geldanamycin (17-AAG). Proc AACR 2000;41:A4581.

256. Kim HR, Kang HS, Kim HD. Geldanamycin induces heat shock protein expression through activation of HSF1 in K562 erythroleukemic cells. IUBMB Life 1999;48:429–433.

257. Nguyen DM, Desai S, Chen A, et al. Modulation of metastasis phenotypes of non-small cell lung cancer cells by 17-allylamino 17-demethoxy geldanamycin. Ann Thorac Surg 2000;70:1853–1860.

258. Mimnaugh EG, Xu W, Vos M, et al. Simultaneous inhibition of hsp 90 and the proteasome promotes protein ubiquitination, causes endoplasmic reticulum-derived cytosolic vacuolization, and enhances antitumor activity. Mol Cancer Ther 2004;3:551–566.

259. Eiseman JL, Grimm A, Sentz DL, et al. Pharmacokinetics and tissue distribution of 17-allylamino(17demethoxy)geldanamycin in SCID mice bearing MDA-MB-453 xenografts and alterations in the expression of p185^erbB2 in xenografts following treatment. Proceeding of the AACR-NCI-EORTC International Conference on Molecular Targets and Cancer Therapeutics. 1999:A536.

260. Basso AD, Solit DB, Rosen N. Ansamycins inhibit AKT activation and induce the 20S proteasomal degradation of AKT protein. Proceeding of the AACR-NCI-EORTC Molecular Targets 2001 Abstracts on CD-ROM. 2001:A611.

261. Solit DB, Munster PN, Basso AD, et al. 17-allyl-amino-geldanamycin induces HER2 degradation and AKT inactivation in a human breast cancer xenograft model. Proceedings of the 11th NCI-EORTC Symposium on New Drugs in Cancer Therapy. 2001:A396.

262. Solit DB, Zheng FF, Drobnjak M, et al. 17-Allylamino-17-demethoxygeldanamycin induces the degradation of androgen receptor and HER-2/neu and inhibits the growth of prostate cancer xenografts. Clin Cancer Res 2002;8:986–993.

263. Yang J, Yang JM, Iannone M, et al. Disruption of the EF-2 kinase/Hsp90 protein complex: a possible mechanism to inhibit glioblastoma by geldanamycin. Cancer Res 2001;61:4010–4016.

264. Enmon R, Yang WH, Ballangrud AM, et al. Combination treatment with 17-N-allylamino-17-demethoxy geldanamycin and acute irradiation produces supra-additive growth suppression in human prostate carcinoma spheroids. Cancer Res 2003;63: 8393–8399.

265. Bisht KS, Bradbury CM, Mattson D, et al. Geldanamycin and 17-allylamino-17-demethoxygeldanamycin potentiate the in vitro and in vivo radiation response of cervical tumor cells via the heat shock protein 90-mediated intracellular signaling and cytotoxicity. Cancer Res 2003;63:8984–8995.

266. Eiseman JL, Sentz DL, Zuhowski EG. Plasma pharmacokinetics and tissue distribution of 17-allylaminogeldanamycin (NSC 330507), a prodrug for geldanamycin, in CD2F1 mice and Fisher 344 rats. Proc AACR 1997;38:A2063.

267. Noker PE, Thompson RB, Smith AC, et al. Toxicity and pharmacokinetics of 17-allylaminogeldanamycin (17-AAG, NSC-330507) in dogs. Proc AACR 1999;40:A804.

268. Banerji U, Walton M, Raynauld F, et al. Validation of pharmacodynamic endpoints for the HSP90 molecular chaperone inhibitor 17-allylamino 17-demethoxygeldanamycin (17AAG) in a human tumor xenograft model. Proc AACR 2001;42:A4473.

269. Banerji U, Maloney A, Asad Y, et al. Pharmacokinetic-pharmacodynamic (PK-PD) relationships for the HSP90 molecular chaperone inhibitor 17-allylamino-17-demethoxygeldanamycin (17AAG) in human ovarian cancer xenografts. Proceedings of the 11th NCI-EORTC Symposium on New Drugs in Cancer Therapy. 2001:A395.

270. Agnew EB, Neckers LM, Hehman HE, et al. Human plasma pharmacokinetics of the novel antitumor agent 17-allylaminogeldanamycin (AAG) using a new HPLC-based analytic assay. Proc AACR 2000;41:A4458.

271. Wilson RH, Takimoto CH, Agnew EB. Phase I pharmacologic study of 17-(allylamino)-17-demethoxygeldanamycin (AAG) in adult patients with advanced solid tumors. Proc ASCO 2001; 20:A325.

272. Agnew EB, Wilson RH, Morrison G, et al. Clinical pharmacokinetics of 17-(allylamino)-17-demethoxygeldanamycin and the

active metabolite 17-(amino)-17-demethoxygeldanamycin given as a one-hour infusion daily for 5 days. Proc AACR 2002;43: A1349.

273. Munster PN, Tong W, Schwartz L. Phase I trial of 17-(ally-lamino)-17-demethoxygeldanamycin (17-AAG) in patients (pts) with advanced solid malignancies. Proc ASCO 2001;20: A326.

274. Erlichman C, Toft D, Reid J. A phase I trial of 17-allyl-amino-gel-danamycin in patients with advanced cancer. Proc AACR 2001;42:A4474.

275. Goetz M, Toft D, Reid J. A phase I trial of 17-allyl-amino-gel-danamycin (17-AAG) in patients with advanced cancer. Eur J Cancer 2002;38 (Suppl 7):S54–S55 (A170).

276. Banerji U, O'Donnell A, Scurr M, et al. A pharmacokinetically (PK)–pharmacodynamically (PD) driven phase I trial of the Hsp90 molecular chaperone inhibitor 17-allylamino 17-demthoxygeldanamycin (17AAG). Proc AACR 2002;43:A1352.

277. Banerji U, O'Donnell A, Scurr M, et al. Phase I trial of the heat shock protein 90 (HSP90) inhibitor 17-allylamino 17-demethoxygeldanamycin (17AAG): pharmacokinetic (PK) profile and pharmacodynamic (PD) endpoints. Proc ASCO 2001; 20:A326.

278. Banerji U, O'Donnell A, Scurr M, et al. A pharmacokinetically (PK)–pharmacodynamically (PD) guided phase I trial of the heat shock protein 90 (HSP90) inhibitor 17-allylamino, 17-demethoxygeldanamycin (17AAG). Proc ASCO 2003;22:A797.

279. Burger AM, Sausville EA, Carmalier RF, et al. Response of human melanomas to 17-AAG is associated with modulation of the molecular chaperone function of Hsp90. Proc AACR 2000; 41:A2844.

Bisphosphonates

26

Matthew R. Smith

INTRODUCTION

Bone metastases are a major cause of morbidity for many patients with advanced-stage cancers. The complications of bone metastases include hypercalcemia, pain, fracture, and spinal cord compression. Most complications of bone metastases result from excessive osteoclast activation.

Bisphosphonates are potent inhibitors of osteoclast-mediated bone resorption. These agents are used to treat benign diseases associated with excessive bone resorption, including Paget's disease and osteoporosis. Bisphosphonates are also an important part of the management for many cancer patients. Bisphosphonates are the treatment of choice for hypercalcemia of malignancy. Bisphosphonates decrease the risk of skeletal complications for patients with multiple myeloma and patients with bone metastases from breast cancer, prostate cancer, and other solid tumors. In addition, bisphosphonates may prevent development of bone metastases in women with high-risk primary breast cancer.

PHARMACOLOGY

Bisphosphonates are synthetic analogs of pyrophosphate characterized by a phosphorus-carbon-phosphorus backbone that renders them resistant to hydrolysis (Fig. 26.1). The properties of bisphosphonates are determined by the R_1 and R_2 carbon side chains.[1] Most bisphosphonates contain a hydroxyl group at the R_1 position that confers high-affinity binding to calcium phosphate. The R_2 side chain is the critical determinant of antiresorptive potency (Table 26.1). Bisphosphonates that contain a primary amino group (pamidronate and alendronate) are approximately 100-fold more potent than first-generation bisphosphonates that do not contain an amino group (etidronate and clodronate). Bisphosphonates that contain a secondary or tertiary amino group (ibandronate, risedronate, and zoledronic acid) are

among the most potent bisphosphonates, with approximately 10,000-fold more activity than etidronate.

Bisphosphonates are poorly absorbed. Bioavailability is less than 1% after oral administration. Bisphosphonates bind calcium, and calcium-containing foods, beverages, and medications alter drug absorption. Oral administration is associated with gastrointestinal toxicity.

Bisphosphonates are not metabolized. They are eliminated by renal excretion. Bisphosphonates have potential renal toxicity related to total drug dose and rate of intravenous administration. Renal toxicity results from the R_1 carbon side chain. Because most bisphosphonates share the same R_1 hydroxyl side chain, renal toxicity is a potential adverse effect of all bisphosphonates.

Bisphosphonates are adsorbed to calcium phosphate (hydroxyapatite) crystals in bone. Approximately one half of an intravenously administered dose accumulates in the skeleton. Bisphosphonates preferentially bind to sites of active bone remodeling. Bisphosphonates become biologically inactive after they are incorporated into quiescent bone, and repetitive administration appears to be required to maintain inhibition of bone resorption.

Etidronate (Didronel), pamidronate disodium (Aredia), and zoledronic acid (Zometa) are marketed for oncology in the United States (Table 26.2). Clodronate (Ostac) and ibandronate (Bondronat) are marketed for oncology in other countries but are not available in the United States.

MECHANISMS OF ACTION

Bisphosphonates inhibit osteoclast-mediated bone resorption by several mechanisms. Etidronate and clodronate are metabolized to cytotoxic analogs of adenosine triphosphate. More potent nitrogen-containing bisphosphonates (risedronate, pamidronate, zoledronic acid) inhibit farnesyl diphosphate synthase, a key enzyme in the mevalonate pathway, and decrease prenylation of essential GTP-binding

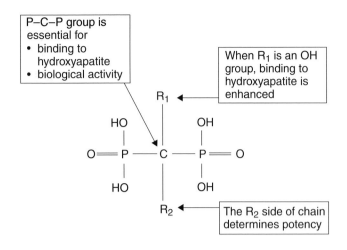

Figure 26.1 General structure of bisphosphonates. The biological activity of bisphosphonates depends on the P-C-P group and the structure of the R_1 and R_2 side chains.

Bisphosphonate	R_1 side chain	R_2 side chain
Etidronate	OH	CH_3
Clodronate	Cl	Cl
Pamidronate	OH	$CH_2CH_2NH_2$
Alendronate	OH	$(CH_2)_3\ NH_2$
Risedronate	OH	CH_2-3-pyridine
Tiludronate	H	CH_2-S-phenyl-Cl
Ibandronate	OH	$CH_2CH_2N(CH_3)$(pentyl)
Zoledronate	OH	CH_2-imidazole

proteins. Bisphosphonates also increase osteoblast secretion of two important cytokines: (1) an inhibitor of osteoclast recruitment and (2) transforming growth factor-β, a signal for osteoclast apoptosis.

The growth of bone metastases involves reciprocal interactions between tumor cells and metabolically active bone.[2] Development and progression of bone metastases involves tumor cell adhesion to bone, invasion, new blood vessel formation, and proliferation. Preclinical studies suggest that bisphosphonates inhibit each of these steps.[3,4] The clinical relevance of the observed antitumor properties of bisphosphonates in preclinical models is not known.

TABLE 26.1
PRECLINICAL POTENCY OF SELECTED BISPHOSPHONATES

Generic Name	Trade Name	Relative Potency
Etidronate	Didronel	1
Clodronate	Ostac	10
Pamidronate	Aredia	100
Ibandronate	Bondronat	10,000
Zoledronic acid	Zometa	10,000

TABLE 26.2
FDA-APPROVED BISPHOSPHONATES FOR ONCOLOGY

Generic Name	Trade Name	Approved Indication(s) in Oncology
Etidronate	Didronel	Hypercalcemia
Pamidronate	Aredia	Hypercalcemia
		Multiple myeloma
		Metastatic breast cancer
Zoledronic acid	Zometa	Hypercalcemia
		Multiple myeloma
		Any solid tumor with bone metastases

HYPERCALCEMIA

Hypercalcemia of malignancy results primarily from increased release of calcium from bone. In the presence of bone metastases, calcium is released from the skeleton by local osteoclast-mediated bone destruction. In addition, hypercalcemia of malignancy may result from tumor secretion of PTHrP.[5] PTHrP causes hypercalcemia by osteoclast activation and decreased renal calcium excretion. Many malignancies produce PTHrP, including breast cancer, squamous cell carcinoma, renal cell carcinoma, multiple myeloma, and some types of lymphoma.

Treatment with intravenous pamidronate disodium (90 mg) achieves normocalcemia in more than 90% of patients with hypercalcemia of malignancy.[6] Pamidronate achieves more complete and longer lasting responses than clodronate. In a double-blind study, 41 patients with hypercalcemia of malignancy persisting after 48 hours of saline rehydration were randomly assigned to receive intravenous pamidronate (90 mg) or intravenous clodronate (1,500 mg).[7] Nineteen of 19 patients (100%) treated with pamidronate achieved normocalcemia compared with 16 of 20 patients (80%) given clodronate. The median duration of normocalcemia was 28 days after pamidronate therapy compared with 14 days after clodronate treatment ($P < .01$).

Ibandronate appears comparable to pamidronate for hypercalcemia of malignancy. Seventy-two patients with hypercalcemia of malignancy (corrected serum calcium > 2.7 mmol) were treated with either ibandronate (2 or 4 mg) or pamidronate (15, 30, 60, or 90 mg).[8] The dose was dependent on the severity of hypercalcemia. The rates of normocalcemia were similar with ibandronate and pamidronate (77% vs. 76%, $P = .30$). The mean decreases in serum calcium were also similar for ibandronate and pamidronate. The median time to increase in serum calcium was longer for ibandronate than pamidronate (14 vs. 4 days, $P = .03$).

Zoledronic acid is superior to pamidronate for hypercalcemia of malignancy. In a double-blind study, 287 patients with moderate to severe hypercalcemia of malignancy (corrected serum calcium 3.0 mmol) were randomly assigned to zoledronic acid (4 or 8 mg) or pamidronate (90 mg).[9] Both doses of zoledronic acid were superior to pamidronate. The rate of normalization of serum calcium at day 10 was 87% for zoledronic acid versus 70% for pamidronate. The median duration of normocalcemia was greater than 30 days for zoledronic acid and 18 days for pamidronate.

Bisphosphonates should be administered to all patients with hypercalcemia of malignancy and a corrected serum calcium level greater than 3.0 mmol.[10] Bisphosphonates should also be administered to symptomatic patients with more moderate hypercalcemia.

MULTIPLE MYELOMA

Multiple myeloma is a malignancy characterized by osteolytic bone lesions and accumulation of mature plasma cells in the bone marrow. Osteoclasts are activated through local release of osteoclast-stimulating factors by myeloma and stromal cells. The growth of myeloma cells in the skeleton is promoted by bone production of interleukin 6 and other growth factors.

Eight large randomized trials of bisphosphonate administration for multiple myeloma have been reported (Table 26.3).

In a Canadian study, 166 patients with previously untreated multiple myeloma were randomly assigned to receive either daily oral etidronate disodium (5 mg/kg) or placebo indefinitely.[11] All patients were treated with intermittent oral melphalan and prednisone. No significant differences were seen in skeletal outcomes (fracture, hypercalcemia, bone pain) between the two groups.

Three randomized studies evaluated the efficacy of oral clodronate in multiple myeloma. In a Finnish study, 336 patients with previously untreated disease were randomly assigned to receive daily oral clodronate (2,400 mg) or placebo for 2 years.[12] All patients were treated with intermittent oral melphalan and prednisolone. No significant differences were noted between the two groups in rates of fracture or hypercalcemia. Bone pain and analgesic usage were also similar in both groups. The proportion of patients with progression of osteolytic bone lesions was lower in the clodronate-treated group than in the control group (12% vs. 24%, $P = .026$).

In an open-label German study, 170 previously untreated patients were randomly assigned to receive daily oral clodronate (1,600 mg) or no bisphosphonate for 1 year.[13] All patients were treated with intravenous melphalan and oral prednisone. Less than one half of the participants completed the 1-year study. No difference was observed in the rate of radiographically apparent disease progression in bone. A trend was seen toward fewer new sites of bone involvement in the clodronate-treated group.

In a Medical Research Council study, 536 patients with previously untreated multiple myeloma were randomly assigned to receive either daily oral clodronate (1,600 mg) or placebo.[14] All patients were treated with primary chemotherapy. Overall survival, time to first skeletal event, hypercalcemia, and need for radiation therapy to bone were no different in the two groups. The proportion of patients with vertebral and nonvertebral fractures was significantly lower in the clodronate-treated group than in the placebo-treated group.

Two randomized studies of pamidronate for multiple myeloma have been reported. In a Danish-Swedish cooperative group study, 300 previously untreated patients were randomly assigned to receive daily oral pamidronate (300 mg) or placebo.[15] All patients were treated with intermittent melphalan and prednisone. Fewer episodes of severe pain were observed in the pamidronate-treated group. After a median of 18 months, the two groups showed no significant differences in skeleton-related morbidity, incidence of hypercalcemia, or survival.

In a Myeloma Aredia Study Group trial, 392 patients with Durie-Salmon stage III multiple myeloma and at least

TABLE 26.3

MAJOR RANDOMIZED CONTROLLED TRIALS OF BISPHOSPHONATES FOR MULTIPLE MYELOMA

Study (Reference)	N	Treatment	Result
Canadian (11)	166	Etidronate vs. placebo	No difference in skeletal morbidity
Finnish (12)	336	Clodronate vs. placebo	No difference in skeletal morbidity
German (13)	170	Clodronate vs. placebo	Trend toward fewer new bone lesions
Medical Research Council (14)	536	Clodronate vs. placebo	Reduced proportion of patients with fracture
Danish-Swedish (15)	300	Pamidronate vs. placebo	No difference in skeletal morbidity; improved pain
Myeloma Aredia Study (16)	377	Pamidronate vs. placebo	38% decrease in skeletal morbidity rate
Myeloma Ibandronate (17)	214	Ibandronate vs. placebo	No differences in skeletal-related events
Zometa Protocol 10 (18)	1,648	Zoledronic acid vs. pamidronate	Noninferiority study in breast and myeloma; similar clinical outcomes overall

one osteolytic lesion were treated with antimyeloma therapy and either placebo or pamidronate (90 mg intravenously every month for 9 months).[16] The proportion of patients who had any skeletal events (pathologic fracture, irradiation of or surgery on bone, or spinal cord compression) was significantly lower in the pamidronate group than in the placebo group (24% vs. 41%, $P < .001$). The patients who received pamidronate had significant decreases in bone pain and improved quality of life. Overall survival was similar for both groups. Among patients receiving second-line chemotherapy at study entry, median survival was significantly longer in the pamidronate-treated group than in the placebo-treated group (21 vs. 14 months, $P = .041$).

A Myeloma Ibandronate Study Group trial assessed the efficacy of ibandronate in patients with advanced-stage multiple myeloma.[17] Two-hundred and fourteen patients with multiple myeloma stage II or III were randomly assigned to receive either intravenous ibandronate (2 mg) or placebo monthly for 12 to 24 months in addition to conventional chemotherapy. The incidence of skeletal-related events, the skeletal morbidity rate, and survival were similar between the ibandronate and placebo groups. In exploratory analyses, strong suppression of bone turnover markers was associated with better clinical outcomes.

Zometa Protocol 10 was designed to demonstrate that zoledronic acid was not inferior to pamidronate for patients with breast cancer or multiple myeloma.[18] Approximately 1,600 patients with either Durie-Salmon stage III multiple myeloma or advanced breast cancer and at least one bone lesion were randomly assigned to treatment with either 4 or 8 mg of zoledronic acid via a 15-minute intravenous infusion or 90 mg of pamidronate via a 2-hour intravenous infusion every 3 to 4 weeks for 12

months.[18] The primary efficacy endpoint was the proportion of patients experiencing at least one skeletal- related event over 13 months. The zoledronic 8-mg group was discontinued because of excess renal toxicity. The proportion of patients with at least one skeletal-related event was similar in all treatment groups. The median time to the first skeletal-related event was approximately 1 year in each treatment group. The skeletal morbidity rate was slightly lower in patients treated with zoledronic acid than in those treated with pamidronate. Safety, including incidence of renal impairment, was similar for the zoledronic acid 4-mg and pamidronate groups.

The American Society of Clinical Oncology has published clinical practice guidelines on the role of bisphosphonates in myeloma.[19] The authors of the guidelines conclude that bisphosphonates provide a meaningful supportive benefit to multiple myeloma patients with lytic bone disease. The authors also conclude that further research is warranted to address the following issues: (1) when to start and stop bisphosphonate therapy, (2) how to integrate its use with other treatments for lytic bone disease, (3) how to evaluate its role in the treatment of myeloma patients without lytic bone involvement, (4) how to distinguish between symptomatic and asymptomatic bony events, and (5) how to better determine the costs and benefits of bisphosphonate therapy.

BREAST CANCER

Several large randomized trials have evaluated the effect of bisphosphonate therapy on skeletal events in women with breast cancer and bone metastases (Table 26.4).

In a double-blind Canadian study, 173 women with breast cancer metastatic to bone were randomly assigned

TABLE 26.4
MAJOR RANDOMIZED CONTROLLED TRIALS OF BISPHOSPHONATES FOR METASTATIC BREAST CANCER

Study (Reference)	N	Treatment	Result
Canadian (20)	173	Clodronate vs. placebo	28% decrease in skeletal events
Netherlands (21)	161	Pamidronate vs. no bisphosphonate	38% reduction in skeletal morbidity rate
Aredia Multinational (22)	224	Pamidronate vs. no bisphosphonate	48% increase in median time to skeletal progression
Aredia Protocol 18 (23)	380	Pamidronate vs. placebo	37% reduction in skeletal morbidity rate
Aredia Protocol 19 (24)	371	Pamidronate vs. placebo	42% reduction in skeletal morbidity rate
Zometa Protocol 10 (18)	1,648	Zoledronic acid vs. pamidronate	Noninferiority study in breast and myeloma; similar clinical outcomes overall; trend toward better outcomes in breast cancer subset
Ibandronate 4265 (26)	466	Ibandronate vs. placebo	Significant improvement in skeletal morbidity period rate
Oral ibandronate (27)	564	Ibandronate vs. placebo	Significant improvement in skeletal morbidity period rate

to receive either daily oral clodronate (1,600 mg) or placebo.[20] No significant difference in survival was found between the two groups. The combined rate of skeletal events was 28% lower in the clodronate-treated group ($P < .001$). Treatment with clodronate resulted in significant reduction in the incidence of hypercalcemia, number of vertebral fractures, and number of vertebral deformities.

In an open-label study in the Netherlands, 161 women with predominantly osteolytic metastases were randomly assigned to receive daily oral pamidronate (300 to 600 mg) or no bisphosphonate.[21] Treatment with pamidronate resulted in a statistically significant 38% reduction in skeletal morbidity. The benefit of treatment appeared to be dose-dependent, although significant gastrointestinal toxicity was observed at the higher dose.

Three randomized studies of intravenous pamidronate therapy have been reported. In an open-label Aredia Multinational Cooperative Group Study, 295 women with progressive bone metastases were randomly assigned to receive either pamidronate (45 mg intravenously every 3 or 4 weeks) or no bisphosphonate until skeletal disease progression.[22] All women were treated with standard chemotherapy. Among 224 evaluable patients, treatment with pamidronate resulted in a statistically significant 48% increase in time to skeletal disease progression. Decreases in other skeleton-related events were not significant. The lack of significant improvements in other skeletal events may reflect the low dose of pamidronate used and the discontinuation of treatment at skeletal disease progression.

In the Protocol 18 Aredia Breast Cancer Study, 372 women who had metastatic breast cancer and at least one lytic bone lesion and who were receiving hormonal therapy were randomly assigned to receive either placebo or pamidronate (90 mg intravenously every 4 weeks) for 24 cycles.[23] The skeletal morbidity rate (ratio of number of skeletal events to time on study) was significantly reduced at 12, 18, and 24 cycles in women treated with pamidronate ($P = .028, .023$, and $.008$, respectively). At 24 cycles, the proportion of patients with any skeletal complication was 56% in the pamidronate group and 67% in the placebo group ($P = .027$). The time to first skeletal complication was longer in patients treated with pamidronate than in those receiving placebo ($P = .049$). No significant difference in survival was seen.

In the Protocol 19 Aredia Breast Cancer Study, 380 women with metastatic breast cancer and at least one lytic bone lesion were treated with cytotoxic chemotherapy and either placebo or pamidronate (90 mg intravenously every month for 12 months).[24] The median time to the occurrence of the first skeletal complication (pathologic fractures, need for radiation to bone or bone surgery, spinal cord compression, and hypercalcemia requiring treatment) was greater in the pamidronate group than in the placebo group (13.1 vs. 7.0 months, $P = .005$). In addition, the proportion of patients in whom any skeletal complication occurred was lower in the pamidronate treatment group (43% vs. 56%,

$P = .008$). The pamidronate group showed significantly less increase in bone pain ($P = .046$) and deterioration of performance status ($P = .027$) than the placebo group.

As noted in the section on multiple myeloma, Zometa Protocol 10 was designed to demonstrate that zoledronic acid was not inferior to pamidronate for patients with breast cancer or multiple myeloma.[18] Approximately 1,600 patients with either Durie-Salmon stage III multiple myeloma or advanced breast cancer and at least one bone lesion were randomly assigned to treatment with either 4 or 8 mg of zoledronic acid via a 15-minute intravenous infusion or 90 mg of pamidronate via a 2-hour intravenous infusion every 3 to 4 weeks for 12 months.[18] The primary efficacy endpoint was the proportion of patients experiencing at least one skeletal-related event over 13 months. The zoledronic 8-mg group was discontinued because of excess renal toxicity. Overall, the incidence of skeletal-related events, time to first skeletal-related event, and skeletal morbidity rate were similar between the groups. In the subset of 1,130 patients with breast cancer, treatment with zoledronic acid was associated with improved outcomes.[25]

Three randomized controlled trials evaluated the efficacy of ibandronate in metastatic breast cancer. In one study, 466 patients with metastatic breast cancer were randomly assigned to intravenous ibandronate (4 mg or 6 mg) versus placebo.[26] The primary efficacy endpoint was the skeletal morbidity period rate (SMPR), defined as the number of 12-week periods with new skeletal related events. Secondary endpoints were bone pain scores and analgesic use. Compared with placebo, no statistically significant differences were noted in any parameter with 4 mg ibandronate. In contrast, subjects in the ibandronate 6 mg group had significantly lower SMPR (-20%, 1.19 vs. 1.48, $P = 0.004$) and longer median time to first SRE (51 vs. 33 weeks, $P = 0.018$) compared to placebo. Using a multivariate Poisson regression model, the mean reduction in the relative risk of SREs was 40% compared with placebo ($P = 0.003$). Secondary endpoints, pain score, analgesic use and QOL deterioration, were also significantly lower for 6 mg ibandronate compared to placebo.

In the two other studies, 564 patients with metastatic breast cancer were randomly assigned to receive oral ibandronate (50 mg/day) or placebo for up to 96 weeks. In pooled analyses of the two studies, the ibandronate group had significant improvement in mean SMPR compared to placebo (0.95 vs. 1.18, $P < 0.004$).[27] By multivariate Poisson's regression analyses, ibandronate significantly reduced the risk of SRE by 38% compared with placebo ($P < 0.001$). The secondary endpoints, bone pain score, analgesic use, and QOL scare reduction, were significantly more favorable in the ibandronate group than in the placebo group ($P = 0.001$, $P < 0.02$ and $P = 0.032$, respectively).

Three randomized controlled trials have evaluated the effect of clodronate on the development of bone metastases on women with high-risk primary breast cancer. Two of the three studies suggest that bisphosphonates reduce the incidence and number of new bony and visceral metastases in women with high-risk primary breast cancer. In one study of 302 women with primary breast cancer and immunohistochemical evidence of tumor cells in the bone marrow, administration of clodronate (1,600 mg by mouth daily for 2 years) reduced the incidence of distant metastases by 50% ($P < .001$).[28] The incidence of both osseous and visceral metastases was significantly lower in the clodronate-treated group than in the control group ($P = .003$). The mean number of bony metastases per patient in the clodronate group was roughly half that in the control group (3.1 vs. 6.3). In another study, 1,069 women with operable breast cancer were randomized to receive oral clodronate (1,600 mg/day) or a placebo for 2 years starting within 6 months of primary treatment.[29] The primary endpoint was relapse in bone, analyzed on an intent-to-treat basis, during the medication period and during the total follow-up period (median follow-up, 2,007 days). During the total follow-up period, there was a nonsignificant reduction in occurrence of bone metastases (hazard ratio, 0.77; 95% CI, 0.56 to 1.08; $P = .13$). During the medication period there was a significant reduction in the occurrence of bone metastases (hazard ratio, 0.44; 95% CI, 0.22 to 0.86; $P = .016$). The occurrence of nonosseous metastases was similar, but there was a significant reduction in mortality in favor of clodronate during the total follow-up period. A third randomized controlled trial failed to demonstrate efficacy of adjuvant clodronate. Two-hundred and ninety-nine women with primary node-positive breast cancer were randomized to clodronate ($n = 149$) or control groups ($n = 150$).[30] Clodronate 1,600 mg daily was given orally for 3 years. The incidence of bone metastases was similar in both groups. Clodronate was associated with greater risk of nonskeletal metastases and shorter disease-free survival. Additional studies are required to evaluate the role of bisphosphonates as adjuvant therapy for breast cancer and other malignancies.

The American Society of Clinical Oncology has published clinical practice guidelines on the role of bisphosphonates in breast cancer.[31] The authors of the guidelines conclude that bisphosphonates provide a supportive, albeit expensive and non-life-prolonging, benefit to many patients with bone metastases. The authors also conclude that additional information is needed about (1) when to stop therapy, (2) alternative doses or schedules for administration, and (3) how to best coordinate bisphosphonates with other palliative therapies.

PROSTATE CANCER

Most bone metastases in men with prostate cancer appear osteoblastic by radiographic imaging. Osteolytic and osteoblastic lesions represent two extremes of a spectrum, however, and morphologic studies suggest that most bone metastases from prostate cancer are characterized by both excess bone formation and bone resorption. Pathological acceleration of bone remodeling results in disorganized bone with impaired biomechanical properties.

Osteoblastic metastases from prostate cancer have increased osteoblast number and activity, increased bone volume, and increased the bone mineralization rate.[32] Osteoclast number and activity are increased in osteoblastic metastases in bone adjacent to metastases and in distant uninvolved bone.[32,33] Biochemical markers of osteoclast activity are elevated in men with osteoblastic metastases from prostate cancer.[34] Although osteoclast activity is increased in men with prostate cancer, it is unclear whether osteoclast activation precedes bone formation, as in normal bone remodeling, or osteoclast activation is secondary to excessive osteoblast activity in the metastases. Markers of osteoclast activity independently predict the risk for subsequent skeletal complications,[35] suggesting that cancer-mediated osteoclast activation not only accompanies bone metastases but also contributes to the clinical complications of metastatic disease. These observations form the rationale for osteoclast-targeted therapy in men with prostate cancer and blastic bone disease.

Three contemporary studies have evaluated the efficacy of bisphosphonates in men with hormone-refractory metastatic prostate cancer (Table 26.5).

In the zoledronic acid 039 study, 643 men with androgen-independent prostate cancer and asymptomatic/minimally symptomatic bone metastases were assigned randomly to zoledronic acid (4 mg intravenously every 3 weeks) or placebo.[36] All men continued androgen-deprivation ther-

TABLE 26.5

CONTEMPORARY RANDOMIZED TRIALS OF BISPHOSPHONATES FOR MEN WITH HORMONE-REFRACTORY METASTATIC PROSTATE CANCER

Study (Reference)	N	Treatment	Result
Zometa 039 (36)	643	Zoledronic acid vs. placebo	Significant decrease in skeletal-related events
Study 032/INT 05 (38)	350	Pamidronate vs. placebo	No significant difference in pain, analgesic use, or skeletal-related events
NCIC Pr06 (37)	204	Mitoxantrone and prednisone ± clodronate	No significant difference in palliative response

apy throughout the study and received additional antineoplastic therapy at the discretion of the investigator. The primary study endpoint was the proportion of men who experienced one or more skeletal-related events (pathological fracture, spinal cord compression, surgery or radiation therapy to bone, or change in antineoplastic treatment to treat bone pain). By fifteen months, at least one skeletal-related event occurred in 44% of men who received placebo and 33% of men who received zoledronic acid ($P = .02$). The median time to first skeletal-related event differed significantly between men who received zoledronic acid and men who received placebo (>420 vs. 321 days; $P = .01$). The study was not designed to evaluate the effect of zoledronic acid on survival. Median time to death, however, was longer in the zoledronic group than in the placebo group (546 vs. 464 days, $P = .09$).

The two other contemporary randomized, controlled trials for men with hormone-refractory prostate cancer were negative. In the National Cancer Institute of Canada Pr06 study, 204 men with androgen-independent prostate cancer and symptomatic bone metastases were assigned randomly to two treatments: mitoxantrone, prednisone, and intravenous clodronate versus mitoxantrone, prednisone, and placebo.[37] The primary study endpoints were pain scores and analgesic use. Pain scores, analgesic use, duration of palliative benefit, and overall survival did not differ significantly between the groups. In a pooled analyses of two multicentered trials, protocol 032 and INT 05, 350 men with androgen-independent prostate cancer and symptomatic bone metastases were assigned randomly to either intravenous pamidronate or placebo every 3 weeks for 27 weeks.[38] Pain scores, analgesic use, proportion of men with at least one skeletal-related event by 27 weeks, and survival were similar in the pamidronate and placebo groups.

Only one study has evaluated the efficacy of bisphosphonates in men receiving initial hormone therapy for metastatic prostate cancer. In the Medical Research Council Pr05 study, 311 men who were starting or responding to primary androgen-deprivation therapy were assigned randomly to either oral clodronate (2,080 mg/day) or placebo.[39] All the men continued primary androgen-deprivation therapy. The relative risk of skeletal disease progression or prostate cancer death was lower in the clodronate group, although the difference was not significant. Adverse events were more common among men treated with clodronate. Gastrointestinal problems and elevated serum concentrations of lactate dehydrogenase were the most common adverse events.

Each of the contemporary randomized, controlled trials in prostate cancer has potential limitations. Inadequate sample size, use of less potent bisphosphonates, and endpoint definition may account for the lack of statistically significant benefits in the MRC Pr05, NCIC Pro6, and Protocol 032/INT 05 studies. In addition, the advanced disease state of subjects in the NCIC Pr06 and Protocol 032/INT 05 may have contributed to the inability to demonstrate any benefit.

OTHER MALIGNANCIES

Only one large randomized controlled trial has evaluated the efficacy of bisphosphonates for patients with bone metastases from other malignancies. In the Zometa Protocol 11 study, 773 patients with bone metastases from lung cancer or other solid tumors (except breast or prostate cancer) were randomly assigned to receive zoledronic acid or placebo every 3 weeks for 9 months.[40] Concurrent antineoplastic therapy was administered at the discretion of the treating physician. The primary efficacy analysis was proportion of patients with at least one skeletal-related event. At 9 months, the proportion of subjects with a skeletal related event was 38% for the zoledronic acid group versus 44% for the placebo group ($P = .13$). The median time to first event was significantly longer for the zoledronic acid group than the placebo group (230 vs. 163 days; $P = .02$). Multiple event analyses showed that the risk of skeletal-related events was significantly decreased with zoledronic acid (hazard ratio, 0.73; $P = .017$). The results of this study contributed to the broad approval of zoledronic acid for the treatment of patients with bone metastases from any solid tumor.

A retrospective analysis of the Zometa Protocol 11 data assessed the efficacy and safety of zoledronic acid in the subset of 74 patients with metastatic renal cell carcinoma.[41] Zoledronic acid (4 mg intravenously every 3–4 weeks) was found to significantly reduce the proportion of patients with skeletal-related event (37% vs. 74% for placebo, $P = .015$). Similarly, zoledronic acid significantly reduced the mean skeletal morbidity rate (2.68 versus 3.38 for placebo, $P = .014$) and extended the time to the first event (median not reached vs. 72 days for placebo, $P = .006$). The median time to progression of bone lesions was significantly longer for patients who were treated with zoledronic acid ($P = .014$).

CONCLUSION

Bisphosphonate therapy has become an important part of supportive care for patients with advanced malignancies. Potent bisphosphonates administered by the intravenous route are the treatment of choice for patients with hypercalcemia of malignancy. Bisphosphonates reduce the skeletal morbidity associated with multiple myeloma and breast cancer with osteolytic bone metastases. Treatment with bisphosphonates reduces pain in patients with symptomatic bone metastases from other primary sites.

In addition to having an established role in supportive care, bisphosphonates show the potential to change the natural history of some cancers. Several studies suggest that adjuvant treatment with bisphosphonates may prevent or delay new bone metastases in women with high-risk primary breast cancer.

REFERENCES

1. Rogers MJ, Watts DJ, Russell RG. Overview of bisphosphonates. Cancer 1997;80:1652–1660.
2. Mundy GR. Metastasis to bone: causes, consequences and therapeutic opportunities. Nat Rev Cancer 2002;2:584–593.
3. Clezardin P. The antitumor potential of bisphosphonates. Semin Oncol 2002;29:33–42,
4. Green JR. Antitumor effects of bisphosphonates. Cancer 2003;97:840–847.
5. Rankin W, Grill V, Martin TJ. Parathyroid hormone-related protein and hypercalcemia. Cancer 1997;80:1564–1571.
6. Body JJ, Dumon JC. Treatment of tumour-induced hypercalcaemia with the bisphosphonate pamidronate: dose-response relationship and influence of tumour type. Ann Oncol 1994;5:359–363.
7. Purohit OP, Radstone CR, Anthony C, et al. A randomised double-blind comparison of intravenous pamidronate and clodronate in the hypercalcaemia of malignancy. Br J Cancer 1995;72:1289–1293.
8. Pecherstorfer M, Steinhauer EU, Rizzoli R, et al. Efficacy and safety of ibandronate in the treatment of hypercalcemia of malignancy: a randomized multicentric comparison to pamidronate. Support Care Cancer 2003;11:539–547.
9. Major P, Lortholary A, Hon J, et al. Zoledronic acid is superior to pamidronate in the treatment of hypercalcemia of malignancy: a pooled analysis of two randomized, controlled clinical trials. J Clin Oncol 2001;19:558–567.
10. Body JJ, Bartl R, Burckhardt P, et al. Current use of bisphosphonates in oncology. International Bone and Cancer Study Group. J Clin Oncol 1998;16:3890–3899.
11. Belch AR, Bergsagel DE, Wilson K, et al. Effect of daily etidronate on the osteolysis of multiple myeloma. J Clin Oncol 1991;9:1397–1402.
12. Lahtinen R, Laakso M, Palva I, et al. Randomised, placebo-controlled multicentre trial of clodronate in multiple myeloma. Finnish Leukaemia Group. Lancet 1992;340:1049–1052.
13. Clemens MR, Fessele K, Heim ME. Multiple myeloma: effect of daily dichloromethylene bisphosphonate on skeletal complications. Ann Hematol 1993;66:141–146.
14. McCloskey EV, MacLennan IC, Drayson MT, et al. A randomized trial of the effect of clodronate on skeletal morbidity in multiple myeloma. MRC Working Party on Leukaemia in Adults. Br J Haematol 1998;100:317–325.
15. Brincker H, Westin J, Abildgaard N, et al. Failure of oral pamidronate to reduce skeletal morbidity in multiple myeloma: a double-blind placebo-controlled trial. Danish-Swedish Co-operative Study Group. Br J Haematol 1998;101:280–286.
16. Berenson JR, Lichtenstein A, Porter L, et al. Efficacy of pamidronate in reducing skeletal events in patients with advanced multiple myeloma. Myeloma Aredia Study Group. N Engl J Med 1996;334:488–493.
17. Menssen HD, Sakalova A, Fontana A, et al. Effects of long-term intravenous ibandronate therapy on skeletal-related events, survival, and bone resorption markers in patients with advanced multiple myeloma. J Clin Oncol 2002;20:2353–2359.
18. Rosen LS, Gordon D, Kaminski M, et al. Zoledronic acid versus pamidronate in the treatment of skeletal metastases in patients with breast cancer or osteolytic lesions of multiple myeloma: a phase III, double-blind, comparative trial. Cancer J 2001;7:377–387.
19. Berenson JR, Hillner BE, Kyle RA, et al. American Society of Clinical Oncology clinical practice guidelines: the role of bisphosphonates in multiple myeloma. J Clin Oncol 2002;20: 3719–3736.
20. Paterson AH, Powles TJ, Kanis JA, et al. Double-blind controlled trial of oral clodronate in patients with bone metastases from breast cancer. J Clin Oncol 1993;11:59–65.
21. van Holten-Verzantvoort AT, Kroon HM, Bijvoet OL, et al. Palliative pamidronate treatment in patients with bone metastases from breast cancer. J Clin Oncol 1993;11:491–498.
22. Conte PF, Latreille J, Mauriac L, et al. Delay in progression of bone metastases in breast cancer patients treated with intravenous pamidronate: results from a multinational randomized controlled trial. The Aredia Multinational Cooperative Group. J Clin Oncol 1996;14:2552–2559.
23. Theriault RL, Lipton A, Hortobagyi GN, et al. Pamidronate reduces skeletal morbidity in women with advanced breast cancer and lytic bone lesions: a randomized, placebo-controlled trial. Protocol 18 Aredia Breast Cancer Study Group. J Clin Oncol 1999;17:846–854.
24. Hortobagyi GN, Theriault RL, Porter L, et al. Efficacy of pamidronate in reducing skeletal complications in patients with breast cancer and lytic bone metastases. Protocol 19 Aredia Breast Cancer Study Group. N Engl J Med 1996;335:1785–1791.
25. Rosen LS, Gordon DH, Dugan W Jr, et al. Zoledronic acid is superior to pamidronate for the treatment of bone metastases in breast carcinoma patients with at least one osteolytic lesion. Cancer 2004;100:36–43.
26. Body JJ, Diel IJ, Lichinitser MR, et al: Intravenous ibandronate reduces the incidence of skeletal complications in patients with breast cancer and bone metastases. Ann Oncol 2003;14:1399–1405.
27. Body JJ, Diel IJ, Lichinitzer M, et al: Oral ibandronate reduces the risk of skeletal complications in breast cancer patients with metastatic bone disease: results from two randomised, placebo-controlled phase III studies. Br J Cancer 2004;90:1133–1137.
28. Diel IJ, Solomayer EF, Costa SD, et al. Reduction in new metastases in breast cancer with adjuvant clodronate treatment. N Engl J Med 1998;339:357–363.
29. Powles T, Paterson S, Kanis JA, et al. Randomized, placebo-controlled trial of clodronate in patients with primary operable breast cancer. J Clin Oncol 2002;20:3219–3224.
30. Saarto T, Blomqvist C, Virkkunen P, et al. Adjuvant clodronate treatment does not reduce the frequency of skeletal metastases in node-positive breast cancer patients: 5-year results of a randomized controlled trial. J Clin Oncol 2001;19:10–17.
31. Hillner BE, Ingle JN, Chlebowski RT, et al. American Society of Clinical Oncology 2003 update on the role of bisphosphonates and bone health issues in women with breast cancer. J Clin Oncol 2003;21:4042–4057.
32. Clarke NW, McClure J, George NJ. Osteoblast function and osteomalacia in metastatic prostate cancer. Eur Urol 1993;24:286–290.
33. Clarke NW, McClure J, George NJ. Morphometric evidence for bone resorption and replacement in prostate cancer. Br J Urol 1991;68:74–80.
34. Garnero P, Sornay-Rendu E, Claustrat B, et al. Biochemical markers of bone turnover, endogenous hormones and the risk of fractures in postmenopausal women: the OFELY study. J Bone Miner Res 2000;15:1526–1536.
35. Berruti A, Dogliotti L, Bitossi R, et al. Incidence of skeletal complications in patients with bone metastatic prostate cancer and hormone refractory disease: predictive role of bone resorption and formation markers evaluated at baseline. J Urol 2000;164:1248–1253.
36. Saad F, Gleason DM, Murray R, et al. A randomized, placebo-controlled trial of zoledronic acid in patients with hormone-refractory metastatic prostate carcinoma. J Natl Cancer Inst 2002;94:1458–1468.
37. Ernst D, Tannock I, Venner P, et al. Randomized placebo controlled trial of mitoxantrone/prednisone and clodronate versus mitoxantrone/prednisone alone in patients with hormone refractory prostate cancer (HRPC) and pain: National Cancer Institute of Canada Clinical Trials Group study [abstract]. Proc ASCO 2002;705:A177.
38. Small EJ, Smith MR, Seaman JJ, et al. Combined analysis of two multicenter, randomized, placebo-controlled studies of pamidronate disodium for the palliation of bone pain in men with metastatic prostate cancer. J Clin Oncol 2003;21.
39. Dearnaley DP, Sydes MR, Mason MD, et al. A double-blind, placebo-controlled, randomized trial of oral sodium clodronate for metastatic prostate cancer (MRC PR05 Trial). J Natl Cancer Inst 2003;95:1300–1311.
40. Rosen LS, Gordon D, Tchekmedyian S, et al. Zoledronic acid versus placebo in the treatment of skeletal metastases in patients with lung cancer and other solid tumors: a phase III, double-blind, randomized trial. Zoledronic Acid Lung Cancer and Other Solid Tumors Study Group. J Clin Oncol 2003;21:3150–3157.
41. Lipton A, Zheng M, Seaman J. Zoledronic acid delays the onset of skeletal-related events and progression of skeletal disease in patients with advanced renal cell carcinoma. Cancer 2003;98:962–969.

Thalidomide and Its Analogs for the Treatment of Hematologic Malignancies, Including Multiple Myeloma and Solid Tumors

27

Paul Richardson   *Constantine S. Mitsiades*
Teru Hideshima   *Kenneth Anderson*

INTRODUCTION

Thalidomide was originally developed in the 1950s for the treatment of pregnancy-associated morning sickness. However, its extensive over-the-counter marketing in Europe was marked by the tragic consequences of teratogenicity and dysmelia (stunted limb growth),[1] which triggered its subsequent withdrawal from the market.[2,3] In addition, the teratogenic properties of thalidomide raised among oncologists the hypothesis that the potent

Disclosure: Dr. Paul Richardson and Dr. Kenneth Anderson are members of the Speakers' Bureau for Celgene Corp. Kenneth Anderson is a member of the Advisory Board of Celgene Corp.

inhibitory effects of this drug on growing fetal tissues, combined with the pathophysiologic similarities linking tumor biology and fetal development, might be redirected towards applications in cancer treatment.[4] In fact, in the early 1960s at least two clinical trials of thalidomide for patients with advanced cancers were reported.[5,6] In one of these trials, thalidomide was administered at daily doses of 300 to 2,000 mg in 71 patients with various types of cancers. No objective clinical responses were observed, except for resolution of a pulmonary metastasis in a patient with renal cell carcinoma.[5] In the second trial, 21 patients with various types of advanced cancer (including 2 patients with multiple myeloma [MM]) received thalidomide at 600 to 2,000 mg daily doses, which led to palliation of symptoms in approximately one third of the patients, while 2 patients had minimal slowing of their tumor's growth.[6] However, these results were not deemed sufficiently encouraging to warrant further clinical development efforts. Thalidomide was therefore not further pursued as a potential anticancer drug for several decades. In the meantime, however, the drug gradually emerged as a therapeutic agent for a range of medical conditions, on the basis of anecdotal clinical evidence and converging supporting research evidence suggesting potential beneficial pharmaco-immunologic effects.[7] For instance, thalidomide was used, within the context of clinical trials or for compassionate use, for the treatment of severe erythema nodosum leprosum (ENL),[8] Behçet's disease,[9] graft versus host disease,[10] and oral ulcers and wasting associated with HIV infection.[11,12] This reemergence of thalidomide was reflected by its FDA approval in 1998 for the short-term treatment of cutaneous manifestations of moderate to severe ENL, together with its use as maintenance therapy to prevent recurrence of cutaneous ENL.[7] This FDA approval was of critical importance for the clinical applications of thalidomide, not only because it has since become a treatment of choice for ENL, but also because it allowed for off-label use of this medication for a wide spectrum of other disease states for which it was speculated that the immunomodulatory and antiangiogenic properties of thalidomide would be beneficial (Table 27.1).[7,13,14] To prevent any occurrence of teratogenic effects, thalidomide is now administered under strict guidelines to prevent fetal exposure to the this medication.[13]

TABLE 27.1

POTENTIAL THERAPEUTIC USES OF THALIDOMIDE CURRENTLY UNDER INVESTIGATION

Cancer and related conditions
   Solid tumors (e.g., brain, breast, renal cell carcinoma)
   Hematologic malignancies (e.g., MM and myelodysplastic
      syndromes [MDS])
Infectious diseases
   HIV/AIDS and related conditions
   Aphthous ulcerations
   Wasting syndrome
   Mycobacterial infections (e.g., tuberculosis)
Autoimmune diseases
   Discoid and systemic lupus erythematosus
   Chronic graft vs. host disease
   Inflammatory bowel disease
   Rheumatoid arthritis
   Multiple sclerosis
Dermatologic diseases
   Behçet's syndrome
   Prurigo nodularis
   Pyoderma gangrenosum
Other disorders
   Sarcoidosis
   Diabetic retinopathy
   Macular degeneration

The interest in the use of thalidomide in the oncologic setting was rekindled in the 1990s with the realization that tumor-associated vasculature is an important therapeutic target in a broad range of neoplasias and that thalidomide possesses substantial antiangiogenic properties in a wide range of in vivo and in vitro models of neovascularization.[15–23]

Indeed, thalidomide inhibited angiogenesis induced by bFGF in the rabbit cornea micropocket assay or by VEGF in a murine model of corneal vascularization.[19,24] Based on these data from D'Amato, Folkman, et al. and the fact that thalidomide is transformed to active metabolites with antiangiogenic activity in humans,[25] thalidomide was evaluated for the treatment of various neoplasias.[26–30] Of particular note was the well-chronicled decision to test thalidomide, at the suggestion of an especially enlightened wife of a MM patient and on the basis of the studies by Folkman et al., in a compassionate use study of three patients with advanced MM at the University of Arkansas. The encouraging evidence of clinical activity in two of these three patients led to a larger phase II effort,[31] which confirmed the clinical activity of thalidomide against MM and was followed by extensive clinical trials of thalidomide-based therapy for MM worldwide as well as other applications in a broad range of other hematologic malignancies and solid tumors. Despite the progress in its use and the fact that thalidomide does not have the classical patterns of toxicities associated with the use of conventional DNA- or microtubule-targeting chemotherapeutics, this is still a drug that is not completely devoid of any adverse effects. This has led to an effort to develop thalidomide analogs that are not only more potent than their parent compound in preclinical models but also retain the clinical activity of thalidomide without some of the serious side effects associated with its use.

In this chapter, we present a comprehensive review of the pharmacology of thalidomide and its analogs, a description of preclinical studies in MM to illustrate the complex putative mechanisms of action of thalidomide, and an overview of clinical studies that have confirmed the activity of thalidomide and its analogs against MM. Studies in other hematologic malignancies and the status of research in solid tumors and in other cancer-related applications are also discussed.

MECHANISM(S) OF ACTION OF THALIDOMIDE AND ITS IMMUNOMODULATORY DERIVATIVES (IMIDS)

Although it was originally hypothesized that the teratogenic and antitumor effects of thalidomide may have a common underlying mechanistic denominator, such as its antiangiogenic effect, the precise mechanisms responsible for the clinical activity of thalidomide remain to be completely elucidated. This can be attributed to a number of reasons: (a) the preclinical in vitro and in vivo studies of thalidomide that are necessary to dissect its mechanisms of action are difficult to perform because of the enantiomeric interconversion and spontaneous cleavage of the drug to multiple metabolites,[32] many of which have been incompletely characterized due to their short half-life; (b) the in vivo activity of thalidomide requires metabolic activation, mainly by the liver, which explains at least in part the discordance between the modest, at best, activity of thalidomide in in vitro assays of antitumor activity[25,33] and the potent in vivo effect; (c) the chemical structure of thalidomide does not offer readily recognizable clues regarding possible intracellular molecular targets that might explain its clinical activity or adverse events; and (d) the species-specific differences in the metabolism and other pharmacokinetic properties of thalidomide complicate the extrapolation of in vivo data from many animal models to the clinical setting in humans.[24]

In regards to the antitumor activity of thalidomide, the biggest wealth of mechanistic information has been acquired in the setting of MM, mainly because this is the disease setting in which thalidomide has demonstrated more impressive clinical activity. Despite the modest activity of thalidomide in antitumor assays in vitro,[34] this drug is currently considered to confer its in vivo anti-MM effects via at least four distinct but potentially complementary types of activity: (a) direct antiproliferative/proapoptotic antitumor activity,[34] probably mediated by one or more of its in vivo metabolites[35]; (b) indirect targeting of tumor cells by abrogation of protective effects conferred on MM tumor cells by bone marrow stromal cells via paracrine or autocrine secretion of cytokines and growth factor or via cell adhesion molecule–mediated interactions[34]; (c) antiangiogenic activity; and (d) immunomodulatory activity that contributes to enhanced antitumor immune response.[36]

The notion that thalidomide possesses direct antitumor effects in MM and other diseases is inferred from a series of converging pieces of evidence from preclinical and clinical studies. Despite the fact that the in vitro effects of thalidomide on proliferation and viability of MM cells are relatively modest,[34] thalidomide derivatives, such as lenalidomide (Revlimid, CC-5013 or IMID-1) and CC-4047 (Actimid),[34,35] have a far more potent in vitro antitumor effect through their antiproliferative and proapoptotic properties than the parent compound in assays performed in the absence of any other cell type (e.g., stromal, endothelial, or liver cells) that could facilitate either thalidomide metabolism or indirect effects on targets other than the tumor cells themselves.[34,35] Therefore, the fact that at least some of the known in vivo thalidomide metabolites can have in vitro activity against tumor cells suggests that thalidomide may confer a direct in vivo antiproliferative/proapoptotic effect via its metabolites. The precise mechanism (or mechanisms) for this direct effect remains

under investigation. Cell cycle analyses, by propidium iodide staining, of thalidomide- and lenalidomide-treated MM cell lines indicate G_0/G_1 growth arrest, subsequently followed by an increased sub-G_1 peak, consistent with induction of MM cell death.[34] Interestingly, clinically relevant doses of thalidomide derivatives, such as lenalidomide or CC-4047, trigger suppression of the transcriptional activity of NF-κB in MM cells.[35] In view of the important role of NF-κB in MM, as well as other neoplasias, in the production of several intracellular antiapoptotic molecules, including the caspase inhibitors FLIP, XIAP, cIAP-2 or the antiapoptotic Bcl-2 family member A1/Bfl-1,[37–39] this effect of thalidomide derivatives supports the notion that thalidomide exerts its in vivo effects, at least in part, by inhibition of NF-κB signaling in MM cells. It is also conceivable that because NF-κB protects MM cells from the proapoptotic effects of steroids or cytotoxic chemotherapeutics,[35,37–39] the effect of thalidomide on NF-κB activity can account for the ability of its combinations with dexamethasone or cytotoxic chemotherapeutics to achieve more potent in vivo antitumor responses than either agent alone.[40–47]

Thalidomide and its derivatives critically modulate the adhesive interactions[48] of MM cells with bone marrow stromal cells (BMSCs). The adhesion of MM cells to BMSCs triggers secretion of proliferative/antiapoptotic cytokines (e.g., IL-6).[49–51] This event is mainly paracrinic, it is mediated by transcriptional activation of NF-κB in BMSCs,[50] and it leads to attenuated sensitivity of MM cells against dexamethasone or cytotoxic chemotherapy.[52] As a result of the effect of thalidomide and its immunomodulatory derivatives (IMiDs) in blocking this MM-stromal paracrine interaction, these agents significantly modify the proliferative and drug resistance properties of MM cells in the bone marrow microenvironment.

Another important property of thalidomide is that it selectively inhibits TNF-α production, while leaving the patient's immune system otherwise intact,[53] which has led to its application in various disorders characterized by increased TNF-α secretion, such as ENL, *Mycobacterium tuberculosis* infection, graft versus host disease, and cancer- and HIV-related cachexia.

The precise mechanism mediating thalidomide-induced inhibition of TNF-α activity has not been fully elucidated, but it is apparently distinct from those of other TNF-α inhibitors, such as pentoxifylline and dexamethasone.[54,55] It has been proposed that thalidomide accelerates the degradation of TNF-α mRNA, thereby substantially (but not necessarily completely) suppressing the production of TNF-α protein.[54,56] Interestingly, thalidomide can decrease the binding of the transcription factor NF-κB to its consensus DNA-binding sites, which include not only the actual TNF-α gene[57] but also other genes that are modulated by TNF-α in an NF-κB-dependent fashion.[35] It has also been proposed that the antiangiogenic properties of thalidomide are mediated, at least in part, by inhibition of TNF-α signaling, in view of the proangiogenic effects of TNF-α itself.[19] However, the absence of a major effect of TNF-α in experimental models of angiogenesis and the inability of (at least some) potent TNFα inhibitors to directly influence angiogenesis suggest that thalidomide's antiangiogenic effects cannot be attributed to TNF-α inhibition alone.[19,24]

Thalidomide and its analogs influence factors that regulate tumor cell proliferation and osteoclast function, including interleukin (IL)-6, IL-1β, IL-10, and TNF-α.[58] Thalidomide also decreases the secretion of vascular endothelial growth factor (VEGF), IL-6,[59] and basic fibroblast growth factor (bFGF) by MM and/or BM stromal cells. These various mechanisms of action are summarized in Figure 27.1. Within the context of characterizing the mechanism underlying the teratogenic effects of thalidomide, D'Amato et al. observed its antiangiogenic properties,[19,24] which involved inhibition of the proangiogenic effects of β-FGF and/or VEGF in their models.[19,24,60] Further in vitro studies have suggested that the antiangiogenic effect of thalidomide is due to its metabolites and not the parent compound.[61]

In regards to the immunomodulatory properties of thalidomide, its precise effects on immune effector cells (e.g., different subpopulations of lymphocytes) have not been consistent across the full spectrum of pertinent studies published to date.[62–64] Although there is evidence that thalidomide does not directly suppress lymphocyte proliferation,[48] there are data indicating differential effects on T-cell stimulation, shifts in T-cell responses, and inhibition of proliferation of already stimulated lymphocytes.[63,65–68] Thalidomide also modifies the expression patterns of cell adhesion molecules on leukocytes, inhibits neutrophil chemotaxis, and modulates the production or function of various cytokines, including not only the inhibition of TNF-α signaling but also the inhibition of IL-12 production, the enhanced synthesis of IL-2, and the inhibition of IL-6.[48,53,69–72] Of particular note for the applications of thalidomide and lenalidomide in MM, thalidomide and its analogs (IMiDs) augment natural killer cell–mediated cytotoxicity in MM.[36] Thalidomide and its IMiDs do not induce T-cell proliferation alone but act as costimulators to trigger proliferation of anti-CD3–stimulated T cells from MM patients, accompanied by an increase in interferon-γ and IL-12 secretion. Importantly, treatment of patient peripheral blood mononuclear cells (PBMCs) with thalidomide or its IMiDs triggers increased lysis of autologous MM cells. Furthermore, PBMCs from MM patients have demonstrated an increase in CD3$^-$CD56$^+$ natural killer cells in response to thalidomide/IMiD therapy.[36]

PHARMACOLOGY OF THALIDOMIDE

Thalidomide or α-N(phthalimido) glutarimide ($C_{13}O_4$ N_2H_9) (gram molecular weight of 258.2)[73] is a glutamic acid derivative that contains two amide rings and a single chiral center (see Fig.27.1).[73] The currently available formulation of thalidomide consists, at physiologic pH, of a nonpolar racemic mixture of S(−) and R(+) isomers, which are cell membrane permeable.[73,74] The S isomer has been associated with thalidomide's teratogenic effect, while the R isomer has been linked with the sedative properties of the drug.[24,74,75] Because of rapidly interconversion

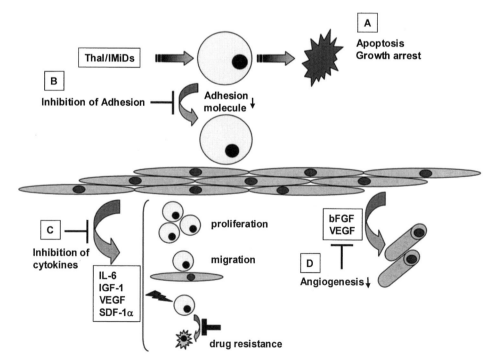

Figure 27.1 Antitumor activity of Thal/IMiDs in the bone marrow milieu. Thal/IMiDs **(A)** induce G$_1$ growth arrest and/or apoptosis in MM cell lines and patient cells resistant to conventional chemotherapy, **(B)** inhibit MM cell adhesion to BMSCs, **(C)** decrease cytokine production and sequelae, and **(D)** decrease angiogenesis in the bone marrow microenvironment.

TABLE 27.2

SINGLE–DOSE PHARMACOKINETIC PARAMETERS OF THALIDOMIDE IN HUMANS[33]

Population	Dose	Mean Apparent Pharmacokinetic Parameters		
		T_{max}	$T_{1/2}$ (hr)	V_d (L)
Elderly patients with hormone	200 mg	3.3*	6.5	66.9
refractory prostate cancer	800 mg	4.4*	18.3	165.8
Patients with HIV infection	300 mg	3.4	5.7	78.2
Healthy female volunteers	200 mg	5.8	4.1	53.0
Healthy male volunteers	200 mg	4.4	8.7	120.7

t_{max}, time to reach maximum concentrations; $t_{1/2}$, elimination half-life; V_d, volume of distribution; HIV, human immunodeficiency virus.
*Median value.
Reproduced with permission from Stirling DI. The pharmacology of thalidomide. Semin Hematol 2000;37:5–14.

of these two isomers at physiologic pH in vivo, any efforts to generate formulations of only the R isomer have failed to neutralize the teratogenic potential of thalidomide.[74,76]

Pharmacokinetics

Pharmacokinetic studies of thalidomide in humans have been limited by the lack of suitable intravenous formulations due to its instability and poor water solubility. Therefore, current knowledge about thalidomide pharmacokinetics is based on animal studies and on clinical trials in human patients receiving oral thalidomide.

As shown in Table 27.2, the pharmacokinetic properties of thalidomide are variable, with the $t_{1/2}$ falling in the range of 4 to 9 hours in most studies

Absorption

Oral administration of thalidomide at a dose of 100mg/kg in animal studies reportedly led to peak serum concentrations within 4 hours.[77] The absorption of thalidomide in these studies appeared independent of administered doses. Subsequent studies in humans indicate a similar pharmacokinetic pattern, with approximately 4 hours mean time to reach peak concentration (C_{max}) with a thalidomide dose of 200 mg.[23–25,29] In particular, single-dose thalidomide trials conducted in healthy volunteers, patients with HIV infection, and patients with hormone-refractory prostate cancer (see Table 27.2) have shown that the time to peak concentration in the peripheral blood ranges between 3 and 6 hours, suggesting slow absorption from the gastrointestinal tract.[78–80] While the area under the curve (AUC) correlates with the thalidomide dose, the maximum concentration (C_{max}) is highly variable, which also reflects the variability of GI absorption.[81,82] Correction for ideal body weight or body surface area does not lessen the variability.[78,79] This variability has further confounded efforts to

delineate the pharmacokinetic properties of thalidomide in humans and define a dose-response relationship in therapeutic trials.

Distribution

In animal studies, thalidomide is widely distributed throughout most tissues and organs,[77] without significant drug binding by plasma proteins.[79,80] Thalidomide is detected in semen of rabbits following oral administration[73,83] and has been shown to be present in semen of patients after a period of 4 weeks of therapy, with levels that seem to correlate with serum levels.[84]

Metabolism

Thalidomide undergoes rapid and spontaneous nonenzymatic hydrolytic cleavage at physiologic pH, generating up to 50 metabolites, 5 of which are considered to be primary metabolites.[25,74,76,77,85] The majority of these metabolites are unstable, and their rapid degradation under physiologic conditions has complicated the research efforts to characterize their biologic properties.[86] Although in vitro studies in rat cells suggested that thalidomide induces cytochrome (CYP) 450 isoenzymes, subsequent evaluation of single- or multiple-dose pharmacokinetic parameters of oral thalidomide at 200 mg daily in healthy volunteers showed that thalidomide does not inhibit or induce its own metabolism over a 21-day period in humans. It is therefore thought that only limited metabolism of thalidomide occurs via the hepatic CYP 450 system.[87–89] No induction of its own metabolism has been noted with prolonged use.[90,91] Importantly, there appear to be substantial species-specific differences in the patterns and profiles of metabolites of thalidomide in mice versus humans.[92–94] This explains why the teratogenic effects of thalidomide in humans were not detected in preclinical murine models

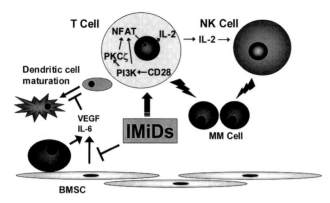

Figure 27.2 Mechanisms of action of IMiDs in augmentation of host immune response. IMiDs augment differentiation of Dendritic Cells (DC) by inhibiting secretion of IL-6 and VEGF from MM and/or BMSCs. IMiDs also stimulate natural killer cell activity by triggering IL-2 secretion from T cells mediated by the CD28/PI3-K/NF-AT2 signaling pathway.

that preceded the first clinical applications of the drug,[1,2] and also why, in immunodeficient mouse models of MM, thalidomide exhibited antitumor activity only in the setting of xenotransplantation of the mice with human liver tissue.[95]

Clearance

The primary mechanism of elimination of thalidomide occurs by the spontaneous hydrolysis in all body fluids, with an apparent mean clearance of 10 L/hour for the (R)-enantiomer and 21 L/h for the (S)-enantiomer in adult subjects.[32] This leads to higher blood concentrations of the (R)-enantiomer than of the (S)-enantiomer. Thalidomide and its metabolites are rapidly excreted in the urine, while the nonabsorbed portion of the drug is excreted unchanged in feces, but clearance is primarily nonrenal, with mean terminal half-lives of the R and S isomers measured in healthy male human volunteers at 4.6 and 4.8 hours, respectively.[77,78,81] After a single dose (200 mg daily), there was minimal intact drug excretion in urine over a 24-hour period.[78] Studies of both single and multiple dosing of thalidomide in elder prostate cancer patients showed a significantly longer half-life at a higher dose (12,00 mg daily) than at a lower dose (200 mg daily).[79] Conversely, no effect of increased age on elimination half-life was identified in the age range of 55 to 80 years.[79] The effect of hepatic dysfunction on drug clearance has not been evaluated.

Drug Interactions

Thalidomide's interactions with other drugs have not been systematically characterized, except for studies that showed a lack of significant interaction with oral contraceptives.[33] Animal studies suggest that thalidomide enhances the sedative effects of barbiturates and alcohol and the catatonic effects of chlorpromazine and reserpine.[96] Conversely,

the CNS stimulatory effects of medications such as methamphetamine and methylphenidate) appear to counteract the depressant effects of thalidomide.[96]

Adverse Effects

Generally, thalidomide is well tolerated at doses below 200 mg daily. Sedation and constipation are the most common adverse effects reported in cancer patients[26,30,33,60] (Table 27.3). The most serious adverse effect is a dose- and time-dependent peripheral sensory neuropathy.[97] An increasing incidence of thromboembolic events in thalidomide-treated patients has been reported, but generally in the context of thalidomide combinations with other drugs, including steroids and particularly anthracycline-based chemotherapy. In fact, these thromboembolic complications, which rarely appear in single-agent thalidomide treatment of MM or other cancer patients, initially triggered closure of studies exploring a combination of thalidomide with liposomal doxorubicin (Doxil) and dexamethasone.[98,99] Possible cardiovascular effects of thalidomide include bradycardia and hypotension. The risk of these adverse cardiovascular events with thalidomide treatment appears to be higher among elderly patients with coronary disease receiving multiple antihypertensive medications.[33] A recent report described for the first time a case of pulmonary hypertension in a MM patient receiving thalidomide.[100]

Safety data from current phase I and II clinical trials of thalidomide in the treatment of solid tumors, MM, and hematologic malignancies suggest peripheral neuropathy occurs in 10 to 30% of patients.[27,29,30,101] Thalidomide-related neuropathy is characterized as asymmetric, painful, peripheral paresthesia with sensory loss.[14,102–105] It commonly presents with numbness of the toes and feet, muscle cramps, weakness, signs of pyramidal tract involvement, and carpal tunnel syndrome.[14,73] The risk of developing

TABLE 27.3

CLINICAL ADVERSE EVENTS REPORTED DURING THALIDOMIDE USE[33]

Neurologic	Dermatologic
Sedation	Exfoliative/erythrodermic
Dizziness	cutaneous reactions
Mood changes	Brittle fingernails
Headaches	Pruritus
Gastrointestinal	**Miscellaneous**
Constipation	Xerostomia
Nausea	Weight gain
Increased appetite	Edema of the face/limbs
	Reduction in thyroid
	hormone secretion
	Hypotension

Reproduced with permission from Stirling DI. The pharmacology of thalidomide. Semin Hematol 2000;37:5–14.

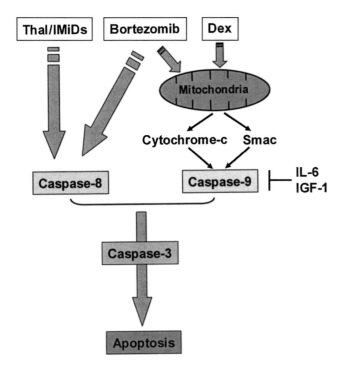

Figure 27.3 Possible apoptotic signaling triggered by Thal/IMiDs and other agents. Thal/IMiDs predominantly induce caspase-8/caspase-3 cleavage. Bortezomib triggers caspase-8 and -9 cleavage, and Dex triggers caspase-9 cleavage, suggesting rationally based combinations of Thal/IMiDs with these agents.

peripheral neuropathy during thalidomide increases with higher cumulative doses of the drug, especially in elderly patients.[73] Although clinical improvement typically occurs upon prompt discontinuation of the drug, long-standing residual sensory loss has been documented.[102–105] It remains to be determined whether the incidence of thalidomide-induced peripheral neuropathy is indeed increased in cancer patients with a history of prior exposure to vinca alkaloids, bortezomib, or other drugs that can cause peripheral neuropathy. In the interim, particular caution and careful monitoring are necessary in cases of cancer patients with a prior history of neuropathy and/or when thalidomide is used in combination with other agents associated with development of neuropathy,[33] especially since there has been little progress in defining effective strategies for alleviation of neuropathic symptoms.

Pharmacology of Thalidomide Derivatives: Focus on Lenalidomide (CC-5013, Revlimid) and CC-4047 (Actimid)

Lenalidomide (or 3-(4′aminoisoindoline-1′-one)-1-piperidine-2,6-dione) is a thalidomide derivative with an empirical formula of $C_{13}H_{13}N_3O_3$ and a molecular weight of 259.25. It constitutes a lead compound in the new class of immunomodulatory thalidomide derivatives (IMiDs) and exhibits a constellation of pharmacological properties, including inhibition of inflammation, stimulation of T

cells and natural killer cells, inhibition of angiogenesis and tumor cell proliferation, as well as modulation of hematopoietic stem cell differentiation.[34,36,58,106] It is an orally administered agent that has been tested in MM and myelodysplastic syndromes (MDS) as well as an expanding array of other clinical settings because of preclinical data suggesting more potent activity and less toxicity than its parent compound, along with a lack of teratogenic effects. The results of single- and multiple-dose studies of lenalidomide administration in healthy male volunteers[33] indicate that this drug is rapidly absorbed following oral administration, with peak plasma levels occurring between 0.6 and 1.5 hours postdose. Coadministration with food delays absorption somewhat but does not alter its actual extent, and the pharmacokinetic disposition of lenalidomide is linear. The C_{max} and AUC values increase proportionately with increasing dose, both over a single-dose range of 5 to 400 mg and after multiple dosing with 100 mg daily.[33] The $t_{1/2}$ increases with dose, from approximately 3 hours at the 5-mg dose to approximately 9 hours at the 400-mg dose (the higher dose is believed to provide a better estimate of the $t_{1/2}$ due to the prolonged elimination phase). Steady-state levels of lenalidomide are achieved by day 4 of administration, and there is no evidence of disproportionate drug accumulation with multiple dosing. Approximately 70% of the orally administered dose of lenalidomide is excreted by the kidney. Ongoing studies are characterizing in detail the adverse event profile of lenalidomide use and are addressing the potential for drug interactions with other agents. The latter consideration is particularly important because the clinical experience with thalidomide to date indicates that the adverse events with this new class of

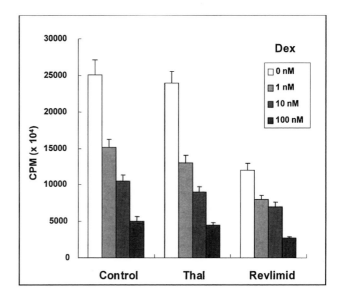

Figure 27.4 Dex augments Thal/IMiDs-induced growth inhibition in MM. MM.1S cells were treated with DMSO control, Thal (1 μM), and Revlimid μM) in the presence of different concentration of Dex for 48 hours. Cell growth was assessed by [³H]-thymidine uptake.

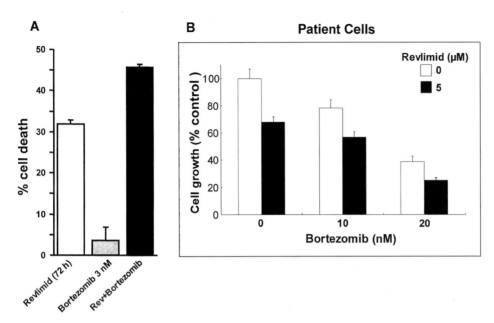

Figure 27.5 Revlimid augments bortezomib-induced cytotoxicity in MM cell lines and patient tumor cells. **A:** MM.1S cells were pretreated with or without 1 μM Revlimid for 48 hours, and then a subtoxic concentration of Bortezomib (3 nM) was added for an additional 24 hours. Revlimid potentiated the apoptotic effect of Bortezomib. **B:** CD138⁺ tumor cells are treated with control or with 10 or 20 nM bortezomib in the presence or absence of 5 μM Revlimid for 24 hours. Cell toxicity was assessed by MTT assay.

agents may be heavily influenced by a broad range of factors, including not only medications administered concomitantly but also "recall" effects of prior exposure to agents causing neurotoxicity; toxicity patterns may also be influenced by the pathophysiology of each disease (e.g., preliminary indication of a higher rate of neuropathy in thalidomide-treated patients with MM versus other disease) and the presence of comorbidities (e.g., possible aggravation of neuropathy in diabetic patients). Therefore, more extensive clinical experience will be required to conclusively determine whether lenalidomide is completely devoid of some of thalidomide's side effects when combined with other drugs and/or used in heavily pretreated patient populations. This is particularly important, because recent studies indicate that other immunomodulatory thalidomide analogs, such as CC-4047 (Actimid), are also active against MM in vivo[107] but maintain thalidomide's potential for teratogenicity[108] and result in a higher incidence of thromboembolic events than either lenalidomide or thalidomide alone,[109] suggesting important differences in the pharmacological properties of different thalidomide derivatives.

CLINICAL STUDIES OF THALIDOMIDE AND ITS DERIVATIVES IN MM

Despite efforts to improve the outcome of MM patients with the use of high-dose chemotherapy and stem cell transplantation, MM remains incurable, necessitating development of more effective therapies based on novel therapeutic targets and corresponding conceptual frameworks that depart from conventional cytotoxic chemotherapy.[110,111] One such approach involves the inhibition of angiogenesis, an approach based on multiple observations that hematologic malignancies, such as MM, are associated

with intense neovascularization of bone marrow.[23,112] Even though the bone marrow sinusoids in normal individuals are endowed with extensive networks of vascular support, the homing of MM cells (or malignant cells from other hematologic neoplasias) to the bone marrow is associated with further increase in its microvascular density (MVD), especially in more advanced cases of his disease.[112–114] This may suggest that the role of bone marrow neoangiogenesis in hematologic malignancies is related less to the sustaining of a sufficient blood supply to tumor cells (since such a supply is always readily available to cells in the bone marrow) than to the generating of a local microenvironment where the activated endothelium of bone marrow neovessels can further support the proliferation, survival, and drug resistance of tumor cells. Nonetheless, because of the extensive data that established neoangiogenesis as a key component in the growth, progression, and metastatic spread of solid tumors,[115] along with the evidence that increased bone marrow blood vessel formation parallels the progression of hematologic malignancies,[31,112,114,116–118] MM and other hematologic neoplasias have frequently been the focus of clinical applications of proposed antiangiogenic therapies.

Vacca and colleagues reported that the extent of bone marrow angiogenesis has high positive correlation with the labeling index (LI) of bone marrow plasma cells as well as disease activity in patients with MM,[112] a finding consistent with subsequent studies confirming extensive bone marrow vascularization in MM.[31,114,117,118] They also observed that a poor prognosis correlates with elevated levels of angiogenic cytokines, such as basic fibroblast growth factor (bFGF) and vascular endothelial growth factor (VEGF), and increased bone marrow levels of mast cells, which secrete a variety of angiogenic factors.[112,117–119] Collectively, these observations provided a rationale for the use of

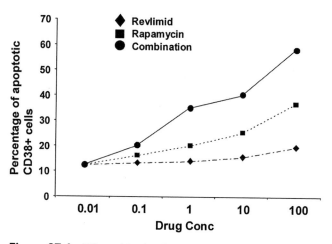

Figure 27.6 Effect of Revlimid, rapamycin, and combination on patient MM cells. A dose-dependent increase in the percentage of apoptotic patient MM cells, evidenced by Apo 2.7 staining of bright CD38 positive cells, was noted after exposure to combination Revlimid and rapamycin treatment.

antiangiogenic drugs to treat MM and other hematologic neoplasias.

Thalidomide therapy for advanced refractory MM was initiated after an encouraging original experience in two patients treated at the University of Arkansas. This prompted a larger phase II study of single-agent thalidomide in 84 patients with relapsed and refractory MM.[31] In this heavily pretreated patient population, 76 of 84 enrolled patients (90%) had relapsed after receiving high-dose chemotherapy; 42% harbored MM tumor cells with deletion of chromosome 13, a cytogenetic abnormality that signifies unfavorable prognosis in patients receiving cytotoxic chemotherapy–based regimens;[31,120] 21% of patients had greater than 50% infiltration of their bone marrow by malignant plasma cells; and 15% had a plasma cell labeling index (PCLI) greater than 1%, which signifies an increased proliferative rate of the malignant plasma cells.

The primary endpoint of this trial was paraprotein response, and additional endpoints included time to response, time to disease progression, event-free survival, overall survival, and improvement in other laboratory parameters. Single-agent thalidomide was administered for a median of 80 days (range, 2 to 465), at a starting dose of 200 mg orally (PO) at nighttime, with subsequent dose escalation by 200 mg every 2 weeks up to a maximum of 800 mg. Most patients received thalidomide daily doses up to 400 mg (86%), with fewer attaining 600 mg/day (68%) and 800 mg/day (55%). Response, which was defined as greater than 25% reduction in serum or urine levels of paraprotein, was seen in 27 patients (32%). Importantly, paraprotein levels in the serum or urine were decreased by greater than 90% in eight patients (including two with complete remission), with median time to paraprotein response of approximately 2 months. In 78% of responding patients, decreases in plasma cell infiltration of bone marrow and

increased hemoglobin values were observed. Interestingly, however, bone marrow microvascular density was not significantly decreased, even among responders to treatment.

In this first experience of thalidomide treatment in MM, adverse events were reported to be generally mild to moderate, with increasing incidence at higher dose levels. Constipation was frequent but manageable with administration of laxatives. Peripheral neuropathy, characterized by paresthesia or numbness, was reported by 12% of patients receiving 200 mg daily. However, its frequency was increased to 28% of patients receiving 800 mg daily. Other mild to moderate side effects included weakness, fatigue, and somnolence, which were reported by 34% of patients receiving 200 mg daily and 43% of those treated at the 800-mg dose level. More severe adverse events were infrequent (occurring in ≤ 10% of patients), and hematologic effects were rare. However, nine patients discontinued thalidomide due to drug intolerance. One responding patient died suddenly on day 37 of treatment, most likely due to sepsis, but a possible relationship to thalidomide could not be ruled out. The incidence of myelosuppression was low, with significant leucopenia, anemia, and/or thrombocytopenia occurring in fewer than 5% of patients. After 12 months of follow-up, Kaplan-Meier estimates of the mean event-free and overall survival for all patients were 22% and 58%, respectively.

Subsequent studies from other centers confirmed that thalidomide is active in MM. In a phase II trial at the MD Anderson Cancer Center, thalidomide was administered in 43 evaluable patients with MM resistant to conventional therapies.[121] Eleven of 43 patients (26%) achieved partial response or better, defined by greater than 50% reduction of serum M-protein and/or greater than 75% reduction of Bence-Jones protein.

In a smaller study from Mayo Clinic, 16 heavily pretreated MM patients received an oral thalidomide dose of 200 mg/day for two weeks, increased by 200 mg/day every 2 weeks to a maximum of 800 mg/day.[122] Four patients (25%) achieved partial responses, lasting between 2 to 10 months. Adverse effects included constipation (25%), excessive sedation (25%), fatigue (25%), and rash (19%). In a multicenter phase II study of relapsed MM patients after high-dose chemotherapy and stem cell transplantation, oral thalidomide was administered with a dose escalation from 200 to 600 mg/day over 12 weeks and a subsequent maintenance phase of 200 mg/day for up to 1 year.[97] The 12-week progression-free survival rate was 67% (95% CI, 48 to 86%). The observed response rate (partial response plus minor response) was 43% (95% CI, 28 to 60%), with a median duration of 6 months. Dose escalation from 200 to 600 mg/d was achieved in 50% of patients. Responses were observed both at lower doses and in patients who completed the dose escalation. These results suggest that the optimal thalidomide dose varies among patients and that the relationship of dose to adverse, dose-limiting toxicity is unpredictable. The dose of thalidomide therapy should be based on the individual patient tolerance.[97] Other reports from Europe have confirmed response rates to thalidomide (at dose ranges of 200 to 800 mg daily) ranging between 36 to 51% in both relapsed and refractory settings.[123,124]

The significant clinical activity of single-agent thalidomide in refractory and relapsed MM, provided a stimulus for trials of combinations of thalidomide with chemotherapy and dexamethasone in view of their nonoverlapping toxicities and different mechanisms of action.

Initial clinical experience incorporating thalidomide into the DCEP (dexamethasone, cyclophosphamide, etoposide, and cisplatinum) regimen revealed a notable capacity to induce complete responses in patients with plasma cell leukemia and MM.[125] Low-dose thalidomide in combination with dexamethasone and also in combination with Biaxin has been reported to be active in relapsed disease in a number of studies,[45] although the effect of Biaxin appears to involve a change in the metabolism of dexamethasone. The combination of dexamethasone and thalidomide has been evaluated in both relapsed and refractory disease as well as in newly diagnosed, previously untreated patients. The importance of addressing such a question in the context of prospective, controlled trials was highlighted by occasional reports of life-threatening toxic epidermal necrolysis associated with the thalidomide-dexamethasone combination.[73] However, a recently reported large phase III randomized trial by ECOG comparing thalidomide in combination with dexamethasone versus high-dose dexamethasone alone showed a significant advantage for the combination (response rate 68% vs. 44%, $P < .0001$). However greater toxicity was observed in the combination arm, including deep venous thrombosis and pulmonary embolism in 16% of patients receiving both drugs. Moreover, there are now extensive reports of thrombotic events resulting from thalidomide treatment when thalidomide is combined not only with dexamethasone but also with anthracyclines, including liposomal doxorubicin (Doxil).[126,127] Because of the significantly lower incidence of thromboembolic events in the setting of thalidomide monotherapy, it is conceivable that thalidomide and/or its metabolites cause a modest increase of hypercoagulability, which is significantly enhanced when the drug is combined with other potentially prothrombotic, antiangiogenic agents.[99]

Therefore, while thalidomide treatment is associated with a promising response rate, its administration is not devoid of significant adverse events, which can, in some cases, be very serious, particularly when thalidomide is administered in combination with other drugs. Dose reductions of thalidomide (or other components of combination therapies), careful selection of patients who will receive these combinations, and comprehensive monitoring of patients may reduce the incidence of such events.

Another approach that has successfully been employed involves the development of thalidomide derivatives that not only are more potent in regards to a least some of the biologically activities of the parent compound but also have fewer side effects.[128] The original efforts to develop such thalidomide analogs yielded two classes of derivatives, the phosphodiesterase type 4 inhibitors, which inhibit TNF-α signaling but have little effect on T-cell activation (so-called selective cytokine-inhibitory drugs, or SelCIDs), and another group of nonphosphodiesterase type 4 inhibitors known as immunomodulatory drugs (IMiDs), which not only inhibit TNFα but also markedly stimulate T-cell proliferation and interferon-γ production.

As described previously, the IMiDs appear to have significantly greater potency than thalidomide, and perhaps a more favorable toxicity profile. On this basis, phase I, II, and III studies of CC-5013 (also known as CDC-5013 or lenalidomide) have been performed in patients with refractory or relapsed MM, with favorable clinical results.[128] The first oncologic setting in which lenalidomide was tested was a phase I dose-escalation study of lenalidomide (at 5, 10, 25, and 50 mg PO daily) in 27 patients (median age, 57 years; range, 40 to 71 years) with relapsed and refractory relapsed MM. In 24 evaluable patients, no dose-limiting toxicity (DLT) was observed in patients treated at any dose level within the first 28 days; however, grade 3 myelosuppression developed after day 28 in all 13 patients at the 50-mg daily dose level. In 12 patients, dose reduction to 25 mg/day was well tolerated and was therefore considered to represent the maximal tolerated dose (MTD). Importantly, no significant somnolence, constipation, or neuropathy was seen in any cohort of that study. Best responses of at least 25% reduction in paraprotein occurred in 17 (71%) of 24 patients (90% CI, 52 to 85%), including 11 patients(46%) who had received prior thalidomide treatment. Stable disease (<25% reduction in paraprotein) was observed in an additional 2 patients (8%). Therefore, 17 (71%) of 24 patients (90% CI, 52 to 85%) demonstrated benefit from treatment with lenalidomide.[128]

These encouraging results provided the stimulus for additional studies of lenalidomide in MM. A phase II multicenter, randomized, controlled, open-label study was conducted comparing oral lenalidomide at either 30 mg once daily or 15 mg twice daily for a total of 6 cycles, each comprising 3 weeks on lenalidomide therapy and 1 week off. That trial showed that a dose of 30 mg once daily is better tolerated than the twice daily regimen and that lenalidomide administered as a part of a 3 weeks on and 1 week off schedule is highly active has a response rate of approximately 35%, has a manageable adverse event profile, results in very little significant neuropathy (<5%), and has a very low incidence of thrombosis (even when combined with dexamethasone). In patients in whom dexamethasone was added to the IMiD, responses were seen in about 40% of cases.

In a phase III trial, a lenalidomide and dexamethasone combination is being compared with dexamethasone plus placebo in relapsed or refractory MM patients. Two randomized studies of high-dose dexamethasone and lenalidomide have now been completed and preliminary results are very encouraging with high response rates that appear remarkably durable, as compared to high dexamethasone and placebo. Toxicities were significant however and notable for a high rate of DVT/PE (~14%) which had not been seen with lenalidomide alone.[200,201]

Finally, a second immunomodulatory thalidomide derivative, CC-4047, has recently entered clinical trials for use in the treatment of MM and other neoplasias. In a phase I dose-escalation study[107] conducted in 24 patients with relapsed and relapsed refractory MM patients, the MTD was identified as 2 mg daily. Neutropenia was the major dose-limiting toxicity and was observed in 58% of patients. Grade 3 deep vein thrombosis was seen in 4 of 24 patients (16%). Other side effects were mild; these included rash, neuropathy, constipation, edema, and hypotension. Importantly, treatment resulted in minor responses (>25% reduction in paraprotein) or better in two thirds of patients, with 4 (16%) of 24 assessable patients achieving complete remission. CC-4047 administration was associated with T-cell activation, with increased RO expression on CD4$^+$ and CD8$^+$ cells, and a concomitant fall in resting CD45RO$^+$ cells seen. Moreover, there were significant increases in serum levels of serum IL-2 receptor and IL-12, possibly indicating activation of T cells.[107] Overall, the results of early CC-4047 clinical studies show important evidence of the antitumor activity of IMiDs as a drug class. Further studies of this orally bioavailable agent in patients with MM and prostate cancer are underway.

CLINICAL STUDIES OF THALIDOMIDE AND THALIDOMIDE DERIVATIVES IN OTHER HEMATOLOGIC NEOPLASIAS OR IN SOLID TUMORS

Other Plasma Cell Dyscrasias

The encouraging clinical results seen with thalidomide and its analogs in MM raised the possibility that MM is more thalidomide responsive than other neoplasias because of pathophysiological features intrinsic to the plasma cell lineage. This suggests by extension that thalidomide may also be active against other plasma cell dyscrasias, including Waldenström's macroglobulinemia (lymphoplasmacytic lymphoma). Indeed, single-agent thalidomide administered in the context of a small phase II study led to a 25% response rate,[129] while a combination of low-dose thalidomide (200 mg daily), dexamethasone (40 mg once weekly), and clarithromycin (500 mg twice daily) showed activity in two trials.[41] In primary systemic amyloidosis, a phase I/II trial of single-agent thalidomide showed hematologic improvement in 5 of 11

patients[130] and disease stabilization in 3 patients. However, as in other reports, substantial toxicities were observed, especially at higher doses of thalidomide.[131] Overall, while thalidomide may be active in some patients who have Waldenström's macroglobulinemia and are refractory to other standard regimens, the use of thalidomide and IMiDs is still investigational for patients with plasma cell dyscrasias other than MM.

Myelodysplastic Syndromes

The increased angiogenesis noted in bone marrow biopsies of at least some cases of myelodysplastic syndromes (MDS) provided the original basis for evaluation of thalidomide as a therapeutic agent for MDS. Bertolini et al. reported clinical responses in 2 of 5 thalidomide-treated MDS patients, with concomitant decreases in bFGF and VEGF in responding patients.[132] In larger studies of 83, 30, and 34 MDS patients, hematologic improvement (e.g., transfusion independence) was observed in approximately 30% of evaluable patients in the first two trials and in 19 of 29 patients (65%) in the third trial.[133-135] Higher platelet counts and lower blast percentage at baseline appeared to be associated with higher probability of response to thalidomide. Additional studies have also documented normalization of counts, with cytogenetic responses, in 3 thalidomide-treated patients with MDS.[136] However, improvement in nonerythroid lineages is not commonly seen,[133] and dose escalation beyond 200 mg daily causes cumulative neurological toxicity without necessarily conferring better hematological responses. Indeed, the North Central Cancer Treatment Group study N998B evaluated the tolerance and activity of an alternate thalidomide schedule of 200 mg daily with escalation to a maximum daily dose of 1,000 mg; there was extensive early patient withdrawal from the study (after a median of less than 2.5 months) due to toxicity.[137] Combination of darbepoetin with thalidomide in patients with MDS was associated with increased thromboembolic events in a small study.[138] However, when tolerated, prolonged drug treatment appears necessary to maximize hematological benefit, since the median time to erythroid response is 16 weeks (range, 12 to 20 weeks), with an erythropoietic response rate of 29% among the patients who completed the minimum 12 weeks of thalidomide treatment in one of the large MDS studies.[133] Subsequent institutional studies have confirmed the ability of thalidomide to lower transfusion requirements. Given the necessity for prolonged administration, its use appears best suited for treatment of patients with lower risk disease.[134,139,140] Investigation of the overall clinical benefit of low-dose thalidomide in MDS is nearing completion in a national randomized, placebo-controlled phase III trial.

The encouraging clinical experience with thalidomide in the treatment of MDS, as well as the favorable profile of manageable side effects of thalidomide analogs in MM, provided a strong impetus for testing lenalidomide in MDS patients.[141,142] Furthermore, lenalidomide inhibits the VEGF-induced trophic response of myeloblasts and endothelial cells while augmenting heterotypic adhesion of hematopoietic progenitors to bone marrow stroma to promote sustained growth arrest and preferential extinction of myelodysplastic clones.[143] In a cohort of 25 MDS patients with symptomatic or transfusion-dependent anemia who completed 8 or more weeks of treatment with lenalidomide, 16 (62%) of patients experienced an erythroid response according to International Working Group (IWG) criteria, with 12 patients experiencing sustained transfusion independence or a 2 g/dL or greater rise in hemoglobin levels.[141,142] Hematopoietic-promoting activity was greater among patients with low-risk or Int-1–risk MDS, with 15 of 21 (71%) experiencing hematological benefit. Erythroid responses to lenalidomide were associated with complete or partial (>50%) reduction in the proportion of abnormal metaphases in 9 of 13 informative patients, as well as improved primitive progenitor outgrowth and reduced grade of cytological dysplasia. Myeloid and platelet toxicity was dose limiting but occurred at all dose levels; it depended on cumulative drug exposure and necessitated either dose reduction or treatment interruption. These preliminary data suggest that lenalidomide is a promising oral agent that may find its clinical niche in the management of ineffective erythropoiesis in MDS patients, and confirmatory trials have recently been completed, with impressive activity in patients with a 5q variant of MDS. Although thalidomide therapy is associated with improvements in cytopenias in patients with MDS, more data are still needed on effects of the drug on the clonal tumor cell population, cytogenetic responses, and progression of MDS to acute myeloid leukemia (AML). Randomized trials are currently ongoing to determine the role of thalidomide and lenalidomide in MDS.

Myelofibrosis with Myeloid Metaplasia

The increased microvascular density in the bone marrow of patients with myelofibrosis/myeloid metaplasia (MMM)[144] also prompted evaluation of thalidomide in this clinical setting. Several studies have shown[145–149] that thalidomide offers, in variable percentages of patients, improvement in hematologic parameters, including increased platelet counts and hemoglobin levels, decreases in spleen size (though usually of moderate degree), increased bone marrow megakaryopoiesis, and decreased bone marrow angiogenesis.[145] Interestingly, however, some of the patients treated with 200 to 400 mg/day developed significant myeloproliferative reactions, including marked leucocytosis and thrombocytosis,[147,148] the precise etiology of which has not been elucidated. Other studies of thalidomide in MMM[150,151] showed improved hemoglobin levels, decreased transfusion requirements or transfusion independence in 29% of patients, increased platelet counts in 38% of

patients with moderate to severe thrombocytopenia, and decreased size of spleen in 41% of patients. On the other hand, more than 60% of patients discontinued the drug within 6 months of starting thalidomide therapy due to side effects, and almost 20% of patients had myeloproliferative reactions with leukocytosis and/or thrombocytosis. However, thalidomide appeared to maintain its clinical activity in MMM even when the daily thalidomide dose was reduced to as low as 50 mg, while most of the side effects appeared to occur at higher doses, suggesting that lower dosing may improve the therapeutic ratio. Furthermore, it appears that the combination of low-dose thalidomide (50 mg daily) with oral prednisone (starting at 0.5 mg/kg per day and tapered over 3 months) is not only well tolerated but also leads to durable objective responses, including improvement in terms of anemia, thrombocytopenia, and spleen size in 62%, 50%, and 19%, respectively, of 21 symptomatic patients (hemoglobin level < 10 g/dL or symptomatic splenomegaly).[152,153] Further trials of thalidomide and lenalidomide in MMM are underway.

Acute Myelogenous Leukemia

The use of thalidomide in acute leukemias was based not only on the putative antiangiogenic effects of this drug and the increased microvascular density of bone marrow of leukemic patients[23] but also on in vitro data suggesting that thalidomide or its derivatives can trigger differentiation or cell death of leukemia cell lines.[154] A phase I/II dose-escalating trial of AML patients[139,140] showed that thalidomide (200 to 400 mg daily for at least 1 month) led to a greater than 50% reduction of blasts in bone marrow, along with improvement in peripheral blood counts, for a median response duration of 3 months (range, 1 to 8 months). Responses were associated with significant decreases in microvascular density and plasma bFGF levels.[37–39,139,140] Overall, however, more data will be required to define the role, if any, that thalidomide should have in the therapeutic management of AML.

Non-Hodgkin's Lymphoma

Similar to other hematologic neoplasias, and despite their ready access to the general circulation, neoplastic lesions of non-Hodgkin's lymphoma (NHL) also present increased microvascular density,[155] while increased serum levels of VEGF and bFGF correlate with poor prognosis.[156] Results from a phase II study of thalidomide (starting dose of 200 mg daily, with dose escalation by 200 mg every week up to a maximum of 800 mg) in 19 patients with recurrent NHL (including patients with small lymphocytic lymphoma; follicular small cleaved, large B-cell lymphoma; mantle-cell lymphoma; mucosa-associated lymphoid tumors (MALTs); and peripheral T-cell lymphoma) and Hodgkin's disease without CNS involvement showed that 1 patient (5%)

with recurrent gastric mucosa–associated lymphoid tissue lymphoma achieved a complete response and 3 patients (16%) achieved stable disease,[157] suggesting that thalidomide has limited single-agent activity in heavily pretreated patients with recurrent or refractory lymphoma. There are also case reports of clinical activity of thalidomide for the treatment of angioimmunoblastic lymphadenopathy,[158,159] but more data will be needed to derive a more conclusive picture on the role of thalidomide, if any, in NHL. A recent phase I/II clinical trial combining thalidomide with fludarabine in treatment-naive CLL patients showed overall response rate of 100% (compared with historical data of response rates of up to ~60% with fludarabine-based regimens), with complete remissions in 55% of patients. At a median follow-up of 15+ months none of the patients had relapsed and median time to disease progression had not yet been reached. Responses were noted at all dose levels. Thalidomide given up to 300 mg per day, concurrently with fludarabine in patients with previously untreated CLL shows encouraging clinical efficacy and acceptable toxicity.[202] More extensive phase II evaluation of the clinical efficacy of this regimen is ongoing.

Clinical Studies of Thalidomide in the Treatment of Solid Tumors and Other Cancer-Related Indications

Kaposi's Sarcoma

Kaposi's sarcoma (KS) was another tumor type that appeared to be a reasonable setting for clinical testing of thalidomide, not only because of the increased vascularity of its lesions but also because of the fortuitous clinical findings of improvement of KS lesions in patients receiving thalidomide for HIV-related oral ulcers. In a phase II trial of male HIV-positive patients with histopathologically diagnosed KS, thalidomide (100 mg PO once nightly for 8 weeks) achieved partial responses in 6 of 17 patients,[160] while a reduction in HHV-8 DNA load to undetectable levels was observed in 3 of the responding patients. These results [161] were also subsequently confirmed in other phase II trials.[162] However, because most patients with HIV-related KS also receive concomitant antiretroviral therapy, caution is warranted in the interpretation of the results, in particular, the degree to which the observed activity reflects the effects of thalidomide. Thalidomide has also shown clinical benefit in non-HIV-related KS, for example, following allogeneic stem cell transplantation,[163] another area of active ongoing investigation.

Renal Cell Cancer

Multiple studies have attempted to address the role of thalidomide in the management of renal cell carcinoma (RCC), a tumor driven by genetic changes (e.g., VHL muta-

tions and constitutive activation of HIF-1a transcriptional activity)[164] that induce angiogenesis. These studies have either involved low-dose thalidomide treatment (≤200 mg daily)[115,165] or higher doses (e.g., 600 mg daily or intrapatient escalation to daily doses as high as 1,200 mg),[166–169]mostly in patients with metastatic RCC. The results have been variable, including partial responses in 3 to 16% of patients, disease stabilization in 16 to 45% of patients, and side effects similar to those seen in other clinical settings. The combination of thalidomide with other immunomodulatory agents, such as IL-2[170,171] or IFN-α, has attracted interest, but the thalidomide–IFN-α combination has led to serious adverse events, including seizures and visual disturbances.[172] Therefore, the precise role of these combinations in the therapeutic management of RCC is uncertain.

Other Solid Tumors

Thalidomide has demonstrated sporadic evidence of activity in a variety of solid tumors, including gliomas,[173–177] melanoma,[115,178,179] and prostate cancer,[180–190] but not in breast carcinoma.[191]

Graft versus Host Disease (GVHD)

The immunomodulatory and anti-inflammatory properties of thalidomide have stimulated interest in the field of GVHD, and over the last decade thalidomide has become established as an adjunctive treatment for chronic GVHD (cGVHD).[192] Vogelsang et al. first demonstrated thalidomide to be safe and effective in 23 patients with cGVHD refractory to conventional treatment and in 21 patients with high-risk GVHD, with complete responses observed in 7 of 23 patients (30%) who were given the drug as salvage treatment and in 7 of 21 patients (33%) who were given it as primary therapy.[193] The median duration of therapy was 240 days, sedation and constipation were the major side effects, and 4 patients discontinued medication because of peripheral neuropathy. Subsequent reports confirmed these results both in adults and in children, with the best responses seen in patients with predominantly mucocutaneous involvement by cGVHD.[194,195] In a larger phase II trial by Parker and colleagues, thalidomide was used as salvage therapy in 80 patients who had refractory cGVHD and had failed to respond to prednisone or prednisone and cyclosporin.[10] Sixteen patients (20%) had a sustained response, with 9 achieving complete responses and 7 partial responses. The median duration of response was 16 months, and most responses were again seen in patients with isolated mouth, skin, and liver GVHD but without severe sclerodermatous manifestations. It should be noted that patients were maintained on prednisone and cyclosporine during thalidomide therapy, and 36% of patients had thalidomide discontinued because of side effects, including sedation, constipation, and neuropathy.

Additional side effects included skin rash and neutropenia, which had not been previously reported in the past studies of cGVHD, and these resulted in discontinuation of the drug in a small number of patients. In a more recent study, response to thalidomide in refractory cGVHD was seen in 38% of patients, and the treatment was well tolerated. However, a separate randomized, placebo-controlled trial found that the duration of thalidomide treatment was too short to assess its efficacy in controlling cGVHD because of side effects, including neutropenia and neuropathy, which led to early discontinuation.[196] At this stage, thalidomide therefore appears to have activity against cGVHD, but whether it should be used for first-line treatment of cGVHD remains to be determined.[28]

Cachexia

Clinical trials of thalidomide in patients with cachexia secondary to terminal cancer are underway, based on encouraging preliminary reports.[197] Interestingly, a recent report has also described beneficial effects of the combination of thalidomide and irinotecan for the treatment of metastatic colorectal cancer, in which abrogation of dose-limiting gastrointestinal toxicity, including diarrhea and nausea, was seen.[198] Finally, studies in the palliative care setting have also looked at the role of thalidomide in chronic nausea, insomnia, and profuse sweating as well as an adjunct in pain control, with symptomatic benefit reported.[199]

CONCLUSION

The tragic experience of the early years of thalidomide use fortunately did not deter a more carefully monitored emergence of its use in diseases where its diverse immunomodulatory and antiangiogenic properties could be beneficial. Importantly, through a combination of careful preclinical study, serendipity, and thoughtful clinical development, thalidomide has become more than a merely promising agent. It is an integral part of the therapeutic management of MM and MDS, but is also used for nonmalignant conditions such as erythema nodosum leprosum (ENL). Importantly, the development of thalidomide derivatives, with more refined biological properties and attenuated potential for specific side effects compared with the parent compound, represents a promising new direction for clinical applications of this class of drugs. It may in fact be appropriate to revise our thinking about thalidomide analogs and view them, not as minor variations of the parent compound, but as a diverse group of structurally related but functionally distinct agents; such revision is indicated, for example, by the different pharmacological and clinical properties of thalidomide and lenalidomide (CC-5013). Even though it remains unclear which of the proposed biological activities of thalidomide and its derivatives account for its effects in MM or other diseases (e.g., their antiangiogenic activity, direct antitumor activity, modulation of tumor-stromal adhesive interactions, or immunomodulatory activity), it is clinically apparent that thalidomide has major activity in patients with MM and MDS. In contrast, the accumulating clinical experience in solid tumors is less encouraging, but patients with certain tumor types may benefit, most likely in the context of thalidomide-containing combination therapies. The uses of thalidomide for the management of certain treatment-related complications (e.g., cGVHD) or for relief of symptoms related to advanced malignancy or its treatment (e.g., cachexia, diarrhea)[197–199] are also noteworthy. The emergence of thalidomide derivatives with considerable potential for improved efficacy and less toxicity provides an exciting platform for future therapies in a wide array of cancers and also non-neoplastic disease settings.

REFERENCES

1. Lenz W. Thalidomide and congenital abnormalities. Lancet 1962;1:45.
2. Lenz W. The susceptible period for thalidomide malformations in man and monkey. Ger Med Mon 1968;4:197–198.
3. Lenz W. Malformations caused by drugs in pregnancy. Am J Dis Child. 1996;2:99–106.
4. Rogerson G. Thalidomide and congenital abnormalities. Lancet 1962;1:691.
5. Grabstald H, Golbey R. Clinical experiences with thalidomide in patients with cancer. Clin Pharmacol Ther 1965;40:298–302.
6. Olson KB, Hall TC, Horton J, et al. Thalidomide (N-phthaloylglutamimide) in the treatment of advanced cancer. Clin Pharmacol Ther 1965;40:292–297.
7. Hales BF. Thalidomide on the comeback trail. Nat Med 1999;5:489–490.
8. Sheskin J. Thalidomide in the treatment of lepra reactions. Clin Pharmacol Ther 1965;6:303–306.
9. Hamuryudan V, Mat C, Saip S, et al. Thalidomide in the treatment of the mucocutaneous lesions of the Behçet syndrome: a randomized, double-blind, placebo-controlled trial. Ann Intern Med 1998;128:443–450.
10. Parker PM, Chao N, Nademanee A, et al. Thalidomide as salvage therapy for chronic graft-versus-host disease. Blood 1995;86:3604–3609.
11. Reyes-Teran G, Sierra-Madero JG, Martinez del Cerro V, et al. Effects of thalidomide on HIV-associated wasting syndrome: a randomized, double-blind, placebo-controlled clinical trial. AIDS 1996;10:1501–1507.
12. Jacobson JM, Greenspan JS, Spritzler J, et al. Thalidomide for the treatment of oral aphthous ulcers in patients with human immunodeficiency virus infection. National Institute of Allergy and Infectious Diseases AIDS Clinical Trials Group. N Engl J Med 1997;336:1487–1493.
13. Zeldis JB, Williams BA, Thomas SD, et al. S.T.E.P.S™: a comprehensive program for controlling and monitoring access to thalidomide. Clin Ther 1999;21:319–330.
14. Stirling DI. Thalidomide and its impact in dermatology. Semin Cutan Med Surg 1998;17:231–242.
15. Folkman J. Tumor angiogenesis: therapeutic implications. N Engl J Med 1971;285:1182–1186.
16. Weidner N, Semple JP, Welch WR, et al. Tumor angiogenesis and metastasis: correlation in invasive breast carcinoma. N Engl J Med 1991;324:1–8.
17. Weidner N, Folkman J, Pozza F, et al. Tumor angiogenesis: a new significant and independent prognostic indicator in early-stage breast carcinoma. J Natl Cancer Inst 1992;84:1875–1887.
18. Weidner N, Carroll PR, Flax J, et al. Tumor angiogenesis correlates with metastasis in invasive prostate carcinoma. Am J Pathol 1993;143:401–409.

19. D'Amato RJ, Loughnan MS, Flynn E, et al. Thalidomide is an inhibitor of angiogenesis. Proc Natl Acad Sci USA 1994;91: 4082–4085.
20. Hlatky L, Tsionou C, Hahnfeldt P, et al. Mammary fibroblasts may influence breast tumor angiogenesis via hypoxia-induced vascular endothelial growth factor up-regulation and protein expression. Cancer Res 1994;54:6083–6086.
21. Folkman J. Angiogenesis in cancer, vascular, rheumatoid and other disease. Nat Med 1995;1:27–31.
22. Folkman J. Clinical applications of research on angiogenesis. N Engl J Med 1995;333:1757–1763.
23. Perez-Atayde AR, Sallan SE, Tedrow U, et al. Spectrum of tumor angiogenesis in the bone marrow of children with acute lymphoblastic leukemia. Am J Pathol 1997;150:815–821.
24. Kenyon BM, Browne F, D'Amato RJ. Effects of thalidomide and related metabolites in a mouse corneal model of neovascularization. Exp Eye Res 1997;64:971–978.
25. Bauer KS, Dixon SC, Figg WD. Inhibition of angiogenesis by thalidomide requires metabolic activation, which is species-dependent. Biochem Pharmacol 1998;55:1827–1834.
26. Eisen T, Boshoff C, Vaughan M, et al. Anti-angiogenic treatment of metastatic melanoma, renal cell, ovarian and breast cancers with thalidomide: a phase II study. Proc Am Soc Clin Oncol 1998;17:441a.
27. Figg WD, Bergan R, Brawley O, et al. Randomized, phase II study of thalidomide in androgen-independent prostate cancer (AIPC). Proc Am Soc Clin Oncol. 1997;16:333a.
28. Fine HA, Loeffler JS, Kyritsis A, et al. A phase II trial of the anti-angiogenic agent, thalidomide, in patients with recurrent high-grade gliomas. Proc Am Soc Clin Oncol 1997;16:385a.
29. Long G, Vredenburgh J, Rizzieri DA, et al. Pilot trial of thalidomide post-autologous peripheral blood progenitor cell transplantation (PBPC) in patients with metastatic breast cancer. Proc Am Soc Clin Oncol 1998;17:181a.
30. Marx GM, Levi JA, Bell DR, et al. A phase I/II trial of thalidomide as an antiangiogenic agent in the treatment of advanced cancer. Proc Am Soc Clin Oncol 1999;18:454a.
31. Singhal S, Mehta J, Desikan R, et al. Antitumor activity of thalidomide in refractory multiple myeloma [see comments] [published erratum appears in N Engl J Med 2000;342:364]. N Engl J Med 1999;341:1565–1571.
32. Eriksson T, Bjorkman S, Hoglund P. Clinical pharmacology of thalidomide. Eur J Clin Pharmacol 2001;57:365–376.
33. Stirling DI. The pharmacology of thalidomide. Semin Hematol 2000;37:5–14.
34. Hideshima T, Chauhan D, Shima Y, et al. Thalidomide and its analogs overcome drug resistance of human multiple myeloma cells to conventional therapy. Blood 2000;96:2943–2950.
35. Mitsiades N, Mitsiades CS, Poulaki V, et al. Apoptotic signaling induced by immunomodulatory thalidomide analogs in human multiple myeloma cells: therapeutic implications. Blood 2002; 99:4525–4530.
36. Davies FE, Raje N, Hideshima T, et al. Thalidomide and immunomodulatory derivatives augment natural killer cell cytotoxicity in multiple myeloma. Blood 2001;210–216.
37. Hideshima T, Chauhan D, Richardson P, et al. NF-kappa B as a therapeutic target in multiple myeloma. J Biol Chem 2002;277: 16639–16647.
38. Mitsiades CS, Mitsiades N, Poulaki V, et al. Activation of NF-kappaB and upregulation of intracellular anti-apoptotic proteins via the IGF-1/Akt signaling in human multiple myeloma cells: therapeutic implications. Oncogene 2002;21:5673–5683.
39. Mitsiades N, Mitsiades CS, Poulaki V, et al. Biologic sequelae of nuclear factor-kappaB blockade in multiple myeloma: therapeutic applications. Blood 2002;99:4079–4086.
40. Dimopoulos MA, Anagnostopoulos A. Thalidomide in relapsed/refractory multiple myeloma: pivotal trials conducted outside the United States. Semin Hematol 2003;40:8–16.
41. Coleman M, Leonard J, Lyons L, et al. Treatment of Waldenstrom's macroglobulinemia with clarithromycin, low-dose thalidomide, and dexamethasone. Semin Oncol 2003;30: 270–274.
42. Srkalovic G, Elson P, Trebisky B, et al. Use of melphalan, thalidomide, and dexamethasone in treatment of refractory and relapsed multiple myeloma. Med Oncol 2002;19:219–226.
43. Rajkumar SV, Hayman S, Gertz MA, et al. Combination therapy with thalidomide plus dexamethasone for newly diagnosed myeloma. J Clin Oncol 2002;20:4319–4323.
44. Garcia-Sanz R, Gonzalez-Fraile MI, Sierra M, et al. The combination of thalidomide, cyclophosphamide and dexamethasone (ThaCyDex) is feasible and can be an option for relapsed/refractory multiple myeloma. Hematol J 2002;3:43–48.
45. Coleman M, Leonard J, Lyons L, et al. BLT-D (clarithromycin [Biaxin], low-dose thalidomide, and dexamethasone) for the treatment of myeloma and Waldenstrom's macroglobulinemia. Leuk Lymphoma 2002;43:1777–1782.
46. Alexanian R, Weber D, Giralt S, et al. Consolidation therapy of multiple myeloma with thalidomide-dexamethasone after intensive chemotherapy. Ann Oncol 2002;13:1116–1119.
47. Palumbo A, Giaccone L, Bertola A, et al. Low-dose thalidomide plus dexamethasone is an effective salvage therapy for advanced myeloma. Haematologica 2001;86:399–403.
48. Geitz H, Handt S, Zwingenberger K. Thalidomide selectively modulates the density of cell surface molecules involved in the adhesion cascade. Immunopharmacology 1996;31:213–221.
49. Uchiyama H, Barut BA, Mohrbacher AF, et al. Adhesion of human myeloma-derived cell lines to bone marrow stromal cells stimulates interleukin-6 secretion. Blood 1993;82:3712–3720.
50. Chauhan D, Uchiyama H, Akbarali Y, et al. Multiple myeloma cell adhesion-induced interleukin-6 expression in bone marrow stromal cells involves activation of NF-kappa B. Blood 1996; 87:1104–1112.
51. Hallek M, Bergsagel PL, Anderson KC. Multiple myeloma: increasing evidence for a multistep transformation process. Blood 1998;91:3–21.
52. Damiano JS, Cress AE, Hazlehurst LA, et al. Cell adhesion mediated drug resistance (CAM-DR): role of integrins and resistance to apoptosis in human myeloma cell lines. Blood 1999;93: 1658–1667.
53. Dunzendorfer S, Schratzberger P, Reinisch N, et al. Effects of thalidomide on neutrophil respiratory burst, chemotaxis, and transmigration of cytokine- and endotoxin-activated endothelium. Naunyn Schmiedebergs Arch Pharmacol 1997;356: 529–535.
54. Moreira AL, Sampaio EP, Zmuidzinas A, et al. Thalidomide exerts its inhibitory action on tumor necrosis factor alpha by enhancing mRNA degradation. J Exp Med 1993;177:1675–1680.
55. Calderon P, Anzilotti M, Phelps R. Thalidomide in dermatology: new indications for an old drug. Int J Dermatol 1997;36: 881–887.
56. Sampaio EP, Sarno EN, Galilly R, et al. Thalidomide selectively inhibits tumor necrosis factor alpha production by stimulated human monocytes. J Exp Med 1991;173:699–703.
57. Turk BE, Jiang H, Liu JO. Binding of thalidomide to 1-acid glycoprotein may be involved in its inhibition of TNF production. Proc Natl Acad Sci USA 1996;93:7552–7556.
58. Corral LG, Haslett PA, Muller GW, et al. Differential cytokine modulation and T cell activation by two distinct classes of thalidomide analogues that are potent inhibitors of TNF- alpha. J Immunol 1999;163:380–386.
59. Gupta D, Treon SP, Shima Y, et al. Adherence of multiple myeloma cells to bone marrow stromal cells upregulates vascular endothelial growth factor secretion: therapeutic applications. Leukemia 2001;1:1950–1961.
60. Kotoh T, Dhar DK, Masunaga R, et al. Anti-angiogenic therapy of human esophageal cancers with thalidomide in nude mice. Surgery 1999;125:536–544.
61. Hastings RC, Trautman JR, Enna CD, et al. Thalidomide in the treatment of erythema nodosum leprosum: with a note on selected laboratory abnormalities in erythema nodosum leprosum. Clin Pharmacol Ther 1970;11:481–487.
62. Fernandez LP, Schlegel PG, Baker J, et al. Does thalidomide affect IL-2 response and production? [published erratum appears in Exp Hematol 1995;23:1324]. Exp Hematol 1995;23: 978–985.
63. Keenan RJ, Eiras G, Burckart GJ, et al. Immunosuppressive properties of thalidomide. inhibition of in vitro lymphocyte proliferation alone and in combination with cyclosporine or FK506. Transplantation 1991;52:908–910.

64. Moncada B, Baranda ML, Gonzalez-Amaro R, et al. Thalidomide: effect on T cell subsets as a possible mechanism of action. Int J Lepr Other Mycobact Dis 1985;53:201–205.

65. Shannon EJ, Ejigu M, Haile-Mariam HS, et al. Thalidomide's effectiveness in erythema nodosum leprosum is associated with a decrease in CD4$^+$ cells in the peripheral blood. Lepr Rev 1992;63:5–11.

66. Haslett P, Hempstead M, Seidman C, et al. The metabolic and immunologic effects of short-term thalidomide treatment of patients infected with the human immunodeficiency virus. AIDS Res Hum Retroviruses 1997;13:1047–1054.

67. McHugh SM, Rifkin IR, Deighton J, et al. The immunosuppressive drug thalidomide induces T helper cell type 2 (Th2) and concomitantly inhibits Th1 cytokine production in mitogen- and antigen-stimulated human peripheral blood mononuclear cell cultures. Clin Exp Immunol 1995;99:160–167.

68. Haslett PA, Corral LG, Albert M, et al. Thalidomide costimulates primary human T lymphocytes, preferentially inducing proliferation, cytokine production, and cytotoxic responses in the CD8+ subset. J Exp Med 1998;187:1885–1892.

69. Nogueira AC, Neubert R, Helge H, et al. Thalidomide and the immune system. simultaneous up- and down-regulation of different integrin receptors on human white blood cells. Life Sci 1994;55:77–92.

70. Rowland TL, McHugh SM, Deighton J, et al. Differential regulation by thalidomide and dexamethasone of cytokine expression in human peripheral blood mononuclear cells. Immunopharmacology 1998;40:11–20.

71. Moller DR, Wysocka M, Greenlee BM, et al. Inhibition of IL-12 production by thalidomide. J Immunol 1997;159:5157–5161.

72. Shannon EJ, Sandoval F. Thalidomide increases the synthesis of IL-2 in cultures of human mononuclear cells stimulated with Concanavalin-A, Staphylococcal enterotoxin A, and purified protein derivative. Immunopharmacology 1995;31:109–116.

73. Tseng S, Pak G, Washenik K, et al. Rediscovering thalidomide: a review of its mechanism of action, side effects, and potential uses. J Am Acad Dermatol 1996;35:969–979.

74. Muller GW. Thalidomide: from tragedy to new drug discovery. Chemtech 1997:21–215.

75. Reist M, Carrupt PA, Francotte E, et al. Chiral inversion and hydrolysis of thalidomide: mechanisms and catalysis by bases and serum albumin, and chiral stability of teratogenic metabolites. Chem Res Toxicol 1998;11:1521–1528.

76. Eriksson T, Bjorkman S, Roth B, et al. Stereospecific determination, chiral inversion in vitro and pharmacokinetics in humans of the enantiomers of thalidomide. Chirality 1995;7:44–52.

77. Faigle JW, Keberle H, Friess W, et al. The metabolic fate of thalidomide. Experientia 1962;18:389–397.

78. Chen TL, Vogelsang GB, Petty BG, et al. Plasma pharmacokinetics and urinary excretion of thalidomide after oral dosing in healthy male volunteers. Drug Metab Dispos 1989;17:402–405.

79. Figg WD, Raje S, Bauer KS, et al. Pharmacokinetics of thalidomide in an elderly prostate cancer population. J Pharm Sci 1999;88:121–125.

80. Piscitelli SC, Figg WD, Hahn B, et al. Single-dose pharmacokinetics of thalidomide in human immunodeficiency virus-infected patients. Antimicrob Agents Chemother 1997;41: 2797–2799.

81. Teo SK, Colburn WA, Thomas SD. Single-dose oral pharmacokinetics of three formulations of thalidomide in healthy male volunteers. J Clin Pharmacol 1999;39:1162–1168.

82. Teo SK, Scheffler MR, Kook KA, et al. Thalidomide dose proportionality assessment following single doses to healthy subjects. J Clin Pharmacol 2001;41:662–667.

83. Ludwak-Mann C, Schmid K, Keberle H. Thalidomide in rabbit semen. Nature 1967;214:1018–1020.

84. Teo SK, Harden JL, Burke AB, et al. Thalidomide is distributed into human semen after oral dosing. Drug Metab Dispos 2001;29:1355–1357.

85. Schumacher H, Smith RL, Williams RT. The metabolism of thalidomide: the spontaneous hydrolysis of thalidomide in solution. Br J Pharmacol 1965;25:324–327.

86. Fabro S, Schumacher H, Smith RL, et al. The metabolism of thalidomide: some biological effects of thalidomide and its metabolites. Br J Pharmacol 1965;25:352–362.

87. Scheffler MR, Colburn W, Kook KA, et al. Thalidomide does not alter estrogen-progesterone hormone single dose pharmacokinetics. Clin Pharmacol Ther 1999;65:483–490.

88. Tsambaos D, Bolsen K, Georgiou S, et al. Effects of oral thalidomide on rat liver and skin microsomal P450 isozyme activities and on urinary porphyrin excretion: interaction with oral hexachlorobenzene. Arch Dermatol Res 1994;286:347–349.

89. Wiener H, Krivanek P, Tuisl E, et al. Induction of drug metabolism in the rat by taglutimide, a sedative-hypnotic glutarimide derivative. Eur J Drug Metab Pharmacokinet 1980;5:93–97.

90. Aweeka F, Trapnell C, Chernoff M, et al. Pharmacokinetics and pharmacodynamics of thalidomide in HIV patients treated for oral aphthous ulcers: ACTG protocol 251. AIDS Clinical Trials Group. J Clin Pharmacol 2001;41:1091–1097.

91. Wohl DA, Aweeka FT, Schmitz J, et al. Safety, tolerability, and pharmacokinetic effects of thalidomide in patients infected with human immunodeficiency virus. AIDS Clinical Trials Group 267. J Infect Dis 2002;185:1359–1363.

92. Lu J, Helsby N, Palmer BD, et al. Metabolism of thalidomide in liver microsomes of mice, rabbits, and humans. J Pharmacol Exp Ther 2004;310:571–577.

93. Lu J, Palmer BD, Kestell P, et al. Thalidomide metabolites in mice and patients with multiple myeloma. Clin Cancer Res 2003;9: 1680–1688.

94. Chung F, Lu J, Palmer BD, et al. Thalidomide pharmacokinetics and metabolite formation in mice, rabbits, and multiple myeloma patients. Clin Cancer Res 2004;10:5949–5956.

95. Yaccoby S, Johnson CL, Mahaffey SC, et al. Antimyeloma efficacy of thalidomide in the SCID-hu model. Blood 2002;100: 4162–4168.

96. Somers GF. Pharmacological properties of thalidomide (α-phthalimido glutarimide), a new sedative hypnotic drug. Br J Pharmacol 1960;15:111–116.

97. Richardson P, Schlossman R, Jagannath S, et al. Thalidomide for patients with relapsed multiple myeloma after high-dose chemotherapy and stem cell transplantation: results of an open-label multicenter phase 2 study of efficacy, toxicity, and biological activity. Mayo Clin Proc 2004;79:875–882.

98. Weber DM, Rankin K, Gavino M. Thalidomide with dexamethasone for resistant multiple myeloma [abstract]. Blood 2000;96:167a.

99. Osman K, Comenzo R, Rajkumar SV. Deep venous thrombosis and thalidomide therapy for multiple myeloma. New Engl J Med 2001;21:1951–1952.

100. Younis TH, Alam A, Paplham P, et al. Reversible pulmonary hypertension and thalidomide therapy for multiple myeloma. Br J Haematol 2003;121:191–192.

101. Singhal S, Mehta J, Eddlemon P, et al. Marked anti-tumor effect from anti-angiogenesis (AA) therapy with thalidomide (T) in high risk refractory multiple myeloma (MM). Blood 1998;92: 318a.

102. Mellin GW, Katzenstein M. The saga of thalidomide (concluded): neuropathy to embryopathy, with case reports of congenital anomalies. N Engl J Med 1962;267:1238–1244.

103. Aronson IK, Yu R, West DP, et al. Thalidomide-induced peripheral neuropathy: effect of serum factor on nerve cultures. Arch Dermatol 1984;120:1466–1470.

104. Clemmensen OJ, Olsen PZ, Andersen KE. Thalidomide neurotoxicity. Arch Dermatol 1984;120:338–341.

105. Fullerton PM, O'Sullivan DJ. Thalidomide neuropathy: a clinical electrophysiological, and histological follow-up study. J Neurol Neurosurg Psychiatry 1968;31:543–551.

106. Corral LG, Kaplan G. Immunomodulation by thalidomide and thalidomide analogues. Ann Rheum Dis 1999;58(Suppl 1):I107–113.

107. Schey SA, Fields P, Bartlett JB, et al. Phase I study of an immunomodulatory thalidomide analog, CC-4047, in relapsed or refractory multiple myeloma. J Clin Oncol 2004;22: 3269–3276.

108. Bartlett JB, Dredge K, Dalgleish AG. The evolution of thalidomide and its IMiD derivatives as anticancer agents. Nat Rev Cancer 2004;4:314–322.

109. Richardson P, Anderson K. Immunomodulatory analogs of thalidomide: an emerging new therapy in myeloma. J Clin Oncol 2004;22:3212–3214.

110. Anderson KC, Hamblin TJ, Traynor A. Management of multiple myeloma today. Semin Hematol 1999;36:3–8.
111. Stevenson F, Anderson KC. Introduction to immunotherapy for multiple myeloma: insights and advances. Semin Hematol 1999;36:1–2.
112. Vacca A, Ribatti D, Roncali L, et al. Bone marrow angiogenesis and progression in multiple myeloma. Br J Haematol 1994;87: 503–508.
113. Vacca A, Di Loreto M, Ribatti D, et al. Bone marrow of patients with active multiple myeloma: angiogenesis and plasma cell adhesion molecules LFA-1, VLA-4, LAM-1, and CD44. Am J Hematol 1995;50:9–14.
114. Vacca A, Ribatti D, Presta M, et al. Bone marrow neovascularization, plasma cell angiogenic potential, and matrix metalloproteinase-2 secretion parallel progression of human multiple myeloma. Blood 1999;93:3064–3073.
115. Eisen T, Boshoff C, Mak I, et al. Continuous low dose thalidomide: a phase II study in advanced melanoma, renal cell, ovarian and breast cancer. Br J Cancer 2000;82:812–817.
116. Munshi N, Wison CS, Penn J, et al. Angiogenesis in newly diagnosed multiple myeloma: poor prognosis with increased microvessel density (MVD) in bone marrow biopsies. Blood 1998;92:92a.
117. Rajkumar SV, Fonseca R, Witzig TE, et al. Bone marrow angiogenesis in patients achieving complete response after stem cell transplantation for multiple myeloma. Leukemia 1999;13: 469–472.
118. Nguyen M, Tran C, Barsky S, et al. Thalidomide and chemotherapy combination: preliminary results of preclinical studies. Int J Oncol 1997;10:965–969.
119. Ribatti D, Vacca A, Nico B, et al. Bone marrow angiogenesis and mast cell density increase simultaneously with progression of human multiple myeloma. Br J Cancer 1999;79:451–455.
120. Barlogie B, Desikan R, Eddlemon P, et al. Extended survival in advanced and refractory multiple myeloma after single-agent thalidomide: identification of prognostic factors in a phase 2 study of 169 patients. Blood 2001;98:492–494.
121. Alexanian R, Webes D. Thalidomide for resistant and relapsing myeloma. Semin Hematol 2000;37:22–25.
122. Rajkumar SV, Fonseca R, Dispenzieri A, et al. Thalidomide in the treatment of relapsed multiple myeloma. Mayo Clin Proc 2000; 75:897–901.
123. Hus M, Dmoszynska A, Soroka-Wojtaszko, et al. Thalidomide treatment of resistant or relapsed multiple myeloma patients. Haematologica 2001;86:404–408.
124. Tosi P, Ronconi S, Zamagni E, et al. Salvage therapy with thalidomide in multiple myeloma patients relapsing after autologous peripheral blood stem cell transplantation. Haematologica 2001;86:409–413.
125. Barlogie B, Desikan R, Munshi N, et al. Single course D.T. PACE anti-angiochemotherapy effects CR in plasma cell leukemia and fulminant multiple myeloma (MM). Blood 1999;92:273b.
126. Zangari M, Anaissie E, Barlogie B, et al. Increased risk of deep-vein thrombosis in patients with multiple myeloma receiving thalidomide and chemotherapy. Blood 2001;98:1614–1615.
127. Zangari M, Siegel E, Barlogie B, et al. Thrombogenic activity of doxorubicin in myeloma patients receiving thalidomide: implications for therapy. Blood 2002;100:1168–1171.
128. Richardson PG, Schlossman RL, Weller E, et al. Immuno-modulatory drug CC-5013 overcomes drug resistance and is well tolerated in patients with relapsed multiple myeloma. Blood 2002;100:3063–3067.
129. Dimopoulos MA, Tsatalas C, Zomas A, et al. Treatment of Waldenstrom's macroglobulinemia with single-agent thalidomide or with the combination of clarithromycin, thalidomide and dexamethasone. Semin Oncol 2003;30:265–269.
130. Seldin DC, Choufani EB, Dember LM, et al. Tolerability and efficacy of thalidomide for the treatment of patients with light chain-associated (AL) amyloidosis. Clin Lymphoma 2003;3: 241–246.
131. Dispenzieri A, Lacy MQ, Rajkumar SV, et al. Poor tolerance to high doses of thalidomide in patients with primary systemic amyloidosis. Amyloid 2003;10:257–261.
132. Bertolini F, Mingrone W, Alietti A, et al. Thalidomide in multiple myeloma, myelodysplastic syndromes and histiocytosis: analysis of clinical results and of surrogate angiogenesis markers. Ann Oncol 2001;12:987–990.
133. Raza A, Meyer P, Dutt D, et al. Thalidomide produces transfusion independence in long-standing refractory anemias of patients with myelodysplastic syndromes. Blood 2001;98:958–965.
134. Zorat F, Shetty V, Dutt D, et al. The clinical and biological effects of thalidomide in patients with myelodysplastic syndromes. Br J Haematol 2001;115:881–894.
135. Strupp C, Germing U, Aivado M, et al. Thalidomide for the treatment of patients with myelodysplastic syndromes. Leukemia 2002;16:1–6.
136. Strupp C, Hildebrandt B, Germing U, et al. Cytogenetic response to thalidomide treatment in three patients with myelodysplastic syndrome. Leukemia 2003;17:1200–1202.
137. Moreno-Aspitia A, Geyer S, Li CY, et al. N998B: multicenter phase II trial of thalidomide (Thal) in adult patients with myelodysplastic syndrome (MDS). Blood 2002;100:96a.
138. Steurer M, Sudmeier I, Stauder R, et al. Thromboembolic events in patients with myelodysplastic syndrome receiving thalidomide in combination with darbepoietin-alpha. Br J Haematol 2003;121:101–103.
139. Steins MB, Bieker R, Padro T, et al. Thalidomide for the treatment of acute myeloid leukemia. Leuk Lymphoma 2003;44: 1489–1493.
140. Steins MB, Padro T, Bieker R, et al. Efficacy and safety of thalidomide in patients with acute myeloid leukemia. Blood 2002;99: 834–839.
141. List AF. New approaches to the treatment of myelodysplasia. Oncologist 2002;7(Suppl 1):39–49.
142. List AF, Kurtin SE, Glinsmann-Gibson BJ, et al. High erythropoietic remitting activity of the immunomodulatory thalidomide analog, CC5013, in patients with myelodysplastic syndrome (MDS). Blood 2002;100:96a.
143. List AF, Tate W, Glinsmann-Gibson BJ, et al. The immunomodulatory thalidomide analog, CC5013, inhibits trophic response to VEGF in AML cells by abolishing cytokine-induced PI3-kinase/Akt activation [abstract]. Blood 2002;100:139a.
144. Mesa RA, Hanson CA, Rajkumar SV, et al. Evaluation and clinical correlations of bone marrow angiogenesis in myelofibrosis with myeloid metaplasia. Blood 2000;96:3374–3380.
145. Elliott MA, Mesa RA, Li CY, et al. Thalidomide treatment in myelofibrosis with myeloid metaplasia. Br J Haematol 2002;117: 288–296.
146. Piccaluga PP, Visani G, Pileri SA, et al. Clinical efficacy and antiangiogenic activity of thalidomide in myelofibrosis with myeloid metaplasia: a pilot study. Leukemia 2002;16: 1609–1614.
147. Barosi G, Grossi A, Comotti B, et al. Safety and efficacy of thalidomide in patients with myelofibrosis with myeloid metaplasia. Br J Haematol 2001;114:78–83.
148. Tefferi A, Elliot MA. Serious myeloproliferative reactions associated with the use of thalidomide in myelofibrosis with myeloid metaplasia. Blood 2000;96:4007.
149. Marchetti M, Barosi G, Balestri F, et al. Low-dose thalidomide ameliorates cytopenias and splenomegaly in myelofibrosis with myeloid metaplasia: a phase II trial. J Clin Oncol 2004;22: 424–431.
150. Merup M, Kutti J, Birgergard G, et al. Negligible clinical effects of thalidomide in patients with myelofibrosis with myeloid metaplasia. Med Oncol 2002;19:79–86.
151. Giovanni B, Michelle E, Letizia C, et al. Thalidomide in myelofibrosis with myeloid metaplasia: a pooled-analysis of individual patient data from five studies. Leuk Lymphoma 2002;43: 2301–2307.
152. Mesa RA, Steensma DP, Pardanani A, et al. A phase 2 trial of combination low-dose thalidomide and prednisone for the treatment of myelofibrosis with myeloid metaplasia. Blood 2003;101:2534–2541.
153. Mesa RA, Elliott MA, Schroeder G, et al. Durable responses to thalidomide-based drug therapy for myelofibrosis with myeloid metaplasia. Mayo Clin Proc 2004;79:883–889.
154. Hatfill SJ, Fester ED, de Beer DP, et al. Induction of morphological differentiation in the human leukemic cell line K562 by exposure to thalidomide metabolites. Leuk Res 1991;15: 129–136.

155. Vacca A, Ribatti D, Roncali L, et al. Angiogenesis in B cell lymphoproliferative diseases: biological and clinical studies. Leuk Lymphoma 1995;20:27–38.

156. Bertolini F, Paolucci M, Peccatori F, et al. Angiogenic growth factors and endostatin in non-Hodgkin's lymphoma. Br J Haematol 1999;106:504–509.

157. Pro B, Younes A, Albitar M, et al. Thalidomide for patients with recurrent lymphoma. Cancer 2004;100:1186–1189.

158. Strupp C, Aivado M, Germing U, et al. Angioimmunoblastic lymphadenopathy (AILD) may respond to thalidomide treatment: two case reports. Leuk Lymphoma 2002;43:133–137.

159. Wilson EA, Jobanputra S, Jackson R, Parker AN, et al. Response to thalidomide in chemotherapy-resistant mantle cell lymphoma: a case report. Br J Haematol 2002;119:128–130.

160. Fife K, Howard MR, Gracie F, et al. Activity of thalidomide in AIDS-related Kaposi's sarcoma and correlation with HHV8 titre. Int J STD AIDS 1998;9:751–755.

161. Abramson N, Stokes PK, Luke M, et al. Ovarian and papillary-serous peritoneal carcinoma: pilot study with thalidomide. J Clin Oncol 2002;20:1147–1149.

162. Little RF, Wyvill KM, Pluda JM, et al. Activity of thalidomide in AIDS-related Kaposi's sarcoma. J Clin Oncol 2000;18:2593–2602.

163. de Medeiros BC, Rezuke WN, Ricci A Jr, et al. Kaposi's sarcoma following allogeneic hematopoietic stem cell transplantation for chronic myelogenous leukemia. Acta Haematol 2000;104:115–118.

164. Kim WY, Kaelin WG. Role of VHL gene mutation in human cancer. J Clin Oncol 2004;22:4991–5004.

165. Motzer RJ, Berg W, Ginsberg M, et al. Phase II trial of thalidomide for patients with advanced renal cell carcinoma. J Clin Oncol 2002;20:302–306.

166. Stebbing J, Benson C, Eisen T, et al. The treatment of advanced renal cell cancer with high-dose oral thalidomide. Br J Cancer 2001;85:953–958.

167. Daliani DD, Papandreou CN, Thall PF, et al. A pilot study of thalidomide in patients with progressive metastatic renal cell carcinoma. Cancer 2002;95:758–765.

168. Escudier B, Lassau N, Couanet D, et al. Phase II trial of thalidomide in renal-cell carcinoma. Ann Oncol 2002;13:1029–1035.

169. Minor DR, Monroe D, Damico LA, et al. A phase II study of thalidomide in advanced metastatic renal cell carcinoma. Invest New Drugs 2002;20:389–393.

170. Amato RJ, Schell J, Thompson N, et al. Phase II study of thalidomide + interleukin-2 (IL-2) in patients with metastatic renal cell carcinoma (MRCC). Proc Am Soc Clin Oncol 2003;22:387a.

171. Olencki T, Malhi S, Mekhail T. Phase I trial of thalidomide and interleukin-2 (IL-2) in patients with metastatic renal cell carcinoma (RCC). Proc Am Soc Clin Oncol 2003:22:387.

172. Nathan PD, Gore ME, Eisen TG. Unexpected toxicity of combination thalidomide and interferon alpha-2a treatment in metastatic renal cell carcinoma. J Clin Oncol 2002;20: 1429–1430.

173. Fine HA, Figg WD, Jaeckle K, et al. Phase II trial of the antiangiogenic agent thalidomide in patients with recurrent high-grade gliomas. J Clin Oncol 2000;18:708–715.

174. Short SC, Traish D, Dowe A, et al. Thalidomide as an anti-angiogenic agent in relapsed gliomas. J Neurooncol 2001;51:41–45.

175. Marx GM, Pavlakis N, McCowatt S, et al. Phase II study of thalidomide in the treatment of recurrent glioblastoma multiforme. J Neurooncol 2001;54:31–38.

176. Parney IF, Chang SM. Current chemotherapy for glioblastoma. Cancer J 2003;9:149–156.

177. Fine HA, Wen PY, Maher EA, et al. Phase II trial of thalidomide and carmustine for patients with recurrent high-grade gliomas. J Clin Oncol 2003;21:2299–2304.

178. Hwu WJ, Krown SE, Menell JH, et al. Phase II study of temozolomide plus thalidomide for the treatment of metastatic melanoma. J Clin Oncol 2003;21:3351–3356.

179. Danson S, Lorigan P, Arance A, et al. Randomized phase II study of temozolomide given every 8 hours or daily with either interferon alfa-2b or thalidomide in metastatic malignant melanoma. J Clin Oncol 2003;21:2551–2557.

180. Figg WD, Dahut W, Duray P, et al. A randomized phase II trial of thalidomide, an angiogenesis inhibitor, in patients with androgen-independent prostate cancer. Clin Cancer Res 2001;7: 1888–1893.

181. Dixon SC, Kruger EA, Bauer KS, et al. Thalidomide up-regulates prostate-specific antigen secretion from LNCaP cells. Cancer Chemother Pharmacol 1999;43(Suppl):S78–84.

182. Pollard M. Thalidomide promotes metastasis of prostate adenocarcinoma cells (PA-III) in L-W rats. Cancer Lett 1996;101:21–24.

183. Drake MJ, Robson W, Mehta P, et al. An open-label phase II study of low-dose thalidomide in androgen-independent prostate cancer. Br J Cancer 2003;88:822–827.

184. Figg WD, Arlen P, Gulley J, et al. A randomized phase II trial of docetaxel (Taxotere) plus thalidomide in androgen-independent prostate cancer. Semin Oncol 2001;28:62–66.

185. Horne MK 3rd, Figg WD, Arlen P, et al. Increased frequency of venous thromboembolism with the combination of docetaxel and thalidomide in patients with metastatic androgen-independent prostate cancer. Pharmacotherapy 2003;23:315–318.

186. Dahut WL, Gulley JL, Arlen PM, et al. Randomized phase II trial of docetaxel plus thalidomide in androgen-independent prostate cancer. J Clin Oncol 2004;22:2532–2539.

187. Behrens RJ, Gulley JL, Dahut WL. Pulmonary toxicity during prostate cancer treatment with docetaxel and thalidomide. Am J Ther 2003;10:228–232.

188. Molloy FM, Floeter MK, Syed NA, et al. Thalidomide neuropathy in patients treated for metastatic prostate cancer. Muscle Nerve 2001;24:1050–1057.

189. Capitosti SM, Hansen TP, Brown ML. Thalidomide analogues demonstrate dual inhibition of both angiogenesis and prostate cancer. Bioorg Med Chem 2004;12:327–336.

190. Ng SS, MacPherson GR, Gutschow M, et al. Antitumor effects of thalidomide analogs in human prostate cancer xenografts implanted in immunodeficient mice. Clin Cancer Res 2004;10: 4192–4197.

191. Baidas SM, Winer EP, Fleming GF, et al. Phase II evaluation of thalidomide in patients with metastatic breast cancer. J Clin Oncol 2000;18:2710–2717.

192. Gaziev D, Galimberti M, Lucarelli G, et al. Chronic graft-versus-host disease: is there an alternative to the conventional treatment? Bone Marrow Transplant 2000;25:689–696.

193. Vogelsang GB, Farmer ER, Hess AD, et al. Thalidomide for the treatment of chronic graft-versus-host disease [see comments]. N Engl J Med 1992;326:1055–1058.

194. Heney D, Norfolk DR, Wheeldon J, et al. Thalidomide treatment for chronic graft-versus-host disease. Br J Haematol 1991;78: 23–27.

195. Rovelli A, Arrigo C, Nesi F, et al. The role of thalidomide in the treatment of refractory chronic graft-versus-host disease following bone marrow transplantation in children. Bone Marrow Transplant 1998;21:577–581.

196. Browne PV, Weisdorf DJ, DeFor T, et al. Response to thalidomide therapy in refractory chronic graft-versus-host diseases. Bone Marrow Transplant 2000.

197. Bruera E, Neumann CM, Pituskin E, et al. Thalidomide in patients with cachexia due to terminal cancer: preliminary report. Ann Oncol 1999;10:857–859.

198. Govindarajan R, Heaton KM, Broadwater R, et al. Effect of thalidomide on gastrointestinal toxic effects of irinotecan [letter]. Lancet 2000;356:566–567.

199. Peuckmann V, Fisch M, Bruera E. Potential novel uses of thalidomide: focus on palliative care [In Process Citation]. Drugs 2000;60:273–292.

200. Dimopoulos M, Weber D, Chen C, et al. Evaluating oral lenalidomide (Revlimid) and dexamethasone versus placebo and dexamethasone in patients with relapsed or refractory multiple myeloma. Haematologica 2005;90(s2):160 (Abstract 0402).

201. Weber D, Dimopoulos M, Chen C et al. Interim results of two international randomized, double-blind phase III studies evaluating oral lenalidomide (Revlimid®) and dexamethasone versus placebo and dexamethasone in patients with relapsed or refractory multiple myeloma. ASCO Scientific Symposium Oral Presentation (2005).

202. Chanan-Khan A, Miller KC, Takeshita K, et al. Thalidomide in combination with fludarabine as initial therapy for patients with treatment-requiring chronic lymphocytic leukemia (CLL). Results of a phase I clinical trial. Blood. 2005 Jul 28; [Epub ahead of print].

Inhibitors of Tumor Angiogenesis

28

Anaadriana Zakarija   William J. Gradishar

Cancer development is a complex process involving the conversion of a normal cell into a cancer cell. In addition to this malignant transformation, a tumor requires a vascular supply. Over 30 years ago, Judah Folkman proposed the theory that tumors are unable to grow beyond a size of 2 to 3 mm in the absence of a new vascular supply.[1] Research has confirmed that a necessary step in the growth of both the primary tumor and metastases is the development of vasculature, termed angiogenesis.[2,3] Normally, this process is tightly regulated by activators and inhibitors of angiogenesis (Table 28.1). Tumors can produce some of these activator molecules or down-regulate expression of inhibitors, therefore altering the balance in favor of an "angiogenic switch."[4,5] Due to the imbalance, these endothelial cells continue to proliferate, unlike normal endothelial cells, which mature and then become quiescent. In addition to an altered growth rate, the cytokine balance results in tumor-associated blood vessels that are structurally abnormal. They are not organized into an intact network of capillaries; the perivascular cells are more loosely associated with the endothelial cells, leading to a leaky basement membrane; and tumor cells can become integrated into the vessel wall.[6] The importance of neoangiogenesis to tumor growth provides a rationale for exploring antiangiogenic therapies in the treatment of cancer.[1]

As understanding of the complex process of angiogenesis in tumors has advanced, many potential strategies for disrupting this process have been identified.[7] Drugs currently in development are grouped into five categories based on mechanism of action: (a) agents that block breakdown of the extracellular matrix, such as matrix metalloproteinase inhibitors (MMPIs); (b) drugs that inhibit endothelial cells; (c) agents that inhibit endothelial cell-specific integrin/survival signaling; (d) drugs that block

activation of angiogenesis, such as anti–vascular endothelial growth factor (VEGF) agents; and (e) drugs with unknown mechanisms of action.[8]

Dozens of agents have been developed and are in various stages of clinical development. This chapter highlights promising agents and the results of clinical trials. To date, the only FDA-approved agent is bevacizumab (Avastin), a recombinant humanized anti-VEGF monoclonal antibody. There have been a number of disappointing clinical trials with a variety of single-agent antiangiogenesis therapies. Due to the complexity of tumorigenesis and angiogenesis, this is not altogether surprising. Future strategies should include combinations of agents that target various processes involved in tumor growth. In addition, correlative studies and measurement of potential targets, such as VEGF or MMP, should be done to better identify the population most likely to benefit or to elucidate whether the desired endpoint is being achieved with a given agent.

MATRIX METALLOPROTEINASE INHIBITORS

MMPs are a family of structurally related zinc-containing endopeptidases that are involved in the degradation of extracellular matrix components (ECM).[9] MMP gene expression and enzymatic activity is an important physiologic process that plays an important role in embryogenesis, wound healing, and the female reproductive cycle.[10] Because MMPs facilitate the breakdown of the basement membrane and the underlying stroma, they have been implicated in tumor invasion and metastasis formation.

Over 20 members of the MMP family have been identified. The MMPs are produced by a variety of different cells,

TABLE 28.1
ANGIOGENIC ACTIVATORS AND INHIBITORS

Activators	Inhibitors
Acidic fibroblast growth factor	Angiostatin*
Angiogenin	Endostatin*
Basic fibroblast growth factor (bFGF)*	Interferons
Epidermal growth factor	Interleukins 12 and 18
Granulocyte colony-stimulating factor	Platelet factor 4
Hepatocyte growth factor	Prolactin, 16-kd fragment
Interleukin 8	Soluble VEGFR-1
Placental growth factor (P1GF)	Thrombospondins 1 and 2*
Platelet-derived endothelial growth factor B (PDGF)	TIMP-1 (tissue inhibitor metalloproteinase-1)
Transforming growth factor α (TGF-α)	TIMP-2
TGF-β	TIMP-3
Tumor necrosis factor α (TNF-α)	TIMP-4
Vascular endothelial growth factor (VEGF)*	

*Most important factors.

including fibroblasts, epithelial cells, inflammatory cells, and endothelial cells.[11] Several studies have demonstrated high levels of MMPs in tumors and in the plasma and urine of patients with malignancy.[9,12] MMP expression is also increased in metastatic tumors as compared with the primary tumor.[13] Physiologic inhibitors known as tissue inhibitors of metalloproteinases (TIMPs) control MMP activity. The TIMP family currently consists of four members: TIMP-1, TIMP-2, TIMP-3, and TIMP-4.[10]

For a primary tumor to progress locally through adjacent normal tissue or for metastases to expand at a site distant from the primary tumor, the ECM must be digested.[14] MMPs are also directly involved in the angiogenic response, as they mediate remodeling and invasion of the ECM by new vessels.[15,16] MMPs promote angiogenesis by regulating endothelial cell attachment, proliferation, and migration.[15,16] These observations suggest that matrix metalloproteinase inhibitors (MMPIs) could inhibit tumor progression at both the primary tumor site and sites of metastases. A concern with the long-term administration of MMPIs is the effect they may have on normal physiologic processes that require MMP activity, such as wound repair or reproduction.[17,18] Several MMPIs have been developed, but results in clinical trials of patients with advanced malignancy have been disappointing; therefore, ongoing studies are limited.

Marimastat

Marimastat is the most extensively tested MMPI. It is a synthetic MMPI that is orally bioavailable and is nonspecific, as it inhibits the activity of MMP-1, -2, -3, -7, and -9.[19] Phase I clinical trials demonstrated that the drug was relatively well tolerated, and musculoskeletal complaints were

the most common adverse effect.[20–22] Marimastat has been evaluated in patients with pancreatic, breast, lung, ovarian, colorectal, gastric, and prostate cancers and glioblastoma. It was tested in a phase III randomized trial as first-line therapy in patients with unresectable pancreatic cancer. A total of 414 patients were randomized to receive 5, 10, or 25 mg bid of marimastat or 1,000 mg/m^2 of gemcitabine.[23] There was evidence of a dose-response, as patients treated with the 25-mg dose had better overall survival than patients treated with the lower doses of marimastat. There was no difference in 1-year survival between patients treated with gemcitabine (19%) and the 25-mg dose of marimastat (20%). Patients treated with gemcitabine had a statistically significant improvement in pain.

A number of phase III trials were performed to test the role of marimastat in patients with metastatic disease who had responded or had stable disease after first-line chemotherapy. These studies included patients with breast cancer, small cell lung cancer, or gastric cancer.[24–26] There was no improvement in overall or disease-free survival in these cohorts. There are a variety of reasons why marimastat may not have been effective. First, only a minority of patients had trough levels of marimastat that were therapeutic. Interestingly, higher levels of marimastat were associated with a higher mortality.[26,27] Higher drug levels were also associated with a rise in the serum concentrations of MMP-9, one of the MMPs associated with tumor grade and metastases. Therefore, despite therapy with an MMPI, other mechanisms overcame inhibition and resulted in stimulation of MMP expression.

More recently marimastat has also been tested in combination with other antiangiogenic therapies. Fifty patients with a variety of advanced malignancies were treated with marimastat, captopril, and dalteparin. One patient with renal cell carcinoma had a prolonged partial remission, while three other patients with renal cell carcinoma had stable disease for 204 to 337 days.[28] There were three major hemorrhagic events, one of which was fatal. In addition, 14% of the patients had grade 3 musculoskeletal toxicity that responded to a reduction in the dose of marimastat; this toxicity has been the most significant in other studies of marimastat.[22,29] It is possible that combination regimens with other antiangiogenic therapies will have more efficacy than single-agent MMPIs.

The disappointing results of phase III trials with marimastat demonstrate the complexities of this targeted therapy. Inhibition of MMP may not achieve the desired effect, and instead MMP expression may be stimulated. This phenomenon highlights the importance of correlative studies in clinical trials. It is necessary to measure the proposed target during therapy to ensure that the desired effect is achieved, for if it is not, this may explain negative results.

Prinomastat and BAY 12-9566 are two additional MMPIs that have shown disappointing results in clinical trials. BAY 12-9566 was found to result in significantly shorter survival times than gemcitabine in a randomized phase III trial in patients with advanced pancreatic cancer.[30] In addition, prinomastat combined with chemotherapy for patients with advanced lung cancer demonstrated a significantly higher incidence of venous thromboembolism than either prinomastat or chemotherapy alone.[31] Due to their lack of efficacy and their toxicity profile, these agents are no longer in development.

BMS-275291

BMS-275291 is another MMPI currently in clinical trials. It is similar in structure to marimastat, is orally bioavailable, and inhibits a number of MMPs, including MMP-1, -2, -7, -9, and -14.[32] It was designed to be specific for the MMPs and not to affect other metalloproteinases, such as sheddases, involved in the release of tumor necrosis factor-α (TNF-α), TNF-α receptor, and interleukin-6 receptor, which were thought to account for musculoskeletal toxicity.[33] In a phase I study in patients with a variety of advanced malignancies, 44 patients were treated with escalating doses of BMS-275291, from 600 to 2,400 mg/day.[33] The maximum tolerated dose was not achieved, as there were no dose-limiting toxicities at 900, 1,800, or 2,400 mg/day. The most common adverse events were grade 1 or 2 myalgias and arthralgias in 59% of patients. Unlike previous trials with MMPIs, the musculoskeletal toxicity did not necessitate discontinuation of the drug. A rash developed in 23% of patients, but in 90% of cases it resolved despite continuation of the drug. The other observed side effects included fatigue (32%), nausea (23%), and headache (16%). The median time on the study was 8 weeks, although 6 patients were treated for over 8 months, and 3 patients were treated for over 1 year. There were no objective partial or complete tumor responses; stable disease was seen in 27% of cases.[33]

The mechanism of action of these drugs suggests that they may be more effective in the setting of small-volume disease or micrometastatic disease. This provides the rationale for treatment in the adjuvant setting. A randomized phase II trial was performed in patients with stage I (T1c) to IIIa breast cancer who were to receive adjuvant therapy with tamoxifen alone, four cycles of doxorubicin and cyclophosphamide (AC), or AC followed by four cycles of paclitaxel.[34] Patients were randomly assigned to receive 1,200 mg of BMS-275291 once daily or placebo for 1 year. Therapy started concurrently with systemic chemotherapy or with tamoxifen if patients were not receiving chemotherapy. The primary objectives of the study were to evaluate rates of drug discontinuation due to intolerance and to ensure that adequate trough levels could be achieved. In the 71 patients treated in the study, the major toxicity was musculoskeletal, seen in 36% of the BMS-275291 group and characterized primarily by tendonitis and bursitis.[34] The symptoms were reversible after drug discontinuation. Two patients in this group developed palpable nontender nodules on tendon surfaces. Musculoskeletal symptoms were seen in 21% of the placebo group, which was not statistically significantly

different. Discontinuation rates at 1 year were similar, 33% in the treatment group and 21% in the placebo group. Only 19% of patients had trough levels that were higher than the IC_{90} for MMP-9 more than half the time. The musculoskeletal toxicity, discontinuation rate, and therapeutic trough levels in a minority of patients resulted in early termination of this study and the conclusion that this drug was not feasible in the adjuvant setting. Clinical trials continue with this agent in other settings, such as hormone-refractory prostate cancer.

DRUGS THAT INHIBIT ENDOTHELIAL CELLS

TNP-470

TNP-470, is a synthetic analog of fumagillin, which is secreted by the fungus *Aspergillus fumigatus Fresenius* and was isolated as a contaminant from an endothelial cell culture.[35] Fumagillin inhibited in vitro endothelial cell proliferation and in vivo tumor growth and angiogenesis but was associated with significant weight loss in mice.[35] TNP-470 is one of the compounds obtained when fumagillin undergoes alkaline hydrolysis and is more potent. TNP-470 blocks endothelial cell proliferation. The potential mechanisms of action include inhibition of the metalloprotease methionine animopeptidase (MetAP-2)[36] and inhibition of protein kinases, including protein kinase C (PKC) and mitogen-activated protein kinase (MAPK).[37] In addition, TNP-470 has been shown to be cytotoxic to cancer cell lines.[38]

Phase I trials of TNP-470 have been conducted in patients with AIDS-related Kaposi's sarcoma, cervical cancer, and other advanced malignancies. Treatment schedules have included drug administration once a week, every other day, or three times a week.[39-41] Pharmacokinetic data from these studies demonstrated a very short half-life for TNP-470 and its metabolites, from 2 to 6 minutes.[40] After the initial trials, the most commonly used dosing regimen has been 60 mg/m^2 infused over 1 hour three times per week.[42,43] The most common toxicity, and the dose-limiting toxicity, in the phase I trials was neurotoxicity.[39,40] Neurotoxicity developed in 44% of patients; it included dizziness/vertigo (43%), ataxia (24%), short-term memory loss (24%), confusion (14%), anxiety/depression (14%), and insomnia (5%).[40] At the highest dose level (235 mg/m^2 once per week), ataxia was the dose-limiting toxicity, with 33% of patients developing grade 3 or 4 toxicity. Other nonneurologic toxicities include nausea (19%), anorexia (19%), and fatigue (19%).[40] A phase II trial was performed in 33 patients with metastatic renal cell cancer; 60 mg/m^2 TNP-470 was infused over 1 hour three times per week.[42] Only 1 patient had a partial response, but 6 others had stable disease for over 6 months. Neurotoxicity was the most common adverse effect (67%); it included cerebellar symptoms, psychiatric changes, and confusion. Other toxicities included fatigue/asthenia (60%), anorexia (36%), and nausea (36%). Fifteen percent of patients discontinued therapy due to neurotoxicity.[42]

TNP-470 has also been tested in combination with traditional chemotherapy. A total of 32 patients with advanced solid tumors were enrolled in a dose-finding study with TNP-470 and paclitaxel.[43] The regimen of paclitaxel 225 mg/m^2 every 3 weeks and TNP-470 60 mg/m^2 three times per week was well tolerated, and TNP-470 did not adversely affect the clearance of paclitaxel.[43] Partial responses were observed in 25% of patients, and 53% had stable disease. The incidence of hematologic toxicities did not appear to be increased with the addition of TNP-470. Nonhematologic toxicities included fatigue (78%), peripheral neuropathy (66%), arthralgias (62%), nausea (59%), diarrhea (41%), dizziness (34%), abnormal vision (34%), and abnormal gait (22%). The neurotoxicity in this study was predominantly mild (grade 1 or 2) and reversible after discontinuation of treatment. Formal neuropsychologic testing was performed as part of this trial and demonstrated that the most commonly seen deficits included decline in executive function, memory, and motor dexterity. In only 9% of cases did function not return to baseline. The addition of carboplatin to a regimen of TNP-470 60 mg/m^2 thrice weekly and paclitaxel 225 mg/m^2 every 3 weeks was evaluated in a clinical trial.[44] Carboplatin at an AUC of 6 was found to be well tolerated, with toxicity similar to that in the previous study by Herbst et al. Responses were also similar; 24% of patients had a partial response and 47% had stable disease.

The responses to date have been relatively modest with TNP-470. Given the short half-life of the drug and its metabolites, a different administration schedule may be more effective. Studies in animal models have demonstrated that daily administration was more effective than thrice weekly administration at inhibiting tumor growth, metastasis, and angiogenesis.[45] Therefore, a phase I trial was designed to determine the feasibility of continuous infusion TNP-470 with or without paclitaxel and carboplatin in patients with advanced solid tumors. The most tolerable regimen when given with paclitaxel (200 mg/m^2) and carboplatin (AUC 5 to 6) was TNP-470 at 2.5 mg/m^2 continuous infusion for 5 days every week.[46] Response data have not been published.

INHIBITION OF ENDOTHELIAL CELL–SPECIFIC INTEGRIN/SURVIVAL SIGNALING

EMD 121974 (Cilengitide)

The interaction between endothelial cells and the extracellular matrix is critical to neoangiogenesis. The integrin $\alpha_V\beta_3$ is expressed on a number of cells, including endothe-lial cells; is responsible for their binding to the extracellular matrix components during angiogenesis; and is up-regulated by basic fibroblast growth factor (bFGF).[47] Apoptosis is induced in vascular cells when this interaction is inhibited.[48] In patients with breast cancer, $\alpha_V\beta_3$ was higher in patients with metastatic tumors and was predictive of relapse-free survival.[49] EMD 121974 is a peptide developed to inhibit the $\alpha_V\beta_3$ receptor.[47] A total of 37 patients with a variety of advanced malignancies were treated in a phase I study.[50] The drug was given intravenously twice a week and was tested at doses from 30 to 1,600 mg/m^2. No hematologic toxicity was seen, and non-hematologic toxicities, including nausea, anorexia, fatigue, and malaise, were mild, with none higher than grade 2.[50] In addition, the plasma half-life is short, 3 to 4 hours. Therefore, the optimal dose and administration schedule have not yet been determined. Further phase I and II studies are ongoing in patients with glioblastoma multiforme, melanoma, acute myeloid leukemia (AML), and other advanced malignancies.

INHIBITION OF ANGIOGENESIS ACTIVATORS

The VEGF signaling family is an important factor in both physiologic and pathologic angiogenesis. The complexities of this system are beyond the scope of this chapter; therefore, only a brief overview is provided, but detailed reviews are available.[51-53] The VEGF family is made up of four main ligands and three tyrosine kinase receptors (see Table 28.2). VEGF-A, also referred to as VEGF, is a primary regulator of angiogenesis. It is important in early endothelial cell survival, but established blood vessels are not VEGF-dependent.[51] Vascular permeability is also mediated by VEGF, which forms fenestrations in blood vessels.[52,53] VEGF expression can be induced by hypoxia and hypoxia-inducible factor 1 (HIF-1); a number of cytokines and growth factors (including fibroblast growth factor-4, platelet-derived growth factor [PDGF], TNF-α, and transforming growth factor-β [TGF-β]); UV-B radiation; and inactivation of the *vHL* (von Hippel Landau) tumor suppressor gene. Natural inhibitors of VEGF include cytokines, such as IL-10 and IL-13.

VEGF-A exerts most of its actions by binding to VEGFR-2, although it also binds to VEGFR-1(flt-1). VEGFR-2 (KDR in humans or flk-1 in the mouse) is expressed on both vascular and lymphatic endothelial cells and is the main regulator of angiogenesis, endothelial cell proliferation and survival, and vascular permeability.[52] The scope of activity of VEGFR-1 varies; if VEGFR-2 is not present, activation of VEGFR-1 will not result in endothelial cell proliferation, yet cell migration is induced. VEGFR-1 may also have an inhibitory role by binding to VEGF-A, thus interfering with its ability to activate VEGFR-2.[51] VEGFR-3 is found predominantly in lymphatics and likely has an important role

TABLE 28.2

VEGF (VASCULAR ENDOTHELIAL GROWTH FACTOR) SIGNALING FAMILY

Receptor	Ligand	Activity
VEGFR-1 (Flt-1)	VEGF-A VEGF-B PlGF	Inhibitory action by binding VEGF-A (early development); induction of MMP-9 and tissue-specific growth factors; monocyte chemotaxis
VEGFR-2 (KDR/Flk-1)	VEGF-A VEGF-C VEGF-D	Angiogenesis; endothelial cell survival and proliferation; vascular permeability
VEGFR-3 (Flt-4)	VEGF-C VEGF-D	Lymphangiogenesis; endothelial cell survival

PlGF, placental growth factor.

in lymphangiogenesis, but can also be induced in tumor-associated endothelial cells.[54]

VEGF and its receptors have been found to be overexpressed in a number of malignant cell lines and tumors, including colorectal, gastric, hepatocellular, lung, breast, and endometrial cancers, AIDS-associated Kaposi's sarcoma, and AML.[55-59] The significance of this overexpression is not completely understood. A number of studies have demonstrated that increased expression of VEGF correlates with an increased vessel density, but the findings on the relationship between VEGFR-2 and vessel density have been mixed.[56,60,61] Retrospective studies to determine whether VEGF or receptor expression correlates with prognosis have not been definitive. In one of the largest series performed, tumors from 259 patients with colorectal cancer were examined, and survival was found to be lower in patients whose tumors were positive for VEGF.[61] Similar

studies in patients with gastric and endometrial cancer, however, did not find VEGF expression to have prognostic significance.[60,62] Despite these uncertainties, animal studies have demonstrated that inhibiting VEGF signaling interrupts tumor growth and invasion.[54,63-66] Therefore, based on evidence for the critical role of VEGF in angiogenesis and preclinical data suggesting that tumor-associated angiogenesis and growth could be altered by targeting this system, a number of agents aimed at the VEGF family have been developed and are presented here (Table 28.3).

Bevacizumab (Avastin)

Bevacizumab is a recombinant humanized monoclonal antibody to VEGF. It binds to VEGF, including a number of its splice variants that are biologically active.[67] In phase I trials, pharmacokinetic studies determined that the half-life

TABLE 28.3

AGENTS TARGETING THE VEGF FAMILY

Drug	Target	Development
Bevacizumab (Avastin)	Monoclonal antibody against VEGF-A	FDA approved in colorectal cancer; phase III trials
VEGF-Trap	Binds VEGF-A	Phase I trials
PTK787/ZK222584 (Vatalanib)	Receptor tyrosine kinase inhibitor of VEGFR-1 and VEGFR-2	Phase II trials
ZD6474	Receptor tyrosine kinase inhibitor of VEGFR-2, VEGFR-3, and EGFR	Phase II trials
IMC-1C11	Monoclonal antibody against VEGFR-2	Phase I trials
SU-5416	Receptor tyrosine kinase inhibitor of VEGFR-2	Development halted due to disappointing phase III trials
SU-6668	Receptor tyrosine kinase inhibitor of VEGFR-2, PDGFR, and FGFR	Phase I trials; future development uncertain

PDGFR, platelet-derived growth factor receptor; EGFR, epidermal growth factor receptor; FGFR fibroblast growth factor receptor.

of the drug is about 21 days at doses greater than 0.3 mg/kg.[67] No patients developed antibodies to the recombinant antibody. Bevacizumab has been tested at doses from 3 to 20 mg/kg. Of interest, the dose-response relationship has not been consistent. In colorectal cancer, a dose of 5 mg/kg was more effective than 10 mg/kg.[68] On the other hand, in renal cell cancer and non–small cell lung cancer, higher doses up to 15 mg/kg are more effective than lower doses.[69,70] A number of clinical trials have been undertaken with bevacizumab either as a single agent or in combination with chemotherapy in a variety of malignancies.

Renal cell carcinoma was felt to be a potentially promising target for bevacizumab, since most clear cell renal carcinomas have a mutation in the *vHL* tumor suppressor gene, leading to HIF-1–mediated VEGF production.[51,69] A randomized phase II trial with single-agent bevacizumab was conducted in patients with metastatic clear cell renal carcinoma who had progressed after immunotherapy. A total of 116 patients were randomly assigned to either placebo, bevacizumab 3 mg/kg every 2 weeks, or bevacizumab 10 mg/kg every 2 weeks.[69] There were no responses in the low-dose group, while a partial response was seen in 10% of patients in the higher dose group. Toxicities seen in this study included proteinuria (53%), hypertension (20%), and epistaxis (17%). There was a difference between progression-free survival in the high-dose group compared with the placebo group (4.8 vs. 2.5 months, $P < .001$), but no improvement in overall survival occurred in any of the cohorts.[69] Single-agent therapy was not felt to be promising in renal cell cancer, and studies were undertaken with combination therapy. Thalidomide plus bevacizumab was also not effective.[71] A phase II trial combined bevacizumab with erlotinib (Tarceva), an epidermal growth factor receptor (EGFR) tyrosine kinase inhibitor.[72] All patients were treated with bevacizumab 10 mg/kg every 2 weeks and erlotinib 150 mg orally daily. Of 57 evaluable patients, a partial response was seen in 25% of patients, and 62% had either minor responses or stable disease.[72] Grade 3 or 4 toxicities included hypertension (11%), diarrhea (9%), and rash (7%). Further studies are warranted to evaluate the role of this combination or others in the treatment of renal cell carcinoma. An ongoing phase III trial randomizes patients to either interferon-α alone or interferon-α plus bevacizumab.[73]

Bevacizumab has been approved by the FDA for use with 5-fluorouracil (5-FU)–based chemotherapy in first-line therapy of patients with metastatic colorectal cancer. This approval was based on two clinical trials in 917 patients with previously untreated metastatic disease.[68,74] In the phase II trial, patients were randomly assigned to one of three treatment regimens: 5-FU/leucovorin (LV), 5-FU/LV plus bevacizumab 5 mg/kg every 2 weeks, or 5FU/LV plus bevacizumab 10 mg/kg every 2 weeks.[68] The 5-FU/LV in all groups was given weekly for the first 6 weeks of an 8-week cycle. The difference in overall median survival was not statistically significant. The time to progression was improved in the 5 mg/kg bevacizumab group when compared with the control group (9 months vs 5.2 months, $P = .005$), as was the overall response (40% vs. 17%, $P = .029$).[68] The time to progression and overall response in the cohort that received the higher dose bevacizumab were no better than for the control group. The phase III trial randomly assigned 411 patients to irinotecan, bolus 5-FU, and LV (IFL) and 402 patients to IFL plus bevacizumab 5 mg/kg every 2 weeks.[74] The group that received bevacizumab had a better overall response rate and improved progression-free and overall survival. The median survival was 15.6 months in the IFL cohort, and 20.3 months in the IFL plus bevacizumab group ($P < .001$).[74] These significant results led to FDA approval of this agent in February 2004.

The toxicities associated with bevacizumab have been similar in these large studies; the most notable have been hypertension, proteinuria, minor and major hemorrhage, wound-healing complications, and gastrointestinal perforation. Hypertension is seen in up to 19% of cases, with grade 3 hypertension seen in 11% of bevacizumab-treated patients in the study of IFL with or without bevacizumab.[74] Patients must be monitored carefully for development of hypertension, and antihypertensive therapy instituted promptly. If significant hypertension develops, the drug should be discontinued. Although rare, hypertensive encephalopathy did develop in 4 patients, of over 1,000 treated in clinical trials (bevacizumab [Avastin] package insert, Genentech, San Francisco, April 2004). Bleeding episodes have also been more frequent with bevacizumab treatment than with chemotherapy alone, 59% versus 11%.[68] The majority of hemorrhagic complications were grade 1 or 2 episodes of epistaxis. In the phase II study by Kabbinavar, 10% of individuals experienced episodes of gastrointestinal hemorrhage, 43% of which were grade 3 or 4;[68] in the larger phase III trial, the incidence of grade 3 or 4 bleeding was not higher than that of the control group.[74] Although rare, the bleeding can be severe. It is important to note that patients with central nervous system metastases were excluded from the clinical trials, and the safety of this therapy in that group has not been established.

The consequences of inhibition of VEGF signaling can be complex, since both hemorrhagic and thrombotic complications have been recognized with bevacizumab. A possible mechanism for these adverse events relates to the decreased ability of endothelial cells to respond to an injury when VEGF is inhibited, thereby leading to a hemorrhagic tendency. On the other hand, if vascular injury occurs, the coagulation system may be activated by exposure of tissue factor, and a thrombotic event may result.[75] In clinical trials to date, thrombotic events have included deep venous thrombosis, pulmonary embolism, catheter-related thrombosis, stroke, and transient ischemic events. On August 4, 2004, Genentech issued a warning notifying physicians of an increased incidence of arterial thromboembolic events, including strokes, transient ischemic attacks, myocardial infarctions, and angina. In addition to bevacizumab exposure, risk factors for these arterial events were history of prior arterial thromboembolism or age greater than 65. If patients develop a thrombosis requiring anticoagulation while on bevacizumab, a recent report suggests that there is no increased risk of bleeding. Patients from the Hurwitz study[74] who developed a thrombosis were placed on full-dose anticoagulation; 55% of patients receiving IFL and 83% of patients treated with IFL plus bevacizumab continued in the study. While on anticoagulation, grade 3 or 4 bleeding developed in 2 of 30 patients (6.7%) on IFL and in 2 of 58 patients (3.8%) receiving bevacizumab.[76] Despite this report, a better understanding of the effects of anti-VEGF therapy on the hemostatic system is necessary before recommendations can be made for safe administration of this therapy with anticoagulation.

Bevacizumab has also shown promise in non–small cell lung cancer. Patients with stage IIIB or IV non–small cell lung cancer were randomized to one of three groups: carboplatin/paclitaxel every 3 weeks or carboplatin/paclitaxel plus bevacizumab 7.5 or 15 mg/kg.[70] The bevacizumab was given after each cycle of carboplatin/paclitaxel. The difference in the median time to progression between the higher dose bevacizumab group and the control arm was statistically significant (7.4 months vs. 4.2 months, $P = .023$).[70] The differences in overall response and survival were not statistically significant. The toxicities were similar to those reported in previous clinical trials with bevacizumab. It is important to note that major life-threatening bleeding occurred in 9% of patients receiving study drug, and fatal hemorrhage, primarily from hemoptysis, occurred in 6% of bevacizumab-treated patients. The bevacizumab doses in both arms of this study were higher than the 5-mg/kg dose that has been approved for the treatment of colorectal cancer.

A randomized phase III study in patients with metastatic breast cancer who had progressed after anthracycline and taxane therapy was conducted, and capecitabine was administered alone or with bevacizumab 15 mg/kg every 3 weeks.[77] The overall response rate was greater in the combination arm (20% vs. 9%), but there was no improvement in progression-free survival. Additional phase III studies are currently being conducted in breast, colorectal, non–small cell lung, and renal cell cancers. In addition, numerous phase II studies are ongoing in patients with small cell lung, head and neck, pancreatic, hepatocellular, and ovarian cancers, melanoma, carcinoid tumors, soft-tissue sarcoma, Kaposi's sarcoma, mesothelioma, non-Hodgkin's lymphoma, chronic myelogenous leukemia, multiple myeloma, and myelodysplastic syndrome (MDS). We await the results of these numerous studies to further define the role of this promising therapy. In addition, an effort should be made to better define a subset of patients who would be more likely to benefit from therapy. In the phase I trials, there was no apparent correlation between baseline levels of serum VEGF and response.[67] Some of the ongoing studies measure biologic surrogates such as serum or urine VEGF levels. Future studies should focus on identifying the utility of biologic markers in predicting response to therapy.

VEGF-Trap

VEGF-Trap is an engineered protein that binds VEGF. It was created by fusing a portion of the extracellular domain of VEGFR1 and VEGFR2 to a human IgG1.[78] It has a very high affinity for all variants of VEGF-A, also binds placental growth factor, and is more efficacious than the VEGFR-2 monoclonal antibodies in binding VEGF.[78] In a neuroblastoma murine model, VEGF-Trap was more effective than an anti-VEGF antibody in inhibiting tumor growth.[79] Phase I trials with this agent are ongoing in patients with advanced malignancies. The dose-escalation study recruited 38 patients who were treated at seven dose levels, from 25 to 800 µg/kg subcutaneously once per week and 800 µg/kg biweekly.[80] A variety of malignancies were represented, including renal cell cancer in 9 patients and colon cancer in 5. The half-life of the drug at the 800 µg/kg per week dose is approximately 25 ± 3 days. The maximum tolerated dose has not yet been achieved. Adverse events of note include proteinuria (14/33), hypertension (5/33, 2 of the 5 with grade 3 or 4 hypertension), grade 3 or 4 thrombosis (2/33), and grade 1 or 2 hemorrhage (1/33). Other grade 1 or 2 toxicities included fatigue, constipation, nausea, vomiting, anorexia, arthralgias, and diarrhea.[81] No patients have developed antibodies to the VEGF-Trap. No responses have been seen, but at the higher dose of 800 µg/kg once or twice per week, 8 of 10 patients demonstrated stable disease after 10 weeks on therapy.

PTK787/ZK 222584 (Vatalanib)

PTK787/ZK 222584 (PTK/ZK) is an oral inhibitor of both VEGF-R1 (Flt-1) and VEGFR-2 (KDR). In animal models, this agent inhibits tumor growth, tumor vessel density, and development of metastases.[82–84] In addition, there is evidence from the preclinical study that treatment resulted in decreased tumor blood flow as detected by color Doppler ultrasound and that this correlated with a decrease in vessel density.[83] In phase I trials of PTK/ZK, this oral agent was well tolerated by patients with a variety of advanced malignancies, including glioblastoma and colorectal cancer.[85,86] Doses have been escalated from 50 to 2,000 mg daily. Toxicities were rare; the only grade 3 toxicities reported to date include deep venous thrombosis, pedal edema, and elevation of liver enzymes.[85] The drug is absorbed within 2 hours, and the average half-life is approximately 6 hours.[86] Dynamic contrast-enhanced magnetic resonance imaging (DCE-MRI) was performed during administration of PTK/ZK in phase I studies in an attempt to identify early biologic response. The reduction in DCE-MRI contrast enhancement was dose-dependent, and there was a correlation between reduction of enhancement and tumor response.[87] Further studies of this technique are required to determine if imaging results will correspond to disease improvement. The potential use for this technique in optimizing dose of antiangiogenic therapy needs to be investigated.

PTK/ZK has also been safely administered with oxaliplatin, 5-FU, and leucovorin (FOLFOX-4) in patients with advanced colorectal cancer.[88] A total of 35 patients who were previously untreated received oral PTK/ZK at doses from 500 to 2,000 mg daily. Dose-limiting toxicities were observed at doses greater than 1,250 mg/day; these included ataxia, dizziness, and expressive dysphasia. For 28 evaluable patients, 1 (4%) had a complete response and 14 (50%) partial responses. As a result of these data, phase III randomized trials are planned in patients with advanced colorectal cancer. Other phase II studies continue in advanced malignancies such as mesothelioma, AML, and MDS.

ZD6474

ZD6474 is an orally bioavailable small-molecule tyrosine kinase inhibitor of VEGFR-2, VEGFR-3, and the epidermal growth factor receptor (EGFR). Early animal studies indicated that this agent was capable of inhibiting VEGF and angiogenesis in bone growth, and a number of tumor xenografts, including lung, colon, breast, and prostate, were inhibited by the ingestion of ZD6474.[89] Due to promising preclinical data, phase I clinical trials were conducted.[90] Doses were escalated from 50 to 600 mg daily in six cohorts. Patients with a variety of advanced malignancies were enrolled (31% of patients had colorectal cancer). The half-life of ZD6474 was estimated to be 120 hours. In normal healthy volunteers, absorption was not found to be affected by concurrent food intake.[91] Toxicities associated with this agent include asymptomatic QTc prolongation, seen in 7 of 49 patients. Grade 3 toxicities included rash (2 patients), diarrhea (2), and thrombocytopenia (1). The maximum tolerated dose was 500 mg per day.[90] A smaller study in Japan displayed similar toxicities, the most common being rash (78%), asymptomatic QTc prolongation (61%), diarrhea (56%), proteinuria (56%), and hypertension (39%).[92] Since ZD6474 is well tolerated, phase II clinical trials have proceeded. A pilot study found no increased toxicity or interactions between docetaxel and ZD6474 in patients with lung cancer.[93] Therefore, a trial is now being conducted that randomly assigns patients with advanced non–small cell lung cancer to either docetaxel with placebo or ZD6474. Other phase II trials are also being conducted that combine ZD6474 with chemotherapy or radiation in patients with lung cancer.

IMC-1C11

IMC-1C11 is a chimeric monoclonal antibody that targets the vascular endothelial growth factor receptor-2 (VEGFR-2),

also known as Flk-1 in mice and KDR in humans. VEGFR-2 is present on endothelial cells and some tumor cells and is thought to be the main mediator of VEGF-stimulated angiogenesis. Animal studies were performed with DC101, a murine monoclonal antibody to VEGFR-2 (flk-1). A variety of tumors, including lung and pancreatic cancers, melanoma, glioblastoma, and lymphoma, were inhibited in mice treated with DC101.[66,94] As a result, chimeric and human anti-VEGFR-2 antibodies were developed.[95] Preclinical studies demonstrated that inhibition of VEGFR-2 by these antibodies decreased leukemia cell migration in vitro and significantly improved survival in a mouse model of leukemia, although leukemia was not eradicated in any of the mice.[95]

IMC-1C11, the chimeric monoclonal antibody, has been tested in a phase I dose-escalation clinical trial in patients with colorectal cancer metastatic to the liver.[96] Fourteen patients were treated with IMC-1C11 at doses from 0.2 to 4 mg/kg weekly, administered intravenously over 1 hour. Pharmacokinetic studies revealed a very short half-life at the lower doses, while at the highest dose (4 mg/kg), the half-life was 3 days.[96] The infusion was well tolerated, with no acute reactions. There were no dose-limiting toxicities in this trial. Minor bleeding, including epistaxis, blood-streaked sputum, and hematuria, was seen in 4 of 14 patients. A human antibody to chimera antibody (HACA) developed in 50% of patients, primarily those who received the lower doses. No patients had a response to therapy, although stable disease was noted in 4. In an attempt to identify surrogate markers for response, this study measured vascular perfusion of the liver metastases by DCE-MRI. Perfusion appeared to decrease with therapy, yet there was no significant radiographic tumor response. This method has been shown to correlate with microvessel density and tumor grade in colorectal cancer.[97] It warrants investigation in larger studies and with other antiangiogenic therapies to determine its role in assessing treatment efficacy. In summary, IMC-1C11 was well tolerated, and further studies with it and other human monoclonal antibodies to VEGFR-2 are planned.

MISCELLANEOUS

Thalidomide

Thalidomide has shown promise as an oral antiangiogenic agent. In the early 1990s, in vivo studies reported that thalidomide inhibited angiogenesis induced by basic fibroblast growth factor (bFGF) in a rabbit corneal micropocket assay.[98] Numerous subsequent preclinical studies demonstrated the antiangiogenic properties of thalidomide, although all the mechanisms of its action are not known. Thalidomide has been shown to down-regulate expression of VEGF and bFGF[99] and inhibit endothelial cell proliferation, which is associated with inhibition of

NF-κB activation.[100] The teratogenic effects of thalidomide have been linked to its generation of reactive oxygen species.[101,102] This free-radical oxidative stress may have a role in thalidomide's tumor antiangiogenic activity. In addition to its antiangiogenic properties, thalidomide has an immunomodulatory effect, which may account for some of its antitumor efficacy. Thalidomide decreases the expression of cell surface adhesion molecules.[103] Also, thalidomide inhibits TNF-α, which may account for its anti-inflammatory effect but may not correlate with antitumor activity.[104] Finally, thalidomide's effect on immune regulation may be due to its action as a costimulator of T cells, primarily of the CD8$^+$ subset.[105]

Thalidomide is a synthetic derivative of glutamic acid and is orally bioavailable. It has low solubility in the gastrointestinal tract, which limits its absorption, but higher doses do result in higher plasma concentrations.[106] The drug undergoes hydrolysis into a number of metabolites, which are renally excreted. At a dose of 200 mg, the half-life is approximately 6 to 7 hours.[106,107]

The first successes with thalidomide as an antitumor agent were described in multiple myeloma. In 1999, Singhal et al. reported activity of thalidomide in previously treated patients with multiple myeloma; 90% of these patients had progressed after high-dose chemotherapy followed by autologous stem cell transplantation.[108] A total of 84 patients were treated with thalidomide starting at a dose of 200 mg per day, and it was escalated as tolerated to a maximum dose of 800 mg, which was achieved in 55% of patients. Ten percent of patients had a complete or near complete response, while 32% had at least a 25% drop in paraprotein levels. Therapy was relatively well tolerated, and grade 3 or 4 toxicities were very rare. This response was encouraging given the advanced nature of disease in this cohort of patients. Further studies have demonstrated similar activity with single-agent thalidomide in both previously treated and untreated multiple myeloma. Overall response rates in these studies are reported to be 25 to 35%.[109–111] Adverse effects are dose-related and have included constipation, fatigue, somnolence, depression, tremor, and sensory neuropathy.[108,109,111] With thalidomide alone, less than 5% of patients developed thrombotic events. Response to thalidomide has not correlated with reduction in angiogenic cytokines such as bFGF, VEGF, and TNF-α.[112] On the other hand, there has been some evidence of reduction in bone marrow microvessel density in patients who respond to thalidomide.[108,113] Therefore, the exact mechanism of thalidomide's action is not well understood.

Other agents such as dexamethasone or combination chemotherapy have been studied with thalidomide in both untreated and previously treated patients with multiple myeloma. The response rates with combination therapy are higher than with thalidomide alone; overall response rates from 55 to 72% have been observed.[111,114–116] It is not clear that overall survival is better with combination therapy, but phase III trials are ongoing. The neurologic toxicities appear to decrease with combination therapy, particularly dexamethasone plus thalidomide, but the incidence of thrombotic events increases significantly. Studies have consistently reported that up to 16% of patients develop deep venous thrombosis with dexamethasone plus thalidomide[111,116,117] and up to 28% with multiagent chemotherapy plus thalidomide.[118] Therefore, prophylactic anticoagulation is warranted with these regimens.

Thalidomide has been evaluated in a number of other hematologic disorders, including AML,[119] myelofibrosis with myeloid metaplasia,[120] and MDS.[121–123] In myelofibrosis with myeloid metaplasia (MMM), thalidomide has shown efficacy in a number of phase II studies. The largest study treated 63 patients with thalidomide, at a dose of 50 mg/day escalated to a maximum of 400 mg/day as tolerated.[120] The median maximum tolerated dose was 100 mg/day. Responses were characterized by an improvement in anemia (26%), platelet increase by more than 50×10^9/L (41%), and 50% reduction in splenomegaly (19%).[120] These results warrant further investigation of thalidomide in MMM.

Responses to thalidomide have also been seen in patients with AML or MDS. In 20 AML patients who were refractory to cytotoxic therapy or who were not candidates for cytotoxic therapy, 25% demonstrated a partial response to single-agent thalidomide.[119] In patients who responded, there was a decrease in bone marrow microvessel density. Studies of single-agent thalidomide have also been promising in patients with MDS; 19 to 55% of patients achieved a hematologic improvement and a subset of patients even became red blood cell transfusion–independent.[121–123] In both the AML and MDS studies, patients experienced significant toxicity, which limited the dose that could be administered. The majority of patients could not tolerate doses above 200 mg/day. The adverse effects were similar to those described in the previous studies, including fatigue, constipation, fluid retention, dizziness, and neuropathy. A study of thalidomide and darbepoetin-α in MDS patients was stopped early due to thromboembolic events in three of the first seven patients, including one fatal pulmonary embolism.[124]

Thalidomide's activity in a number of solid tumors has also been investigated. Single-agent thalidomide or combination therapy has demonstrated antitumor activity in glioblastoma multiforme, melanoma, renal cell cancer, and prostate cancer. Patients with glioblastoma multiforme were treated with either thalidomide alone (19 patients) or thalidomide with temozolomide (25 patients) after resection and irradiation.[125] Although this was not a randomized study, overall survival was significantly better in the combination arm, 103 weeks versus 63 weeks. Temozolomide is an oral alkylating agent that is well tolerated. Only 1 patient of 25 had grade 3 myelosuppression. Other toxicities were those commonly reported with thalidomide in particular, sedation and thrombotic events.[125] The combination of thalidomide and temozolomide has also been effective in metastatic melanoma, as demonstrated in two separate phase II studies.[126,127] Danson and colleagues randomized patients with metastatic melanoma to either temozolomide alone (59), temozolomide and interferon α-2b (62), or temozolomide and thalidomide (60); objective responses were observed in 9%, 18%, and 15% of patients, and median survival was 5.3, 7.7, and 7.3 months, respectively. The temozolomide-thalidomide arm was better tolerated due to the low frequency of hematologic adverse events.[127] The treatment doses in this study were 100 mg of thalidomide daily with temozolomide 150 mg/m² daily for 5 days during the first cycle, increased to 200 mg/m² daily for 5 days in each subsequent cycle. Higher doses of thalidomide are also tolerated in this patient population; 200 mg daily of thalidomide was escalated to 400 mg daily, and the temozolomide dose was 75 mg/m² daily for 6 weeks followed by a 2-week rest.[126] The response rate in this single-arm phase II trial was 32%, including a complete response lasting over 25 months. Further studies to determine the optimal dosing and treatment schedule are necessary in this group of patients.

Renal cell carcinoma is another vascular tumor in which thalidomide has been tested. When thalidomide was used as a single agent, responses were modest, with rare partial responses and a small subset of patients with stable disease.[128,129] In these studies, thalidomide was dose escalated from 400 to 1,200 mg daily. Significant toxicity, particularly neurotoxicity, was observed. In addition, venous thromboembolic events, which have been rare in other studies with single-agent thalidomide, occurred in 9 of 40 patients (23%) in the study by Escudier and colleagues.[128] Better results have been seen when thalidomide was combined with interferon-α, but the studies have been small. Among 30 patients treated with interferon-α 1.2 million units three times daily and thalidomide 300 mg once daily, 20% had a partial response, and 63% had stable disease for at least 3 months.[130] The added benefit of thalidomide in this group of patients is not clear, and results from randomized phase III trials are anticipated.

In hormone-refractory prostate cancer, thalidomide at low doses (100 to 200 mg daily) has shown some activity as a single agent, resulting in PSA decline.[131,132] Thalidomide has been successfully combined with docetaxel in this same population. Patients were randomly assigned to receive either docetaxel alone (30 mg/m² weekly for 3 weeks of a 4-week cycle) or docetaxel plus thalidomide (200 mg daily).[133] Overall survival at 18 months was 43% in the docetaxel arm versus 68% in the docetaxel-thalidomide arm ($P = .11$). The therapy was relatively well tolerated; only 8% of patients had grade 3 hematologic toxicity in the combination group. Thromboembolic events were significantly increased in the combination group. Twelve of the first 43 patients in this group developed a venous thrombosis (9) or transient ischemic event/stroke (3). The subsequent 6 patients treated on the combination arm received prophylactic low molecular weight heparin during therapy.

The role of thalidomide in these diseases is promising but needs to be better defined. Ongoing studies continue with thalidomide in a variety of other solid tumors, including small and non–small cell lung cancer, ovarian cancer, sarcoma, and hepatocellular cancer.

IMiDs: CC-5013 (Revlamid) and CC-4047 (Actimid)

A number of thalidomide derivatives have been developed, and these make up at least two new classes of drugs: immunomodulatory drugs (IMiDs) and selective cytokine-inhibitory drugs (SelCIDs). They exhibit effects on immune regulation, cytokine production, angiogenesis, and tumor growth in the preclinical setting that are similar to or more potent than those of thalidomide.[134–138] T-cell stimulation is observed only in the IMiD class. Antiangiogenic activity, which has been seen in both classes *in vivo* and *in vitro*, appears to be distinct from the immunomodulatory effects.[138] Phase I studies of the IMiDs that show better tolerability and potential efficacy (CC-5013 and CC-4047) have been conducted.[139–141]

To date, most clinical experience has been with CC-5013 (Revlamid). Pharmacokinetic studies in patients with multiple myeloma have demonstrated that the drug is absorbed within 2 hours and that the elimination half-life is between 3 and 6 hours.[139,142] The maximum tolerated dose in patients with multiple myeloma is 25 mg daily. Myelosuppression, predominantly neutropenia and thrombocytopenia, is the dose-limiting toxicity. Lethargy, constipation, and neuropathy have not been observed. In 17 of 24 patients (71%), the paraprotein concentration decreased by at least 25%, and the decrease was seen in 11 patients who had previously received thalidomide.[139] Preliminary results in patients with MDS are very promising. A total of 45 patients who were transfusion-dependent or had symptomatic anemia were treated with one of three doses of CC-5013: 25 mg daily, 10 mg daily, or 10 mg daily for 3 weeks followed by a 1-week break.[143] In this study, 88% of patients were in the Low/Intermediate-1 International Prognostic Scoring System (IPSS) group. A major hematologic response was seen in 19 patients. In addition, cytogenetic responses were observed in 11 patients, with 10 patients converting to a normal karyotype. Myelosuppression was the most common and significant adverse event. Phase I studies have also been conducted in patients with malignant melanoma, high-grade gliomas, and other advanced solid tumors.[140,144] CC-5013 is safe and tolerable in this cohort. We await the results of ongoing studies to define the efficacy of CC-5013 and its role in treatment algorithms for multiple myeloma, MDS, and other malignancies.

The experience with CC-4047 (Actimid) is less extensive. In a phase I clinical trial in 24 patients with multiple myeloma, CC-4047 was well tolerated.[141] It is orally bioavailable, with an elimination half-life of about 7 hours. The maximum tolerated dose was determined to be 2 mg per day. Myelosuppression, primarily neutropenia, was the dose-limiting toxicity. In addition, 4 patients developed a deep venous thrombosis while receiving doses of 1, 2, or 5 mg. Four patients achieved a complete response, while 9 had a partial response. The results from this phase I study are encouraging, and further studies are being conducted in multiple myeloma, MDS, prostate cancer, and other solid tumors.

AE-941 (Neovostat)

AE-941 is an antiangiogenic agent that has been purified from shark cartilage. In animal studies, this agent decreased both angiogenesis and metastases.[145] It exerts its effects through a number of mechanisms. In vitro and in vivo animal studies have demonstrated that AE-941 competitively inhibits binding of VEGF to the VEGF receptor-2.[146] In addition, AE-941 inhibits MMP-2, -9, and -12[147] and induces endothelial cell apoptosis.[148] It is an orally bioavailable agent and has been well tolerated in a number of trials that have included over 800 patients total.[149]

A phase I/II dose escalation study was conducted in patients who had advanced non–small cell lung cancer and were refractory to previous therapy. No dose-limiting toxicity was identified in the 80 patients.[150] The most common side effects included nausea (9%), pruritus (5%), anorexia (4%), and emesis (4%). Although there were no tumor responses with therapy, 26% of patients in the highest dose group (240 mL/day) had stable disease, as compared with 14% in the lower dose groups. A phase III trial of induction chemoradiotherapy with or without AE-941 in unresectable non–small cell lung cancer continues to accrue patients.

Results of using this agent in patients with renal cell cancer have shown promise. A phase II trial was reported in patients with advanced renal cell cancer.[151] Initially patients were treated with AE-941 60 mL per day; due to results from other trials, 14 months into the study the dose was increased to 240 mL per day, given in a divided dose. A total of 22 patients were enrolled, and 14 received the higher dose. Median survival was improved in the cohort that received 240 mL per day (16.3 vs. 7.1 months, $P =$ .01)[151] The regimen was well tolerated, and the most common adverse event was altered taste (14% of patients). The only grade 3 event was peripheral edema in one patient. A phase III trial in over 300 renal cell cancer patients has been completed and results are pending.[152]

Angiostatin

A series of experiments performed by O'Reilly and colleagues identified an endogenous inhibitor of tumor growth and angiogenesis, angiostatin.[153] It was found to be a 38-kd fragment composed of the first four kringle domains of plasminogen. The antiangiogenic effect was unique to angiostatin and was not demonstrated by treatment with intact plasminogen.[153] The mechanism of action of angiostatin is not well understood, but three endothelial cell surface receptors have been identified. These include ATP synthase, angiomotin, and integrin $\alpha_v\beta_3$.[154] Angiostatin binding likely results in apoptosis. In preclinical investigations, recombinant angiostatin administered to mice inhibited the growth of both primary tumors and metastases.[155,156]

Recombinant human angiostatin (rhAngiostatin) has been developed and is in early clinical trials. The first reported trial included 15 patients with a variety of advanced malignancies.[157] rhAngiostatin was administered daily as an intravenous infusion, at doses from 15 to 120 mg/m^2, with no dose-limiting toxicities observed. VEGF and bFGF levels decreased in some of the treated patients.[157] A subsequent study treated 24 patients with twice daily subcutaneous injections of rhAngiostatin, at doses of either 7.5, 15, or 30 mg/m^2 per day.[158] The therapy was well tolerated, and the most commonly observed toxicity was grade 1 or 2 erythema at the injection site (54% of patients). Other significant toxicities included 2 patients with hemorrhage into brain metastases and 2 patients who developed a deep venous thromboembolism. Twenty-five percent of patients had stable disease for over 6 months. In this study, treatment did not decrease serum or urine bFGF or VEGF levels. A phase II trial of combination chemotherapy plus rhAngiostatin is currently underway in patients with advanced non–small cell lung cancer.[159] Patients with stage IIIB or IV disease who had never previously received chemotherapy participated. Treatment included paclitaxel 175 mg/m^2 and carbolplatin AUC 5 on day 1, with administration of rhAngiostatin at either 15 or 60 mg subcutaneously twice daily for a maximum of six cycles. If patients responded or had stable disease on this therapy, they continued to receive maintenance rhAngiostatin until progression. Patients received rhAngiostatin for a median of 125 days. The most commonly observed adverse effect was a skin rash (grade 1 to 3) in 92% of patients. Grade 3 or 4 toxicities included: neutropenia (42%), fatigue (42%), and dyspnea (25%). There were no complete responses, but 39% of the patients (9) had a partial response, and stable disease occurred in 39%.[159] This study demonstrated the feasibility of rhAngiostatin administration with combination chemotherapy. Further studies will be necessary to determine whether these results are better than those attainable with chemotherapy alone.

Endostatin

Endostatin is an endogenous inhibitor of angiogenesis and tumor growth first discovered by O'Reilly and colleagues.[160] It is a 20-kd fragment of collagen XVIII. In mouse models, endostatin administered subcutaneously resulted in tumor regression.[161] Recombinant human endo-statin (rh-Endostatin) has been produced in yeast and has been tested in phase I clinical trials. In three clinical trials, rh-Endostatin was administered to 61 patients as a daily intravenous infusion over either 20 or 60 minutes.[162-164] Doses were escalated from 15 to 600 mg/m^2 daily and were all well tolerated. Doses over 300 mg/m^2 daily resulted in an AUC that was therapeutic in preclinical studies.[162,164] Grade 3 toxicities were rare; they included anemia, deep venous thrombosis, and dyspnea each in only one patient.[162] No significant clinical tumor responses were observed in these studies. There was no consistent reduction of VEGF or bFGF levels in patients treated with endostatin.[162,164] In addition, tumor blood flow analysis by PET scan and biopsies to assess tumor and endothelial cell apoptosis were performed in patients treated with endostatin.[165] Further studies will be required to demonstrate whether these measures correlate to tumor response. Based on preclinical mouse tumor mod-els suggesting that efficacy is improved with continuous infusion,[166] new clinical trials were designed to administer endostatin continuously. Preliminary results are also available from a phase II study of 41 patients with advanced neuroendocrine tumors. Rh-Endostatin, was administered as a subcutaneous injection at a dose of 30 mg/m^2 twice a day.[167] Only 5% of patients had a minor radiographic response, and 62% had stable disease. Results in the clinical trials have been disappointing, as they did not reflect the promising results observed in preclinical models.

CONCLUSION

A number of agents with antiangiogenic activity show promise in the treatment of a wide variety of malignancies. One of the challenges facing clinical researchers interested in an agent that may inhibit angiogenesis is determining the optimal way to assess the clinical efficacy of the agent.[168] The traditional approach for evaluating a new cytotoxic agent is to perform a phase I dose-escalation trial that identifies the maximal tolerated dose (MTD) of drug. With conventional cytotoxic agents, the MTD frequently correlates with maximal antitumor activity. With agents that inhibit angiogenesis, however, tumor regression may or may not be observed. As a result, the MTD may not accurately reflect the optimal biologic effect of the drug. Although identifying both acute and long-term toxicities associated with any new agent is important, an angiogene-sis inhibitor may have a defined optimal biologic dose that is very different from the MTD.

Identifying plasma concentrations of the angiogenesis inhibitor in animals that are optimal for the desired bio-logic effect is important. Because angiogenesis inhibitors may not cause tumor shrinkage when administered alone, the clinical development of an agent may be abandoned if surrogate endpoints that reflect the activity of the agent are not incorporated into the trial design. Potential biologic

markers for antiangiogenic activity have included measure-ment of serum markers of angiogenesis (VEGF, bFGF, VCAM-1 [vascular cell adhesion molecule], E-selectin) or circulating endothelial cells, assessment of endothelial cell and tumor cell apoptosis on biopsy, PET scan assessment of tumor blood flow, and DCE-MRI contrast enhancement as a reflection of microvessel density. Whether these effects of a new agent legitimately reflect the antiangiogenic or antitumor activity remains unclear. Yet these or other sur-rogate markers will likely be important in assessing the activity of angiogenesis inhibitors in early clinical trials.

REFERENCES

1. Folkman J. Tumor angiogenesis: therapeutic implications. N Engl J Med 1971;285:1182–1186.
2. Folkman J. Angiogenesis in cancer, vascular, rheumatoid and other disease. Nat Med 1995;1:27–31.
3. Hanahan D, Weinberg RA. The hallmarks of cancer. Cell 2000;100:57–70.
4. Folkman J, Shing Y. Angiogenesis. J Biol Chem 1992;267:10931–10934.
5. Hanahan D, Folkman J. Patterns and emerging mechanisms of the angiogenic switch during tumorigenesis. Cell 1996;86:353–364.
6. Bergers G, Benjamin LE. Tumorigenesis and the angiogenic switch. Nat Rev Cancer 2003;3:401–410.
7. Scappaticci FA. Mechanisms and future directions for angiogene-sis-based cancer therapies. J Clin Oncol 2002;20:3906–3927.
8. Rak J, Kerbel RS. Prospects and progress in the development of anti-angiogenic agents. In: Updates Rosenberg SA, ed. Principles and Practice of Biologic Therapy of Cancer. 3rd ed. Philadelphia: Lippincott Williams & Wilkins, 2002, updates, volume 3(2): 2002 p1–16.
9. Hidalgo M, Eckhardt SG. Development of matrix metallopro-teinase inhibitors in cancer therapy. J Natl Cancer Inst 2001;93:178–193.
10. Stetler-Stevenson WG. Matrix metalloproteinases in angiogene-sis: a moving target for therapeutic intervention. J Clin Invest 1999;103:1237–1241.
11. Werb Z. ECM and cell surface proteolysis: regulating cellular ecology. Cell 1997;91:439–442.
12. Zucker S, Hymowitz M, Conner C, et al. Measurement of matrix metalloproteinases and tissue inhibitors of metalloproteinases in blood and tissues: clinical and experimental applications. Ann NY Acad Sci 1999;878:212–227.
13. Sutinen M, Kainulainen T, Hurskainen T, et al. Expression of matrix metalloproteinases (MMP-1 and -2) and their inhibitors (TIMP-1, -2 and -3) in oral lichen planus, dysplasia, squamous cell carcinoma and lymph node metastasis. Br J Cancer 1998;77:2239–2245.
14. Liotta LA, Tryggvason K, Garbisa S, et al. Metastatic potential cor-relates with enzymatic degradation of basement membrane col-lagen. Nature 1980;284:67–68.
15. Mignatti P, Rifkin DB. Biology and biochemistry of proteinases in tumor invasion. Physiol Rev 1993;73:161–195.
16. Stetler-Stevenson WG, Hewitt R, Corcoran M. Matrix metallopro-teinases and tumor invasion: from correlation and causality to the clinic. Semin Cancer Biol 1996;7:147–154.
17. Brenner CA, Adler RR, Rappolee DA, et al. Genes for extracellu-lar-matrix-degrading metalloproteinases and their inhibitor, TIMP, are expressed during early mammalian development. Genes Dev 1989;3:848–859.
18. Wolf C, Chenard MP, Durand de Grossouvre P, et al. Breast-cancer-associated stromelysin-3 gene is expressed in basal cell carcinoma and during cutaneous wound healing. J Invest Dermatol 1992;99:870–872.
19. Wojtowicz-Praga SM, Dickson RB, Hawkins MJ. Matrix metallo-proteinase inhibitors. Invest New Drugs 1997;15:61–75.

20. Millar AW, Brown PD, Moore J, et al. Results of single and repeat dose studies of the oral matrix metalloproteinase inhibitor marimastat in healthy male volunteers. Br J Clin Pharmacol 1998; 45:21–26.

21. Wojtowicz-Praga S, Torri J, Johnson M, et al. Phase I trial of marimastat, a novel matrix metalloproteinase inhibitor, administered orally to patients with advanced lung cancer. J Clin Oncol 1998;16:2150–2156.

22. Tierney GM, Griffin NR, Stuart RC, et al. A pilot study of the safety and effects of the matrix metalloproteinase inhibitor marimastat in gastric cancer. Eur J Cancer 1999;35:563–568.

23. Bramhall SR, Rosemurgy A, Brown PD, et al. Marimastat as first-line therapy for patients with unresectable pancreatic cancer: a randomized trial. J Clin Oncol 2001;19:3447–3455.

24. Shepherd FA, Giaccone G, Seymour L, et al. Prospective, randomized, double-blind, placebo-controlled trial of marimastat after response to first-line chemotherapy in patients with small-cell lung cancer: a trial of the National Cancer Institute of Canada Clinical Trials Group and the European Organization for Research and Treatment of Cancer. J Clin Oncol 2002;20: 4434–4439.

25. Bramhall SR, Hallissey MT, Whiting J, et al. Marimastat as maintenance therapy for patients with advanced gastric cancer: a randomised trial. Br J Cancer 2002;86:1864–1870.

26. Sparano JA, Bernardo P, Gradishar WJ, et al. Randomized phase III trial of marimastat versus placebo in patients with metastatic breast cancer who have responding or stable disease after first-line chemotherapy: an Eastern Cooperative Oncology Group trial (E2196) [abstract]. Proc Annu Meet Am Soc Clin Oncol 2002;21:173.

27. Sparano JA, Gray R, Giantonio B, et al. Evaluating antiangiogenesis agents in the clinic: the Eastern Cooperative Oncology Group Portfolio of Clinical Trials. Clin Cancer Res 2004;10:1206–1211.

28. Jones PH, Christodoulos K, Dobbs N, et al. Combination antiangiogenesis therapy with marimastat, captopril and Fragmin in patients with advanced cancer. Br J Cancer 2004;91:30–36.

29. Miller KD, Gradishar W, Schuchter L, et al. A randomized phase II pilot trial of adjuvant marimastat in patients with early-stage breast cancer. Ann Oncol 2002;13:1220–1224.

30. Moore MJ, Hamm J, Dancey J, et al. Comparison of gemcitabine versus the matrix metalloproteinase inhibitor BAY 12-9566 in patients with advanced or metastatic adenocarcinoma of the pancreas: a phase III trial of the National Cancer Institute of Canada Clinical Trials Group. J Clin Oncol 2003;21:3296–3302.

31. Behrendt CE, Ruiz RB. Venous thromboembolism among patients with advanced lung cancer randomized to prinomastat or placebo, plus chemotherapy. Thromb Haemost 2003;90:734–737.

32. Naglich JG, Jure-Kunkel M, Gupta E, et al. Inhibition of angiogenesis and metastasis in two murine models by the matrix metalloproteinase inhibitor, BMS-275291. Cancer Res 2001;61: 8480–8485.

33. Rizvi NA, Humphrey JS, Ness EA, et al. A phase I study of oral BMS-275291, a novel nonhydroxamate sheddase-sparing matrix metalloproteinase inhibitor, in patients with advanced or metastatic cancer. Clin Cancer Res 2004;10:1963–1970.

34. Miller KD, Saphner TJ, Waterhouse DM, et al. A randomized phase II feasibility trial of BMS-275291 in patients with early stage breast cancer. Clin Cancer Res 2004;10:1971–1975.

35. Ingber D, Fujita T, Kishimoto S, et al. Synthetic analogues of fumagillin that inhibit angiogenesis and suppress tumour growth. Nature 1990;348:555–557.

36. Sin N, Meng L, Wang MQ, Wen JJ, et al. The anti-angiogenic agent fumagillin covalently binds and inhibits the methionine aminopeptidase, MetAP-2. Proc Natl Acad Sci USA 1997;94: 6099–6103.

37. Tudan C, Jackson JK, Pelech SL, et al. Selective inhibition of protein kinase C, mitogen-activated protein kinase, and neutrophil activation in response to calcium pyrophosphate dihydrate crystals, formyl-methionyl-leucyl-phenylalanine, and phorbol ester by O-(chloroacetyl-carbamoyl) fumagillol (AGM-1470; TNP-470). Biochem Pharmacol 1999;58:1869–1880.

38. Sedlakova O, Sedlak J, Hunakova L, et al. Angiogenesis inhibitor TNP-470: cytotoxic effects on human neoplastic cell lines. Neoplasma 1999;46:283–289.

39. Kudelka AP, Levy T, Verschraegen CF, et al. A phase I study of TNP-470 administered to patients with advanced squamous cell cancer of the cervix. Clin Cancer Res 1997;3:1501–1505.

40. Bhargava P, Marshall JL, Rizvi N, et al. A phase I and pharmacokinetic study of TNP-470 administered weekly to patients with advanced cancer. Clin Cancer Res 1999;5:1989–1995.

41. Moore JD, Dezube BJ, Gill P, et al. Phase I dose escalation pharmacokinetics of O-(chloroacetylcarbamoyl) fumagillol (TNP-470) and its metabolites in AIDS patients with Kaposi's sarcoma. Cancer Chemother Pharmacol 2000;46:173–179.

42. Stadler WM, Kuzel T, Shapiro C, et al. Multi-institutional study of the angiogenesis inhibitor TNP-470 in metastatic renal carcinoma. J Clin Oncol 1999;17:2541–2545.

43. Herbst RS, Madden TL, Tran HT, et al. Safety and pharmacokinetic effects of TNP-470, an angiogenesis inhibitor, combined with paclitaxel in patients with solid tumors: evidence for activity in non-small-cell lung cancer. J Clin Oncol 2002;20: 4440–4447.

44. Tran HT, Blumenschein GR Jr, Lu C, et al. Clinical and pharmacokinetic study of TNP-470, an angiogenesis inhibitor, in combination with paclitaxel and carboplatin in patients with solid tumors. Cancer Chemother Pharmacol 2004;54:308–314.

45. Inoue K, Chikazawa M, Fukata S, et al. Frequent administration of angiogenesis inhibitor TNP-470 (AGM-1470) at an optimal biological dose inhibits tumor growth and metastasis of metastatic human transitional cell carcinoma in the urinary bladder. Clin Cancer Res 2002;8:2389–2398.

46. Blumenschein GR, Fossella FV, Pisters KM, et al. A phase I study of TNP-470 continuous infusion alone or in combination with paclitaxel and carboplatin in adult patients with NSCLC and other solid tumors [abstract]. Proc Annu Meet Am Soc Clin Oncol 2002;21:1254.

47. Dechantsreiter MA, Planker E, Matha B, et al. N-methylated cyclic RGD peptides as highly active and selective alpha(V)beta(3) integrin antagonists. J Med Chem 1999;42:3033–3040.

48. Ruoslahti E, Reed JC. Anchorage dependence, integrins, and apoptosis. Cell 1994;77:477–478.

49. Gasparini G, Brooks PC, Biganzoli E, et al. Vascular integrin alpha(v)beta3: a new prognostic indicator in breast cancer. Clin Cancer Res 1998;4:2625–2634.

50. Eskens FA, Dumez H, Hoekstra R, et al. Phase I and pharmacokinetic study of continuous twice weekly intravenous administration of Cilengitide (EMD 121974), a novel inhibitor of the integrins alphavbeta3 and alphavbeta5 in patients with advanced solid tumours. Eur J Cancer 2003;39:917–926.

51. Ferrara N, Gerber HP, LeCouter J. The biology of VEGF and its receptors. Nat Med 2003;9:669–676.

52. Neufeld G, Cohen T, Gengrinovitch S, et al. Vascular endothelial growth factor (VEGF) and its receptors. FASEB J 1999;13:9–22.

53. Ferrara N. Role of vascular endothelial growth factor in physiologic and pathologic angiogenesis: therapeutic implications. Semin Oncol 2002;29(6 Suppl 16):10–14.

54. Kubo H, Fujiwara T, Jussila L, et al. Involvement of vascular endothelial growth factor receptor-3 in maintenance of integrity of endothelial cell lining during tumor angiogenesis. Blood 2000;96:546–553.

55. Ferrara N. Vascular endothelial growth factor as a target for anticancer therapy. Oncologist 2004;9(Suppl 1):2–10.

56. Padro T, Bieker R, Ruiz S, et al. Overexpression of vascular endothelial growth factor (VEGF) and its cellular receptor KDR (VEGFR-2) in the bone marrow of patients with acute myeloid leukemia. Leukemia 2002;16:1302–1310.

57. Skobe M, Brown LF, Tognazzi K, et al. Vascular endothelial growth factor-C (VEGF-C) and its receptors KDR and flt-4 are expressed in AIDS-associated Kaposi's sarcoma. J Invest Dermatol 1999;113:1047–1053.

58. Yoshiji H, Gomez DE, Shibuya M, et al. Expression of vascular endothelial growth factor, its receptor, and other angiogenic factors in human breast cancer. Cancer Res 1996;56:2013–2016.

59. Guidi AJ, Abu-Jawdeh G, Tognazzi K, et al. Expression of vascular permeability factor (vascular endothelial growth factor) and its receptors in endometrial carcinoma. Cancer 1996;78:454–460.

60. Tanigawa N, Amaya H, Matsumura M, et al. Correlation between expression of vascular endothelial growth factor and tumor

vascularity, and patient outcome in human gastric carcinoma. J Clin Oncol 1997;15:826–832.

61. Harada Y, Ogata Y, Shirouzu K. Expression of vascular endothelial growth factor and its receptor KDR (kinase domain-containing receptor)/Flk-1 (fetal liver kinase-1) as prognostic factors in human colorectal cancer. Int J Clin Oncol 2001;6:221–228.

62. Fine BA, Valente PT, Feinstein GI, et al. VEGF, flt-1, and KDR/flk-1 as prognostic indicators in endometrial carcinoma. Gynecol Oncol 2000;76:33–39.

63. Kim KJ, Li B, Winer J, et al. Inhibition of vascular endothelial growth factor-induced angiogenesis suppresses tumour growth in vivo. Nature 1993;362:841–844.

64. Millauer B, Longhi MP, Plate KH, et al. Dominant-negative inhibition of Flk-1 suppresses the growth of many tumor types in vivo. Cancer Res 1996;56:1615–1620.

65. Skobe M, Rockwell P, Goldstein N, et al. Halting angiogenesis suppresses carcinoma cell invasion. Nat Med 1997;3:1222–1227.

66. Prewett M, Huber J, Li Y, et al. Antivascular endothelial growth factor receptor (fetal liver kinase 1) monoclonal antibody inhibits tumor angiogenesis and growth of several mouse and human tumors. Cancer Res 1999;59:5209–5218.

67. Gordon MS, Margolin K, Talpaz M, et al. Phase I safety and pharmacokinetic study of recombinant human anti-vascular endothelial growth factor in patients with advanced cancer. J Clin Oncol 2001;19:843–850.

68. Kabbinavar F, Hurwitz HI, Fehrenbacher L, et al. Phase II, randomized trial comparing bevacizumab plus fluorouracil (FU)/leucovorin (LV) with FU/LV alone in patients with metastatic colorectal cancer. J Clin Oncol 2003;21:60–65.

69. Yang JC, Haworth L, Sherry RM, et al. A randomized trial of bevacizumab, an anti-vascular endothelial growth factor antibody, for metastatic renal cancer. N Engl J Med 2003;349:427–434.

70. Johnson DH, Fehrenbacher L, Novotny WF, et al. Randomized phase II trial comparing bevacizumab plus carboplatin and paclitaxel with carboplatin and paclitaxel alone in previously untreated locally advanced or metastatic non-small-cell lung cancer. J Clin Oncol 2004;22:2184–2191.

71. Elaraj DM, White DE, Steinberg SM, et al. A pilot study of antiangiogenic therapy with bevacizumab and thalidomide in patients with metastatic renal cell carcinoma. J Immunother 2004;27:259–264.

72. Hainsworth JD, Sosman JA, Spigel DR, et al. Phase II trial of bevacizumab and erlotinib in patients with metastatic renal carcinoma [abstract]. Proc Annu Meet Am Soc Clin Oncol 2004;23:4502.

73. Rini BI, Halabi S, Taylor J, et al. Cancer and Leukemia Group B 90206: a randomized phase III trial of interferon-alpha or interferon-alpha plus anti-vascular endothelial growth factor antibody (bevacizumab) in metastatic renal cell carcinoma. Clin Cancer Res 2004;10:2584–2586.

74. Hurwitz H, Fehrenbacher L, Novotny W, et al. Bevacizumab plus irinotecan, fluorouracil, and leucovorin for metastatic colorectal cancer. N Engl J Med 2004;350:2335–2342.

75. Kilickap S, Abali H, Celik I. Bevacizumab, bleeding, thrombosis, and warfarin. J Clin Oncol 2003;21:3542; author reply 3543.

76. Hambleton J, Novotny WF, Hurwitz H, et al. Bevacizumab does not increase bleeding in patients with metastatic colorectal cancer receiving concurrent anticoagulation [abstract]. Proc Annu Meet Am Soc Clin Oncol 2004;23:3528.

77. Miller KD, Rugo HS, Cobleigh MA, et al. Phase III trial of capecitabine (Xeloda) plus bevacizumab (Avastin) versus capecitabine alone in women with metastatic breast cancer previously treated with an anthracycline and a taxane [abstract]. Breast Cancer Res Treat 2002;76:36.

78. Holash J, Davis S, Papadopoulos N, et al. VEGF-Trap: a VEGF blocker with potent antitumor effects. Proc Natl Acad Sci USA 2002;99:11393–11398.

79. Kim ES, Serur A, Huang J, et al. Potent VEGF blockade causes regression of coopted vessels in a model of neuroblastoma. Proc Natl Acad Sci USA 2002;99:11399–11404.

80. Dupont J. Phase I and pharmacokinetic study of VEGF Trap administered subcutaneously (sc) to patients with advanced solid malignancies. Proc Annu Meet Am Soc Clin Oncol 2004. Available at: www.asco.org/ac/1,1003,_12-002511-00_18-0026-00_19-009645,00.asp.

81. Dupont J, Schwartz L, Koutcher J, et al. Phase I and pharmacokinetic study of VEGF Trap administered subcutaneously (sc) to patients with advanced solid malignancies [abstract]. Proc Annu Meet Am Soc Clin Oncol 2004;23:3009.

82. Wood JM, Bold G, Buchdunger E, et al. PTK787/ZK 222584, a novel and potent inhibitor of vascular endothelial growth factor receptor tyrosine kinases, impairs vascular endothelial growth factor-induced responses and tumor growth after oral administration. Cancer Res 2000;60:2178–2189.

83. Drevs J, Hofmann I, Hugenschmidt H, et al. Effects of PTK787/ZK 222584, a specific inhibitor of vascular endothelial growth factor receptor tyrosine kinases, on primary tumor, metastasis, vessel density, and blood flow in a murine renal cell carcinoma model. Cancer Res 2000;60:4819–4824.

84. Goldbrunner RH, Bendszus M, Wood J, et al. PTK787/ZK222584, an inhibitor of vascular endothelial growth factor receptor tyrosine kinases, decreases glioma growth and vascularization. Neurosurgery 2004;55:426–432; discussion 432.

85. Yung WKA, Friedman H, Jackson E, et al. A phase I trial of PTK787/ZK 222584 (PTK/ZK), a novel oral VEGFF TK inhibitor in recurrent glioblastoma [abstract]. Proc Annu Meet Am Soc Clin Oncol 2002;21:315.

86. Drevs J, Schmidt-Gersbach CI, Mross K, et al. Surrogate markers for the assessment of biological activity of the VEGF-receptor inhibitor PTK787/ZK 222584 (PTK/ZK) in two clinical phase I trials [abstract]. Proc Annu Meet Am Soc Clin Oncol 2002;21:337.

87. Morgan B, Thomas AL, Drevs J, et al. Dynamic contrast-enhanced magnetic resonance imaging as a biomarker for the pharmacological response of PTK787/ZK 222584, an inhibitor of the vascular endothelial growth factor receptor tyrosine kinases, in patients with advanced colorectal cancer and liver metastases: results from two phase I studies. J Clin Oncol 2003;21:3955–3964.

88. Steward WP, Thomas A, Morgan B, et al. Expanded phase I/II study of PTK787/ZK 222584 (PTK/ZK), a novel, oral angiogenesis inhibitor, in combination with FOLFOX-4 as first-line treatment for patients with metastatic colorectal cancer [abstract]. Proc Annu Meet Am Soc Clin Oncol 2004;23:3556.

89. Wedge SR, Ogilvie DJ, Dukes M, et al. ZD6474 inhibits vascular endothelial growth factor signaling, angiogenesis, and tumor growth following oral administration. Cancer Res 2002;62:4645–4655.

90. Hurwitz H, Holden SN, Eckhardt SG, et al. Clinical evaluation of ZD6474, an orally active inhibitor of VEGF signaling, in patients with solid tumors [abstract]. Proc Annu Meet Am Soc Clin Oncol 2002;21:325.

91. Smith RP, Kennedy S, Robertson J, et al. The effect of food on the intra-subject variability of the pharmacokinetics of ZD6474, a novel antiangiogenic agent, in healthy subjects [abstract]. J Clin Oncol, Proc Annu Meet Am Soc Clin Oncol 2004;23:3167(abst).

92. Minami H, Ebi H, Tahara M, et al. A phase I study of an oral VEGF receptor tyrosine kinase inhibitor ZD6474, in Japanese patients with solid tumors [abstract]. J Clin Oncol, Proc Annu Meet Am Soc Clin Oncol 2003;22:778(abst).

93. Heymach JV, Dong R-P, Dimery I, et al. ZD6474, a novel antiangiogenic agent, in combination with docetaxel in patients with NSCLC: Results of the run-in phase of a two-part, randomized phase II study [abstract]. Proc Annu Meet Am Soc Clin Oncol 2004;23:3051.

94. Wang ES, Teruya-Feldstein J, Wu Y, et al. Targeting autocrine and paracrine VEGF receptor pathways inhibits human lymphoma xenografts in vivo. Blood 2004;epub.

95. Zhu Z, Hattori K, Zhang H, et al. Inhibition of human leukemia in an animal model with human antibodies directed against vascular endothelial growth factor receptor 2: correlation between antibody affinity and biological activity. Leukemia 2003;17:604–611.

96. Posey JA, Ng TC, Yang B, et al. A phase I study of anti-kinase insert domain-containing receptor antibody, IMC-1C11, in patients with liver metastases from colorectal carcinoma. Clin Cancer Res 2003;9:1323–1332.

97. Tuncbilek N, Karakas HM, Altaner S. Dynamic MRI in indirect estimation of microvessel density, histologic grade, and prognosis in colorectal adenocarcinomas. Abdom Imaging 2004;29: 166–172.

98. D'Amato RJ, Loughnan MS, Flynn E, et al. Thalidomide is an inhibitor of angiogenesis. Proc Natl Acad Sci USA 1994;91: 4082–4085.

99. Li X, Liu X, Wang J, et al. Thalidomide down-regulates the expression of VEGF and bFGF in cisplatin-resistant human lung carcinoma cells. Anticancer Res 2003;23(3B):2481–2487.

100. Moreira AL, Friedlander DR, Shif B, et al. Thalidomide and a thalidomide analogue inhibit endothelial cell proliferation in vitro. J Neurooncol 1999;43:109–14.

101. Parman T, Wiley MJ, Wells PG. Free radical-mediated oxidative DNA damage in the mechanism of thalidomide teratogenicity. Nat Med 1999;5:582–585.

102. Sauer H, Gunther J, Hescheler J, et al. Thalidomide inhibits angiogenesis in embryoid bodies by the generation of hydroxyl radicals. Am J Pathol 2000;156:151–158.

103. Geitz H, Handt S, Zwingenberger K. Thalidomide selectively modulates the density of cell surface molecules involved in the adhesion cascade. Immunopharmacology 1996;31(2-3):213–221.

104. D'Amato RJ, Lentzsch S, Anderson KC, et al. Mechanism of action of thalidomide and 3-aminothalidomide in multiple myeloma. Semin Oncol 2001;28:597–601.

105. Haslett PA, Corral LG, Albert M, et al. Thalidomide costimulates primary human T lymphocytes, preferentially inducing proliferation, cytokine production, and cytotoxic responses in the CD8+ subset. J Exp Med 1998;187:1885–1892.

106. Teo SK, Colburn WA, Tracewell WG, et al. Clinical pharmacokinetics of thalidomide. Clin Pharmacokinet 2004;43:311–327.

107. Figg WD, Raje S, Bauer KS, et al. Pharmacokinetics of thalidomide in an elderly prostate cancer population. J Pharm Sci 1999;88:121–125.

108. Singhal S, Mehta J, Desikan R, et al. Antitumor activity of thalidomide in refractory multiple myeloma. N Engl J Med 1999;341:1565–1571.

109. Barlogie B, Desikan R, Eddlemon P, et al. Extended survival in advanced and refractory multiple myeloma after single-agent thalidomide: identification of prognostic factors in a phase 2 study of 169 patients. Blood 2001;98:492–494.

110. Rajkumar SV, Gertz MA, Lacy MQ, et al. Thalidomide as initial therapy for early-stage myeloma. Leukemia 2003;17:775–779.

111. Weber D, Rankin K, Gavino M, et al. Thalidomide alone or with dexamethasone for previously untreated multiple myeloma. J Clin Oncol 2003;21:16–19.

112. Neben K, Moehler T, Kraemer A, et al. Response to thalidomide in progressive multiple myeloma is not mediated by inhibition of angiogenic cytokine secretion. Br J Haematol 2001;115: 605–608.

113. Kumar S, Witzig TE, Dispenzieri A, et al. Effect of thalidomide therapy on bone marrow angiogenesis in multiple myeloma. Leukemia 2004;18:624–627.

114. Dimopoulos MA, Zervas K, Kouvatseas G, et al. Thalidomide and dexamethasone combination for refractory multiple myeloma. Ann Oncol 2001;12:991–995.

115. Kropff MH, Lang N, Bisping G, et al. Hyperfractionated cyclophosphamide in combination with pulsed dexamethasone and thalidomide (HyperCDT) in primary refractory or relapsed multiple myeloma. Br J Haematol 2003;122:607–616.

116. Rajkumar SV, Hayman S, Gertz MA, et al. Combination therapy with thalidomide plus dexamethasone for newly diagnosed myeloma. J Clin Oncol 2002;20:4319–4323.

117. Rajkumar SV, Blood E, Vesole DH, et al. A randomized phase III trial of thalidomide plus dexamethasone versus dexamethasone in newly diagnosed multiple myeloma (E1A00): a trial coordinated by the Easter Cooperative Oncology Group [abstract]. Proc Annu Meet Am Soc Clin Oncol 2004;23:6508.

118. Zangari M, Anaissie E, Barlogie B, et al. Increased risk of deep-vein thrombosis in patients with multiple myeloma receiving thalidomide and chemotherapy. Blood 2001;98:1614–1615.

119. Steins MB, Padro T, Bieker R, et al. Efficacy and safety of thalidomide in patients with acute myeloid leukemia. Blood 2002;99: 834–839.

120. Marchetti M, Barosi G, Balestri F, et al. Low-dose thalidomide ameliorates cytopenias and splenomegaly in myelofibrosis with myeloid metaplasia: a phase II trial. J Clin Oncol 2004;22: 424–431.

121. Raza A, Meyer P, Dutt D, et al. Thalidomide produces transfusion independence in long-standing refractory anemias of patients with myelodysplastic syndromes. Blood 2001;98:958–965.

122. Zorat F, Shetty V, Dutt D, et al. The clinical and biological effects of thalidomide in patients with myelodysplastic syndromes. Br J Haematol 2001;115:881–894.

123. Strupp C, Germing U, Aivado M, et al. Thalidomide for the treatment of patients with myelodysplastic syndromes. Leukemia 2002;16:1–6.

124. Steurer M, Sudmeier I, Stauder R, et al. Thromboembolic events in patients with myelodysplastic syndrome receiving thalidomide in combination with darbepoietin-alpha. Br J Haematol 2003;121:101–103.

125. Baumann F, Bjeljac M, Kollias SS, et al. Combined thalidomide and temozolomide treatment in patients with glioblastoma multiforme. J Neurooncol 2004;67:191–200.

126. Hwu WJ, Krown SE, Menell JH, et al. Phase II study of temozolomide plus thalidomide for the treatment of metastatic melanoma. J Clin Oncol 2003;21:3351–3356.

127. Danson S, Lorigan P, Arance A, et al. Randomized phase II study of temozolomide given every 8 hours or daily with either interferon alfa-2b or thalidomide in metastatic malignant melanoma. J Clin Oncol 2003;21:2551–2557.

128. Escudier B, Lassau N, Couanet D, et al. Phase II trial of thalidomide in renal-cell carcinoma. Ann Oncol 2002;13:1029–1035.

129. Minor DR, Monroe D, Damico LA, et al. A phase II study of thalidomide in advanced metastatic renal cell carcinoma. Invest New Drugs 2002;20:389–393.

130. Hernberg M, Virkkunen P, Bono P, et al. Interferon alfa-2b three times daily and thalidomide in the treatment of metastatic renal cell carcinoma. J Clin Oncol 2003;21:3770–3776.

131. Drake MJ, Robson W, Mehta J, et al. An open-label phase II study of low-dose thalidomide in androgen-independent prostate cancer. Br J Cancer 2003;88:822–827.

132. Figg WD, Dahut W, Duray P, et al. A randomized phase II trial of thalidomide, an angiogenesis inhibitor, in patients with androgen-independent prostate cancer. Clin Cancer Res 2001;7: 1888–1893.

133. Dahut WL, Gulley JL, Arlen PM, et al. Randomized phase II trial of docetaxel plus thalidomide in androgen-independent prostate cancer. J Clin Oncol 2004;22:2532–2539.

134. Lentzsch S, LeBlanc R, Podar K, et al. Immunomodulatory analogs of thalidomide inhibit growth of Hs Sultan cells and angiogenesis in vivo. Leukemia 2003;17:41–44.

135. Hideshima T, Chauhan D, Shima Y, et al. Thalidomide and its analogs overcome drug resistance of human multiple myeloma cells to conventional therapy. Blood 2000;96:2943–2950.

136. Davies FE, Raje N, Hideshima T, et al. Thalidomide and immunomodulatory derivatives augment natural killer cell cytotoxicity in multiple myeloma. Blood 2001;98:210–216.

137. Mitsiades N, Mitsiades CS, Poulaki V, et al. Apoptotic signaling induced by immunomodulatory thalidomide analogs in human multiple myeloma cells: therapeutic implications. Blood 2002; 99:4525–4530.

138. Dredge K, Marriott JB, Macdonald CD, et al. Novel thalidomide analogues display anti-angiogenic activity independently of immunomodulatory effects. Br J Cancer 2002;87:1166–1172.

139. Richardson PG, Schlossman RL, Weller E, et al. Immunomodulatory drug CC-5013 overcomes drug resistance and is well tolerated in patients with relapsed multiple myeloma. Blood 2002;100:3063–3067.

140. Bartlett JB, Michael A, Clarke IA, et al. Phase I study to determine the safety, tolerability and immunostimulatory activity of thalidomide analogue CC-5013 in patients with metastatic malignant melanoma and other advanced cancers. Br J Cancer 2004;90:955–961.

141. Schey SA, Fields P, Bartlett JB, et al. Phase I study of an immunomodulatory thalidomide analog, CC-4047, in relapsed or refractory multiple myeloma. J Clin Oncol 2004;22: 3269–3276.

142. Wu A, Scheffler MR. Multiple-dose pharmacokinetics and safety of CC-5013 in 15 multiple myeloma patients [abstract]. Proc Annu Meet Am Soc Clin Oncol. 2004;23:2056.

143. List AF, Kurtin S, Glinsmann-Gibson B, et al. Efficacy and safety of CC5013 for treatment of anemia in patients with myelodysplastic syndromes [abstract]. Blood 2003;102:184 (abst. 641).

144. Fine HA, Kim L, Royce C, et al. A phase I trial of CC-5013, a potent thalidomide analog, in patients with recurrent high-grade gliomas and other refractory CNS malignancies [abstract]. Proc Annu Meet Am Soc Clin Oncol 2003;22:418.

145. Dupont E, Falardeau P, Mousa SA, et al. Antiangiogenic and antimetastatic properties of Neovastat (AE-941), an orally active extract derived from cartilage tissue. Clin Exp Metastasis 2002; 19:145–153.

146. Beliveau R, Gingras D, Kruger EA, et al. The antiangiogenic agent Neovastat (AE-941) inhibits vascular endothelial growth factor-mediated biological effects. Clin Cancer Res 2002;8:1242–1250.

147. Gingras D, Renaud A, Mousseau N, et al. Matrix proteinase inhibition by AE-941, a multifunctional antiangiogenic compound. Anticancer Res 2001;21(1A):145–155.

148. Gingras D, Mousseau N, Gaumont-Leclerc MF. AE-941 (Neovastat) induces endothelial cell apoptosis through activation of caspase-3 activity [abstract]. Proc Am Assoc Cancer Res 2001;42:3892.

149. Gingras D, Boivin D, Deckers C, et al. Neovastat: a novel antiangiogenic drug for cancer therapy. Anticancer Drugs 2003;14: 91–96.

150. Latreille J, Batist G, Laberge F, et al. Phase I/II trial of the safety and efficacy of AE-941 (Neovastat) in the treatment of non-small-cell lung cancer. Clin Lung Cancer 2003;4:231–236.

151. Batist G, Patenaude F, Champagne P, et al. Neovastat (AE-941) in refractory renal cell carcinoma patients: report of a phase II trial with two dose levels. Ann Oncol 2002;13:1259–1263.

152. Bukowski RM. AE-941, a multifunctional antiangiogenic compound: trials in renal cell carcinoma. Expert Opin Investig Drugs 2003;12:1403–1411.

153. O'Reilly MS, Holmgren L, Shing Y, et al. Angiostatin: a novel angiogenesis inhibitor that mediates the suppression of metastases by a Lewis lung carcinoma. Cell 1994;79:315–328.

154. Wahl ML, Moser TL, Pizzo SV. Angiostatin and anti-angiogenic therapy in human disease. Recent Prog Horm Res 2004;59: 73–104.

155. O'Reilly MS, Holmgren L, Chen C, et al. Angiostatin induces and sustains dormancy of human primary tumors in mice. Nat Med 1996;2:689–692.

156. Sim BK, O'Reilly MS, Liang H, et al. A recombinant human angiostatin protein inhibits experimental primary and metastatic cancer. Cancer Res 1997;57:1329–1334.

157. DeMoraes ED, Fogler WE, Grant D, et al. Recombinant human angiostatin (rhA): a phase I clinical trial assessing safety, pharmacokinetics(PK), and pharmacodynamics(PD) [abstract]. Proc Annu Meet Am Soc Clin Oncol 2001;20:10.

158. Beerepoot LV, Witteveen EO, Groenewegen G, et al. Recombinant human angiostatin by twice-daily subcutaneous injection in advanced cancer: a pharmacokinetic and long-term safety study. Clin Cancer Res 2003;9:4025–4033.

159. Hanna NH, Estes D, Cress A, et al. Recombinant human angiostatin (rhAngiostatin) in combination with paclitaxel and carboplatin in patients with advanced NSCLC: preliminary results of a phase II trial [abstract]. Proc Annu Meet Am Soc Clin Oncol 2004;23:7105.

160. O'Reilly MS, Boehm T, Shing Y, et al. Endostatin: an endogenous inhibitor of angiogenesis and tumor growth. Cell 1997;88: 277–285.

161. Boehm T, Folkman J, Browder T, et al. Antiangiogenic therapy of experimental cancer does not induce acquired drug resistance. Nature 1997;390:404–407.

162. Herbst RS, Hess KR, Tran HT, et al. Phase I study of recombinant human endostatin in patients with advanced solid tumors. J Clin Oncol 2002;20:3792–3803.

163. Eder JP Jr, Supko JG, Clark JW, et al. Phase I clinical trial of recombinant human endostatin administered as a short intravenous infusion repeated daily. J Clin Oncol 2002;20: 3772–3784.

164. Thomas JP, Arzoomanian RZ, Alberti D, et al. Phase I pharmacokinetic and pharmacodynamic study of recombinant human endostatin in patients with advanced solid tumors. J Clin Oncol 2003;21:223–231.

165. Herbst RS, Mullani NA, Davis DW, et al. Development of biologic markers of response and assessment of antiangiogenic activity in a clinical trial of human recombinant endostatin. J Clin Oncol 2002;20:3804–3814.

166. Kisker O, Becker CM, Prox D, et al. Continuous administration of endostatin by intraperitoneally implanted osmotic pump improves the efficacy and potency of therapy in a mouse xenograft tumor model. Cancer Res 2001;61:7669–7674.

167. Kulke M, Bergsland E, Ryan DP, et al. A phase II, open-label, safety, pharmacokinetic, and efficacy study of recombinant human endostatin in patients with advanced neuroendocrine tumors [abstract]. Proc Annu Meet Am Soc Clin Oncol 2003;22:958.

168. Gradishar WJ. Endpoints for determination of efficacy of antiangiogenic agents in clinical trials. In: Teicher BA, ed. Antiangiogenic agents in cancer therapy. Totowa, NJ: Humana Press, 1999:341–353.

Proteasome Inhibitors

29

Owen A. O'Connor

In 2004, Ciechanover, Hershko, and Rose were awarded the Nobel Prize in Chemistry for their seminal work regarding the discovery of an ATP-dependent ubiquitin-mediated protein degradation pathway.[1-7] Only a year before, in May of 2003, bortezomib, the very first drug capable of inhibiting the ubiquitin-proteasome pathway (UPP), was approved by the US Food and Drug Administration (FDA) for the treatment of a disease universally characterized by an overaccumulation of protein in the body. The approval of bortezomib in multiple myeloma has now underscored the therapeutic merits of targeting this novel pathway in the treatment of cancer. It has become evident that targeting the ubiquitin-proteasome pathway is associated with a seemingly infinite array of different biological effects on the cell. These effects are not only providing new treatment options but are teaching us much about how and why cancer cells behave the way they do.

Intracellular proteolytic mechanisms may not seem like the most obvious target for anticancer drug development. Such processes are ubiquitous in all cells in the body. Drugs that affect such a "common" target might not have a therapeutic index or sufficient tumor specificity. While lysosomal pathways of protein degradation by acid hydrolases have been well clarified in eukaryotes for decades, it was a focus on protein dynamics in denervated muscle that provided some of the first clues to a nonlysosomal pathway for intracellular protein degradation.[8] The observation that the rate of protein degradation, and not protein synthesis, was the basis for muscle wasting and cachexia spawned major research initiatives on how cells maintain protein homeostasis.[9] In the early 1970s, work by Goldberg and others[10,11] revealed the presence of a soluble ATP-dependent proteolytic system that mediated the breakdown of intracellular proteins in *Escherichia coli*. While the basis for the energy requirements remained elusive for many years, Ciechanover, Hershko, and Rose made the critical observation that ATP was an absolute necessity for the covalent linkage of ubiquitin (a small 76 amino acid [~8,000 MW]

heat-stable protein) to the protein substrate targeted for degradation.

Ubiquitin-conjugating reactions are a simple cellular strategy for "tagging" or earmarking specific protein substrates for proteolytic degradation at the proteasome. The structure and function of the 26S proteasome (a grouping of proteolytic enzymes into a cell organelle) had been alluded to over the years in the literature by a variety of different groups in a variety of ways.[12-16] In about 1990, the three essential elements of the pathway came together when it was demonstrated that, in the presence of ATP, the 20S proteasome was a component of the larger 26S proteasome, which was responsible for the proteolysis of the ubiquitin-conjugated proteins. Eighty percent to 90% of all intracellular proteins are degraded by the ubiquitin-proteasome pathway, including both short-lived and long-lived proteins.

The generation of early inhibitors of the proteasome proteases, mostly aldehyde-based peptides, soon led to the identification of a panoply of different unexpected biological effects. For example, Palombella et al.[17] showed that the proteasome was important in the activation of NF-κB, which plays a major role in inflammation and malignant cell growth. The proteasome also plays a major role in regulating at least five major categories of proteins. These include (1) proteins involved in cell cycle regulation; (2) proteins involved in regulating apoptosis; (3) IκB, an inhibitor of the transcription factor NF-κB; and (4) the processing of proteins in antigen-presenting cells (APCs), peptides of which are loaded into MHC molecules for presentation to T cells; and(s) proteins involved in cell adhesion. Thus, targeting this pathway could alter a broad spectrum of cellular functions.

CHEMISTRY

The very first inhibitors of the proteasome were potent inhibitors of other proteases, some of which possess enzymatic functions similar to that of the proteasome. Four

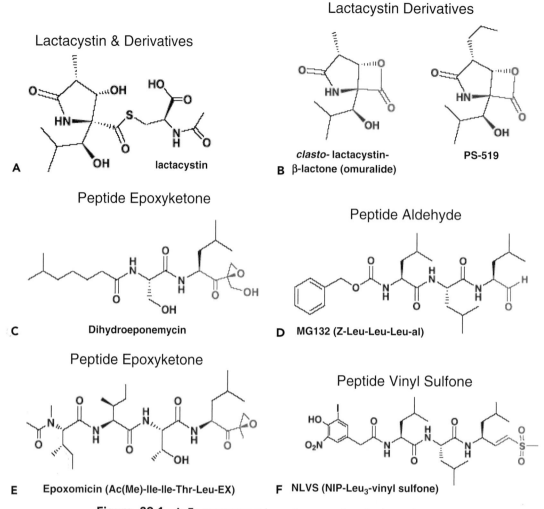

Figure 29.1 A–F: Representative classes of select proteasome

broad classes of compounds that inhibit the proteasome have been identified (Fig. 29.1 and Table 29.1), including (1) natural products (e.g., lactacystin, eponemycin, gliotoxin, epoxomicin); (2) synthetic peptide-based aldehyde inhibitors (e.g., MG132, MG 115; calpain inhibitors I and II, PSI, dipeptide aldehyde, glyoxal, CEP 1612, and bifunctional aldehydes); (3) synthetic reversible inhibitors of peptide amides and boronates (e.g., benzamide, dipeptidyl boronic esters, α-ketoamide, and bortezomib); and (4) synthetic irreversible inhibitors that are derivatives of vinyl sulfones and epoxyketones.

While several *natural product inhibitors* have been used and studied in the laboratory, none of these compounds has emerged to become a commercially viable therapeutic. One of these compounds, known as lactacystin, is a metabolite produced by the microorganism *Streptomyces lactacystinaeus*. Lactacystin and its derivative *clasto*-lactacystin β-lactone are structurally complex compounds unrelated to any of the peptide-based inhibitors (Fig. 29.1), which makes its total synthesis and clinical application more difficult and expensive.[18] The β-lactone derivative of lactacystin covalently modifies the amino-terminal threo-

nine residues of the β-subunits in the 20S proteasome, interfering with the primary mechanism of catalysis for both the tryptic-like and chymotryptic-like proteases.[19] Unfortunately, like many of the compounds known as "proteasome inhibitors," lactacystin derivatives inhibit a host of other proteases, limiting their specificity and therapeutic potential. These compounds have been shown to have significant antitumor effects and are capable of inhibiting cell cycle progression in sarcoma cell lines.[20,21] Isolation of an unidentified strain of actinomycete (Q996-17) in the early 1990s by Hanada et al.[22] led to the isolation and characterization of a family of compounds known as "peptidyl epoxyketones," including one derivative called "epoxomicin." The subsequent total synthesis of epoxomicin[23] eventually led to the demonstration that this compound is a highly specific inhibitor of the 20S proteasome. While these two molecules are among the best-known natural product inhibitors of the proteasome, most other natural product compounds have been shown to be less specific inhibitors, including some cyclic hexapeptides produced from other strains of *Streptomyces*.

TABLE 29.1

SELECT PROTEASOME INHIBITORS AND THEIR KI FOR INHIBITING THE 26S PROTEASOME.

Compound	CT-L (k obs / [I] (m/s))	T-L (k obs / [I] (m/s))	PGPH (k obs / [I] (m/s))	In Vivo Activity	Cross-reactivity	Reference
A. Synthetic Peptide Aldehyde Inhibitors						
MG132	K_i = 4.0 nM	K_i = 2,760 nM	K_i = 900 nM	0.4 μM[a]	Calpain, cathepsins	Kisselev et al. (38) Fevig et al. (131) Loidl et al. (132)
Bifunctional aldehyde	IC_{50} > 100 μM	IC_{50} = 0.5 μM	IC_{50} > 100 μM	ND	ND	Myung et al. (133)
B. Synthetic Reversible Inhibitors: Peptide Amides and Boronates						
Benzamide	IC_{50} = 0.14 μM	IC_{50} > 20 μM	IC_{50} > 20 μM	IC_{50} = 8 μM[a]	No calpain I	Lum et al. (134)
Dipeptidyl boronic ester	IC_{50} = 8 nM	No inhibition up to 1 μM	ND	ND	100-fold selective vs. chymotrypsin	Iqbal (135)
Bortezomib	53,000 IC_{50} = 0.62 nM	150	3,200	0.02 μM[b]	None found	Adams et al. (30) Harding et al. (136)
Cbz-LLL-boronic acid	K_i = 0.03 nM	ND	ND	0.04 μM[b]	ND	Adams et al. (31) Harding et al. (136)
C. Synthetic Irreversible Inhibitors: Vinyl Sulfones and Epoxyketones						
NLVS	5000	3.4	4.0	8 μM[a]	Cathepsin S and B	Bogyo et al. (137)
D. Natural Product Inhibitors						
Lactacystin	1,500	110	17	4 μM[a]	Cathepsin A, TPPII	Bogyo et al. (138)
Clasto-lactacystin β-lactone	7,400	68	47	ND	Cathepsin A, TPPII	Elofsson et al. (139)
Epoxomicin	20,000	300	40	0.03 μM[a]	None found	Myung et al. (133)
Dihydroeponemycin	114	17	217	2 μM[b]	Cathepsin (weak)	Meng et al. (140) Myung et al. (133)

CT-L, chymotrypsin-like; T-L, trypsin-like; PGPH, post-glutamyl peptide hydrolase; ND, not determined; K_i inhibition constant.

[a]Eighty-percent growth inhibition of EL4 cells

[b]For intracellular proteolysis of proteasome substrate and MHC1 processing.

Adapted from Kim KB, Crews CM. Natural product synthetic proteasome inhibitors. In: Adams J, ed. Proteasome Inhibitors in Cancer Therapy. Totowa, NJ: Humana Press, 2004:47–63.

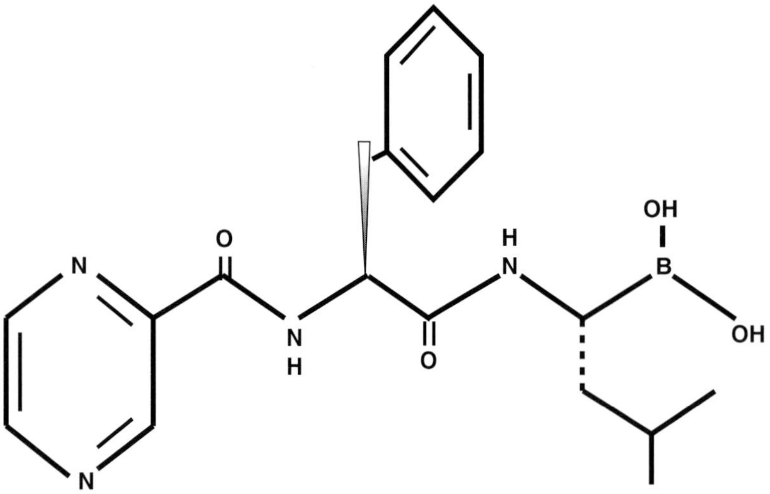

N-Pyrazinecarbonyl-L-phenylalanine-L-leucineboronic acid

(PS-341; Bortezomib; Velcade)

Figure 29.2 Chemical structure of bortezomib.

Like lactacystin, peptides containing a C-terminal vinyl sulfone moiety have been shown to covalently modify the N-terminal active site on the threonine of the β-subunits. These compounds are typically irreversible inhibitors and were originally introduced as cysteine proteases. Subsequent efforts to refine their structure to generate analogs with increased selectivity and potency succeeded only in generating compounds with dual inhibitor properties (i.e., they inhibited both threonine proteases and cysteine proteases).[24,25] As a result, while these compounds still serve as valuable tools in the laboratory, their lack of specificity has relegated them to experimental use only.

Several classes of reversible and irreversible synthetic inhibitors of the proteasome have been described. The *synthetic peptide-based aldehydes* were among the first potent reversible inhibitors described. Their structures have provided a model upon which many new analogs have been synthesized with even better and more selective inhibitory effects against the 20S proteasome. For example, leupeptin is a well-known inhibitor of serine proteases (e.g., trypsin and plasmin) and cysteine proteases (papain and cathepsin B) and is also a relatively potent inhibitor of the trypsin-like activity in the 20S proteasome.[26] In contrast, the calpain inhibitors have been shown to be potent inhibitors of the chymotrypsin-like activity.[12,27] Many of these compounds, including MG115 (acetyl-Leu-leu-norleucinal, also known as Calpain Inhibitor I or ALLN) and MG132 (Cbz-leu-leu-leucinal), are tripeptide aldehydes with potent inhibitory activity against the chymotryptic-like component of the 20S proteasome.[28] MG132 exhibits a K_i against the chymotrypsin-like, trypsin-like, and peptidyl glutamyl hydrolase enzymes, of 4, 2,760, and 900 nM, respectively (Table 29.1).

Most aldehyde-based proteasome inhibitors were found to be relatively nonspecific.[29] Chemical synthetic efforts to develop novel compounds with more selective properties eventually led to the identification of a new class of chemicals that were synthetic reversible peptide amide and boronic acid derivatives. Early efforts focused on altering the chemically interactive moiety of the inhibitor (or "warhead") that interfaces with the active site of the proteasome. A series of peptidyl aldehyde compounds that were derivatives of boronic acid were found to display dramatically enhanced potency inhibiting the chymotryptic-like enzymatic activities.[30] To date, a variety of boronic acid peptide inhibitors have been developed and studied,[30,31] of which bortezomib (formerly known as PS-341) was selected as a lead compound (Fig. 29.2). Independently, Lowe et al.[32] determined the x-ray crystallographic structure of the 20S proteasome from an archaebacterial species. These pivotal studies revealed a unique mode of catalysis in the proteasome, a mechanism that centered around a threonine residue.[32] Targeting the unique threonine residue within the proteasome proteases provided the selectivity of the aldehyde boronic acid derivatives. N-pyrazinecarbonyl-L-phenylalanine-L-leucineboronic acid (Fig. 29.2; formerly known as PS-341, now known as bortezomib and Velcade) selectively inhibited the threonine residue on the chymotryptic-like enzyme ($K_i \sim 0.6$ nM) specifically through the boronic acid moiety (Table 29.2) and did not inhibit other important proteases in the cell, including chymotrypsin ($K_i \sim 320$ nM), thrombin ($K_i \sim 13,000$ nM), and trypsin.

MECHANISM OF ACTION

How inhibiting the proteasome leads to cell death is still an area of intensive research. What is clear is that there is a remarkable diversity of biological processes that are

TABLE 29.2
THE K_i (nM) FOR BORTEZOMIB AGAINST SELECT INTRACELLULAR PROTEASES

Specific Protease	Bortezomib (K_i app) [nM]
20S proteasome	0.62
Chymotrypsin	970
Trypsin	>10,000
Cathepsin B	>10,000
Elastase	5,700
Calpain I	>10,000
Calpain II	>10,000
Angiotensin-converting enzyme (ACE)	490
Thrombin	>10,000
Factor XIIa	>10,000
Tissue plasminogen activator (TPA)	>10,000
Papain	>10,000

affected by proteasome inhibition. The sentinel event leading to cell death could be distinct in different diseases.

The Ubiquitin-Proteasome Pathway (UPP)

The ubiquitin-proteasome pathway (UPP) consists of two major components: the ubiquitinating enzyme complex and the proteasome. Three enzymes make up the ubiquitinating enzyme complex, the ubiquitin-activating enzyme (E1), the ubiquitin-conjugating enzyme (E2) and the ubiquitin protein ligase (E3). E1 is a generic enzyme used by the pathway regardless of the protein substrate targeted. In contrast, there are 20 to 30 different ubiquitin-conjugating enzymes (E2) and likely hundreds of ubiquitin protein ligases (E3). The ligase step is the point where the specificity

of the ubiquitylation process is controlled, with most protein substrates having their own distinct ubiquitin protein ligase.[33-35] Each of these enzymes represents a potential therapeutic target, offering unique ways to selectively inhibit the degradation of very specific proteins or groups of proteins. The initial step of this process involves the binding of this three-enzyme complex, known also as the ubiquitinating enzyme complex (UEC), to the N-terminus of the target protein (Fig. 29.3). This enzyme complex catalyzes the covalent linkage of ubiquitin molecules to the ε-amino moieties of internal lysine residues in a processive manner. These ATP-dependent catalytic reactions eventually lead to the generation of a branched polyubiquitylated protein. This ubiquitylation process is the fundamental means by which the cell "tags" or "earmarks" specific proteins for proteolytic degradation at the 26S proteasome.

The second major component of the pathway includes the proteasome proper (Fig. 29.4). The proteasome is composed of two components, the 20S proteasome (720 kd) and the 19S regulatory subunit (890 kd). Collectively, they form a complex called the 26S proteasome.[36] The isolated 20S proteasome exhibits no proteolytic activity in the absence of the 19S regulatory subunit. The 19S subunit mediates the ATP-dependent process of denaturing and unfolding the ubiquitin conjugates. The 26S proteasome is a very large (2.5 MDa) structure composed of 44 distinct polypeptides. The proteases within the proteasome possess different mechanisms of catalysis relative to other proteases. Specifically, they are threonine proteases, not the usual serine and cysteine proteases. In addition, the proteasome proteases are known to be highly processive. Normally, most proteases cleave their substrate once, generating two new fragments. In contrast, the proteasome, by virtue of the fact that its is a redundant multicatalytic enzyme, cleaves polypeptides at multiple sites, releasing very small peptides

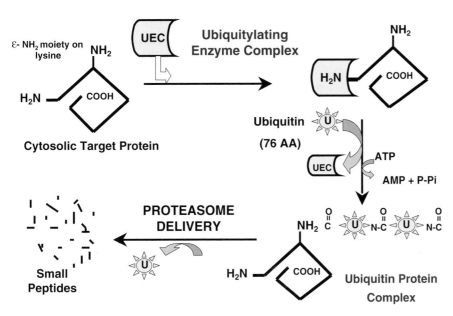

Figure 29.3 Schematic of the ubiquitin-proteasome pathway.

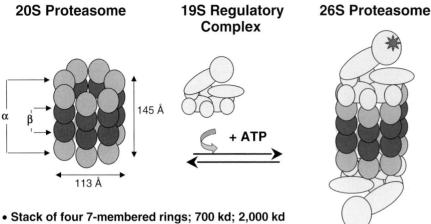

20S Proteasome

α   β

113 Å

145 Å

19S Regulatory Complex

+ ATP

26S Proteasome

- Stack of four 7-membered rings; 700 kd; 2,000 kd
- 700 kDa
- 14 distinct subunits
- Broad substrate specificity
- Catalytic nucleophile: Thr¹of β subunit

- 2,000 kDa
- Degrades ubiquitinated proteins
- Proteolysis is ATP-dependent

Figure 29.4 Structure of the 26S proteasome and its assembly.

ranging in length from 2 to 24 amino acids, with a median size of six to seven residues each.[37-39]

The 19S regulatory subunit consists of at least nine polypeptides, including multiple isopeptidases that disassemble and unfold the polyubiquitin conjugates. It also plays a major role in facilitating and regulating the many ATP-dependent processes used by the proteasome. In fact, this energy-consuming process requires ATP for a number of functions including complex formation resulting from the 20S and 19S assembly; protein unfolding; ubiquitylation; the actual translocation of ubiquitin conjugates into the 20S lumen; the opening of the regulatory "gate" that allows the protein to enter the 26S lumen; and the action of the isopeptidases, which result in the recycling of the ubiquitin molecules.[40]

The 20S proteasome (720 kd) consists of four rings, each containing seven individual globular proteins. As can be seen from Figure 29.4, the assembly of the four rings forms a central lumen through which proteins are funneled. The two outer or flanking layers of the 20S proteasome are referred to as the α-layers and are basically a structural feature that allows anchorage of the 19S regulatory subunit. The two inner rings are referred to as the β-layers and contain the distinct proteases that account for the proteolytic activity of the proteasome. The 19S regulatory subunit sits on the top and bottom of the 20S subunit, controlling the entry of ubiquitylated proteins into the core of the proteasome.[40] Once the protein enters the lumen of the proteasome, the proteases digest the protein into smaller peptide fragments. The activity of these proteases can be quantitatively assessed by using specific fluorogenic peptides that are substrates for only one of these proteases. These assays have provided a valuable tool by which biochemists can decipher which of the three different

proteolytic functions are being affected by test inhibitors. To date, at least three different enzymatic activities have been ascribed to the β-layers, including (1) *a peptidylglutamyl activity* (β1) that cleaves proteins near glutamate residues; (2) *a tryptic-like function* (β2) that cleaves proteins next to the basic amino acids lysine and arginine; and (3) *a chymotryptic-like function* (β5) that cleaves proteins near the aromatic amino acids phenylalanine, tyrosine, and tryptophan.[36,41-44] Bortezomib is a reversible and selective inhibitor of the chymotryptic-like protease found in the 26S proteasome (Fig. 29.5).

Influencing the NF-κB Pathway

The early discovery by Palombella et al.[17] that proteasome inhibition could lead to inactivation of NF-κB helped

Cross-sectional view of the β ring

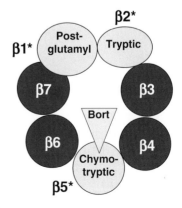

β2*

β1*   Post-glutamyl   Tryptic

β7   β3

Bort

β6   β4

Chymo-tryptic

β5*

Figure 29.5 Cross-sectional view of the B-ring and the binding of bortezomib (Bort) to the chymotryptic-like protease.

formulate the hypothesis that inhibitors of this pathway could have effects on a vast array of biological processes. NF-κB is the prototype for a family of dimeric transcription factors involved in the inflammatory and immune responses, promotion of cell growth, and blocking of apoptosis. Constitutive activation of NF-κB has been described in a number of solid tumors, including pancreatic and colorectal cancer, as well as several hematological malignancies. Its role in drug resistance and oncogenesis has now been firmly established.

Five members of the NF-κB family—p65/RelA, c-Rel, Rel B, p52/100, and p50/105—have been defined, all capable of forming a number of different homodimeric or heterodimeric complexes.[45,46] The activation of NF-κB is tightly regulated through its inhibitor IκB. IκB, in fact, belongs to a family of proteins that includes IκBα, IκBβ, IκBε, and Bcl-3. The interaction of IκB with the dimeric transcription factors blocks the nuclear translocation of NF-κB, preventing access of the transcription factor to DNA. Activation of NF-κB typically involves the induction of IκB kinase (IKK), leading to the phosphorylation of IκB, followed by its ubiquitylation and eventual degradation by the 26S proteasome. Interestingly, a number of different stimuli have been shown to induce IκB, including tumor necrosis factor-α (TNF-α), lipopolysaccharide, various interleukins (ILs) and interferons, hypoxia, and even cytotoxic drug exposure.[45,47–50] Liberation of free NF-κB leads to its translocation into the nucleus, where it binds to the promoter region of several genes, resulting in transcriptional activation. If serine residues on IκB are mutated to alanine, which cannot be phosphorylated, IκB cannot be degraded, and it permanently sequesters NF-κB in the cytoplasm. This mutated form of IκB has proven to be a model for mimicking the effect of proteasome inhibition.[51]

One of the first clues that NF-κB was important in cancer biology came in the mid-1980s, when Sen and Baltimore[52] first described the protein as a B-cell transcription factor that bound a site in the immunoglobulin enhancer. Subsequently, these same authors demonstrated that NF-κB could be activated in a variety of other cells following exposure to assorted stimuli like phorbol esters and that the activation of NF-κB was independent of protein synthesis.[53] The range of NF-κB inducers has continued to grow beyond those typically associated with immune function. The variety of stimuli known to induce NF-κB[47] are enormous and are known to include (a) *a number of immune effector proteins,* such as tumor necrosis factor (TNF-α), lymphotoxin, IL-1 and -2, granulocyte/macrophage colony-stimulating factor (GM-CSF), allogeneic stimulation, lectins, phorbol ester, diacylglycerol, CD40 ligand, leukotriene B4, and prostaglandin E2; (b) *physical stresses,* such as UV irradiation, ionizing radiation, and hypoxia; oxidative stresses like hydrogen peroxide, oxidized lipids, and butyl peroxide; (c) *many different chemical agents,* such as conventional chemotherapy drugs and protein synthesis inhibitors; and (d) *a host of infectious agents,* including bacterial products,

viruses, and some parasites. These stimuli have been shown to activate NF-κB primarily through the induced degradation of IκB, allowing for transcriptional activation within minutes of exposure.

Perhaps even more daunting are the number of NF-κB responsive genes,[47] which include (a) *a host of cytokines and growth factors,* such as IL-1, IL-2, IL-6, IL-8, TNF-α, GM-CSF, G-CSF, and interferon-β; (b) *a number of immunoreceptors,* such as immunoglobulin κ light chains, the T-cell receptor β-chain, major histocompatibility complex class I and II (MHC-I and II), and β2 microglobulin; (c) *several adhesion molecules,* such as endothelial-leukocyte adhesion molecule-1 (ELAM-1), vascular endothelial adhesion molecule-1 (VCAM-1), and intracellular cell adhesion molecule-1 (ICAM-1); and (d) a number of transcription factors, such as Rel, p105, IκB-α, c-myc, and interferon regulatory factor-1. These lists suggest the complex biology influenced by NF-κB. While targeting this pathway may be a fruitful strategy in drug development, it is also clear that identifying a singular mechanism of action across different diseases will likely remain elusive. Furthermore, it provides credence to the idea that inhibitors of the proteasome that can influence such complex signaling cascades are likely to be associated with a multitude of biological consequences and that inhibition of NF-κB alone is not likely to be the sole mechanism of action in any disease. The broad range of biological effects of NF-κB and its ubiquitous expression also raise concerns about undesired effects of NF-κB inhibition.

Effects on Cell Cycle Regulation

Control of cell cycle transition points depends heavily on both transcriptional and posttranscriptional mechanisms. The timely degradation of essential regulatory proteins through the UPP allows for the coordinated progression of a cell through the cell cycle. Inhibition of the degradation of any of the host of proteins that play a role in orchestrating this process can have a profound influence on cell cycle kinetics. For example, p21 and p27 are members of the Cip/kip family of cyclin-dependent kinase inhibitors, which halt cell cycle progression at the G_1-S junction by inactivating the cyclin/cdk complexes.[54] The cdk inhibitor $p21^{WAF/CIP1}$, a transcriptional target of p53, is thought to be what couples cellular differentiation with cell cycle arrest. Treatment of the human colon cancer cell lines RKO and HCT-116 with the proteasome inhibitor lactacystin results in cell cycle arrest mediated by p21 accumulation.[55] Another well-established cell cycle control mechanism revolves around the expression of cyclin B, the synthesis of which begins very early in the S phase, accumulating to its highest levels during G_2 and early mitosis (M phase). During these phases of growth, cyclin B is complexed with the CDK/cdc2, with specific phosphorylation and dephosphorylation of cdc2 governing the activity of the complex.[56] Progression into and through anaphase is tightly dependent on the degradation of cyclin B, which is tightly controlled through its ubiquitylation and proteolytic degradation by the 26S proteasome.[57] Similarly, entrance into the S phase from G_1 is controlled by the cyclin E-CDK2 complex. Association of this complex with p27 is responsible for inhibiting the kinase activity, leading to cell cycle arrest.[58,59] Degradation of the cell cycle inhibitory protein p27, allows the cell to pass the G_1/S transition, allowing for DNA synthesis within only hours. This critical event is also tightly controlled through the ubiquitylation- and proteasome-mediated degradation of p27.[58,60,61] Hence, one important mechanism of action of proteasome inhibitors is to dysregulate normal cell cycle kinetics, usually by inducing cell cycle arrest.

The significance of these particular changes was underscored in an evaluation of several forms of non-Hodgkin's lymphoma (NHL), in which most mantle cell lymphomas (91 of 112) and diffuse large B-cell lymphomas (12 of 19) were shown to have lost expression of p27.[62,63] In contrast, small lymphocytic lymphoma and extranodal marginal zone lymphomas were found to have ample p27 expression.[62] Mantle cell lymphomas actually had normal p27 mRNA expression but increased p27 protein degradation through the ubiquitin-proteasome pathway. Interestingly, overexpression of p53 and/or loss of p27 in patients with MCL correlated with a statistically significant reduction in overall survival.[63] While the mechanism of p27 loss is not entirely clear, some have suggested sequestration with cyclins D1 and D3, while others have suggested that the level of Skp2, a component of the p27^{Kip1} ubiquitin ligase, may be important in select NHLs.[62] The basis for the involvement of Skp2 revolves around the observation that high Skp2 levels correlate with greater E3 activity and hence greater proteasome-mediated degradation of the target protein (i.e., p27), establishing an inverse relationship between the two. In aggressive lymphomas and blastic MCL, high Skp2 levels were associated with a low p27^{Kip1} level, suggesting increased proteasome-mediated degradation of p27^{Kip1}.[62] Loss of p27 identified a poorer outcome among the p53 negative cases and established this pathway as an important high-risk marker in these patients, potentially providing a therapeutic rationale for proteasome inhibitors in mantle cell lymphoma. Furthermore, MCL cell lines (i.e., Granta 519 and NCEB) treated with lactacystin failed to accumulate cyclin D1 or cdk4 (despite the overexpression mediated by the t[11:14] translocation), though cell cycle arrest and induction of apoptosis was accompanied by accumulation of the cdk inhibitor p21 and p27 in both cell lines.[64] These observations have been corroborated in human non–small cell lung cancer (NSCLC) cell lines as well, where a pronounced G_2-M phase arrest was associated with the inhibited degradation of p21$^{cip/waf-1}$.[65] There is much to be learned about how proteasome inhibition affects the cell cycle regulation and whether those actions will translate into a specific antitumor effect.

Induction of Apoptosis

Proteasome inhibition can lead to apoptosis through both direct and indirect influences.[66] NF-κB mediates an anti-apoptotic effect. For example, Beg and Baltimore[67] and Van Antwerp et al.[68] have shown that activation of NF-κB suppressed TNF-α–induced apoptosis. NF-κB also protects cells exposed to either ionizing radiation or daunorubicin from death. The inhibition of NF-κB nuclear translocation has been found to enhance apoptotic killing by radiation or chemotherapy.[69] This represents one mechanism through which proteasome inhibitors can influence cell death signaling.

Other more direct influences of proteasome inhibition on the induction of apoptosis have been shown in leukemic cells following exposure to the proteasome inhibitor lactacystin. Marshansky et al.[70] demonstrated in both Jurkat (T-cell tumor) and Namala (B-cell tumor) cell lines that inhibition of the proteasome differentially up-regulated a proapoptotic Bcl-2 family member known as Bik by decreasing its proteolytic degradation. Interestingly, other family members in this model, including Bax, Bak, and Bad, were not similarly affected. Up-regulation and accumulation of Bik was shown to be sufficient for inducing apoptosis in these leukemic cells. Additionally, these authors showed that proper functioning of the electron transport chain is dependent on proteasome activity and that interruption of protein turnover adversely influenced the transmitochondrial membrane potential, leading to the induction of apoptosis. It was shown that Bik and the anti-apoptotic member Bcl-$_{XL}$ coprecipitated, leading to the hypothesis that excess Bik could trap and theoretically nullify the influences of Bcl-$_{XL}$, since the level of Bcl-$_{XL}$ is not changed following proteasome inhibition. This "trapping" of the Bcl-$_{XL}$ then offers a theoretical mechanism for overriding the antiapoptotic effects of Bcl-$_{XL}$, leading to cell death.

The temporal sequence of events following exposure to the proteasome inhibitor bortezomib on Bcl-2 was shown by Ling et al.[71] Treatment of the H460 cell line with bortezomib resulted in a both a time-dependent and concentration-dependent set of effects on Bcl-2 phosphorylation and cleavage. For example, treatment of the cells with bortezomib resulted in cleavage of Bcl-2, with the identification of a unique cleavage product (Mr 25,000). The generation of this cleavage product was not prevented by caspase inhibitors, which was the case with the Mr 23,000 cleavage product typically seen following exposure to conventional cytotoxic therapies, suggesting the possibility of a caspase-independent pathway. The Bcl-2 cleavage products accumulated in the mitochondrial membrane early, usually 12 hours after exposure, while poly(ADP-ribose) polymerase (PARP) cleavage and DNA fragmentation were seen about 36 hours post exposure. The authors concluded that inhibition of the proteasome resulted in a prompt phosphorylation of Bcl-2, leading to the formation of a unique cleavage product that was associated with G_2-M arrest and the induction of apoptosis.[71]

A link between the NF-κB and apoptotic pathways was also established by Heckman et al.,[72] and it may provide some insight into one of the possible mechanisms of action in follicular lymphoma. Follicular lymphomas are well characterized by the translocation of the bcl-2 proto-oncogene from chromosome 18q21 to the immunoglobulin heavy chain locus (IgH) at chromosome 14q32.[73-75] The resulting translocation, t(14:18), is the sine qua non lesion seen in follicular lymphoma and leads to the overexpression of the antiapoptotic bcl-2 protein, protecting cells from apoptosis. In addition, lymphoma cells carrying the t(14:18) also overexpress NF-κB. These authors demonstrated that cell lines expressing an IκBα super-repressor exhibited marked reductions in bcl-2 protein, implying a role for NF-κB in cells carrying this translocation. These observations could provide a rationale for employing proteasome inhibitors in follicular lymphoma.[72] While the impact of the NF-κB signaling pathway in these studies was not analyzed, it is reasonable to suggest that the pathways leading to the induction of apoptosis in cancer cells will involve both direct and indirect influences on the mitochondria. The ultimate pathway leading to cell death is likely to depend on the molecular perturbations that drive the behavior of that malignant clone. For example, in mantle cell lymphoma, inhibition of the constitutive activation of NF-κB leads to the induction of both cell cycle arrest and apoptosis through the down-regulation of bcl-2 family members and the activation of caspases.[76]

The Unfolded Protein Response

One of the lesser recognized mechanisms that may lead to cell death or injury following inhibition of the ubiquitin-proteasome pathway is based on the cell's need to "protect" itself from misfolded or damaged intracellular proteins. Such mechanisms for damaged protein elimination have been established in prokaryotes long before the discovery of the ubiquitin-proteasome pathway was discovered in eukaryotes.[11,77] Misfolded or damaged proteins can arise in any cell through errors in DNA repair or spontaneous mutation. In addition, there are a host of other physical and chemical factors that can lead to damaged intracellular protein, including denaturing conditions at high temperatures; the presence of oxidizing agents or high redox conditions; activated proteases or kinases, high salt concentrations, which may favor disaggregation of large multimeric complexes; or the presence of detergents. Resulting proteins can be highly noxious to the cell and are capable of inducing cell death. This mechanism of cell death, though not well defined, is likely due to the ability of these damaged proteins to form insoluble aggregates. Such protein inclusions have been seen in a variety of inherited and neurodegenerative disease, strongly pointing towards a failure of the cell to break down intracellular protein as the basis for the underlying pathology.

Lee et al.[78] have provided some valuable insight into this process, especially in multiple myeloma. Using a variety of myeloma cell lines they demonstrated that the transcription factor XBP-1 is an important inducer of plasma cell differentiation. XBP-1 is a major regulator of this unfolded protein response in plasma cells. Treatment of myeloma cells with proteasome inhibitors resulted in impaired production of XBP-1, leading to the induction of their apoptosis.[78] When unfolded proteins accumulate inside cells, they tend to saturate the proteolytic capacity of the cell (as might occur following treatment with any proteasome inhibitor), leading to the activation of the heat shock response[42,79] and the induction of more proteasome biosynthesis.[80] The continued accumulation of these proteins eventually triggers the activation of Jnk kinases and apoptosis.[81,82] Blocking the cell's mechanisms for protecting itself against damage by misfolded proteins with proteasome inhibitors alone or in combination with agents that inhibit heat shock proteins may provide new therapeutic opportunities for both malignant and nonmalignant diseases.

PRECLINICAL PHARMACOLOGY

Proteasome inhibitors have potent anticancer properties. Imajoh-Ohmi et al.[83] demonstrated that the microbial metabolite lactacystin induced cell death in U937 cells at concentrations of about 5 μM. These insights were broadened when several groups reported that tripeptide inhibitors of the proteasome but not lysosomal protease inhibitors induced apoptosis in Rat-1 and PC12 cells in a p53-dependent manner.[84] Normal cells were found to be more resistant to proteasome inhibitors than transformed cells. For example, the proteasome inhibitor CEP1612 induced apoptosis selectively in simian virus 40 (SV-40)–transformed cells but not in normal human fibroblasts.[85] Orlowski et al.[86] demonstrated that fibroblasts transformed with ras and myc, lymphoblasts transformed by c-myc alone, and a Burkitt's lymphoma cell line that overexpresses c-myc were up to 40-fold more susceptible to apoptosis induced by proteasome inhibitors than were primary rodent fibroblasts or immortalized nontransformed human lymphoblasts. The explanation for these observations remains unclear.

Boronate proteasome inhibitors have been shown to kill tumor cells in culture, as demonstrated by their activity in the NCI tumor cell line screen.[31] Data from this well-characterized cell line screen established an excellent correlation between the intrinsic potency of different proteasome inhibitors (the K_i [nM]) and their cytotoxicity.[31,87] Using data from the NCI's algorithm COMPARE, the analysis established that the mechanism of cytotoxicity of bortezomib was markedly different from any of the other 60,000 compounds already in the library. The average growth inhibition of (GI50%) for bortezomib was 7 nM across the entire panel of cells. More detailed in vitro and in vivo data were obtained using the prostate cancer cell line PC-3, in which bortezomib was found to result in an accumulation of cells in G2-M, which was attributed to the accumulation of CDK inhibitors p21 and p27. Cell death was noted at 20 and 100 nM for cells incubated for 24 and 48 hours in the presence of bortezomib.[31] In a nude mouse model with PC-3, bortezomib was found to kill the tumor in a dose-dependent manner.

Intravenous dosing with radiolabeled [^{14}C]-bortezomib in rats followed by whole-body autoradiography revealed that the highest radioactivity levels 10 minutes after drug administration were in the adrenal glands, renal cortex, liver, prostate, and spleen. Lower levels were found throughout other organs, including skeletal muscle, skin, and blood, while no detectable drug could be found crossing the blood-brain barrier (brain, eye, testes). Sixty-six percent of the radiolabeled drug was recovered from the bile, while the remainder was recovered from the urine.[31]

Multiple myeloma is one disease where significant activity has been seen in both clinical and preclinical models.[88–90] In vivo models of drug-resistant human myeloma have shown that twice weekly schedules of bortezomib administration resulted both in tumor shrinkage and prolonged median survival of treated mice.[89–91] Preclinical models of multiple myeloma have shown that proteasome inhibitors induce the down-regulation of the cytokine-induced expression of E-selectin, vascular cell-adhesion molecule-1 (VCAM-1), and intracellular cell adhesion molecule 1.[92] VCAM-1 is essential for facilitating the interactions between the myeloma cells and the bone marrow stromal cells, an interaction that leads to the protection of the myeloma cells from apoptosis.[93,94] Second, the inhibition of NF-κB reduces the transcription of the NF-κB–responsive IL-6 gene. IL-6 is a growth and survival factor for multiple myeloma cells lines.[89] Most recently, lactacystin, bortezomib, and MG262 have been shown to have antiangiogenic properties and may help to reduce the degree of neovascularization in the bone marrow, adversely affecting the survival of the myeloma cells.[95–99] Obviously, many of these latter effects would not be appreciated in the standard in vivo or in vitro models of anticancer drug screening.

CLINICAL PHARMACOLOGY

Pharmacokinetic (PK) Profiles and Metabolism

Studies in nonhuman primates have shown that the tissue distribution is extensive, though the drug does not appear to cross the blood-brain or blood-testes barriers. After a single intravenous dose of bortezomib, plasma concentrations decline in a classic biphasic manner, which is charac-

PLASMA PHARMACOKINETICS

1.0 vs. 1.3 mg/m^2

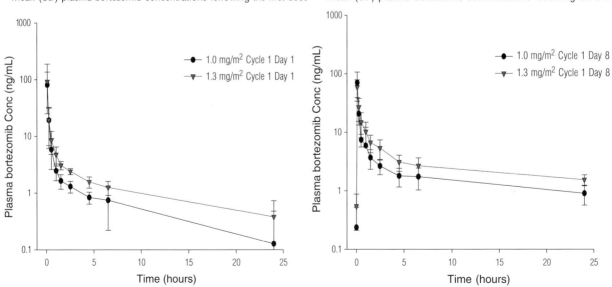

Figure 29.6   Plasma pharmacokinetics of the 1.0 and 1.3 mg/m^2

MAJOR METABOLITES OF BOTEZOMIB

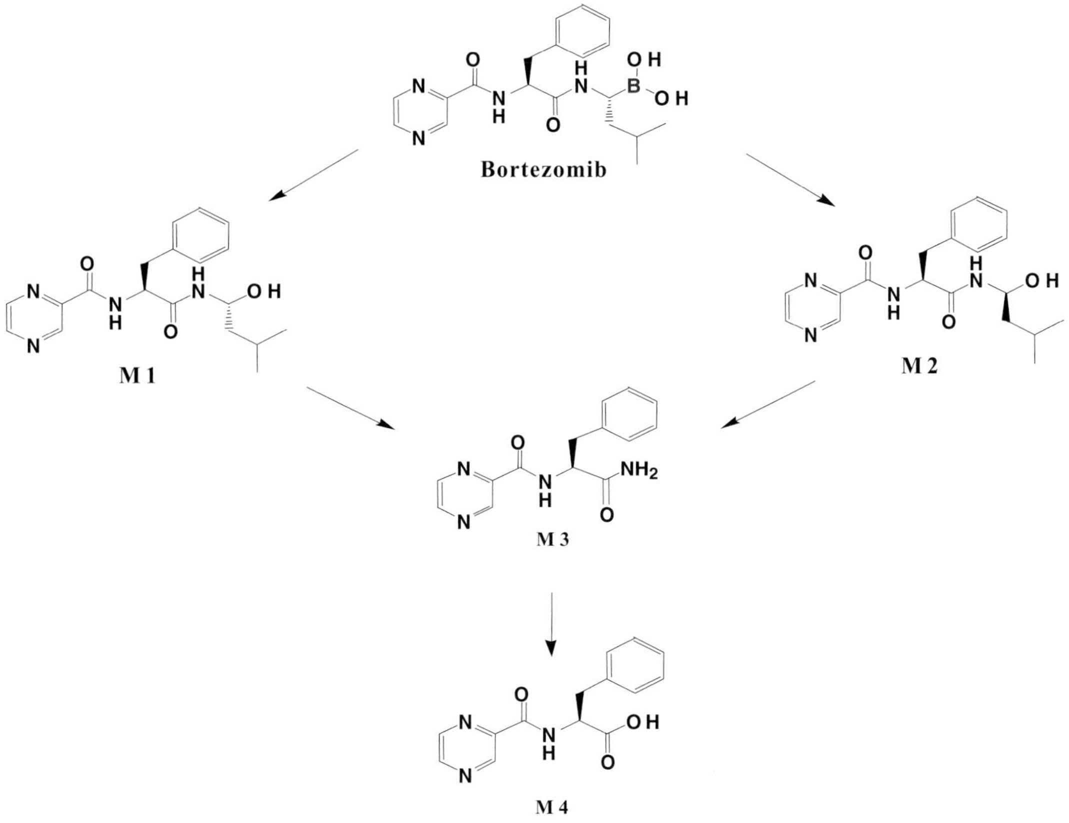

Figure 29.7 Major metabolites of borte-

terized by a very rapid distribution period, with a $t_{1/2}\alpha$ of approximately 10 minutes.[100] The terminal elimination phase in humans has been estimated between 5 and 15 hours. Figure 29.6 presents a plot of the mean plasma concentrations of bortezomib following a single and one-repeat dose of bortezomib in patients receiving 1.0 or 1.3 mg/m². Multiple doses of drug appear to result in some decrease in clearance, with a resulting increase in the terminal elimination half-life and AUC, but they have no effect on the estimated C_{max} or distribution half-life. For example, in patients with solid tumor malignancies, the mean terminal half-life increased from 5.45 to 19.7 hours, while the AUC increased from 30.1 after the first dose to 54 hr × ng/mL after the third dose of the first cycle (MPI, on file, 2004). These pharmacokinetic profiles have also been observed in preclinical studies in rodents and cynomolgus monkeys and do not appear to result in increased toxicity from accumulation of the drug with repeat dosing. The overall disposition of bortezomib is most consistent with a two-compartment PK model.

The principal pathway of elimination of bortezomib is through oxidative deboronation (Fig. 29.7). Based on in vitro studies, the major phase 1 metabolic reactions are mediated by cytochrome P450 isoforms 3A4 and 2C19,

while the major phase 2 conjugation pathways do not appear to play any major role in elimination.[101] The inactive deboronated metabolites then undergo a series of hydroxylations, leading to their elimination. Radiolabeled studies using [14C]-bortezomib have confirmed elimination of some metabolites through both renal and hepatic routes (approximately 66% of the initial drug load), though only a small quantity of intact bortezomib is recovered from the urine (MPI, on file, 2004).

Pharmacodynamic Endpoints

The critical pharmacodynamic endpoint for bortezomib is proteasome inhibition in vivo. As shown in Figure 29.8, 20S proteasome inhibition was quantified as a function of both dose and time.[102–105] Blood samples were collected before therapy and then 1, 6, and 24 hours after each dose of bortezomib in the first cycle for measurement of the 20S proteasome activity. The degree of proteasome inhibition was measured by quantitating the rate of hydrolysis of sample fluorogenic peptide substrates relative to the normalized chymotryptic activity. Bortezomib induced a dose-dependent inhibition of the 20S proteasome compared with pretreatment controls, with the 0.40, 1.04, 1.20, and

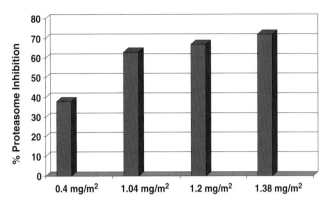

Figure 29.8   Proteasome inhibition as a function of dose.

bition. At 72 hours post bortezomib infusion, there is little to no residual inhibition of the proteasome. Figure 29.9 shows that the plasma levels of bortezomib predict the level of proteasome inhibition. This pharmacodynamic endpoint has helped to establish the clinical basis for the once-every-72-hours dosing strategy, along with the recognition that dosing bortezomib more frequently would lead to a "stacking" of the proteasome inhibition, eventually leading to complete inhibition of the proteasome. Based on several in vivo models, complete inhibition of the proteasome is not compatible with life, while about 60 to 70% inhibition of the proteasome may be required for the bulk of the anticancer activity.

Single-Agent Phase I Experience

To date, three phase I experiences with bortezomib have been completed (Table 29.3), with one of these devoted to patients with hematologic malignancies.[102–104] These phase I experiences have explored weekly and twice-weekly intravenous bolus schedules. In general, the pattern of toxicity paralleled what was noted in the preclinical findings. In the phase I study conducted by Papandreou et al.,[104] bortezomib was administered weekly × 4 weeks every 6 weeks, establishing 1.6 mg/m² as the maximum tolerated dose (MTD) on this schedule. The authors noted that hypoten-

1.38 mg/m² doses producing inhibition levels of 36%, 60%, 65%, and 74%, respectively. Doses of bortezomib less than 0.4 mg/m² produce marginal inhibition of the proteasome. The majority of the proteasome inhibition is attained at about 1 hour post drug infusion, after which proteasome inhibition decays with a half-life of about 24 hours. The data exhibit a classic sigmoidal maximal effect distribution, where larger increases in dose produce correspondingly smaller interval increases in proteasome inhi-

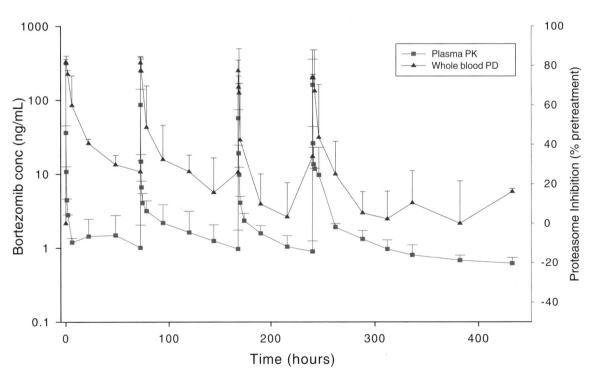

Figure 29.9   Plot of the plasma pharmacokinetic profile and the kinetics of proteasome inhi-

TABLE 29.3
PHASE I STUDIES OF BORTEZOMIB

Schedule	Length of Cycle (weeks)	Doses of Bortezomib (mg/m²)	No. of Patients	MTD (mg/m²)	DLT	Study
Weekly × 4 weeks	6	0.13–2	53	1.6	Hypotension, syncope	Papandreou et al. (104)
Twice weekly × 2 weeks	3	0.4–1.5	43	1.3[a]	Diarrhea, neuropathy	Aghajanian et al. (103)
Twice weekly × 4 weeks	6	0.4–1.38	27	1.04	Hyponatremia, hypokalemia, malaise	Orlowski et al. (102)

MTD, maximum tolerated dose; DLT, dose-limiting toxicity.
[a]MTD in publication noted to be 1.56 mg/m²; generally accepted MTD based on available studies with this schedule is 1.3 mg/m².

sion and syncope were dose-limiting toxicities on the weekly schedule up to 2 mg/m². In what has now emerged as the "standard schedule" for bortezomib in most of the early phase II studies done to date, Aghajanian et al.[103] conducted a phase I study of bortezomib in a range from 0.4 to 1.5 mg/m² twice weekly for 2 weeks every 3 weeks. On this schedule, diarrhea and neuropathy were the dose-limiting toxicities. While there is some debate about the MTD established in this study (1.3 vs. 1.5 mg/m²), most have adopted 1.3 mg/m² as the MTD on this schedule.

The phase I study reported by Orlowski et al.[102] was the only one devoted to patients with hematologic malignancies. This multicenter study conducted by investigators at the University of North Carolina and Memorial Sloan-Kettering Cancer Center included 27 heavily pretreated patients with a variety of hematologic malignancies, including Hodgkin's disease ($n = 4$), small lymphocytic lymphoma/chronic lymphocytic leukemia ($n = 2$), diffuse large B-cell lymphoma ($n = 2$), mantle cell lymphoma ($n = 3$), Waldenstrom's macroglobulinemia ($n = 1$), and multiple myeloma ($n = 11$). The patients had received a median of 3 prior forms of chemotherapy (range, 1 to 12), and over one third ($n = 10$) had had prior high-dose chemotherapy and peripheral blood stem cell transplantation. The drug was administered twice a week for 4 consecutive weeks every 6 weeks at dose levels of 0.4, 1.04, 1.2, or 1.38 mg/m² . The major dose-limiting toxicities included thrombocytopenia, which was observed at every dose level; hyponatremia; hypokalemia; fatigue; and malaise. This twice-weekly schedule for 4 of 6 weeks established a slightly lower MTD of 1.04 mg/m². Interestingly, among the nine fully assessable patients with heavily pretreated plasma cell dyscrasias completing at least one cycle of therapy, one achieved a complete remission, and eight other patients demonstrated a major reduction in paraprotein levels and/or bone marrow plasma cells. In addition, one of three patients with mantle cell lymphoma achieved a durable partial remission, as did one patient with follicular lymphoma.

Phase II Experience

A variety of single-agent studies have been conducted in patients with solid tumors and hematologic malignancies. A summary of these experiences is presented in Table 29.4. The promising activity seen in multiple myeloma has led to FDA approval for that disease. Other studies focusing on lymphoma, NSCLC, and renal cell carcinoma have also been reported.

Multiple Myeloma

Based on the responses seen in multiple myeloma in the phase I study, a large multicenter, open-label, nonrandomized phase II trial of bortezomib for patients with relapsed or refractory multiple myeloma was initiated (the Summit trial). Patients were required to have relapsed and progressive disease following conventional chemotherapy and to have disease refractory to salvage chemotherapy, as defined by progression of disease during treatment or within 60 days of completion of their therapy. Two hundred and two patients were registered to the study. Treatment consisted of bortezomib administered at a dose of 1.3 mg/m² as an intravenous push given on days 1, 4, 8, and 11 every 21 days. The study was conducted in a very heavily pretreated population of patients with a median of 6 lines of prior treatment, which included high-dose chemotherapy and stem cell transplantation in almost two thirds of patients. Based on the report of Richardson et al.[106] and the analysis by the FDA,[107] the overall response rate according to the stringent Blade criteria was 27.7%, with 2.7% ($n = 5$) of patients meeting criteria for complete remission (complete disappearance of paraprotein). The median time to response was 38 days (range, 30 to 127 days), and the median duration of response was 365 days (range, 41 to 509 days). Interestingly, these responses were independent of the number and type of previous therapies, performance status, β2 microglobulin level, chromosome 13 deletion status, or type of myeloma. The most common adverse effects (all grades) included nausea (64%), diarrhea (49%),

TABLE 29.4
SUMMARY OF SELECT EFFICACY STUDIES OF BORTEZOMIB

Disease[1]	n	ORR	CR	Duration of Response (months)	Comments	Reference
Multiple myeloma (Summit study)	202	35%	4%	12	Median overall survival was 16 months	Richardson et al. (106)
Multiple myeloma (Crest study)	54	1.3 mg/m² = 38% 1.1 mg/m² = 30%	3.7%	ND	Compared 1.3 vs. 1.1 mg/m²	Jagannath et al. (108)
Indolent and mantle cell lymphoma	25 59	61% 54%	4% 10%	6–19 months	Marked differences among the different subtypes of NHL; marked activity in MCL	O'Connor et al. (110) O'Connor et al. (109)
B-cell lymphoma	60	41% in MCL and 15% in all other B-cell neoplasms	20% in MCL	6 months MCL	Significant activity in MCL, minimal in other subtypes, though heavily treated population of patients	Goy et al. (112)
Mantle cell lymphoma	30	33%	3%	2.5–14.8 months	10 patients received no prior therapy, 14 had prior therapy; minimal difference between the two	Belch et al. (141)
Non–small cell lung cancer	27	4%	0%	NR	12 patients experienced stabilization of their disease	Stevenson (115)
Renal cell carcinoma	21	5%	0%	2 months	Allowed dose escalations to 1.7 mg/m² with no clear benefit	Davis et al. (113)
Renal cell carcinoma	37	11%	0%	8–20+ months	Median survival was 7.5 months	Kondagunta et al. (112)

ORR, overall response rate; CR, complete remissions.

fatigue (49%), thrombocytopenia (44%), constipation (43%), vomiting (36%), anorexia (34%), and sensory neuropathy (34%). Overall, most of these adverse effects were grade 1 or 2. Severe adverse events (>grade 3) included thrombocytopenia (29%), peripheral neuropathy (14%), neutropenia (15%), asthenia (11%), and anemia (9%). The frequency and severity of the diarrhea appeared to be dose-dependent. Based on these data, bortezomib was approved by the FDA for the treatment of relapsed or refractory multiple myeloma in May 2003.

Following the Summit trial, a second dose-response phase II study of bortezomib in myeloma was launched (the Crest study). This trial was an open-label, randomized phase II dose-response study in 54 patients who received bortezomib at a dose of 1.3 or 1.0 mg/m² on days 1, 4, 8, and 11 every 21 days.[108] The median number of prior therapies was three for both cohorts, with about 48% of all patients having received prior stem cell transplantation. In the Crest study, no grade 4 adverse events were reported, and the side effect profile was similar to what had been seen in the Summit trial. The overall response rate according to the European Group for Blood and Marrow Transplantation criteria (cases of complete remission plus cases of partial remission) was 38% and 30% in the 1.3 mg/m² (n = 26) and 1.0 mg/m² (n = 28) cohorts, respectively. One complete remission was noted at each dose level (about a 3.7%

complete remission rate). There was no statistically significant difference in response rate between the two cohorts. As expected, the incidence of adverse effects was less at the 1.0 mg/m² dose level, with less overall peripheral neuropathy, fewer neuropathic pain syndromes, less weakness, and less neutropenia being noted. This study, while not statistically powered to address the issue of equivalency between these two dose cohorts, clearly demonstrated that a lower dose of bortezomib was effective in myeloma and had a more favorable adverse effects profile.

The promising single-agent activity in patients with relapsed or refractory multiple myeloma has prompted a multitude of clinical trials studying the activity of bortezomib as primary treatment as well as in the relapsed setting in combination with other active drugs. For example, the APEX study randomly assigned patients to receive dexamethasone at a dose of 40 mg/day orally on days 1 to 4, 9 to 12, and 17 to 20 every 5 weeks or bortezomib at a dose of 1.3 mg/m² on the typical schedule used in the Summit study. Patients in the bortezomib arm experienced a 58% improvement in median time to progression (5.7 months) compared with patients receiving dexamethasone (3.6 months); the difference was statistically significant. Jagannath et al.[108] reported a phase II study in which untreated patients with myeloma received bortezomib as in the Summit study; however, for those patients who did not achieve partial remission or remission, dexamethasone was added. Of 24 evaluable patients, 6 patients attained either a complete remission or near complete remission, while 13 attained a partial remission, for an overall response rate of 79%. Of the 14 patients who received additional dexamethasone, 8 demonstrated an improvement in their response.

Non-Hodgkin's Lymphoma

Based upon the activity seen in the phase I study, a single-agent phase II study of bortezomib in patients with indolent and mantle cell lymphoma was initiated.[109,110] This study was limited to patients with follicular lymphoma, mantle cell lymphoma, small lymphocytic lymphoma/chronic lymphocytic leukemia, and marginal zone lymphoma. Unlike in the Summit study, all patients were initially treated with a dose of 1.5 mg/m^2 on days 1, 4, 8, and 11 every 21 days, with criteria for dose reduction to 1.3 and 1.1 mg/m^2. Patients were required to have three or fewer lines of prior therapy and were allowed to have been treated with prior radioimmunotherapy and/or peripheral stem cell transplantation.[109,110] The median age of the 59 patients was 62, with a median KPS of 90%, with a slight male predominance. Thirty patients (51%) had mantle cell lymphoma, 18 (31%) had follicular lymphoma, 6 had marginal zone lymphoma, and 5 had small lymphocytic lymphoma. Overall the drug was well tolerated, with only one half of all patients requiring a dose reduction to 1.3 mg/m^2, mostly for issues related to thrombocytopenia, asthenia, and neuropathy. The median number of prior therapies was three, and virtually all patients had received rituximab, about half having received multiple courses of rituximab. The different forms of lymphoma had quite variable overall response rates and time to response. Overall, the response rate was 54%. Sixty-five percent of patients with follicular lymphoma achieved a response, with 2 patients meeting criteria for complete response or unconfirmed complete response. Among patients with mantle cell lymphoma, 54% of these patients achieved a major response, with 4 meeting criteria for complete response or unconfirmed complete response. Interestingly, patients with follicular lymphoma tended to respond later, on average after cycle 3 or 4, while patients with mantle cell lymphoma typically responded by the second cycle. In all cases, the responses were durable, with most patients having a duration of remission that exceeded that seen with the last treatment before receiving the study drug. Following this study, a second study of bortezomib in B-cell lymphomas was launched, which included patients with any subtype of B-cell non-Hodgkin's lymphoma, with no cap on the number of prior therapies. Adopting virtually the same study design, this study initially established cohorts for patients with mantle cell lymphoma alone and patients with other types of B-cell neoplasms. Overall, the patients reported in the study by Goy et al.[111] were more heavily pretreated. Of 29 patients with MCL, 12 met the criteria for a major response, with 6 attaining a complete remission. Among the patients with other B-cell neoplasms, 12 had diffuse large B-cell lymphoma, of which only 1 attained a partial remission. Overall, the experience in NHL is encouraging; however, response rates will need to be defined for each histologic form of lymphoma.

Solid Tumors

Early clues to the activity of bortezomib in solid tumors were seen in the two phase I studies of the drug. In one of these phase I studies, Aghajanian et al.[103] treated 43 patients on days 1, 4, 8, and 11 every 21 days, with doses ranging from 0.13 to 1.56 mg/m^2. In this heavily treated patient population, one patient with NSCLC (bronchioloalveolar type) achieved a partial remission. The remission lasted about three months. In the second single-agent phase I experience, a weekly schedule of bortezomib administration at doses ranging from 0.13 to 2 mg/m^2 was studied. Responses were seen in patients with androgen-independent prostate cancer (AIPCa) but not in patients with renal cell carcinoma or transitional cell carcinoma.[104] Two (4%) of the 47 patients with AIPCa had a greater than 50% decline in serum prostate-specific antigen (PSA) while 9 (19%) of 47 patients had stable PSA measurements over the study period. Two patients with measurable disease attained partial remission, with shrinkage of their retroperitoneal lymphadenopathy. One of these responses was seen at a dose of 0.4 mg/m^2, the other at a dose of 1.6 mg/m^2.

Some suggestion of activity has also been reported in patients with metastatic renal cell carcinoma. Thirty-seven patients were treated at a dose of 1.5 mg/m^2 on days 1, 4, 8, and 11.[112] Four of these patients achieved a partial remission, while another 14 were found to have stable disease after having documented disease progression at the time of enrollment. The remissions were durable, lasting 8, 8+, 15+, and 20+ months. With a median follow-up of 11.7 months, the proportion of patients alive at one year was 36%, and the median survival time was 7.5 months. In contrast, a second phase II study in patients with renal cell carcinoma reported on 21 assessable patients, of which only 1 partial remission was reported.[113] Interestingly, a large retrospective study of over 251 patients with renal cell carcinoma enrolled in 29 consecutive clinical trials at Memorial Sloan Kettering Cancer Center between 1975 and 2002 demonstrated that patients treated after 1990 showed slightly longer survival compared with patients treated prior to 1990.[114] More importantly, the authors established three major prognostic factors for this patient population that adversely affect outcome: low Karnofsky performance status, low hemoglobin, and a high corrected serum calcium level. The median time to death in patients with zero risk factors was 22 months. In comparison, the median time to death for patients with one or two to three risk factors was 11.9 and 5.4 months, respectively. This kind of analysis is essential for deciphering the true benefit of novel drugs in the single-agent phase II setting.

Based on the response seen in the original phase I experience, a single-agent study of bortezomib inpatients with advanced NSCLC was initiated using a dose of 1.5 mg/m2 on days 1, 4, 8, and 11 every 21 days. Among 27 evaluable patients, 1 achieved partial remission, and 12 had stable disease.[115] It is not clear what biological features separate responding from nonresponding patients with NSCLC. Additional phase II studies to define activity in other tumor types are underway or planned.

Combination Phase I/II Experiences

The natural evolution of most drug treatment strategies is to explore integration into standard chemotherapy regimens. The rationale for integrating drugs that target the ubiquitin-proteasome pathway, in particular, the NF-κB signaling pathways, is that there is a strong theoretical basis for drug synergy with this class of molecules. Many types of environmental stress, including chemotherapy exposure, hypoxia, and radiation exposure, are known to activate NF-κB, presumably as part of a survival response. For example, irinotecan (CPT-11) has been shown to markedly increase NF-κB levels, which leads to the increased transcription of anti-apoptotic factors and cell survival.[116,117] If all the cells within in any tumor population are not completely eradicated with a given cytotoxic drug, then those cells left behind will activate various survival pathways to overcome the antitumor activity of the cytotoxic agent. If one could block the induction of this survival response by inhibiting NF-κB, then one might overcome some of these survival strategies and improve antitumor efficacy.

A number of studies have documented synergistic effects by combining bortezomib with a host of conventional drugs, including irinotecan, paclitaxel, doxorubicin, rituximab, bcl-2 antisense, cyclophosphamide, and several other drugs.[36,118–123] This sort of approach is now being studied in a variety of combination phase I and II studies in both hematologic and solid tumor malignancies. The results of such studies are eagerly anticipated.

Some encouraging clinical data in support of synergistic interactions have been reported by Orlowski et al.[124] (2005), who have explored a combination of bortezomib and pegylated liposomal doxorubicin (PegLD). The basis of this particular synergistic interaction is derived from the observation that proteasome inhibitors transcriptionally induce the MKP-1 phosphatases a process which is antiapoptotic through its inactivation of JNK, while anthracyclines like doxorubicin appear to down-regulate MKP-1.[125,126] In the phase I experience with this combination, bortezomib was administered on days 1, 4, 8, and 11 at doses ranging from 0.9 to 1.5 mg/m², while the PegLD was administered at a fixed dose of 30 mg/m² on day 4 every 21 days. The MTD was determined to be 1.3 mg/m2 of bortezomib with 30 mg/m² of PegLD. Based on 22 evaluable patients, 8

patients with advanced multiple myeloma had a complete remission or near complete remission, including several with anthracycline-resistant myeloma. Another 8 myeloma patients experienced a partial remission. Additionally, one patient with refractory T-cell lymphoma achieved a complete remission, one patient with acute myeloid leukemia achieved a partial remission, and one patient with non-Hodgkin's lymphoma achieved a partial remission. The remarkable activity seen in myeloma has now led to what will likely be a large cooperative group trial of this combination in multiple myeloma.

The future development of bortezomib will depend on the toxicity and efficacy of this agent in combination with other conventional and investigational agents. Preclinical data support the notion that proteasome inhibitors may be synergistic with other novel classes of drugs, including histone deacetylase inhibitors, cyclin-dependent kinase inhibitors like flavopiridol, and the bcl-2 antisense molecule G3139 (Genasense).[123,127,128] What remains to be clarified from a pharmacologic perspective is the importance of scheduling these agents and defining the optimal concentrations of these drugs for inhibiting their principal targets. For example, in some in vivo models of non-Hodgkin's lymphoma, the activity of the bcl-2 antisense molecule G3139 with cyclophosphamide and bortezomib was found to be very schedule dependent. Better results were seen using antisense bcl-2 first followed by cyclophosphamide and then followed 24 hours later by bortezomib.[123] Combinations of many standard chemotherapy drugs are often given together. Such approaches, while certainly more convenient for the patient, often disregard compelling preclinical evidence of schedule dependency. The onus is now on both laboratory and physician scientists to understand these scheduling phenomena and then to elucidate the biological basis for the schedule dependency. In addition to sorting out these critical pharmacologic questions with this new class of molecules, it is apparent that understanding the molecular basis for the response or nonresponse of certain patients will be absolutely critical in the development of new classes of drugs.

FUTURE DIRECTIONS

Investigators have begun to explore the relationships between the response and gene expression profile of a particular myeloma. For example, in a recent study presented by Barlow et al.,[129] different subsets of genes were identified that could be used to predict survival and event-free survival in myeloma patients receiving bortezomib. A subset of 10 genes were then identified that could predict poor survival, including genes involved in cell cycle control like CDC2, TYMS, BUBI, TOP2A, and Ki-67. Additional data presented by Richardson et al.[130] have also established that both clinical and molecular information can be used to identify relatively good-risk and poor-risk populations of patients with respect to their ability to respond to bortezomib. The identification of patients most likely to benefit from a particular therapeutic approach is an important goal and may one day allow oncologists to construct drug cocktails capable of producing the best effects in particular patients.

REFERENCES

1. Hershko A, Ciechanover A, Rose IA. Resolution of the ATP-dependent proteolytic system from reticulocytes: a component that interacts with ATP. Proc Natl Acad Sci USA 1979;76: 3107–3110.
2. Ciechanover A, Heller H, Elias S, et al. ATP-dependent conjugation of reticulocyte proteins with the polypeptide required for protein degradation. Proc Natl Acad Sci USA 1980;77:1365–1368.
3. Hershko A, Ciechanover A, Heller H, et al. Proposed role of ATP in protein breakdown: conjugation of protein with multiple chains of the polypeptide of ATP-dependent proteolysis. Proc Natl Acad Sci USA 1980;77:1783–1786.
4. Ciechanover A, Elias S, Heller H, et al. Characterization of the heat-stable polypeptide of the ATP-dependent proteolytic system from reticulocytes. J Biol Chem 1980;255:7525–7528.
5. Ciechanover A, Heller H, Katz-Etzion R, et al. Activation of the heat-stable polypeptide of the ATP-dependent proteolytic system. Proc Natl Acad Sci USA 1981;78:761–765.
6. Hershko A, Ciechanover A, Rose IA. Identification of the active amino acid residue of the polypeptide of ATP-dependent protein breakdown. J Biol Chem 1981;256:1525–1528.
7. Ciechanover A. The ubiquitin-proteasome proteolytic pathway. Cell 1994;79:13–21.
8. Goldberg AL. Protein turnover in skeletal muscle, II: effects of denervation and cortisone on protein catabolism in skeletal muscle. J Biol Chem 1969;244:3223–3229.
9. Mitch WE, Goldberg AL. Mechanisms of muscle wasting: the role of the ubiquitin-proteasome pathway. N Engle J Med 1996;335: 1897–1905.
10. Goldberg AL. A role of aminoacyl-tRNA in the regulation of protein breakdown in Escherichia coli. Proc Natl Acad Sci USA 1971; 68:362–366.
11. Goldberg AL. Degradation of abnormal proteins in Escherichia coli (protein breakdown-protein structure-mistranslation-amino acid analogs-puromycin). Proc Natl Acad Sci USA 1972;69: 422–426.
12. Orlowski M. The multicatalytic proteinase complex, a major extralysosomal proteolytic system. Biochemistry 1990;29: 10289–10297.
13. Arrigo AP, Tanaka K, Goldberg AL, et al. Identity of the 19S "prosome" particle with the large multifunctional protease complex of mammalian cells (the proteasome). Nature 1988;331: 192–194.
14. Matthews W, Driscoll J, Tanaka K, et al. Involvement of the proteasome in various degradative processes in mammalian cells. Proc Natl Acad Sci USA 1989;86:2597–2601.
15. Eytan E, Ganoth D, Armon T, et al. ATP-dependent incorporation of 20S protease into the 26S complex that degrades proteins conjugated to ubiquitin. Proc Natl Acad Sci USA 1989;86: 7751–7755.
16. Driscoll J, Goldberg AL. The proteasome (multicatalytic protease) is a component of the 1500-kDa proteolytic complex which degrades ubiquitin-conjugated proteins. J Biol Chem 1990;265:4789–4792.
17. Palombella VJ, Rando OJ, Goldberg AL, et al. The ubiquitin-proteasome pathway is required for processing the NF-κ B1 precursor protein and the activation of NF-κ B. Cell 1994; 78: 773–785.
18. Corey EJ, Li WD. Total synthesis and biological activity of lactacystin, omuralide and analogs. Chem Pharm Bull (Tokyo) 1999;47:1–10.
19. Fenteany G, Standaert RF, Lane WS, et al. Inhibition of proteasome activities and subunit-specific amino-terminal threonine modification by lactacystin. Science 1995;268:726–731.
20. Fenteany G, Standaert RF, Reichard GA, et al. A beta-lactone related to lactacystin induces neurite outgrowth in a neuroblastoma cell line and inhibits cell cycle progression in an osteosarcoma cell line. Proc Natl Acad Sci USA 1994;91:3358–3362.
21. Katagiri M, Hayashi M, Matsuzaki K, et al. The neuritogenesis inducer lactacystin arrests cell cycle at both G0/G1 and G2 phases in neuro 2a cells. J Antibiot (Tokyo) 1995;48:344–346.
22. Hanada M, Sugawara K, Kaneta K, et al. Epoxomicin, a new antitumor agent of microbial origin. J Antibiot (Tokyo) 1992;45: 1746–1752.
23. Sin N, Kim KB, Elofsson M, et al. Total synthesis of the potent proteasome inhibitor epoxomicin: a useful tool for understanding proteasome biology. Bioorg Med Chem Lett 1999;9: 2283–2288.
24. Bogyo M, McMaster JS, Gaczynska M, et al. Covalent modification of the active site threonine of proteasomal beta subunits and the Escherichia coli homolog HslV by a new class of inhibitors. Proc Natl Acad Sci USA 1997;94:6629–6634.
25. Bogyo M, Shin S, McMaster JS, et al. Substrate binding and sequence preference of the proteasome revealed by active-site–directed affinity probes. Chem Biol 1998;5:307–320.
26. Wilk S, Orlowski M. Evidence that pituitary cation-sensitive neutral endopeptidase is a multicatalytic protease complex. J Neurochem 1983;40:842–849.
27. Figueiredo-Pereira ME, Berg KA, Wilk S. A new inhibitor of the chymotrypsin-like activity of the multicatalytic proteinase complex (20S proteasome) induces accumulation of ubiquitin-protein conjugates in a neuronal cell. J Neurochem 1994;63: 1578–1581.
28. Rock KL, Gramm C, Rothstein L, et al. Inhibitors of the proteasome block the degradation of most cell proteins and the generation of peptides presented on MHC class I molecules. Cell 1994;78:761–771.
29. Vinitsky A, Cardozo C, Sepp-Lorenzino L, et al. Inhibition of the proteolytic activity of the multicatalytic proteinase complex (proteasome) by substrate-related peptidyl aldehydes. J Biol Chem 1994;269:29860–29866.
30. Adams J, Behnke M, Chen S, et al. Potent and selective inhibitors of the proteasome: dipeptidyl boronic acids. Bioorg Med Chem Lett 1998;8:333–338.
31. Adams J, Palombella VJ, Sausville EA, et al. Proteasome inhibitors: a novel class of potent and effective antitumor agents. Cancer Res 1999;59:2615–2622.
32. Lowe J, Stock D, Jap B, et al. Crystal structure of the 20S proteasome from the archaeon T. acidophilum at 3.4 A resolution. Science 1995;268:533–539.
33. Hershko A, Ciechanover A. The ubiquitin system for protein degradation. Annu Rev Biochem 1992;61:761–807.
34. Rechsteiner M, Hoffman L, Dubiel W. The multicatalytic and 26 S proteases. J Biol Chem 1993;268:6065–6068.
35. Adams J. Potential for proteasome inhibition in the treatment of cancer. Drug Discov Today 2003;8:307–315.
36. Adams J, Palombella VJ, Elliott PJ. Proteasome inhibition: a new strategy in cancer treatment. Invest New Drugs 2000;18:109–121.
37. Nussbaum AK, Dick TP, Keilholz W, et al. Cleavage motifs of the yeast 20S proteasome beta subunits deduced from digests of enolase 1. Proc Natl Acad Sci USA 1998;95:12504–12509.
38. Kisselev AF, Akopian TN, Woo KM, et al. The sizes of peptides generated from protein by mammalian 26 and 20 S proteasomes: implications for understanding the degradative mechanism and antigen presentation. J Biol Chem 1999;274: 3363–3371.
39. Holzl H, Kapelari B, Kellermann J, et al. The regulatory complex of Drosophila melanogaster 26S proteasomes: subunit composition and localization of a deubiquitylating enzyme. J Cell Biol 2000;150:119–130.
40. Voges D, Zwickl P, Baumeister W. The 26S proteasome: a molecular machine designed for controlled proteolysis. Annu Rev Biochem 1999;68:1015–1068.
41. Ciechanover A. The ubiquitin-proteasome pathway: on protein death and cell life. EMBO J 1998;17:7151–7160.
42. Lee DH, Goldberg AL. Proteasome inhibitors: valuable new tools for cell biologists. Trends Cell Biol 1998;8:397–403.
43. Spataro V, Norbury C, Harris AL. The ubiquitin-proteasome pathway in cancer. Br J Cancer 1998;77:448–455.

44. Zwickl P, Baumeister W, Steven A. Dis-assembly lines: the protea-some and related ATPase-assisted proteases. Curr Opin Struct Biol 2000;10:242–250.

45. Baeuerle PA, Baltimore D. NF-kappa B: ten years after. Cell 1996;87:13–20.

46. Baldwin AS Jr. The NF-kappa B and I kappa B proteins: new dis-coveries and insights. Annu Rev Immunol 1996;14:649–683.

47. Siebenlist U, Franzoso G, Brown K. Structure, regulation and function of NF-kappa B. Annu Rev Cell Biol 1994;10:405–455.

48. Andreakos E, Sacre SM, Smith C, et al. Distinct pathways of LPS-induced NF-kappa B activation and cytokine production in human myeloid and nonmyeloid cells defined by selective uti-lization of MyD88 and Mal/TIRAP. Blood 2004;103:2229–2237.

49. Guo Z, Zhang M, An H, et al. Fas ligation induces IL-1beta–dependent maturation and IL-1beta–independent survival of dendritic cells: different roles of ERK and NF-kappaB signaling pathways. Blood 2003;102:4441–4447.

50. O'Neil J, Ventura JJ, Cusson N, et al. NF-kappaB activation in premalignant mouse tal-1/scl thymocytes and tumors. Blood 2003;102:2593–2596.

51. Voorhees PM, Dees C, O'Neil B et al. The proteasome as a target for cancer therapy. Clinical Cancer Research; 9:6316–6325.

52. Sen R, Baltimore D. Multiple nuclear factors interact with the immunoglobulin enhancer sequences. Cell 1986;46:705–716.

53. Sen R, Baltimore D. Inducibility of kappa immunoglobulin enhancer-binding protein Nf-kappa B by a posttranslational mechanism. Cell 1986;47:921–928.

54. Harper JW, Adami GR, Wei N, et al. The p21 Cdk-interacting pro-tein Cip1 is a potent inhibitor of G1 cyclin-dependent kinases. Cell 1993;75:805–816.

55. Blagosklonny MV, Wu GS, Omura S, et al. Proteasome-depen-dent regulation of p21$^{WAF1/CIP1}$ expression. Biochem Biophys Res Commun 1996;227:564–569.

56. Tassan JP, Schultz SJ, Bartek J, et al. Cell cycle analysis of the activ-ity, subcellular localization, and subunit composition of human CAK (CDK-activating kinase). J Cell Biol 1994;127:467–478.

57. Glotzer M, Murray AW, Kirschner MW. Cyclin is degraded by the ubiquitin pathway. Nature 1991;349:132–138.

58. Polyak K, Lee MH, Erdjument-Bromage H, et al. Cloning of p27Kip1, a cyclin-dependent kinase inhibitor and a potential mediator of extracellular antimitogenic signals. Cell 1994;78:59–66.

59. Toyoshima H, Hunter T. p27, a novel inhibitor of G1 cyclin-Cdk protein kinase activity, is related to p21. Cell 1994;78:67–74.

60. Machiels BM, Henfling ME, Gerards WL, et al. Detailed analysis of cell cycle kinetics upon proteasome inhibition. Cytometry 1997;28:243–252.

61. Pagano M, Tam SW, Theodoras AM, et al. Role of the ubiquitin-proteasome pathway in regulating abundance of the cyclin-dependent kinase inhibitor p27. Science 1995;269:682–685.

62. Lim MS, Adamson A, Lin Z, et al. Expression of Skp2, a p27(Kip1) ubiquitin ligase, in malignant lymphoma: correlation with p27(Kip1) and proliferation index. Blood 2002;100:2950–2956.

63. Chiarle R, Budel LM, Skolnik J, et al. Increased proteasome degradation of cyclin-dependent kinase inhibitor p27 is associ-ated with a decreased overall survival in mantle cell lymphoma. Blood 2000;95:619–626.

64. Bogner C, Ringshausen I, Schneller F, et al. Inhibition of the pro-teasome induces cell cycle arrest and apoptosis in mantle cell lymphoma cells. Br J Haematol 2003;122:260–268.

65. Ling YH, Liebes L, Jiang JD, et al. Mechanisms of proteasome inhibitor PS-341–induced G(2)-M-phase arrest and apoptosis in human non-small cell lung cancer cell lines. Clin Cancer Res 2003;9:1145–1154.

66. Vaskivuo TE, Stenback F, Tapanainen JS. Apoptosis and apoptosis-related factors Bcl-2, Bax, tumor necrosis factor-alpha, and NF-kappaB in human endometrial hyperplasia and carcinoma. Cancer 2002;95:1463–1471.

67. Beg AA, Baltimore D. An essential role for NF-kappaB in prevent-ing TNF-alpha–induced cell death. Science 1996;274:782–784.

68. Van Antwerp DJ, Martin SJ, Kafri T, et al. Suppression of TNF-alpha–induced apoptosis by NF-kappaB. Science 1996;274:787–789.

69. Wang CY, Mayo MW, Baldwin AS Jr. TNF- and cancer therapy-induced apoptosis: potentiation by inhibition of NF-kappaB. Science 1996;274:784–787.

70. Marshansky V, Wang X, Bertrand R, et al. Proteasomes modulate balance among proapoptotic and antiapoptotic Bcl-2 family members and compromise functioning of the electron transport chain in leukemic cells. J Immunol 2001;166:3130–3142.

71. Ling YH, Liebes L, Ng B, et al. PS-341, a novel proteasome inhibitor, induces Bcl-2 phosphorylation and cleavage in associ-ation with G2-M phase arrest and apoptosis. Mol Cancer Ther 2002;1:841–849.

72. Heckman CA, Mehew JW, Boxer LM. NF-kappaB activates Bcl-2 expression in t(14;18) lymphoma cells. Oncogene 2002;21:3898–3908.

73. Cleary ML, Smith SD, Sklar J. Cloning and structural analysis of cDNAs for bcl-2 and a hybrid bcl-2/immunoglobulin tran-script resulting from the t(14;18) translocation. Cell 1986;47:19–28.

74. Tsujimoto Y, Gorham J, Cossman J, et al. The t(14;18) chromo-some translocations involved in B-cell neoplasms result from mistakes in VDJ joining. Science 1985;229:1390–1393.

75. Tsujimoto Y, Croce CM. Analysis of the structure, transcripts, and protein products of bcl-2, the gene involved in human follicular lymphoma. Proc Natl Acad Sci USA 1986;83:5214–5218.

76. Pham LV, Tamayo AT, Yoshimura LC, et al. Inhibition of consti-tutive NF-kappa B activation in mantle cell lymphoma B cells leads to induction of cell cycle arrest and apoptosis. J Immunol 2003;171:88–95.

77. Goldberg AL. Protein degradation and protection against mis-folded or damaged proteins. Nature 2003;426:895–899.

78. Lee AH, Iwakoshi NN, Anderson KC, et al. Proteasome inhibitors disrupt the unfolded protein response in myeloma cells. Proc Natl Acad Sci USA 2003;100:9946–9951.

79. Kisselev AF, Goldberg AL. Proteasome inhibitors: from research tools to drug candidates. Chem Biol 2001;8:739–758.

80. Meiners S, Heyken D, Weller A, et al. Inhibition of proteasome activity induces concerted expression of proteasome genes and de novo formation of mammalian proteasomes. J Biol Chem 2003;278:21517–21525.

81. Meriin AB, Yaglom JA, Gabai VL, et al. Protein-damaging stresses activate c-Jun N-terminal kinase via inhibition of its dephospho-rylation: a novel pathway controlled by HSP72. Mol Cell Biol 1999;19:2547–2555.

82. Sherman MY, Goldberg AL. Cellular defenses against unfolded proteins: a cell biologist thinks about neurodegenerative dis-eases. Neuron 2001;29:15–32.

83. Imajoh-Ohmi S, Kawaguchi T, Sugiyama S, et al. Lactacystin, a specific inhibitor of the proteasome, induces apoptosis in human monoblast U937 cells. Biochem Biophys Res Commun 1995;217:1070–1077.

84. Lopes UG, Erhardt P, Yao R, et al. p53-dependent induction of apoptosis by proteasome inhibitors. J Biol Chem 1997;272:12893–12896.

85. An B, Goldfarb RH, Siman R, et al. Novel dipeptidyl proteasome inhibitors overcome Bcl-2 protective function and selectively accumulate the cyclin-dependent kinase inhibitor p27 and induce apoptosis in transformed, but not normal, human fibroblasts. Cell Death Differ 1998;5:1062–1075.

86. Orlowski RZ, Eswara JR, Lafond-Walker A, et al. Tumor growth inhibition induced in a murine model of human Burkitt's lym-phoma by a proteasome inhibitor. Cancer Res 1998;58:4342–4348.

87. Boyd MR, Paull D. Some practical considerations and applica-tions of the National Cancer Institute in vitro anticancer drug discovery screen. Drug Devel. Res. 34:91–109,1995.

88. Mitsiades N, Mitsiades CS, Richardson PG, et al. The proteasome inhibitor PS-341 potentiates sensitivity of multiple myeloma cells to conventional chemotherapeutic agents: therapeutic applications. Blood 2003;101:2377–2380.

89. Hideshima T, Richardson P, Chauhan D, et al. The proteasome inhibitor PS-341 inhibits growth, induces apoptosis, and over-comes drug resistance in human multiple myeloma cells. Cancer Res 2001;61:3071–3076.

90. Hideshima T, Mitsiades C, Akiyama M, et al. Molecular mechanisms mediating antimyeloma activity of proteasome inhibitor PS-341. Blood 2003;101:1530-1534.

91. LeBlanc R, Catley LP, Hideshima T, et al. Proteasome inhibitor PS-341 inhibits human myeloma cell growth in vivo and prolongs survival in a murine model. Cancer Res 2002;62:4996-5000.

92. Read MA, Neish AS, Luscinskas FW, et al. The proteasome pathway is required for cytokine-induced endothelial-leukocyte adhesion molecule expression. Immunity 1995;2:493-506.

93. Nefedova Y, Landowski TH, Dalton WS. Bone marrow stromal-derived soluble factors and direct cell contact contribute to de novo drug resistance of myeloma cells by distinct mechanisms. Leukemia 2003;17:1175-1182.

94. Damiano JS, Cress AE, Hazlehurst LA, et al. Cell adhesion mediated drug resistance (CAM-DR): role of integrins and resistance to apoptosis in human myeloma cell lines. Blood 1999;93:1658-1667.

95. Mitsiades N, Mitsiades CS, Poulaki V, et al. Molecular sequelae of proteasome inhibition in human multiple myeloma cells. Proc Natl Acad Sci USA 2002;99:14374-14379.

96. Sunwoo JB, Chen Z, Dong G, et al. Novel proteasome inhibitor PS-341 inhibits activation of nuclear factor-kappa B, cell survival, tumor growth, and angiogenesis in squamous cell carcinoma. Clin Cancer Res 2001;7:1419-1428.

97. Vacca A, Ribatti D, Presta M, et al. Bone marrow neovascularization, plasma cell angiogenic potential, and matrix metalloproteinase-2 secretion parallel progression of human multiple myeloma. Blood 1999;93:3064-3073.

98. Oikawa T, Sasaki T, Nakamura M, et al. The proteasome is involved in angiogenesis. Biochem Biophys Res Commun 1998;246:243-248.

99. Mezquita J, Mezquita B, Pau M, et al. Down-regulation of Flt-1 gene expression by the proteasome inhibitor MG262. J Cell Biochem 2003;89:1138-1147.

100. Supko JG, Eder JP, Lynch TJ, et al. Pharmacokinetics of gemcitabine and the proteasome inhibitor bortezomib (formerly PS-341) in adult patients with solid malignancies. Annual Meeting Proceedings–American Society of Clinical Oncology, 2003, Volume 22, Abstract 544.

101. Nix D, Pien C, Newman R, et al. Clinical Development of a proteasome inhibitor, PS-341, for the treatment of cancer. Annual Meeting Proceedings–American Society of Clinical Oncology, 2001, Volume 20, Abstract 339.

102. Orlowski RZ, Stinchcombe TE, Mitchell BS, et al. Phase I trial of the proteasome inhibitor PS-341 in patients with refractory hematologic malignancies. J Clin Oncol 2002a;20:4420-4427.

103. Aghajanian C, Soignet S, Dizon DS, et al. A phase I trial of the novel proteasome inhibitor PS341 in advanced solid tumor malignancies. Clin Cancer Res 2002;8:2505-2511.

104. Papandreou CN, Daliani DD, Nix D, et al. Phase I trial of the proteasome inhibitor bortezomib in patients with advanced solid tumors with observations in androgen-independent prostate cancer. J Clin Oncol 2004;22:2108-2121.

105. Logothetis CJ. Dose-dependent inhibition of 20S proteasome results in serum Il-6 and PSA decline in patients (PTS) with androgen-independent prostate cancer (AIPCa) treated with the proteasome inhibitor PS-341. Proc Am Soc Clin Oncol 2001; Abstract 740.

106. Richardson PG, Barlogie B, Berenson J, et al. A phase 2 study of bortezomib in relapsed, refractory myeloma. N Engl J Med 2003;348:2609-2617.

107. Kane RC, Bross PF, Farrell AT, et al. Velcade: U.S. FDA approval for the treatment of multiple myeloma progressing on prior therapy. Oncologist 2003;8:508-513.

108. Jagannath S, Barlogie B, Berenson J, et al. A phase 2 study of two doses of bortezomib in relapsed or refractory myeloma. Br J Haematol 2004;127:165-172.

109. O'Connor OA. The emerging role of bortezomib in the treatment of indolent non-Hodgkin's and mantle cell lymphomas. Curr Treat Options Oncol 2004;5:269-281.

110. O'Connor OA, Wright J, Moskowitz C, et al. Phase II clinical experience with the novel proteasome inhibitor bortezomib in patients with indolent non-Hodgkin's lymphoma and mantle cell lymphoma. J Clin Oncol 2005; Feb 1;23(4):676-684.

111. Goy A, Younes A, McLaughlin P, et al. Phase II study of proteasome inhibitor bortezomib in relapsed or refractory B-cell non-Hodgkin's lymphoma. J Clin Oncol 2005; Feb 1;23(4)667-75.

112. Kondagunta GV, Drucker B, Schwartz L, et al. Phase II trial of bortezomib for patients with advanced renal cell carcinoma. J Clin Oncol 2004;22:3720-3725.

113. Davis NB, Taber DA, Ansari RH, et al. Phase II trial of PS-341 in patients with renal cell cancer: a University of Chicago phase II consortium study. J Clin Oncol 2004;22:115-119.

114. Motzer RJ, Bacik J, Schwartz LH, et al. Prognostic factors for survival in previously treated patients with metastatic renal cell carcinoma. J Clin Oncol 2004;22:454-463.

115. Stevenson JP, Nho CW, Johnson SW, et al. Effects of bortezomib (PS-341) on NF-KB activation in peripheral blood mononuclear cells (PBMCs) of advanced non-small lung cancer (NSCLC) patients: a phase II/pharmacodynamic trial. Annual Meeting Proceedings. American Society of Clinical Oncology 2004;23, Abstract 2346.

116. Wang CY, Cusack JC Jr, Liu R, et al. Control of inducible chemoresistance: enhanced anti-tumor therapy through increased apoptosis by inhibition of NF-kappaB. Nat Med 1999;5:412-417.

117. Cusack JC Jr, Liu R, Houston M, et al. Enhanced chemosensitivity to CPT-11 with proteasome inhibitor PS-341: implications for systemic nuclear factor-kappaB inhibition. Cancer Res 2001;61:3535-3540.

118. Orlowski RZ, Baldwin AS Jr. NF-kappaB as a therapeutic target in cancer. Trends Mol Med 2002;8:385-389.

119. Ma MH, Yang HH, Parker K, et al. The proteasome inhibitor PS-341 markedly enhances sensitivity of multiple myeloma tumor cells to chemotherapeutic agents. Clin Cancer Res 2003;9:1136-1144.

120. Teicher BA, Ara G, Herbst R, et al. The proteasome inhibitor PS-341 in cancer therapy. Clin Cancer Res 1999;5:2638-2645.

121. Wang CY, Guttridge DC, Mayo MW, et al. NF-kappaB induces expression of the Bcl-2 homologue A1/Bfl-1 to preferentially suppress chemotherapy-induced apoptosis. Mol Cell Biol 1999; 19:5923-5929.

122. Desai SD, Liu LF, Vazquez-Abad D, et al. Ubiquitin-dependent destruction of topoisomerase I is stimulated by the antitumor drug camptothecin. J Biol Chem 1997;272:24159-24164.

123. O'Connor O, Wright J, Moskowitz C, et al. Promising activity of the proteasome inhibitor bortezomib (Velcade) in the treatment of indolent non-Hodgkin's lymphoma and mantle cell lymphoma. Blood 2003;102(11) Abstract 7145.

124. Orlowski RZ, Voorhes PM, Garcia RA, et al. Phase I trial of the proteasome inhibitor bortezomib and pegylated liposomal doxorubicin in patients with advanced hematologic malignancies Blood, 2005;105(8):3058-3065.

125. Orlowski RZ, Small GW, Shi YY. Evidence that inhibition of p44/42 mitogen–activated protein kinase signaling is a factor in proteasome inhibitor–mediated apoptosis. J Biol Chem 2002; 277:27864-27871.

126. Small GW, Somasundaram S, Moore DT, et al. Repression of mitogen-activated protein kinase (MAPK) phosphatase-1 by anthracyclines contributes to their antiapoptotic activation of p44/42-MAPK. J Pharmacol Exp Ther 2003;307:861-869.

127. Gao N, Dai Y, Rahmani M, et al. Contribution of disruption of the nuclear factor-kappaB pathway to induction of apoptosis in human leukemia cells by histone deacetylase inhibitors and flavopiridol. Mol Pharmacol 2004;66:956-963.

128. Dai Y, Rahmani M, Pei XY, et al. Bortezomib and flavopiridol interact synergistically to induce apoptosis in chronic myeloid leukemia cells resistant to imatinib mesylate through both Bcr/Abl-dependent and -independent mechanisms. Blood 2004; 104:509-518.

129. Barlow W, Fenghuang Z, Huang Y, et al. Predicting event-free and overall survival after treatment of myeloma with the proteasome inhibitor bortezomib with pre-treatment and 48-hour post-therapy gene expression patterns. Blood 2004;104(11), Abstract 1481.

130. Richardson P, Chanan-Khan A, Schlossman R, et al. Prognostic factors associated with response in patients with relapsed and

refractory mutiple myeloma (MM) treated with bortezomib Blood, 2004;109:(11) Abstract 336.

131. Fevig JM, Buriak J Jr, Cacciola J, et al. Rational design of boropeptide thrombin inhibitors: beta, beta-dialkyl-phenethylglycine P2 analogs of DuP 714 with greater selectivity over complement factor I and an improved safety profile. Bioorg Med Chem Lett 1998;8:301–306.
132. Loidl G, Groll M, Musiol HJ, et al. Bifunctional inhibitors of the trypsin-like activity of eukaryotic proteasomes. Chem Biol 1999;6:197–204.
133. Myung J, Kim KB, Lindsten K, et al. Lack of proteasome active site allostery as revealed by subunit-specific inhibitors. Mol Cell 2001;7:411–420.
134. Lum RT, Nelson MG, Joly A, et al. Selective inhibition of the chymotrypsin-like activity of the 20S proteasome by 5-methoxy-1-indanone dipeptide benzamides. Bioorg Med Chem Lett 1998;8:209–214.
135. Iqbal M, Chatterjee S, Kauer JC, et al. Potent inhibitors of proteasome. J Med Chem 1995;38:2276–2277.
136. Harding CV, France J, Song R, et al. Novel dipeptide aldehydes are proteasome inhibitors and block the MHC-I antigen-processing pathway. J Immunol 1995;155:1767–1775.
137. Bogyo M, McMaster JS, Gaczynska M, et al: Covalent modification of the active site threonine of proteasomal beta subunits and the Escherichia coli homolog HslV by a new class of inhibitors. Proc Natl Acad Sci USA 1997;94:6629–34.
138. Bogyo M, Shin S, McMaster JS, et al: Substrate binding and sequence preference of the proteasome revealed by active-site-directed affinity probes. Chem Biol 1998;5:307–20.
139. Elofsson M, Splittgerber U, Myung J, et al. Towards subunit-specific proteasome inhibitors: synthesis and evaluation of peptide alpha′,beta′-epoxyketones. Chem Biol 1999;6:811–822.
140. Meng L, Kwok BH, Sin N, et al. Eponemycin exerts its antitumor effect through the inhibition of proteasome function. Cancer Res 1999;59:2798–2801.
141. Belch A, Kouroukis CT, Crump M, et al. Phase II Trial of Bortezomib in Mantle Cell Lymphoma Blood, 2004;104:11, Abstract 608.

Molecular Targeted Drugs and Growth Factor Receptor Inhibitors

30

Jeffrey W. Clark

INTRODUCTION

From the first identification of mutations unique to neoplastic cells, the dream has been that targeting those mutations would provide a means of specifically killing malignant cells while sparing normal tissues. Discoveries in biological mechanisms of cancer cells at the DNA, RNA, and protein level are continuing to lead to rapid improvements in understanding the specific processes important for the survival, proliferation, and metastasis of different types of neoplastic cells. By combining these with technologic advances that allow sophisticated manipulation and analysis of nucleic acids and proteins, agents that target proteins or genes critical to the neoplastic process have been identified and further developed. A variety of compounds, including designed small molecules, monoclonal antibodies (mAbs), peptidomimetics, siRNAs, antisense oligonucleotides, and expressed genes, and other molecularly targeted therapies are being evaluated for potential treatment of cancer (Table 30.1). An increasing number of these have sufficient clinical activity to be important components of current therapy for a number of different malignancies (Table 30.2). Approved mAbs include trastuzumab (Herceptin) for breast cancer; rituximab, ibritumomab tiuxetan (Zevalin with Yttrium-90), and tositumomab + I131 (Bexxar) for follicular B-cell non-Hodgkin's lymphomas (NHLs); alemtuzamab for B-cell chronic lymphocytic leukemia (B-CLL); gemtuzumab ozogamicin for acute myelogenous leukemia (AML); and bevacizumab and cetuximab for colorectal cancer. Targeted small molecules

include imatinib (Gleevec) for chronic myeloid leukemia (CML) and gastrointestinal stromal tumors (GISTs) and gefitinib (Iressa) and erlotinib (Tarceva) for non–small cell lung cancer (NSCLC). The immunotoxin denileukin diftitox (diphtheria toxin-interleukin 2 [IL-2] fusion protein, DAB486IL-2) is approved for the treatment of cutaneous T-cell lymphomas. A schematic representation of signaling through growth factor receptors and, where currently approved, targeted anticancer agents that inhibit this process is shown in Figure 30.1. A large number of other agents are in clinical trials, and this list is certain to grow.

Conceptually, targeting a specific gene or protein appears straightforward. Theoretically, antitumor agents can be designed based on known sequence data, obviating the need to empirically screen a large number of compounds. However, many issues in the successful development of these agents remain to be addressed. It is important that the targeted protein in the neoplastic cell either be sufficiently different (if mutant) to provide a specific target or else not be critical for the survival of normal cells in order to decrease the risk of serious toxicity. Targeting one gene or protein may have limited effects on growth of neoplastic cells unless that gene or protein is vital for the proliferation or survival of those cells. In many cases, which gene (or genes) should be targeted is unclear. Genes important for the process by which a cell becomes a neoplastic cell may not be important for the continued proliferation or survival of the cell and therefore may be irrelevant targets for treating established malignancies. Inhibition of many genes, even if they are important for neoplastic cell growth, may only be cytostatic. It would be

TABLE 30.1

TYPES OF MOLECULARLY TARGETED COMPOUNDS

Agent	Potential Target(s)
Antisense oligonucleotides	RNA, DNA, proteins
SiRNA	RNA
Gene therapy	Neoplastic cells, immune mediator cells, and normal cells (to produce proteins)
Ribozymes	RNA and DNA in tumor cells
Monoclonal antibodies	Growth factor receptors, cell surface antigens, and other cellular proteins
Modified peptides	Growth factor receptors, cell surface antigens, extra- and intracellular proteins (e.g., enzymes and signal transduction molecules)
Small molecules	All of the above targets

more useful to target genes whose inhibition (or stimulation) induces cell death (i.e., by apoptosis) or terminal differentiation.[1] Ultimately, these approaches must be capable of eliminating (or at least leading to prolonged growth suppression of) all tumor cells, either by themselves or in combination with other agents, if they are to be effective in curing patients. Agents with cytostatic effects might need to be used in combination with other therapy.

These are all important issues that need to be addressed for successful development of targeted therapies. Despite the difficulties, strategies using each of the just-mentioned approaches have been shown to be effective in animal models, and, as outlined above, a number of targeted molecules have significant clinical activity against several human tumors. Clearly, a number of genes could be targeted simultaneously or sequentially, and combinations of approaches inhibiting certain genes (e.g., oncogenes) or their protein products and enhancing expression of others (e.g., tumor suppressor genes) may ultimately be used. Continued analysis of the human genome and improved understanding of complex interactions among different genes and proteins will continue to provide a large range of potential targets in the coming decades. With numerous potential targets, determining at an early stage which of these are most fruitful to pursue in treating cancer remains an important challenge.

RATIONALE FOR TARGETING GROWTH FACTOR RECEPTORS AND DOWNSTREAM SIGNALING PATHWAYS

Until the past decade, cancer therapy primarily used drugs that lack selectivity for tumor cells. These agents are predominantly cytotoxins, lethal for both neoplastic and normal cells, with a narrow therapeutic index. They were discovered through cytotoxic screens rather than efforts to exploit targets that are specific for malignant cells. They have improved treatment of many solid tumors and have cured some hematologic malignancies and selected solid tumors, but with significant toxicity to normal tissues. They have also improved cure rates for several malignancies when used in the adjuvant setting or in combination with radiation therapy. However, they have not been curative for the majority of patients with metastatic solid tumors. Therefore, new approaches for the treatment of the majority of cancers are needed.

The rapid growth in knowledge of cancer biology has led to a more rational approach to therapeutic discovery through the targeting of pathways and proteins that are essential for

TABLE 30.2

APPROVED MOLECULARLY TARGETED AGENTS

Type of Compound	Agent	Target	Indication
Uncoupled monoclonal antibodies	Alemtuzumab	CD52	B-CLL
	Bevacizumab	VEGF	Colorectal cancer
	Cetuximab	EGFR	Colorectal cancer
	Herceptin	Her-2	Breast cancer
	Rituximab	CD20	B-cell NHL
Monoclonal antibodies coupled to radioactive or cytotoxic agents	Ibritumomab tiuxetan Y-90	CD20	B-cell NHL
	Tositumomab I-131	CD20	B-cell NHL
	Gemtuzimab ozogamicin	CD33	AML
Small molecules	Gefitinib	EGFR	NSCLC
	Imatinib	BCR-ABL	CML
	Imatinib	KIT	GIST
	Erlotinib	EGFR	NSCLC

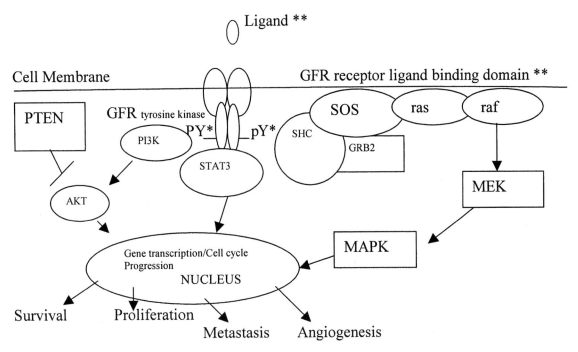

Figure 30.1 Schematic of growth factor ligand binding to cell surface receptors and the subsequent downstream signaling cascade that leads to biological effects such as survival, proliferation, metastasis, and angiogenesis. Double asterisks indicate steps at which approved monoclonal antibodies inhibit the process. Single asterisks indicate steps at which small tyrosine kinase molecules inhibit the process.

the survival of cancer cells and, either quantitatively or qualitatively, unique to cancer.[1-7] Studies in cancer biology have revealed a number of such pathways and proteins. Many of these are either overexpressed or in some way altered in cancer cells. Possible targets include the overexpression of growth factors or their receptors, such as the epidermal growth factor receptor (EGFR) family, including the *HER-2-neu* tyrosine kinase; angiogenic pathways (e.g., vascular endothelial growth factor [VEGF] or platelet-derived growth factor [PDGF]–mediated angiogenesis) that provide a blood supply for the expanding tumor; antiapoptotic mechanisms that antagonize cell death, such as overexpression of Bcl-2 or decreased BAX expression; and enhanced activity of intracellular signaling pathways that promote growth, impede apoptosis, or both.[1-7] The most unique targets on cancer cells are mutant genes. Examples of mutations of growth factor receptors themselves include c-KIT in GIST and EGFR in certain cases of NSCLC, both of which have proven clinically useful targets for small molecular inhibitors of their tyrosine kinase activity. Mutations of genes in signaling pathways downstream of growth factor receptors, such as activation of one of the ras family of proteins, can lead to unrestrained growth. In addition, or alternatively, important brakes on proliferation induced by stimulation of constitutively active mutant growth factor receptors can be lost, such as by mutations or other processes that inhibit the function of p53, retinoblastoma (RB), or the phosphate and tensin homolog (PTEN), which regulates the PI3-kinase pathway.[5-8]

Recognition of a potential target for drug discovery is only the first step. The target requires "validation" if it is to warrant the extensive efforts required to develop a clinically effective antitumor agent. A number of theoretical and practical questions must be answered before the investment is justified. Among the most relevant questions are the following:

1. Are the subject gene and its protein found in human tumors, and is there selective expression in tumors versus normal tissues?
2. Is function of the overexpressed or mutated target essential to the transformed behavior of the malignant cells? Does inhibition of the gene product change the phenotype of these cells? Does inhibition lead to the desired result (such as a decrease in metastasis) in an animal model? Experiments evaluating the biological effects when the subject gene is mutated, deleted, or neutralized with short RNAs with specific sequence that have been shown to selectively inhibit expression of genes within cells (small interfering or siRNAs) are important for addressing these questions. The discovery of the ability of siRNAs to inhibit specific genes within cells has provided a powerful tool for analyzing the role those genes play in the biology of the cell. Not only has this revolutionized the study of the effects of silencing specific genes because of its relative ease of use technically compared to the other techniques, but siRNAs also have

potential as therapeutic agents. This is an area that is being actively investigated.

3. In the case of an overexpressed (as opposed to mutant) protein in a tumor, is the protein also expressed in key proliferating normal tissues, such as intestinal epithelium and bone marrow progenitors, or even nonproliferating tissues, such as heart, kidney, or brain, and does the protein therefore carry the risk for significant toxicity if targeted? Patterns of drug toxicity are often difficult to predict, but the profile of gene expression in normal tissues may provide helpful clues about potential toxicity of an agent directed against that target gene. Does a knockout of the gene have fatal consequences for the host (in animal models), indicating that inhibition of that gene or its protein product might lead to significant toxicity?

4. Are there closely related proteins that are essential for normal tissue function and survival of the host and that might be cross-targeted by the agent, making it nonselective as a molecularly targeted inhibitor?

These considerations are paramount in determining the choice of a target and the probability of success. Obviously, even the most validated target may not be amenable to a drug discovery strategy for a number of reasons. Unanticipated toxicities, interactions with previously inapparent receptors or proteins, pharmacologic problems in drug distribution, and unfavorable pharmacokinetic (PK) properties may defeat the most rational strategy.

A number of excellent reviews of high-priority molecular targets for cancer therapy are available.[1-7] Angiogenesis inhibitors and mAbs are covered elsewhere in this book. The following is a brief review of several of the growth factor receptor and downstream signaling pathways that have yielded substantial new leads for cancer treatment.

POTENTIAL MOLECULAR TARGETS

The current choice of a molecular target for anticancer therapy is often dictated by an important practical consideration. It is vastly easier to design an inhibitor of the function of a protein that is either constitutively activated by mutation or has increased functional activity by another mechanism, such as by being overexpressed, than it is to replace an inactive or deleted function. Thus, although mutations in tumor suppressor genes, such as those affecting the p53 or RB pathways, play a prominent role in tumorigenesis, it is difficult to restore the function of these proteins without restoring a fully functional gene. In those cases where protein function is suppressed as opposed to mutated, such as by the binding of MDM2 to p53, inhibitors of that binding might be able to restore function, but in this case the target is the inhibitor of the normal function of these genes. Thus, at the present time, the primary choices for targeting remain proteins that are either activated by a mutation or have increased activity by being overexpressed.[1]

APPROACHES TO IDENTIFYING AND SYNTHESIZING MODULATORS FOR MOLECULAR TARGETS

The diversity of approaches to developing inhibitors or modulators for identified targets in cancers is large, although small molecules, antibodies, and modified peptides are the agents with clearly established clinical value at this time.

One approach to developing agents targeting specific genes or proteins is to empirically screen a large number of compounds for activity and subsequently design better ones based on the structure of the active compound (this is the approach by which most anticancer agents have been developed). High-throughput screens allowing rapid evaluation of a large number of compounds have enhanced the utility of this approach. Alternatively, compounds can be designed based on the structure of the specific region being targeted, using known sequence and other information available about the gene or protein (e.g., x-ray crystallography, nuclear magnetic resonance [NMR] imaging, computer molecular modeling, and analysis). Clearly, some combination of these two approaches might be most useful—for example, lead identification by random high-throughput screening followed by lead optimization through structural studies of the inhibitor and target. This allows more rational design of antineoplastic molecules and, at the same time, efficient screening of potentially therapeutic agents with a wide range of structures.

The complexity of molecular structures and the frequent interaction between proteins and other proteins or molecules makes designing compounds based on actual structure (as opposed to DNA sequence) a significant undertaking that requires sophisticated technology (e.g., x-ray crystallography, extensive computer analysis, and molecular modeling). Certain proteins, such as growth factor receptors (GFRs), which are among the most attractive targets for anticancer therapy because of their accessibility and potential importance in proliferation and survival pathways, are large and therefore still difficult to analyze even with current analytic approaches. It is not yet possible to predict which properties of an agent might influence subsequent development of resistance (which remains a major obstacle to the ultimate effectiveness of any treatment), because mechanisms of resistance to the compound cannot be fully predicted beforehand. Nonetheless, knowledge of the critical surface for ligand interaction with the target and how this might be modified by changes in the protein or interacting proteins may allow the design of a series of compounds that could overcome resistance due to mutations in the targeted protein or in the proteins with which it interacts. These could be given either simultaneously, to prevent the selection of resistant cells, or possibly sequentially, to maintain the response for a longer time. The complexity of the body's handling of compounds makes predicting toxicology and PKs difficult. At the present time, pharmacologic features can only be determined from careful preclinical and clinical studies.

As with all forms of systemic cancer therapy, the ultimate usefulness of these treatment approaches depends on the ability to effectively deliver the agent to tumor cells; adequate binding to neoplastic cells (in the case of mAbs or other compounds used to activate the immune system or deliver radioactive compounds) or uptake by neoplastic cells; the presence or expression of the agent on or within cells for a sufficient time to lead to death or differentiation of those cells; a high gradient of concentration for the compound in malignant versus normal cells; the rate of elimination of the agent from normal and malignant cells; and the toxicity of the agent for normal tissues, acutely and chronically. Heterogeneity of neoplastic cells within tumors limits single-drug therapy and is also a problem for single molecularly targeted therapy. Therefore, approaches that target heterogeneous cell populations, including mechanisms for overcoming resistance, need to be part of the strategic plan in designing therapeutic use of these compounds.

There are a number potential negative pharmacologic factors for certain classes of targeted compounds, such as mAbs, antisense oligonucleotides, and modified peptides. These include relatively large size, which makes delivery more difficult; complex structure, which contributes to decreased absorption, enhanced hepatic clearance, and decreased permeation from blood into tissues; natural nucleases and proteases that rapidly break down unmodified compounds; specific receptors for these agents that circulate in the blood or are expressed on normal cells and that alter their distribution; and potential immunogenicity, because these compounds often have features that make them directly immunogenic or inducers of host cytokine release, a property that can limit their long-term use.

SPECIFIC TARGETS

Growth Factor Receptors

Growth factor receptors or their ligands represent some of the most attractive molecular targets for cancer therapy. They are overexpressed on a number of malignancies, mutated in several, and in both cases have increased activity, so that they are targets for inhibition. The importance of growth factors and downstream signaling pathways in a number of cellular processes essential for proliferation and survival of cells has been demonstrated. Studies have established the importance of growth factors (such as VEGF in the angiogneic process for a number of malignances) or their receptors (such as HER-2 in breast cancer) in the neoplastic process. There is significant evidence for the role of growth factors and their receptors (such as VEGF, VEGFR, EGF ligands, and EGFR) in the metastatic process.[9,10] Their presence on the cell surface makes them

more readily accessible than many proteins. Thus, the rationale for targeting growth factors and their receptors for anticancer therapy is well established.

The members of the EGFR family of receptors, including HER-2, are especially attractive targets. The majority of cancers arise from epithelial cells that express EGFR. As outlined, EGFR family members have been shown to have a role in tumor cell survival and proliferation as well as the metastatic process. Inhibition of EGFR in certain preclinical models leads to death of malignant cells and significant antitumor response. As discussed above, mutant proteins provide the most specific target in cancer. EGFR are mutated in a subset of NSCLC tumors with adenocarcinoma or adenocarcinoma with bronchoalveolar cancer histology.[11,12] Mutations in c-KIT are found frequently in GIST tumors, and their targeting by imatinib has been very successful clinically.[13,14] Growth factor receptors have been shown to be overexpressed in certain malignances. These include overexpression of VEGF/VEGFR in a number of malignancies, platelet-derived growth factor receptors (PDGFRs) in brain tumors, and EGFRs in head and neck cancer as well as a number of other epithelial malignancies.[15-17]

Downstream Signaling Pathways of Growth Factor Receptors

A number of signaling pathways downstream of growth factor receptors have been identified and shown to play important roles in cancers. The potential for targeting these pathways directly either alone or in combination with anti–growth factor receptor agents as a means of treating cancer continues to be actively investigated.

Ras Pathways

One of the first oncogenes to be recognized in human tumors was the mutation and constitutive activation of *ras*.[18] Ras proteins play central roles in transducing signals important for a variety of critical processes in cells, including proliferation and differentiation.[18] One of the key roles played by Ras proteins is in transmitting signals from GFRs to downstream signaling molecules. A scheme for *ras* function is shown in Figure 30.1. The ras protein family (K-*ras*, N-*ras*, and H-*ras*) are activated by upstream signaling from tyrosine kinase receptors, such as the EGFRs. Ras proteins are activated by binding guanosine triphosphate (GTP), and subsequently they activate downstream targets in the signaling cascade, including the raf kinase. In the process, GTP is hydrolyzed to guanosine diphosphate, and *ras* is inactivated. Mutations at codons 12, 13, or 61 of the *ras* genes constitutively activate *ras* by locking it in the GTP-bound state. This leads to activation of raf and the signal transduction pathway in the absence of growth factor stimulation. Ras must be bound to the plasma membrane to activate raf. In concert with other mutations, *ras* is transforming in normal cells. *Ras* mutations occur relatively frequently in a number of malignancies. For example, K-*ras* mutations are found in approximately 40 to 50% of colon cancers, 70 to 90% of pancreatic cancers, and 30% of adenocarcinomas of the lung. [18-20] N-*ras* is mutated in approximately 20 to 30% of acute nonlymphocytic leukemias. [13] H-*ras* is mutated in a minority of bladder and head and neck cancers. Thus, as a molecular target, *ras* has attractive features.

There are several potential methods of inhibiting ras. The unprocessed native protein is inactive and requires sequential posttranslational modification to allow insertion in the plasma membrane, which is required for its active signaling function. [18] It must first be farnesylated (attachment of a 15-carbon, lipophilic group) by soluble prenylation enzymes. The carbon terminal (C-terminal) CAAX motif of ras then directs the prenylated protein to the endoplasmic reticulum and Golgi, in which the C-terminal AAX residues are cleaved by a specific protease. The terminal prenylcysteine is then methylated by a prenyl cysteine methyl transferase found in the endomembrane system. The final product is exported to its active site in the plasma membrane. In the case of N- and H-*ras*, this occurs after further lipid attachment (palmitic acid) to another cysteine or cysteines. K-*ras*, which possesses a polybasic region upstream from the C-terminal peptide, does not require palmitoylation to localize in the plasma membrane. [18-21]

Initial attempts to develop compounds blocking *ras* function have been devoted to the discovery of inhibitors of the farnesylation reaction, [22] although there has also been interest in exploring inhibition of prenyl cysteine methyl transferase and the *ras* proteases. In addition, targeting of downstream effectors of *ras*, such as the raf kinase, are also being pursued. [23] Potent and selective farnesyl transferase inhibitors (FTIs) with preference for H-*ras* inhibition have been isolated by selecting lead compounds in high-throughput screening. With subsequent structural refinement, a number of compounds entered clinical trial. Although some limited antitumor activity has been seen with several of these compounds, the ultimate clinical use of any of these compounds remains uncertain.

Experience with the FTIs taught valuable lessons about targeted drug discovery. A number of initial assumptions have proven to be invalid: (a) Contrary to what was initially believed, it is now clear that an ever growing number of proteins other than ras proteins undergo farnesylation. One or more other farnesylated proteins, such as RhoB, may be the critical targets in the inhibition of tumor cell growth by FTIs. [24] (b) K-*ras* can be inserted into the cell membrane and thus activated through geranyl-geranylation, bypassing FTI inhibition. (c) *Ras* plays a role in signaling via a complex set of pathways in cells, and it is not always clear what effects might be produced by inhibition of its function in different cellular circumstances. [21-25] Not surprisingly, given these facts, antitumor activity of FTIs in

cell culture does not necessarily correlate with the presence of *ras* mutation. In addition, the FTIs as a class are not selective for tumors but demonstrate a spectrum of toxicities in humans, including diarrhea, hepatotoxicity, neurotoxicity, cardiac conduction abnormalities, and myelosuppression.

Other targets within the ras pathway are also being attacked. As mentioned above, the raf kinase is an immediate downstream target of ras. Raf inhibition has been shown to have significant antitumor effects in preclinical models and remains a potentially valid target. [23] A molecule designed to target the raf kinase, BAY 43-9006, has had sufficient antitumor activity to be tested in clinical trials for a number of malignancies. [23,26] This compound is not entirely specific for the raf kinase. It has significant inhibiting activity for another potentially important target (VEGFR-2), making it difficult to determine what role the inhibition of raf is playing in its antitumor activity. Other inhibitors of raf as well as inhibitors of further downstream targets (such as ERK) in the ras pathway are also undergoing study.

Retinoblastoma Pathway

A second prominent target that modifies signaling from growth factor receptors is the RB pathway. [6] This pathway is named for the critical role played by the product of the RB gene, a protein that in its underphosphorylated state inhibits E2F, a transcription factor that promotes synthesis of messenger RNAs (mRNAs) for a number of proteins involved in DNA synthesis. The function of RB is, in turn, tightly controlled by a complex sequence of protein interactions that regulate its phosphorylation state. Two of the responsible kinases, cdk4 and cdk6, are activated by cyclin D and inhibited by p16 and p21. Multiple sites of mutation or alteration in this pathway can be involved in the neoplastic process; essentially any mutation or modification that eliminates or inactivates RB function (including by phosphorylation) will activate E2F and allow cell cycle progression. These alterations include loss of RB itself in patients with retinoblastoma; activation of cdk4 in melanoma; overexpression of cyclin D in many human tumors; and loss of p16 function (such as by mutation), which can occur in a number of malignancies. Most human tumors display an alteration of at least one component of this pathway, most frequently p16 deletion or cyclin D overexpression. Experimental models of RB loss or inactivation have confirmed the tumorigenic effect of mutations in this pathway. Thus, antitumor therapy targeted at inhibiting RB phosphorylation is rational.

An inhibitor of cdk4, flavopiridol, has entered clinical trials. Thus far it has had modest antitumor activity in phase I and early phase II studies, although it has had moderate activity against B-CLL. [7] It fulfills many of the hypothesized advantages of molecularly targeted therapies. It has limited toxicity for normal proliferating tissues, induces apoptosis in tumor cells, and enhances cytotoxicity of traditional drugs. However, its mechanism of action, competitive inhibition of the adenosine triphosphate–binding site of the kinase, is characteristic of compounds that are not highly selective for only one kinase. This is true for a number of kinase inhibitors, including imatinib.

In fact, although flavoperidol inhibits cdk4, it lacks specificity for cdk4 in that it inhibits cdk1, cdk2, cdk7, cdk9, and, at higher (micromolar) concentrations, a number of other kinases. In addition, it suppresses expression of cyclin D1, the important activator of cdk4. Thus, whether its antitumor effects are attributable to inhibition of RB phosphorylation is unclear. This question can only be answered by detailed studies of the correlation of changes in RB phosphorylation status in tumors with the response of those malignancies to flavoperidol. The fact that flavoperidol has some antitumor activity (especially against B-CLL), that it potently induces apoptosis in various human tumor cells in a p53-independent manner, and that it has synergy with cytotoxins is reason enough to pursue its clinical development and that of related compounds.[7]

Mutant Proteins That Lead to Unrestrained Growth of Malignant Cells

Bcr-Abl Kinase

The 9:22 translocation in CML has proven to be a particularly attractive target.[27] The translocation places the Abl tyrosine kinase activity on chromosome 9 in juxtaposition to the breakpoint cluster region of chromosome 22. The resulting protein has a complex variety of functions, including a constitutively active tyrosine kinase that affects a number of signaling pathways within the cell. It is capable of cell transformation in mice. Antisense to the *bcr-abl* gene reverses the malignant phenotype and induces apoptosis in CML cells in vitro. Thus, a large body of preclinical data argues that *bcr-abl* inhibition should produce significant anti-CML effect. In fact, imatinib, a potent inhibitor of the tyrosine kinase activity of Bcr-Abl, is highly effective against CML, as discussed elsewhere in this chapter.

Other Targets

Few mutations or biological processes associated with human cancer provide such a clear target for drug development as the bcr-abl protein. Most epithelial cancers represent the evolution of multiple mutations, and targeting different genes may be necessary to kill individual clones of cells within a given cancer. Mutations or cellular processes that might be good candidates for targeting neoplastic cells more effectively include apoptosis, telomerase, critical growth factor signaling pathways [e.g., EGFR and HER-2-neu receptor], PTEN gene mutations and deletion in the PI3-kinase pathway, and various angiogenic targets, such as the VEGF and its receptor (see Chapter 35).[16,17,28–30] Clinical responses in patients treated with mAbs to HER-2-neu (using trastuzumab) or the EGFR (using cetuximab) and with EGFR small molecule inhibitors (gefitinib and erlotinib) have shown that interruption of growth signals can be a useful strategy for drug design.[11,12,29–31] The success of bevacizumab in combination with chemotherapy in treating colorectal cancer has established the benefit of inhibiting VEGF, a critical molecule in tumor angiogenesis. Approaches targeting each of the other proteins or pathways discussed earlier are under active investigation.

SPECIFIC TARGETING AGENTS OF GROWTH FACTOR RECEPTORS, CELL SURFACE PROTEINS, AND DOWNSTREAM SIGNALING PATHWAYS

Monoclonal Antibodies

The ability to generate highly specific antibodies against the antigen of choice makes such antibodies excellent targeting agents. They can be used alone or to deliver radionuclides, toxins, or chemotherapy to malignant cells or specific tissues. MAbs directed against growth factor receptors (GFRs) and other cell surface antigens have undergone extensive testing in treatment of a number of cancers.[32] Those that have been approved for treating patients include trastuzumab against the HER-2 member of the EGFR family (for breast cancer); bevicizumab against VEGF and cetuximab against EGFR (for colorectal cancer); three antibodies directed against the CD20 antigen: rituximab, zevalin (coupled to yttrium 90 to deliver radiation therapy), and tositumomab (coupled to I131 to deliver radiation therapy) (Bexxar) (for B-cell NHL); alemtuzamab, which binds to CD52 (for B-CLL); and gemtuzamab ozogomicin (Mylotarg), which binds to CD33 and contains a cytotoxic agent (for AML). A number of others are currently undergoing clinical evaluation. Continued improvements utilizing antibodies to target agents, such as radioactive compounds or chemotherapeutic agents, in an attempt to selectively kill tumor cells continue to be explored. Combinations of antibodies and radiation therapy or chemotherapeutic agents are also being investigated. Radiolabeled antibodies are also useful as imaging agents for cancer. This is an area of continuing study directed toward enhancing specificity and sensitivity in imaging tumors. See Chapter 31 for a more complete discussion of monoclonal antibodies.

Small Molecules

The ability to rapidly screen and iteratively redesign a large number of molecules, in combination with favorable pharmacokinetic (PK) properties compared to other compounds, make small molecules among the most attractive agents for targeted therapy in cancer. The approach used by Drucker and colleagues in identifying the activity of imatinib in the 1990s is a prototypic example of the potential development of small molecules for molecular targeting.[27] Using high-throughput screening against recombinant bcr-abl protein, they identified a peptidomimetic molecule (imatinib) that has a high affinity for the adenosine triphosphate–binding site of the Abl tyrosine kinase and is capable of suppressing proliferation and inducing apoptosis of bcr-abl transfected tumor cells in vitro and in vivo.[27] The subsequent clinical development of this compound to treat CML and GIST has paved the way for further development of small molecular inhibitors targeted at aberrant tyrosine kinase activity in tumors.

Imatinib

Mechanism of Action

Imatinib's structure is given in Figure 30.2. It is a member of the two-phenylaminopyrimidine class of tyrosine kinase inhibitors. Imatinib mesylate is a potent inhibitor of certain protein tyrosine kinases, including bcr-abl, which is constitutively active in CML; c-KIT, which is frequently mutated in GIST; and PDGFR-alpha, which is overexpressed in a number of malignant cells.[32–35]

Cellular Pharmacology and Metabolism

Imatinib is orally active and freely soluble in water. It is rapidly taken up by cells. It undergoes extensive hepatic metabolism. The major enzyme that metabolizes it is the Cyp3A4 member of P450 family of enzymes in the liver involved in the metabolism of many drugs. Minor metabolism occurs by other P450 enzymes. The elimination half-

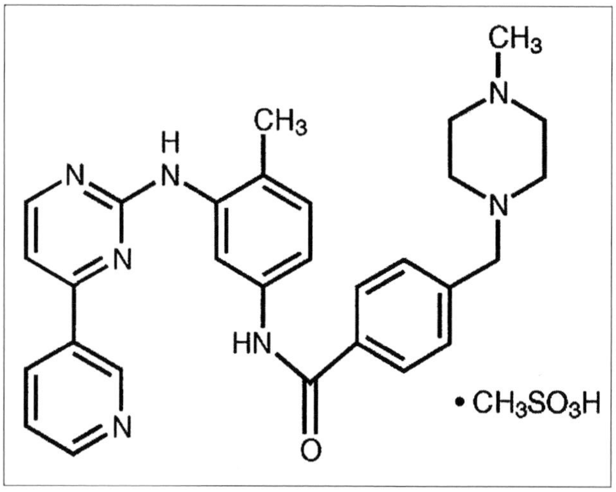

Imatinib mesylate

Figure 30.2 Structure of imatinib mesylate, a tyrosine kinase inhibitor.

life is approximately 14–20 hours for the parent compound and 40 hours for the major active metabolite, N-demethylated piperazine derivative (N-desmethyl-imatinib). This metabolite has approximately the same potency as the parent compound. Elimination is primarily in the feces, approximately 85 to 90%, with approximately 10 to 15% in the urine. The majority of the drug is secreted within 7 days, with unchanged imatinib accounting for approximately 25% of the dose. Clearance varies by about 40% between patients, which means that it is important to monitor for toxicity in individual patients.

In vitro, imatinib has been shown to be a potent inhibitor of a number of P450 enzymes and, especially, cyp3A4. There is significant increase in imatinib exposure (with increases in both maximum concentration [C_{max}] and the area under the curve [AUC]) when imatinib is given with cyp3A4 inhibitors such as ketoconazole. Similarly, imatinib significantly increases the concentration of simvastatin, another cyp3A4 substrate, when they are given together. Inducers of cyp3A4, such as phenytoin, significantly decrease imatinib exposure.

Clinical Pharmacology

After oral administration, the drug is relatively quickly absorbed (within 2 to 4 hours) and exhibits high bioavailability (98%). It is 95% bound to plasma proteins, primarily albumin and alpha 1-acid glycoprotein. The AUC increases proportionally with increasing dose. There is no significant change in PK with repeated dosing. There is a 1.5- to 2.5-fold accumulation at the steady state when the dose is given daily. It has poor penetration into the CSF.

Toxicity

The major toxicities seen with imatinib include

- hematological toxicity with neutropenia, thrombocytopenia, and anemia
- hepatotoxicity, usually manifested by elevated liver enzymes (toxicity can be decreased by holding or adjusting the dose, but occasionally it can be severe, especially if the agent is given with acetaminophen; thus, acetaminophen should be used with caution in patients who are taking imatinib)
- fluid retention or edema (often periorbital edema, which is usually manageable though occasionally serious, with a low incidence of ascites, pleural effusions, and brain edema)
- musculoskeletal pains and cramps
- rash
- occasional diarrhea
- GI irritation (imatinib should be taken with food and a large glass of water)
- GI bleeding or intratumoral bleeding (especially in patients with GIST), which can be significant

Holding of doses or appropriate dose modification should be done for toxicities as necessary. Dose modifications are dependent on the specific disease being treated (PDR). For example, for chronic phase CML or GIST, dose should be held for ANC $< 1 \times 10^9$ or platelets $< 50 \times 10^9$ and then resumed at the same dose (the CML starting dose is 400 mg/day; the GIST starting dose is 400 or 600 mg/day) once ANC has recovered to 1.5×10^9 and platelets to $\geq 75,000$. If hematological toxicity recurs, then the dose should be reduced to 300 mg if the starting dose was 400 mg or reduced to 400 mg if starting dose was 600 mg once counts have returned to the parameters outlined above. For patients with CML in accelerated phase, when the ANC $< .5 \times 10^9$ or platelets $< 10,000$, then bone marrow should be checked. If the decreased ANC is not disease related, then imatinib should be reduced to 400 mg/day (from the starting dose of 600 mg/day). If cytopenias persist for 2 weeks, then dose should be further reduced to 300 mg/day. If cytopenias persist at 4 weeks, imatinib should be held until ANC $\geq 1 \times 10^9$ and platelets $\geq 20,000$, then the dose should be resumed at 300 mg/day. For hepatotoxicity, imatinib should be held for T. Bili more than three times the upper limit of normal or transaminases more than five times the upper limit of normal. The dose should then be resumed after reduction (100-mg reduction for 400-mg dose or 200-mg reduction for 600-mg dose) once the bilirubin has decreased to less than 1.5 times the normal and the transaminases have decreased to less than 2.5 times the normal. Of course the PDR package insert should be followed for appropriate standard dose modifications of any drug.

As discussed above, because imatinib is metabolized by cyp3A4, it is important to modify the dose when given with cyp3A4 inhibitors (e.g., itraconazole, erythromycin, clarithromycin). Similarly, exposure to imatinib may be decreased by inducers of cyp3A4 (e.g., dexamethasone, phenytoin, carbamazepine, rifampin, or phenobarbital). Drugs that might have increased exposure when given with imatinib include simvastatin, cyclosporine, pimozide, warfarin, and certain HMG coA reductase inhibitors. Whenever possible, alternate drugs that do not interact with cyp3A4 should be utilized, such as low molecular weight heparin instead of warfarin. Grapefruit and grapefruit juice inhibit cyp3A4 and should be avoided. In addition, a number of compounds used as alternative therapies might influence cyp3A4 function and should be avoided.

Clinical Effectiveness

CML

Imatinib is approved for treatment of patients with CML. It produces clinical hematologic responses in the majority of patients (approximately 90 to 95%) with CML in chronic phase either previously untreated or refractory to interferon, at doses that have acceptable toxicity (400 mg/m^2

TABLE 30.3
KEY FEATURES OF IMATINIB MESYLATE

2-Phenylaminopyrimidine class of tyrosine kinase inhibitor
Inhibits adenosine triphosphate binding
Selective inhibitor of tyrosine kinase activity of bcr-abl kinase, c-KIT and platelet-derived growth factor receptor
Daily oral therapy
Half-life approximately 18 hr
Acceptable toxicity at clinically effective doses
Hematologic and cytogenetic responses in majority of chronic phase patients with CML
Responses in majority of patients with GIST

per day). It produces cytogenetic complete remission in approximately 54% of previously untreated patients and 32% of those with previous interferon therapy. The median time to cytogenetic response is approximately 1 month. At higher dose (600 mg/m^2 per day), it also has activity against CML in accelerated phase, with approximately 28 to 37% complete hematological response and 20% major cytogenetic response. Although less active in patients with blast crisis, when used at the 600 mg/m^2 per day dose level, it still produces a small percentage of complete hematological responses (4 to 7%) and major cytogenetic responses (14 to 15%). It has had less clinical activity in patients with acute lymphoblastic leukemia who have the 9:22 translocation, possibly because of a greater role for src family kinases, although the actual mechanism remains to be fully elucidated. The drug's key features are given in Table 30.3.

GIST

Gastrointestinal stromal tumors (GIST) are the most common mesenchymal tumors arising from the GI tract.[36,37] They originate from the interstitial cell of Cajal, an intestinal pacemaker cell. Although they can arise from anywhere in the gastrointestinal tract or even the omentum, mesentery, or retroperitoneum, they most commonly occur in the stomach, followed by the intestine. Many of these tumors were formerly called "leiomyosarcomas." The primary therapy for GIST is surgical resection. However, a fairly high rate of recurrence or metastatic disease is noted. Historically, these tumors have been largely unresponsive to standard chemotherapeutic agents, including those active against sarcomas.

Imatinib has significant inhibitory effects on the tyrosine kinase activity of the c-KIT receptor and the PDGF receptor (PDGFR).[38] Immunohistochemical staining for c-KIT is usually positive in GIST tumors. Furthermore, the c-KIT receptor is mutated in a high proportion of patients with GIST (approximately 85%). A number of different mutations in the c-KIT receptor in GIST tumors have been identified (Table 30.4). The clinical antitumor activity of imatinib against GIST correlates with specific mutations in

TABLE 30.4
C-KIT MUTATIONS AND RESPONSE TO IMATINIB

Mutation	Response to Imatinib Therapy (PR)
c-KIT exon 11	84%
c-KIT exon 9	48%
c-KIT exon 13	100%*
c-KIT exon 17	50%*
PDGFRA sensitive	67%*
PDGFRA resistant	0%*
No c-KIT or PDGFRA mutations	0%

*Based on very small numbers, with large margin for error.
Adopted with permission from Heinrich MC, et al. Kinase mutations and imatinib response in patients with metastatic gastrointestinal stromal tumors. J Clin Oncol 2003;21:4342–4349; Table 1.

c-KIT, as shown in Table 30.4. The most common mutation is in exon 11, which occurs in approximately two thirds of patients. The highest response rates are seen in patients with exon 11 mutations. The second most common mutation is in exon 9, which occurs in approximately 17% of cases. These mutations so far have only been found in tumors that originate in either the small bowel or colon. Mutations also occur occasionally in exons 13 or 17. In those GIST tumors with wild-type c-KIT, the PDGFR-α is mutated in approximately 40% of cases.[36,37]

The approved dose of imatinib for GIST is 400 mg/day or 600 mg/day. The potential benefit of dose escalation for those who stop responding to imatinib is uncertain at the present time, although no responses were seen in a small group of patients who were escalated to the higher dose after they stopped responding to 400 mg/day. Ongoing clinical trials are evaluating imatinib against PDGFR-expressing tumors, such as gliomas and prostate cancer.

Gefitinib

Mechanism of Action

Gefitinib's structure is shown in Figure 30.3. It is a member of the anilinoquinazoline class of tyrosine kinase inhibitors. Gefitinib (Iressa) is a specific inhibitor of the EGFR tyrosine kinase (Table 30.5).[11,12,39–45] Similar to imatinib, which inhibits the bcr-abl tyrosine kinase, it is targeted at the ATP-binding site of the EGFR tyrosine kinase. Since EGFR signaling is involved in the survival and proliferation of certain neoplastic cells, inhibition of the tyrosine kinase activity leads to inhibition of cell proliferation and apoptosis of these cells in vitro.

Cellular Pharmacology and Metabolism

Gefitinib is rapidly taken up by cells and leads to inhibition of the intracellular tyrosine kinase domain of the EGFR. Pharmacodynamic data using skin biopsies at 1

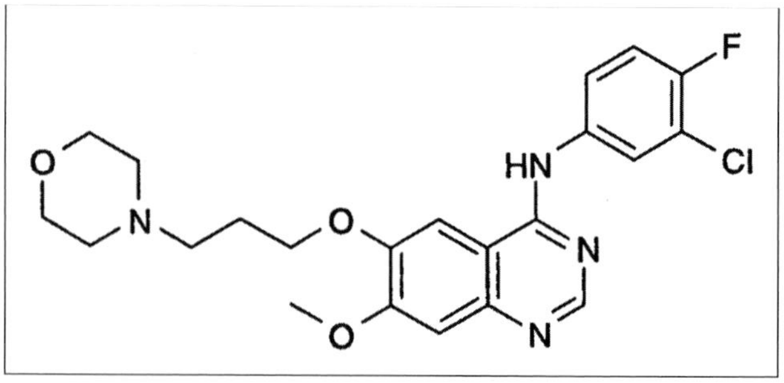

Gefitinib

Figure 30.3 Structure of gefitinib EGFR tyrosine kinase inhibitor.

month into treatment have shown that significant inhibition of EGFR activation occurred at all doses greater than 150 mg/day, and inhibition of downstream signaling (such as through map kinase) was also noted with increased cyclin-dependant kinase expression and apoptosis.

Clinical Pharmacology

Gefitinib is orally bioavailable. Its uptake is slow and not significantly affected by food. It is distributed extensively, with maximal plasma concentration between 3 and 7 hours after dose. It is approximately 60% bioavailable. The terminal half-life is approximately 40–50 hours with multiple dosing, and the steady-state level is reached by 7 to 10 days. It is dose proportional with increasing dose. There is interpatient variability of up to 56% and intrapatient variability of up to 30%. Ninety-one percent of the drug is plasma protein bound. Gefitinib does not alter the PKs of the chemotherapeutic agents with which it has been used to date, but gefitinib exposure is increased when it is given with carboplatin and paclitaxel.[43] However, this has not significantly altered toxicity.

Gefitinib undergoes extensive hepatic metabolism. The metabolism of gefitinib is complex, with at least five identified metabolites and three sites of biotransformation. None of the metabolites are thought to be bioactive. It is primarily cleared through the bile, with approximately 86% cleared in feces and less than 4% cleared in urine.

TABLE 30.5
KEY FEATURES OF GEFITINIB

Anilinoquinazoline class of tyrosine kinase inhibitors
Inhibits adenosine triphosphate binding
Selective inhibitor of EGFR
Daily oral therapy
Elimination half-life approximately 40–50 hr
Acceptable toxicity at clinically effective doses
Responses in 10–12% of patients with NSCLC (adenocarcinoma or bronchoalveolar carcinoma, especially those with EGFR mutations)

Similar to imatinib, it is processed by cyp3A4, with all the same potential drug interactions mentioned in the discussion of imatinib. For example, activation of cyp3A4 (e.g., by barbiturates) increases clearance, whereas inhibitors of cyp3A4 (e.g., ketoconazole) increase exposure to gefitinib. It is also an inhibitor of cyp2D6 and therefore increases levels of coadministered cyp2D6 substrates such as amitriptyline and codeine.

Toxicity

Diarrhea (occurring in 37 to 50 % of patients) and skin rash, often acneiform (occurring in approximately 40 to 50% of patients), are the most common toxicities. Nausea, pruritus, elevated liver function tests, and asthenia all can be seen. Uncommon but potentially serious toxicities include eye changes (corneal erosion or ulcer) and interstitial pneumonitis, which can be life-threatening or fatal.

Clinical Effectiveness

Gefitinib has activity against approximately 10 to 12% of NSCLCs that have progressed after two lines of chemotherapy. Gefitinib's antitumor activity does not correlate with intensity of immunohistochemical staining for EGFR in the tumor, suggesting that the level of EGFR expression does not predict response. However, similar to the situation for imatinib mesylate, which has increased activity against GIST tumors with specific c-KIT mutations, the activity of gefitinib appears to correlate with somatic mutations that are clustered around the ATP-binding pocket of the intracellular catalytic tyrosine kinase domain of the EGFR.[11,12,39–45] These mutations increase both EGF-induced activation as well as gefitinib inhibition of the receptor. The mutations are heterozygous, and thus the mutant protein appears to have a dominant effect. In two studies, 13 of 14 of the responding patients had a mutation in EGFR, versus no mutations in 11 nonresponders.[11,12] To date, all of the mutations have been found in tumors that are adenocarcinomas with or without bronchoalveolar features. Mutations are found more frequently in patients who are nonsmokers, women, and Japanese. The reason for the association of EGFR mutations with these features is currently unknown. In addition, mutational status does not appear to account for all of the clinical activity. Studies are ongoing to deliniate this further.

Gefitinib did not increase the clinical activity of chemotherapy when used in combination in large trials.[42,43] This was also true for erlotinib, an EGFR inhibitor similar to gefitinib, when used with chemotherapy in treatment of NSCLC (see next section). Both of these agents are currently being evaluated for potential treatment of other malignancies alone and in combination with chemotherapy or other agents. The absence of survival advantage for patients who received gefitinib has led to restriction of its use to patients already benefiting from it.

The small molecules approved for tyrosine kinase targeted therapy to date have so far shown significant clinical

activity primarily against mutant proteins (bcr-abl and c-KIT in the case of imatinib, EGFR in the case of gefitinib and erlotinib). This provides greater antitumor selectivity but also potentially decreases the population that might benefit. Whether this is going to be generally true for clinically active small molecular inhibitors of tyrosine kinases is not known. However, as noted above, mutational status of EGFR is only part of the mechanism defining effectiveness of erlotinib. This remains an active area of investigation.

Erlotinib

Mechanism of Action

Erlotinib (Tarceva) is a potent specific inhibitor of the EGFR tyrosine kinase.[46,47] Similar to gefitinib, it is targeted at the ATP-binding site of the molecule.

Cellular Pharmacology and Metabolism

Erlotinib is orally active. Similar to gefitinib, it is metabolized by cyp3A4, with all the potential drug interactions and other caveats discussed in the section on gefitinib.

Clinical Pharmacology

PK studies have shown it to be dose proportional with increasing dose; to have a half-life of approximately 36 hours; to have increased C_{max} and AUC when taken with food, along with a delayed T_{max}; and to have relatively low interpatient variability (range less than twofold). The maximum tolerated dose is 150 mg/day.

Toxicity

The toxicities are similar to those seen with gefitinib. At the recommended dose of 150 mg/day, these include skin changes, including rash, dermatitis, and pruritus, totaling 83% overall, with 13% grade 3 or 4; diarrhea (38% overall, 6% grade 3), nausea (33%), fatigue (18%), and rare cases of interstitial pneumonitis, which can be life-threatening (PDR).

Clinical Effectiveness

Erlotinib has a level of activity similar to that of gefitinib against NSCLC (approximately 12% response rate).[46–48] This was associated with prolongation of survival in patients who had previously failed two previous chemotherapy regimens for metastatic lung cancer.[48] As with gefitinib, the response rate is higher in patients who have adenocarcinoma with or without bronchoalveolar features and whose tumors contain the mutation in the ATP-binding pocket of the catalytic domain of the EGFR.[49] However, survival did not correlate with EGFR mutational status. The FDA has approved Tarceva for potential treatment of NSCLC.

Two other targeted small molecular inhibitors that are in clinical trial have sufficient activity against renal cell cancer that they are currently in pivotal trials. These are

Bayer 43-4009 and SU-011248.[23,26,50,51] Bayer 43-4009 is an orally available compound that was initially developed as an inhibitor of the raf kinase. As discussed earlier, the raf protein is one of the immediate downstream targets of ras in signal transduction, and thus inhibiting raf could inhibit proliferative signaling from growth factor receptors. However, subsequent evaluation has shown that it has activity against a number of other kinases, including the VEGFR2 tyrosine kinase. Thus, it has potential as an antiangiogenic agent in addition to its potential activity directly against malignant cells by blocking the ras-raf pathway. It is not known at present exactly which inhibitory effect or effects are responsible for Bayer 43-4009's antitumor activity. In any case, early clinical trials showed it to have antitumor activity against a number of malignancies, especially renal cell cancer, with acceptable toxicity. Preliminary data from a phase III trial evaluating the potential clinical efficacy of Bayer 43-9006 against renal cell cancer have shown that it prolongs progression free survival compared with placebo.[51a] Participants in the study are currently being followed for overall survival. A number of other studies are evaluating its efficacy against other malignancies.

SU-011248 is an orally available small molecular inhibitor of the tyrosine kinase activity of the VEGFR-2, PDGFR, and KIT receptors. As with BAY43-9006, it exhibited some antitumor activity against a number of malignancies in phase I studies, including against renal cell cancer, also with acceptable toxicity. It is also currently in clinical trials against a number of malignancies, including renal cell cancer but also GIST tumors that have progressed during imatinib treatment.

A large number of other small molecules targeting a variety of tyrosine kinases are currently undergoing clinical investigation. Some of these are chosen to have greater specificity for specific kinases, whereas others have activity against a number of kinases. At present, it is not known whether having specific activity (and potentially combining different agents each with specific activity) or having broader activity will be more clinically effective. Both strategies are being pursued in the development of kinase inhibitors. Strategies for combining different classes of targeted agents (e.g., mAbs and small molecules) are also being pursued.

A number of issues remain that need to be addressed through further investigation of small molecular inhibitors of kinases as anticancer agents, including these:

- The three malignancies that have been responsive to small molecular tyrosine kinase inhibitors to date (CML, GIST, and lung adenocarcinoma with or without bronchoalveolar features) have all had specific mutations in the protein being targeted (bcr-abl in CML, KIT in GIST, and EGFR in lung adenocarcinoma). Efforts are being made to identify other potentially mutated tyrosine kinases in other tumors that might be targets for therapy. A corollary question is whether small molecular inhibitors of tyrosine kinase activity might be clinically active in tumors that

have overexpressed but not mutated tyrosine kinases (such as the EGFR in head and neck cancer).

- Might combinations of monoclonal antibodies and small molecular inhibitors directed against the same target have greater activity in combination than when used alone? Although conceptually these combinations might appear to be redundant and therefore no more active, because they attach to different sites on the molecule, they could have enhanced activity.

- What is the best way to target multiple steps in GFR pathways, and will there be increased antitumor activity or clinical benefit from targeting multiple steps in the best way possible?

- How can multiple receptors or pathways be most effectively targeted?

- How can resistance to the targeted agent (which remains a significant problem) best be prevented or overcome?

Research is addressing each of these issues.

Other Modified Peptides and Peptidomimetics

As discussed in the sections on imatinib mesylate and gefitinib, modified peptides or peptidomimetic compounds designed to bind to and inhibit the active sites of proteins are natural candidates for effective inhibitors of protein function. The ubiquitous presence of proteases, the extremely short half-lives of most naturally occurring peptides, and their rapid hepatic and renal clearance make unmodified molecules impractical for clinical use. Therefore, modified compounds or, more commonly, small organic molecules that mimic peptides functionally, so-called peptidomimetics, have been the major focus of study. Modifications include incorporation of altered amino acids (e.g., phosphonates) that are less prone to degradative attack, incorporation of compounds (e.g., benzodiazepine analogs) that structurally mimic amino acids but are not targets of proteases, and use of totally synthetic polymers that structurally mimic peptides but are not targets for enzymatic degradation.

For these agents to be effective, a target that is therapeutically relevant must be chosen (Table 30.6). This is an obvious but critical point that can be forgotten in the excitement of knowing the sequence or structure of a gene that may not be an ideal candidate from the standpoint of tumor biology. Defining the best genes to target is especially important given the large number of potential targets and the high cost of evaluating each of them. Continued studies are helping to define the properties of optimal targets. Structures of the appropriate active sites of the target protein must be known. Ideally, structures of the specific regions being targeted are known from x-ray crystallography, allowing initial evaluation of potential binding compounds by computer analysis. Short peptidomimetics can be synthesized based on known sequences of active

TABLE 30.6

MODIFIED PEPTIDE TARGETS

Target	Examples
Cell surface growth factor	Growth factor analogs or receptor antagonists, growth factor–toxin conjugates
Cell surface binding proteins	Laminin peptide antagonists
Enzymes	Farnesyltransferase inhibitors, inhibitors of angiogenesis, metalloproteinase inhibitors, telomerase inhibitors
Protein interaction sites[a]	SH2 and SH3 domains

SH, Src homology.
[a]To date, it has been difficult to synthesize effective specific inhibitors of protein interaction sites that are readily taken up into cells.

binding sites critical for the function of target proteins. Those predicted to have the best binding properties can be synthesized. Thus, the process requires the production, purification, and crystallization of the known protein, followed by x-ray crystallographic and computer analysis.

These can be used for initial screening and provide the basis for subsequent modifications to improve efficacy. Clinically, the most extensively studied of the modified peptide compounds to date have been somatostatin analogs.[52,53] Thus, to illustrate pharmacological features of these compounds, somatostatin analogs are discussed as prototypical examples of synthetic peptide or peptide-like structures. Where appropriate, other peptidomimetics or general features of these types of compounds are discussed. Peptide analogs of luteinizing hormone–releasing hormone (LHRH) are also extensively used clinically, but because the antitumor effect is mediated via hormonal manipulation, these are discussed under hormonal therapies.

Mechanisms of Action

Uncoupled Modified Peptides

Somatostatins are, in general, growth inhibitory for a wide variety of cells, including neoplasms.[52–56] Receptors for somatostatin have been found on a number of tumors, including lung, colon, pancreas, breast, and neuroendocrine tumors. Most animal models suggest that the biologic effects of these compounds (or analogs) are mediated via binding to receptors, although a few studies have not shown a direct correlation between receptor numbers and the biologic effects of the compound.

Somatostatin itself has too short a half-life (approximately 3 minutes) to be clinically useful. In addition, withdrawal of somatostatin can produce rapid rebound effects. Therefore, a number of analogs have been developed that have greater stability, have more selectivity, and possibly induce less of a rebound effect than somatostatin itself.[52–56]

Somatostatin analogs that are significantly more active than the parent compound have been studied extensively. They vary in potency for different somatostatin effects, suggesting some specificity of different analogs. For example, sandostatin is 45 times more potent than somatostatin in inhibiting GH release, 11 times more potent in inhibiting glucagon, and 1.3 times more potent in inhibiting insulin.[52–56] Binding of various somatostatin analogs varies between different tissues, suggesting that there are possibly different subtypes of receptors.[52–56] Antiproliferative effects of somatostatin analogs appear to be mediated by a number of mechanisms. One mechanism is inhibition of centrosomal separation and cell proliferation induced by epidermal growth factor (EGF).[57] This may be due, at least in part, to stimulating a tyrosine phosphatase that inhibits signaling via the EGFR pathway, although additional studies are necessary to further define the mechanism.[58] A large number of potential indirect mechanisms of tumor inhibition by somatostatin analogs exist, including suppression of growth hormone (GH) and prolactin, which can be growth stimulatory for breast cancer; inhibition of GH, with subsequent suppression of a number of growth factors (e.g., insulin-like growth factor I) that are important for tumor cell growth; and suppression of plasma-EGF levels.[52–56] Somatostatin analogs have been shown to inhibit tumor growth in vitro and in a number of animal model systems.[52–56] The effect appears to be primarily cytostatic, with return of tumor growth once analogs are removed.

Peptide analogs that recognize the binding site of other receptors also have been synthesized to bind to and inhibit receptor function directly. These have been shown to be effective in vitro, and if these or modified peptides that would be more stable in vivo can be effectively delivered to tumors, then they might be clinically useful.[57–59]

In addition to development of peptidomimetics targeted to cell surface receptors, much of the current interest in these molecules is focused on their potential as inhibitors of specific steps in signal transduction pathways from cell surface to nucleus. The identification of the mammalian target for rapamycin (mTOR, which is a downstream effector in the phosphatidylinositol 3-kinase/Akt pathway that is involved in controlling cell cycle progression and proliferation) has led to the development of a number of analogs that are currently in clinical evaluation.[60] Clearly, a large number of other potential targets for peptidomimetics are present within cells, including proteins involved in other signaling pathways, enzymes, or sequences important for protein-protein interactions.[61] Many of these are being actively pursued as potential therapeutic targets.

Targeting Cytotoxic Agents via Modified Peptides

Similar to mAbs directed against GFRs, peptide growth factors can be used to target toxic compounds to cells. Given the rapid degradation of growth factors once they are internalized, peptide growth factors are most useful for targeting toxic compounds.[62,63] This approach has been shown to be effective in inhibiting the growth of neoplastic cell lines in culture and tumors in animal models, with tolerable toxicity. Human trials also have shown efficacy for this approach using an IL-2–diphtheria hybrid toxin (denileukin diftitox) to treat cutaneous T-cell lymphomas (CTCLs) and other hematological malignancies that express the CD25 component of the IL-2 receptor. It is approved for the treatment of persistent or recurrent CTCL that expresses the CD25 antigen.[64]

Given the immunogenicity of toxins, the short plasma half-life of most small peptides, and the tendency of many peptides (e.g., growth factors) administered in vivo to concentrate in organs, such as the liver and kidney, these compounds must be modified to make them consistently useful therapeutic agents for systemic therapy. A potential means of decreasing systemic side effects and increasing the amount delivered to tumor cells is to deliver therapy locally. Approaches to doing this, such as intravesicular therapy or hepatic arterial infusion, are being pursued.

Peptides can be modified in a number of ways to enhance their potential as effective therapeutic agents. One of these is coupling them to compounds, such as dextran, that prevent the extremely rapid degradation of peptides that normally occurs in cells and therefore allow longer retention in these cells.[65] If these constructs are coupled with radioactive or cytotoxic compounds, they can provide a potentially effective system for delivering the toxic compound to malignant cells.

Cellular Pharmacology and Metabolism

The factors important for the cellular pharmacologic properties of modified peptides targeted to GFRs (or other cell surface antigens) are similar to those for mAbs. The activity, half-life, and metabolism of these peptides are dependent on whether the ligand-receptor complex is internalized. Internalization is not necessarily essential and might be pharmacologically detrimental for compounds that bind to and inhibit the receptor directly or are ligated to radionuclides. On the other hand, for toxin or chemotherapy conjugates, internalization is essential. Furthermore, some agonist ligands that promote the growth of normal cells paradoxically produce growth arrest and apoptosis in tumor cells (CD40, CD25). Modified peptides targeted at intracellular proteins clearly need to be delivered into cells. As discussed earlier for *ras*, compounds with these properties can be constructed. It is impossible to generalize the pharmacologic properties of different modified peptides because they are affected by the presence, concentration, and properties (e.g., internalization) of the proteins to which they bind in plasma as well as on the cell surface.

Clinical Pharmacology

Somatostatin analogs are rapidly absorbed after subcutaneous injection. The peak plasma concentrations are seen in approximately 25 to 30 minutes. The $t_{1/2}\alpha$ values are approximately 10 to 15 minutes, and $t_{1/2}\beta$ values are approximately 100 to 115 minutes when the dose is given by subcutaneous injection and approximately half as long when given by intravenous bolus. Approximately one third of the dose is excreted unchanged in the urine. A number of analogs have different biologic and pharmacologic effects. Somatuline, which has been studied in the treatment of pancreatic cancer, has a plasma half-life of approximately 90 minutes.[66] The short half-life of initially developed somatostatin analogs meant that, in order to have sufficient concentrations for therapeutic effect for any duration, they had to be given by subcutaneous injection three to four times per day or continuously either intravenously or subcutaneously. Therefore, a long-acting somatostatin analog, an LAR depot form for intramuscular use given once monthly, was developed and has been approved for clinical use. Steady-state octreotide serum concentrations are achieved after the third dose. Although effective in treating the carcinoid syndrome and for controlling symptoms related to GH and prolactin-secreting pituitary tumors, it has been only minimally evaluated in other tumor settings.

Denileukin diftitox is usually administered as intravenous therapy over at least 15 minutes once daily for 5 days in a row, with treatment repeated every 21 days. It is rapidly cleared from the serum, with a short distribution phase of 2 to 5 minutes and a terminal half-life of 70 to 80 minutes.[67] There is not a significant difference in PKs between bolus and 90-minute infusion schedules. As with antibodies, there is significant interpatient variability in PKs. The majority of patients developed antibodies against the toxin, against the IL-2, or against both by the third cycle of therapy, and the specific types of antibodies that develop may enhance clearance rates, which tend to be two to three times more rapid by the third course.

Given the short half-lives of peptides, a number of approaches to improving their in vivo pharmacologic properties have been investigated. For example, polyethylene glycol conjugated to peptides might improve their PKs by a number of mechanisms, including prolonged plasma half-life, decreased immunogenicity (although occasionally it may actually enhance immunogenicity), increased solubility, resistance to proteolysis, and better coupling to liposomes. Innovative approaches, such as controlled-release polymers, may enhance peptide delivery for a prolonged period.[61] Additionally, mathematical models have been developed to define parameters required for in vivo use of targeted therapies, and these might be useful in attempting to optimize the design of compounds for clinical use.[68] Ultimately, clinical trials are necessary to define PK properties and toxicity for any given compound.

Toxicity

Somatostatin analogs are quite nontoxic, with median lethal dose values not being reached in rats. There is no evidence of chronic toxicity in studies conducted up to 2 years in dogs.[66] In addition, they have been given to patients for many years with no discernible long-term side effects. Side effects include pain at the injection site, abdominal pain, cramps, and diarrhea. Chololithiasis can occur.

Denileukin diftitox is moderately well tolerated.[64,67] Constitutional (flu-like) and gastrointestinal symptoms (low-grade fevers and chills, asthenia, anorexia, nausea/vomiting, headache, diarrhea, arthralgias/myalgias) develop in approximately 90% of patients but usually can be treated symptomatically. Hypersensitivity reactions (dyspnea, chest tightness, hypotension, back pain, pruritus and flushing) occur in approximately 60% of patients, but, again, most of these are controllable or preventable by slowing the rate or temporarily interrupting the infusion and/or symptomatic therapy with antihistamines and acetaminophen. Occasionally, glucocorticoids have been necessary. Vascular leak syndrome occurs in about one quarter of patients. It usually is self-limited and can be treated symptomatically. Rashes occur in approximately one third of patients. A significant number of patients have some elevations of hepatic enzymes, but this is not accompanied by other liver abnormalities. Renal insufficiency defined the maximum tolerated dose. Anemia, thrombocytopenia, hemolysis, and proteinuria are also seen.

The toxicity profiles of new modified peptides will be defined by the results of trials using those agents.

Clinical Effectiveness

Unconjugated Peptidomimetics

Clearly, somatostatin analogs have activity in controlling symptoms related to GH and prolactin-secreting pituitary tumors, GI neuroendocrine tumors (especially carcinoid tumors), and diarrhea related to certain chemotherapeutic agents.[66,68] Clinical trials have demonstrated minor activity against prostate cancer, minimal activity in breast and pancreatic cancer, and no activity against small cell lung cancer.[66,69–71] High-dose therapy using somatuline (in the range of 12 mg/day by continuous infusion subcutaneously) has biologic activity as measured by suppression of GH and IGF-I, but the evaluation of clinical effectiveness against different tumors is still in progress. As new, potentially more potent somatostatin analogs are developed, they continue to be evaluated for treating malignancies.[66,71]

Given the relatively low level of antitumor activity of these agents used alone, combinations with other agents have been evaluated in several trials. RC-160 (somatostatin analog) and SB-75 (LH-RH antagonist) inhibit the growth of human pancreatic xenograft in a mouse model.[72] However, no beneficial effects were seen in a large trial using LH-RH (not the antagonist) and somatostatin, alone or in combination, to treat patients with pancreatic cancer, and the LH-RH agonist goserelin plus hydrocortisone produced no responses.[73] Somatostatin analogs appear to enhance the antitumor effects of tamoxifen in preclinical studies.[74] A randomized study suggests that the combination of a somatostatin analog, an antiprolactin agent, and tamoxifen produced a higher response rate and time to disease progression than tamoxifen alone for patients with metastatic breast cancer.[75] However, there was no difference in overall survival. The evaluation of combinations of somatostatin analogs and other agents or approaches, including chemotherapy and radiation therapy, is ongoing.[76]

Conjugated Modified Peptides

In addition to combination therapy, a potentially promising approach is to use modified peptides to deliver cytotoxic agents to tumors expressing high receptor levels. This approach has been studied utilizing radionuclide-coupled somatostatin analogs to treat neuroendocrine tumors.[52,56,76–79] The only significant toxicities to date have been reversible myelosuppression, especially anemia; decreases in lymphocyte counts; mild thrombocytopenia; and mild increases in creatinine. Although this approach has produced some antitumor activity, this activity has not yet been sufficient to establish the approach as clinically useful. Efforts to improve these agents are ongoing. Other analogs coupled to radionuclides, chemotherapeutic agents, and toxins are also being developed and evaluated as potential therapeutic as well as imaging agents.[80–82]

Denileukin diftitox has shown effectiveness against a number of hematopoietic malignancies, including Hodgkin's disease and lymphomas (including cutaneous T-cell lymphomas [CTCLs]).[64] It is approved for use in the treatment of patients with advanced or refractory CTCL.

To date, clinically useful targeted compounds have come from one of the three classes of agents already discussed. However, significant research is ongoing to evaluate the following classes of compounds for potential utility as anticancer agents.

Antisense Oligonucleotides

Antisense oligonucleotides (oligos) are modified single-stranded DNA molecules usually between 15 and 25 nucleotides in length. They are synthesized to have nucleotide sequences complementary to DNA or mRNA sequences of the specific gene being targeted for inhibition. As drugs, oligos have inherent disadvantages, including large size, significant charge, difficult synthesis, and poor penetration of cells. In part for these reasons, they still have not fulfilled their promise as therapeutic agents. However, development is ongoing, with the hope that they will prove useful after a better understanding is achieved of their clinical pharmacology and how to optimize their modification of gene expression.

Mechanism of Action

When therapy is directed at mRNA, it is based on one of the fundamental features of biology, the specificity of Watson and Crick base pairing. By means of binding an

TABLE 30.7

POTENTIAL MECHANISMS OF MESSENGER RNA (mRNA) FUNCTION OR mRNA MODIFICATION TARGETED BY ANTISENSE OLIGONUCLEOTIDES

Inhibition of mRNA
Translational arrest
Splicing
5' Capping
3' Polyadenylation
Transport
Degradation
Activation of RNaseH, an enzyme present ubiquitously in cells, which degrades RNA complexed to DNA

mRNA, the synthesis of the specific protein encoded by that mRNA is ultimately inhibited, and its function blocked. Using mRNA as the target, a number of specific mechanisms can be invoked[83-87] (Table 30.7), including the activation of the RNA-degrading enzyme, RNaseH.

Alternatively, specific DNA or protein sequences can be targeted by oligos. The major target in DNA is Hoogsteen and anti-Hoogsteen base pairing in the major groove to produce triple-helical structures, leading to inhibition of transcription. Oligos can be coupled to a number of antineoplastic compounds to specifically target them, especially to DNA.

Hybridization to RNA or DNA is a relatively slow process, and, in general, the association rates of oligos determine their efficacy.[83-87] The minimum size of oligos required to provide necessary specificity and affinity for these purposes appears to be 15 to 18 bases. A caveat to this specificity is that mismatched oligos can induce degradation of target mRNA, so it is certainly possible that cleavage of nontarget mRNA sequences might occur when specific oligos are used in vivo.

The binding of proteins (e.g., transcription factors) to specific DNA or RNA sequences can be targeted. The sequence length required depends on the precise protein-DNA (or RNA) interaction site.[83-87] Proteins that do not normally bind to DNA or RNA can also potentially be inhibited by binding to oligos specifically and nonspecifically. An approach to designing specific oligos for this purpose is protein epitope targeting. A large number of partially random oligos are used to screen for binding to a target protein. This allows identification of oligos that bind to specific epitopes. The bound oligos can be amplified by polymerase chain reaction. Identified sequences can then be used to develop improved oligos for targeting the protein therapeutically.

Cellular Pharmacology and Metabolism

Necessary requirements for oligos to be useful therapeutically are outlined in Table 30.8. Oligos appear to bind to the cell surface through receptors, although the exact nature of these receptors remains to be defined. This process is saturable. However, it is not clear whether this saturability of uptake will be important for systemic use of oligos. Once bound to the cell surface, oligo uptake into cells appears to occur primarily by pinocytosis, adsorptive endocytosis, or both.[83-87] Although certain studies suggest that a significant proportion of oligos remain in endosomes, the consensus is that retention in endosomes is not a major limitation in their effectiveness. Binding by cellular proteins may modify the PKs and efficacy of oligos.[83-87]

Uptake of oligos varies among different cell types (studies suggest greater uptake in carcinoma than leukemic cells) and among cells in the same culture. Various factors (e.g., number of oligo receptors, cell cycle stage, rate of division) can explain differences in oligo uptake. Increased cell density decreases uptake of phosphorothioate oligos.[88] As would be expected, differences in the intracellular degradation of oligos by cells can have a profound effect on their efficacy.[89] Exocytosis also occurs and is a potentially important determinant of the concentration of oligos within cells over time and therefore of their efficacy. Thus, a number of aspects of cellular pharmacology are critical in determining the activity of these compounds.

Clinical Pharmacology

Oligos present a special problem as in vivo compounds because of the ubiquitous presence of nucleases that rapidly degrade unmodified constructs.[89] Fortunately, the potential clinical use of oligos can be enhanced by medicinal chemical approaches.[83-87] Certain modifications make them potentially better for some purposes but not as good for others. Modifications can be designed to prevent rapid metabolism, increase cellular uptake, increase targeting to tumor cells, stabilize binding of oligos to the target structure, or increase inhibitory efficacy. Oligos can be conjugated with ribozymes (with catalytic RNase activity; see "Ribozymes, Other Nucleases, and Proteases") or other reagents that cleave specific nucleic acid sequences.[90]

TABLE 30.8

REQUIREMENTS FOR OLIGONUCLEOTIDES TO BE THERAPEUTICALLY USEFUL

Stability in vivo
Uptake into and retention in neoplastic cells
Specific and relatively stable interaction with target sequences in RNA, DNA, or protein, or a combination of the three, without nonspecific inhibition of other cellular molecules
Absence of significant toxicity to normal cells or organ systems
Limited potential for mutagenicity
Lack of significant immunogenicity
Favorable pharmacokinetics (distribution, metabolism, and excretion) in vivo to allow sufficient delivery to tumor cells to inhibit their multiplication

Peptide nucleic acids can inhibit DNA and RNA function. Attachment of toxic compounds to oligos can target those agents to DNA and enhance cell killing, such as using antisense bcr-abl constructs to target compounds specifically to DNA in CML cells.

The most important modifications for in vivo use have been chemical alterations of the bases used to construct oligos. This includes using methylphosphonates or phosphorothioates as the phosphodiester backbone, a change that prevents their destruction by nucleases.[83-87] Phosphorothioates appear to be the more advantageous of these analogs, because they have higher affinity than dimethyl phosphonates for nucleic acids, and they are more effective in activating RNaseH. Therefore, phosphorothioates have been the most extensively studied modified oligos. Many other modifications to oligos, including incorporation of methylene, carbonate (or carbamate), sulfonamide, amino acid, peptide, phosphorodithioate, C-5 propyne analogs of cytidine and uridine, and pyrimidines modified at the 5 and 6 positions, also have significant activity in vitro.[83-87,91] However, these have not yet been extensively developed for clinical use.

A number of methods have been used to increase specificity of delivery of oligos to tumor cells and uptake by those cells. Molecules such as porphyrin, cholesterol (or cholesteryl), poly-L-lysine, and transferrin-polylysine significantly enhance uptake and retention, although they also reduce the time of the interaction with mRNA or DNA.[83-87] Liposomes (e.g., pH-sensitive liposomes) may provide an effective way of delivering oligos into cells.[92] Complexes of liposomes with compounds (e.g., the Sendai virus protein coat) can significantly enhance their uptake by cells. Coupling of liposomes (with encapsulated oligos) to targeting peptides (i.e., mAbs directed against antigens expressed on the cell surface) offers another means of specific targeting.[93]

Ex vivo use of oligonucleotides does not have many of the problems associated with in vivo use. Oligos by themselves, as well as in combination with chemotherapy, are highly effective in inhibiting tumor cell growth ex vivo. These strategies may be useful in purging bone marrow of leukemic or other malignant cells.[94] Small molecule alternatives to antisense, with more favorable PK properties, could potentially inhibit site-specific interactions between RNA and proteins or nucleotides.[95] This is an area of active study.

Pharmacokinetics

In the excitement over the potential use of antisense therapy for the treatment of cancer, the PKs of these agents in vivo have received relatively little attention and study. Until the last decade, the paucity of PK data was at least partially due to the high cost of producing sufficient amounts of the compounds for careful PK studies, even in mice. Fortunately, the cost of producing oligos has decreased

dramatically with continued improvements in technology. A second problem has been assay methodology for separation of the parent compound and its stepwise oligo cleavage products. These problems have been sufficiently solved for PK studies of oligos to be performed.

Several animal models have been used for evaluating the targeting, pharmacology, and effectiveness of these compounds. Most studies suggest that oligos are fairly rapidly cleared from the circulation (phosphorothioate analogs, which are resistant to nucleases, water soluble, and readily taken up by cells, have been primarily studied; methylphosphonates have been studied to a lesser extent).[96-105] Most studies in animals have shown that $t_{1/2}\alpha$ ranges from 5 minutes to several hours after bolus administration; human studies to date have been more variable, with $t_{1/2}\alpha$ ranging from 30 minutes to as long as 26 hours after bolus administration and approximately 7 hours after subcutaneous administration.[96-105] In any case, overall oligos have relatively short half-lives, arguing for the need for frequent administration if continued inhibition of the target is to be maintained.

Oligonucleotides are distributed to the majority of tissues, including malignancies. In the absence of central nervous system abnormalities, brain takes up little of systemically delivered phosphorothioate or methylphosphonate oligos.[96-105] Oligo length (at least within the 20 to 50 base range), base sequence, and dose (at least in the range up to 150 mg/kg) do not appear to significantly affect the rate of plasma clearance.[99-105] However, the specific base analog used in constructing the oligos does affect their PKs.[96-105]

Given the relatively slow uptake of oligos by cells, rapid clearance from the circulation makes delivery of oligos to tumor cells difficult. Mechanisms for enhancing delivery are important considerations if oligos are to be used successfully as systemic agents. In normal tissues, the highest concentrations accumulate in the kidney and liver, with up to 40% in the liver at 12 hours.[96-105] This can induce some degree of hepatic inflammation, as indicated by elevations in lactate dehydrogenase and transaminases.[96-104] To a lesser extent, accumulation occurs in other tissues, including intestine, spleen, lung, heart, and muscle.[96-104] Route of administration may affect organ distribution, with subcutaneous injection possibly favoring accumulation in spleen and muscle. Oligos are stable in most tissues but are more rapidly metabolized in kidney and liver.[96-105] Degradation in blood and tissues appears to be primarily due to 3'-exonucleases.[99] Rate of degradation does not appear to be dose-dependent, as would be expected given the large amount of nucleases present. The $t_{1/2}\beta$ of total-body clearance is approximately 30 to 40 hours.[96-105] Clearance of methylphosphonate and unmodified oligos is more rapid than clearance of phosphorothioates.[99] Most of the dose is excreted in urine in 2 to 3 days (with approximately 30% in the first 24 hours) and significantly less via the GI tract.[96-105] Most oligos that are excreted are degraded, so only a small proportion of intact oligos are found in the urine. Modifications to the oligos, including addition of bases, can occur in several tissues, including liver, kidney, and GI tract.[96-105] Interactions with other drugs are poorly understood; there continues to be a need for careful evaluation of PKs in the setting of coadministered drugs. However, most studies have not shown significant PK interactions between oligos and chemotherapeutic drugs (see below for further discussion).

Toxicity

Although antisense molecules differ in their sequence and target, they seem to share similar PK and toxicologic properties, independent of effects on the target sequence itself. Although a single dose of 640 mg/kg of anti-HIV phosphorothioate was lethal, single doses of up to 150 mg/kg have been well tolerated in mice.[105] Antisense molecules that are cytostatic may require prolonged administration, making potential chronic toxicity an important consideration. Doses up to 100 mg/kg of phosphorothioate oligos for 14 days do not appear to produce serious toxic effects.[96-105] In rhesus monkeys, continuous infusions of oligos at doses up to 1,500 mg for periods as long as 15 days did not produce significant toxicities.[106] Mild elevations in liver func-

tions were seen in the majority of animals, and mild neutropenia was seen in one third. Many oligos seem to produce complement activation and thrombocytopenia as their dose-limiting toxicities in animals. Oligos can also accumulate in kidneys, with the potential for nephrotoxicity, although significant nephrotoxicity is primarily seen at higher doses.[44-50]

Most of the clinical trials in humans have indicated that oligonucleotides are generally safe. The most common toxicities have been thrombocytopenia, asthenia, fevers, hypotension, hyperglycemia, and minor changes in renal function (Table 30.9).[100-104] All of these are usually mild and rapidly reverse when the oligonucleotide is discontinued. Local skin reactions are also seen when oligos are delivered subcutaneously. Less common toxicities have included activation of complement and clotting abnormalities.

Clinical Effectiveness

The in vivo effectiveness of antisense oligos has been demonstrated in a number of animal model systems.[96-105] Longer exposure of animals to oligos appears to produce a greater antitumor effect.[96] These results indicate that suffi-

---

TABLE 30.9

TOXICITIES OF SOME OF THE OLIGONUCLEOTIDES IN CLINICAL TRIALS FOR CANCER PATIENTS

Compound	Toxicities
Antisense to bcl-2	Fatigue, flu-like symptoms (myalgias, arthralgias), transaminitis
Antisense to c-raf-1	Fever, complement activation, prolonged PTT
Antisense to H-ras	Flu-like symptoms, fatigue, nausea, self- limiting hemolytic uremic syndrome
Antisense to protein kinase C-α	Fever, flu-like symptoms, transaminitis, complement activation, prolonged PT, prolonged PTT, decreased platelets, hemorrhage

PT, prothrombin time; PTT, partial prothrombin time.
Adapted from Chen H, Ness E, Marshall J, et al. Phase I trial of a second generation oligonucleotide (GEM 123) targeted at type I protein kinase A in patients with refractory solid tumors. Proc ASCO 1999;18:159a; Mani S, Shulman K, Kunkel K, et al. Phase I trial of protein kinase-Ca antisense oligonucleotide (ISIS 3521; ISI 641A) with 5-fluorouracil (5-FU) and leucovorin (LV) in patients with advanced cancer. Proc ASCO 1999;18; Advani R, Fisher A, Grant P, et al. A phase I trial of an antisense oligonucleotide targeted to protein kinase Ca (ISIS 3521/ISI641A) delivered as a 24-hour continuous infusion (CI). Proc ASCO 1999;18; Dorr A, Bruce J, Monia B, et al. Phase I and pharmacokinetic trial of ISIS 2503, a 20-Mer antisense oligonucleotide against H-RAS, by 14-day continuous infusion (CIV) in patients with advanced cancer. Proc ASCO 1999;18:157a; Gordon MS, Sandler AB, Holmlund JT, et al. A phase I trial of ISIS 2503, an antisense inhibitor of H-RAS, administered by a 24-hour (hr) weekly infusion to patients (pts) with advanced cancer. Proc ASCO 1999;18:157a; Holmlund JT, Rudin CM, Mani S, et al. Phase I trial of ISIS 5132/ODN 698A, a 20-Mer phosphorothioate antisense oligonucleotide inhibitor of C-RAF kinase, administered by a 24-hour weekly intravenous (IV) infusion to patients with advanced cancer. Proc ASCO 1999;18:157a; Daugherty CK, Goh BC, Ratain M, et al. The standard phase II trial design is not acceptable to most patients (pts). Proc ASCO 2000;19; Alavi JB, Grossman SA, Supko J, et al. Efficacy, toxicity and pharmacology of an antisense oligonucleotide directed against protein kinase C-a (ISIS 3521) delivered as a 21 day continuous intravenous infusion in patients with recurrent high grade astrocytomas (HGA). Proc ASCO 2000;19; Yuen A, Advani R, Fisher G, et al. A phase I/II trial of ISIS 3521, an antisense inhibitor of protein kinase C Alpha, combined with carboplatin and paclitaxel in patients with non-small cell lung cancer. Proc ASCO 2000; Chi KN, Gleave ME, Klasa R, et al. A phase I trial of an antisense oligonucleotide to BCL-2 (6139) mitoxantrone in patients with metastatic hormone refractory prostate (HRPC). Proc ASCO 2000;19; Scher HI, Morris MJ, Tong W, et al. A phase I trial of G3139, a bcl2 antisense drug, by continuous infusion (CI) as a single agent and with weekly taxol. Proc ASCO 2000;19:199a.

cient quantities of oligos can be delivered over time to a variety of tumors in mice to achieve an antitumor effect at doses that do not produce significant toxicity.

Clinical trials have been completed using antisense constructs alone and in combination with chemotherapy.[96–105] Antisense constructs to other mutated cancer genes, including *p53* and *bcr-abl*, as well as to HIV (in patients with HIV-associated malignancies), have been performed. These have shown the following: (a) Target genes can be inhibited in peripheral blood cells and malignant cells in lymph nodes at achievable concentrations of oligonucleotides. (b) Occasional patients have had responses (including a complete response seen in a patient with B-cell NHL treated with Bcl-2 antisense).[101–104] A proportion of patients have had stable disease. However, most patients have not responded. (c) Combinations of oligonucleotides with chemotherapy can be delivered with acceptable toxicity. In addition, these have not indicated significant PK interactions between oligos and chemotherapeutic agents. Although this remains a potential concern, it does not occur commonly. Additional clinical trials are ongoing, and the results will indicate whether sufficient clinical efficacy can be achieved in humans (either efficacy of oligonucleotides themselves or in combination with chemotherapy) for this approach to be of value in treating cancer patients. Other routes of administration (ex vivo, intraperitoneal, transcutaneous, intrathecal) are also being explored. A number of antisense constructs against growth factor receptors, especially the EGFR, have been evaluated in a number of preclinical models and are being considered for clinical trials.

Posttranscriptional Gene Silencing via RNA Interference Other Than by Use of Antisense DNA Compounds

The discovery of the mechanism of RNA interference in which double-stranded RNAs are processed to small interfering RNAs (siRNAs) that ultimately bind to complementary RNA molecules, leading to their cleavage and the posttranscriptional gene silencing (PTSG) of the gene, has provided a very powerful tool for studying the effects of silencing specific genes.[107–109] Although double-stranded RNAs trigger the antiviral response in mammalian cells that interferes with the ability to use them to silence specific genes, siRNAs can bypass this response and can be utilized for this purpose. A large number of studies have utilized siRNAs to evaluate the effects of silencing specific genes on cellular phenotype and function. This is critical in assessing the potential effects of agents targeted to a specific gene. Although still in the early stages of development as therapeutic agents, the potential delivery of siRNAs as therapeutic agents to silence specific genes is actively being evaluated. The identification of the related microRNAs (miRNAs), which are single-stranded RNA molecules processed from stem-looped precursors and are thought to

be involved in gene regulation in a variety of organisms (including humans), has provided further insight into the importance of PTSG in regulating gene expression and the potential utility of these agents for targeting the expression of specific genes.[110]

Ribozymes, Other Nucleases, and Proteases

Ribozymes are RNAs that can catalyze a variety of RNA or DNA cleavage reactions (i.e., splicing or site-specific cleavage) via their tertiary structures, and therefore they function as enzymes or possibly drugs.[111–116] Their advantage over protein enzymes is that one can, through sequence and structure changes, modify ribozymes to carry out specific functions much more readily than can be done in the case of proteins. As with oligos, they need to be modified to make them nuclease resistant to be useful for in vivo purposes. The stability of the RNA being targeted and the turnover rate of ribozyme-substrate interaction are important determinants of the potential usefulness of ribozymes. They can be targeted to cells by coupling with proteins, genetic vectors, or other compounds to be most useful. The pharmacology of these coupled compounds for the most part resembles that of the targeting agent to which they are coupled. The most extensively studied of the ribozymes as anticancer agents to date has been angiozyme.[114–116] Angiozyme is a ribozyme directed against the FLT-1 (VEGFR-1) receptor. It has been shown to down-regulate the FLT-1 receptor in vivo and to have antitumor and antimetastatic activity in an animal tumor model. Phase I studies showed it to be well tolerated when given as a subcutaneous injection, with the major toxicity being mild to moderate local skin reactions. Bioavailability after subcutaneous injection is estimated at greater than 74%. It has an approximately 6-hour half-life after subcutaneous injection. Approximately 10 to 20% of the drug is excreted unchanged in the urine. It has been evaluated in a phase I study in combination with chemotherapy for colorectal cancer. It was well tolerated, and initial results were encouraging, although it is impossible to know whether angiozyme added to the effectiveness of chemotherapy in this setting. Further development of angiozyme is currently being considered. Studies evaluating other ribozymes as possible antiviral agents as well as antitumor agents are ongoing.

Gene Therapy

Gene therapy uses the insertion of new genetic information into cells and its expression in those cells to alter their biologic behavior for the purpose of achieving therapeutic benefit. The initial promise of gene therapy (and still an important area of investigation) lay in the placement of a normal critical gene into cells that either do not express the gene at all or have a mutated form of the gene. Such placement could also potentially suppress the abnormal function of a mutated gene. This strategy is being pursued for inherited genetic disorders and for introducing tumor suppressor genes into neoplastic cells. However, a number of significant hurdles remain to be overcome if malignancies are to be treated using this approach. These include the need to transfect at least the vast majority of malignant cells for this to be clinically useful, the inefficiency of gene transfer into cells, the difficulties of in vivo delivery to neoplastic cells, and the problem of maintaining continued expression of the transduced gene in those cells over time.

Therefore, much of the emphasis in gene therapy as an approach to treating neoplasms has shifted to making cells more immunogenic in order to activate host-mediated killing of the cells. A number of animal model systems suggest that modification of a subpopulation of tumor cells may lead to an "innocent bystander effect" (by mechanisms that have not been fully elucidated but presumably are, at least in part, immune mediated) whereby nontransfected tumor cells are also eliminated. This approach would not require transfecting every cell to be effective.[117-125] The fact that the innocent bystander effect is seen with a wide variety of transferred genes suggests that the mechanism or mechanisms involved in mediating this effect may not be immunologic (or some may not), but much more study is required to determine why this occurs and how it might be best used. Alternatively, genes that protect normal cells against toxicity of therapeutic agents used to treat the malignancy could be used to protect the host and allow higher-dose delivery of the toxic agents.

Difficulties remain in ensuring that expression of the transfected gene is appropriately controlled in tumor cells, maintaining expression in these cells during a prolonged period (expression of most genes tends to decrease with time) while preventing deleterious function in normal cells. These need to be adequately addressed for gene therapy to be therapeutically useful.

Mechanism of Action

Introduced genetic material can be used to inhibit or augment gene function or produce proteins beneficial to the host by a number of potential mechanisms (Table 30.10).[117-125] For example, such material can be used:

- as RNA decoys (multiple copies of a sequence can be transcribed and compete with other intracellular sequences for protein binding)
- as transdominant altered proteins that can suppress specific protein function in cells (if these happen to be critical proteins for a signal transduction pathway [e.g., ras or raf], one could potentially disrupt the entire pathway)
- in the production of intracellular toxins, leading to cell death
- in the intracellular production of antibodies to block the function of specific proteins

TABLE 30.10
POTENTIAL APPLICATIONS OF GENE THERAPY

RNA decoys
Transdominant altered proteins
Intracellular toxins
Intracellular antibodies
Ribozymes
Proteins that make tumor cells more immunogenic
Proteins that make tumor cells susceptible to killing by specific drugs
Proteins that make normal cells resistant to cytotoxic agents
Proteins beneficial to host expressed in immune effector or other host cells

- as ribozymes to catalyze the cleavage of specific RNA or DNA sequences
- in the expression of proteins that make tumor cells more immunogenic and therefore prone to elimination by the host's immune system and that generate a systemic immune response against the tumor
- in the expression of genes that make cells susceptible to killing by specific drugs (e.g., the herpesvirus thymidine kinase [TK] gene, which makes cells susceptible to killing by ganciclovir, or the cytosine deaminase gene, which activates 5-fluorocytosine)
- in the expression of a gene (e.g., the dihydrofolate reductase or multiple drug resistance type 1 gene) in normal cells that makes them more resistant to killing by cytotoxic agents or radiation therapy
- to produce proteins beneficial to the host in an ongoing and controllable manner, either in immune-effector or other host cells, such as fibroblasts

Cellular Pharmacology and Metabolism

Two major methods for introducing genetic material into cells are (a) physical approaches, such as via liposomal delivery, DNA-ligand complexes, ballistic techniques (in which multiple pellets coated with DNA are rapidly injected into cells), and direct injection of DNA itself, and (b) viral-mediated transfer. Defective retroviral vectors were the initial ones studied for use as a means of getting genes into and expressed in mammalian cells.[117-119] However, they have a number of limitations for therapeutic use, which has led to the development of other viral vectors for this purpose. Limitations of retroviral vectors include these: it is necessary to have active cell division for retroviral vectors to integrate into chromosomes; cells must have the appropriate receptors to take up the vectors; the integration of viral DNA into random chromosomal sites raises concerns about the potential activation of endogenous genes, which might be transforming, or the inactivation of genes important in controlling cell proliferation; and the vectors may become inactivated, such as by complement, when used in vivo. In fact, the activation of the T-cell oncogene LMO2 after gene therapy for X-linked immunodeficiency, with resultant uncontrolled T-cell proliferation, has confirmed this potential risk.[125]

For these reasons, construction of other viral vectors that might not carry the same degree of risk for mutagenesis or induction of host genes has been actively pursued. These viral vectors include vaccinia (and other poxviruses), polio, Sindbis (and other RNA viruses), adenovirus, adeno-associated viruses, herpesvirus vectors (e.g., herpes simplex virus 1), and HIV-1, which have all been modified for use in gene therapy.[117–125] As with retroviral vectors, each of these has its potential benefits but also potential problems as delivery systems for gene therapy. There is an ongoing effort to improve each of these vectors in order to achieve better vector systems for therapeutic use. As an example, a possible method for making these vectors safer is by incorporating the TK gene, rendering the cells they infect susceptible to ganciclovir and therefore susceptible to elimination, should this be desired. This approach has been explored to control graft versus host disease mediated by alloreactive donor T cells; however, donor cells have occasionally become leukemic as a consequence of insertional mutagenesis.[126]

Physical methods of gene transfer not requiring modified viral vectors also have been used, including liposomal delivery, direct injection of genetic material, in vivo lipofection with cationic lipid–DNA complexes, ballistic techniques to "microinject" large amounts of DNA-coated pellets into cells, and targeted DNA-ligand complexes via cell endocytosis.[117–119] Examples of ligands used for this purpose include liver-specific asialoglycoprotein receptors and transferrin receptors. Special efforts have to be made to inhibit lysosomal degradation of introduced DNA. Chloroquine is one of the compounds used for this purpose. Viral particles (e.g., adenovirus, which can disrupt endosomes) provide another means of preventing DNA degradation. These approaches have not been toxic in animal models. Ultimately, combinations of different delivery systems using the advantages of each may provide the most useful approach to gene therapy.

Clinical Pharmacology

Gene delivery can either be ex vivo or in vivo. Advantages of ex vivo delivery include high efficiency, ability to enrich infected cells, and ability to assess for presence of the transduced gene before reinfusing the cells.[117–125] Cells can be labeled fluorescently for in vivo tracking, which allows a means of following the fate of ex vivo transfected cells.[117–125] Targeting vectors to cells via specific receptors is also currently being studied.[117–125] In addition, DNA can be injected directly into tissues to produce desired proteins, such as activators of the immune system.[117–125] Direct injection of the genes for enzymes that activate prodrugs into

malignant cells, followed by treatment with prodrugs, is another approach. Many of the current trials evaluating the efficacy of gene therapy in treating cancer involve ex vivo introduction of a gene (usually an immunomodulatory molecule, such as granulocyte-macrophage colony-stimulating factor [GM-CSF]) into tumor cells (either autologous or allogeneic), with reintroduction of modified, inactivated cells (inactivated usually by irradiation) into the patient as cancer vaccines.

In vivo, a number of approaches can be used to enhance gene delivery to tumors in specific settings.[117–125] Liposomal delivery can be used to target cells, such as in the liver or lung. Methods of getting compounds across the blood-brain barrier, such as using the high concentration of transferrin receptors in brain capillary endothelial cells, also might be useful for delivery to lesions in the central nervous system. Cationic liposomes may offer an advantage for targeting delivery to specific tissues. Each of these approaches can be combined with tissue-specific promoter-enhancer elements to limit expression of the gene to tissues of interest (see below).[117–125] A number of factors may be important in the expression of transgenes in vivo, including composition of the liposomal lipid, the DNA-liposome ratio, and the promoter-enhancer elements that control the expression of the gene.[117–125] Combinations of viral and physical systems offer yet another approach.

Controlling the expression of genes in vivo remains an important issue. The expression of genes can be limited to target tissues by using tissue-specific transcriptional regulatory sequences upstream of the gene. An example of this is targeting the active form of a drug by virally directed enzyme prodrug therapy; in this method, tissue-specific transcriptional regulatory sequences are placed upstream of the drug-activating gene so that its expression is restricted in a tissue-specific manner.[101,102] The expression of most genes has been relatively low and declines with time due to the death of transfected cells as well as the loss of gene activity by mechanisms that are not yet well delineated but may involve nucleases.

Although there have been a large number of clinical trials evaluating gene therapy for cancer treatment in humans, a significantly smaller number of these have evaluated the PKs of virus, especially delivered systemically. Two recent trials in humans have evaluated the PKs of virus and vector DNA when injected intratumorally.[127,128] Both trials used adenoviral vectors (replication defective in one case and replication competent in the other) and had similar results inasmuch as there was no detectable intact infectious adenovirus in the blood at any time point although vector DNA was detected in the blood. In both trials, an immune response to the vector was induced. In one trial, tumors were resected between 3 and 8 days after the injection and showed the presence of virus in approximately 20% of cells at the dose of 1×10^{11} virus particles.[127] Viral particles were seen in tumor cells but also in other cells, including mostly macrophages but also lymphocytes and fibroblasts. In the other trial, biopsies were obtained over time to evaluate the persistence of transgene expression in the target tissue (prostate) in a small number of patients. Expression was seen in 3 of 3 patients at 2 weeks, 1 of 3 patients at 3 weeks, and 0 of 3 patients at 4 weeks.[128] As the authors point out, biopsies have the potential for sampling error that might underestimate the persistence of expression elsewhere in the organ. These trials illustrate features that have been commonly found in studies: antibody responses to vectors occur in a significant percentage of patients, infectious particles are not commonly detectable in secreted fluids or blood when the vectors are delivered directly into tumors, viral replication occurs and is detectable for 1 to 2 weeks after delivery, and persistence of expression of the gene of interest over time remains a problem to be solved.

Toxicity

As regards the toxicity of gene therapy, the main concern is the potential toxicity of different viral vectors and the potential for serious toxicity to an organ (such as the liver or lung) from marked immune response or viral replication as well as the possible risk of malignancy from the insertion of retroviral vectors in critical areas of the genome. In fact, the death of a patient from overwhelming toxicity (particularly hepatotoxicity) after receiving a modified adenoviral vector and the development of uncontrolled clonal proliferation of mature T cells in two children with X-SCID treated with the common γ chain of the interleukin-2 receptor delivered via a modified retroviral vector that inserted near the proto-oncogene LMO2 promoter showed that these risks are real.[127,129] These two events have led to significant reevaluation of how gene therapy can be made safer as well as heightened oversight of gene therapy trials.

Clinical Effectiveness

It has been shown that the transfection of tumor cells with a wide spectrum of cytokines, antisense constructs, foreign major histocompatibility complex genes, or other genes important in mediating various aspects of the immune response, as well as the reintroduction of these cells into animals, has significant antitumor effects, putatively by immune-mediated mechanisms.[117–125,128,130,131] Most studies suggest that a proportion of tumor cells are killed by an innocent bystander effect (presumably immunologically mediated). However, this effect is seen even with approaches that would not be expected to generate a strong immune response, and the actual mechanisms for the innocent bystander effect remain undetermined.

Gene therapy is undergoing extensive clinical evaluation in humans.[117–125] Approaches demonstrated to be effective in animal studies and currently undergoing clinical trials include (a) inhibition of an oncogene (e.g., K-ras or raf); (b) replacement of a functional tumor suppressor gene (e.g., p53); (c) transfection of activating enzymes for prodrugs (e.g., hTK gene) into tumor cells, followed by treatment with the prodrugs (e.g., ganciclovir); (d) transfer of protecting genes (e.g., MDR1) into normal (especially hematopoietic) cells, followed by high-dose chemotherapy; (e) transduction of immune effector cells with cytokine genes (e.g., TNF or IL-2) to enhance their effectiveness in killing tumor cells; (f) transduction of tumor cells with immunomodulatory molecules (GM-CSF, IL-2, IL-4, HLA-B7) to make them more susceptible to immunologic destruction, as well as to generate a systemic immune response against the tumor; and (g) use of vectors expressing antisense messages to inhibit the function of critical genes for tumor cell survival, proliferation, or metastasis, such as growth factors or their receptors or angiogenic factors (e.g., VEGF) or their receptors.[77,103,105–112] There are extensive ongoing efforts to optimize dendritic cell activation by those approaches using immunomodulatory molecules, such as GM-CSF and IL-4. These approaches have all been successful in treating tumors in animal models, but clearly their potential use in patients is in the early stages of development. To date, these approaches for treating cancer patients have been shown to be feasible but have had limited clinical efficacy. Efforts to enhance and prolong the expression of transduced genes in vivo, as well as other approaches for enhancing the therapeutic efficacy of these approaches, are being evaluated in ongoing studies.

CONCLUSION

Sufficient understanding of the biology of cellular processes exists, and tools are now available to manipulate molecular systems for therapeutic benefit, to allow the rational design and delivery of molecules directed at specific proteins or genes important for the survival or growth of malignant cells. Over the past decade, a number of molecularly targeted agents have been developed and are now part of the standard anticancer armamentarium. Targets include mutant proteins, proteins overexpressed on malignant cells, and angiogenic factors. These include growth factor receptors and their ligands as well as proteins involved in the signaling processes downstream from growth factor receptors. Most targeted therapies have been designed to inhibit the target directly, although several deliver cytotoxic compounds to malignant cells. Agents that have been approved include mAbs for treatment of breast cancer, colorectal cancer, AML, B-CLL, and B-cell NHL as well as an immunotoxin for treatment of CTCL; the small molecule bcr-abl and the KIT tyrosine kinase inhibitor imatinib mesylate for CML and GIST, respectively; and the small molecules gefitinib and erlotinib for treatment of patients with NSCLC. A number of other targeted agents are in late clinical development, and the list will continue to grow.

This is an exciting time in the development of rationally targeted therapies. However, there is still a significant amount of study necessary to develop additional clinically useful antitumor approaches using targeted agents. Continued improvement in our understanding of the critical processes in cancer development, growth, and metastasis should provide new targets and new agents for attacking these. Technological advances allowing much more sophisticated evaluation of intracellular and intercellular processes, such as utilization of siRNAs and analysis of protein-protein interactions, will play an increasingly important role. As more information is gathered about the immensely complex interaction of proteins in cells, this effort will require the use of mathematical evaluation by powerful computers. However, carefully performed toxicity and pharmacologic studies to determine how to best deliver these therapies to patients remain critical to the successful clinical development of any of these agents. Because there is no current method for adequately modeling these by in vitro studies, analysis (e.g., by computer models), well-designed and well-performed animal and, most importantly, human clinical studies remain essential to the development of these compounds as therapeutic agents. Knowledge gained from the successful development of targeted agents and also from failed attempts will provide insights into how to best identify and develop new compounds. As studies continue to identify new targets, there will be an ongoing effort to develop new and improved targeted agents against them to improve the treatment of different cancers. Gradually, the dream of targeted therapy is being turned into reality.

REFERENCES

1. Abou-Jawde R, Choueiri T, Alemany C, et al. An overview of targeted treatments in cancer. Clin Ther 2003;25:2121–2137.
2. Guillemard V, Sargovi HU. Novel approaches for targeted cancer therapy. Curr Cancer Drug Targets 2004;4:313–326.
3. Finley RS. Overview of targeted therapies for cancer. Am J Health Syst Pharm 2003;60:S4–10.
4. Strausberg RL, Simpson AJ, Old IJ, et al. Oncogenomics and the development of cancer therapies 2004;429:469–474.
5. Brugarolas J, Clark JW, Chabner B. Using "rationally designed drugs" rationally. Lancet 2003;9371:1758–1759.
6. Lundberg AS, Weinberg RA. Control of the cell cycle and apoptosis. Science 1999;35:1886–1894.
7. Swanton C. Cell-cycle targeted therapies. Lancet Oncol 2004;5:27–36.
8. Wu X, Senechal K, et al. The PTEN/MMAC1 tumor suppressor phosphatase functions as a negative regulator of the phosphoinositide 3-kinase/AKT pathway. Proc Natl Acad Sci USA 1998;95: 15587–15591.
9. Alessi P, Ebbinghaus C, Neri D. Molecular targeting of angiogenesis. Biochim Biophys Acta 2004;1654:39–49.
10. Mosesson Y, Yarden Y. Oncogenic growth factor receptors: implications for signal transduction therapy. Semin Cancer Biol 2004;14:262–270.
11. Lynch TJ, Bell DW, Sordella R, et al. Activating mutations in the epidermal growth factor receptor underlying responsiveness of non-small-cell lung cancer to gefitinib. N Engl J Med 2004; 350:2191–2193
12. Paez JG, Janne PA, Lee JC, et al. EGFR mutations in lung cancer: correlation with clinical response to gefitinib therapy. Science 2004;304:1497–1500.
13. Sattler M, Salgia R. Targeting c-KIT mutations: basic science to novel therapies. Leuk Res 2004;28(Suppl):S11–20.
14. Joensuu H, Kindblom LG. Gastrointestinal stromal tumors: a review. Acta Orthop Scand Suppl 2004;75:62–71.
15. Sakorafas GH, Tsiotou AG, Tsiotos GG. Molecular biology of pancreatic cancer: oncogenes, tumour suppressor genes, growth factors, and their receptors from a clinical perspective. Cancer Treat Rev 2000;26:29–52.
16. Leenders WP. Targeting VEGF in anti-angiogenic and anti-tumor therapy: where are we now? Int J Exp Pathol 1998;79:339–346.
17. Gibbs JB. Anticancer drug targets: growth factors and growth factor signaling. J Clin Invest 2000;105:9–13.
18. Yamamoto T, Taya S, Kaibuchi K. Ras-induced transformation and signaling pathway. J Biochem 1999;126:799–803.
19. Gao HG, Chen J, et al. Distribution of p53 and K-ras mutations in human lung cancer tissues. Carcinogenesis 1997;18:473–478.
20. Breivik J, Meling G, et al. K-ras mutations in colorectal cancer: relations to patient age, sex, and tumor source. Br J Cancer 1994; 69:367–371.
21. Baupre DM, Kurzrock R. Ras and leukemia: from basic mechanisms to gene directed therapy. J Clin Oncol 1999;17:1071–1079.
22. End DW. Farnesyl protein transferase inhibitors and other therapies targeting the Ras signal transduction pathway. Invest New Drugs 1999;18:241–258.
23. Bollag G, Freeman S, Lyons JF, et al. Raf pathway inhibitors in oncology. Curr Opin Investig Drugs 2003;4:1436–1441.
24. Lebowitz PF, Pendergast GC. Non-ras targets of farnesyltransferase inhibitors: focus on Rho. Oncogene 1998;17:1439–1445.
25. Waddick KG, Uckum FM. Innovative treatment programs against cancer, I: ras oncoprotein as a molecular target. Biochem Pharmacol 1998;56:1411–1426.
26. Wong KK, Eder JP, Clark J, et al. Final results of a phase I study to determine the safety, maximum tolerated dose, pharmacokinetics, and pharmacodynamics of BAY 43-9006 in repeated cycles of 1 week on/1 week off in patients with advanced, refractory solid tumors. Proc ASCO 2003;22:244 (abst. 976).
27. Drucker BJ, Lydon NB. Lessons learned from the development of an Abl tyrosine kinase inhibitor for chronic myelogenous leukemia. J Clin Invest 2000;105:3–7.
28. Hahn WC, Stewart S, et al. Inhibition of telomerase limits the growth of human cancer cells. Nat Med 1999;5:1164–1170.
29. Cunningham D, Humblet Y, Siena S, et al. Cetuximab monotherapy and cetuximab plus irinotecan in irinotecan-refractory metastatic colorectal cancer. M Engl J Med 2004;351: 337–345.
30. Seidman AD, Fornier M, et al. Weekly trastuzumab and paclitaxel therapy for metastatic breast cancer with analysis of efficacy by HER2 immunophenotype and gene amplification. J Clin Oncol 2001;19:2587–2595.
31. Perea-Soler R. The role of erlotinib (Tarceva, OSI 774) in the treatment of non-small cell lung cancer. Clin Cancer Res 2004;10:4238s–4240s.
32. Harris M. Monoclonal antibodies as therapeutic agents for cancer. Lancet Oncol 2004;5:292–302.
33. Peng B, Hayes M, et al. Pharmacokinetics and pharmacodynamics of imatinib in a phase I trial with chronic myeloid leukemia patients. J Clin Oncol 2004;22:935–942.
34. le Coutre P, Kreuzer K, et al. Pharmacokinetics and cellular uptake of imatinib and its main metabolite CGP74588. Cancer Chemother Pharmacol 2004;53:313–323.
35. O'Brien SG, Meinhardt P, et al. Effects of imatinib mesylate (ST1571, Glivec) on the pharmacokinetics of simvastatin, a cytochrome P450 3A4 substrate, in patients with chronic myelogenous leukemia. Br J Cancer 2003;89:1855–1859.
36. de Jong FA, Verweij J. Role of imatinib mesylate (Gleevec/Glivec) in gastrointestinal stromal tumors. Expert Rev Anticancer Ther 2003;3:757–766.
37. Heinrich MC, et al. Kinase mutations and imatinib response in patients with metastatic gastrointestinal stromal tumors. J Clin Oncol 2003;21:4342–4349.
38. Demetri GD. Targeting the molecular pathophysiology of gastrointestinal stromal tumors with imatinib: mechanisms,

successes, and challenges to rational drug development. Hematol Oncol Clin North Am 2002;16:115–124.

39. Baselga J. Combining the anti-EGFR agent gefitinib with chemotherapy in non-small-cell lung cancer: how do we go from INTACT to impact? J Clin Oncol 2004;22:759–761.

40. Wolf M, Swaisland H, Averbuch S. Development of the novel biologically targeted anticancer agent gefitinib: determining the optimum dose for clinical efficacy. Clin Cancer Res 2004;10: 4607–4613.

41. Cersosimo RJ. Gefitinib: a new antineoplastic for advanced non-small-cell lung cancer. Am J Health Syst Pharm 2004;61: 889–898.

42. Thomas SM, Grandis JR. Pharmacokinetic and pharmacodynamic properties of EGFR inhibitors under clinical investigation. Cancer Treat Rev 2004;30:255–268.

43. Hammond LA. Pharmacokinetic evaluation of gefitinib when administered with chemotherapy. Clin Lung Cancer 2003; 5(Suppl 1):S18–21.

44. Liu CY, Seen S. Gefitinib therapy for advanced non-small-cell lung cancer. Ann Pharmacother 2003;37:1644–1653.

45. Ransom M, Wardell S. Gefitinib, a novel, orally administered agent for the treatment of cancer. J Clin Pharm Ther 2004;29: 95–103.

46. Hidalgo M, Bloedow D. Pharmacokinetics and pharmacodynamics: maximizing the clinical potential of erlotinib (Tarceva). Semin Oncol 2003;30:25–33.

47. Sandler A. Clinical experience with the HER1/EGFR tyrosine kinase inhibitor erlotinib. Oncology 2003;17:17–22.

48. Shepherd F, Pereira J, Ciuleanu T, et al. A randomized placebo-controlled trial of erlotinib in patients with advanced non-small cell lung cancer (NSCLC) following failure of 1st or 2nd line chemotherapy: a National Cancer Institute of Canada Clinical Trials Group (NCIC CTG) trail [abstract]. Proc ASCO 2004;23:A7022.

49. Henrick MC, Corless CL, Demetri GD, et al. Kinase mutations and imatinib response in patients with metastic gastrointestinal stromal tumor. J Clin Oncol 2003;21:4342–4349.

50. Maki RG. Gastrointestinal stromal tumors respond to tyrosine kinase-targeted therapy. Curr Treat Options Gastroenterol 2004; 7:13–17.

51. Demetri GD, Desai J, Fletcher J, et al. SU11248, a multi-targeted tyrosine kinase inhibitor, can overcome imatinib (IM) resistance caused by diverse genomic mechanisms in patients (pts) with metastatic gastrointestinal stromal tumor (GIST). Proc ASCO 2004;23:195 (abst. 3001).

51a Escudier B, Szczylik C, Eisen T, et al. Randomized phase III trial of the Raf kinase and VEGFR inhibitor sorafenib (BAY 43-9006) in patients with advanced renal cell carcinoma (RCC). J Clin Oncol (Meeting Abstracts) 2005;23:LBA4510.

52. Grotzinger C, Wiedenmann B. Somatostatin receptor targeting for tumor imaging and therapy. Ann NY Acad Sci 2004;1014: 258–264.

53. Pollak MN, Schally AV. Mechanisms of antineoplastic action of somatostatin analogs. Proc Soc Exp Biol Med 1998;217: 143–152.

54. Gillespie TJ, Erenberg A, et al. Novel somatostatin analogs for the treatment of acromegaly and cancer exhibit improved in vivo stability and distribution. J Pharmacol Exp Ther 1998;285:95–104.

55. O'Byrne KJ, Dobbs N, et al. Phase II study of RC-160 (vapreotide), an octapeptide analog of somatostatin, in the treatment of metastatic breast cancer. Br J Cancer 1999;79:1413–1418.

56. Woltering EA. Development of targeted somatostatin-based antiangiogenic therapy: a review and future perspectives. Cancer Biother Radiopharm 2003;18:601–609.

57. Moscardo R, Sherline P. Somatostatin inhibits rapid centrosomal separation and cell proliferation induced by epidermal growth factor. Endocrinology 1982;3:1394.

58. Liebow C, Reilly C, et al. Somatostatin analogs inhibit growth of pancreatic cancer by stimulating tyrosine phosphatase. Proc Natl Acad Sci USA 1989;86:2003–2007.

59. Shadid M, Sioud M. Selective targeting of cancer cells using synthetic peptides. Drug Resist Updat 2003;6:363–371.

60. Mitsiades CS, Mitsiades N, Koutsilieris M. The Akt pathway: molecular targets for anti-cancer drug development. Curr Cancer Drug Targets 2004;4:235–256.

61. Rowinsky EK. Signal events: cell signal transduction and its inhibition in cancer. Oncologist 2003;8(Suppl 3):5–17.

62. Schally AV, Nagy A. Cancer chemotherapy based on targeting of cytotoxic peptide conjugates to their receptors on tumors. Eur J Endocrinol 1999;141:1–14.

63. Yang D, Kuan C, et al. Recombinant heregulin-*Pseudomonas* exotoxin fusion proteins: interactions with the heregulin receptors and antitumor activity in vivo. Clin Cancer Res 1998;4:993–1004.

64. Kreitman RJ. Recombinant toxins for the treatment of cancer. Curr Opin Mol Ther 2003;5:44–51.

65. Behe M, Du J, et al. Biodistribution, blood half-life, and receptor binding of a somatostatin-dextran conjugate. Med Oncol 2001;18: 59–64.

66. Parmar H, Phillips RH, Lightman SL. Somatostatin analogs: mechanisms of action. Recent Results Cancer Res 1993;129:1–24.

67. Olsen E, Duvic M, et al. Pivotal phase III trial of two dose levels of denileukin diftitox for the treatment of cutaneous T-cell lymphoma. J Clin Oncology 2001;19:376–388.

68. Buchanan KD. Effects of sandostatin on neuroendocrine tumours of the gastrointestinal system. Rec Results Cancer Res 1993;129:45–55.

69. Reubi JC. Peptide receptors as molecular targets for cancer diagnosis and therapy. Endocr Rev 2003;24:389–427.

70. Prevost G, Israel L. Somatostatin and somatostatin analogs in human breast carcinoma. Rec Results Cancer Res 1993;129:63–70.

71. Canobbio L, Boccardo F, et al. Treatment of advanced pancreatic carcinoma with the somatostatin analog BIM 23014: preliminary results of a pilot study. Cancer 1992;69:648–650.

72. Radulovic S, Comaru-Schally A, et al. Somatostatin analog RC-160 and LH- RH antagonist SB-75 inhibit growth of MIA PaCa-2 human pancreatic cancer xenografts in nude mice. Pancreas 1993;8:88–97.

73. Philip PA, Carmichael J, et al. Hormonal treatment of pancreatic carcinoma: a phase II study of LHRH agonist goserelin plus hydrocortisone. Br J Cancer 1993;67:379–382.

74. Pollak M. Enhancement of the anti-neoplastic effects of tamoxifen by somatostatin analogs. Digestion 1996;57:29– 33.

75. Bontenbal M, Foekens J, et al. Feasibility, endocrine and antitumour effects of a triple endocrine therapy with tamoxifen, a somatostatin analog and an antiprolactin in post-menopausal metastatic breast cancer: a randomized study with long-term follow-up. Br J Cancer 1998;77:115–122.

76. Robbins RJ. Somatostatin and cancer. Metab Clin Exp 1996;45: 98–100.

77. Kwekkeboom DJ, Krenning EP. Radiolabeled somatostatin analog scintigraphy in oncology and immune diseases: an overview. Eur Radiol 1997;7:1103–1109.

78. Schally AV, Nagy A. Cancer chemotherapy based on targeting of cytotoxic peptide conjugates to their receptors on tumors. Eur J Endocrinol 1999;141:1–14.

79. De Jong M, Breeman W, et al. Therapy of neuroendocrine tumors with radiolabeled somatostatin analogs. Q J Nucl Med 1999;43: 356–366.

80. Pagamelli G, Zoboli S, et al. Receptor-mediated radionuclide therapy with 90Y-DOTA-D-Tyr3-Octreotide: preliminary report in cancer patients. Cancer Biother Radiopharm 1999;14:477– 483.

81. Saleh MN, LeMaistre C, et al. Antitumor activity of DAB389IL-2 fusion toxin in mycosis fungoides. J Am Acad Dermatol 1998;39:63–73.

82. LeMaistre CF, Saleh M, et al. Phase I trial of a ligand fusion-protein (DAB389IL-2) in lymphomas expressing the receptor for interleukin-2. Blood 1998;91:399–405.

83. Marcusson EG, Yacyshyn B, et al. Preclinical and clinical pharmacology of antisense oligonucleotides. Mol Biotech 1999;12:1–11.

84. Curcio LD, Bouffard DY, Scanlon KJ. Oligonucleotides as modulators of cancer gene expression. Pharmacol Ther 1997;74:317–332.

85. Dachs GU, Dougherty G, et al. Targeting gene therapy to cancer: a review. Oncol Res 1997;9:313–325.

86. Alama A, Barbieri F, et al. Antisense oligonucleotides as therapeutic agents. Pharmacol Res 1997;36:171–178.

87. Calogero A, Hospers GA, Mulders NH. Synthetic oligonucleotides: useful molecules? A review. Pharm World Sci 1997;19:264–268.

88. Iwanaga T, Ferriola PC. Cellular uptake of phosphorothioate oligodeoxynucleotides is negatively affected by cell density in a transformed rat tracheal epithelial cell line: implication for

antisense approaches. Biochem Biophys Res Commun 1993;191: 1152–1157.

89. Ryte A, Morelli S, et al. Oligonucleotide degradation contributes to resistance to antisense compounds. Anticancer Drugs 1993;4: 197–200.

90. Sarver N, et al. Ribozymes as potential anti-HIV-1 therapeutic agents. Science 1990;247:1222–1225.

91. Sanghvi YS, et al. Antisense oligodeoxynucleotides: synthesis, biophysical and biological evaluation of oligodeoxynucleotides containing modified pyrimidines. Nucleic Acids Res 1993;21: 3197–3203.

92. Pagnan A, et al. Delivery of c-myb antisense oligonucleotides to human neuroblastoma cells via disialoganglioside GD(2)-targeted immunoliposomes: antitumor effects. J Natl Cancer Inst 2000;92:253–261.

93. Penichet ML, et al. An antibody-avidin fusion protein specific for the transferrin receptor serves as a vehicle for effective brain targeting: initial applications in anti-HIV antisense therapy in the brain. J Immunol 1999;163:4421–4426.

94. Bergan RC. Ex vivo bone marrow purging with oligonucleotides. Antisense Nucleic Acid Drug Dev 1997;7:251–255.

95. Zapp ML, Stern S, Green MR. Small molecules that selectively block RNA binding of HIV-1 Rev protein inhibit Rev function and viral production. Cell 1993;74:969–978.

96. Ratajczak MZ, et al. In vivo treatment of human leukemia in a SCID mouse model with c-myb antisense oligodeoxynucleotides. Proc Natl Acad Sci USA 1992;89:11823–11827.

97. Iversen P. In vivo studies with phosphorothioate oligonucleotides: pharmacokinetics prologue. Anticancer Drug Design 1991;6:531–538.

98. Levin AA. A review of the issues in the pharmacokinetics and toxicology of phosphorothioate antisense oligonucleotides. Biochim Biophys Acta 1999;1489:69–84.

99. Vlassov V, Yakubov L. Oligonucleotides in cells and organisms: pharmacological considerations. In: Wickstrom E, ed. Prospects for Antisense Nucleic Acid Therapy of Cancer and AIDS. New York: Wiley, 1991;243.

100. Gewirtz AM. Oligonucleotide therapeutics: a step forward. J Clin Oncol 2000;18:1809–1811.

101. Waters JS, et al. Phase I clinical and pharmacokinetic study of Bcl-2 antisense oligonucleotide therapy in patients with non-Hodgkin's lymphoma. Science 1992;258:1792–1795.

102. O'Dwyer PJ, et al. C-raf-1 depletion and tumor responses in patients treated with raf-1 antisense oligodeoxynucleotide ISIS 5132 (CGP 69846A). Clin Cancer Res 1999;5:647–661.

103. Yuen AR, Sikic BI. Clinical studies of antisense therapy in cancer. Front Biosci 2000;5:D588–593.

104. Galderisi U, Cascino A, Giordano A. Antisense oligonucleotides as therapeutic agents. J Cell Physiol 1999;81:251–257.

105. Agrawal S, Zhang R. Pharmacokinetics of oligonucleotides. Ciba Found Symp 1997;209:60–75

106. Spinolo J, et al. Toxicity of human p53 antisense oligonucleotide infusions in rhesus macacca. Proc AACR 1993;33:3125.

107. Montgomery MK. RNA interference: historical overview and significance. Methods Mol Biol 2004;265:3–21.

108. Ichim TE, et al. RNA interference: a potent tool for gene-specific therapeutics. Am J Transplant 2004;4:1227–1236.

109. Dorsett Y, Tuschl T. siRNAs: applications in functional genomics and potential as therapeutics. Nat Rev Drug Discov 2004;3:318–329.

110. He L, Hannon GJ. MicroRNAs: small RNAs with a big role in gene regulation. Nat Rev Genet 2004;5:522–531.

111. Norris JS, et al. Design and testing of ribozymes for cancer gene therapy. Adv Exp Med Biol 2000;465:293–301.

112. Parry TJ, et al. Ribozyme pharmacokinetic screening for predicting pharmacodynamic dosing regimens. Curr Issues Mol Biol 2000;2:113–118.

113. Usman N, Blatt LM. Nuclease-resistant synthetic ribozymes: developing a new class of therapeutics. J Clin Invest 2000;106: 1197–1202.

114. Weng DE, Usman N. Angiozyme: a novel angiogenesis inhibitor. Curr Oncol Rep 2001;3:141–146.

115. Sandberg JA, et al. Pharmacokinetics and tolerability of an antiangiogenic ribozyme (ANGIOZYME) in healthy volunteers. J Clin Pharmacol 2000;40:1462–1469.

116. Basche M, et al. Angiozyme, an anti-VEGFR1 ribozyme, carboplatin, and paclitaxel: results of a phase I study [abstract]. Proc ASCO 2002;A445.

117. Scanlon KJ. Cancer gene therapy: challenges and opportunities. Anticancer Res 2004;24:501–504.

118. Nabel GJ. Cancer gene therapy: present status and future directions. Ernst Schering Res Found Workshop 2003;43: 81–88.

119. Scanlon I, et al. Gene regulation in cancer gene therapy strategies. Curr Med Chem 2003;10:2175–2184

120. Kanerva A, Hemminki A. Modified adenoviruses for cancer gene therapy. Int J Cancer 2004;110:475–480.

121. Acres B, et al. Therapeutic cancer vaccines. Curr Opin Mol Ther 2004;6:40–47.

122. McNeish IA, Bell SJ, Lemoine NR. Gene therapy progress and prospects: cancer gene therapy using tumor suppressor genes. Gene Ther 2004;11:497–503.

123. Waxman DJ, Schwarz PS. Harnessing apoptosis for improved anticancer gene therapy. Cancer Res 2003;63:8563–8572.

124. Kamiya H, Akita H, Harashima H. Pharmacokinetic and pharmacodynamic considerations in gene therapy. Drug Discov Today 2003;8:990–996.

125. Neumanaitis J. Selective replicating viral vectors: potential for use in cancer gene therapy. BioDrugs 2003;17:251–262.

126. Hacein-Bay-Abina S, et al. LMO2-associated clonal T-cell proliferation in two patients after gene therapy for SCID-X1. Science 2003;302:415–419.

127. McCormack MP, Rabbitts TH. Activation of the T-cell oncogene LMO2 after gene therapy for X-linked combined immunodeficiency. N Engl J Med 2004;350:913–922.

128. Palmer DH, et al. Virus-directed enzyme prodrug therapy: intratumoral administration of a replication-deficient adenovirus encoding nitroreductase to patients with respectable liver cancer. J Clin Oncology 2004:22:1546–1552.

129. Grilly BJ, Gee AP. Gene transfer: regulatory issues and their impact on the clinical investigator and the good manufacturing production facility. Cytotherapy 2003;5:197–207.

130. Freytag SO, et al. Phase I study of replication-competent adenovirus-mediated double-suicide gene therapy in combination with conventional-dose three-dimensional conformal radiation therapy for the treatment of newly diagnosed, intermediate- to high-risk prostate cancer. Cancer Res 2003;63: 7497–7506.

131. Soiffer R, et al. Vaccination with irradiated, autologous melanoma cells engineered to secrete granulocyte-macrophage colony-stimulating factor by adenoviral-mediated transfer augments antitumor immunity in patients with metastatic melanoma. J Clin Oncol 2003;21:3343–3350.

Antibody Therapies of Cancer

31

David A. Scheinberg   *Deborah A. Mulford*

Joseph G. Jurcic   *George Sgouros*   *Richard P. Junghans*

Monoclonal antibodies (mAbs) are remarkably versatile agents with potential therapeutic applications in a number of human diseases, including cancer. There are now eight FDA-approved mAbs for the treatment of cancer. MAbs have long promised to offer a safe, specific approach to therapy. Over more than a decade, preclinical evaluation and human clinical trials have identified new strategies for the use of mAbs, as well as a number of obstacles to their effective application. Although the use of antibodies as targeting agents dates to the 1950s,[1] clinical investigation of antibodies as a potential treatment for cancer could not be initiated until the mid-1970s, when efficient and reliable methods for the production of mAbs were developed.[2]

Five approaches to mAb therapy are used in humans. First, mAbs can be used to focus an inflammatory response against a target cell. The binding of a mAb to a target cell can result in the fixation of complement, which yields cell lysis or results in opsonization that marks the cell for lysis by various effector cells, such as natural killer (NK) cells, neutrophils, and monocytes. Second, mAbs may be used as carriers to deliver another small molecule, atom, radionuclide, peptide, or protein to a specific site in vivo. Third, mAbs may be directed at critical hormones, growth factors, interleukins, or other regulatory molecules or their receptors to control growth or other cell functions. Fourth, anti-idiotypic mAbs may be used as vaccines to generate an active immune response. Finally, mAbs may be used to speed the clearance of other drugs or toxins or fundamentally alter the pharmacokinetic properties of other therapeutic agents. For example, mAbs may be fused to drugs or factors to increase their plasma half-life, change their biodistribution, or render them multivalent. Alternatively, mAbs may be used to clear previously infused mAbs from the circulation.

Despite the diversity of approaches, significant problems remain that are peculiar to mAbs. The mAbs are large, immunogenic proteins, often of rodent origin, that rapidly generate neutralizing immune responses in patients within days or weeks after their first injection. The sheer size of mAbs—150 kd for immunoglobulin G to 950 kd for immunoglobulin M, 100 times larger than that of typical drugs—makes their pharmacology (particularly diffusion into bulky tumors or other extravascular areas) problematic for effective use. Many early mAbs or mAb constructs were either poorly cytotoxic or relatively nonspecific, which rendered them ineffective. Moreover, the high degree of mAb specificity that is routinely achievable may allow tumor cells that do not bear the specific antigen target to escape from cytotoxic effects.

Nonetheless, mAbs still have great potential to be safe and effective anticancer agents. Recent clinical investigations have highlighted several areas in which mAbs can be effective, either alone or in combination with other, more conventional agents.

This chapter reviews the basic biochemical and biologic properties of mAbs and the most commonly used derivatives (immunotoxins, radioimmunoconjugates, mAb fragments), discusses the pharmacologic issues peculiar to mAbs, and outlines some of the important clinical results obtained with mAbs. Potential solutions to the most difficult issues in the use of mAbs are presented. Because mAbs and conjugates of mAbs represent many different drugs with characteristics that result from their origin (rodent or human), their isotypes, their structure, or the various conjugated toxic agents, generalizations about the properties of mAbs often may not be possible. Treatment of cancer with mAbs is a new and rapidly changing field, and readers are encouraged to consult other reviews for more comprehensive discussions of individual areas.[3]

IMMUNOGLOBULIN STRUCTURES

Immunoglobulins are separated into five classes or isotypes based on structure and biologic properties: immunoglobulin M (IgM), immunoglobulin D (IgD), immunoglobulin E (IgE), immunoglobulin A (IgA), and immunoglobulin G (IgG). IgM is the primordial antibody whose expression by the B cell on its surface represents the commitment of that cell to a particular but broad recognition space that subsequently narrows as part of the maturation response induced by antigen interactions.[4] In some cases, the antibodies interact with specialized receptors that link their action to host cellular defenses; in others, the antibodies interact with the humoral complement system. IgG is further divided into four subclasses, and IgA into two subclasses. Heritable deficiencies in individual immunoglobulin classes or IgG subclasses are associated with susceptibility to particular infections and autoimmune disorders.[5] Table 31.1 summarizes various features of the antibodies discussed in this section.

The fundamental structural elements of all antibodies are indicated by size as heavy and light chains of 55 to 75 kd and 22 kd, respectively (Fig. 31.1). Light chains are either κ or λ and are each distributed among all immunoglobulin subclasses. Heavy chains are μ, δ, γ, ε, and α, corresponding to IgM, IgD, IgG, IgE, and IgA and the biologic characteristics of each antibody class. The amino-terminal domain of each chain is the variable (V_H or V_L) region that mediates antigen recognition; the remaining domains are constant regions designated C_L for light chain and C_H1, C_H2, and C_H3 for heavy chain (and C_H4 for μ and ε). Between C_H1 and C_H2 is the hinge region, which confers flexibility on the antibody "arms" and susceptibility to proteases (see later), except in IgM and IgE, in which the C_H2 domain itself serves this role.

Heavy (H) and light (L) chains are normally paired 1:1 with each other, but the smallest stable unit is a four-chain $(HL)_2$ structure (Fig. 31.1), for a nominal total mass of 150 to 160 kd for IgG and higher for other isotypes (Table 31.1). IgE and IgG are composed of a single $(HL)_2$ unit, whereas IgM exists as a pentamer of $(HL)_2$ units joined by disulfide bonding with a third J-chain component. IgA exists mainly as a monomer in serum, but in secretions it exists primarily as a dimer plus trimer and higher forms in which the oligomers are linked by J chain as well as the fragment of secretory chain (secretory piece) that is involved in the mucosal transport.

The V region itself is composed of subdomains—relatively conserved framework regions interdigitated with the complementarity-determining regions (CDRs; also termed "hypervariable segments" [HVSs]) that make primary contact with antigen (Fig. 31.1).[6] Three CDRs are found in

TABLE 31.1

PROPERTIES OF ANTIBODY CLASSES

Property	IgG	IgA	IgM	IgD	IgE
Usual molecular form	Monomer	Monomer, dimer, etc.	Pentamer	Monomer	Monomer
Molecular formula	$\gamma_2\kappa_2$ or $\gamma_2\lambda_2$	$(\alpha_2\kappa_2)n$ or $(\alpha_2\lambda_2)n$	$(\mu_2\kappa_2)5$ or $(\mu_2\lambda_2)5$	$\delta_2\kappa_2$ or $\delta_2\lambda_2$	$\varepsilon_2\kappa_2$ or $\varepsilon_2\lambda_2$
Heavy-chain domains	V, C_H1–3	V, C_H1–3	V, C_H1–4	V, C_H1–3	V, C_H1–4
Other chains	—	J chain, S piece	J chain	—	—
Subclasses	IgG1, IgG2, IgG3, IgG4	IgA1, IgA2	—	—	—
Heavy-chain allotypes	Gm (~30)	Am (2)	Mm (2)	—	—
Molecular weight (Da)	150,000	160,000	950,000	175,000	190,000
Sedimentation constant (S)	6.6	7, 9, 11, 14	19	7	8
Carbohydrate content (%)	3	7	10	9	13
Serum level (mg/100 mL)	1,250 ± 300	210 ± 50	125 ± 50	4	0.03
Percentage of total serum Ig	75–85	7–15	5–10	0.3	0.003
Half-life (days)	23 (IgG3, 7)	5.8	5.1	2.8	2.5
Antibody valence	2	2, 4, 6, . . .	10	1 or 2	2
Complement fixation (classic)	+ (Ig G1, G2, G3)	—	++	—	—
Fc receptors	FcγR-I, FcγR-II, FcγR-III				FcεR-I, FcεR-II
Binding to cells	Monocyte macrophages, neutrophils, LGLs	—	?	—	Mast cells
Other biologic properties	Secondary Ab response; placental transfer	Secretory antibody	Primary Ab response; B-cell surface Ig, rheumatoid factor	B-cell surface Ig	Homocytotropic Ab; anaphylaxis; allergy

+, active; ++, strongly active; Ab, antibody; CH, constant region of the heavy chain; Ig, immunoglobulin; LGLs, large granular lymphocytes; V, variable region.

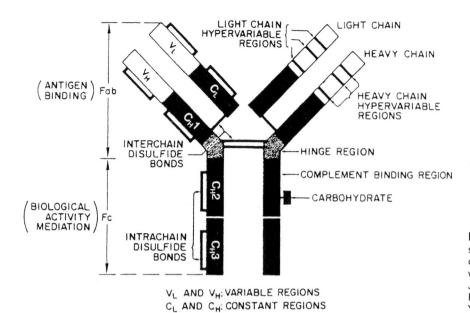

V_L AND V_H: VARIABLE REGIONS
C_L AND C_H: CONSTANT REGIONS

Figure 31.1 Antibody structure. The structural relationships and functions of domains of immunoglobulin G. (Reproduced with permission from Wasserman RL, Capra JD. Immunoglobulins. In: Horowitz MI, Pigman W, eds. The Glycoconjugates. New York: Academic Press, 1977:323.)

each heavy and light chain that may participate in antigen binding. The V regions should be seen as juxtaposed three-fingered gloves, with the CDRs covering the tips (Fig. 31.2), arrayed in a broad contact surface with antigen (Fig. 31.3).

Antibodies are glycoproteins. Glycosylation of proteins plays various roles related to solubility, transport, conformation, function, and stability. Carbohydrate is located mainly in antibody C domains, with a lower frequency in V regions (see data on M195 later).[7] IgG contains a major conserved glycosylation site in C_H2 that contributes to the conformation of this domain, which is crucial to the functional ability to bind to complement and to Fcγ receptors.

The IgG antibody "unit" has been defined in terms of susceptibility to proteases that cleave in the exposed, non-folded regions of the antibody (Fig. 31.1). A summary of antibody fragments and engineered or synthetic products is presented in Table 31.2. Fab contains the V region and first C domain of the heavy chain ($V_H + C_H1 = Fd$) and the entire light chain (L); Fab' includes in addition a portion of the H chain hinge region and one or more free cysteines (Fd'); Fabc2 is a dimer of Fab' linked through hinge disulfide(s); and Fv is a semistable antibody fragment that includes only $V_H + V_L$, the smallest antigen-binding unit. Fc is the C-terminal crystallizable fragment that includes the complement and Fc receptor–binding domains (see later). Genetically engineered products include the δ constructs; these lack the second C domain of heavy chain and behave like Fab'2, with bivalence, abbreviated survival and lack of interaction with host effector systems, but they do not require enzymic processing.[8] Another genetically engineered product, sFv (single-chain Fv), is Fv with a peptide linkage engineered to join the C-terminus of one chain to the N-terminus of the other for improved stability. More advanced products have been designed that conceptually represent the antigen-binding domain in a single peptide product[9]; this is not related structurally to an antibody and is therefore considered an antibody mimic.

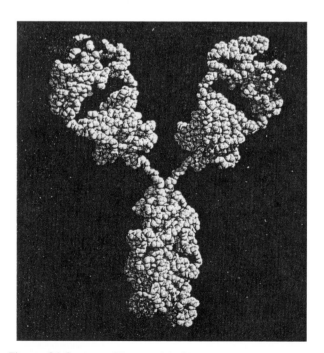

Figure 31.2 Space-filling model of human immunoglobulin G1 antibody with complementarity-determining regions in color representing anti–Tac-H; human myeloma protein Eu with complementarity-determining regions grafted from murine anti-Tac. (Photo provided courtesy of Dr. C. Queen.)

ONTOGENY

Antibodies possibly represent the most strikingly evolved, adaptive system in all of biology. The most diverse representation of classes and functions is found in Mammalia.

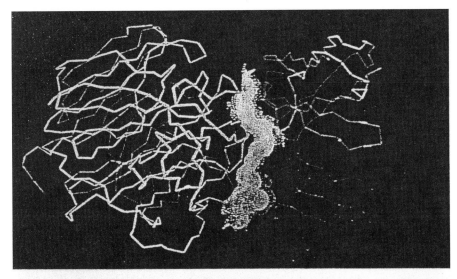

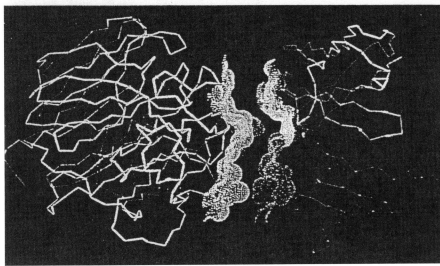

Figure 31.3 Antigen-antibody binding surface juxtaposition. The variable (V) region (Fv) of antibody (*right*) binds to influenza virus protein neuraminidase (*left*) in the top panel. The V_H (*red*) and V_L (*blue*) regions are separately colored to show their respective binding contributions. The bottom panel offsets the two molecules by 8 Å to show the complementarity of surfaces that promotes the binding interaction. The stippled surface of the neuraminidase defines the antigen "epitope." (Photo provided courtesy of Drs. P.M. Colman and W.R. Tulip, CSIRO Australia.)

The power of antigen recognition begins with an inherited array of duplicated and diversified germ-line V genes, a random mutational process that creates novel CDRs, a combinatorial selection process that amplifies the germline capabilities, and a controlled and directed mutational process that hones the specificity and matures the antibody into a high-affinity, antigen-specific reagent.

The biologic expression of antibody begins with the B-cell progenitor, which undergoes a series of maturation steps that begin with V gene selection for heavy chain followed by light chain V selection that yields surface expression and secretion by the mature B cell. On interaction with antigen, the B cells are activated to proliferate, secrete antibody, undergo CDR mutagenesis and affinity maturation, and finally undergo chain switch and plasma cell conversion. Plasma cells remain in tissues, spleen, or lymph nodes and secrete large quantities of antibody, which is the sole function of this terminally differentiated cell.[4]

The genes of heavy and light chains share important features of structure and maturation. Each gene locus contains widely separated V, C, and minigene domains that are placed into juxtaposition by DNA recombination mechanisms. The minigenes—diversity (D) and joining (J) regions for heavy chain and J regions for light chain—contribute to or constitute, with modifications, the CDR3.[10] The κ and λ light chain loci are located on chromosomes 2 and 22, respectively, but all heavy chains are contained within a single massive locus on chromosome 14.

Germ-line diversity is essential to the generation of the antibody repertoire. On the heavy chain locus are an estimated 80 functional V_H genes, 12 D regions, and 6 J regions for a potential of 6,000 combinations (Fig. 31.4).[10–12] Roughly 80 Vκ light chain and 5 Jκ domains are found, which, randomly associated, can generate 400 combinations (the λ locus contains a smaller number of distinct V genes). A simple arithmetical calculation suggests that VκV_H combinations alone could generate a diversity of approximately 2×10^6. Yet even this number is conservative, because this diversity is amplified in turn by errors in recombination and processes called N and P nucleotide

TABLE 31.2

ANTIBODY FRAGMENT DEFINITIONS

Designation	Representation	Description
Fabc		Complete immunoglobulin G
Enzyme-generated products		
Fab	Fd / L	Papain digest; Fd + L
Fab'	Fd' / L	Pepsin digest monomer; Fd' + L
Fab'2	Fab'	Pepsin digest dimer
Fv	V_H / V_L	V region digestion fragment; $V_H + V_L$
Fc (or Fc')	CH_2 / CH_3	C region digestion fragment; crystallizable fragment
pFc (or pFc')	CH_2 / CH_3	Smaller fragments of Fc
Genetically engineered products		
δC_H2	CH_3	Deleted C_H2 domain; dimer of $V - C_H1 - C_H3 + L$
SFv	V_H / V_L	Single-chain Fv; V_H and V_L joined by peptide linker
Synthetic products		
ABU		Antigen-binding unit; peptide mimic

C, constant region; CH, constant region of the heavy chain; L, light chain; V, variable; VH, variable region of the heavy chain; VL, variable region of the light chain.

addition in CDR3, which add enormously to the potential complexity, in theory exceeding the total lifetime B-cell output by several orders of magnitude.[10] Many authors, however, have cautioned that the mathematical diversity does not allow for the redundancy in configurations that could provide equivalent binding domains; in terms of antigen binding, the practical diversity is probably in range of 1×10^7.

V gene selection is based on random expression followed by specific amplification. The argument has been made on physicochemical grounds that 10^5 different antibody molecules are sufficient to create a topologic set that recognizes any antigen surface with an affinity of 10^5 to 10^6 M^{-1},[13] a weak but biologically important number that corresponds to recognition affinities of naive antibody-antigen contacts that are often broadly polyreactive. B cells express antibody, principally IgM and IgD, on their membranes. On contacting antigen, these cells are stimulated to divide and undergo CDR mutations. Subsequent binding and stimulation are in proportion to the strength of the

binding reaction; hence, an in vivo selection occurs for mutations that enhance the affinity of the antibody for the antigen, a process termed "affinity maturation."[14] Simultaneous with this increased affinity is a narrowing of the specificity, with the antibody shedding its early polyreactive phenotype. The cell then undergoes "class switch" to one of the mature antibodies (IgG, IgA, IgE) by deleting DNA between the VDJ region and the new C region of the heavy chain, which brings this new C domain in juxtaposition with the V region (Fig. 31.4). (The light chain is unchanged.) Some time after commitment to a mature antibody, the cell ceases its CDR mutagenesis, affinity maturation is completed, and the B cell undergoes morphogenesis to a tissue-resident plasma cell.[4]

ANTIGEN-ANTIBODY INTERACTIONS

Affinity is a quantitative measure of the strength of the interaction between an antibody and its cognate antigen,

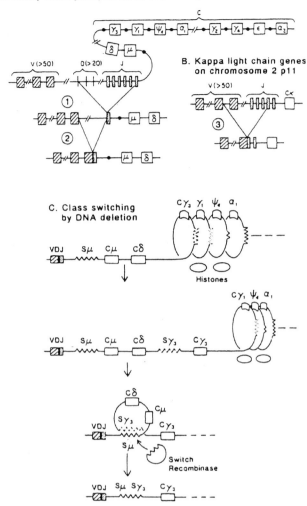

A. Heavy chain genes on chromosome 14 p32

B. Kappa light chain genes on chromosome 2 p11

C. Class switching by DNA deletion

Figure 31.4 Generation of diversity. VJ and VDJ joining occur in L chain and H chain by excision of intervening DNA in the genome. Class switch involves deletion of intervening constant (C) domains (C_μ, $C\delta$, etc.) and transcription through the new proximal C region. C is finally joined to the V gene by splicing of the messenger RNA. (C, constant; J, joining; V, variable.) (Reproduced with permission from Cooper MD. Current concepts: B lymphocytes—normal development. *N Engl J Med* 1987;317:1452.)

analogous to the equilibrium constant in the chemical mass action equation:

$$[AB] = K_a [A] [B] \qquad [31.1]$$

The equilibrium or affinity constant (K_a) is represented in units of M^{-1}. In most instances studied by x-ray crystallography, contacts between antibody and protein antigen are dominated by noncovalent hydrogen bonds (O—H), with a lower frequency of salt bridges (COO— + H_3N), for a total of 15 to 20 contacts. The effect of adding a new H–bond can be estimated from the free energy gain (0.5 to 1 kcal per mole $\alpha 10°C$) and from $\Delta G = -RT \ln K_a$ to yield affinity increases of threefold to tenfold. Therefore, the affinity maturation that takes place (or affinity that may be *lost* in antibody engineering) changes quickly with a rela-

tively small change in the number of bonds; that is, creating as few as three new hydrogen bonds may generate an affinity enhancement of more than 100-fold. This has been borne out by affinity changes that accompanied productive amino acid substitutions in V region engineering (see later). Of note, antibody affinities are generally much higher for protein antigens than for carbohydrate antigens, which may have less opportunity for hydrogen-bonding interactions (but are also "T-independent" antigens).

Although affinity and K_a directly express the binding potential of the antibody and are the most suitable measures for comparing affinities, the inverse of K_a, termed K_d or the *dissociation constant*, is expressed in molar units and indicates the concentration that is the middle of the range for the biologic action of the antibody:

$$1/K_d = K_a \qquad [31.2]$$

That is, K_d is the concentration of free antibody at which antigen is 50% saturated; if the antibody is in large excess, the input antibody concentration approximates the *free concentration*. K_d is a frequently used term, but its relationship to affinity must always be borne in mind; that is, low affinity equals high K_d, and high affinity equals low K_d. For example, a K_a of 2×10^9 M^{-1} implies a K_d of 0.5×10^{-9} mol/L (0.5 nmol/L), or approximately 0.1 μg/mL antibody concentration for IgG. If antigen is in the picomolar (10^{-12} mol/L) range, this concentration of antibody will have half of the antigen saturated, and half of the antigen will remain "free." At 10-fold higher antibody concentration (1 μg/mL, $10 \times K_d$), antigen will be 90% saturated and 10% free, and at 10-fold higher concentration (10 mg/mL, $100 \times K_d$), antigen will be 99% saturated and only 1% unbound. *A key point of understanding is that the ratio of antibody to antigen has very little impact on the degree of antigen saturation when antibody is in excess.* If antibody concentration is 1 nmol/L with a K_d of 1 nmol/L, it does not matter whether antigen is 0.1 nmol/L at the K_d, 0.1 pmol/L, or 0.1 fmol/L; antigen in each case is 50% bound, although the ratio of antibody to antigen is 10, 10^4, and 10^7, respectively. *Only the relation of free antibody to its K_d determines the degree of antigen saturation.*

The affinity constant K_a is itself composed of two terms that describe the on-rate (forward; units of $M^{-1} S^{-1}$) and off rate (back; units of S^{-1}) of the reaction:

$$K_a = k_f - k_b \qquad [31.3]$$

To a first approximation, the forward rate is diffusion limited and is comparable for many antibodies reacting with macromolecules or cell-bound structures. Reactions of antibodies with haptens and other small molecules in solution are dominated by the faster linear and rotational diffusion rates of the smaller component.[15] For example, when 0.1 nmol/L of dinitrophenyl-lysine (0.1 ng/mL) or 0.1 nmol/L of cell-bound HLA-A2 (50 ng/mL) is mixed with specific IgG antibody at 10 μg/mL (65 nmol/L), 0.1 second is required for the antibody to react with 50% of the antigen for the hapten but 4 minutes is required to react with the surface protein. Yet they have virtually the same affinity constant.[15] This is due to the fact that the fast association rate is balanced by a fast dissociation rate for the hapten (clearance half-time [$t_{1/2}$] = 0.7 seconds) whereas stability is longer for the protein antigen ($t_{1/2}$ = 6 minutes).

Although exceptions exist, the on-rates of antibodies to protein and cell-bound antigens are primarily in this range and inversely proportional to antibody concentration for antibody in excess of antigen (i.e., at 1 µg/mL, the 50% on time would be on the order of 0.5 to 1 hour). Accordingly, differences in affinity between antibodies to the same cellular antigen are in many instances reflective of the off-rate (k_b). For most purposes, an antibody is generally considered of "good" affinity if its K_a is equal to or greater than 10^9 M^{-1}, where off-rate $t_{1/2}$ values of an hour or more at 4°C are common. Association and dissociation times at 37°C are both accelerated relative to the times at 4°C, on the order of 5 or more, frequently with a net decrease in antibody affinity of 2-fold to 10-fold. This must be explicitly tested, however, because in some instances protein-ligand affinities have been found to be enhanced by higher temperature.[16]

The foregoing expresses basic principles of binding processes. A further important feature of antibodies is their multivalent structures. Although the on-rates for monovalent Fab and bivalent Fab'2 constructs are comparable, the bivalent off-times may be 10-fold longer than for the monovalent constructs, which yield affinities that are similarly enhanced.[15] To discriminate the affinity that is intrinsic to the V region antigen interaction from the effective affinity in a bivalent or multivalent interaction, the latter is often referred to as *avidity*. For monovalent interactions, avidity equals affinity; for multivalent interactions, avidity is greater than or equal to affinity. Theory predicts avidity enhancements that vastly exceed observed numbers, but structural constraints undoubtedly restrain the energy advantage of multivalent binding.[17,18] In the extreme, steric factors constrain some bivalent antibodies (e.g., anti-Tac)[19] to bind only monovalently to antigens on cell surfaces although they will bind bivalently to antigen in solution. When antigens are presented multivalently on the surfaces of cells, viruses, or other pathogens, even the low-affinity IgM interactions can yield a high-avidity, stable binding to such targets in vivo.

PHARMACOKINETICS AND PHARMACODYNAMICS

The metabolism of immunoglobulins determines the duration of usefulness of antibodies in vivo. Under normal conditions, the serum levels of endogenous immunoglobulins are determined by a balance between synthetic and catabolic rates.[20] When antibodies are administered as therapeutics, these catabolic rates effectively specify the dose and schedule necessary to maintain therapeutic blood levels when steady-state exposures are targeted. Table 31.1 lists the half-lives of human antibody survival in humans. IgG has the longest survival, 23 days (this value is

for IgG1, IgG2, and IgG4; IgG3 survival is 7 days). A key element in the regulation of IgG catabolism is the Brambell receptor (FcRB), named after its discoverer, F. W. R. Brambell, who described this receptor more than 30 years ago (see ref. 21 for a review). This receptor is located in endosomes of endocytically active tissues, primarily vascular endothelium, which is mainly responsible for the catabolism of plasma proteins, including IgG. There, FcRB binds IgG, recycling it to the cell surface and diverting it from the pathway to lysosomes and the catabolism that is the fate of other, nonprotected proteins. In this role, FcRB is also termed the IgG protection receptor (FcRp). Yet FcRB is also responsible for transmission of IgG from mother to young, via yolk sac, placenta, or newborn intestine; in this manifestation, it is termed the IgG neonatal transport receptor (FcRn) for neonatal intestine, the tissue from which the receptor was initially cloned.

A substantial body of knowledge exists on the metabolism of immunoglobulins in various disease states. Conditions of protein wasting (enteropathies, vascular leak syndromes, burns), febrile states, hyperthyroidism, hypergammaglobulinemia, and inflammatory disorders are accompanied by significant acceleration of immunoglobulin catabolism.[20] This information is of importance for understanding in vivo survival data in various clinical applications. In fact, the controlled conditions of testing immunoglobulin metabolism are rarely duplicated in practice, with antibody survivals typically shorter than suggested by the numbers above. Typically, murine antibody survival $t_{1/2}$ values are in the range of less than 1 to 3 days, and antibodies with human gamma Fc domains (chimeric or humanized) have $t_{1/2}$ values in the range of 1 to 15 days. Some of this acceleration in clearance is clearly due to disease-associated catabolic factors and to antigen binding in vivo, but subtle changes in the drug structure during product preparation may have a role in this acceleration as well. The influence of antigen expression on antibody clearance in vivo is considered later.

Antibody fragments have been studied because of their abbreviated survival and because their small size may translate into better tissue penetration. Fab and Fab'2 have survivals in vivo of 2 to 5 hours in mice, with comparable values in humans, and survival is dependent largely on kidney filtration mechanisms.[20] This is not based on size alone, because the Fc fragment, which is comparable in size to Fab, is not filtered and has an in vivo survival of 10 days in humans. These rapidly catabolized fragments, like other filtered proteins, are largely absorbed in the proximal tubule and degraded to amino acids, which are returned to circulation. No intact immunoglobulin or fragments reenter circulation once filtered.[22] In normal kidney, less than 5% of filtered light chain is excreted intact, whereas this fraction increases in the setting of renal tubular disease.[23]

A recently active area of investigation has been the role of circulating antigen in the setting of antitumor therapies. This was first encountered in anti-idiotype therapies directed at the surface Ig on B-cell lymphomas, some of which secreted high levels of idiotype.[24] This prevented access of administered antibody to the idiotype on tumor cells, which effectively neutralized the drug, unless very high doses were given to overwhelm the secreted quantities of idiotype. Subsequent further studies showed that other tumor antigens, including carcinoembryonic antigen (CEA),[25] gangliosides GD2 and GD3,[26,27] and Tac,[28] could achieve significant levels that might require adjustments to therapy.

Key observations include that there is (a) a direct relationship between the soluble antigen levels and the dose necessary to attain 50% (or 90% or 99%) bindability of administered antibody and (b) a predictable relationship between the rate of antigen synthesis and the time to antibody saturation.[28] The actual partitioning of antibody between soluble and cellular antigen depends on several features, including the effective avidity of antibody for antigen on cells (which may be higher than for soluble antigen) and other factors influencing tumor penetration.

A special concern in this setting is that many soluble forms of antigen have short $t_{1/2}$ values once shed from tumor cell surfaces, and the interaction with antibody may prolong their in vivo survival and increase their level in the whole body. When the target itself is a cytokine or cytokine receptor, adverse consequences conceivably could derive from the antibody treatment if the antigen retains activity in the antibody complex, as shown for interleukin-3, interleukin-4, and interleukin-7 complexes in vivo.[29] If the antigen does not retain activity in complex, then this problem causes no concern because the free concentration of antigen cannot be *increased* by the presence of antibody, even after antibody is fully saturated with excess antigen. A different potential consequence of antigen load is that it may reduce transport of radioantibody to tumor for imaging or therapy. Studies have shown, however, that antibody can partition sufficiently between soluble and cellular antigen to yield targeting adequate for tumor-imaging purposes (CEA,[25] Tac[28]).

BIOLOGIC FUNCTIONS

Antibodies mediate several actions of potential therapeutic interest, some of which are part of the normal biologic function of antibodies and some of which are adapted in novel ways to the needs of specific settings.

Complement-Dependent Cytotoxicity

The complement (C′) system is at least as primitive evolutionarily as antibodies. One view is that the alternate (antibody-independent) pathway is the primordial system, which diversified to create the classic pathway to collaborate with antibody to direct the attack complex (C5–C9) against antibody-coated targets. The most effective mediator of complement-dependent cytotoxicity (CDC) is IgM. Single IgM molecules can fix and activate complement on cell surfaces. In contrast, IgG-mediated CDC depends on the juxtaposition of pairs of IgG molecules to bind com-

plement to cells,[30] with substantially lower complement fixation and reduced killing efficiency relative to IgM. Human IgG1 and IgG3; mouse IgG2a, IgG2b, and IgG3; rat IgG2a; and rabbit IgG all fix and activate complement, whereas human IgG2 fixes C′ poorly, and human IgG4 and murine IgG1 normally do not fix C′.[31] (Complement fixation depends on conserved residues in the C_H2 domain; short hinge regions are thought to hinder C1q access and binding with these latter isotypes.) Although human IgG3 fixes human C′ better than IgG1, actual target lysis may be better with IgG1 due to more efficient activation of C4.[32] For the most part, human and murine antibodies function comparably well in directing CDC with rabbit C′ in in vitro tests and in fixing human or rabbit C′. Some cases may exist, however, in which murine IgG3 is more potent owing to the unique feature of Fc polymerization on cell surfaces apparently not being similarly available to human IgG.[33]

Despite these considerations, the impact of C′ fixation and CDC in therapeutic applications against cancer is uncertain. Two considerations may be relevant: First, the complete first component of human complement is very large (approximately 800 kd) and, like IgM,[20] probably has limited extravascular penetration. Second, the cells to which complement has ready access (e.g., cells of the hematopoietic system and vascular endothelium) are endowed with potent phosphoinositol-linked membrane protease activities, decay-accelerating factor (DAF, CD55), and homologous restriction factor (HRF, CD59), which act as steps subsequent to C1 fixation to inactivate the human complement cascade.[34,35] Rabbit, guinea pig, or other heterologous sera can kill cells in vitro that are resistant to human C′ because they bypass the human species restriction of these protease activities.

Antibody-Dependent Cellular Cytotoxicity

In antibody-dependent cellular cytotoxicity (ADCC), target cells are coated with antibody and engage effector cells equipped with Fc receptors (FcRs) that bind to the Fc region of IgG, release cytolysins, and lead to cell killing. The only classes demonstrated to mediate ADCC are IgE and IgG. Because of the dangers of anaphylaxis that would be associated with IgE use, antitumor IgE antibodies are not likely to be developed, and further discussion therefore focuses on IgG.

Classically, cells that mediated ADCC were called "K (killer) cells," and all bear FcRs on their surfaces. Among these, there are at least three IgG FcRs and two IgE FcRs. Table 31.3 lists the FcRs for IgG and their properties.[36–38] All FcRs are capable of directing the ADCC of effectors against appropriate antibody-coated targets. Cytolytic mechanisms include perforins, a system closely related to the C9 protein of the complement attack complex (C5−C9), serine proteases (granzymes) in large granular lymphocytes (LGLs); superoxides, free radicals, proteases, and lysozymes in monocytes-macrophages and granulocytes; tumor necrosis factor; and other components. As far

TABLE 31.3

FCγ RECEPTORS: PROPERTIES AND BINDING CHARACTERISTICS

Receptor	Size (kd)	K_a	Cells	Mouse IgG	Human IgG
FcRI (CD64)	72	10^8	Mono, mac, act. PMN, eos	2a, 3	3 > 1 > 4
FcRII (CD32)	40	10^6	Mono, mac, gran, B cell, plt	2a, 2b, 1 (immune complexes or aggregates)	3, 1
FcRIII (CD16A) transmembrane (CD16B) PI-linked	50–70	5×10^5	LGL/NK, mac, few T, act. mono PMN, act. eos	3, 2a > 1	3, 1 > 2, 4

act., activated; eos, eosinophile; gran, granulocyte; LGL, large granular lymphocytes; mac, macrocytes; mono, monocytes; NK, natural killer cells; plt, platelet; PMN, polymorphonuclear leukocyte.
Adapted from Van de Winkel GJ, Capel JA. Human IgG Fc receptor heterogeneity: molecular aspect and clinical implications. Immunol Today 1993;14:215; Simmons D, Seed B. The Fcγ receptor of natural killer cells is a phosphoinositol-linked membrane protein [later shown not PI-linked]. Nature 1988;333:568; Walker MR, Woof JM, Bruggemann M, et al. Interaction of human IgG chimeric antibodies with the human FcR1 and FcR11 receptors: requirements for antibody-mediated host cell-target cell interaction. Mol Immunol 1989;26:403.

as is known, the lytic mechanisms of LGLs and cytotoxic lymphocytes are similar or identical, and the monocyte-macrophage and granulocyte mechanisms also share numerous features. The monocyte-granulocyte mechanisms are probably adapted to killing and engulfment of microorganisms, whereas T cells, the closest lineage relative of LGL-NK cells, have the role of killing cells of self-origin that express foreign or neoantigens. In general, the most potent of the mediators of cellular killing in circulation have been the LGLs. These cells also perform natural killing (NK cells), which is an antibody-independent lectin-like ligand interaction system.[39] Other effectors, for example, monocytes and granulocytes, have been shown to mediate ADCC against nucleated targets,[40] but in most direct comparisons with LGLs, the LGLs were more potent than these numerically more dominant cells.[41] Nevertheless, the most effective approaches may include a multipronged attack that enlists the collaboration of more than a single cellular system to kill antibody-coated tumor targets.

Among the features that influence the amount of killing in ADCC are (1) the species origin of the antibody, (2) the IgG subclass, (3) the number of antibody molecules bound per target cell, (4) the ratio of effector cells to targets, (5) the activation state of effectors, (6) the presence of irrelevant IgG, and, perhaps, (7) the presence of tumor cell protective factors and (8) different classes of Fc receptors that enhance or inhibit effective activity.[42–44] These are discussed in turn.

1. The species origin appears to have a significant influence on the ability of an antibody to recruit human effectors to kill human tumors. Although human and rat antibodies mediate ADCC with human effectors, murine antibodies are often less potent in this role. Long ago, isologous antiserum was determined to be more effective with any species' effector cells,[45] which suggests that the match of antibody to effector cell Fc receptor is a significant feature of ADCC.

2. In principle, all IgG subclasses are capable of ADCC. However, the IgG1 subclass of humans, the IgG2a and IgG3 subclasses of the mouse, and the IgG2b and IgG3 subclasses

of the rat have been inferred to be the most active with human cells. This does not always parallel the order of FcR binding affinity, and other factors of Fc-FcR binding must be postulated that influence the induction of cytolysis.[46]

3. The selection of highly expressed target antigens has a direct impact on the likelihood that the cell can be killed with ADCC. The control of the number of antibody molecules bound reveals that a nearly linear relationship exists with cytolysis.[47] A corollary of this phenomenon is that the modulation of antigen by antibody binding (antigen-antibody complex internalization or shedding) reduces target susceptibility even when baseline antigen is highly expressed.

4. Higher effector-to-target ratios yield increased killing, although a plateau in efficacy typically is achieved at higher ratios.[45,48] In vivo, the ratio of effector cells to targets is not so readily controlled, except by stimulating proliferation or supplementing effectors, but this effect may provide a stronger rationale for treatment in adjuvant settings when the tumor burden is small, that is, after debulking surgery or induction chemotherapy.

5. The activation state of effectors has been shown in several systems, both in vitro and in vivo, to play an important role in the lysis of targets. This activation is achieved with any of several agents and by the expression of different classes of activating or inhibiting Fc receptors.[42–44] Evaluation of the application of cytokines specific to the range of potential effectors is beyond the scope of this review, but in each instance cytolytic capacity has been strongly correlated with the degree of effector cell activation. Only LGLs (NK cells) appear to have significant antitumor potency in ADCC in the absence of cytokine activation, but here, too, activation with cytokines also increases ADCC killing (Fig. 31.5).[48] Interleukin-2 (IL-2) activation of LGLs has been the most widely applied in clinical trials to date (see Chapter 36).

6. The presence of circulating IgG is probably the most problematic of features for exploiting ADCC in vivo. Clearly, the very existence of FcRs and the presence of

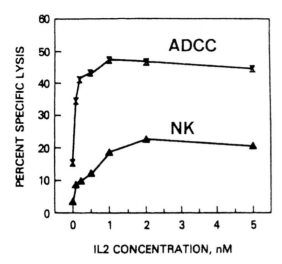

Figure 31.5 Impact of interleukin 2 (IL-2) on antibody-dependent cellular cytotoxicity (ADCC) after 16 hours of activation of peripheral blood lymphocytes. (NK, natural killer cells.) (Reproduced with permission from Junghans RP. A strategy for evaluating lymphokine activation and novel monoclonal antibodies in antibody-dependent cell-mediated cytotoxicity and effector cell retargeting assays. Cancer Immunol Immunother 1990;31:207.)

cytolytic granules are teleologic indications of the relevance of this capability to biology. Although one might argue that monocytes-macrophages and granulocytes are adapted to combat microorganisms, the sole role of T cells is to kill nucleated cells of self that present viral or other abnormal peptides, for which they use distinct cytolytic mechanisms. As stated above, LGLs apparently duplicate the cytolytic mechanisms of T cells but in addition possess FcRs to enable them to interact with antibodies that will direct them to these targets through non–major histocompatibility complex mechanisms. The problem with this interaction is that monomeric Fc of IgG has an affinity of approximately $5 \times 10^5 \, M^{-1}$ ($K_d = 2$ mmol/L) for the dominant FcR on LGLs (Table 31.3). At a 1 g/dL in vivo concentration, IgG is 65 mmol/L and 30-fold above this K_d, which implies that more than 95% of the FcR on LGLs is occupied with IgG Fc. (The occupancy fraction on monocytes-macrophages with higher-affinity FcR type I is still higher.) Countering this in the biologic interaction is that the affinity of specific IgG for antigen is typically much higher than this, which yields a stable multivalent surface presentation of IgG Fc on the target that in turn may interact in a multivalent manner with the effector cell FcR. In practice, however, most ADCC assays are markedly inhibited by added human serum. (Assays using fetal calf serum are not so affected because IgG is absent due to lack of placental transport in ungulates.)[20] Whether the longer-term in vivo incubations of days versus the brief duration (approximately 3 hours) of in vitro assays allow a therapeutic effect in a treatment program requires further study. However, observed clinical responses to antibody therapies (see later) suggest that ADCC may in some instances be operative in vivo.

7. Interest has recently focused on *tumor-based* factors that may mediate *resistance* to ADCC. One such factor is the complement regulatory protein HRF. HRF was originally defined as acting at C2 and C9 of the complement cascade. The cytolytic protein perforin I that is released by LGL-NK cells and cytotoxic lymphocytes is also referred to as C9-related protein and is likewise subject to proteolysis by HRF, which thereby neutralizes the lytic power of the killer cell.[49] (The observation has been made, however, that HRF-related protein Ly6 [CD59] does not protect against perforin lysis.) HRF is present at high levels on activated T cells and NK cells and is thought to play a role in protecting these cells from autolysis during lysis of intended targets. Cells that are resistant to ADCC could be induced to become sensitive by blocking with anti-HRF antibodies.[34] Another factor that may contribute to cellular resistance is the secretion of mucins, which inhibit the penetration of antibodies and other macromolecules to the cell surfaces. Other issues of tumor penetration are discussed later.

8. Finally, the relevance of the in vitro ADCC assay to in vivo function is much discussed. Only in a few instances has this been examined by comparing ADCC-competent and ADCC-*in*competent antibodies.[44,50] In a complement-deficient leukemic AKR mouse model, a leukemia-specific IgG monoclonal antibody suppressed tumor, whereas an IgM antibody of the same specificity was ineffective.[51] This suggested that binding to antigen was not sufficient and that C' played no role. Other reports of studies in mice showed that the only antibody to induce an in vivo response was that which showed ADCC activity in vitro.[52] Several studies have shown that antibody plus IL-2 activation of effectors was much more effective than either alone, which implicates cooperation between the cellular and humoral immune systems that is the sine qua non of ADCC. Human trials in which a leukemic patient received human IgG Fc coupled to a murine antibody showed a more effective response than when the antibody was without human Fc.[53] A further human trial with class/isotype-switched CAMPATH-1 anti-lymphocyte antibody showed a dramatic response in patients with B-cell chronic lymphocytic leukemia only for the one isotype that mediates ADCC in vitro.[54]

PHAGOCYTOSIS

Antibody-dependent phagocytosis may be performed by cells of the granulocytic and monocyte-macrophage lineages. Furthermore, these cells have receptors for C3 fragments, which enhance binding of antibody-coated targets that also activate complement, leading to C3 fixation. Only *activated* macrophages, however, are capable of engulfing antibody-coated erythrocytes. The ability to engulf larger tumor cells has been uncertain, but one in vitro evaluation of activated monocytes demonstrated phagocytosis of melanoma and neuroblastoma targets when assays were appropriately monitored.[55] Nevertheless, phagocytic cells in the liver (i.e., Kupffer cells) and spleen probably are the primary mediators of circulatory clearance of antibody-coated platelets in alloimmune and autoimmune settings[56] and in the instances in which rapid clearance of leukemic cells was observed during antibody therapies. Whether these cells are trapped and then lysed by ADCC mechanisms rather than phagocytosis is uncertain.

RECEPTOR BLOCKADE

Antibody binding occurs without cooperation of other elements of the immune system. Therefore, just as antitoxin can prevent a toxin from acting at its target site in the body, antibody can also deny access of growth factors to tumors whose proliferation is factor dependent. This approach has been applied more widely in nonmalignant settings for the suppression of immune responses in autoimmune and alloimmune settings.[57] This approach is limited in malignancy because most tumors appear to be autonomous. In principle, an antibody directed against a cytokine should have the same result. However, the short half-lives of most cytokines and the locally high antibody concentrations required may make this approach more difficult. Such autocrine or paracrine loops may be better interrupted by an antireceptor than by an anticytokine antibody. One report has documented a marked *enhancement* of cytokine activity by antibody to cytokine via $t_{1/2}$ prolongation, which runs counter to the goal of suppressing cytokine activity.[29]

Design of such applications also must consider the receptor occupancy that is necessary for cell survival and proliferation. Only 10% occupancy of the receptor for granulocyte-macrophage colony-stimulating factor is sufficient to induce maximal activation of granulocytes.[58] Similarly, one must block more than 90% of the α chain of IL-2 receptor with antibody to have a significant impact on IL-2–dependent, antigen-induced T-cell proliferation.[47]

APOPTOSIS

Apoptosis is a process by which signals are transmitted through cell surface receptors to induce autoenzyme-mediated cell death or by which downstream events are accessed to achieve the same result. This has been demonstrated most persuasively during development and in the programming of T-cell precursors in the thymus. The Fas antigen is probably the natural membrane receptor for this process and is expressed in liver, heart, thymus, lung, and ovary, although other antigens may exert similar effects. Anti-Fas antibody administration resulted in an extraordinarily complete and rapid tissue destruction in animal studies.[59] One report suggests that part of the killing mechanism of T cells is to engage this receptor on target cells.[60] Some

hematologic malignant cells, like their normal counterparts, are Fas-positive and are potential targets of antibody therapy (a) if these antibodies are not cross-reactive for normal tissue, (b) if ways of engaging the receptor can be selectively achieved (i.e., bifunctional anti-Fas antitumor antibody), or (c) if other antigens unique to tumors can be found that also access this cellular process. To date, such tumor-specific, apoptosis-inducing antigens have not been described, but lineage-associated, apoptosis-inducing antigens have been targeted in the treatment of lymphoma (see later section).

Ab2 VACCINES

Antibody recognition of antigen entails the presentation of a molecular surface that is the complement in space of the antigen (Fig. 31.3), termed a "mirror image." In the Jerne network nomenclature, the designation of antigen and antibody becomes arbitrary. The antigen is Ab0, the antibody is Ab1, the antibody to the antibody idiotype is Ab2, and so forth. Although antibody can react with idiotype in many ways, a subset of Ab2 is still considered to exist that mimics Ab0 (antigen), and a fraction of Ab3 raised against Ab2 mimics Ab1 and reacts with Ab0 (antigen).[61] Therefore, a tumor antigen may not be immunogenic in the human host that carries it, but a murine antibody (Ab1) can be raised to this antigen, and a goat antibody (Ab2) can be raised to this. This Ab2 antibody includes epitopes that mimic antigen but presents them in a novel context in which they may be immunogenic in the original host. Such Ab2s have been used as vaccines to induce Ab3 antibody responses in the host that can cross-react with antigen (Ab0) on tumor. Antibody therapy in this sense is applied to induce an endogenous antibody and occasionally a T-cell response against tumor.[62,63]

ANTIBODY MODIFICATIONS FOR THERAPY

As discussed later, despite all the functions that antibodies perform in vivo, not all antibodies are therapeutically successful. Two major factors have been the focus of research efforts considered in this section: (a) immunogenicity and (b) lack of therapeutic and cytolytic potency. The approaches to improve potency have themselves been twofold: (a) to improve the collaboration of antibodies with the other components of the immune system and (b) to use the antibody as a vector to deliver toxic agents (toxins or radioactivity) to tumor cells. This latter approach essentially abandons the immunologic collaboration of antibodies with the remainder of the immune system.

Reduction of Immunogenicity

Immunogenicity derives from the fact that most antibodies are of non-human origin and as such are foreign proteins in the human host. The human antiglobulin response to mouse antibodies is directed mainly against the C domains of the murine antibody, with typically lower titers against the V domains. To address this problem, three versions of the foreign protein have been prepared. First, there is a chimeric version, in which the mouse C domains are replace by human C domains. Second, there is a "humanized" or hyperchimeric version, in which the murine framework regions are replaced by human framework sequences (Fig. 31.4). Third, entirely "human" IgG produced *in vivo* (in transgenic mice).[64,65]

The first humanized antibody for cancer therapy was the panlymphocyte antibody CAMPATH-1H.[66] Since that time, many others have been prepared and tested in humans. The hyperchimeric and humanized antibodies have been much more successful in avoiding antiglobulin[67] responses, with an incidence of 4% with CAMPATH-1H and comparably low antiglobulin response rates with anti–Tac-H[68] and HuM195.[69,70] The less extensively substituted chimeric antibodies have been more widely applied, with anti–V-region responses observed.[61,71,72] Further experience is required to ascertain the rules governing these responses. The innovation of human combinatorial phage display libraries[70,73] is also being applied for deriving antiself and antitumor human antibodies. Efforts to suppress human antimurine antibody with immunosuppressive drugs have not been successful to date.

Human IgG C domains (specifically C_H2) can confer a longer in vivo $t_{1/2,}$ on the order of 23 days, for human IgG in humans versus the 1- to 3-day $t_{1/2}$ of murine antibody in humans.[20] One study compared a chimeric anti-idiotype antibody with the parental murine antibody, demonstrating a prolonged in vivo survival (with $t_{1/2}$ longer than 10 days for a nonreactive chimeric construct).[47] Other studies involving chimeric antibodies against colon carcinoma yielded survival $t_{1/2}$ values of 3 to 6 days and 4 to 12 days.[71,72] The humanized CAMPATH-1H had survival $t_{1/2}$ values of 1 to 6 days,[67] and anti–Tac-H had values of 2 to 15 days.[68] Thus, observed survivals fall short of those expected from controlled studies in normal volunteers. Some of this acceleration in clearance is clearly due to disease-associated catabolic factors,[20] but in vivo antigen binding and product preparation may also play a role in rapid clearance of the antibody. Further studies are necessary to better understand the various factors that determine the $t_{1/2}$ of the antibody *in vivo*.

Binding Affinity of Engineered Antibodies

The affinity for substrate (antigen) is an intrinsic characteristic of an antibody conferred by the particular amino acid sequence and spatial presentation of the CDRs. In the past, the affinity that was retrieved from a given hybridoma was an immutable feature of the antibody; it could be altered only by reducing the valence of the product (i.e., Fab vs. Fab'2, IgG vs. IgM), which only reduced affinity. More recent

efforts in the preparation of IgG dimers, however, have shown a marked increase in affinity of up to 1,000-fold,[74] which may accentuate the improvement in Fc-dependent functions with such constructs. With CDR manipulation in the humanization of antibodies, a major disturbance sometimes occurred in the affinity for antigen. Search for causes of this affinity loss revealed the importance of single, critical residues or carbohydrates to total affinity.[75-77]

Novel procedures using phage display technology offer powerful new procedure to improve affinities by mutating the CDR's. Fab molecules are expressed on the surface of phage and are selected against immobilized antigen and enriched in proportion to their affinity. This enabled a random CDR mutagenesis-selection procedure that recapitulates in vitro the in vivo process of affinity selection and maturation.[78] By this procedure, the affinity for antigen of any low-affinity antibody can be enhanced 1,000-fold or more in a simple selection procedure. Finally, the issue of valence has been addressed to reduce the likelihood of antigen modulation during therapy by preparing *univalent* IgG that still retains the Fc effector domains and Fc-dependent functions.[79,80]

Complement-Dependent Cytotoxicity

The opportunities and problems of CDC as a means of killing tumors were outlined earlier. The humanization of antibodies has in some instances shown an improvement in cellular killing with heterologous complement, but for the most part, the effect has not been dramatic and is not sufficiently potent to kill human tumor cells with human complement when murine antibodies failed. On the other hand, the principle of the relative advantage of human over mouse antibodies has been clearly violated by occasional observations of failure to fix C' with chimeric human IgG1 and IgG3 molecules when the murine antibodies have fixed C', first noted by Junghans et al.[47] and since corroborated by others.[77,81] In any case, the impact of humanization of IgG antibodies is not expected to render them as effective as IgM antibodies for CDC killing. In addition, the possibility exists that the murine IgG3 may be more potent than any human IgG given its capacity for polymerization on cell membranes with enhanced C' fixation and lysis.[33] Finally, dimeric forms of human IgG1 antibodies have been engineered that are far more effective in fixing complement than monomeric versions,[82,83] but none has yet been tested for these effects in humans.

Antibody-Dependent Cellular Cytotoxicity

In contrast to CDC, ADCC with human antibodies show a fairly consistent advantage of over mouse antibodies by their improved efficacy of their interaction with human effector cells. In several tests, a marked increase is seen in the potency of cellular killing in the chimeric constructs with human Fc domains. Of the human isotypes, IgG1 has been consistently the most effective, and chimeric and humanized antibodies are equivalent when normalized to molecules bound per target cell.[47] Bifunctional antibodies (BFAs), discussed later, appear to have the best opportunity to enhance this killing activity, although clinical data are very limited at this point. Another approach has been to apply anti–homologous restriction factor (anti-HRF) antibodies to block the inhibitory effects of HRF on ADCC (see earlier), which has been demonstrated in vitro[34] but to date has not been not tested in in vivo models.

FEATURES OF SPECIFIC MODIFICATIONS

Humanized Antibodies

Winter and collaborators showed that the CDRs of antibodies could be transferred from murine to human frameworks with maintenance of binding specificity,[84,85] albeit with losses in affinity of 1.6- to 15-fold. Such affinity losses became a recurrent concern with these constructs (Fig. 31.6). Subsequently, this group humanized a rat antibody, CAMPATH-1, which is directed at a human panlymphocyte antigen, with the intention of therapeutic application in leukemias and lymphomas (see "Clinical Trials of Monoclonal Antibodies in Cancer Therapy" later in the chapter). The second antibody to be humanized for therapy, anti–Tac-H, was derived from the murine anti–human IL-2 receptor antibody anti-Tac for use in alloimmune and autoimmune settings and in Tac-expressing leukemias and lymphomas (Fig. 31.2).[47,86] The manipulations to create this antibody also had a modest impact on affinity, which was reduced from 9×10^9 to 3×10^9 M^{-1} [47], but another humanized antibody, HuM195, actually showed increased affinity after engineering.[75] Since that time, several antibodies have been humanized, and humanization effectively reduces immunogenicity.

Immunoadhesins

Another type of chimeric antibody genetically couples a natural ligand with an immunoglobulin Fc domain to confer in vivo survival characteristics of antibodies and recruitment of host effector functions. The prototypical immunoadhesin was CD4IgG, which was used to target gp120-expressing cells infected with human immunodeficiency virus[87] but may plausibly be extended to human tumor antigens for which ligands can be derived or for which effector cell antigens can be recruited (see the following section).

Bifunctional Antibodies

(BFAs) were devised to address two problems of ADCC. First, effector-target conjugate formation is inefficient due to competition with circulating Fc for FcR binding. Second, mouse antibodies, as noted, often fail to promote ADCC with natural human targets, even in the absence of competing IgG,[45] a difficulty partially addressed by "humanization" of antibodies.

BFAs improve conjugate formation by creating molecules that have dual specificities, one to the target cell and one to an "activator" antigen of the killer cell (Fig. 31.7).[88] BFAs direct killer cells—both NK cells *and* T cells—to lyse targets dictated by the antibody specificity in a function called "effector cell retargeting." In the case of NK cells, the BFA substitutes through its anti-FcR (anti-CD16) moiety a high-affinity antigen-antibody interaction for a low-affinity, nonspecific Fc-FcR interaction, causing a marked improvement in conjugate formation and target cell lysis, even in the presence of human serum. In the case of T cells, the BFA recruits an entirely new cell class into antibody-directed killing. With the binding of anti-CD3 to the CD3 antigen, the T cell is stimulated into a killing mode, bypassing the normal major histocompatibility complex and antigen-specific restrictions of T-cell killing.

CD16 and CD3 each involve proteins that are central to the killing mechanisms of LGLs and cytotoxic T lymphocytes, respectively. The CD3 antibodies are mainly directed against the ε chain of the CD3 complex. Other surface antigens on these cells also have been used, generally to less effect,[88,89] although promising results with *tri*functional antibodies that are also anti-CD28 have been obtained.[90] Other FcRs have been targeted on monocytes-macrophages.[40]

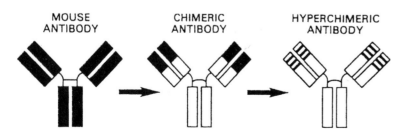

MOUSE ANTIBODY   CHIMERIC ANTIBODY   HYPERCHIMERIC ANTIBODY

■ MOUSE
□ HUMAN

Figure 31.6 Schematic of chimeric versus hyperchimeric (humanized) antibodies. See also Figure 31.2. (Reproduced with permission from Junghans RP, Waldmann TA, Landolfi NF, et al. Anti Tac-H, a humanized antibody to the interleukin 2 receptor with new features for immunotherapy in malignant and immune disorders. Cancer Res 1990; 50:1495.)

1) heteroconjugate

complete immunoglobulins,
chemically cross-linked,
multimeric form,
multivalent

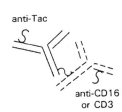

anti-Tac

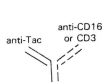

anti-CD16
or CD3

TARGET   EFFECTOR

Tac   CD16 or CD3

Tac   CD16 or CD3

Tac

2) bispecific

hemi globulins,
native disulfide linkage,
(hybrid hybridomas or
disulfide exchange)
monomeric form,
bivalent

anti-Tac   anti-CD16
or CD3

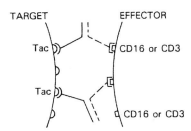

TARGET   EFFECTOR

Tac   CD16 or CD3

Tac

CD16 or CD3

Figure 31.7 Schematic of bifunctional antibodies as conjugates versus quadroma (hybrid hybridoma) products.

Bifunctional constructs are generated by chemical processes, by chemical cross-linking (heteroaggregates) of complete IgG, by chain shuffling, by cross-linking of Fab' molecules, or by hybrid hybridoma (quadroma) technology.[91] These latter products are the most useful for therapy because they provide a continuous supply of monomeric IgG products with normal in vivo survivals; however, because 10 combinations of heavy and light chains are predicted from the parental antibodies in the mix, of which only one is the desired BFA, purification by standard chromatographic methods may not be able to provide a pure BFA preparation.[92] On the other hand, aggregates and fragments prepared with high yield by other methods have abbreviated survivals in vivo. Newer genetic constructs are in preparation—single-chain BFAs, *fos-jun*–linked Fabs, immunoadhesin with antitumor antibody, and so on—whose efficacy and advantages will be determined in the near future. Bifunctional immunoadhesin antibody constructs have linked anti-CD3 antibody with hormones or cytokines to interact with receptor-bearing cells on tumor targets,[93,94] and other work is underway using B7 as an immunoadhesin in BFAs to recruit effector cells through CD28.

Typically, these constructs are markedly more active than the parental antibodies in net lysis of tumor cell targets (the difference is particularly great in the presence of human serum). BFAs can cure or prevent tumors in animal hosts in which unmodified antitumor antibodies are inactive.[95–97] Although this approach is promising, clinical trials have been limited.

Antibody as Vector for Toxic Agents

Many of the deficiencies of antibodies in recruitment of host effector functions are being addressed by the methods described previously. Other approaches have bypassed this effort by exploiting the specificity and affinity of antibodies to direct cytotoxic agents against tumor cells. These toxic agents include chemotoxins, biotoxins, and radioisotopes. Radioimmunotherapies are discussed later in this chapter.

Chemotoxins

Conjugates of antibody with anthracyclines and other chemotherapy agents have the potential to permit delivery of high doses of drug to antigen-expressing tumor cells while sparing nonexpressor normal cells from the toxic effects of the drug. Several studies have shown efficacy in animal models in which antibody alone and drug alone were ineffective.[98,99] As a rule, chemotoxins and biotoxins are expected to be more effective in cases in which the antigen is known to be internalized after antibody binding, as with the Lewis Y antigen targeted by BR96-doxorubicin conjugates.[98] This approach has been taken furthest with the anti-CD33 targeting of leukemia cells in patients using a humanized Ig conjugated to calicheamicin, a small-molecule toxin. (see "Clinical Trials of Monoclonal Antibodies in Cancer Therapy").

A merging of BFA technology with chemotherapy delivery has been developed that displays an enzymatic activity that converts prodrug to active agent at the site of the tumor,[100] called "antibody-dependent enzyme-prodrug therapy" (ADEPT). The design of this therapy is dictated by a problem common to all antibody-toxin/radioisotope approaches: the high body burden of toxin and nonspecific toxic effects at sites away from tumor. To circumvent this problem, antibody in the form of enzyme-conjugated antibody (ECA) is allowed to equilibrate to obtain optimal tumor penetration (Fig. 31.8). When antigen saturation is achieved and the tumor to normal tissue ratio of ECA is optimal, then a low molecular weight prodrug is injected. Rapid tumor penetration occurs, and prodrug is then converted to active drug, thereby killing tumor cells. To accentuate this effect, the unbound ECA may be cleared from circulation by a second antibody to exaggerate the tumor to plasma ratio of ECA and minimize prodrug conversion

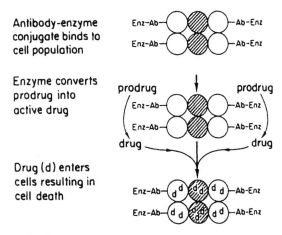

Antibody-enzyme conjugate binds to cell population

Enzyme converts prodrug into active drug

Drug (d) enters cells resulting in cell death

Figure 31.8 Schematic of antibody-dependent enzyme-prodrug therapy (ADEPT). (Reproduced with permission from Senter PD. Activation of prodrugs by antibody-enzyme conjugates: a new approach to cancer therapy. FASEB J 1990;4:188.)

except at sites of antibody binding. Optimizations of this strategy have been analyzed by Jain and coworkers.[101] Analogous approaches with radiolabeled antibodies are under development.[102]

Several animal studies have validated the principles of this approach, and clinical studies have been initiated.[103] In pioneering work by Pastan, Vitetta, and others, the application of extremely potent biotoxins to clinical cancer therapy was explored. The first-generation products were chemically cross-linked conjugates of antibody with unmodified toxins. Early studies determined that whole toxin molecules coupled with antibody were too toxic due to nonspecific uptake.[104] Molecular analysis of toxin domains was done for the purpose of designing molecules that were less nonspecifically toxic. Three domains corresponded to specific functions, as exemplified by work with the *Pseudomonas* exotoxin (PE): *adherence,* causing nonspecific binding and uptake, mainly by liver; *translocation,* responsible for moving the toxin from the endosomic vesi-

cle to the cytoplasm; and *adenosine diphosphate ribosylation,* the enzymic activity that is responsible for inactivating elongation factor 2 and arresting protein synthesis.[105] In principle, a single molecule of toxin is sufficient to kill the cell. Studies were performed with diphtheria toxin, which acts like PE, and with ricin, which inhibits protein synthesis by acting on the ribosome directly.

Modifications were made to eliminate or block the adherence domain, which led to a marked reduction in nonspecific toxicity. In addition, the discovery was made that the chemical coupling of toxins to antibody could be accompanied by a loss of specific activity of the toxin due to preferential use of key active-site lysines by the linkage. To bypass this, a genetic construct of PE was prepared that put into a single chain the antigen-recognition domain of the antibody (single-chain Fv) and a truncated version of the toxin (Fig. 31.9).[106] This construct, anti-Tac (single-chain Fv)–PE40, had high toxicity for antigen-expressing cells and no toxicity for antigen-negative cells; the concentration causing 50% inhibition (IC_{50}) was higher for lower-expressing cells, but in each case the IC_{50} corresponded to binding of approximately 100 antibody molecules per cell. Another construct was designed with truncated PE and an anti-CD22 variable domain (Fv).[107] Sixteen patients with cladribine-refractory hairy-cell leukemia (a leukemia whose malignant cells are strongly positive for CD22) were treated with this immunotoxin, BL22. Two patients experienced hemolytic uremic syndrome, but otherwise the treatment was well tolerated. Despite the poor prognosis of these heavily pretreated and refractory patients, 11 patients (69%) achieved a complete remission, and 10 of these had elimination of minimal residual disease by immunohistochemical analysis of the bone marrow. Several additional toxin constructs have been prepared with similar in vitro profiles of activity, including B4-blocked ricin[108] and CD22-ricin A for treating B-cell chronic lymphocytic leukemia and purging leukemic cells from autologous marrow grafts.[109,110] Excellent summaries of these applications are available.[104,111]

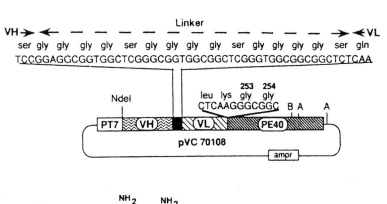

Figure 31.9 Single-chain Fv-PE40 toxin. (PE40, truncated version of *Pseudomonas* exotoxin; VH, variable region of the heavy chain; VL, variable region of the light chain.) (Reproduced with permission from Chaudhary VK, Queen C, Junghans RP, et al. A recombinant immunotoxin consisting of two antibody variable domains fused to *Pseudomonas* exotoxin. Nature 1989; 339:394.)

Antibody as a Vector for Radioactivity

Labeling of antibodies with radioactive atoms is another major approach to antibody-based cancer treatment that has received considerable attention. This approach remains promising and benefits from some inherent advantages over direct (passive) or toxin-based immunotherapy. These advantages result from the use of radiation as the primary cytotoxic agent. The cytotoxic activity of radiolabeled antibodies is the result of electron (beta-particle) or alpha-particle emissions that occur when the radionuclide decays while attached to an antibody that is bound to tumor-associated antigen. These emissions travel a distance that depends on their type (electron or alpha particle) and energy. As they travel, they deposit energy along their paths. If an adequate number of such emissions traverse a given tumor cell nucleus, the total energy deposited within the nucleus will kill the cell by causing an irreparable number of DNA strand breaks. A radiolabeled antibody attached to a particular tumor cell may also, because of the range and random direction of its emissions, kill adjacent tumor cells that do not express the antigen or that have not been reached by the radiolabeled antibody. Because of the range of the emissions, tumor cell kill is not necessarily dependent on internalization of the antigen-bound antibody, nor does it depend on any specific metabolic process of the tumor cell.

As a further distinguishing feature of radiolabeled antibody therapy, the loss of cytotoxic activity over time due to radioactive decay has important implications for its use in comparison with the use of passive or toxin-based immunotherapy. Depending on the clearance kinetics of the antibody and of the free radionuclide after detachment from the antibody, radionuclide loss due to decay may be either advantageous or disadvantageous. If the half-life of the radionuclide matches the uptake kinetics of the target tissue, and the antibody remains tumor-associated for a sufficient period of time, the decrease in radioactivity reduces normal tissue exposure once the antibody dissociates or is catabolized. A radionuclide that is cleared too rapidly will deliver the largest fraction of its decay energy to normal tissue before reaching the tumor. Alternatively, a radionuclide with a prolonged residence time will deliver a small fraction of its decay energy to the tumor, because the time during which it is tumor-associated is a small proportion of its total decay lifetime.

The radionuclide half-life also determines the rate at which radiation is delivered to the target cells (the dose rate). Depending on the repair rate of the target cells, this value may be more important than the total dose. A very long-lived radionuclide (i.e., one with a very low dose rate) may be incapable of eradicating tumor cells that exhibit a rapid repair capacity, because the cells may be capable of repairing the radiation-induced damage as it occurs. This phenomenon does not apply to alpha-particle emitters, because the damage to DNA from the energy deposited along each alpha-particle track is far greater than the repair capacity of cells.

Although it is not essential for tumor cell kill, an additional feature of some radionuclides that has permitted a detailed investigation of the in vivo pharmacokinetics of radiolabeled antibodies is the release of photons in addition to electrons and alpha particles during decay. Relative to electrons and alpha particles, photons deposit very little energy within tissue, and those that emit sufficient energy, between 100 and 400 keV, can be imaged externally. Images of the spatial distribution of radiolabeled antibody within a patient may be obtained using nuclear medicine scanners. After a low level of radioactivity is administered, such pharmacokinetic information can be used to assess antibody targeting and to determine the likelihood of tumor eradication or normal tissue morbidity before a therapeutic dose is given.

This brief introduction to the unique aspects of antibody therapy combined with radionuclides reveals some of the complexity of radioimmunotherapy. A large number of parameters must be chosen for the implementation of this approach. The optimal treatment strategy for one set of circumstances (disease type, location, radiosensitivity, patient treatment history) may not apply under a different set of conditions. The following section reviews some of the pharmacologic and dosimetric considerations associated with the implementation of radioimmunotherapy.

Pharmacology and Pharmacokinetics of Radiolabeled Monoclonal Antibodies

The pharmacokinetics of radiolabeled antibodies is difficult to describe in terms of average or typical kinetics. In general, in vivo behavior depends on the antibody, the target antigen, the radiolabel, and the patient's prior treatment history (e.g., exposure to mouse-derived antibody). The kinetics may change depending on whether the antibody is an intact IgG or a fragment and whether it cross-reacts with normal tissue. Antigens shed into the circulation also may affect antibody kinetics by complexing with and increasing the clearance rate of circulating antibody. Internalization of a cell-bound antibody-antigen complex may lead to catabolism of the complex, followed by release of the radionuclide. Depending on the technique used to label the antibody, radionuclide also may be released while the antibody is in circulation. The kinetics of the free radionuclide reflect the pharmacokinetics of the parent element rather than that of the administered antibody. Additionally, if previous antibody exposure produces a human immune reaction, the pharmacokinetics are profoundly affected. Mouse-derived antibodies elicit human antimouse activity (HAMA), and humanized antibodies may elicit human antihuman activity (HAHA). The effect in both cases is usually rapid complexing with administered antibody, followed by rapid clearance of the complex from the circulation. This phenomenon may eliminate the therapeutic activity of radiolabeled antibody and thereby greatly reduce the applicability of radioimmunotherapy. A human immune reaction (HAMA or HAHA) usually precludes the use of multiple courses of radioimmunotherapy or the retreatment of patients who have undergone radioimmunotherapy.

Macroscopic Pharmacokinetics

As indicated earlier, the photon emissions of most radionuclides used in radioimmunotherapy allow for a detailed assessment of antibody pharmacokinetics. Measurement of the radioactivity in sequential blood samples is generally combined with gamma camera imaging and with whole-body, urine measurements, or both. Imaging is rarely performed after a therapeutic administration, however, because the radioactivity in the patient exceeds the imaging (or counting) capacity of most nuclear medicine imaging devices. Imaging information obtained from a trace-labeled administration of antibody is used instead to project the kinetics of the therapeutic administration.

The distinction between a therapeutic and a tracer administration of antibody lies in the amount of radioactivity and the type of radionuclide administered. Radioactivity, expressed in megabecquerels (MBq, or millions of decays per second), may vary from a diagnostic administration of 20 to 200 MBq to a therapeutic administration of 2,000 to 15,000 MBq for iodine-131 (^{131}I), one of the most commonly used radionuclides in radioimmunotherapy. The very large range of values for therapy reflects the diversity of antibodies used and the range of patient responses. Doses as low as 1,000 MBq have elicited patient responses in B-cell lymphoma.[112] Alternatively, doses as high as 22,000 MBq have been used in the treatment of B-cell lymphoma. Therapeutic doses of the radiolabeled conjugate depend on the choice of antibody and antigen target.

A number of studies have examined the relationship between the amount of antibody administered and the resulting pharmacokinetics.[113–119] In most cases, a (non–statistically significant) trend toward longer plasma clearance half-times is observed with increasing milligram dose. In those cases in which a statistically significant effect is observed,[25,113,119,120] the results may be due to diminished binding and removal of antibody from the circulation once target antigen sites are saturated. The relationship between serum pharmacokinetics and antibody dose is therefore likely to depend on the available antigen sites and their distribution relative to the milligram amount of administered antibody. Antibodies that exhibit such dependence generally yield improved diagnostic[119] and therapeutic results[120] when the dose is increased.

The plasma clearance half-times of antibodies that target hematologic malignancies are generally shorter than those of solid tumor antibodies. In hematologic malignancies, the half-time of the first component of plasma clearance is on the order of 1 to 3 hours.[112,117,121] This is thought to reflect rapid binding of antibody to circulating and therefore readily available target antigen sites. Except for

antibodies that target antigen that is also released in circulation, the plasma clearance curves for solid tumor antibodies are generally fit by a single-exponential or double-exponential curve in which the half-time of the rapid component is on the order of 3 to 10 hours.

Due to the high molecular weight of most radioimmunoconjugates, the initial distribution of intravenously administered antibody is generally confined to the vascular space and to the extracellular space of tissues that lack a fully developed capillary basal lamina (e.g., marrow, liver, spleen, and other tissues of the reticuloendothelial system).[122,123] In a 70-kg man, this volume is approximately 4 L; that is, it modestly exceeds plasma volume. In this way, significantly higher "apparent" distribution volumes may be observed when targeting tumor cells that are rapidly accessible to intravenously administered radiolabeled antibody.[121] In such cases, antibody binding to tumor cells provides an alternative mechanism for the rapid reduction in plasma concentration.

Microscopic Pharmacokinetics

The larger molecular weight of antibodies raises issues that are not generally relevant to the targeting of chemotherapeutic agents. The molecular weight of the IgG antibody, the isotype most commonly used for cancer treatment, is 150 kd, which is 150 times heavier than most chemotherapeutic agents. In order to target antigen-positive cells, intravenously administered antibody must cross the capillary basal lamina and then traverse the extravascular space of solid tumor.

In most normal organs, the capillary basal lamina presents a substantial barrier to traversal of a 150-kd protein.[124] Due to the "leaky" nature of tumor vasculature,[124–126] this barrier is greatly diminished in tumors, and passage of antibodies is close to that of low molecular weight chemotherapeutic agents. The vascular permeability coefficient of tumor capillaries for methotrexate, for example, ranges from 1 to 10×10^{-6} cm/second[127]; the corresponding value for IgG is 0.6×10^{-6} cm/second.[124] Once the antibody reaches the extravascular side of the capillary, it must cross the interstitial space to bind antigen-positive cells. For most chemotherapeutic agents, such transport occurs by diffusion.[127] A typical low molecular weight cytotoxic agent (350 Da) has a diffusion coefficient in the interstitial space of tumor of approximately 6.4×10^{-6} cm^2/second.[128] The corresponding value for IgG antibody ranges from 0.005 to 0.015×10^{-6} cm^2/second.[129] These values translate into 4 seconds (for the low molecular weight cytotoxic agent) versus 0.5 to 1 hour (for the antibody) to achieve 16% of the source concentration at a 100-mm distance. Antibody transport across the interstitial space is therefore primarily dependent on bulk fluid flow or convection. Such flow relies on a positive pressure difference between the periphery and the tumor center.

Interstitial pressure is consistently higher in solid tumors than in normal tissues.[130,131] This pressure is thought to arise because solid tumors do not have completely developed lymphatic drainage. In normal tissues, vascular fluid that filters into the interstitial space and is not reabsorbed into the microvascular network is taken up by lymphatic vessels. In solid tumors, such vessels may not exist or may be inadequate to reabsorb excess interstitial fluid rapidly.[132] Additionally, interstitial pressure increases with the size of the tumor. Such interstitial fluid pressure presents a significant physiologic barrier to antibody penetration of large solid tumors and may help explain the highly nonuniform distribution of antibody in solid tumors as well as observations of increased antibody uptake in smaller tumor cell clusters.[133]

A further barrier to antibody penetration of a cluster of antigen-positive cells is the *binding-site barrier phenomenon*.[134,135] The binding-site barrier arises as a result of the low antibody concentration in the tumor interstitial space relative to the local antigen concentration. (The local concentration of antigen sites depends on the number of antigen sites per cell [typically 10^4 to 10^6] and the number of cells per unit volume.) The antibody is, in effect, prevented from diffusing to the interior of the solid tumor until the antigen sites in the periphery are occupied. In systems in which interstitial pressure is not of concern (e.g., in vitro tumor cell spheroids or micrometastases), the binding-site barrier may, depending on the concentration of antibody, yield a highly nonuniform distribution of antigen-bound, radiolabeled antibody, with very high concentrations in the periphery and negligible amounts in the center.[136,137]

CONSIDERATIONS SPECIFIC TO RADIOIMMUNOTHERAPY

Dosimetry

Dose in the context of chemotherapy is fundamentally different from the therapeutically relevant quantity in radioimmunotherapy. The quantity of a cytotoxic agent that is delivered to a patient in the chemotherapeutic context is generally the amount in milligrams or the area under a blood time × concentration curve. The latter provides a measure of the drug's residence time in the circulation. The radioimmunotherapeutic equivalents are *activity* (also often referred to as *dose*) in megabecquerels and *cumulated activity* in megabecquerels × seconds (total number of radionuclide decays). The cumulated activity need not be limited to blood circulation. For solid tumors in particular, one is interested in the cumulated activity in the tumor. Using external imaging at various times after antibody administration to obtain a time-activity curve that is then integrated over time, one may obtain the cumulated activity for tumor or other tissues. The therapeutically relevant quantity for radioimmunotherapy, however, is the *absorbed dose* (also often referred to as the *dose*) in grays (energy absorbed per unit mass of tissue). This value is

obtained by multiplying the total number of decays that have occurred in a given tissue (i.e., the cumulated activity) by the total energy released per radionuclide decay and by a factor that accounts for the fraction of emitted energy that is absorbed within the tissue. This fraction depends on the tissue's geometry and the energy (or range) of each radionuclide emission. Dividing by the mass of the target tissue yields the absorbed dose. The resulting absorbed-dose estimate only accounts for emissions that occur within the given tissue. Depending on the range and type of radionuclide emissions, radioactivity in other organs also may contribute to the total absorbed dose of a given target organ. Contributions from other organs are calculated as described earlier, except that the geometric factor reflects the fraction of emitted energy in a source organ that is absorbed by the given target organ. The total target tissue absorbed dose is then obtained by adding the absorbed dose contributions from all the source organs to the target tissue self-dose. The procedure described here was developed by the Medical Internal Radiation Dose Committee.[138] The absorbed dose to a given organ is a much more precise measure of cytotoxic potential than the administered activity or the cumulated activity, because the pharmacokinetics and the radionuclide properties are accounted for by the absorbed-dose value.

The red marrow is the dose-limiting organ in most implementations of intravenously administered radiolabeled antibody.[139,140] Marrow vasculature, unlike that of most normal organs, is fenestrated and does not present a significant barrier to antibody penetration. The red marrow is composed of cells that are continuously undergoing cell division and that are therefore more radiosensitive.[141] These two factors—easy accessibility and enhanced radiosensitivity—account for the marrow toxicity that is observed in almost all radiolabeled-antibody dose-escalation studies.

The marrow absorbed dose from radiolabeled antibody that does not bind to components of the marrow, blood, or bone is generally obtained by assuming that marrow kinetics is the same as that of blood and multiplying by a factor to account for the different antibody concentrations in the two volumes.[139,142] In hematologic disease, antibody binding to specific blood or marrow components occurs and must be considered in determining the red marrow absorbed dose.[143] In this case, imaging of a marrow-rich, low-background region (e.g., head and neck of the femur), in combination with one or more bone marrow biopsies, is generally used to obtain a time-activity curve for red marrow dosimetry.[143,144]

Several of the radioimmunotherapy protocols for patients with hematologic diseases include hematopoietic stem cell transplantation. In such protocols, the red marrow is no longer the dose-limiting organ, and preliminary results suggest that lung, liver, or renal toxicity may limit the total dose that can be administered.[69,145,146] In such cases, determination of the spatial distribution of absorbed dose and a dose-volume histogram for the actual organ volume of each patient are necessary to assess the probability of normal tissue morbidity. Although techniques for determining the spatial distribution of absorbed dose by performing three-dimensional dosimetry have been developed,[147,148] a key obstacle to their clinical implementation has been the difficulty of obtaining accurate, patient-specific, three-dimensional biodistribution data. Ongoing improvements in quantitative imaging with single-photon emission computed tomography may eventually overcome this difficulty.

Radionuclide Choice

The choice of an appropriate isotope depends on a variety of factors, including the physical and biological half-life of the nuclide and its emission characteristics, the labeling efficiency of the isotope, and the pharmacology of the immunoconjugate. Because of their long range, beta particles can destroy target cells without antigen-antibody complex internalization and may also kill antigen-negative tumor cells. The gamma emissions from ^{131}I allow dosimetry studies to be performed easily, but treatment at high doses requires patient isolation and can result in significant radiation exposure to hospital staff. Additionally, the 8-day half-life poses a waste hazard. Radiolabeling with ^{131}I can also cause loss of biological function, particularly at high specific activities. This decrease in immunoreactivity is directly related to the number of tyrosine residues in the hypervariable region of the mAb to which radioiodine attaches.[149]

Yttrium-90 (^{90}Y) is a pure β-emitter; its lack of gamma emissions allows outpatient administration of high doses and reduces radiation exposure risk to hospital staff, and the high-energy beta allows a low effective dose.[150-151] If the targeted antigen undergoes modulation, ^{90}Y is more likely to be retained intracellularly than [131]I.[152] Moreover, if ^{90}Y dissociates from the mAb complex in vivo, the isotope is likely to be deposited in bone, potentially delivering additional radiation to leukemic cells in the marrow. Therapy with ^{90}Y, however, poses several difficulties: (a) unlike ^{131}I, ^{90}Y cannot be directly conjugated to a mAB but must be linked to the antibody by a bifunctional chelate, and (b) because of the absence of gamma emissions, biodistribution and dosimetry studies require administration of mAb trace-labeled with a second isotope, usually Indium-111 (^{111}In). The biodistribution of ^{90}Y and ^{111}In is not identical; studies have shown, however, that it is similar enough that the prediction of safe doses of radiolabeled antibody with maximal antitumor effect is possible.[153] The use of quantitative positron emission tomography (PET) following the administration of [86]Y-labeled mAb may permit more precise dose estimates, thereby maximizing the antitumor effect and minimizing toxicity.[154] Other radiometals, such as rhenium-186, rhenium-188, and copper-67, have been studied.

Alpha particle–emitting isotopes, such as [212]Bi, [213]Bi, and [211]At, have also displayed potent antitumor effects.[155] Because of their high linear energy transfer, as few as one to two alpha particles can destroy a target cell. The 50 to 80 μm range of these particles could result in decreased toxicity to surrounding normal bystander cells. The potential for specific antitumor effects makes targeted alpha-particle therapy an attractive approach for the treatment of micrometastatic disease or minimal residual disease.

TABLE 31.4

INCIDENCE OF HUMAN ANTIMOUSE ACTIVITY (HAMA) RESPONSES IN CLINICAL TRIALS OF MONOCLONAL ANTIBODIES (mAbs)

Population of Patients	No. of Trials	No. of Patients	Incidence of HAMA (%)
Patients with solid tumors given murine mAb	9	167	74
Patients with hematopoietic tumors given rodent mAbs			
Lymphoid neoplasms	7	124	9
Myeloid neoplasms	3	32	54
Patients with solid tumors given chimeric mAbs	4	45	46
Patients with hematopoietic tumors given CDR-grafted mAbs			
Lymphoid neoplasms	1	2	0
Myeloid neoplasms	2	28	0

CDR, complementarity-determining region.
From P. Chapman, D.A. Scheinberg, unpublished research.

The safety and feasibility of targeted alpha-particle therapy was first demonstrated using humanized anti-CD33 HuM195 labeled with[213]Bi in patients with myeloid leukemia.[156] Fourteen of the 18 patients had a reduction in the percentage of bone marrow blasts after therapy; however, there were no complete remissions, demonstrating the difficulty of targeting one or two [213]Bi atoms to each leukemic blast at the specific activities used in this trial. Subsequently, remissions have been observed in some patients treated with [213]Bi-HuM195 after partial cytoreduction with cytarabine.[157]

[225]Ac decays by alpha emission, with a 10-day half-life through three atoms, each of which also emits an alpha particle, yielding a total of four alpha particles, and it can be conjugated to a variety of antibodies using derivatives of the macrocyclic ligand 1,4,7,10-tetraazacyclododecane tetraacetic acid (DOTA). Therefore, [225]Ac-DOTA can act as an atomic nanogenerator, delivering an alpha-particle cascade to a cancer cell when coupled to an internalizing antibody. As a result of these properties, [225]Ac immunoconjugates are approximately 1,000 times more potent than [213]Bi-containing conjugates.[158] Although this increased potency could make [225]Ac more effective than other α-emitters, the possibility of free daughter radioisotopes in circulation after decay of [225]Ac raises concerns about the potential toxicity of this isotope. In nude mice bearing human prostate carcinoma and lymphoma xenografts, single nanocurie doses of [225]Ac-labeled, tumor-specific antibodies prolonged survival compared with controls and cured a substantial proportion of animals.[158]

Produced by the bombardment of bismuth with alpha particles in a cyclotron, the halogen [211]At emits two alpha particles in its decay to stable [107]Pb.[159] Due to its long 7.2-hour half-life, [211]At-labeled constructs can be used even when the targeting molecule does not gain immediate access to tumor cells. Additionally, its daughter, polonium-211 ([211]Po), emits K x-rays that permit photon counting of samples and external imaging for biodistribution studies.

Investigators at Duke University have extensively studied [211]At-81C6, a chimeric astatine-labeled antibody that targets tenascin, a glycoprotein overexpressed on gliomas relative to normal brain tissue. Early results of a phase I dose-escalation trial of [211]At-81C6 in patients with malignant gliomas following surgical resection of the tumor suggest that adjuvant therapy with [211]At-81C6 prolongs survival in these patients compared with historic controls.[160]

Like [225]Ac, radium-223 ([223]Ra) emits four alpha particles over its decay scheme. Because of its bone-seeking properties, unconjugated cationic [223]Ra is a promising candidate for delivery of high-LET radiation to cancer cells on bone surfaces. Preliminary results of a clinical phase I study demonstrated reduction in pain intensity and tumor marker levels in the treatment of skeletal metastases in patients with prostate and breast cancer.[161]

Pretargeting Methods

In an effort to reduce radiation doses to normal organs and improve tumor to normal organ dose ratios, pretargeted methods of radioimmunotherapy have been developed. First, a monoclonal antibody or engineered targeting molecule conjugated to streptavidin is given. After administration of a biotinylated N-acetylgalactosamine–containing "clearing agent" to remove excess circulating antibody, therapeutically radiolabeled biotin is infused. The radiolabeled biotin can bind specifically to "pretargeted" streptavidin at the tumor, while unbound radiolabeled biotin is rapidly excreted in the urine.[162]

This approach has been applied to a mouse model of adult T-cell leukemia (ATL) that expresses the cell-surface marker CD25.[163] After treatment with a streptavidin-labeled, humanized anti-CD25 antibody and the clearing agent, immunodeficient mice with human ATL received DOTA-biotin labeled with either [213]Bi or [90]Y. Treatment with [213]Bi reduced the levels of the surrogate tumor markers human β$_2$-microglobulin and soluble CD25 and improved survival compared with controls. Treatment with ^{90}Y, however, did not improve survival compared with controls. Mice treated with [213]Bi using the pretargeting approach survived longer than those treated with [213]Bi labeled directly to anti-Tac. This approach was also studied using an anti-CD25 single-chain Fv-streptavidin fusion protein, followed by radiolabeled biotin. Significant antitumor effects were seen after administration of [213]Bi-DOTA-biotin to leukemic mice, and when the [213]Bi-DOTA-biotin was combined with unconjugated anti-Tac, 7 of 10 mice were cured. In a recent phase I trial, 15 patients with relapsed or refractory CD20-positive B-cell NHL received an anti-CD20 second-generation fusion protein (B9E9FP), followed by a synthetic clearing agent 48 or 72 hours later to remove the unbound B9E9FP.[164] Twenty-four hours later, ^{90}Y-DOTA-biotin or ^{111}In-DOTA-biotin was injected. In this trial, the clearing agent was very effective in removing the B9E9FP, and the radioimmunoconjugate was rapidly absorbed at the tumor sites. Both the nonhematologic and hematologic toxicities were minimal, and three patients had a response.

Another pretargeting approach that has yielded promising results in animal studies and clinical trials uses a bifunctional antibody in which one arm binds to tumor antigen and the other to a radiolabeled ligand. In some implementations, the radiolabeled ligand is designed to be multivalent and therefore capable of attaching to the ligand-binding arm of two different bifunctional antibodies.[165]

TOXICITY OF ANTIBODY THERAPIES

Most native Abs, whether rodent or human, are remarkably nontoxic. Maximum tolerated doses (MTDs) are generally not reached in therapeutic trials of mAbs. However, reaching an MTD may be irrelevant, since the goal of mAb therapy is usually to saturate available target sites, thereby achieving the maximum biologic response in the tumor. Hence, further increases in delivered doses may not improve cell kill and may have the theoretical adverse consequences of increased immunogenicity and rapid modulation (loss) of cell surface protein targets.

The mAbs with the most potent activities in vitro (CDC or ADCC) tend to have the most prominent toxicities. Administration of CAMPATH-1H and rituximab (anti-CD20), each a potent activator of the human immune system, results in fever, chills, and rigors in a dose-dependent manner. Usually the infusion-related reaction follows the first dose of antibody only.[67] Release of cytokines from targeted cells also may contribute to toxicity. In principle, one would expect that toxicities of mAbs should relate to targeted tissues, neoplastic or normal. Hence, the more specific a mAb, the fewer toxic effects expected. For example, the antibody 3F8, a potent activator of human complement, targets GD2 on neuroblastoma but also binds to GD2 on peripheral nerve, which results in a severe pain syndrome.[166] CAMPATH-1H, which targets both normal as well as malignant lymphoid cells, is associated with a high rate of opportunistic infections in treated patients, including infections with herpes viruses, cytomegalovirus, and *Pneumocystis carinii*.[67]

HAMA is sometimes characterized as an adverse effect, but it is generally not defined as a treatment-related toxicity (Table 31.4). Treatment of patients with an active HAMA response does not appear to increase toxicity; it can lead to adverse consequences for pharmacokinetics due to rapid clearing of antibody and the development of serum sickness.[167] Anaphylaxis has been reported in fewer than 1% of infused patients.

Toxicities associated with conjugated mAbs are generally a consequence of the cytotoxic agent carried by the mAb. With radioimmunoconjugates, myelosuppression is prominent in all studies in which dose escalation is applied.[145,151,167–171] Autologous or allogeneic bone marrow transplantation is often required as a rescue in treated patients.[145,167] Toxin conjugates pose a special problem, and some unusual toxicities have been observed. Temporary hepatic injury, as evidenced by elevations in liver enzyme function test results, and vascular leak syndromes, characterized by weight gain, edema, and hypoalbuminemia, are also seen.[105,108,109] Neurologic toxicity has been observed, but this effect may be due to targeting of neural tissues.[172] The long-term consequences of therapy with mAb constructs are entirely unknown but are not expected to differ from those of the cytotoxic agent carried by the mAb.

CLINICAL TRIALS OF MONOCLONAL ANTIBODIES IN CANCER THERAPY

Numerous therapeutic and radioimmunodiagnostic trials with mAbs or mAb constructs have been reported. Those that illustrate important aspects of mAb therapy or describe pivotal trials that have altered the standard of care for a certain malignancy are addressed in this chapter (Table 31.5).

In early trials, the majority of the monoclonal antibodies were of murine origin. These antibodies were safe, even

TABLE 31.5
FDA-APPROVED MONOCLONAL ANTIBODIES, TARGETS, INDICATIONS, AND OTHER USES

Antibody	Trade Name	Target Antigen	Antibody Type	FDA Indication	Other Potential Uses
Rituximab	Rituxan	CD20	Chimeric	B-NHL	CLL[a]; WM[a]
[90]Y-ibritumomab tiuxetan	Zevalin	CD20	Murine radiolabeled	Rel/ref FL and transf B-NHL	Upfront FL; upfront DLBCL[a]
[131]I-tositumomab	Bexxar	CD20	Murine radiolabeled	Rel/ref FL and transf B-NHL	Upfront FL[a]; upfront DLBCL[a]
Alemtuzumab	Campath	CD52	Humanized	CLL[b]	T-cell PLL[a]
Gemtuzumab ozogamicin	Mylotarg	CD33	Humanized *with toxin*	AML	
Bevacizumab	Avastin	EGFR	Humanized	Metastatic CRC	RCC; first-line rx for stage 3b/4 NSCLC[a]
Cetuximab	C225	EGFR	Humanized	CPT-11 ref metastatic CRC	Adv H/N Ca (with XRT)[c]; pancreatic ca[a]; NSCLC[a]
Trastuzumab	Herceptin	HER2/neu	Humanized	Metastatic Br CA	Adjuvant Br CA[c]

Adv H/N Ca, advanced head and neck cancer; AML, acute myeloid leukemia; B-NHL, B-cell non-Hodgkin's lymphoma; Br CA, breast carcinoma; CLL, chronic lymphocytic leukemia; CRC, colorectal carcinoma; DLBCL, diffuse large B-cell lymphoma; EGFR, epidermal growth factor receptor; FL, follicular lymphoma; MCL, mantle cell lymphoma; NSCLC, non–small cell lung cancer; PLL, prolymphocytic leukemia; ref, refractory; RCC, renal cell carcinoma; rel, relapsed; transf, transformed; WM, Waldenström's macroglobulinemia.
[a]Phase II clinical trial is ongoing or completed.
[b]Fludarabine and alkylator therapy failure.
[c]Phase III clinical trial is ongoing.

at high doses. However, the usefulness of rodent mAb was limited due to the high rate of HAMA, which developed in most patients following the first dose of antibody. Additionally, murine isotypes are sometimes not capable of effector activity. Genetic engineering has led to the production of partially human (chimeric), more fully human (humanized), and fully human antibodies in order to improve therapeutic efficacy. Dozens of these chimeric or humanized mAbs have been investigated in clinical trials. Several showed significant activity against their targets, minimal toxicity, and a marked reduction in HAMA compared with their murine counterparts.

To date, eight mAbs have been approved by the US Food and Drug Administration for human use in the treatment of specific malignancies. Rituximab (Rituxan) was the first mAb approved by the FDA in 1997 for the treatment of relapsed or refractory low-grade or follicular CD20-positive B-cell non-Hodgkin's lymphoma (B-NHL). Today, rituximab is used in patients with many types of CD20-positive B-NHL. Based on an overall response rate of 33% in heavily pretreated chronic lymphocytic leukemia (CLL) patients, alemtuzumab (Campath-1H) was approved by the FDA for the treatment of fludarabine-refractory B-cell CLL. Patients with metastatic Her-2 Neu overexpressing metastatic breast carcinoma can receive targeted therapy with trastuzumab (Herceptin). Bevacizumab and cetuximab recently received FDA approval for the treatment of metastatic colorectal carcinoma. Gemtuzumab ozogamicin (Mylotarg), an antibody-drug conjugate, was approved by the FDA in 2000 for the treatment of CD33-positive, relapsed acute myeloid leukemia (AML) patients who are 60 years of age or older. ^{90}Y-ibritumomab tiuxetan (Zevalin) was the first radiolabeled antibody approved for cancer therapy. Subsequently, ^{131}I-tositumomab (Bexxar) was approved by the FDA for the treatment of relapsed or refractory low-grade follicular or transformed CD20-positive B-cell NHL.

Rituximab

Rituximab, a chimeric IgG1 anti-CD20 antibody, represents an important advance in the treatment of B-cell NHL. Multiple mechanisms of action of rituximab have been proposed, including complement fixation, ADCC, and direct cytotoxicity via apoptotic pathways activated by binding to CD20.[173] In the phase II trial that led to its approval by the FDA, the overall rate of response to single-agent rituximab in patients with heavily pretreated, relapsed low-grade lymphoma was 48%, with a 12-month median duration of response.[174] Similarly, phase II studies of relapsed or refractory intermediate and high-grade lymphoma demonstrated a 32% overall rate of response to rituximab alone. Patients with untreated indolent NHL achieved an overall response rate of 73%, a complete response rate of 37%, and a median progression-free survival of 34 months with rituximab therapy.[175] Hainsworth et al. administered rituximab weekly for 4 weeks at 6-month

intervals. A Swiss research group investigated the benefit of maintenance rituximab.[176] In this study, all patients received four weekly doses of rituximab. At week 12, patients with responding or stable disease were then randomized to no further treatment or a prolonged course of rituximab (one dose of antibody at 2-month intervals for a total of four times). The median event-free survival was increased from 12 months in the control arm to 23 months in the study group.

The impressive single-agent activity of rituximab led to the exploration of its use in combination with standard chemotherapy for treatment of indolent and aggressive NHL. Czuczman et al. established the safety and efficacy of rituximab and cyclophosphamide, doxorubicin, vincristine sulfate, and prednisone (CHOP) chemotherapy in a phase II trial of patients with previously treated and newly diagnosed low-grade NHL.[177] In a large multicenter, randomized phase III trial, the addition of rituximab to cyclophosphamide, vincristine, and prednisone (CVP) significantly improved the overall response rate (81% vs. 57%), complete response rate (40% vs. 10%), and time to treatment failure (27 vs. 7 months).[178] The benefit of rituximab in combination with chemotherapy for elderly patients with untreated diffuse large B cell lymphoma (DLBCL) was investigated in a randomized phase III trial.[179] With a median follow-up of 3 years, those who were treated with rituximab and CHOP (R-CHOP) had significantly higher rates of complete response (76% vs. 63%), event-free survival (53% vs. 35%, $P = .00008$), and overall survival (62% vs. 51%, $P = .008$) than those treated with chemotherapy alone. In another phase III multicenter trial,[180] a similar patient population ($N = 632$) was randomized to R-CHOP versus CHOP, followed by a second randomization to maintenance (Hainsworth schedule)[175] or no further therapy. There were no statistically significant differences in overall survival. However, the patients who received CHOP and maintenance rituximab had a statistically significant improvement in time to treatment failure. The Mabthera International trial (MinT study), a randomized phase III trial investigating the efficacy of R-CHOP versus CHOP in untreated, younger (less than 60 years), good-prognosis patients with DLBCL was closed to patient accrual in December 2003. The trial ended early because a preplanned interim analysis demonstrated a significant improvement in time to treatment failure, a primary endpoint of the study. In all of the aforementioned studies, the combination of rituximab and standard chemotherapy did not result in an increase in toxicity. As a result of these and other studies, rituximab has become a common part of many lymphoma treatment regimens.

Many studies, some mentioned in earlier in this section, have focused on the issue of maintenance therapy in patients with lymphoma. In the Hainsworth trial, untreated patients with indolent NHL received four weekly doses of rituximab, followed by maintenance rituximab.[175] Patients who had stable disease or an objective tumor response received weekly rituximab for four doses at 6-month intervals (maximum of four courses of rituximab). At 6 weeks, only 7% of these patients achieved a complete response, whereas 37% had a complete response following at least one course of maintenance treatment. A Swiss research group also investigated the benefit of maintenance rituximab.[176] As in the previous trial, all patients received four weekly doses of rituximab. At week 12, patients with responding or stable disease were then randomized to no further treatment versus maintenance rituximab (one dose of antibody at 2-month intervals for a total of four times). The median EFS was increased from 12 months in the control arm to 23 months in the study group.

A number of studies using weekly rituximab at 375 mg/m^2 demonstrated an inferior response rate for patients with small lymphocytic leukemia (SLL) or CLL compared with the 48% response rate associated with relapsed advanced follicular NHL.[174,181–184] One possible explanation for the inferior results in this malignancy is due to the low density of CD20 expression on tumor cells. A previous study discovered a correlation between CD20 antigen density and response rates in patients with NHL.[184] Pharmacokinetics may also point to another reason for its lack of activity in CLL and SLL. Since mean plasma antibody concentration is strongly correlated with response to rituximab, the high intravascular tumor burden in CLL and SLL may result in rapid intravascular clearance of the antibody, leading to decreased efficacy. Because of this finding, a thrice weekly dosing schedule was further explored for rituximab monotherapy. A phase I/II trial demonstrated that this schedule was safe and more effective than the weekly administration.[185] Alternatively, O'Brien et al. demonstrated that higher doses of weekly rituximab, ranging from 500 to 2,250 mg/m2, were associated with an overall response rate of 36%. Response rates from 44% to 75% were seen at the higher dose levels.[186] Data from these two trials have established that single-agent rituximab is both a safe and an effective treatment for patients with CLL or SLL as long as a modified dose or schedule is utilized. Currently, the use of rituximab in combination with cyclophosphamide and a nucleoside analog is currently being investigated in both upfront and relapsed CLL.[187,188]

The use of rituximab for the treatment of mantle-cell lymphoma appears more useful in the setting of minimal residual disease. Progression-free survival was not prolonged in patients with untreated mantle-cell lymphoma who received R-CHOP.[189] However, the number of molecular remissions in patients with mantle-cell lymphoma seems to increase following each antibody administration in the post–autologous bone-marrow transplantation setting.[190]

Rituximab has also shown some activity in other malignancies or autoimmune disorders. Patients with refractory hairy-cell leukemia can achieve complete remissions following rituximab.[191] A response rate of 20% has been demonstrated in patients with multiple myeloma whose tumors overexpress CD20.[192] An overall response rate of approximately 50% has been observed in several small studies of patients with relapsed or refractory immune thrombocytopenic purpura. Similarly, rituximab is used to treat relapsed or refractory pure red-cell aplasia and autoimmune hemolytic anemia.[193,194]

Alemtuzumab

Alemtuzumab is humanized monoclonal antibody that targets CD52, a glycoprotein highly expressed on both B-CLL cells and normal B and T cells. The mechanism of action of alemtuzumab is not well understood, but it is presumed to work via ADCC, CDC, and/or apoptosis. Initial studies demonstrated that this agent was effective at clearing tumor cells from the blood and bone marrow of patients with NHL but did not result in significant diminution of bulky lymphadenopathy.[66] Therefore, CLL seemed the optimal setting for this new agent, as it is primarily a malignancy of the peripheral blood and bone marrow.

Based on the results of a multicenter study, alemtuzumab (Campath-1H) was approved by the FDA for the treatment of B-cell CLL unsuccessfully treated by alkylating agents and fludarabine. In a pivotal multicenter phase II trial,[195] heavily pretreated patients in whom fludarabine had failed ($N = 93$) achieved an overall response rate of 33% and a complete response rate of 2% with 12 weeks of intravenous alemtuzumab. The median time to progression was 4.7 months (9.5 months for responders), and the median survival was 16 months (32 months for responders). Side effects were frequent and included infusion-related reactions (occurring mostly within the first week of therapy) and infection (26% of patients had a grade 3 or 4 infection). Nine deaths (9.6%) occurred on study, which compares favorably with the death rate of 22% reported in fludarabine trials.[196]

In a phase II trial, untreated, symptomatic patients with B-cell CLL were treated with subcutaneous alemtuzumab.[197] The overall response rate and complete remission rate were 87% and 19%, respectively, which were similar to published results for treatment with fludarabine in untreated patients. Significant clearance of tumor cells was noted in the blood, bone marrow, and nonbulky lymphadenopathy. None of the patients with a large lymph node (measuring greater than 5 cm) achieved a complete response. Using a dose-escalation approach for the first week of therapy, alemtuzumab was well tolerated. Although 20% of patients had grade 4 neutropenia (ANC $< 0.5 \times 10^9$/L), none of the 38 patients had fever and neutropenia. Ten percent of patients had CMV reactivation, which responded promptly to intravenous antibiotics.

In order to increase response rates, time to progression, and median survival, alemtuzumab is also being investigated in combination with other agents, such as purine analogs and rituximab. A German group treated relapsed or refractory CLL patients ($N = 14$) with alemtuzumab and fludarabine. Preliminary results from 11 evaluable patients revealed a 64% response rate (8 complete responses; 1 partial response) and an acceptable safety profile.[198] In a phase II study of previously treated patients with lymphoid malignancies, combination therapy with rituximab was also well tolerated and produced an improved overall response rate of 52% (complete response, 8%; nodular partial response, 4%; partial response, 40%).[199] Further investigation of combined treatment programs using one or more monoclonal antibodies with fludarabine and/or alkylator-based chemotherapeutics in CLL are ongoing and may continue to demonstrate improved response rates and overall survival.

Alemtuzumab is active against T-prolymphocytic leukemia (T-PLL), a disease that is resistant to most chemotherapeutic agents. In a retrospective analysis of 76 patients with heavily pretreated T-PLL, Keating et al. demonstrated a 51% overall response rate and a 39.5% complete response rate following alemtuzumab treatment.[200] The median time to progression (4.5 months) was double that of the first-line therapy. In a prospective phase II trial, patients with relapsed T-PLL who were treated with alemtuzumab achieved a 76% overall response rate and a 60% complete response rate.[201] The median disease-free interval was 7 months, a significant improvement over the brief response (3 months) typically associated with conventional CHOP therapy or pentostatin. Further prospective studies are needed to define how alemtuzumab should be utilized in T-PLL, whether as a single agent or in combination with cytotoxic chemotherapeutics in the upfront, relapsed, or peritransplant setting.

Graft versus host disease (GVHD) is a major contributor to transplant-related mortality following allogeneic stem cell transplantation. Alemtuzumab is also utilized for both in vitro and in vivo depletion of T-cells in order to reduce the incidence of acute GVHD. Since it also eliminates host T cells, graft rejection is minimized. Sixty-five patients with lymphoproliferative disorders were treated with a nonmyeloablative allogeneic stem cell transplantation following BEAM-alemtuzumab conditioning.[202] The incidence of acute GVHD was 17%, and only grade I-II acute GVHD was observed. Sustained donor engraftment occurred in most patients (97%), and a high rate of complete remission (70%) was seen. In a retrospective analysis comparing the results from two prospective nonmyeloablative transplants, the incidence of acute and chronic GVHD was significantly reduced in those patients receiving alemtuzumab/cyclosporin compared with the cyclosporin A/methotrexate group.[203] Many of the alemtuzumab-treated patients required donor-lymphocyte infusions, but there were no significant differences between the two groups in both event-free and overall survival. Further studies with alemtuzumab are ongoing, with the goal of minimizing acute and chronic GVHD without compromising the overall response rate.

Herceptin

Trastuzumab (Herceptin) is a humanized IgG1 antibody that targets the HER2/neu antigen, which is overexpressed in 25 to 30% of breast carcinomas. In 1998, it was approved by the FDA for treatment of her-2/Neu positive metastatic breast carcinoma. Like rituximab, trastuzumab appears to act via multiple mechanisms, including down-regulation of her-2/Neu expression, induction of G_1 arrest and downstream cell regulatory signals, initiation of ADCC and CDC, and promotion of apoptosis.[204] Trastuzumab is well tolerated and has single-agent activity in her-2/Neu overexpressors lasting approximately 9 months.[205,206] In combination with a chemotherapeutic agent, such as paclitaxel, docetaxel, or doxorubicin, the response rate, time to progression, and overall survival are significantly improved.[207,208] However, this survival benefit was not observed in patients with her-2 negative tumors assessed by fluorescence in situ hybridization or immunohistochemical analysis (score less than 3, NE+). Based on these positive findings, trastuzumab is being studied in combination with chemotherapy in the adjuvant setting or in conjunction with other targeted therapies. Its use in other her-2/Neu–overexpressing, epithelial tumors is another active research focus. Further discussion of trastuzumab is covered in Chapter 30.

Bevacizumab

Bevacizumab, a humanized monoclonal antibody against vascular endothelial growth factor (VEGF), has shown promising activity in a variety of solid tumors in early phase I and II trials and was approved by the FDA in 2004 for the treatment of metastatic colorectal cancer. VEGF is overexpressed in cancer cells of many solid tumors and hematologic malignancies. Increased expression of VEGF is commonly observed in tumors associated with poorer prognosis and decreased rates of disease-free and overall survival.[209] Antibodies that target the VEGF receptor and/or neutralize VEGF were developed in the hope of blocking this important regulator of tumor angiogenesis. Preclinical studies confirmed that infusion of VEGF neutralizers resulted in an inhibition of tumor growth in multiple human cancer xenograft models.

A randomized phase III trial comparing irinotecan, bolus fluorouracil, and leucovorin (IFL) with and without bevacizumab was conducted in 813 patients with untreated metastatic colorectal cancer.[210] Patients who received bevacizumab and IFL therapy had a significant improvement in median duration of survival (20.3 vs. 15.6 months, $P < .001$) and progression-free survival (10.6 vs. 6.2 months, $P < .001$). Overall, the treatment was not associated with more toxicity than treatment with IFL, except for an increased incidence of grade 3 hypertension (11% vs. 2.3%). Based on these data, bevacizumab plus fluorouracil-based chemotherapy has become a standard treatment regimen for metastatic colorectal cancer.

Clinical development of bevacizumab is being investigated in numerous solid tumors and hematologic malignancies as monotherapy and in combination with other cytotoxic agents. In a prospective, double-blind, placebo-controlled phase II trial, an interim analysis demonstrated a significant prolongation of time to progression in patients with metastatic renal cell carcinoma who received bevacizumab compared with placebo ($P < .001$).[211] Preliminary data from a phase II trial in pancreatic cancer shows an impressive response rate of 24%.[212] A phase I dose-escalation study is ongoing to evaluate the use of bevacizumab in combination with chemoradiation for locally advanced or recurrent head and neck cancer. Other trials are planned or ongoing in sarcoma, melanoma, hepatocellular carcinoma, esophageal carcinoma, multiple myeloma, myelodysplastic syndrome, AML, NHL, and CML. There has been one negative trial thus far, using bevacizumab with capecitabine in patients with previously treated metastatic breast cancer.[213] It remains to be seen whether this agent will be an effective treatment for the multiple solid and hematologic malignancies that overexpress VEGF. Refer to chapter 30 for a more detailed discussion of bevacizumab.

Cetuximab

Overexpression of the epidermal growth factor receptor (EGFR), a regulator of cellular growth and survival, has been observed in multiple epithelial tumors and is a potential target for cetuximab, a chimeric monoclonal antibody against EGFR. In a recent phase II trial,[214] patients with irinotecan-refractory, EGFR-positive metastatic colorectal cancer were randomized to receive either cetuximab and irinotecan or cetuximab monotherapy. The response rate (23% vs. 10.8%, $P = .007$) and median time to progression (4.1 vs. 1.5 months, $P < .001$) were significantly improved in the combination therapy arm versus the monotherapy arm. There was also a trend towards an increase in median survival in the cetuximab and irinotecan group (8.6 vs 6.9 months). Unlike the trastuzumab data, which demonstrated a relationship between Her-2/Neu overexpression and efficacy, the level of EGFR expression did not correlate with response. However, the previously reported association between skin reactions following cetuximab and higher response rates was confirmed in this study. Based on these data and previous studies, cetuximab was approved by the FDA for the treatment of irinotecan-refractory metastatic colorectal cancer.

The activity of cetuximab in head and neck cancer with radiation therapy is very encouraging.[215] In a phase III study of radiation therapy with or without cetuximab in locally advanced squamous cell carcinoma of the head and neck, the combined modality treatment arm was not associated with increased toxicity compared with the control group, except for a higher incidence of grade 3/4 skin reactions. Median survival was prolonged from 28 to 54

months by adding cetuximab to high doses of radiation therapy. The combination of cetuximab and platinum-based chemotherapy in platinum-refractory advanced head and neck cancer resulted in an 11% response rate. These data suggest that cetuximab can reverse platinum-resistance in some head and neck cancer patients. Based on phase II data, cetuximab also enhances the activity of standard chemotherapy in patients with pancreatic cancer and non–small cell lung cancer. The use of cetuximab is currently being investigated in multiple epithelial tumors. Chapter 30 contains a more detailed discussion of cetuximab.

Gemtuzumab Ozogamicin

Gemtuzumab ozogamicin (GO, Mylotarg) consists of a recombinant, humanized anti-CD33 monoclonal antibody conjugated to calicheamicin, a potent antitumor antibiotic. Within the acidic environment of lysosomes after internalization, calicheamicin dissociates from the antibody and migrates to the nucleus, where it binds within the minor groove of DNA and causes double-stranded DNA breaks. In a phase I trial, 8 of 40 patients with relapsed or refractory AML treated with escalating doses of gemtuzumab ozogamicin had reductions in the percentage of bone marrow blasts to below 5%, and complete remission was achieved in three patients.[216]

Subsequently, 142 patients with AML in first relapse were treated with two doses of gemtuzumab ozogamicin (9 mg/m^2) 2 weeks apart in three phase II trials.[217–219] Patients with secondary AML or prior MDS were excluded. Complete remission was achieved in 23 patients (16%), and 19 patients (13%) had a complete response without complete platelet recovery. The response rate was not significantly influenced by age or duration of prior remission. Response durations, however, were brief unless patients received additional chemotherapy or hematopoietic stem cell transplantation. Grade 3 or 4 hyperbilirubinemia developed in 23% of patients, and elevated levels of serum transaminases were seen in 17%. Hepatic veno-occlusive disease (VOD) developed in 4% of patients. Other toxicities included pulmonary edema and acute respiratory distress syndrome, particularly in patients with high leukocyte counts.

Recent phase II studies have reported higher rates of VOD associated with gemtuzumab ozogamicin. Among 46 patients who received gemtuzumab ozogamicin in first relapse and then underwent stem cell transplantation, 8 (17%) developed VOD, and there were 5 fatal cases.[220] In a report from the Dana-Farber Cancer Institute, 9 of 14 patients (64%) who received gemtuzumab ozogamicin before allogeneic stem cell transplantation developed VOD, compared with 4 of 48 patients (8%) without prior exposure to gemtuzumab ozogamicin ($P < .0001$).[221] Another study noted that 11 of 23 patients (48%) treated with gemtuzumab ozogamicin after stem cell transplantation developed liver injury suggestive of VOD.[222] In a series of 119 patients treated with gemtuzumab ozogamicin at the MD Anderson Cancer Center, 14 (12%) developed VOD in the absence of stem cell transplantation, but the majority of these patients received gemtuzumab ozogamicin in combination with other agents or at more frequent intervals than originally described.[223]

Combination therapy that includes gemtuzumab ozogamicin is now under investigation for newly diagnosed AML. Because of its toxicity profile, however, administration of full-dose gemtuzumab ozogamicin with other agents has been difficult. In a study conducted by the Medical Research Council, 64 patients with newly diagnosed AML received one of three standard induction regimens along with gemtuzumab ozogamicin.[224] The maximum tolerated dose of gemtuzumab ozogamicin was a single infusion of 3 mg/m^2. Hepatotoxicity and delayed hematopoietic recovery prevented delivery of higher doses for induction or repeated administration during subsequent chemotherapy courses. Overall, the complete remission rate was 86%. Similarly, DeAngelo and colleagues found that a 6 mg/m^2 dose of gemtuzumab ozogamicin could be given safely with cytarabine and daunorubicin in younger patients with newly diagnosed AML.[225] Grade 3 or 4 liver function abnormalities were seen in 16% of patients, and none of the patients developed VOD. Among 43 evaluable patients, 36 (84%) achieved a complete remission.[226] Since CD33 is universally expressed by APL cells, including the leukemic stem cell, the use of gemtuzumab ozogamicin is particularly attractive for treating this disease.[227] Preliminary results suggest that gemtuzumab ozogamicin in combination with ATRA can produce high molecular remission rates as first-line therapy and that its use as consolidation could potentially eliminate the need for standard anthracycline-based consolidation.[228]

Radioimmunotherapy for Hematopoietic Cancers

Hematopoietic cancers have been treated successfully with radiolabeled mAbs in a number of systems. This is due to the accessibility of the cells in the vasculature, their relative radiosensitivity, and the large number of differentiation antigens available as cell surface targets. Current technology and pharmacologic issues have limited the success of this approach for the treatment of solid tumors or for intraperitoneal (regional) infusions.[229,230] Alternatively, antitumor activity was demonstrated in the majority of patients with leukemia and lymphoma in the early radioimmunotherapeutic trials.

The isotope used most widely has been ^{131}I, not because it is the most effective but because it is inexpensive and is readily conjugated to mAbs through simple chemistry. It also emits a gamma particle for imaging and quantitative dosimetry, in addition to its cytotoxic beta emission. The agent ^{131}I-BC8 (anti-CD45) appears to be effective at clearing the bone marrow of normal and leukemic cells before allogeneic bone marrow transplantation.[231] Long-term survival has been seen in a significant fraction of patients treated in this manner. A high-dose approach also has been taken with ^{131}I-M195 (anti-CD33) and HuM195[151] and with another anti-CD33 mAb, p67,[232] in the treatment of myeloid leukemia. ^{131}I-M195 mAb specifically targets the marrow and kills 99% of leukemia cells at high doses, even with tumor burdens as high as 1 kg. In early phase I trials in which conventional allogeneic bone marrow transplantation was performed after ^{131}I-M195 ablation in patients with refractory leukemia, high response rates (90%) were achieved, with little apparent toxicity above that expected from an allogeneic transplant.[151] At lower doses, this agent appears active against minimal disease in myeloid leukemia as well.[233]

Nonmyeloablative use of an ^{131}I anti-CD20 murine antibody, ^{131}I-tositumomab (Bexxar), is well tolerated and highly effective in the treatment of relapsed or refractory low-grade, follicular, or transformed B-cell NHL (B-NHL). Based on promising data from two earlier trials, a multicenter, nonrandomized phase III study was conducted to evaluate the efficacy of ^{131}I-tositumomab in patients with relapsed (relapse within 6 months of completion of last chemotherapy) or refractory low-grade or transformed B-NHL.[234] Although the primary toxicity was hematologic, only one patient was hospitalized for fever and neutropenia. Four heavily pretreated patients developed myelodysplasia, but it is uncertain whether this condition was secondary to the ^{131}I-tositumomab or due to previous alkylating agent exposure. The overall and complete response rates were 65% and 20%, respectively. Five ^{131}I-tositumomab trials involving 250 patients have been conducted since 1990.[235] Thirty percent of these patients with relapsed, refractory, and transformed B-NHL have had durable responses lasting 60 months. The majority of these long-term responders had many high-risk features, including advanced stage, poor response to last treatment, bulky disease, and bone marrow involvement. Based on these data, ^{131}I-tositumomab was approved by the FDA for the treatment of CD20-positive follicular NHL (with or without transformation) in patients whose disease is refractory to rituximab and has relapsed following chemotherapy. Additionally, encouraging results have been seen with myeloablative doses of ^{131}I-tositumomab in relapsed B-cell lymphoma.[236]

Administration of the radioimmunoconjugate ^{90}Y-ibritumomab tiuxetan (Zevalin) is safe and leads to a significantly prolonged time to progression in patients with newly diagnosed or pretreated low-grade or transformed NHL. Over the past 9 years, over 770 patients have tolerated this treatment, with minimal side effects. Since there is an increased rate of myelosuppression with increased lymphomatous bone marrow involvement, use of this radioimmunoconjugate is restricted to patients who have less than 25% malignant infiltration of the bone marrow.[237] The annual rate of MDS/AML is 0.62% per year following ^{90}Y-ibritumomab tiuxetan. This rate is similar to the incidence of MDS/AML for patients with NHL who are being treated with standard dose chemotherapy.[237,238] The results from a phase I/II trial conducted in patients with relapsed or refractory follicular or relapsed aggressive NHL were recently updated with a median follow-up of 63 months for responders.[239] Fifty-one patients were treated with escalating doses of ^{90}Y-ibritumomab tiuxetan. The median time to progression for patients who achieved either a complete response or an unconfirmed complete response was 28.3 months. The subset of complete responders (confirmed or unconfirmed complete response) who received the maximum tolerated dose (0.4 mCi/kg) had a median time to progression of 45 months. Overall response rates in the range of 74 to 83% were even seen in rituximab-refractory patients.[240] A phase III trial was designed to compare ^{90}Y-ibritumomab tiuxetan to rituximab in the same patient population. One hundred forty-three patients were randomized to either the study arm or the control arm. The study group had a better overall response rate (80% vs. 56%; $P = .002$) than the control group. The complete response rate of the study group was nearly double that of the control group (30% vs. 16%; $P = .04$). The differences in time to progression, however, were not statistically significant. Randomized trials comparing ^{131}I-tositumomab and ^{90}Y-ibritumomab tiuxetan have not been done.

Conclusions Drawn from Clinical Studies

Many mAbs have been proven to be both safe and effective anticancer therapies. More antineoplastic mAbs are still at the phase I and early phase II stages of investigation. Several generalizations can be made regarding their use and efficacy from published data. First, many mAbs can be administered safely and can reach their target tissues. The most efficient delivery appears to occur with hematopoietic neoplasms and with small tumor burdens. Second, and perhaps more important, rodent mAbs are highly immunogenic, and neutralizing human antibody responses develop in most patients except those who are very immunosuppressed. The advent of humanized and chimeric antibodies has enabled more effective delivery of mAbs.

Third, mAbs without potent effector functions in vitro are not likely to be active against tumors in vivo. As a corollary, mAbs that are highly active work via ADCC, CDC, or apoptosis or via a conjugate, such as a radioisotope or toxin. Fourth, the pharmacodynamics and kinetics of the large IgG structure are significant obstacles to the effective use of radiolabeled mAbs to treat solid tumors. Use of mAbs in solid tumors may be most appropriate in settings of minimal residual disease or as an adjuvant. These studies will require large randomized studies to confirm activity. In

contrast, radioimmunoconjugates can reduce or eliminate large tumor burdens consisting of leukemia or lymphoma cells.

CURRENT OBSTACLES TO MONOCLONAL ANTIBODY CANCER THERAPY

A number of significant obstacles have slowed successful therapeutic applications of mAbs (Table 31.6). Better chemical methods for attaching radionuclides or toxins to mAbs appear to be resolving some of the issues of biochemical stability. New approaches using antibody fragments or genetically engineered single-chain binding proteins may improve delivery to tumors, but the pharmacologic difficulties may still be significant. Rapid modulation of cell surface immune complexes, a phenomenon that reduces ADCC and CDC, can be used to advantage by coupling toxins or isotopes that require entry into the cell. Efficient delivery of the toxin to the appropriate subcellular compartment and retention of radionuclides within cells still pose problems. New methods of engineering rodent mAbs into humanized mAbs or of producing true human mAbs resolves many of the issues related to HAMA (Table 31.4), but it is unclear whether anti-idiotype responses will be seen after repeated doses. One of the paradoxes of mAb-based therapies is that increasing the specificity of the agents may yield more avenues of tumor cell escape. Because native mAbs target and kill individual cells based on the presence of antigen, tumor cells that have little or no antigen may be spared any cytocidal effects. Antigen-negative cells are thus selected for later relapse.[241] In contrast, radioimmunoconjugates with long-range beta

TABLE 31.6
CURRENT OBSTACLES TO MONOCLONAL ANTIBODY (mAb) TREATMENT OF CANCER

Biochemical and biologic instability
    Of the immunoglobulin
    Of the radionuclide or radiometal chelate
    Of the immunotoxin linkage
Difficulties in pharmacology
Poor extravascular diffusion and penetration into tumors
Rapid cell surface modulation of immune complexes
Long half-lives (may also be an advantage with native mAb)
Immunogenicity of rodent-derived (and human?) mAb
Specificity and tumor heterogeneity
Inadequate specificity and targeting of normal cells
Excessive specificity and sparing of antigen-negative cells
Inadequate potency of native mAb
Toxicity
Bystander cell kill by radioconjugates
Normal cell kill by immunotoxins
Allergic reactions (rare)

emissions may kill antigen-negative bystander cells[242] but will consequently have greater toxicity.

CONCLUSION

Monoclonal antibodies are versatile anticancer agents with wide-ranging potential for therapy. As of late 2004, eight mAbs have already been approved by the FDA for the treatment of specific malignancies. These mAbs are also being investigated for use in other hematologic and solid tumors. Many other mAbs or their constructs remain in the early stages of clinical development. MAbs are of great interest primarily because of their specificity and potential for reduced toxicity compared with cytotoxic chemotherapy. In addition, their long half-lives and ability to kill cells via a variety of mechanisms also make them attractive drugs. Nonimmunogenic, humanized, and chimeric mAbs of appropriate specificity have been genetically engineered to block a certain receptor or to lyse tumor cells via ADCC or CDC. When the antibody is conjugated to radioisotopes or toxins, this treatment can reduce or eliminate bulky tumors. Unconjugated mAbs are ideally suited for the treatment of minimal residual disease, in either the consolidation or adjuvant setting. Finally, mAbs are likely to be most effective when integrated into combination therapeutic strategies involving chemotherapy, radiation therapy, and biologic therapy.

REFERENCES

1. Pressman D, Korngold L. The in vivo localization of anti-Wagner osteogenic sarcoma antibody. Cancer 1953;6:619.
2. Kohler G, Milstein C. Continuous cultures of fused cells secreting antibody of predefined specificity. Nature 1975;256:495–497.
3. Harris M. Monoclonal antibodies as therapeutic agents for cancer. Lancet Oncol 2004;5:292–302.
4. Burrows PD, Cooper MD. B-cell development in man. Curr Opin Immunol 1993;5(2):201–206.
5. Rosen FS, Cooper MD, Wedgwood RJ. The primary immunodeficiencies (1). N Engl J Med 1984;311:235–242.
6. Petersen JG, Dorrington KJ. An in vitro system for studying the kinetics of interchain disulfide bond formation in immunoglobulin G. J Biol Chem 1974;249:5633–5641.
7. Morrison SL, Wright A. Antibody variable region glycosylation. Semin Immunopathol 1993;15:259–273.
8. Mueller BM, Reisfeld RA, Gillies SD. Serum half-life and tumor localization of a chimeric antibody deleted of the CH2 domain and directed against the disialoganglioside GD2. Proc Natl Acad Sci U S A 1990;87:5702–5705.
9. Welling GW, Geurts T, van Gorkum J, et al. Synthetic antibody fragment as ligand in immunoaffinity chromatography. J Chromatogr 1990;512:337–343.
10. Hunkapiller T, Hood L. Diversity of the immunoglobulin gene superfamily. Adv Immunol 1989;44:1–63.
11. Walter MA, Surti U, Hofker MH, et al. The physical organization of the human immunoglobulin heavy chain gene complex. EMBO J 1990;9:3303–3313.
12. Max EE. Immunoglobulins: Molecular Genetics. In: Paul WE, ed. Fundamental Immunology. New York: Raven Press; 1989.
13. Perelson A. Immune network theory. Immunol Rev 1989;110:5–36.
14. Tonegawa S. Somatic generation of antibody diversity. Nature 1983;302:575–581.
15. Mason DW, Williams AF. The kinetics of antibody binding to membrane antigens in solution and at the cell surface Biochem J 1980;187:1–20.
16. Moore JP, McKeating JA, Huang YX, et al. Virions of primary human immunodeficiency virus type 1 isolates resistant to soluble CD4 (sCD4) neutralization differ in sCD4 binding and glycoprotein gp120 retention from sCD4-sensitive isolates. J Virol 1992;66:235–243.
17. Kaufman EN, Jain RK. Effect of bivalent interaction upon apparent antibody affinity: experimental confirmation of theory using fluorescence photobleaching and implications for antibody binding assays. Cancer Res 1992;52:4157–4167.
18. Dower SK, Ozato K, Segal DM. The interaction of monoclonal antibodies with MHC class I antigens on mouse spleen cells, I: analysis of the mechanism of binding. J Immunol 1984;132: 751–758.
19. Robb RJ, Greene WC, Rusk CM. Low and high affinity cellular receptors for interleukin 2: implications for the level of Tac antigen. J Exp Med 1984;160:1126–1146.
20. Waldmann TA, Strober W. Metabolism of immunoglobulins. Prog Allergy 1969;13:1–110.
21. Junghans RP. Finally! The Brambell receptor (FcRB): mediator of transmission of immunity and protection from catabolism for IgG. Immunol Res 1997;16:29–57.
22. Mogielnicki RP, Waldmann TA, Strober W. Renal handling of low molecular weight proteins, I: L-chain metabolism in experimental renal disease. J Clin Invest 1971;50:901–909.
23. Waldmann TA, Strober W, Mogielnicki RP. The renal handling of low molecular weight proteins, II: disorders of serum protein catabolism in patients with tubular proteinuria, the nephrotic syndrome, or uremia. J Clin Invest 1972;51:2162–2174.
24. Meeker TC, Lowder J, Maloney DG, et al. A clinical trial of anti-idiotype therapy for B cell malignancy. Blood 1985;65: 1349–1363.
25. Sharkey RM, Goldenberg DM, Goldenberg H, et al. Murine monoclonal antibodies against carcinoembryonic antigen: immunological, pharmacokinetic, and targeting properties in humans. Cancer Res 1990;50:2823–2831.
26. Sela B-A, Ilipoulos D, Gheurry D, et al. Levels of disialogangliosides in sera of melanoma patients monitored by sensitive thin layer chromatography and immunostaining. J Natl Cancer Inst 1989;81:1489–1492.
27. Schulz G, Cheresh DA, Varki NM, et al. Detection of ganglioside GD2 in tumor tissues and sera of neuroblastoma patients. Cancer Res 1984;44:5914–5920.
28. Junghans RP, Carrasquillo JA, Waldmann TA. Impact of antigenemia on the bioactivity of infused anti-Tac antibody: implications for dose selection in antibody immunotherapies. Proc Natl Acad Sci USA 1998;95:1752–1757.
29. Finkelman FD, Madden KB, Morris SC, et al. Anti-cytokine antibodies as carrier proteins: prolongation of in vivo effects of exogenous cytokines by injection of cytokine–anti-cytokine antibody complexes. J Immunol 1993;151:1235–1244.
30. Borsos T, Rapp HJ. Complement fixation on cell surfaces by 19S and 7S antibodies. Science 1965;150:505–506.
31. Prodinger WM, Wurner R, Stoiber H, Dierich MP. Complement. In: Paul WF, ed. Fundamental Immunology, 5th ed. Philadelphia Lippincott, Williams & Wilkins, 2003:1077–1104.
32. Bindon CI, Hale G, Bruggemann M, et al. Human monoclonal IgG isotypes differ in complement activating function at the level of C4 as well as C1q. J Exp Med 1988;168:127–142.
33. Greenspan NS, Cooper LJ. Intermolecular cooperativity: a clue to why mice have IgG3? Immunol Today 1992;13:164–168.
34. Martin DE, Zalman LS, Muller-Eberhard HJ. Induction of expression of cell-surface homologous restriction factor upon anti-CD3 stimulation of human peripheral lymphocytes. Proc Natl Acad Sci USA 1988;85:213–217.
35. Davitz MA. Decay-accelerating factor (DAF): a review of its function and structure. Acta Med Scand Suppl 1987;715:111–121.
36. Van de Winkel JG, Capel PJ. Human IgG Fc receptor heterogeneity: molecular aspect and clinical implications. Immunol Today 1993;14:215–221.
37. Simmons D, Seed B. The Fc gamma receptor of natural killer cells is a phospholipid-linked membrane protein. Nature 1988;333: 568–570.

38. Walker MR, Woof JM, Bruggemann M, et al. Interaction of human IgG chimeric antibodies with the human FcR1 and FcR11 receptors: requirements for antibody-mediated host cell–target cell interaction. Mol Immunol 1989;26:403–411.

39. Giorda R, Rudert WA, Vavassori C, et al. NKR-P1, a signal transduction molecule on natural killer cells. Science 1990;249:1298–1300.

40. Fanger MW, Shen L, Graziano RF, et al. Cytotoxicity mediated by human Fc receptors for IgG. Immunol Today 1989;10:92–99.

41. Ortaldo JR, Woodhouse C, Morgan AC, et al. Analysis of effector cells in human antibody-dependent cellular cytotoxicity with murine monoclonal antibodies. J Immunol 1987;138:3566–3572.

42. Katz HR. Inhibitory receptors and allergy. Curr Opin Immunol 2002;14:698–704.

43. Davis RS, Dennis G Jr, Odom MR, et al. Fc receptor homologs: newest members of a remarkably diverse Fc receptor gene family. Immunol Rev 2002;190:123–136.

44. Clynes RA, Towers TL, Presta LG, et al. Inhibitory Fc receptors modulate in vivo cytoxicity against tumor targets. Nat Med 2000;6:443–446.

45. Lovchik JC, Hong R. Antibody-dependent cell-mediated cytolysis (ADCC): analyses and projections. Prog Allergy 1977;22:1–44.

46. Gergely J, Sarmay G. The two binding-site models of human IgG binding Fc gamma receptors. FASEB J 1990;4:3275–3283.

47. Junghans RP, Waldmann TA, Landolfi NF, et al. Anti-Tac-H, a humanized antibody to the interleukin 2 receptor with new features for immunotherapy in malignant and immune disorders. Cancer Res 1990;50:1495–1502.

48. Junghans RP. A strategy for evaluating lymphokine activation and novel monoclonal antibodies in antibody-dependent cell-mediated cytotoxicity and effector cell retargeting assays. Cancer Immunol Immunother 1990;31:207–212.

49. Zalman LS, Brothers MA, Strauss KL. Inhibition of cytolytic lymphocytes by homologous restriction factor: lack of species restriction. J Immunol 1991;146:4278–4281.

50. Houghton AN, Scheinberg DA. Monoclonal antibody therapies: a "constant" threat to cancer. Nat Med 2000;6:373–374.

51. Bernstein ID, Tam MR, Nowinski RC. Mouse leukemia: therapy with monoclonal antibodies against a thymus differentiation antigen. Science 1980;207:68–71.

52. Buchsbaum DJ, Wahl RL, Normolle DP, et al. Therapy with unlabeled and 131I-labeled pan-B-cell monoclonal antibodies in nude mice bearing Raji Burkitt's lymphoma xenografts. Cancer Res 1992;52:6476–6481.

53. Hamblin TJ, Cattan AR, Glennie MJ, et al. Initial experience in treating human lymphoma with a chimeric univalent derivative of monoclonal anti-idiotype antibody. Blood 1987;69:790–797.

54. Dyer MJ, Hale G, Hayhoe FG, et al. Effects of CAMPATH-1 antibodies in vivo in patients with lymphoid malignancies: influence of antibody isotype. Blood 1989;73:1431–1439.

55. Munn DH, Cheung NK. Phagocytosis of tumor cells by human monocytes cultured in recombinant macrophage colony-stimulating factor. J Exp Med 1990;172:231–237.

56. Mylvaganam R, Sprinz PG, Ahn YS, et al. An animal model of alloimmune thrombocytopenia, I: the role of the mononuclear phagocytic system (MPS). Clin Immunol Immunopathol 1984;31:163–170.

57. Kirkman RL, Shapiro ME, Carpenter CB, et al. A randomized prospective trial of anti-Tac monoclonal antibody in human renal transplantation. Transplantation 1991;51:107–113.

58. Begley CG, Nicola NA, Metcalf D. Proliferation of normal human promyelocytes and myelocytes after a single pulse stimulation by purified GM-CSF or G-CSF. Blood 1988;71:640–645.

59. Ogasawara J, Watanabe-Fukunaga R, Adachi M, et al. Lethal effect of the anti-Fas antibody in mice. Nature 1993;364:806–809.

60. Rouvier E, Luciani MF, Golstein P. Fas involvement in Ca(2+)-independent T cell-mediated cytotoxicity. J Exp Med 1993;177:195–200.

61. Bona C. Fundamental Immunology. New York: Raven Press, 1989.

62. Coelho M, Gauthier P, Pugniere M, et al. Isolation and characterization of a human anti-idiotypic scFv used as a surrogate tumour antigen to elicit an anti-HER-2/neu humoral response in mice. Br J Cancer 2004;90:2032–2041.

63. Saha A, Chatterjee SK, Foon KA, et al. Murine dendritic cells pulsed with an anti-idiotype antibody induce antigen-specific protective antitumor immunity. Cancer Res 2003;63:2844–2854.

64. Green LL, Hardy MC, Maynard-Currie CE, et al. Antigen-specific human monoclonal antibodies from mice engineered with human Ig heavy and light chain YACs. Nat Genet 1994;7:13–21.

65. Ishida I, Tomizuka K, Yoshida H, et al. Production of human monoclonal and polyclonal antibodies in TransChromo animals. Cloning Stem Cells 2002;4:91–102.

66. Hale G, Dyer MJ, Clark MR, et al. Remission induction in non-Hodgkin lymphoma with reshaped human monoclonal antibody CAMPATH-1H. Lancet 1988;2:1394–1399.

67. Clendeninn N, Hethersell A, Scott J. Phase I/II trials of Campath-1H, a humanized anti-lymphocyte monoclonal antibody (MoAb), in non-Hodgkin's lymphoma (NHL) and chronic lymphocytic leukemia (CLL). Blood 1992;80(Suppl 1):158a.

68. Anasetti C, Hansen J, Waldmann H. Treatment of acute graft-versus-host disease with a humanized monoclonal antibody specific for the IL-2 receptor. Blood 1992;80(Suppl 1):373a.

69. Caron PC, Jurcic JG, Scott AM, et al. A phase 1B trial of humanized monoclonal antibody M195 (anti-CD33) in myeloid leukemia: specific targeting without immunogenicity. Blood 1994;83:1760–1768.

70. Winter G, Griffiths AD, Hawkins RE, et al. Making antibodies by phage display technology. Annu Rev Immunol 1994;12:433–455.

71. LoBuglio AF, Wheeler RH, Trang J, et al. Mouse/human chimeric monoclonal antibody in man: kinetics and immune response. Proc Natl Acad Sci USA 1989;86:4220–4224.

72. Khazaeli MB, Saleh MN, Liu TP, et al. Pharmacokinetics and immune response of 131I-chimeric mouse/human B72.3 (human gamma 4) monoclonal antibody in humans. Cancer Res 1991;51:5461–5466.

73. Barbas CF 3rd, Kang AS, Lerner RA, et al. Assembly of combinatorial antibody libraries on phage surfaces: the gene III site. Proc Natl Acad Sci USA 1991;88:7978–7982.

74. Wolff EA, Esselstyn J, Maloney G, et al. Human monoclonal antibody homodimers: effect of valency on in vitro and in vivo antibacterial activity. J Immunol 1992;148:2469–2474.

75. Caron PC, Co MS, Bull MK, et al. Biological and immunological features of humanized M195 (anti-CD33) monoclonal antibodies. Cancer Res 1992;52:6761–6767.

76. Riechmann L, Clark M, Waldmann H, et al. Reshaping human antibodies for therapy. Nature 1988;332:323–327.

77. Carter P, Presta L, Gorman CM, et al. Humanization of an anti-p185HER2 antibody for human cancer therapy. Proc Natl Acad Sci USA 1992;89:4285–4289.

78. Gram H, Marconi LA, Barbas CF 3rd, et al. In vitro selection and affinity maturation of antibodies from a naive combinatorial immunoglobulin library. Proc Natl Acad Sci USA 1992;89:3576–3580.

79. Stevenson G, Glennie M, Hamblin T. Problems and prospects in the use of lymphoma idiotypes as therapeutic targets. Int J Cancer 1988;3(Suppl):9–12.

80. Cobbold SP, Waldmann H. Therapeutic potential of monovalent monoclonal antibodies. Nature 1984;308:460–462.

81. Sims MJ, Hassal DG, Brett S, et al. A humanized CD18 antibody can block function without cell destruction. J Immunol 1993;151:2296–2308.

82. Shopes B. A genetically engineered human IgG mutant with enhanced cytolytic activity. J Immunol 1992;148:2918–2922.

83. Caron PC, Laird W, Co MS, et al. Engineered humanized dimeric forms of IgG are more effective antibodies. J Exp Med 1992;176:1191–1195.

84. Verhoeyen M, Milstein C, Winter G. Reshaping human antibodies: grafting an antilysozyme activity. Science 1988;239:1534–1536.

85. Jones PT, Dear PH, Foote J, et al. Replacing the complementarity-determining regions in a human antibody with those from a mouse. Nature 1986;321:522–525.

86. Queen C, Schneider WP, Selick HE, et al. A humanized antibody that binds to the interleukin 2 receptor. Proc Natl Acad Sci USA 1989;86:10029–10033.

87. Byrn RA, Mordenti J, Lucas C, et al. Biological properties of a CD4 immunoadhesin. Nature 1990;344:667–670.

88. Segal DM, Wunderlich JR. Targeting of cytotoxic cells with heterocrosslinked antibodies. Cancer Invest 1988;6:83–92.

89. Scott CF Jr, Blattler WA, Lambert JM, et al. Requirements for the construction of antibody heterodimers for the direction of lysis of tumors by human T cells. J Clin Invest 1988;81:1427–1433.

90. Tutt A, Stevenson GT, Glennie MJ. Trispecific F(ab')3 derivatives that use cooperative signaling via the TCR/CD3 complex and CD2 to activate and redirect resting cytotoxic T cells. J Immunol 1991;147:60–69.

91. Lanzavecchia A, Scheidegger D. The use of hybrid hybridomas to target human cytotoxic T lymphocytes. Eur J Immunol 1987;17:105–111.

92. Tada H, Toyoda Y, Iwasa S. Bispecific antibody-producing hybrid hybridoma and its use in one-step immunoassays for human lymphotoxin. Hybridoma 1989;8:73–83.

93. Liu MA, Nussbaum SR, Eisen HN. Hormone conjugated with antibody to CD3 mediates cytotoxic T cell lysis of human melanoma cells. Science 1988;239:395–398.

94. Gillies SD, Wesolowski JS, Lo KM. Targeting human cytotoxic T lymphocytes to kill heterologous epidermal growth factor receptor-bearing tumor cells: tumor-infiltrating lymphocyte/hormone receptor/recombinant antibody. J Immunol 1991;146:1067–1071.

95. Garrido MA, Perez P, Titus JA, et al. Targeted cytotoxic cells in human peripheral blood lymphocytes. J Immunol 1990;144:2891–2898.

96. Titus JA, Perez P, Kaubisch A, et al. Human K/natural killer cells targeted with hetero-cross-linked antibodies specifically lyse tumor cells in vitro and prevent tumor growth in vivo. J Immunol 1987;139:3153–3158.

97. Titus JA, Garrido MA, Hecht TT, et al. Human T cells targeted with anti-T3 cross-linked to antitumor antibody prevent tumor growth in nude mice. J Immunol 1987;138:4018–4022.

98. Trail PA, Willner D, Lasch SJ, et al. Cure of xenografted human carcinomas by BR96-doxorubicin immunoconjugates. Science 1993;261:212–215.

99. Pietersz GA, McKenzie IF. Antibody conjugates for the treatment of cancer. Immunol Rev 1992;129:57–80.

100. Senter PD. Activation of prodrugs by antibody-enzyme conjugates: a new approach to cancer therapy. FASEB J 1990;4:188–193.

101. Yuan F, Baxter LT, Jain RK. Pharmacokinetic analysis of two-step approaches using bifunctional and enzyme-conjugated antibodies. Cancer Res 1991;51:3119–3130.

102. Stickney DR, Anderson LD, Slater JB, et al. Bifunctional antibody: a binary radiopharmaceutical delivery system for imaging colorectal carcinoma. Cancer Res 1991;51:6650–6655.

103. Bagshawe KD, Sharma SK, Springer CJ, et al. Antibody directed enzyme prodrug therapy (ADEPT): clinical report. Dis Markers 1991;9:233–238.

104. Vitetta ES, Thorpe PE, Uhr JW. Immunotoxins: magic bullets or misguided missiles? Immunol Today 1993;14:252–259.

105. Pastan I, FitzGerald D. Recombinant toxins for cancer treatment. Science 1991;254:1173–1177.

106. Chaudhary VK, Queen C, Junghans RP, et al. A recombinant immunotoxin consisting of two antibody variable domains fused to *Pseudomonas* exotoxin. Nature 1989;339:394–397.

107. Kreitman RJ, Wilson WH, Bergeron K, et al. Efficacy of the anti-CD22 recombinant immunotoxin BL22 in chemotherapy-resistant hairy-cell leukemia. N Engl J Med 2001;345:241–247.

108. Grossbard ML, Lambert JM, Goldmacher VS, et al. Anti-B4-blocked ricin: a phase I trial of 7-day continuous infusion in patients with B-cell neoplasms. J Clin Oncol 1993;11:726–737.

109. Vitetta ES, Stone M, Amlot P, et al. Phase I immunotoxin trial in patients with B-cell lymphoma. Cancer Res 1991;51:4052–4058.

110. Lambert JM, Goldmacher VS, Collinson AR, et al. An immunotoxin prepared with blocked ricin: a natural plant toxin adapted for therapeutic use. Cancer Res 1991;51(23 Pt 1):6236–6242.

111. Ghetie MA, Tucker K, Richardson J, et al. Eradication of minimal disease in severe combined immunodeficient mice with disseminated Daudi lymphoma using chemotherapy and an immunotoxin cocktail. Blood 1994;84:702–707.

112. Goldenberg DM, Horowitz JA, Sharkey RM, et al. Targeting, dosimetry, and radioimmunotherapy of B-cell lymphomas with iodine-131-labeled LL2 monoclonal antibody. J Clin Oncol 1991;9:548–564.

113. Rosenblum MG, Murray JL, Lamki L, et al. Comparative clinical pharmacology of [111In]-labeled murine monoclonal antibodies. Cancer Chemother Pharmacol 1987;20:41–47.

114. Murray JL, Rosenblum MG, Lamki L, et al. Clinical parameters related to optimal tumor localization of indium-111-labeled mouse antimelanoma monoclonal antibody ZME-018. J Nucl Med 1987;28:25–33.

115. Hnatowich DJ, Rusckowski M, Brill AB, et al. Pharmacokinetics in patients of an anti-carcinoembryonic antigen antibody radiolabeled with indium-111 using a novel diethylenetriamine pentaacetic acid chelator. Cancer Res 1990;50:7272–7278.

116. Patt YZ, Lamki LM, Haynie TP, et al. Improved tumor localization with increasing dose of indium-111-labeled anti-carcinoembryonic antigen monoclonal antibody ZCE-025 in metastatic colorectal cancer. J Clin Oncol 1988;6:1220–1230.

117. Scheinberg DA, Straus DJ, Yeh SD, et al. A phase I toxicity, pharmacology, and dosimetry trial of monoclonal antibody OKB7 in patients with non-Hodgkin's lymphoma: effects of tumor burden and antigen expression. J Clin Oncol 1990;8:792–803.

118. Welt S, Divgi CR, Real FX, et al. Quantitative analysis of antibody localization in human metastatic colon cancer: a phase I study of monoclonal antibody A33. J Clin Oncol 1990;8:1894–1906.

119. Carrasquillo JA, Abrams PG, Schroff RW, et al. Effect of antibody dose on the imaging and biodistribution of indium-111 9.2.27 anti-melanoma monoclonal antibody. J Nucl Med 1988;29:39–47.

120. Eary JF, Press OW, Badger CC, et al. Imaging and treatment of B-cell lymphoma. J Nucl Med 1990;31:1257–1268.

121. Scheinberg DA, Lovett D, Divgi CR, et al. A phase I trial of monoclonal antibody M195 in acute myelogenous leukemia: specific bone marrow targeting and internalization of radionuclide. J Clin Oncol 1991;9:478–490.

122. Zamboni L, Pease DC. The vascular bed of red bone marrow. J Ultrastruct Res 1961;5:65–85.

123. Renkin EM. Multiple pathways of capillary permeability. Circ Res 1977;41:735–743.

124. Gerlowski LE, Jain RK. Microvascular permeability of normal and neoplastic tissues. Microvasc Res 1986;31:288–305.

125. Thomas GD, Chappell MJ, Dykes PW, et al. Effect of dose, molecular size, affinity, and protein binding on tumor uptake of antibody or ligand: a biomathematical model. Cancer Res 1989;49:3290–3296.

126. Dvorak HF, Nagy JA, Dvorak JT, et al. Identification and characterization of the blood vessels of solid tumors that are leaky to circulating macromolecules. Am J Pathol 1988;133:95–109.

127. Jain RK. Barriers to drug delivery in solid tumors. Sci Am 1994;271(1):58–65.

128. Nugent LJ, Jain RK. Extravascular diffusion in normal and neoplastic tissues. Cancer Res 1984;44:238–244.

129. Clauss MA, Jain RK. Interstitial transport of rabbit and sheep antibodies in normal and neoplastic tissues. Cancer Res 1990;50:3487–3492.

130. Butler TP, Grantham FH, Gullino PM. Bulk transfer of fluid in the interstitial compartment of mammary tumors. Cancer Res 1975;35(11 Pt 1):3084–3088.

131. Jain RK, Baxter LT. Mechanisms of heterogeneous distribution of monoclonal antibodies and other macromolecules in tumors: significance of elevated interstitial pressure. Cancer Res 1988;48(24 Pt 1):7022–7032.

132. Jain RK. Transport of molecules in the tumor interstitium: a review. Cancer Res 1987;47:3039–3051.

133. Williams LE, Duda RB, Proffitt RT, et al. Tumor uptake as a function of tumor mass: a mathematic model. J Nucl Med 1988;29:103–109.

134. Fujimori K, Covell DG, Fletcher JE, et al. A modeling analysis of monoclonal antibody percolation through tumors: a binding-site barrier. J Nucl Med 1990;31:1191–1198.

135. Fujimori K, Covell DG, Fletcher JE, et al. Modeling analysis of the global and microscopic distribution of immunoglobulin G, F(ab')2, and Fab in tumors. Cancer Res 1989;49:5656–5663.

136. Juweid M, Neumann R, Paik C, et al. Micropharmacology of monoclonal antibodies in solid tumors: direct experimental evidence for a binding site barrier. Cancer Res 1992;52:5144–5153.

137. Langmuir V, Mendonca H. The role of radionuclide distribution in the efficacy of I-131-labeled antibody as modeled in multicell spheroids. Antibody Immunocon Radiopharmacol 1992;5:273.

138. Loevinger R, Budinger T, Watson E. MIRD Primer for Absorbed Dose Calculations. New York: Society of Nuclear Medicine, 1989.

139. Behr TM, Behe M, Sgouros G. Correlation of red marrow radiation dosimetry with myelotoxicity empirical factors influencing the radiation-induced myelotoxicity of radio labeled antibodies, fragments, and peptides in preclinical and clinical settings. Cancer Biother Radiopharm 2002;17:445–464.

140. Zanzonico PB. Internal radionuclide radiation dosimetry: a review of basic concepts and recent developments. J Nucl Med 2000;41:297–308.

141. IEAE/WHO Manual on Radiation Hematology. Technical report series no. 123. Vienna: International Atomic Energy Agency and the World Health Organization, 1971.

142. Sgouros G. Bone marrow dosimetry for radioimmunotherapy: theoretical considerations. J Nucl Med 1993;34:689–694.

143. Sgouros G, Stabin M, Erdi Y, et al. Red marrow dosimetry for radiolabeled antibodies that bind to marrow, bone or blood components. Med Phys 2000; 27:2150–2164.

144. Sgouros G, Graham MC, Divgi CR, et al. Modeling and dosimetry of monoclonal antibody M195 (anti-CD33) in acute myelogenous leukemia. J Nucl Med 1993;34:422–430.

145. Press OW, Eary JF, Badger CC, et al. Treatment of refractory non-Hodgkin's lymphoma with radiolabeled MB-1 (anti-CD37) antibody. J Clin Oncol 1989;7:1027–1038.

146. Bunjes D, Buchmann I, Duncker C, et al. Rhenium 188-labeled anti-CD66 (a, b, c, e) monoclonal antibody to intensify the conditioning regimen prior to stem cell transplantation for patients with high-risk acute myeloid leukemia or myelodysplastic syndrome: results of a phase I-II study. Blood 2001;98:565–572.

147. Sgouros G, Barest G, Thekkumthala J, et al. Treatment planning for internal radionuclide therapy: three-dimensional dosimetry for nonuniformly distributed radionuclides. J Nucl Med 1990;31:1884–1891.

148. Roberson PL, Buchsbaum DJ, Heidorn DB, et al. Three-dimensional tumor dosimetry for radioimmunotherapy using serial autoradiography. Int J Radiat Oncol Biol Phys 1992;24:329–334.

149. Nikula TK, Bocchia M, Curcio MJ. Impact of the high tyrosine fraction in complementarity determining regions: measured and predicted effects of radioiodination on IgG immunoreactivity. Mol Immunol 1995;32:865–872.

150. Jurcic JG, Divgi CR, McDevitt MR, et al. Potential for myeloablation with Yttrium-90-HuM195 (anti-CD33) in myeloid leukemia [abstract]. Proc Am Soc Clin Oncol 2000:A24.

151. Burke JM, Caron PC, Papadopoulos EB, et al. Cytoreduction with iodine-131-anti-CD33 antibodies before bone marrow transplantation for advanced myeloid leukemias. Bone Marrow Transplant 2003;32:549–556.

152. Scheinberg DA, Strand M. Kinetic and catabolic considerations of monoclonal antibody targeting in erythroleukemic mice. Cancer Res 1983;43:265–272.

153. Carrasquillo JA, White JD, Paik CH, et al. Similarities and differences in ^{111}In- and ^{90}Y-labeled 1B4M-DTPA antiTac monoclonal antibody distribution. J Nucl Med 1999;40:268–276.

154. Lovqvist A, Humm JL, Sheikh A, et al. PET imaging of (86)Y-labeled anti-Lewis Y monoclonal antibodies in a nude mouse model: comparison between (86)Y and (111)In radiolabels. J Nucl Med 2001;42:1281–1287.

155. McDevitt MR, Sgouros G, Finn RD, et al. Radioimmunotherapy with alpha-emitting nuclides. Eur J Nucl Med 1998;25: 1341–1351.

156. Jurcic JG, Larson SM, Sgouros G, et al. Targeted alpha particle immunotherapy for myeloid leukemia. Blood 2002;100: 1233–1239.

157. Burke JM, Jurcic JG, Chaitanya RD, et al. Sequential cytarabine and alpha-particle immunotherapy with bismuth-213-labeled anti-CD33 monoclonal antibody HuM195 in acute myeloid leukemia (AML) [abstract]. Blood 2002;100:339a.

158. McDevitt MR, Ma D, Lai LT, et al. Tumor therapy with targeted atomic nanogenerators. Science 2001;294:1537–1540.

159. Zalutsky MR, Narula AS. Astatation of proteins using an N-succinimidyl tri-n-butylstannyl benzoate intermediate. Int J Rad Appl Instrum [A] 1988;39:227–232.

160. Zalutksy M, Cokgor I, Akabani G. Phase I trial of alpha-particle-emitting astatine-211 labeled chimeric anti-tenascin antibody in recurrent malignant glioma patients [abstract]. Proc Am Assoc Cancer Res 2000;41:544.

161. Nisson S, Larson RH, Fossen SD, et al. First clinical experience with alpha-emittings radium-223 in the treatment of skeletal metastases. Clin Cancer Res 2005; 11:4451–4459.

162. Axworthy DB, Reno JM, Hylarides MD, et al. Cure of human carcinoma xenografts by a single dose of pretargeted yttrium-90 with negligible toxicity. Proc Natl Acad Sci USA 2000;97: 1802–1807.

163. Zhang M, Zhang Z, Garmestani K, et al. Pretarget radiotherapy with an anti-CD25 antibody-streptavidin fusion protein was effective in therapy of leukemia/lymphoma xenografts. Proc Natl Acad Sci USA 2003;100:1891–1895.

164. Forero A, Weiden PL, Vose JM, et al. Phase 1 trial of a novel anti-CD20 fusion protein in pretargeted radioimmunotherapy for B-cell non-Hodgkin lymphoma. Blood 2004;104:227–236.

165. Chang CH, Sharkey RM, Rossi EA, et al. Molecular advances in pretargeting radioimmunotherapy with bispecific antibodies. Mol Cancer Ther 2002;1:553–563.)

166. Cheung NK, Lazarus H, Miraldi FD, et al. Ganglioside GD2 specific monoclonal antibody 3F8: a phase I study in patients with neuroblastoma and malignant melanoma. J Clin Oncol 1987;5:1430–1440.

167. Schwartz MA, Lovett DR, Redner A, et al. Dose-escalation trial of M195 labeled with iodine 131 for cytoreduction and marrow ablation in relapsed or refractory myeloid leukemias. J Clin Oncol 1993;11:294–303.

168. Czuczman MS, Straus DJ, Divgi CR, et al. Phase I dose-escalation trial of iodine 131-labeled monoclonal antibody OKB7 in patients with non-Hodgkin's lymphoma. J Clin Oncol 1993; 11:2021–2029.

169. DeNardo SJ, DeNardo GL, O'Grady LF, et al. Treatment of B cell malignancies with 131I Lym-1 monoclonal antibodies. Int J Cancer Suppl 1988;3:96–101.

170. DeNardo GL, Mahe MA, DeNardo SJ, et al. Body and blood clearance and marrow radiation dose of 131I-Lym-1 in patients with B-cell malignancies. Nucl Med Commun 1993;14: 587–595.

171. Papadopoulos E, Caron P, Casto-Malaspina H. Results of allogeneic bone marrow transplant following 131-IM195/-busulfan/cyclophosphamide (Bu/Cy) in patients with advanced/refractory myeloid malignancies. Blood 1993; 82(Suppl):80a.

172. Pai LH, Bookman MA, Ozols RF, et al. Clinical evaluation of intraperitoneal *Pseudomonas* exotoxin immunoconjugate OVB3-PE in patients with ovarian cancer. J Clin Oncol 1991;9: 2095–2103.

173. Shan D, Ledbetter JA, Press OW. Apoptosis of malignant human B cells by ligation of CD20 with monoclonal antibodies. Blood 1998;91:1644–1652.

174. McLaughlin P, Grillo-Lopez AJ, Link BK, et al. Rituximab chimeric anti-CD20 monoclonal antibody therapy for relapsed indolent lymphoma: half of patients respond to a four-dose treatment program. J Clin Oncol 1998;16:2825–2833.

175. Hainsworth JD, Litchy S, Burris HA 3rd, et al. Rituximab as first-line and maintenance therapy for patients with indolent non-Hodgkin's lymphoma. J Clin Oncol 2002;20:4261–4267.

176. Ghielmini M, Schmitz S-FH, Cogliatti SB, et al. Prolonged treatment with rituximab in patients with follicular lymphoma significantly increases event-free survival and response duration compared with the standard weekly × 4 schedule. Blood 2004;103:4416–4423.

177. Czuczman MS, Grillo-Lopez AJ, White CA, et al. Treatment of patients with low-grade B-cell lymphoma with the combination of chimeric anti-CD20 monoclonal antibody and CHOP chemotherapy. J Clin Oncol 1999;17:268–276.

178. Marcus R, Imrie K, Belch A, et al. An international multi-centre, randomized, open-label, phase III trial comparing rituximab added to CVP chemotherapy to CVP chemotherapy alone in untreated stage III/IV follicular non-Hodgkin's lymphoma [abstract]. Blood 2003;102:28a.

179. Coiffier B, Herbrecht R, Tilly H, et al. GELA study comparing CHOP and R-CHOP in elderly patients with DLCL: 3-year

median follow-up with an analysis according to co-morbidity factors [abstract]. Proc Am Soc Clin Oncol 2003;22:596.

180. Habermann T, Weller E, Morrison V. Phase III trial of rituximab-CHOP (R-CHOP) vs. CHOP with a second randomization to maintenance rituximab (MR) or observation in patients 60 years of age and older with diffuse large B-cell lymphoma (DLBCL) [abstract]. Blood 2003;102:8a.

181. Foran JM, Rohatiner AZ, Cunningham D, et al. European phase II study of rituximab (chimeric anti-CD20 monoclonal antibody) for patients with newly diagnosed mantle-cell lymphoma and previously treated mantle-cell lymphoma, immunocytoma, and small B-cell lymphocytic lymphoma. J Clin Oncol 2000;18:317–324.

182. Berinstein NL, Grillo-Lopez AJ, White CA, et al. Association of serum rituximab (IDEC-C2B8) concentration and anti-tumor response in the treatment of recurrent low-grade or follicular non-Hodgkin's lymphoma. Ann Oncol 1998;9:995–1001.

183. Winkler U, Jensen M, Manzke O, et al. Cytokine-release syndrome in patients with B-cell chronic lymphocytic leukemia and high lymphocyte counts after treatment with an anti-CD20 monoclonal antibody (rituximab, IDEC-C2B8). Blood 1999;94:2217–2224.

184. Nguyen DT, Amess JA, Doughty H, et al. IDEC-C2B8 anti-CD20 (rituximab) immunotherapy in patients with low-grade non-Hodgkin's lymphoma and lymphoproliferative disorders: evaluation of response on 48 patients. Eur J Haematol 1999;62:76–82.

185. Byrd JC, Murphy T, Howard RS, et al. Rituximab using a thrice weekly dosing schedule in B-cell chronic lymphocytic leukemia and small lymphocytic lymphoma demonstrates clinical activity and acceptable toxicity. J Clin Oncol 2001;19:2153–2164.

186. O'Brien SM, Kantarjian H, Thomas DA, et al. Rituximab dose-escalation trial in chronic lymphocytic leukemia. J Clin Oncol 2001;19:2165–2170.

187. Wierda W, O'Brien SM, Faderl S, et al. Improved survival in patients with relapsed-refractory chronic lymphocytic leukemia (CLL) treated with fludarabine, cyclophosphamide, and rituximab (FCR) combination [abstract]. Blood 2003;102:110.

188. Weiss M, Lamanna N, Jurcic J, et al. Pentostatin, cyclophosphamide, and rituximab (PCR therapy): a new active regimen for previously treated patients with chronic lymphocytic leukemia (CLL) [abstract]. Blood 2003;102:673a.

189. Howard OM, Gribben JG, Neuberg DS, et al. Rituximab and CHOP induction therapy for newly diagnosed mantle-cell lymphoma: molecular complete responses are not predictive of progression-free survival. J Clin Oncol 2002;20:1288–1294.

190. Brugger W, Hirsch J, Repp R. Treatment of follicular and mantle-cell non-Hodgkin's lymphoma with anti-CD antibody rituximab after high-dose chemotherapy with autologous CD34+ enriched peripheral-blood stem cell transplantation [abstract]. Blood 2000;96:A482.

191. Hsi E, Hussein M, Elson P. Biologic and clinical evaluation of Rituxan in the management of newly diagnosed multiple myeloma patients: an update [abstract]. Proc Am Soc Clin Oncol 2001;20:298a.

192. Cooper N, Stasi R, Cunningham-Kundles S, et al. The efficacy and safety of B-cell depletion with anti-CD20 monoclonal antibody in adults with chronic immune thrombocytopenic purpura. Br J Hacmatol 2004;125:232–239.

193. Ahrens N, Kingreen D, Seltsam A, et al. Treatment of refractory autoimmune haemolytic anaemia with anti-CD20 (rituximab). Br J Haematol 2001;114:244–245.

194. Ghazal H. Successful treatment of pure red cell aplasia with rituximab in patients with chronic lymphocytic leukemia. Blood 2002;99:1092–1094.

195. Keating MJ, Flinn I, Jain V, et al. Therapeutic role of alemtuzumab (Campath-1H) in patients who have failed fludarabine: results of a large international study. Blood 2002;99:3554–3561.

196. Insert. Physician's Desk Reference. Montvale NJ. Thomson PDR, 1999:724–726.

197. Lundin J, Kimby E, Bjorkholm M, et al. Phase II trial of subcutaneous anti-CD52 monoclonal antibody alemtuzumab (Campath-1H) as first-line treatment for patients with B-cell chronic lymphocytic leukemia (B-CLL). Blood 2002;100:768–773.

198. Elter T, Borchman P, Schulz M, et al. Development of a new, four-weekly schedule (FluCam) with concomitant application of Campath-1H and fludarabine in patients with relapsed/refractory CLL [abstract]. Blood 2002;100:803a.

199. Faderl S, Thomas DA, O'Brien S, et al. Experience with alemtuzumab plus rituximab in patients with relapsed and refractory lymphoid malignancies. Blood 2003;101:3413–3415.

200. Keating MJ, Cazin B, Coutre S, et al. Campath-1H treatment of T-cell prolymphocytic leukemia in patients for whom at least one prior chemotherapy regimen has failed. J Clin Oncol 2002;20:205–213.

201. Dearden CE, Matutes E, Cazin B, et al. High remission rate in T-cell prolymphocytic leukemia with CAMPATH-1H. Blood 2001;98:1721–176.

202. Faulkner RD, Craddock C, Byrne JL, et al. BEAM-alemtuzumab reduced-intensity allogeneic stem cell transplantation for lymphoproliferative diseases: GVHD, toxicity, and survival in 65 patients. Blood 2004;103:428–434.

203. Perez-Simon JA, Kottaridis PD, Martino R, et al. Nonmyeloablative transplantation with or without alemtuzumab: comparison between 2 prospective studies in patients with lymphoproliferative disorders. Blood 2002;100:3121–3127.

204. Nahta R, Esteva FJ. HER-2-targeted therapy: lessons learned and future directions. Clin Cancer Res 2003;9:5078–5084.

205. Baselga J, Tripathy D, Mendelsohn J, et al. Phase II study of weekly intravenous recombinant humanized anti-p185HER2 monoclonal antibody in patients with HER2/neu-overexpressing metastatic breast cancer. J Clin Oncol 1996;14:737–744.

206. Cobleigh MA, Vogel CL, Tripathy D, et al. Multinational study of the efficacy and safety of humanized anti-HER2 monoclonal antibody in women who have HER2-overexpressing metastatic breast cancer that has progressed after chemotherapy for metastatic disease. J Clin Oncol 1999;17:2639–2648.

207. Slamon DJ, Leyland-Jones B, Shak S, et al. Use of chemotherapy plus a monoclonal antibody against HER2 for metastatic breast cancer that overexpresses HER2. N Engl J Med 2001;344:783–792.

208. Esteva FJ, Valero V, Booser D, et al. Phase II study of weekly docetaxel and trastuzumab for patients with HER-2-overexpressing metastatic breast cancer. J Clin Oncol 2002;20:1800–1808.

209. Rosen LS. Clinical experience with angiogenesis signaling inhibitors: focus on vascular endothelial growth factor (VEGF) blockers. Cancer Control 2002;9(Suppl 2):36–44.

210. Hurwitz H, Fehrenbacher L, Novotny W, et al. Bevacizumab plus irinotecan, fluorouracil, and leucovorin for metastatic colorectal cancer. N Engl J Med 2004;350:2335–2342.

211. Yang JC, Haworth L, Sherry RM, et al. A randomized trial of bevacizumab, an anti-vascular endothelial growth factor antibody, for metastatic renal cancer. N Engl J Med 2003;349:427–434.

212. Kindler HL, Friberg G, Stadler WM et al. Bevacizumab plus gemcitabine is an active combination in patients with advanced pancreatic cancer: interim results of an ongoing phase II trial from the University of Chicago Phase II Consortium. In: Proceedings of the 2004 Gastrointestinal Cancers Symposium Alexandia, VA: Am Soc Clin Oncol 2004:86.

213. Miller K, Rugo H, Cobleig M et al. Phase III trial of capecitabine (Xeloda) plus bevacizumab (Avastin) versus capecitabine alone in women with metastatic breast cancer (MBC) previously treated with an anthracycline and a taxane. San Antonio Breast Cancer Res and Treatment 2002;76(Suppl):537.

214. Cunningham D, Humblet Y, Siena S, et al. Cetuximab monotherapy and cetuximab plus irinotecan in irinotecan-refractory metastatic colorectal cancer. N Engl J Med 2004;351:337–345.

215. Baselga J, Trigo J, Bouthis J. Cetuximab (C225) plus cisplatin/carboplatin is active in patients with recurrent/metastatic squamous-cell carcinoma of the head and neck progressing on a same dose and schedule platinum-based regimen [abstract]. Proc Am Soc Clin Oncol 2002;21:226a.

216. Sievers EL, Appelbaum FR, Spielberger RT, et al. Selective ablation of acute myeloid leukemia using antibody-targeted chemotherapy: a phase I study of an anti-CD33 calicheamicin immunoconjugate. Blood 1999;93:3678–3684.

217. Bross PF, Beitz J, Chen G, et al. Approval summary: gemtuzumab ozogamicin in relapsed acute myeloid leukemia. Clin Cancer Res 2001;7:1490–1496.

218. Larson RA, Boogaerts M, Estey E, et al. Antibody-targeted chemotherapy of older patients with acute myeloid leukemia in first relapse using Mylotarg (gemtuzumab ozogamicin). Leukemia 2002;16:1627–1636.

219. Sievers EL. Efficacy and safety of gemtuzumab ozogamicin in patients with CD33-positive acute myeloid leukaemia in first relapse. Expert Opin Biol Ther 2001;1:893–901.

220. Sievers E, Larson R, Estey E. Final report of prolonged disease-free survival in patients with acute myeloid leukemia in first relapse treated with gemtuzumab ozogamicin followed by hematopoietic stem cell transplantation [abstract]. Blood 2002;100:89a.

221. Wadleigh M, Richardson PG, Zahrieh D, et al. Prior gemtuzumab ozogamicin exposure significantly increases the risk of veno-occlusive disease in patients who undergo myeloablative allogeneic stem cell transplantation. Blood 2003;102:1578–1582.

222. Rajvanshi P, Shulman HM, Sievers EL, et al. Hepatic sinusoidal obstruction after gemtuzumab ozogamicin (Mylotarg) therapy. Blood 2002;99:2310–2314.

223. Giles FJ, Kantarjian HM, Kornblau SM, et al. Mylotarg (gemtuzumab ozogamicin) therapy is associated with hepatic venooclusive disease in patients who have not received stem cell transplantation. Cancer 2001;92:406–413.

224. Kell WJ, Burnett AK, Chopra R, et al. A feasibility study of simultaneous administration of gemtuzumab ozogamicin with intensive chemotherapy in induction and consolidation in younger patients with acute myeloid leukemia. Blood 2003;102:4277–4283.

225. DeAngelo D, Schiffer C, Stone R. Interim analysis of a phase II study of the safety and efficacy of gemtuzumab ozogamicin (Mylotarg) given in combination with cytarabine and daunorubicin in patients less than 60 years old with untreated acute myeloid leukemia [abstract]. Blood 2002;100:198a–199a.

226. Deangelo D, Liu D, Stone R. Preliminary report of a phase 2 study of gemtuzumab ozogamicin in combination with cytarabine and daunorubicin in patients less than 60 years of age with de novo acute myeloid leukemia [abstract]. Proc Am Soc Clin Oncol 2002;22:578a.

227. Bonnet D, Dick JE. Human acute myeloid leukemia is organized as a hierarchy that originates from a primitive hematopoietic cell. Nat Med 1997;3:730–737.

228. Estey EH, Giles FJ, Beran M, et al. Experience with gemtuzumab ozogamycin ("Mylotarg") and all-trans retinoic acid in untreated acute promyelocytic leukemia. Blood 2002;99:4222–4224.

229. Stewart JS, Hird V, Snook D, et al. Intraperitoneal radioimmunotherapy for ovarian cancer: pharmacokinetics, toxicity, and efficacy of I-131 labeled monoclonal antibodies. Int J Radiat Oncol Biol Phys 1989;16:405–413.

230. Epenetos AA, Munro AJ, Stewart S, et al. Antibody-guided irradiation of advanced ovarian cancer with intraperitoneally administered radiolabeled monoclonal antibodies. J Clin Oncol 1987;5:1890–1899.

231. Matthews DC, Appelbaum FR, Eary JF, et al. Phase I study of (131)I-anti-CD45 antibody plus cyclophosphamide and total body irradiation for advanced acute leukemia and myelodysplastic syndrome. Blood 1999;94:1237–1247.

232. Appelbaum FR, Matthews DC, Eary JF, et al. The use of radiolabeled anti-CD33 antibody to augment marrow irradiation prior to marrow transplantation for acute myelogenous leukemia. Transplantation 1992;54:829–833.

233. Jurcic JG, Caron, PC, Miller WH Jr, et al. Sequential targeted therapy for relapsed acute promyelocytic leukemia with all-trans retinoic acid and anti-CD33 monoclonal antibody M195. Leukemia 1995; 9:244–248.

234. Kaminski MS, Zelenetz AD, Press OW, et al. Pivotal study of iodine I 131 tositumomab for chemotherapy-refractory low-grade or transformed low-grade B-cell non-Hodgkin's lymphomas. J Clin Oncol 2001;19:3918–3928.

235. Kashyap A, Zelenetz A, Vose J. Tositumomab and iodine I 131 tositumomab produces a meaningful therapeutic benefit for patients with relapsed, refractory, and transformed low-grade (LG) NHL: summary of the long-term response population (LTRP) [abstract]. Proc Am Soc Clin Oncol 2003;22:576a.

236. Liu SY, Eary JF, Petersdorf SH, et al. Follow-up of relapsed B-cell lymphoma patients treated with iodine-131-labeled anti-CD20 antibody and autologous stem-cell rescue. J Clin Oncol 1998;16:3270–3278.

237. Witzig TE, White CA, Gordon LI, et al. Safety of yttrium-90 ibritumomab tiuxetan radioimmunotherapy for relapsed low-grade, follicular, or transformed non-Hodgkin's lymphoma. J Clin Oncol 2003;21:1263–1270.

238. Kantarjian HM, Keating MJ. Therapy-related leukemia and myelodysplastic syndrome. Semin Oncol 1987;14:435–443.

239. Gordon LI, Molina A, Witzig T, et al. Durable responses after ibritumomab tiuxetan radioimmunotherapy for CD20$^+$ B-cell lymphoma: long-term follow-up of a phase 1/2 study. Blood 2004;103:4429–4431.

240. Witzig TE, Gordon LI, Cabanillas F, et al. Randomized controlled trial of yttrium-90-labeled ibritumomab tiuxetan radioimmunotherapy versus rituximab immunotherapy for patients with relapsed or refractory low-grade, follicular, or transformed B-cell non-Hodgkin's lymphoma. J Clin Oncol 2002;20:2453–2463.

241. Levy R, Miller RA. Therapy of lymphoma directed at idiotypes. J Natl Cancer Inst Monogr 1990:61–68.

242. Nourigat C, Badger CC, Bernstein ID. Treatment of lymphoma with radiolabeled antibody: elimination of tumor cells lacking target antigen. J Natl Cancer Inst 1990;82:47–50.

Interferons

32

Daniel J. Lindner   *Kevin L. Taylor*   *Frederic J. Reu*
Paul A. Masci   *Ernest C. Borden*

INTRODUCTION

Interferon-α (IFN-α) was the first human protein effective for cancer treatment and the first economically important clinical product for cancer developed from recombinant DNA technology. IFNs have been prototypes for the clinical development of other immunomodulatory and growth-regulatory cytokines. IFN-α2, one IFN-α family member, has proven effective not only as an antitumor protein but also for antiviral therapy. The complex biologic and therapeutic activities of IFNs include virus inhibition, immunomodulation, slowing of cell proliferation, oncogene suppression, angiogenesis inhibition, alterations in differentiation, and induction of other cytokines (Table 32.1). Reflecting the pleiotropic biological effects, IFN-β has proven effective for slowing disease progression and relapses in multiple sclerosis and IFN-γ for intracellular pathogens.[1-4]

Modulation of gene expression, which is reviewed below, must underlie the clinical activities of IFNs. An important regulatory pathway for gene induction, the Janus kinase/signal transducers and activators of transcription (JAK-STAT) pathway, was originally elucidated by the study of IFNs but has proven to be critical for signaling by other cytokines and growth factors. Dissection of signal transduction pathways has enabled beginning dissection of the mechanisms of therapeutic resistance. The IFN-induced proteins that mediate these activities have only been partially identified.[5]

In seven malignancies, IFN-α2 results in regression or control of disease processes (Table 32.2). The spectrum of single-agent activity of IFNs compares favorably with other systemic cancer treatment modalities. The antitumor effects of IFNs can be enhanced in experimental tumor models by cytotoxic compounds, radiation, and other biologics. Greater clinical benefit will undoubtedly result through the use of IFNs in combination with other treatments, a topic beyond the scope of this chapter but dependent on understanding IFNs' effects as single agents.

INTERFERONS: THEIR STRUCTURE AND INDUCERS

Like many other cytokines, the IFNs are a family of proteins that include more than a dozen different members encoded on human chromosome 9p (except IFN-γ which is encoded on human chromosome 12q) (Table 32.3). The biologic and clinical significance of the individual proteins encoded by the approximately 15 distinct nonallelic IFN-α genes has barely been studied. These individual proteins differ over a 50-fold range in their potency in eliciting antiproliferative, immunomodulatory, and antiviral cellular effects.[6] Other than IFN-α2, the only IFN-α gene product generated for clinical research trial has been IFN-α1, which has proven to be better tolerated than IFN-α2.[7] The three major classes of IFNs (α, β, γ) were initially defined on the basis of their chemical, antigenic, and biologic variation. These variations result from differences in their primary amino acid sequences. Complete nucleotide sequences have been determined for almost 20 human IFNs.[8-11] IFN-α and IFN-β have approximately 45% nucleotide homology and 29% amino acid homology. Each of the nonallelic human IFN-α genes differs by approximately 10% in nucleotide sequence and 15 to 25% in amino acid sequence (Table 32.3). IFN-γ, 143 amino acids in length, is located on chromosome 12[11,12] and has only minimal sequence homology with IFN-α or IFN-β. Three additional IFN classes, ω, λ, and τ, have been defined. IFN-ω and IFN-λ bind to the same receptor as IFN-α and IFN-β and mediate similar biologic effects.[13,14] IFN-τ is a novel class of IFN, identified in domestic

The authors would like to acknowledge the support of the National Institutes of Health and the National Cancer Institute (CA095020 to DJL; CA89344 and CA90914 to ECB).

TABLE 32.1
BIOLOGIC EFFECTS OF INTERFERONS

Microbial inhibition
RNA viruses
DNA viruses
Intracellular pathogens
Immunomodulatory
T cell (major histocompatibility complex restricted)
Natural/lymphokine-activated killer cell (non–major histocompatibility complex restricted)
Monocytes
Dendritic cells
Antiproliferative effects and apoptosis
Oncogene depression
Slow mitotic cycle
Differentiation
Protein induction
Cell surface proteins
Enzymes
Cytokines
Apoptosis
Antigen processing
Vascular
Angiogenesis inhibition
Lipoprotein reduction
Antitumor
Mouse
Human

ruminants but not humans, that maintains the appropriate milieu in the endometrium for trophoblastic implantation.[15,16] Despite the glycosylation of endogenous IFN-β and IFN-γ, the biologic effects of the unglycosylated proteins produced in *Escherichia coli* have been shown to be similar.[17] The glycosylated and unglycosylated IFNs inhibit the replication of RNA and DNA viruses. Second-generation IFN molecules, bioengineered for potentially desirable

TABLE 32.2
INTERFERONS: INTERNATIONALLY APPROVED INDICATIONS

Malignancies
Hairy cell leukemia
Chronic myelogenous leukemia
Myeloma
Follicular lymphoma
Renal cell carcinoma
Kaposi's sarcoma
Melanoma
Viral diseases
Hepatitis C
Hepatitis B
Herpetic keratitis
Papillomas
Genital
Laryngeal
Immunomodulation
Multiple sclerosis
Chronic granulomatous disease

TABLE 32.3
MOST COMMON INTERFERON FAMILY MOLECULES

Family	Chromosome (Human)	Types (*n*)	Amino Acids	Homology[a] (%)
Alpha	9	12	166	75–85
Beta	9	1	166	30
Gamma	12	1	143	1

[a] Compared to IFN-α.
Note: The IFN licensed for clinical use and produced by recombinant DNA technology is IFN-α. IFN-α2a (Hoffmann LaRoche) differs from IFN-α2b (Schering-Plough) by a single amino acid at position 23 (lysine in IFN-α2a, arginine in IFN-α2b). IFN-α2 is 165 amino acids, with a deletion of an aspartate residue at amino acid 44 when compared to other members of the IFN-α family.

effects, have now entered clinical trials in oncology. One of these has been approved for use in chronic active hepatitis.[18–20]

In addition to the direct administration of IFNs, chemically defined IFN inducers may have several therapeutic applications. They may possess advantageous pharmacokinetics for IFN induction, directly induce additional cytokines, activate immune effector cells, and, if administered orally, be more convenient. In some clinical settings, they might prove more effective as therapeutic agents, in addition to potentially being chemopreventive. The first chemically defined inducers of IFNs were double-stranded polyribonucleotides, such as polyriboinosinic-polyribocytidilic acid (poly I:poly C), now known to induce IFNs through activation of toll-like receptor 3 (TLR3). Although potent IFN inducers and immunomodulators in mice, poly I:poly C and various modifications do not consistently induce IFN or have any antitumor activity in humans at clinically tolerable doses.[21] Subsequently, low molecular weight organic compounds, such as tilorone, halopyrimidinones, acridines, substituted quinolones, and flavone acetic acid, were identified as inducers of IFNs in different animal species. Several IFN inducers have been introduced into human clinical trials, and some induce substantial amounts of IFN and activate the IFN system.[22–26] Imiquimod, a low molecular weight compound, and CpG7909, a phosphorothioate oligodeoxyribonucleotide, activate TLR8 and TLR9, respectively.[27–30] Emerging data suggest that these IFN and cytokine inducers may have clinically useful therapeutic activity.

INTERFERON SIGNALING AND RESISTANCE MECHANISMS

Signal Transduction and Control of Interferon-Stimulated Gene Expression

Cellular responses to IFNs are initiated by ligand binding to specific plasma membrane receptors.[31] These receptors have been characterized using genetic, biochemical, and molecular biologic approaches.[32] The following sections focus on IFN receptors, the mechanisms by which IFN-stimulated genes (ISGs) are induced, and the genes regulated by IFNs.

IFN receptors lack intrinsic enzymatic activity[31] but instead are associated with cytoplasmic tyrosine kinases of the JAK family (JAK kinases, including JAK1, JAK2, JAK3, and Tyk2).[31,33] Following IFN binding to its receptor, the JAK kinases phosphorylate tyrosine residues on latent cytoplasmic transcriptional factors, designated "signal transducers and activators of transcription" (STATs), which migrate to the nucleus and induce transcription of IFN-stimulated genes (Fig. 32.1).[31,34]

Interferon Receptors

IFN-α, IFN-β and IFN-ω bind to a common IFN receptor (type I), whereas IFN-γ binds to a distinct receptor (type II).[35] The two types of IFN receptors are found on the cells of all normal and malignant tissues[36] and possess equilibrium dissociation constants (K_D) between 10^{-11} and 10^{-9} M. The number of receptors is between 100 and 2,000 per cell. Type I and type II receptors are transmembrane glycoproteins (Fig. 32.1).

Two subunits of the type I IFN receptor, IFNAR-1[37] and IFNAR-2[38,39] have been cloned. They associate with Tyk2 (tyrosine kinase 2) and JAK1 kinases, respectively.[40,41] The genes encoding the two subunits are located in the q22.1 region of human chromosome 21.[40–42] Human IFNAR-1 and IFNAR-2, when expressed in mouse cells, confer

antiviral activity in response to type I human IFNs.[43] The failure of human IFNAR-1 and IFNAR-2 to confer on mouse cells the antiproliferative activity of human type I IFNs suggests the involvement of additional molecules in the receptor complex.[43]

The IFN-γ receptor has two subunits, IFNGR-1 and IFNGR-2,[44–46] which are associated with the JAK1 and JAK2 kinases, respectively.[47,48] In humans, IFNGR-1 is located on chromosome 6q.[44] IFN-γ binds to IFNGR-1, inducing IFNGR-1 dimerization and association with IFNGR-2 to activate the receptor-coupled JAK1 and JAK2 kinases in transducing signals.[47]

Signal Transduction

IFNs, like many other cytokines, activate protein tyrosine kinases to transduce signals. The lack of protein tyrosine kinase domains in IFN receptors indicated that additional receptor or nonreceptor protein tyrosine kinases must be involved.[38,39,44–46] Complementation of IFN-resistant mutant cell lines by genes coding for members of the JAK kinases provided direct evidence that JAK1, JAK2, and Tyk2 are required for signal transduction. A mutant cell line that lacked the ability to respond to IFN-α or IFN-γ became responsive to IFNs when the JAK1 kinase was expressed in the mutant,[49] indicating the central role of JAK1 in IFN-α and IFN-γ signaling pathways. Complementation of an IFN-γ nonresponsive mutant (IFN-α and IFN-β response intact) with the gene for JAK2 demonstrated the requirement for JAK2 in the IFN-γ response.[50] Complementation of an IFN-α nonresponsive mutant (IFN-γ response intact)

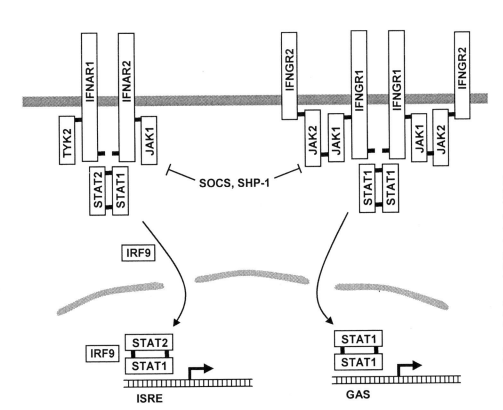

Figure 32.1 Components of the interferon (IFN) signaling pathways. The major components responsible for relaying IFN-mediated signals from the cell surface to the regulatory elements of IFN-stimulated genes are represented. GAS, IFN-γ activated site; IFNAR, IFN-α receptor; IFNGR, IFN-γ receptor; ISRE, IFN-stimulated response element; JAK, Janus kinase; SHP, src-homology 2 domain–containing protein tyrosine phosphatase; SOCS, suppressor of cytokine signaling; STAT, signal transducer and activator of transcription; Tyk, JAK family kinase. Small black bars represent tyrosine residues that become phosphorylated and induce complex formation.

with the gene for Tyk2 demonstrated that Tyk2 is essential for the IFN-α response.[51] Biochemical studies demonstrated that each subunit of the IFN receptors associates specifically with a JAK family kinase (Fig. 32.1) that is activated by IFN binding to the receptors, resulting in phosphorylation of tyrosine residues of cellular proteins, including STATs.

The STAT family of proteins transduce signals from a variety of cell surface receptors to the nucleus and activate transcription by binding to DNA regulatory elements.[31] Each of the STATs has a dimerization domain at its N-terminal region, an IFN-regulatory factor (IRF)–binding domain, a DNA-binding domain, SH2 and SH3 domains, and a C-terminal transcription activation domain.[34] The JAK kinases, when activated by IFN binding to the receptors, undergo autophosphorylation, transphosphorylate each other, and phosphorylate the receptor subunits.[33] The phosphorylated tyrosine residues in these proteins provide binding sites for the SH2 domains of STATs, resulting in STAT recruitment to the receptor and JAK complexes and the phosphorylation of tyrosine residues in the STATs.[31] This leads to STAT dimerization, translocation to the nucleus, and binding to promoter elements to control the transcription of IFN-stimulated genes.[31,33,34]

To date, seven STAT proteins (STAT1–4, 5a, 5b, 6) have been cloned and characterized.[52] Two isoforms of STAT1 (STAT1a and STAT1b) are produced through alternative splicing and differ at their C-termini.[53] Unlike STAT1a, STAT1b lacks the transcriptional activation domain and thus functions as a signal transducer but not a transcriptional activator. Complementation of STAT-deficient mutant cells demonstrates that STAT1 is essential for IFN-α, -β, and -γ signal transduction, whereas STAT2 is required for IFN-α and -β signaling only.[54,55] The functional importance of STAT1 in IFN signaling has been further supported by the failure of STAT1-deficient mice to respond to IFNs and by the heightened susceptibility of these mice to viral and microbial infections.[56,57]

Two types of regulatory DNA elements are recognized by IFN-activated STATs and control the transcription of IFN-stimulated genes. The IFN-stimulated response element (ISRE) is a highly conserved enhancer that responds to IFN-α and -β.[31] Genes stimulated by IFN-γ contain a cis-acting element called the IFN-γ activated site (GAS).[34] The core sequence of the ISRE is a direct repeat of GAAA spaced by one or two nucleotides: GAAAN(N)GAAA. Mutational analysis of ISRE reporter constructs defined the minimal element that is necessary and sufficient for IFN responsiveness.[58] The ISRE is recognized by three DNA-binding complexes designated IFN-stimulated gene factor 1 (ISGF-1), IRF-1, and ISGF-3. Unlike ISGF-1, which is constitutively expressed, IRF-1 and ISGF-3 are induced by IFNs.[59] ISGF-3 is a heterotrimeric complex of STAT1, STAT2, and p48/IRF-9.[52] STAT1 and STAT2, activated via tyrosine phosphorylation, associate with p48/IRF-9, translocate to the nucleus, bind the ISRE and activate transcription.[60] The GAS consensus

sequence is AANNNNNTT.[31] The GAS element is conserved between species and can be contained within the ISRE. IFN-γ stimulation induces tyrosine phosphorylation of STAT1a, which forms homodimers (also called "gamma activated factor" [GAF]) and binds to GAS to activate transcription.[32]

Phosphatases play a key role in turning off IFN signaling. Src-homology 2 domain–containing protein tyrosine phosphatase-1 (SHP-1) and SHP-2 are protein tyrosine phosphatases that contain SH2 domains.[61] SHP-1 can dephosphorylate JAK family kinases and terminate signaling.[62] Its negative regulatory role in IFN signaling is demonstrated by a heightened response to IFNs in SHP-1–deficient cells.[63] Similarly, SHP-2–deficient cells show augmented STAT activation and reduction of cell viability in response to IFNs.[64] Other protein tyrosine phosphatases also regulate JAK and STAT proteins and may down-regulate IFN signaling.[43,65–67]

A family of suppressor of cytokine signaling (SOCS, also known as "CIS-cytokine-inducible SH2") proteins has been identified.[68,69] These proteins have a central SH2 domain and a conserved C-terminal SOCS box (also known as "CIS-homology domain" or "CH domain"). Most SOCS proteins are induced by several different cytokines, and some of them have been shown to negatively regulate cytokine signaling through binding and inactivation of JAKs and STATs,[70] targeting the protein for degradation, or both.[71] Importantly, SOCS proteins are induced by IFNs.[72,73] Stable expression of SOCS1 or SOCS3 blocks IFN-mediated antiviral effects and IFN-induced growth arrest.[72,73] Thus, these SOCS proteins may be the effectors of a negative feedback mechanism that terminates the IFN response (Fig. 32.1).

Although JAK-STAT pathways play an essential role in IFN signaling, other kinases and transcriptional factors are also involved. The antiproliferative activity of IFN-α in T cells requires components of the T-cell receptor signaling pathway, including the Lck and ZAP-70 protein tyrosine kinases.[74] IRF-1 and IRF-2, transcriptional factors related to p48,[75] regulate ISG expression by binding to ISREs.[76,77] IRF-1 acts as a positive regulator of IFN-α-induced, IFN-β-induced, and IFN-γ-induced genes, whereas IRF-2 represses the effects of IRF-1.[78,79] These antagonistic factors may play a role in oncogenesis. Forced expression of IRF-2 resulted in transformation and enhanced tumorigenicity of NIH3T3 cells, which was reversed by expression of IRF-1.[80] Transgenic mice deficient in IRF-1 or IRF-2 confirm their important regulatory roles.[81] The IFN consensus sequence-binding protein (ICSBP) is another negative regulatory factor that binds to the ISRE of many IFN-regulated genes, including the major histocompatibility complex (MHC) class I genes.[82] Expression of ICSBP is restricted to cells of the hematopoietic lineage and is induced by IFN-γ but not by IFN-α and IFN-β.[83] Yeast two-hybrid screens have identified the protein inhibitor of activated STATs (PIAS) gene family.[84] PIASs bind to STAT1 and STAT3 dimers, thereby blocking their DNA-binding activity.

Mechanism of Interferon Resistance

Despite the successful application of IFNs to the treatment of several malignancies, the potential of the IFNs in antitumor therapies has not yet been fully realized. So far, the mechanism of IFN resistance in human cancer patients has been little studied. Although IFN-α results in an excellent hematologic response in 75% of patients with chronic myelogenous leukemia (CML), it induces complete cytogenetic remission in fewer than 20%. This suggests the presence of partial or complete primary IFN resistance in nonresponding patients.[85] On the other hand, development of acquired IFN resistance in vivo appears to be common and is indicated by loss of IFN responsiveness in some patients who were initially responsive to IFNs. This is illustrated by a patient with T-cell lymphoma whose initial positive response to IFN therapy was followed by rapid progression, due to the appearance of a subpopulation of IFN-resistant malignant cells.[86]

Interferon Signaling Molecules in Interferon Resistance

Cell lines unresponsive to IFNs have been generated by mutagenesis, and these lack distinct IFN signaling molecules, including components of IFN receptors, JAK kinases, or STATs.[32] Complementation of the mutant cell lines with the corresponding signaling molecules restores the IFN response.[32] Defects of signaling molecules in human tumor cells have also been reported. An IFN-resistant human leukemia cell line lacked IFN receptor expression.[87] In vivo sensitivity and resistance of CML cells to IFN-α correlated with reduced receptor binding.[88] A IFN-resistant human tumor CTLL cell line (Hut78R) lacks STAT1 expression.[89] IFN-α-resistance of renal carcinoma cell lines was associated with defects in STAT1 induction.[90] These observations indicate that defects in the IFN receptor and STAT1 may exist in certain IFN-resistant human tumor cells and may block IFN antitumor activity. Interestingly, in contrast to the antiproliferative effect of IFN-α on the parental cells, increased concentrations of IFN-α caused a marked stimulation of growth in the IFN-resistant Hut78R cells.[89] Thus, STAT defects might also be involved in tumor progression.

SHP-1 involvement in human leukemia is suggested by the localization of the SHP-1 gene at chromosome 12p13,[91] a region frequently affected in acute lymphoblastic leukemia (ALL), and by the deletion of the SHP-1 gene in some ALL cases with 12p abnormalities.[92] Given the negative regulatory role of SHP-1 in IFN signaling,[63] ALL cases with reduced or absent SHP-1 expression could be predicted to be more sensitive to IFNs and are potential candidates for IFN therapy. Increased expression of SOCS proteins can potentially block IFN signaling.[69]

The biologic activity of IFNs depends on the induction of specific genes that affect cell morphology, cell viability, cell cycle progression, differentiation, and intercellular interactions. Defects in IFN-induced gene expression were detected in IFN-resistant primary leukemia cells.[93] The identification of novel ISGs using the DNA-chip technique will help to further assess the involvement of ISGs in IFN resistance.[94] Microarray analysis identified changes in gene expression following development of IFN resistance in cutaneous T-cell lymphoma in vitro.[95] The parental IFN-sensitive line and the resultant IFN-resistant line both displayed normal STAT1 activation and ISG induction. The gene *MAL* was overexpressed in resistant cells and was highly expressed in tumor biopsies of patients with cutaneous T-cell lymphoma.

Besides proteins that are intrinsic components of the IFN-signaling pathways, a number of other cellular factors may also participate in IFN resistance. IFN resistance correlated with heightened expression of the *bcl-2* proto-oncogene in primary myeloma cells.[96] As induction of apoptosis may be important in IFN-mediated antitumor activity,[97] overexpression of bcl-2 protein may protect the tumor cells from IFN-induced apoptosis and confer IFN resistance. Viruses produce factors that block IFN responses. Adenovirus, Epstein-Barr virus, and hepatitis B virus have all been implicated in the pathogenesis of human malignancies. The E1A and virus-associated (VA) I RNA of adenovirus, the EBNA-2 protein of Epstein-Barr virus, and the terminal protein of hepatitis B virus inhibit cellular responses to IFN.[93,98,99] Therefore, IFN resistance in virus-associated human tumors may be mediated, at least in part, by the expression of specific viral proteins.

ANTITUMOR MECHANISMS: CELLULAR AND MOLECULAR

Angiogenesis

Angiogenesis is the process of new blood vessel formation from existing vessels and is a requirement for tumor growth.[100] IFNs inhibit angiogenesis by altering the angiogenic potential of tumor cells as well as inhibiting the angiogenic capacity of endothelial cells. Following IFN treatment, tumor vessels undergo coagulation necrosis—a sign of disrupted blood flow.[101] Inhibition of angiogenesis by IFNs precedes the antiproliferative effects on tumor cells and can be detected within 24 hours of tumor cell inoculation.[102] Tumor progression studies of IFN-sensitive and IFN-resistant bladder carcinoma cell lines in mice show that systemic administration of IFN-α reduces tumor cell growth in the IFN-sensitive cells by directly regulating the expression of basic fibroblast growth factor (bFGF), an angiogenic growth factor.[103] IFN-α and IFN-β both downregulated bFGF in other human carcinoma cells, including in the prostate, colon, and breast.[104] This down-regulation correlated with reduced vascularization and tumor growth.[103] Knockout studies in tumor cell lines showed that STAT1 was necessary for IFN modulation of bFGF signaling.[105]

In addition to its action on bFGF, IFN can inhibit angiogenesis by acting on other angiogenesis mediators. IFN inhibited VEGF mRNA and protein expression in neuroendocrine tumors by regulating VEGF promoter activity.[106] IL-8 is a potent mediator of angiogenesis[107] and consequently tumorigenesis.[108] IL-8 protein production can be inhibited by IFN-α2b[109] and IFN-β.[110] IL-8 is a member of the C-X-C chemokine family and contains the ELR binding motif.[111] Other IFN-stimulated genes in the chemokine family that lack the ELR motif include I-TAC, Mig, and IP-10, all of which function as angiogenic inhibitors[111] are also IFN-stimulated genes.[94] GTPases are a family of proteins that function as molecular switches in signal transduction pathways. Several GTPase families are induced by IFNs. These include the Mx proteins (discussed later in "Direct Antitumor Mechanisms") and the guanylate-binding proteins (GBPs). These GTPases have a distinct hydrolysis profile, since they bind GTP, GDP, and GMP with similar affinity and can hydrolyze GTP to GDP or GMP.[112,113] To date, five human GBPs (hGBP1–5) and five murine GBPs (mGBP1–5) have been identified. They are closely related and have similar tissue expression patterns during infection.[114] In endothelial cells, hGBP1 functions as an inflammatory response factor that can inhibit endothelial proliferation[115] and angiogenesis.[116] Thus, in addition to its antiviral activity, GBP1 may have antitumor effects through inhibition of angiogenesis. The third family of GTPases includes IRG-47,[117] LRG-47,[118] TGTP/Mg21,[119,120] and IGTP,[121] all approximately 47 kd, and they may exert antiviral effects by regulating intracellular membrane trafficking.[122,123]

Clinically, IFN-α2b has proven effective in the treatment of infantile hemangiomas,[124] hemangioblastomas,[125] and giant cell tumor of the mandible.[126] Clinical efficacy in all three instances correlated with decreased bFGF protein. Kaposi's sarcoma, a neoplastic disease of endothelial origin, is the most common neoplasm in AIDS patients and responds to treatment with IFN-α2b.[127] Physiologic and pathologic angiogenesis is believed to be regulated by the balance between angiogenic activators and inhibitors. The "angiogenic switch" occurs when the level of activators exceeds that of the inhibitors.[128] Endogenous IFN-α/β signaling plays a role as a negative regulator, keeping the angiogenic switch in the off position. IFN-α/β receptor knockout mice have increased angiogenesis and tumorigenesis compared with wild-type mice.[129]

Immune Effects

The in vivo antitumor activity of IFN may be mediated by activation of immune cells as well as enhance the immunogenicity of tumor cells. IFNs enhance the activity of cytotoxic and helper T cells,[130,131] natural killer (NK) cells,[132] macrophages,[133] and dendritic cells.[134] IFN-γ promotes cytotoxic T cell expansion by up-regulating IL-2 gene expression.[135] IFNs activate NK cells and macrophages both in vitro and in vivo.[136] Furthermore, IFNs can induce expression of Apo2L/TRAIL on immune effector cell surfaces, sensitizing tumor cells to T cell–mediated and NK cell–mediated cytotoxicity.[137] Treatment of both immunocompetent and athymic-nude mice with IFN-α–blocking or IFN-β–blocking antibodies enhances the growth of several different murine tumors,[138] suggesting a role for immune cells in IFN antitumor effects. In addition to stimulating immune effector cells, IFNs up-regulate the expression of major histocompatibility (MHC) antigens, which facilitates activation of CD8+ cytotoxic T cells.[139–142] IFNs not only up-regulate the transcription of MHC class I genes but also coordinately induce expression of additional proteins required for the surface expression of the mature MHC class I complex.[139,140,143] This complex contains the MHC class I polypeptide, β2-microglobulin, and an 8– to 10–amino acid antigenic peptide bound to the MHC polypeptide. As nascent class I molecules are synthesized, they associate with β2-microglobulin, also an ISG, in the endoplasmic reticulum for transport to the cell surface. The generation of antigenic peptides for loading onto class I molecules occurs in the proteasome.[144] The three subunits, low molecular weight protein-2 (LMP-2), LMP-7, and MECL/LMP-10, that make up the proteasome are all ISGs.[145,146] In addition, the transporter associated with antigen processing (TAP) is induced by IFN-γ.[147] TAP transports the processed peptides from cytosol to the ER for loading onto class I molecules. Two additional proteins involved in MHC class I antigen presentation, tapasin and the ER protein gp96, are induced by IFN-γ.[139] IFNs also induce MHC class II proteins,[139] which present peptide antigens to CD4+ T helper cells.[148] The MHC class II transactivator factor (CIITA) is considered the master regulator of MHC class II expression and is induced by IFN-γ.[149] In addition, three of the cathepsins, proteolytic enzymes located in the lysosome and thought to be partly responsible for peptide antigen processing and loading onto MHC class II protein,[150] are also up-regulated by IFN-γ.[139]

IFNs induce tumor-associated antigens,[151] such as carcinoma embryonic antigen[152] and Tag-72,[151] and Fc receptors[153] on the surface of tumor cells, subjecting them to enhanced immune surveillance. IFNs induce a number of growth factors and cytokines. ISG-15, a secreted protein induced by IFN-α and IFN-β, induces IFN-γ synthesis by T cells and proliferation of NK and lymphokine-activated killer (LAK) cells.[154] Chemokines are low molecular weight, secreted proteins that function as chemoattractants. IFN-induced chemokines include RANTES,[155] IP-10,[156] MCP-1,[157] MIP-1α, MIG,[158] and I-TAC.[159] These proteins are chemoattractive to both lymphocytes and monocytes and play a crucial role in recruiting these cells into tissues.

Direct Antitumor Mechanisms

The pleiotropic cellular effects induced by IFNs are mediated primarily by the diverse activities of interferon-stimulated genes (ISGs). In the last few years, DNA microarrays have identified hundreds of new ISGs (Table 32.4). These oligonucleotide arrays identified genes induced by IFN-α, IFN-β, or IFN-γ[94] (http://www.lerner.ccf.org/labs/ williams/ der.html). Although type I and II IFNs regulate a number of unique genes, there is significant overlap in the genes regulated by both classes.[94,141]

Some ISGs initially found to mediate antiviral activity were subsequently implicated in the antiproliferative and immunomodulatory effects of IFNs.[160,161] One of these proteins is the double-stranded RNA-dependent protein kinase (dsRNA-PKR). PKR is induced by type I and II IFNs, and upon activation, it slows cellular and viral proliferation by phosphorylating the eukaryotic initiation factor-2, which inhibits protein synthesis.[160] PKR can also be activated in a dsRNA-independent mechanism by the protein PACT.[162] In the absence of viral infection, PKR can induce or enhance apoptosis but also may be required for normal cell proliferation. PKR enhances Apo2L/TRAIL-induced apoptosis by preventing protein synthesis following Apo2L/TRAIL binding to its receptor.[160]

The family of 2'-5'-oligoadenylate synthetases (2-5 synthetase) exert antiviral activity.[163] Following activation by dsRNA, these enzymes polymerize ATP into 2'-5'-oligoadenylates. These 2'-5'-oligoadenylates in turn activate the enzyme RNaseL. RNaseL inhibits protein synthesis by degrading single-stranded RNA. Recently, this gene was found to be a strong candidate for the hereditary prostate cancer allele.[164] RNaseL induces apoptosis in prostate carcinoma cells treated with 2'-5'-oligoadenylate analogs; mutations in the RNaseL gene prevent apoptosis.[165]

The best characterized GTPases are the Mx proteins, MxA and MxB, which belong to the dynamin superfamily of large GTPases.[141,166,167] Mx proteins are induced by type I but not type II IFNs. MxA has antiviral activity against negative-strand RNA viruses, including the influenza virus.[166] Animal studies have shown that MxA is sufficient to block viral replication in the absence of IFN.[167] Genetic studies indicate that MxA has antiviral activity against many RNA viruses, but to date MxB has not been shown to exert any antiviral activity.[141] IFN-γ–mediated microbial and tumor cell killing is mediated by nitric oxide (NO). NO and its reactive intermediates activate both neutrophils and macrophages and have been included here because their products can enhance tumor cell killing. The NO synthetase (NOS) family of enzymes catalyze NAPDH-dependent oxidation of arginine to yield NO. One of these family members, inducible NOS (iNOS), is induced by IFN-γ.[141] IFN-induced iNOS can suppress tumor formation as well as metastasis by regulating genes related to survival, metastasis, and angiogenesis.[154]

The interferon p200 family of proteins, induced by both type I and II IFNs, play a role in cellular growth regulation and differentiation. The p200 family of proteins contain a unique 200-amino acid domain and include six murine members (p202a, p202b, p202c, p203, p204, and p205) and three human members (IFI-16, myeloid cell

TABLE 32.4
INTERFERON (IFN)-REGULATED GENE PRODUCTS AND FUNCTIONS

Antiviral
Guanylate binding protein (GBP)-1
MxA
TGTP
Antigen processing and presentation
β$_2$-microglobulin
Cathepsins B, H, and S
CIITA
Invariant chain
Low molecular weight protein (LMP)-2, LMP-7, LMP-10
MHC class I
MHC class II
Proteasome accelerator 28
Cytokines and chemokines
β-R1/TAC
IP-10
RANTES
ISG-15
Signal transduction
IFN consensus sequence–binding protein
IFI 16
IFN-regulatory factor (IRF)-1
IRF-2
Protein synthesis inhibition
2',5'-oligoA synthetase
PKR
Tryptophan metabolism
Tryptophanyl-transfer RNA synthase
Indoleamine 2,3-dioxygenase
Respiratory burst/nitric oxide metabolism
gp91-phox
GTP cyclohydroxylase
Nitric oxide synthase
p47-phox
GTPases
GBP-2
MxB
Cell activation
Natural killer cell cytotoxicity
Monocyte
Nonspecific cytotoxicity
Antibody-dependent cell-mediated cytotoxicity
Peroxide generation
Miscellaneous
Carcinoembryonic antigen
Fc-γ receptor
ISG-20
Myeloid cell nuclear differentiation antigen
Promyelocytic leukemia
SP-100
Interleukin-1 receptor antagonist
Tumor necrosis factor–soluble receptor
TAG-72

nuclear differentiation antigen [MNDA], and absent in melanoma 2 [AIM2]).[168] IFI-16, AIM2, and p202 inhibit cell proliferation.[168] The murine p202a gene inhibits proliferation by binding the tumor suppressor gene *RB*,[169]

TABLE 32.5
PHARMACOKINETICS OF INTERFERONS

Route of Administration	Dose (mU)	Serum Concentration (U/mL)	Peak Time	Duration (from–to)	IFN Type	Reference
IFN-α						
I.M.	72	300	2–8 hr	0.5 to >48 hr	α2a	26
	3,108	400	8 hr	0.5 to >48 hr		
	198	1,000	2 hr	0.5 to >48 hr		
	3–36	20–200	2–8 hr	<0.5–24 hr		
I.M.	50	2,000 pg/mL	6 hr	<0.5 to >24 hr	α2a	286
	36	1,000 pg/mL	6 hr	<0.5–24 hr		
	18	500 pg/mL	6 hr	<0.5–24 hr		
I.M.	3	60	6 hr	<24 hr	Cantell buffy coat	287
	9	230	2 hr	>24 hr		
I.M	1	80	6 hr		α Lymphoblastoid	288
	3	400	6 hr			
	10	1,200	6 hr			
I.M.	9–18	100	6–8 hr	<0.5–12 hr	α2a	289
	36–50	200	6–8 hr	<0.5–24 hr		
	68	500	6–8 hr	<0.5 to >4 hr		
	86	600	6–8 hr			
Continuous I.V. infusion	5–10 mU/m^2	100–800	<24 hr	Continuous	α2a	290
	10–50	10^3	<24 hr	Continuous		
	100–200	10^3–10^4	<24 hr	Continuous		
Continuous S.C. infusion	2–5	20–60	Steady state	24–72 hr	α2b	291
IFN-β						
I.V.	4–10	10–300	30 min		Fibroblast β	292
	40–80	200–10,000	30 min			
	160–320	2,000–20,000	30 min			
S.C.	90	10^2		1–8 hr	β1b	246
I.V.	90	10^3	5 min	5 min–12 hr		
I.V. 4-h infusion	0.01–1.00	<10			β1b	293
	10	25–30	6 hr	0.5–24 hr		
	30	140	4 hr	0.05–24 hr		
I.V.	45	350	5 min		β1b	294
	180	1,800	5 min			
S.C.	45	0				
	180	25				
IFN-γ						
I.V. 10-min infusion	0.01–20.00	0			γ	242
		30	15 min	<0.5–12 hr		
		75	15 min	<0.5–24 hr		
I.V. 6-hr infusion	0.5 mg/m^2	3 ng/mL	6 hr	2–8 hr	γ	295
	1 mg/m^2	6 ng/mL	6 hr	<1–8		
S.C.	1 mU	4 mg/mL	13 hr		γ	296

p53,[170] and the transcription factor E2F.[171,172] This inhibition of proliferation results in loss of the transformed phenotype[173] and decreased tumor formation in mouse models.[174]

Nuclear bodies (NBs) are multiprotein complexes in the nucleus that are associated with human diseases, including acute promyelocytic leukemia, AIDS, and viral infections.[175] The promyelocytic (PML) protein, the NB organizer protein,[176] is also an ISG. Studies in PML knockout mice indicate that PML is necessary for apoptosis.[177] Other proteins that make up NBs (sp100, sp140, sp110, and ISG-20) are also ISGs. Thus, proteins that make up NBs may play a

TABLE 32.6
INTERFERON SIDE EFFECTS

Initial injections
Chills and rigors
Fevers
Malaise
Myalgias
Mild neutropenia
Chronic administration
Fatigue
Anorexia
Mild neutropenia
Transaminase elevations
Weight loss
Depression
General
At least partly result from receptor-triggered effects
Individual patient variability
Correlated with dose and duration
Chronic anorexia and fatigue most limiting
Reversible side effects resolve off treatment

role in the IFN response to cancer, apoptosis, and immunomodulation.[176]

IFN-α decreased the activities of cyclins and cyclin-dependent kinases (CDKs) by induction of CDK inhibitors p21[WAF1] and p15, with associated prevention of retinoblastoma protein (Rb) hyperphosphorylation, thus keeping this tumor suppressor in the active state. Activated Rb binds and inactivates transcription factors like E2F that are required for cell cycle progression.[178–182] Induction of the CDK inhibitor p21[WAF1] by IFN-α in Daudi Burkitt's lymphoma cells leads to cell cycle arrest, differentiation, and apoptosis.[178]

Unlike apoptosis induced by camptothecin, programmed cell death in response to IFNs is a late effect, requiring 48 hours of exposure. Underlying this latency is the requirement for gene induction. Gene array experiments have identified apoptosis-promoting ISGs.[183] In CML[184] and multiple myeloma cells,[185] induction of the death receptor Fas/CD95 by IFN-α resulted in apoptosis through recruitment of FADD (Fas associated death domain) and subsequent activation of caspase-8/FLICE. Intralesional administration of IFN-α into basal cell carcinomas increased Fas expression and led to regression.[186] Cholangiocarcinoma cells were sensitized to Fas-mediated apoptosis by pretreatment with IFN-γ.[187] Similarly, IFN-γ increased susceptibility of melanoma cells to apoptosis by Fas activators.[188] IFN-β induced Apo2L/TRAIL (TNF-related apoptosis-inducing ligand) in melanoma cells more potently than did IFN-α.[189] In myeloma cells, IFN-α induced Apo2L/TRAIL expression; apoptosis was inhibited by expression of the dominant negative mutant death receptor 5 (DR5Δ), which binds Apo2L/TRAIL without eliciting intracellular signals.[190] Promoter mapping, RNA interference, and ChIP studies suggested that Apo2L/TRAIL induction in breast cancer cells by IFN and retinoic acid (RA) is mediated through IRF-1 activa-

tion of the Apo2L/TRAIL promoter.[191] Combination treatment with IFN and RA synergistically induced Apo2L/TRAIL, which may explain synergistic anticancer effects.[191] Induced by IFN-β in melanoma cells,[192] XAF-1 promotes apoptosis by interfering with the apoptosis inhibitor XIAP,[193] thus preventing inactivation of caspase-3, -7, and -9.[194] XAF-1 overexpression in A375 melanoma cells by itself did not result in apoptosis but sensitized cells to Apo2L/TRAIL-induced apoptosis.[192]

Caspases are key apoptotic enzymes that are activated by either external signals via death receptors or internal stresses via mitochondria. In the final common pathway, activation of caspase-3 brings about ordered breakdown of the cell.[195–197] IFN-γ sensitized breast cancer cells to death receptor–mediated apoptosis, associated with up-regulation of caspase-8 expression and IRF-1 induction.[198,199] In astrocytoma cells, IFN-γ increased expression of caspase-1, -4, and -7,[200] whereas caspases-3, -4, -7, and -8 were increased in colon cancer cells.[201] Type I IFNs induced caspase-4 in melanoma[161] and fibrosarcoma cells.[202]

Mice lacking IRF-8 develop a disease similar to CML. Interestingly, overexpression of IRF-8 in Bcr-Abl–transformed cells inhibited leukemogenesis as well as resistance to chemotherapy with imatinib, which correlated with reduced bcl-2 expression.[203] IRF 5, inducible by both p53 and type I IFNs, was recently described to have a p53-independent tumor suppressor function in lymphoma cells.[204]

Inositol hexakisphosphate kinase2 (IHPK2) was identified as a regulator of IFN-induced death in ovarian cancer cells by an antisense technical knockout approach.[205] It is located on chromosome 3p21, a region frequently affected by loss of heterozygosity and chromosomal rearrangements in human cancer. Overexpression of IHPK2 sensitized tumor cell lines to apoptosis in response to a variety of chemotherapeutics and ionizing radiation, suggesting a role in a central apoptotic pathway.[206]

Inducible by IFN-α, SCF, G-CSF, and EGF, phospholipid scramblase 1 (PLSCR1) localizes to the plasma membrane[207–211] but can translocate to the nucleus via nuclear membrane receptors.[207] It may play a role in trans-bilayer movement of phospholipids during apoptosis, thereby providing macrophages with a signal for engulfment.[212–214] Ovarian cancer cells overexpressing PLSCR1 grew slower in nude mice compared to vector-transfected cells, and the resultant tumors were infiltrated by neutrophils and macrophages.[215] Thus, by inducing PLSCR 1, IFNs might facilitate tumor cell phagocytosis by macrophages.

Identified as mediators of IFN-γ–induced apoptosis, gene,[216] death-associated protein kinases (DAPK) are serine threonine kinases with ankyrin and death domains that induce caspase-independent cell death.[217] Reduced expression correlated with malignant behavior while restoration of expression led to apoptosis of mouse lung tumors.[218] Their expression is frequently silenced in human malignancies, especially in lymphoid tumors,[219] further supporting their role as tumor suppressors. DAPK7, also called ZIP kinase, phosphorylated MDM2 and p21[WAF1], with resultant prolongation of the p21[WAF1] half-life, providing a DAPK– mediated link between the p53 and IFN pathways.[220]

In summary, IFNs increase expression of a number of cell cycle inhibitory and apoptotic genes. These direct effects on tumor cells likely contribute to the anticancer effect in vivo. In some instances, addition of another drug is required for full activation of apoptotic pathways, providing a rationale for combination trials. Combination of IFNs with inhibitors of survival genes, like epidermal growth factor receptor,[221,222] may prove beneficial.

Clinical Pharmacology of Interferons

IFNs can be measured in serum using bioassays, which measure protection from viral cytopathic effect, or with more direct immunological tests. Both methods have sensitivities around 5 U/mL, while reproducibility may be higher for the latter. Most studies used bioassays and generally confirmed higher maximum serum levels of IFN-α compared to IFN-β or -γ after subcutaneous administration (Table 32.5). Additionally, a number of biological effects that result from gene induction by IFNs (e.g., neopterin or β_2-microglobulin serum levels, mononuclear cell 2-5 A synthetase production, and NK cell activation) have been measured both to document in vivo activity and in an attempt to predict response. Unfortunately, the latter aim has not been achieved, but 2-5 A synthetase has correlated to IFN dose and serum level in some studies,[223] which may explain why some studies suggested a correlation between 2-5 A levels and response.

IFN-α

When given subcutaneously or intramuscularly to humans, approximately 80% of IFN-α is absorbed.[223] While local effects of oral IFN-α seem possible in Sjogren's disease[224,225] and measles,[226] the promising antimelanoma effect observed in mice[227] could not be demonstrated in limited clinical evaluation for human cancer.[228] After intra-

muscular or subcutaneous administration of IFN-α, the serum or plasma levels peak at 1 to 8 hours, and IFN-α remains detectable for at least 4 to 24 hours. Clearance varies between 4.8 to 48 L/hour, and the terminal elimination half-life is 4 to 16 hours.[223] The Kirkwood schedule of high-dose IFN-α2b therapy for melanoma (20 million IU/m^2 intravenously per day 5 days a week for 4 weeks, followed by 10 million IU/m^2 subcutaneously three times a week)[229] may yield peak serum levels of 2,500 IU/mL at the end of the intravenous phase and 150 IU/mL after subcutaneous administration.[223,230]

IFN-α2 has been chemically modified in order to increase its serum half-life. A monopegylated IFN-α2b has been developed by Schering Plough (Kenilworth, NJ). It has reduced renal clearance and retains approximately 27% of the in vitro antiviral activity of native IFN-α2b. Hoffmann-La Roche (Nutley, NJ) similarly has developed a monopegylated species of IFN-α2a. This species has a 70-fold increase in serum half-life compared with native IFN-α2a.[231] Linkage of a 40-kd branched polyethylene glycol (PEG) molecule to IFN-α2a or a 12-kd linear PEG moiety to IFN-α2b markedly altered the pharmacokinetic profile and increased activity against hepatitis C in a direct clinical comparison of once weekly subcutaneous PEG-IFN with the parent compound given subcutaneously. three times a week.[232] The larger PEG moiety of PEG–IFN-α2a leads to the slowest absorption half-life and the longest elimination half-life (Table 32.7).[233]

PEG-IFN-α2b at 1 µg/kg per week induced a biological response (increase in serum neopterin and mononuclear cell 2-5 A synthetase activity) similar to that of IFN-α2b at 3 million IU administered subcutaneously three times a week.[234] The efficacy of PEG–IFN-α2b has been clinically studied in patients with chronic myelogenous leukemia (CML) and those with advanced solid organ malignancies, particularly melanoma and renal cell carcinoma. A phase I dose-escalation trial of PEG–IFN-α2b administered once weekly was conducted in 27 patients with chronic phase CML who had been previously treated with native IFN-α2b.[235] Thirteen of the patients (48%) achieved a complete hematologic or improved cytogenetic response.

TABLE 32.7
PHARMACOKINETICS OF PEGYLATED PARENTAL IFN-ALPHAS

	IFN-α2a	PEG IFN-α2a	IFN-α2b	PEG IFN-α2b
Volume of distribution	31–73 L	8–12 L	1.4 L/kg	0.99 L/kg
Absorption t½	2.3 hr	50 hr	2.3 hr	4.6 hr
Elimination t½	3–8 hr	65 hr	4 hr	~40 hr
Time to max. conc.	7.3–12 hr	80 hr	7.3–12 hr	15–44 hr
Peak/trough		1.5		>10

t½, half-life; max. conc., maximal concentration; ∞, infinitesimal.
Pegylation of IFN-α 2a with a 40-kd branched molecule or pegylation of IFN-α2b with a 20-kd linear polyethylene glycol moiety alters pharmacokinetics in humans (ref. 233).

Accumulation of serum levels of PEG–IFN-α2b was observed in several dose cohorts at week 4. No dose-limiting toxicities were observed in any of the cohorts through the 4-week study period, but they did occur in those patients treated with higher doses on an extended study protocol.[235] After encouraging results for PEG–IFN-α2b in CML patients who had failed IFN-α treatment,[236] it was directly compared with the parent drug as initial treatment for chronic phase CML in a phase III study, where it showed efficacy and toxicity at 6 μg/kg per week similar to those of IFN-α2b at 5 million IU/m^2 per day.[237] Anticancer activity against solid tumors was demonstrated in a phase I/II trial of PEG–IFN-α2b, which determined 6 μg/kg per week as the maximal tolerated dose (MTD) and showed evidence of drug accumulation with an area under the curve (AUC) of 374 pg/hour per mL for week 1, compared with 480 pg/hour per mL at week 4 for patients treated with the MTD.[238] In a phase II study of pegylated IFN-α2a given subcutaneously at 450 μg once a week to patients with advanced renal cancer, peak levels in the first week (mean 19 ng/mL) were reached 48 hours after the first injection and were maintained for the remainder of week 1. Over the following 5 to 9 weeks, a rise to a plateau (54 ng/mL) was observed. Toxicity and efficacy were comparable to historical controls treated with the parental compound.[239] A small randomized trial of PEG–IFN-α2b given at 1 μg/kg once or twice a week showed improved pharmacokinetics and viral kinetics with twice a week dosing.[240] Whether PEG–IFN-α will increase antitumor activity must be addressed in future studies. Additionally, other members of the IFN-α family, such as IFN-α1, which is currently undergoing clinical evaluation, may provide the same clinical benefits with fewer side effects.[241]

IFN-β

A single species in humans, IFN-β exists as a 23-kd glycoprotein containing 166 amino acids, with an isoelectric point between 6.8 and 7.8, and an N-linked glycosylation site at asn80. Animal studies suggest IFN-β is metabolized primarily in the liver.[223] After intravenous injection, the terminal elimination half-life is about 1 to 2 hours, and IFN-β remains measurable for up to 4 hours (Table 32.5). In contrast, after a single subcutaneous or intramuscular injection, serum IFN-β is barely detectable.[223] However, intravenous and subcutaneous administration of the same dose elicited similar pharmacodynamic responses, including 2-5 A synthetase induction.[242] Oral IFN-β1a had no effect on disease or neopterin levels in multiple sclerosis patients, suggesting proteolysis in the intestinal tract.[243] While in vitro and animal data suggest greater antitumor activity of IFN-β compared with IFN-α,[189,244,245] there have only been a limited number of clinical trials utilizing IFN-β. IFN-β intravenous dosing 2 or 4 times per week resulted in clinical responses in 5 out of 25 patients with advanced malignancies in phase I and I/II trials.[246,247] In a phase I trial of IFN-β1a given to

patients with malignancies unresponsive to standard therapy, 2-5 A synthetase levels remained elevated throughout the 28-day subcutaneous dosing phase; there was no correlation of serum level with IFN dose (1.5 to 24 million IU/m^2). Out of 29 patients, 5 had stabilization of disease.[248]

Three avenues of improving IFN-β pharmacokinetics are being pursued and have generated encouraging preclinical data. Albuferon is a recombinant protein resulting from fusion of the IFN-β peptide with albumin. In monkeys, the bioavailability of subcutaneous Albuferon was 87%, plasma clearance was reduced by 140-fold, and the terminal half-life increased 5-fold, while in vitro and in vivo activity was preserved.[249] Fusion of IFN-β to soluble recombinant type I IFN receptor subunit (sIFNAR-2) prolonged the half-life and increased antitumor activity in mice.[250] Finally, pegylation of IFN-β1a with a linear 20-kd molecule increased the maximum serum concentration achieved 4-fold, while the AUC increased 10-fold and the half-life increased 3-fold.[251]

IFN-γ

After subcutaneous or intramuscular administration, 30 to 70% of IFN-γ is absorbed, and the terminal elimination half-life is 25 to 35 minutes; after intravenous injection, IFN-γ remains detectable in serum up to 4 hours (Table 32.5). Like IFN-β, IFN-γ appears to be metabolized primarily by the liver.[223] A phase I trial in colon cancer patients achieved IFN-γ concentrations greater than 5 U/mL for more than 6.5 hours following 100 μg/m^2 given subcutaneously.[252] Pegylation increased the half-life of PEG–IFN-γ in rats, and activity was preserved,[253] but this molecule has not yet been evaluated in patients.

IFN Fusion Molecules

Gene constructs have made possible protein fusion molecules. Albuferon is a novel hybrid protein produced by the genetic fusion of human serum albumin and a recombinant IFN-α to form a single polypeptide molecule.[241,254] In vitro studies suggest comparable and in some cases improved antiproliferative activity compared with native IFN-α2b.[241] Studies in primates demonstrate a markedly longer circulating half-life than that of IFN-α2b. This increase in half-life correlates with significant and prolonged increases in mRNA transcripts of oligoadenylate synthase, a known IFN-stimulated gene product.[254]

Gene-Shuffled IFNs

Recombinant technology allows the production of sequence-altered IFNs.[255] In vitro studies of several gene-shuffled IFN products show promising results and may lead to translational studies of IFNs with improved efficacy and reduced side effects.[241]

Toxicities

IFNs cause several consistent acute and chronic side effects influenced by dose, route, and schedule.[256,257] The acute side effects are mainly constitutional. Nearly all patients experience fever, chills, malaise, myalgias, arthralgias, and headache beginning 2 to 3 hours after the first dose and lasting approximately 6 to 8 hours (Table 32.6). Fever and chills can be attenuated with the use of acetaminophen and narcotics, respectively. Nausea and vomiting may occur as part of the acute side effects, but they are infrequent.[258] Tachyphylaxis to the acute side effects develops quickly with subsequent doses. However, the symptoms may recur if treatment is interrupted even for a few days.[259]

Elevation of hepatocellular enzymes may occur acutely but is usually mild and reversible. Dose modifications, however, are recommended with significant increases of hepatocellular enzymes, since fatal hepatotoxicity has occurred in rare instances.[260] Serious hepatocellular injury may occur in those patients with preexisting liver disease.[260] Changes in serum lipids consisting of an increase in triglycerides with or without a decrease in total cholesterol may be observed in some patients. Marked hypertriglyceridemia may respond to treatment with gemfibrozil.[261]

Acute hematologic toxicity is often observed.[258] The hematologic effects most commonly observed are neutropenia and thrombocytopenia. Neutropenia is rapidly reversible because it results not from maturation arrest of granulocyte precursors but from impaired release of granulocytes from the bone marrow. No increase in infectious complications has occurred during IFN-induced neutropenia.

The chronic side effects of fatigue, weight loss, and mood alteration can be difficult to control and are the main reasons for discontinuation of IFN-α2b therapy.[260] Dosing delays or dose reductions due to toxicity during maintenance treatment with IFN-α2b were required in 36 to 52% of patients enrolled in the three intergroup trials that evaluated adjuvant high-dose IFN for high-risk melanoma.[258] These chronic effects are generally not observed with the administration of IFN-β.

Fatigue and anorexia are the dose-limiting toxicities with chronic administration of IFN-α.[262] The mechanisms are poorly understood, but weight loss may be significant (greater than 10%) with the use of IFN-α[263,264] Both weight loss and fatigue are uncommon with chronic administration of IFN-β[265,266] Therapy with high-dose IFN-α may lead to a syndrome of altered mood, memory impairment, and cognitive slowing.[267] Depressed mood and occasionally symptoms of major clinical depression may prevail and are the most commonly identified neuropsychiatric toxicity in patients receiving IFN-α2b.[258] Although the mechanisms of IFN-induced mood changes are poorly understood, recent data demonstrate significant increases in serum tryptophan degradation products and neopterin concentrations in patients who were receiving IFN-α and developed depression when compared with those patients who were receiving IFN-α but did not develop depression.[268] Patients with a history of a mood disorder or depression may still be considered candidates for treatment with IFN-α if necessary, but they may be at higher risk for developing depression while being treated.[267] A recent clinical trial suggested that the use of paroxetine can prevent depression and the early discontinuation of IFN-α2b in patients receiving adjuvant therapy for high-risk melanoma.[269]

Changes in creatinine levels are not reported with the use of IFNs. However, mild proteinuria is commonly described, with nephrotic syndrome and acute renal insufficiency being rarely reported.[270, 271] Occasional patients have developed alterations in thyroid function, but no residual toxicities in parenchymal organ function have been identified.[259,272]

CONCLUSION

IFNs have activity for both hematologic malignancies and solid tumors. In CML, IFN-α2 has demonstrated sustained clinical and cytogenetic responses.[273] The median survival for responding patients who show some, although not complete, evidence of cytogenetic response is approximately 6 years. More than 90% of cytogenetic complete responders will be in remission at 10 years.[274] Addition of cytosine arabinoside to IFN-α2 has resulted in a further increase in major cytogenetic responses and further prolongation of survival.[275,276] Emerging resistance to imatinib has resulted in initiation of combination trials, supported by preclinical evidence of synergistic interaction. For B-cell neoplasms, the significant single-agent activity of IFN-α2 can be integrated with effective chemotherapy for low-grade and intermediate-grade non-Hodgkin's lymphoma,[277,278] with prolonged disease-free survival and overall survival. For myeloma, some, but not all, phase II and III studies have suggested that, for induction or maintenance, IFN-α2 may add to effectiveness.[279–281] Prolongation of disease-free survival has emerged from use of IFN-α2 as an adjuvant to surgery for high-risk patients with primary melanoma and metastatic renal cell carcinoma.[282–285]

Clinical trials have thus defined therapeutic effectiveness in hematologic malignancies and solid tumors. Therapeutic applications will likely broaden in the next decade (Table 32.8). A combination of biochemical and genetic approaches has led to the identification of a new cellular signal transduction pathway and more than 300

TABLE 32.8

INTERFERON SYSTEM: CHALLENGES IN 2005–2015

Expand therapeutic usefulness
Individual types
Inducers
Combinations
Define mechanisms of action

IFN-stimulated genes. Further exploration of signal transduction and the genes induced should enhance the understanding of the biologic and pharmacologic effects of IFNs, the focus of this chapter. In the next decade, the clinical benefits of this potent and pleiotropic family of cytokines for the treatment of malignancy will be even more completely realized.

REFERENCES

1. PRISMS. Randomised double-blind placebo-controlled study of interferon beta-1a in relapsing/remitting multiple sclerosis. PRISMS (Prevention of Relapses and Disability by Interferon beta-1a Subcutaneously in Multiple Sclerosis) Study Group. Lancet 1998;352:1498–1504.
2. European Study Group on Interferon beta-1b in Secondary Progressive MS. Placebo-controlled multicentre randomised trial of interferon beta-1b in treatment of secondary progressive multiple sclerosis. Lancet 1998;352:1491–1497.
3. International Chronic Granulomatous Disease Cooperative Study Group. A controlled trial of interferon gamma to prevent infection in chronic granulomatous disease. N Engl J Med 1991;324:509–516.
4. Badaro R, Falcoff S, Badaro FS, et al. Treatment of visceral leishmaniasis with pentavalent antimony and interferon gamma. N Engl J Med 1990;322:16–21.
5. Pfeffer, LM, Dinarello CA, Herberman RB, et al. Biological properties of recombinant alpha-interferons: 40th anniversary of the discovery of interferons. Cancer Res 1998;58:2489–2499.
6. Pestka, S. The human interferon-alpha species and hybrid proteins. Semin Oncol 1997;24:S9-4–9-17.
7. Hawkins MJ, Borden EC, Merritt JA, et al. Comparison of the biologic effects of two recombinant human interferons alpha (rA and rD) in humans. J Clin Oncol 1984;2:221–226.
8. Nagata S, Mantei N, Weissmann C. The structure of one of the eight or more distinct chromosomal genes for human interferon-alpha. Nature 1980;287:401–408.
9. Goeddel DV, Leung DW, Dull TJ, et al. The structure of eight distinct cloned human leukocyte interferon cDNAs. Nature 1981;290:20–26.
10. Streuli M, Nagata S, Weissmann C. At least three human type alpha interferons: structure of alpha 2. Science 1980; 209: 1343–1347.
11. Jay E, MacKnight D, Lutze-Wallace C, et al. Chemical synthesis of a biologically active gene for human immune interferon-gamma: prospect for site-specific mutagenesis and structure-function studies. J Biol Chem 1984;259:6311–6317.
12. Gray PW, Goeddel DV. Structure of the human immune interferon gene. Nature 1982;298:859–863.
13. Adolf GR. Antigenic structure of human interferon omega 1 (interferon alpha II1): comparison with other human interferons. J Gen Virol 1987;68(Pt 6):1669–1676.
14. Capon DJ, Shepard HM, Goeddel DV. Two distinct families of human and bovine interferon-alpha genes are coordinately expressed and encode functional polypeptides. Mol Cell Biol 1985;5:768–779.
15. Roberts RM, Cross JC, Leaman DW. Unique features of the trophoblast interferons. Pharmacol Ther 1991;51:329–345.
16. Leaman DW, Cross JC, Roberts RM. Multiple regulatory elements are required to direct trophoblast interferon gene expression in choriocarcinoma cells and trophectoderm. Mol Endocrinol 1994; 8:456–468.
17. Liberati AM, Garofani P, De Angelis V, et al. Double-blind randomized phase I study on the clinical tolerance and pharmacodynamics of natural and recombinant interferon-beta given intravenously. J Interferon Res 1994;14:61–69.
18. Lee WM, Reddy KR, Tong MJ, et al. Early hepatitis C virus-RNA responses predict interferon treatment outcomes in chronic hepatitis C. Consensus Interferon Study Group. Hepatology 1998;28:1411–1415.
19. Pockros PJ, Tong M, Lee WM, et al. Relationship between biochemical and virological responses to interferon therapy in chronic hepatitis C infection. Consensus Interferon Study Group. J Viral Hepat 1998;5:271–276.
20. Tong MJ, Blatt LM, Resser KJ, et al. Treatment of chronic hepatitis C virus infection with recombinant consensus interferon. J Interferon Cytokine Res 1998;18:81–86.
21. Hawkins MJ, Levin M, Borden EC. An Eastern Cooperative Oncology Group phase I-II pilot study of polyriboinosinic-polyribocytidylic acid poly-L-lysine complex in patients with metastatic malignant melanoma. J Biol Response Mod 1985;4: 664–668.
22. Litton GJ, Hong R, Grossberg SE, et al. Biological and clinical effects of the oral immunomodulator 3,6-bis(2-piperidinoethoxy)acridine trihydrochloride in patients with malignancy. J Biol Response Mod 1990;9:61–70.
23. Rios A, Stringfellow DA, Fitzpatrick FA, et al. Phase I study of 2-amino-5-bromo-6-phenyl-4(3H)-pyrimidinone (ABPP), an oral interferon inducer, in cancer patients. J Biol Response Mod 1986;5:330–338.
24. Urba WJ, Longo DL, Lombardo FA, et al. Enhancement of natural killer activity in human peripheral blood by flavone acetic acid. J Natl Cancer Inst 1988;80:521–525.
25. Goldstein, D, Hertzog P, Tomkinson E, et al. Administration of imiquimod, an interferon inducer, in asymptomatic human immunodeficiency virus-infected persons to determine safety and biologic response modification. J Infect Dis 1998;178:858–861.
26. Witt PL, Ritch PS, Reding D, et al. Phase I trial of an oral immunomodulator and interferon inducer in cancer patients. Cancer Res 1993;53:5176–5180.
27. Schon MP, Schon M. Immune modulation and apoptosis induction: two sides of the antitumoral activity of imiquimod. Apoptosis 2004;9:291–298.
28. Akira S, Hemmi H. Recognition of pathogen-associated molecular patterns by TLR family. Immunol Lett 2003;85:85–95.
29. Hemmi H, Takeuchi O, Kawai T, et al. A toll-like receptor recognizes bacterial DNA. Nature 2000;408:740–745.
30. Okamoto M, Sato M. Toll-like receptor signaling in anti-cancer immunity. J Med Invest 2003;50:9–24.
31. Darnell JE Jr, Kerr IM, Stark GR. Jak-STAT pathways and transcriptional activation in response to IFNs and other extracellular signaling proteins. Science 1994;264:1415–1421.
32. Stark GR, Kerr IM, Williams BR, et al. How cells respond to interferons. Ann Rev Biochem 1998;67:227–264.
33. Ihle JN. Cytokine receptor signalling. Nature 1995;377: 591–594.
34. Ihle JN. STATs: signal transducers and activators of transcription. Cell 1996;84:331–334.
35. Branca AA, Baglioni C. Evidence that types I and II interferons have different receptors. Nature 1981;294:768–770.
36. Merlin G, Falcoff E, Aguet M. 125I-labelled human interferons alpha, beta and gamma: comparative receptor-binding data. J Gen Virol 1985;66 (Pt 5):1149–1152.
37. Uze G, Lutfalla G, Gresser I. Genetic transfer of a functional human interferon alpha receptor into mouse cells: cloning and expression of its cDNA. Cell 1990;60:225–234.
38. Novick D, Cohen B, Rubinstein M. The human interferon alpha/beta receptor: characterization and molecular cloning. Cell 1994;77:391–400.
39. Domanski P, Witte M, Kellum M, et al. Cloning and expression of a long form of the beta subunit of the interferon alpha beta receptor that is required for signaling. J Biol Chem 1995; 270:21606–21611.
40. Lutfalla G, Gardiner K, Proudhon D, et al. The structure of the human interferon alpha/beta receptor gene. J Biol Chem 1992;267:2802–2809.
41. Colamonici OR, Domanski P. Identification of a novel subunit of the type I interferon receptor localized to human chromosome 21. J Biol Chem 1993;268:10895–10899.
42. Cleary CM, Donnelly RJ, Soh J, et al. Knockout and reconstitution of a functional human type I interferon receptor complex. J Biol Chem 1994;269:18747–18749.
43. Platanias LC, Domanski P, Nadeau OW, et al. Identification of a domain in the beta subunit of the type I interferon (IFN) receptor that exhibits a negative regulatory effect in the growth inhibitory action of type I IFNs. J Biol Chem 1998;273:5577–5581.

44. Aguet M, Dembic Z, Merlin G. Molecular cloning and expression of the human interferon-gamma receptor. Cell 1988; 55:273–280.

45. Soh J, Donnelly RJ, Kotenko S, et al. Identification and sequence of an accessory factor required for activation of the human interferon gamma receptor. Cell 1994;76:793–802.

46. Hemmi, S, Bohni R, Stark G, et al. A novel member of the interferon receptor family complements functionality of the murine interferon gamma receptor in human cells. Cell 1994;76: 803–810.

47. Greenlund AC, Farrar MA, Viviano BL, et al. Ligand-induced IFN gamma receptor tyrosine phosphorylation couples the receptor to its signal transduction system (p91). EMBO J 1994;13:1591–1600.

48. Igarashi K, Garotta G, Ozmen L, et al. Interferon-gamma induces tyrosine phosphorylation of interferon-gamma receptor and regulated association of protein tyrosine kinases, Jak1 and Jak2, with its receptor. J Biol Chem 1994;269: 14333–14336.

49. Muller M, Briscoe J, Laxton C, et al. The protein tyrosine kinase JAK1 complements defects in interferon-alpha/beta and -gamma signal transduction. Nature 1993;366:129–135.

50. Watling D, Guschin D, Muller M, et al. Complementation by the protein tyrosine kinase JAK2 of a mutant cell line defective in the interferon-gamma signal transduction pathway. Nature 1993;366:166–170.

51. Velazquez L, Fellous M, Stark GR, et al. A protein tyrosine kinase in the interferon alpha/beta signaling pathway. Cell 1992;70:313–322.

52. Kisseleva T, Bhattacharya S, Braunstein J, et al. Signaling through the JAK/STAT pathway: recent advances and future challenges. Gene 2002;285:1–24.

53. Schindler C, Fu XY, Improta T, et al. Proteins of transcription factor ISGF-3: one gene encodes the 91-and 84-kDa ISGF-3 proteins that are activated by interferon alpha. Proc Natl Acad Sci USA 1992;89:7836–7839.

54. Muller M, Laxton C, Briscoe J, et al. Complementation of a mutant cell line: central role of the 91 kDa polypeptide of ISGF3 in the interferon-alpha and -gamma signal transduction pathways. EMBO J 1993;12:4221–4228.

55. Leung S, Qureshi SA, Kerr IM, et al. Role of STAT2 in the alpha interferon signaling pathway. Mol Cell Biol 1995;15:1312–1317.

56. Meraz MA, White JM, Sheehan KC, et al. Targeted disruption of the Stat1 gene in mice reveals unexpected physiologic specificity in the JAK-STAT signaling pathway. Cell 1996;84:431–442.

57. Durbin JE, Hackenmiller R, Simon MC, et al. Targeted disruption of the mouse Stat1 gene results in compromised innate immunity to viral disease. Cell 1996;84:443–450.

58. Williams BR. Transcriptional regulation of interferon-stimulated genes. Eur J Biochem 1991;200:1–11.

59. Levy DE, Kessler DS, Pine R, et al. Interferon-induced nuclear factors that bind a shared promoter element correlate with positive and negative transcriptional control. Genes Dev 1988; 2:383–393.

60. Schindler C, Shuai K, Prezioso VR, et al. Interferon-dependent tyrosine phosphorylation of a latent cytoplasmic transcription factor. Science 1992;257:809–813.

61. Adachi M, Fischer EH, Ihle J, et al. Mammalian SH2-containing protein tyrosine phosphatases. Cell 1996;85:15.

62. Jiao H, Berrada K, Yang W, et al. Direct association with and dephosphorylation of Jak2 kinase by the SH2-domain-containing protein tyrosine phosphatase SHP-1. Mol Cell Biol 1996;16:6985–6992.

63. David M, Chen HE, Goelz S, et al. Differential regulation of the alpha/beta interferon-stimulated Jak/Stat pathway by the SH2 domain-containing tyrosine phosphatase SHPTP1. Mol Cell Biol 1995;15:7050–7058.

64. You M, Yu DH, Feng GS. Shp-2 tyrosine phosphatase functions as a negative regulator of the interferon-stimulated Jak/STAT pathway. Mol Cell Biol 1999;19:2416–2424.

65. Igarashi K, David M, Finbloom DS, et al. In vitro activation of the transcription factor gamma interferon activation factor by gamma interferon: evidence for a tyrosine phosphatase/kinase signaling cascade. Mol Cell Biol 1993;13:1634–1640.

66. Wang D, Stravopodis D, Teglund S, et al. Naturally occurring dominant negative variants of Stat5. Mol Cell Biol 1996; 16:6141–6148.

67. Haque SJ, Wu Q, Kammer W, et al. Receptor-associated constitutive protein tyrosine phosphatase activity controls the kinase function of JAK1. Proc Natl Acad Sci USA 1997;94:8563–8568.

68. Yoshimura A. The CIS/JAB family: novel negative regulators of JAK signaling pathways. Leukemia 1998;12:1851–1857.

69. Nicholson SE, Hilton D J. The SOCS proteins: a new family of negative regulators of signal transduction. J Leukoc Biol 1998; 63:665–668.

70. Yasukawa H, Misawa H, Sakamoto H, et al. The JAK-binding protein JAB inhibits Janus tyrosine kinase activity through binding in the activation loop. EMBO J 1999;18:1309–1320.

71. Zhang JG, Farley A, Nicholson SE, et al. The conserved SOCS box motif in suppressors of cytokine signaling binds to elongins B and C and may couple bound proteins to proteasomal degradation. Proc Natl Acad Sci USA 1999;96:2071–2076.

72. Sakamoto H, Yasukawa H, Masuhara M, et al. A Janus kinase inhibitor, JAB, is an interferon-gamma-inducible gene and confers resistance to interferons. Blood 1998;92:1668–1676.

73. Song MM, Shuai K. The suppressor of cytokine signaling (SOCS) 1 and SOCS3 but not SOCS2 proteins inhibit interferon-mediated antiviral and antiproliferative activities. J Biol Chem 1998;273:35056–35062.

74. Petricoin EF 3rd, Ito S, Williams BL, et al. Antiproliferative action of interferon-alpha requires components of T-cell-receptor signalling. Nature 1997;390:629–632.

75. Veals SA, Schindler C, Leonard D, et al. Subunit of an alpha-interferon-responsive transcription factor is related to interferon regulatory factor and Myb families of DNA-binding proteins. Mol Cell Biol 1992;12:3315–3324.

76. Miyamoto M, Fujita T, Kimura Y, et al. Regulated expression of a gene encoding a nuclear factor, IRF-1, that specifically binds to IFN-beta gene regulatory elements. Cell 1988;54:903–913.

77. Harada H, Fujita T, Miyamoto M, et al. Structurally similar but functionally distinct factors, IRF-1 and IRF-2, bind to the same regulatory elements of IFN and IFN-inducible genes. Cell 1989;58:729–739.

78. Fujita T, Kimura Y, Miyamoto M, et al. Induction of endogenous IFN-alpha and IFN-beta genes by a regulatory transcription factor, IRF-1. Nature 1989;337:270–272.

79. Harada H, Willison K, Sakakibara J, et al. Absence of the type I IFN system in EC cells: transcriptional activator (IRF-1) and repressor (IRF-2) genes are developmentally regulated. Cell 1990;63:303–312.

80. Harada H, Kitagawa M, Tanaka N, et al. Anti-oncogenic and oncogenic potentials of interferon regulatory factors-1 and -2. Science 1993;259:971–974.

81. Matsuyama, T, Kimura T, Kitagawa M, et al. Targeted disruption of IRF-1 or IRF-2 results in abnormal type I IFN gene induction and aberrant lymphocyte development. Cell 1993;75:83–97.

82. Driggers PH, Ennist DL, Gleason S L, et al. An interferon gamma-regulated protein that binds the interferon-inducible enhancer element of major histocompatibility complex class I genes. Proc Natl Acad Sci USA 1990;87:3743–3747.

83. Politis AD, Sivo J, Driggers PH, et al. Modulation of interferon consensus sequence binding protein mRNA in murine peritoneal macrophages: induction by IFN-gamma and down-regulation by IFN-alpha, dexamethasone, and protein kinase inhibitors. J Immunol 1992;148:801–807.

84. Shuai K. Modulation of STAT signaling by STAT-interacting proteins. Oncogene 2000;19:2638–2644.

85. Gutterman JU. Cytokine therapeutics: lessons from interferon alpha. Proc Natl Acad Sci USA 1994;91:1198–1205.

86. Heyman M, Nordgren A, Jeddi-Tehrani M, et al. A T cell lymphoblastic lymphoma patient with two malignant cell populations carrying different 9p deletions including the p16INK4 and p15INK4B genes: clinical response to interferon-alpha therapy in one of the subclones. Leukemia 1996;10:909–917.

87. Colamonici OR, Uyttendaele H, Domanski P, et al. p135tyk2, an interferon-alpha-activated tyrosine kinase, is physically associated with an interferon-alpha receptor. J Biol Chem 1994;269:3518–3522.

88. Rosenblum MG, Maxwell BL, Talpaz M, et al. In vivo sensitivity and resistance of chronic myelogenous leukemia cells to alpha-interferon: correlation with receptor binding and induction of 2′,5′-oligoadenylate synthetase. Cancer Res 1986;46: 4848–4852.

89. Sun WH, Pabon C, Alsayed Y, et al. Interferon-alpha resistance in a cutaneous T-cell lymphoma cell line is associated with lack of STAT1 expression. Blood 1998;91:570–576.

90. Brinckmann A, Axer S, Jakschies D, et al. Interferon-alpha resistance in renal carcinoma cells is associated with defective induction of signal transducer and activator of transcription 1 which can be restored by a supernatant of phorbol 12-myristate 13-acetate stimulated peripheral blood mononuclear cells. Br J Cancer 2002;86:449–455.

91. Yi TL, Cleveland JL, Ihle JN. Protein tyrosine phosphatase containing SH2 domains: characterization, preferential expression in hematopoietic cells, and localization to human chromosome 12p12-p13. Mol Cell Biol 1992;12:836–846.

92. Komuro H, Valentine MB, Rubnitz JE, et al. p27KIP1 deletions in childhood acute lymphoblastic leukemia. Neoplasia 1999; 1:253–261.

93. Kanda K, Decker T, Aman P, et al. The EBNA2-related resistance towards alpha interferon (IFN-alpha) in Burkitt's lymphoma cells effects induction of IFN-induced genes but not the activation of transcription factor ISGF-3. Mol Cell Biol 1992; 12:4930–4936.

94. Der SD, Zhou A, Williams BR, et al. Identification of genes differentially regulated by interferon alpha, beta, or gamma using oligonucleotide arrays. Proc Natl Acad Sci USA 1998;95: 15623–15628.

95. Tracey L, Villuendas R, Ortiz P, et al. Identification of genes involved in resistance to interferon-alpha in cutaneous T-cell lymphoma. Am J Pathol 2002;161:1825–1837.

96. Sangfelt O, Osterborg A, Grander D, et al. Response to interferon therapy in patients with multiple myeloma correlates with expression of the Bcl-2 oncoprotein. Int J Cancer 1995; 63:190–192.

97. Sangfelt O, Erickson S, Castro J, et al. Induction of apoptosis and inhibition of cell growth are independent responses to interferon-alpha in hematopoietic cell lines. Cell Growth Diff 1997;8:343–352.

98. Foster GR, Ackrill AM, Goldin RD, et al. Expression of the terminal protein region of hepatitis B virus inhibits cellular responses to interferons alpha and gamma and double-stranded RNA. Proc Natl Acad Sci USA 1991;88:2888–2892.

99. Reich N, Pine R, Levy D, et al. Transcription of interferon-stimulated genes is induced by adenovirus particles but is suppressed by E1A gene products. J Virology 1988;62:114–119.

100. Folkman J, Klagsbrun M. Angiogenic factors. Science 1987; 235:442–447.

101. Dvorak HF, Gresser I. Microvascular injury in pathogenesis of interferon-induced necrosis of subcutaneous tumors in mice. J Natl Cancer Inst 1989;81:497–502.

102. Sidky YA, Borden EC. Inhibition of angiogenesis by interferons: effects on tumor- and lymphocyte-induced vascular responses. Cancer Res 1987;47:5155–5161.

103. Dinney CP, Bielenberg DR, Perrotte P, et al. Inhibition of basic fibroblast growth factor expression, angiogenesis, and growth of human bladder carcinoma in mice by systemic interferon-alpha administration. Cancer Res 1998;58:808–814.

104. Singh RK, Gutman M, Bucana CD, et al. Interferons alpha and beta down-regulate the expression of basic fibroblast growth factor in human carcinomas. Proc Natl Acad Sci USA 1995; 92:4562–4566.

105. Huang S, Bucana CD, Van Arsdall M, et al. Stat1 negatively regulates angiogenesis, tumorigenicity and metastasis of tumor cells. Oncogene 2002;21:2504–2512.

106. von Marschall Z, Scholz A, Cramer T, et al. Effects of interferon alpha on vascular endothelial growth factor gene transcription and tumor angiogenesis. J Natl Cancer Inst 2003;95:437–448.

107. Koch AE, Polverini PJ, Kunkel SL, et al. Interleukin-8 as a macrophage-derived mediator of angiogenesis. Science 1992; 258:1798–1801.

108. Arenberg DA, Kunkel SL, Polverini PJ, et al. Inhibition of interleukin-8 reduces tumorigenesis of human non-small cell lung cancer in SCID mice. J Clin Invest 1996;97:2792–2802.

109. Reznikov LL, Puren AJ, Fantuzzi G, et al. Spontaneous and inducible cytokine responses in healthy humans receiving a single dose of IFN-alpha2b: increased production of interleukin-1 receptor antagonist and suppression of IL-1-induced IL-8. J Interferon Cytokine Res 1998;18:897–903.

110. Singh RK, Gutman M, Llansa N, et al. Interferon-beta prevents the upregulation of interleukin-8 expression in human melanoma cells. J Interferon Cytokine Res 1996;16:577–584.

111. Strieter RM, Polverini PJ, Kunkel SL, et al. The functional role of the ELR motif in CXC chemokine-mediated angiogenesis. J Biol Chem 1995;270:27348–27357.

112. Cheng YS, Patterson CE, Staeheli P. Interferon-induced guanylate-binding proteins lack an N(T)KXD consensus motif and bind GMP in addition to GDP and GTP. Mol Cell Biol 1991;11: 4717–4725.

113. Schwemmle M, Staeheli P. The interferon-induced 67-kDa guanylate-binding protein (hGBP1) is a GTPase that converts GTP to GMP. J Biol Chem 1994;269:11299–11305.

114. Nguyen TT, Hu Y, Widney DP, et al. Murine GBP-5, a new member of the murine guanylate-binding protein family, is coordinately regulated with other GBPs in vivo and in vitro. J Interferon Cytokine Res 2002;22:899–909.

115. Guenzi E, Topolt K, Cornali E, et al. The helical domain of GBP-1 mediates the inhibition of endothelial cell proliferation by inflammatory cytokines. EMBO J 2001;20:5568–5577.

116. Guenzi E, Topolt K, Lubeseder-Martellato C, et al. The guanylate binding protein-1 GTPase controls the invasive and angiogenic capability of endothelial cells through inhibition of MMP-1 expression. EMBO J 2003;22:3772–3782.

117. Gilly M, Wall R. The IRG-47 gene is IFN-gamma induced in B cells and encodes a protein with GTP-binding motifs. J Immunol 1992;148:3275–3281.

118. Sorace JM, Johnson RJ, Howard DL, et al. Identification of an endotoxin and IFN-inducible cDNA: possible identification of a novel protein family. J Leukoc Biol 1995;58:477–484.

119. Carlow DA, Marth J, Clark-Lewis I, et al. Isolation of a gene encoding a developmentally regulated T cell-specific protein with a guanine nucleotide triphosphate-binding motif. J Immunol 1995;154:1724–1734.

120. Lafuse WP, Brown D, Castle L, et al. Cloning and characterization of a novel cDNA that is IFN-gamma-induced in mouse peritoneal macrophages and encodes a putative GTP-binding protein. J Leukoc Biol 1995;57:477–483.

121. Taylor GA, Jeffers M, Largaespada DA, et al. Identification of a novel GTPase, the inducibly expressed GTPase, that accumulates in response to interferon gamma. J Biol Chem 1996; 271:20399–20405.

122. MacMicking JD, Taylor GA, McKinney JD. Immune control of tuberculosis by IFN-gamma-inducible LRG-47. Science 2003; 302:654–659.

123. Taylor GA, Stauber R, Rulong S, et al. The inducibly expressed GTPase localizes to the endoplasmic reticulum, independently of GTP binding. J Biol Chem 1997;272:10639–10645.

124. Chang E, Boyd A, Nelson CC, et al. Successful treatment of infantile hemangiomas with interferon-alpha-2b. J Pediatr Hematol Oncol 1997;19:237–244.

125. Niemela M, Maenpaa H, Salven P, et al. Interferon alpha-2a therapy in 18 hemangioblastomas. Clin Cancer Res 2001;7:510–516.

126. Kaban LB, Mulliken JB, Ezekowitz RA, et al. Antiangiogenic therapy of a recurrent giant cell tumor of the mandible with interferon alfa-2a. Pediatrics 1999;103:1145–1149.

127. Krown SE, Li P, Von Roenn JH, et al. Efficacy of low-dose interferon with antiretroviral therapy in Kaposi's sarcoma: a randomized phase II AIDS Clinical Trials Group study. J Interferon Cytokine Res 2002;22:295–303.

128. Folkman J, Hanahan D. Switch to the angiogenic phenotype during tumorigenesis. Princess Takamatsu Symp 1991;22:339–347.

129. McCarty MF, Bielenberg D, Donawho C, et al. Evidence for the causal role of endogenous interferon-alpha/beta in the regulation of angiogenesis, tumorigenicity, and metastasis of cutaneous neoplasms. Clin Exp Metastasis 2002;19:609–615.

130. von Hoegen P. Synergistic role of type I interferons in the induction of protective cytotoxic T lymphocytes. Immunol Lett 1995;47:157–162.

131. McAdam AJ, Pulaski BA, Storozynsky E, et al. Analysis of the effect of cytokines (interleukins 2, 3, 4, and 6, granulocyte-monocyte colony-stimulating factor, and interferon-gamma) on generation of primary cytotoxic T lymphocytes against a weakly immunogenic tumor. Cell Immunol 1995;165:183–192.

132. Zarling JM, Eskra L, Borden EC, et al. Activation of human natural killer cells cytotoxic for human leukemia cells by purified interferon. J Immunol 1979;123:63–70.

133. Pace JL, Russell SW, Torres BA, et al. Recombinant mouse gamma interferon induces the priming step in macrophage activation for tumor cell killing. J Immunol 1983;130: 2011–2013.

134. Luft T, Pang KC, Thomas E, et al. Type I IFNs enhance the terminal differentiation of dendritic cells. J Immunol 1998; 161:1947–1953.

135. Siegel JP. Effects of interferon-gamma on the activation of human T lymphocytes. Cell Immunol 1988;111:461–472.

136. Edwards BS, Hawkins MJ, Borden EC. Comparative in vivo and in vitro activation of human natural killer cells by two recombinant alpha-interferons differing in antiviral activity. Cancer Res 1984;44:3135–3139.

137. Sato K, Hida S, Takayanagi H, et al. Antiviral response by natural killer cells through TRAIL gene induction by IFN-alpha/ beta. Eur J Immunol 2001;31:3138–3146.

138. Gresser I, Belardelli F, Maury C, et al. Injection of mice with antibody to interferon enhances the growth of transplantable murine tumors. J Exp Med 1983;158:2095–2107.

139. Boehm U, Klamp T, Groot M, et al. Cellular responses to interferon-gamma. Annu Rev Immunol 1997;15:749–795.

140. Pamer E, Cresswell P. Mechanisms of MHC class I-restricted antigen processing. Annu Rev Immunol 1998;16:323–358.

141. Samuel CE.. Antiviral actions of interferons. Clin Microbiol Rev 2001;14:778–809.

142. Rock KL, York IA, Saric T, et al. Protein degradation and the generation of MHC class I-presented peptides. Adv Immunol 2002;80:1–70.

143. Min W, Pober JS, Johnson DR. Kinetically coordinated induction of TAP1 and HLA class I by IFN-gamma: the rapid induction of TAP1 by IFN-gamma is mediated by Stat1 alpha. J Immunol 1996;156:3174–3183.

144. Rock KL, Gramm C, Rothstein L, et al. Inhibitors of the proteasome block the degradation of most cell proteins and the generation of peptides presented on MHC class I molecules. Cell 1994;78:761–771.

145. Nandi D, Jiang H, Monaco JJ. Identification of MECL-1 (LMP-10) as the third IFN-gamma-inducible proteasome subunit. J Immunol 1996;156:2361–2364.

146. Foss GS, Larsen F, Solheim J, et al. Constitutive and interferon-gamma-induced expression of the human proteasome subunit multicatalytic endopeptidase complex-like 1. Biochim Biophys Acta 1998;1402:17–28.

147. Ma W, Lehner PJ, Cresswell P, et al. Interferon-gamma rapidly increases peptide transporter (TAP) subunit expression and peptide transport capacity in endothelial cells. J Biol Chem 1997;272:16585–16590.

148. Benham A, Tulp A, Neefjes J. Synthesis and assembly of MHC-peptide complexes. Immunol Today 1995;16:359–362.

149. Steimle V, Siegrist CA, Mottet A, et al. Regulation of MHC class II expression by interferon-gamma mediated by the transactivator gene CIITA. Science 1994;265:106–109.

150. Watts C. Capture and processing of exogenous antigens for presentation on MHC molecules. Annu Rev Immunol 1997;15: 821–850.

151. Sivinski CL, Lindner DJ, Borden EC, et al. Modulation of tumor-associated antigen expression on human pancreatic and prostate carcinoma cells in vitro by α- and β-interferons. J Immunother Emphasis Tumor Immunol 1995;18:156–165.

152. Roselli M, Guadagni F, Buonomo O, et al. Systemic administration of recombinant interferon alpha in carcinoma patients upregulates the expression of the carcinoma-associated antigens tumor-associated glycoprotein-72 and carcinoembryonic antigen. J Clin Oncol 1996;14:2031–2042.

153. Daeron M. Fc receptor biology. Annu Rev Immunol 1997; 15:203–234.

154. Xie K, Fidler IJ. Therapy of cancer metastasis by activation of the inducible nitric oxide synthase. Cancer Metastasis Rev 1998;17: 55–75.

155. Marfaing-Koka A, Devergne O, Gorgone G, et al. Regulation of the production of the RANTES chemokine by endothelial cells: synergistic induction by IFN-gamma plus TNF-alpha and inhibition by IL-4 and IL-13. J Immunol 1995;154:1870–1878.

156. Taub DD, Lloyd AR, Conlon K, et al. Recombinant human interferon-inducible protein 10 is a chemoattractant for human monocytes and T lymphocytes and promotes T cell adhesion to endothelial cells. J Exp Med 1993;177:1809–1814.

157. Rollins BJ, Yoshimura T, Leonard EJ, et al. Cytokine-activated human endothelial cells synthesize and secrete a monocyte chemoattractant, MCP-1/JE. Am J Pathol 1990;136:1229–1233.

158. Liao F, Rabin RL, Yannelli JR, et al. Human Mig chemokine: biochemical and functional characterization. J Exp Med 1995; 182:1301–1314.

159. Cole KE, Strick CA, Paradis TJ, et al. Interferon-inducible T cell alpha chemoattractant (I-TAC): a novel non-ELR CXC chemokine with potent activity on activated T cells through selective high affinity binding to CXCR3. J Exp Med 1998; 187:2009–2021.

160. Clemens MJ. Targets and mechanisms for the regulation of translation in malignant transformation. Oncogene 2004; 23:3180–3188.

161. Leaman DW, Chawla-Sarkar M, Jacobs B, et al. Novel growth and death related interferon-stimulated genes (ISGs) in melanoma: greater potency of IFN-beta compared with IFN-alpha2. J Interferon Cytokine Res 2003;23:745–756.

162. Patel RC, Sen GC. PACT, a protein activator of the interferon-induced protein kinase, PKR. EMBO J 1998;17:4379–4390.

163. Hovanessian AG. Interferon-induced and double-stranded RNA-activated enzymes: a specific protein kinase and 2′,5′-oligoadenylate synthetases. J Interferon Res 1991;11:199–205.

164. Silverman RH. Implications for RNase L in prostate cancer biology. Biochemistry 2003;42:1805–1812.

165. Xiang Y, Wang Z, Murakami J, et al. Effects of RNase L mutations associated with prostate cancer on apoptosis induced by 2′,5′-oligoadenylates. Cancer Res 2003;63:6795–6801.

166. Obar RA, Collins CA, Hammarback JA, et al. Molecular cloning of the microtubule-associated mechanochemical enzyme dynamin reveals homology with a new family of GTP-binding proteins. Nature 1990;347:256–261.

167. Arnheiter H, Frese M, Kambadur R, et al. Mx transgenic mice: animal models of health. Curr Top Microbiol Immunol 1996; 206:119–147.

168. Asefa B, Klarmann KD, Copeland NG, et al. The interferon-inducible p200 family of proteins: a perspective on their roles in cell cycle regulation and differentiation. Blood Cells Mol Dis 2004;32:155–167.

169. Choubey D, Lengyel P. Binding of an interferon-inducible protein (p202) to the retinoblastoma protein. J Biol Chem 1995;270:6134–6140.

170. Datta B, Li B, Choubey D, et al. p202, an interferon-inducible modulator of transcription, inhibits transcriptional activation by the p53 tumor suppressor protein, and a segment from the p53-binding protein 1 that binds to p202 overcomes this inhibition. J Biol Chem 1996;271:27544–27555.

171. Choubey D, Li SJ, Datta B, et al. Inhibition of E2F-mediated transcription by p202. EMBO J 1996;15:5668–5678.

172. Choubey D, Gutterman JU. Inhibition of E2F-4/DP-1-stimulated transcription by p202. Oncogene 1997;15:291–301.

173. Yan DH, Wen Y, Spohn B, et al. Reduced growth rate and transformation phenotype of the prostate cancer cells by an interferon-inducible protein, p202. Oncogene 1999;18:807–811.

174. Wen Y, Yan DH, Spohn B, et al. Tumor suppression and sensitization to tumor necrosis factor alpha-induced apoptosis by an interferon-inducible protein, p202, in breast cancer cells. Cancer Res 2000;60:42–46.

175. Borden KL. Pondering the promyelocytic leukemia protein (PML) puzzle: possible functions for PML nuclear bodies. Mol Cell Biol 2002;22:5259–5269.

176. Regad T, Chelbi-Alix MK. Role and fate of PML nuclear bodies in response to interferon and viral infections. Oncogene 2001;20:7274–7286.

177. Wang ZG, Ruggero D, Ronchetti S, et al. PML is essential for multiple apoptotic pathways. Nat Genet 1998;20:266–272.

178. Subramaniam PS, Cruz PE, Hobeika AC, et al. Type I interferon induction of the Cdk-inhibitor p21WAF1 is accompanied by ordered G1 arrest, differentiation and apoptosis of the Daudi B-cell line. Oncogene 1998;16:1885–1890.

179. Tiefenbrun N, Melamed D, Levy N, et al. Alpha interferon suppresses the cyclin D3 and cdc25A genes, leading to a reversible G0-like arrest. Mol Cell Biol 1996;16:3934–3944.

180. Kumar R, Atlas I. Interferon alpha induces the expression of retinoblastoma gene product in human Burkitt lymphoma Daudi cells: role in growth regulation. Proc Natl Acad Sci USA 1992;89:6599–6603.

181. Balkwill F, Taylor-Papadimitriou J. Interferon affects both G1 and S+G2 in cells stimulated from quiescence to growth. Nature 1978;274:798–800.

182. Sangfelt O, Erickson S, Castro J, et al. Molecular mechanisms underlying interferon-alpha-induced G0/G1 arrest: CKI-mediated regulation of G1 Cdk-complexes and activation of pocket proteins. Oncogene 1999;18:2798–2810.

183. Chawla-Sarkar M, Lindner DJ, Liu YF, et al. Apoptosis and interferons: role of interferon-stimulated genes as mediators of apoptosis [review]. Apoptosis 2003;8:237–249.

184. Selleri C, Sato T, Del Vecchio L, et al. Involvement of Fas-mediated apoptosis in the inhibitory effects of interferon-alpha in chronic myelogenous leukemia. Blood 1997;89:957–964.

185. Spets H, Georgii-Hemming P, Siljason J, et al. Fas/APO-1 (CD95)-mediated apoptosis is activated by interferon-gamma and interferon-alpha in interleukin-6 (IL-6)-dependent and IL-6-independent multiple myeloma cell lines. Blood 1998;92:2914–2923.

186. Buechner SA, Wernli M, Harr T, et al. Regression of basal cell carcinoma by intralesional interferon-alpha treatment is mediated by CD95 (Apo-1/Fas)-CD95 ligand-induced suicide. J Clin Invest 1997;100:2691–2696.

187. Ahn EY, Pan G, Vickers SM, et al. IFN-gamma upregulates apoptosis-related molecules and enhances Fas-mediated apoptosis in human cholangiocarcinoma. Int J Cancer 2002;100: 445–451.

188. Ugurel S, Seiter S, Rappl G, et al. Heterogenous susceptibility to CD95-induced apoptosis in melanoma cells correlates with bcl-2 and bcl-x expression and is sensitive to modulation by interferon-gamma. Int J Cancer 1999;82:727–736.

189. Chawla-Sarkar M, Leaman DW, Borden EC. Preferential induction of apoptosis by interferon (IFN)-beta compared with IFN-alpha2: correlation with TRAIL/Apo2l induction in melanoma cell lines. Clin Cancer Res 2001;7:1821–1831.

190. Chen Q, Gong B, Mahmoud-Ahmed AS, et al. Apo2L/TRAIL and Bcl-2-related proteins regulate type I interferon-induced apoptosis in multiple myeloma. Blood 2001;98:2183–2192.

191. Clarke N, Jimenez-Lara AM, Voltz E, et al. Tumor suppressor IRF-1 mediates retinoid and interferon anticancer signaling to death ligand TRAIL. EMBO J 2004;23:3051–3060.

192. Leaman DW, Chawla-Sarkar M, Vyas K, et al. Identification of X-linked inhibitor of apoptosis-associated factor-1 as an interferon-stimulated gene that augments TRAIL Apo2L-induced apoptosis. J Biol Chem 2002;277:28504–28511.

193. Liston P, Fong WG, Kelly NL, et al. Identification of XAF1 as an antagonist of XIAP anti-caspase activity. Nat Cell Biol 2001;3:128–133.

194. Deveraux QL, Takahashi R, Salvesen GS, et al. X-linked IAP is a direct inhibitor of cell-death proteases. Nature 1997;388: 300–304.

195. Earnshaw WC, Martins LM, Kaufmann SH. Mammalian caspases: structure, activation, substrates, and functions during apoptosis. Annu Rev Biochem 1999;68:383–424.

196. Ashkenazi A, Dixit VM. Death receptors: signaling and modulation. Science 1998;281:1305–1308.

197. Thornberry NA, Lazebnik Y. Caspases: enemies within. Science 1998;281:1312–1316.

198. Ruiz de Almodovar C, Lopez-Rivas A, Ruiz-Ruiz C.. Interferon-gamma and TRAIL in human breast tumor cells. Vitam Horm 2004;67:291–318.

199. Ruiz-Ruiz C, Ruiz de Almodovar C, Rodriguez A, et al. The up-regulation of human caspase-8 by interferon-gamma in breast tumor cells requires the induction and action of the transcription factor interferon regulatory factor-1. J Biol Chem 2004; 279:19712–19720.

200. Choi C, Jeong E, Benveniste EN. Caspase-1 mediates Fas-induced apoptosis and is up-regulated by interferon-gamma in human astrocytoma cells. J Neurooncol 2004;67:167–176.

201. Geller J, Petak I, Szucs KS, et al. Interferon-gamma-induced sensitization of colon carcinomas to ZD9331 targets caspases, downstream of Fas, independent of mitochondrial signaling and the inhibitor of apoptosis survivin. Clin Cancer Res 2003; 9:6504–6515.

202. de Veer MJ, Holko M, Frevel M, et al. Functional classification of interferon-stimulated genes identified using microarrays. J Leukoc Biol 2001;69:912–920.

203. Burchert A, Cai D, Hofbauer LC, et al. Interferon consensus sequence binding protein (ICSBP; IRF-8) antagonizes BCR/ABL and down-regulates bcl-2. Blood 2004;103:3480–3489.

204. Barnes BJ, Kellum MJ, Pinder KE, et al. Interferon regulatory factor 5, a novel mediator of cell cycle arrest and cell death. Cancer Res 2003;63:6424–6431.

205. Morrison BH, Bauer JA, Kalvakolanu DV, et al. Inositol hexakisphosphate kinase 2 mediates growth suppressive and apoptotic effects of interferon-β in ovarian carcinoma cells. J Biol Chem 2001;276:24965–24970.

206. Morrison BH, Bauer JA, Hu J, et al. Inositol hexakisphosphate kinase 2 sensitizes ovarian carcinoma cells to multiple cancer therapeutics. Oncogene 2002;21:1882–1889.

207. Ben-Efraim I, Zhou Q, Wiedmer T, et al. Phospholipid scramblase 1 is imported into the nucleus by a receptor-mediated pathway and interacts with DNA. Biochemistry 2004;43: 3518–3526.

208. Zhou Q, Zhao J, Wiedmer T, et al. Normal hemostasis but defective hematopoietic response to growth factors in mice deficient in phospholipid scramblase 1. Blood 2002;99:4030–4038.

209. Zhou Q, Zhao J, Al-Zoghaibi F, et al. Transcriptional control of the human plasma membrane phospholipid scramblase 1 gene is mediated by interferon-alpha. Blood 2000;95:2593–2599.

210. Sun J, Nanjundan M, Pike LJ, et al. Plasma membrane phospholipid scramblase 1 is enriched in lipid rafts and interacts with the epidermal growth factor receptor. Biochemistry 2002; 41:6338–6345.

211. Sun J, Zhao J, Schwartz MA, et al. c-Abl tyrosine kinase binds and phosphorylates phospholipid scramblase 1. J Biol Chem 2001;276:28984–28990.

212. Fadok VA, Bratton DL, Henson PM.. Phagocyte receptors for apoptotic cells: recognition, uptake, and consequences. J Clin Invest 2001;108:957–962.

213. Fadok VA, Xue D, Henson P. If phosphatidylserine is the death knell, a new phosphatidylserine-specific receptor is the bell-ringer. Cell Death Differ 2001;8:582–587.

214. Frasch SC, Henson PM, Kailey JM, et al. Regulation of phospholipid scramblase activity during apoptosis and cell activation by protein kinase Cdelta. J Biol Chem 2000;275: 23065–23073.

215. Silverman RH, Halloum A, Zhou A, et al. Suppression of ovarian carcinoma cell growth in vivo by the interferon-inducible plasma membrane protein, phospholipid scramblase 1. Cancer Res 2002;62:397–402.

216. Deiss LP, Feinstein E, Berissi H, et al. Identification of a novel serine/threonine kinase and a novel 15-kd protein as potential mediators of the gamma interferon-induced cell death. Genes Develop 1995;9:15–30.

217. Inbal B, Bialik S, Sabanay I, et al. DAP kinase and DRP-1 mediate membrane blebbing and the formation of autophagic vesicles during programmed cell death. J Cell Biol 2002;157:455–468.

218. Inbal B, Cohen O, Polak-Charcon S, et al. DAP kinase links the control of apoptosis to metastasis. Nature 1997;390:180–184.

219. Esteller M, Corn PG, Baylin SB, et al. A gene hypermethylation profile of human cancer. Cancer Res 2001;61:3225–3229.

220. Burch LR, Scott M, Pohler E, et al. Phage-peptide display identifies the interferon-responsive, death-activated protein kinase family as a novel modifier of MDM2 and p21WAF1. J Mol Biol 2004;337:115–128.

221. Yang JL, Qu XJ, Russell PJ, et al. Regulation of epidermal growth factor receptor in human colon cancer cell lines by interferon alpha. Gut 2004;53:123–129.

222. Caraglia M, Tagliaferri P, Marra M, et al. EGF activates an inducible survival response via the RAS-> Erk-1/2 pathway to counteract interferon-alpha-mediated apoptosis in epidermoid cancer cells. Cell Death Differ 2003;10:218–229.

223. Wills RJ. Clinical pharmacokinetics of interferons. Clin Pharmacokinet 1990;19:390–399.

224. Khurshudian AV. A pilot study to test the efficacy of oral administration of interferon-alpha lozenges to patients with Sjogren's syndrome. Oral Surg Oral Med Oral Pathol Oral Radiol Endod 2003;95:38–44.

225. Ship JA, Fox PC, Michalek JE, et al. Treatment of primary Sjogren's syndrome with low-dose natural human interferon-alpha administered by the oral mucosal route: a phase II clinical trial. IFN Protocol Study Group. J Interferon Cytokine Res 1999;19:943–951.

226. Lecciones JA, Abejar NH, Dimaano EE, et al. A pilot double-blind, randomized, and placebo-controlled study of orally administered IFN-alpha-n1 (Ins) in pediatric patients with measles. J Interferon Cytokine Res 1998;18:647–652.

227. Fleischmann WR Jr, Masoor J, Wu TY, et al. Orally administered IFN-alpha acts alone and in synergistic combination with intraperitoneally administered IFN-gamma to exert an antitumor effect against B16 melanoma in mice. J Interferon Cytokine Res 1998;18:17–20.

228. Dhingra K, Duvic M, Hymes S, et al. A phase-I clinical study of low-dose oral interferon-alpha. J Immunother 1993;14:51–55.

229. Kirkwood JM, Manola J, Ibrahim J, et al. A pooled analysis of Eastern Cooperative Oncology Group and intergroup trials of adjuvant high-dose interferon for melanoma. Clin Cancer Res 2004;10:1670–1677.

230. Tagliaferri P, Caraglia M, Budillon A, et al. New pharmacokinetic and pharmacodynamic tools for interferon-alpha (IFN-alpha) treatment of human cancer. Cancer Immunol Immunother 2004.

231. Bailon P, Palleroni A, Schaffer CA, et al. Rational design of a potent, long-lasting form of interferon: a 40 kDa branched polyethylene glycol-conjugated interferon alpha-2a for the treatment of hepatitis C. Bioconjug Chem 2001;12:195–202.

232. Karnam US, Reddy KR. Pegylated interferons. Clin Liver Dis 2003;7:139–148.

233. Zeuzem S, Welsch C, Herrmann E. Pharmacokinetics of peginterferons. Semin Liver Dis 2003;23(Suppl 1):23–28.

234. Glue P, Fang JW, Rouzier-Panis R, et al. Pegylated interferon-alpha2b: pharmacokinetics, pharmacodynamics, safety, and preliminary efficacy data. Hepatitis C Intervention Therapy Group. Clin Pharmacol Ther 2000;68:556–567.

235. Talpaz M, O'Brien S, Rose E, et al. Phase 1 study of polyethylene glycol formulation of interferon alpha-2B (Schering 54031) in Philadelphia chromosome-positive chronic myelogenous leukemia. Blood 2001;98:1708–1713.

236. Thompson JA, Cox WW, Lindgren CG, et al. Subcutaneous recombinant gamma interferon in cancer patients: toxicity, pharmacokinetics, and immunomodulatory effects. Cancer Immunol Immunother 1987;25:47–53.

237. Michallet M, Maloisel F, Delain M, et al. Pegylated recombinant interferon alpha-2b vs recombinant interferon alpha-2b for the initial treatment of chronic-phase chronic myelogenous leukemia: a phase III study. Leukemia 2004;18:309–315.

238. Bukowski R, Ernstoff MS, Gore ME, et al. Pegylated interferon alfa-2b treatment for patients with solid tumors: a phase I/II study. J Clin Oncol 2002;20:3841–3849.

239. Motzer RJ, Rakhit A, Thompson J, et al. Phase II trial of branched peginterferon-alpha 2a (40 kDa) for patients with advanced renal cell carcinoma. Ann Oncol 2002;13: 1799–1805.

240. Eid P, Meritet JF, Maury C, et al. Oromucosal interferon therapy: pharmacokinetics and pharmacodynamics. J Interferon Cytokine Res 1999;19:157–169.

241. Masci P, Bukowski RM, Patten PA, et al. New and modified interferon alphas: preclinical and clinical data. Curr Oncol Rep 2003;5:108–113.

242. Goldstein D, Sielaff KM, Storer BE, et al. Human biologic response modification by interferon in the absence of measurable serum concentrations: a comparative trial of subcutaneous and intravenous interferon-beta serine. J Natl Cancer Inst 1989;81:1061–1068.

243. Polman C, Barkhof F, Kappos L, et al. Oral interferon beta-1a in relapsing-remitting multiple sclerosis: a double-blind randomized study. Mult Scler 2003;9:342–348.

244. Borden EC. Effects of interferons in neoplastic diseases of man. Pharmacol Ther 1988;37:213–229.

245. Johns TG, Mackay IR, Callister KA, et al. Antiproliferative potencies of interferons on melanoma cell lines and xenografts: higher efficacy of interferon beta. J Natl Cancer Inst 1992; 84:1185–1190.

246. Abdi EA, Kamitomo VJ, McPherson TA, et al. Extended phase I study of human beta-interferon in human cancer. Clin Invest Med 1986;9:33–40.

247. Rinehart JJ, Young D, Laforge J, et al. Phase I/II trial of interferon-beta-serine in patients with renal cell carcinoma: immunological and biological effects. Cancer Res 1987; 47:2481–2485.

248. Ravandi F, Estrov Z, Kurzrock R, et al. A phase I study of recombinant interferon-beta in patients with advanced malignant disease. Clin Cancer Res 1999;5:3990–3998.

249. Sung C, Nardelli B, LaFleur DW, et al. An IFN-beta-albumin fusion protein that displays improved pharmacokinetic and pharmacodynamic properties in nonhuman primates. J Interferon Cytokine Res 2003;23:25–36.

250. McKenna SD, Vergilis K, Arulanandam AR, et al. Formation of human IFN-beta complex with the soluble type I interferon receptor IFNAR-2 leads to enhanced IFN stability, pharmacokinetics, and antitumor activity in xenografted SCID mice. J Interferon Cytokine Res 2004;24:119–129.

251. Pepinsky RB, LePage DJ, Gill A, et al. Improved pharmacokinetic properties of a polyethylene glycol-modified form of interferon-beta-1a with preserved in vitro bioactivity. J Pharmacol Exp Ther 2001;297:1059–1066.

252. Schwartzberg LS, Petak I, Stewart C, et al. Modulation of the Fas signaling pathway by IFN-gamma in therapy of colon cancer: phase I trial and correlative studies of IFN-gamma, 5-fluorouracil, and leucovorin. Clin Cancer Res 2002;8:2488–2498.

253. Kita Y, Rohde MF, Arakawa T, et al. Characterization of a polyethylene glycol conjugate of recombinant human interferon-gamma. Drug Des Deliv 1990;6:157–167.

254. Osborn BL, Olsen HS, Nardelli B, et al. Pharmacokinetic and pharmacodynamic studies of a human serum albumin-interferon-alpha fusion protein in cynomolgus monkeys. J Pharmacol Exp Ther 2002;303:540–548.

255. Kurtzman AL, Govindarajan S, Vahle K, et al. Advances in directed protein evolution by recursive genetic recombination: applications to therapeutic proteins. Curr Opin Biotechnol 2001;12:361–370.

256. Borden EC, Parkinson D. A perspective on the clinical effectiveness and tolerance of interferon-alpha. Semin Oncol 1998; 25:3–8.

257. Jonasch E, Haluska FG. Interferon in oncological practice: review of interferon biology, clinical applications, and toxicities. Oncologist 2001;6:34–55.

258. Kirkwood JM, Bender C, Agarwala S, et al. Mechanisms and management of toxicities associated with high-dose interferon alfa-2b therapy. J Clin Oncol 2002;20:3703–3718.

259. Quesada JR, Talpaz M, Rios A, et al. Clinical toxicity of interferons in cancer patients: a review. J Clin Oncol 1986;4:234–243.

260. Kirkwood JM, Strawderman MH, Ernstoff MS, et al. Interferon alfa-2b adjuvant therapy of high-risk resected cutaneous melanoma: the Eastern Cooperative Oncology Group Trial EST 1684. J Clin Oncol 1996;14:7–17.

261. Sgarabotto D, Vianello F, Stefani PM, et al. Hypertriglyceridemia during long-term interferon-alpha therapy in a series of hematologic patients. J Interferon Cytokine Res 1997;17:241–244.

262. Weiss K. Safety profile of interferon-alpha therapy. Semin Oncol 1998;25:9–13.

263. Licinio J, Kling MA, Hauser P. Cytokines and brain function: relevance to interferon-alpha-induced mood and cognitive changes. Semin Oncol 1998;25:30–38.

264. Plata-Salaman CR. Cytokines and anorexia: a brief overview. Semin Oncol 1998;25:64–72.

265. Borden EC, Rinehart JJ, Storer BE, et al. Biological and clinical effects of interferon-beta ser at two doses. J Interferon Cytokine Res 1990;10:559–570.

266. Hawkins M, Horning S, Konrad M, et al. Phase I evaluation of a synthetic mutant of beta-interferon. Cancer Res 1985;45: 5914–5920.

267. Valentine AD, Meyers CA, Kling M, et al. Mood and cognitive side effects of interferon-alpha therapy. Semin Oncol 1998; 25:39–47.

268. Capuron L, Neurauter G, Musselman DL, et al. Interferon-alpha-induced changes in tryptophan metabolism: relationship to depression and paroxetine treatment. Biol Psychiatry 2003;54:906–914.

269. Musselman DL, Lawson DH, Gumnick JF, et al. Paroxetine for the prevention of depression induced by high-dose interferon alfa. N Engl J Med 2001;344:961–966.

270. Averbuch SD, Austin HA 3rd, Sherwin SA, et al. Acute interstitial nephritis with the nephrotic syndrome following recombinant leukocyte A interferon therapy for mycosis fungoides. N Engl J Med 1984;310:32–35.

271. Selby P, Kohn J, Raymond J, et al. Nephrotic syndrome during treatment with interferon. Br Med J (Clin Res Ed) 1985; 290:1180.

272. Burman P, Totterman TH, Oberg K, et al. Thyroid autoimmunity in patients on long term therapy with leukocyte-derived interferon. J Clin Endocrinol Metab 1986;63:1086–1090.

273. Kantarjian HM, Deisseroth A, Kurzrock R, et al. Chronic myelogenous leukemia: a concise update. Blood 1993;82:691–703.

274. Italian Cooperative Study Group on Chronic Myeloid Leukemia. Long-term follow-up of the Italian trial of interferon-alpha versus conventional chemotherapy in chronic myeloid leukemia. Blood 1998;92:1541–1548.

275. Guilhot F, Chastang C, Michallet M, et al. Interferon alfa-2b combined with cytarabine versus interferon alone in chronic myelogenous leukemia. French Chronic Myeloid Leukemia Study Group. N Engl J Med 1997;337:223–229.

276. Kantarjian HM, O'Brien S, Smith TL, et al. Treatment of Philadelphia chromosome-positive early chronic phase chronic myelogenous leukemia with daily doses of interferon alpha and low-dose cytarabine. J Clin Oncol 1999;17:284–292.

277. Smalley RV, Andersen JW, Hawkins MJ, et al. Interferon alfa combined with cytotoxic chemotherapy for patients with non-Hodgkin's lymphoma. N Engl J Med 1992;327:1336–1341.

278. Solal-Celigny P, Lepage E, Brousse N, et al. Recombinant interferon alfa-2b combined with a regimen containing doxorubicin in patients with advanced follicular lymphoma. Groupe d'Etude des Lymphomes de l'Adulte. N Engl J Med 1993; 329:1608–1614.

279. Mandelli F, Avvisati G, Amadori S, et al. Maintenance treatment with recombinant interferon alfa-2b in patients with multiple myeloma responding to conventional induction chemotherapy. N Engl J Med 1990;322:1430–1434.

280. Osterborg A, Bjorkholm M, Bjoreman M, et al. Natural interferon-alpha in combination with melphalan/prednisone versus melphalan/prednisone in the treatment of multiple myeloma stages II and III: a randomized study from the Myeloma Group of Central Sweden. Blood 1993;81:1428–1434.

281. Oken MM. Multiple myeloma: prognosis and standard treatment. Cancer Invest 1997;15:57–64.

282. Kirkwood JM, Ibrahim JG, Sosman JA, et al. High-dose interferon alfa-2b significantly prolongs relapse-free and overall survival compared with the GM2-KLH/QS-21 vaccine in patients with resected stage IIB-III melanoma: results of intergroup trial E1694/S9512/C509801. J Clin Oncol 2001;19:2370–2380.

283. Pehamberger H, Soyer HP, Steiner A, et al. Adjuvant interferon alfa-2a treatment in resected primary stage II cutaneous melanoma. Austrian Malignant Melanoma Cooperative Group. J Clin Oncol 1998;16:1425–1429.

284. Grob JJ, Dreno B, de la Salmoniere P, et al. Randomised trial of interferon alpha-2a as adjuvant therapy in resected primary melanoma thicker than 1.5 mm without clinically detectable node metastases. French Cooperative Group on Melanoma. Lancet 1998;351:1905–1910.

285. Medical Research Council Renal Cancer Collaborators. Interferon-alpha and survival in metastatic renal carcinoma: early results of a randomised controlled trial. Lancet 1999; 353:14–17.

286. Gutterman JU, Fine S, Quesada J, et al. Recombinant leukocyte A interferon: pharmacokinetics, single-dose tolerance, and biologic effects in cancer patients. Ann Intern Med 1982;96: 549–556.

287. Quesada JR, Gutterman JU. Clinical study of recombinant DNA-produced leukocyte interferon (clone A) in an intermittent schedule in cancer patients. J Natl Cancer Inst 1983; 70:1041–1046.

288. Maluish AE, Reid JW, Crisp EA, et al. Immunomodulatory effects of poly(I,C)-LC in cancer patients. J Biol Response Mod 1985; 4:656–663.

289. Robins HI, Sielaff KM, Storer B, et al. Phase I trial of human lymphoblastoid interferon with whole body hyperthermia in advanced cancer. Cancer Res 1989;49:1609–1615.

290. Quesada JR, Hawkins M, Horning S, et al. Collaborative phase I-II study of recombinant DNA-produced leukocyte interferon (clone A) in metastatic breast cancer, malignant lymphoma, and multiple myeloma. Am J Med 1984;77:427–432.

291. Rohatiner AZ, Balkwill FR, Griffin DB, et al. A phase I study of human lymphoblastoid interferon administered by continuous intravenous infusion. Cancer Chemother Pharmacol 1982; 9:97–102.

292. Dorr RT, Salmon SE, Robertone A, et al. Phase I-II trial of interferon-alpha 2b by continuous subcutaneous infusion over 28 days. J Interferon Res 1988;8:717–725.

293. Chiang J, Gloff CA, Soike KF, et al. Pharmacokinetics and antiviral activity of recombinant human interferon-beta ser17 in African green monkeys. J Interferon Res 1993;13:111–120.

294. Grunberg SM, Kempf RA, Venturi CL, et al. Phase I study of recombinant beta-interferon given by four-hour infusion. Cancer Res 1987;47:1174–1178.

295. Rinehart JJ, Malspeis L, Young D, et al. Phase I/II trial of human recombinant interferon gamma in renal cell carcinoma. J Biol Response Mod 1986;5:300–308.

296. Vadhan-Raj S, Al-Katib A, Bhalla R, et al. Phase I trial of recombinant interferon gamma in cancer patients. J Clin Oncol 1986;4:137–146.

Adoptive Cellular Therapies

33

Carl H. June

INTRODUCTION

Adoptive immunotherapy is the isolation, ex vivo activation, and infusion of antigen-specific or antigen-nonspecific lymphocytes. Adoptive cellular therapy can be considered a strategy aimed at tumor elimination through direct antineoplastic effects or through indirect effects such as immune-mediated antiangiogenic effects. Adoptive cellular therapy may also have a role in replacing, repairing, or enhancing the immune function damaged as a consequence of cytotoxic therapy by means of autologous or allogeneic cell infusions. Genetic engineering can be used to enhance the function, engraftment, or persistence of the adoptively transferred cells. The analysis of the presently available clinical results suggests that, despite some disappointments, there is room for optimism that both adoptive immunotherapy and active immunotherapy (vaccination) may eventually become part of the therapeutic arsenal and help prevent or combat cancer in a more efficient way. Although adoptive immunotherapy has thus far added little to the routine treatment of most human cancer, it can now be considered "front-line" therapy for patients with chronic myeloid leukemia in relapse after allogeneic stem cell or marrow transplantation and for certain Epstein-Barr virus (EBV)–related tumors. This chapter describes the history of using adoptive cellular therapies for the treatment of cancer, the rationale for such use, and current clinical and experimental approaches.

HISTORY

The seminal discovery made by William B. Coley in the 1890s—that patients with certain malignancies responded to the intratumoral inoculation of live bacterial organisms or bacterial toxins—became the impetus for the development of immunotherapy for cancers.[1] In a series of experiments addressing mechanisms of skin allograft rejection, Bellingham and coworkers first coined the term "adoptive immunity" to describe the transfer of lymphocytes to mediate an effector function.[2] Based on these studies, immunologists have categorized immunotherapies as either active or passive. Active immunizations require an intact host immune system and are typically delivered as prophylactic or therapeutic vaccines. In contrast, passive or adoptive immunotherapies transfer serum, antibodies, or lymphocytes to the host and do not require an intact host immune system to generate the response. One characteristic of an adoptively transferred immune response is that the host has never experienced the primary immune response. This is particularly attractive for patients with late-stage tumors who may not have the time or capability to mount a primary immune response. However, as noted later, with the advent of dendritic cell transfer therapies, in a practical sense the distinction between active and passive (or adoptive) cellular therapy is blurring.

The concept of adoptive cellular therapy for tumor allografts was first reported for rodents over 45 years ago by Mitchison.[3] The cloning of T-cell growth factors made possible the first ex vivo expansion of tumor-specific T cells for adoptive immunotherapy in mouse syngeneic tumor models.[4] There are several excellent reviews of the rationale and experimental basis for adoptive T-cell therapy of tumors.[5-8] In early clinical trials, patients were given adoptive transfers of autologous, allogeneic, and xenogeneic lymphocytes for a variety of tumors. The results of these early trials were not promising, and this is not surprising, since they were carried out before the principles of T-cell biology and tumor antigens were understood. The field of adoptive cellular therapy during its first 25 years was reviewed by Rosenberg and Terry.[9]

TUMOR IMMUNOLOGY AND CELL BIOLOGY

Rational use of adoptive cellular therapy is predicated upon an understanding of the relevant principles of cellular and molecular immunology and cancer cell biology. The reasons for the shortcomings of many previous forms of adoptive cellular therapy are now clear, based on current advances in the basic sciences.

Immunosurveillance and Immunoediting

Sir MacFarlane Burnet proposed a theory of immunological surveillance.[10] The concept of immunosurveillance remains controversial; the basic idea is that a function of the immune system is to control the outgrowth of cancer cells by eliminating cells bearing malignant mutations. Thus, immunocompromised humans do have a propensity to develop tumors, and the tumors are often found in immunologically privileged sites such as the brain. However, there is evidence that goes against this concept. For example, athymic nude mice do not develop tumors with greater frequency than normal mice.[11] However, more immunosuppressed mice that lack interferon-γ, interferon-γ receptors, or perforin, as well as mice deficient in the recombinase-activating gene 2, have an increased incidence of spontaneous or methylcholanthrene-induced tumors.[12,13] In humans, patients with melanoma frequently have tumor-specific T-cell immunity that developed spontaneously.[14] The most direct evidence to support immunosurveillance in human tumors is from studies that provide a clear demonstration that patients with advanced ovarian carcinoma can expect to have much longer overall and progression-free survival if the tumor is infiltrated by T cells than if it lacks infiltrating T cells.[15] Furthermore, as discussed later, the occurrence of certain immunologically mediated paraneoplastic syndromes also provides strong support for tumor immunosurveillance in some circumstances. In retrospect, the theory of immunosurveillance appears to have been largely correct; however, sophisticated mechanisms used by tumors in many instances probably thwart the natural immune response.

Immune Escape Mechanisms

Current immunologic dogma is that tumor cells are antigenic but not immunogenic. The fact that tumors frequently survive and prosper in the face of measurable immune responses underscores the importance of regarding living tumors as complex entities rather than clonal aggregates of transformed cells. There are multiple means that tumors use to escape or prevent immune-mediated elimination.[16,17] These are broadly classified as (a) mechanisms leading to decreased immunogenicity and (b) mechanisms leading to tolerance or immunosuppression. Tumor cells often have low expression of MHC class I molecules, and absent or low density of peptide/MHC complexes may cause lack of recognition, a phenomenon termed immune ignorance. Tumor cells themselves are poor antigen-presenting cells (APCs), as the lack of cell surface costimulatory molecules such as B7 may induce T-cell anergy. Ineffective presentation of tumor antigens by the tumor itself as well as by APCs leads to a failure to provide the necessary costimulatory signals required to activate antigen-specific T cells and then to a subsequent functional clonal inactivation of tumor-specific T cells.

Multiple tumor immunosuppressive events may also blunt or eliminate a tumor-specific immune response. For example, tumor cells often secrete suppressive cytokines such as TGF-β or IL-10, which can down-regulate T-cell responses. Tumor cells may also express an enzyme termed indoleamine 2,3-dioxygenase, leading to the catabolism of tryptophan and the subsequent inhibition of T-cell proliferation.[18] Finally, to sustain an ongoing T-cell response, a continued production of IL-2 is required; other cytokines such as IL-15 may also play a role.[19] In the absence of cytokines, cytotoxic T lymphocytes (CTLs) undergo a few cell divisions and die. CTLs require helper T cells to supply these cytokines, and the tumor microenvironment is generally deficient in helper T cells.

Tumor Antigens

Adoptive cellular therapy is based on the premise that tumor cells possess intracellular or surface antigens that are qualitatively or quantitatively distinct from those present on normal cells. Furthermore, the adoptively transferred T cells must be able to recognize the tumor antigens. The initial successes of adoptive T cell therapy in the 1950s were discredited when it was realized that the tumors were allogeneic and that tumor rejection was simply a form of allograft rejection. However, Klein and Hellström provided strong evidence for specific tumor immunity by demonstrating that after resection of a methylcholanthrene-induced tumor, the host could subsequently reject challenge with its own resected tumor.[20] Indeed, tumor immunology was not considered a respectable field until the last decade, when a clear molecular understanding of the nature of antigenic targets presented by tumors became available. The present consensus is that most, if not all, human tumors express tumor antigens.[21]

Tumor antigens can be classified according to the type of immune response they elicit: humoral, cellular, CD4+, or CD8+, CTL responses. Humoral antigens must be expressed on the surface of the tumor cells for it to be a therapeutic target, whereas T-cell antigens may be derived from cytosolic as well as membrane proteins. A classification of human tumor rejection antigens was proposed.[22] Tumor antigens include the following:

- Nonself tumor antigens such as transforming proteins of viral origin for tumors caused by viruses. For example, a number of human cancers are caused by transforming viruses such as EBV and human papillomavirus.
- Mutated "self" antigens occur because tumor cells have genetic instability and may accumulate mutations or chromosomal translocations.
- Overexpressed mutated oncogene products, of which the best examples are p53 and Her-2/neu.
- In addition, tumor antigens may be normal self-tumor antigens such as reexpressed embryonic antigens, which were not expressed during the development of the immune system; differentiation antigens that are transiently expressed in tissue development and may be reexpressed in tumor cells; and reexpressed retroviral gene products encoded in the mammalian genome (these have been identified for mouse tumors but not yet for human tumors); as well as tissue-specific antigens that may be from immunologically privileged sites or from so-called dispensable tissue.
- Self-antigens modified chemically by carcinogens such as methylcholanthrene in the mouse.
- "Silent" genes, which are cellular genes that are not normally expressed but become transcriptionally active in tumor cells, such as cytochrome P450 subfamily 1 (CYP1B1).[23]

There is currently an explosive growth in the understanding of human tumor antigens and the immune response to tumors. This is based on the development of technologies to identify human tumor rejection antigens.[24,25] A second major advance in the understanding of the human tumor immune response has been the development of tetramers and other immunoglobulin-based reagents that display antigen-specific binding to T-cell receptors. These reagents permit for the first time the tracking and quantification of tumor-specific T cells. Initial studies with tetramers of the MHC class I restricted CD8 T-cell response in patients with melanoma indicate that tumor-specific or tissue-specific T cells are present in most patients with ovarian cancer and melanoma.

Dispensable Tissues: A New Paradigm for Tumor Immunotherapy?

For decades the goal of most cancer immunotherapy centered on the induction of immune responses against tumor-specific "neoantigens." However, the coalescence of results from many laboratories now indicates that the generation of tissue-specific autoimmune responses represents an alternate approach to cancer immunotherapy that is gaining momentum.[26,27] This is because it is now clear that for most tumors there is no special set of tumor proteins targets; tumor antigens are by and large normal self proteins.

Furthermore, for many and perhaps most tumor proteins, active immunologic tolerance has not been induced, as these proteins have simply been ignored previously by the immune system because they have not been presented in an immunogenic form.[28]

For common tumors derived from "dispensable tissues" such as prostate, pancreas, breast, ovary, and skin, an acceptable toxicity could include the immune-mediated damage or destruction of normal as well as neoplastic tissue. Given that many common cancers such as melanoma, prostate cancer, pancreatic cancer, and breast cancer are derived from dispensable tissues, the induction of immune responses against tissue-specific antigens shared by these tumors might represent an immunotherapy approach whose autoimmune side effects would represent acceptable "collateral damage." Thus, a new hypothesis in cancer therapy is that the ability to induce tissue-specific autoimmunity could permit the treatment of many important cancers.

The rationale for the induction of tissue-specific rather than tumor-specific responses is derived from several observations. First, in the 1980s immunologists learned that, for many peripheral tissues, T-cell tolerance to self antigens is not maintained purely by clonal deletion of autoreactive T cells in the thymus but also by peripheral mechanisms that result in the functional silencing of the T cells or ignorance to the peripheral tissue. Autoimmunity is the disruption of this mechanism and leads to the loss of self-tolerance to tissues. Second, in the 1990s it was discovered that patients who experienced immune-based rejection of tumors often had responses that were directed against normal self antigens. For example, Brichard and colleagues[29] discovered that the target for a melanoma-specific CD8$^+$ T-cell clone isolated from a melanoma patient was wild-type tyrosinase, a melanosomal enzyme selectively expressed in melanocytes and responsible for one of the steps in melanin biosynthesis. Additional evidence for the relevance of tissue-specific responses in melanoma immunotherapy came from the finding that patients whose tumors responded to IL-2–based immunotherapy occasionally developed vitiligo, an autoimmune depigmentation of patches of skin, whereas vitiligo was essentially never seen among melanoma patients who failed to respond to immunotherapy.[30] Third, recent therapeutic vaccine trials and adoptive transfer studies in melanoma patients indicate that it is now routinely possible to induce vitiligo.[31] Thus, the ability to break self-tolerance does not appear to require rare MHC backgrounds or other unusual polymorphisms.

The ability of adoptive cellular therapies to "break" tolerance to tissue-specific antigens for cancer therapy will probably depend on the antigenic target as well as other host-specific genetic elements that set immune trigger sensitivity such as the patient's MHC background and CTLA-4 alleles.[32] It is likely that both the specific antigen as well as the form of immunologic adjuvant will be critical in defining the qualitative and quantitative nature of immune responses generated. Under physiologic circumstances, the level of endogenous immunity against an antigen is below a critical threshold necessary for clinical autoimmunity or antitumor immunity. A successful antitumor response would require the elevation of immunity against a particular antigen above a critical threshold. The stringency of tolerance against a particular antigen will dictate how potent the vaccination strategy will have to be to raise the immune response above the threshold level. For antigens that are difficult to elicit responses against, approaches to interfere with the normal down-regulation of the immune responses, such as blocking CTLA-4 or PD-1 interactions, might be required for the induction of clinically evident antitumor immunity.[33–35]

Paraneoplastic Syndromes

One premise for adoptive immunotherapy, especially when using an autologous source of T cells for infusion is that T-cell immunity occurs in response to tumors and that clinically evident tumors have developed the means to escape or overwhelm the cellular response. Unfortunately, it has been extraordinarily difficult to demonstrate naturally occurring T-cell immunity to most human tumors. Other than recent tetramer data, paraneoplastic syndromes provide perhaps the clearest examples of naturally occurring tumor immunity in humans. A recent series of studies in a rare subset of patients with occult carcinomas indicates that spontaneous and potent T-cell immunity in fact occurs in some human tumors. Studies indicate that patients with paraneoplastic neurologic disorders often harbor systemic tumors that express proteins whose normal expression is restricted to the central nervous system. Thus, the expression of these antigens by tumors outside of the normal immunologically privileged site of expression allows for their recognition by the immune system and, consequently, the fortuitous antitumor response. A Purkinje neuronal protein termed "cdr2" has been identified as a target that is responsible for paraneoplastic cerebellar degeneration (PCD) in patients with ovarian and breast tumors.[36] Cdr2 mRNA is expressed in almost all tissues, whereas the protein is expressed only in the brain and testis.[37] Previous studies had shown that although tumor immunity and autoimmune neuronal degeneration in PCD correlates with a specific antibody response to the tumor and brain antigen cdr2, this humoral response has not been shown to be pathogenic. Darnell and coworkers have detected expanded populations of MHC class I–restricted cdr2-specific CTLs in the blood of PCD patients.[38] Thus, it is likely that tumor-induced peripheral activation of cdr2-specific CTLs contributes to the subsequent development of the autoimmune neuronal degeneration in the central nervous system. These studies raise the hope that therapeutically induced immunity to this antigen and perhaps other similar "self" antigens might be an effective immune-based therapy for a variety of carcinomas.

They also raise the possibility that effective immunotherapy against some carcinomas could be subject to CNS toxicity, as they may share immunodominant antigens with CNS tissue.

Principles of T-Cell Growth

Adoptive cellular therapy depends on the ability to optimally select or genetically produce cells with the desired antigenic specificity and then induce cellular proliferation while preserving the effector function, engraftment, and homing abilities of the lymphocytes. Unfortunately, many previous clinical trials were carried out with adoptively transferred cells that were propagated in what are now understood to be suboptimal conditions that impair the essential functions of the adoptively transferred cells. Our understanding of T-cell activation through cell surface receptors and proteins now indicates that this is a complex multistaged process of recognition, adhesion, and stimulation. In vivo, the generation of antigen-specific T cells requires the interaction of dendritic cells and naïve T cells in a secondary lymphoid organ, usually a lymph node.[39]

For over a half a century, immunologists have sought to understand how self-tolerance is induced and maintained. Bretscher and Cohn first proposed a two-signal model of B lymphocyte activation that was later modified by Lafferty and Cunningham for T-cell activation and allograft rejection.[40] The essential features of these models were that activation of lymphocytes requires an antigen-specific signal 1 as well as a second antigen-nonspecific event termed "signal 2." Moreover, these theories and later modifications proposed that signal 1 in the absence of the costimulatory signal 2 led to tolerance or apoptosis. Indeed, in some instances, the binding of tumor antigen presented to the T-cell receptor in the absence of costimulation not only fails to activate the cell but also leads to functional inactivation.[41] Antigenic stimulation of T cells leads to at least three distinct outcomes: (a) activation, clonal expansion, and differentiation to produce cells that secrete distinct subsets of cytokines or to express lytic machinery; (b) induction of an unresponsive state termed "anergy," and (c) induction of apoptosis.[42,43]

The most appropriate methods of ex vivo T-cell activation and propagation mimic the physiologic processes whereby dendritic cells generate a constellation of antigen-specific and costimulatory signals in the T cells. Polyclonal T-cell proliferation can be induced by mimicking the antigen signal by anti–T-cell receptor antibodies or anti-CD3 antibodies.[44,45] However, anti-CD3 stimulation without the addition of IL-2 or another costimulus is not sufficient for full activation of T cells and long-term growth.[46] Enhanced polyclonal T-cell activation and proliferation results when cells are stimulated via the T-cell receptor as well as the CD28 receptor.[47] This culture system has been adapted for clinical use, and starting with an initial apheresis product, it is possible to generate the total number of mature T cells found in adults within 2 weeks of ex vivo culture.[48,49] Antigen-specific T-cell proliferation can be induced by the addition of autologous dendritic cells that have been loaded with the desired antigen or by the use of tetramers to activate the T cells with the desired specificity.[50,51] Dendritic cells are most efficient for the activation of naïve T cells; however, other forms of APC may suffice for previously primed T cells. Schultze and coworkers have shown that CD40-stimulated B cells are an efficient means to propagate antigen-specific T cells.[52]

In addition, cell lines and beads can be engineered to create artificial APC in order to generate antigen-specific T cells and avoid the need to use autologous APC for patient-specific cultures.[53] General approaches have been to produce artificial APC, either by coating beads with peptide:MHC "tetramer" complexes or by transfecting MHC-negative cells with MHC molecules and costimulatory molecules. Magnetic beads were coated with MHC class I molecules loaded with specific peptide, the beads were used as a substrate for T-cell capture, and, following isolation and expansion, the recovered cells specifically killed target cells in vitro and displayed antiviral therapeutic effects in vivo in a rodent model.[54] Others have used nonmagnetic microspheres coated with complexes of recombinant MHC molecules to successfully generate CTLs ex vivo from naïve precursor cells.[55] Peptide-MHC tetramers specific for the melanoma proteins MART-1 and gp100 have been used to isolate high-avidity tumor-reactive CD8[+] T cells from a heterogeneous population by flow cytometry. The tetramer reactive cells could be cloned, and they retained their functional activity on reexpansion.[56,57] Sadelain and colleagues engineered APC that could be used to stimulate the T cells of any patient with a given HLA type.[58] Mouse fibroblasts were retrovirally transduced with a single HLA class I molecular complex along with the human accessory molecules CD80 (B7.1), CD54 (ICAM-1), and CD58 (LFA-3). These artificial APCs consistently elicited and expanded CTLs specific for the melanoma tumor antigens gp100 and MART-1. Our approach has been to create artificial APCs based on expression of the 4-1BB ligand[59]; such APCs efficiently expand human central memory CD8 T cells.[60]

Other T cell culture techniques have been developed to selectively activate and/or clonally expand tumor-specific T cells, with the goal of retaining in vivo antitumor reactivity, trafficking, and engraftment potential. The identification of tumor antigens has permitted the expansion of antigen-specific CTLs that can specifically lyse tumor cells. Theoretically, oligoclonal T-cell lines are preferred to CTL clones for treatment, because a more broadly directed response is likely to minimize the emergence of tumor cells that fail to express the targeted epitope. They are also less costly to develop. However, CTL clones represent a powerful tool for identifying the precise sequence of tumor or viral epitopes, and by virtue of their specificity, they are the least likely cell preparations to trigger adverse effects

such as autoimmunity. Initial studies have used dendritic cells or other APC loaded with antigen to activate and expand T-cell clones or lines. The limited general availability of autologous tumor cells to serve as a source of antigen for repeated in vitro stimulation of T cells is a practical limitation for clinical therapy. This approach is also not desirable because many tumor cells secrete immunosuppressive cytokines such as TGF-β or IL-10. When tumor cells themselves are used as APCs, only MHC class I reactive T cells are usually obtained. Obtaining sufficient autologous dendritic cells for repeated pulsing of the T cells is also a practical limitation. However, this limitation may be circumvented with the advent of flt3 ligand–mediated dendritic cell mobilization protocols. APCs should be autologous or MHC-matched for propagation of tumor-specific T cells. The most widely used method currently employed for the generation of CTLs in vitro is to pulse dendritic cells with tumor-specific peptides that are presented by the appropriate MHC-restricting allele. It is critical that the correct concentration of peptide be used to pulse the dendritic cells. Berzofsky and colleagues showed that if high peptide concentrations are used in vitro, only low-avidity T cells are propagated because the high-avidity T cells die by apoptosis,[61] suggesting that a submaximal concentration of peptides may be required for in vitro induction of tumor-reactive CTLs. Furthermore, CTLs generated with peptide-pulsed APCs are often peptide-reactive but not reactive with tumors that express the gene of interest due to low-level expression or impaired antigen processing by the tumor cells. To circumvent this, Greenberg and colleagues have used recombinant vaccinia virus encoding the tyrosinase gene to infect autologous APCs and have generated tyrosinase-specific and melanoma-reactive CTL cells from the peripheral blood of five out of eight patients with melanoma.[62] Tyrosinase-specific CD4[+] T-cell clones were isolated from six of the eight patients by stimulation with autologous APCs infected with recombinant vaccinia virus, and all of these clones were capable of recognizing autologous tumor cells.

An obstacle to adoptive T-cell therapy with antigen-specific T cells is that each T-cell culture is patient-specific and tumor-specific. Thus, if universal tumor antigens could be identified that are presented by most MHC types, are expressed and presented in most tumors, have limited expression in normal tissues, and are directly involved in the malignant phenotype of the tumor, a more widely applicable form of cellular therapy could be developed. Several candidates for universal tumor antigens have been identified, including the catalytic subunit of telomerase (hTERT), cytochrome P450 isoform 1B1, survivin, WT-1, and MDM2.

Limitations to Adoptive Cellular Therapy

The major rationale for the use of T cells is that these cells have the capacity to specifically kill tumor cells, proliferate, and persist after transfer, and therefore they could completely eliminate all residual tumor cells or newly emerging tumor cells. Mathematical modeling suggests that adoptive transfer of CTLs should augment antitumor immunity in a variety of scenarios.[63] T-cell survival and replication in the host is essential for efficacy, as irradiation of adoptively transferred T cells before their transfer abrogates therapeutic efficacy in most animal models.[64,65] Factors leading to failure or suboptimal efficacy of adoptive cellular therapies can be classified as those due to intrinsic limitations of the infused cells and as immunosuppressive conditions in the tumor-bearing host (Table 33.1). Large tumor burdens present qualitative and quantitative problems for immunotherapy, and as with all therapies, cell transfer therapy has most promise when conducted in the setting of minimal residual disease. Immunologists have long observed a process termed "tumor sneaking through," by which is meant that small tumors grow progressively, medium-sized tumors are rejected, and large ones break through again. De Boer and colleagues developed mathematical models studying tumor kinetics in the setting of adoptively transferred T cells.[66] In De Boer's model, the magnitude of the cytotoxic effector cell response depends on the time at which helper T cells become activated: early helper activity steeply increases the magnitude of the immune response. Thus, tumor rejection is most favored if the tumor-specific CD4 helper T cells are induced early, as this helps to magnify the induction of CTLs. Recent studies have shown DeBoer's work to be remarkably prescient, as there is an emerging consensus that one of the primary

limitations in the immune response to tumors is the failure to develop antigen-specific CD4[+] helper T cells.[67] Given the accumulating evidence that CD4[+] T cells are critical participants in effective antitumor immune responses, a number of potential roles have been suggested. While it had long been known that CD4[+] T cells provide help for the priming of CTLs,[68] more recent evidence has indicated that CD4 cells are required to maintain the optimal effector function of CD8 cells throughout their lifespans.[69]

Another host-specific factor that can prevent therapeutic efficacy of adoptively transferred T cells is the inactivation of the T cells in the immunosuppressive environment of the host. The priming of tumor antigen–specific T cells is critical for the initiation of successful antitumor immune responses, yet the fate of such cells during tumor progression is unknown. In a lymphoma model in mice, when naive CD4[+] T cells specific for an antigen expressed by tumor cells were transferred into tumor-bearing mice, transient clonal expansion occurred early after transfer. The adoptively transferred cells then developed a diminished tumor-specific response, suggesting that tolerance to tumor antigens may impose a significant barrier to therapeutic vaccination, at least in the case of tumors that express MHC class II antigens.[70] T cells from patients with Hodgkin's disease have defects in activation that are reversible in vitro by stimulation with anti-CD3 and anti-CD28.[71] Numerous strategies are being tested in animal models to overcome limitations to adoptive immunotherapy.[72–75] With the exception of homeostatic proliferation, these strategies have yet to be tested clinically.

TABLE 33.1

POTENTIAL EXPLANATIONS FOR LACK OF EFFICACY OF ADOPTIVE T-CELL THERAPY

Limitations of the infused cells

Ex vivo expanded T cell population approaches or reaches replicative senescence or loss of CD28 expression

Tumor antigen–specific T cells have been deleted or tolerized in the donor by previous chemotherapy or by the tumor itself

Ex vivo expansion of T cell population introduces failure to home to tumor or lymph nodes

Culture process renders transferred T cells immunogenic, leading to failure of sustained engraftment

Limitations in the host

Unrealistic effector to target ratio: host tumor burden exceeds killing capacity of adoptively transferred cells

Poor engraftment of adoptively transferred CTLs: lack of CD4 T cell help, cytokine "addiction"

Infertile soil: previous chemotherapy or radiotherapy has ablated stroma and lymph nodes, leading to impaired survival signals and lack of "niche"

Regulatory cells in the host kill or inactivate adoptively transferred T cells

Tumor cells kill or inactivate adoptively transferred T cells

Transferred T cells do not recognize tumor-associated antigens due to loss of tumor antigen expression

Lack of tumor costimulation induces anergy or apoptosis of adoptively transferred cells

ADOPTIVE CELLULAR THERAPY FOR HUMAN TUMORS

Natural Killer (NK) and Lymphokine-Activated Killer (LAK) Cell Adoptive Therapy

Unlike T cells or B cells, which recognize antigen using clonally restricted receptors generated by gene rearrangement, natural killer (NK) cells appear to use a variety of different, non-rearranging receptors to initiate cytolytic activity and cytokine production. NK cells are cytolytic for targets even in the absence of MHC class I expression, and inhibitory receptors expressing immunoreceptor tyrosine-based inhibition (ITIM) motifs prevent NK cells from harming tissues expressing normal levels of MHC class I. This latter characteristic, the ability to cause non-MHC–restricted lysis, is a major feature of NK cells that distinguishes them from T cells. Many receptors have been implicated in NK cell activation, including NKG2D, CD94/NKG2C, NKR-P1, CD2, and CD16.[76] NK cells, unlike T cells, do not have an extensive replicative potential, perhaps due to the fact that telomerase is expressed at much lower levels in NK cells than in T cells.[77] Tumors may shed soluble ligands for NK receptors as a means of promoting immune evasion.[78]

Human lymphocytes that mediate non-MHC–restricted cytotoxicity can be divided into multiple subpopulations. The physiologic basis for this is the differential expression of multiple killer receptors at the single cell level. For example, T cells develop NK-like cytotoxicity after activation with anti-CD3 or cytokines, and the most likely explanation for this phenomenon is the de novo expression of one or more NK receptors. The ability of NK and LAK cells to kill a variety of tumor cell targets in vitro made them attractive candidates for adoptive cellular therapy. This T-cell receptor-independent form of cellular cytotoxicity was originally reported to spare normal tissues; however, autologous human lymphocytes and cultured normal human kidney cells can be killed by LAK cells.[79,80] Another major drawback of NK and LAK cells is their relative inability to traffic to the tumor.

The availability of recombinant IL-2 permitted the first clinical trials of adoptively transferred autologous NK cells.[81] An extensive series of trials has demonstrated clinical responses in a minority of patients, particularly those with melanoma and renal cell carcinoma.[82,83] Randomized studies at the National Cancer Institute with LAK cells have failed to show clinical efficacy.[84] Subsequent analysis has shown that the IL-2 that was administered concomitant with the LAK cells accounted for the majority of the clinical responses that were observed. Human MHC-unrestricted cytotoxic NK cell leukemia lines have been shown to display antitumor effects and can be grown ex vivo for clinical use.[85] For example, the xenogeneic adoptive transfer of human TALL-104 killer cells into a dog with metastatic mammary adenocarcinoma resulted in a 50% reduction of the largest lung metastasis and stabilization of the other lesions for 10 weeks, accompanied by the development of tumor-specific immune responses.[86] A phase I trial with TALL-104 cells in patients with metastatic breast carcinoma demonstrated safety and showed some indications of anti-tumor efficacy.[87]

At present, adoptive therapy with NK cells has been largely abandoned. However, it is likely that variations of this form of therapy will be explored again, given that adoptively transferred T cells can not kill MHC class I negative tumors and also given that T-cell therapy will likely select for tumor cell loss variants of this phenotype. Furthermore, NK cells express both activating and inhibitory receptors. The same NK cell can express both inhibitory and activating receptors. Because of the expression of inhibitory receptors (KIRs) for certain major histocompatibility complex (MHC) class I allotypes, a person's NK cells will not recognize and will therefore kill cells from individuals lacking their own KIR epitopes. Recently "alloreactive" NK cells were shown to mediate antileukemic effects against acute myeloid leukemia after mismatched transplantation when KIR ligand incompatibility existed in the direction of graft versus host disease (GVHD) (i.e., MHC class I KIR ligand that is absent in the recipient but present in the donor).[88] This beneficial antitumor effect does not appear to occur against acute lymphoblastic leukemia. Alloreactive NK cells are cytotoxic for melanoma and renal cell cancer cells in vitro,[89] suggesting that HLA-mismatched hematopoietic stem cell transplantation may be a setting to exploit NK cell adoptive therapies for patients with solid tumors. Once the complexity of the NK system is better understood, it is likely that clinical trials using combinations of tumor-specific T cells and NK cells will be done.[90,91]

Adoptive T-Cell Therapy

The principles of adoptive immunotherapy established in animal models have formed the basis for the testing of therapeutic strategies for human tumors. The primary attraction of the use of T cells for adoptive therapy is their ability to specifically target tumor cells that express small peptides, even if the intact target protein itself is not expressed on the cell surface. A second attraction is the potentially long clonal lifespan of T cells. Finally, unlike NK and LAK cells, adoptively transferred human T cells have been shown to traffic to tumor.[92]

Autologous T-Cell Therapy

In mice, nearly all successful immunotherapies have required the use of large numbers of T cells derived from multiple immunized syngeneic animals. In humans, it is not possible to use this approach, and therefore a central issue for the development of clinical adoptive immunotherapy strategies has been the development of culture systems that produce adequate numbers of effector T cells. Two

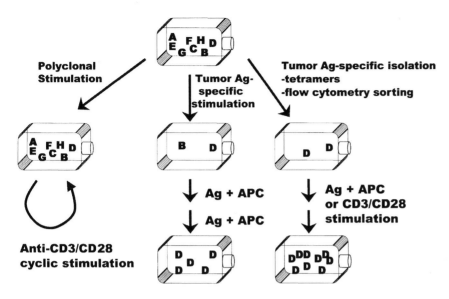

Figure 33.1 General approaches for ex vivo T cell expansion. The initial T cells are obtained from peripheral blood, TIL, or draining lymph nodes. The starting T-cell repertoire can be expanded by polyclonal stimulation via CD3/CD28 stimulation or other methods to generate cells with enhanced effector function or to maintain the TCR repertoire of the initial population (left). Antigen-specific CTLs can be generated without prior selection or enrichment by repeated stimulation with antigen-pulsed antigen-presenting cells (APC) or tumor cells. This process usually requires several rounds of stimulation (middle). Selection of CTLs via tetramers can improve the efficiency of antigen-specific T-cell generation, and several methods can be used for ex vivo expansion of these antigen-specific cells (right). At least 27 cell divisions are required from a single precursor T cell in order to generate 1 billion clonal T cells.

basic approaches are being tested (Fig. 33.1). In one case, polyclonal ex vivo activation of the T cells is done, based on results from mouse syngeneic tumor models.[44,93] This approach is based on the assumptions that tumor-specific T cells are present in the patient but that they have not been primed in the patient and/or that the in vivo function of the cells in the patient is impaired. The cells are activated polyclonally by various means in vitro and are then reinfused to the patient in the hope that they will now respond directly to tumor or to tumor antigen presented by APCs in the patient. The second approach is to isolate and activate antigen-specific T cells or tumor-infiltrating lymphocytes (TILs) in vitro and then clonally expand antigen-specific cells in vitro by various approaches.

As to the first approach, one of the first human trials of activated autologous polyclonal T cell transfers was done by Mazumder and colleagues at the National Cancer Institute.[94] They and others had shown that the in vitro activation of T cells from cancer patients with the lectin phytohemagglutinin (PHA) generated cells that were lytic for fresh autologous tumor. In a phase I clinical protocol, 10 patients with late-stage cancers were given repeated infusions of up to 10^{11} autologous T cells after in vitro culture in PHA for 2 days. Ten patients were treated, and the toxicities encountered included fever and chills in 10 of 10 patients, headaches in 5 of 10, and nausea and vomiting in 3 and 10. No tumor regressions were seen.

Investigators have used mouse tumor models to show that antibodies that bind to the CD3 complex can mimic antigen, and even though all T cells are activated ex vivo nonspecifically, it has been demonstrated that subsequent specific antitumor responses can be enhanced. For example, tumor-specific T cells from the spleens of mice immunized with the FBL-3 leukemic cell line could be expanded in number in vitro by culture with anti-CD3 and IL-2.[44] In a related approach, Osband and colleagues developed a technique termed "autolymphocyte therapy for activating

human T cells ex vivo." Peripheral blood mononuclear cells are activated ex vivo for 5 days by low doses of the mitogenic monoclonal antibody OKT3 in conditioned medium, a mixture of previously prepared culture supernatant that contains autologous cytokines in the presence of cimetidine and indomethacin.[95]

In a phase I trial in patients with advanced cancer, Curti and coworkers tested autologous adoptive transfers of T cells activated with anti-CD3 ex vivo for 4 days.[96] They showed that the anti-CD3–activated $CD4^+$ T cells could traffic to tumor sites in vivo and mediate antitumor effects. Of four lymphoma patients in this study, three had tumor regressions, one of which was a complete response. Patients in this trial were given IL-2 infusions following the T-cell infusion, so that it is not possible to distinguish the relative contributions of the adoptively transferred T cells and the IL-2 to the clinical responses. Repeated ex vivo stimulation with anti-CD3 may cause cell death in vitro and preferential expansion of $CD8^+$ T cells.[97] Using a related approach, based on the idea that anti-CD3 and anti-CD28 can more efficiently activate T cells ex vivo[46,47] and that tumor-draining lymph node cells cultured with anti-CD3 and anti-CD28 can mediate antitumor effects in mice,[98] encouraging results have been observed in several phase I trials in which the adoptive transfer of anti-CD3–activated and anti-CD28–activated autologous T cells was performed in patients with refractory lymphoma, chronic lymphocytic leukemia, myeloma, and renal cell cancer.[99-101] This T-cell culture process has been scaled up for clinical testing[48] and commercial development.[102]

In the second general approach—activation and expansion of tumor-specific T cells ex vivo—infusions of TILs have been tested most extensively. This approach is based on the hypothesis that tumor-specific T cells will be preferentially present in the resected tumor specimens.[103] TIL reactivity to tumor is enhanced compared to unselected peripheral blood T cells, and the antitumor response is generally MHC class I restricted. Furthermore, the TILs are relatively more specific to the tumor of origin. TILs are generated by in vitro culture of dissociated tumor cell preparations in the presence of high concentrations of IL-2. In mice, TILs are 50- to 100-fold more potent than NK cells in several tumor models.[104] TILs have proven to be very useful for the identification of tumor antigens.[105] The failure to consistently generate TILs from tumor specimens has limited widespread clinical application of the approach.[106] Furthermore, clinical studies with TILs have shown poor engraftment efficiencies in patients.[92] Gene-marked TILs have been infused in patients with melanoma and renal cell carcinoma, and selective trafficking of the TILs to the tumor site could not be demonstrated.[107,108] It is likely that the poor clinical results initially obtained with TILs were in part due to the prolonged 4- to 6-week in vitro culture time, which leads to replicative senescence and loss of homing abilities in the TILs. It is also possible that TIL trials have been disappointing because the populations of TIL cells infused also contain regulatory T cells that inhibit the antitumor response.[109,110] Finally, it is possible that the TIL populations that were tested have only contained effector cells and that the response is limited by a lack of tumor-specific T helper and central memory cells.[111]

Shu and Chang have developed an approach that should circumvent many of the limitations posed by TIL therapy. They and others have shown in mice that tumor-draining lymph nodes harbor T cells that are not capable of mediating tumor rejection in adoptive transfer experiments. In contrast, if the draining lymph node cells are activated in vitro with anti-CD3 and IL-2, the cells are now capable of mediating tumor rejection after adoptive transfer.[8] They have shown that for mouse T cells optimal generation of effector T cells occurs when anti-CD3 is added to the culture for the first 2 days and IL-2 is added subsequently on days 3 to 5 of culture.[93] In further studies, T cells were isolated from vaccine-primed lymph nodes obtained from patients with melanoma, renal cell, and head and neck cancer. In the absence of antigen-presenting cells, activation with anti-CD3 and anti-CD28 greatly enhanced subsequent T-cell expansion in IL-2 (>100-fold), compared with anti-CD3 alone.[112] Thus, these results define conditions in which tumor-draining lymph node cells could be stimulated in the absence of tumor antigen to develop into specific therapeutic effector cells during an abbreviated period of cell culture. Based on these preclinical studies, Chang and coworkers carried out a phase I trial in patients with late-stage melanoma and renal cell carcinoma.[113] Patients were given intradermal vaccination with irradiated autologous tumor cells and bacille Calmette-Guérin (BCG) as an adjuvant. The draining lymph nodes were harvested 7 to 10 days later, and the vaccine-primed T cells cultured with anti-CD3 and IL-2. Among the 11 melanoma patients, 1 had a partial tumor response, and there were two complete and two partial responses among the 12 patients with renal cell carcinoma. Thus there may be some clinical activity with this

approach in patients with metastatic renal cell carcinoma. One potential limitation of this approach is that the infused T cells may be immunogenic with this particular culture process, as they will contain the murine anti-CD3 OKT3 antibody that is bound to the T cells.

The clinical utility of tumor-specific CTLs has not yet been extensively evaluated. In one study, CTLs were induced in vitro by repeated stimulation with inactivated autologous tumor cells, and the CTL lines were administered intravenously to 11 patients with advanced cancers once every 2 weeks for 10 weeks. The cell infusions were not toxic, and tumor reduction or decreased tumor markers were observed in 4 patients.[114] In another study, autologous CTLs were generated against primary-cultured malignant gliomas from peripheral blood mononuclear cells in vitro in 4 patients.[115] The CTLs specifically recognized the corresponding autologous glioma in vitro. The CTLs were injected 3 times into the primary tumor–resected cavity via an Ommaya tube, and reduction of the tumor volume was observed in 3 of the 4 patients. These results suggest that adoptive immunotherapy with autologous CTLs may be a promising approach for malignant gliomas; however, further testing will be required to establish whether there is clinical benefit.

Tumor-specific CTLs generated ex vivo with the rapid expansion method[116] appear to have substantial activity in melanoma, as 8 of 10 patients with refractory, metastatic melanoma had minor, mixed, or stable responses.[117] However, recent studies at the NCI indicate that host conditioning can increase the response to adoptive immunotherapy with TILs. When 13 patients with progressive metastatic melanoma were given cyclophosphamide and fludarabine, a regimen that is immunosuppressive but does not have antimelanoma efficacy, 6 patients had partial responses as judged by RECIST criteria, and 4 others had mixed responses.[31] Significantly, the patients had prolonged engraftment with the adoptively transferred TILS, and the levels of engraftment correlated with the clinical responses.[31,118] In contrast, 34% of patients with melanoma who were treated with TIL administration and high-dose IL-2 therapy and who received no prior conditioning therapy to induce lymphodepletion achieved objective clinical responses[119]; most of the responses were transient, and the patients had limited persistence of the transferred cells.[92] Adverse effects included opportunistic infections and the frequent induction of vitiligo and uveitis, presumably due to autoimmunity. If confirmed, these results indicate that induction of immunosuppression in the host is essential to improve the antitumor efficacy of adoptive immunotherapy.

Virally Induced Lymphomas

Virally induced lymphomas that retain some expression of the inciting viral genome are likely to present a good target for adoptive cellular therapy. Unlike in the case of most spontaneous tumors, the repertoire of T-cell receptors contains receptors with a high affinity for the viral protein as a consequence of the lack of deletion of these T cells in the thymus. In patients recovering from allogeneic bone marrow transplantation, a severe defect in the cellular immune system exists, and this often results in the death of the patients from reactivation of systemic CMV or EBV infection. Donor-derived, CMV antigen–specific $CD8^+$ CTLs have been administered to the patients, and an extremely promising restoration of immune function has been noted.[120,121] EBV often reactivates after bone marrow or organ transplantation, resulting in aggressive lymphoma. Infusions of allogeneic peripheral blood T cells (DLI) have proved effective, as have infusions of EBV-specific T-cell lines. The latter approach has the benefit of reduced risk of inducing or exacerbating GVHD, since the T cells with allospecificity are eliminated or greatly reduced before infusion. In vitro cultured T-cell lines or clones that recognize viral antigens can be effective in suppressing EBV-associated lymphoproliferative disorders. Even relatively modest doses of T cells (1×10^6 cells/kg) are an effective treatment or prophylaxis for EBV-associated lymphoma, with complete remissions recorded in most patients.[122,123] Pneumonitis and tumor swelling with respiratory obstruction have been reported as adverse events following CTL infusion for lymphoma.[123] EBV-specific CTLs are safe and have significant antitumor activity in Hodgkin's disease and nasopharyngeal carcinoma associated with EBV infection.[124,125]

A single patient with an aggressive EBV-associated lymphoma treated with adoptive immunotherapy using autologous LAK cells was reported.[126] The patient had leukapheresis, autologous peripheral blood mononuclear cells were cultured in IL-2 for 10 days, and the IL-2–activated LAK cells were returned to the patient in the absence of systemic IL-2 therapy. The patient experienced a complete response.

Donor Lymphocyte Infusions and Allogeneic T-Cell Therapy

The first form of human adoptive T-cell therapy was given "inadvertently" as passenger T cells contained in stem cell infusions from bone marrow harvests. The bone marrow infusions were given to patients receiving allogeneic marrow grafts using myeloablative regimens as therapy for leukemia. At the time, the T cells were regarded as "contaminants" of the stem cell grafts. Weiden and coworkers performed a retrospective analysis of a series of patients treated with total body irradiation and high-dose cyclophosphamide,[127] and to their surprise they discovered that the probability of tumor recurrence was significantly lower in patients receiving allografts than in those who had syngeneic (twin) grafts. Later studies showed that the probability of tumor recurrence was inversely related to the occurrence of GVHD. Resting donor peripheral blood T cells are now given routinely to patients with chronic myeloid leukemia who relapse following a marrow allograft, and this procedure results in the induction of molecular complete remissions in a high proportion of cases.[128–131] This

form of therapy is now termed "donor lymphocyte infusion" (DLI).

The mechanisms of DLI-mediated antitumor effects are not yet well understood. It is likely that T cells and/or dendritic cells are involved and that the antigenic targets are minor histocompatibility antigens or leukemia-specific antigens. It is noteworthy that the kinetics of the clinical response are delayed, as clinical response following DLI takes weeks to months, and often 6 to 8 months are required for maximal antileukemic effects; these kinetics are typical of an acquired immune response that is mediated by T cells. Recently, Falkenburg and coworkers used T-cell leukemia-reactive CTL lines generated from a patient's HLA-identical donor to induce a complete remission in a patient with chronic myelogenous leukemia (CML).[132] The CTLs did not react with normal lymphocytes from the donor or recipient and did not affect donor hematopoietic progenitor cells. The CTL lines were infused at 5-week intervals at a cumulative dose of 3.2×10^9 CTLs, and following the third infusion, a complete eradication of the leukemic cells was observed. The interpretation of the clinical benefit in this experiment is difficult, since the patient had been given previous DLI that was terminated due to failure to induce a response and the onset of GVHD. If the clinical response that was eventually observed was in fact due to the infused CTLs, then it is likely that the CTLs engrafted and proliferated in vitro. This is due to the fact that the initial effector to target ratio was only $\sim 1:1,000$ in vivo immediately after the CTL infusion, given the patient's estimated leukemic burden of 1×10^{12} to 3×10^{12} cells.

One critical issue with DLI is that it often results in the induction of chronic GVHD. Under some experimental conditions in transgenic mice, high-avidity T cells reactive for tumor antigens as well as self antigens are deleted, and the remaining low-avidity T cells appear to be sufficient to provide protection against subsequent tumor challenge but do not suffice to provoke autoimmunity.[133] This may explain why clinically evident GVHD does not appear necessary for clinically evident antitumor effects. However, clinical trials are evaluating whether depletion of $CD8^+$ T cells from the adoptively transferred cell population might reduce GVHD while retaining the antileukemic effects.[134,135] Given the early results of these trials, it is likely that $CD8^+$ T lymphocytes are important as effectors of GVHD but may not be essential for the DLI-mediated antitumor effect. Another limitation of DLI is that, though it is very effective for CML, it is much less effective for other forms of leukemia, and it is not yet known if DLI will have a role in treating solid tumors. Limited but impressive data indicate that potent allogeneic antitumor effects can be observed in selected patients with renal cell carcinoma, ovarian cancer, and breast cancer.[136–139]

It is possible that the antitumor effects of donor leukocytes can be used for therapeutic benefit outside the setting of allogeneic transplantation. Xenogeneic and allogeneic adoptive T-cell therapy has the obvious advantage that the in vivo antitumor effect is not dependent on the condition that all tumor cells express tumor-specific antigens, since alloantigens or minor histocompatibility antigens can serve as targets. Furthermore, the donor repertoire has not been contracted by previous chemotherapy, and therefore it is more likely to contain naïve T cells reactive with tumor antigens. Xenogeneic adoptive lymphocyte transfers have been done in humans by Symes and coworkers.[140] Pigs were immunized with transitional cell carcinoma fragments, and later the draining porcine lymph node cells were harvested and injected into patients with bladder carcinoma. Two of seven patients had objective responses, and no significant toxicity was observed, in part because of the rapid rejection of the porcine allograft that likely occurred.

Allogeneic MHC-mismatched human lymphocytes have also been transferred to patients in a variety of settings without the myeloablative or immunosuppressive conditioning required to permit engraftment. As can be seen in Figure 33.2, the general design of some of these early trials was remarkably similar to current approaches. In spite of the limitations of these early trials due to the failure to obtain engraftment of the adoptively transferred cells, objective tumor regressions were observed when patients were given infusions of allogeneic MHC-mismatched lymphocytes from donors immunized with the recipient's tumor.[141,142] However, in the absence of MHC matching, it is unlikely that allogeneic or xenogeneic T cells can mediate tumor-specific responses, and it is possible that the responses observed in these early trials were due to NK cells.

Terasaki and coworkers performed the first adoptive transfers of HLA-matched allogeneic lymphocytes and observed objective responses in two of six patients with advanced cancers.[143] Haploidentical lymphocytes have been given in conjunction with cyclophosphamide to a small group of patients with various tumors as primary therapy without inducing GVHD.[144] Six patients received

infusions of lymphocytes after alloactivation and expansion in vitro, and this resulted in a complete response in one patient with lymphoma. More recently, MHC-matched allogeneic DLI has been given to patients without minimal immunosuppressive conditioning[145,146]; remission has been induced in a significant fraction of patients with refractory hematologic malignancies. Slavin and coworkers have obtained similar results in patients with breast cancer given allogeneic lymphocyte infusions following autologous stem cell transplants.[147] The main limitations of these approaches are the generally short-term engraftment, the suboptimal response rate, and the unpredictable onset of GVHD in a subset of patients.

In order for the full antitumor potential of allogeneic T cells to be realized, it is necessary to achieve long-term donor engraftment. Previously, this was only possible in young patients who could survive the rigorous myeloablative protocols. This fact largely precluded the use of allografting for patients older than 55 years or for younger patients with certain kinds of preexisting organ damage. A major step toward decreasing the rigors of allogeneic stem cell transplants occurred with the development of nonmyeloablative stem cell transplantation (NMSCT), a procedure where the preparative regimen is designed only to provide sufficient immunosuppression to achieve engraftment of an allogeneic stem cell graft.[148,149] The nonmyeloablative regimen does not by itself completely eliminate residual host hematopoietic cells, but rather the allogeneic T cells over the period of weeks to months may either maintain partial hematopoietic chimerism or eliminate all residual host elements and achieve full donor chimerism. Barrett and coworkers have studied the kinetics of engraftment in patients receiving NMSCT consisting an allogeneic peripheral blood stem cell transplant from an HLA-matched donor after a preparative regimen of cyclophosphamide and fludarabine.[150] Donor myeloid chimerism

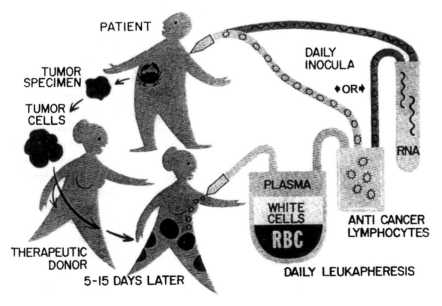

Figure 33.2 A clinical adoptive transfer approach used by Nadler and Moore in the 1960s.[141] MHC unrelated patients with cancer were immunized with viable tumors by subcutaneous injection. The allogeneic donor was then subjected to leukapheresis, and the buffy coat given as a form of donor leukocyte infusion (DLI) to another cancer-bearing patient. (Reproduced with permission from Nadler SH, Moore GE. Immunotherapy of malignant disease. Arch Surg 1969;99:376.) This approach is not endorsed by the author or by the editors, and this experiment is illustrated simply to indicate the general similarity to currently ongoing clinical trials.

gradually supplanted recipient hematopoiesis, and the myeloid compartment became fully donor in all survivors by 200 days after transplantation. In contrast, T-cell engraftment was more rapid, with full chimerism occurring in some patients by day 30 and in other patients by day 200 after cyclosporine withdrawal and DLI. Ten of 14 patients surviving more than 30 days had delayed tumor regression, consistent with a T cell–mediated tumor rejection.

An unanticipated benefit of NMSCT is that the incidence of acute GVHD is markedly decreased, permitting allogeneic marrow grafts to be done in much older patients. This is likely due to the absence of chemotherapy-induced mucositis, which leads to the secretion of cytokines, the generation of other danger signals, and the subsequent activation of allogeneic donor T cells. Another attractive feature of NMSCT is that adoptive cell transfers can be given to patients later, once the graft has been established, creating an ideal platform for adoptive immunotherapy with allogeneic T cells and dendritic cells. Now that older patients can undergo allogeneic adoptive transfers, it will be possible for the first time to determine the efficacy of this approach in patients with the common solid tumors that occur in this age group. Thus, it is likely that a resurgence of interest in allogeneic adoptive cell therapy will occur due to the advent of NMSCT. NMSCT provides a platform to minimize acute GVHD and to circumvent the difficulties with autologous T cell therapy in patients who have had previous repertoire contractions due to chemotherapy.

RANDOMIZED CLINICAL TRIALS

A number of randomized controlled clinical trials testing the efficacy of adoptively transferred cells have been reported (Table 33.2). The first tumors in humans treated with adoptive immunotherapy to be subjected to randomized controlled trials were melanoma and renal cell carcinoma. Renal cell carcinoma and melanoma are relatively highly immunogenic tumors that have proven resistant to standard cytotoxic chemotherapy but have shown reproducible responses to immune-based therapy. Infusions of NK cells, LAK cells isolated from peripheral blood, and polyclonal T cell populations isolated from TILs and nonspecifically expanded in vitro with IL-2 suggested the therapeutic potential of tumor-reactive T cells in humans. However, the low response rates and the severe toxicity due to the high doses of IL-2 injected to maintain cell survival dampened the early enthusiasm. Indeed, randomized studies using this approach have not demonstrated efficacy of the adoptively transferred cell populations. The responses observed can be attributed to cytokine-mediated antitumor effects alone. Similarly, positive effects in randomized trials of patients with advanced renal cell carcinoma treated with anti-CD3–activated peripheral blood mononuclear cells cultured in conditioned medium were also reported;[151]

however, a larger, multicenter phase III trial failed to confirm the earlier studies. While further trials are ongoing, thus far these approaches have not consistently shown benefit in comparison with standard immune-based treatment with biologic response modifiers, most importantly, high-dose bolus IL-2. In a randomized phase I trial by Fenton and colleagues at the NCI,[152] more than half of the patients with advanced renal cell carcinoma entering the trial were found to be anergic to recall antigens, confirming other studies indicating that patients with late-stage tumors can be significantly immunosuppressed and that this may present a significant barrier to overcome if immunotherapy is to be successful. For reasons that remain unclear and may reflect the lack of immunosurveillance and trafficking to the eye, some investigators have reported that metastatic ocular melanoma is much less responsive than cutaneous melanoma to adoptive cellular transfers.[153] It is likely that other approaches will be required to establish the usefulness of adoptive immunotherapy in melanoma and renal cell carcinoma, but its promise for these difficult diseases is already evident.

Randomized trials suggest that other tumors may also be responsive to immunotherapy. A single randomized trial of adoptive immunotherapy with TIL and IL-2 infusions indicated a survival advantage for patients with non–small cell lung carcinoma, particularly those with stage IIIB.[154] Similarly, in another randomized trial of patients with non–small cell lung carcinoma, LAK cell infusions plus IL-2 therapy in combination with standard therapy was shown to be superior to standard therapy alone.[155] In both of these trials, it was not possible to discern if the adoptively transferred cells contributed to the beneficial effects due to the confounding effects of the concomitant IL-2 infusions. Finally, patients with hepatoma may have immunogenic tumors that are targets for adoptively transferred cells.[156] Although some intriguing clinical results have been noted, no published randomized controlled trials have convincingly demonstrated clinical benefit from adoptively transferred cells. Currently, adoptive immunotherapy does not represent the standard of care for any disease except for patients with chronic myeloid leukemia who relapse following an allogeneic marrow grafting procedure.

ADOPTIVE CELLULAR THERAPY: TOXICITY, DOSE, AND SCHEDULING ISSUES

Information on the dose and schedule dependence of adoptively transferred cells is widely scattered in the literature, and from this literature one concludes that there is no standardized dose system. In nonlymphopenic hosts, fractionated doses of adoptively transferred T cells are superior to a single infusion of T cells.[157] The ideal dose of transferred cells is related to the tumor burden and the homing

TABLE 32.2

RANDOMIZED CLINICAL TRIALS OF ADOPTIVE IMMUNOTHERAPY

Indication	Description	Reference
Metastatic renal cell cancer and melanoma	Patients were randomly assigned to receive either systemic IL-2 alone or IL-2 plus adoptively transferred lymphokine-activated killer cells. Twenty-three patients with renal cell carcinoma and 20 with melanoma were entered into the protocol. No objective responses were noted.	193
Metastatic renal cell cancer and melanoma	Patients were randomly assigned to receive either systemic IL-2 alone or IL-2 plus adoptively transferred lymphokine-activated killer cells. The results suggested a trend toward increased survival when IL-2 was given with LAK cells in patients with melanoma ($P = .09$), but no trend was observed for patients with renal cell cancer.	84
Metastatic renal cell cancer	Adoptive autologous polyclonal T therapy after activation with anti-CD3 and conditioned medium. Ninety patients with metastatic renal cell carcinoma were randomly assigned to receive 6 monthly infusions of autologous activated peripheral blood lymphocytes plus oral cimetidine or cimetidine alone. Positive results were reported, but later trials did not confirm the initial results.	151, 194
Advanced renal cell cancer	A randomized phase III trial compared continuous intravenous infusion IL-2 alone with IL-2 plus LAK cell adoptive transfers. Seventy-one patients were treated, 36 on the IL-2 arm and 35 on the IL-2 plus LAK arm. Four patients (6%) had major responses (2 complete, 2 partial). The addition of LAK cells did not improve the response rate ($P = .61$) or survival ($P = .67$).	195
Advanced renal cell cancer	A randomized phase I trial was done to determine whether subcutaneous administration of IL-2 in combination with an autologous renal cell vaccine is feasible and can augment tumor immunity. Seventeen patients with metastatic renal cell carcinoma underwent surgical resection with preparation of an autologous tumor cell vaccine. Patients were vaccinated intradermally twice with 10e7 irradiated tumor cells plus bacille Calmette-Guerin and once with 10e7 tumor cells alone. Patients were randomly assigned to one of three groups: no adjuvant IL-2, low-dose IL-2, or high-dose IL-2. Four patients developed cellular immunity specific for autologous tumor cells as measured by DTH responses. IL-2 did not have a major effect on the DTH response. Prospective testing of response to recall antigens indicated that 7 of 12 tested patients were anergic.	152
Metastatic renal cell cancer	A multicenter randomized trial to test the efficacy of TILs in combination with low-dose IL-2 compared with IL-2 alone after radical nephrectomy in 178 patients with metastatic renal cell carcinoma was done. Intent-to-treat analysis demonstrated objective response rates of 9.9% vs. 11.4% and 1-year survival rates of 55% vs. 47% in the TIL/rIL-2 and rIL-2 control groups, respectively. Treatment with TILs did not improve response rate or survival in patients treated with low-dose rIL-2 after nephrectomy.	196
Myeloma	The primary objective of this study was to determine whether T-cell infusions could accelerate lymphocyte reconstitution and restore the ability to immunize patients after high-dose chemotherapy and autologous stem cell rescue. The randomized primary endpoint data show that the groups of patients on day 42 after transplant who were assigned to early (day 14) T-cell infusions had significantly higher CD4 counts than the group assigned to delayed T-cell infusions and that the antipneumococcal humoral and cellular vaccine response to Prevnar (protein-conjugated pneumococcal polysaccharide) was augmented in recipients of adoptively transferred T cells.	197
Hepatocellular carcinoma	Patients were treated with spleen-derived LAK cells cultured for 3 to 30 days in recombinant interleukin-2. These autologous activated spleen cells were administered to patients 2 days after the intraarterial infusion of doxorubicin. Patients randomly assigned to receive splenic LAK cells had a lower recurrence rate that did not reach statistical significance.	156
Non–small cell lung cancer	A phase II randomized study tested the efficacy of TIL plus IL2 infusions in 113 patients with stage II, IIIa, or IIIb NSCLC. Three-year survival was significantly better for patients given TIL therapy than for controls.	154
Non–small cell lung cancer	One hundred and seventy-four patients in a phase III trial were randomly assigned to receive either combined immunotherapy with IL-2 and LAK cells or no adjuvant therapy, or radiotherapy or chemotherapy. There were statistically improved survival rates in the immunotherapy group; however, it is difficult to interpret the results due to changes in study design that occurred during the trial.	155, 198, 199

and persistence (memory) characteristics of the infused cells.[158] Doses of adoptively transferred cells are usually reported as the total number of viable cells administered or as the total number of viable cells per kilogram body weight or per square meter body surface area. However, total lymphocyte numbers do not correlate well with body surface area but rather display a stronger inverse correlation with age. Other variables add to the complexity, particularly the fact that, in the case of T cells or other adoptively transferred cells with high replicative potential, the infused dose may not relate well to the steady-state number of cells. Therefore, dose considerations are more complex than in other areas of transfusion medicine, where, for example, the maximal level of transfused red cells or platelets occurs immediately following infusion. In our studies of adoptively transferred autologous CD4[+] T cells, we often find that the highest number of cells in the host peaks 2 weeks after infusion of the cells. This is because the engraftment potential and the replicative potential of the infused cells depends on complex host variables such as the number of niches available in the host for engraftment and the antigenic stimulus for clonal expansion or deletion. In most rodent tumor models, T-cell proliferation in the host after transfer is obligatory for therapeutic efficacy (reviewed in ref. 5).

Cytokines given to the host can also have major impact on the persistence of adoptively transferred T cells. Others have found that the persistence of adoptively transferred CD8[+] T cells is enhanced by coadministration of IL-2;[159] however, we have found that when autologous human CD4[+] T cells are also given, that persistence is not increased by concomitant IL-2 therapy.[160] Finally, IL-2 can induce proliferation and maintain effector CD8[+] T cells but may actually delete memory cells, while IL-15 and IL-7 appear to select for the persistence of memory CD8[+] T cells.[19] Thus, it may be desirable to provide IL-2 at early times in immunotherapy when tumor cytoreduction is the issue but to remove IL-2 and/or provide IL-7 and IL-15 signaling later in therapy in order to promote antitumor memory.

Immunotherapy has often been advertised as a "nontoxic therapy" when compared with cytotoxic chemotherapy. However, it is instructive to recall that William Coley's first therapeutic vaccines were accompanied by life-threatening toxicity.[1] Furthermore, anyone who has experienced the fatigue and malaise that accompanies systemic viral infections such as infectious mononucleosis would not be surprised to learn that cellular therapies have many of the same toxicities. Thus, one would expect that, in the setting of therapeutic immunization to treat established malignancy, systemic toxicity will be an expected response and that prophylactic immunization strategies in cases with no or minimal residual disease would be accompanied by less toxicity.

Many types of adverse events have been reported following infusion of human autologous or allogeneic lymphocytes or dendritic cells. The toxicities can be classified as (1) those due to extrinsic factors present in the culture process, (2) those due to accompanying cytokines that may be coinfused with the cells, and (3) those that are intrinsic to the cells themselves. With regard to the first type of toxicity, with the earlier cell manufacturing techniques many cell products were cultured in sources of foreign proteins such as fetal calf serum. In such cases, patients often developed febrile transfusion reactions that were sometimes severe and could include anaphylaxis. These reactions were usually encountered in cases of multiple cell infusions to the same patient, but instances have occurred where patients were presensitized to bovine proteins, and the patients have had severe reactions even on the occasion of the first cellular infusion. Hepatitis A has been reported due to the contamination of the culture medium with infectious pooled human serum.[84] With the widespread use of serum-free culture medium, a substantial reduction has been seen in the incidence of immediate-type allergic responses, febrile transfusion reactions, and infectious complications. Similarly, with the development of closed cell culturing and manufacturing processes, the potential for microbial contamination has been substantially decreased.[161]

Many patients have been given infusions of IL-2 at the time of and following cellular adoptive transfer. IL-2 has a well-known dose-dependent and schedule-dependent toxicity. IL-2 given in high doses and by intravenous bolus injection induces multiorgan dysfunction due to a capillary leak syndrome that is directly mediated by local production of nitric oxide by cells of the monocyte-macrophage lineage. In contrast, low doses and subcutaneous injections of IL-2 induce an influenza-like syndrome, and this can be ameliorated by giving the IL-2 at night. Laboratory abnormalities induced at high and low doses of IL-2 include anemia, lymphopenia with rebound lymphocytosis, and eosinophilia.[162]

The spectrum of adverse effects intrinsic to the cellular therapy is still being defined and appears to be related to whether the cell product is genetically engineered. For cell products that have not been genetically engineered, the adverse effects are limited and are similar to those observed with therapeutic vaccines. Respiratory obstruction has been reported following CTL infusion for EBV-related lymphomas.[123] This is probably due to a T cell–induced inflammatory response that results in tumor edema and necrosis. T cells infused under conditions that lead to long-term engraftment produce only mild toxicities. In over 200 infusions of autologous activated CD4[+] and CD8[+] T cells given to patients with lymphoma or HIV infection in the absence of concomitant IL-2 infusions, we have observed a dose-dependent induction of fever and headaches in a substantial proportion of patients. These symptoms are self-limited, and they typically resolve within 36 hours following the infusion. The onset of the symptoms is delayed and does not occur immediately upon infusion of the cells but rather several hours following the infusion. The etiology of the symptoms is likely related to secretion of cytokines by the infused cells. These symptoms are not due to allergy to the infused cells, because subsequent infusions of cells do not engender more severe adverse effects. Modest eosinophilia occurs in some patients, and this is likely related to an indirect effect of secretion of IL-2 by the infused T cells. As was mentioned previously, eosinophilia occurs in patients treated with systemic IL-2.

Effector functions of infused T cells can be expected to include tissue damage similar to that encountered in T-cell mediated autoimmune diseases. In the case of allogeneic lymphocyte infusions (DLIs), GVHD and marrow aplasia often occur.[128] Autoimmune thyroiditis with hypothyroidism has been reported to occur following LAK cell and IL-2 infusions.[163] The passive transfer of antibodies with shared specificities between normal and malignant tissues can also induce autoimmune pathology.[164] Theoretic toxicities associated with T-cell transfer also include leukemia or lymphoma if transformation is induced consequent to the in vitro culture process. T-cell lymphomas have developed in nonhuman primates following transplantation with gene-modified stem cells.[165] The etiology of the lymphomas appears to be due to insertional mutagenesis from the presence of replication-competent retrovirus that was generated from recombination from the viral vector that was used to transduce the stem cells. T-cell leukemia due to insertional mutagenesis in the LMO-2 oncogene has occurred in children following retrovirally modified CD34 cell infusion to correct common gamma chain deficiency.[166] In human trials involving genetically modified T cells, no cases of malignant transformation of the infused T cells have been reported to date.

Schedule-dependent efficacy and adverse effects from adoptively transferred cells have been reported. Many studies in rodent tumor models show that the administration of cytotoxic therapy can enhance the effects of adoptively transferred cells. Cyclophosphamide is the preferred drug, and the mechanism is not thought to be consequent to tumor cytoreduction. The mechanism is likely due to multiple causes, including (a) killing of host regulatory lymphocytes that suppress antitumor immune responses,[7,110] (b) creating "space" in the host so that the adoptively transferred cells can engraft,[158] and perhaps (c) enhanced cross-priming of tumor antigens. Cyclophosphamide and/or fludarabine is generally given several days before the adoptively transferred T cells.[31,110] Curti and colleagues[96] have examined a related issue concerning the optimal time to harvest autologous CD4$^+$ T cells in relation to the timing of cyclophosphamide administration in patients with advanced cancers. T cells were harvested at steady state, when on the decline, or when on recovery from the cyclophosphamide-induced leukopenia. From that study, they concluded that the best time to harvest autologous T cells was not at steady state but rather just before the leukopenic nadir that occurred following administration of cyclophosphamide. The best in vivo expansion of the infused CD4$^+$ T cells occurred when the cells had been harvested as patients entered the cyclophosphamide-induced nadir. Most of the clinical antitumor responses also occurred in patients treated on this schedule. These results are generally consistent with animal models that predicted a need to ablate immunosuppressive lymphocytes for efficient engraftment and subsequent in vivo expansion of adoptively transferred CD4$^+$ T cells.

In a study of patients with stage III non–small cell lung cancer, investigators tested the sequence of adoptive therapy with autologous TIL and IL-2, followed by standard chemotherapy and radiotherapy; perhaps not surprisingly, they found that the sequence of immunotherapy followed by chemotherapy is not effective.[167]

In patients with early-stage cancers who have not yet had cytotoxic chemotherapy, it is probably best to harvest autologous T cells before initiation of chemotherapy. Adults have limited capacity to generate new T cells from the thymus, and therefore the repertoire remains contracted for long periods of time and in many cases never recovers.[168,169] Naïve T cells are most sensitive to the effects of cytotoxic chemotherapy, and their numbers are severely depleted in heavily pretreated patients. It is not yet known whether the tumor-specific T cells are derived from primed or naïve T cells in the host, and this likely varies depending on the intrinsic immunogenicity of the tumor. Studies with tetramers that can identify tumor antigen–specific T cells show that in some patients chemotherapy can ablate the tumor-specific T cells that have an effector phenotype while sparing memory cells.[14] The mechanism for this is unknown, but the authors speculated that the effector cells were in the active phases of the cell cycle and were therefore relatively susceptible to the cytotoxic effects of the chemotherapy. If these results are confirmed, they would argue that patients should have their repertoire "archived" by apheresis before undergoing chemotherapy.

Anecdotal evidence suggests that immunotherapy may in some circumstances restore tumors to a chemotherapy-sensitive state. Several of our patients had platinum-resistant ovarian cancer and were then treated with adoptive cellular therapies or therapeutic vaccines. The patients had responses to the immunotherapy; however, they subsequently experienced disease progression. Interestingly, when chemotherapy was recommenced, they appeared to have tumor that was more sensitive to the drugs than when they had previously been treated. If this observation is confirmed, this would suggest a need for further study of this interesting scheduling issue between cytotoxic chemotherapy and immunotherapy. Data in mouse syngeneic tumor models support this concept.[170,171]

Finally, there are dose-dependent and schedule-dependent effects that have been observed with DLI in connection with the induction of GVHD. Early studies showed that the infusion of donor T cells soon after a myeloablative transplant conditioning regimen resulted in the marked augmentation of acute GVHD.[172] It has been well established by the work of O'Reilly and colleagues that the initial dose of infused T cells in the setting of allogeneic marrow transplantation has a major effect on the incidence and severity of acute GVHD.[173] As was discussed earlier, it has only recently been appreciated that donor T cells can be infused with relative freedom from acute GVHD in the setting of NMSCT.[148] Studies by Goldman and colleagues showed that in the steady-state setting of relapsed CML, infusions of resting T cells result in a decreased incidence of GVHD when given by dose fractionation, starting with low doses of donor cells and escalating subsequent doses as required.[130] In a nonrandomized trial, the researchers compared a bulk, single-infusion DLI (average 1.5×10^8 CD3$^+$ cells/kg) to an escalating dose regimen of DLI, where increasing numbers of cells (average total 1.9×10^8 CD3$^+$ cells/kg) were given at 20-week average intervals between infusion. They found that antileukemic effects were preserved but that the incidence of GVHD was much lower using the escalating dose regimen of DLI.

T REGULATORY CELL ADOPTIVE THERAPY

CD4$^+$CD25$^+$ T regulatory (Treg) cells have been shown to regulate self-tolerance in mice. Initially they were described to be critical for the control of autoimmunity[174] and were found on adoptive transfer to prevent experimental autoimmune diseases.[175] More recently, Treg cells have been shown to suppress allogeneic immune responses[176] and can prevent transplant rejection.[177] Studies of human Treg have been hindered by the low numbers present in peripheral blood and the fact that the cells were initially thought to have poor replicative capacity in vitro.[178] However, it was later shown that Tregs have substantial replicative capacity in vivo.[179] We and others have developed improved ex vivo culture conditions that should permit pilot trials of Treg adoptive immunotherapy for the prevention or therapy of GVHD.[180]

GENETICALLY MODIFIED CELLULAR THERAPY

Genetic modification of T cells and dendritic cells ex vivo to engineer an improved antitumor effect is an attractive strategy for many settings. Unlike hematopoietic stem cells, currently available vectors provide high-level expression of transgenes in T cells and dendritic cells. The first use of genetically modified T cells was to demonstrate that adoptively transferred cells could persist in the host and traffic to tumor, albeit with low efficiency.[92] A principal limitation of immunotherapy for some tumors is that the tumors are poorly antigenic, in that no T cells are available that have high avidity for tumor-specific antigens or that no T cells remaining in the patient after chemotherapy have the desired specificity. To address this problem, some clinical trials attempt to endow T cells with novel receptor constructs by the introduction of "T bodies," chimeric receptors that have antibody-based external receptor structures and cytosolic domains that encode signal transduction modules of the T-cell receptor.[181] These constructs can function to retarget T cells in vitro in an MHC-unrestricted manner. The major issues with the approach currently

involve improved receptor design and the immunogenicity of the T body construct. T cells are also being transduced to express natural TCR receptor alpha beta heterodimers of known specificity and avidity for tumor antigens[182]; however, this approach is of limited general value for humans because each TCR will be specific for a given MHC allele such that each vector would be patient-specific.

A major limitation to adoptive transfer of CTLs is that they have short-term persistence in the host in the absence of antigen-specific T helper cells. Greenberg and coworkers have transduced human CTLs with chimeric GM-CSF/IL-2 receptors that deliver an IL-2 signal on binding GM-CSF. Stimulation of the CTLs with antigen caused GM-CSF secretion and resulted in an autocrine growth loop such that the CTL clones proliferated in the absence of exogenous cytokines. This type of genetic modification has potential for increasing the circulating half-life and, by extension, the efficacy of ex vivo–expanded CTLs. A related strategy to rejuvenate T cell function is to engineer T cells to ectopically express CD28 or the catalytic subunit of telomerase.[183,184] To date, there is limited clinical experience with engineered T cells; however, in certain instances such T cells have been shown to persist after adoptive transfer in humans for years.[160,185]

As was noted, severe and potentially lethal GVHD represents a frequent complication of allogeneic DLI. The promising results with DLI have created increased interest in developing T cells with an inducible suicide phenotype. Expression of herpes simplex virus thymidine kinase (HSV TK) in T cells provides a means of ablating transduced T cells in vivo by the administration of acyclovir or ganciclovir.[186] Using this strategy, Bordignon and colleagues infused donor lymphocytes into 12 patients who, after receiving allogeneic bone marrow transplants, had suffered complications such as cancer relapse or virus-induced lymphomas.[187] The lymphocytes survived for up to a year, and complete or partial tumor remissions in five of the eight patients were achieved. Tumor regressions coincided with the onset of GVHD, and in most cases the GVHD was abrogated when ganciclovir was given. Thus, GVHD associated with the therapeutic infusion of donor lymphocytes after allogeneic marrow transplantation could be efficiently controlled by these novel suicide gene strategies in allogeneic lymphocytes. However, subsequent studies have indicated problems with this approach, in that the HSV TK gene confers immunogenicity to the transfused cells, leading to impaired survival and the inability to retreat a patient with DLI should the tumor recur. Future experiments will be required to develop vectors that are less immunogenic and able to confer even higher ganciclovir sensitivity to transduced human lymphocytes. Investigators have developed suicide systems composed of fusion proteins containing a Fas or caspase death domain and a modified FKBP.[188,189] These approaches have the advantage that the suicide switches are expected to be nonimmunogenic. T cells expressing these modified chimeric proteins are induced to undergo apoptosis when exposed to a drug that dimerizes the modified FKBP.[190,191] Finally, the advent of lentiviral vectors has greatly increased the efficiency of T-cell engineering, and it is likely that adoptive therapies with lentiviral engineered T cells will become a clinical reality.[192]

SUMMARY

The basis for tumor immunology is the premise that the immune system is capable of recognizing tumor cells together with the premise that the activated immune system can lead to the subsequent rejection of tumors. While the former premise is now well accepted, the latter remains controversial. As we complete nearly 50 years of research into adoptive immunity for tumors, there are no forms of cellular therapy that have been approved by the Food and Drug Administration. Allogeneic DLI is being incorporated into the practice of medicine as a valuable and potentially curative indication for selected patients with CML. However, there are several obstacles that investigators must overcome before adoptive immunotherapy can become a more generally applicable and successful a form of prophylaxis or treatment for human tumors. Concerns about the costs of cellular therapy should eventually be overcome if it achieves curative potential or long-lasting tumor immunity for patients with indications that are otherwise chemotherapy refractory. Finally, it is likely that adoptive immunotherapy will be used not alone but in combination with other forms of immunotherapy and chemotherapy.

REFERENCES

1. Coley WB. The treatment of malignant tumors by repeated inoculations of erysipelas: with a report of ten original cases. Am J Med Sci 1893;105:487–511.
2. Billingham RE, Brent L, Medawar PB. Quantitative studies on tissue transplantation immunity, II: the origin, strength and duration of actively and adoptively acquired immunity. Proc R Soc 1954;143:58–80.
3. Mitchison NA. Studies on the immunological response to foreign tumor transplants in the mouse, I: the role of lymph node cells in conferring immunity by adoptive transfer. J Exp Med 1955; 102:157–177.
4. Cheever MA, Greenberg PD, Fefer A. Specific adoptive therapy of established leukemia with syngeneic lymphocytes sequentially immunized in vivo and in vitro and nonspecifically expanded by culture with interleukin 2. J Immunol 1981;126:1318–1322.
5. Greenberg PD. Adoptive T cell therapy of tumors: mechanisms operative in the recognition and elimination of tumor cells. Adv Immunol 1991;49:281–355.
6. Cheever MA, Chen W. Therapy with cultured T cells: principles revisited. Immunol Rev 1997;157:177–194.
7. Melief CJ. Tumor eradication by adoptive transfer of cytotoxic T lymphocytes. Adv Cancer Res 1992;58:143–175.
8. Strome SE, Krauss JC, Chang AE, et al. Strategies of lymphocyte activation for the adoptive immunotherapy of metastatic cancer: a review. J Hematother 1993;2:63–73.
9. Rosenberg SA, Terry WD. Passive immunotherapy of cancer in animals and man. Adv Cancer Res 1977;25:323–388.
10. Burnet FM. The concept of immunological surveillance. Prog Exp Tumor Res 1970;13:1–27.
11. Rygaard J, Povlsen CO. The nude mouse vs. the hypothesis of immunological surveillance. Transplant Rev 1976;28:43–61.
12. Shankaran V, Ikeda H, Bruce AT, et al. IFNgamma and lymphocytes prevent primary tumour development and shape tumour immunogenicity. Nature 2001;410:1107–1111.
13. Dunn GP, Old LJ, Schreiber RD. The immunobiology of cancer immunosurveillance and immunoediting. Immunity 2004; 21:137–148.
14. Lee PP, Yee C, Savage PA, et al. Characterization of circulating T cells specific for tumor-associated antigens in melanoma patients. Nat Med 1999;5:677–685.
15. Zhang L, Conejo-Garcia JR, Katsaros D, et al. Intratumoral T cells, recurrence, and survival in epithelial ovarian cancer. N Engl J Med 2003;348:203–213.
16. Marincola FM, Jaffee EM, Hicklin DJ, et al. Escape of human solid tumors from T-cell recognition: molecular mechanisms and functional significance. Adv Immunol 2000;74:181–273.
17. Rivoltini L, Carrabba M, Huber V, et al. Immunity to cancer: attack and escape in T lymphocyte–tumor cell interaction. Immunol Rev 2002;188:97–113.
18. Hwu P, Du MX, Lapointe R, et al. Indoleamine 2,3-dioxygenase production by human dendritic cells results in the inhibition of T cell proliferation. J Immunol 2000;164:3596–3599.
19. Ku CC, Murakami M, Sakamoto A, et al. Control of homeostasis of CD8$^+$ memory T cells by opposing cytokines. Science 2000; 288:675–678.
20. Klein G. Tumor antigens. Annu Rev Microbiol 1966;20:223–252.
21. van der Bruggen P., Zhang Y, Chaux P, et al. Tumor-specific shared antigenic peptides recognized by human T cells. Immunol Rev 2002;188:51–64.
22. Gilboa E. The makings of a tumor rejection antigen. Immunity 1999;11:263–270.
23. Maecker B, Sherr DH, Vonderheide RH, et al. The shared tumor-associated antigen cytochrome P450 1B1 is recognized by specific cytotoxic T cells. Blood 2003;102:3287–3294.
24. Lurquin C, Van Pel A, Mariame B, et al. Structure of the gene of tum- transplantation antigen P91A: the mutated exon encodes a peptide recognized with Ld by cytolytic T cells. Cell 1989; 58:293–303.
25. Wang RF, Wang X, Atwood AC, et al. Cloning genes encoding MHC class II–restricted antigens: mutated CDC27 as a tumor antigen. Science 1999;284:1351–1354.
26. Nanda NK, Sercarz EE. Induction of anti-self-immunity to cure cancer. Cell 1995;82:13–17.
27. Pardoll DM. Inducing autoimmune disease to treat cancer. Proc Natl Acad Sci USA 1999;96:5340–5342.
28. Lanzavecchia A. How can cryptic epitopes trigger autoimmunity? J Exp Med 1995;181:1945–1948.
29. Brichard V, Van Pel A, Wolfel T, et al. The tyrosinase gene codes for an antigen recognized by autologous cytolytic T lymphocytes on HLA-A2 melanomas. J Exp Med 1993;178:489–495.
30. Rosenberg SA, White DE. Vitiligo in patients with melanoma: normal tissue antigens can be targets for cancer immunotherapy. J Immunother Emphasis Tumor Immunol 1996;19:81–84.
31. Dudley ME, Wunderlich JR, Robbins PF, et al. Cancer regression and autoimmunity in patients after clonal repopulation with antitumor lymphocytes. Science 2002;298:850–854.
32. Ueda H, Howson JM, Esposito L, et al. Association of the T-cell regulatory gene CTLA4 with susceptibility to autoimmune disease. Nature 2003;423:506–511.
33. Hurwitz AA, Yu TF, Leach DR, et al. CTLA-4 blockade synergizes with tumor-derived granulocyte-macrophage colony-stimulating factor for treatment of an experimental mammary carcinoma. Proc Natl Acad Sci USA 1998;95:10067–10071.
34. Zha YY, Blank C, Gajewski TF. Negative regulation of T-cell function by PD-1. Crit Rev Immunol 2004;24:229–238.
35. Dong H, Strome SE, Salomao DR, et al. Tumor-associated B7-H1 promotes T-cell apoptosis: a potential mechanism of immune evasion. Nat Med 2002;8:793–800.
36. Sakai K, Mitchell DJ, Tsukamoto T, et al. Isolation of a complementary DNA clone encoding an autoantigen recognized by an anti-neuronal cell antibody from a patient with paraneoplastic cerebellar degeneration. Ann Neurol 1990;28: 692–698.

37. Corradi JP, Yang C, Darnell JC, et al. A post-transcriptional regulatory mechanism restricts expression of the paraneoplastic cerebellar degeneration antigen cdr2 to immune privileged tissues. J Neurosci 1997;17:1406–1415.
38. Albert ML, Darnell JC, Bender A, et al. Tumor-specific killer cells in paraneoplastic cerebellar degeneration. Nat Med 1998;4:1321–1324.
39. Banchereau J, Steinman RM. Dendritic cells and the control of immunity. Nature 1998;392:245–252.
40. Bretscher P, Cohn M. A theory of self-nonself discrimination. Science 1970;169:1042–1049.
41. Chen L, Ashe S, Brady WA, et al. Costimulation of antitumor immunity by the B7 counterreceptor for the T lymphocyte molecules CD28 and CTLA-4. Cell 1992;71:1093–1102.
42. June CH, Bluestone JA, Nadler LM, et al. The B7 and CD28 receptor families. Immunol Today 1994;15:321–331.
43. Lenschow DJ, Walunas TL, Bluestone JA. CD28/B7 system of T cell costimulation. Annu Rev Immunol 1996;14:233–258.
44. Crossland KD, Lee VK, Chen W, et al. T cells from tumor-immune mice nonspecifically expanded in vitro with anti-CD3 plus IL-2 retain specific function in vitro and can eradicate disseminated leukemia in vivo. J Immunol 1991;146:4414–4420.
45. Katsanis E, Xu Z, Anderson PM, et al. Short-term ex vivo activation of splenocytes with anti-CD3 plus IL-2 and infusion post-BMT into mice results in in vivo expansion of effector cells with potent anti-lymphoma activity. Bone Marrow Transplant 1994;14:563–572.
46. Levine BL, Bernstein W, Craighead N, et al. Effects of CD28 costimulation on long term proliferation of CD4+ T cells in the absence of exogenous feeder cells. J Immunol 1997;159:5921–5930.
47. Levine BL, Mosca J, Riley JL, et al. Antiviral effect and ex vivo CD4+ T cell proliferation in HIV-positive patients as a result of CD28 costimulation. Science 1996;272:1939–1943.
48. Levine BL, Cotte J, Small CC, et al. Large scale production of CD4+ T cells from HIV-infected donors following CD3/CD28 stimulation. J Hematother 1998;7:437–448.
49. Garlie NK, LeFever AV, Siebenlist RE, et al. T cells coactivated with immobilized anti-CD3 and anti-CD28 as potential immunotherapy for cancer. J Immunother 1999;22:336–345.
50. Rogers J, Mescher MF. Augmentation of in vivo cytotoxic T lymphocyte activity and reduction of tumor growth by large multivalent immunogen. J Immunol 1992;149:269–276.
51. Altmann DM, Hogg N, Trowsdale J, et al. Cotransfection of ICAM-1 and HLA-DR reconstitutes human antigen-presenting cell function in mouse L cells. Nature 1989;338:512–514.
52. Schultze JL, Michalak S, Seamon MJ, et al. CD40-activated human B cells: an alternative source of highly efficient antigen presenting cells to generate autologous antigen-specific T cells for adoptive immunotherapy. J Clin Invest 1997;100:2757–2765.
53. Kim JV, Latouche JB, Riviere I, et al. The ABCs of artificial antigen presentation. Nat Biotechnol 2004;22:403–410.
54. Luxembourg AT, Borrow P, Teyton L, et al. Biomagnetic isolation of antigen-specific CD8+ T cells usable in immunotherapy. Nat Biotechnol 1998;16:281–285.
55. Lone YC, Motta I, Mottez E, et al. In vitro induction of specific cytotoxic T lymphocytes using recombinant single-chain MHC class I/peptide complexes. J Immunother 1998;21:283–294.
56. Dunbar PR, Chen JL, Chao D, et al. Cutting edge: rapid cloning of tumor-specific CTL suitable for adoptive immunotherapy of melanoma. J Immunol 1999;162:6959–6962.
57. Yee C, Savage PA, Lee PP, et al. Isolation of high avidity melanoma-reactive CTL from heterogeneous populations using peptide-MHC tetramers. J Immunol 1999;162:2227–2234.
58. Latouche JB, Sadelain M. Induction of human cytotoxic T lymphocytes by artificial antigen-presenting cells. Nat Biotechnol 2000;18:405–409.
59. Maus MV, Thomas AK, Leonard D, et al. Ex vivo expansion of polyclonal and antigen-specific cytotoxic T lymphocytes by artificial APCs expressing ligands for the T cell receptor, CD28 and 4-1BB. Nat Biotechnol 2002;20:143–148.
60. Maus MV, Kovacs B, Kwok WW, et al. Extensive replicative capacity of human central memory T cells. J Immunol 2004;172:6675–6683.
61. Alexander-Miller MA, Leggatt GR, Berzofsky JA. Selective expansion of high- or low-avidity cytotoxic T lymphocytes and efficacy for adoptive immunotherapy. Proc Natl Acad Sci USA 1996;93:4102–4107.
62. Yee C, Gilbert MJ, Riddell SR, et al. Isolation of tyrosinase-specific CD8+ and CD4+ T cell clones from the peripheral blood of melanoma patients following in vitro stimulation with recombinant vaccinia virus. J Immunol 1996;157:4079–4086.
63. Takayanagi T, Ohuchi A. A mathematical analysis of the interactions between immunogenic tumor cells and cytotoxic T lymphocytes. Microbiol Immunol 2001;45:709–715.
64. Fefer A. Adoptive chemoimmunotherapy of a Moloney lymphoma. Int J Cancer 1971;8:364–373.
65. Wong RA, Alexander RB, Puri RK, et al. In vivo proliferation of adoptively transferred tumor-infiltrating lymphocytes in mice. J Immunol 1991;10:120–130.
66. de Boer RJ, Hogeweg P, Dullens HF, et al. Macrophage T lymphocyte interactions in the anti-tumor immune response: a mathematical model. J Immunol 1985;134:2748–2758.
67. Pardoll DM, Topalian SL. The role of CD4+ T cell responses in antitumor immunity. Curr Opin Immunol 1998;10:588–594.
68. Schoenberger SP, Toes RE, van der Voort EI, et al. T-cell help for cytotoxic T lymphocytes is mediated by CD40-CD40L interactions. Nature 1998;393:480–483.
69. Bevan MJ. Helping the CD8(+) T-cell response. Nat Rev Immunol 2004;4:595–602.
70. Staveley-O'Carroll K, Sotomayor E, Montgomery J, et al. Induction of antigen-specific T cell anergy: an early event in the course of tumor progression. Proc Natl Acad Sci USA 1998;95:1178–1183.
71. Renner C, Ohnesorge S, Held G, et al. T cells from patients with Hodgkin's disease have a defective T-cell receptor zeta chain expression that is reversible by T-cell stimulation with CD3 and CD28. Blood 1996;88:236–241.
72. Matsui K, O'Mara LA, Allen PM. Successful elimination of large established tumors and avoidance of antigen-loss variants by aggressive adoptive T cell immunotherapy. Int Immunol 2003;15:797–805.
73. Lou Y, Wang G, Lizee G, et al. Dendritic cells strongly boost the antitumor activity of adoptively transferred T cells in vivo. Cancer Res 2004;64:6783–6790.
74. Klebanoff CA, Finkelstein SE, Surman DR, et al. IL-15 enhances the in vivo antitumor activity of tumor-reactive CD8+ T cells. Proc Natl Acad Sci USA 2004;101:1969–1974.
75. Overwijk WW, Theoret MR, Finkelstein SE, et al. Tumor regression and autoimmunity after reversal of a functionally tolerant state of self-reactive CD8+ T cells. J Exp Med 2003;198:569–580.
76. Lanier LL. Turning on natural killer cells. J Exp Med 2000;191:1259–1262.
77. Mariani E, Meneghetti A, Formentini I, et al. Telomere length and telomerase activity: effect of ageing on human NK cells. Mech Ageing Dev. 2003;124:403–408.
78. Groh V, Wu J, Yee C, et al. Tumour-derived soluble MIC ligands impair expression of NKG2D and T-cell activation. Nature 2002;419:734–738.
79. Sondel PM, Hank JA, Kohler PC, et al. Destruction of autologous human lymphocytes by interleukin 2–activated cytotoxic cells. J Immunol 1986;137:502–511.
80. Miltenburg AM, Meijer-Paape ME, Daha MR, et al. Lymphokine-activated killer cells lyse human renal cancer cell lines and cultured normal kidney cells. Immunology 1988;63:729–731.
81. Rosenberg SA, Lotze MT, Muul LM, et al. A progress report on the treatment of 157 patients with advanced cancer using lymphokine-activated killer cells and interleukin-2 or high-dose interleukin-2 alone. N Engl J Med 1987;316:889–897.
82. Urba WJ, Longo DL. Adoptive cellular therapy. Cancer Chemother Biol Response Modif 1990;11:265–280.
83. Chang AE, Geiger JD, Sondak VK, et al. Adoptive cellular therapy of malignancy. Arch Surg 1993;128:1281–1290.
84. Rosenberg SA, Lotze MT, Yang JC, et al. Prospective randomized trial of high-dose interleukin-2 alone or in conjunction with lymphokine-activated killer cells for the treatment of patients with advanced cancer. J Natl Cancer Inst 1993;85:622–632.

85. Tam YK, Martinson JA, Doligosa K, et al. Ex vivo expansion of the highly cytotoxic human natural killer-92 cell-line under current good manufacturing practice conditions for clinical adoptive cellular immunotherapy. Cytotherapy 2003;5:259–272.

86. Visonneau S, Cesano A, Jeglum KA, et al. Adoptive therapy of canine metastatic mammary carcinoma with the human MHC non-restricted cytotoxic T-cell line TALL-104. Oncol Rep 1999; 6:1181–1188.

87. Visonneau S, Cesano A, Porter DL, et al. Phase I trial of TALL-104 cells in patients with refractory metastatic breast cancer. Clin Cancer Res 2000;6:1744–1754.

88. Ruggeri L, Capanni M, Urbani E, et al. Effectiveness of donor natural killer cell alloreactivity in mismatched hematopoietic transplants. Science 2002;295:2097–2100.

89. Igarashi T, Wynberg J, Srinivasan R, et al. Enhanced cytotoxicity of allogeneic NK cells with killer immunoglobulin-like receptor ligand incompatibility against melanoma and renal cell carcinoma cells. Blood 2004;104:170–177.

90. Ruggeri L, Capanni M, Martelli MF, et al. Cellular therapy: exploiting NK cell alloreactivity in transplantation. Curr Opin Hematol 2001;8:355–359.

91. Farag SS, Fehniger TA, Ruggeri L, et al. Natural killer cell receptors: new biology and insights into the graft-versus-leukemia effect. Blood 2002;100:1935–1947.

92. Rosenberg SA, Aebersold P, Cornetta K, et al. Gene transfer into humans: immunotherapy of patients with advanced melanoma, using tumor-infiltrating lymphocytes modified by retroviral gene transduction. N Engl J Med 1990;323:570–578.

93. Yoshizawa H, Chang AE, Shu S. Specific adoptive immunotherapy mediated by tumor-draining lymph node cells sequentially activated with anti-CD3 and IL-2. J Immunol 1991;147: 729–737.

94. Mazumder A, Eberlein TJ, Grimm EA, et al. Phase I study of the adoptive immunotherapy of human cancer with lectin activated autologous mononuclear cells. Cancer 1984;53:896–905.

95. Gold JE, Zachary DT, Osband ME. Adoptive transfer of ex vivo–activated memory T-cell subsets with cyclophosphamide provides effective tumor-specific chemoimmunotherapy of advanced metastatic murine melanoma and carcinoma. Int J Cancer 1995;61:580–586.

96. Curti BD, Ochoa AC, Powers GC, et al. A phase I trial of anti-CD3 stimulated CD4$^+$ T cells, infusional interleukin-2 and cyclophosphamide in patients with advanced cancer. J Clin Oncol 1998;16:2752–2760.

97. Curti BD, Ochoa AC, Urba WJ, et al. Influence of interleukin-2 regimens on circulating populations of lymphocytes after adoptive transfer of anti-CD3-stimulated T cells: results from a phase I trial in cancer patients. J Immunother Emphasis Tumor Immunol 1996;19:296–308.

98. Harada M, Okamoto T, Omoto K, et al. Specific immunotherapy with tumour-draining lymph node cells cultured with both anti-CD3 and anti-CD28 monoclonal antibodies. Immunology 1996;87:447–453.

99. Lum LG, LeFever AV, Treisman JS, et al. Immune modulation in cancer patients after adoptive transfer of anti-CD3/anti-CD28-costimulated T cells: phase I clinical trial. J Immunother 2001;24:408–419.

100. Laport GG, Levine BL, Stadtmauer EA, et al. Adoptive transfer of costimulated T cells induces lymphocytosis in patients with relapsed/refractory non-Hodgkin lymphoma following CD34$^+$-selected hematopoietic cell transplantation. Blood 2003; 102:2004–2013.

101. Thompson JA, Figlin RA, Sifri-Steele C, et al. A phase I trial of CD3/CD28-activated T cells (Xcellerated T cells) and interleukin-2 in patients with metastatic renal cell carcinoma. Clin Cancer Res 2003;9:3562–3570.

102. Kalamasz D, Long SA, Taniguchi R, et al. Optimization of human T-cell expansion ex vivo using magnetic beads conjugated with anti-CD3 and anti-CD28 antibodies. J Immunother 2004; 27:405–418.

103. Rosenberg SA, Spiess P, Lafreniere R. A new approach to the adoptive immunotherapy of cancer with tumor-infiltrating lymphocytes. Science 1986;233:1318–1321.

104. Spiess PJ, Yang JC, Rosenberg SA. In vivo antitumor activity of tumor-infiltrating lymphocytes expanded in recombinant interleukin-2. J Natl Cancer Inst 1987;79:1067–1075.

105. van der Bruggen P, Traversari C, Chomez P, et al. A gene encoding an antigen recognized by cytolytic T lymphocytes on a human melanoma. Science 1991;254:1643–1647.

106. Hoffman DM, Gitlitz BJ, Belldegrun A, et al. Adoptive cellular therapy. Semin Oncol 2000;27:221–233.

107. Merrouche Y, Negrier S, Bain C, et al. Clinical application of retroviral gene transfer in oncology: results of a French study with tumor-infiltrating lymphocytes transduced with the gene of resistance to neomycin. J Clin Oncol 1995;13:410–418.

108. Economou JS, Belldegrun AS, Glaspy J, et al. In vivo trafficking of adoptively transferred interleukin-2 expanded tumor-infiltrating lymphocytes and peripheral blood lymphocytes: results of a double gene marking trial. J Clin Invest 1996;97:515–521.

109. Dye ES, North RJ. T cell–mediated immunosuppression as an obstacle to adoptive immunotherapy of the P815 mastocytoma and its metastases. J Exp Med 1981;154:1033–1042.

110. North RJ. Models of adoptive T-cell–mediated regression of established tumors. Contemp Top Immunobiol 1984;13:243–257.

111. Sallusto F, Lenig D, Forster R, et al. Two subsets of memory T lymphocytes with distinct homing potentials and effector functions. Nature 1999;401:708–712.

112. Li Q, Furman SA, Bradford CR, et al. Expanded tumor-reactive CD4$^+$ T-cell responses to human cancers induced by secondary anti-CD3/anti-CD28 activation. Clin Cancer Res 1999;5: 461–469.

113. Chang AE, Aruga A, Cameron MJ, et al. Adoptive immunotherapy with vaccine-primed lymph node cells secondarily activated with anti-CD3 and interleukin-2. J Clin Oncol 1997;15: 796–807.

114. Soda H, Koda K, Yasutomi J, et al. Adoptive immunotherapy for advanced cancer patients using in vitro activated cytotoxic T lymphocytes. J Surg Oncol 1999;72:211–217.

115. Tsurushima H, Liu SQ, Tuboi K, et al. Reduction of end-stage malignant glioma by injection with autologous cytotoxic T lymphocytes. Jpn J Cancer Res 1999;90:536–545.

116. Riddell S.R., and Greenberg, P.D. 1998. Rapid expansion method ("REM") for in vitro propagation of T lymphocytes. US Patent #5,827,642.

117. Yee C, Thompson JA, Byrd D, et al. Adoptive T cell therapy using antigen-specific CD8$^+$ T cell clones for the treatment of patients with metastatic melanoma: in vivo persistence, migration, and antitumor effect of transferred T cells. Proc Natl Acad Sci USA 2002;99:16168–16173.

118. Robbins PF, Dudley ME, Wunderlich J, et al. Cutting edge: persistence of transferred lymphocyte clonotypes correlates with cancer regression in patients receiving cell transfer therapy. J Immunol 2004;173:7125–7130.

119. Rosenberg SA, Yannelli JR, Yang JC, et al. Treatment of patients with metastatic melanoma with autologous tumor-infiltrating lymphocytes and interleukin 2. J Natl Cancer Inst 1994;86: 1159–1166.

120. Riddell SR, Watanabe KS, Goodrich JM, et al. Restoration of viral immunity in immunodeficient humans by the adoptive transfer of T cell clones. Science 1992;257:238–241.

121. Walter EA, Greenberg PD, Gilbert MJ, et al. Reconstitution of cellular immunity against cytomegalovirus in recipients of allogeneic bone marrow by transfer of T-cell clones from the donor. N Engl J Med 1995;333:1038–1044.

122. Heslop HE, Ng CY, Li C, et al. Long-term restoration of immunity against Epstein-Barr virus infection by adoptive transfer of gene-modified virus-specific T lymphocytes. Nat Med 1996; 2:551–555.

123. Heslop HE, Rooney CM. Adoptive cellular immunotherapy for EBV lymphoproliferative disease. Immunol Rev 1997;157: 217–222.

124. Bollard CM, Aguilar L, Straathof KC, et al. Cytotoxic T lymphocyte therapy for Epstein-Barr virus$^+$ Hodgkin's disease. J Exp Med 2004;200:1623–1633.

125. Straathof KC, Bollard CM, Popat U, et al. Treatment of nasopharyngeal carcinoma with Epstein-Barr virus–specific T lymphocytes. Blood 2004;105:1898–1904.

126. Li PK, Tsang K, Szeto CC, et al. Effective treatment of high-grade lymphoproliferative disorder after renal transplantation using autologous lymphocyte activated killer cell therapy. Am J Kidney Dis 1998;32:813–819.

127. Weiden PL, Flournoy N, Thomas ED, et al. Antileukemic effect of graft-versus-host disease in human recipients of allogeneic-marrow grafts. N Engl J Med 1979;300:1068–1073.

128. Kolb HJ, Mittermuller J, Clemm C, et al. Donor leukocyte transfusions for treatment of recurrent chronic myelogenous leukemia in marrow transplant patients. Blood 1990;76:2462–2465.

129. Porter DL, Roth MS, McGarigle C, et al. Induction of graft-versus-host disease as immunotherapy for relapsed chronic myeloid leukemia. N Engl J Med 1994;330:100–106.

130. Dazzi F, Szydlo RM, Craddock C, et al. Comparison of single-dose and escalating-dose regimens of donor lymphocyte infusion for relapse after allografting for chronic myeloid leukemia. Blood 2000;95:67–71.

131. Collins RH Jr, Shpilberg O, Drobyski WR, et al. Donor leukocyte infusions in 140 patients with relapsed malignancy after allogeneic bone marrow transplantation. J Clin Oncol 1997;15:433–444.

132. Falkenburg JH, Wafelman AR, Joosten P, et al. Complete remission of accelerated phase chronic myeloid leukemia by treatment with leukemia-reactive cytotoxic T lymphocytes. Blood 1999;94:1201–1208.

133. Morgan DJ, Kreuwel HT, Fleck S, et al. Activation of low avidity CTL specific for a self epitope results in tumor rejection but not autoimmunity. J Immunol 1998;160:643–651.

134. Giralt S, Hester J, Huh Y, et al. CD8-depleted donor lymphocyte infusion as treatment for relapsed chronic myelogenous leukemia after allogeneic bone marrow transplantation. Blood 1995;86:4337–4343.

135. Alyea EP, Soiffer RJ, Canning C, et al. Toxicity and efficacy of defined doses of CD4(+) donor lymphocytes for treatment of relapse after allogeneic bone marrow transplant. Blood 1998;91:3671–3680.

136. Childs RW, Clave E, Tisdale J, et al. Successful treatment of metastatic renal cell carcinoma with a nonmyeloablative allogeneic peripheral-blood progenitor-cell transplant: evidence for a graft-versus-tumor effect. J Clin Oncol 1999;17:2044.

137. Ueno NT, Rondon G, Mirza NQ, et al. Allogeneic peripheral-blood progenitor-cell transplantation for poor-risk patients with metastatic breast cancer. J Clin Oncol 1998;16:986–993.

138. Bishop MR, Fowler DH, Marchigiani D, et al. Allogeneic lymphocytes induce tumor regression of advanced metastatic breast cancer. J Clin Oncol 2004;22:3886–3892.

139. Bay JO, Fleury J, Choufi B, et al. Allogeneic hematopoietic stem cell transplantation in ovarian carcinoma: results of five patients. Bone Marrow Transplant 2002;30:95–102.

140. Feneley RC, Eckert H, Riddell AG, et al. The treatment of advanced bladder cancer with sensitized pig lymphocytes. Br J Surg 1974;61:825–827.

141. Nadler SH, Moore GE. Clinical immunologic study of malignant disease: response to tumor transplants and transfer of leukocytes. Ann Surg 1966;164:482–490.

142. Nadler SH, Moore GE. Immunotherapy of malignant disease. Arch Surg 1969;99:376–381.

143. Yonemoto RH, Terasaki PI. Cancer immunotherapy with HLA-compatible thoracic duct lymphocyte transplantation: a preliminary report. Cancer 1972;30:1438–1443.

144. Kohler PC, Hank JA, Exten R, et al. Clinical response of a patient with diffuse histiocytic lymphoma to adoptive chemoimmunotherapy using cyclophosphamide and alloactivated haploidentical lymphocytes: a case report and phase I trial. Cancer 1985;55:552–560.

145. Porter DL, Connors JM, Van Deerlin VM, et al. Graft-versus-tumor induction with donor leukocyte infusions as primary therapy for patients with malignancies. J Clin Oncol 1999;17:1234–1243.

146. Ballen KK, Becker PS, Emmons RV, et al. Low-dose total body irradiation followed by allogeneic lymphocyte infusion may induce remission in patients with refractory hematologic malignancy. Blood 2002;100:442–450.

147. Or R, Ackerstein A, Nagler A, et al. Allogeneic cell-mediated immunotherapy for breast cancer after autologous stem cell transplantation: a clinical pilot study. Cytokines Cell Mol Ther 1998;4:1–6.

148. Giralt S, Estey E, Albitar M, et al. Engraftment of allogeneic hematopoietic progenitor cells with purine analog-containing chemotherapy: harnessing graft-versus-leukemia without myeloablative therapy. Blood 1997;89:4531–4536.

149. Slavin S, Nagler A, Naparstek E, et al. Nonmyeloablative stem cell transplantation and cell therapy as an alternative to conventional bone marrow transplantation with lethal cytoreduction for the treatment of malignant and nonmalignant hematologic diseases. Blood 1998;91:756–763.

150. Childs R, Clave E, Contentin N, et al. Engraftment kinetics after nonmyeloablative allogeneic peripheral blood stem cell transplantation: full donor T-cell chimerism precedes alloimmune responses. Blood 1999;94:3234–3241.

151. Osband ME, Lavin PT, Babayan RK, et al. Effect of autolymphocyte therapy on survival and quality of life in patients with metastatic renal-cell carcinoma. Lancet 1990;335:994–998.

152. Fenton RG, Steis RG, Madara K, et al. A phase I randomized study of subcutaneous adjuvant IL-2 in combination with an autologous tumor vaccine in patients with advanced renal cell carcinoma. J Immunother Emphasis Tumor Immunol 1996;19:364–374.

153. Keilholz U, Scheibenbogen C, Brado M, et al. Regional adoptive immunotherapy with interleukin-2 and lymphokine-activated killer (LAK) cells for liver metastases. Eur J Cancer 1994;30A:103–105.

154. Ratto GB, Zino P, Mirabelli S, et al. A randomized trial of adoptive immunotherapy with tumor-infiltrating lymphocytes and interleukin-2 versus standard therapy in the postoperative treatment of resected nonsmall cell lung carcinoma. Cancer 1996;78:244–251.

155. Kimura H, Yamaguchi Y. A phase III randomized study of interleukin-2 lymphokine-activated killer cell immunotherapy combined with chemotherapy or radiotherapy after curative or noncurative resection of primary lung carcinoma. Cancer 1997;80:42–49.

156. Uchino J, Une Y, Kawata A, et al. Postoperative chemoimmunotherapy for the treatment of liver cancer. Semin Surg Oncol 1993;9:332–336.

157. Kircher MF, Allport JR, Graves EE, et al. In vivo high resolution three-dimensional imaging of antigen-specific cytotoxic T-lymphocyte trafficking to tumors. Cancer Res 2003;63:6838–6846.

158. Freitas AA, Rocha B. Peripheral T cell survival. Curr Opin Immunol 1999;11:152–156.

159. Cheever MA, Greenberg PD, Fefer A, et al. Augmentation of the anti-tumor therapeutic efficacy of long-term cultured T lymphocytes by in vivo administration of purified interleukin 2. J Exp Med 1982;155:968–980.

160. Mitsuyasu RT, Anton P, Deeks SG, et al. Prolonged survival and tissue trafficking following adoptive transfer of CD4ζ gene-modified autologous CD4$^+$ and CD8$^+$ T cells in HIV-infected subjects. Blood 2000;96:785–793.

161. Carter CS, Leitman SF, Cullis H, et al. Development of an automated closed system for generation of human lymphokine-activated killer (LAK) cells for use in adoptive immunotherapy. J Immunol Methods 1987;101:171–181.

162. Ettinghausen SE, Moore JG, White DE, et al. Hematologic effects of immunotherapy with lymphokine-activated killer cells and recombinant interleukin-2 in cancer patients. Blood 1987;69:1654–1660.

163. Atkins MB, Mier JW, Parkinson DR, et al. Hypothyroidism after treatment with interleukin-2 and lymphokine-activated killer cells. N Engl J Med 1988;318:1557–1563.

164. Livingston PO, Ragupathi G, Musselli C. Autoimmune and anti-tumor consequences of antibodies against antigens shared by normal and malignant tissues. J Clin Immunol 2000;20:85–93.

165. Donahue RE, Kessler SW, Bodine D, et al. Helper virus induced T cell lymphoma in nonhuman primates after retroviral mediated gene transfer. J Exp Med 1992;176:1125–1135.

166. Hacein-Bey-Abina S, von Kalle C, Schmidt M, et al. A serious adverse event after successful gene therapy for X-linked severe combined immunodeficiency. N Engl J Med 2003;348:255–256.

167. Ratto GB, Cafferata MA, Scolaro T, et al. Phase II study of combined immunotherapy, chemotherapy, and radiotherapy in the

postoperative treatment of advanced non-small-cell lung cancer. J Immunother 2000;23:161–167.

168. Mackall CL, Fleisher TA, Brown MR, et al. Age, thymopoiesis, and CD4+ T-lymphocyte regeneration after intensive chemotherapy. N Engl J Med 1995;332:143–149.

169. Mackall CL, Gress RE. Pathways of T-cell regeneration in mice and humans: implications for bone marrow transplantation and immunotherapy. Immunol Rev 1997;157:61–72.

170. Hermans IF, Chong TW, Palmowski MJ, et al. Synergistic effect of metronomic dosing of cyclophosphamide combined with specific antitumor immunotherapy in a murine melanoma model. Cancer Res 2003;63:8408–8413.

171. Dillman RO. Rationales for combining chemotherapy and biotherapy in the treatment of cancer. Mol Biother 1990;2: 201–207.

172. Sullivan KM, Storb R, Buckner CD, et al. Graft-versus-host disease as adoptive immunotherapy in patients with advanced hematologic neoplasms. N Engl J Med 1989;320:828–834.

173. Kernan NA, Collins NH, Juliano L, et al. Clonable T lymphocytes in T cell–depleted bone marrow transplants correlate with development of graft-v-host disease. Blood 1986;68:770–773.

174. Sakaguchi S, Sakaguchi N, Shimizu J, et al. Immunologic tolerance maintained by CD25+ CD4+ regulatory T cells: their common role in controlling autoimmunity, tumor immunity, and transplantation tolerance. Immunol Rev 2001;182:18–32.

175. Tang Q, Henriksen KJ, Bi M, et al. In vitro–expanded antigen-specific regulatory T cells suppress autoimmune diabetes. J Exp Med 2004;199:1455–1465.

176. Taylor PA, Lees CJ, Blazar BR. The infusion of ex vivo activated and expanded CD4(+)CD25(+) immune regulatory cells inhibits graft-versus-host disease lethality. Blood 2002;99:3493–3499.

177. Wood KJ, Sakaguchi S. Regulatory T cells in transplantation tolerance. Nat Rev Immunol 2003;3:199–210.

178. Jonuleit H, Schmitt E, Stassen M, et al. Identification and functional characterization of human CD4(+)CD25(+) T cells with regulatory properties isolated from peripheral blood. J Exp Med 2001;193:1285–1294.

179. Yamazaki S, Iyoda T, Tarbell K, et al. Direct expansion of functional CD25+ CD4+ regulatory T cells by antigen-processing dendritic cells. J Exp Med 2003;198:235–247.

180. Godfrey WR, Spoden DJ, Ge Ying, et al. In vitro expanded human CD4+CD25+ T regulatory cells markedly inhibit allogeneic dendritic cell stimulated MLR cultures. Blood 2004; 104:453–461.

181. Eshhar Z, Bach N, Fitzer-Attas CJ, et al. The T-body approach: potential for cancer immunotherapy. Springer Semin Immunopathol 1996;18:199–209.

182. Arca MJ, Mule JJ, Chang AE. Genetic approaches to adoptive cellular therapy of malignancy. Semin Oncol 1996;23:108–117.

183. Topp MS, Riddell SR, Akatsuka Y, et al. Restoration of CD28 expression in CD28− CD8+ memory effector T cells reconstitutes antigen-induced IL-2 production. J Exp Med 2003;198:947–955.

184. Hooijberg E, Ruizendaal JJ, Snijders PJ, et al. Immortalization of human CD8(+) T cell clones by ectopic expression of telomerase reverse transcriptase. J Immunol 2000;165:4239–4245.

185. Blaese RM, Culver KW, Miller AD, et al. T lymphocyte–directed gene therapy for ADA-SCID: initial trial results after 4 years. Science 1995;270:475–480.

186. Helene M, Lake-Bullock V, Bryson JS, et al. Inhibition of graft-versus-host disease: use of a T cell–controlled suicide gene. J Immunol 1997;158:5079–5082.

187. Bonini C, Ferrari G, Verzeletti S, et al. HSV-TK gene transfer into donor lymphocytes for control of allogeneic graft-versus-leukemia. Science 1997;276:1719–1724.

188. Clackson T, Yang W, Rozamus LW, et al. Redesigning an FKBP-ligand interface to generate chemical dimerizers with novel specificity. Proc Natl Acad Sci USA 1998;95:10437–10442.

189. Straathof KC, Spencer DM, Sutton RE, et al. Suicide genes as safety switches in T lymphocytes. Cytotherapy 2003;5: 227–230.

190. Thomis DC, Marktel S, Bonini C, et al. A Fas-based suicide switch in human T cells for the treatment of graft-versus-host disease. Blood. 2001;97:1249–1257.

191. Berger C, Blau CA, Huang ML, et al. Pharmacologically regulated Fas-mediated death of adoptively transferred T cells in a nonhuman primate model. Blood 2004;103:1261–1269.

192. Sadelain M, Riviere I, Brentjens R. Targeting tumours with genetically enhanced T lymphocytes. Nat Rev Cancer 2003;3:35–45.

193. Koretz MJ, Lawson DH, York RM, et al. Randomized study of interleukin 2 (IL-2) alone vs IL-2 plus lymphokine-activated killer cells for treatment of melanoma and renal cell cancer. Arch Surg 1991;126:898–903.

194. Graham S, Babayan RK, Lamm DL, et al. The use of ex vivo-activated memory T cells (autolymphocyte therapy) in the treatment of metastatic renal cell carcinoma: final results from a randomized, controlled, multisite study. Semin Urol 1993;11:27–34.

195. Law TM, Motzer RJ, Mazumdar M, et al. Phase III randomized trial of interleukin-2 with or without lymphokine-activated killer cells in the treatment of patients with advanced renal cell carcinoma. Cancer 1995;76:824–832.

196. Figlin RA, Thompson JA, Bukowski RM, et al. Multicenter, randomized, phase III trial of CD8(+) tumor-infiltrating lymphocytes in combination with recombinant interleukin-2 in metastatic renal cell carcinoma. J Clin Oncol 1999;17:2521–2529.

197. Rapoport AP, Stadtmauer EA, Levine BL, et al. Adoptive transfer of ex vivo costimulated autologous T-cells after autotransplantation for myeloma accelerates post-transplant T-cell recovery. Blood 2004;104:abstract 439.

198. Kimura H, Yamaguchi Y. Adjuvant immunotherapy with interleukin 2 and lymphokine-activated killer cells after noncurative resection of primary lung cancer. Lung Cancer 1995;13:31–44.

199. Kimura H, Yamaguchi Y. Adjuvant chemo-immunotherapy after curative resection of stage II and IIIA primary lung cancer. Lung Cancer 1996;14:301–314.

Cancer Vaccines

34

Glenn Dranoff

INTRODUCTION

Significant progress towards elucidating the requirements for effective antitumor immunity has invigorated efforts to develop cancer immunotherapies. Novel genetic, biochemical, and bioinformatics technologies have uncovered a large number of tumor-associated gene products that evoke immune recognition. A critical function for endogenous host reactions in modulating spontaneous tumor formation and progression has been revealed through studies of mice rendered immune-deficient by gene-targeting techniques in embryonic stem cells. Specific types of human antitumor immune responses have been linked to improved patient outcomes in diverse cancers. The importance of dendritic cell activation in priming potent antitumor reactions and the key role of immune regulatory networks in attenuating antitumor immunity have been delineated.

Together, these powerful insights provide a rich scientific foundation for crafting therapeutic strategies aimed at augmenting antitumor immunity. Whereas the passive transfer of antitumor antibodies and T cells already has proven efficacious for some hematologic and solid malignancies, the active immunization of cancer patients has become a dynamic investigative enterprise. Multiple cancer vaccination schemes have achieved impressive antitumor effects in preclinical models, and the major requirements for tumor rejection have been clarified. Many of these approaches have been translated into early stage clinical evaluation, and preliminary evidence of immunologic activity, safety, and tumor destruction has been obtained in several phase I studies. A small number of immunization strategies have progressed further to definitive efficacy testing in ongoing randomized phase III trials. Indeed, cancer vaccines have entered the mainstream of clinical investigation in oncology. In this review, I discuss recent progress in cancer immunology and highlight the ways in which a deeper understanding of the antitumor response has improved the prospects for realizing therapeutic and prophylactic cancer vaccines.

ENDOGENOUS ANTITUMOR RESPONSES

Tumors emerge from and are sculpted by a microenvironment composed of stroma, vascular elements, and immune cells.[1] Cross-talk among these populations modulates tumor growth, survival, invasion, and metastasis. Cytokines produced in response to transformation play a key role in disease pathogenesis, in part through triggering immune reactions aimed at minimizing cellular stress and tissue damage.[2]

Infiltrating immune cells recognize cancers through two major pathways. Innate immune effectors, which include granulocytes, mast cells, macrophages, dendritic cells, and natural killer (NK) cells, detect tumor cells directly. NK cells and phagocytes express NKG2D molecules that function as receptors for stress-related genes, such as *MICA* and *MICB*, which are induced as a consequence of cellular transformation.[3] NK cells further scan for the loss of MHC class I molecules on the surface of tumor cells.[4] Dendritic cells employ a variety of scavenger receptors to accomplish the phagocytosis of dying tumor cells.[5]

The adaptive immune system, composed of CD4[+] and CD8[+] T cells and B cells, recognizes cancer initially through an indirect pathway termed cross-priming. In this scheme, dendritic cells process tumor cell debris and migrate to regional lymph nodes to stimulate CD4[+] and CD8[+] T cells[6]; these specific lymphocytes react with major histocompatibility complex (MHC)–restricted tumor peptides derived from mutated proteins, aberrantly expressed gene

Work on this chapter was supported by NIH grants CA74886, CA66996, and CA092625 and by the Leukemia and Lymphoma Society.

products, and normal differentiation antigens.[7] Primed T cells acquire the capacity to detect tumor cells directly in an MHC-restricted fashion. CD4[+] T cells also contribute to B-cell production of antibodies directed against amplified or mutated tumor-associated gene products.[8]

The outcomes of cancer immune recognition have been explored through the use of immune-deficient mice generated through gene-targeting technologies. Mice with defective interferon-γ(IFN-γ) function manifested more tumors and a shorter latency (time to develop cancer) in response to chemical carcinogens compared to wild type controls.[9] Similarly, mice lacking the adaptive immune response showed an increased susceptibility to methylcholanthrene exposure.[10] Mice doubly deficient in IFN-γ and adaptive immunity succumbed to spontaneous adenocarcinomas of the colon, breast, and lung,[10] whereas mice lacking IFN-γ and granulocyte-macrophage colony-stimulating factor (GM-CSF) developed diverse hematological and solid neoplasms in a background of chronic infection and inflammation.[11]

Together, these studies reveal an important role for host responses in attenuating tumor growth in experimental models. Consistent with these findings, dense intratumoral lymphocyte infiltrates in early-stage neoplasms are strongly correlated with reduced frequencies of metastasis and improved patient survival in multiple cancer types.[12,13] Moreover, lymphocyte infiltrates predict for subsequent responsiveness to standard oncologic therapy, particularly in advanced ovarian carcinoma.[14] Viewed in this light, the development of clinically evident cancers indicates a failure of host immunity. Some of the mechanisms responsible for loss of immune control include tumor-derived immunosuppressive factors, regulatory pathways that maintain immune tolerance to self-antigens, inefficient cross-priming, and tumor genomic instability, which might promote the emergence of escape variants.[15]

In contrast to this protective role, however, tumor cells can in some cases exploit host responses to promote disease progression. In this context, unresolved inflammation elicits cell turnover in an effort to restore tissue homeostasis, which together with carcinogen-induced or phagocyte-induced DNA damage can eventually culminate in transformation.[16] Studies of immune-deficient mice underscore the ways in which tumor cells subvert immune reactions. Mice deficient in tumor necrosis factor-α and interleukin-6 (IL-6) were protected from the development of skin tumors and lymphomas by chemical carcinogens, establishing critical roles for these cytokines in promoting tumor formation.[17,18] Similarly, mice lacking macrophage colony-stimulating factor, a key growth and differentiation factor for monocyte/macrophages, showed impaired breast cancer invasion and metastasis.[19] Innate immune cells were required for the development of squamous cell carcinomas in mice transgenic for human papilloma virus, in part through the production of matrix metalloproteinase-9, an important cofactor for angiogenesis.[20] Moreover, tumor cells use the expression of chemokine receptors to subvert the normal signals for cell migration, thus fostering metastasis.[21] Consistent with the idea of immune subversion, the attenuation of chronic inflammation with cyclooxygenase-2 inhibitors suppresses tumor formation in multiple murine models and in patients with diverse malignancies.[22]

Collectively, these studies of endogenous host reactions to tumors illuminate a dual role for immunity in cancer initiation and progression. The mechanisms that dictate whether a host will develop a beneficial or permissive response remain to be established but are likely to include the mixture of cytokines produced in the tumor microenvironment. While this dual role needs to be considered in designing immunotherapy, altering the cytokine balance, as discussed later, can prove therapeutic by promoting the generation of protective antitumor reactions.

CANCER VACCINE MODELS

Experiments with murine transplantable tumors have provided important insights into the mechanisms underlying immune-mediated tumor destruction. In syngeneic models of chemically-induced neoplasms, tumor cell death, accomplished by irradiation or surgical excision, can serve as a vaccine that engenders protective immunity against subsequent wild-type tumor challenge.[23] Tumor elimination involves T-cell and B-cell responses directed against mutated cancer-associated gene products.[24] Rejection of this class of neoplasms is highly specific, reflecting the random targeting of distinct genes by chemical carcinogens.[25] The autochthonous host can similarly mount an effective response against these relatively immunogenic tumors.[26] In contrast, vaccination against spontaneous neoplasms is significantly more stringent and therefore not easily achieved by surgical excision or vaccination with irradiated tumor cells. Nonetheless, exposing tumor cells to mutagens before immunization can evoke protection against subsequent wild-type tumor challenge; in this scenario, mutated gene products trigger initial immune recognition, which subsequently spreads to other gene products expressed by wild-type tumor cells.[27] Thus, once a threshold for effective immune priming is overcome, the activated effectors are capable of destroying even poorly immunogenic tumors.

The efficient priming of antitumor immunity depends on proper stimulation of professional antigen-presenting cells, particularly dendritic cells. An improved understanding of dendritic cell development and maturation has catalyzed a large number of studies exploring the use of these cells for cancer vaccination.[28] In one approach, dendritic cells are expanded ex vivo from hematopoietic progenitors (by culture in GM-CSF and other cytokines), loaded with tumor antigens, and then transplanted into tumor-bearing hosts to enhance cancer immunity. Whole tumor cell lysates, tumor cell fusions, and defined tumor antigens (in the form of RNA, DNA, peptides, or proteins) have all augmented tumor rejection in various models.[29] In a second scheme, dendritic cell function is modulated in vivo, resulting in improved tumor antigen presentation. The inoculation of naked DNA encoding defined tumor antigens promotes dendritic cell activation in situ, primarily through engagement of toll-like receptor-9 by unmethylated CpG oligonucleotides.[30] Tumor-derived heat shock proteins also trigger dendritic cell maturation while chaperoning partially digested tumor moieties into dendritic cell antigen presentation pathways.[31] Tumor antigen–expressing recombinant viral vectors derived from adenovirus, herpes simplex virus, and pox viruses present an additional approach to stimulate dendritic cell function in vivo.[32]

Manipulating the cytokine milieu can further regulate dendritic cell activities. The systemic administration of Flt3 ligand induces a marked increase in dendritic cell numbers in many tissues and thereby improves tumor antigen presentation.[33] Altering the mixture of cytokines present in the tumor microenvironment similarly shifts the outcome of the host response. Forni and colleagues were the first to show that the peritumoral injection of specific cytokines, such as IL-2, provoked tumor rejection through the recruitment and activation of neutrophils, eosinophils, macrophages, NK cells, dendritic cells, and lymphocytes.[34] The application of gene transfer techniques for the stable modification of tumor cells significantly advanced this line of inquiry by enabling a comparison of the relative abilities of multiple cytokines to stimulate tumor rejection. Of a large number of gene products examined, IL-12 and GM-CSF proved to be the most potent in multiple tumor models.[35] IL-12 induced antitumor effects involving Th1 responses (characterized by robust IFN-γ production), increased lymphocyte cytotoxicity, and angiogenesis inhibition.[36] GM-CSF enhanced the local activation of dendritic cells, macrophages, granulocytes, and NKT cells, resulting in a coordinated humoral and cellular response that mediated tumor destruction.[37]

Immunotherapy has also been explored for transgenic murine systems in which tumor formation is driven by the expression of defined oncogenes. These models recapitulate the multiple stages of tumor progression and provide a more physiologic context to examine spontaneous and elicited antitumor host reactions. The strains that have been productively analyzed include Min mice, which harbor a mutation in the *APC* tumor suppressor gene that results in gastrointestinal carcinomas[38]; TRAMP mice, which express the SV40 early T and t genes in the prostate epithelium and thereby develop metastatic prostate adenocarcinomas[39]; and BALB-neuT mice, which express a mutated rat *HER2/neu* oncogene in the breast epithelium and thus generate multiple breast carcinomas.[40] Remarkably, when dendritic cell or cytokine-secreting tumor cell vaccines are administered to animals manifesting precursor stages of disease (i.e., atypical hyperplasia or dysplasia), progression to invasive carcinoma can be abrogated.[41,42] Vaccine-induced antitumor humoral and cellular responses inhibit tumor progression through a coordinated attack on transformed cells, vasculature, and stroma. These provocative findings serve as a strong foundation for initiating clinical trials of prophylactic vaccination in patients harboring inherited mutations that confer a high risk of cancer development.[43]

CANCER ANTIGEN–BASED VACCINES

The investigations in murine tumor models indicate that potent immunotherapy involves efficient tumor antigen presentation by activated dendritic cells and a coordinated effector response that includes antibodies and multiple innate and adaptive cell types. The translation of these principles into clinical trials of immunotherapy has been supported by the development of several informative techniques for immunologic monitoring. When defined cancer antigens are used for vaccination, these methods allow for detailed analysis of elicited B-cell and T-cell responses. Antibody titers and isotypes can be readily measured with ELISAs that use recombinant protein produced in bacteria or insect cells.[8] Bioinformatic algorithms facilitate the identification of cancer antigen–derived, MHC-restricted peptide epitopes that are the targets of CD4$^+$ and CD8$^+$ tumor-specific T cells. These peptides can be incorporated into fluorochrome-labeled, soluble MHC tetramers for the detection and quantification of tumor antigen–specific T cells.[44] Tetramer binding cells can be further characterized phenotypically for activation status and tissue-trafficking patterns. Functional analysis of tumor-specific T cells can be performed with ELISPOT (cytokine production) and cytotoxicity (killing) assays. The immunohistochemistry of resected lesions can identify types of tumor-infiltrating leukocytes and determine tumor antigen expression.

The advantages afforded by these techniques have promoted the undertaking of a large number of clinical trials based on defined cancer antigens.[45] Because of space limitations, a comprehensive review of all these efforts is not possible; rather, selected approaches will be highlighted to illustrate the breadth of investigation. A key issue for all studies using specific antigens is target selection.[7] Unfortunately, the criteria for choosing the optimal target currently remain unclear; paradoxically, definition of the "best" antigens might need to await the validation of a particular target and vaccination strategy in large patient studies that employ standard clinical endpoints (prolonged survival and/or regression). In view of this limited information, several classes of antigens have entered clinical testing. One group, exemplified by the idiotype of B-cell malignancies, encompasses gene products with expression limited to neoplastic cells.[46] These targets might be most advantageous for vaccination, since they should be subjected to less stringent tolerance mechanisms that delete self-reactive cells. A second group includes genes with high-level expression in tumors but restricted expression in normal tissues (typically testes and placenta); intensively studied examples are MAGE-3 and NY-ESO-1.[47] These genes likely manifest intermediate susceptibilty to tolerance pathways. A third class of targets are nonmutated differentiation antigens that are expressed in both tumors and their normal tissue counterparts; members of this large group include Her2/neu and the melanosomal pigmentation proteins MART-1, gp100, and tyrosinase.[48] These gene products should stimulate the strongest tolerizing mechanisms yet confer the greatest risk for autoimmunity.

As multiple strategies to enhance tumor antigen presentation have been successful in experimental models, a wide array of vaccination strategies are being tested clinically. Whereas immunization with MAGE-3–derived peptides alone can evoke some antitumor effects,[49] most peptide-based vaccinations incorporate adjuvants to improve antigen presentation. A number of cytokines, including GM-CSF, Flt3 ligand, IL-12, and IL-2, augment immunity to various peptides in melanoma, breast, and ovarian cancer patients.[50–52] Although the relative immunostimulatory activities of these molecules remain to be clarified in humans, preliminary evidence suggests that GM-CSF might be more effective than Flt3 ligand as an adjuvant.[53]

Several trials of ex vivo expanded dendritic cells pulsed with peptides similarly demonstrated the consistent induction of T-cell responses and occasional tumor regressions.[28] However, key issues regarding the optimal source of hematopoietic progenitors for dendritic cell expansion (peripheral blood mononuclear cells, bone marrow, purified CD34$^+$ cells, with or without prior systemic treatment with Flt3 ligand), the best method for inducing dendritic cell maturation (i.e., tumor necrosis factor, poly I-C, CD40 ligation) and the optimal dose and route of administration remain to be clarified. Moreover, the relative immunogenicity of peptide-pulsed dendritic cells versus peptides plus cytokine needs to be defined. An excellent study that directly compared vaccination with a mixture of four peptides derived from gp100 and tyrosinase, either in an emulsion with GM-CSF and Montanide ISA-51 (a saponin-type adjuvant) or with monocyte-derived dendritic cells, demonstrated a stronger overall immune response in the GM-CSF arm.[54]

Whereas peptide vaccines can target specific MHC molecules, whole gene product immunizations should be broadly applicable to a population with diverse MHC haplotypes. Idiotype vaccinations, either with GM-CSF as an adjuvant or with pulsed dendritic cells, elicit cellular and humoral responses associated with tumor regressions in patients with non-Hodgkin's lymphoma[55,56]; these encouraging findings have motivated current phase III trials. Immunization with NY-ESO-1 protein admixed with ISCOMATRIX, a novel saponin-type adjuvant, consistently resulted in a broad response consisting of high titer antibodies, delayed-type hypersensitivity reactions, and specific

CD4$^+$ and CD8$^+$ T cells.[57] Vaccination with dendritic cells pulsed with a fusion protein composed of prostatic acid phosphatase and GM-CSF triggered immune reactivity in advanced prostate cancer patients.[58] Similarly, recombinant viruses expressing full-length tumor antigens manifest biologic activity in humans. Prime-boost regimens with vaccinia and fowl pox vectors (which elicit non-cross-reactive responses) encoding prostate-specific antigen enhance immunity and may delay tumor progression in relapsed prostate cancer patients.[59]

Glycolipid antigens can also be effectively incorporated into vaccines. The inoculation of a mucin-related O-linked glycopeptide, α-N-acetylgalatosamine-O-serine/threonine emulsified in the saponin QS-21, stimulated high-titer antibodies in prostate cancer patients.[60] Moreover, the injection of dendritic cells pulsed with α-galactosylceramide, a glycolipid that binds to the MHC class I–related gene CD1d, triggered invariant NKT-cell activation and subsequent adaptive immune responses in patients with diverse malignanices.[61]

CELL-BASED CANCER VACCINES

While defined cancer antigen–based vaccinations augment tumor immunity and mediate tumor destruction, they might be currently limited by incomplete knowledge of the most immunogenic targets. The evolution of antigen-loss variants under immune selection further suggests that a diversified response encompassing multiple targets might evoke a more durable antitumor effect. These considerations underlie the application of whole tumor cells as vaccines. In this approach, if antigens shared among multiple tumors are sufficiently immunogenic, then standardized cancer cell vaccines might prove broadly efficacious. Alternatively, if tumor-specific, mutated gene products (generated as a consequence of cancer genomic instability) confer greater immunostimulation, then patient-specific vaccines might be preferable, despite the increased manufacturing complexity.

Several standardized cellular vaccine strategies are under active investigation. Allogeneic melanoma cell lines admixed with BCG appear to prolong survival in patients with fully resected stage IV melanoma, although the results of ongoing randomized Phase III trials are required to resolve this issue definitively.[62] Vaccination with allogeneic pancreatic cancer cells engineered to secrete GM-CSF elicited surprisingly long survival in a minority of patients with advanced disease, and larger studies to define efficacy are underway.[63] Immunization with GM-CSF–secreting, allogeneic prostate carcinoma cells also might be associated with improved survival in patients with metastatic disease, and phase III studies to clarify this finding are in progress.[64] Lysates of allogeneic melanoma cell lines pulsed onto ex vivo expanded dendritic cells similarly evoked significant antitumor immunity.[65]

Multiple autologous tumor cell vaccines are in various stages of clinical development. Melanoma cells that have been coupled to haptens, small chemical moieties that provoke hypersensitivity reactions, might prolong survival in resected stage III patients, particularly when delayed-type hypersensitivity responses to unmodified tumor cells are elicited.[66] Vaccination with autologous solid tumor lysates pulsed onto dendritic cells and fusions of autologous breast carcinomas or renal cell carcinomas with dendritic cells augmented tumor immunity and accomplished tumor destruction in some patients with advanced disease.[67,68] The pulsing of dendritic cells with RNA derived from autologous renal cell carcinomas stimulated cellular responses to a diverse array of target antigens and was associated with unexpectedly prolonged survival.[69] Immunization with heat shock proteins isolated from autologous melanomas provoked strong cellular responses and some tumor regressions, and phase III trials of this approach have been initiated.[70] The use of adenoviral vectors to engineer autologous GM-CSF–secreting melanoma cell vaccines consistently stimulated immunity in stage IV patients and might be associated with prolonged survival.[71] The same immunization strategy in stage IV non–small cell lung carcinoma patients mediated some durable complete responses, and large phase II studies to validate these findings are underway.[72,73]

IMMUNE REGULATORY NETWORKS

Many cancer antigen–based and whole cell–based vaccines augment tumor immunity in patients with advanced tumors, but most subjects eventually succumb to progressive disease. An important mechanism that restrains tumor immunity involves regulatory circuits that normally function to maintain tolerance to self-antigens. A critical role for cytotoxic T lymphocyte–associated antigen-4 (CTLA-4) has emerged in this context.[74] Upon T-cell activation, surface expression of CTLA-4 is up-regulated, whereupon engagement by B7-1 or B7-2 results in cell cycle arrest and diminished cytokine production.[75] Furthermore, regulatory T cells, a distinct population devoted to modulating effector T-cell activities, constitutively express CTLA-4.[76] The importance of this pathway for immune homeostasis was underscored by the development of a lethal lymphoproliferative disease in young CTLA-4–deficient mice.[77] Nonetheless, the transient inhibition of CTLA-4 function with blocking antibodies improved the efficacy of tumor vaccines in murine models, albeit with a loss of tolerance to some normal antigens.[78]

To obtain an initial assessment of the biologic activity of antagonizing CTLA-4 function in humans, we administered a single infusion of the humanized CTLA-4–blocking monoclonal antibody MDX-CTLA4 (3 mg/kg) to nine previously vaccinated metastatic melanoma or ovarian carcinoma patients.[79] Tolerance was partially compromised by

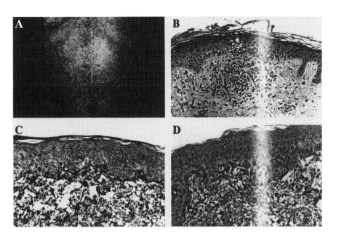

Figure 34.1 MDX-CTLA4 compromises tolerance to normal melanocytes. **A:** Reticular erythematous rash. **B:** Perivascular lymphocyte infiltrate extending into epidermis with interface dermatitis. **C:** CD4$^+$ T cells apposed to dying melanocytes. **D:** CD8$^+$ T cells apposed to dying melanocytes. (Reprinted with permission from Hodi FS, Mihm MC, Soiffer RJ et al. Biologic activity of cytotoxic T lymphocyte–associated antigen 4 antibody blockade in previously vaccinated metastatic melanoma and ovarian carcinoma patients. Proc Natl Acad Sci USA 2003;100:4712–4717.)

therapy, as manifested by low titers of autoantibodies in four patients and rashes due to CD4$^+$ and CD8$^+$ T cells directed against normal melanocytes in five patients (Fig. 34-1). Nonetheless, MDX-CTLA4 provoked extensive tumor necrosis with lymphocyte and granulocyte infiltrates in three of three metastatic melanoma patients and a reduction or stabilization of CA-125 levels in two of two metastatic ovarian carcinoma patients previously vaccinated with irradiated, autologous GM-CSF–secreting tumor cells. In contrast, MDX-CTLA4 did not elicit tumor necrosis in four of four metastatic melanoma patients previously immunized with defined melanosomal antigens. Pathologic examination of the responding metastases revealed CD4$^+$ and CD8$^+$ T cells, CD20$^+$ B cells producing immunoglobulin, and granulocytes leading to tumor destruction (Fig. 34-2). Moreover, a striking circumferential lymphoid infiltrate was also detected in occluded tumor blood vessels, resulting in extensive ischemic necrosis. Since these pathologic features were similar to those previously observed in patients responding to GM-CSF–secreting tumor vaccines, they raise the possibility that MDX-CTLA4 may amplify a long-lived memory response.

Additional studies examined serial infusions of MDX-CTLA4 together with melanosomal antigen–derived peptide vaccines.[80] Of 14 patients tested, 3 achieved objective tumor responses, while 6 developed serious autoimmune disorders, including enterocolitis, hepatitis, dermatitis, and hypophysitis. This work highlights the potential for CTLA-4 antibody blockade to elicit serious autoimmune toxicities, thereby underscoring the need to determine optimal dosages and schedules for selective tumor destruction.

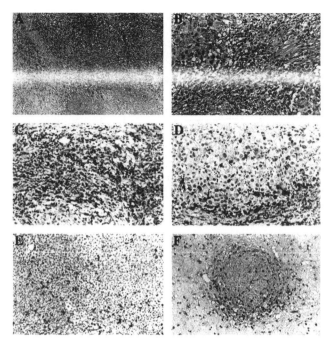

Figure 34.2 MDX-CTLA4 provokes extensive tumor necrosis. **A, B:** Tumor necrosis with granulocytes and lymphocytes. **C:** CD4$^+$ T cells. **D:** CD8$^+$ T cells. **E:** CD20$^+$ B cells. **F:** Vasculopathy with perivascular and intramural lymphoid infiltrates associated with luminal thrombosis. (Reprinted with permission from Hodi FS, Mihm MC, Soiffer RJ et al. Biologic activity of cytotoxic T lymphocyte–associated antigen 4 antibody blockade in previously vaccinated metastatic melanoma and ovarian carcinoma patients. Proc Natl Acad Sci USA 2003;100: 4712–4717.)

CONCLUSION

An improved understanding of the mechanisms underlying antitumor immunity provides a strong foundation for undertaking detailed clinical studies of cancer vaccination. The development of new technologies to measure antitumor immune responses with precision substantially elevates the scientific rigor that can be applied to investigations in human cancer immunology. Indeed, several promising strategies to improve dendritic cell–mediated tumor antigen presentation have been validated in patients with diverse cancers. Moreover, initial trials of CTLA-4 antibody blockade have illuminated the therapeutic potential of interrupting tolerance networks that otherwise attenuate tumor immunity, albeit with a risk for autoimmunity. Determining the proper balance of immune stimulation and inhibition of negative regulation poses a significant clinical challenge, but one that the maturing field of tumor immunology most welcomes.

REFERENCES

1. Hanahan D, Weinberg RA. The hallmarks of cancer. Cell 2000;100: 57–70.
2. Dranoff G. Cytokines in cancer pathogenesis and cancer therapy. Nat Rev Cancer 2004;4:11–22.
3. Diefenbach A, Raulet D. The innate immune response to tumors and its role in the induction of T-cell immunity. Immunol Rev 2002;188:9–21.
4. Karre K. NK cells, MHC class I molecules and the missing self. Scan J Immunol 2002;55:221–228.
5. Albert M, Pearce S, Francisco L, et al. Immature dendritic cells phagocytose apoptotic cells via a$_v$b$_5$ and CD36, and cross-present antigens to cytotoxic T lymphocytes. J Exp Med 1998;188: 1359–1368.
6. Banchereau J, Steinman R. Dendritic cells and the control of immunity. Nature 1998;392:245–252.
7. Gilboa E. The makings of a tumor rejection antigen. Immunity 1999;11:263–270.
8. Old L, Chen Y-T. New paths in human cancer serology. J Exp Med 1998;187:1163–1167.
9. Kaplan D, Shankaran V, Dighe A, et al. Demonstration of an interferon γ–dependent tumor surveillance system in immunocompetent mice. Proc Natl Acad Sci USA 1998;95:7556–7561.
10. Shankaran V, Ikeda H, Bruce AT, et al. IFN-γ and lymphocytes prevent primary tumour development and shape tumour immunogenicity. Nature 2001;410:1107–1111.
11. Enzler T, Gillessen S, Manis JP, et al. Deficiencies of GM-CSF and interferon-gamma link inflammation and cancer. J Exp Med 2003;197:1213–1219.
12. Clark W, Elder D, Guerry D, et al. Model predicting survival in stage I melanoma based on tumor progression. J Natl Cancer Inst 1989;81:1893–1904.
13. Naito Y, Saito K, Shiiba K, et al. CD8$^+$ T cells infiltrated within cancer cell nests as a prognostic factor in human colorectal cancer. Cancer Res 1998;58:3491–3494.
14. Zhang L, Conejo-Garcia J, Katsaros D, et al. Intratumoral T cells, recurrence, and survival in epithelial ovarian cancer. N Engl J Med 2003;348:203–213.
15. Marincola FM, Jaffee EM, Hicklin DJ, et al. Escape of human solid tumors from T-cell recognition: molecular mechanisms and functional significance. Adv Immunol 2000;74:181–273.
16. Ames BN, Gold LS, Willett WC. The causes and prevention of cancer. Proc Natl Acad Sci USA 1995;92:5258–5265.
17. Moore RJ, Owens DM, Stamp G, et al. Mice deficient in tumor necrosis factor-a are resistant to skin carcinogenesis. Nature Med 1999;5:828–831.
18. Hilbert DM, Kopf M, Mock BA, et al. Interleukin 6 is essential for in vivo development of B lineage neoplasms. J Exp Med 1995;182:243–248.
19. Lin E, Nguyen A, Russell R, et al. Colony-stimulating factor 1 promotes progression of mammary tumors to malignancy. J Exp Med 2001;193:727–739.
20. Coussens LM, Tinkle CL, Hanahan D, et al. MMP-9 supplied by bone marrow–derived cells contributes to skin carcinogenesis. Cell 2000;103:481–490.
21. Muller A, Homey B, Soto H, et al. Involvement of chemokine receptors in breast cancer metastasis. Nature 2001;410:50–56.
22. Wang D, DuBois RN. Cyclooxygenase 2–derived prostaglandin E2 regulates the angiogenic switch. Proc Natl Acad Sci USA 2004; 101:415–416.
23. Prehn RT, Main JM. Immunity to methylcholanthrene-induced sarcomas. J Natl Cancer Inst 1957;18:769–778.
24. Ikeda H, Ohta N, Furukawa K, et al. Mutated mitogen–activated protein kinase: a tumor rejection antigen of mouse sarcoma. Proc Natl Acad Sci USA 1997;94:6375–6379.
25. Basombrio MA. Search for common antigenicity among twenty-five sarcomas induced by methylcholanthrene. Cancer Res 1970;30:2458–2462.
26. Klein G, Sjogren HO, Klein E, et al. Demonstration of resistance against methylcholanthrene-induced sarcomas in the primary autochtonous host. Cancer Res 1960;20:1561–1572.
27. Van Pel A, Boon T. Protection against a non-immunogenic mouse leukemia by an immunogenic variant obtained by mutagenesis. Proc Natl Acad Sci USA 1982;79:4718–4722.
28. Cerundolo V, Hermans IF, Salio M. Dendritic cells: a journey from laboratory to clinic. Nat Immunol 2004;5:7–10.
29. Young JW, Inaba K. Dendritic cells as adjuvants for class I major histocompatibility complex–restricted antitumor immunity. J Exp Med 1996;183:7–11.

30. Krieg AM. CpG motifs: the active ingredient in bacterial extracts? Nat Med 2003;9:831–835.

31. Suto R, Srivastava PK. A mechanism for the specific immunogenicity of heat shock protein–chaperoned peptides. Science 1995;269:1585–1588.

32. Pardoll DM. Spinning molecular immunology into successful immunotherapy. Nat Rev Immunol 2002;2:227–238.

33. Lynch D, Andreasen A, Maraskovsky E, et al. Flt3 ligand induces tumor regression and antitumor immune responses in vivo. Nature Med 1997;3:625–631.

34. Forni G, Fujiwara H, Martino F, et al. Helper strategy in tumor immunology: expansion of helper lymphocytes and utilization of helper lymphokines for experimental and clinical immunotherapy. Cancer Metast Rev 1988;7:289–309.

35. Mach N, Dranoff G. Cytokine-secreting tumor cell vaccines. Curr Opin Immunol 2000;12:571–575.

36. Cavallo F, Signorelli P, Giovarelli M, et al. Antitumor efficacy of adenocarcinoma cells engineered to produce interleukin 12 (IL-12) or other cytokines compared with exogenous IL-12. J Natl Cancer Inst 1997;89:1049–1058.

37. Dranoff G. GM-CSF–based cancer vaccines. Immunol Rev 2002; 188:147–154.

38. Haigis KM, Hoff PD, White A, et al. Tumor regionality in the mouse intestine reflects the mechanism of loss of Apc function. Proc Natl Acad Sci USA 2004.

39. Greenberg NM, Demayo F, Finegold MJ, et al. Prostate cancer in a transgenic mouse. Proc Natl Acad Sci USA 1995;92:3439–3443.

40. Nanni P, Nicoletti G, De Giovanni C, et al. Combined allogeneic tumor cell vaccination and systemic interleukin 12 prevents mammary carcinogenesis in HER-2/neu transgenic mice. J Exp Med 2001;194:1195–1205.

41. Iinuma T, Homma S, Noda T, et al. Prevention of gastrointestinal tumors based on adenomatous polyposis coli gene mutation by dendritic cell vaccine. J Clin Invest 2004;113:1307–1317.

42. De Giovanni C, Nicoletti G, Landuzzi L, et al. Immunoprevention of HER-2/neu transgenic mammary carcinoma through an interleukin 12–engineered allogeneic cell vaccine. Cancer Res 2004;64: 4001–4009.

43. Finn OJ, Forni G. Prophylactic cancer vaccines. Curr Opin Immunol 2002;14:172–177.

44. Altman J, Moss P, Goulder P, et al. Direct visualization and phenotypic analysis of virus-specific T lymphocytes in HIV-infected individuals. Science 1996;274:94–96.

45. Finn OJ. Cancer vaccines: between the idea and the reality. Nat Rev Immunol 2003;3:630–641.

46. Kwak LW, Campbell MJ, Czerwinski DK, et al. Induction of immune responses in patients with B-cell lymphoma against the surface-immunoglobulin idiotype expressed by their tumors. N Engl J Med 1992;327:1209–1215.

47. Boon T, van der Bruggen P. Human tumor antigens recognized by T lymphocytes. J Exp Med 1996;183:725–729.

48. Rosenberg SA. Progress in human tumour immunology and immunotherapy. Nature 2001;411:380–384.

49. Marchand M, van Baren N, Weynants P, et al. Tumor regressions observed in patients with metastatic melanoma treated with an antigenic peptide encoded by gene MAGE-3 and presented by HLA-A1. Int J Cancer 1999;80:219–230.

50. Disis ML, Schiffman K, Guthrie K, et al. Effect of dose on immune response in patients vaccinated with an her-2/neu intracellular domain protein–based vaccine. J Clin Oncol 2004;22: 1916–1925.

51. Peterson AC, Harlin H, Gajewski TF. Immunization with Melan-A peptide–pulsed peripheral blood mononuclear cells plus recombinant human interleukin-12 induces clinical activity and T-cell responses in advanced melanoma. J Clin Oncol 2003;21: 2342–2348.

52. Rosenberg S, Yang J, Schwartzentruber D, et al. Immunologic and therapeutic evaluation of a synthetic peptide vaccine for the treatment of patients with metastatic melanoma. Nature Med 1998;4: 321–327.

53. Disis ML, Rinn K, Knutson KL, et al. Flt3 ligand as a vaccine adjuvant in association with HER-2/neu peptide–based vaccines in patients with HER-2/neu–overexpressing cancers. Blood 2002;99: 2845–2850.

54. Slingluff CL Jr, Petroni GR, Yamshchikov GV, et al. Clinical and immunologic results of a randomized phase II trial of vaccination using four melanoma peptides either administered in granulocyte-macrophage colony-stimulating factor in adjuvant or pulsed on dendritic cells. J Clin Oncol 2003;21:4016–4026.

55. Bendandi M, Gocke C, Kobrin C, et al. Complete molecular remissions induced by patient-specific vaccination plus granulocyte-monocyte colony-stimulating factor against lymphoma. Nature Med 1999;5:1171–1177.

56. Timmerman JM, Czerwinski DK, Davis TA, et al. Idiotype-pulsed dendritic cell vaccination for B-cell lymphoma: clinical and immune responses in 35 patients. Blood 2002;99:1517–1526.

57. Davis ID, Chen W, Jackson H, et al. Recombinant NY-ESO-1 protein with ISCOMATRIX adjuvant induces broad integrated antibody and CD4(+) and CD8(+) T cell responses in humans. Proc Natl Acad Sci USA 2004;101:10697–10702.

58. Small EJ, Fratesi P, Reese DM, et al. Immunotherapy of hormone-refractory prostate cancer with antigen-loaded dendritic cells. J Clin Oncol 2000;18:3894–3903.

59. Kaufman HL, Wang W, Manola J, et al. Phase II randomized study of vaccine treatment of advanced prostate cancer (E7897): a trial of the Eastern Cooperative Oncology Group. J Clin Oncol 2004;22: 2122–2132.

60. Slovin SF, Ragupathi G, Musselli C, et al. Fully synthetic carbohydrate-based vaccines in biochemically relapsed prostate cancer: clinical trial results with alpha-N-acetylgalactosamine-O-serine/threonine conjugate vaccine. J Clin Oncol 2003;21:4292–4298.

61. Nieda M, Okai M, Tazbirkova A, et al. Therapeutic activation of Valpha24+Vbeta11+ NKT cells in human subjects results in highly coordinated secondary activation of acquired and innate immunity. Blood 2004;103:383–389.

62. Hsueh EC, Essner R, Foshag LJ, et al. Prolonged survival after complete resection of disseminated melanoma and active immunotherapy with a therapeutic cancer vaccine. J Clin Oncol 2002;20:4549–4554.

63. Jaffee E, Hruban R, Biedrzycki B, et al. Novel allogeneic granulocyte-macrophage colony-stimulating factor–secreting tumor vaccine for pancreatic cancer: a phase I trial of safety and immune activation. J Clin Oncol 2001;19:145–156.

64. Simons J, Mikhak B, Chang JF, et al. Induction of immunity to prostate cancer antigens: results of a clinical trial of vaccination with irradiated autologous prostate tumor cells engineered to secrete granulocyte-macrophage colony-stimulating factor using ex vivo gene transfer. Cancer Res 1999;59:5160–5168.

65. Nestle F, Alijagic S, Gilliet M, et al. Vaccination of melanoma patients with peptide- or tumor lysate-pulsed dendritic cells. Nature Med 1998;4:328–332.

66. Berd D, Sato T, Maguire HC Jr, et al. Immunopharmacologic analysis of an autologous, hapten-modified human melanoma vaccine. J Clin Oncol 2004;22:403–415.

67. Stift A, Friedl J, Dubsky P, et al. Dendritic cell–based vaccination in solid cancer. J Clin Oncol 2003;21:135–142.

68. Avigan D, Vasir B, Gong J, et al. Fusion cell vaccination of patients with metastatic breast and renal cancer induces immunological and clinical responses. Clin Cancer Res 2004;10:4699–4708.

69. Su Z, Dannull J, Heiser A, et al. Immunological and clinical responses in metastatic renal cancer patients vaccinated with tumor RNA–transfected dendritic cells. Cancer Res 2003;63:2127–2133.

70. Belli F, Testori A, Rivoltini L, et al. Vaccination of metastatic melanoma patients with autologous tumor-derived heat shock protein gp96–peptide complexes: clinical and immunologic findings. J Clin Oncol 2002;20:4169–4180.

71. Soiffer R, Hodi FS, Haluska F, et al. Vaccination with irradiated, autologous melanoma cells engineered to secrete granulocyte-macrophage colony-stimulating factor by adenoviral-mediated gene transfer augments antitumor immunity in patients with metastatic melanoma. J Clin Oncol 2003;21:3343–3350.

72. Salgia R, Lynch T, Skarin A, et al. Vaccination with irradiated autologous tumor cells engineered to secrete granulocyte-macrophage colony-stimulating factor augments antitumor immunity in some patients with metastatic non-small-cell lung carcinoma. J Clin Oncol 2003;21:624–630.

73. Nemunaitis J, Sterman D, Jablons D, et al. Granulocyte-macrophage colony-stimulating factor gene-modified autologous tumor vaccines in non-small-cell lung cancer. J Natl Cancer Inst 2004;96:326–331.

74. Chambers CA, Kuhns MS, Egen JG, et al. CTLA-4–mediated inhibition in regulation of T cell responses: mechanisms and manipulation in tumor immunotherapy. Annu Rev Immunol 2001;19: 565–594.

75. Salomon B, Bluestone JA. Complexities of CD28/B7: CTLA-4 costimulatory pathways in autoimmunity and transplantation. Annu Rev Immunol 2001;19:225–252.

76. Shevach EM, McHugh RS, Piccirillo CA, et al. Control of T-cell activation by CD4$^+$ CD25$^+$ suppressor T cells. Immunol Rev 2001;182:58–67.

77. Tivol EA, Borriello F, Schweitzer AN, et al. Loss of CTLA-4 leads to massive lymphoproliferation and fatal multiorgan tissue destruction, revealing a critical negative regulatory role of CTLA-4. Immunity 1995;3:541–547.

78. van Elsas A, Hurwitz A, Allison J. Combination immunotherapy of B16 melanoma using anti-cytotoxic T lymphocyte–associated antigen 4 (CTLA-4) and granulocyte/macrophage colony-stimulating factor (GM-CSF)–producing vaccines induces rejection of subcutaneous and metastatic tumors accompanied by autoimmune depigmentation. J Exp Med 1999;190: 355–366.

79. Hodi FS, Mihm MC, Soiffer RJ, et al. Biologic activity of cytotoxic T lymphocyte–associated antigen 4 antibody blockade in previously vaccinated metastatic melanoma and ovarian carcinoma patients. Proc Natl Acad Sci USA 2003;100:4712–4717.

80. Phan GQ, Yang JC, Sherry RM, et al. Cancer regression and autoimmunity induced by cytotoxic T lymphocyte–associated antigen 4 blockade in patients with metastatic melanoma. Proc Natl Acad Sci USA 2003;100:8372–8377.

Hematopoietic Growth Factors

35

William P. Petros

INTRODUCTION

Hematopoietic growth factors (HGFs) are an important therapeutic class of agents for patients being treated with cytotoxic chemotherapy. Appropriate prescribing of these compounds has resulted in reductions in transfusion requirements and prevention of myelosuppression-related complications. The primary function of these acidic glycoprotein molecules is augmentation of the production and activation of hematopoietic cells. They may also play a role in immune response.

The HGFs have many uses in oncology (Table 35.1). The focus of this chapter is on evaluating the cytokines with known clinical importance for hematopoiesis in the patient with cancer. Most of the justification for the current role of HGFs in therapeutics is directly linked to both the degree of interpatient variability in chemotherapy-induced myelosuppression and the role of dose intensity in the treatment of a particular malignancy. At the present time, these agents should not be used to increase chemotherapy doses indiscriminately and without scientific justification.

CHEMISTRY AND PHARMACEUTICS

Chemically, the HGFs are glycoproteins typically consisting of a primary chain of over 100 amino acids that are intermittently bridged by disulfide bonds. The tertiary structure of the protein plays an important role in its biologic activity. Some HGFs circulate as dimers. The molecular weight of these molecules (approximately 19 to 90 kd) is dependent on both the primary chemical structure and the extent of glycosylation. Several endogenous forms of a particular HGF may be found in the circulation varying by

the degree of glycosylation—a posttranscriptional event. Recombinant HGFs may be glycosylated depending on the type of expression system used in their manufacture. Three expression systems have been used in HGF synthesis: bacterial, yeast, and mammalian cell lines. Bacterial systems, such as *E. coli*, do not produce glycosylated products; whereas yeast cells do provide some degree of glycosylation. Mammalian cells produce glycosylation that is more similar to the human pattern. It is not yet clear if differences in glycosylation translate into clinically important effects. In vitro studies suggest that glycosylation may alter the receptor binding, the elimination patterns, and/or the immunogenicity of cytokines.[1,2] Thus individual generic names have been assigned depending on the expression vector used in the manufacturing process (e.g., see GM-CSF in Table 35.2). The unknown clinical significance of variations in glycosylation and the use of different activity assay methods by the various manufacturers make dosage comparisons difficult even between generic types of an HGF.

EPO is a good example of how glycosylation can alter the pharmacologic properties of an HGF. Site-directed mutagenesis of the gene encoding EPO was utilized; the mutation added two N-glycosylation sites, producing the product darbepoetin.[3] This resulted in a 23% increase in molecular weight compared with recombinant EPO but a threefold prolongation of the serum circulation time due to protection from metabolic degradation.[4]

Another approach to increasing the circulation time of recombinant proteins involves increasing the molecular size or hydrodynamic volume by conjugation with polyethylene glycol (PEG). This effectively constrains renal filtration of the drug and thus circumvents much of the metabolic degradation typically occurring during tubular reabsorption. Using this approach, a currently marketed

TABLE 35.1

CURRENT AND POTENTIAL USES OF HEMATOPOIETIC GROWTH FACTORS IN ONCOLOGY

Aid to hematopoietic reconstitution following myelosuppressive therapy
Bone marrow failure
Drug-induced (not chemotherapy-induced) neutropenia
Regional therapy for localized infections
Immunostimulation
In vivo cellular expansion of hematopoietic stem cells
Ex vivo cellular expansion
Generation of immune effector cells (e.g., dendritic cells)
Immune thrombocytopenic purpura
Transporters for toxins to treat hematologic malignancies

form of G-CSF, pegfilgrastim, was created by covalently binding a 20-kd PEG molecule to the N-terminal methionine residue.

HEMATOPOIETIC GROWTH FACTOR RECEPTORS

Polymorphisms in genes that regulate HGF receptors have been reported, and some data suggest this type of variability has physiologic significance.[5] Glycoprotein receptors for HGFs are transcribed and expressed in a variety of hematologic and nonhematologic cells, including many cancer cell lines. The clinical implications of HGF receptor expression on malignant cells are unknown; however, one study showed that the ability of multiple malignant cell lines to transcribe genes encoding for a cytokine receptor is, by itself, insufficient to render these cells responsive to cytokine stimulation.[6] Numerous clinical trials of G-CSF and GM-CSF for prevention or reversal of chemotherapy-associated neutropenia assessed the effect of these cytokines on patient survival, but not as much attention has been paid to the effects of EPO until recently. It is known that EPO activates antiapoptotic pathways and has a role in angiogenesis. Functional receptors for the cytokine are present in breast, prostate, and various pediatric tumors.[7,8] Placebo-controlled clinical trials of EPO in patients with breast cancer or head and neck found worse cancer control in those receiving EPO; unfortunately, the studies were not powered to address this issue in a prospective manner.[9,10] Additional studies focusing on the effects of EPOs on cancer progression are underway.

HGF receptors contain either one subunit (e.g., EPO, G-CSF, TPO) or multiple subunits (e.g., GM-CSF, IL-3, IL-6), and frequently subunits are shared between HGF receptors. Most common is a unique α subunit and a shared β subunit, with the latter essential for both high-affinity binding

and signal transduction. Cytokine binding to cell surface receptors results in receptor clustering (oligomerization), activation, and generation of intracellular signals. In general, the HGF receptors lack intrinsic tyrosine kinase domains (except for M-CSF, SCF, and FLT-3); however, cytoplasmic tyrosine kinases have been implicated in signal transduction pathways for some of these cytokines.[11] HGF receptor density is both cell and maturation specific. For a particular HGF, occupancy of only a small percentage of available receptors is required to adequately stimulate a hematopoietic cell.[12] Exposure to exogenously administered cytokines may result in altered regulation of that cytokine's receptor or the receptors of other cytokines, leading to synergistic or antagonistic effects.[13]

The ultimate physiologic effect of circulating HGFs is determined by both the cytokine concentration in blood and the presence of receptor antagonists and/or inhibitors (Fig. 35.1). A number of studies have investigated the relevance of soluble forms of the HGF receptors.[14] The potential biologic effects of these molecules are numerous and include ligand stabilization before binding, receptor competition for ligand, receptor down-regulation, and cell sensitization that enhances the response to a ligand (Fig. 35.2).[15] Diverse biologic responses to soluble receptors may be a function of their concentration. The level of these molecules is tightly regulated and thought to be primarily produced by proteolytic cleavage of the transmembrane receptor's extracellular ligand-binding domain or by alternative splicing of a truncated mRNA for the receptor.[16] Receptor antagonists that block cell-surface receptors and compounds that down-modulate cell surface receptors may also inhibit cytokine activity. Elevated serum concentrations of various soluble receptors have been associated with inflammation or malignant diseases.

MECHANISM OF ACTION AND BIOLOGIC EFFECTS

Multiple biologic and biochemical effects are influenced by HGFs; thus, an overall paradigm as to their mechanism(s) of action is not well established. In addition to their ability to augment activation and proliferation, these cytokines aid in committing cells to a restricted differentiation pathway as well as increase the survival of some cells. The interpretation of biologic effects resulting from administering an HGF is sometimes complex because these effects may be attributable to the HGF's ability to alter the endogenous concentrations of other cytokines.

Animal models that are genetically deficient in a particular HGF have helped define the putative roles of HGFs. For example, homozygous G-CSF–deficient mice are viable, fertile, and superficially healthy but display chronic neutropenia, whereas those rendered GM-CSF–deficient do not have altered hematopoiesis.[17,18]

TABLE 35.2
PHARMACEUTICAL CHARACTERISTICS OF HEMATOPOIETIC GROWTH FACTORS

Cytokine	Other Names	Generic Names	Expression Vector	Brand Names	No. of Amino Acids	Human Chromosome Location	Normal Endogenous Sources
G-CSF	Granulocyte colony-stimulating factor	Filgrastim Lenograstim	E. coli CHO	Neupogen (Amgen) Granocyte (Chugai)	174	17	Monocytes/macrophages, fibroblasts, endothelial cells, keratinocytes
GM-CSF	Granulocyte-macrophage colony-stimulating factor	Sargramostim Molgramostim Regramostim	Yeast E. coli CHO	Leukine (Immunex) Leucomax (Schering)	127	5	T-lymphocytes, monocytes/macrophages, fibroblasts, endothelial cells, osteoblasts, epithelial cells
EPO	Erythropoietin	Epoetin-α Epoetin-α Epoetin-β Darbepoetin-α	CHO CHO CHO CHO	Epogen (Amgen) Procrit/Eprex (Ortho) NeoRecormon (Roche) Aranesp (Amgen)	165	7	Renal cells, hepatocytes
IL-11	Interleukin-11	Oprelvekin	E. coli	Neumega (Genetics Institute)	178	19	Stromal fibroblasts, trophoblasts
SCF	Stem cell factor, steel factor, mast cell growth factor, c-kit ligand	Ancestim	E. coli	Stemgen (Amgen)	165	12	Endothelial cells, fibroblasts, circulating mononuclears, bone marrow stromal cells
TPO	Thrombopoietin, megakaryocyte growth and development factor				332	3	Liver, kidney

CHO, Chinese hamster ovary cells; CSF, colony-stimulating factor.

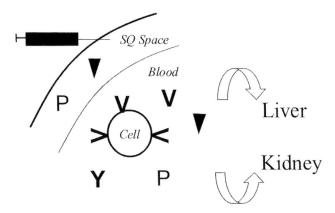

Figure 35.1 Potential routes of cytokine action and clearance. (▼, cytokine receptor antagonist; P, protease; V, receptors for cytokine [soluble or attached to cell membrane]; Y, antibodies to cytokine.)

Figure 35.3 depicts the hematopoietic effects elicited by the various HGFs. Although such representation is useful as a basic learning tool, the true nature of the system, which produces hundreds of billions of cells per day in steady-state conditions, is undoubtedly much more complex than shown here. Interactions between recombinant and endogenous cytokines may play an important role in their biologic effects.[19]

Best established are the effects of HGFs such as EPO and G-CSF on the terminal differentiation of erythrocytes and neutrophils, respectively. The in vitro sensitivity of bone marrow cells to stimulation by G-CSF may be related to the patient's age, with a lower sensitivity noted in older subjects.[20] Other important effects include a reduction in the time taken for newly produced neutrophils to be released from the bone marrow into the circulation and increases in antibody-dependent cytotoxic capacity. The former effect occurs primarily with G-CSF, as compared with GM-CSF.[21] Administration of G-CSF following chemotherapy stimulates primitive hematopoietic progenitors to appear in the peripheral blood to such a degree that they may exceed the concentrations of these cells in normal bone marrow.[22] Interestingly, G-CSF receptor expression appears not to be required for mobilization of early hematopoietic progenitor cells by that cytokine.[23] Molecules such as G-CSF also enhance responses such as membrane depolarization, release of arachidonic acid, and generation of superoxide anions by neutrophils.

The therapeutic effects of EPO include maintenance of the induction, proliferation, and differentiation of erythroid progenitors from the bone marrow. Clearly, the primary effects of EPO are on the erythroid lineage; however, it may also play a role in the stimulation of early multipotent progenitors.[24] Its erythropoietic activity may be at least partly attributable to induction of heme synthetic enzymes such as porphobilinogen deaminase. Other data suggest EPO may act by suppressing apoptosis of colony-forming units.

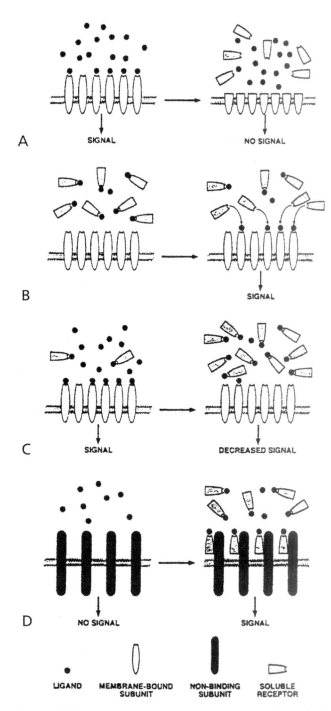

Figure 35.2 Some potential pharmacologic interactions of soluble colony-stimulating factor receptors. **A:** Proteolytic cleavage of soluble receptors results in a down-modulation of the membrane-bound receptor. **B:** Ligand binding to soluble receptor results in prolongation of ligand effect by stabilizing it in extracellular space. **C:** Competition between soluble and membrane-bound receptors for ligand results in decreased signal. **D:** Association of soluble receptors with ligand and nonbinding receptor subunits produces ligand sensitivity in cells without expression of membrane-bound receptor. (Reproduced with permission from Heaney ML, Golde DW. Soluble cytokine receptors. Blood 1996;87:847–857.)

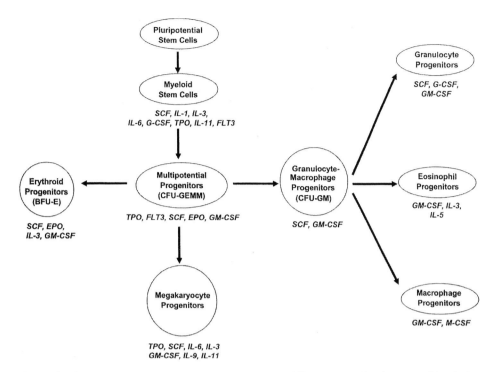

Figure 35.3   Representation of myeloid hematopoietic differentiation. Cytokines capable of stimulating specific cells are listed below such cells. See Table 35.2 for other names of cytokines shown here. (BFU-E, burst-forming unit, erythroid; CFU-GEMM, colony-forming unit–granulocyte-erythrocyte-megakaryocyte macrophage; CFU-GM, colony-forming unit–granulocyte-macrophage; EPO, erythropoietin; G-CSF, granulocyte colony-stimulating factor; GM-CSF, granulocyte-macrophage colony-stimulating factor; IL, interleukin; M-CSF, macrophage colony-stimulating factor; SCF, stem cell factor; TPO, thrombopoietin.)

The primary effect of GM-CSF on hematopoietic cells lies in its ability to augment the survival and proliferation of cells in the granulocytic and macrophage lineages as well as maintain megakaryocyte progenitors at high concentrations. In vitro studies have shown that GM-CSF increases the proportion of hematopoietic cells entering the S phase of the cell cycle and results in a dose-dependent shortening in the length of the cell cycle. Increases in granulocyte life span, metabolic functional activity, and antibody-dependent cellular cytotoxicity have been noted with in vitro incubations. These may be particularly important for the monocyte/macrophage cell lines because production of other cytokines seems to be an important function of these cells. HGFs may display both acute and subacute effects on the peripheral blood concentrations of myeloid cells. For example, leukocyte concentrations initially decline following administration of GM-CSF, most likely as a result of margination of cells induced to express Mo1 leukocyte cell surface adhesion antigen.[25] Other alterations of cellular function by GM-CSF include inhibition of neutrophil migration to sterile inflammatory fields.[26] GM-CSF is a potent stimulator (in vitro and in vivo) of dendritic cells, which are important initiators of primary immune responses.[27] The clinical implications of these effects are under study.

The glycoprotein thrombopoietin (TPO), also known as the "c-mpl ligand" or "megakaryocyte growth and development factor" (MGDF), is thought to play a very important, early, and relatively specific role in the regulation of platelet production. Mice deficient in mpl have mature, functional platelets, albeit at a concentration 15% of normal.[28] TPO has been shown to stimulate blast colony formation in cells obtained from patients with acute myelogenous leukemia (AML), but solid tumors do not routinely express the mpl receptor.[29] Production of TPO is thought to occur predominantly in the liver at a constant rate, whereas circulating concentrations are regulated by platelet receptor–mediated clearance of the cytokine. One negative aspect of TPO is its potential to inhibit platelet release from mature megakaryocytes.[30]

IL-11 is known for its properties as a stimulator of megakaryopoiesis, perhaps interacting at a later stage than TPO. However, it also has been shown to synergistically act with early and later acting cytokines in various stages of hematopoiesis. In addition, it is expressed and has activity in many other tissues, including those of the CNS, GI tract, and testes.

SCF is a very early acting cytokine that is a ligand for the oncogene *c-kit*. Stimulation of in vitro proliferation has been demonstrated in mast cells as well as early and intermediate bone marrow progenitors. SCF can also protect hematopoietic cells from radiation-induced damage.

CLINICAL PHARMACOLOGY

Endogenous production of HGFs occurs in a wide variety of both hematopoietic and nonhematopoietic cells (Table 35.2). Some of these cytokines are found in detectable quantities in blood; however, many factors may influence their concentrations, including concurrent drug therapy, disease, and cell homeostasis.[31,32] For example, concentrations of G-CSF and TPO increase during periods of neutropenia and thrombocytopenia, respectively. This initially led to speculation that such cytopenias cause enhanced production of these cytokines. However, the effect was a result of the reduction of the receptor-based HGF clearance (see later). Exogenously administered cytokines or other drugs may also influence endogenous cytokine concentrations in patients with cancer. We have noted relatively higher concentrations of M-CSF, IL-6, and TNF-α in patients receiving GM-CSF than in those on G-CSF following autologous bone marrow transplantation.[33] These observations are in accordance with in vitro studies indicating that recombinant GM-CSF can induce neutrophil and macrophage production of multiple cytokines.[34] Blood obtained following administration of G-CSF to human volunteers has been shown to yield an increase in the concentrations of anti-inflammatory cytokines upon ex vivo stimulation.[35] Endogenous cytokine concentrations have also been helpful in evaluating the efficacy[19,33] and toxicity[33] of HGF therapy.

Assay Methodology

Most published pharmacokinetic studies of HGFs are conducted by ELISA or RIA quantitative techniques. Use of an automated plate reader with these immunoassays allows the measurement of approximately 75 samples in several hours or less. ELISA assays provide easy and sensitive quantitative measurement of cytokine concentrations; however, they determine the immunoactivity, not necessarily the biological activity, of proteins. False-positive results are possible when a molecule that has been rendered biologically inactive remains intact at the assay's antibody binding site. However, currently used biological assays are often too cumbersome, costly, and variable for extensive studies of cytokines at multiple sample time points. Furthermore, endogenous inhibitors sometimes found in clinical samples may influence them. Neither assay type can distinguish endogenous HGFs from an exogenously administered recombinant forms, although approaches capable of distinguishing them are emerging.[36]

Pharmacokinetics

A variety of processes may influence the pharmacokinetic disposition of recombinant proteins such as the HGFs, as summarized in Figure 35.1. Some characteristics may be predictable by the molecular weight and/or glycosylation, while others may vary depending on receptor concentrations at particular time points.

Absorption

Subcutaneous administration of HGFs generally has been shown to produce lower bioavailability. This effect is thought to be secondary to degradation of the recombinant protein by subcutaneous proteases. Conversely, subcutaneous administration may result in greater clinical efficacy than short intravenous infusions. One explanation for these effects may be secondary to the low yet prolonged blood concentrations achieved with subcutaneous delivery. A study evaluating this effect through a clinical comparison of intravenous and subcutaneous administration of GM-CSF was conducted in patients with myelodysplasia.[37] Twenty patients were randomly assigned to receive GM-CSF (yeast) either by 2-hour IV infusion or subcutaneously every 12 hours. Treatment lasted for 2 weeks, followed by a 2-week washout; thereafter patients were crossed over to the alternative administration route. Optimal hematopoietic stimulation occurred with the subcutaneous route. Severe toxicity occurred at a similar rate in each group.

Distribution

HGFs typically display relatively small volumes of distribution, approximating that of the plasma volume. As expected, studies that are designed to evaluate multiple compartment pharmacokinetics have described rapid distribution phases, followed by more prolonged elimination. Peak concentrations generally follow a linear dose-dependency.

Metabolism/Excretion

Serum HGF concentrations may be influenced by exogenous drug administration, increased endogenous production, or reduced elimination. Decay of HGFs from the circulation may occur via a variety of possible mechanisms, including: attachment of the ligand to the cell surface receptor, with subsequent endocytosis; metabolism by proteolytic enzymes (especially in the liver); and urinary excretion by glomerular filtration, followed by reabsorption and catabolism (Fig. 35.1). The pattern and elimination pathways of exogenously administered cytokines may be affected by the dose; the administration route and schedule; the degree of glycosylation/pegylation of the recombinant protein; the specific receptors available; the production of antibodies; and, in some cases, renal function. Receptors for G-CSF are

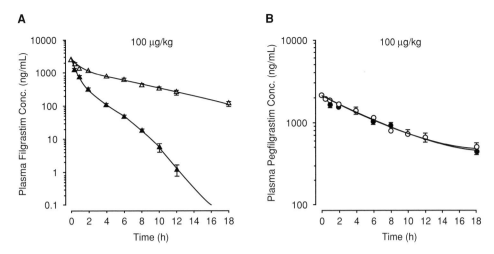

Figure 35.4   Influence of the kidney on pharmacokinetics of pegylated versus nonpegylated proteins. Plasma disposition of filgrastim (Panel A) or pegfilgrastim (Panel B) following IV administration of 100 µg/kg to either normal (closed symbols) or nephrectomized (open symbols) rats. (Data from Yang B-B, Lum PK, Hayashi MM, et al. Polyethylene glycol modification of filgrastim results in decreased renal clearance of the protein in rats. J Pharm Sci 2004;93:1367–1373.)

of sufficient quantity in patients with a normal or recovering WBC count to provide an important mechanism of clearing the protein. These effects are more pronounced with the pegylated form of filgrastim, since the additional molecular size hinders the protein's renal filtration and thus its subsequent availability for metabolism (Fig. 35.4).[38] In addition, it appears that administration of G-CSF during neutropenia up-regulates the number of receptors per cell and thus enhances its own clearance.[39] Therefore, the serum profile of filgrastim shows greater fluctuation (peak to trough) during times when the patient is starting to recover from neutropenia than in the midst of neutropenia. Disposition of the pegylated form of filgrastim shows comparatively little decay during neutropenia until the WBC count begins its rebound.

The presence of other proteins, such as receptor antagonists or modulators of receptor expression, may also significantly affect receptor-mediated clearance. Dramatic reductions in the systemic clearance of a cytokine have been observed to follow concurrent administration of antibodies to that cytokine.[40] This result may seem paradoxical; however, the substantially higher molecular weight of the antibody-HGF complex could limit its ability to be filtered by the glomerulus.

A summary of the pharmacokinetic parameters from published studies of selected CSFs is provided in Table 35.3. Factors potentially affecting the variability in the studies include assay methods, patient age, CSF dosage, receptor concentrations (e.g., WBC count), and the expression vector of the recombinant protein.

The effects of organ dysfunction on the pharmacokinetics of these proteins have not been extensively evaluated. It has previously been reported that systemic clearance and urinary excretion of regramostim is altered in bone marrow transplant patients with increased serum creatinine levels following an ablative regimen that included cisplatin.[41]

The hypothesis was that the tubular toxicity produced by cisplatin alters the renal metabolism of regramostim and that this is modified further by reduced creatinine clearance. It is of importance to note that even though the data in Table 35.3 are summarized for multiple recombinant forms of each product (with different degrees of glycosylation) for purposes of comparing different CSFs, one cannot necessarily extrapolate such data to other GM-CSF molecules with different degrees of glycosylation.

Limited clinical data are available that evaluate the effects of glycosylation on these molecules. For example, it has been firmly established that EPO needs terminal sialic acid residues on the oligosaccharides to protect the molecule from immediate proteolytic attack.[42] However, other HGFs, such as GM-CSF, do not require glycosylation to be of practical clinical use. Hovgaard et al. published a comparison between molgramostim (*E. coli*-derived and nonglycosylated) and regramostim (Chinese hamster ovary-derived and glycosylated) in a small series of patients.[43] This non-crossover study found a significantly shorter distributional half-life, a higher peak serum concentration, and a lower AUC in patients receiving intravenous molgramostim. Comparison of the products following subcutaneous administration yielded a quicker time to peak concentration and a shorter duration of detectable levels with molgramostim (Fig. 35.5). While a pharmacodynamic study will need to be completed, the data thus far suggest that differences in glycosylation may limit interchangeability of dosing data for products such as these.

CLINICAL DATA FOR INDIVIDUAL DRUGS

A number of factors must be taken into consideration when interpreting the clinical results of HGF trials. Neutrophil recovery is obviously influenced by the

TABLE 35.3

SUMMARY OF PHARMACOKINETIC STUDIES OF HEMATOPOIETIC GROWTH FACTORS

CSF	Route	N	Half-life (hr)	T_{max} (hr)	Cl (mL/min/kg)
G-CSF	SQ	37	2.5–5.8	4–8	19–56
Peg G-CSF	SQ	10	27–47	72–120	0.04–0.68
G-CSF	IV	58	(α 8[a], β 1.8) 1.3–5.1	NA	4–21
GM-CSF	SQ	55	1.6–5.8	2.7–20	249–312
GM-CSF	IV	63	(α 5–20[a], β 1.1–2.5) 1.1–2.4	NA	9.9–178
EPO	SQ	125	9–38	12–28	N/A
EPO	IV	135	4–11.2	NA	2.8–6.7
DARBO	SQ	14	33–49	54–86	0.062
DARBO	IV	28	18–25	NA	0.027–0.033
IL-11	SQ	18	6.9	3.2	NA[b]

Cl, systemic clearance (values are "apparent" for SQ route); CSF, colony-stimulating factor; DARBO, darbepoetin alpha; EPO, erythropoietin; G-CSF, granulocyte colony-stimulating factor; GM-CSF, granulocyte-macrophage colony-stimulating factor; IL, interleukin; N, number of patients; NA, not applicable; Peg, pegylated; T_{max}, time of maximal concentration after SQ injection.
Data presented are ranges of mean values in the reviewed studies (refs. 41, 43, 173, 175)
[a]Values are in minutes.
[b]Clearance of IL-11 in infants and children is 1.2-fold to 1.6-fold higher than in adults or adolescents.

chemotherapy regimen and dosages selected. Individual patient factors are also important, as evidenced by descriptions of reduced HGF efficacy in patients with extensive prior myelosuppressive therapy. Likewise HGFs such as G-CSF or GM-CSF, which are thought to act primarily on more mature cell types, may not be very effective in patients receiving even low doses of stem cell toxins such as thiotepa.[44] Early HGF studies typically did not include concomitant administration of prophylactic antibiotics, a practice that is currently more common.

Administration of stem cell transfusions obviously influences reconstitution. The number and type of cells (e.g., CD34$^+$ selected peripheral blood progenitors, umbilical cord blood, etc.) can also cause sufficient heterogeneity in reconstitution so as to make any comparisons difficult.

Caution needs to be exercised in the use of these products, since concomitant administration of cycle-specific chemotherapy and G-CSF or GM-CSF has led to enhanced myelosuppression with some regimens.[45,46]

Erythropoietin

Multiple factors may account for anemia in patients with cancer, although the predominant causes are thought related to the cancer itself or to cytotoxic chemotherapy. The etiology can be explained by both increased red cell destruction and reduced red cell production. Erythropoiesis is inversely correlated to disease stage in malignancies, such as multiple myeloma, where deficient red cell production is thought to be the primary mechanism.[47] Chemotherapy may obviously alter the bone marrow's

ability to produce erythrocytes while also eliciting toxic effects to the kidney. Renal toxicity is important because almost all endogenous EPO is produced in the peritubular interstitial cells of the kidney and is regulated by an oxygen sensor (Fig. 35.6). Although the etiology of these effects is thought to be related to platinum analog toxicity, some data suggest that alternative mechanisms are important.[48] More specifically, investigators have noted an apparent deficiency in endogenous serum EPO associated with malignancy-related anemia that is not entirely explained by clinically apparent renal dysfunction. Platinum-associated anemia may be due to reduced EPO production secondary to toxic effects on EPO-producing renal cells or possibly effects of platinum on cytochrome P450 hemoproteins.[49] Both inappropriately low and surprisingly high EPO concentrations have been reported following chemotherapy.[50,51] Such variability may be partly due to acute paradoxical elevations of endogenous EPO concentrations immediately following chemotherapy.[52] The measurement of endogenous concentrations of EPO may be used to select anemic cancer patients who would achieve the greatest therapeutic benefit from administration of the recombinant protein. However, this practice is no longer common.[53,54] Efficacy of EPO is dependent on adequate iron stores. Aggressive therapy with intravenous iron has been shown to improve the hemoglobin response in cancer patients treated with recombinant EPO.[55]

Abels summarized the results from a randomized, placebo-controlled study that used recombinant EPO for anemia (HCT < 32%) in patients with cancer.[56,57] Recombinant EPO (100 to 150 U/kg per day) was administered

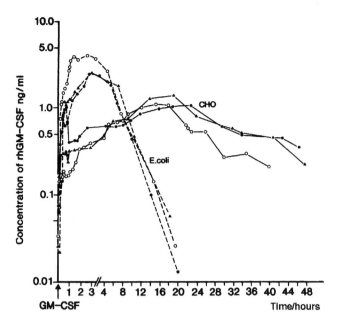

Figure 35.5 Serum disposition of molgramostim (derived from *Escherichia coli*) (*dashed line*) and regramostim (derived from Chinese hamster ovary cells) (*solid line*) after subcutaneous injection in patients treated with 5.5 or 8.0 μg/kg per day, respectively. (GM-CSF, granulocyte-macrophage colony-stimulating factor; rhGM-CSF, recombinant human granulocyte-macrophage colony-stimulating factor.) (Reproduced with permission from Hovgaard D, Mortensen BT, Schifter S, et al. Comparative pharmacokinetics of single-dose administration of mammalian and bacterially derived recombinant human granulocyte-macrophage colony-stimulating factor. Eur J Haematol 1993;50:32–36.)

three times weekly for 8 to 12 weeks or until the patient's hematocrit reached 38 to 40%. Patients were divided into three cohorts depending on whether they were receiving chemotherapy and whether the regimen included cisplatin. The criteria for RBC transfusion were not standard-

ized but appeared similar between the groups. As shown in Table 35.4, the patients treated with EPO in each group demonstrated statistically significant increases in HCT and a higher frequency of correction of anemia; however, the transfusion requirements were not significantly different. When the two cohorts that received chemotherapy were combined, significant reductions in the number of patients transfused (28% vs. 46%) and the number of units transfused per patient (1.04 vs. 1.81) were evident following the first month of therapy in the EPO group. Others have confirmed these findings.[58]

Randomized trials of prophylactic EPO therapy have also demonstrated efficacy in the prevention of anemia during treatment with a cyclophosphamide, epirubicin, and fluorouracil combination chemotherapy regimen for breast cancer or a platinum-based combination for small cell lung cancer.[59,60] Similar results have also been found with the use of the longer-acting darbepoetin analog in prevention of cancer/chemotherapy-associated anemia.[61,62]

A randomized (but not placebo-controlled) evaluation of EPO therapy following allogeneic BMT has been reported in 28 patients with leukemia.[63] EPO (100 to 150 U/kg per day) was administered for 30 days posttransplant. EPO therapy significantly accelerated the appearance of reticulocytes and reduced the RBC transfusion requirements (12 units in the control group vs. 4 units in the treatment group); however, median hemoglobin levels were unaffected. Interestingly, patients in the EPO group also demonstrated significantly quicker platelet recovery, which translated into a reduction in the number of platelet transfusions; however, more patients in the control group experienced venoocclusive disease, thus complicating the interpretation. Some preclinical studies indicate that chronic administration of high-dose EPO may produce competition

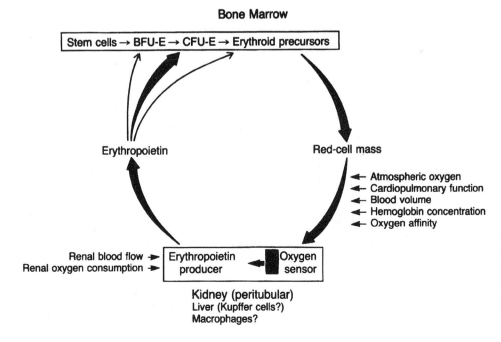

Figure 35.6 Feedback control of erythropoietin and erythrocyte production. (BFU-E, burst-forming unit, erythroid; CFU- E, colony-forming unit, erythroid.) (Reproduced with permission from Erslev AJ. Erythropoietin. N Engl J Med 1991;324: 1339–1344.)

TABLE 35.4

RESULTS OF RANDOMIZED, PLACEBO-CONTROLLED TRIAL OF EPO IN PATIENTS WITH MALIGNANCIES

	EPO			Placebo		
	I	II	III	I	II	III
Number of patients	63	79	64	55	74	61
Change in HCT (mg/dL)	+2.8[a]	+6.9[a]	+6.0[a]	−0.1	+1.1	+1.3
Correction of anemia (% with HCT (38)	20.6[a]	40.5[a]	35.9[a]	3.6	4.1	1.6
Patients transfused (%)	33.3	40.5	53.1	38.2	48.6	68.9
Mean transfusions per patient	1.52	2.03	3.56	2.19	2.75	4.01

HCT, hematocrit.
Patients in group I were not receiving chemotherapy. Patients in group II received nonplatinum-based chemotherapy. Patients in group III underwent chemotherapy regimens that included cisplatin.
[a]Values significantly different from placebo group.
Reproduced with permission from Abels RI. Use of recombinant human erythropoietin in the treatment of anemia in patients who have cancer. Semin Oncol 1992;19(Suppl 8):2935.

between erythrocytic and megakaryocytic cell lines, resulting in thrombocytopenia.[64] Subsequent randomized trials in the allogeneic and autologous BMT settings have failed to show a substantial prophylactic benefit from EPO administration.[65,66]

Guidelines suggest a trigger hemoglobin value of 10 g/dL for the initiation of EPO; however, comorbid factors such as cardiac disease should be taken into account and may indicate a lower target.[67] A 6- to 8-week trial of EPO-based therapy is typically sufficient for the assessment of response (1 to 2 g/dL rise in hemoglobin).

A variety of EPO dosing schedules have been evaluated. Studies conducted in healthy volunteers suggest that the thrice weekly subcutaneous regimen provides better erythropoietic response than the same total dose given once weekly;[68] however, the initial report of a large, open-label, once weekly EPO regimen in cancer patients did demonstrate efficacy.[69] The most common regimen in current use for cancer patients is 40,000 units per week administered subcutaneously.

Darbepoetin was initially approved as a once weekly injection. However, subsequent data support extending the interval to every 2 weeks (200 μg subcutaneously), and this is the most common darbepoetin regimen in use today. Further extension of the dosing interval is being explored, along with more complicated regimens (frontloading). The goal of the latter trials is to accelerate the hemoglobin response by use of weekly darbepoetin administration and then extend the interval to every 3 weeks or longer once a target hemoglobin is achieved.

Granulocyte Colony-Stimulating Factor

Clinical data from phase I/II studies of G-CSF or GM-CSF have been reviewed.[70] Many randomized, placebo-controlled phase III clinical trials have evaluated the efficacy of using G-CSF as a prophylactic for febrile neutropenia following myelosuppressive chemotherapy (Table 35.5).[71–82] In general, these trials have demonstrated a significant acceleration of neutrophil recovery using an HGF, with some trials leading to a reduction in hospitalization for neutropenic fever (Fig. 35.7). One must realize that chemotherapy regimens expected to produce substantial myelosuppression were selected for many of these studies in order to optimize potential differences between the groups. In some trials, prophylaxis with G-CSF also improved other events related to myelosuppression, such as infections and mucositis.

Most published HGF clinical trials were not designed to evaluate differences achieved in chemotherapy dose intensity. Nonrandomized and randomized studies have demonstrated an increased ability to give chemotherapy cycles on the planned time schedule with use of G-CSF or GM-CSF prophylaxis.[83–87] Some phase I studies of new cytotoxic agents with myelosuppression as the dose-limiting toxicity have been successful in achieving additional dose escalations with the aid of prophylactic HGFs.[88] The European randomized study of filgrastim with CAE (cyclophosphamide, Adriamycin, etoposide) in small cell lung cancer[75] differed from the US trial[72] in that it did not allow patients on the placebo arm to receive filgrastim if they became neutropenic and febrile on a previous cycle. This enabled evaluation of the effect of filgrastim on the dose intensity of CAE. Twenty-nine percent of patients treated with filgrastim had chemotherapy doses reduced secondary to myelosuppression, compared with 61% of patients receiving placebo. While this difference was statistically significant, the median percentage of the prescribed dose given (mg/m² per week) was approximately 88% for the patients on placebo, compared with 96% for patients treated with filgrastim. The results of this and other studies[89] demonstrate that HGFs alone will probably not allow

TABLE 35.5

RESULTS OF RANDOMIZED, PLACEBO-CONTROLLED CLINICAL TRIALS OF G-CSF OR GM-CSF PROPHYLAXIS AFTER CHEMOTHERAPY IN PATIENTS NOT RECEIVING HEMATOPOIETIC CELLULAR SUPPORT

Reference	Cancer Diagnosis	Chemotherapy	CSF Given	N	N+	H+	Ab+	ID
71	Leukemias	ME	G-CSF (*E. coli*)	108	↓	NR	NR	↓
72	SCLC	CAE	G-CSF (*E. coli*)	211	↓	↓	↓	NR
73	Urogenital	Various	G-CSF (*E. coli*)	77	↓	NR	NR	NR
75	SCLC	CAE	G-CSF (*E. coli*)	130	↓	↓	↓	NC
74	NHL	VAPEC-B	G-CSF (*E. coli*)	80	↓	NC	NC	NC
76	Pediatric ALL	Standard + VP16/ARAC	G-CSF (*E. coli*)	164	↓	↓	NC	↓
77	Solid tumors, lymphoma	Various	G-CSF (*E. coli*)[a]	138	↓	NC	NC	NC
78	Breast	FEC	G-CSF (CHO)	120	↓	↓	↓	↓
79	AML	DNM, ARA-C	G-CSF (CHO)	173	↓	NR	NR	NC
80	AML (>54 yr)	DNM, ARA-C	G-CSF (*E. coli*)	234	↓	NC	↓	NC
81	AML	DNM, ARA-C, VP-16	G-CSF (*E. coli*)	521	↓	↓	↓	NC
129	NHL	COP-BLAM	GM-CSF (*E. coli*)	182	↓	↓	↓	↓
128	Ovarian	CC	GM-CSF (CHO)	15	↓	NR	NR	NR
130	NSCLC	MVP	GM-CSF (NR)	52	↓	NR	NR	NR
131	AML (>59 yr)	DNM, ARA-C	GM-CSF (*E. coli*)	388	↓	NC	NR	NC
133	AML (>55 yr)	DNM, ARA-C	GM-CSF (yeast)	124	↓	NC	NR	↓
132	Breast	FAC	GM-CSF (yeast)	142	↓	NC	NR	NR

↓, decreased; Ab+, use of antibiotics; ALL, acute lymphoblastic leukemia; AML, acute myelogenous leukemia; ARA-C, cytosine arabinoside; BLAM, bleomycin sulfate, doxorubicin hydrochloride, and procarbazine; CAE, cyclophosphamide, doxorubicin hydrochloride, and etoposide; CC, carboplatin and cyclophosphamide; COP, cyclophosphamide, vincristine sulfate, prednisone; CSF, colony-stimulating factor; DNM, daunomycin; FAC, 5-fluorouracil, doxorubicin hydrochloride, and cyclophosphamide; FEC, fluorouracil, etoposide, and cisplatin; G-CSF, granulocyte colony-stimulating factor; GM-CSF, granulocyte-macrophage colony-stimulating factor; H+, duration of hospitalization; ID, frequency of infectious complications; ME, behenoylcytosine arabinoside and etoposide; MVP, mitomycin, vinblastine sulfate, and cisplatin; N, number of patients; N+, duration of neutropenia; NC, no significant change; NHL, non-Hodgkin's lymphoma; NR, not reported or no data provided regarding statistical significance; NSCLC, non–small cell lung cancer; SCLC, small cell lung cancer; VAPEC-B, vincristine, doxorubicin, prednisolone, etoposide, cyclophosphamide, bleomycin; VP-16, etoposide.
[a]CSF initiated when absolute neutrophil count was <500/mm^3.

substantial increases in dose intensity unless some type of cellular support is incorporated into the regimen. However, it does appear that HGFs may facilitate compression of chemotherapy schedules (i.e., improve dose density).[90]

A randomized, open-label study of filgrastim during part of the induction chemotherapy (cyclophosphamide, cytarabine, methotrexate, 6-MP) for 76 patients with acute lymphoblastic leukemia (ALL) found substantial

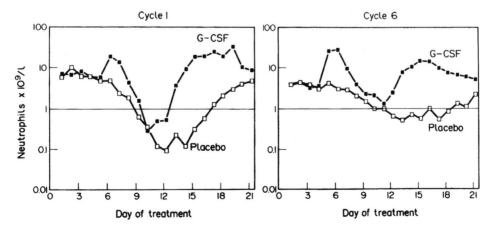

Figure 35.7   Neutrophil concentrations in 129 patients randomly assigned to receive either granulocyte colony-stimulating factor (G-CSF) or placebo after cyclophosphamide, doxorubicin hydrochloride, and etoposide (CAE) chemotherapy. (Reproduced with permission from Trillet-Lenoir V, Green J, Manegold C, et al. Recombinant granulocyte colony stimulating factor reduces the infectious complications of cytotoxic chemotherapy. Eur J Cancer 1993;29A:319–324.)

improvement in the duration of neutropenia, fewer interruptions in the chemotherapy schedule, and no change in disease-free survival at a median of 20 months follow-up.[91] Interestingly, a randomized study of lenograstim as part of induction chemotherapy (cytarabine plus idarubicin or amsacrine) in 640 patients with AML found improvements in disease-free survival among patients who were on lenograstim and had standard-risk disease.[92]

The most common administration technique for filgrastim (and one that is approved by the FDA) is to initiate the drug approximately 24 hours following chemotherapy. Some relatively small trials have attempted to delay the initiation for several days, without obvious negative effects.[93] A single administration of pegfilgrastim (100 mcg/kg or 6 mg total dose) following chemotherapy appears to be equivalent to the full 10- to 14-day course of daily (5 mcg/kg) filgrastim injections, based on randomized, double-blind trials.[94,95] Delay in the institution of filgrastim prophylaxis for afebrile patients until the ANC is $500/mm^3$ or lower has been shown to shorten the period of neutropenia but not change the rate or duration of hospitalization.[77]

Use of G-CSF (or placebo) to *treat* febrile neutropenia was assessed in a double-blind, randomized trial of 218 patients who were also receiving standard antibiotic therapy. Use of G-CSF was associated with an acceleration of neutrophil recovery and a shortening in the duration of neutropenic fever; however, the overall hospitalization duration was unaffected.[96]

G-CSF has been used in several phase I, II, and III trials for acceleration of hematopoietic recovery following stem cell transplantation (Table 35.6).[97–100] In general, these trials indicate that G-CSF administered following high-dose chemotherapy and autologous bone marrow transplantation will improve the rate of peripheral blood neutrophil recovery once it begins, but G-CSF has no substantial effect on the approximately 8 day period of absolute leukopenia or on platelet recovery. The proportion of patients with febrile neutropenia has not been substantially altered, although the number of days of febrile neutropenia has been reduced with G-CSF. Studies have also administered G-CSF for several days before BMT in order to produce high concentrations of progenitor cells in the peripheral blood (PBPCs) for subsequent reinfusion.[101–103] The premise is that the PBPCs will express receptors for terminally acting HGFs (such as G-CSF) and thus be immediately able to proliferate, providing some neutrophils during the 8-day period of absolute leucopenia. G-CSF is the most common cytokine utilized to generate in vivo production of PBPCs, either alone or following administration of myelosuppressive standard-dose chemotherapy (Table 35.6). A somewhat unexpected benefit of this therapy is a reduction in platelet transfusion requirements. Such effects may be explained in part by a dose-dependent increase in the early peripheral blood myeloid progenitors ($CD34^+$) noted in the PBPC product.

Administration of G-CSF following autologous PBPC reinfusion aids engraftment.[104–108] Most of the original investigations initiated HGF therapy immediately following administration of the bone marrow; however, some studies have suggested that a 5- to 6-day delay in G-CSF use may achieve similar efficacy.[109,110] Caution should be exercised in translating these data to situations where progenitor cells are being administered, due to their quicker hematopoietic reconstitution and potentially different interactions with HGFs; however, both similar or conflicting results have been found in other trials.[111–113] Use of G-CSF following allogeneic transplantation is controversial. A large retrospective evaluation and a meta-analysis agree that HGFs accelerate myeloid recovery. However, some data suggest a detrimental effect on platelet recovery and graft versus host disease.[114,115] Effects on the latter could vary depending on the stem cell source.[116,117]

Other controversial issues being studied include the optimal timing of leukapheresis and the concomitant use of other cytokines to aid trilineage engraftment. HGF-primed PBPCs have also been used to compress the schedule of multicyclic cytotoxic chemotherapy regimens such as those involving treatment with ifosfamide, carboplatin, and etoposide (ICE).[118]

Determining the optimal schedule, dose, and combination of G-CSF with other cytokines is a focus of interest among institutions. A randomized chemotherapy-based priming study evaluated sequential administration of GM-CSF followed by G-CSF compared with either agent alone. The G-CSF–containing arms yielded better mobilization and more beneficial outcomes (less transfusions, myelosuppression, etc.) compared with the GM-CSF–treated patients.[119] A combination of G-CSF with cyclophosphamide is routinely used to increase the generation of $CD34^+$ cells; however, a randomized study found greater efficacy and less toxicity with G-CSF alone in patients with multiple myeloma.[120] A randomized, crossover study of progenitor cell mobilization with chemotherapy (high-dose cyclophosphamide) plus G-CSF versus GM-CSF plus G-CSF demonstrated more efficient generation of progenitors with the chemotherapy combination.[121] Several studies have shown that combining G-CSF with the early acting cytokine SCF results in more efficient progenitor cell mobilization and reduces apheresis requirements.[122]

A wide variety of G-CSF doses and administration techniques have been used in clinical trials. One randomized study of over 100 patients was not able to demonstrate differences in filgrastim doses of 5 versus 10 μg/kg per day for PBPC mobilization.[123] The most common filgrastim dose for prophylaxis of myelosuppression following standard or high-dose chemotherapy is 5 μg/kg per day. Lower doses of lenograstim (2 μg/kg per day) appear to have efficacy similar to that of standard doses (5 μg/kg per day).[124] A crossover study of filgrastim (*E. coli*-derived) and lenograstim (CHO-derived) suggests higher hematopoietic activity of the former with equimolar dosing.[125] Discontinuation

TABLE 35.6

RESULTS OF RANDOMIZED CLINICAL TRIALS OF G-CSF OR GM-CSF IN ASSOCIATION WITH HIGH-DOSE CHEMOTHERAPY AND STEM CELL TRANSPLANTATION

Reference	Cancer Type	Stem Cell Source	CSF Given Post Cells	N	WBC Recovery	Days ANC >500 vs. Control	PLT Recovery	Fever
136	Leukemia	Allo-BM	GM-CSF (CHO)	20[a]	−	3	NC	↑
137	Lymphoma	Auto-BM	GM-CSF (Yeast)	128[a]	+	7	NC	NC
138	Lymphoma/ALL	Auto-BM	GM-CSF (E. coli)	81[a]	+	13	NC	NC
139	Lymphoma	Auto-BM	GM-CSF (E. coli)	61[a]	+	7	NC	NC
140	Lymphoma	Auto-BM	GM-CSF (E. coli)	69[a]	+	4	NC	NR
141	Leukemia/etc.	Allo-BM	GM-CSF (CHO)	57[a]	+	4	NC	NC
142	NHL	Auto-BM	GM-CSF (E. coli)	91[a]	+	7	NC	NC
143	Hodgkin's	Auto-BM	GM-CSF (E. coli)	24[a]	+	NR	+	NR
144	Various	Allo-BM	GM-CSF (Yeast)	109[a]	+	4	NC	NC
145	Various	Allo-BM	GM-CSF (E. coli)	53[a]	+	4	NC	NC
97	NR	Allo-BM	G-CSF (CHO)	53[a]	+	10	NR	NR
100	Various	Allo-PBPC	G-CSF (E. coli)	54[a]	+	4	NC	NR
117	Various	Allo-PBPC	G-CSF (E. coli)	42[a]	+	3	NC	NR
99	Lymphoma	Auto-BM	G-CSF (E. coli)	43	+	8	NC	↓
98	Lymphoma	Auto-BM	G-CSF (E. coli)	54	+	7	NC	NC
150	Various	Auto-PBPC	GM-CSF (E. coli)	50[a]	NC	NR	NC	↑
105	Various	Auto-PBPC	G-CSF (NR)	41	+	5.5	NC	NC
108	Lymphoma	Auto-PBPC	G-CSF (E. coli)	23	+	3.5	NC	NC
106	Various (peds)	Auto-PBPC	G-CSF (E. coli)	63	+	1	NC	NC
107	Lymphoma/ myeloma	Auto-PBPC	G-CSF (E. coli)	38[a]	+	4	NC	NC
174	Various	Auto-PBPC	G-CSF (NR) + GM-CSF (NR)	37[a]	+	6	NC	NC

+, augmented; −, worsened; ↑, increased; ↓, decreased; ALL, acute lymphoblastic leukemia; allo-BM, allogeneic bone marrow transplant; ANC, absolute neutrophil count; auto-BM, autologous bone marrow transplant; auto-PBPC, autologous peripheral blood progenitor cells; CHO, Chinese hamster ovary; CSF, colony-stimulating factor; G-CSF, granulocyte colony-stimulating factor; GM-CSF, granulocyte-macrophage colony-stimulating factor; NC, no significant change; NHL, non-Hodgkin's lymphoma; NR, not reported or no data provided regarding statistical significance; PLT, platelet; WBC, white blood cell count.
[a]Placebo-controlled.

of G-CSF during its use in the recovery phase following myelosuppressive chemotherapy will typically result in a rebound depression of the WBC count by approximately 50% within 24 hours. Pegfilgrastim can be given as a fixed dose (6 mg) once per chemotherapy cycle. The current labeling indicates that the drug should be given 24 hours after chemotherapy and at least 14 days before the next cycle of chemotherapy. Studies are ongoing to evaluate administration of pegfilgrastim on the same day as select chemotherapy.

Some evidence suggests that use of G-CSF in children with ALL during intensive therapy with etoposide may be associated with a higher frequency of secondary myeloid malignancies.[126] This potential effect should be prospectively evaluated as trials attempt to increase dose density with use of growth factors in other diseases. Other adverse effects thought secondary to G-CSF administration have been fairly mild in the clinical trials reported. Bone pain is the most frequent complaint, often occurring near the time

of maximal hematopoiesis. Concurrent administration of G-CSF with cycle-specific chemotherapy may paradoxically worsen myelosuppressive effects.[127]

Granulocyte-Macrophage Colony-Stimulating Factor

GM-CSF has been used in numerous phase I, II, and III trials following standard doses of myelosuppressive chemotherapy, where it does seem to reduce the occurrence of febrile neutropenia (Table 35.5).[128–132] A large phase III placebo-controlled study of sargramostim as prophylaxis for neutropenic fever was conducted in elderly patients with AML. In addition to the benefit of enhanced neutrophil recovery and reduction of infections, the sargramostim-treated group also displayed significantly longer survival.[133]

A randomized, placebo-controlled study that evaluated the initiation of molgramostim in patients only at the onset of chemotherapy-induced febrile neutropenia could not demonstrate substantial clinical or monetary benefit.[134]

In another randomized, placebo-controlled study of molgramostim, 240 patients with AML were given the cytokine (or placebo) during and after induction chemotherapy (idarubicin plus cytarabine).[135] Treatment with GM-CSF shortened the time to neutrophil recovery and improved disease-free survival in those 55 to 64 years old.

Randomized, placebo-controlled clinical trials involving GM-CSF have also been conducted in the setting of high-dose chemotherapy with stem cell support (Table 35.6).[136-145] The results demonstrate that GM-CSF has an ability to accelerate neutrophil recovery after a few days of absolute leukopenia when bone marrow alone is used as the sole stem cell source (Fig. 35.8). Patients who were previously exposed to drugs that deplete stem cells (e.g., carmustine or busulfan) experienced less benefit from GM-CSF.[146] Most studies could not discern an effect of the HGF on the rate of documented bacterial infections. The impact of GM-CSF on platelet recovery is inconsistent, and use of GM-CSF has generally not solved the problem of transfusion dependence. GM-CSF therapy has shown no significant effect on the incidence or severity of graft versus host disease in patients receiving allogeneic transplants.

As with G-CSF, a number of nonrandomized and randomized trials have found GM-CSF (alone or following chemotherapy) useful to prime PBPCs for subsequent leukapheresis.[101,147-150] Kritz et al. randomly assigned patients to receive GM-CSF–primed PBPCs or no cellular support following cytotoxic chemotherapy, with autologous marrow rescue given if needed on day 15. The study was stopped early due to a substantial difference in myeloid and platelet recovery between the groups, in favor of the PBPC-treated patients.[151] While this study was small and had short follow-up, it demonstrated the potential

ability of GM-CSF to improve hematopoiesis through PBPCs alone.

Filgrastim and molgramostim appear to produce similar yields of CD34$^+$ PBPCs when used in conjunction with chemotherapy for priming. However, filgrastim may shorten this process.[152] Caballero et al. randomly assigned 42 patients with breast cancer to receive open-label filgrastim or molgramostim following STAMP I or V high-dose chemotherapy and autologous, filgrastim-stimulated PBPCs.[153] All patients also received acetaminophen before the HGF doses and prophylactic antibiotics. The only differences noted between the arms were slightly faster platelet recovery and shorter hospitalization (by 2 days) in the filgrastim arm.

Dose-related adverse effects with GM-CSF include capillary leak syndrome, central vein thrombosis, and hypotension. Effects seen over a variety of doses include fever, pleuritis, myalgia, bone pain, pulmonary infiltrates, rash, and thrombophlebitis. Some patients have experienced a syndrome of transient hypoxia and hypotension following the first dose but not subsequent doses of GM-CSF.[154] Most randomized studies that used the standard dose (250 mcg/m^2 per day) and the currently marketed sargramostim version (vs. molgramostim) have shown only mild adverse effects. GM-CSF is a known inducer of other endogenous cytokines, which are thought to account for at least some of the adverse effects. As with G-CSF, the simultaneous administration of GM-CSF and cycle-specific chemotherapy or radiation therapy has worsened myelosuppression.[155,156]

Clinical Synopsis of G-CSF AND GM-CSF

Introduction of G-CSF, and to a lesser extent GM-CSF, into routine clinical practice has profoundly influenced the treatment of chronic neutropenias and the generation of PBPCs for collection and subsequent reinfusion following high-dose chemotherapy. However, the most frequent use of these agents has been in prophylaxis of chemotherapy-induced neutropenic fever, an indication for which the outcome data are less clear. There is still not much evidence that administration of an HGF improves disease-free or overall survival, even for tumor types typically thought to be chemosensitive. Thus, routine HGF use (i.e., as primary prophylaxis) is not justified for most patients. Attempts to define the populations that benefit from HGFs are underway. For example, elderly patients are more likely to have chemotherapy dose reductions, probably as a result of myelosuppression.[157] HGFs are being evaluated in this clinical setting. The majority of current HGF prescriptions are for secondary prophylaxis (i.e., written for patients who experienced myelosuppression on a previous cycle of chemotherapy.) There are even less data showing any effect of HGFs on disease-free or overall survival for such an indication. Use of HGFs in the treatment of neutropenic fever is unlikely to improve patient outcome.

Use of HGFs for priming PBPCs does decrease toxicity, both in the priming period and posttransplant, in addition

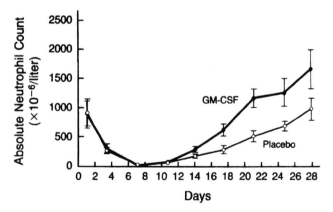

Figure 35.8 Neutrophil concentrations in 129 patients randomly assigned to receive either granulocyte-macrophage colony-stimulating factor (GM-CSF) or placebo after high-dose chemotherapy with autologous bone marrow transplantation. (Reproduced with permission from Nemunaitis J, Rabinowe SN, Singer JW, et al. Recombinant granulocyte-macrophage colony-stimulating factor after autologous bone marrow transplantation for lymphoid cancer. N Engl J Med 1991;324:1773–1778.)

to reducing length of hospital stay and cost of therapy. There is probably some benefit to the administration of HGFs following stem cell infusion; however, the degree of the effect is most likely dependent on the quality and quantity of the cells infused. Older studies that report differences in hospitalization should be interpreted with caution, given the changes in the outpatient treatment of neutropenic fever, even following high-dose chemotherapy.

Interleukin-11

Preclinical and in vitro studies indicate that IL-11 directly stimulates megakaryocytes. Oprelvekin (recombinant IL-11) was the first cytokine to reach the market for the prevention of chemotherapy-induced thrombocytopenia, and this occurred only 3 years after the initial research application. Phase I evaluations in patients with cancer demonstrated an impressive ability to increase steady-state platelet counts by over twofold.[158]

The ability of recombinant IL-11 to prevent thrombocytopenia was evaluated in a randomized, placebo-controlled trial of 77 patients with breast cancer who had not previously experienced severe chemotherapy-induced thrombocytopenia. Patients received two cycles of doxorubicin/cyclophosphamide followed by G-CSF and study drug on each cycle. Using the limit of 20,000 platelets/μL, 43% of patients on placebo and 30% on IL-11 required a platelet transfusion. The mean number of transfusions was 2.2 for the placebo group versus 0.8 for the IL-11 group.[159]

A randomized, placebo-controlled evaluation of IL-11 for secondary prophylaxis of thrombocytopenia was conducted in 93 patients with cancer who previously received platelet transfusions for chemotherapy-induced toxicity. As expected, greater than 90% of the patients in the placebo arm required a platelet transfusion, compared with 72% of the IL-11–treated patients. The mean number of transfusions was 3.3 for the placebo group versus 2.2 for the IL-11 group.[160]

Administration of IL-11 did not appear to substantially alter platelet recovery or transfusion requirements in 80 patients with breast cancer enrolled in a randomized, placebo-controlled study following high-dose chemotherapy and infusion with G-CSF–primed PBPCs.[161]

Approximately 60% of patients treated with IL-11 experience some degree of generalized edema, thought to be secondary to increased retention of sodium. In addition, atrial arrhythmias, tachycardia, conjunctival injection, and worsening of effusions can occur. Constitutional symptoms such as myalgia, arthralgia, and fatigue were the dose-limiting toxicities during phase I trials.

Thrombopoietin

Murine studies suggested a complex thrombopoietin (TPO) dose versus platelet response curve, perhaps due to inhibitory effects on platelet progenitors at high doses.[162]

Murine and nonhuman primate studies demonstrated a synergism between TPO and G-CSF in the acceleration of neutrophil and platelet recovery following myelosuppressive chemotherapy, with no evidence of lineage competition.

Clinical studies of recombinant TPO were initially conducted with either the full-length glycosylated TPO molecule (rTPO, Genetech/Pfizer) or a truncated, pegylated derivative (rMGDF, Amgen). A clinical study of rMGDF in 17 patients with cancer (not currently receiving chemotherapy) demonstrated a dose-dependent increase in platelet counts. Those receiving the highest doses achieved from a 51 to 584% increase in platelet counts. The effect was clinically evident following 6 days of therapy, and the counts continued to rise several days after drug discontinuation.[163] Platelets generated in these patients appeared to have normal function based on in vitro assays. Similar data were found with the full-length rTPO molecule.[164]

Two other studies administered recombinant rMGDF to a total of 94 patients with lung cancer both prior to and following a carboplatin/cyclophosphamide regimen. A significant shortening in the time to platelet nadir and a quicker platelet recovery were noted.[165,166] Similar effects were seen in a gynecologic cancer population being treated with carboplatin and the full-length rTPO molecule.[167] A placebo-controlled trial of rMGDF in patients being treated for AML was not able to demonstrate an impact on thrombocytopenia.[168] Utilization of rMGDF following autologous bone marrow transplantation demonstrated that its thrombopoietic effects were delayed and not impressive.[169]

rTPO and rMGDF were generally well tolerated in these early studies, with essentially no evidence of dose-limiting adverse effects, nor were any fever or flu-like symptoms discernable; however, a few patients did experience thrombotic events. The role of the study drug in such processes is unclear.

Clinical development of rMGDF was halted when some patients in cancer trials and normal, healthy volunteers given the cytokine began to demonstrate neutralizing antibodies to TPO. A similar phenomenon has occurred when some other recombinant growth factors, molgramostim and PIXY321 (an IL-3/GM-CSF fusion protein), have been used without immunosuppressive chemotherapy, resulting in abrogation of their hematopoietic activities.[170,171] Novel peptide and nonpeptide, potentially less immunogenic molecules are also being investigated.[172]

REFERENCES

1. Moonen P, Mermod JJ, Ernst JM, et al. Increased biological activity of deglycosylated recombinant human granulocyte/macrophage colony-stimulating factor produced by yeast or animal cells. Proc Natl Acad Sci 1987;84: 4428–4431.
2. Fukuda M, Sasaki H, Fukuda MN. Erythropoietin metabolism and the influence of carbohydrate structure. Contrib Nephrol 1989;76:8–89.

3. Elliott S, Lorenzini T, Asher S, et al. Enhancement of therapeutic protein in vivo activities through glycoengineering. Nat Biotechnol 2003;21:414–421.

4. Allon M, Kleinman K, Walczyk M, et al. Pharmacokinetics and pharmacodynamics of darbepoetin alfa and epoetin in patients undergoing dialysis. Clin Pharmacol Ther 2002;72:546–555.

5. Zeng SM, Murray JC, Widness JA, et al. Association of single nucleotide polymorphisms in the thrombopoietin-receptor gene, but not the thrombopoietin gene, with differences in platelet count. Am J Hematol 2004;77:12–21.

6. Guillaume T, Sekhavat M, Rubinstein DB, et al. Transcription of genes encoding granulocyte-macrophage colony-stimulating factor, interleukin 3, and interleukin 6 receptors and lack of proliferative response to exogenous cytokines in nonhematopoietic human malignant cell lines. Cancer Res 1993; 53:3139–3144.

7. Arcasoy MO, Amin K, Karayal AF, et al. Functional significance of erythropoietin receptor expression in breast cancer. Lab Invest 2002;82:911–918.

8. Batra S, Perelman N, Luck LR, et al. Pediatric tumor cells express erythropoietin and a functional erythropoietin receptor that promotes angiogenesis and tumor cell survival. Lab Invest 2003;83:1477–1487.

9. Leyland-Jones B; BEST Investigators and Study Group. Breast cancer trial with erythropoietin terminated unexpectedly. Lancet Oncol 2003;4:459–460.

10. Henke M, Laszig R, Rube C, et al. Erythropoietin to treat head and neck cancer patients with anaemia undergoing radiotherapy: randomised, double-blind, placebo-controlled trial. Lancet 2003 18;362:1255–1260.

11. Miyajima A, Mui ALF, Ogorochi T, et al. Receptors for granulocyte-macrophage colony-stimulating factor, interleukin-3, and interleukin-5. Blood 1993;82:1960–1974.

12. Park LS, Urdal DL. Colony-stimulating factor receptors. Trans Proc 1989;21:54–56.

13. Jacobsen SEW, Ruscetti FW, Dubois CM, et al. Induction of colony-stimulating factor receptor expression on hematopoietic progenitor cells: proposed mechanism for growth factor synergism. Blood 1992;80:678–687.

14. Sayani, F, Montero-Julian FA, Ranchin V, et al. Identification of the soluble granulocyte-macrophage colony stimulating factor receptor protein in vivo. Blood 2000;95:461–469.

15. Heaney ML, Golde DW. Soluble hormone receptors. Blood 1993;82:1945–1948.

16. Porteu F, Nathan C. Shedding of tumor necrosis factor receptors by activated human neutrophils. J Exp Med 1990; 172: 599–607.

17. Lieschke GJ, Grail D, Hodgson G, et al. Mice lacking granulocyte colony-stimulating factor have chronic neutropenia, granulocyte and macrophage progenitor cell deficiency, and impaired neutrophil mobilization. Blood 1994;84:1737–1746.

18. Dranoff G, Crawford AD, Sadelain M, et al. Involvement of granulocyte-macrophage colony-stimulating factor in pulmonary homeostasis. Science 1994;264:713–716.

19. Petros WP, Rabinowitz J, Gibbs JP, et al. Effect of endogenous TNF-alpha on recombinant G-CSF stimulated hematopoiesis in mice and humans. Pharmacotherapy 1998;18:816–823.

20. Chatta GS, Andrews RG, Rodger E, et al. Hematopoietic progenitors and aging: alterations in granulocytic precursors and responsiveness to recombinant human G-CSF, GM-CSF, and IL-3. J Gerontol 1993;48:M207–212.

21. Lord BI, Gurney H, Chang J, et al. Haemopoietic cell kinetics in humans treated with rGM-CSF. Int J Cancer 1992;50:26–31.

22. Pettengell R, Testa NG, Swindell R, et al. Transplantation potential of hematopoietic cells released into the circulation during routine chemotherapy for non-Hodgkin's lymphoma. Blood 1993;82:2239–2248.

23. Liu F, Poursine-Laurent J, Link DC. Expression of the G-CSF receptor on hematopoietic progenitor cells is not required for their mobilization by G-CSF. Blood 2000;95:3025–3031.

24. Jaar B, Baillou C, Viron B, et al. Long-term effects of recombinant human erythropoietin on bone marrow progenitor cells. Nephrol Dial Transplant 1993;8:614–620.

25. Arnaout MA, Wang EA, Clark SC, et al. Human recombinant granulocyte-macrophage colony-stimulating factor increases cell-cell adhesion and surface expression of adhesion-promoting surface glycoproteins on mature granulocytes. J Clin Invest 1986;7:597–601.

26. Peters WP, Stuart A, Affronti ML, et al. Neutrophil migration is defective during recombinant human granulocyte-macrophage colony-stimulating factor infusion after autologous bone marrow transplantation in humans. Blood 1988;72:1310–1315.

27. Demir G, Klein HO, Tuzuner N. Low dose daily rhGM-CSF application activates monocytes and dendritic cells in vivo. Leuk Res 2003;27:1105–1108.

28. Gurney AL, Carver-Moore K, de Sauvage FJ, et al. Thrombocytopenia in c-mpl–deficient mice. Science 1995;265: 1445–1447.

29. Graf G, Dehmel U, Drexler HG. Expression of TPO and TPO receptor MPL in human leukemia-lymphoma and solid tumor cell lines. Leuk Res 1996;20:831–838.

30. Choi ES, Hokom MM, Chen JL, et al. The role of megakaryocyte growth and development factor in terminal stages of thrombopoiesis. Br J Haematol 1996;95:227–233.

31. Rabinowitz J, Petros WP, Peters WP. Cytokine kinetics: clinical pharmacology studies complementing recombinant growth factor trials. Cancer Bull 1994;46:40–47.

32. Milsits K, Beyer J, Siegert W. Serum concentrations of G-CSF during high-dose chemotherapy with autologous stem cell rescue. Bone Marrow Transplant 1993;11:372–377.

33. Rabinowitz J, Petros WP, Stuart AR, et al. Characterization of endogenous cytokine concentrations after high-dose chemotherapy with autologous bone marrow support. Blood 1993; 81:2452–2459.

34. Lindemann A, Riedel D, Oster W, et al. Granulocyte-macrophage colony-stimulating factor induces cytokine secretion by human polymorphonuclear leukocytes. J Clin Invest 1989; 83:1308–1312.

35. Hartung T, Docke W-D, Gantner F, et al. Effect of granulocyte colony-stimulating factor treatment on ex vivo blood cytokine response in human volunteers. Blood 1995;85:2482–2489.

36. Pascual JA, Belalcazar V, de Bolos C, et al. Recombinant erythropoietin and analogues: a challenge for doping control. Ther Drug Monit 2004;26:175–179.

37. Rosenfeld CS, Sulecki M, Evans C, et al. Comparison of intravenous versus subcutaneous recombinant human granulocyte-macrophage colony-stimulating factor in patients with primary myelodysplasia. Exp Hematol 1991;19:273–277.

38. Johnston E, Crawford J, Blackwell S, et al. Randomized, dose-escalation study of SD/01 compared with daily filgrastim in patients receiving chemotherapy. J Clin Oncol 2000;18: 2522–2528.

39. Terashi K, Oka M, Ohdo S, et al. Close association between clearance of recombinant human granulocyte colony-stimulating factor (G-CSF) and G-CSF receptor on neutrophils in cancer patients. Antimicrob Agents Chemother 1999;43:21–24.

40. Tomlinson-Jones A, Ziltener HJ. Enhancement of the biologic effects of interleukin-3 in vivo by anti-interleukin-3 antibodies. Blood 1993;82:1133–1141.

41. Petros WP, Rabinowitz J, Stuart AR, et al. Disposition of recombinant human granulocyte-macrophage colony-stimulating factor in patients receiving high-dose chemotherapy and autologous bone marrow support. Blood 1992;80:1135–1140.

42. Fukuda M, Sasaki H, Fukuda MN. Erythropoietin metabolism and the influence of carbohydrate structure. Contrib Nephrol 1989;76:78–89.

43. Hovgaard D, Mortensen BT, Schifter S, et al. Comparative pharmacokinetics of single-dose administration of mammalian and bacterially-derived recombinant human granulocyte-macrophage colony-stimulating factor. Eur J Haematol 1993; 50:32–36.

44. O'Dwyer PJ, LaCreta FP, Schilder R, et al. Phase I trial of thiotepa in combination with recombinant human granulocyte-macrophage colony-stimulating factor. J Clin Oncol 1992;10: 1352–1358.

45. Petros WP, Crawford J. Safety of concomitant use of granulocyte colony-stimulating factor or granulocyte-macrophage colony-stimulating factor with cytotoxic chemotherapy agents. Curr Opinion Hematol 1997;4:213–216.

46. Tjan-Heijnen VCG, Biesma B, Festen J, et al. Enhanced myelotoxicity due to granulocyte colony-stimulating factor administration until 48 hours before the next chemotherapy course in patients with small-cell lung carcinoma. J Clin Oncol 1998; 16:2708–27014.

47. Beguin Y, Yerna M, Loo M, et al. Erythropoiesis in multiple myeloma: defective red cell production due to inappropriate erythropoietin production. Br J Haematol 1992;82:648–653.

48. Miller CB, Jones RJ, Piantadosi S, et al. Decreased erythropoietin response in patients with the anemia of cancer. N Engl J Med 1990;322:1689–1692.

49. Fandrey J, Seydel FP, Siegers CP, et al. Role of cytochrome P450 in the control of the production of erythropoietin. Life Sci 1990;47:127–134.

50. Smith DH, Goldwasser E, Volkes EE. Serum immunoerythropoietin levels in patients with cancer receiving cisplatin-based chemotherapy. Cancer 1991;68:1101–1105.

51. Birgegard G, Wide L, Simonsson B. Marked erythropoietin increase before fall in Hb after treatment with cytostatic drugs suggests mechanism other than anaemia for stimulation. Br J Haematol 1989;72:462–466.

52. Schapira M, Antin JH, Ransil BJ, et al. Serum erythropoietin levels in patients receiving intensive chemotherapy and radiotherapy. Blood 1990;76:2354–2359.

53. Osterborg A, Boogarets MA, Cimino R, et al. Recombinant human erythropoietin in transfusion-dependent anemic patients with multiple myeloma and non-Hodgkin's lymphoma: a randomized multicenter study. Blood 1996; 87:2675–2682.

54. Ludwig H, Fritz E, Leitgeb C, et al. Prediction of response to erythropoietin treatment in chronic anemia of cancer. Blood 1994;84:1056–1063.

55. Auerbach M, Ballard H, Trout JR, et al. Intravenous iron optimizes the response to recombinant human erythropoietin in cancer patients with chemotherapy-related anemia: a multicenter, open-label, randomized trial. J Clin Oncol 2004; 22: 1301–1307.

56. Abels RI. Use of recombinant human erythropoietin in the treatment of anemia in patients who have cancer. Semin Oncol 1992;19(Suppl 8):29–35.

57. Case DC, Bukowski RM, Carey RW, et al. Recombinant human erythropoietin therapy for anemic cancer patients on combination chemotherapy. J Natl Cancer Inst 1993;85:801–806.

58. Cascinu S, Fedeli A, Del Ferro E, et al. Recombinant human erythropoietin treatment in cisplatin-associated anemia: a randomized, double-blind trial with placebo. J Clin Oncol 1994; 12:1058–1062.

59. Del Mastro L, Venturini M, Lionetto R, et al. Randomized phase III trial evaluating the role of erythropoietin in the prevention of chemotherapy-induced anemia. J Clin Oncol 1997; 15:2715–2721.

60. De Campos E, Radford J, Steward W, et al. Clinical and in vitro effects of recombinant human erythropoietin in patients receiving intensive chemotherapy for small-cell lung cancer. J Clin Oncol 1995;13:1623–1631.

61. Hedenus M, Adriansson M, San Miguel J, et al. Efficacy and safety of darbepoetin alfa in anaemic patients with lymphoproliferative malignancies: a randomized, double-blind, placebo-controlled study. Darbepoetin Alfa 20000161 Study Group. Br J Haematol 2003;122:394–403.

62. Vansteenkiste J, Pirker R, Massuti B, et al. Double-blind, placebo-controlled, randomized phase III trial of darbepoetin alfa in lung cancer patients receiving chemotherapy. Aranesp 980297 Study Group. J Natl Cancer Inst 2002;94:1211–1220.

63. Steegmann JL, Lopez J, Otero MJ, et al. Erythropoietin treatment in allogeneic BMT accelerates erythroid reconstitution: results of a prospective controlled randomized trial. Bone Marrow Transplant 1992;10:541–546.

64. McDonald TP, Clift RE, Cottrell MB. Large, chronic doses of erythropoietin cause thrombocytopenia in mice. Blood 1992; 80:352–358.

65. Biggs JC, Atkinson KA, Booker V, et al. Prospective randomised double-blind trial of the in vivo use of recombinant human erythropoietin in bone marrow transplantation from HLA-identical sibling donors. Bone Marrow Transplant 1995;15:129–134.

66. Chao NJ, Schriber JR, Long GD, et al. A randomized study of erythropoietin and granulocyte colony-stimulating factor (G-CSF) versus placebo and G-CSF for patients with Hodgkin's and non-Hodgkin's lymphoma undergoing autologous bone marrow transplantation. Blood 1994; 83:2823–2828.

67. Rizzo JD, Lichtin AE, Woolf SH, et al. Use of epoetin in patients with cancer: evidence-based clinical practice guidelines of the American Society of Clinical Oncology and the American Society of Hematology. J Clin Oncol. 2002; 20:4083–4107.

68. Cheung WK, Goon BL, Guilfoyle MC, et al. Pharmacokinetics and pharmacodynamics of recombinant human erythropoietin after single and multiple subcutaneous doses to healthy subjects. Clin Pharmacol Ther 1998;64:412–423.

69. Gabrilove JL, Cleeland CS, Livingston RB, et al. Clinical evaluation of once-weekly dosing of epoetin alfa in chemotherapy patients: improvements in hemoglobin and quality of life are similar to three-times-weekly dosing. J Clin Oncol 2001; 19:2875–2882.

70. Lieschke GJ, Burgess AW. Granulocyte colony-stimulating factor and granulocyte-macrophage colony-stimulating factor [pt. 2]. N. Engl J Med 1992;327:99–106.

71. Ohno R, Tomonaga M, Kobayashi T, et al. Effect of G-CSF after intensive induction therapy in relapsed or refractory acute leukemia. N Engl J Med 1990;323:871–877.

72. Crawford J, Ozer H, Stoller R, et al. Reduction by granulocyte colony-stimulating factor of fever and neutropenia induced by chemotherapy in patients with small-cell lung cancer. N Engl J Med 1991;325:164–170.

73. Kotake T, Miki T, Akaza H, et al. Effect of recombinant granulocyte colony-stimulating factor on chemotherapy-induced neutropenia in patients with urogenital cancer. Cancer Chemother Pharmacol 1991;27:2553–2557.

74. Pettengell R, Gurney H, Radford JA, et al. Granulocyte colony-stimulating factor to prevent dose-limiting neutropenia in non-Hodgkin's lymphoma: a randomized controlled trial. Blood 1992;80:1430–1436.

75. Trillet-Lenoir V, Green J, Manegold C, et al. Recombinant granulocyte colony stimulating factor reduces the infectious complications of cytotoxic chemotherapy. Eur J Cancer 1993;29A: 319–324.

76. Pui C-H, Boyett JM, Hughes WT, et al. Human granulocyte colony-stimulating factor after induction chemotherapy in children with acute lymphoblastic leukemia. N Engl J Med 1997; 336:1781–1787.

77. Hartmann LC, Tschetter LK, Habermann TM, et al. Granulocyte colony-stimulating factor in severe chemotherapy induced afebrile neutropenia. N Engl J Med 1997;336:1776–1780.

78. Chevallier B, Chollet P, Merrouche Y, et al. Lenograstim prevents morbidity from intensive induction chemotherapy in the treatment of inflammatory breast cancer. J Clin Oncol 1995; 13:1564–1571.

79. Dombret H, Chastang C, Fenaux P, et al. A controlled study of recombinant human granulocyte colony-stimulating factor in elderly patients after treatment for acute myelogenous leukemia. N Engl J Med 1995;332:1678–1683.

80. Godwin JE, Kopecky KJ, Head DR, et al. A double-blind placebo-controlled trial of granulocyte colony-stimulating factor in elderly patients with previously untreated acute myeloid leukemia: a Southwest Oncology Group study (9031). Blood 1998;91: 3607–3615.

81. Heil G, Hoelzer D, Sanz MA, et al. A randomized, double-blind, placebo-controlled, phase III study of filgrastim in remission induction and consolidation therapy for adults with de novo acute myeloid leukemia. Blood 1997; 90:4710–4713.

82. Harousseau JL, Witz B, Lioure B, et al. Granulocyte colony-stimulating factor after intensive consolidation chemotherapy in acute myeloid leukemia: results of a randomized trial of the Groupe Ouest-Est Leucemies Aigues Myeloblastiques. J Clin Oncol 2000;18:780–787.

83. Gabrilove JL, Jakubowski A, Scher H, et al. Effect of granulocyte colony-stimulating factor on neutropenia and associated morbidity due to chemotherapy for transitional cell carcinoma of the urothelium. N Engl J Med 1988;318:1414–1422.

84. Bronchud MH, Howell A, Crowther D, et al. The use of granulocyte colony-stimulating factor to increase the intensity of treatment with doxorubicin in patients with advanced breast and ovarian cancer. Br J Cancer 1989;60:121–125.

85. Scinto AF, Ferraresi V, Campioni N, et al. Accelerated chemotherapy with high-dose epirubicin and cyclophosphamide plus r-met-HUG-CSF in locally advanced and metastatic breast cancer. Ann Oncol 1995; 6:665–671.

86. Piccart MJ, Bruning P, Wildiers J, et al. An EORTC pilot study of filgrastim (recombinant human granulocyte colony stimulating factor) as support to a high dose-intensive epiadriamycin-cyclophosphamide regimen in chemotherapy-naïve patients with locally advanced or metastatic breast cancer. Ann Oncol 1995;6:673–677.

87. Michel G, Landman-Parker J, Auclerc MF, et al. Use of recombinant human granulocyte colony-stimulating factor to increase chemotherapy dose-intensity: a randomized trial in very high-risk childhood acute lymphoblastic leukemia. J Clin Oncol 2000;18:1517–1524.

88. Rowinsky EK, Grochow LB, Sartorius SE, et al. Phase I and pharmacologic study of high doses of the topoisomerase I inhibitor topotecan with granulocyte colony-stimulating factor in patients with solid tumors. J Clin Oncol 1996;14:1224–1235.

89. Doorduijn JK, van der Holt B, van Imhoff GW, et al. CHOP compared with CHOP plus granulocyte colony-stimulating factor in elderly patients with aggressive non-Hodgkin's lymphoma. J Clin Oncol 2003;21:3041–3050.

90. Citron ML, Berry DA, Cirrincione C, et al. Randomized trial of dose-dense versus conventionally scheduled and sequential versus concurrent combination chemotherapy as postoperative adjuvant treatment of node-positive primary breast cancer: first report of Intergroup Trial C9741/Cancer and Leukemia Group B Trial 9741. J Clin Oncol 2003;21:1431–1439.

91. Ottmann OG, Hoelzer D, Gracien E, et al. Concomitant granulocyte colony-stimulating factor and induction chemoradiotherapy in adult acute lymphocytic leukemia: a randomized phase III trial. Blood 1995;86:444–450.

92. Lowenberg B, van Putten W, Theobald M, et al. Effect of priming with granulocyte colony-stimulating factor on the outcome of chemotherapy for acute myeloid leukemia. Dutch-Belgian Hemato-Oncology Cooperative Group; Swiss Group for Clinical Cancer Research. N Engl J Med 2003;349:743–752.

93. Rahiala J, Perkkio M, Riikonen P. Prospective and randomized comparison of early versus delayed prophylactic administration of granulocyte colony-stimulating factor (filgrastim) in children with cancer. Med Pediatr Oncol 1999;32:326–330.

94. Green MD, Koelbl H, Baselga J, et al. A randomized double-blind multicenter phase III study of fixed-dose single-administration pegfilgrastim versus daily filgrastim in patients receiving myelosuppressive chemotherapy. International Pegfilgrastim 749 Study Group. Ann Oncol 2003;14:29–35.

95. Holmes FA, O'Shaughnessy JA, Vukelja S, et al. Blinded, randomized, multicenter study to evaluate single administration pegfilgrastim once per cycle versus daily filgrastim as an adjunct to chemotherapy in patients with high-risk stage II or stage III/IV breast cancer. J Clin Oncol 2002;20:727–731.

96. Mahr DW, Lieschke GJ, Green M, et al. Filgrastim in patients with chemotherapy-induced febrile neutropenia. Ann Intern Med 1994;121:492.

97. Asano S, Masaoka T, Takaku F. Beneficial effect of human glycosylated granulocyte colony-stimulating factor in marrow-transplanted patients: results of multicenter phase II-III studies. Transplant Proc 1991;23:1701–1703.

98. Schmitz N, Dreger P, Zander AR, et al. Results of a randomized, controlled, multicentre study of recombinant human granulocyte colony-stimulating factor (filgrastim) in patients with Hodgkin's disease and non-Hodgkin's lymphoma undergoing autologous bone marrow transplantation. Bone Marrow Transplant 1995;15:261–266.

99. Stahel RA, Jost LM, Cerny T, et al. Randomized study of recombinant human granulocyte colony-stimulating factor after high-dose chemotherapy and autologous bone marrow transplantation for high-risk lymphoma malignancies. J Clin Oncol 1994;12:1931–1938.

100. Bishop MR, Tarantolo SR, Geller RB, et al. A randomized, double-blind trial of filgrastim (granulocyte colony-stimulating factor) versus placebo following allogeneic blood stem cell transplantation. Blood 2000;96:80–85.

101. Peters WP, Rosner G, Ross M, et al. Comparative effects of granulocyte-macrophage colony-stimulating factor and granulocyte colony-stimulating factor on priming peripheral blood progenitor cells for use with autologous bone marrow after high-dose chemotherapy. Blood 1993;81:1709–1719.

102. Chao NJ, Schriber JR, Grimes K, et al. Granulocyte colony-stimulating factor "mobilized" peripheral blood progenitor cells accelerate granulocyte and platelet recovery after high-dose chemotherapy. Blood 1993;81:2031–2035.

103. Sheridan WP, Begley CG, Juttner CA, et al. Effect of peripheral-blood progenitor cells mobilised by filgrastim (G-CSF) on platelet recovery after high-dose chemotherapy. Lancet 1992;339:640–644.

104. Shimazaki C, Oku N, Uchiyama H, et al. Effect of granulocyte colony-stimulating factor on hematopoietic recovery after peripheral blood progenitor cell transplantation. Bone Marrow Transplant 1994;13:271.

105. Klumpp TR, Magan KF, Goldberg SL, et al. Granulocyte colony-stimulating factor accelerates neutrophil engraftment following peripheral-blood stem-cell transplantation: a prospective, randomized trial. J Clin Oncol 1995;13:1323–1327.

106. Kawano Y, Takaue Y, Mimaya J, et al. Marginal benefit/disadvantage of granulocyte colony-stimulating factor therapy after autologous blood stem cell transplantation in children: results of a prospective randomized trial. Blood 1998;92:4040–4046.

107. McQuaker IG, Hunter AE, Pacey S, et al. Low-dose filgrastim significantly enhances neutrophil recovery following autologous peripheral-blood stem-cell transplantation in patients with lymphoproliferative disorders: evidence for clinical and economic benefit. J Clin Oncol 1997;15:451–457.

108. Lee SM, Radford JA, Dobson L, et al. Recombinant human granulocyte colony-stimulating factor (filgrastim) following high-dose chemotherapy and peripheral blood progenitor cell rescue in high-grade non-Hodgkin's lymphoma: clinical benefits at no extra cost. Br J Cancer 1998;77:1294–1299.

109. Torres Gomez A, Jimenez MA, Alvarez MA, et al. Optimal timing of granulocyte colony-stimulating factor (G-CSF) administration after bone marrow transplantation: a prospective randomized study. Ann Hematol 1995;71:65–70.

110. Vey N, Molnar S, Faucher C, et al. Delayed administration of granulocyte colony-stimulating factor after autologous bone marrow transplantation: effect on granulocyte recovery. Bone Marrow Transplant 1994;14:779–782.

111. Faucher C, Le Corroller AG, Chabannon C, et al. Administration of G-CSF can be delayed after transplantation of autologous G-CSF–primed blood stem cells: a randomized study. Bone Marrow Transplant 1996;17:533–536.

112. Hornedo J, Sola C, Solano C, et al. The role of granulocyte colony-stimulating factor (G-CSF) in the post-transplant period. SOLTI Group. Bone Marrow Transplant 2002; 29: 737–743.

113. de Azevedo AM, Nucci M, Maiolino A, et al. A randomized, multicenter study of G-CSF starting on day +1 vs day +5 after autologous peripheral blood progenitor cell transplantation. Bone Marrow Transplant 2002;29:745–751.

114. Ho VT, Mirza NQ, Junco D, Okamura T, Przepiorka D. The effect of hematopoietic growth factors on the risk of graft-vs-host disease after allogeneic hematopoietic stem cell transplantation: a meta-analysis. Bone Marrow Transplant 2003;32: 771–775.

115. Ringden O, Labopin M, Gorin NC, et al. Treatment with granulocyte colony-stimulating factor after allogeneic bone marrow transplantation for acute leukemia increases the risk of graft-versus-host disease and death: a study from the Acute Leukemia Working Party of the European Group for Blood and Marrow Transplantation. J Clin Oncol 2004;22:416–423.

116. Morton J, Hutchins C, Durrant S. Granulocyte-colony-stimulating factor (G-CSF)–primed allogeneic bone marrow: significantly less graft-versus-host disease and comparable engraftment to G-CSF-mobilized peripheral blood stem cells. Blood 2001;98:3186–3191.

117. Przepiorka D, Smith TL, Folloder J, et al. Controlled trial of filgrastim for acceleration of neutrophil recovery after allogeneic blood stem cell transplantation from human leukocyte antigen-matched related donors. Blood 2001;97:3405–3410.

118. Pettengell R, Wall P, Thatcher N, et al. Multicyclic, dose-intensive chemotherapy supported by sequential reinfusion of hematopoietic progenitors in whole blood. J Clin Oncol 1995; 13:148–156.

119. Weaver CH, Schulman KA, Wilson-Relyea B, et al. Randomized trial of filgrastim, sargramostim, or sequential sargramostim and filgrastim after myelosuppressive chemotherapy for the harvesting of peripheral-blood stem cells. J Clin Oncol 2000; 18:43–53.

120. Desikan KR, Barlogie B, Jagannath S, et al. Comparable engraftment kinetics following peripheral-blood stem-cell infusion mobilized with granulocyte colony-stimulating factor with or without cyclophosphamide in multiple myeloma. J Clin Oncol 1998;16;1547–1553.

121. Koc ON, Gerson SL, Cooper BW, et al. Randomized cross-over trial of progenitor-cell mobilization: high-dose cyclophosphamide plus granulocyte colony-stimulating factor (G-CSF) versus granulocyte-macrophage colony-stimulating factor plus G-CSF. J Clin Oncol 2000;18:1824–1830.

122. Stiff P, Gingrich R, Luger S, et al. A randomized phase 2 study of PBPC mobilization by stem cell factor and filgrastim in heavily pretreated patients with Hodgkin's disease or non-Hodgkin's lymphoma. Bone Marrow Transplant 2000;26:471–481.

123. Andre M, Baudoux E, Bron D, et al. Phase III randomized study comparing 5 or 10 microg per kg per day of filgrastim for mobilization of peripheral blood progenitor cells with chemotherapy, followed by intensification and autologous transplantation in patients with nonmyeloid malignancies. Transfusion 2003; 43:50–57.

124. Toner GC, Shapiro JD, Laidlaw CR, et al. Low-dose versus standard-dose lenograstim prophylaxis after chemotherapy: a randomized, crossover comparison. J Clin Oncol 1998;16; 3874–3879.

125. Carlsson G, Ahlin A, Dahllof G, et al. Efficacy and safety of two different rG-CSF preparations in the treatment of patients with severe congenital neutropenia. Br J Haematol 2004;126: 127–132.

126. Relling MV, Boyett JM, Blanco JG, et al. Granulocyte colony-stimulating factor and the risk of secondary myeloid malignancy after etoposide treatment. Blood 2003;101:3862 – 3867.

127. Meropol NJ, Miller LL, Korn EL, et al. Severe myelosuppression resulting from concurrent administration of granulocyte colony-stimulating factor and cytotoxic chemotherapy. J Natl Cancer Inst 1992;84:1201–1203.

128. de Vries, EGE, Biesma B, Willemese PHB, et al. A double-blind placebo-controlled study with granulocyte-macrophage colony-stimulating factor during chemotherapy for ovarian carcinoma. Cancer Res 1991;51:116–122.

129. Gerhartz HH, Engelhard M, Meusers P, et al. Randomized, double-blind, placebo-controlled, phase III study of recombinant human granulocyte-macrophage colony-stimulating factor as adjunct to induction treatment of high-grade malignant non-Hodgkin's lymphomas. Blood 1993;82:2329–2339.

130. Eguchi K, Kabe J, Kudo S, et al. Efficacy of recombinant human granulocyte-macrophage colony-stimulating factor for chemotherapy-induced leukemia in patients with non-small-cell lung cancer. Cancer Chemother Pharmacol 1994; 34:37–43.

131. Stone RM, Berg DT, George SL, et al. Granulocyte-macrophage colony-stimulating factor after initial chemotherapy for elderly patients with primary acute myelogenous leukemia. N Engl J Med 1995;332:1671–1677.

132. Jones SE, Schottstaedt MW, Duncan LA, et al. Randomized double-blind prospective trial to evaluate the effects of sargramostim versus placebo in a moderate-dose fluorouracil, doxorubicin, and cyclophosphamide adjuvant chemotherapy program for stage II and III breast cancer. J Clin Oncol 1996; 14:2976–2983.

133. Rowe JM, Andersen JW, Mazza JJ, et al. A randomized placebo-controlled phase III study of granulocyte-macrophage colony-stimulating factor in adult patients (>55 to 70 years of age) with acute myelogenous leukemia: a study of the Eastern Cooperative Oncology Group (E1490). Blood 1995; 86:457–462.

134. Vellenga E, Uyl-de Groot CA, de Wit R, et al. Randomized placebo-controlled trial of granulocyte-macrophage colony-stimulating factor in patients with chemotherapy-related febrile neutropenia. J Clin Oncol 1996;14:619–627.

135. Witz F, Sadoun A, Perrin MC, et al. A placebo-controlled study of recombinant human granulocyte-macrophage colony-stimulating factor administered during and after induction treatment for de novo acute myelogenous leukemia in elderly patients. Groupe Ouest Est Leucemies Aigues Myeloblastiques (GOELAM). Blood 1998;91:2722–2730.

136. Powles R, Smith C, Milan S, et al: Human recombinant GM-CSF in allogeneic bone-marrow transplantation for leukemia: double-blind, placebo-controlled trial. Lancet 1990; 336:1417–1420.

137. Nemunaitis J, Rabinowe SN, Singer JW, et al. Recombinant granulocyte-macrophage colony-stimulating factor after autologous bone marrow transplantation for lymphoid cancer. N Engl J Med 1991; 324:1773–1778.

138. Link H, Boogaerts MA, Carella AM, et al. A controlled trial of recombinant human granulocyte-macrophage colony-stimulating factor after total body irradiation, high-dose chemotherapy, and autologous bone marrow transplantation for acute lymphoblastic leukemia or malignant lymphoma. Blood 1992; 80:2188–2195.

139. Khwaja A, Linch DC, Goldstone AH, et al. Recombinant human granulocyte-macrophage colony-stimulating factor after autologous bone marrow transplantation for malignant lymphoma: a British National Lymphoma Investigation double-blind, placebo-controlled trial. Br J Haematol 1992; 82:317–323.

140. Advani R, Chao NJ, Horning SJ, et al. Granulocyte-macrophage colony-stimulating factor as an adjunct to autologous hemopoietic stem cell transplantation for lymphoma. Ann Intern Med 1992;116:183–189.

141. De Witte T, Gratwohl A, Van Der Lely N, et al. Recombinant human granulocyte-macrophage colony-stimulating factor accelerates neutrophil and monocyte recovery after allogeneic T-cell–depleted bone marrow transplantation. Blood 1992; 79:1359–1365.

142. Gorin NC, Coiffier B, Hayat M, et al. Recombinant human granulocyte-macrophage colony-stimulating factor after high-dose chemotherapy and autologous bone marrow transplantation with unpurged and purged marrow in non-Hodgkin's lymphoma: a double-blind placebo-controlled trial. Blood 1992; 80:1149–1157.

143. Gulati SC, Bennett CL. Granulocyte-macrophage colony-stimulating factor as adjunctive therapy in relapsed Hodgkin disease. Ann Intern Med 1992;116:177–182.

144. Nemunaitis J, Rosenfeld CS, Ash R, et al. Phase III randomized, double-blind placebo-controlled trial of rhGM-CSF following allogeneic bone marrow transplantation. Bone Marrow Transplant 1995;15:949.

145. Hiraoka A, Masaoka T, Mizoguchi H, et al. Recombinant human non-glycosylated granulocyte-macrophage colony stimulating factor in allogeneic bone marrow transplantation: double-blind placebo-controlled phase III clinical trial. Jpn J Clin Oncol 1994; 24:205–211.

146. Rabinowe SN, Neuberg D, Bierman PJ, et al. Long-term follow-up of a phase III study of recombinant human granulocyte-macrophage colony-stimulating factor after autologous bone marrow transplantation for lymphoid malignancies. Blood 1993;81:1903–1908.

147. Boiron JM, Marit G, Faberes C, et al. Collection of peripheral blood stem cells in multiple myeloma following single high-dose cyclophosphamide with and without recombinant human granulocyte-macrophage colony-stimulating factor. Bone Marrow Transplant 1993; 12:49–55.

148. Elias AD, Ayash L, Anderson KC, et al. Mobilization of peripheral blood progenitor cells by chemotherapy and granulocyte-macrophage colony-stimulating factor for hematopoietic support after high-dose intensification for breast cancer. Blood 1992;79:3036–3044.

149. Huan SD, Hester J, Spitzer G, et al. Influence of mobilized peripheral blood cells on the hematopoietic recovery by autologous marrow and recombinant human granulocyte-macrophage colony-stimulating factor after high-dose cyclophosphamide, etoposide, and cisplatin. Blood 1992; 79:3388–3393.

150. Legros M, Fleury J, Bay JO, et al. RhGM-CSF vs placebo following rhGM-CSF-mobilized PBPC transplantation: a phase III double-blind randomized trial. Bone Marrow Transplant 1997; 19:209–213.

151. Kritz A, Crown JP, Motzer RJ, et al. Beneficial impact of peripheral blood progenitor cells in patients with metastatic breast cancer treated with high-dose chemotherapy plus granulocyte-macrophage colony-stimulating factor: a randomized trial. Cancer 1993;71:2515–2521.

152. Ballestrero A, Ferrando F, Garuti A, et al. Comparative effects of three cytokine regimens after high-dose cyclophosphamide: granulocyte colony-stimulating factor, granulocyte-macrophage colony-stimulating factor, and sequential interleukin-3 and GM-CSF. J Clin Oncol 1999; 17:1296–1303.

153. Caballero MD, Vazquez L, Barragan JM, et al. Randomized study of filgrastim versus molgramostim after peripheral stem cell transplant in breast cancer. Haematologica 1998; 83:514–518.

154. Lieschke GJ, Cebon J, Morstyn G. Characterization of the clinical effects after the first dose of bacterially synthesized recombinant human granulocyte-macrophage colony-stimulating factor. Blood 1989; 74:2634–2643.

155. Shaffer DW, Smith LS, Burris HA, et al. A randomized phase I trial of chronic oral etoposide with or without granulocyte-macrophage colony-stimulating factor in patients with advanced malignancies. Cancer Res 1993;53:5929–5933.

156. Bunn PA, Crowley J, Kelly K, et al. Chemoradiotherapy with or without granulocyte-macrophage colony-stimulating factor in the treatment of limited-stage small-cell lung cancer: a prospective phase III randomized study of the Southwest Oncology Group. J Clin Oncol 1995;13:1632–1641.

157. Lyman GH, Dale DC, Crawford J. Incidence and predictors of low dose-intensity in adjuvant breast cancer chemotherapy: a nationwide study of community practices.J Clin Oncol 2003; 21:4524–4531.

158. Gordon MS, McCaskill-Stevens WJ, Battiato LA, et al. A phase I trial of recombinant human interleukin-11 (Neumega rhIL-11 growth factor) in women with breast cancer receiving chemotherapy. Blood 1996; 87:3615–3624.

159. Isaacs C, Robert NJ, Bailey A, et al. Randomized placebo-controlled study of recombinant human interleukin-11 to prevent chemotherapy-induced thrombocytopenia in patients with breast cancer receiving dose-intensive cyclophosphamide and doxorubicin. J Clin Oncol 1997;15:3368–3377.

160. Tepler I, Elias L, Smith JW, et al. A randomized placebo-controlled trial of recombinant human interleukin-11 in cancer patients with severe thrombocytopenia due to chemotherapy. Blood 1996;87:3607–3614.

161. Hussein A, Vredenburgh J, Elkordy M, et al. Randomized, placebo-controlled study of recombinant human interleukin eleven (Neumega rhIL-11 growth factor) in patients with breast cancer following high-dose chemotherapy with autologous hematopoietic progenitor cell support. Exp Hemetol 1996; 24:634a.

162. Choi ES, Hokom MM, Chen JL, et al. The role of MGDF in terminal stages of thrombopoiesis. Br J Haematol 1996; 95:227–233.

163. Basser RL, Rasko JE, Clarke K, et al. Thrombopoietic effects of pegylated recombinant human megakaryocyte growth and development factor in patients with advanced cancer. Lancet 1996;348;1270–1281.

164. Vadhan-Raj S, Murray LJ, Bueso-Ramos C, et al. Stimulation of megakaryocyte and platelet production by a single dose of recombinant human thrombopoietin in patients with cancer. Ann Intern Med 1997;126:673–681.

165. Fanucchi M, Glaspy J, Crawford J, et al. Effects of polyethylene glycol-conjugated recombinant human megakaryocyte growth and development factor on platelet counts after chemotherapy for lung cancer. N Engl J Med 1997;336:404–409.

166. Basser RL, Rasko JEJ, Clarke K, et al. Randomized, blinded, placebo-controlled phase I trial of pegylated recombinant human megakaryocyte growth and development factor with filgrastim after dose-intensive chemotherapy in patients with advanced cancer. Blood 1997;89:3118–3128.

167. Vadhan-Raj S, Verschraegen CF, Bueso-Ramos C, et al. Recombinant human thrombopoietin attenuates carboplatin-induced severe thrombocytopenia and the need for platelet transfusions in patients with gynecologic cancer. Ann Intern Med 2000;132:364–368.

168. Schiffer CA, Miller K, Larson RA, et al. A double-blind, placebo-controlled trial of pegylated recombinant human megakaryocyte growth and development factor as an adjunct to induction and consolidation therapy for patients with acute myeloid leukemia. Blood 2000; 95:2530–2535.

169. Schuster MW, Beveridge R, Frei-Lahr D, et al. The effects of pegylated recombinant human megakaryocyte growth and development factor (PEG-rHuMGDF) on platelet recovery in breast cancer patients undergoing autologous bone marrow transplantation. Exp Hematol 2002;30:1044–1050.

170. Ragnhammar P, Friesen H-J, Frodin J-E, et al. Induction of anti-recombinant human granulocyte-macrophage colony-stimulating factor (*Escherichia coli*-derived) antibodies and clinical effects in nonimmunocompromised patients. Blood 1994; 84:4078–4087.

171. Miller LL, Korn EL, Stevens DS, et al. Abrogation of the hematological and biological activities of the interleukin-3/granulocyte-macrophage colony-stimulating factor fusion protein PIXY321 by neutralizing anti-PIXY321 antibodies in cancer patients receiving high-dose carboplatin. Blood 1999; 93: 3250–3258.

172. Bussel, JB, George JN, Kuter DJ, et al. An open-label, dose-finding study evaluating the safety and platelet response of a novel thrombopoietic protein (AMG 531) in thrombocytopenic adult patients with immune thrombocytopenic purpura [abstract]. Blood 2003;102;293.

173. Petros WP, Rabinowitz J, Stuart A, Peters WP. Clinical pharmacology of filgrastim following high-dose chemotherapy and autologous bone marrow transplantation. Clin Cancer Res 1997;3:705–11.

174. Spitzer G, Adkins D, Mathews M, et al. Randomized comparison of G-CSF+GM-CSF vs G-CSF alone for mobilization of peripheral blood stem cells: effects on hematopoietic recovery after high-dose chemotherapy. Bone Marrow Transplant. 1997;20:921–30.

Interleukins

36

Gheath Alatrash   *Ronald M. Bukowski*
Charles S. Tannenbaum   *James H. Finke*

The study of cytokines has evolved from the description of protein factors mediating particular cellular functions to studies at the molecular level using recombinant proteins that allow definitive identification of their structures and functions. The biologic activities of these molecules are complex, with pleiotropic and redundant actions common. Cytokines are often part of a cascade that can then lead to the synthesis and production of other mediators and result in either positive or negative regulatory effects. The antitumor activities of various cytokines have led to their use in patients with malignancy, and a large body of data now exists on their clinical effects and pharmacology. This chapter discusses six different factors, all of which have been used clinically and demonstrate the difficulties encountered in evaluating biologic agents with complex functions in vivo.

INTERLEUKIN-2

The recognition in 1965 that soluble mitogenic factors were present in conditioned supernatants from mixed lymphocyte cultures[1] provided the initial observation indicating the existence of lymphokines that could stimulate cell division. In 1976, Morgan et al.[2] demonstrated that normal human T lymphocytes obtained from bone marrow could be maintained in culture for periods of up to 1 year by using media from phytohemagglutinin (PHA)–stimulated mononuclear cells. Shortly thereafter, this media was also found to sustain the proliferation of antigen-specific cytolytic T cells.[3] This cytokine was ultimately designated as IL-2 (Second Annual Lymphokine Workshop, 1979), and the cDNA encoding human IL-2 was isolated.[4]

Structure and Mechanisms of Action

IL-2 is a 15-kd glycoprotein that varies in degree of glycosylation and sialylation.[5,6] It contains a carbohydrate-binding domain that is thought to be involved in the clearance and intracellular distribution of this protein.[7] In structure, IL-2 is similar to GM-CSF and IL-4.[5,6] IL-2 has four major amphipathic α helices that are arranged in an antiparallel manner (Fig. 36.1).[5,6] One disulfide bridge exists in the IL-2 protein; it provides stability of the tertiary structure and is necessary for biologic activity.[8]

T cells are the primary source of IL-2, and among mature T cells most of the IL-2 is produced by the CD4$^+$ subset. In murine systems, IL-2 is produced by unprimed CD4$^+$ cells (T$_H$0) and by the T$_H$1 subset of helper cells involved in delayed-type hypersensitivity responses.[9]

IL-2 is not constitutively produced but is induced on T-cell activation.[10] Two signals are required for IL-2 gene expression. One is provided by stimulation through the T-cell receptor (TCR)/CD3 complex. The second signal appears to be provided by accessory cells that express the cell surface molecule B7, which is the ligand for CD28 or CTLA-4 molecules that are present on T cells.[11] The stimulation of T cells via the TCR in the absence of costimulation (B7/CD28) can induce T-cell anergy, a state of T-cell unresponsiveness, and involves a block in IL-2 gene transcription.[12] When both signals are provided, IL-2 gene expression occurs, with peak levels of IL-2 mRNA accumulation within 6 hours of stimulation.[13] The induction of IL-2 gene expression is under the control of a transcriptional enhancer located approximately 300 base pairs upstream of the transcription site.[14] This region contains binding sites for several DNA-binding proteins that are required for the transcription of the IL-2 gene, including nuclear factor AT (NFAT), activating protein 1 (AP-1), NF-κB, AP-3, and Oct.[13]

IL-2 mediates its biologic effects by binding to the IL-2 receptor (IL-2R), which is composed of three distinct chains, α (55 kd), β (75 kd), and γ (64 kd).[5,15] All three chains have external domains of similar length, whereas the cytoplasmic domains vary. The β subunit (286 residues)

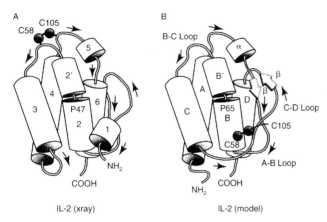

IL-2 (xray)   **IL-2 (model)**

Figure 36.1 Comparison of x-ray–derived and model folds of interleukin-2 (IL-2). **A:** Schematic drawing of the IL-2 x-ray helix bundle (3). Cylindrical helices are marked 1 to 6. Loops are drawn as loose ribbons; Pro[47] (P47) is marked. The disulfide bond is noted by linked spheres. **B:** In the granulocyte-macrophage colony-stimulating factor–IL-4–like IL-2 model, the chain through the core helices is retraced and reconnected, the disulfide bridge is relocated, and the existence of a small β sheet is proposed; Pro[65] (P65) is marked. Only helix D remains fully equivalent in sequence to x-ray helix 6. (Reproduced with permission from Bazan JF. Unraveling the structure of IL-2. Science 1992;257:410–413.)

has the largest internal domain, and the α chain has the smallest (13 residues).[15–18] The IL-2R that binds IL-2 with high affinity (K_d [dissociation constant] = 10 pmol/L) requires the presence of all three chains.[5] Cells that express both the β and γ chains but are missing the α chain have an intermediate-affinity receptor (approximately 100-fold less than the high-affinity receptor) that is capable of signal transduction. The expression of only the α chain results in cells with a low IL-2–binding affinity and no intracellular signaling.[15]

Signaling via the IL-2R requires oligomerization of the β and γ chains.[19–21] Neither of these chains has intrinsic

kinase activity; however, they appear to be substrates for protein tyrosine kinases (PTKs), which associate with the IL-2R after IL-2 binding (Fig. 36.2). Multiple PTKs are involved, each associated with a specific region of the intracytoplasmic tails of the γ and β chains.[21,22] This interaction results in the activation of PTKs and the phosphorylation of multiple substrates that include the γ and β chains themselves.[22] The binding of Janus kinase 3 (Jak3) to the γ chain is critical to transducing the proliferative signal via the IL-2R.[23–25] The importance of Jak3 and γ chain function is illustrated by the fact that loss of either Jak3 or the γ chain results in severe combined immunodeficiency syndrome in humans.[26] The proximal region of the IL-2Rβ chain, which is rich in serine residues, is also important for proliferation and cell survival through the induction of c-myc and Bcl-2/Bcl-XL, respectively.[22] This region is required for activation of phosphatidylinositol 3 kinase (PI3K) and the downstream kinase Akt, which are likely involved in the expression of c-myc and Bcl-2.[27,28] Both the Zap-70 kinase, Syk, and Janus kinase 1 (Jak1) bind to the serine-rich region, and although Syk appears to be involved in c-myc induction, the role of Jak1 is not defined.[29,30] The acidic region of the IL-2Rβ chain appears to be responsible for the signaling pathway leading to c-fos and c-jun induction.[31,32] The src kinase p56lck constitutively associates with this region and is activated by IL-2 binding.[31,32] Evidence is growing of a linkage between p56lck and the Ras pathway, which is involved in the IL-2–dependent activation of c-fos and c-jun and T-cell proliferation.[21,33–35] The carboxy-terminal domain of the IL-2Rβ chain appears to be involved in signal transduction and transcription-activating factor 5 (STAT5).[36,37] STAT5 may regulate T-cell proliferation partly through the induction of the high-affinity IL-2Rα chain.[38]

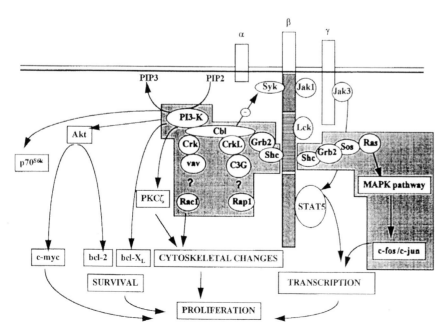

Figure 36.2 Schematic diagram of the interleukin-2 signal transduction cascade. (MAPK, mitogen-activated protein kinase; PI3K, phosphatidylinositol 3 kinase; PKC, protein kinase C; STAT, signal transduction and transcription–activating factor.) (Reproduced with permission from Gesbert F, Delespine-Carmagnat M, Bertoglio J. Recent advances in the understanding of interleukin-2 signal transduction. J Clin Immunol 1998;18:307–320.)

Several cell types involved in inflammation and immunity express IL-2R.[5,39-41] The IL-2Rβ chain is constitutively expressed on monocytes/macrophages and certain lymphoid cells such as natural killer (NK) cells. The majority of NK cells (90%) express the intermediate-affinity IL-2R; only a subset has the high-affinity receptor.[41] Activation of T cells via the T-cell receptor complex up-regulates IL-2Rβ and induces IL-2Rα chain expression, which leads to formation of the high-affinity receptor.[42] B cells can also be induced to express IL-2R and become IL-2 responsive after cross-linking of surface immunoglobulin.[43] IL-2 stimulation also leads to activation of other kinases, including the serine/threonine-specific kinase Raf-1.[44,45] Evidence also exists that IL-2 binding to its receptor on T cells leads to the phosphorylation of the retinoblastoma-susceptibility gene product p110Rb, a process that is important for cell cycle progression.[46]

Cellular Pharmacology

IL-2 is a major growth factor for lymphoid cells, including T cells and NK cells.[2,5,47] IL-2 binding to IL-2R on activated T cells promotes clonal expansion of antigen-specific cells, an important component in the development of host immunity. It also plays an important role in potentiating cytotoxic activity of lymphocytes, including antigen-specific major histocompatibility complex (MHC)–restricted cytotoxic CD8$^+$ and CD4$^+$ T lymphocytes.[48,49] IL-2 can also enhance the cytolytic activity of NK cells, which are responsible for what has been referred to as "LAK cell activity."[50] The potentiation of cytotoxic activity is likely due to IL-2 up-regulation of the expression of proteins involved in the lytic process. IL-2 alone or in combination with other stimuli can up-regulate mRNA levels for perforin and granzyme B in both T and NK cells.[5,51] Macrophage cytotoxicity is also potentiated by IL-2.[49] IL-2 is also known to stimulate cytokine secretion from mononuclear cells, including NK cells, T cells, and macrophages.[49] NK cells cultured with IL-2 secrete cytokines (TNF-α, IFN-γ, GM-CSF), which can facilitate inflammation and immunity by acting on monocytes and macrophages.[5,49] IL-2 can also cooperate with TCR triggering to induce IFN-γ secretion from T lymphocytes.[49]

IL-2 may also have a negative regulatory effect on the immune response.[52,53] IL-2 plays an important role in promoting apoptosis in T cells, a major mechanism of controlling immune responses. This concept is supported by the observation that knockout mice missing IL-2 or the α or β chains of the IL-2R display autoimmunity and lymphadenopathy.[54-56] Thus, mice deficient in IL-2R signaling have abnormal accumulation of activated T cells with impaired TCR-induced apoptosis. IL-2 enhances activation-induced cell death (AICD) mediated through the Fas pathway.[52-56] Crossing IL-2 knockout mice with TCR transgenic mice demonstrated that activated T cells from these animals were impaired in Fas-mediated AICD.[57] IL-2 augments

AICD by increasing the transcription of Fas ligand in antigen-stimulated T cells, partly through the induction of STAT5.[53,58] IL-2 also inhibits the transcription of the inhibitor of the Fas pathway, FLIP (FADD-like IL-1β–converting enzyme [FLICE] inhibitory protein).[58] In the potentiation of AICD, IL-2 cannot be replaced by other cytokines such as interleukin-7 (IL-7) or IL-4. Thus, although IL-2 serves as a growth signal during the early phase of an immune response, it can potentiate apoptosis in T cells after repeated antigen activation, which results in termination of an immune response. IL-2 is also important for the induction of passive apoptosis in T cells. This form of apoptosis results when there is no further antigen stimulation and the induction of IL-2 and IL-2R ceases, resulting in lymphokine withdrawal.[52,53] This pathway of apoptosis is distinct from Fas-mediated AICD. Passive apoptosis results from an increase in mitochondrial permeability and cytochrome *c* release and can be blocked by Bcl-2.[52,53]

Clinical Pharmacokinetics

Clinical assessment of the immunopharmacology of IL-2 has been assisted by the availability of a sensitive bioassay procedure, development of ELISAs,[59] and the use of cytolytic (NK- and LAK-cell) assays to define the biologic effects of IL-2 administration. The bioassay assesses the capacity of the sera or supernatant in question to maintain the growth of an IL-2–dependent T-cell clone.

Initial studies with IL-2 used material produced by the Jurkat T-cell tumor line and purified by affinity chromatography.[60] Doses of 14 to 2,000 μg were administered, and serum levels were measured using a bioassay.[61] The biologic half-life varied from 6 to 10 minutes after a bolus infusion. Sustained serum levels during continuous infusion were also noted.

Several recombinant preparations of IL-2 (rIL-2) have been used clinically and are outlined in Table 36.1. They are nonglycosylated and produced in *Escherichia coli*. The Chiron preparation[62] differs from natural human IL-2; the cysteine residue at amino acid 125 is replaced by serine, and it also lacks the N-terminal alanine. These alterations permit correct folding and maintenance of the biologic activity of this agent. Amgen rIL-2[63] has a similar serine substitution at position 125 and in addition has an N-terminal methionine residue. The Hoffmann-La Roche rIL-2 preparation[64] lacks the amino acid substitution at position 125, has an additional N-terminal methionine residue, and has a specific activity similar to that of natural IL-2. These molecules can form only one disulfide bridge and belong to the class of proteins known as muteins, or mutationally altered and biologically active products.

Confusion has arisen because of the definitions used for units of activity and the methods used to calculate dosage (body surface area versus kilogram). At present, the accepted definition for a unit is based on an international standard described by the World Health Organization.[68] A

TABLE 36.1

RECOMBINANT INTERLEUKIN-2 (rIL-2) PREPARATIONS

Source	Formulation	Activity	Study
Chiron	Des-alanye, serine-125 rIL-2	16.5×10^6 IU/mg	Lotze et al. (62)
Amgen	r-met HuIL-2 (ala 125)	9.4×10^6 IU/mg	Sarna et al. (63)
Hoffmann-La Roche	r-met IL-2	$12–15 \times 10^6$ IU/mg	Sosman et al. (64)
Chiron	PEG rIL-2	4×10^6 IU/mg	Zimmerman et al. (65)
Roussel-Uclaf	rIL-2	$1.2 \pm 0.6 \ 10^7$ IU/mg	Tursz et al. (66), Tzannis et al. (67)

PEG rIL-2, polyethylene glycol interleukin-2; r-met HuIL-2, recombinant methionyl human interleukin-2; r-met IL-2, recombinant methionyl interleukin-2.

unit of IL-2 is defined as the reciprocal of the dilution that produces 50% of the maximal proliferation of murine HT2 cells in a short-term tritium-labeled thymidine incorporation assay. One milligram of Chiron rIL-2 contains 16.3 IU/mg of drug. In the past, a Cetus unit was commonly used to express doses of this cytokine, with 3×10^6 Cetus units equaling 1 mg of rIL-2. Hoffmann-La Roche rIL-2 contained 15.0×10^6 U/mg of protein. One Hoffmann-La Roche unit was reported as equivalent to one Biological Response Modifiers Program (BRMP) unit[69] and approximately 3.0 IU. This situation has produced confusion in the comparing of dosages and toxicity among studies that used the various rIL-2 preparations.

The clinical and in vitro activities of these two rIL-2 preparations have been compared by Hank et al.[70] Equivalent international units of each cytokine were used, and quantitative differences were noted. A dosage of 1.5×10^6 IU/m^2 per day of Roche rIL-2 was equivalent in toxicity to 4.5×10^6 IU/m^2 per day of Chiron rIL-2. Equivalent amounts also differed in the induction of proliferation by various T-cell lines and binding to IL-2 receptors. These findings suggested that 3 to 6 IU of Chiron rIL-2 are required for induction of the biologic effects produced by 1 IU of Hoffmann-La Roche rIL-2.

The only preparation currently available for clinical use in the United States is Chiron rIL-2. Findings such as these suggest that one must be cautious when using doses and schedules developed with alternative preparations. The reasons for these differences in biologic activity may be related to structural and solubility differences between these proteins. Two other IL-2 preparations used clinically are natural human IL-2 (nIL-2) and Sanofi rIL-2; however, limited information is available concerning these agents.

The clinical pharmacokinetics of both the Chiron and Hoffmann-La Roche preparations have been studied, and the features of the latter more fully characterized. Like many other cytokines, rIL-2 has a short half-life. Various parameters for Jurkat cell–derived IL-2 and recombinant IL-2 preparations are outlined in Table 36.2. When rIL-2 is administered as an intravenous (i.v.) bolus, its pharmacokinetics are approximately linear, and the resulting serum levels are proportional to the dose.[71] Injection of 6×10^6 IU/m^2 produces serum levels of 1,950 IU/mL. The levels decrease with a $t_{1/2}\alpha$ of 12.9 minutes, followed by a slower phase with a $t_{1/2}\beta$ of 85 minutes. Figure 36.3 illustrates the serum levels obtained after injection of an i.v. bolus of 6×10^6 IU/m^2.[72] The reported clearance rate of 117 mL/minute is consistent with renal filtration being the major route of elimination.

The variables influencing rIL-2 pharmacokinetics have been studied in animal models.[33,73,74] The biodistribution of ^{125}I-radiolabeled rIL-2 was studied in Sprague-Dawley rats.[33] The most significant uptake was found in the kidney

TABLE 36.2

PHARMACOKINETICS OF INTERLEUKIN-2 PREPARATIONS AFTER INTRAVENOUS BOLUS ADMINISTRATION

IL-2 Preparation	Source	Serum $t_{1/2}$ (min)		AUC (U × min/mL)	Clearance (mL/min)
		$t_{1/2}\alpha$	$t_{1/2}\beta$		
Recombinant IL-2 (rIL-2) (62)	Chiron	13.8 ± 7.7	86 ± 34	$18,200 \pm 15,900$	117
PEG IL-2 (71)	Chiron	183	740	NS	4.50
Native IL-2 (60)	Dupont	5–7	30	NS	NS
rIL-2 (64)	Amgen	13.4 (8.5–18.8)	NS	NS	NS

AUC, area under the concentration-time curve; NS, not stated; PEG IL-2, polyethylene glycol interleukin-2; $t_{1/2}$, half-life.

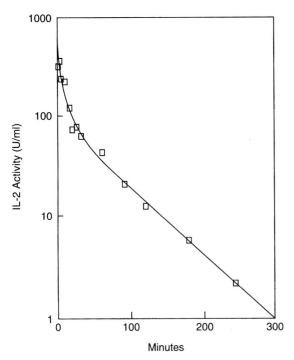

Figure 36.3 Interleukin-2 (IL-2) serum clearance after an i.v. bolus. A dose of 1.0 MU/m² was given as a 5-minute i.v. bolus. Serum samples were taken, and the IL-2 bioactivity was determined. A biexponential curve has been fitted to the assay values, minimizing the sum of the squares of the percentage of deviation of the curve from the data. (Reproduced with permission from Konrad MW, Hemstreet G, Hersh EM, et al. Pharmacokinetics of recombinant interleukin 2 in humans. Cancer Res 1990;50:2009–2017.)

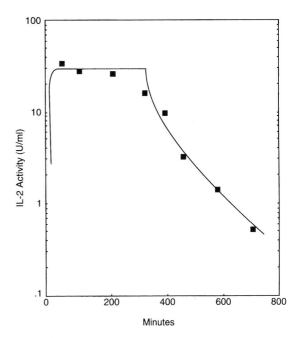

Figure 36.4 Serum levels during and after a 6-hour i.v. infusion of interleukin-2 (IL-2). The patient received 1 MU/m² over 6 hours, and the steady-state level of approximately 28 U/mL is close to the dose-normalized median level seen in all patients. Because the first blood sample was taken 60 minutes after the start of the infusion, the rising phase of the curve was not accurately determined, and the curve seen here is somewhat symbolic of the actual time course expected. (Reproduced with permission from Konrad MW, Hemstreet G, Hersh EM, et al. Pharmacokinetics of recombinant interleukin 2 in humans. Cancer Res 1990;50:2009–2017.)

and liver, with the kidney cortex demonstrating the highest activity. Irradiated and splenectomized mice have been used to assess the potential role of rIL-2 binding to lymphoid cells.[74] The rIL-2 was injected intravenously, and no alterations were found. In addition, the half-life of rIL-2 in nephrectomized animals rose from 2.5 to 3.5 minutes to 84 minutes, and ureteral ligation had minimal effect on the rIL-2 half-life. Finally, active IL-2 is not excreted in the urine, which implies renal tubular catabolism.

Other schedules of i.v. rIL-2 administration, such as continuous infusion, have also been investigated. Infusion times have varied from 2 to 24 hours, and steady-state levels are generally achieved within 2 hours (Fig. 36.4). Median steady-state levels of 123 IU/mL are produced by infusion of 6 × 10⁶ IU/m² over 6 hours, and the levels then fall rapidly after termination of rIL-2 infusion. The clearance rate after i.v. infusion resembles that seen with bolus administration.

The pharmacokinetics of very low doses of rIL-2 may be different than that observed with higher doses. Saturable pathways, binding to serum proteins or receptors and internalization of the receptor-ligand complex may play significant roles in altering distribution. Continued administration of rIL-2 and the accompanying lymphocytosis with increased IL-2 receptor density may potentially result in an increase of rIL-2 metabolism. In addition,

alterations in renal function may change clearance of this cytokine.

Most frequently, rIL-2 is administered as a subcutaneous (s.c.) injection.[72] Time to peak concentration varies from 120 to 360 minutes, and with doses of 6 × 10⁶ IU/m², median peak serum levels of 32.1 IU/mL and 42 IU/mL have been reported. The kinetics of lower-dose s.c. rIL-2 are different than those of high-dose i.v. administration. Studies demonstrate that IL-2 serum levels are 50- to 100-fold less than with i.v. administration.[72] Some studies[75] do suggest alternative clearance mechanisms at lower doses. Interleukin-2 may be bound to proteins such as soluble IL-2R (sIL-2R), α_2-macroglobulin, and immunoglobulins with saturable processes in operation.[75] Administration to an anephric patient on dialysis produced slightly higher IL-2 concentrations, but the pharmacokinetics of s.c. rIL-2 appeared similar to those in patients with normal renal function.[75] Kirchner et al.[76] examined the pharmacokinetics of subcutaneously administered rIL-2. Two schedules were investigated (20 MIU/m² daily and 10 MIU/m² twice daily). For the once-daily schedule, the 24-hour area under the concentration × time curve (AUC) was 627 IU/mL × 1 hour, and for the twice-daily schedule 1,130 IU/mL × 1 hour. The highest observed concentration for both schedules was similar. By 72 hours, the levels of sIL-R increased, with some reductions in AUC seen. The authors concluded that two daily doses of rIL-2 provide superior bioavailability.

TABLE 36.3

DOSES AND SCHEDULES OF RECOMBINANT INTERLEUKIN-2 (rIL-2) IN TRIALS INVOLVING PATIENTS WITH RENAL CELL CARCINOMA

Study	rIL-2 Source	Dose and Schedule of rIL-2	No. Patients	Response (CRs + PRs)
Fisher et al. (80)	Chiron	600,000 IU/kg q8h × 5 d, i.v.b. (repeated in 1 wk)	255	15% (17 CRs)
Bukowski et al. (81)	Chiron	60×10^6 IU/m^2 t.i.w. (i.v.b.)	41	9.7% (1 CR)
Palmer et al. (82)	Chiron	18×10^6 IU/m^2 c.i.v. d 1–5	225	15% (7 CRs)
Sleijfer et al. (83)	Chiron	18×10^6 IU/m^2 s.c. d 1–5 (wk 1) and d 1 & 2 (wk 2–6), followed by 9×10^6 IU/m^2 s.c. d 3–5 (wk 2–6).	47	19% (2 CRs)
Negrier et al. (84)	Chiron	18×10^6 IU/m^2 c.i.v. d 1–5, 12–16	138	6.5% (2 CRs)

c.i.v., continuous intravenous infusion; CR, complete response; i.v.b., intravenous bolus; PR, partial response.

Clinical Effects and Toxicity

The variables influencing serum levels and biologic activity have led to the clinical investigation of multiple schedules and doses (Table 36.3). Among the solid tumors, malignant melanoma and renal cell carcinoma (RCC) (predominantly clear cell histologic subtype)[77] appear to be the most responsive to rIL-2 therapy, and in both tumor types, rIL-2 has been approved for treatment. Rosenberg et al.[78] used dosages of 1.8 to 6.0×10^5 IU/kg every 8 hours for 5 days. This approach using high doses of rIL-2 administered frequently is associated with severe and life-threatening toxicity. These doses were investigated when initial studies using lower doses or less frequent administration produced limited antitumor effects. The response and survival data for this type of schedule and dose of rIL-2 in patients with renal cancer are summarized in Table 36.4. Approximately 5% of patients experienced durable complete responses.[79] A comparison of results reported with various schedules and routes of rIL-2 administration is provided in Table 36.5.

The short half-life of i.v. bolus rIL-2 prompted investigation of continuous intravenous (c.i.v.) administration of this cytokine. The majority of reports have used 18.0 MIU/m^2 per day. Response rates between studies vary, but in a group of 922 patients (Table 36.5), the overall response rate was 13.3%. Complete regressions occur, and in some series[87] the rates are similar to those reported with high-dose bolus rIL-2.

In one trial[84] patients with metastatic renal cancer were randomly assigned to receive either c.i.v. rIL-2 (18.0 MIU/m^2 per day on days 1 through 5 and 12 through 16), IFN-α, or the combination. The response rate in the 138 patients receiving c.i.v. rIL-2 was 6.5%. Sixty-nine percent of individuals developed hypotension resistant to vasopressor agents. A retrospective analysis from four open-label, nonrandomized phase II trials of rIL-2 in patients with metastatic RCC showed no significant differences in overall response rate, duration, or survival between s.c. or c.i.v. routes of rIL-2 administration.[88] S.c. administration was associated with a significantly lower incidence of adverse events and fewer dose reductions. Thus, the toxicity of single-agent high-dose rIL-2 given as a c.i.v. infusion is substantial. Lower doses of rIL-2 administered as a c.i.v. infusion produce less toxicity. Caligiuri et al.[89] administered 0.05 to 0.6 MIU/m^2 per day c.i.v. for up to 90 days; the clinical activity of this approach is unclear.

S.c. administration of rIL-2 in patients with RCC has also been examined. In the group of 290 patients (for which the data are summarized in Table 36.5), a response rate of 16.8% was noted. In the report by Buter et al.,[90] two complete responses lasting 29 months and longer than 35 months were seen in patients with metastatic renal cancer, which suggests that some of these responses may be durable. Lissoni et al.[91] reported a 5-year survival time in

TABLE 36.4

CLINICAL RESULTS WITH HIGH-DOSE RECOMBINANT INTERLEUKIN-2 IN PATIENTS WITH RENAL CELL CARCINOMA

No. patients	255
Median age (range)	52 (18–71)
Sex (male/female)	178/77
ECOG performance status	
0	166
1	80
≤2	9
Prior therapy	
Nephrectomy	218
Chemotherapy	8
Responses (CRs + PRs)	36 (14%)
CR	12
Median response duration (mo)	
CR	Not reached
PR	19.0
CR + PR	20.3

CR, complete response; ECOG, Eastern Cooperative Oncology Group; PR, partial response.
From Fisher RI, Rosenberg SA, Sznol M, et al. High-dose aldesleukin in renal cell carcinoma: long-term survival update. Cancer J Sci Am 1997;3(Suppl 1):S70–72.

TABLE 36.5

RESULTS OF SINGLE-AGENT RECOMBINANT INTERLEUKIN-2 (rIL-2) TREATMENT OF METASTATIC RENAL CELL CARCINOMA

Method of rIL-2 Administration	No. of Patients	No. of CRs (%)	No. of PRs (%)	Overall Percentage (%)
Subcutaneous (85)	290	8 (3.0)	40 (13.8)	16.8
Continuous intravenous infusion (85)	922	25 (2.7)	98 (10.6)	13.3
Intravenous bolus (86)	733	38 (5.2)	86 (11.3)	16.5
Total	1,945	71 (3.7)	221	15.0

CR, complete response; PR, partial response.

response to low-dose s.c. IL-2 to be similar to that obtained with higher doses of IL-2; as expected, responding patients live longer than patients with progressive disease. Yang et al.[92] conducted a prospective randomized trial to determine the effectiveness of s.c. rIL-2 compared with bolus rIL-2. Regimens used include the following: high-dose bolus (720,000 IU/kg), low-dose bolus (72,000 IU/kg), and s.c. administration (250,000 IU/kg per day for 5 of 7 days in week 1, followed by 125,000 IU/kg per day for 5 of 7 days in weeks 2 to 6). A higher response proportion was noted with high-dose IL-2 than with low-dose i.v. and s.c. IL-2. The response rate for s.c. IL-2 was similar to that for the low-dose group. This, however, did not produce an overall survival benefit.

To determine whether synergism with IFN-α would affect the dosing level of IL-2, McDermott et al.[93] compared the administration of high-dose IL-2 with low-dose IL-2 plus IFN-α in patients with metastatic RCC. Significantly higher response rates were noted with high-dose IL-2 than with low-dose IL-2/IFN-α, especially in patients with bone or liver metastases or primary tumor in place. Furthermore, median and overall response durations were longer in the high-dose IL-2 group; however, this did not meet statistical significance. Similarly, Atkins et al.[94] reported more responses with high-dose IL-2 than with lower-dose IL-2/IFN-α in advanced RCC, and they concluded that high-dose IL-2 is the treatment of choice in selected patients with advanced RCC. In a systematic review of 92 studies using different IL-2 routes of administration (i.v., c.i.v., or s.c.) in metastatic renal cancer, Baaten et al.[95] concluded that high-dose bolus i.v. IL-2 is superior to other doses and routes of administration. Although these reports suggest that high-dose IL-2 should be the preferred IL-2 regimen for appropriately selected patients, no survival benefits have been demonstrated between the various IL-2 dosing levels in the treatment of RCC.[96,97]

Because of the observed differences in response rates among the various studies of IL-2 in RCC, many investigators have documented numerous factors that correlate with disease outcome following IL-2 therapy. These include, but are not limited to, the following: prior nephrectomy and time from nephrectomy to relapse[98,99]; number of organs with metastases[84]; presence of metastases to liver, bone, or lymph nodes[94,100]; degree of treatment-related thrombocytopenia[101]; lymphocyte count and rebound lymphocytosis[102]; thyroid dysfunction[103]; erythropoietin production[104]; and absence of prior IFN therapy.[101] Despite attempts to develop models to predict response to IL-2 therapy, factors that determine disease progression and resistance to IL-2 treatment remain unclear at this time.

Administration of nebulized IL-2 via inhalation has also been investigated. Aerosol therapy produces high pulmonary drug concentrations and low systemic drug levels and thereby enhances the therapeutic index.[105] Huland et al.[106] reported on the use of natural IL-2 administered via nebulizer. Aerosol IL-2 100,000 U was delivered five times daily and was combined with systemic IL-2 and IFN-α. The toxicity of inhaled IL-2 was reported as minimal, which allowed administration in the outpatient department, and antitumor responses were reported. These results have been updated in 116 patients with pulmonary or mediastinal metastatic disease (or both).[107] Three different IL-2 formulations were used: natural nIL-2, glycosylated rIL-2 (Sanofi, Montpellier, France), and nonglycosylated rIL-2 (Chiron). Thirty-six, 12, and 68 patients received these IL-2 preparations, respectively, via inhalation. Eleven percent received only inhaled IL-2; 33% received concomitant s.c. rIL-2; and 56% were given concomitant rIL-2 and IFN-α. In 105 patients with pulmonary metastases, 16 patients responded (15.2%), of whom 3 showed complete responses. The median response duration was 15.5 months. The administration of inhaled rIL-2 has also been reported by Lorenz et al.[108] and Nakamoto et al.[109] In these studies, 16 patients with renal cancer were treated, and four responses (including one complete response) were noted. In another study by Huland et al.[110] comparing 94 high-risk patients with RCC and pulmonary metastases treated with inhaled plus concomitant low-dose s.c. rhIL-2 to 103 comparable historical controls given IL-2 systemically, longer overall survival and progression-free survival durations were observed in the inhaled rhIL-2 group. However, the contribution of inhaled IL-2 in these studies is unclear in view of the concurrent administration systemic IL-2 as well as the administration of other cytokines. In a small study comprising

40 patients with pulmonary metastases of RCC, Merimsky et al.[111] reported feasibility, tolerability, and disease-progression arrest following the administration of inhaled IL-2 alone. Nevertheless, to more accurately assess the value of this approach, randomized trials comparing results in patients receiving only inhaled cytokine with results in patients receiving systemic therapy with and without inhaled cytokine are required. The delivery of liposome-encapsulated rIL-2 was noted to be well tolerated in humans.[112] This method may in the future provide an alternative delivery system. Other routes of delivery for rIL-2, such as intraarterial,[108] intrapleural,[113] and intraperitoneal,[114] have also been examined. Results remain preliminary.

Administration of rIL-2 produces functional alterations in most organ systems. A decrease in lymphocytes occurs initially and then resolves. Subsequently, the peripheral blood lymphocyte pool ($CD3^+$, $CD56^+$) expands. Soluble IL-2R levels increase in the circulation, and IL-2R–positive lymphocytes also are seen.[115,116] Cytolytic activity of peripheral blood lymphocytes may be enhanced during continuous infusion of high doses, which results in increased NK cell activity and the appearance of LAK cells in the circulation.[117] The effects of rIL-2 on lymphocytes are mediated through specific cell surface receptors on the various subsets. The expression of high-affinity receptors and their saturation by prolonged low-dose infusion of rIL-2 has been reported.[118] The possibility that these cytolytic mononuclear cells mediate the antitumor effects of systemically administered rIL-2 has been investigated. The inability to demonstrate correlations of response and development of cytolytic activity in patients treated with rIL-2, however, does not support this hypothesis.

Although most applications have been in the treatment of solid malignancies, IL-2 has also shown promise in the primary therapy of hematologic malignancies as well as in the setting of stem cell transplantation. Myeloid and lymphoid leukemic cells have been reported to be susceptible to IL-2–induced LAK activity[119,120] and have been shown to lack proliferative responses to IL-2, even when expressing the IL-2 receptor.[121] Various trials demonstrated the induction of complete and partial remissions in acute myeloid leukemia following rIL-2 therapy.[122–124] Furthermore, IL-2 has been successfully used in conjunction with bone marrow transplantation (BMT) for the treatment of residual malignant hematologic disease in both humans and animals. Studies with rIL-2 following BMT and donor lymphocyte infusions increased survival, induced remissions, and decreased relapse rates in various hematologic malignancies, including acute and chronic myeloid leukemias, non-Hodgkin's lymphoma, and multiple myeloma.[125–128] RIL-2 administration following BMT is believed to increase graft-versus-leukemia effects, possibly leading to the observed improvements in frequency and durations of remission rates.[129,130]

Other effects of rIL-2 include endothelial cell activation, with increased expression of adhesion molecules such as intercellular adhesion molecule 1 (ICAM-1) and endothelial-leukocyte adhesion molecule 1 (ELAM-1).[131] Secondary cytokine production (TNF-α, IFN-γ, IL-6) and increased C-reactive protein levels[132–134] also have been noted. Finally, rIL-2 may be immunosuppressive in certain circumstances, with decreased delayed hypersensitivity[135] and neutrophil chemotaxis reported.[136]

The severity and nature of rIL-2 side effects are related to the dose and schedule used. The toxicities of bolus, c.i.v., and s.c. rIL-2 are outlined in Table 36.6. Uniformly, patients develop chills, fever, and malaise. A vascular leak syndrome occurs with higher dosages of rIL-2 and is characterized by weight gain, oliguria, tachycardia, and hypotension.[137]

TABLE 36.6

TOXICITY PRODUCED BY VARIOUS SCHEDULES AND DOSES OF RECOMBINANT INTERLEUKIN-2 (rIL-2)

	Yang et al. (141)	Buter et al. (90)	Negrier et al. (84)
rIL-2 dose level & schedule	720,000 MIU/kg i.v.b. q8h × 5 d	18 MIU/m² s.c. d 1–5 (wk 1), 9.0 MIU/m² s.c. d 1 & 2, then 18 MIU/m² d 3–5 (wk 2–6)	18 MIU/m² c.i.v. d 1–5, 12–16
Type of toxicity	% >grade 3[a]	% any grade[b]	% >grade 3[b]
Nausea/vomiting	19%	96%	34%
Diarrhea	11%	55%	27.5%
Elevated creatinine level	2% (>8 mg/dL)	9% (>200 μmol/L)	3.6%
Renal effects	21% (oliguria < 80 mL/8 h)	NS	15.2%
Hypotension	43%	26% (11% < 90 mm Hg)	68% (vasopressor resistant)
Neuropsychiatric effects	14%	21%	12.3%
Elevated bilirubin level	4%	2%	1%
Cardiac effects	5%	4%	12.3%
Anemia	NS	NS	17.4%
Thrombocytopenia	9%	0	3.6%

c.i.v., continuous intravenous; i.v.b., intravenous bolus; NS, not stated.
[a]Expressed as percent of courses.
[b]Expressed as percent of patients.

When this syndrome is present, supplemental i.v. fluids, vasopressors, and diuretics may be required for management. Cardiac toxicities, including arrhythmias and myocardial infarction, and pulmonary side effects, including dyspnea and pleural effusions, may develop. Cardiovascular toxicities include not only vascular leak syndrome and hypotension but direct effects on the myocardium. Hemodynamic studies[138] have demonstrated decreased mean arterial pressure and systemic vascular resistance consistent with changes noted during septic shock. Myocardial injury with creatine phosphokinase elevations[139] and myocarditis secondary to lymphocyte infiltration[140] have also been noted.

Hematopoietic findings include anemia, thrombocytopenia, and leukopenia,[142] and an increased frequency of sepsis in patients requiring central venous lines has been reported.[143] This latter complication may relate to the previously noted granulocyte defect.[135] Hepatic toxicities characterized by increases in serum bilirubin levels and minimal changes in transaminase levels are common. Fisher et al.[80] investigated this phenomenon using technetium-labeled disofenin and noted delayed excretion and uptake consistent with cholestasis. Return to baseline levels within 4 to 6 days of rIL-2 discontinuation is usual. Gastrointestinal toxicities includes nausea, vomiting, diarrhea, and mucositis. Colon dilation,[144] perforation,[145] and ischemic necrosis[146] have also been seen but represent uncommon manifestations of rIL-2 toxicity.

Neurologic and neuropsychiatric effects can develop acutely or chronically during rIL-2 administration. Patients receiving high-dose intensive therapy may become agitated, disoriented, and occasionally comatose.[147] Increases in peritumoral edema in a series of patients with gliomas receiving rIL-2[137] and increases of brain water content[148] indicate that cerebral edema may be responsible. These effects are generally transient and resolve with drug discontinuation. Neuropsychiatric effects, including a decrease in cognitive function and impaired memory, have been reported in patients receiving c.i.v. rIL-2.[149] These latter findings resemble the chronic central nervous system toxicity associated with IFN-α.[150]

Miscellaneous toxicities include dermatologic complications such as erythema, pruritus, and generalized erythroderma.[151] In patients with preexisting dermatologic conditions such as psoriasis, exacerbation of the underlying condition has been described.[152] Finally, hypothyroidism or hyperthyroidism has also been seen.[153] The cause of this complication is uncertain, but the development of autoimmune thyroiditis secondary to induction of class II antigens in thyroid tissue has been proposed.[154] The suggestion has also been made that patients developing this complication are more likely to respond.[155]

The etiology of rIL-2–related toxicity is uncertain but may involve interstitial lymphocyte infiltrates, vascular leaks, and secondary production of cytokines such as TNF-α.[134] The side effects are generally self-limited and resolve rapidly on discontinuation of rIL-2 therapy. Rapid resolution with use of systemic glucocorticoids has also been reported.[156,157] Attempts to diminish rIL-2–related toxicity by coadministration of agents such as the phosphoesterase inhibitor pentoxifylline,[158] soluble TNF-α receptor,[159] and soluble IL-1 receptor[160] have not been successful. In contrast, Samlowski et al.[161] demonstrated a decrease in IL-2–induced dose-limiting hypotension after the administration of the superoxide dismutase mimetic (M40403) to mice. Furthermore, the coadministration of agents that either increase the sensitivity of malignant cells to IL-2 or synergize with IL-2 antitumor activities, such as thalidomide,[162] IL-18,[163] or IL-12,[164] may allow the use of lower doses of IL-2 and thereby decrease some of the toxic effects of this cytokine (see next section).

Drug Interactions

Initial studies with rIL-2 involved single-agent therapy with or without coadministration of ex vivo–activated peripheral blood lymphocytes (LAK cells)[165] or tumor-infiltrating lymphocytes.[166] These studies were based on preclinical investigations demonstrating benefit of adoptive immunotherapy.[167] Randomized trials comparing use of rIL-2 alone with administration of rIL-2 together with LAK or tumor-infiltrating lymphocytes have not, however, demonstrated significant increases in response rates or survival in patients with RCC or melanoma.[106,167]

Cytokine combinations involving rIL-2 and a variety of other lymphokines based on studies in animal models have also been used clinically. The cytokines combined with rIL-2 have included IFN-α, interferon-β (IFN-β), IFN-γ, IL-1, IL-4, IL-12, and TNF-α.[78,164,168–172] Although the combination of rIL-2 and IFN-α has been the most widely investigated and may produce higher response rates in patients with RCC[173,174] than rIL-2 alone,[84] Tourani et al. concluded from a multicenter trial that the coadministration of IFN-α does not improve response or survival rates in patients with metastatic renal cancer compared with s.c. IL-2 alone.[175] These observations were also reported by others.[93,94]

The combination of chemotherapy and rIL-2 has also been studied. In RCC, administration of vinblastine sulfate and rIL-2 did not produce enhanced antitumor effects.[176] The preclinical finding of synergistic effects for doxorubicin hydrochloride and rIL-2[177] led to a series of phase I trials investigating different schedules and doses of these two agents.[178,179] Additive toxicity and no immunomodulatory interactions were seen. Finally, cyclophosphamide has been administered before rIL-2 at doses of 350 or 1,000 mg/m[2].[180,181] The rationale involves the possible immunomodulatory effects of cyclophosphamide.[182] No convincing evidence for enhancement of responses to rIL-2 has been seen.

Multiagent biochemotherapy combinations including rIL-2 have been investigated in patients with RCC and malignant melanoma. In patients with RCC, the combination of rIL-2, IFN-α, and fluorouracil has been used. Atzpodien et al.[183] initially reported regression rates over 35%; however, response rates of 1.8%[113] and 8.2%[184] have been noted. Olencki et al.[185] reported a 28% response rate in patients with metastatic renal cancer, but the addition of fluorouracil to rIL-2 and IFN-α significantly increased the toxicity of this therapy. Allen et al.[186] also reported significant efficacy but manageable toxicity following the combination of IL-2, IFN-α, and fluorouracil in patients with metastatic renal cancer. In a similar patient population with metastatic RCC, Dutcher et al.[187] noted that the addition of fluorouracil to IL-2/IFN-α failed to increase the efficacy and added new toxicity. The benefit of this regimen remains unclear.

In patients with malignant melanoma, combinations of rIL-2, IFN-α, and chemotherapy consisting of imidazole carboximide, carmustine (bischloroethylnitrosourea [BCNU]), and tamoxifen have been used.[188] Response rates over 50% have been reported. Despite the high overall response rates noted using biochemotherapy, no survival benefits have been noted in patients with malignant melanoma.[189]

Other Recombinant Interleukin-2 Preparations

The clinical antitumor effects and toxicity of rIL-2 and its immunomodulatory activities have prompted development of different rIL-2 formulations in an attempt to diminish toxicity and enhance efficacy. Covalent binding of rIL-2 to polyethylene glycol (PEG) at amino acid sites results in an rIL-2 preparation with persistent antitumor activity in murine models.[190] Phase I[71] and phase II[191] trials have been completed. The maximum tolerated dose (MTD) of PEG–IL-2 given as an i.v. bolus once weekly is 20×10^6 IU/m^2. Pharmacokinetic studies have demonstrated a prolonged $t_{1/2}\alpha$ (183 minutes) and $t_{1/2}\beta$ (740 minutes). Serum levels of 15,000 IU/mL were seen, and the clearance was 4.5 mL/minute per m^2. The prolonged half-life and decreased clearance were predicted by animal models[73] and may be secondary to elimination of renal clearance because of the large hydrodynamic size of PEG–IL-2. The clinical toxicity reported resembles that seen with rIL-2, and antitumor responses were noted in patients with metastatic RCC (2/31 patients). The advantages of weekly administration for an agent such as rIL-2 make the pegylated formulation attractive; however, delayed and unpredictable toxicities have been seen.

Another method of limiting the toxicity of rIL-2 is to incorporate it into liposomes. This produces altered distribution, metabolism, and elimination of the cytokine. A phase I trial of liposome-encapsulated rIL-2 has been initiated and uses escalating doses given as an i.v. bolus. Mild toxicity has been noted,[192] and immunologic activity, including elevated serum IL-2R levels, NK activity, and numbers of CD16$^+$CD56$^+$ cells, was seen. Use of this preparation may result in a decrease in overall side effects

related to rIL-2 while maintaining its immunomodulatory activities. Finally, Yao et al.[193] investigated the role of albumin-conjugated IL-2 in the treatment of solid tumors in an animal model and reported a significantly longer circulation time, lower kidney uptake, and increased drug localization in liver, spleen, and lymph nodes, suggesting the potential for improved efficacy and reduced toxicity using this form of IL-2.

INTERLEUKIN-4

IL-4 is a cytokine with pleiotropic actions that was first described in 1982 as a T-cell–derived factor with B-lymphocyte stimulatory activity.[194,195] Since its initial description, IL-4 has been reported to affect a wide variety of cell types[196] and to have both stimulatory and suppressive effects on various responses. The genes encoding murine and human IL-4 have been cloned[197,198] and expressed in *E. coli*. In vivo and in vitro antitumor effects have been found, and initial trials of recombinant IL-4 are under way in patients with various malignancies.

Structure and Mechanisms of Action

IL-4 is a glycoprotein with a molecular weight between 15 and 19 kd. The human and murine forms share extensive homology;[197,199] however, unlike other cytokines, they are species specific.[200] The cDNA for human IL-4 encodes a protein of 153 amino acids, which is then cleaved to yield a mature protein containing 129 amino acids.[197] The IL-4 gene is on band q23-31 of chromosome 5[201] and is located in the vicinity of the genes encoding interleukin 3 (IL-3) and GM-CSF.[202] This gene occurs as a single copy and contains four exons and three introns.[199]

The human IL-4 gene has been expressed in *E. coli* (Schering-Plough), and milligram quantities are available. Recombinant IL-4 (Schering-Plough) has a molecular weight of 14.9 kd and contains 129 amino acids. It contains two potential glycosylation sites and six cysteine residues that form three disulfide bonds.[203] The three-dimensional topology of recombinant human IL-4 (rhuIL-4) has been investigated,[204] and interestingly it is similar to that described for recombinant human GM-CSF.[205]

The Sterling preparation of rhuIL-4 also has 129 amino acid residues and differs from the natural protein at six sites.[206] It was expressed in a yeast strain (*Saccharomyces cerevisiae*), and amino acids 1 to 4 (Glu-Ala-Glu-Ala) are not in natural IL-4 but are a consequence of the expression system. Asp38 and Asp105 are substituted for asparagine to preclude glycosylation. These changes result in a recombinant molecule that has the same biologic activity as the fully glycosylated rhuIL-4. In vitro comparative studies of the two preparations of rhuIL-4 are not available.

IL-4 produces its effects by interaction with cell surface receptors (IL-4Rs) that are present on various hematopoietic and nonhematopoietic cells. IL-4R is up-regulated by cytokines such as IL-2, IL-4,[207,208] IFN-γ, and IL-6.[209,210] IL-4 signaling depends on binding to the IL-4R, which is composed of two chains. IL-4 actually binds the 140-kd IL-4Rα chain with high affinity (K_d 20 to 3,000 pmol/L).[211-214] The IL-4Rα chain is a member of the hematopoietin receptor superfamily and also serves a part of the interleukin-13 receptor.[211,215-217] IL-4 bound to the IL-4Rα then heterodimerizes with the common γ chain, which does not change the affinity of IL-4 for the receptor but is necessary for initiating signal transduction.[218,219] Activation of the IL-4R leads to tyrosine phosphorylation of the α chain at multiple sites.[220] Three Janus kinase members are activated by the IL-4Rα chain.[221-223] Studies using deletion mutants of the IL-4Rα chain indicate that different cytoplasmic regions have distinct functions, which include binding to Janus kinases, initiation of proliferation, and induction of gene expression.[214,224-227] The IL-4–dependent pathway leading to proliferation is initiated by the phosphorylation of insulin receptor substrate 1 (IRS-1) by Jak1 and possibly by Janus kinase 2 (Jak2) after IRS-1 interaction with the IL-4Rα chain (residues 437–557).[211,228-230] PI3K, which is composed of an 85-kd regulatory unit and a 110-kd catalytic subunit, then binds to the phosphorylated IRS-1.[229,231,232] This lipid kinase initiates the generation of the second messenger molecules phosphatidylinositol-(3,4,5)-triphosphate and phosphatidylinositol-(3,4)-bisphosphate.[233,234] These molecules are involved in the downstream activation

of protein kinase C and Akt kinase.[235,236] The IL-4 stimulation of PI3K and Akt kinase is also thought to enhance the survival of hematopoietic cells.[211,235,236] The phosphorylation of IRS-1 by IL-4 is also known to activate the Ras/MAPK pathway, although not consistently in all cell lines tested.[211] The region between residues 557 and 657 of the IL-4Rα chain is responsible for IL-4–dependent gene expression through the activation of STAT6.[211,227] In IL-4–treated cells, nuclear translocation of this transcription factor results in the expression of a number of genes, including class II MHC molecules, select immunoglobulins, and CD23.[211,214,227,237,238]

Cellular Pharmacology

IL-4 is produced by activated T helper cells[239] and mast cells[240] and has pleiotropic effects both in vitro and in vivo (Table 36.7). Stimulation of B- and T-cell functions has been recognized, and a wide range of effects on diverse cell populations have also been reported. IL-4–deficient mice produced by genetic manipulation have provided some insights into its function.[241] These animals have normal T- and B-lymphocyte development, but serum levels of immunoglobulin G1 and immunoglobulin E are decreased. Transgenic mice overexpressing IL-4,[241] in contrast, have elevated levels of serum immunoglobulin G1 and immunoglobulin E.[242] Thus, IL-4 may play a critical role in the development of humoral immunity, particularly

TABLE 36.7
BIOLOGIC EFFECTS OF INTERLEUKIN-4 ON HUMAN CELLS

Cell Type	Responses	
	Stimulation	**Inhibition**
T and NK/LAK cells	T-cell, TIL, CTL proliferation	IL-2–induced T-cell proliferation, IL-2–induced NK/LAK cytotoxicity, T-cell IFN-γ secretion
B cells	Proliferation, IgG and IgM secretion, IgE and IgG class switch, CD23/FcR expression	Antigen-specific Ig secretion, IL-2–induced proliferation
Monocytes	Class I expression, G-CSF	IL-1, TNF, IL-6, and GM-CSF production, FcR and CD23 expression
Hematopoietic progenitors	G-CSF–supported CFU-GM	IL-3–induced CFU-GM, EPO–induced BFU-E, and M-CSF–induced CFU-M
Mast cells	Proliferation, ICAM-1 expression	
Endothelial cells	IL-6 production, T-cell adhesion, ICAM-1 and ELAM-1 expression	

BFU-E, burst-forming unit, erythroid; CFU-GM, colony-forming unit granulocyte-macrophage; CFU-M, colony-forming unit macrophage; CTL, cytolytic T lymphocyte; ELAM-1, endothelial-leukocyte adhesion molecule 1; EPO, erythropoietin; FcR, Fc receptor; G-CSF, granulocyte colony-stimulating factor; GM-CSF, granulocyte-macrophage colony-stimulating factor; ICAM-1, intercellular adhesion molecule 1; IFN, interferon; Ig, immunoglobulin; IL, interleukin; LAK, lymphokine-activated killer; M-CSF, macrophage colony-stimulating factor; NK, natural killer; TIL, tumor-infiltrating lymphocyte; TNF, tumor necrosis factor.
Adapted with permission from Puri RK, Siegel JP. Interleukin-4 and cancer therapy. Cancer Invest 1993;11:473–486.

TABLE 36.8

RECOMBINANT INTERLEUKIN-4 PREPARATIONS

Source	Molecular Weight (kd)	Number of Amino Acids	Expression Vector	Activity	Clinical Trials
Schering-Plough (256)	14.9	129	*Escherichia coli*	NA	Phase I and II
Immunex/Sterling (257)	15.4	129	*Saccharomyces cerevisiae*	1.8 + 0.7 107 μg/mg[a]	Phase I

NA, not applicable.
[a] One unit of recombinant human interleukin-4 is defined as the amount that stimulates 50% of maximum uptake of tritium-labeled thymidine in human tonsil B-cell assay.

immunoglobulin E. Studies with IL-4R knockout mice and STAT6 knockout mice revealed that IL-4–producing T cells play an important role in the development of an immune response to infections with helminths and other parasites. IL-4 has other functions related to the immune system, including up-regulation of the expression of MHC class II molecules on B cells. It also functions in inflammatory responses by increasing the expression of vascular cell adhesion molecule 1 (VCAM-1) on endothelial cells.

In addition to these pleiotropic immunoregulatory activities, IL-4 is involved in the proliferation and maturation of dendritic cells. These cells represent antigen-processing cells that in vivo capture, process, and present foreign antigenic peptides to T lymphocytes. A variety of steps in the maturation and functioning of these cells have been identified, and in vitro a variety of cytokines are involved in their generation. The combination of GM-CSF and IL-4 generates functional dendritic cells that can endocytose antigens and stimulate T cells.[243] This property of IL-4 and its control of dendritic cell proliferation are being used for the production of these cells for use in current vaccination approaches.

Antitumor activity has also been attributed to IL-4 and is suggested by a series of observations. Various murine epithelial tumor cells express IL-4R,[244] and in vivo administration to mice with fibrosarcomas or spontaneous adenocarcinomas has antitumor effects. Tepper et al.[245]

demonstrated that IL-4 gene transfection into murine tumor cells resulted in their rejection. This appeared to correlate with the degree of eosinophil and macrophage infiltration. In another model, IL-4–producing tumor cells[246] induced systemic immunity against murine spontaneous renal carcinoma cells (RENCA).

Studies with human tumors have demonstrated that rhuIL-4 inhibits the in vitro growth of various tumor cells.[247-249] These include hematopoietic tumors as well as various solid tumors, such as breast cancer, ovarian cancer, and head and neck tumors.[250,251] Various reports indicate that the effects of IL-4 may be mediated by inhibition of autocrine growth factors such as IL-6[252] and GM-CSF[253] IL-4 may have both direct and indirect effects on hematopoietic malignancies. Solid tumors may also contain IL-4R, and in vitro inhibition by IL-4 of cell growth in a wide variety of tumors has been reported.[254,255]

Clinical Pharmacokinetics

Two recombinant IL-4 preparations have been evaluated and are outlined in Table 36.8. They have been produced after expression of the IL-4 gene in either *E. coli* or yeast. The results of reported phase I trials using these preparations are summarized in Table 36.9.

Serum assays for IL-4 are performed using both biologic and ELISA methods. The traditional assay involves

TABLE 36.9

PHASE I CLINICAL TRIALS OF INTERLEUKIN-4 (IL-4)

Study	IL-4 Preparation	Dose Range	Schedule	MTD	$t_{1/2}\alpha$	$t_{1/2}\beta$
Lotze (256)	Sterling	1–30 μg/kg	i.v. q.d. or t.i.d.	20 μg/kg	8 min	48 min
Markowitz et al. (258)	Sterling	20–1,280 μg/m²/d	i.v. q.d. d 1, d 4–17	NS	NS	NS
Taylor et al. (259)	Sterling	40–1,200 μg/m²/d	s.c. d 1–5	500 μg/m²	NS	NS
Atkins et al. (260)	Sterling	10, 15 μg/kg	i.v. t.i.d. d 1–5, 15–19	10 μg/kg	NS	NS
Prendiville et al. (261)	Sterling	40, 120, 280, 400 μg/m²	i.v. q.d. d 1, 24-h c.i. d 4–5, s.c. d 8–22	400 μg/m²	15–22 min	NS
Gilleece et al. (262)	Schering-Plough	0.5, 1.0, 5.0 μg/kg	s.c. d 1, 8–17, 29–57	>1.0 and <5.0 μg/kg	NS	NS
Maher et al. (263)	Schering-Plough	0.25, 1.0, 5.0 μg/kg	s.c. d 1, 8–17, 28–57	Not reached	NS	NS

c.i., continuous infusion; MTD, maximum tolerated dose; NS, not stated; $t_{1/2}$, half-life.

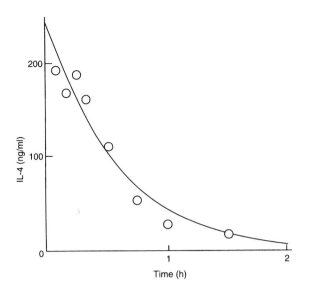

Figure 36.5 Concentration of interleukin-4 (IL-4) over time in the serum of a patient receiving 400 μg/m² of IL-4 as an i.v. bolus. (Reproduced with permission from Prendiville J, Thatcher N, Lind M, et al. Recombinant human interleukin-4 [rhu IL-4] administered by the i.v. and s.c. routes in patients with advanced cancer: a phase I toxicity study and pharmacokinetic analysis. Eur J Cancer 1993;29A:1700–1707.)

proliferation of human tonsillar B lymphocytes in the presence of cross-linking antibodies to immunoglobulin M. A variation[264] involves induction of CD23 expression in various Burkitt's lymphoma and Epstein-Barr virus–transformed B-cell lines by IL-4. Serum may inhibit this assay and therefore must be used as a control. Finally, an ELISA using purified rabbit anti–IL-4 antibodies is available.[257]

The pharmacokinetic behavior of IL-4 has been investigated in a variety of studies. Lotze et al.[256] used a biologic assay and estimated an α distribution phase of 8 minutes and a β clearance phase of 48 minutes. Ghosh et al.[257] and Prendiville et al.[261] investigated the serum levels and pharmacokinetic behavior of rhuIL-4 (Sterling) after a single i.v. bolus dose, a 24-hour infusion, or s.c. administration. Serum IL-4 levels were determined using an ELISA. After

i.v. bolus administration, serum levels of IL-4 increased with increasing doses, and the agent was rapidly cleared (Fig. 36.5 and Table 36.10). The half-life was between 15 and 22 minutes, and peak serum levels achieved after s.c. administration of rhuIL-4 (Fig. 36.6) were 10-fold less than after comparable i.v. administration. Serum levels produced were dose-dependent, and after s.c. administration of 400 μg/m², rhuIL-4 bioavailability was 71% ± 14.[257] A linear relationship between IL-4 dose level and AUC was found, which indicates linear pharmacokinetics for the dose ranges investigated.[261] The rapid clearance and low distribution volume are consistent with binding to IL-4R on peripheral lymphocytes. The short half-life observed for rhuIL-4 is similar to that seen for other cytokines.

Clinical Effects and Toxicity

Preclinical evaluation of rhuIL-4 has demonstrated a wide range of pharmacologic and toxicologic effects in target organs, including the cardiac system, liver, spleen, and bone marrow.[265] These effects were dose-related and included death, cardiac inflammation and necrosis, and hepatitis. These were seen at doses greater than 25 μg/kg per day in cynomolgus monkeys. In human trials, rhuIL-4 was safe and well tolerated at dose levels of up to 5 μg/kg per day administered subcutaneously.

The toxicity of rhuIL-4 in humans is dose-dependent. S.c. administration at low dose produces fever, headache, sinus congestion, nausea, and elevated hepatic enzyme levels.[262] Anorexia, fatigue, and flu-like symptoms also are seen and generally resolve within 24 hours of rhuIL-4 discontinuation.[262] Dose-limiting toxicities reported at 5 μg/kg per day include headaches and arthralgias.

At higher dose levels and with i.v. administration,[256,260] toxicity is more severe. Nasal congestion, periorbital and peripheral edema, weight gain, diarrhea, and dyspnea have been seen.[256,260] A vascular leak syndrome resembling that produced by rIL-2 has been reported,[256] and gastritis with gastric ulceration was also seen.[266]

TABLE 36.10

PHARMACOKINETICS OF INTERLEUKIN-4 AFTER INTRAVENOUS BOLUS INJECTION

Dose rhuIL-4 (μg/m²/d)	AUC (ng × h/mL)	t_{1/2} (min) (mL/min)	Cl_{tot}	V_d (L)
40	5.76	15.69	202.63	4.65
120	22.34	20.04	240.06	7.17
280	74.21	19.39	153.03	4.24
400	108.95	22.13	108.80	3.41

AUC, area under concentration-time curve; Cl_{tot}, total plasma clearance; rhuIL-4, recombinant human interleukin-4; t_{1/2}, elimination half-life; V_d, apparent volume of distribution.
Adapted with permission from Prendiville J, Thatcher N, Lind M, et al. Recombinant human interleukin 4 (rhu IL-4) administered by the intravenous and subcutaneous routes in patients with advanced cancer: a phase I toxicity study and pharmacokinetic analysis. Eur J Cancer 1993;29A:1700–1707.

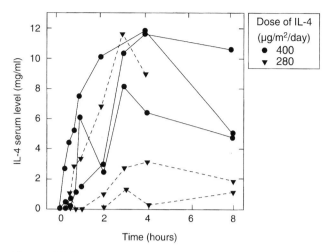

Figure 36.6 Serum levels of interleukin-4 (IL-4) following s.c. injection in patients receiving recombinant human IL-4. (Reproduced with permission from Ghosh AK, Smith NK, Prendiville J, et al. A phase I study of recombinant human interleukin-4 administered by the i.v. and s.c. route in patients with advanced cancer: immunological studies. Eur Cytokine Netw 1993;4:205–211.)

In a series of phase II trials involving patients with melanoma or RCC,[260] rhuIL-4 was administered at a dose of 600 to 800 μg/m² by i.v. bolus every 8 hours on days 1 through 5. With this high-dose intensive schedule, four patients developed cardiac toxicity characterized by electrocardiographic changes consistent with infarction and elevated creatine phosphokinase-MB fractions. One patient expired, and at autopsy myocardial infiltration by polymorphonuclear leukocytes, including eosinophils and mast cells, was observed. These findings appear to be related to frequent high-dose administration of rhuIL-4 above the recognized MTD.

The immunologic effects of rhuIL-4 are quite variable. Absolute lymphocyte counts decrease during rhuIL-4 therapy[260]; however, flow cytometry studies have not demonstrated consistent and reproducible changes in the distribution of lymphocyte phenotypes.[257,260,262] Lymphocyte cytolytic activities (NK, LAK) are not augmented or induced, and occasional increases in proliferative responses produced by mitogens or rIL-2 have been reported.[257]

Administration of high doses of rhuIL-4 is not associated with increases in serum TNF-α or IL-1β levels but does produce significant elevations of IL-1ra.[260] Soluble CD23 levels also increase with rhuIL-4 therapy.[260] No alterations in serum immunoglobulin levels have been noted,[260] and antibody production to rhuIL-4 has not been seen.

In the phase I trials reported to date, no responses have been seen in patients with solid tumors. In patients with hematologic malignancies, tumor regression has been reported in individual patients with Hodgkin's disease and non-Hodgkin's lymphoma.[263] Experience to date is limited, however. Phase II studies involving patients with malignant melanoma, non–small cell lung cancer, and acquired immunodeficiency syndrome–related Kaposi's sarcoma have been reported. The results of these studies are summarized in Table 36.11. Limited activity of rhuIL-4 has been noted, and no further investigation of its antitumor activities is planned.

TUMOR NECROSIS FACTOR

The discovery by Dr. William Coley that patients who developed streptococcal infections occasionally had clinical tumor regressions and his use of bacterial extracts to treat patients with advanced malignancies[270] constituted one of the earliest applications of biologic therapy as a treatment for cancer. Shear et al.[271] used an extract of *Serratia marcescens* and noted hemorrhagic necrosis in mice bearing transplanted tumors. The responsible ingredient was identified as an LPS from bacterial cell walls. Carswell and colleagues[272] then identified in the sera of mice receiving LPS a factor, termed "tumor necrosis factor," that produced hemorrhagic necrosis in transplanted murine Meth A sarcoma tumors. An in vitro bioassay using cytotoxicity of these sera for specific tumor cell lines was developed, followed by purification and cloning of human TNF and subsequent large-scale production of recombinant TNF-α.

Coincidentally, lymphotoxin, a cytolytic protein produced by lymphocytes, was recognized.[273] It shows 30% homology with TNF-α and appears to share the same receptor.[274] This cytokine has been termed "tumor necrosis factor β" (TNF-β) and, along with TNF-α has been implicated in monocyte-mediated and lymphocyte-mediated tumor cell killing.[275]

TABLE 36.11
PHASE II TRIALS WITH RECOMBINANT HUMAN INTERLEUKIN-4 (rhuIL-4)

Study	Malignancy	Dose and Schedule of rhuIL-4	No. of Patients	CRs + PRs
Whitehead et al. (267)	Malignant melanoma	5 μg/kg s.c. d 1–28	34	1 (CR)
Vokes et al. (268)	Non–small cell lung cancer	0.25, 1.0 μg/kg t.i.w. s.c.	22 (0.25 μg/kg); 41 (1.0 μg/kg)	1 (PR)
Tulpule et al. (269)	AIDS-related Kaposi's sarcoma	1 μg/kg/d s.c.	18	1 (PR)

AIDS, acquired immunodeficiency syndrome; CR, complete response; PR, partial response.

Structure and Mechanisms of Action

The TNF-α gene is located on chromosome 6 in the 6p23 segment.[276] It is approximately 3 kb in length and comprises four exons, the last of which encodes over 80% of the secreted protein. TNF-α production is a two-step process, with gene transcription and translation tightly controlled. The basal level of TNF gene expression in human monocytes is minimal[277] and is enhanced by agents such as LPS[278] or 12-O-tetradecanoylphorbol 13-acetate. PGE$_2$ and cyclic nucleotides appear to be mediators of TNF gene regulation,[279] and phosphoesterase inhibitors such as pentoxifylline block TNF production.[280] Secretion of TNF-α protein is regulated by a separate process and appears to require additional signals.[281] A variety of inducers have been identified and include endotoxin, calcium ionophores, and Fc-receptor cross-linking.[282,283] Inhibitors of the secretory process have also been found and include botulinum D toxin.[284]

Secreted TNF-α contains 154 to 157 amino acids and one disulfide bridge. It is initially synthesized as a proprotein containing 230 amino acids[285] and may exist as a transmembrane surface protein that is cytotoxic to TNF-sensitive cells. Cleavage of the proprotein results in the secretion of a mature TNF protein containing 157 amino acids. Purified natural or recombinant TNF exists in solution as a trimer and under denaturing condition has a molecular weight of 17 kd.[286,287]

As with other cytokines, TNF acts through specific cell surface receptors that bind both TNF-α and TNF-β.[274] Most cells contain TNF receptors (TNFRs); however, the number varies from 200 to 7,000.[288] Once TNF binds to its receptor, the complex is internalized and degraded.[289] Studies have identified two receptor proteins (TNFR1 and TNFR2) with molecular weights of 55 kd and 75 kd[290] that are also shed into the circulation. TNFR1 (p55) can trigger either an apoptotic or an antiapoptotic pathway. The binding of TNF-α to TNFR1 causes the dimerization of receptor death domains in the cytoplasmic tail.[291] The adaptor molecule TNFR-associated death domain (TRADD) interacts with the activated receptor.[292] This interaction then leads to the recruitment of TNF-associated factor 2 (TRAF-2) and receptor-interacting protein (RIP), which results in the activation of the transcription factors NF-κB and JNK/AP-1.[292–294] The signaling pathway for the activation of NF-κB via TNFR1, in which TRAF-2 and RIP can activate the NF-κB kinase NIK, which then activates the IKKα, β, γ has been relatively well characterized.[292,294,295] This enzyme complex is responsible for the phosphorylation of the IκBα and IκBβ inhibitors, which leads to their polyubiquitinylation and degradation by the 26S proteasome.[296] Activation of the death pathway results from the recruitment by TNFR1-bound TRADD of another death domain–containing protein, FADD.[292,296] FADD couples the TNFR1-TRADD complex with the activation of procaspase 8 to the active form, which in turn activates effector caspases and results in apoptosis.[296] Unlike with TNFR1, the cytoplasmic domains of TNFR2 directly bind TRAF to induce NF-κB activation and promote cell survival.[293,294,296] Because TNFR2 does not bind TRADD family members, it does not appear to play a major role in the induction of apoptosis.[296] The density of TNF receptors on cells is also regulated. Type I interferons and IFN-γ increase expression,[297,298] and agents such as LPS and IL-1 down-regulate this protein.[299]

The probable role of TNF-α in the pathogenesis of various disease such as rheumatoid arthritis and in the toxicity produced by cytokines such as rIL-2 led to investigation of approaches to decrease toxicity. One of these uses administration of soluble TNF receptors (sTNFRs). Etanercept produced by Immunex (Seattle, WA) is a genetically engineered fusion protein consisting of two identical chains of recombinant TNFR p75 monomer fused with the Fc domain of human immunoglobulin G1.[300] This preparation binds and inactivates TNF. It has been shown to be effective therapy for rheumatoid arthritis.[301,302] In addition, it has been used unsuccessfully in patients receiving high-dose rIL-2 to ameliorate toxicity.[67]

Cellular Pharmacology

The in vitro activities of TNF are pleiotropic. The best recognized are antiproliferative effects on a wide range of human and murine tumor cell lines.[303] Cytolytic and cytostatic effects have both been described. The antiproliferative effects are measured in vitro by growth inhibition or cytotoxicity assays,[304] which are also used to define a unit of TNF activity. Cell surface receptors are required for these activities, but the receptor density does not correlate with the sensitivity of cells to TNF-α effects.[305]

In some cell types, TNF-α can induce apoptosis; however, most cells are protected from apoptosis due to the expression of NF-κB–regulated antiapoptotic genes.[306,307] The inhibition of protein synthesis of the selective inhibitors of the antiapoptotic genes makes cells susceptible to TNF-α–mediated apoptosis.[296] TNF-α also can affect differentiation of various cell types. One early observation indicated that TNF-α reversed adipocyte differentiation, which resulted in "dedifferentiation."[308] Proliferation of hematopoietic precursors such as colony-forming unit granulocyte erythroid monocyte-megakaryocyte (CFU-GEMM), colony-forming unit granulocyte-macrophage (CFU-GM), and erythroid burst-forming unit is inhibited,[309,310] and in HL-60 cells monocyte differentiation is promoted.[311] TNF also has mitogenic properties and in normal fibroblast cultures increases DNA synthesis.[312] The growth of a wide variety of other human tumor cells is stimulated by TNF.[313]

The immunomodulatory effects of TNF-α have also been well studied and include variable effects on T and B lymphocytes, mononuclear phagocytes, and neutrophils. Table 36.12 summarizes some of the reported effects. TNF-α appears to act as an activation signal for various classes of leukocytes during the inflammatory response.

TABLE 36.12

IMMUNOMODULATORY EFFECTS OF TUMOR NECROSIS FACTOR α (TNF-α)

Cell Type	Effect
Monocytes	TNF-α production, secretion of cytokines (IL-1, IL-6, G-CSF, GM-CSF)
Macrophages	Superoxide production, secretion of chemoattractants, increased HLA-DR expression, increased proliferation, secretion of PGE_2, secretion of thromboxane
Lymphocytes	Increased IL-2R, enhanced proliferation, increased production of G-CSF/GM-CSF/M-CSF, increased LAK activity, decreased NK activity, TNFR up-regulated, immunoglobulin secretion
Neutrophils	Increased H2O2 production, increased phagocytic activity, enhanced adherence, enhanced ADCC

ADCC, antibody-dependent cell-mediated cytotoxicity; G-CSF, granulocyte colony-stimulating factor; GM-CSF, granulocyte-macrophage colony-stimulating factor; IL, interleukin; IL-2R, interleukin-2 receptor; LAK, lymphokine-activated killer cells; M-CSF, macrophage colony-stimulating factor; NK, natural killer cells; PGE2, prostaglandin E2; TNFR, tumor necrosis factor receptor.
Based on Logan TF, Gooding WE, Whiteside TL, et al. Biologic response modulation by tumor necrosis factor alpha (TNF alpha) in a phase Ib trial in cancer patients. J Immunother 1997;20:387–398; Spriggs DR. Tumor necrosis factor: basic principles and preclinical studies. In: DeVita VT Jr, Hellman S, Rosenberg SA, eds. Biologic Therapy of Cancer. Philadelphia: JB Lippincott, 1989:361–370.

Finally, TNF-α up-regulates a variety of different molecules on the surface of endothelial cells, including class I MHC antigens[314] and leukocyte adhesion molecules (ELAM-1, ICAM-1).[315,316] Production of various inflammatory mediators such as IL-1[317] platelet-activating factor,[318] and IL-6.[319] are also enhanced by TNF-α.

Clinical Pharmacokinetics

In view of the hemorrhagic necrosis produced by TNF preparations and the multiple in vitro effects suggesting potential antitumor properties of this agent, initial clinical trials were performed in patients with advanced malignancies. Because of endotoxin contamination of purified natural TNF-α, the various recombinant preparations listed in Table 36.13 have been used. They contain from 155 to 157 amino acid residues and have specific activities from 2.2×10^6 to 4.0×10^7 U per milligram of protein. Two varieties of recombinant TNF-α (rTNF-α) are found, one containing 155 and the other 157 amino acid residues. The two types are identical except for the addition of a Val-Arg sequence at the N-terminus of the smaller molecule. The biologic activities of these preparations are similar[287]; however, specific activities vary.

Phase I trials of rTNF-α preparations involving over 500 patients have been conducted and have used a variety of administration routes and schedules. These are summarized in Table 36.14. The MTD identified in most trials is less than 200 $\mu g/m^2$ per day and may vary with the route of administration.

The measurement of TNF-α in bodily fluids has been performed using several different methods. Bioassays for detecting cytotoxicity in various cell lines, including L-M cells,[320] L-929 cells,[321] and WEHI-164 cells,[322] have been used and can detect TNF-α concentrations in sera as low as 50 pg/mL. Cell lysis is measured by either crystal violet dye uptake by residual viable cells[320] or tritium-labeled thymidine incorporation.[321] In addition, ELISA assays using

TABLE 36.13

RECOMBINANT TUMOR NECROSIS FACTOR α PREPARATIONS USED IN CLINICAL TRIALS

Source	Amino Acid Residues	Specific Activity (U/mg protein)	Nature of Product
Dainippon Pharmaceutical	155	3×10^6	Lyophilized
Asahi	155	2.2×10^6	Lyophilized
Genentech	157	4×10^7	Liquid
Cetus	157	25×10^6	Liquid
Knoll	157	8.2×10^6	Lyophilized

Adapted with permission from Taguchi T, Sohmura Y. Clinical studies with TNF. Biotherapy 1991;3:177–186.

TABLE 36.14

PHASE I CLINICAL TRIALS OF RECOMBINANT HUMAN TUMOR NECROSIS FACTOR α

Total no. patients	529	
Routes/schedules used	i.v.b. × 1 d	
	0.5- to 120-h i.v. infusion over 1–5 d	
	i.m.	
	s.c.	
	Alternating s.c.–i.v. or i.m.–i.v.	
Dose ranges	1–818 $\mu g/m^2/d$	
Maximum tolerated doses	Schedule	Dose ($\mu g/m^2$)
	i.v. single bolus	227–818 $\mu g/m^2$
	24-h i.v. × 1 d	200 $\mu g/m^2$
	24-h i.v. × 5 d	160 $\mu g/m^2$
	i.m. 3 × 1 wk	150 $\mu g/m^2$
	s.c. 5 × 1 wk	150 $\mu g/m^2$

i.v.b., intravenous bolus.
Adapted from Taguchi T, Sohmura Y. Clinical studies with TNF. Biotherapy 1991;3:177–186; Mittelman A, Puccio C, Gafney E, et al. A phase I pharmacokinetic study of recombinant human tumor necrosis factor administered by a 5-day continuous infusion. Invest New Drugs 1992;10:183–190.

polyclonal antibodies to TNF-α have been developed and can detect TNF-α at levels from 100 to 2,800 pg/mL.[322] Comparison of both methods for the detection of serum levels of rTNF-α in several clinical studies[322,323] has demonstrated that they provide similar results.

Pharmacokinetic studies in rats and nonhuman primates have been performed. Pang et al.[324] administered ^{125}I-labeled and unlabeled rTNF-α (Genentech) to Sprague-Dawley rats. A biexponential clearance was found, with a $t_{1/2}\alpha$ of 5 minutes and a $t_{1/2}\beta$ of 30 minutes for unlabeled TNF-α. The ^{125}I-labeled cytokine had a prolonged β phase of 280 minutes, which suggests altered receptor binding and degradation in vivo. Similar results have been reported in mice.[325] In rhesus monkeys,[326] short-term infusion (0.5 hour) of rTNF-α (Genentech) at various doses was administered, and two different elimination mechanisms were found. At low doses, a saturable specific process was evident. At higher dose levels, a nonspecific nonsaturable process was found. This latter process was felt probably to represent glomerular filtration of TNF-α. Similarly, in nephrectomized rats, clearance of rTNF-α was significantly reduced.[327]

In humans, rTNF-α has been administered by a variety of routes and schedules. Table 36.15 summarizes pharmacokinetic data for trials using i.v. administration. In the report by Blick et al.,[322] rTNF-α was given as an i.v. bolus, and the half-life did not appear to change with increasing doses. The volume of distribution decreased, however, and the AUC increased when doses were escalated (Table 36.16). These data suggest a one-compartment model, as illustrated in Figure 36.7. In the reports by Moritz et al.[323] and Kimura et al.,[328] serum half-life and clearance increased

TABLE 36.15

PHARMACOKINETICS OF HUMAN RECOMBINANT TUMOR NECROSIS FACTOR α (rHuTNF-α) AFTER INTRAVENOUS ADMINISTRATION

Study	rHuTNF-α Preparation	Schedule	Levels	$t_{1/2}$	C_{max}
Chapman et al. (331)	Genentech	i.v.b.	1–200 $\mu g/m^2$	20 min	2.5–80.0 ng/mL
Feinberg et al. (332)	Genentech	30-min i.v. infusion	5–200 $\mu g/m^2$	NS	20 pg/mL
Moritz et al. (323)	Knoll	10-min i.v. infusion	40–280 $\mu g/m^2$	11–70 min	12 ng/mL
Blick et al. (322)	Genentech	i.v.b.	1–150 $\mu g/m^2$	13.9–18.0 min	500–8,000 pg/mL
Creaven et al. (333)	Asahi	1-h i.v. infusion	1–48 × 10^4 U/m^2	0.20–0.72 h	NS
Mittelman et al. (329)	Knoll	24-h infusion	40–200 $\mu g/m^2$	20–30 min	300–500 pg/mL
Spriggs et al. (330)	Asahi	24-h infusion	4.5–645 $\mu g/m^2$	NS	90–900 pg/mL
Kimura et al. (328)	Asahi	30-min i.v. infusion	116 105 U/m^2	1,080 min	4.8896.0 U/mL

C_{max}, highest observed concentration; i.v.b., intravenous bolus; NS, not stated; $t_{1/2}$, elimination half-life.

TABLE 36.16

PHARMACOKINETICS OF RECOMBINANT TUMOR NECROSIS FACTOR α (rTNF-α) AFTER INTRAVENOUS BOLUS ADMINISTRATION

rTNF-α Dose (μg/m²)	$t_{1/2}$ (min)	V_d (L)	AUC (ng × min/mL)
25	15.9 + 3.6	66 + 30	10.5 + 2.7
35	13.9 + 1.0	13.3 + 5.0	19.7 + 5.3
50	16.0 + 2.0	13.4 + 1.1	89.6 + 13.9
60	18.0 + 0.4	17.7 + 4.0	114.6 + 26.5
100	17 + 2	12 + 4	224.8 + 69.0

AUC, area under the concentration time curve; $t_{1/2}$, elimination half-life; V_d, volume of distribution.
Values are expressed as mean + standard error of the mean.
Adapted with permission from Saks S, Rosenblum S. Recombinant human TNF-α: preclinical studies and results from early clinical trials. Immunol Ser 1992;56:567–587.

with higher doses, which is consistent with a saturable receptor-mediated clearance mechanism. Administration of rTNF-α as a 24-hour continuous infusion[329] did not yield detectable serum TNF-α concentrations except at the highest dose levels (160 and 200 μg/m² per day). Serum levels were undetectable after 60 minutes. The influence of TNFR levels in serum and tissues on rTNF-α pharmacokinetics is uncertain; however, as with other cytokines, these may play a role in determining which clearance mechanisms are operative. Induction of TNF-α clearance mechanisms is also suggested by the observations during 24-hour continuous infusion of rTNF-α.[329,330]

The intramuscular (i.m.) and s.c. routes of administration for rTNF-α have also been investigated.[334] Blick et al.[322]

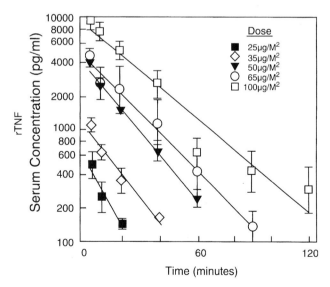

Figure 36.7 Serum disappearance of recombinant tumor necrosis factor (rTNF) after i.v. administration as measured by enzyme-linked immunosorbent assay. Symbols represent the mean blood levels for each dose for all patients at that dose. Standard error bars are shown unless insufficient data points were available. (Reproduced with permission from Blick M, Sherwin SA, Rosenblum M, et al. Phase I study of recombinant tumor necrosis factor in cancer patients. Cancer Res 1987;47:2986–2989.)

administered doses from 5 to 200 μg/m². Unlike in the case of the i.v. route, serum rTNF-α levels were not consistently detected until doses were higher than 150 μg/m². Peak serum levels were noted at 2 hours and occasionally persisted for 24 hours. Zamkoff et al.[335] administered rTNF-α (Chiron) subcutaneously at doses from 5 to 150 μg/m² per day. No serum rTNF-α levels were detected, even at the highest doses. Thus, these routes of administration produce lower or undetectable serum levels compared with the i.v. route.

Other modes of administration such as intratumoral, intraperitoneal, and regional have also been studied. These approaches were suggested by animal studies indicating that high levels of TNF are required for antitumor effects.[336] Pfreundschuh et al.[337] administered escalating doses of rTNF-α as a single intralesional injection to cancer patients. The MTD was 391 μg/m², and detectable serum levels of rTNF-α were found at higher doses, consistent with systemic absorption. Intraperitoneal instillation of rTNF-α in patients with advanced gastrointestinal tumors and ovarian carcinoma has been reported.[338] Prolonged TNF-α levels in ascitic fluid without detectable serum levels were seen.

Finally, intraarterial administration of rTNF has been investigated. Hepatic artery infusion of TNF-α[339] produced tumor regressions in 14% of patients with liver metastases, but the MTD of TNF-α was not altered compared with i.v. administration. Use of TNF-α in isolated limb perfusion in an attempt to increase local TNF-α concentrations without systemic exposure has also been studied.[340] The rTNF-α was administered to three patients at doses of 2.0, 3.0, and 4.0 μg for 90 minutes via isolated extremity perfusion. Serum levels of TNF-α during perfusion never exceeded 62 ng/mL. Perfusate levels of TNF-α varied between 970 and 2,000 ng/mL (ELISA), with no apparent decay. Higher, more stable levels of TNF-α appear to be maintained using this route of administration than with systemic administration. When TNF-α is administered in this fashion, doses exceeding the MTD can be given; however, severe systemic toxicity occurs. The stable concentrations maintained in the perfusate are therefore of interest.

Clinical Effects and Toxicity

The role of TNF in homeostasis predicts that a sepsis-like clinical syndrome would result from its administration. In humans, the toxicity seen is dose-related except for fever and chills, which have occurred even at low doses. The fever appears rapidly after administration and generally resolves within several hours.[322,323] Additional systemic toxicities include anorexia, fatigue, malaise, and myalgia.

The initial hemodynamic effects of i.v. TNF-α include tachycardia and hypertension, followed within several hours by hypotension. This has been the dose-limiting toxicity reported in most trials, and it becomes less severe with repeated administration. The mechanisms responsible for the hypotension are unclear but may include myocardial depression,[341] vascular endothelial changes,[342] and secondary secretion of IL-1 and IL-6.[343,344]

Hematologic toxicity includes thrombocytopenia, which has been dose-limiting in several reports.[328,335,345] This is generally mild, and in all instances recovery occurred within 24 to 48 hours after rTNF-α discontinuation. Leukopenia has been noted at 30 to 90 minutes after injection,[327,328] and the leukocyte count quickly returns to baseline or higher (neutrophilia). These findings resemble those reported with other cytokines such as GM-CSF. The changes in leukocyte and platelet counts have generally not been associated with either bleeding or infection. Coagulation parameters such as prothrombin time and activated partial thromboplastin time remain normal, and mild elevations of fibrin degradation products have been seen.[346]

Hepatic toxicity is also common, with increased levels of transaminase, alkaline phosphatase, and total bilirubin reported.[287] These levels have generally returned to normal or baseline during continued therapy. In several instances,[328,347] however, these changes were dose-limiting. Mild renal toxicity in the form of slight elevation of blood urea nitrogen and creatinine may occur,[323,328] but it is felt to be of little clinical significance.

Other less frequent toxicities reported include confusion, somnolence, hallucinations, and speech defects.[322,348] Pulmonary toxicity is rare, with occasional reports of dyspnea[349,350] and decreased carbon monoxide diffusing capacity.[350] The metabolic changes developing during rTNF-α therapy include increases in serum triglycerides and reciprocal decreases in cholesterol.[332] Although weight loss has been noted in animal studies with rTNF-α,[351] this has not been a significant finding in human studies.

Administration of rTNF as a s.c. or i.m. injection has a similar toxicity spectrum.[331,335,352,353] In contrast to i.v. injection, these routes are also associated with pain and induration at the injection sites. S.c. administration also induces erythema and vesiculation associated with neutrophil and mononuclear cell infiltration.[331,335]

Regional rTNF-α administration has similar toxicity. Hepatic artery infusion produces effects resembling those seen during i.v. administration. Isolated limb perfusion with doses of rTNF-α from 2.0 to 4.0 μg also produces systemic side effects, with hypotension, tachycardia, fever, chills, and renal toxicity noted.[340] Use of hydration with prophylactic dopamine in these patients has controlled the cardiovascular complications, however.

The immunologic effects of rTNF-α administration in humans have been well characterized. Chapman et al.[331] reported mild elevation of the acute-phase reactant C-reactive protein during rTNF-α administration. Delayed hypersensitivity to various antigens has been examined in 26 patients, 6 of whom were anergic before rTNF-α therapy.[353] Three of these latter patients then developed positive skin tests during therapy. NK and LAK activity in peripheral blood has also been studied.[76,352,354] Significant depression at 48 hours was noted during a 120-hour continuous infusion of rTNF-α, with subsequent increases above baseline.[352,354] Decreases in IL-2–inducible LAK cells have also been reported.[355] Monocyte studies[356] have demonstrated increases in hydrogen peroxide production after i.v. therapy with rTNF-α. Studies of lymphocyte subsets demonstrate decreases in the percentages of CD8+ and CD56+ cells, with increases in CD4+ and CD19+ subsets.[355] Secondary increases in IL-6,[302] G-CSF,[357] and macrophage colony-stimulating factor (M-CSF)[357] serum concentrations after TNF-α administration have also been noted. The increases in these latter two hematopoietic growth factors coincided temporally with the leukocytosis seen during TNF-α infusion.

In contrast to the hemorrhagic necrosis of tumors seen in murine tumor models, the clinical antitumor effects of systemically administered rTNF have been minimal. Responses have been reported in phase I trials in patients with non-Hodgkin's lymphoma,[358] gastric carcinoma,[287] hepatoma,[287] RCC,[347] breast cancer,[330] and pancreatic cancer.[358] Phase II trials of rTNF treatment of most of these malignancies,[359] however, have not demonstrated significant clinical activity. The apparent differences between the effects in murine and human tumors may be related to the tolerance of mice to much larger doses of rTNF-α than are tolerated by humans. Estimates are that a dose of 5 μg, which produces hemorrhagic necrosis of murine tumors, is equivalent to 1,000 μg/m^2 of rTNF-α in humans.[360] This represents a fivefold greater dose than the MTD of rTNF-α in humans, which is 200 μg/m^2. The responses seen with intratumor injection of rTNF-α appear more frequent[287] and would suggest that this differential tolerance may be an important factor in the lack of antitumor effects clinically.

The local administration of TNF-α has been investigated as a strategy to minimize systemic toxicity and serum levels, increase local concentrations, and concomitantly increase the antitumor effects of this cytokine. Intraperitoneal administration in patients with ascites and ovarian carcinoma has been evaluated in a small randomized trial.[361] The recombinant human TNF-α was given at a dose of 0.06 mg/m² intraperitoneally after paracentesis at weekly intervals (×3) and compared with paracentesis alone. Intraperitoneal instillation was well tolerated, with pain in 42.1% of patients, fever and chills in 36.9%, and hypotension in 5.3%. Responses were not seen in either group.

TNF-α has also been used to perfuse extremities and the hepatic circulation. Limb perfusion using IFN-γ, TNF-α, and melphalan in patients with nonresectable sarcomas has been reported.[362] In a series of 55 patients, complete responses were seen in 18%, partial responses in 64%, and no change in 18%. Limb salvage was achieved in 84%. Systemic side effects were moderate. Another study investigating the role of TNF-α and melphalan in the therapy of soft tissue sarcoma and melanoma reported a response rate of 76% and a limb-salvage rate of 76% in the soft tissue sarcoma group and a 100% response rate and a 93% limb-salvage rate in the melanoma group, following isolated limb perfusion with TNFα and melphalan.[363] In advanced limb melanoma, the presence of regional lymph node or distant metastases was associated with an increased risk of death within 1 year, even after limb perfusion.[364] Hohenberger[365] reported extensive tumor necrosis of recurrent synovial sarcoma tumor beds in two children following limb perfusion with high-dose recombinant TNF-α combined with melphalan. Similarly, Noorda et al.[366] demonstrated a 63% overall tumor response rate and a 57% local control rate with limb preservation in patients who had unresectable soft tissue sarcomas of the limbs and underwent ILP with TNF-α and melphalan, followed by resection of the tumor remnant when possible. There has also been success in the treatment of liver metastasis with isolated hepatic perfusion (IHP) using TNF-α in combination with other agents. Numerous trials[367-370] have been conducted using IHP with TNF-α in combination with melphalan and other agents in the treatment of hepatic metastases. A response rate of up to 75% was demonstrated by hepatic tumor regression in patients with liver metastases following IHP with TNF-α in combination with other agents. The use of TNF-α perfusion techniques has also been explored for primary RCC,[371] with uncertain clinical utility.

Drug Interactions

Preclinical studies have indicated that combining rTNF-α with other cytokines or chemotherapeutic agents may enhance the results. IFN-γ produces an up-regulation of TNFR on various cells in vitro,[274] and therefore rTNF-α and IFN-γ have been combined in phase I studies. Dose-limiting toxicity has included hyperbilirubinemia,[372] hypotension,[373] and acute dyspnea with hypoxemia.[373] The MTD for rTNF-α in these trials is less than 156 μg/m² per day,

which suggests synergistic toxicity. In murine models, the combination of rTNF-α and rIL-2 has had significant antitumor effects.[374,375] Clinical trials of this combination have been conducted to determine toxicity.[78] In addition, rTNF-α has been administered with rIL-2 and IFN-α in a phase I trial.[376] Patients received 40 to 120 μg/m² of rTNF-α on days 1 through 5 and fixed doses of rIL-2 (1 to 3 × 10⁶ IU/m² on days 1 through 5, days 8 through 12, and days 15 through 19) and IFN-α (9 × 10⁶ IU/m² three times a week). Systemic toxicity was substantial, but outpatient administration was felt to be possible.

TNF-α shows synergy with a variety of chemotherapeutic compounds in vitro, including doxorubicin[377] and cisplatin.[378] Synergistic in vitro cytotoxicity against tumor cells has also been noted with combinations of rTNF-α and topoisomerase II inhibitors such as etoposide and dactinomycin (actinomycin D or DACT).[379,380] Phase I trials of rTNF-α and etoposide have also been conducted.[381] Results of these combinations suggest some clinical activity; however, more studies are needed to elucidate further the clinical utility of these combinations.

INTERLEUKIN-11

Unlike the other cytokines discussed in this chapter, which are primarily utilized for their direct antitumor actions, interleukin-11 (IL-11) has shown benefits in managing chemotherapy-induced toxicity, specifically hematopoietic toxicity. IL-11 is member of the IL-6–type cytokine family, which also includes IL-6, leukemia inhibitory factor, oncostatin M, and ciliary neurotropic factor.[382-384] IL-11 was first detected in the conditioned media from the immortalized primate bone marrow stromal cell line PU-34.[385] IL-11 is a megakaryocytopoietic cytokine that offers an alternative to the short-lived effects of platelet transfusion therapy in the treatment of chemotherapy-induced thrombocytopenia.

Structure and Mechanism of Action

Human IL-11 is a 199–amino acid protein, including a 21–amino acid leader sequence, with a molecular weight of approximately 19 kd.[386] It is encoded by a 7-kb genomic sequence consisting of five exons and four introns.[387] The IL-11 gene has been localized to the long arm of human chromosome 19 at band 19q13.3-q13.4.[387] The human and murine forms of IL-11 demonstrate significant structural similarities, sharing 80% and 88% sequence homologies at the nucleotide and protein levels, respectively.[388] Recombinant human IL-11 (rhIL-11) (Oprelvekin, Neumega), developed by the Genetics Institute (Cambridge, MA), has 177 amino acids, differing from the 178–amino acid native protein in that it lacks the amino-terminal proline residue. It is produced in E. coli by standard recombinant DNA methods. Similar to the native protein, the recombinant form also has a molecular mass of approximately 19 kd.

The three-dimensional structure of IL-11 has been well characterized, resembling the structures of hGH[389] and human granulocyte colony-stimulating factor.[390] It is composed of four α-helices connected by loops of variable lengths.[383] This structure, which is also noted in IL-2,[6] IL-4,[391] granulocyte-macrophage colony-stimulating factor,[392] macrophage colony-stimulating factor (M-CSF),[393] and IL-5,[394] is believed to play a role in preserving the interactions of these cytokines with specific cellular receptors.

IL-11 signaling is mediated through a hexameric receptor complex composed of two molecules of IL-11, the IL-11 receptor α-chain (IL-11Rα) and the transmembrane signal transducer glycoprotein gp130.[395] Signaling in response to IL-11 is restricted to cells expressing gp130 in addition to IL-11Rα.[396,397] The requirement of gp 130 in the IL-11/IL11Rα multisubunit receptor complex is not unique to IL-11 and is shared among the other members of IL-6–type cytokines, including IL-6, leukemia inhibitory factor, oncostatin M, and ciliary neurotropic factor.[398-400] The use of gp130 by these different cytokines may contribute to the observed overlapping of biological activities.[401,402] Signaling through the IL-11 receptor leads to the activation of numerous proteins, including the Janus kinase signal transducer and activator of transcription (Jak-STAT) pathway,[400,403] as well as Ras and mitogen-activated protein kinase (MAPK). This activation is followed by downstream activation of various cytokine-responsive and primary response genes. Depending on the cell type, signaling through the IL-11 receptor complex can modify various cellular functions, including the production of the proinflammatory cytokines IL-1β, interferon-γ, TNF, and IL-12,[404,405] as well as cell survival through the regulation of numerous proteins involved in apoptosis and cell protection, such as NF-κB, Bcl-2, and heat shock protein.[384,406]

Cellular Pharmacology

IL-11 has pleiotropic effects in various tissues, including hematopoietic tissues, where it exerts its effects on primitive stem cells as well as mature progenitor cells.[407,408] IL-11 induces the proliferation and differentiation of primitive stem cells, including multipotential and committed hematopoietic progenitor cells from various tissues such as bone marrow and cord and peripheral blood.[409-411] These effects are mediated in synergy with other cytokines and growth factors, including thrombopoietin (TPO), stem cell factor (SCF), granulocyte colony-stimulating factor (GSF), granulocyte-macrophage colony-stimulating factor (GM-CSF), and interleukin-3, -4, -6, -7, -12, and -13.[412-419]

Of the various hematopoietic cell types, megakaryocytes and their precursors appear to be particularly responsive to the effects of IL-11, as demonstrated by human and animal models reporting increased proliferation and maturation of megakaryocytes after stimulation by IL-11.[420-422] Synergy with TPO and SCF appear to be critical for IL-11–mediated megakaryocytopoiesis. This is highlighted by studies reporting up to 90% reduction in megakaryocytic colony formation after blocking TPO with anti-TPO antiserum or soluble TPO receptor c-Mpl[423] and compete abrogation of the proliferation of hematopoietic progenitors after blocking the SCF receptor c-kit.[424]

Although not approved as an erythropoietic or leukopoietic agent, in addition to its role in thrombopoiesis, IL-11 has also been shown to be a stimulator of erythropoiesis and leukopoiesis. Unlike in the case of megakaryocytopoiesis, which requires IL-11 synergy with other growth factors and cytokines, IL-11 as a single agent may exert effects on erythropoiesis directly, although synergy with other cytokines has also been reported.[425,426] IL-11 exerts its effects on burst-forming unit-erythroid (BFU-E) early in erythroid development in combination with IL-3, while it can act alone later in erythroid differentiation to support the development of erythroid colony-forming units (CFU-E).[425] Further supporting the role of IL-11 in erythropoiesis are observations noting a 6.4-fold increase in IL-11 levels in patients with polycythemia vera.[427] Animal models have demonstrated various effects of IL-11 on the differentiation and maturation of lymphoid and myeloid progenitors. In combination with SCF, IL-11 promotes the development of B-lymphocytes and stimulates the proliferation of myeloid colonies, while the addition of IL-4 or IL-13 directs colony differentiation toward a macrophage cell lineage.[416,428] Other cell types affected by IL-11 include bone marrow stromal cells and fibroblasts,[429] pulmonary and GI epithelial cells,[430,431] osteoclasts,[432] osteoblasts,[433] and various neuronal cells.[434]

Clinical Pharmacokinetics

The pharmacokinetics of rhIL-11 following i.v. and s.c. infusions has been characterized by Aoyama et al., who found linear pharmacokinetics for both forms of drug administration.[435] Using an ELISA method developed by the Genetics Institute specifically for the detection of rhIL-11, Aoyama et al. were able to analyze blood and urine concentrations of rhIL-11 after s.c. and i.v. administrations. Following single i.v infusion at 10, 25, and 50 μg/kg, the mean plasma concentration of rhIL-11 was 53.8, 49.7, and 120 ng/mL, respectively.[435] Furthermore, the bioavailability of rhIL-11 following s.c. administration at 3, 10, 25, and 50μg/kg was 67%, 65%, 62%, and 65%, respectively, when calculated on the basis of AUC after an i.v. dose of 50 μg/kg.[435] The half-life following i.v. and s.c. administration was approximately 2 hours and 8 hours, respectively, irrespective of dose, indicative of absorption rate–limited pharmacokinetics after s.c. administration.[435]

RhIL-11 appears to be eliminated primarily by the kidney following degradation and metabolism.[436,437] Aoyama et al. failed to detect immunoreactive rhIL-11 in the urine of healthy volunteers.[435] These data, in addition to results from animal models demonstrating 1% urinary excretion of intact radiolabeled rhIL-11,[436] point toward degradation mechanisms accounting for the elimination of rhIL-11 before renal excretion.

Clinical Effects and Toxicity

Numerous studies to date have evaluated the toxicity and efficacy of rhIL-11 when used following chemotherapy to reduce thrombocytopenia-related complications. Toxicity related to rhIL-11 is dose-dependent and involves multiple organ systems, ranging from constitutional symptoms such as headaches, nausea, vomiting, and myalgias to more serious side effects primarily involving the cardiovascular system. In a phase I trial of rhIL-11 in patients with breast cancer, Gordon et al. determined the MTD for rhIL-11 to be 75 µg/kg per day, primarily limited by grade 2 constitutional symptoms, including arthralgias/myalgias and fatigue.[438] Another phase I trial using low doses of s.c. rhIL-11 (5-15µg/kg per week) reported the most common side effects occurring in greater than 10% of patients to be (in descending order) reaction at injection site, headache, pharyngitis, nausea, asthenia, and rhinitis.[439]

The most serious side effect related to rhIL-11 reported by Antin et al. was severe fluid retention resistant to diuresis, which contributed to early mortality.[440] Although several reports noted edema and fluid retention following rhIL-11 therapy,[438,439,441,442] these side effects were mild and responded partially to diuretics.[443] Fluid retention with rhIL-11 therapy is believed to contribute to the dilutional anemia that is noted following therapy with rhIL-11. Plasma volume expansion is believed to be secondary to rhIL-11–mediated reduced sodium excretion, a mechanism similar to that noted following interleukin-6 administration.[443-445] RhIL-11 has also been noted to increase levels of the acute-phase proteins CRP, fibrinogen, von Willebrand's factor, ferritin, and haptoglobin in a dose-related manner; levels returned to normal after discontinuation of therapy.[437,438,443] It has been suggested by Gordon et al. that such increases in acute-phase proteins can serve as a marker of rhIL-11 activity.[438] Finally, rhIL-11 has been associated with cardiac side effects, including palpitations and atrial arrhythmias,[441,446,447] although these are believed to be secondary to the volume expansion and overload induced by rhIL-11.[447]

Many trials have demonstrated the therapeutic efficacy of rhIL-11 in the treatment of chemotherapy-induced thrombocytopenia in cancer patients, as well as in nonmalignant diseases, including aplastic anemia, MDS, and liver cirrhosis.[441,442,448] The efficacy of rhIL-11 is dose-dependent between 10 and 75 µg/kg per day,[438] with increasing platelet counts documented at doses as low as 10 µg/kg per day.[438,442] In a randomized, placebo-controlled study in patients with advanced breast cancer receiving dose-intensive cyclophosphamide and doxorubicin, rhIL-11 decreased the requirement for platelet transfusions and also decreased time to platelet recovery when administered at 50 µg/kg per day subcutaneously for 10 to 17 days.[446] In another randomized, double-blinded, placebo-controlled trial in patients with a variety of solid malignancies and lymphoma, 14- to 21-day therapy with s.c. rhIL-11 at 50 µg/kg per day was noted to decrease the need for platelet transfusions in the same patients during subsequent chemotherapeutic cycles, compared with rhIL-11 at 25 µg/kg per day of placebo.[441] In both studies, the threshold for platelet transfusions was less than 20,000/µL. RhIL-11 has also shown potential therapeutic efficacy in the treatment of nonmalignant diseases, including Crohn's disease, mucositis, psoriasis, and rheumatoid arthritis. Demonstration of mucosal antiinflammatory properties in animal models[449-451] led to human studies that showed efficacy of rhIL-11 in the treatment of Crohn's colitis.[452,453] Because mechanisms similar to those of intestinal mucosal damage are believed to play a role in chemotherapy-associated oral mucosal injury, rhIL-11 may also decrease the severity of oral mucositis,[454-457] although to date no large placebo-controlled studies have demonstrated this. Even though its antiinflammatory properties, which include reducing macrophage activity and down-regulating the production of proinflammatory mediators (e.g., TNF, IL-12, and IFN-γ), have been well documented,[458] rhIL-11 has shown minimal clinical efficacy in the therapy of psoriasis and rheumatoid arthritis.[439,459] While the use of rhIL-11 in nonmalignant diseases has shown some promise, the current therapeutic indications remain for the amelioration of severe thrombocytopenia and the reduction of platelet transfusions following myelosuppressive chemotherapy. Further studies are required to clarify the utility of this cytokine in nonmalignant disease processes.

INTERLEUKIN-12

Interleukin-12 (IL-12), originally named "natural killer cell stimulatory factor" (NKSF)[460] and "cytotoxic lymphocyte maturation factor" (CLMF)[461] by the groups identifying its multiple activities, was first isolated as a molecule secreted from Epstein-Barr virus–transformed B-cell lines. Early characterization revealed that this protein could act synergistically with IL-2 to augment cytotoxic lymphocyte responses,[462] could cause the proliferation of mitogen-activated peripheral blood lymphoblasts,[463] and could induce IFN-γ secretion by resting peripheral blood lymphocytes.[464]

Structure and Mechanisms of Action

On purification, IL-12 was determined to be a 70-kd disulfide-linked heterodimeric protein composed of two polypeptides with approximate molecular weights of 35 kd and 40 kd.[460,465,466] Characterization of the cDNAs encoding the subunits revealed that the p35 component was a 219–amino acid polypeptide containing seven cysteine residues and three potential *N*-glycosylation sites, whereas the p40 molecule was composed of 328 amino acids, ten of which are cysteines, with four possible glycosylation sites.[467–469] The mature protein encoded by the p35 cDNA has an actual molecular weight of 27,500 kd but appears larger on sodium dodecyl sulfate polyacrylamide gel electrophoresis (SDS-PAGE) due to its extensive glycosylation. Mature p40 has a calculated molecular weight of 34,700 kd and is comparatively less glycosylated than the mature p35 molecule.[467–469]

The heterodimeric structure of IL-12 is unique among the cytokines.[470] Although transfection of cell lines with cDNAs encoding either the p35 or p40 IL-12 polypeptides results in synthesis and secretion of the individual molecules, expression of active, secreted IL-12 requires that the same cell be cotransfected with both cDNAs.[471] Interestingly, expression studies suggest that the p35 gene is synthesized by numerous cell types of both hematopoietic and non-hematopoietic origin[471,472] but that active IL-12 is secreted by only those cells that also transcribe p40.[471] Thus p40 likely is required for the efficient export of the p70 molecule. The p40 polypeptide is produced in large excess of the IL-12 heterodimer.[472] Secreted p40 homodimers may even act as IL-12 antagonists.[473] The actual physiologic significance of p40 overexpression and homodimerization, however, remains largely unknown.

The genes encoding the p40 and p35 subunits are completely unrelated and have been mapped to different chromosomes.[474] The p35 gene maps to human chromosome band 3p12-3q13.2.[474] It has a primary amino acid sequence that is suggestive of a richly α-helical protein and hence in this regard is similar to most other cytokines.[471] Indeed, many of the amino acid positions conserved between IL-6 and GM-CSF are also shared by the IL-12 p35 subunit.[475] The p40 gene has been mapped to human chromosome band 5q31-q33 and, though not homologous to any known cytokines, does strongly resemble members of the hematopoietic cytokine receptor family.[474] The p40 sequence has particularly strong homologies with the extracellular regions of receptors for IL-6 and ciliary neurotropic factor[468,476] and is closely linked genetically to the M-CSF receptor.[474] The p70 heterodimer thus has the characteristics of a disulfide-linked complex between a cytokine and a receptor.[471]

Cellular Pharmacology

A number of different cell types are important sources of IL-12. Among normal peripheral blood mononuclear cells, monocytes and monocyte-derived macrophages are perhaps the most significant producers of the cytokine,[472,477] although the production of IL-12 by dendritic cells during antigen presentation is the crucial signal for induction of a

T$_H$1 response pattern and effective cell-mediated immunity.[471,477–479] Some studies now also suggest that IL-12 is the requisite "third signal" that participates with class I MHC/antigen complexes and B7 to induce the proliferation and activation of naïve CD8$^+$ T cells[480] and hence the cytolytic component of antitumor function. Neutrophils have also been shown to make IL-12,[481] although some controversy exists as to whether nontransformed B cells are also a physiological source of the molecule.[481,482] Langerhans cells,[483] murine mast cells,[484] and keratinocytes[485] have also been reported to produce IL-12 under some stimulatory conditions.

The most potent inducers of IL-12 are bacteria, microbial components such as LPS, and intracellular parasites.[472,478,479] IL-12 production was found to be significantly enhanced when peripheral blood mononuclear cells were stimulated with Gram-positive and Gram-negative bacteria, endotoxin, *Mycobacterium tuberculosis*, *Mycobacterium leprae*, and *Toxoplasma gondii*.[472] LPS has also been shown to induce IL-12 synthesis by polymorphonuclear leukocytes.[479]

In addition to being modulated by the components of pathogens, IL-12 synthesis is also positively and negatively regulated by various cytokines. IFN-γ and GM-CSF are both capable of stimulating IL-12 production by phagocytic cells,[486] although, interestingly, the p35 and p40 polypeptide components of IL-12 seem to be differentially induced: although IFN-γ directly stimulates the accumulation of p35 mRNA by monocytes and neutrophils, it can only augment the LPS-induced synthesis of p40 mRNA by those same cell types.[486,487] Among the cytokines with inhibitory effects on IL-12 are IL-10, IL-4, and TGF-β.[488,489] These products mediate their effects at the level of both RNA and protein, as they inhibit the secretion of the p70 heterodimeric protein as well as the accumulation of mRNAs encoding the p35 and p40 polypeptides.[488,489] The IL-10–mediated inhibition of IFN-γ production by T and NK cells occurs indirectly through the ability of IL-10 to prevent IL-12 synthesis by phagocytic cells.[470,488]

Membrane-bound ligands present on activated T lymphocytes also stimulate phagocytes to synthesize and secrete IL-12.[490–492] Although they are not yet fully defined, at least several receptor-ligand interactions have been characterized that mediate this induction. Perhaps most significant in this regard is the augmented production of IL-12 by antigen-presenting cells on engagement of their CD40 receptor by CD40 ligand (CD40L) expressed on antigen (phytohemagglutinin [PHA])–stimulated T cells.[490,492] The importance of this CD40/CD40L binding in mediation of IL-12 induction has been demonstrated for both murine and human cells. In human peripheral blood mononuclear cells, CD40/CD40L interactions stimulated IFN-γ production via an IL-12–dependent mechanism when the mononuclear cells were first optimally prestimulated with PHA.[492] Direct CD28 engagement can also stimulate IFN-γ production and does so in an IL-12–dependent fashion by two different mechanisms: either by increasing CD40L expression on T cells, which then stimulate CD40 receptors and IL-12 synthesis by antigen-presenting cells, or by augmenting the levels of the IL-12 receptor β1 (IL-12Rβ1) chain on T cells and hence the capacity of IL-12 to bind to their receptors.[492] CD28/B7 interactions can also enhance IFN-γ synthesis independently of IL-12. Evidence for cooperation of the CD40L/CD40 and B7/CD28 pathways for stimulating IL-12 expression comes from studies performed under conditions of low B7 expression (inadequate antigen or PHA concentrations), in which CD40L-stimulated IL-12 production was found to be enhanced by anti-CD28.[492]

Cells expressing IL-12 receptors (IL-12Rs) were originally identified using fluorescent anti–IL-12 antibodies to detect the cell-bound cytokine. Using this technique, IL-12Rs were observed on activated NK cells and T cells but not on B cells or resting T cells.[493] When IL-12 was added to peripheral blood mononuclear cells and cross-linked after binding, anti–IL-12 antibodies immunoprecipitated a single protein of approximately 110 kd that was purported to be the IL-12 receptor.[493] Subsequent expression cloning studies identified what were believed to be two distinct low-affinity IL-12 receptors, which together reportedly formed a high-affinity binding site.[494] Each was characterized as having the general composition of a β-type cytokine receptor subunit and as being a gp130-like member of the cytokine receptor family.[494] Thus, the functional high-affinity IL-12 receptor was originally thought to be composed of these two subunits, each of which independently exhibited a low affinity for IL-12.[495]

Additional studies have determined that the functional IL-12 receptor is a heterodimer composed of a β1 and β2 polypeptide and that each mediates a specific activity requisite for IL-12 responsiveness.[496,497] IL-12Rβ1 is the polypeptide that binds IL-12,[498] and the β2 chain is the component that transduces the IL-12 signal into the nucleus.[497,499,500] Normal T_H1 cells express both chains and hence are fully IL-12 responsive. T_H2 cells express only the IL-12Rβ1 chain, and although they thus bind IL-12 with high affinity, no reactivity to the cytokine is exhibited with the absence of signal transduction capacity.[497,501] Indeed, the selective loss of IL-12Rβ2 expression is an important correlate of T_H2 cell differentiation,[496] and ongoing T_H1 responses can be inhibited by immunosuppressive cytokines that act by negatively regulating that molecule.[502–504] IFN-γ and IFN-α have been shown to induce IL-12Rβ2 expression in the mouse and human, respectively.[499] Others have reported that the expression of both IL-12Rβ1 and IL-12Rβ2 mRNA is increased in the lymph nodes of naïve mice after systemic administration of recombinant IL-12.[496] The notion that the IL-12 inductive effect on IL-12Rβ2 mRNA is mediated indirectly through IFN-γ was suggested by the observation that in IFN-γ receptor −/− mice, β2 mRNA levels were significantly lower than in wild-type mice after IL-12 treatment.[505]

Several pathologic conditions are characterized by predominantly T_H2 cell populations, and lymphocytes from such individuals display no IL-12Rβ2 chains due to their high production of IL-4, interleukin-5 (IL-5), IL-10, and TGF-β.[497,504] Antibodies to TGF-β and IL-10 restore IL-12Rβ2 chain synthesis and IFN-γ production[504] by these peripheral blood lymphocytes in vitro, which supports the notion that T_H1 protective responses are highly dependent on adequate expression levels of IL-12 receptor components. It is perhaps because of its potent immunostimulatory effects that IL-12 has its activity stringently regulated at both the agonist level (see earlier) and the receptor level.

The binding of IL-12 to its receptor induces dimerization of the component IL-12Rβ1 and IL-12Rβ2 chains, which leads to the interaction of their receptor-associated Jak2 tyrosine kinases.[506] These kinases mediate each other's transactivation,[507] which allows the now functional enzymes to phosphorylate tyrosine residue 800 in the IL-12Rβ2 chain cytoplasmic region.[500] Signal transduction and transcription-activating factor 4 (STAT4) has specificity for the resulting unique phosphorylated peptide sequence on IL-12Rβ2 (GpYLPSNID, where pY represents phosphotyrosine, and the core G-pY[800]-L is the critical motif for binding),[500,508] and it itself is phosphorylated by Jak2 on binding by its SH2 domain to this receptor site.[508] Phosphorylated STAT4 molecules dimerize and migrate to the nucleus, where they bind specific DNA sequences and activate transcription of proinflammatory genes that stimulate T_H1 responses.[509,510] The requirement for STAT4 in IL-12–mediated responses was demonstrated by experiments indicating that IL-12–dependent increases in IFN-γ production, cellular proliferation, and NK cell cytotoxicity were abrogated in lymphocytes from STAT4-deficient mice.[511] The involvement of both Jak2 and tyrosine kinase 2 (Tyk2) in the IL-12 pathway[506,507,512,513] is circumstantially supported by the finding that TGF-β inhibits IL-12–induced phosphorylation of Jak2, Tyk2, and STAT4 and that TGF-β also inhibits IL-12–induced IFN-γ production.[513] The possibility that Jak2 or Tyk2 molecules can independently mediate STAT4 phosphorylation is suggested by data indicating that tyrosine phosphorylation of STAT4 is not abrogated when either Tyk2 alone or Jak2 alone is inhibited.[512]

As discussed briefly above, IL-12 was originally isolated as a cytokine that induced the proliferation and cytolytic activity of NK cells, LAK cells, and cytolytic T lymphocytes. This stimulatory activity is now known to be specific to T cells and NK cells preactivated with either antireceptor antibody,[514] mitogens, or IL-2,[463] as freshly isolated peripheral blood T cells exhibit minimal responsiveness to IL-12.[514] The requirement for activation is related to the absence of IL-12Rs on resting cells[514] and their induction on mitogenic stimulation.[514–516] T-cell activation is also necessary to induce components of the transduction pathway (STAT4) required for IL-12 signaling.[514] Use of purified T-cell clones and PHA-stimulated T-cell subpopulations indicates that both CD4$^+$ and CD8$^+$ T-cell subsets are susceptible to IL-12 stimulation.[460,462,466,517-520]

IL-12 has a pivotal role in establishing the T$_H$1 versus T$_H$2 balance of a developing immune response.[521-523] Dendritic cells processing foreign antigens in peripheral tissues migrate to lymph nodes and, by secreting IL-12, induce IFN-γ production by NK cells and IFN-γ and IL-2 synthesis by antigen-stimulated T cells.[470,521-525] Dendritic cell–derived IL-12 is also capable of acting synergistically with the induced IFN-γ to steer naïve T-cell precursors towards T$_H$1 cellular immune responses[481] and of acting synergistically with IL-2 to further augment IFN-γ production and cytotoxic lymphocyte responses.[460,463,466]

In addition to stimulating T$_H$1 activity by naïve cells,[470] IL-12 also has been shown to transform preexisting T$_H$2 responses into responses with an effective T$_H$1 cellular component. Such activity was particularly noteworthy in a murine infectious disease model in which the characteristic detrimental T$_H$2 response was converted into a predominantly curative cellular response after systemic administration of IL-12.[526] That IL-12 can reverse T$_H$2 responses is somewhat paradoxical, as T$_H$2 cells secrete large quantities of IL-4, IL-5, and IL-10,[470] cytokines known to strongly down-regulate the signaling IL-12Rβ2 chain of the IL-12 receptor. Whether this reversal is mediated by the purported capacity of IL-12 to induce transient, low-level production of IFN-γ by T$_H$2 clones[526-528] or rather by the initiation of an overlapping T$_H$1 immune response capable of dominating the preexisting T$_H$2 activity is unclear. The determination that IFN-γ inhibits IL-4, IL-5, and IL-10 synthesis by T$_H$2 cells suggests the possibility that IL-12 mediates its anti-T$_H$2 effects indirectly via stimulation of IFN-γ production by NK cells.[529]

IL-12 has been shown to be an effective antitumor agent in a number of murine models, including the renal cell carcinoma RENCA,[530,531] CT-26 colon adenocarcinoma,[531,532] MCA-105 sarcoma,[533] M5076 reticulum cell sarcoma, B16-F10 melanoma,[530] MC38/colon carcinoma,[533] KA 31 sarcoma,[534] OV-HM ovarian carcinoma,[535] HTH-K breast carcinoma,[536] MBT-2 bladder carcinoma,[537] and MB-48 transitional cell carcinoma,[537] among others. Numerous studies have now demonstrated that IL-12 therapy results in inhibition of tumor growth, reduction of metastatic lesions, increased survival time, and in some models regression of and resistance to secondary challenge with the same tumor.[530,537] IL-12 is distinctive among cytokines displaying antitumor activity in that it often has proven effective even when therapy is initiated weeks after establishment of a significant tumor burden.[530,531,537,538] An exception to this pattern is the HTH-K breast carcinoma model, against which IL-12 mediated measurable antitumor activity only when administered 3 days but not 7 days after tumor cell inoculation.[536]

IL-12 has no direct cytotoxicity or antiproliferative effect on cultured tumor cells, which indicates that its antitumor effect is mediated indirectly through IL-12–inducible cellular and molecular intermediates.[530] One molecule induced by and central to IL-12 activity is IFN-γ, as antibodies to that protein essentially abrogate IL-12–mediated antitumor function.[533,539,540] Interestingly, although IFN-γ is required for IL-12 activity, administration of exogenous IFN-γ does not mediate the potent antitumor function characteristic of IL-12.[541] Several factors may explain this paradox, including the differential half-lives of the two cytokines and the more limited capacity of IFN-γ to reach the tumor site: whereas IFN-γ receptors are ubiquitously expressed on numerous cell types outside the tumor environment, IL-12 receptors are limited to NK cells and activated T cells.[541] Thus, compared with IFN-γ, systemically administered IL-12 is much less apt to be completely consumed by cells irrelevant to the antitumor immune response before reaching the specific effector cell types that will ultimately mediate function.[541]

Many investigators have shown that IL-12 enhances NK and cytolytic T-lymphocyte activity, stimulates antigen-primed T cells to proliferate and differentiate into T$_H$1 cells, and induces NK cells and sensitized T cells to secrete IFN-γ. One study demonstrated that a preexisting CD8 and NK cell tumor infiltrate is required for maximal efficacy of IL-12–mediated antitumor therapy.[541] The suggestion was made that these IL-12–responsive cells synthesize IFN-γ within the tumor bed, which induces the local molecular events required for tumor eradication.[541] This hypothesis would explain why established tumors are often more susceptible to IL-12 administration than nascent tumors, because large immunogenic tumors are more apt than small ones to contain significant inflammatory infiltrates.

Data support at least three distinct mechanisms of IL-12–mediated antitumor activity, each of which requires IFN-γ as an induced molecular intermediate to execute the response. Tannenbaum et al. demonstrated that a molecular correlate of effective IL-12 antitumor activity in the murine RENCA model is the expression of two chemokines, monokine induced by IFN-γ (MIG) and IFN-γ–inducible protein 10 (IP-10), within the regressing tumor.[542] These molecules have since been determined to be chemotactic for NK and activated T cells, which correlates well with immunohistologic data indicating a tremendous influx of CD8$^+$ and CD4$^+$ cells into the treated tumor.[531,542] The tumors undergoing therapy were also characterized by elevated levels of the cytotoxins perforin and granzyme B, which may be among the terminal effector molecules of the infiltrating CD8 T cells in this system.[531,542,543] An integral role for the IFN-γ–inducible chemokines in IL-12–mediated antitumor activity was indicated by subsequent studies in which antibodies to MIG and IP-10 abrogated all correlates of IL-12–mediated tumor eradication: tumor shrinkage, the T-cell infiltrate, and perforin expression within the tumor bed.[531] When explants of human renal tumors were treated in vitro with IL-12, a sequence of molecular events similar to those observed in the murine model was observed: explanted RCC synthesized IFN-γ and IP-10 mRNA in response to the IL-12 treatment.[544] These results were also consistent with the authors' findings that biopsied renal tumors from patients enrolled in a phase I IL-12 trial variably expressed augmented levels of those molecules after therapy.[544] The conclusion was thus that, as in the murine system, recombinant human IL-12 treatment of patients with RCC has the potential to induce the expression of gene products within the tumor bed that may contribute to the development of a successful immune response.

Numerous other studies support the role of enhanced cellular immunity in the IL-12 antitumor effect. Early experiments performed with this cytokine demonstrated a strict requirement for T cells, as IL-12 antitumor function was essentially abrogated in nude mice and in mice depleted of CD8 T cells.[530] A negligible role for NK cells was suggested, however, by the finding that IL-12 antitumor function remained basically normal when therapy was performed in beige mice or wild-type mice depleted of NK cells by treatment with anti-asialo GM1.[530] Multiple laboratories also reported a rapid and significant infiltration of IL-12–treated tumors by macrophages,[542,545] and additional studies determined that tumor-infiltrating polymorphonuclear leukocytes are also an important component of the IL-12 response.[546] Perforin knockout mice have been shown to be unresponsive to IL-12 antitumor therapy,[543] a result that supports the correlation originally found between IL-12 efficacy and intratumoral perforin expression.[542]

When the antitumor activities of intratumorally and intraperitoneally administered IL-12 were compared, both therapeutic modalities were found to lead to similar immune responses at the tumor site: both augmented IFN-γ expression, cytokine expression, chemokine expression, and inflammatory cell infiltration into the tumor bed. Systemic therapy orchestrated these responses more quickly and with greater efficacy than did local IL-12 treatment.[546] Compared with systemic therapy, which immediately activated and rendered peripheral cells responsive to chemotactic signals simultaneously induced at the target site,[546] locally administered IL-12 required additional time to diffuse and stimulate the same sequence of events. The greater rapidity and intensity of the global immune response after systemic IL-12 treatment was thus associated with a more favorable cure rate for large subcutaneous tumors.[546]

A second mechanism by which IL-12–induced IFN-γ mediates antitumor activity is through its stimulation of other molecules with cytotoxic function, including nitric oxide synthase. Nitric oxide synthase is produced by endothelial cells, neurons, epithelial cells, macrophages, and tumor cells themselves, and it catalyzes the production of nitric oxide.[547] Nitric oxide is known to be an important contributor to macrophage antitumor activity, and its central role in the protective process has been demonstrated by the ability of the nitric oxide inhibitor N^G-monomethyl-

L-arginine to abrogate IL-12 antitumor efficacy.[547] IFN-γ has also been shown to induce the tryptophan degradation enzyme indolamine 2,3-dioxygenase within the tumor bed, which converts L-tryptophan to N-formyl L-kynurenine.[548] RNA encoding this enzyme has been detected in IL-12–treated regressing tumor masses, and the enzyme effectively starves the tumor of that required amino acid.

A third mechanism purported to be involved in IL-12–mediated antitumor function is the IFN-γ–dependent induction of various antiangiogenic factors.[549-551] Growing tumors require ongoing neovascularization for nourishment, expansion, and metastatic spread.[552] Several molecules, including the IFN-inducible chemokines MIG, IP-10, and platelet factor 4, have been demonstrated to inhibit IL-8–stimulated angiogenic activity in the rabbit corneal pocket assay[550,553] and in several other in vivo models[549,554-557] and in vitro correlates[549,558,559] of blood vessel formation. One reported determinant of whether a specific CXC chemokine mediates angiogenic or antiangiogenic activity is the amino acid composition of its N-terminal region.[560] The presence of Glu-Leu-Arg, the ELR motif, in the N-terminus of a CXC chemokine endows the molecule with chemotactic activity for neutrophils[561] and angiogenic activity.[556,560] CXC chemokines lacking this motif, on the other hand, such as IP-10, MIG, and PF4, have been found not only to lack chemotactic function but also to inhibit neovascularization.[560] The mechanisms by which these non-ELR CXC chemokines mediate antiangiogenic function is not certain, but in vitro studies show that nanogram concentrations of IP-10 can inhibit endothelial cell chemotaxis,[558] proliferation,[559] and differentiation into tubelike structures.[549] The actual contribution the antiangiogenic molecules make to IL-12–mediated antitumor activity is uncertain; some workers find that IL-12 efficacy is abrogated in T-cell–depleted animals[530,546] and that IP-10 is an effective antitumor agent in euthymic but not in nude mice. Several reports have nonetheless supported a significant role for MIG and IP-10 in tumor necrosis and damage to tumor vasculature when these molecules are injected directly into the tumors of nude mice or induced in those lesions by local or systemic IL-12 therapy.[562,563]

Clinical Pharmacokinetics

Recombinant human IL-12 manufactured by the Genetics Institute is available for clinical trials. It is a lyophilized product and is reconstituted with sterile water. Phase I trials using either i.v. or s.c. administration have been performed.

Motzer et al.[564] performed a phase I trial in which IL-12 was administered subcutaneously at a fixed dose weekly for 3 weeks. An MTD of 0.5 μg/kg per week was identified, with hepatic, hematopoietic, and pulmonary toxicity being dose-limiting. The toxicities seen with IL-12 are summarized

TABLE 36.17
INTERLEUKIN-12 TOXICITY

Constitutional
Fever and chills
Headaches
Nausea and vomiting
Fatigue
Hematologic
Anemia
Leukopenia
Thrombocytopenia
Dose limiting
Leukopenia
Hepatic toxicity
Pulmonary toxicity
Stomatitis

in Table 36.17. A second phase of this trial involved gradual escalation of the IL-12 dose level after an initial dose of 0.1 μg/kg. In this portion, the MTD identified was 1.25 μg/kg.

Intravenous IL-12 has also been investigated in a phase I trial. Forty patients, including 20 with renal cancer, 12 with melanoma, and 5 with colon cancer, were enrolled.[565] Two weeks after a single injection of IL-12 (3 to 1,000 ng/kg), patients received an additional 6-week course of i.v. IL-12 therapy, administered 5 consecutive days every 3 weeks. The MTD was 0.5 μg/kg per day, and the toxicities included fever and chills, fatigue, nausea, and headaches. Laboratory findings included anemia, neutropenia, lymphopenia, hyperglycemia, thrombocytopenia, and hypoalbuminemia.

A phase II trial of i.v. IL-12 was then initiated using 0.5 μg/kg per day for 5 days.[566] Seventeen patients were entered, and due to unexpectedly severe toxicity, the study was abandoned. The data from both the s.c. and i.v. phase I trials suggest that a single predose of IL-12 may be associated with a decrease in toxicity and permits escalation to high dosages. The antitumor effects of IL-12 in early clinical trials are summarized in Table 36.18. Responses have been seen in patients with renal cancer and melanoma but are infrequent.

Table 36.19 outlines serum IL-12 levels in patients receiving IL-12 subcutaneously.[564,567] Studies were also performed during weeks 1 and 7 of drug administration and demonstrate a decrease in IL-12 levels after prolonged administration. This has been termed an adaptive response and has been attributed to either antibody formation or an immunoregulatory feedback response. Antibody formation in response to IL-12 has not been found.[564] Rakhit et al.[567] examined this issue in murine models and noted down-regulation of serum IL-12 levels correlated with up-regulation of IL-12R expression, which was not observed in IL-12Rβ −/− mice. These observation suggest that receptor-mediated clearance is operative and that increases in IL-12R enhance clearance of IL-12.

In preclinical studies, IL-12 induces secretion of IFN-γ by a variety of lymphoid cells. After s.c. or i.v. administration, increases in serum levels of this cytokine are also observed. Rakhit et al.[567] reported that 0.5 μg/kg of IL-12 produces peak levels of 250 pg/mL, with the maximum concentration occurring approximately 24 hours after administration. IFN-γ levels then gradually decreased to baseline over the next 7 days and are minimally elevated with continuous administration of IL-12 (Table 36.20). In patients receiving escalating doses of cytokine, 1.0 μg/kg produced lower serum IFN-γ levels on day 15.[564] In patients receiving i.v. IL-12, dose-dependent increases in serum IFN-γ levels have also been reported.[568] Other surrogate markers such as neopterin also increase, with peak concentrations noted between 72 and 96 hours after administration of a single IL-12 dose.[564] In addition to these effects, administration of IL-12 increases serum levels

TABLE 36.18
ANTITUMOR EFFECTS OF INTERLEUKIN-12 IN PHASE I AND II TRIALS

Tumor Type	No. of Patients Treated	CRs/PRs	Comments
Renal cell cancer	118	2/2	CR durations > 18 mo.
Melanoma	22	0/1	Regressions of subcutaneous and liver lesions reported in 3 patients.
Miscellaneous	8	0/0	Five of 8 patients had colon cancer.

CR, complete response; PR, partial response.
Adapted from Motzer RJ, Rakhit A, Schwartz LH, et al. Phase I trial of subcutaneous recombinant human interleukin-12 in patients with advanced renal cell carcinoma. Clin Cancer Res 1998;4:1183–1191; Atkins MB, Robertson MJ, Gordon M, et al. Phase I evaluation of intravenous recombinant human interleukin 12 in patients with advanced malignancies. Clin Cancer Res 1997;3:409–417; Bajetta E, Del Vecchio M, Mortarini R, et al. Pilot study of subcutaneous recombinant human interleukin 12 in metastatic melanoma. Clin Cancer Res 1998;4:75–85.

TABLE 36.19

PHARMACOKINETICS OF INTERLEUKIN-12 AFTER SUBCUTANEOUS ADMINISTRATION: WEEK 1 VERSUS WEEK 7

Parameter	0.5 μg/kg		1.0 μg/kg	
	Week 1	Week 7	Week 1	Week 7[a]
C_{max} (pg/mL)	321 ± 46	128 ± 422	1,092 ± 275	352 ± 1,693
T_{max} (h)	13.00 ± 1.65	14.0 ± 2.7	16.0 ± 2.7	8.0 ± 0.9
AUC (pg h/mL)	7,043 ± 1,325	1,473 ± 604[b]	26,589 ± 6,633	3,597 ± 1,300[c]

AUC, area under the concentration-time curve; C_{max}, highest observed concentration; T_{max}, sampling time of C_{max}.
[a]Dose reduced to 50%; data are for 0.5 μg/kg given in weeks 2–7.
[b]$P < .001$ for week 7 versus week 1.
[c]$P < .005$ for week 7 versus week 1.
Adapted from Rakhit A, Yeon MM, Ferrante J, et al. Down-regulation of the pharmacokinetic-pharmacodynamic response to interleukin-12 during long-term administration to patients with renal cell carcinoma and evaluation of the mechanism of this "adaptive response" in mice. Clin Pharmacol Ther 1999;65:615–629.

of IL-10,[567] which results in activation of a complex immunoregulatory cytokine network (Table 36.20).

Following IL-12 administration, significant lymphopenia is observed after 24 hours.[568] This involves all the major lymphocyte subsets, with NK cells the most severely affected.[568,569] Augmented NK cytolytic activity and T-cell proliferative responses have also been noted.[568]

Bukowski et al.[544] have investigated the expression of a variety of genes in peripheral blood mononuclear cells after s.c. administration of IL-12 to patients with RCC. Rapid induction of IFN-γ mRNA was found and was accompanied by subsequent induction of mRNA for IP-10 and MIG. These chemokines are IFN-γ inducible and mediate chemotaxis of T lymphocytes.[542] In addition, IP-10 appears to have antiangiogenic effects and decreases proliferation of endothelial cells. Other investigators[559] have also suggested that the antitumor effects of IL-12 may involve inhibition of angiogenesis.[556,559]

Although no overwhelming clinical responses have been noted to date, IL-12 has shown promise in the therapy of various malignancies, including melanoma,[164,570] RCC,[164,571,572] head and neck squamous cell carcinoma,[573] cervical cancer,[574] transitional cell carcinoma of the bladder,[575] lymphoma,[576,577] and hematologic malignancies.[578] In these trials, various methods of administration have been employed, including subcutaneous,[570–572] intravenous,[164,570,574] intratumoral,[573] and intravesical.[575]

Because of its lack of efficacy when given as a single agent, combinations of cytokines have been tested. The combination of IL-12 with IL-2 or IFN-α has been shown to enhance the antitumor effects in melanoma and RCC. Alatrash et al.[572] reported tolerability of subcutaneously administered IL-12 and IFN-α2b and noted the MTD for s.c. IL-12 and IFN-α2b to be 500 ng/kg and 1.0 MU/m², respectively. The addition of IL-12 lowered the MTD for IFN-α2b by up to eightfold compared with prior studies using IFN-α2b either as a single agent or in combination with chemotherapeutic drugs.[579–582] The effects of this combination on cytokine expression (i.e., of IP-10, Mig, IL-5, and IFN-γ) by peripheral blood lymphocytes were similar

TABLE 36.20

INTERFERON γ (IFN-γ) AND INTERLEUKIN-10 (IL-10) LEVELS AFTER SUBCUTANEOUS ADMINISTRATION OF INTERLEUKIN-12 (0.5 μg/kg)[a]

Cycle[b]	IFN-γ (pg/mL)		IL-10 (pg/mL)	
	1	2	1	2
C_{max} (pg/mL)	267 ± 53	34 ± 4	80 ± 13	35 ± 17
T_{max} (h)	24 (24–72)	24 (24)	24 (24–96)	24 (24–48)

[a]Patients with renal cancer ($n = 5$).
[b]Data for cycle 1 collected on day 1 of weekly (weeks 16) subcutaneous administration of IL-12; data for cycle 2 collected in week 7.
Adapted from Rakhit A, Yeon MM, Ferrante J, et al. Down-regulation of the pharmacokinetic-pharmacodynamic response to interleukin-12 during long-term administration to patients with renal cell carcinoma and evaluation of the mechanism of this "adaptive response" in mice. Clin Pharmacol Ther 1999;65:615–629.

to those noted using IL-12 alone in human[571] and murine models.[531] When given in conjunction with s.c. IL-2, i.v. IL-12 was well tolerated at an MTD of 500 ng/kg.[164] The addition of IL-2 after approximately 3 weeks of IL-12 therapy led to the restoration and maintenance of IFN-γ and IP-10 levels in patient blood samples, which were otherwise noted to decrease to below those at the initiation of IL-12 therapy. The activation and expansion of NK cell populations was also noted with this combination. Although some disease stabilizations and partial responses were noted, phase II studies need to be conducted to further define the role of these combinations in RCC and melanoma.

REFERENCES

1. Kasakura S, Lowenstein L. A factor stimulating DNA synthesis derived from the medium of leukocyte cultures. Nature 1965; 208:794–795.
2. Morgan DA, Ruscetti FW, Gallo R. Selective in vitro growth of T lymphocytes from normal human bone marrows. Science 1976;193:1007–1008.
3. Gillis S, Union NA, Baker PE, et al. The in vitro generation and sustained culture of nude mouse cytolytic T-lymphocytes. J Exp Med 1979;149:1460–1476.
4. Taniguchi T, Matsui H, Fujita T, et al. Structure and expression of a cloned cDNA for human interleukin-2 [1983 classic article]. Biotechnology 1992;24:304–309.
5. Smith KA. Lowest dose interleukin-2 immunotherapy. Blood 1993;81:1414–1423.
6. Bazan JF. Unraveling the structure of IL-2 [letter]. Science 1992;257:410–413.
7. Sherblom AP, Sathyamoorthy N, Decker JM, et al. IL-2, a lectin with specificity for high mannose glycopeptides. J Immunol 1989;143:939–944.
8. Landgraf BE, Williams DP, Murphy JR, et al. Conformational perturbation of interleukin-2: a strategy for the design of cytokine analogs. Proteins 1991;9:207–216.
9. Mosmann TR, Cherwinski H, Bond MW, et al. Two types of murine helper T cell clone, I: definition according to profiles of lymphokine activities and secreted proteins. J Immunol 1986; 136:2348–2357.
10. Kroemer G, Helmberg A, Bernot A, et al. Evolutionary relationship between human and mouse immunoglobulin kappa light chain variable region genes. Immunogenetics 1991;33:42–49.
11. Linsley PS, Clark EA, Ledbetter JA. T-cell antigen CD28 mediates adhesion with B cells by interacting with activation antigen B7/BB-1. Proc Natl Acad Sci USA 1990;87:5031–5035.
12. Mueller DL, Jenkins MK, Schwartz RH. Clonal expansion versus functional clonal inactivation: a costimulatory signalling pathway determines the outcome of T cell antigen receptor occupancy. Annu Rev Immunol 1989;7:445–480.
13. Lindstein T, June CH, Ledbetter JA, et al. Regulation of lymphokine messenger RNA stability by a surface-mediated T cell activation pathway. Science 1989;244:339–343.
14. Ullman KS, Northrop JP, Verweij CL, et al. Transmission of signals from the T lymphocyte antigen receptor to the genes responsible for cell proliferation and immune function: the missing link. Annu Rev Immunol 1990;8:421–452.
15. Takeshita T, Asao H, Ohtani K, et al. Cloning of the gamma chain of the human IL-2 receptor. Science 1992;257:379–382.
16. Leonard WJ, Depper JM, Crabtree GR, et al. Molecular cloning and expression of cDNAs for the human interleukin-2 receptor. Nature 1984;311:626–631.
17. Nikaido T, Shimizu A, Ishida N, et al. Molecular cloning of cDNA encoding human interleukin-2 receptor. Nature 1984;311: 631–635.
18. Hatakeyama M, Tsudo M, Minamoto S, et al. Interleukin-2 receptor beta chain gene: generation of three receptor forms by cloned human alpha and beta chain cDNA's. Science 1989;244: 551–556.
19. Nakamura Y, Russell SM, Mess SA, et al. Heterodimerization of the IL-2 receptor beta- and gamma-chain cytoplasmic domains is required for signalling. Nature 1994;369:330–333.
20. Nelson BH, Lord JD, Greenberg PD. Cytoplasmic domains of the interleukin-2 receptor beta and gamma chains mediate the signal for T-cell proliferation. Nature 1994;369:333–336.
21. Gesbert F, Delespine-Carmagnat M, Bertoglio J. Recent advances in the understanding of interleukin-2 signal transduction. J Clin Immunol 1998;18:307–320.
22. Miyazaki T, Liu ZJ, Kawahara A, et al. Three distinct IL-2 signaling pathways mediated by bcl-2, c-myc, and lck cooperate in hematopoietic cell proliferation: critical role of the interleukin 2 (IL-2) receptor gamma-chain–associated Jak3 in the IL-2–induced c-fos and c-myc, but not bcl-2, gene induction. Proc Natl Acad Sci USA 1995;92:8724–8728.
23. Nosaka T, van Deursen JM, Tripp RA, et al. Defective lymphoid development in mice lacking Jak3 [published erratum appears in Science 1996;271:17]. Science 1995;270:800–802.
24. Chen M, Cheng A, Chen YQ, et al. The amino terminus of JAK3 is necessary and sufficient for binding to the common gamma chain and confers the ability to transmit interleukin 2–mediated signals. Proc Natl Acad Sci USA 1997;94:6910–6915.
25. Kawahara A, Kobayashi T, Nagata S. Inhibition of Fas-induced apoptosis by Bcl-2. Oncogene 1998;17:2549–2554.
26. Noguchi M, Yi H, Rosenblatt HM, et al. Interleukin-2 receptor gamma chain mutation results in X-linked severe combined immunodeficiency in humans. Cell 1993;73:147–157.
27. Kanazawa T, Keeler ML, Varticovski L. Serine-rich region of the IL-2 receptor beta-chain is required for activation of phosphatidylinositol 3-kinase. Cell Immunol 1994;156:378–388.
28. Ahmed NN, Grimes HL, Bellacosa A, et al. Transduction of interleukin-2 antiapoptotic and proliferative signals via Akt protein kinase. Proc Natl Acad Sci USA 1997;94:3627–3632.
29. Minami Y, Nakagawa Y, Kawahara A, et al. Protein tyrosine kinase Syk is associated with and activated by the IL-2 receptor: possible link with the c-myc induction pathway. Immunity 1995; 2:89–100.
30. Miyazaki T, Kawahara A, Fujii H, et al. Functional activation of Jak1 and Jak3 by selective association with IL-2 receptor subunits. Science 1994;266:1045–1047.
31. Hatakeyama M, Kono T, Kobayashi N, et al. Interaction of the IL-2 receptor with the src-family kinase p56lck: identification of novel intermolecular association. Science 1991;252:1523–1528.
32. Minami Y, Kono T, Yamada K, et al. Association of p56lck with IL-2 receptor beta chain is critical for the IL-2–induced activation of p56lck. EMBO J 1993;12:759–768.
33. Gennuso R, Spigelman MK, Vallabhajosula S, et al. Systemic biodistribution of radioiodinated interleukin-2 in the rat. J Biol Response Mod 1989;8:375–384.
34. Evans GA, Goldsmith MA, Johnston JA, et al. Analysis of interleukin-2–dependent signal transduction through the Shc/Grb2 adapter pathway: interleukin-2–dependent mitogenesis does not require Shc phosphorylation or receptor association. J Biol Chem 1995;270:28858–28863.
35. Satoh T, Minami Y, Kono T, et al. Interleukin 2–induced activation of Ras requires two domains of interleukin 2 receptor beta subunit, the essential region for growth stimulation and Lck-binding domain. J Biol Chem 1992;267:25423–25427.
36. Gaffen SL, Lai SY, Ha M, et al. Distinct tyrosine residues within the interleukin-2 receptor beta chain drive signal transduction specificity, redundancy, and diversity. J Biol Chem 1996;271: 21381–21390.
37. Fujii H, Nakagawa Y, Schindler U, et al. Activation of Stat5 by interleukin 2 requires a carboxyl-terminal region of the interleukin 2 receptor beta chain but is not essential for the proliferative signal transmission. Proc Natl Acad Sci USA 1995;92:5482–5486.
38. Nakajima H, Liu XW, Wynshaw-Boris A, et al. An indirect effect of Stat5a in IL-2–induced proliferation: a critical role for Stat5a in IL-2–mediated IL-2 receptor alpha chain induction. Immunity 1997;7:691–701.

39. Siegel JP, Sharon M, Smith PL, et al. The IL-2 receptor beta chain (p70): role in mediating signals for LAK, NK, and proliferative activities. Science 1987;238:75–78.

40. Tsudo M, Goldman CK, Bongiovanni KF, et al. The p75 peptide is the receptor for interleukin 2 expressed on large granular lymphocytes and is responsible for the interleukin 2 activation of these cells. Proc Natl Acad Sci USA 1987;84:5394–5398.

41. Caligiuri MA, Zmuidzinas A, Manley TJ, et al. Functional consequences of interleukin 2 receptor expression on resting human lymphocytes: identification of a novel natural killer cell subset with high affinity receptors. J Exp Med 1990;171:1509–1526.

42. Cantrell DA, Smith KA, Muraguchi A, et al. Transient expression of interleukin 2 receptors: consequences for T cell growth. J Exp Med 1985;161:181–197.

43. Muraguchi A, Kehrl JH, Longo DL, et al. Interleukin 2 receptors on human B cells: implications for the role of interleukin 2 in human B cell function. J Exp Med 1985;161:181–197.

44. Turner B, Rapp U, App H, et al. Interleukin 2 induces tyrosine phosphorylation and activation of p72-74 Raf-1 kinase in a T-cell line. Proc Natl Acad Sci USA 1991;88:1227–1231.

45. Zmuidzinas A, Mamon HJ, Roberts TM, et al. Interleukin-2–triggered Raf-1 expression, phosphorylation, and associated kinase activity increase through G1 and S in CD3-stimulated primary human T cells. Mol Cell Biol 1991;11:2794–2803.

46. Evans GA, Wahl LM, Farrar WL. Interleukin-2–dependent phosphorylation of the retinoblastoma-susceptibility-gene product p110-115RB in human T-cells. Biochem J 1992;282:759–764.

47. Baker PE, Gillis S, Smith KA. Monoclonal cytolytic T-cell lines. J Exp Med 1979;149:273–278.

48. Baker PE, Gillis S, Ferm MM, et al. The effect of T cell growth factor on the generation of cytolytic T cells. J Immunol 1978;121:2168–2173.

49. Kroemer G, Andreu JL, Gonzale JA, et al. Interleukin-2, autotolerance and autoimmunity. Adv Immunology 1991;50: 147–235.

50. Grimm EA, Mazumder A, Zhang HZ, et al. Lymphokine-activated killer cell phenomenon: lysis of natural killer–resistant fresh solid tumor cells by interleukin 2–activated autologous human peripheral blood lymphocytes. J Exp Med 1982;155:1823–1841.

51. Liu CC, Rafii S, Granelli-Piperno A, et al. Perforin and serine esterase gene expression in stimulated human T cells: kinetics, mitogen requirements, and effects of cyclosporin A. J Exp Med 1989;170:2105–2118.

52. Lenardo M, Chan KM, Hornung F, et al. Mature T lymphocyte apoptosis-immune regulation in a dynamic and unpredictable antigenic environment. Annu Rev Immunol 1999;17:221–253.

53. Refaeli Y, Van Parijs L, Abbas AK. Genetic models of abnormal apoptosis in lymphocytes. Immunol Rev 1999;169:273–282.

54. Willerford DM, Chen J, Ferry JA, et al. Interleukin-2 receptor alpha chain regulates the size and content of the peripheral lymphoid compartment. Immunity 1995;3:521–530.

55. Suzuki H, Kundig TM, Furlonger C, et al. Deregulated T cell activation and autoimmunity in mice lacking interleukin-2 receptor beta. Science 1995;268:1472–1476.

56. Sadlack B, Merz H, Schorle H, et al. Ulcerative colitis-like disease in mice with a disrupted interleukin-2 gene: interleukin-2 programs mouse alpha beta T lymphocytes for apoptosis. Nature 1991;353:858–861.

57. Lenardo MJ. Interleukin-2 programs mouse alpha beta T lymphocytes for apoptosis. Nature 1991;353:858–861.

58. Refaeli Y, Van Parijs L, London CA, et al. Biochemical mechanisms of IL-2–regulated Fas-mediated T cell apoptosis. Immunity 1998;8:615–623.

59. Bocci V, Carraro F, Zeuli M, et al. The lymphatic route, VIII: distribution and plasma clearance of recombinant human interleukin-2 after SC administration with albumin in patients [published erratum appears in Biotherapy 1993;6:233]. Biotherapy 1993;6:73–77.

60. Lotze MT, Matory YL, Ettinghausen SE, et al. In vivo administration of purified human interleukin 2, II: half life, immunologic effects, and expansion of peripheral lymphoid cells in vivo with recombinant IL 2 T cell growth factor: parameters of production and a quantitative microassay for activity. J Immunol 1978;120:2027–2032.

61. Gillis S, Ferm MM, Ou W, et al. T cell growth factor: parameters of production and a quantitative microassay for activity. J Immunol 1978;120:2027–2032.

62. Lotze MT, Matory YL, Rayner AA, et al. Clinical effects and toxicity of interleukin-2 in patients with cancer. Cancer 1986;58:2764–2772.

63. Sarna GP, Figlin RA, Pertcheck M, et al. Systemic administration of recombinant methionyl human interleukin-2 (Ala 125) to cancer patients: clinical results. J Biol Response Mod 1989;8:16–24.

64. Sosman JA, Kohler PC, Hank JA, et al. Repetitive weekly cycles of interleukin-2, II: clinical and immunologic effects of dose, schedule, and addition of indomethacin. J Natl Cancer Inst 1988;80:1451–1461.

65. Zimmerman RJ, Aukerman SL, Katre NV, et al. Schedule dependency of the antitumor activity and toxicity of polyethylene glycol–modified interleukin 2 in murine tumor models. Cancer Res 1989;49:6521–6528.

66. Tursz T. [Interleukin 2: present and future role in cancerology (editorial)]. Presse Med 1991;20:241–243.

67. Tzannis ST, Hrushesky WJ, Wood PA, et al. Irreversible inactivation of interleukin 2 in a pump-based delivery environment. Proc Natl Acad Sci USA 1996;93:5460–5465.

68. Gearing AJ, Thorpe R. The international standard for human interleukin-2: calibration by international collaborative study. J Immunol Methods 1988;114:3–9.

69. Rossio JL, Thurman GB, Long C, et al. The BRMP IL-2 reference reagent. Lymphokine Res 1986;5(Suppl 1):S13–18.

70. Hank JA, Surfus J, Gan J, et al. Distinct clinical and laboratory activity of two recombinant interleukin-2 preparations. Clin Cancer Res 1999;5:281–289.

71. Meyers FJ, Paradise C, Scudder SA, et al. A phase I study including pharmacokinetics of polyethylene glycol conjugated interleukin-2. Clin Pharmacol Ther 1991;49:307–313.

72. Konrad MW, Hemstreet G, Hersh EM, et al. Pharmacokinetics of recombinant interleukin 2 in humans. Cancer Res 1990;50:2009–2017.

73. Knauf MJ, Bell DP, Hirtzer P, et al. Relationship of effective molecular size to systemic clearance in rats of recombinant interleukin-2 chemically modified with water-soluble polymers. J Biol Chem 1988;263:15064–15070.

74. Donohue JH, Rosenberg SA. The fate of interleukin-2 after in vivo administration. J Immunol 1983;130:2203–2208.

75. Banks RE, Forbes MA, Hallam S, et al. Treatment of metastatic renal cell carcinoma with subcutaneous interleukin 2: evidence for non-renal clearance of cytokines. Br J Cancer 1997;75:1842–1848.

76. Kirchner GI, Franzke A, Buer J, et al. Pharmacokinetics of recombinant human interleukin-2 in advanced renal cell carcinoma patients following subcutaneous application: natural history and therapy of metastatic renal cell carcinoma: the role of interleukin-2. Cancer 1997;80:1198–1220.

77. Upton MP, Parker RA, Youmans A, et al. Histologic predictors of renal cell carcinoma (RCC) response to interleukin-2–based therapy [abstract]. Proc Am Soc Clin Oncol 2003;22:851 (abstr. 3420).

78. Rosenberg SA, Lotze MT, Yang JC, et al. Experience with the use of high-dose interleukin-2 in the treatment of 652 cancer patients. Ann Surg 1989;210:474–484; discussion.

79. Fisher RI, Rosenberg SA, Sznol M, et al. High-dose aldesleukin in renal cell carcinoma: long-term survival update: recent advances in the understanding of interleukin-2 signal transduction. J Clin Immunol 1998;18:307–320.

80. Fisher B, Keenan AM, Garra BS, et al. Interleukin-2 induces profound reversible cholestasis: a detailed analysis in treated cancer patients. J Clin Oncol 1989;7:1852–1862.

81. Bukowski RM, Goodman P, Crawford ED, et al. Phase II trial of high-dose intermittent interleukin-2 in metastatic renal cell carcinoma: a Southwest Oncology Group study. J Natl Cancer Inst 1990;82:143–146.

82. Palmer PA, Vinke J, Philip T, et al. Prognostic factors for survival in patients with advanced renal cell carcinoma treated with recombinant interleukin-2. Ann Oncol 1992;3:475–480.

83. Sleijfer DT, Janssen RA, Buter J, et al. Phase II study of subcutaneous interleukin-2 in unselected patients with advanced renal

cell cancer on an outpatient basis. J Clin Oncol 1992;10: 1119–1123.

84. Negrier S, Escudier B, Lasset C, et al. Recombinant human interleukin-2, recombinant human interferon alfa-2a, or both in metastatic renal-cell carcinoma. Groupe Francais d'Immunotherapie. N Engl J Med 1998;338:1272–1278.

85. Bukowski RM, Dutcher JD, Low dose interleukin-2: single agent and combination regimens. In: Scardino PT, Shipley W, Cobbey DS, eds. Comprehensive Textbook of Genitourinary Oncology. Philadelphia: Lippincott Williams & Wilkins, 2000: 218–233.

86. Bukowski RM. Natural history and therapy of metastatic renal cell carcinoma: the role of interleukin-2. Cancer 1997;80: 1198–1220.

87. Escudier B, Ravaud A, Fabbro M, et al. High-dose interleukin-2 two days a week for metastatic renal cell carcinoma: a FNCLCC multicenter study. J Immunother Emphasis Tumor Immunol 1994;16:306–312.

88. Geertsen PF, Gore ME, Negrier S, et al. Safety and efficacy of subcutaneous and continuous intravenous infusion rIL-2 in patients with metastatic renal cell carcinoma. Br J Cancer 2004;90: 1156–1162.

89. Caligiuri MA. Low-dose recombinant interleukin-2 therapy: rationale and potential clinical applications. Semin Oncol 1993; 20:3–10.

90. Buter J, Sleijfer DT, van der Graaf WT, et al. A progress report on the outpatient treatment of patients with advanced renal cell carcinoma using subcutaneous recombinant interleukin-2. Semin Oncol 1993;20:16–21.

91. Lissoni P, Bordin V, Vaghi M, et al. Ten-year survival results in metastatic renal cell cancer patients treated with monoimmunotherapy with subcutaneous low-dose interleukin-2. Anticancer Res 2002;22(2B):1061–1064.

92. Yang JC, Sherry RM, Steinberg SM, et al. Randomized study of high-dose and low-dose interleukin-2 in patients with metastatic renal cancer. J Clin Oncol 2003;21:3127–3132.

93. McDermott DF, Flaherty L, Clark J. A randomized phase III trial of high-dose interleukin-2 (HD IL2) versus subcutaneous (SC) IL2/interferon (IFN) in patients with metastatic renal cell carcinoma [abstract]. Proc Am Soc Clin Oncol 2001;20:172a.

94. Atkins MB, Sparano J, Fisher RI, et al. Randomized phase II trial of high-dose interleukin-2 either alone or in combination with interferon alfa-2b in advanced renal cell carcinoma. J Clin Oncol 1993;11:661–670.

95. Baaten G, Voogd AC, Wagstaff J. A systematic review of the relation between interleukin-2 schedule and outcome in patients with metastatic renal cell cancer. Eur J Cancer 2004;40: 1127–1144.

96. McDermott DF, Atkins MB. Application of IL-2 and other cytokines in renal cancer. Expert Opin Biol Ther 2004;4: 455–468.

97. Coppin C, Porzsolt F, Kumpf J, et al. Immunotherapy for advanced renal cancer. Cochrane Database Syst Rev 2000;(3):CD001425.

98. Figlin R, Gitlitz B, Franklin J, et al. Interleukin-2–based immunotherapy for the treatment of metastatic renal cell carcinoma: an analysis of 203 consecutively treated patients. Cancer J Sci Am 1997;3(Suppl 1):S92–97.

99. McDermott DF, Parker R, Youmans A. The effect of recent nephrectomy on treatment with high-dose interleukin-2 (HD IL-2) or subcutaneous (SC) IL-2/interferon alfa-2b (IFN) in patients with metastatic renal cell carcinoma [abstract]. Proc Am Soc Clin Oncol 2003;22:385.

100. Negrier S, Caty A, Lesimple T, et al. Treatment of patients with metastatic renal carcinoma with a combination of subcutaneous interleukin-2 and interferon alfa with or without fluorouracil. Groupe Francais d'Immunotherapie, Federation Nationale des Centres de Lutte Contre le Cancer. J Clin Oncol 2000;18: 4009–4015.

101. Royal RE, Steinberg SM, Krouse RS, et al. Correlates of response to IL-2 therapy in patients treated for metastatic renal cancer and melanoma. Cancer J Sci Am 1996;2:91.

102. Fumagalli LA, Vinke J, Hoff W, et al. Lymphocyte counts independently predict overall survival in advanced cancer patients: a

biomarker for IL-2 immunotherapy. J Immunother 2003;26: 394–402.

103. Atkins MB, Mier JW, Parkinson DR, et al. Hypothyroidism after treatment with interleukin-2 and lymphokine-activated killer cells. N Engl J Med 1988;318:1557–1563.

104. Janik JE, Sznol M, Urba WJ, et al. Erythropoietin production: a potential marker for interleukin-2/interferon-responsive tumors. Cancer 1993;72:2656–2659.

105. Newman SP, Clarke SW. Therapeutic aerosols 1: physical and practical considerations. Thorax 1983;38:881–886.

106. Huland E, Huland H, Heinzer H. Interleukin-2 by inhalation: local therapy for metastatic renal cell carcinoma. J Urol 1992; 147:344–348.

107. Huland E, Heinzer H, Mir TS, et al. Inhaled interleukin-2 therapy in pulmonary metastatic renal cell carcinoma: six years of experience. Cancer J Sci Am 1997;3(Suppl 1):S98–105.

108. Lorenz J, Wilhelm K, Kessler M, et al. Phase I trial of inhaled natural interleukin 2 for treatment of pulmonary malignancy: toxicity, pharmacokinetics, and biological effects. Clin Cancer Res 1996;2:1115–1122.

109. Nakamoto T, Kasaoka Y, Mitani S, et al. Inhalation of interleukin-2 combined with subcutaneous administration of interferon for the treatment of pulmonary metastases from renal cell carcinoma. Int J Urol 1997;4:343–348.

110. Huland E, Burger A, Fleischer J, et al. Efficacy and safety of inhaled recombinant interleukin-2 in high-risk renal cell cancer patients compared with systemic interleukin-2: an outcome study. Folia Biol (Praha), 2003;49:183–190.

111. Merimsky O, Gez E, Weitzen R, et al. Targeting pulmonary metastases of renal cell carcinoma by inhalation of interleukin-2. Ann Oncol, 2004;15:610–612.

112. Skubitz KM, Anderson PM. Inhalational interleukin-2 liposomes for pulmonary metastases: a phase I clinical trial. Anticancer Drugs 2000;11:555–563.

113. Ravaud A, Audhuy B, Gomez F, et al. Subcutaneous interleukin-2, interferon alfa-2a, and continuous infusion of fluorouracil in metastatic renal cell carcinoma: a multicenter phase II trial. Groupe Francais d'Immunotherapie. J Clin Oncol 1998;16: 2728–2732.

114. Freedman RS, Gibbons JA, Giedlin M, et al. Immunopharmacology and cytokine production of a low-dose schedule of intraperitoneally administered human recombinant interleukin-2 in patients with advanced epithelial ovarian carcinoma. J Immunother Emphasis Tumor Immunol 1996;19: 443–451.

115. Kolitz JE, Welte K, Wong GY, et al. Expansion of activated T-lymphocytes in patients treated with recombinant interleukin 2. J Biol Response Mod 1987;6:412–429.

116. Gambacorti-Passerini C, Radrizzani M, Marolda R, et al. In vivo activation of lymphocytes in melanoma patients receiving escalating doses of recombinant interleukin 2. Int J Cancer 1988; 41:700–706.

117. Thompson JA, Lee DJ, Lindgren CG, et al. Influence of dose and duration of infusion of interleukin-2 on toxicity and immunomodulation. J Clin Oncol 1988;6:669–678.

118. Caligiuri MA, Murray C, Robertson MJ, et al. Selective modulation of human natural killer cells in vivo after prolonged infusion of low dose recombinant interleukin 2. J Clin Invest 1993;91:123–132.

119. Oshimi K, Oshimi Y, Akutsu M, et al. Cytotoxicity of interleukin 2–activated lymphocytes for leukemia and lymphoma cells. Blood 1986;68:938–948.

120. Fierro MT, Liao XS, Lusso P, et al. In vitro and in vivo susceptibility of human leukemic cells to lymphokine activated killer activity. Leukemia 1988;2:50–54.

121. Foa R, Caretto P, Fierro MT, et al. Interleukin 2 does not promote the in vitro and in vivo proliferation and growth of human acute leukaemia cells of myeloid and lymphoid origin. Br J Haematol 1990;75:34–40.

122. Meloni G, Foa R, Vignetti M, et al. Interleukin-2 may induce prolonged remissions in advanced acute myelogenous leukemia. Blood 1994;84:2158–2163.

123. Foa R, Meloni G, Tosti S, et al. Treatment of acute myeloid leukaemia patients with recombinant interleukin 2: a pilot study. Br J Haematol 1991;77:491–496.

124. Maraninchi D, Blaise D, Viens P, et al. High-dose recombinant interleukin-2 and acute myeloid leukemias in relapse. Blood 1991;78:2182–2187.

125. Slavin S, Naparstek E, Nagler A, et al. Allogeneic cell therapy for relapsed leukemia after bone marrow transplantation with donor peripheral blood lymphocytes. Exp Hematol 1995;23:1553–1562.

126. Soiffer RJ, Murray C, Gonin R, et al. Effect of low-dose interleukin-2 on disease relapse after T-cell–depleted allogeneic bone marrow transplantation. Blood 1994;84:964–971.

127. Nadal E, Fowler A, Kanfer E, et al. Adjuvant interleukin-2 therapy for patients refractory to donor lymphocyte infusions. Exp Hematol 2004;32:218–223.

128. Van Besien K, Mehra R, Wadehra N, et al. Phase II study of autologous transplantation with interleukin-2–incubated peripheral blood stem cells and posttransplantation interleukin-2 in relapsed or refractory non-Hodgkin lymphoma. Biol Blood Marrow Transplant 2004;10:386–394.

129. Weiss L, Reich S, Slavin S. Use of recombinant human interleukin-2 in conjunction with bone marrow transplantation as a model for control of minimal residual disease in malignant hematological disorders, I: treatment of murine leukemia in conjunction with allogeneic bone marrow transplantation and IL-2–activated cell-mediated immunotherapy. Cancer Invest 1992; 10:19–26.

130. Slavin S, Ackerstein A, Weiss L, et al. Immunotherapy of minimal residual disease by immunocompetent lymphocytes and their activation by cytokines. Cancer Invest 1992;10:221–227.

131. Cotran RS, Pober JS, Gimbrone MA Jr, et al. Endothelial activation during interleukin 2 immunotherapy: a possible mechanism for the vascular leak syndrome. J Immunol 1988;140:1883–1888.

132. Gemlo BT, Palladino MA Jr, Jaffe HS, et al. Circulating cytokines in patients with metastatic cancer treated with recombinant interleukin 2 and lymphokine-activated killer cells. Cancer Res 1988;48:5864–5867.

133. Mier JW, Vachino G, van der Meer JW, et al. Induction of circulating tumor necrosis factor (TNF alpha) as the mechanism for the febrile response to interleukin-2 (IL-2) in cancer patients. J Clin Immunol 1988;8:426–436.

134. Kasid A, Director EP, Rosenberg SA. Induction of endogenous cytokine-mRNA in circulating peripheral blood mononuclear cells by IL-2 administration to cancer patients. J Immunol 1989;143:736–739.

135. Wiebke EA, Rosenberg SA, Lotze MT. Acute immunologic effects of interleukin-2 therapy in cancer patients: decreased delayed type hypersensitivity response and decreased proliferative response to soluble antigens. J Clin Oncol 1988;6: 1440–1449.

136. Klempner MS, Noring R, Mier JW, et al. An acquired chemotactic defect in neutrophils from patients receiving interleukin-2 immunotherapy. N Engl J Med 1990;322:959–965.

137. Parkinson DR. Interleukin-2 in cancer therapy. Semin Oncol 1988;15:10–26.

138. Gaynor ER, Vitek L, Sticklin L, et al. The hemodynamic effects of treatment with interleukin-2 and lymphokine-activated killer cells. Ann Intern Med 1988;109:953–958.

139. Nora R, Abrams JS, Tait NS, et al. Myocardial toxic effects during recombinant interleukin-2 therapy. J Natl Cancer Inst 1989;81:59–63.

140. Osanto S, Cluitmans FH, Franks CR, et al. Myocardial injury after interleukin-2 therapy [letter]. Lancet 1988;2:48–49.

141. Yang JC, Rosenberg SA. An ongoing prospective randomized comparison of interleukin-2 regimens for the treatment of metastatic renal cell cancer. Cancer J Sci Am 1997;3(Suppl 1):S79–84.

142. Ettinghausen SE, Moore JG, White DE, et al. Hematologic effects of immunotherapy with lymphokine-activated killer cells and recombinant interleukin-2 in cancer patients. Blood 1987;69:1654–1660.

143. Snydman DR, Sullivan B, Gill M, et al. Nosocomial sepsis associated with interleukin-2. Ann Intern Med 1990;112:102–107.

144. Post AB, Falk GW, Bukowski RM. Acute colonic pseudo-obstruction associated with interleukin-2 therapy. Am J Gastroenterol 1991;86:1539–1541.

145. Schwartzentruber D, Lotze MT, Rosenberg SA. Colonic perforation: an unusual complication of therapy with high-dose interleukin-2. Cancer, 1988;62:2350–2353.

146. Rahman R, Bernstein Z, Vaickus L, et al. Unusual gastrointestinal complications of interleukin-2 therapy. J Immunother 1991;10:221–225.

147. Denicoff KD, Rubinow DR, Papa MZ, et al. The neuropsychiatric effects of treatment with interleukin-2 and lymphokine-activated killer cells. Ann Intern Med 1987;107:293–300.

148. Saris SC, Patronas NJ, Rosenberg SA. The effect of intravenous interleukin-2 on brain water content. J Neurosurg 1989;71:169–174.

149. Caraceni A, Martini C, Belli F, et al. Neuropsychological and neurophysiological assessment of the central effects of interleukin-2 administration. Eur J Cancer 1993;29A:1266–1269.

150. Adams F, Quesada JR, Gutterman JU. Neuropsychiatric manifestations of human leukocyte interferon therapy in patients with cancer. JAMA 1984;252:938–941.

151. Gaspari AA, Lotze MT, Rosenberg SA, et al. Dermatologic changes associated with interleukin 2 administration. JAMA 1987;258:1624–1629.

152. Lee RE, Gaspari AA, Lotze MT, et al. Interleukin 2 and psoriasis. Arch Dermatol 1988;124:1811–1815.

153. Atkins MB, Mier JW, Parkinson DR, et al. Hypothyroidism after treatment with interleukin-2 and lymphokine-activated killer cells. N Engl J Med 1988;318:1557–1563.

154. Pichert G, Jost LM, Zobeli L, et al. Thyroiditis after treatment with interleukin-2 and interferon alpha-2a. Br J Cancer 1990;62:100–104.

155. Franzke A, Peest D, Probst-Kepper M, et al. Autoimmunity resulting from cytokine treatment predicts long-term survival in patients with metastatic renal cell cancer. J Clin Oncol 1999;17:529–533.

156. Papa MZ, Vetto JT, Ettinghausen SE, et al. Effect of corticosteroid on the antitumor activity of lymphokine-activated killer cells and interleukin 2 in mice. Cancer Res 1986;46:5618–5623.

157. Mier JW, Vachino G, Klempner MS, et al. Inhibition of interleukin-2–induced tumor necrosis factor release by dexamethasone: prevention of an acquired neutrophil chemotaxis defect and differential suppression of interleukin-2–associated side effects. Blood 1990;76:1933–1940.

158. Margolin K, Atkins M, Sparano J, et al. Prospective randomized trial of lisofylline for the prevention of toxicities of high-dose interleukin 2 therapy in advanced renal cancer and malignant melanoma. Clin Cancer Res 1997;3:565–572.

159. Du Bois JS, Trehu EG, Mier JW, et al. Randomized placebo-controlled clinical trial of high-dose interleukin-2 in combination with a soluble p75 tumor necrosis factor receptor immunoglobulin G chimera in patients with advanced melanoma and renal cell carcinoma. J Clin Oncol 1997;15:1052–1062.

160. McDermott DF, Trehu EG, Mier JW, et al. A two-part phase I trial of high-dose interleukin 2 in combination with soluble (Chinese hamster ovary) interleukin 1 receptor. Clin Cancer Res 1998;4:1203–1213.

161. Samlowski WE, Petersen R, Cuzzocrea S, et al. A nonpeptidyl mimic of superoxide dismutase, M40403, inhibits dose-limiting hypotension associated with interleukin-2 and increases its antitumor effects. Nat Med 2003;9:750–755.

162. Kedar I, Mermershtain W, Ivgi H. Thalidomide reduces serum C-reactive protein and interleukin-6 and induces response to IL-2 in a fraction of metastatic renal cell cancer patients who failed IL-2–based therapy. Int J Cancer 2004;110:260–265.

163. Redlinger RE Jr, Mailliard RB, Lotze MT, et al. Synergistic interleukin-18 and low-dose interleukin-2 promote regression of established murine neuroblastoma in vivo. J Pediatr Surg 2003;38:301–307.

164. Gollob JA, Veenstra KG, Parker RA, et al. Phase I trial of concurrent twice-weekly recombinant human interleukin-12 plus low-dose IL-2 in patients with melanoma or renal cell carcinoma. J Clin Oncol 2003;21:2564–2573.

165. Rosenberg SA, Lotze MT, Muul LM, et al. A progress report on the treatment of 157 patients with advanced cancer using lymphokine-activated killer cells and interleukin-2 or high-dose interleukin-2 alone. N Engl J Med 1987;316:889–897.

166. Bukowski RM, Sharfman W, Murthy S, et al. Clinical results and characterization of tumor-infiltrating lymphocytes with or without recombinant interleukin 2 in human metastatic renal cell carcinoma. Cancer Res 1991;51:4199–4205.

167. Papa MZ, Mule JJ, Rosenberg SA. Antitumor efficacy of lymphokine-activated killer cells and recombinant interleukin 2 in vivo: successful immunotherapy of established pulmonary metastases from weakly immunogenic and nonimmunogenic murine tumors of three district histological types. Cancer Res 1986;46:4973–4978.

168. Rosenberg SA, Lotze MT, Yang JC, et al. Combination therapy with interleukin-2 and alpha-interferon for the treatment of patients with advanced cancer. J Clin Oncol 1989;7:1863–1874.

169. Redman BG, Flaherty L, Chou TH, et al. A phase I trial of recombinant interleukin-2 combined with recombinant interferon-gamma in patients with cancer. J Clin Oncol 1990;8:1269–1276.

170. Krigel RL, Padavic-Shaller KA, Rudolph AR, et al. Renal cell carcinoma: treatment with recombinant interleukin-2 plus beta-interferon. J Clin Oncol 1990;8:460–467.

171. Triozzi P, Martin E, Kim J, et al. Phase 1b trial of interleukin-1b (IL-1b)/interleukin-2 (IL-2) in patients with metastatic cancer [abstract]. Proc Am Soc Clin Oncol 1993;12:290.

172. Olencki T, Finke J, Tubbs R, et al. Immunomodulatory effects of interleukin-2 and interleukin-4 in patients with malignancy. J Immunother Emphasis Tumor Immunol 1996;19:69–80.

173. Ilson DH, Motzer RJ, Kradin RL, et al. A phase II trial of interleukin-2 and interferon alfa-2a in patients with advanced renal cell carcinoma. J Clin Oncol 1992;10:1124–1130.

174. Budd GT, Murthy S, Finke J, et al. Phase I trial of high-dose bolus interleukin-2 and interferon alfa-2a in patients with metastatic malignancy. J Clin Oncol 1992;10:804–809.

175. Tourani JM, Pfister C, Tubiana N, et al. Subcutaneous interleukin-2 and interferon alfa administration in patients with metastatic renal cell carcinoma: final results of SCAPP III, a large, multicenter, phase II, nonrandomized study with sequential analysis design. Subcutaneous Administration Propeukin Program Cooperative Group. J Clin Oncol 2003;21:3987–3994.

176. Kuebler JP, Whitehead RP, Ward DL, et al. Treatment of metastatic renal cell carcinoma with recombinant interleukin-2 in combination with vinblastine or lymphokine-activated killer cells. J Urol 1993;150:814–820.

177. Gautam SC, Chikkala NF, Ganapathi R, et al. Combination therapy with Adriamycin and interleukin 2 augments immunity against murine renal cell carcinoma. Cancer Res 1991;51:6133–6137.

178. Bukowski RM, Sergi JS, Budd GT, et al. Phase I trial of continuous infusion interleukin-2 and doxorubicin in patients with refractory malignancies. J Immunother 1991;10:432–439.

179. Paciucci PA, Bekesi JG, Ryder JS, et al. Immunotherapy with IL2 by constant infusion and weekly doxorubicin. Am J Clin Oncol 1991;14:341–348.

180. Dillman RO, Church C, Oldham RK, et al. Inpatient continuous-infusion interleukin-2 in 788 patients with cancer: the National Biotherapy Study Group experience. Cancer 1993;71:2358–2370.

181. Mitchell MS. Chemotherapy in combination with biomodulation: a 5-year experience with cyclophosphamide and interleukin-2. Semin Oncol 1992;19:80–87.

182. Berd D, Maguire HC Jr, Mastrangelo MJ. Potentiation of human cell-mediated and humoral immunity by low-dose cyclophosphamide. Cancer Res 1984;44:5439–5443.

183. Atzpodien J, Kirchner H, Hanninen EL, et al. Interleukin-2 in combination with interferon-alpha and 5-fluorouracil for metastatic renal cell cancer. Eur J Cancer 1993;29A(Suppl 5):S6–8.

184. Negrier S, Escudier B, Dovillard JY. Randomized study of interleukin 2 (IL-2) and interferon (IFN) with or without 5-FU (FUCY study) in metastatic renal cell carcinoma (MRCC) [abstract]. Proc Am Soc Clin Oncol 1997;16:326a.

185. Olencki T, Peereboom D, Wood L, et al. Phase I and II trials of subcutaneously administered rIL-2, interferon alfa-2a, and fluorouracil in patients with metastatic renal carcinoma. J Cancer Res Clin Oncol 2001;127:319–324.

186. Allen MJ, Vaughan M, Webb A, et al. Protracted venous infusion 5-fluorouracil in combination with subcutaneous interleukin-2 and alpha-interferon in patients with metastatic renal cell cancer: a phase II study. Br J Cancer 2000;83:980–985.

187. Dutcher JP, Logan T, Gordon M, et al. Phase II trial of interleukin 2, interferon alpha, and 5-fluorouracil in metastatic renal cell cancer: a Cytokine Working Group study. Clin Cancer Res 2000;6:3442–3450.

188. Legha SS, Ring S, Eton O, et al. Development and results of biochemotherapy in metastatic melanoma: the University of Texas M.D. Anderson Cancer Center experience. Cancer J Sci Am 1997;3(Suppl 1):S9–15.

189. El-Maraghi R, Verma S, Charette M, et al. A meta-analysis of biochemotherapy (BCT) for the treatment of metastatic malignant melanoma (MM) [abstract]. Proc Am Soc Clin Oncol 2004;23:714 (abstr. 7529).

190. Katre NV, Knauf MJ, Laird WJ. Chemical modification of recombinant interleukin 2 by polyethylene glycol increases its potency in the murine Meth A sarcoma model. Proc Natl Acad Sci USA 1987;84:1487–1491.

191. Bukowski RM, Young J, Goodman G, et al. Polyethylene glycol conjugated interleukin-2: clinical and immunologic effects in patients with advanced renal cell carcinoma. Invest New Drugs 1993;11:211–217.

192. Gause B, Longo DL, Janik J. A phase I study of liposome-encapsulated IL-2 (LE-IL-2). Proc Am Soc Clin Oncol 1993;12:293.

193. Yao Z, Dai W, Perry J, et al. Effect of albumin fusion on the biodistribution of interleukin-2. Cancer Immunol Immunother 2004;53:404–410.

194. Isakson PC, Pure E, Vitetta ES, et al. T cell–derived B cell differentiation factor(s): effect on the isotype switch of murine B cells. J Exp Med 1982;155:734–748.

195. Howard M, Farrar J, Hilfiker M. Identification of a T cell–derived B cell stimulatory factor distinct from IL-2. J Exp Med 1982;155:914–923.

196. Puri RK, Siegel JP. Interleukin-4 and cancer therapy. Cancer Invest 1993;11:473–486.

197. Yokota T, Otsuka T, Mosmann T, et al. Isolation and characterization of a human interleukin cDNA clone, homologous to mouse B-cell stimulatory factor 1, that expresses B-cell– and T-cell–stimulating activities. Proc Natl Acad Sci USA 1986;83:5894–5898.

198. Lee F, Yokota T, Otsuka T, et al. Isolation and characterization of a mouse interleukin cDNA clone that expresses B-cell stimulatory factor 1 activities and T-cell– and mast-cell–stimulating activities. Proc Natl Acad Sci USA 1986;83:2061–2065.

199. Arai N, Nomura D, Villaret D, et al. Complete nucleotide sequence of the chromosomal gene for human IL-4 and its expression. J Immunol 1989;142:274–282.

200. Ohara J, Coligan JE, Zoon K, et al. High-efficiency purification and chemical characterization of B cell stimulatory factor-1/interleukin 4. J Immunol 1987;139:1127–1134.

201. Le Beau MM, Lemons RS, Espinosa R, et al. Interleukin-4 and interleukin-5 map to human chromosome 5 in a region encoding growth factors and receptors and are deleted in myeloid leukemias with a del(5q). Blood 1989;73:647–650.

202. van Leeuwen BH, Martinson ME, Webb GC, et al. Molecular organization of the cytokine gene cluster, involving the human IL-3, IL-4, IL-5, and GM-CSF genes, on human chromosome 5. Blood 1989;73:1142–1148.

203. Yokota T, Arai N, de Vries J, et al. Molecular biology of interleukin 4 and interleukin 5 genes and biology of their products that stimulate B cells, T cells and hemopoietic cells. Immunol Rev 1988;102:137–187.

204. Walter MR, Cook WJ, Zhao BG, et al. Crystal structure of recombinant human interleukin-4. J Biol Chem 1992;267:20371–20376.

205. Walter MR, Cook WJ, Ealick SE, et al. Three-dimensional structure of recombinant human granulocyte-macrophage colony-stimulating factor. J Mol Biol 1992;224:1075–1085.

206. Dorr RT, Von Hoff DD. Interleukin-4 drug monograph. In: Dorr RT, Von Hoff DD, eds. Cancer Chemotherapy Handbook. East Norwalk, CT: Appleton & Lange, 1994; 601–605.

207. Ohara J, Paul WE. Receptors for B-cell stimulatory factor-1 expressed on cells of haematopoietic lineage. Nature 1987;325:537–540.

208. Ohara J, Paul WE. Up-regulation of interleukin 4/B-cell stimulatory factor 1 receptor expression. Proc Natl Acad Sci USA 1988; 85:8221–8225.

209. Wagteveld AJ, van Zanten AK, Esselink MT, et al. Expression and regulation of IL-4 receptors on human monocytes and acute myeloblastic leukemic cells. Leukemia 1991;5:782–788.

210. Feldman GM, Finbloom DS. Induction and regulation of IL-4 receptor expression on murine macrophage cell lines and bone marrow–derived macrophages by IFN-gamma. J Immunol 1990;145:854–859.

211. Nelms K, Keegan AD, Zamorano J, et al. The IL-4 receptor: signaling mechanisms and biologic functions. Annu Rev Immunol 1999;17:701–738.

212. Lai SY, Molden J, Liu KD, et al. Interleukin-4–specific signal transduction events are driven by homotypic interactions of the interleukin-4 receptor alpha subunit. EMBO J 1996;15: 4506–4514.

213. Fujiwara H, Hanissian SH, Tsytsykova A, et al. Homodimerization of the human interleukin 4 receptor alpha chain induces Cepsilon germline transcripts in B cells in the absence of the interleukin 2 receptor gamma chain. Proc Natl Acad Sci USA 1997;94:5866–5871.

214. Reichel M, Nelson BH, Greenberg PD, et al. The IL-4 receptor alpha-chain cytoplasmic domain is sufficient for activation of JAK-1 and STAT6 and the induction of IL-4–specific gene expression. J Immunol 1997;158:5860–5867.

215. Obiri NI, Debinski W, Leonard WJ, et al. Receptor for interleukin 13: interaction with interleukin 4 by a mechanism that does not involve the common gamma chain shared by receptors for interleukins 2, 4, 7, 9, and 15: the IL-13 receptor structure differs on various cell types and may share more than one component with IL-4 receptor. J Immunol 1997;158:756–764.

216. Miloux B, Laurent P, Bonnin O, et al. Cloning of the human IL-13R alpha1 chain and reconstitution with the IL4R alpha of a functional IL-4/IL-13 receptor complex. FEBS Lett 1997;401: 163–166.

217. Obiri NI, Leland P, Murata T, et al. The IL-13 receptor structure differs on various cell types and may share more than one component with IL-4 receptor. J Immunol 1997;158:756–764.

218. Letzelter F, Wang Y, Sebald W. The interleukin-4 site-2 epitope determining binding of the common receptor gamma chain. Eur J Biochem 1998;257:11–20.

219. Russell SM, Keegan AD, Harada N, et al. Interleukin-2 receptor gamma chain: a functional component of the interleukin-4 receptor. Science 1993;262:1880–1883.

220. Kammer W, Lischke A, Moriggl R, et al. Homodimerization of interleukin-4 receptor alpha chain can induce intracellular signaling. J Biol Chem 1996;271:23634–23637.

221. Witthuhn BA, Silvennoinen O, Miura O, et al. Involvement of the Jak-3 Janus kinase in signalling by interleukins 2 and 4 in lymphoid and myeloid cells: phosphorylation and activation of the Jak-3 Janus kinase in response to interleukin-2. Nature 1994;370:151–153.

222. Murata T, Noguchi PD, Puri RK. IL-13 induces phosphorylation and activation of JAK2 Janus kinase in human colon carcinoma cell lines: similarities between IL-4 and IL-13 signaling. J Immunol 1996;156:2972–2978.

223. Johnston JA, Kawamura M, Kirken RA, et al. Phosphorylation and activation of the Jak-3 Janus kinase in response to interleukin-2. Nature 1994;370:151–153.

224. Keegan AD, Nelms K, Wang LM, et al. Interleukin 4 receptor: signaling mechanisms. Immunol Today 1994;15:423–432.

225. Koettnitz K, Kalthoff FS. Human interleukin-4 receptor signaling requires sequences contained within two cytoplasmic regions. Eur J Immunol 1993;23:988–991.

226. Seldin DC, Leder P. Mutational analysis of a critical signaling domain of the human interleukin 4 receptor. Proc Natl Acad Sci USA 1994;91:2140–2144.

227. Ryan JJ, McReynolds LJ, Keegan A, et al. Growth and gene expression are predominantly controlled by distinct regions of the human IL-4 receptor: common elements in interleukin 4 and insulin signaling pathways in factor-dependent hematopoietic cells. Proc Natl Acad Sci USA 1993;90: 4032–4036.

228. Wang LM, Myers MG Jr, Sun XJ, et al. IRS-1: essential for insulin- and IL-4–stimulated mitogenesis in hematopoietic cells. Science 1993;261:1591–1594.

229. Sun XJ, Wang LM, Zhang Y, et al. Role of IRS-2 in insulin and cytokine signalling. Nature 1995;377:173–177.

230. Wang LM, Keegan AD, Li W, et al. Common elements in interleukin 4 and insulin signaling pathways in factor-dependent hematopoietic cells. Proc Natl Acad Sci USA 1993;90:4032–4036.

231. Sun XJ, Crimmins DL, Myers MG Jr, et al. Pleiotropic insulin signals are engaged by multisite phosphorylation of IRS-1. Mol Cell Biol 1993;13:7418–7428.

232. Dhand R, Hiles I, Panayotou G, et al. PI 3-kinase is a dual specificity enzyme: autoregulation by an intrinsic protein-serine kinase activity. EMBO J 1994;13:522–533.

233. Stephens LR, Jackson TR, Hawkins PT. Agonist-stimulated synthesis of phosphatidylinositol(3,4,5)-trisphosphate: a new intracellular signalling system? Biochim Biophys Acta 1993;1179:27–75.

234. Auger KR, Serunian LA, Soltoff SP, et al. PDGF-dependent tyrosine phosphorylation stimulates production of novel polyphosphoinositides in intact cells. Cell 1989;57:167–175.

235. Franke TF, Kaplan DR, Cantley LC, et al. Direct regulation of the Akt proto-oncogene product by phosphatidylinositol-3, 4-bisphosphate. Science 1997;275:665–668.

236. Franke TF, Kaplan DR, Cantley LC. PI3K: downstream AKTion blocks apoptosis. Cell 1997;88:435–437.

237. Delphin S, Stavnezer J. Regulation of antibody class switching to IgE: characterization of an IL-4-responsive region in the immunoglobulin heavy-chain germline epsilon promoter. Ann NY Acad Sci 1995;764:123–135.

238. Takeda K, Tanaka T, Shi W, et al. Essential role of Stat6 in IL-4 signalling. Nature 1996;380:627–630.

239. Mossmann TR, Cherwinski H, Bond MW. Two types of murine helper T cell clones: definition according to profiles of lymphokines, activities, and secreted proteins. J Immunol 1986; 136:2348–2357.

240. Plaut M, Pierce JH, Watson CJ, et al. Mast cell lines produce lymphokines in response to cross-linkage of Fc epsilon RI or to calcium ionophores. Nature 1989;339:64–67.

241. Kuhn R, Rajewsky K, Muller W. Generation and analysis of interleukin-4 deficient mice. Science 1991;254:707–710.

242. Tepper RI, Levinson DA, Stanger BZ, et al. IL-4 induces allergic-like inflammatory disease and alters T cell development in transgenic mice. Cell 1990;62:457–467.

243. Tarte K, Lu ZY, Fiol G, et al. Generation of virtually pure and potentially proliferating dendritic cells from non-CD34 apheresis cells from patients with multiple myeloma. Blood 1997;90: 3482–3495.

244. Puri RK, Ogata M, Leland P, et al. Expression of high-affinity interleukin 4 receptors on murine sarcoma cells and receptor-mediated cytotoxicity of tumor cells to chimeric protein between interleukin 4 and *Pseudomonas* exotoxin. Cancer Res 1991;51: 3011–3017.

245. Tepper RI, Pattengale PK, Leder P. Murine interleukin-4 displays potent anti-tumor activity in vivo. Cell 1989;57:503–512.

246. Golumbek PT, Lazenby AJ, Levitsky HI, et al. Treatment of established renal cancer by tumor cells engineered to secrete interleukin-4. Science 1991;254:713–716.

247. Karray S, DeFrance T, Merle-Beral H, et al. Interleukin 4 counteracts the interleukin 2–induced proliferation of monoclonal B cells. J Exp Med 1988;168:85–94.

248. DeFrance T, Fluckiger AC, Rossi JF, et al. Antiproliferative effects of interleukin-4 on freshly isolated non-Hodgkin malignant B-lymphoma cells. Blood 1992;79:990–996.

249. Taylor CW, Grogan TM, Salmon SE. Effects of interleukin-4 on the in vitro growth of human lymphoid and plasma cell neoplasms. Blood 1990;75:1114–1118.

250. Gooch JL, Lee AV, Yee D. Interleukin 4 inhibits growth and induces apoptosis in human breast cancer cells. Cancer Res 1998;58:4199–4205.

251. Mehrotra R, Varricchio F, Husain SR, et al. Head and neck cancers, but not benign lesions, express interleukin-4 receptors in situ. Oncol Rep 1998;5:45–48.

252. Herrmann F, Andreeff M, Gruss HJ, et al. Interleukin-4 inhibits growth of multiple myelomas by suppressing interleukin-6 expression. Blood 1991;78:2070–2074.

253. Akashi K, Shibuya T, Harada M, et al. Interleukin 4 suppresses the spontaneous growth of chronic myelomonocytic leukemia cells. J Clin Invest 1991;88:223–230.

254. Tungekar MF, Turley H, Dunnill MS, et al. Interleukin 4 receptor expression on human lung tumors and normal lung. Cancer Res 1991;51:261–264.

255. Toi M, Bicknell R, Harris AL. Inhibition of colon and breast carcinoma cell growth by interleukin-4. Cancer Res 1992;52:275–279.

256. Lotze MT. Role of IL-4 in the anti-tumor response. In: Spitz, H, ed. IL-4: Structure and Function. CRC Press, Boca Raton FL 1992:237–262.

257. Ghosh AK, Smith NK, Prendiville J, et al. A phase I study of recombinant human interleukin-4 administered by the intravenous and subcutaneous route in patients with advanced cancer: immunological studies. Eur Cytokine Netw 1993;4:205–211.

258. Markowitz A, Kleinerman E, Hudson M. Phase I study of recombinant IL-4 in patients with advanced cancer. Blood 1989;74(Suppl):146a.

259. Taylor CW, Hultquist KE, Taylor AM. Immunopharmacology of recombinant human interleukin-4 administered by the subcutaneous route in patients with malignancy. Blood 1992;76(Suppl):221a.

260. Atkins MB, Vachino G, Tilg HJ, et al. Phase I evaluation of thrice-daily intravenous bolus interleukin-4 in patients with refractory malignancy. J Clin Oncol 1992;10:1802–1809.

261. Prendiville J, Thatcher N, Lind M, et al. Recombinant human interleukin-4 (rhu IL-4) administered by the intravenous and subcutaneous routes in patients with advanced cancer:·a phase I toxicity study and pharmacokinetic analysis. Eur J Cancer 1993;29A:1700–1707.

262. Gilleece MH, Scarffe JH, Ghosh A, et al Recombinant human interleukin 4 (IL-4) given as daily subcutaneous injections: a phase I dose toxicity trial. Br J Cancer 1992;66:204–210.

263. Maher D, Boyd A, McKendrick J. Rapid response of B cell malignancies induced by interleukin 4. Blood 1990;76(Suppl):152a.

264. Custer MC, Lotze MT. A biologic assay for IL-4: rapid fluorescence assay for IL-4 detection in supernatants and serum. J Immunol Methods 1990;128:109–117.

265. Leach MW, Rybak ME, Rosenblum IY. Safety evaluation of recombinant human interleukin-4, II: clinical studies. Clin Immunol Immunopathol 1997;83:12–14.

266. Rubin JT, Lotze MT. Acute gastric mucosal injury associated with the systemic administration of interleukin-4. Surgery 1992;111:274–280.

267. Whitehead RP, Unger JM, Goodwin JW, et al. Phase II trial of recombinant human interleukin-4 in patients with disseminated malignant melanoma: a Southwest Oncology Group study. J Immunother 1998;21:440–446.

268. Vokes EE, Figlin R, Hochster H, et al. A phase II study of recombinant human interleukin-4 for advanced or recurrent non-small cell lung cancer. Cancer J Sci Am 1998;4:46–51.

269. Tulpule A, Joshi B, DeGuzman N, et al. Interleukin-4 in the treatment of AIDS-related Kaposi's sarcoma. Ann Oncol 1997;8:79–83.

270. Coley WB. The treatment of malignant tumors by repeated inoculations of erysipelas, with a report of ten original cases [1893 classic article]. Clin Orthop Relat Res 1991;(262):3–11.

271. Shear MJ, Turner FC, Perrault A. Chemical treatment of tumors, V: isolation of the hemorrhage producing fraction from *Serratia marcescens* culture filtrates. J Natl Cancer Inst 1943;4:81–97.

272. Carswell EA, Old LJ, Kassel RL, et al. An endotoxin-induced serum factor that causes necrosis of tumors. Proc Natl Acad Sci USA 1975;72:3666–3670.

273. Aggarwal BB, Moffat B, Harkins RN. Human lymphotoxin: production by a lymphoblastoid cell line, purification, and initial characterization. J Biol Chem 1984;259:686–691.

274. Aggarwal BB, Eessalu TE, Hass PE. Characterization of receptors for human tumour necrosis factor and their regulation by gamma-interferon. Nature 1985;318:665–667.

275. Ruddle NH. Tumor necrosis factor (TNF-alpha) and lymphotoxin (TNF-beta). Curr Opin Immunol 1992;4:327–332.

276. Nedwin GE, Naylor SL, Sakaguchi AY, et al. Human lymphotoxin and tumor necrosis factor genes: structure, homology and chromosomal localization. Nucleic Acids Res 1985;13:6361–6373.

277. Sariban E, Imamura K, Luebbers R, et al. Transcriptional and post-transcriptional regulation of tumor necrosis factor gene expression in human monocytes. J Clin Invest 1988;81:1506–1510.

278. Shakhov AN, Collart MA, Vassalli P, et al. Kappa B-type enhancers are involved in lipopolysaccharide-mediated transcriptional activation of the tumor necrosis factor alpha gene in primary macrophages. J Exp Med 1990;171:35–47.

279. Kunkel SL, Spengler M, May MA, et al. Prostaglandin E2 regulates macrophage-derived tumor necrosis factor gene expression. J Biol Chem 1988;263:5380–5384.

280. Strieter RM, Remick DG, Ward PA, et al. Cellular and molecular regulation of tumor necrosis factor-alpha production by pentoxifylline. Biochem Biophys Res Commun 1988;155:1230–1236.

281. Hibbs JB Jr, Taintor RR, Chapman HA Jr, et al. Macrophage tumor killing: influence of the local environment. Science 1977;197:279–282.

282. Debets JM, Van der Linden CJ, Dieteren IE, et al. Fc-receptor cross-linking induces rapid secretion of tumor necrosis factor (cachectin) by human peripheral blood monocytes. J Immunol 1988;141:1197–1201.

283. Kornbluth RS, Gregory SA, Edgington TS. Initial characterization of a lymphokine pathway for the immunologic induction of tumor necrosis factor-alpha release from human peripheral blood mononuclear cells. J Immunol 1988;141:2006–2015.

284. Imamura K, Spriggs D, Ohno T, et al. Effects of botulinum toxin type D on secretion of tumor necrosis factor from human monocytes. Mol Cell Biol 1989;9:2239–2243.

285. Muller R, Marmenout A, Fiers W. Synthesis and maturation of recombinant human tumor necrosis factor in eukaryotic systems. FEBS Lett 1986;197:99–104.

286. Smith RA, Baglioni C. The active form of tumor necrosis factor is a trimer. J Biol Chem 1987;262:6951–6954.

287. Taguchi T, Sohmura Y. Clinical studies with TNF. Biotherapy 1991;3:177–186.

288. Creasey AA, Doyle LV, Reynolds MT, et al. Biological effects of recombinant human tumor necrosis factor and its novel muteins on tumor and normal cell lines. Cancer Res 1987;47:145–149.

289. Watanabe N, Kuriyama H, Sone H, et al. Continuous internalization of tumor necrosis factor receptors in a human myosarcoma cell line. J Biol Chem 1988;263:10262–10266.

290. Hohmann HP, Remy R, Brockhaus M, et al. Two different cell types have different major receptors for human tumor necrosis factor (TNF alpha). J Biol Chem 1989;264:14927–14934.

291. Ware CF, VanArsdale S, VanArsdale TL. Apoptosis mediated by the TNF-related cytokine and receptor families. J Cell Biochem 1996;60:47–55.

292. Hsu H, Shu HB, Pan MG, et al. TRADD-TRAF2 and TRADD-FADD interactions define two distinct TNF receptor 1 signal transduction pathways. Cell 1996;84:299–308.

293. Rothe M, Pan MG, Henzel WJ, et al. The TNFR2-TRAF signaling complex contains two novel proteins related to baculoviral inhibitor of apoptosis proteins. Cell 1995;83:1243–1252.

294. Rothe M, Sarma V, Dixit VM, et al. TRAF2-mediated activation of NF-kappa B by TNF receptor 2 and CD40. Science 1995;269:1424–1427.

295. Woronicz JD, Gao X, Cao Z, et al. IkappaB kinase-beta: NF-kappaB activation and complex formation with IkappaB kinase-alpha and NIK. Science 1997;278:866–869.

296. Wickremasinghe RG, Hoffbrand AV. Biochemical and genetic control of apoptosis: relevance to normal hematopoiesis and hematological malignancies. Blood 1999;93:3587–3600.

297. Tsujimoto M, Feinman R, Vilcek J. Differential effects of type I IFN and IFN-gamma on the binding of tumor necrosis factor to receptors in two human cell lines. J Immunol 1986;137:2272–2276.

298. Ruggiero V, Tavernier J, Fiers W, et al. Induction of the synthesis of tumor necrosis factor receptors by interferon-gamma. J Immunol 1986;136:2445–2450.

299. Holtmann H, Wallach D. Down regulation of the receptors for tumor necrosis factor by interleukin 1 and 4 beta-phorbol-12-myristate-13-acetate. J Immunol 1987;139:1161–1167.

300. Etanercept. Soluble tumour necrosis factor receptor, TNF receptor fusion protein, TNFR-Fc, TNR 001, Enbrel. Drugs R D 1999;1:258–261.

301. Moreland LW, Baumgartner SW, Schiff MH, et al. Treatment of rheumatoid arthritis with a recombinant human tumor necrosis factor receptor (p75)-Fc fusion protein. N Engl J Med 1997;337: 141–147.

302. Moreland LW, Schiff MH, Baumgartner SW, et al. Etanercept therapy in rheumatoid arthritis: a randomized, controlled trial. Ann Intern Med 1999;130:478–486.

303. Sugarman BJ, Aggarwal BB, Hass PE, et al. Recombinant human tumor necrosis factor-alpha: effects on proliferation of normal and transformed cells in vitro. Science 1985;230:943–945.

304. Dealtry GB, Balkwill FR, Cell growth inhibition by interferons and tumor necrosis factor. In: Lymphokines and Interferons: A Practical Approach. Washington, DC: IRL Press, 1987: 371–372.

305. Tsujimoto M, Yip YK, Vilcek J. Tumor necrosis factor: specific binding and internalization in sensitive and resistant cells. Proc Natl Acad Sci USA 1985;82:7626–7630.

306. Chu ZL, McKinsey TA, Liu L, et al. Suppression of tumor necrosis factor–induced cell death by inhibitor of apoptosis c-IAP2 is under NF-kappaB control. Proc Natl Acad Sci USA 1997;94: 10057–10062.

307. Van Antwerp DJ, Martin SJ, Kafri T, et al. Suppression of TNF-alpha–induced apoptosis by NF-kappaB. Science 1996;274: 787–789.

308. Torti FM, Dieckmann B, Beutler B, et al. A macrophage factor inhibits adipocyte gene expression: an in vitro model of cachexia. Science 1985;229:867–869.

309. Murase T, Hotta T, Saito H, et al. Effect of recombinant human tumor necrosis factor on the colony growth of human leukemia progenitor cells and normal hematopoietic progenitor cells. Blood 1987;69:467–472.

310. Broxmeyer HE, Williams DE, Lu L, et al. The suppressive influences of human tumor necrosis factors on bone marrow hematopoietic progenitor cells from normal donors and patients with leukemia: synergism of tumor necrosis factor and interferon-gamma. J Immunol 1986;136:4487–4495.

311. Peetre C, Gullberg U, Nilsson E, et al. Effects of recombinant tumor necrosis factor on proliferation and differentiation of leukemic and normal hemopoietic cells in vitro: relationship to cell surface receptor. J Clin Invest 1986;78:1694–1700.

312. Vilcek J, Palombella VJ, Henriksen-DeStefano D, et al. Fibroblast growth enhancing activity of tumor necrosis factor and its relationship to other polypeptide growth factors. J Exp Med 1986;163:632–643.

313. Sidhu RS, Bollon AP. Tumor necrosis factor activities and cancer therapy: a perspective. Pharmacol Ther 1993;57:79–128.

314. Pober JS, Gimbrone MA Jr. Expression of Ia-like antigens by human vascular endothelial cells is inducible in vitro: demonstration by monoclonal antibody binding and immunoprecipitation. Proc Natl Acad Sci USA 1982;79:6641–6645.

315. Collins T, Lapierre LA, Fiers W, et al. Recombinant human tumor necrosis factor increases mRNA levels and surface expression of HLA-A,B antigens in vascular endothelial cells and dermal fibroblasts in vitro. Proc Natl Acad Sci USA 1986;83:446–450.

316. Bevilacqua MP, Stengelin S, Gimbrone MA Jr, et al. Endothelial leukocyte adhesion molecule, I: an inducible receptor for neutrophils related to complement regulatory proteins and lectins. Science 1989;243:1160–1165.

317. Kurt-Jones EA, Fiers W, Pober JS. Membrane interleukin 1 induction on human endothelial cells and dermal fibroblasts. J Immunol 1987;139:2317–2324.

318. Bussolino F, Camussi G, Baglioni C. Synthesis and release of platelet-activating factor by human vascular endothelial cells treated with tumor necrosis factor or interleukin 1 alpha. J Biol Chem 1988;263:11856–11861.

319. Lapierre LA, Fiers W, Pober JS. Three distinct classes of regulatory cytokines control endothelial cell MHC antigen expression: interactions with immune gamma interferon differentiate the effects of tumor necrosis factor and lymphotoxin from those of leukocyte alpha and fibroblast beta interferons. J Exp Med 1988; 167:794–804.

320. Kramer SM, Carver ME. Serum-free in vitro bioassay for the detection of tumor necrosis factor. J Immunol Methods 1986;93: 201–206.

321. Garrelds IM, Zijlstra FJ, Tak CJ, et al. A comparison between two methods for measuring tumor necrosis factor in biological fluids. Agents Actions 1993;38(Special Issue):C89–C91.

322. Blick M, Sherwin SA, Rosenblum M, et al. Phase I study of recombinant tumor necrosis factor in cancer patients. Cancer Res 1987;47:2986–2989.

323. Moritz T, Niederle N, Baumann J, et al. Phase I study of recombinant human tumor necrosis factor alpha in advanced malignant disease. Cancer Immunol Immunother 1989;29:144–150.

324. Pang XP, Hershman JM, Pekary AE. Plasma disappearance and organ distribution of recombinant human tumor necrosis factor-alpha in rats. Lymphokine Cytokine Res 1991;10:301–306.

325. Beutler BA, Milsark IW, Cerami A. Cachectin/tumor necrosis factor: production, distribution, and metabolic fate in vivo. J Immunol 1985;135:3972–3977.

326. Greischel A, Zahn G. Pharmacokinetics of recombinant human tumor necrosis factor alpha in rhesus monkeys after intravenous administration. J Pharmacol Exp Ther 1989;251:358–361.

327. Ferraiolo BL, McCabe J, Hollenbach S, et al. Pharmacokinetics of recombinant human tumor necrosis factor-alpha in rats: effects of size and number of doses and nephrectomy. Drug Metab Dispos 1989;17:369–372.

328. Kimura K, Taguchi T, Urushizaki I, et al. Phase I study of recombinant human tumor necrosis factor. Cancer Chemother Pharmacol 1987;20:223–229.

329. Mittelman A, Puccio C, Gafney E, et al. A phase I pharmacokinetic study of recombinant human tumor necrosis factor administered by a 5-day continuous infusion. Invest New Drugs 1992; 10:183–190.

330. Spriggs DR, Sherman ML, Michie H, et al. Recombinant human tumor necrosis factor administered as a 24-hour intravenous infusion: a phase I and pharmacologic study. J Natl Cancer Inst 1988;80:1039–1044.

331. Chapman PB, Lester TJ, Casper ES, et al. Clinical pharmacology of recombinant human tumor necrosis factor in patients with advanced cancer. J Clin Oncol 1987;5:1942–1951.

332. Feinberg B, Kurzrock R, Talpaz M, et al. A phase I trial of intravenously-administered recombinant tumor necrosis factor-alpha in cancer patients. J Clin Oncol 1988;6:1328–1334.

333. Creaven PJ, Plager JE, Dupere S, et al. Phase I clinical trial of recombinant human tumor necrosis factor. Cancer Chemother Pharmacol 1987;20:137–144.

334. Saks S, Rosenblum S. Recombinant human TNF-a: preclinical studies and results from early clinical trials. Immunol Ser 1992; 56:567–587.

335. Zamkoff KW, Newman NB, Rudolph AR, et al. A phase I trial of subcutaneously administered recombination tumor necrosis factor to patients with advanced malignancy. J Biol Response Mod 1989;8:539–552.

336. Van de Wiel PA, Bloksma N, Kuper CF, et al. Macroscopic and microscopic early effects of tumour necrosis factor on murine Meth A sarcoma, and relation to curative activity. J Pathol 1989;157:65–73.

337. Pfreundschuh MG, Steinmetz HT, Tuschen R, et al. Phase I study of intratumoral application of recombinant human tumor necrosis factor. Eur J Cancer Clin Oncol 1989;25:379–388.

338. Raeth U, Schmid H, Hofman J. Intraperitoneal application of recombinant tumor necrosis factor as an effective palliative treatment of malignant ascites from ovarian and gastroenteropancreatic carcinomas [abstract]. Proc Am Soc Clin Oncol 1989; 8:181.

339. Mavligit GM, Zukiwski AA, Charnsangavej C, et al. Regional biologic therapy. Hepatic arterial infusion of recombinant human tumor necrosis factor in patients with liver metastases. Cancer 1992;69:557–561.

340. Lienard D, Ewalenko P, Delmotte JJ, et al. High-dose recombinant tumor necrosis factor alpha in combination with interferon gamma and melphalan in isolation perfusion of the limbs for melanoma and sarcoma. J Clin Oncol 1992;10:52–60.

341. Suffredini AF, Fromm RE, Parker MM, et al. The cardiovascular response of normal humans to the administration of endotoxin. N Engl J Med 1989;321:280–287.

342. Bevilacqua MP, Pober JS, Majeau GR, et al. Recombinant tumor necrosis factor induces procoagulant activity in cultured human

vascular endothelium: characterization and comparison with the actions of interleukin 1. Proc Natl Acad Sci USA 1986;83: 4533–4537.

343. Jablons DM, Mule JJ, McIntosh JK, et al. IL-6/IFN-beta-2 as a circulating hormone: induction by cytokine administration in humans. J Immunol 1989;142:1542–1547.

344. Dinarello CA, Cannon JG, Wolff SM, et al. Tumor necrosis factor (cachectin) is an endogenous pyrogen and induces production of interleukin 1. J Exp Med 1986;163:1433–1450.

345. Sherman ML, Spriggs DR, Arthur KA, et al. Recombinant human tumor necrosis factor administered as a five-day continuous infusion in cancer patients: phase I toxicity and effects on lipid metabolism. J Clin Oncol 1988;6:344–350.

346. Logan TF, Bontempo FA, Kirkwood JM. Evidence for the presence of fibrin degradation products in patients on a phase 1 trial with tumor necrosis factor. Proc Am Assoc Cancer Res 1988;29:370.

347. Creaven PJ, Brenner DE, Cowens JW, et al. A phase I clinical trial of recombinant human tumor necrosis factor given daily for five days. Cancer Chemother Pharmacol 1989;23:186–191.

348. Lenk H, Tanneberger S, Muller U, et al. Human pharmacological investigation of a human recombinant tumor necrosis factor preparation (PAC-4D) a phase-I trial. Arch Geschwulstforsch 1988;58:89–97.

349. Moldawer NP, Figlin RA. Tumor necrosis factor: current clinical status and implications for nursing management. Semin Oncol Nurs 1988;4:120–125.

350. Figlin R, deKernion J, Sarna G. Phase II study of recombinant tumor necrosis factor in patients with metastatic renal cell carcinoma and malignant melanoma [abstract]. Proc Am Soc Clin Oncol 1988;7:169.

351. Tracey KJ, Wei H, Manogue KR, et al. Cachectin/tumor necrosis factor induces cachexia, anemia, and inflammation. J Exp Med 1988;167:1211–1227.

352. Kist A, Ho AD, Rath U, et al. Decrease of natural killer cell activity and monokine production in peripheral blood of patients treated with recombinant tumor necrosis factor. Blood 1988;72:344–348.

353. Bartsch HH, Nagel GA, Mule R. Tumor necrosis factor in man: clinical and biologic observations. Br J Cancer 1987;56:803–808.

354. Charnetsky PS, Greisman RA, Salmon SE, et al. Increased peripheral blood leukocyte cytotoxic activity in cancer patients during the continuous intravenous administration of recombinant human tumor necrosis factor. J Clin Immunol 1989;9:34–38.

355. Logan TF, Gooding WE, Whiteside TL, et al. Biologic response modulation by tumor necrosis factor alpha (TNF alpha) in a phase Ib trial in cancer patients. J Immunother 1997;20: 387–398.

356. Conkling PR, Chua CC, Nadler P, et al. Clinical trials with human tumor necrosis factor: in vivo and in vitro effects on human mononuclear phagocyte function. Cancer Res 1988; 48:5604–5609.

357. Logan TF, Gooding W, Kirkwood JM, et al. Tumor necrosis factor administration is associated with increased endogenous production of M-CSF and G-CSF but not GM-CSF in human cancer patients. Exp Hematol 1996;24:49–53.

358. Creagan ET, Kovach JS, Moertel CG, et al. A phase I clinical trial of recombinant human tumor necrosis factor. Cancer 1988;62: 2467–2471.

359. Hersh EM, Metch BS, Muggia FM, et al. Phase II studies of recombinant human tumor necrosis factor alpha in patients with malignant disease: a summary of the Southwest Oncology Group experience. J Immunother 1991;10:426–431.

360. Spriggs DR, Tumor Necrosis Factor: Basic Principles and Preclinical Studies. In: DeVita VT, Hellman S, eds. Biologic Therapy of Cancer. Philadelphia: Lippincott, 1995; 361–370.

361. Hirte HW, Miller D, Tonkin K, et al. A randomized trial of paracentesis plus intraperitoneal tumor necrosis factor-alpha versus paracentesis alone in patients with symptomatic ascites from recurrent ovarian carcinoma. Gynecol Oncol 1997;64:80–87.

362. Eggermont AM, Schraffordt Koops H, Klausner JM, et al. Isolated limb perfusion with tumor necrosis factor and melphalan for limb salvage in 186 patients with locally advanced soft tissue extremity sarcomas: the cumulative multicenter European experience. Ann Surg 1996;224:756–764.

363. van Etten B, van Geel AN, de Wilt JH, et al. Fifty tumor necrosis factor–based isolated limb perfusions for limb salvage in patients older than 75 years with limb-threatening soft tissue sarcomas and other extremity tumors. Ann Surg Oncol 2003; 10:32–37.

364. Noorda EM, Vrouenraets BC, Nieweg OE, et al. Prognostic factors for survival after isolated limb perfusion for malignant melanoma. Eur J Surg Oncol 2003;29:916–921.

365. Hohenberger P, Tunn PU. Isolated limb perfusion with rhTNF-alpha and melphalan for locally recurrent childhood synovial sarcoma of the limb. J Pediatr Hematol Oncol 2003;25: 905–909.

366. Noorda EM, Vrouenraets BC, Nieweg OE, et al. Isolated limb perfusion with tumor necrosis factor-alpha and melphalan for patients with unresectable soft tissue sarcoma of the extremities. Cancer 2003;98:1483–1490.

367. Alexander HR, Libutti SK, Bartlett DL, et al. A phase I-II study of isolated hepatic perfusion using melphalan with or without tumor necrosis factor for patients with ocular melanoma metastatic to liver. Clin Cancer Res 2000;6:3062–3070.

368. Libutti SK, Barlett DL, Fraker DL, et al. Technique and results of hyperthermic isolated hepatic perfusion with tumor necrosis factor and melphalan for the treatment of unresectable hepatic malignancies. J Am Coll Surg 2000;191:519–530.

369. Nakamoto T, Inagawa H, Takagi K, et al. A new method of anti-tumor therapy with a high dose of TNF perfusion for unresectable liver tumors. Anticancer Res 2000;20(6A):4087–4096.

370. Bartlett DL, Libutti SK, Figg WD, et al. Isolated hepatic perfusion for unresectable hepatic metastases from colorectal cancer. Surgery 2001;129:176–187.

371. Walther MM, Jennings SB, Choyke PL, et al. Isolated perfusion of the kidney with tumor necrosis factor for localized renal-cell carcinoma. World J Urol 1996;14(Suppl 1):S2–7.

372. Abbruzzese JL, Levin B, Ajani JA, et al. Phase I trial of recombinant human gamma-interferon and recombinant human tumor necrosis factor in patients with advanced gastrointestinal cancer. Cancer Res 1989;49:4057–4061.

373. Demetri GD, Spriggs DR, Sherman ML, et al. A phase I trial of recombinant human tumor necrosis factor and interferon-gamma: effects of combination cytokine administration in vivo. J Clin Oncol 1989;7:1545–1553.

374. McIntosh JK, Mule JJ, Merino MJ, et al. Synergistic antitumor effects of immunotherapy with recombinant interleukin-2 and recombinant tumor necrosis factor-alpha. Cancer Res 1988;48: 4011–4017.

375. McIntosh JK, Mule JJ, Krosnick JA, et al. Combination cytokine immunotherapy with tumor necrosis factor alpha, interleukin 2, and alpha-interferon and its synergistic antitumor effects in mice. Cancer Res 1989;49:1408–1414.

376. Eskander ED, Harvey HA, Givant E, et al. Phase I study combining tumor necrosis factor with interferon-alpha and interleukin-2. Am J Clin Oncol 1997;20:511–514.

377. Safrit JT, Belldegrun A, Bonavida B. Sensitivity of human renal cell carcinoma lines to TNF, Adriamycin, and combination: role of TNF mRNA induction in overcoming resistance. J Urol 1993; 149:1202–1208.

378. Mutch DG, Powell CB, Kao MS, et al. In vitro analysis of the anti-cancer potential of tumor necrosis factor in combination with cisplatin. Gynecol Oncol 1989;34:328–333.

379. Alexander RB, Isaacs JT, Coffey DS. Tumor necrosis factor enhances the in vitro and in vivo efficacy of chemotherapeutic drugs targeted at DNA topoisomerase II in the treatment of murine bladder cancer. J Urol 1987;138:427–429.

380. Alexander RB, Nelson WG, Coffey DS. Synergistic enhancement by tumor necrosis factor of in vitro cytotoxicity from chemotherapeutic drugs targeted at DNA topoisomerase II. Cancer Res 1987;47:2403–2406.

381. Lush R, Schwartz R, Logan T. Phase I and pharmacological evaluation of tumor necrosis factor (rHuTNF) administered in combination with etoposide [abstract]. Proc Am Soc Clin Oncol 1993;12:158.

382. Zhang XG, Gu JJ, Lu ZY, et al. Ciliary neurotropic factor, interleukin 11, leukemia inhibitory factor, and oncostatin M are growth factors for human myeloma cell lines using the inter-

leukin 6 signal transducer gp130. J Exp Med 1994;179: 1337–1342.

383. Czupryn MJ, McCoy JM, Scoble HA. Structure-function relationships in human interleukin-11: identification of regions involved in activity by chemical modification and site-directed mutagenesis. J Biol Chem 1995;270:978–985.

384. Kiessling S, Muller-Newen G, Leeb SN, et al. Functional expression of the interleukin-11 receptor alpha-chain and evidence of antiapoptotic effects in human colonic epithelial cells. J Biol Chem 2004;279:10304–10315.

385. Paul SR, Bennett F, Calvetti JA, et al. Molecular cloning of a cDNA encoding interleukin 11, a stromal cell-derived lymphopoietic and hematopoietic cytokine. Proc Natl Acad Sci USA 1990;87:7512–7516.

386. Ohsumi J, Miyadai K, Kawashima I, et al. Adipogenesis inhibitory factor: a novel inhibitory regulator of adipose conversion in bone marrow. FEBS Lett 1991;288:13–16.

387. McKinley D, Wu Q, Yang-Feng T, et al. Genomic sequence and chromosomal location of human interleukin-11 gene (IL11). Genomics 1992;13:814–819.

388. Morris JC, Neben S, Bennett F, et al. Molecular cloning and characterization of murine interleukin-11. Exp Hematol 1996;24: 1369–1376.

389. de Vos AM, Ultsch M, Kossiakoff AA. Human growth hormone and extracellular domain of its receptor: crystal structure of the complex. Science 1992;255:306–312.

390. Hill CP, Osslund TD, Eisenberg D. The structure of granulocyte-colony-stimulating factor and its relationship to other growth factors. Proc Natl Acad Sci USA 1993;90:5167–5171.

391. Walter MR, Cook WJ, Zhao BG, et al. Crystal structure of recombinant human interleukin-4. J Biol Chem 1992;267: 20371–20376.

392. Diederichs K, Boone T, Karplus PA. Novel fold and putative receptor binding site of granulocyte-macrophage colony-stimulating factor. Science 1991;254:1779–1782.

393. Pandit J, Bohm A, Jancarik J, et al. Three-dimensional structure of dimeric human recombinant macrophage colony-stimulating factor. Science 1992;258:1358–1362.

394. Milburn MV, Hassell AM, Lambert MH, et al. A novel dimer configuration revealed by the crystal structure at 2.4: a resolution of human interleukin-5. Nature 1993;363:172–176.

395. Barton VA, Hall MA, Hudson KR, et al. Interleukin-11 signals through the formation of a hexameric receptor complex. J Biol Chem 2000;275:36197–36203.

396. Nandurkar HH, Hilton DJ, Nathan P, et al. The human IL-11 receptor requires gp130 for signalling: demonstration by molecular cloning of the receptor. Oncogene 1996;12:585–593.

397. Hilton DJ, Hilton AA, Raicevic A, et al. Cloning of a murine IL-11 receptor alpha-chain: requirement for gp130 for high affinity binding and signal transduction. EMBO J 1994;13:4765–4775.

398. Fourcin M, Chevalier S, Lebrun JJ, et al. Involvement of gp130/interleukin-6 receptor transducing component in interleukin-11 receptor. Eur J Immunol 1994;24:277–280.

399. Taga T, Kishimoto T. Gp130 and the interleukin-6 family of cytokines. Annu Rev Immunol 1997;15:797–819.

400. Heinrich PC, Behrmann I, Muller-Newen G, et al. Interleukin-6–type cytokine signalling through the gp130/Jak/STAT pathway. Biochem J 1998;334(Pt 2):297–314.

401. Yin T, Taga T, Tsang ML, et al. Involvement of IL-6 signal transducer gp130 in IL-11–mediated signal transduction. J Immunol 1993;151:2555–2561.

402. Liu J, Modrell B, Aruffo A, et al. Interleukin-6 signal transducer gp130 mediates oncostatin M signaling. J Biol Chem 1992;267: 16763–16766.

403. Ihle JN. STATs: signal transducers and activators of transcription. Cell 1996;84:331–334.

404. Leng SX, Elias JA. Interleukin-11 inhibits macrophage interleukin-12 production. J Immunol 1997;159:2161–2168.

405. Peterson RL, Wang L, Albert L, et al. Molecular effects of recombinant human interleukin-11 in the HLA-B27 rat model of inflammatory bowel disease. Lab Invest 1998;78:1503–1512.

406. Ropeleski MJ, Tang J, Walsh-Reitz MM, et al. Interleukin-11–induced heat shock protein 25 confers intestinal epithelial-specific cytoprotection from oxidant stress. Gastroenterology 2003;124:1358–1368.

407. Du X, Williams DA. Interleukin-11: review of molecular, cell biology, and clinical use. Blood 1997;89:3897–3908.

408. Du X, Everett ET, Wang G, et al. Murine interleukin-11 (IL-11) is expressed at high levels in the hippocampus and expression is developmentally regulated in the testis. J Cell Physiol 1996; 168:362–372.

409. Bertolini F, Lazzari L, Lauri E, et al. Cord blood plasma-mediated ex vivo expansion of hematopoietic progenitor cells. Bone Marrow Transplant 1994;14:347–353.

410. van de Ven C, Ishizawa L, Law P, et al. IL-11 in combination with SLF and G-CSF or GM-CSF significantly increases expansion of isolated CD34$^+$ cell population from cord blood vs. adult bone marrow. Exp Hematol 1995;23:1289–1295.

411. Sato N, Sawada K, Koizumi K, et al. In vitro expansion of human peripheral blood CD34$^+$ cells. Blood 1993;82: 3600–3609.

412. Musashi M, Yang YC, Paul SR, et al. Direct and synergistic effects of interleukin 11 on murine hemopoiesis in culture. Proc Natl Acad Sci USA 1991;88:765–769.

413. Jacobsen FW, Keller JR, Ruscetti FW, et al. Direct synergistic effects of IL-4 and IL-11 on proliferation of primitive hematopoietic progenitor cells. Exp Hematol 1995;23:990–995.

414. Ikebuchi K, Clark SC, Ihle JN, et al. Granulocyte colony-stimulating factor enhances interleukin 3-dependent proliferation of multipotential hemopoietic progenitors. Proc Natl Acad Sci USA 1988;85:3445–3449.

415. Ploemacher RE, van Soest PL, Boudewijn A, et al. Interleukin-12 enhances interleukin-3 dependent multilineage hematopoietic colony formation stimulated by interleukin-11 or steel factor. Leukemia 1993;7:1374–1380.

416. Jacobsen SE, Okkenhaug C, Veiby OP, et al. Interleukin 13: novel role in direct regulation of proliferation and differentiation of primitive hematopoietic progenitor cells. J Exp Med 1994;180: 75–82.

417. Ikebuchi K, Wong GG, Clark SC, et al. Interleukin 6 enhancement of interleukin 3–dependent proliferation of multipotential hemopoietic progenitors. Proc Natl Acad Sci USA 1987;84: 9035–9039.

418. Lemoli RM, Fogli M, Fortuna A, et al. Interleukin-11 stimulates the proliferation of human hematopoietic CD34$^+$ and CD34$^+$CD33$^-$DR$^-$ cells and synergizes with stem cell factor, interleukin-3, and granulocyte-macrophage colony-stimulating factor. Exp Hematol 1993;21:1668–1672.

419. Broudy VC, Lin NL, Kaushansky K. Thrombopoietin (c-mpl ligand) acts synergistically with erythropoietin, stem cell factor, and interleukin-11 to enhance murine megakaryocyte colony growth and increases megakaryocyte ploidy in vitro. Blood 1995;85: 1719–1726.

420. Neben TY, Loebelenz J, Hayes L, et al. Recombinant human interleukin-11 stimulates megakaryocytopoiesis and increases peripheral platelets in normal and splenectomized mice. Blood 1993;81:901–908.

421. Yonemura Y, Kawakita M, Masuda T, et al. Effect of recombinant human interleukin-11 on rat megakaryopoiesis and thrombopoiesis in vivo: comparative study with interleukin-6. Br J Haematol 1993;84:16–23.

422. Teramura M, Kobayashi S, Hoshino S, et al. Interleukin-11 enhances human megakaryocytopoiesis in vitro. Blood 1992;79: 327–331.

423. Kaushansky K, Broudy VC, Lin N, et al. Thrombopoietin, the Mp1 ligand, is essential for full megakaryocyte development. Proc Natl Acad Sci USA 1995;92:3234–3238.

424. Ku H, Yonemura Y, Kaushansky K, et al. Thrombopoietin, the ligand for the Mpl receptor, synergizes with steel factor and other early acting cytokines in supporting proliferation of primitive hematopoietic progenitors of mice. Blood 1996;87: 4544–4551.

425. Quesniaux VF, Clark SC, Turner K, et al. Interleukin-11 stimulates multiple phases of erythropoiesis in vitro. Blood 1992;80: 1218–1223.

426. Rodriguez MH, Arnaud S, Blanchet JP. IL-11 directly stimulates murine and human erythroid burst formation in semisolid cultures. Exp Hematol 1995;23:545–550.

427. Hermouet S, Godard A, Pineau D, et al. Abnormal production of interleukin (IL)-11 and IL-8 in polycythaemia vera. Cytokine 2002;20:178–183.

428. Hirayama F, Clark SC, Ogawa M. Negative regulation of early B lymphopoiesis by interleukin 3 and interleukin 1 alpha. Proc Natl Acad Sci USA 1994;91:469–473.

429. Krieger MS, Nissen C, Wodnar-Filipowicz A. Stem-cell factor in aplastic anemia: in vitro expression in bone marrow stroma and fibroblast cultures. Eur J Haematol 1995;54:262–269.

430. Booth C, Potten CS. Effects of IL-11 on the growth of intestinal epithelial cells in vitro. Cell Prolif 1995;28:581–594.

431. Elias JA, Zheng T, Einarsson O, et al. Epithelial interleukin-11: regulation by cytokines, respiratory syncytial virus, and retinoic acid. J Biol Chem 1994;269:22261–22268.

432. Girasole G, Passeri G, Jilka RL, et al. Interleukin-11: a new cytokine critical for osteoclast development. J Clin Invest 1994; 93:1516–1524.

433. Romas E, Udagawa N, Zhou H, et al. The role of gp130-mediated signals in osteoclast development: regulation of interleukin 11 production by osteoblasts and distribution of its receptor in bone marrow cultures. J Exp Med 1996;183:2581–2591.

434. Fann MJ, Patterson PH. Neuropoietic cytokines and activin A differentially regulate the phenotype of cultured sympathetic neurons. Proc Natl Acad Sci USA 1994;91:43–47.

435. Aoyama K, Uchida T, Takanuki F, et al. Pharmacokinetics of recombinant human interleukin-11 (rhIL-11) in healthy male subjects. Br J Clin Pharmacol 1997;43:571–578.

436. Takagi A, Yabe Y, Oka Y, et al. Renal disposition of recombinant human interleukin-11 in the isolated perfused rat kidney. Pharm Res 1997;14:86–90.

437. Schwertschlag US, Trepicchio WL, Dykstra KH, et al. Hematopoietic, immunomodulatory and epithelial effects of interleukin-11. Leukemia 1999;13:1307–1315.

438. Gordon MS, McCaskill-Stevens WJ, Battiato LA, et al. A phase I trial of recombinant human interleukin-11 (Neumega rhIL-11 growth factor) in women with breast cancer receiving chemotherapy. Blood 1996;87:3615–3624.

439. Moreland L, Gugliotti R, King K, et al. Results of a phase-I/II randomized, masked, placebo-controlled trial of recombinant human interleukin-11 (rhIL-11) in the treatment of subjects with active rheumatoid arthritis. Arthritis Res 2001;3:247–252.

440. Antin JH, Lee SJ, Neuberg D, et al. A phase I/II double-blind, placebo-controlled study of recombinant human interleukin-11 for mucositis and acute GVHD prevention in allogeneic stem cell transplantation. Bone Marrow Transplant 2002;29: 373–377.

441. Tepler I, Elias L, Smith JW II, et al. A randomized placebo-controlled trial of recombinant human interleukin-11 in cancer patients with severe thrombocytopenia due to chemotherapy. Blood 1996;87:3607–3614.

442. Kurzrock R, Cortes J, Thomas DA, et al. Pilot study of low-dose interleukin-11 in patients with bone marrow failure. J Clin Oncol 2001;19:4165–4172.

443. Dykstra KH, Rogge H, Stone A, et al. Mechanism and amelioration of recombinant human interleukin-11 (rhIL-11)–induced anemia in healthy subjects. J Clin Pharmacol 2000;40:880–888.

444. Atkins MB, Kappler K, Mier JW, et al. Interleukin-6–associated anemia: determination of the underlying mechanism. Blood 1995;86:1288–1291.

445. Vredenburgh JJ, Hussein A, Fisher D, et al. A randomized trial of recombinant human interleukin-11 following autologous bone marrow transplantation with peripheral blood progenitor cell support in patients with breast cancer. Biol Blood Marrow Transplant 1998;4:134–141.

446. Isaacs C, Robert NJ, Bailey FA, et al. Randomized placebo-controlled study of recombinant human interleukin-11 to prevent chemotherapy-induced thrombocytopenia in patients with breast cancer receiving dose-intensive cyclophosphamide and doxorubicin. J Clin Oncol 1997;15:3368–3377.

447. Smith JW II. Tolerability and side-effect profile of rhIL-11. Oncology (Huntingt) 2000;14(9 Suppl 8):41–47.

448. Ghalib R, Levine C, Hassan M, et al. Recombinant human interleukin-11 improves thrombocytopenia in patients with cirrhosis. Hepatology 2003;37:1165–1171.

449. Greenwood-Van Meerveld B, Tyler K, Keith JC Jr. Recombinant human interleukin-11 modulates ion transport and mucosal inflammation in the small intestine and colon. Lab Invest 2000; 80:1269–1280.

450. Venkova K, Keith JC Jr, Greenwood-Van Meerveld B. Oral treatment with recombinant human interleukin-11 improves mucosal transport in the colon of human leukocyte antigen-B27 transgenic rats. J Pharmacol Exp Ther 2004;308:206–213.

451. Du XX, Doerschuk CM, Orazi A, et al. A bone marrow stromal-derived growth factor, interleukin-11, stimulates recovery of small intestinal mucosal cells after cytoablative therapy. Blood 1994;83:33–37.

452. Sands BE, Winston BD, Salzberg B, et al. Randomized, controlled trial of recombinant human interleukin-11 in patients with active Crohn's disease. Aliment Pharmacol Ther 2002;16:399–406.

453. Sands BE, Bank S, Sninsky CA, et al. Preliminary evaluation of safety and activity of recombinant human interleukin 11 in patients with active Crohn's disease. Gastroenterology 1999;117:58–64.

454. Sonis S, Muska A, O'Brien J, et al. Alteration in the frequency, severity and duration of chemotherapy-induced mucositis in hamsters by interleukin-11. Eur J Cancer B Oral Oncol 1995; 31B:261–266.

455. Sonis S, Edwards L, Lucey C. The biological basis for the attenuation of mucositis: the example of interleukin-11. Leukemia 1999;13:831–834.

456. Sonis ST, Peterson RL, Edwards LJ, et al. Defining mechanisms of action of interleukin-11 on the progression of radiation-induced oral mucositis in hamsters. Oral Oncol 2000;36:373–381.

457. Filicko J, Lazarus HM, Flomenberg N. Mucosal injury in patients undergoing hematopoietic progenitor cell transplantation: new approaches to prophylaxis and treatment. Bone Marrow Transplant 2003;31:1–10.

458. Trepicchio WL, Ozawa M, Walters IB, et al. Interleukin-11 therapy selectively downregulates type I cytokine proinflammatory pathways in psoriasis lesions. J Clin Invest 1999;104:1527–1537.

459. Walmsley M, Butler DM, Marinova-Mutafchieva L, et al. An anti-inflammatory role for interleukin-11 in established murine collagen-induced arthritis. Immunology 1998;95:31–37.

460. Kobayashi M, Fitz L, Ryan M, et al. Identification and purification of natural killer cell stimulatory factor (NKSF), a cytokine with multiple biologic effects on human lymphocytes. J Exp Med 1989;170:827–845.

461. Gately MK, Wilson DE, Wong HL. Synergy between recombinant interleukin 2 (rIL 2) and IL 2–depleted lymphokine-containing supernatants in facilitating allogeneic human cytolytic T lymphocyte responses in vitro. J Immunol 1986;136:1274–1282.

462. Gately MK, Wolitzky AG, Quinn PM, et al. Regulation of human cytolytic lymphocyte responses by interleukin-12. Cell Immunol 1992;143:127–142.

463. Gately MK, Desai BB, Wolitzky AG, et al. Regulation of human lymphocyte proliferation by a heterodimeric cytokine, IL-12 (cytotoxic lymphocyte maturation factor). J Immunol 1991;147: 874–882.

464. Chan SH, Perussia B, Gupta JW, et al. Induction of interferon gamma production by natural killer cell stimulatory factor: characterization of the responder cells and synergy with other inducers. J Exp Med 1991;173:869–879.

465. Podlaski FJ, Nanduri VB, Hulmes JD, et al. Molecular characterization of interleukin 12. Arch Biochem Biophys 1992;294: 230–237.

466. Stern AS, Podlaski FJ, Hulmes JD, et al. Purification to homogeneity and partial characterization of cytotoxic lymphocyte maturation factor from human B-lymphoblastoid cells. Proc Natl Acad Sci USA 1990;87:6808–6812.

467. Wolf SF, Temple PA, Kobayashi M, et al. Cloning of cDNA for natural killer cell stimulatory factor, a heterodimeric cytokine with multiple biologic effects on T and natural killer cells. J Immunol 1991;146:3074–3081.

468. Schoenhaut DS, Chua AO, Wolitzky AG, et al. Cloning and expression of murine IL-12. J Immunol 1992;148:3433–3440.

469. Gubler U, Chua AO, Schoenhaut DS, et al. Coexpression of two distinct genes is required to generate secreted bioactive cytotoxic lymphocyte maturation factor. Proc Natl Acad Sci USA 1991;88: 4143–4147.

470. Murphy EE, Terres G, Macatonia SE, et al. B7 and interleukin 12 cooperate for proliferation and interferon gamma production by mouse T helper clones that are unresponsive to B7 costimulation. J Exp Med 1994;180:223–231.

471. Trinchieri G. Interleukin-12: a cytokine produced by antigen-presenting cells with immunoregulatory functions in the generation of T-helper cells type 1 and cytotoxic lymphocytes. Blood 1994; 84:4008–4027.

472. D'Andrea A, Rengaraju M, Valiante NM, et al. Production of natural killer cell stimulatory factor (interleukin 12) by peripheral blood mononuclear cells. J Exp Med 1992;176:1387–1398.

473. Mattner F, Fischer S, Guckes S, et al. The interleukin-12 subunit p40 specifically inhibits effects of the interleukin-12 heterodimer. Eur J Immunol 1993;23:2202–2208.

474. Sieburth D, Jabs EW, Warrington JA, et al. Assignment of genes encoding a unique cytokine (IL12) composed of two unrelated subunits to chromosomes 3 and 5. Genomics 1992;14:59–62.

475. Merberg DM, Wolf SF, Clark SC. Sequence similarity between NKSF and the IL-6/G-CSF family [letter]. Immunol Today 1992;13:77–78.

476. Gearing DP, Cosman D. Homology of the p40 subunit of natural killer cell stimulatory factor (NKSF) with the extracellular domain of the interleukin-6 receptor [letter]. Cell 1991;66: 9–10.

477. Macatonia SE, Hsieh CS, Murphy KM, et al. Dendritic cells and macrophages are required for Th1 development of CD4+ T cells from alpha beta TCR transgenic mice: IL-12 substitution for macrophages to stimulate IFN-gamma production is IFN-gamma- dependent. Int Immunol 1993;5:1119–1128.

478. Macatonia SE, Hosken NA, Litton M, et al. Dendritic cells produce IL-12 and direct the development of Th1 cells from naive CD4+ T cells. J Immunol 1995;154:5071–5079.

479. Cassatella MA, Meda L, Gasperini S, et al. Interleukin-12 production by human polymorphonuclear leukocytes. Eur J Immunol 1995;25:1–5.

480. Curtsinger JM, Schmidt CS, Mondino A, et al. Inflammatory cytokines provide a third signal for activation of naive CD4+ and CD8+ T cells. J Immunol 1999;162:3256–3262.

481. Hall SS. IL-12 at the crossroads. Science 1995;268:1432–1434.

482. Guery JC, Ria F, Galbiati F, et al. Normal B cells fail to secrete interleukin-12. Eur J Immunol 1997;27:1632–1639.

483. Kang K, Kubin M, Cooper KD, et al. IL-12 synthesis by human Langerhans cells. J Immunol 1996;156:1402–1407.

484. Smith TJ, Ducharme LA, Weis JH. Preferential expression of interleukin-12 or interleukin-4 by murine bone marrow mast cells derived in mast cell growth factor or interleukin-3. Eur J Immunol 1994;24:822–826.

485. Muller G, Saloga J, Germann T, et al. Identification and induction of human keratinocyte-derived IL-12. J Clin Invest 1994; 94:1799–1805.

486. Kubin M, Chow JM, Trinchieri G. Differential regulation of interleukin-12 (IL-12), tumor necrosis factor alpha, and IL-1 beta production in human myeloid leukemia cell lines and peripheral blood mononuclear cells. Blood 1994;83:1847–1855.

487. Snijders A, Kalinski P, Hilkens CM, et al. High-level IL-12 production by human dendritic cells requires two signals. Int Immunol 1998;10:1593–1598.

488. D'Andrea A, Aste-Amezaga M, Valiante NM, et al. Interleukin 10 (IL-10) inhibits human lymphocyte interferon gamma–production by suppressing natural killer cell stimulatory factor/IL-12 synthesis in accessory cells. J Exp Med 1993;178:1041–1048.

489. D'Andrea A, Ma X, Aste-Amezaga M, et al. Stimulatory and inhibitory effects of interleukin (IL)-4 and IL-13 on the production of cytokines by human peripheral blood mononuclear cells: priming for IL-12 and tumor necrosis factor alpha production. J Exp Med 1995;181:537–546.

490. Shu U, Kiniwa M, Wu CY, et al. Activated T cells induce interleukin-12 production by monocytes via CD40-CD40 ligand interaction. Eur J Immunol 1995;25:1125–1128.

491. Hunter CA, Ellis-Neyer L, Gabriel KE, et al. The role of the CD28/B7 interaction in the regulation of NK cell responses during infection with *Toxoplasma gondii*. J Immunol 1997;158: 2285–2293.

492. McDyer JF, Goletz TJ, Thomas E, et al. CD40 ligand/CD40 stimulation regulates the production of IFN-gamma from human peripheral blood mononuclear cells in an IL-12- and/or CD28-dependent manner. J Immunol 1998;160:1701–1707.

493. Chizzonite R, Truitt T, Desai BB, et al. IL-12 receptor, I: characterization of the receptor on phytohemagglutinin-activated human lymphoblasts. J Immunol 1992;148:3117–3124.

494. Gubler U, Presky DH. Molecular biology of interleukin-12 receptors. Ann NY Acad Sci 1996;795:36–40.

495. Presky DH, Yang H, Minetti LJ, et al. A functional interleukin 12 receptor complex is composed of two beta-type cytokine receptor subunits. Proc Natl Acad Sci USA 1996;93:14002–14007.

496. Thibodeaux DK, Hunter SE, Waldburger KE, et al. Autocrine regulation of IL-12 receptor expression is independent of secondary IFN-gamma secretion and not restricted to T and NK cells. J Immunol 1999;163:5257–5264.

497. Showe LC, Fox FE, Williams D, et al. Depressed IL-12–mediated signal transduction in T cells from patients with Sézary syndrome is associated with the absence of IL-12 receptor beta 2 mRNA and highly reduced levels of STAT4. J Immunol 1999;163: 4073–4079.

498. Wang X, Wilkinson VL, Podlaski FJ, et al. Characterization of mouse interleukin-12 p40 homodimer binding to the interleukin-12 receptor subunits. Eur J Immunol 1999;29: 2007–2013.

499. Murphy KM, Ouyang W, Szabo SJ, et al. T helper differentiation proceeds through STAT1-dependent, STAT4-dependent and STAT4-independent phases. Curr Top Microbiol Immunol 1999;238:13–26.

500. Naeger LK, McKinney J, Salvekar A, et al. Identification of a STAT4 binding site in the interleukin-12 receptor required for signaling. J Biol Chem 1999;274:1875–1878.

501. Rogge L, Papi A, Presky DH, et al. Antibodies to the IL-12 receptor beta 2 chain mark human Th1 but not Th2 cells in vitro and in vivo. J Immunol 1999;162:3926–3932.

502. Wu C, Warrier RR, Wang X, et al. Regulation of interleukin-12 receptor beta1 chain expression and interleukin-12 binding by human peripheral blood mononuclear cells. Eur J Immunol 1997;27:147–154.

503. Szabo SJ, Jacobson NG, Dighe AS, et al. Developmental commitment to the Th2 lineage by extinction of IL-12 signaling. Immunity 1995;2:665–675.

504. Zhang F, Nakamura T, Aune TM. TCR and IL-12 receptor signals cooperate to activate an individual response element in the IFN-gamma promoter in effector Th cells. J Immunol 1999;163: 728–735.

505. Mountford AP, Coulson PS, Cheever AW, et al. Interleukin-12 can directly induce T-helper 1 responses in interferon-gamma (IFN-gamma) receptor-deficient mice, but requires IFN-gamma signalling to downregulate T-helper 2 responses. Immunology 1999;97:588–594.

506. Yamamoto K, Shibata F, Miura O, et al. Physical interaction between interleukin-12 receptor beta 2 subunit and Jak2 tyrosine kinase: Jak2 associates with cytoplasmic membrane–proximal region of interleukin-12 receptor beta 2 via amino-terminus. Biochem Biophys Res Commun 1999;257:400–404.

507. Bacon CM, Petricoin EF, Ortaldo JR, et al. Interleukin 12 induces tyrosine phosphorylation and activation of STAT4 in human lymphocytes. Proc Natl Acad Sci USA 1995;92:7307–7311.

508. Yao BB, Niu P, Surowy CS, et al. Direct interaction of STAT4 with the IL-12 receptor. Arch Biochem Biophys 1999;368:147–155.

509. Akira S. Functional roles of STAT family proteins: lessons from knockout mice. Stem Cells 1999;17:138–146.

510. Ouyang W, Jacobson NG, Bhattacharya D, et al. The Ets transcription factor ERM is Th1-specific and induced by IL-12 through a STAT4-dependent pathway. Proc Natl Acad Sci USA 1999;96:3888–3893.

511. Kaplan MH, Sun YL, Hoey T, et al. Impaired IL-12 responses and enhanced development of Th2 cells in STAT4–deficient mice. Nature 1996;382:174–177.

512. Bright JJ, Du C, Sriram S. Tyrphostin B42 inhibits IL-12–induced tyrosine phosphorylation and activation of Janus kinase-2 and prevents experimental allergic encephalomyelitis. J Immunol 1999;162:6255–6262.

513. Pardoux C, Ma X, Gobert S, et al. Downregulation of interleukin-12 (IL-12) responsiveness in human T cells by transforming growth factor-beta: relationship with IL-12 signaling. Blood 1999; 93:1448–1455.

514. Gollob JA, Schnipper CP, Orsini E, et al. Characterization of a novel subset of CD8(+) T cells that expands in patients receiving interleukin-12. J Clin Invest 1998;102:561–575.

515. Gately MK, Renzetti LM, Magram J, et al. The interleukin-12/interleukin-12-receptor system: role in normal and pathologic immune responses. Annu Rev Immunol 1998;16:495–521.

516. Adorini L. Interleukin-12, a key cytokine in Th1-mediated autoimmune diseases [In Process Citation]. Cell Mol Life Sci 1999;55:1610–1625.

517. Aste-Amezaga M, Ma X, Sartori A, et al. Molecular mechanisms of the induction of IL-12 and its inhibition by IL-10. J Immunol 1998;160:5936–5944.

518. Trinchieri G, Wysocka M, D'Andrea A, et al. Natural killer cell stimulatory factor (NKSF) or interleukin-12 is a key regulator of immune response and inflammation. Prog Growth Factor Res 1992;4:355–368.

519. Soiffer RJ, Robertson MJ, Murray C, et al. Interleukin-12 augments cytolytic activity of peripheral blood lymphocytes from patients with hematologic and solid malignancies. Blood 1993;82:2790–2796.

520. Robertson MJ, Soiffer RJ, Wolf SF, et al. Response of human natural killer (NK) cells to NK cell stimulatory factor (NKSF): cytolytic activity and proliferation of NK cells are differentially regulated by NKSF. J Exp Med 1992;175:779–788.

521. Mosmann TR, Coffman RL. Heterogeneity of cytokine secretion patterns and functions of helper T cells. Adv Immunol 1989;46:111–147.

522. Mosmann TR, Coffman RL. TH1 and TH2 cells: different patterns of lymphokine secretion lead to different functional properties. Annu Rev Immunol 1989;7:145–173.

523. Scott P. IL-12: initiation cytokine for cell-mediated immunity [comment]. Science 1993;260:496–497.

524. Heufler C, Koch F, Stanzl U, et al. Interleukin-12 is produced by dendritic cells and mediates T helper 1 development as well as interferon-gamma production by T helper 1 cells. Eur J Immunol 1996;26:659–668.

525. Manetti R, Gerosa F, Giudizi MG, et al. Interleukin 12 induces stable priming for interferon gamma (IFN-gamma) production during differentiation of human T helper (Th) cells and transient IFN-gamma production in established Th2 cell clones. J Exp Med 1994;179:1273–1283.

526. Meyaard L, Hovenkamp E, Otto SA, et al. IL-12–induced IL-10 production by human T cells as a negative feedback for IL-12–induced immune responses. J Immunol 1996;156:2776–2782.

527. Jung T, Witzak K, Dieckhoff K, et al. IFN-gamma is only partially restored by co-stimulation with IL-12, IL-2, IL-15, IL-18 or engagement of CD28. Clin Exp Allergy 1999;29:207–216.

528. Yssel H, Fasler S, de Vries JE, et al. IL-12 transiently induces IFN-gamma transcription and protein synthesis in human CD4+ allergen-specific Th2 T cell clones. Int Immunol 1994;6:1091–1096.

529. Huang T, MacAry PA, Wilke T, et al. Inhibitory effects of endogenous and exogenous interferon-gamma on bronchial hyperresponsiveness, allergic inflammation and T-helper 2 cytokines in brown-Norway rats [In Process Citation]. Immunology 1999;98:280–288.

530. Brunda MJ, Luistro L, Warrier RR, et al. Antitumor and antimetastatic activity of interleukin 12 against murine tumors. J Exp Med 1993;178:1223–1230.

531. Tannenbaum CS, Tubbs R, Armstrong D, et al. The CXC chemokines IP-10 and Mig are necessary for IL-12–mediated regression of the mouse RENCA tumor. J Immunol 1998;161:927–932.

532. Martinotti A, Stoppacciaro A, Vagliani M, et al. CD4 T cells inhibit in vivo the CD8-mediated immune response against murine colon carcinoma cells transduced with interleukin-12 genes. Eur J Immunol 1995;25:137–146.

533. Nastala CL, Edington HD, McKinney TG, et al. Recombinant IL-12 administration induces tumor regression in association with IFN-gamma production. J Immunol 1994;153:1697–1706.

534. Gately MK, Gubler U, Brunda MJ, et al. Interleukin-12: a cytokine with therapeutic potential in oncology and infectious diseases. Ther Immunol 1994;1:187–196.

535. Mu J, Zou JP, Yamamoto N, et al. Administration of recombinant interleukin 12 prevents outgrowth of tumor cells metastasizing spontaneously to lung and lymph nodes. Cancer Res 1995;55:4404–4408.

536. Dias S, Thomas H, Balkwill F. Multiple molecular and cellular changes associated with tumour stasis and regression during IL-12 therapy of a murine breast cancer model. Int J Cancer 1998;75:151–157.

537. Brunda MJ, Luistro L, Rumennik L, et al. Antitumor activity of interleukin 12 in preclinical models. Cancer Chemother Pharmacol 1996;38(Suppl):S16–21.

538. Fujiwara H, Hamaoka T, Dias S, et al. Antitumor and antimetastatic effects of interleukin 12: multiple molecular and cellular changes associated with tumour stasis and regression during IL-12 therapy of a murine breast cancer model. Int J Cancer 1998;75:151–157.

539. Brunda MJ, Luistro L, Hendrzak JA, et al. Role of interferon-gamma in mediating the antitumor efficacy of interleukin-12. J Immunother Emphasis Tumor Immunol 1995;17:71–77.

540. Seder RA, Gazzinelli R, Sher A, et al. Interleukin 12 acts directly on CD4+ T cells to enhance priming for interferon gamma production and diminishes interleukin 4 inhibition of such priming. Proc Natl Acad Sci USA 1993;90:10188–10192.

541. Colombo MP, Vagliani M, Spreafico F, et al. Amount of interleukin 12 available at the tumor site is critical for tumor regression. Cancer Res 1996;56:2531–2534.

542. Tannenbaum CS, Wicker N, Armstrong D, et al. Cytokine and chemokine expression in tumors of mice receiving systemic therapy with IL-12. J Immunol 1996;156:693–699.

543. Hashimoto W, Osaki T, Okamura H, et al. Differential antitumor effects of administration of recombinant IL-18 or recombinant IL-12 are mediated primarily by Fas-Fas ligand- and perforin-induced tumor apoptosis, respectively. J Immunol 1999;163:583–589.

544. Bukowski RM, Rayman P, Molto L, et al. Interferon-gamma and CXC chemokine induction by interleukin 12 in renal cell carcinoma: inflammatory cytokines provide a third signal for activation of naive CD4+ and CD8+ T cells. J Immunol 1999;162:3256–3262.

545. Ha SJ, Lee SB, Kim CM, et al. Rapid recruitment of macrophages in interleukin-12–mediated tumour regression. Immunology 1998;95:156–163.

546. Cavallo F, Di Carlo E, Butera M, et al. Immune events associated with the cure of established tumors and spontaneous metastases by local and systemic interleukin 12. Cancer Res 1999;59:414–421.

547. Wigginton JM, Kuhns DB, Back TC, et al. Interleukin 12 primes macrophages for nitric oxide production in vivo and restores depressed nitric oxide production by macrophages from tumor-bearing mice: implications for the antitumor activity of interleukin 12 and/or interleukin 2. Cancer Res 1996;56:1131–1136.

548. Yu WG, Yamamoto N, Takenaka H, et al. Molecular mechanisms underlying IFN-gamma–mediated tumor growth inhibition induced during tumor immunotherapy with rIL-12. Int Immunol 1996;8:855–865.

549. Angiolillo AL, Sgadari C, Tosato G. A role for the interferon-inducible protein 10 in inhibition of angiogenesis by interleukin-12. Ann NY Acad Sci 1996;795:158–167.

550. Kerbel RS, Hawley RG. Interleukin 12: newest member of the antiangiogenesis club [editorial; comment]. J Natl Cancer Inst 1995;87:557–559.

551. Sgadari C, Angiolillo AL, Tosato G. Inhibition of angiogenesis by interleukin-12 is mediated by the interferon-inducible protein 10. Blood 1996;87:3877–3882.

552. O'Reilly MS, Boehm T, Shing Y, et al. Endostatin: an endogenous inhibitor of angiogenesis and tumor growth. Cell 1997;88:277–285.

553. Voest EE, Kenyon BM, O'Reilly MS, et al. Inhibition of angiogenesis in vivo by interleukin 12. J Natl Cancer Inst 1995;87:581–586.

554. Sgadari C, Angiolillo AL, Cherney BW, et al. Interferon-inducible protein-10 identified as a mediator of tumor necrosis in vivo. Proc Natl Acad Sci USA 1996;93:13791–13796.

555. Keane MP, Arenberg DA, Lynch JP, et al. The CXC chemokines, IL-8 and IP-10, regulate angiogenic activity in idiopathic pulmonary fibrosis. J Immunol 1997;159:1437-1443.

556. Arenberg DA, Kunkel SL, Polverini PJ, et al. Interferon-gamma–inducible protein 10 (IP-10) is an angiostatic factor that inhibits human non-small cell lung cancer (NSCLC) tumorigenesis and spontaneous metastases. J Exp Med 1996;184:981–992.

557. Strieter RM, Polverini PJ, Arenberg DA, et al. The role of CXC chemokines as regulators of angiogenesis. Shock 1995;4:155–160.

558. Strieter RM, Kunkel SL, Arenberg DA, et al. Interferon gamma–inducible protein 10 (IP-10), a member of the C-X-C chemokine family, is an inhibitor of angiogenesis. Biochem Biophys Res Commun 1995;210:51–57.

559. Luster AD, Greenberg SM, Leder P. The IP-10 chemokine binds to a specific cell surface heparan sulfate site shared with platelet factor 4 and inhibits endothelial cell proliferation. J Exp Med 1995;182:219–231.

560. Strieter RM, Polverini PJ, Arenberg DA, et al. Role of C-X-C chemokines as regulators of angiogenesis in lung cancer. J Leukoc Biol 1995;57:752–762.

561. Clark-Lewis I, Dewald B, Geiser T, et al. Platelet factor 4 binds to interleukin 8 receptors and activates neutrophils when its N terminus is modified with Glu-Leu-Arg. Proc Natl Acad Sci USA 1993;90:3574–3577.

562. Sgadari C, Farber JM, Angiolillo AL, et al. Mig, the monokine induced by interferon-gamma, promotes tumor necrosis in vivo. Blood 1997;89:2635–2643.

563. Kanegane C, Sgadari C, Kanegane H, et al. Contribution of the CXC chemokines IP-10 and Mig to the antitumor effects of IL-12. J Leukoc Biol 1998;64:384–392.

564. Motzer RJ, Rakhit A, Schwartz LH, et al. Phase I trial of subcutaneous recombinant human interleukin-12 in patients with advanced renal cell carcinoma. Clin Cancer Res 1998;4:1183–1191.

565. Atkins MB, Robertson MJ, Gordon M, et al. Phase I evaluation of intravenous recombinant human interleukin 12 in patients with advanced malignancies. Clin Cancer Res 1997;3:409–417.

566. Mier J, Dollob JA, Atkins M. Interleukin 12, a new antitumor cytokine. Int J Immunopath Pharm 1998;11:109–115.

567. Rakhit A, Yeon MM, Ferrante J, et al. Down-regulation of the pharmacokinetic-pharmacodynamic response to interleukin-12 during long-term administration to patients with renal cell carcinoma and evaluation of the mechanism of this "adaptive response" in mice. Clin Pharmacol Ther 1999;65:615–629.

568. Robertson MJ, Cameron C, Atkins MB, et al. Immunological effects of interleukin 12 administered by bolus intravenous injection to patients with cancer. Clin Cancer Res 1999;5:9–16.

569. Bajetta E, Del Vecchio M, Mortarini R, et al. Pilot study of subcutaneous recombinant human interleukin 12 in metastatic melanoma. Clin Cancer Res 1998;4:75–85.

570. Cebon J, Jager E, Shackleton MJ, et al. Two phase I studies of low dose recombinant human IL-12 with Melan-A and influenza peptides in subjects with advanced malignant melanoma. Cancer Immun 2003;3:7.

571. Motzer RJ, Rakhit A, Thompson JA, et al. Randomized multicenter phase II trial of subcutaneous recombinant human interleukin-12 versus interferon-alpha 2a for patients with advanced renal cell carcinoma. J Interferon Cytokine Res 2001;21:257–263.

572. Alatrash G, Hutson TE, Molto L, et al. Clinical and immunologic effects of subcutaneously administered interleukin-12 and interferon alfa-2b: phase I trial of patients with metastatic renal cell carcinoma or malignant melanoma. J Clin Oncol 2004;22:2891–2900.

573. Van Herpen CM, Huijbens R, Looman M, et al. Pharmacokinetics and immunological aspects of a phase Ib study with intratumoral administration of recombinant human interleukin-12 in patients with head and neck squamous cell carcinoma: a decrease of T-bet in peripheral blood mononuclear cells. Clin Cancer Res 2003;9:2950–2956.

574. Wadler S, Levy D, Frederickson HL, et al. A phase II trial of interleukin-12 in patients with advanced cervical cancer: clinical and immunologic correlates. Eastern Cooperative Oncology Group study E1E96. Gynecol Oncol 2004;92:957–964.

575. Weiss GR, O'Donnell MA, Loughlin K, et al. Phase 1 study of the intravesical administration of recombinant human interleukin-12 in patients with recurrent superficial transitional cell carcinoma of the bladder. J Immunother 2003;26:343–348.

576. Ansell SM, Witzig TE, Kurtin PJ, et al. Phase 1 study of interleukin-12 in combination with rituximab in patients with B-cell non-Hodgkin lymphoma. Blood 2002;99:67–74.

577. Rook AH, Zaki MH, Wysocka M, et al. The role for interleukin-12 therapy of cutaneous T cell lymphoma. Ann NY Acad Sci 2001;941:177–184.

578. Robertson MJ, Pelloso D, Abonour R, et al. Interleukin 12 immunotherapy after autologous stem cell transplantation for hematological malignancies. Clin Cancer Res 2002;8:3383–3393.

579. McHutchison JG, Gordon SC, Schiff ER, et al. Interferon alfa-2b alone or in combination with ribavirin as initial treatment for chronic hepatitis C. Hepatitis Interventional Therapy Group. N Engl J Med 1998;339:1485–1492.

580. Flanigan RC, Salmon SE, Blumenstein BA, et al. Nephrectomy followed by interferon alfa-2b compared with interferon alfa-2b alone for metastatic renal-cell cancer. N Engl J Med 2001;345:1655–1659.

581. Perez-Zincer F, Olencki T, Budd GT, et al. A phase I trial of weekly gemcitabine and subcutaneous interferon alpha in patients with refractory renal cell carcinoma. Invest New Drugs 2002;20:305–310.

582. Kriegmair M, Oberneder R, Hofstetter A. Interferon alfa and vinblastine versus medroxyprogesterone acetate in the treatment of metastatic renal cell carcinoma. Urology 1995;45:758–762.

Hormonal Therapy for Breast Cancer

37

Peter F. Lebowitz   Sandra M. Swain

INTRODUCTION

The hormonal treatment of breast cancer was first used over 100 years ago and now plays a critical role in the prevention and treatment of the disease at all stages.[1] The correct application and further development of this therapy requires an appreciation of (a) estrogen synthesis and metabolism, (b) the endocrine regulation of these processes, (c) the molecular basis of estrogen signaling through the estrogen receptors, (d) the response of cancer cells to the modulation of estrogen receptor signaling, and (e) the pharmacology of the growing number of hormonal therapeutics. This chapter aims to provide a reference source on this basis, focusing on hormonal therapies that affect the estrogen and progesterone nuclear hormone receptors to achieve control of tumor growth.

HISTORICAL PERSPECTIVE

Early Clinical Observations

In 1896, Dr. George Beatson reported on the first successful use of estrogen deprivation to treat breast cancer.[2] Based on observations in farm animals that the ovaries have effects on lactation, he hypothesized that the removal of the ovaries might lead to decreased growth of breast tumors. His report describes the treatment of a premenopausal patient with advanced breast cancer who underwent a bilateral oophorectomy and experienced marked regression of her tumor. While ovarian ablation was used over the next few decades to treat breast cancer, the scientific underpinnings of these early clinical observations were just beginning to be understood.

Discovery of Estrogen and the Estrogen Receptor (ER)

The demonstration by Knauer in 1900 that ovarian transplants prevented uterine atrophy and loss of sexual function accompanying ovariectomy established the hormonal nature of ovarian function in regulating reproductive function.[3] Over 20 years later, in 1923, Allen and Doisy developed a rat bioassay for assessing changes in the vaginal smear induced by ovarian extracts.[4] The identification of a female sex hormone in the blood of various species was demonstrated in 1925, and in 1926 Loewe and Lange discovered a hormone in the urine of menstruating women that varied in concentration with the phase of the menstrual cycle.[5,6] This hormone was also found in large amounts in the urine of pregnant women.[7] This finding led to the isolation and crystallization of an active substance, later identified and synthesized as estradiol.[8]

While the identification of estradiol was critical in the further study of this hormonal system, it took another few decades before the second major component of this system was identified, the estrogen receptor (ER). In 1963, Jensen and Jacobsen used radioactively labeled estradiol to determine the target tissues of the "hormone of estrus."[9] This, eventually, lead to the discovery and characterization of the ER by Toft and Gorski.[10,11] In 1971, Jensen built on this discovery with the development of an ER assay that could predict clinical response to hormonal manipulation.[12]

The First Antiestrogens

Around the time of the seminal work resulting in the identification of the ER, scientists at ICI Pharmaceuticals were

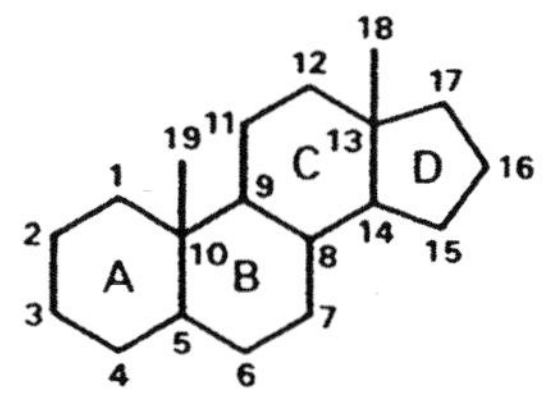

Figure 37.1 The structure and numbering of the cyclopentane-perhydrophenanthrene nucleus.

developing the first antiestrogens. The trans-isomer of triphenylethylene, initially named "ICI 46,474," was discovered in an attempt to use antiestrogens for postcoital contraception. Ironically, this compound, eventually named "tamoxifen," was later marketed as a fertility treatment. In the early 1970s, tamoxifen was shown to induce breast cancer regression.[13] Since then, it has become a prototype drug for the hormonal treatment of cancer, with use in prevention and treatment of all stages of breast cancer. Tamoxifen is not a steroid and is associated with a better side effect profile than high-potency estrogen treatment, the contemporary treatment for advanced breast cancer at the time when tamoxifen was introduced.[14] Because long-term tamoxifen administration is safe and well tolerated, clinical use in the adjuvant and prevention settings is possible.[15] Indeed, the introduction of tamoxifen likely contributed to the recent decline in breast cancer mortality observed in high-incidence Western countries.[16]

Since the 1970s, the armamentarium of medical hormonal therapies has expanded considerably with aromatase inhibitors, luteinizing hormone-releasing hormone (LHRH) agonists, progestins, and selective estrogen down-regulators. A growing number of clinical trials are ongoing to improve the safety and efficacy of endocrine therapy for breast cancer.

ESTROGEN STRUCTURE, BIOSYNTHESIS, TRANSPORT, AND METABOLISM

Structure of Estrogen

Estrogens, like all steroids, have a hydrated four-ring structure (cyclopentane-perhydro-phenanthrene), in which a five-sided cyclopentane ring (designated the D ring) is attached to three six-sided phenanthrene rings (desig-

nated the A, B, and C rings) (Figures 37.1 and 37.2). The carbon atoms that form these rings are numbered 1 to 17. Additional side chain carbons in sex steroids are attached to either carbon atom 10 or 13 and carbon atom 18 for estrogens. Corticoids and progestins are characterized by a two-carbon side chain (carbons 21 and 22) attached to carbon atom 17.

The three endogenous estrogens are estradiol, estrone, and estriol. Estradiol is readily formed from estrone and can also be formed directly by aromatization of testosterone. Hydroxylation of estrone at the 16 position results in the formation of estriol, the other biologically important estrogen in humans. These compounds are shown in Figure 37.3. The trivial (or common) and systematic names of selected steroidal hormones used for cancer therapy are shown in Figure 37.2, together with their structures. Table 37.1 provides a list of the derivative names for compounds available to manipulate estrogen action for therapeutic effect. Detailed chemical descriptions and steroid nomenclature are available from a number of sources.[17-20] The physiologic effects of estrogens are summarized in Table 37.2.

Estrogen Biosynthesis

The ultimate source of estrogens, like all endogenous steroid molecules, is cholesterol, which derives directly from the diet or via endogenous synthesis. All tissues, except possibly the adult brain, can synthesize cholesterol, although quantitatively the liver is the most important source. Cholesterol binds to lipoprotein receptors and is then taken up by steroid-producing cells, where it is transferred to the inner membrane of the mitochondria. In this location, the cytochrome P-450 enzymes begin to convert cholesterol to different steroid hormones via alteration of side chains on the molecule.[21] Figure 37.4 provides a schematic of the enzymatic steps in steroid biosynthesis.

The final step in estrogen synthesis is aromatization, which is catalyzed by the P-450 aromatase monooxygenase enzyme complex located in the endoplasmic reticulum. The aromatase enzyme complex consists of the P-450 cytochrome, P-450 arom, and a flavoprotein, nicotinamide adenine dinucleotide phosphate cytochrome P-450 reductase, that regenerates active aromatase after completion of the aromatization reaction.[21] The active site of aromatase contains a heme complex responsible for the nucleophilic attack on the androgenic precursor C19 methyl group that

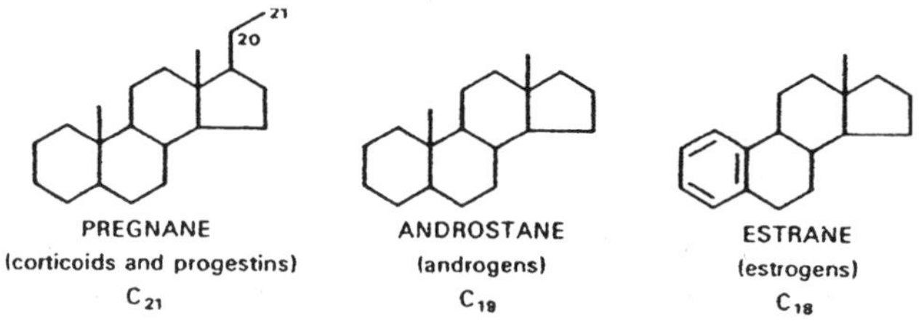

PREGNANE
(corticoids and progestins)
C_{21}

ANDROSTANE
(androgens)
C_{19}

ESTRANE
(estrogens)
C_{18}

Figure 37.2 The structure and names of the five major steroid hormones. (Trivial name is followed by systematic.) Cortisol, 4-pregnen-11β,17α, 21-triol-3,20-dione; aldosterone, 4-pregnen-11β,21-diol-18-al-3,20-dione; progesterone, 4-pregnen-3,20-dione; testosterone, 4-androsten-17β-ol-3-one; estradiol, 1,3,5(10)-estratrien-3,17β-diol.

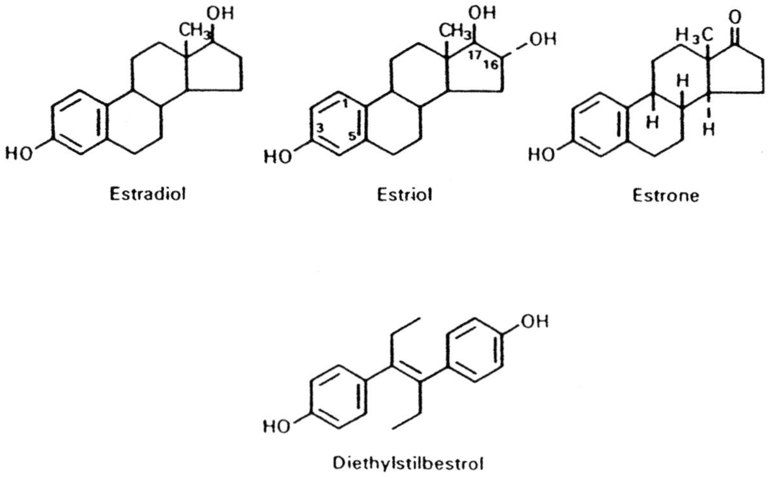

Figure 37.3 Endogenous and synthetic estrogens.

generates formic acid and an aromatized A ring characteristic of estrogenic steroids (Fig. 37.5).[22]

The gene encoding the cytochrome component of aromatase, cytochrome P-450 (CYP) 19, has low homology with other members of the CYP family and has been mapped to chromosome 15.[23] The hormonal regulation of the CYP19 gene, which spans 120 kb, is intricate, primarily due to a complex promoter structure, with regulatory elements targeted by gonadotrophins, glucocorticoids,

growth factors, cytokines, and the intracellular signaling molecule cAMP.[24–26] Examples of peptide growth factors that may increase local estrogen production are the insulin-like growth factors (IGF-I and IGF-II), key players in breast cancer pathogenesis and ER function.[27] IGF-I and IGF-II promote aromatase activity in stromal cells and the conversion of estrone to the more active molecule estradiol.[28] There are a number of unique promoters that direct expression of the gene in a tissue-specific manner. In ovar-

TABLE 37.1

TRIVIAL AND SYSTEMATIC NAMES FOR CLINICALLY RELEVANT ESTROGENS, ANTIESTROGENS, PROGESTINS, AND ANTIPROGESTINS

Trivial	Systematic
Estrogens and antiestrogens	
Steroidal	
Estradiol	1,3,5-Estratriene-3,17β-diol
Estradiol benzoate	1,3,5-Estratriene-3,17β-diol-3 benzoate
Estriol	1,3,5-Estratriene-3,16α,17β-triol
Estrone	1,3,5-Estratriene-3-ol-17-one
Ethinyl estradiol	17α-Ethinyl-1,3,5-estratriene-3,17β-diol
Faslodex (fulvestrant)	7α-[9-(4,4,5,5,5-Pentafluoropentylsulfinyl)nonyl]estra-1,3,5, (10)-triene-3,17β-diol
Nonsteroidal	
Diethylstilbestrol	3,4-Di-p-hydroxyphenylhex-3-ene
Tamoxifen	trans-1-(p-β-Dimethylaminoethoxyphenyl)-1,2-diphenylbut-1-ene
Toremifene	4-Chloro-1,2-diphenyl-1-{4-[2-N,N-dimethylamino)ethoxy]-phenyl}-1-butane
Raloxifene	[6-Hydroxy-2(4-hydroxyphenyl)benzo[b]thien-3-yl]{4-[2-(1-piperidinyl)ethoxy]phenyl}methanone-hydrochloride
Progesterones	
Medroxyprogesterone acetate	6α-Methyl-4-pregnon-17-ol-3,20-dione acetate
Megestrol acetate	6-Methyl-4,6-pregnadien-17-ol-3,20-dione acetate
Aromatase inhibitors	
Aminoglutethimide	3-(4-Aminophenyl)-3-ethylpiperidine-2,6-dione
Letrozole	[4,4'-(1H-1,2,4-Triazol-1-yl-methylene)-bis-benzonitrile]
Anastrozole	2,2'-[5-(1H-1,2,4-Triazol-1-ylmethyl)-1,3-phenylene]bis (2-methyl-propiononitrile)
Exemestane	6-Methylenandrosta-1,4-diene-3,17-dione

TABLE 37.2
PHYSIOLOGIC EFFECTS OF ESTROGENS

Growth and maintenance of female genitalia
Pubertal expression of female secondary sex characteristics
Breast enlargement
Increase in size and pigmentation of nipple and areolae
Molding of body contour with alteration of subcutaneous fat deposition
Promotion of female psyche formation
Alteration in skin texture
Maintenance of pregnancy (in concert with progestins)
Sodium retention

ian tissue, the proximal promoter II drives CYP19 expression and is regulated by FSH through cyclic AMP.[29] Aromatase is also regulated by LH during the menstrual cycle.[30] In adipose tissue, on the other hand, the distal promoter I.4 regulates CYP19 expression under the control of glucocorticoids and TNFα.[30] In tumor tissues, a switch in the aromatase gene promoters, from promoter II to promoter I.4, can occur, leading to increased aromatase activity and possibly to tumor initiation and/or promotion.[30]

The pathways of estrogen synthesis described above are carried out in a number of different tissues. In premenopausal women, the principle source of estrogens consists of the ovaries, which primarily produce estradiol. Total blood concentrations of estradiol range from a low of approximately 10 pg/mL in the early follicular phase to as high as 500 pg/mL during midcycle. This peak is quite sharp and usually precedes the ovulatory gonadotropin surge.[31] A second rise in serum estrogen occurs during the luteal phase and is lower but more prolonged. The cyclic nature of ovarian steroidogenesis occurs due to the cyclic secretory patterns of FSH and LH established by GnRH (LHRH) release from the arcuate nucleus of the hypothalamus. Steroidogenesis in the ovary is initiated by the binding of LH to LH receptors on theca interna cells, with the activation of adenylate cyclase, the formation of cAMP, and the activation of PKA. Uniquely, ovarian estrogens are synthesized by the cooperative action of two cell types. Androgens (either androstenedione or testosterone) are synthesized by ovarian thecal cells and converted to estrogens in the neighboring granulosa cells by aromatase.

In postmenopausal women, estrogens are not directly produced by the ovaries but are instead formed from the extragonadal conversion of ovarian and adrenal androgens via aromatase. Androgens from the ovaries and adrenal glands are released into the circulation and converted to estrogens in tissues with aromatase activity, including adipose tissue and muscle.[32] Thus, in the postmenopausal state, estrogens may act primarily as paracrine factors, with much higher concentrations in local environments with high aromatase activity. This model is supported by findings of high aromatase activity in breast tumors.[30]

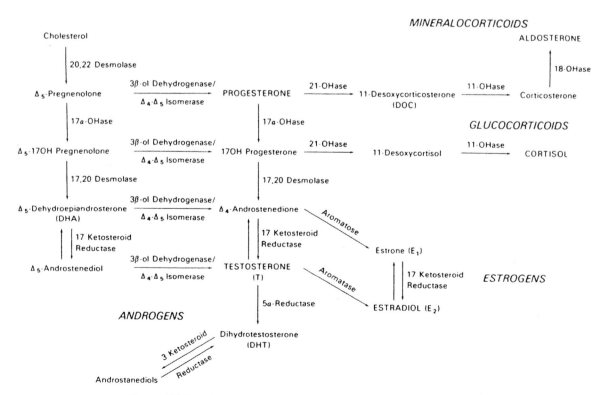

Figure 37.4 Enzymatic steps in the biosynthesis of the steroid hormone.

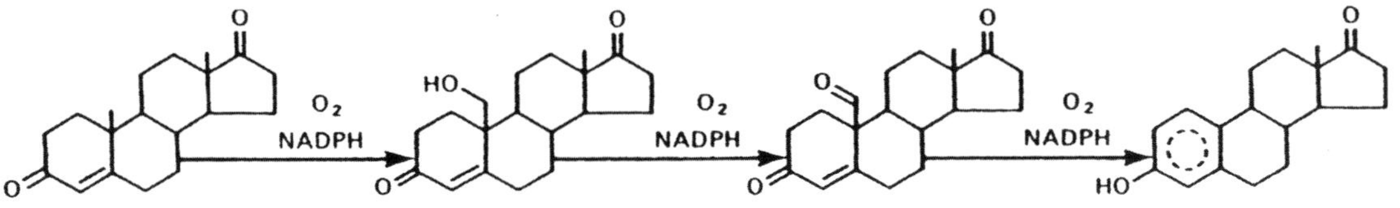

Figure 37.5 Aromatase reaction. (NADPH, nicotinamide adenine dinucleotide phosphate.)

Estrogen Metabolism

Estrogen metabolism occurs primarily in the liver, where there is free interconversion between estrone and estradiol.[33] Equilibrium slightly favors estrone, which probably serves as the main precursor for the hydroxylated estrogen metabolites in the urine.[34] Endogenous estrogens are excreted in the urine predominantly as glucuronides and sulfates, although numerous other water-soluble metabolites have been identified.[35] These conjugates undergo enterohepatic recirculation via hydrolysis by bacteria in the intestine and then reabsorption into the enteric blood supply. More than half of the estrogen metabolites and one third of the progesterone metabolites are excreted in the bile shortly after the administration of radioactive hormone. Eventually, 50 to 80% of an administered dose is excreted as metabolites in the urine within 4 to 6 days, and up to 18% may be found in the feces. In the liver, two systems for sulfation exist, one for the estrogens and the other for 3β-hydroxy steroids. Glucuronides are formed from diphosphoglucuronic acid by the microsomal enzyme glucuronyl transferase.[35]

Estrogens also undergo hydroxylation and methylation in the liver and other tissues, resulting in the formation of catechol and methoxylated estrogen metabolites. These metabolic pathways are important because the resultant products are active compounds with differing biologic properties. Hydroxylation of estrogens leads to the formation of 2-hydroxyestrogens (2-HE), 4-hydroxyestrogens (4-HE), and 16α-hydroxyestrogens (16α-HE).[21,36] Both 4-HE and 16α-HE are known to be estrogenic and are hypothesized to be carcinogenic due to their ability to form DNA adducts and create gene mutations.[37] In contrast, methylation of 2-HEs and 4-HEs yields a number of anticarcinogenic methoxylated metabolites. Thus, the proportion of carcinogenic versus anticarcinogenic metabolites generated from estrogens appears to be a balance between the 2-HE and 16α-HE reactions. Genetic polymorphisms affecting these metabolic pathways have been linked to an alteration of breast cancer risk.[36,38,39] Further details of estrogen metabolism and physiology can be found in other sources.[40,41]

Estrogen Transport

Estrogens, like other steroids, circulate in the bloodstream predominantly bound to albumin and steroid-binding globulins. The estrogens and androgens are transported via testosterone and estradiol-binding globulin (TEBG) or sex steroid–binding globulin.[41] The unbound, or free, hormone, which make up only 2 to 3% of total circulating estrogens, enters the cell by a non- energy-dependent process, the cell membrane providing a favorable lipid-rich environment for passage of the hormone by diffusion.[21] Once inside the cell, estrogens bind to the estrogen receptor (ER), thereby starting a complex series of signaling events in the target cell.

THE ESTROGEN RECEPTOR

ER Structure

The ER is a member of the nuclear hormone receptor superfamily that includes the progesterone receptor (PgR), androgen receptor (AR), glucocorticoid receptor (GR), and mineralocorticoid receptor. This receptor family also includes receptors for nonsteroidal nuclear hormones such as the retinoids (retinoid alpha receptor and retinoid X receptor), vitamin D or deltanoids, and thyroid hormone. The amino acid homologies that define this receptor family are illustrated in Figure 37.6.

The ER, like most nuclear hormone receptors, operates as a ligand-dependent transcription factor that binds to DNA at estrogen response elements to direct changes in gene expression in response to hormone binding.[21,42] The ER protein structure includes six domains, designated A to E (Fig. 37.6). Estradiol binds to the ligand-binding site in the E domain. The E domain also mediates ER dimerization, with assistance from residues in domain C. The sequence-specific DNA-binding function resides in domain C. Domain D contains a nuclear localization signal required for transfer of the ER from the cytoplasm to the nucleus. Domains that promote transcription, or activation functions (AFs), are present in domains A and B (AF1) and domain E (AF2). The basic structure and functional components of steroid hormones follow the same pattern, with a hormone-binding site, a dimerization domain, transactivation domain(s), and a nuclear localization signal.[43]

ER Subtypes: ERα and ERβ

The first identified ER, now known as "ERα," was discovered in the late 1960s, and the gene was cloned in 1986. The second ER, named "ERβ," was first reported in 1996[44] and has provided a further layer of complexity to our understanding of estrogen-regulated gene expression.[45]

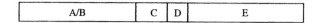

A/B   AF-1 transactivation domain
C   DNA Binding and homodimerization domain
D   NLS and HSP90 binding domain
E   AF-2 transactivation domain

% amino acid homology in relation to GR

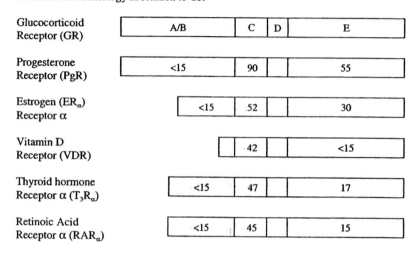

Figure 37.6 Examples of amino acid homology between nuclear hormone receptors. (A/B, activation function 1 transactivation domain; C, DNA-binding and homodimerization domain; D, nuclear localization signal and heat shock protein 90–binding domain; E, activation function 2 transaction domain.)

Furthermore, each subtype of ER exists in several isoforms. While ERα has been studied more extensively, the role of ERβ in breast cancer and endocrine therapy sensitivity is beginning to be elucidated.[45]

At the amino acid level, ERα and ERβ are highly homologous in the DNA-binding domain (96%), but the homology in the ligand-binding domain (LBD) is only 58%. This structural comparison suggests that the two subtypes would recognize and bind to similar DNA sites. However, the differences in the LBD suggests that responses to different ligands may be more distinct than anticipated from primary sequence analysis,[46] Experimental data have shown that affinities for estrogens and antiestrogens do vary significantly between ERα and ERβ.[47]

In contrast to the hormone- and DNA-binding domains, ERα and ERβ are not homologous in the N-terminal A and B (transactivation) domains, and, as a result, the transcriptional properties of ERα and ERβ are dissimilar, as discussed later in the "Hormonal Resistance" section.

Consensus on the clinical significance of ERβ expression in breast cancer has been elusive, with some conflicting findings in many different studies. However, Speirs et al. have observed that breast cancers that coexpress ERα and ERβ tend to be node-positive and a higher grade than tumors that express ERα alone,[48] and Dotzlaw et al. noted a tendency for ERβ-expressing tumors to be PgR-negative.[49] These correlations suggest an adverse effect of ERβ expression on prognosis. Other work, on the other hand, suggests that decreased levels of ERβ may be associated with increased tumorigenesis.[45]

Another major difference between ERα and ERβ is tissue expression. ERα is primarily expressed in classical estrogen target tissues such as the uterus, mammary gland, placenta, liver, CNS, cardiovascular system, and bone. ERβ is highly expressed in nonclassical estrogen target tissues such as prostate, testis, ovary, pineal gland, thyroid, parathyroid, adrenals, pancreas, gallbladder, skin, urinary tract, lymphoid, and erythroid tissues.[50] As might be expected, ERβ is therefore less important than ERα for normal reproductive organ development and function in mouse models.[51] As further study of this ER subtype progresses, however, additional actions of estrogens may be better understood.

CLASSICAL ER SIGNAL TRANSDUCTION

Ligand-dependent ER Signaling

The well-described classical ER signaling pathway is illustrated in Figure 37.7. Estrogens bind to the LBD of the ER, leading to the release of the receptor from heat shock protein (HSP) 90. This ligand binding is then followed by phosphorylation of the receptor at specific serine residues, ER dimerization, and then sequence-specific DNA binding to a sequence referred to as an "estrogen response element" (ERE). In the presence of estrogen, messenger RNA (mRNA) transcription is promoted though AF2. Residues in AF1 also promote transcription, although the function of AF1 does not require the presence of estrogen.[50] The

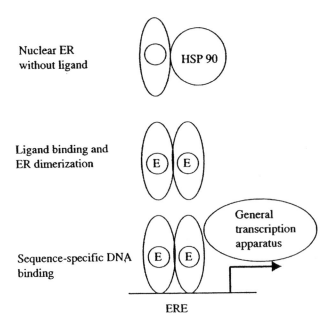

Figure 37.7 Simplified operational details of nuclear hormone action, using the estrogen receptor as an example. (E, estrogen-occupied ligand-binding site; ER, estrogen receptor; ERE, estrogen response element; HSP, heat shock protein.)

TR, ER, RAR receptors

8bp core motif

ERE	TCAGGTCAnnnTGACCTGA	P
RARE	TCAGGTCAnnnnnTCAGGTCA	DR
T$_3$RE	ACTGGACTnnnnAGTCCAGT	IP
	TCAGGTCAnnnnTCAGGTCA	DR
VDRE	TCAGGTCAnnnTCAGGTCA	DR

GR, PgR, AR

Core motif: AGAACA

ARE, GRE	GGTACAnnnTGTTCT	P
PRE	GGGACAnnnTGTCCC	P

Flanking sequences around the core motif of AR and GR may contribute to receptor specificity

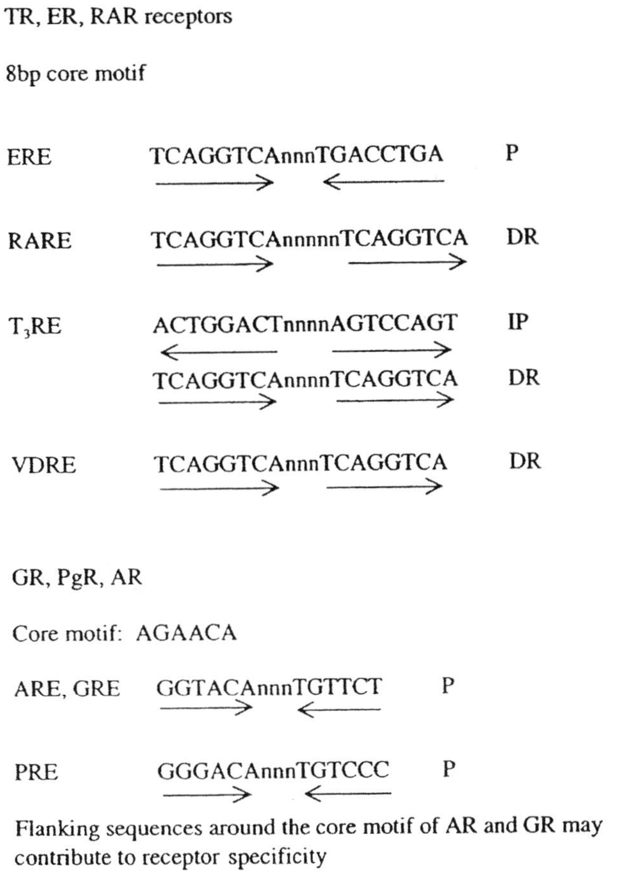

Figure 37.8 Consensus core response element motifs for nuclear hormone receptors. (AR, androgen receptor; ARE, androgen receptor response element; DR, direct repeat; ER, estrogen receptor; ERE, estrogen response element; GR, glucocorticoid receptor; GRE, glucocorticoid response element; IP, inverted palindrome; n, any nucleotide; P, palindrome; PgR, progesterone receptor; PRE, progesterone receptor response element; RAR, retinoic acid receptor; RARE, retinoic acid receptor response element; T$_3$RE, triiodothyronine receptor response element; VDRE, vitamin D receptor response element.)

consensus sequence GGTCAnnnTGACC has been defined as the ERE. Like other steroid hormone response elements, this is a palindromic sequence separated by a spacer sequence, which varies in length according to the cognate receptor. The consensus DNA binding sites for each of the nuclear hormones are illustrated in Figure 37.8. While the ER binds most strongly to the ERE consensus sequence, it is also capable of promoting transcription through sequences that have only partial homology to a classic ERE. In these cases, nearby response elements for other transcription factors (e.g., SP-1) contribute to ER activity.[50–52] The characteristics of the target gene promoter are critical to the specific nuclear actions of the activated ER. Other factors that are critical are the structure of the bound ligand and, as discussed later, the balance of coactivators and corepressors associated with the ER-ligand complex. In addition, ERα and ERβ can either homodimerize or heterodimerize, and this has an impact on their activity at the DNA binding site.[53]

ER Coactivators and Corepressors

Ligand-bound receptors interact with a family of "coactivator" and "corepressor" proteins that are sensitive to the conformational changes that occur in the LBD of each receptor. These coregulatory proteins interact with the ER to either increase or decrease transcriptional activity at a promoter site. One key mechanism for the coactivator and corepressor modulation of ER transcription likely involves alteration of histone acetylation.[54] On ligand binding, a histone deacetylase–containing corepressor complex is displaced from the nuclear receptor in

exchange for a histone acetyltransferase–containing coactivator complex. As their name implies, histone acetyltransferases catalyze the acetylation of histones, thereby altering chromatin structure. When histones become acetylated in the vicinity of the liganded nuclear receptor, DNA becomes unwound, or open, allowing access to the RNA polymerase complex, and transcription is initiated.[55] In addition to alteration of chromatin structure and histone acetylation, coactivators may also promote interactions between the nuclear hormone receptor and the basal transcriptional machinery to activate gene transcription.[43]

An increasing number of proteins have been described with coactivator properties. Some ER coactivators actually possess intrinsic histone acetyltransferase activity. Other coactivators, such as p160 coactivators, augment ER-mediated transcription by recruiting other proteins with chromatin-modifying activity. There are three p160 coactivators,

NCoA-1 (SRC-1), NCoA-2 (TIF2, GRIP1), and NCoA-3 (AIB1, ACTR, RAC3, p/CIP, TRAM-1).[43] The p160 coactivators recruit other transcriptional coactivators and histone acetyltransferases such as p300, CBP (CREB–binding protein), and pCAF (p300/CBP-associated factor).[56] The complex of proteins assembled around the ER promotes histone acetylation to allow gene transcription to occur. An additional group of coactivators, including TRAP220 (thyroid hormone receptor–associated protein, DRIP205), PGC-1, SNURF, PELP1, and NCoA-7, bind to the ER and allow interaction with transcriptional machinery.[43]

Corepressors have the opposite function and negatively regulate transcription via recruitment of histone deacetylases.[57] The list of corepressors is shorter but is also growing and includes the nuclear receptor corepressor (N-CoR) and silencing mediator for retinoid and thyroid receptors (SMRT). Other recently identified corepressors, such as SHP, DAX-1, and ER-specific corepressor, act by competing with p160 coactivators for binding to the ER.[58]

In general, coactivators and corepressors appear to be expressed at similar levels in many different tissues, suggesting that the responses to estrogen agonists and antagonists are not determined simply by the relative abundance of these cofactors. Instead, it appears that differential regulation of coactivator activity occurs through other signal transduction pathways.[54]

NONCLASSICAL ER SIGNAL TRANSDUCTION

ER Activation by Other Signal Transduction Pathways

The classical ER signaling pathway, as described earlier, is perhaps the best-studied mechanism of ER signal transduction, but recently other pathways have been described (Fig. 37.9). It is important to emphasize that nuclear hormones are not simply receptors for lipid-soluble hormones but are also critical signaling targets for protein phosphorylation–dependent second messenger pathways.[59] These functional relationships, or cross-talk, with growth factor pathways suggest that nuclear hormone receptors have an integration function that ultimately determines the cellular response to a complex set of extracellular signals.

ER expression and function are strongly influenced by growth factor signaling (Fig. 37.9B). As a result, ER expression levels correlate with distinct patterns of growth factor receptor overexpression. When ErbB2 or EGFR is activated in experimental systems, ER expression is suppressed. For example, chronic activation with heregulin, a ligand for the ErbB family of receptors, can lead to ER down-regulation and the acquisition of an ER-negative phenotype.[60,61] These data suggest that EGFR and ErbB2 signaling can bypass the

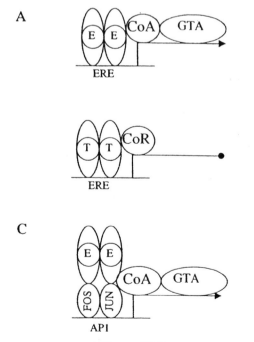

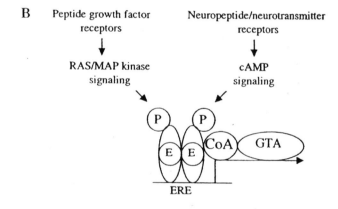

Figure 37.9 More complex models of estrogen receptor (ER) models. **A:** Estrogen (E) promotes coactivator (CoA) interactions that activate the general transcription apparatus (GTA). Tamoxifen (T) promotes corepressor (CoR) interactions that prevent activation of the general transcription apparatus. **B:** Estrogen receptor is phosphorylated by protein kinases activated by growth factors and neurotransmitters. **C:** ER interacts with other DNA-binding transcription factors to modulate the transcription of genes that do not possess an ERE. (cAMP, cyclic adenosine monophosphate; ERE, estrogen response element; MAP, mitogen-activated protein kinase; P, phosphate.)

requirement for estrogen for breast cancer cell growth and drive breast cancer cells into an ER-negative, endocrine therapy– resistant state.[62]

In other circumstances, EGFR and Erb2 signaling can activate the ER in a estrogen-independent manner. Signaling of these growth factors through the mitogen-activated protein (MAP) kinase cascade leads to phosphorylation of the Ser118 residue in the ERα AF-1 domain.[63,64] This, in turn, leads to recruitment of coactivators, allowing ligand-independent gene transcription by the ER.[60–62]

In a similar manner, signaling through the IGF-I receptor provides another example of a positive interaction between growth factor signaling and ER function. Several key components of the IGF system (e.g., the IGF-I receptor and the signaling intermediate insulin receptor substrate-I) are regulated by estrogen. As a result, IGF-I and estrogen synergistically promote the growth of breast cancer cells.[65,66] The angiogenic fibroblast growth factor family also regulates ER function, with induction of tamoxifen resistance, in an animal model.[67] Finally, the neurotransmitter dopamine and the second messenger cAMP also influence ER function through phosphorylation.[59] Interestingly, activation of cAMP leads to phosphorylation in the AF2 domain, altering the agonist and antagonist response to tamoxifen. This suggests a role for cAMP in modulating the tissue-specific effects of tamoxifen.[59] As discussed in the "Hormonal Resistance" section, insights into the cross-talk between the ER and other signal transduction pathways provide a potential strategy for novel therapeutic combinations as well as an approach to new predictive tests for endocrine therapy sensitivity.

Interaction of the ER with Other Transcription Factors

In another departure from the classical ER signaling model, ER-mediated transcription can also occur without direct contact with DNA (Fig. 37.9C). In these instances, the ER operates in conjunction with a second transcription factor that provides the sequence-specific DNA-binding function. Through this indirect mechanism, the ER can influence transcription through a greater variety of promoter sequences. Examples include the AP1 site (a target for many signals involved in cellular proliferation),[68,69] NFκB sites,[70] and a polypurine tract in the transforming growth factor-beta promoter referred to as a "raloxifene response element."[44] Because AP1 transcription factors, such as c-fos and c-jun, are key regulators of cell growth, ER-dependent AP1 activation may be critical to estrogen-dependent cell cycle progression. Furthermore, new classes of antiestrogen do not have the same profile of activities at AP1 sites as tamoxifen, which may help to explain differences in the clinical activity between compounds.[68]

Plasma Membrane ER Signal Transduction

With classical ER signaling pathways, the induction of gene transcription by estrogen can take 30 to 45 minutes, with another few hours required to see protein translation.[71,72] The observation that some estrogen effects can occur within seconds to minutes suggests a nongenomic component to ER signaling. In 1977, Pietras and Szego demonstrated that a plasma membrane form of the ER is present in cells, and this receptor was shown to respond to estradiol.[73,74] Over the past several years, this plasma membrane ER signaling pathway has received increasing attention.

Within a few seconds, estradiol can stimulate an intracellular calcium increase, adenylate cyclase activation, and phospholipase C activation.[71] These events occur through activation of the membrane ER, leading to association with G proteins. In endothelial cells, this interaction leads to generation of nitric oxide, with resulting vasodilation.[71] In addition, plasma membrane ER signaling can lead to the activation of EGFR, with subsequent activation of the Ras-Raf-MAPK signaling cascade.[75] The observation that the membrane ER can activate the EGFR-Ras-Raf-MAPK cascade is particularly interesting and suggests a feed-forward signaling circuit where the ER on the plasma membrane activates the EGFR pathway, which then increases ER activity in the nucleus. This interlaced complexity of estrogen signaling suggests the possibility of potentiating hormonal therapy through concomitant signal transduction inhibition.

ESTROGEN THERAPY

Background

High-dose estrogen therapy was the first medical treatment for metastatic breast and prostate carcinoma and has been used for nearly 6 decades.[76] While the antiandrogenic actions of estrogen explain the activity of estrogen against prostate cancer, the mechanism for antitumor activity in breast cancer remains unclear. Physiologic dosages of estradiol stimulate receptor-positive tumor cell growth in vitro[77,78] and in vivo.[79] However, high dosages inhibit breast cancer growth in vitro[80] and in vivo.[81] There are a number of possible explanations for the paradoxical inhibitory effects of high-dose estrogens. One possibility is that excess estrogen causes an imbalance of estrogen-ER complex and coactivators that are critical to ER activity. Thus the altered stoichiometry of the estrogen-ER complex with coactivators causes the number of active ER complexes to decrease.[82] In addition, it has been observed that high-dose estrogens cause a decrease in the level of ER in the cell; this also may explain the inhibitory effect on breast cancer cells.[78] Finally, one study suggested that estrogens promote chromosomal nondisjunction, which could cause loss of cellular viability.[83]

Estrogen Preparations

Several different estrogens have been used in clinical trials in the treatment of breast and prostate cancer. These include polyestradiol phosphate, micronized 17β-estradiol, ethinyl estradiol, conjugated equine estrogenic hormones, DES diphosphate, estradiol undecylate, stilbestrol, and DES.[84] The most widely used agent has been DES, a nonsteroidal synthetic estrogen; however, this agent is no longer freely available in the United States. Nonetheless, these agents are briefly discussed, as the therapeutic value of high-dose estrogen continues to be explored even after exhausting the many different hormonal therapies for metastatic breast cancer.[85]

The relative potency of several estrogens has been assayed by determining their effects on plasma FSH, a measure of the systemic effect, and by measuring increases in SHBG, CBG, and angiotensinogen, all of which indicate the hepatic effect. Piperazine estrone sulfate and micronized estradiol were equipotent with respect to increases in SHBG, whereas conjugated estrogens were 3.2-fold more potent, DES was 28.4-fold more potent, and ethinyl estradiol was 600-fold more potent. With respect to decreased FSH, conjugated estrogens were 1.4-fold, DES was 3.8-fold, and ethinyl estradiol was 80- to 200-fold more potent than piperazine estrone sulfate. The dose equivalents for ethinyl estradiol (50 µg) and DES (1 mg) reflect these relative potencies.[86] Intravaginal administration of creams containing either conjugated estrogens or 17β-estradiol results in substantial pharmacologic levels of estradiol and estrone, with subsequent decreases in LH and FSH.[87] Therefore, vaginal creams containing estrogens should be used with caution for patients who are at high risk of developing breast cancer or who have a history of early breast cancer.

Diethylstilbestrol

DES, a potent synthetic estrogen (see Fig. 37.12), is absorbed well after an oral dosage. Patients given 1 mg of DES daily had plasma concentrations at 20 hours ranging from 0.9 to 1.9 ng/mL. The initial half-life of DES is 80 minutes, with a secondary half-life of 24 hours.[88] The principal pathways of metabolism are conversion to the glucuronide and oxidation. The oxidative pathways include aromatic hydroxylation of the ethyl side chains and dehydrogenation to (Z,Z)-dienestrol, producing transient quinone-like intermediates that react with cellular macromolecules and cause genetic damage in eukaryotic cells.[89] Metabolic activation of DES may explain its well-established carcinogenic properties.[90]

Ethinyl Estradiol

Ethinyl estradiol, a more potent estrogen than DES, has a biologic half-life in plasma of approximately 28 hours. It is excreted in urine as a glucuronide and as unchanged drug. It is 600-fold more potent than piperazine estrone sulfate and 22-fold more effective than DES in increasing sex hormone–binding globulin (SHBG), a parameter of estrogen potency.[86] The usual dosage is 1 mg three times a day for female breast cancer and 150 µg per day for prostate cancer.

Toxicity

Despite substantial response rates in breast cancer, serious complications of estrogen therapy, including exacerbation of ischemic heart disease, hypertension, congestive heart failure, venous thromboembolic disease, and cerebral ischemia, have limited the value of this treatment approach.[14,91] These side effects are dose-dependent and most troublesome with DES doses of 5 mg daily. In addition, estrogens induce increased platelet aggregation and increases in factor VII and plasminogen, as well as decreased antithrombin III.[92–94] Hypertension is believed to result from estrogen-related fluid retention. Other side effects of exogenous estrogens include nausea and vomiting, diarrhea, abdominal cramps, anorexia, and glucose intolerance. Chloasma, erythema multiforme, erythema nodosum, hirsutism, and alopecia have been reported.[94,95] Estrogens cause various central nervous system side effects, including dizziness, headache, and depression. Keratoconus, or change in the corneal curvature, has been noted, with resultant intolerance to contact lenses for patients treated with estrogens. Hypercalcemia and increased bone pain are associated with a greater likelihood of subsequent antitumor response. Women may develop pigmentation of the nipples, vaginal bleeding, urinary urgency, and incontinence. Premenopausal women report mastodynia, venous dilatation of the breast, amenorrhea, and dysmenorrhea. Men develop gynecomastia and mastodynia. The risk of gallbladder disease is higher in postmenopausal women taking conjugated estrogens.[96] Elevated liver function tests and cholestatic jaundice have been seen. Hepatocellular adenomas have been reported in oral contraceptive users.[97] The use of conjugated estrogens without a progestational agent is associated with an increased risk of endometrial carcinoma.[98] Estrogens are rarely used to treat premenopausal breast cancer, but they should never be administered to pregnant patients. Vaginal adenosis is found in 66.8%, and vaginal or cervical ridges are found in 40% of DES-exposed offspring.[99] Also, the occurrence of clear cell adenocarcinoma of the vagina has been determined to correlate with DES exposure in utero.[100] A recent analysis of DES-exposed offspring reveals a risk through age 34 of 1 case per 1,000 women. In addition there is an association between intrauterine DES exposure and testicular cancer in men.[101,102]

Drug Interactions

Inducers of the hepatic microsomal enzymes, such as rifampin, barbiturates, carbamazepine, phenylbutazone, phenytoin, and primidone, enhance the metabolism of estrogen and decrease estrogenic activity. Estrogens have been reported to decrease the activity of oral anticoagulants because of the induction of the synthesis of clotting factors. Estrogens increase the half-life and pharmacologic effects of glucocorticoids but induce the metabolism and anticonvulsant activity of phenytoin and other hydantoin anticonvulsants.

TAMOXIFEN

Background

Tamoxifen is a nonsteroidal triphenylethylene first synthesized in 1966. Activity in metastatic breast cancer was first described in the early 1970s, and tamoxifen rapidly became the drug of choice for advanced disease, with response rates ranging from 16 to 56%.[103-105] Tamoxifen became the preferred drug not because it proved better than contemporary alternatives but because it was found to be safe and easy to tolerate.[14,106,107] In fact, the tolerability of tamoxifen was one of the chief reasons for the success of tamoxifen adjuvant and prevention trials, as patients are able to take the drug for prolonged periods of time with acceptable levels of toxicity.

Tamoxifen: The First Selective Estrogen Receptor Modulator (SERM)

Tamoxifen affects organ systems besides the breast. Organs affected by tamoxifen administration include the endometrium (endometrial cancer and hypertrophy),[108-110] the coagulation system (thrombosis),[111,112] bone (modulation of mineral density),[113,114] and liver (alterations of blood lipid profile).[115,116] In the organ systems listed here, tamoxifen generally acts as an agonist, mimicking the effect of estrogen, in contrast to its action on breast epithelial cells, where it generally acts as an antagonist. Therefore, tamoxifen is correctly described as a selective estrogen receptor modulator (SERM) with organ site–specific mixed agonist and antagonist effects. The agonist properties of tamoxifen also manifest in the treatment of advanced breast cancer. Flare reactions, withdrawal responses, and the experimental demonstration of breast tumor growth stimulated by tamoxifen (see the "Hormonal Resistance" section) are evidence that tamoxifen can operate as an agonist in breast tissue under certain circumstances.

Tamoxifen Metabolism

The metabolism of tamoxifen is complex and has been extensively studied by thin-layer chromatography, high-pressure liquid chromatography, and gas chromatography.[117] Ten major metabolites have been identified in patient sera (Fig. 37.10 and Table 37.3).[118-120] An excellent review of tamoxifen and its metabolism is available that presents in schematic form the proposed metabolic pathways of tamoxifen.[121] Originally, it was believed that 4-hydroxytamoxifen was the major metabolite,[117] but Adam et al., by using a different solvent system, found that

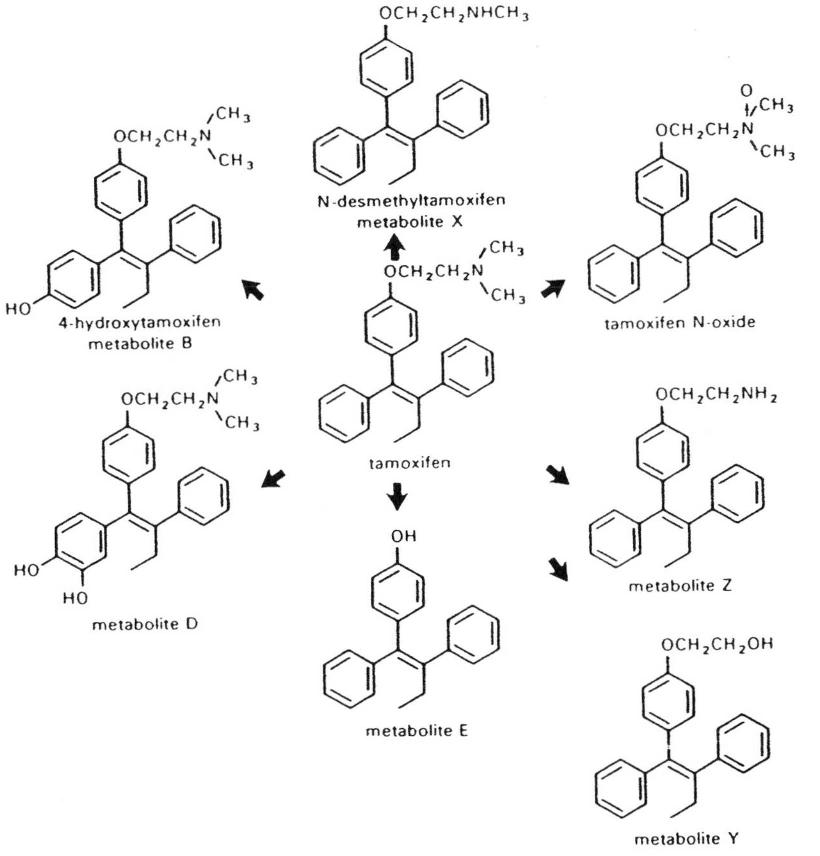

Figure 37.10 Tamoxifen and metabolites. (Adapted with permission from Lyman SD, Jordan VC. Metabolism of nonsteroidal antiestrogens. In: Jordan VC, ed. Estrogen/Antiestrogen Action and Breast Cancer Therapy. Madison: University of Wisconsin Press, 1986:191.)

TABLE 37.3
TAMOXIFEN PHARMACOLOGY

Mechanism of action	Changes folding of the steroid-binding domain, preventing gene activation of estrogen receptor
	Blocks cells in mid-G_1, may be mediated by cyclin D1
	Blocks estrogen-stimulated progesterone receptor synthesis, 52-K protein synthesis, DNA polymerase activity, and tritiated thymidine incorporation
	Stimulates production of T-cell growth factor β, decreases insulin-like growth factor-I
Metabolism	Metabolite B: 4-hydroxytamoxifen
	Metabolite E: (loss of basic side chain)-phenol
	Tamoxifen *N*-oxide
	Metabolite X: *N*-desmethyltamoxifen
	Metabolite Y: primary alcohol
	Metabolite Z: desdimethyltamoxifen
	Metabolite BX: 4-hydroxy-*N*-desmethyltamoxifen
	Metabolites A, C, D, F: (tentative)
Relative binding affinity for estrogen receptor	17β-Estradiol = 100
	Tamoxifen = 6
	Metabolite B = 280
	Metabolite E = 3
	Tamoxifen *N*-oxide = 6
	Metabolite X = 4
	Metabolite Y = 0.5
Pharmacokinetics	Tamoxifen
	$t_{1/2\alpha}$ 4–14 hr
	$t_{1/2\alpha}$ > 7 d
	Steady state, 4–16 wk
	N-Desmethyltamoxifen
	$t_{1/2}$ 9.8–14 d
	Steady state, 8 wk
Elimination	Conjugation with biliary excretion
Drug interactions	Potentiates mild hepatotoxicity induced by chronic allopurinol treatment
	Medroxyprogesterone acetate and aminoglutethimide affect metabolism
	? Inhibition of warfarin metabolism
Toxicity	Rat oncogenicity study—hepatocellular carcinoma at doses of 5–35 mg/kg/d and increased incidence of cataracts
	Intraretinal opacities, primarily paramacular, and optic neuritis
	Venous thrombosis and pulmonary embolism
	Hepatitis, fatty liver, two cases of hepatic carcinoma
	Thrombocytopenia (2–5%)
	Increased incidence of endometrial carcinoma
	Severe lipemia in patients with prior history of hypertriglyceridemia
	Anovulation

$t_{1/2}$, half-life.

the major plasma metabolite was *N*-desmethyltamoxifen.[122] Metabolism of tamoxifen is mediated in the liver by cytochrome P-450–dependent oxidases. The metabolites are excreted largely in the bile as conjugates, with little tamoxifen eliminated in the unchanged form. In two subjects given 14C-labeled tamoxifen, Fromson et al. found that 74 to 78% of the radioactivity was recovered in the feces and 9 to 14% was recovered in the urine.[123] Sutherland et al. reported that impaired renal function does not result in elevated blood levels of tamoxifen.[124]

Also, metabolite BX, or 4-hydroxy-*N*-desmethyl-tamoxifen, has been detected in serum from patients receiving tamoxifen; its biologic significance is unknown at the present time.[125,126]

The estrogen agonist and antagonist effects of the metabolites of tamoxifen have been tested in the rat and mouse systems.[118,127,128] Agonist effects are seen as positive uterotropic effects, and antagonist actions as blocking the uterotropic effects of estrogen.[118] It must be mentioned, however, that tamoxifen acts as an estrogen agonist in mice but as a partial agonist in rats and that the metabolite effects differ in these species. Metabolite B, or 4-hydroxytamoxifen, is an estrogen agonist in mice but a mixed agonist and antagonist in rat uteri. Metabolite D is an estrogen antagonist in rat uteri and a mixed agonist and antagonist in mice. Metabolite E is the only metabolite that has no antagonist properties in any system but acts as a pure agonist. Metabolites X and Y are mixed estrogen agonists and antagonists. Metabolite A has antiuterotrophic effects in rats. Finally, tamoxifen-N-oxide acts as a pure estrogen antagonist for MCF-7 cell proliferation.[128]

Tamoxifen Pharmacokinetics

Data concerning steady-state plasma levels and the relative potency of binding to the ER suggest that the biologic actions of tamoxifen are exerted by the parent compound and its 4-hydroxy metabolite.[129–134] Estradiol is present in plasma in the range of 15 to 48 pg/mL. Tamoxifen equilibrates at levels of 300 ng/mL, its N-desmethyl metabolite at 470 ng/mL, and 4-hydroxytamoxifen at 7 ng/mL.[127,134] Because 4-hydroxytamoxifen binds to the ER with 25 to 50 times the affinity of tamoxifen and with an affinity equal to that of estradiol, tamoxifen and 4-hydroxy-tamoxifen may exert an equal biologic action. N-desmethyltamoxifen is probably a minor contributor to the therapeutic effect of tamoxifen, because, despite a higher plasma concentration in plasma, its binding affinity for ER is 1,250 less than that of 4-hydroxytamoxifen. Another active metabolite, 4-hydroxy-N-desmethyl-tamoxifen, was recently identified which is present in the plasma at an average of 12.4 ng/mL in women on chronic tamoxifen therapy.[126] The plasma levels of tamoxifen and metabolites remain roughly proportional to dosage over the therapeutic dosage range, indicating no saturation of metabolic pathways.[133,135]

The initial plasma half-life of tamoxifen ranges from 4 to 14 hours, depending on the study, with a secondary half-life of approximately 7 days.[117,123,130,136] Steady-state concentrations of tamoxifen are achieved after 4 to 16 weeks of treatment.[130] The biologic half-life of the metabolite N-desmethyltamoxifen is 14 days, with a steady-state concentration reached at 8 weeks. These long half-lives reflect the high level of plasma binding to protein (greater than 99%) and enterohepatic recirculation.[130] Only free tamoxifen or metabolites can bind to ERs. Tamoxifen persists in the plasma of patients for at least 6 weeks after discontinuation of treatment.[136] Because of the long plasma half-life of tamoxifen, at least 4 weeks are required to reach steady-state levels in plasma, leading several investigators to explore the use of loading doses. In general, these investigators aimed at achieving plasma levels of 150 ng/mL, the lowest steady-state concentration observed for patients responding to the drug. Loading doses of 80 mg/m² twice daily yielded levels of 225 ng/mL at 3 hours after the first dose, whereas 50 mg/m² twice daily yielded proportionately lower levels, barely exceeding 150 ng/mL. Another study using 100 mg/m² over 24 hours on day 1 confirmed that peak concentrations of tamoxifen exceeded 150 ng/mL by the end of day 1 and could be maintained above that level by a daily dose of 20 mg.[136,137] Although studies of loading doses are of theoretical interest, their clinical relevance is uncertain. It is likely that tamoxifen and its 4-hydroxy metabolite are present in excess at all dosage levels used clinically. A thorough analysis indicates that a single dose of 20 mg a day is the most appropriate approach to tamoxifen administration.[136] Because most tamoxifen is bound to serum proteins, tamoxifen is present in low concentrations in the cerebrospinal fluid,[138] suggesting the response to tamoxifen is likely to be poor in leptomeningeal disease and central nervous system metastasis.

Intratumoral Tamoxifen Metabolism

Osborne et al. measured tamoxifen metabolites in 14 breast tumors.[139] The metabolite 4-hydroxytamoxifen exists in the trans (potent antiestrogen) and cis (weak antiestrogen) forms. In nonresponding patients, all except one had reduced tumor tamoxifen levels or a high cis-trans ratio of the metabolite. It was suggested that these metabolic abnormalities might contribute to tamoxifen resistance. Another group investigated this hypothesis in an animal system; it concluded that the metabolism and isomerization of tamoxifen to more estrogenic compounds were not mechanisms of tamoxifen resistance.[140] Levels have been measured in tumor biopsy specimens after a daily dose of 40 mg.[134] The mean concentration of tamoxifen was 25.1 ng; of N-desmethyltamoxifen, 52 ng; and of 4-hydroxytamoxifen, 0.53 ng per mg of protein. These concentrations are sufficient to prevent specific binding of estradiol to ER in human tumors in vitro.

Drug Interactions

The CYP3A family is responsible for N-demethylation of tamoxifen. Many other drugs are substrates for this enzyme family, such as erythromycin, nifedipine, cyclosporine, testosterone, diltiazem, and cortisol. The combination of tamoxifen with any of these drugs could potentially interfere with tamoxifen metabolism.[141] Mani et al. found tamoxifen N-demethylation is catalyzed in humans by CYP3A enzymes, whereas 4-hydroxylation is catalyzed by CYP2D6.[142,143] None of the inducers of P-450 tested was able to elevate the rate of 4-hydroxylation. Inducers of P-450 enzymes do enhance N-demethylation, but the clinical relevance of this information is unknown at this time. CYP2D6 is commonly involved in drug hydroxylation. There is an absence of hepatic CYP2D6 in 8% of Caucasians, defining a group in which 4-hydroxytamoxifen would not be produced efficiently.

The activity of CYP2D6 is also reduced by serotonin selective reuptake inhibitor antidepressants (SSRIs).[144] In view of the widespread use of SSRIs in patients with a history of breast cancer, a detailed study was done to determine the effects on tamoxifen metabolites.[145] Levels of 4-hydroxy-*N*-desmethyl-tamoxifen, a metabolite generated via CYP3A4 and CYP2D6 activity, was 64% lower in women taking SSRIs. While the clinical significance of this finding is unclear, it does raise the possibility that a common combination of drugs may alter clinical results. Tamoxifen also lowers plasma levels of the aromatase inhibitor letrozole, indicating that these two agents should not be administered together.[146] Medroxyprogesterone acetate has been found to alter the metabolism of tamoxifen.[147] Also, serum concentrations of tamoxifen and the metabolites Y, B, BX, X, and Z are reduced with the use of aminoglutethimide combined with tamoxifen.

Finally, reports of an interaction between warfarin and tamoxifen have prompted the manufacturer to list concurrent warfarin use as a contraindication.[148] Supratherapeutic effects of warfarin have been reported with tamoxifen use; however, the number of cases is small. The mechanism of this interaction is likely inhibition of hepatic metabolism of warfarin by tamoxifen. While in some clinical settings, the potential benefits of tamoxifen may outweigh the risks, it is critical to monitor coagulation indices closely when warfarin and tamoxifen are prescribed together.[148]

Tamoxifen Side Effects

Although tamoxifen remains the first-line endocrine therapy for early-stage and advanced breast cancer, important side effects should be considered. The tamoxifen chemoprevention trial, National Surgical Adjuvant Breast Project (NSABP) P01, established one of the most accurate sources of information on tamoxifen toxicity, because the true incidence of tamoxifen side effects was not obscured by tumor-related medical problems.[149] In NSABP P01, the excess incidence of serious adverse events (pulmonary embolus, deep venous thrombosis, cerebrovascular accident, cataract, and endometrial cancer) for patients receiving tamoxifen therapy was five to six events per 1,000 patient years of treatment. Less serious but troublesome side effects of tamoxifen included hot flashes, nausea, and vaginal discharge. Depression is also considered a side effect of tamoxifen, although there was no clear evidence of this association for women who received tamoxifen or placebo in NSABP P01. In summary, tamoxifen therapy is usually well tolerated and safe, and serious side effects occur in approximately 1 in 200 patients annually.

Ophthalmologic Side Effects

Tamoxifen retinopathy, with macular edema and loss of visual acuity, was first reported in patients receiving 120 to 160 mg per day. Three of the four originally reported patients also had corneal opacities.[150] The retinal lesions are superficial, white, refractile bodies 3 to 10 μm in diameter in the macula and 30 to 35 μm in diameter in the para-

macular tissues, and they occur in the nerve fiber layer, suggesting that they are products of axonal degeneration.[151] Additional cases have been described among patients receiving 30 to 180 mg per day.[152] Other ophthalmologic findings reported include optic neuritis, macular edema, crystalline macular deposits with reduced visual acuity, intraretinal crystals with noncystoid macular edema, refractile deposits in the paramacular areas with progressive retinal pigment atrophy, bilateral optic disc edema with visual impairment and retinal hemorrhages, tapetoretinal degeneration, and two cases of superior ophthalmic vein thrombosis.[152-155] It is worth emphasizing that, in the chemoprevention study, the only significant optic toxicity at increased incidence compared with placebo was cataract.[149]

Thrombosis

The increased risk of thrombosis associated with tamoxifen therapy may be associated with decreased levels of antithrombin III levels. Enck and Rios found a decreased functional activity of antithrombin III in 42% of tamoxifen-treated patients.[111] Pemberton et al. found reduced antithrombin III and protein C levels in women taking tamoxifen.[156] The incidence of venous thrombosis in this study was 5.62%, compared with 0% in controls. The generally accepted rate is lower. In the P01 prevention trial, the average annual rates per 1,000 women of stroke, pulmonary embolism, and deep venous thrombosis were increased by 0.53, 0.46, and 0.50 cases respectively.[149] The NSABP B-14 study reported thromboembolic events in 12 patients (0.9%), with one fatal pulmonary embolus, compared with two thromboemboli (0.2%) in controls,[157] a rate similar to that occurring in the P01 prevention trial.[149]

Hematologic Side Effects

Thrombocytopenia occurs in 5% of patients and is usually transient, resolving after the first week of treatment. Leukopenia is less frequent and is also transient.[158]

Lipoproteins

Changes in serum lipoproteins have been noted in patients taking tamoxifen. Changes occur that are indicative of an estrogenic effect of tamoxifen: an increase in total triglycerides, a decrease in total cholesterol, an increase in low-density lipoprotein (LDL) triglycerides, and a decrease in LDL cholesterol. Many other studies substantiate the effect of tamoxifen on lowering total cholesterol and, in most cases, LDL cholesterol and apolipoprotein B.[159-161] Despite these potentially favorable effects, there was no evidence of an improvement in the rate of cardiovascular mortality in either the Oxford metaanalysis[15] or the NSABP P01 prevention trial.[149]

Hepatic Toxicity

Tamoxifen has been associated with various hepatic abnormalities, including cholestasis, jaundice, peliosis hepatitis, and hepatitis. Carcinogenicity studies in rats reveal hepatocellular carcinoma in dosages ranging from 5 to 35 mg/kg per day.[162] A dose of 20 to 40 mg given to humans is 5 to 10 times less than the 5 mg/kg dose, and an increase in hepatocellular carcinoma in humans taking tamoxifen has not been reported. This is significant because tamoxifen forms adducts with DNA and could be mutagenic and carcinogenic.[163]

Bone Side Effects

The effect of tamoxifen on bone mineral content in postmenopausal women can be considered an advantageous side effect, with substantial data supporting an estrogen agonistic activity of tamoxifen on bone.[164,165] In the P01 study, a nonsignificant decrease in fracture rate was documented; further follow-up of this study should clarify this issue.[149] In premenopausal women, bone mineral density is decreased. Presumably in a high-estrogen environment, tamoxifen operates predominantly as an antagonist.[166,164]

Gynecologic Side Effects

Many premenopausal patients notice a change in the duration of menses or heaviness of flow, and there have been suggestions of an increased incidence of ovarian cysts in these patients.[167] In postmenopausal women, endometrial cancer is increased, but screening for endometrial cancer is complicated by tamoxifen-induced benign endometrial hyperplasia and polyp formation. Data from the pilot British Breast Cancer Prevention Trial found that 39% of women taking tamoxifen had histologic endometrial changes, 16% with atypical hyperplasia and 8% with endometrial polyps. These results compared with 10% abnormalities in placebo-treated patients, with no atypical hyperplasia and 2% with polyps. Transvaginal ultrasonography was used, with an endometrial thickness of 8 mm or more predictive for atypical hyperplasia or polyps.[168] The risk of endometrial cancer relates to age and duration of tamoxifen treatment. In the original Swedish report, 13 endometrial cancers were diagnosed in 695 tamoxifen patients, for a frequency of 0.9% among patients receiving 2 years of drug treatment versus 3% among those receiving 5 years of treatment. The frequency for the controls was similar to that for patients receiving 2 years of treatment, whereas the highest frequency occurred among those treated for 5 years. The increased frequency appeared in the third and fourth years of follow-up. It should be noted that the Swedish patients received the high dose of 40 mg daily. The same investigators later described the histology of 17 cases of tamoxifen-linked endometrial cancer, 16 of which were grade 1 or 2, although three

patients from the group died of the uterine malignancy.[168] These frequencies are similar to those reported for the P01 study, with an increase in endometrial cancer but overall a low rate of death from the disease. Recently a case-control study found that exposure to tamoxifen interacts with other risk factors for endometrial cancer, namely, a history of hormone replacement therapy and higher body mass index.[169]

In addition to endometrial cancer, recent reports shown that the risk of uterine sarcoma, a very rare malignancy, is also increased by tamoxifen. A recent update from six NSABP trials in which over 17,000 women were randomized to tamoxifen or placebo shows that the rate of uterine sarcoma was increase to 0.17 per 1,000 women-years versus 0 per 1,000 women years in women taking tamoxifen versus placebo.[170]

Recommendations for gynecologic follow-up of patients taking tamoxifen have varied from observation to yearly vaginal ultrasound to yearly endometrial biopsy, with no solid data supporting any of these approaches. Yearly pelvic examinations and rapid investigation of postmenopausal bleeding, but not radiologic or biopsy screening, are currently recommended. Particular attention should be given to patients at higher risk.[169] Cyclic progestins have been considered to obviate the estrogenic effect of tamoxifen on the endometrium. Preclinical data suggest that progesterone may reverse the antitumor effect of tamoxifen in the dimethylbenzanthracene-induced rat mammary tumor model.[171] There continues to be concern about the safety of cyclic progestins. Furthermore, many postmenopausal women find regular "withdrawal" bleeding inconvenient.

Endocrine Effects

The effects of tamoxifen on circulating hormones through feedback effects on the pituitary-hypothalamus axis, through effects on plasma steroid-binding proteins, or through end-organ effects vary according to gender and menopausal status. In postmenopausal women, most investigators have found a decrease in prolactin, LH, and FSH, although all three remain within the normal range.[172-175] Thyrotropin-releasing hormone induction of prolactin secretion is suppressed.[176] Plasma estrone and estradiol remain unchanged in most studies, although one study reported a minor decrease in plasma estrogens and an increased urinary excretion of glucuronide conjugates, suggesting an increase in metabolism or renal clearance of endogenous estrogens.[177] In premenopausal women, estradiol, estrogen, and progesterone have been reported to be increased after tamoxifen.[175] Many women continue to ovulate while taking tamoxifen, and in those who do, supraphysiologic levels of estradiol have been seen.[178] Tamoxifen causes an elevation of serum cortisol due to an increase in transcortin,[179] as well as increases in sex hormone–binding globulin, thyroxine-binding globulin, and apolipoprotein AI.[180-182] Because tamoxifen is a weak estrogen, it binds to ER and has estrogenic effects on normal hormone-responsive organs. In postmenopausal women, it causes an increase in cornification of the vaginal epithelium[183] and induces PgR in the endometrium[184] and in breast tumors.[185] In men, the only consistent finding seems to be an increase in progesterone in plasma,[132] whereas levels of LH, estradiol, and other hormones remain unchanged in most studies.[132,134] IGF-I or somatomedin C levels have been shown to be decreased with the use of tamoxifen.[186-188] Because exogenous estrogens are known to decrease IGF-I levels in postmenopausal women, it is possible that the effect seen with tamoxifen is an estrogen agonistic effect.[189]

Pregnancy

The effect of tamoxifen on offspring is unknown. There was one case report of a mother on tamoxifen giving birth to a baby with Goldenhar's syndrome, an oculoauriculovertebral syndrome.[190] This woman also had smoked marijuana and ingested cocaine, so the effect of tamoxifen is unclear. In the same case report, there is a discussion of 50 pregnancies on file at AstraZeneca Pharmaceuticals in women taking tamoxifen. These resulted in 19 normal births, 8 terminated pregnancies, 13 unknown outcomes, and 10 infants with a fetal and neonatal disorder, 2 of which had craniofacial defects. In another report, 85 women taking tamoxifen for prevention of breast cancer became pregnant; none of these pregnancies resulted in fetal abnormalities.[191] Another case of an infant born with ambiguous genitalia after in utero exposure through 20 weeks has also been reported.[192] The evidence for the teratogenicity of tamoxifen is primarily derived from animal studies, in which reproductive organ abnormalities and increased susceptibility to carcinogens were found.[193] Despite this evidence in animals, in humans only anecdotal reports of abnormalities, without an established definitive causal link to tamoxifen, have been reported. However, given the possibility of harmful effects, women should be told to use mechanical contraception while on this drug.

Male Breast Cancer

There have been case reports of impotence[194] and of nocturnal priapism[195] in male breast cancer patients receiving tamoxifen. Another series reported a decrease in libido in 29.2% of male breast cancer patients.[196] The issue of impotence in men treated with tamoxifen has been studied in men treated with tamoxifen for male infertility. One paper reports a loss of libido in four cases (9%),[197] whereas studies that reported an increase in testosterone levels with tamoxifen did not report an increase in impotence.[198] These data suggest that the effect of tamoxifen on sexual function is minimal and is probably not the cause of impotence.

Flare Reactions

A transient exacerbation of symptoms, or "flare reaction," was first observed during the treatment of postmenopausal women with high-dose estrogen. A clinical flare reaction is characterized by a dramatic increase in bone pain and an increase in the size and number of metastatic skin nodules with erythema.[199] Typically, symptoms occur from 2 days to 3 weeks after starting treatment and can be accompanied by hypercalcemia, which occurs in approximately 5% of patients.[200] Tumor regression may occur as the reaction subsides.

In this context, two further manifestations of flare need to be taken into consideration, tumor marker flare and bone scintigraphic flare. Tumor marker analysis should be interpreted with caution in the first months after starting tamoxifen, because up to 75% of patients beginning a new therapy for metastatic disease will exhibit a rise in tumor marker levels that subsequently return to baseline or below. Bone scans can also show flare, with an increase in uptake 2 to 4 months after the initiation of systemic therapy, which may confuse a radiographic evaluation of flare-like symptoms.[201,202] Plain film radiography is helpful here, as the presence of sclerosis, suggesting healing, may be documented in previously purely lytic lesions.

Withdrawal Response

Between 25% and 35% of patients treated with estrogens have a secondary response if estrogen is stopped when disease progression is diagnosed.[14,203] The same phenomena can be observed on withdrawal of tamoxifen and progestins.[204] Convincing withdrawal responses only occur for patients who have experienced tumor regression followed by subsequent recurrence of tumor.

OTHER SERMs

Background

The structures of SERMs and antiestrogens that have been recently approved or are under investigation are provided in Figure 37.11. Although pure antiestrogen therapy, as discussed later with fulvestrant, is a logical approach to the treatment of advanced breast cancer, drugs devoid of all estrogenic activities might be problematic in the adjuvant and prevention settings, because secondary hormone replacement therapy–like benefits of tamoxifen are considered worthwhile for postmenopausal women. This concern stimulated the development of alternative antiestrogens with a modified mixed agonist and antagonist profile. Ideally, these drugs are antiestrogenic in the breast and endometrial but retain beneficial effects on bone mineralization. Although, historically, estrogenic effects on lipids and other cardiovascular markers were felt to be beneficial,

Nonsteroidal

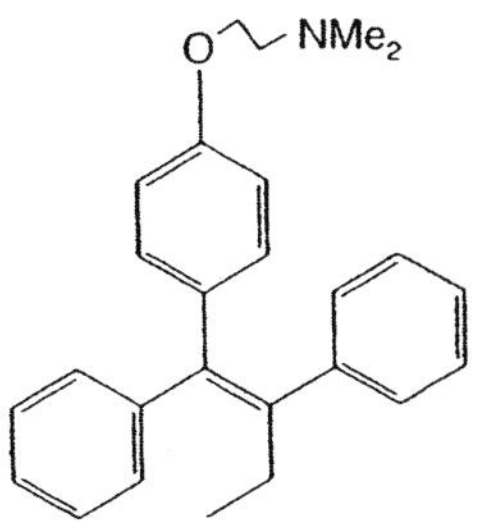

Tamoxifen

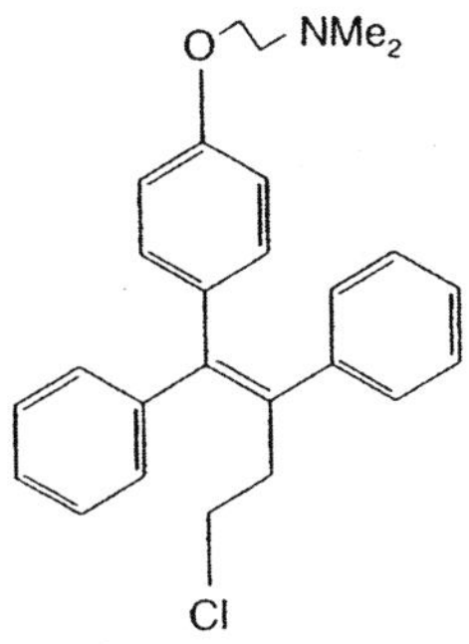

Toremifene

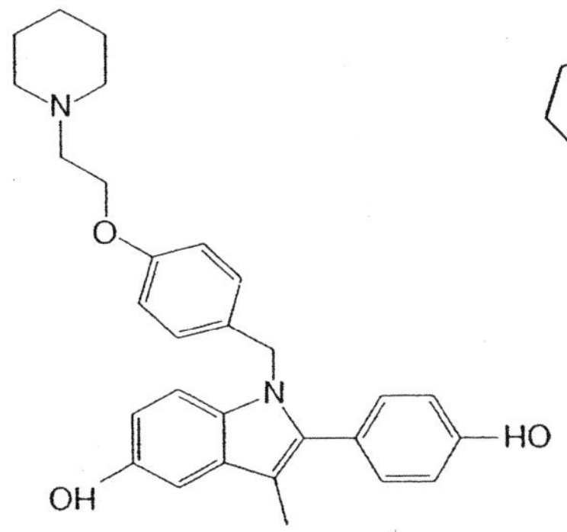

ERA-923

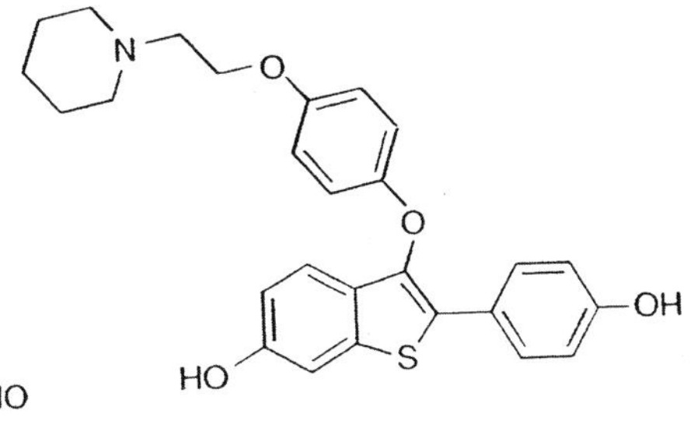

Raloxifene

Steroidal

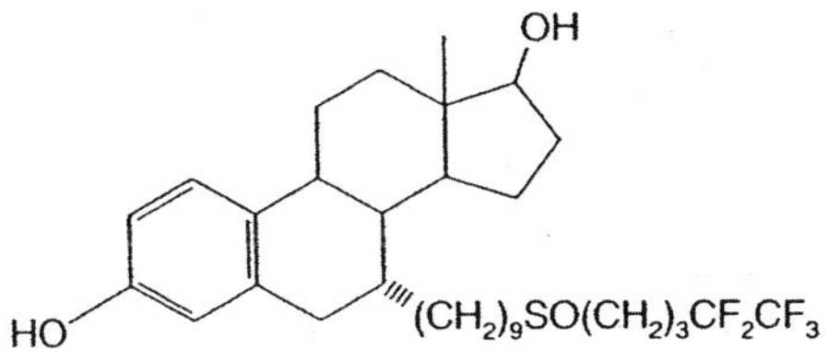

Faslodex

Figure 37.11 Antiestrogens. (SERM, selective estrogen receptor modulator.)

a recent large randomized study, the Women's Health Initiative, has demonstrated that hormone replacement did not improve cardiovascular outcomes.[205] As a result, the optimal balance of agonism versus antagonism for cardiovascular endpoints remains a issue of debate.

It is also important to emphasize that although ideal SERMs may represent a small advance in terms of safety, they are not necessarily more efficacious. In general, antiestrogens that exhibit a mixed agonist and antagonist profile, even if modified in a way that improves tissue-specific toxicities, are likely to exhibit resistance and toxicity profiles that overlap those of tamoxifen.[206] This may be because any antiestrogen that triggers ER dimerization and DNA binding is prone to the same coactivator-based resistance mechanisms that may limit the activity of tamoxifen.

Raloxifene

Raloxifene [6-hydroxy-2-(4-hydroxyphenyl)-benzo[b]thien-3-yl]–[4-[2-(1-piperidinyl) ethoxy] phenyl] is the first approved drug to exhibit a "modified" SERM profile; however, the indication for raloxifene is osteoporosis, not breast cancer.[207] An early evaluation of activity in tamoxifen-resistant breast cancer (when the drug was referred to as "keoxifene" or "LY156758") was disappointing.[208] Consequently, raloxifene should not be used for the treatment of either early stage or advanced breast cancer. However, there is continued interest in this drug in the prevention setting, because a decrease in breast cancer incidence was seen in raloxifene osteoporosis trials.[209] The current NSABP prevention study compares raloxifene to tamoxifen in women at high risk of the disease.[210] A raloxifene-related drug, currently referred to as "arzoxifene," has a profile similar to that of raloxifene but with greater ER antagonist activity in breast cancer models.

Mechanism of Action

While raloxifene has agonist and antagonist activity that is similar to tamoxifen in breast tissue and bones, its antagonist effects in the endometrial provide a distinct advantage. The molecular mechanisms of this endometrial activity are now fairly well understood. Raloxifene is a benzothiophene with a structure that includes a flexible "hinge" region that results in a nearly orthogonal orientation of its side chains. This is markedly different from tamoxifen, which has a rigid triphenylethylene structure.[211] Although both drugs bind to the ER, their structural differences lead to dissimilar conformations of the ER-ligand complex[212]; this conformation difference may partly account for differential recruitment of co activators and co repressors. In the Ishikawa endometrial carcinoma cell line, tamoxifen, but not raloxifene, induces recruitment of coactivators SRC-1, AIB1, and CBP to the c-Myc and IGF-1 promoters.[213] This recruitment of coactivators is critical to tamoxifen's transactivating ability and agonist activity in the endometrium. The comparative inability of raloxifene to assemble this coactivator complex appears to account for its antagonist activity in the endometrium.

Pharmacology and Metabolism

Raloxifene binds to the ER with a K_d of about 50 pmol/L, which is comparable to the value for estradiol.[214] The drug is given at 60 mg per day, and after oral administration it is rapidly absorbed, reaching its maximal concentration in about 30 minutes.[215] While absorption of 60% is seen, first-pass glucuronidation limits the drug's bioavailability to 2%. After absorption, raloxifene is distributed widely throughout the body and is bound to plasma proteins, including albumin. The half-life of the drug is 27.7 hours.[215]

Metabolism of raloxifene, as mentioned, is primarily via first-pass metabolism in the liver, where it is glucuronidated. The agent does not appear to be metabolized by the CYP enzyme systems, and there are no other known metabolites.[215] Elimination occurs primarily through bile and feces, with just a small amount found in the urine.

Drug Interactions

Cholestyramine causes a 60% reduction in raloxifene absorption and enterohepatic circulation.[215] Unlike tamoxifen, raloxifene has a minor interaction with warfarin, with just a 10% decrease in prothrombin time. Concomitant therapy with ampicillin reduced the raloxifene peak concentration by 28%, which was felt to be clinically insignificant.[216]

Skeletal Effects

Raloxifene has been demonstrated to have estrogen agonist activity in bone in both animal models and in clinical trials. Promotion of bone density may occur through inhibition of osteoclast activity and stimulation of osteoblasts. In an ovariectomized rat model, raloxifene protected against bone loss and resulted in augmentation of bone strength.[211] Furthermore, in rats with intact ovarian function, the drug does not antagonize estrogen effects on bone density.

Results in human clinical trials have demonstrated similar effects. Bone remodeling studies show that raloxifene inhibits bone resorption.[216] This activity results in increased bone density in postmenopausal women with and without osteoporosis. The largest raloxifene trial reported to date, the MORE study, enrolled 7,705 women with osteoporosis to determine if the drug could decrease the rate of fractures.[217] While vertebral fractures were reduced by 30%, nonvertebral fracture were not significantly different. However, bone mineral density was increased in both the spine and femoral neck.

Endometrial Effects

Unlike estrogen and tamoxifen, raloxifene does not have stimulatory activity in the uterus. In rat models, uterine weight and endothelial height were unchanged with raloxifene exposure.[218] Similarly, a number of clinical trials have carefully evaluated endometrial thickness, endometrial hyperplasia, vaginal bleeding, and endometrial cancer. All studies have found that raloxifene does not promote uterine proliferation.[218] The 4-year update of the MORE trial further confirmed this finding over a longer time frame. In this study, the rates of vaginal bleeding and endometrial cancer in patients taking raloxifene have been the same as those on placebo.[219]

Cardiovascular Effects

Raloxifene has also been shown to have estrogen agonist effects on the cardiovascular system, with reduction of serum cholesterol levels by 70% in postmenopausal rat models.[218] In clinical trials, raloxifene has been shown to reduce serum LDL, fibrinogen, lipoprotein (a), homocysteine, and C-reactive protein. Unlike tamoxifen, however, raloxifene does not affect triglycerides or HDL. Despite these findings, which would argue for a possible cardiovascular protective effect, there is only limited data indicating that raloxifene has clinical benefit in this regard.[218] While in the MORE trial, there was no difference in cardiovascular events and cerebrovascular events in the overall cohort, subgroup analysis with multiple comparisons revealed that women with increased cardiovascular risk had a relative risk reduction in cardiac events of 40% when taking raloxifene.[209] This finding, however, must be confirmed in other trials, given the exploratory nature of the analysis. In addition, the

Women's Health Initiative, a large prospective, randomized trial that assigned women to hormone-replacement therapy or placebo, showed no decrease in cardiovascular disease with estrogen alone, so it is possible that similar results may be found with raloxifene.[205] The RUTH (Raloxifene Use for the Heart) trial is currently enrolling patients and was specifically designed to evaluate cardiovascular endpoints.[220]

Other Side Effects

Other major side effects of raloxifene compared to placebo in the MORE trial included hot flashes (9.7% vs. 6.4%), leg cramps (5.5% vs. 1.9%), and thromboembolic events (1.4% vs. 0.47%).[217] The etiology of leg cramps is unclear, but they were generally mild and did not result in discontinuation.[211] The increased risk of thromboembolic events is similar to that seen with tamoxifen and is perhaps the side effect of most concern when the drug is used in clinical practice. In addition, raloxifene has been demonstrated to be teratogenic in animal studies.[211] Given this risk and the lack of clinical data in the premenopausal setting, raloxifene should only be used in postmenopausal women outside of a clinical trial.

Toremifene

Toremifene was the first new antiestrogen since tamoxifen to be approved in the United States, and it provides an alternative to tamoxifen for first-line treatment of advanced breast cancer.[221] Toremifene is reported to have antiestrogenic activity similar to that of tamoxifen.[222] The drug acts as almost a pure antiestrogen in rats and is partially agonistic in mice. Unlike tamoxifen, however, this drug has no hepatocarcinogenicity or DNA adduct-forming ability in rats.[222] It was hoped, therefore, that toremifene would provide a safer SERM for long-term use, such as in the adjuvant setting, although studies comparing the two drugs have shown no clear advantage over tamoxifen. As a result, toremifene's use in the clinic has been somewhat limited. The major metabolites of toremifene are N-demethyl-toremifene and 4-hydroxytoremifene. The mean terminal half-life of toremifene and these metabolites is from 5 to 6 days.[223] The side effects are similar to those of tamoxifen, with hot flashes being the most common. Five patients developed leukopenia, with the lowest white blood cell count being 2,500. One patient had to discontinue therapy because of tremor. Toremifene is cross-resistant with tamoxifen and should not be used in tamoxifen-resistant disease.[222]

FULVESTRANT: A PURE ANTIESTROGEN

Background

Given findings that resistance to tamoxifen may sometimes be due to its partial agonist effects, pure antiestrogens without agonist activity were developed as hormonal agents. Fulvestrant, which is the only approved pure antiestrogen, is a 7α-alkylamide analog of 17β-estradiol (Fig. 37.11). This drug is also often called a "selective estrogen receptor down-regulator" (SERD), because it has been demonstrated to decrease the level of ER protein in the cell.[224]

Mechanism of Action

Fulvestrant is a steroidal antiestrogen that acts in a distinctly different manner than tamoxifen and other SERMs. The drug binds the ER, like SERMs, but its long, bulky alkylamide side chain at the 7α position prevents ER dimerization due to steric effects. The result is that the ER cannot bind DNA, and in addition it is eliminated more rapidly via proteosome degradation, leading to a marked reduction in ER protein levels.[225,226] In this way, fulvestrant blocks ER-mediated gene transcription completely. In vitro, this results in inhibition of tamoxifen-resistant breast cancer cell lines by fulvestrant. In addition, the drug has no growth stimulatory effect in a tamoxifen-stimulated MCF-7 breast cancer xenograft model.[225] In primate studies, fulvestrant also acts as a pure antiestrogen outside of the breast, with complete inhibition of estrogen stimulation of uterine tissue.[227]

The antiproliferative effects of fulvestrant may be augmented by its ability to suppress insulin-like growth factor receptor signaling. This appears to occur both in vitro and in animal models. Finally, fulvestrant also has activity as an aromatase inhibitor, although it is not known how much this property contributes to the clinical activity of the drug.[228]

The effects of fulvestrant on ER, PgR, proliferation, and apoptosis have been examined in benign endometrial tissue and malignant breast tissue. When fulvestrant was given for a week before hysterectomy, it was found to decrease a Ki67-based proliferation assay; however, ER and PgR levels were not affected. In contrast, short-term exposure to fulvestrant before breast surgery decreased ER and PgR expression and proliferation and increased apoptosis.[229,230] These data suggest that, as in the case of other antiestrogens, there may be differences in the action of fulvestrant at different organ sites.

While current experience with fulvestrant in breast cancer is limited to postmenopausal women, there have been trials with benign gynecologic conditions that demonstrate its antiestrogenic properties in premenopausal women.[225,231]

Pharmacology

In vitro, fulvestrant has an ER-binding affinity that is 100-fold greater than that of tamoxifen.[225] Because the drug is not reliably absorbed orally, it is formulated as a monthly depot intramuscular injection. With this preparation, peak levels of fulvestrant occur at a median of 8 to 9 days after dosing and decline thereafter, but the levels remain above the projected therapeutic threshold at day 28. In pharmacokinetic studies, the AUC was 140 ng per day in the first month and 208 ng per day after 6 months, suggesting some drug accumulation.[232] Because a single injection of the 5-mL volume can be difficult in some patients, the drug is often given as two 2.5-mL injections; this alternative method of delivery has no effect on the pharmacokinetics of the drug.[233]

Metabolism

While published data on the metabolism of fulvestrant are sparse, the drug is known to undergo oxidation, hydroxylation, and conjugation with glucuronic acid and/or sulphate in the liver, with negligible renal excretion. The half-life of the drug is approximately 40 days.[234]

Side Effects

In preclinical studies, fulvestrant has been reported to cause decreased bone mineral density in adult female rats, suggesting that osteoporosis might be a side effect.[235] Clinically, there is not yet enough data to determine if fulvestrant leads to osteoporosis. Preclinical results also show that fulvestrant differs from tamoxifen in its effects on bovine lenses maintained in vitro. While these experiments suggest that fulvestrant might have decreased ocular effects as compared with tamoxifen, large randomized trials would be required to determine differences in this rare complication.[225]

In other preclinical studies, fulvestrant was found to allow the uptake of [^{3}H]-estradiol in the brain, suggesting that the drug might have decreased CNS effects compared with other hormonal approaches. Interestingly, in early human studies, no clear effect on FSH levels and LH levels have been documented, indicating that fulvestrant has no impact on pituitary function.[225] Despite these findings, the frequency of hot flashes with fulvestrant in clinical trials has been similar to the frequency with aromatase inhibitors. However, a recent trial comparing fulvestrant and tamoxifen in the metastatic setting suggested decreased hot flashes with fulvestrant.[236] There were no other side effect in this trial that were statistically different between the two drugs.

In early clinical studies, fulvestrant did not cause a change in sex hormone–binding globulin, prolactin, or lipids.[224] In addition, there was no increase in endometrial thickness in patients undergoing hysterectomy.[231] In more recent clinical trials for metastatic breast cancer, fulvestrant has been well tolerated, with hot flashes and gastrointestinal disturbances as the most common adverse events. Tolerability was similar between fulvestrant and anastrozole in two phase III trials, with a treatment-related withdrawal rate of 2.5%.[225]

Fulvestrant in Premenopausal Women

While breast cancer trials with fulvestrant have focused on postmenopausal women, the drug has also been used in premenopausal women with uterine fibroids and endometriosis. In these studies, fulvestrant had pure antagonizing effects in endometrial tissue.[225]

Other Pure Antiestrogens

Clinical development programs have recently been activated for other "pure" antiestrogens. EM 652 has a nonsteroidal structure and is theoretically interesting because of an inhibitory action against ERα and ERβ whether these receptors are operating through a classic ERE or an AP1 site.[237]

ERA923 is another nonsteroidal antiestrogen in early clinical trials. No preclinical information on this compound has been released.

AROMATASE INHIBITORS

Aromatase Background

Postmenopausal Estrogen

The therapeutic effect of reducing estrogen levels for patients with breast cancer was originally restricted to patients with functioning ovaries. However, as discussed earlier, postmenopausal women still produce significant amounts of estrogen through aromatization of circulating adrenal androgens in peripheral normal tissues, such as fat, muscle, liver, and the epithelial and stromal components of the breast.[237,238] Peripheral aromatization is increased in certain medical conditions, including obesity, hepatic disease, and hyperthyroidism, but is independent of pituitary hormone secretion. The relative proportion of estrogens synthesized in extragonadal sites increases with age, and eventually nonovarian estrogens predominate in the circulation.[239]

Intratumoral Aromatase

Expression of aromatase in the breast led to the hypothesis that local synthesis of estrogens contributes to breast cancer growth in postmenopausal women.[240,241] In support of this theory, the decline in estrogen concentrations after menopause is less marked in breast tissue than in plasma due to a combination of aromatase activity and preferential estrogen uptake from the circulation.[28] Furthermore, aromatase activity has been shown to correlate with a marker of breast cancer cell proliferation, and quadrants of the breast bearing a breast cancer have more aromatase expression than those not bearing tumors.[242] It is unclear whether an increase in aromatase expression precedes breast cancer development or is a direct consequence of the presence of a tumor. However, aromatase activity in the breast is an attractive resolution to the paradox that breast cancer increases with age although overall estrogen levels decline.[28]

Development of Aromatase Inhibitors

Steroidal versus Nonsteroidal

The pivotal role of aromatase in the development of breast cancer defines this enzyme as a key therapeutic target. Two distinct solutions evolved to the problem of designing potent, specific, and safe aromatase inhibitors.[243] One strategy was to develop "steroidal" aromatase inhibitors that are resistant to aromatase action and that bind aromatase and block conversion of androgenic substrates (Type 1 inhibitors). An alternative was to develop a family of "nonsteroidal" inhibitors that disrupt the aromatase active site by coordinating within the heme complex without affecting the active sites of other steroidogenic enzymes (Type 2 inhibitors). Both approaches led to the successful introduction into clinical practice of potent and specific aromatase inhibitors.

Early Aromatase Inhibitors

In 1973, Griffiths et al. first demonstrated the activity of aminoglutethimide, an inhibitor of cholesterol conversion to pregnenolone in the treatment of metastatic breast cancer.[244] Subsequently, it was appreciated that inhibition of aromatase, rather than suppression of general steroidogenesis, was key to the therapeutic action of aminoglutethimide.[245,246] Although the drug has well-documented efficacy in the metastatic setting, its side effect profile is troublesome. Unfortunately, even at the lowest dosages effective against breast cancer, aminoglutethimide inhibits the formation of corticosteroids by blocking P-450 enzymes involved in cholesterol side chain cleavage.[247] This lack of specificity exposes patients to the risk of glucocorticoid deficiency. Furthermore, the clinical utility of aminoglutethimide is limited by troublesome side effects, including rash, nausea, somnolence (aminoglutethimide was originally developed as a sedative), and blood dyscrasias.[247,248]

These observations provided a strong rationale for the development of more potent and selective aromatase inhibitors. While second-generation aromatase inhibitors, such as fadrozole and formestane, had improved potency and selectivity, the third-generation aromatase inhibitors were soon found to provide superior clinical results. These newer aromatase inhibitors have now rendered both aminoglutethimide and the second-generation drugs obsolete in breast cancer therapeutics.

Exemestane: Steroidal Aromatase Inhibitor

Background

A large number of androstenedione derivatives were screened in aromatase inhibition assays, and two com-

pounds, formestane (4-hydroxyandrostenedione) and exemestane (6-methylenandrosta-1, 4-diene-3, 17-dione), emerged as drugs suitable for clinical development.[249] Given the superior potency and clinical activity of exemestane, the use of formestane, which is available in Europe but not the United States, has declined precipitously. As shown in Figure 37.12, the structures of these compounds retain androgenic properties but have side chain substitutions that prevent conversion to estrogenic metabolites. Although not intrinsically reactive, exemestane exhibits tight or even irreversible binding to the aromatase active site.[28] The compound is therefore considered a "mechanism-based" or "suicide" inhibitor because it permanently inactivate aromatase. Recovery of aromatase activity after treatment with a suicide inhibitor therefore requires the synthesis of new aromatase protein. In vivo, the pharmacokinetics of suicide inhibition is characterized by persistently low aromatase activity despite complete drug clearance. Because suicide inhibition prolongs drug action, intermittent dosing should be possible, potentially improving the side effect to benefit ratio. However, in clinical practice, this benefit remains largely theoretical, because exemestane has been administered daily with a favorable toxicity profile.[28]

Pharmacology

Exemestane (Fig. 37.12) has potent aromatase activity with a K_i of 26 nM and no cholesterol side chain cleavage (desmolase) or 5-reductase activity. An oral dose is rapidly absorbed, with peak plasma concentrations reached within 2 hours of administration. The absorption of exemestane is enhanced by high-fat foods, and it is recommended that the drug be taken after eating.[250] Plasma concentrations fall below the limit of detection 4 hours later (for the approved 25-mg dose), although inhibition of the enzyme persists for at least 5 days.[250] Steady-state levels are achieved within 7 days with daily dosing, and the time to maximal estradiol suppression is 3 to 7 days.[251] The smallest dosage found to have maximal suppression of plasma estrone, estradiol, and estrone sulfate and urinary estrone and estradiol was 25 mg, now the recommended daily dosage. This dosage inactivates peripheral aromatase by 98% and reduces basal plasma estrone, estradiol, and estrone sulphate levels by 85 to 95%.[252] Other endocrine parameters, such as cortisol, aldosterone, dehydroepiandrosterones, 17-OH-progesterone, FSH, and LH, were not significantly affected by 25 mg of exemestane.[253]

Metabolism

Exemestane is extensively metabolized, with rapid oxidation of the methylene group at position 6 and reduction of the 17-keto group, along with subsequent formation of many secondary metabolites. The drug is excreted in both the urine and feces. As a consequence, clearance is affected by

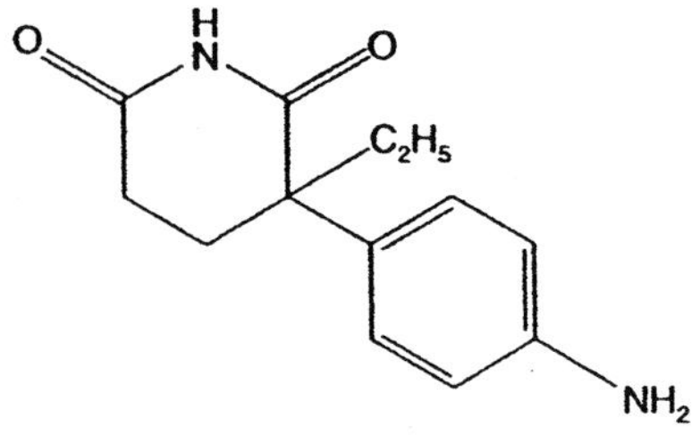

Aminoglutethimide

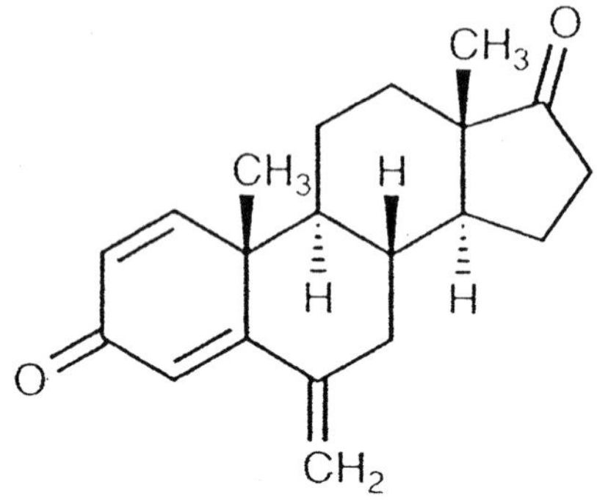

Exemestane

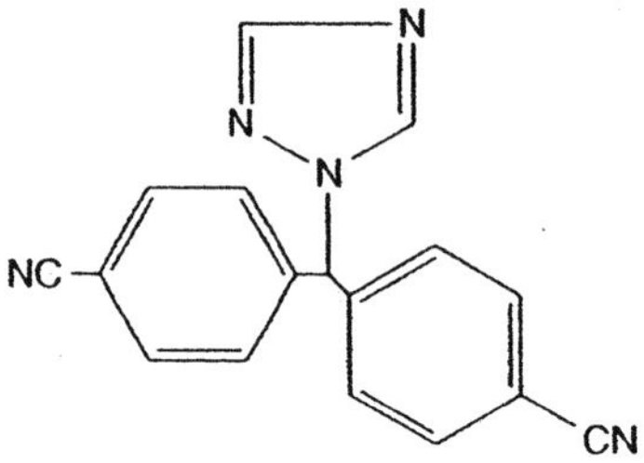

Letrozole

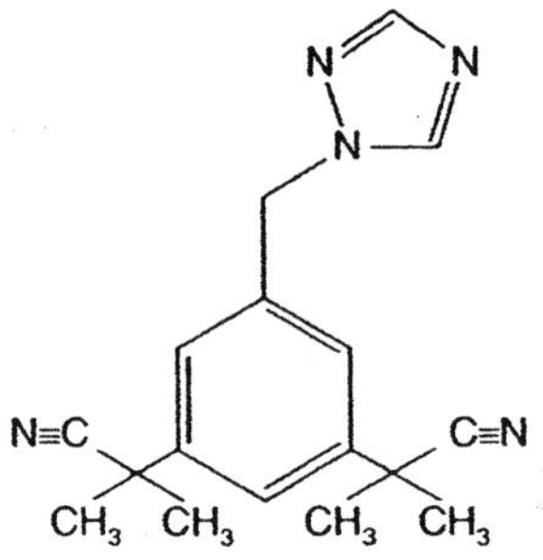

Anastrozole

Figure 37.12 Aromatase inhibitors.

both renal and hepatic insufficiency, with threefold elevations in the AUC under either condition. Metabolism occurs through CYP3A4 and aldoketoreductases, and the activity of the major CYP enzymes is unaffected.[251,254] While exemestane does not bind to the ER and only weakly binds to the AR, with an affinity of 0.28% relative to DHT, the binding affinity of the 17-dihydrometabolite is 100 times that of the parent compound.[255] As a result, there is slight androgenic activity in the rat with this drug. A screen of potential metabolites for aromatase activity did not reveal any compounds with inhibitory activity greater than exemestane.[256]

Toxicities

In clinical studies, exemestane has been well tolerated and has had a treatment-related discontinuation rate of less than 3%.[254] At high doses in rat studies, exemestane has been observed to have androgenic effects. Similarly, at high doses in clinical trials, androgenic side effects, including hypertrichosis, hair loss, hoarseness, and acne, have been reported in 4% of patients.[254] Other reported side effects include hot flashes, increased sweating, and nausea.

With all aromatase inhibitors, bone loss is a significant concern. However, the androgenic properties of exemestane metabolites might mitigate this effect. In ovariectomized rat studies, exemestane treatment provided protection from bone loss in comparison with untreated animals.[257] Initial studies in postmenopausal women using bone turnover biomarkers suggest that exemestane has a significantly smaller impact on bone formation and bone resorption than letrozole.[258] Despite these findings, results of the Intergroup Exemestane Study showed that postmenopausal patients on exemestane experience more osteoporosis than those on tamoxifen.[259]

Other side effects that were increased in the exemestane group in this trial included visual disturbances, arthralgia, and diarrhea. Conversely, patients on tamoxifen experienced more gynecologic symptoms, vaginal bleeding, thromboembolic disease, and cramps.[259]

Drug Interactions

Given that exemestane is extensively metabolized by CYP3A4, interference with other drugs affected by this P-450 enzyme may occur. Interestingly, however, ketoconazole does not significantly influence the pharmacokinetics of exemestane, suggesting that with CYP3A4 inhibition exemestane may be metabolized via a different route.[251]

Nonsteroidal Aromatase Inhibitors

The nonsteroidal approach to aromatase inhibition has yielded two compounds with significant clinical impact, anastrozole and letrozole. In attempts to find potent nonsteroidal inhibitors, research focused on a series of imidazole and triazole derivatives with "molecular shapes" that efficiently coordinate within the aromatase heme complex. Progress was assisted by new systems for rapid drug screening, and out of these screens came three drugs with the desired profile: anastrozole, letrozole, and vorozole (Fig. 37.12).[260] Because vorozole is not available for further clinical trials despite good clinical activity,[261] our discussion focuses on letrozole and anastrozole.

Anastrozole

Pharmacokinetics

Anastrozole [2,2'-[5-(1H-1,2,4-triazol-1-ylmethyl)-1,3-phenylene]bis(2-methyl-propiononitrile)] is a competitive aromatase inhibitor with high potency and was the first selective aromatase inhibitor approved in North America and Europe. It inhibits human placental aromatase and has an IC50 (the concentration that inhibits enzyme activity by 50%) of 15 nM.[262] Anastrozole is rapidly absorbed, with the maximum level occurring within 2 hours after administration, and it is 40% bound to plasma proteins. The mean peak plasma concentration at the 1-mg dose was 13.1 ng/mL.[262] Pharmacodynamic studies reveal that subjects receiving 1 mg per day orally achieved 96.7% aromatase inhibition, with maximal estradiol suppression and a decrease of estradiol ranging from 78 to 86% from baseline. Suppression is maintained long term, and there is no compensatory rise in androstenedione levels. The drug has a half-life of 40.6 hours and reaches steady-state levels in 7 days, with maximal estrogen suppression within 3 to 4 hours.[251] There is no effect on glucocorticoid or mineralocorticoid secretion as tested by ACTH stimulation.[262] In addition, anastrozole at a dosage of 1 mg daily does not have an effect on gonadotrophins or

follicle-stimulating hormone. Importantly, even at higher doses (5 to 10 mg), anastrozole administration does not affect basal or ACTH-stimulated cortisol and aldosterone levels.[251]

Metabolism

Elimination of anastrozole is primarily by metabolic degradation, and less than 10% of the drug is cleared as unchanged drug. Degradation occurs through N-dealkylation, hydroxylation, and glucuronidation, and metabolites are excreted predominantly in the urine. The plasma elimination half-life with the 0.5- and 1.0-mg multiple doses ranges from 38 to 61 hours.[262]

Anastrozole has no effect on CYP2A6 but does inhibit CYP1A2 and CYP2C8, with an IC50 of 30 μmol/L and 48 μmol/L, respectively. In clinical use, the drug is present at much lower levels than are required to inhibit these enzymes.[251]

Toxicity

Growing clinical experience with anastrozole in the metastatic and adjuvant settings shows that it is well tolerated even with extended use.[263] In comparison with megestrol acetate in metastatic disease, anastrozole is associated with less weight gain. In contrast, nausea and vomiting were more common with anastrozole. However, gastrointestinal toxicities were less troublesome with the 1-mg dose, and gastrointestinal problems rarely led to interruption of therapy.[264,265] In the ATAC (Arimidex, Tamoxifen Alone or in Combination) trial, a large adjuvant trial comparing anastrozole versus tamoxifen versus their combination, anastrozole demonstrated a favorable toxicity profile with prolonged use.[263] Compared with patients taking tamoxifen, patients in the anastrozole arm of the study experienced less vaginal bleeding (4.8% vs. 8.7%), vaginal discharge (3.0% vs. 12.2%), endometrial malignancy (0.1% vs. 0.7%), ischemic cerebrovascular events (1.1% vs. 2.3%), and venous thromboembolic events (2.2% vs. 3.8%). Anastrozole, however, did result in an increase in fractures (7.1% vs. 4.4%) and in musculoskeletal complaints (30.3% vs. 23.7%). Given that there was no placebo control in this trial, it is not clear if the increased incidence of fractures is due to deleterious effects of anastrozole or protective effects of tamoxifen.

Drug Interactions

To date, clinically significant drug interactions with anastrozole have been minimal. Coadministration with tamoxifen has been shown to lead to a 27% decrease in steady-state levels of anastrozole.[251] However, given the ATAC trial findings that combining tamoxifen and anastrozole provides inferior clinical outcomes compared with anastrozole alone, the combination of these drugs should not be used clinically in the future. It is unclear whether this pharmacokinetic interaction might partially account for the inferiority of the combination arm in ATAC.

Letrozole

Pharmacokinetics

Letrozole (4,4'-[(1H-1,2,4-triazol-1-yl)methylene]bisbenzonitrile) was the second nonsteroidal selective aromatase inhibitor approved for the treatment of advanced breast cancer. The drug has a profile similar to anastrozole, combining high potency, selectivity, and good clinical activity against breast cancer.[260] The IC50 for placental aromatase is 11.5 nM, so it is marginally more potent than anastrozole or exemestane. For comparison, the IC50 for aminoglutethimide is 1,900 nM. Oral absorption is rapid, with high bioavailability that is only minimally affected by food.[251] Aromatase inhibition at the recommended 2.5-mg dose of letrozole reaches 98.9%,[251] and both letrozole doses examined in phase III trials, 0.5 mg and 2.5 mg, suppress estrogen levels over 90% (less than 0.5 pmol/L).[266] Letrozole reaches peak concentration within 2 hours, and steady-state levels are achieved within 14 to 40 days.[251] Maximal estrogen suppression occurs within 2 to 3 days, and the half-life of the drug is 2 to 4 days.[251]

Although letrozole has high specificity for aromatase, two studies have shown effects on either cortisol levels or aldosterone levels; however, these two studies had conflicting results.[267,268] In addition, changes in glucocorticoid and mineralocorticoid levels were small and do not appear to be clinically meaningful. In these studies, no changes were found in 11-deoxycortisol, 17-hydroxyprogesterone, ACTH, or plasma renin levels. In addition, plasma androgens, thyroid function, LH, and FSH remained unchanged.

Comparison with Anastrozole

While letrozole appears to have characteristics similar to those of anastrozole, comparison of the drugs at the recommended doses has revealed minor differences in potency. In a preclinical model of aromatase-dependent breast cancer growth, letrozole had greater antitumor activity than did anastrozole and tamoxifen.[269] In a double-blind, cross-over study, letrozole was found to suppress aromatization by greater than 99.1%, versus 97.3% for anastrozole ($P = .0022$). In addition, suppression of plasma estrone sulfate was greater with letrozole treatment.[270] The clinical implications of these differences is not yet clear; however, preliminary data from a study in metastatic disease revealed no difference between the two drugs.[271]

Metabolism

As with anastrozole, metabolic clearance of letrozole is mainly through the liver, and the half-life of 50 hours

allows a once-a-day dosing schedule. CYP3A4 and CYP2A6 catalyze letrozole to its major metabolite, 4,4'-methanolbisbenzonitrile, which is then subjected to glucuronidation. Letrozole can be safely prescribed for patients with renal insufficiency, because only 5% of the drug is cleared in the urine. However, the drug should be used with caution in treating patients with severe liver impairment.[251] There are no known drug interactions with erythromycin, warfarin, or cimetidine. As with anastrozole, coadministration of tamoxifen reduces letrozole levels by 37%; in the case of letrozole, this is likely due to the induction of CYP3A4.[146]

Toxicity

Like anastrozole, letrozole is extremely well tolerated, with only 2% of patients discontinuing the drug due to adverse events; in comparison, megestrol acetate has an 8% discontinuation rate.[272] A recently reported large adjuvant trial using letrozole versus placebo in patients who had completed 5 years of tamoxifen treatment has provided data on toxicities associated with long-term letrozole use.[273] With a median follow-up of 2.4 years, patients on letrozole experienced an increased incidence of hot flashes (47.2% vs. 40.5%), arthritis (5.6% vs. 3.5%), arthralgias (21.3% vs. 16.6%), and myalgias (11.8% vs. 9.5%). In addition, there was a trend towards increased osteoporosis (5.8% vs. 4.5%). Compared with placebo, patients on letrozole had less vaginal bleeding (4.3% vs 6.0%). Discontinuations rates were nearly identical for placebo and letrozole.

Aromatase Inhibitors in Premenopausal Women

Hereditary aromatase deficiency, due to inherited loss-of-function mutations in the aromatase gene, is associated with a syndrome of hypergonadotropic hypogonadism, multicystic ovaries, virilism, and bone demineralization in childhood. These problems are reversible with low-dose estrogens.[274,275] Polycystic ovary syndrome in adult women has a less well defined etiology, although low aromatase activity is believed to play a part.[276] Treatment of premenopausal women with aromatase inhibitors may therefore be complicated by polycystic ovaries and virilization. To circumvent these problems, the treatment of premenopausal women with advanced breast cancer with an LHRH analog and selective aromatase inhibitor combination is under investigation. Aminoglutethimide treatment of premenopausal women does not suppress estrogen levels, so the indication for this drug was restricted to patients without ovarian function.[277] However, more potent aromatase inhibitors are able to suppress ovarian aromatase activity. For example, in a small pharmacokinetic study, a combination of formestane and an LHRH agonist produced more effective inhibition of premenopausal estradiol levels than the LHRH agonist alone.[278] This is also the case for the nonsteroidal aromatase vorozole, because the combination of vorozole and goserelin was markedly more effective in reducing estrogen levels than goserelin alone.[279] Further investigations will be required to determine whether the extremely low estrogen levels achieved with an LHRH-A and a third-generation aromatase inhibitor will translate into increased clinical benefit. Outside of clinical trials, the use of selective aromatase inhibitors continues to be restricted to postmenopausal women for adjuvant treatment or metastatic disease.

PROGESTINS

Historical Perspective

In 1897, Beard postulated that the corpus luteum was essential for pregnancy.[280] Support for this hypothesis was provided by Fraenkel in 1905, who demonstrated that destruction of the corpora lutea in pregnant rabbits caused abortion, an event that could be prevented by the injection of luteal extracts.[281] Although progesterone, the active principle in corpus lutea extracts, was isolated in 1929 from the corpora lutea of sows by Corner and Allen,[282] the limited amounts of available hormone hampered further studies until the 1950s, when progesterones with prolonged activity were synthesized. Since that time, progestins have been widely used as oral contraceptives. High-dose progestin therapy is the last synthetic sex steroid routinely used in the treatment of advanced breast cancer. Until recently, megestrol acetate was a favored second-line therapy for patients with tamoxifen-resistant disease. However, megestrol acetate has been relegated to third- or fourth-line therapy, with the emergence of third-generation aromatase inhibitors and fulvestrant, which both have better side effect and efficacy profiles.[22,265]

Progesterone Physiology

Progesterone is secreted mainly by the corpus luteum of the ovary during the second half of the menstrual cycle. The principal physiologic target organ for progesterone is the uterine endometrium. Progesterone secretion begins just before ovulation, coincident with the LH surge, and derives from the follicle that becomes the corpus luteum once the ovum is released.[48] Progesterone is synthesized from cholesterol and pregnenolone in all steroid-producing tissues: the ovary, testis, adrenal cortex, and placenta. Although the luteotroph varies with the species, in humans LH is the primary stimulator of progesterone synthesis.[49] The production rate of progesterone varies from a few milligrams per day during the follicular phase to 10 to 20 mg per day during the luteal phase (reaching blood levels of 10 ng/mL), increasing to several hundred milligrams daily during the latter parts of pregnancy. Rates of 1 to 5 mg per day have been measured in men and are comparable to the values in women during the follicular phase of the cycle.[283] Once secreted into the bloodstream, progesterone is either bound to CBG (with an affinity roughly equal to that of cortisol) or rapidly cleared from the circulation within a few minutes, predominantly by the liver, where glucuronidation or sulfation occurs before excretion in the urine. The isomers of pregnanediol are the principal metabolites.[35,284] In total, 50 to 60% of the progesterone C-14 given is excreted in the urine. A small and probably physiologically insignificant proportion is stored in body fat, from which it is slowly released. The enhanced biologic potency of such synthetic progestins as medroxyprogesterone acetate (6α-methyl 17α-hydroxyprogesterone acetate) may be explained by a lower metabolic clearance rate than progesterone[285] and by the greater affinity for the PgR.[286] The biologic roles of progesterone are listed in Table 37.4. Although progestins act principally through the PgR, these agents have some antiandrogenic (or sometimes weakly androgenic) and antimineralocorticoid-like properties on the basis of their low affinity for androgen and mineralocorticoid receptors.

Mechanism of Action in Breast Cancer Therapy

A variety of progestins have been used for patients with hormone-dependent cancer. These include the C-21, 17-acetoxysteroids, such as medroxyprogesterone acetate and megestrol acetate, and the 19-carbon steroids, such as norethisterone (Fig. 37.13). Historically, the rate of response to progestins was quoted as approximately 27 to 35% and as positively correlated with estrogen and PgR expression.[158] This has been confirmed in large phase III studies in comparison with selective aromatase inhibitors, if patients who experience disease stabilization (lack of progression at 24 weeks) are included.[265,272]

The mechanism of the anticancer action of the progestins is not established, in part because these agents act

TABLE 37.4
PHYSIOLOGIC EFFECTS OF PROGESTINS

Establishment and maintenance of pregnancy
Promotion of development of secretory epithelium of uterine
  endometrium after estrogen priming
Alterations in vaginal epithelium, causing change from abundant
  watery secretions to scant viscid material
Proliferation and engorgement of mammary acini (in concert with
  estrogens)
Thermogenesis
Weakly antiandrogenic
Weakly antimineralocorticoid

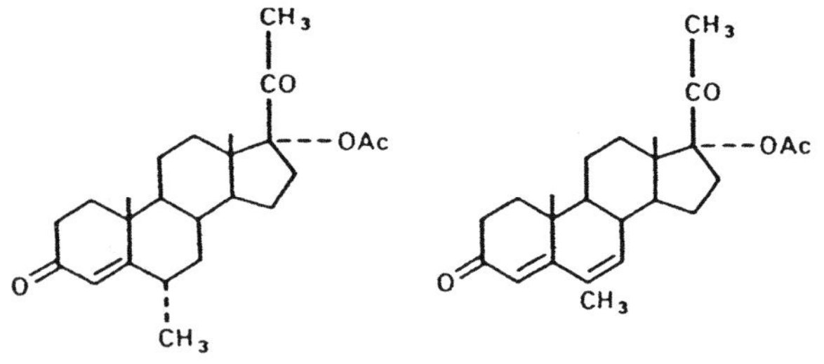

Figure 37.13 Progestins.

not only through the PgR but also through the AR and ER. Although progestins may have a direct antitumor action,[287] progestins also suppress basal and GnRH-simulated gonadotropin secretion, cortisol, dehydroepiandrosterone, and estradiol in a dose-dependent manner.[288] In the normal menstrual cycle, breast epithelial cell proliferation is maximal during the luteal phase (days 20 to 28), when progesterone levels are highest.[289] These data suggest that progestins stimulate the growth of normal mammary epithelium. Antiprogestins induce apoptosis in mammary tumor models,[290] suggesting that progesterone is an important stimulatory factor during mammary tumorigenesis. Also, progestins regulate metastasis-related cell surface receptors, such as the laminin receptor for adhesion molecules,[291] which may result in increased metastases. A direct antitumor action is supported by data, suggesting that progestins alter signaling through peptide growth factor receptors. Vignon et al. showed that R5020, a progestin, decreases the production of a mitogenic 52-kd glycoprotein.

Progestin treatment results in a decrease in FSH and LH levels[293,294] Also, cortisol and ACTH levels are depressed, and the ACTH response to metyrapone is blunted.[295] The cortisol decrease is ACTH-dependent. Estrone levels are decreased in postmenopausal women by 82% compared with pretreatment,[294] as are the levels of dehydroepiandrostenedione sulfate and androstenedione.[296] Suppression of postmenopausal estrogen is therefore likely to be a predominant mode of action of progestins.

Medroxyprogesterone Acetate

Medroxyprogesterone acetate (MPA) was once commonly used for treating breast and endometrial cancer. The usual route of administration was intramuscular (i.m.). As a result, when oral progestins such as megestrol acetate became available, the use of MPA declined. MPA is extensively metabolized, and less than 1% of an intravenous (i.v.) dosage is recovered intact in the urine.[284,297] However, there were no clear correlations between plasma MPA and efficacy or between dosage and efficacy. There has been at least one study in which MPA was administered orally at a dose of 400 mg per day, with a 53% response rate in 30 patients.[158,298]

Megestrol Acetate

Megestrol acetate (MA) is the synthetic progestin most commonly prescribed for advanced breast cancer. The pharmacokinetics differ from MPA, because MA has a shorter half-life (4 hours), greater renal excretion (56 to 78%, with 12% excreted as parent compound), and higher plasma levels.[284,299] The metabolites of MA are shown in Table 37.5. With oral dosages of 400 mg per day, plasma concentrations reach 400 ng/mL, with considerable interpatient variation. The recommended dosage is 40 mg four times each day or a single daily dose of 160 mg. MPA and MA probably have equivalent activities in breast cancer, but patients on MPA have a higher incidence of side effects[300]

Toxicity

Pannuti et al. noted increased toxicity with high i.m. dosages of MPA, with little increase in efficacy.[301] These side effects include gluteal abscesses in 15% of patients receiving 1,500 mg intramuscularly per day, moon-shaped facies in 11%, fine tremors in 19%, and leg cramps in 19%; there is a much lower incidence of each of these effects with the 500-mg i.m. dose. Other side effects with MPA include sweating, vaginal discharge, and amenorrhea.[158] Another significant side effect is weight gain, largely due to increased adipose tissue in the abdominal and cervicodorsal regions.[299] Weight gain ranged from 3 to 10 kg in 56% of patients treated with 1,000 to 1,500 mg intramuscularly per day. Because there is no difference in efficacy with different dosages or routes of administration, 400 to 500 mg orally per is probably an adequate dosage. Crona et al. reported decreases in high-density lipoprotein (HDL) cholesterol and apolipoprotein A1 and an increase in triglycerides in patients receiving 1,000 mg intramuscularly per week.[302] These results suggest that the risk of cardiovascular disease could be increased in patients taking MPA. Side

TABLE 37.5
MEGESTROL ACETATE PHARMACOLOGY

Mechanism of action	Unknown
Metabolism	17α-Acetoxy-6-hydroxymethyl-pregna-4,6-diene-3,20-dione
	2α-Hydroxy-6-hydroxymethyl-pregna-4,6-diene-3,20-dione
	17α-Acetoxy-6-hydroxymethyl-pregna-4,6-diene-3,20-dione
	2α-Hydroxy-6-hydroxymethyl-pregna-4,6-diene-3,20-dione
	17α-Acetoxy-21-hydroxy-6α-methylpregna-4,6-diene-3,20-dione
Pharmacokinetics	Half-life = 4 hr
Elimination	Renal excretion, 56–78%, fecal excretion, 7.7–30.0%

effects with MA include increased appetite, weight gain of 5 to 20 kg, elevated liver function tests, thromboembolism, vaginal bleeding, hot flashes, fluid retention, nausea and vomiting, hypercalcemia and flare, and rash.[299] In addition, megestrol acetate has shown activity in cancer patients as a treatment for anorexia and weight loss.[303] This activity appears to result from suppression of cytokines that induce tumor cachexia.[304] Megestrol acetate in low dosages (20 mg per day) is also active in the treatment of postmenopausal hot flashes in breast cancer patients.[305]

LUTEINIZING HORMONE-RELEASING HORMONE AGONISTS

Background

Oophorectomy has been a standard therapy option for breast cancer for more than 100 years. As adjuvant therapy for premenopausal women, oophorectomy is associated with a marked reduction in relapse and death from breast cancer.[306] The development of LHRH agonists has provided the option of reversible medical ovarian ablation. The only randomized comparison between ovariectomy and LHRH agonist therapy was underpowered, but it did not reveal significant differences between these two approaches to estrogen deprivation.[307] Because premenopausal women treated with LHRH agonists have plasma estradiol concentrations typical for postmenopausal women, surgical oophorectomy and treatment with LHRH agonists are generally held to be equivalent.[307-309] Premenopausal women with breast cancer treated with LHRH agonists have objective response rates of between 36% and 44%.[309] Medical castration using LHRH agonists is currently used in premenopausal women in both the adjuvant and metastatic setting, with or without tamoxifen. Despite the fact that a number of LHRH agonists have been tested in breast cancer, goserelin acetate (Zoladex, AstraZeneca) is the only one approved for this disease and is therefore the LHRH agonist of choice for breast cancer patients. The general characteristics and amino acid sequence of different LHRH agonists are detailed in Table 37.6 and Figure 37.14.

Mechanism of Action

LHRH agonists reduce circulating concentrations of estrogens in premenopausal women via an inhibitory effect on the hypothalamic-pituitary-gonadal axis. The drugs bind to the LHRH receptors on the pituitary gland, leading to an initial stimulation of FSH and LH production during the first few days of treatment.[308] After this initial stimulation, the ligand-receptor complexes cluster and get sequestered in the cell; this leads to a reduction in the number of active receptors on the surface. This mechanism accounts for the paradoxical inhibition of pituitary gonadotropic cells with

TABLE 37.6

PHARMACOLOGY OF LUTEINIZING HORMONE–RELEASING HORMONE AGONISTS

Mechanisms of action	Inhibition of gonadotropin secretion with resultant castration levels of testosterone in men and estrogens in women
	Direct inhibitory effects on steroidogenesis through blockade of 17,20-desmolase and 17α-hydroxylase enzymes
	Direct antitumor effect on human mammary cancer in vitro
Pharmacokinetics	Gonadotropin-releasing hormone $t_{1/2a}$, 2–8 min
	$t_{1/2b}$, 15–60 min
	Goserelin s.c. 4.9 h
	Triptorelin s.c. 2.8 h
Elimination	Enzymatic degradation by pyroglutamate aminopeptidase, endopeptidase, and post-proline-cleaving enzymes and renal excretion
Drug interactions	None known
Toxicity	Hot flashes
	Reduced libido
	Impotence
	Local irritation at the injection site
	Polyuria and polydipsia
	Gastrointestinal problems, such as indigestion, nausea and vomiting, and constipation
	Taste sensations
	Peripheral edema
	Rash
	Gynecomastia and mastodynia
	Disease flare
	General allergic reaction
Precautions	Because there is an initial surge of luteinizing hormone, follicle-stimulating hormone, and testosterone, an acute exacerbation of disease may be seen

$t_{1/2}$, half-life.

GnRH

pyro Glu-His-Trp-Ser-Tyr-Gly-Leu-Arg-Pro-Gly-NH2

Goserelin

pyro Glu-His-Trp-Ser-Tyr-D-Ser (tert Butyl)-Leu-Arg-Pro-Azgly

Tripterelin

pyro Glu-His-Trp-Ser-Tyr-D-Trp-Leu-Arg-Pro-Gly-NH2

Figure 37.14 Gonadotropin-releasing hormone (GnRH) and analogs. (Arg, arginine; Glu, glucose; Gly, glycerol; His, histidine; Leu, leucine; Pro, proline; Ser, serine; Trp, tryptophan; Tyr, tyrosine.)

continuous instead of pulsatile LHRH agonism.[310] As a result, after a few days of stimulation, FSH and LH levels fall and remain persistently suppressed, reaching levels comparable to the postmenopausal state within 21 days.[310] Plasma progesterone, estrone, estrone sulfate, and estradiol levels decrease to postmenopausal levels after 6 weeks of treatment. There is no change in androstenedione, prolactin, or cortisol levels.

Goserelin: Pharmacology and Metabolism

Goserelin is a synthetic decapeptide analog of LHRH that is administered as a subcutaneous depot, providing gradual release of the drug. A 3.6-mg depot formulation is given once a month. In addition, a 10.8-mg depot is given once every 3 months, although this formulation is approved only for prostate cancer, not breast cancer.

When administered as a solution subcutaneously, goserelin has been observed to have a half-life of about 4 hours.[311] After administration of the 3.6-mg depot, there is an initial, short-duration peak of goserelin in the serum at 8 hours. A more prolonged peak then occurs at about 14 days. There is no accumulation of the drug with multiple administration of the depots. After administration of the 10.8-mg depot, the serum concentration profile is notably different than for the 3.6-mg depot. After an initial release over a few days, the profile shows a downward trend, with a shallow second peak at 5 weeks.

Elimination of goserelin is primarily in the urine (93%), with only 2% found in the feces. Excretion occurs fairly rapidly, with greater than 75% of a dose being excreted within 12 hours.[311] In the urine, approximately 20% of the drug is excreted unchanged, and the remaining products are fragments of the decapeptide. With renal impairment, goserelin clearance decreases, and there is a corresponding increase in half-life. With hepatic impairment, differences in the pharmacokinetic parameters of goserelin were minimal, with a small increase in C_{max} but not AUC as compared with controls.[311] Given the wide therapeutic window of goserelin, it is not considered necessary to alter dosing in patients with either renal or hepatic insufficiency.

Following an initial dose of the 3.6-mg depot, LH and FSH levels rise to a peak at about 48 hours.[311] In women with benign gynecologic conditions, the levels then rapidly decline to below baseline by day 3. The levels are greatly reduced after day 8. Estradiol levels rise transiently at 3 days, followed by a decrease of estradiol; similar results are seen with progesterone. Estradiol levels return to normal within 3 months of stopping goserelin. With the 10.8-mg depot, there is an initial increase in LH and FSH in the first week, and castrate range is achieved within 21 days.

While ovarian ablation is achieved in most patients treated with LHRH agonists, there are reports of failure with normal treatment doses.[312] In a study with three different LHRH analogs, residual ovarian estrogen production was detected in 5 of 40 patients at 3 months despite profound suppression of LH in all patients.[313] In addition, up to 9% of patients treated for endometriosis had persistence of uterine bleeding episodes at 6 months.[314]

Triptorelin: Pharmacology and Metabolism

Triptorelin is a synthetic decapeptide analog of LHRH that is not yet approved for use in breast cancer treatment; however, there are currently two large adjuvant studies using this drug in premenopausal women.[315] Both trials, the IBCSG Tamoxifen and Exemestane Trial (TEXT) and the IBCSG Suppression of Ovarian Function Trial (SOFT), will use the drug in combination with either exemestane or tamoxifen.

The drug can be administered as an intramuscular injection of a suspension of microspheres at a dose of 3, 3.2, or 3.75 mg once a month or 11.25 mg every 3 months.[316] With the monthly formulation, peak serum levels of the drug occur during the first week and then remain at a detectable plateau level for about 4 weeks. As with goserelin, initially levels of LH and FSH increase but fall to low levels after 1 to 2 weeks,[317] and estradiol levels reach nadir levels by 21 days.[316] Studies in patients with hepatic and renal insufficiency show that clearance of the drug decreases by about half under both conditions. Given the generous therapeutic window of triptorelin, however, dose modification does not appear to be necessary.[318]

LHRH Agonist Toxicity

Side effects in women include hot flashes, nausea and vomiting, headache, dizziness, vaginitis, sweating, emotional lability, breast atrophy, tumor flare, diarrhea, local reaction, irritability, hives, and severe polydipsia and polyuria in one patient.[131,308,319] Also, amenorrhea is induced in all women. Bone mineral density is reduced in the lumbar spine and femur after 4 months of treatment with goserelin and does not normalize after discontinuation of treatment.[320] In the adjuvant breast cancer setting, this may be of concern, and treatment with bisphosphonates may be appropriate. Total serum cholesterol, LDL cholesterol, and LDL to HDL cholesterol ratios were higher, whereas HDL cholesterol was lower in polycystic ovary patients treated with goserelin for 6 months.[321] Measurement of antithrombin III concentrations after treatment with goserelin revealed no change.[322] This suggests there may be no increased risk of thromboembolic episodes with this therapy. There are limited data available on known drug-drug interactions.

HORMONAL RESISTANCE

Despite the proven clinical efficacy of hormonal therapy in all stages of breast cancer, hormone-refractory breast cancer remains a formidable challenge. Many ER-positive tumors are intrinsically resistant, and all patients with ER-positive metastatic disease ultimately become refractory to hormonal treatments. From a clinical standpoint, hormone-refractory breast cancer can be considered to exhibit either primary resistance (no response to hormones) or secondary resistance (progression after disease regression or stability). Approximately one third of patients with secondary resistance obtain clinical benefit from subsequent endocrine therapy. The molecular mechanisms of resistance can be divided into three groups: (1) ER mutation, splice variants, and isoform ratio; (2) coactivator and corepressor effects; and (3) activation of other signaling pathways.

ER Mutation, Splice Variants, and Isoform Ratio

One hypothesis to explain the variable clinical response to hormones in ER-positive breast cancer invokes ER gene mutation or splice variants.[323–325] ER mutations that allow ligand-independent activity have been described in human tumors. Specifically, a missense mutation substituting tyrosine 537 in the ligand-binding domain for asparagine was equally active in the absence of ligand, with tamoxifen or with estradiol.[326] However, evaluation of primary breast tumors has established that somatic mutations in ER are rare, occurring in fewer than 1% of either ER-positive or ER-negative breast cancers.[327] Therefore, it does not appear that mutations in ER explain the majority of instances of tamoxifen resistance.[323,328]

Another potential alteration of ER function may occur through changes in the ERα-ERβ ratio. Steroidal antiestrogens have been shown to activate ERβ-mediated transcription while they repress ERα activity.[68] Although the biologic significance of this remains unclear, this observation suggests that increased ERβ might counter inhibitory effects of antiestrogens, but there is conflicting data regarding this issue. In support of this hypothesis, a relatively small study demonstrated that ERβ mRNA levels were twice as high as ERα mRNA levels in tamoxifen-resistant tumors compared with tamoxifen-responsive tumors.[329] Other studies, however, suggest that ERβ-positive tumors are less likely to be responsive to tamoxifen.[330]

ERα and ERβ splice variants may also play a role in hormonal resistance. Alternatively spliced ER mRNA variants have also been commonly identified in normal and malignant breast tissues.[45] An ERα transcript that has received particular attention lacks exon 5; exon 4 directly splices into exon 6, with preservation of the reading frame.[331] The exon 5–deleted variant binds to DNA but not to estrogen, and it activates transcription in an estrogen-independent manner (a dominant positive receptor). These properties imply a role in estrogen-independent growth. However, coexpression of the exon 5–deleted variant with an intact ER did not alter the transcriptional response to estrogen, arguing against a critical role in breast cancer pathogenesis.[332]

At least five isoforms and one tyrosine mutant of ERβ have been identified; however their role in hormone-resistance is not clear.[45] The most interesting ERβ variant is ERβcx, which lacks amino acid residues important for ligand binding. Although ERβcx does not bind estrogen, is does heterodimerize with ERα and inhibits DNA binding. This, in turn, results in a dominant negative effect on ligand-dependent transcription of the ER.[50] Higher levels of ERβcx in tumors have been correlated with resistance to tamoxifen; however, confirmatory studies are required.[45]

Coactivators and Corepressors

Given the role of coactivators and corepressors in regulating ER activity, it is not surprising that they might also contribute to hormonal response. NCoA3 (AIB1) was initially identified based on its amplification in breast cancer.[328] When expressed in cultured cells, AIB1 promotes tamoxifen's agonist activity, suggesting a role in hormonal resistance.[333] Overexpression of another coactivator, NCoA1, similarly increases tamoxifen's agonist activity, indicating a role in tamoxifen resistance.[334]

Conversely, decreased activity of corepressors has also been implicated as a mechanism of resistance. In a mouse model of tamoxifen resistance, NCoR1 levels were decreased, suggesting a role in hormonal response.[328] Together, these findings suggest that alteration of the coactivator-corepressor balance can result in conversion of tamoxifen from an antagonist to an agonist.

Growth Factor Signaling Pathways

As previously discussed, ER function is strongly influenced by peptide growth factor signaling, including EGFR, ERBB2, and IGF-1-R, that leads to stimulation of ER activity in the absence of estrogen. These mitogenic pathways lead to downstream activation of kinases that phosphorylate the ER and/or ER coregulators.[335] In this way, these growth factor pathways can allow the ER to function in the absence of ligand.

EGF has been shown to mimic the effect of estrogens on uterine cell proliferation in ovariectomized mice, and tumors overexpressing EGFR are less likely to be sensitive to hormonal therapy.[335] Similar results have been demonstrated with overexpression of ERBB2.[335] Several groups have evaluated response to hormonal therapy with respect to ErbB2 tumor status or circulating ErbB2 levels.[336–338] These studies have found a markedly decreased response to hormones in patients with ErbB2-overexpressing tumors.

Strategies to Combat Hormonal Resistance

There has been remarkable growth in the number of hormone therapies available for the treatment of breast cancer. With more hormonal options, the clinical efficacy of hormonal therapy has improved; however, the improvement has been incremental in nature. While hormone resistance remains the primary obstacle, the combination of hormonal agents with new signal transduction inhibitors may provide new avenues of success. The inhibition of multiple growth pathways simultaneously could potentially combat the redundancy and cross-talk of growth signals, thereby providing effective, well-tolerated therapy.

FUTURE DIRECTIONS

With the advent of advanced techniques, such as DNA microarrays and proteomic technologies, the characterization of different types of tumors will continue to make major strides. With regard to hormonal therapy, significant achievements have already been made. Several groups have demonstrated that supervised cluster analysis of DNA microarray data allows identification of a set of genes that can distinguish between ER-positive and ER-negative breast tumors.[339,340] The marked difference in the gene expression profile of these breast cancer subtypes suggests the possibility of distinct precursor cells. Interestingly, only a small number of genes that discriminate between ER-positive and ER-negative tumors are involved in ER signaling.[341]

Further classification of tumors will continue to be achieved. Recently, genes that predict patient benefit from adjuvant tamoxifen treatment have been identified.[342] Given that resistance to hormonal agents does not entirely overlap, further work with other agents will likely show different resistance and sensitivity patterns associated with various hormonal therapies. This will undoubtedly help define how to use different hormonal agents. Furthermore, as signal transduction inhibitors are tested in combination with hormonal therapy, DNA microarrays will be critical in determining which targeted drug cocktail to use against a specific tumor.

In addition to predicting the ER status of tumors and their response to therapy, gene expression profiling has the potential to help elucidate which signaling pathways are critical in tumors and thus provide strategies to improve treatment. It is important to note that, with DNA microarray analysis, the delineation of differences in signaling pathways between tumors is only inferential. While these advanced analytic procedures can help generate hypotheses, the findings from these studies still require testing with more traditional laboratory techniques. A number of laboratories have identified and characterized changes in gene expression that occur with various hormonal agents.[343,344] Ontology mapping, whereby genes are classified into various functional categories, has been helpful in describing major cellular events that occur. However, constructing a detailed and integrated picture of differences in signaling pathways will require further work. Proteomic technologies, which are beginning to allow large-scale interrogation of signaling pathways, will be critical in achieving this goal. Integration of these technologies into clinical trial design is essential.

The determination of predictive biomarkers for targeted therapy is currently a major goal in the oncology community. Interestingly, the use of hormonal therapy for ER/PR-positive breast cancer provides the oldest paradigm for this approach. In addition, this history gives a glimpse of the promise and limitations of targeted therapy. Hormonal resistance remains a problem that we are only beginning to address in the clinic. However, with the development of new technologies and new drugs, hormonal therapy can be a foundation on which to build more effectively tailored and targeted treatments.

REFERENCES

1. Love RR, Philips J. Oophorectomy for breast cancer: history revisited. J Natl Cancer Inst 2002;94:1433–1434.
2. Beatson CT. On treatment of inoperable cases of carcinoma of the mamma: suggestions for a new method of treatment with illustrative cases. Lancet 1896;2:104–107.
3. Knauer E. Die Ovarien-Transplantation. Arch Gynaekol 1900;60:322–376.
4. Allen E, Doisy EA. An ovarian hormone: preliminary report on its localization, extraction, and partial purification, and action in test animals. JAMA 1923;819–821.
5. Loewe S, Lange F. Der gehalt des frauenharns an brur sterzengenden stoffen in abhangigkeit von ovariellen zylkus. Klin Wochenschr 1926;5:1038–1039.
6. Frank RT, Frank ML, Gustavosn RG. Demonstration of the female sex hormone in the circulating blood. JAMA 1925;85:510.
7. Zondek B. Darstellung des weiblichem sexualhormon aus dem harn. Klin Wochenschr 1928;7:485.

8. Butenandt A. Uber progynon ein crystallisiertes, weibliches sexualhormon. Naturwissenschaften 1929;7:879.
9. Jensen EV, Jacobson HI. Basic guides to the mechanism of estrogen actions. Recent Prog Hormone Res 1962;18:387–414.
10. Toft D, Shyamala G, Gorski J. A receptor molecule for estrogens: studies using a cell-free system. Proc Natl Acad Sci USA 1967;57:1740–1743.
11. Toft D, Gorski J. A receptor molecule for estrogens: isolation from the rat uterus and preliminary characterization. Proc Natl Acad Sci USA 1966;55:1574–1581.
12. Jensen EV, Block GE, Smith S, et al. Estrogen receptors and breast cancer response to adrenalectomy. Natl Cancer Inst Monogr 1971;34:55–70.
13. Furr BJ, Jordan VC. The pharmacology and clinical uses of tamoxifen. Pharmacol Ther 1984;25:127–205.
14. Ingle JN, Ahmann DL, Green SJ, et al. Randomized clinical trial of diethylstilbestrol versus tamoxifen in postmenopausal women with advanced breast cancer. N Engl J Med 1981;304:16–21.
15. Tamoxifen for early breast cancer: an overview of the randomised trials. Early Breast Cancer Trialists' Collaborative Group. Lancet 1998;351:1451–1467.
16. Hermon C, Beral V. Breast cancer mortality rates are levelling off or beginning to decline in many western countries: analysis of time trends, age-cohort and age-period models of breast cancer mortality in 20 countries. Br J Cancer 1996;73:955–960.
17. IUPAC Commission on the Nomenclature of Organic Chemistry (CNOC) and IUPAC-IUB Commission on Biochemical Nomenclature (CBN). The nomenclature of steroids: revised tentative rules. Eur J Biochem 1969;10:1–19.
18. Briggs MJ. Steroid Biochemistry and Pharmacology. London: Academic Press, 1970.
19. Brotherton J. Sex Hormone Pharmacology. London: Academic Press, 1976.
20. Briggs MJ, Christie GA. Advances in steroid biochemistry and pharmacology. London: Academic Press, 1977.
21. Gruber CJ, Tschugguel W, Schneeberger C, et al. Production and actions of estrogens. N Engl J Med 2002;346:340–352.
22. Brodie A. Aromatase inhibitors in breast cancer. Trends Endocrinol Metab 2002;13:61–65.
23. Chen SA, Besman MJ, Sparkes RS, et al. Human aromatase: cDNA cloning, Southern blot analysis, and assignment of the gene to chromosome 15. DNA 1988;7:27–38.
24. Agarwal VR, Bulun SE, Leitch M, et al. Use of alternative promoters to express the aromatase cytochrome P450 (CYP19) gene in breast adipose tissues of cancer-free and breast cancer patients. J Clin Endocrinol Metab 1996;81:3843–3849.
25. Santner SJ, Pauley RJ, Tait L, et al. Aromatase activity and expression in breast cancer and benign breast tissue stromal cells. J Clin Endocrinol Metab 1997;82:200–208.
26. Zhou D, Clarke P, Wang J, et al. Identification of a promoter that controls aromatase expression in human breast cancer and adipose stromal cells. J Biol Chem 1996;271:15194–15202.
27. Ellis MJ, Jenkins S, Hanfelt J, et al. Insulin-like growth factors in human breast cancer. Breast Cancer Res Treat 1998;52:175–184.
28. Johnston SR, Dowsett M. Aromatase inhibitors for breast cancer: lessons from the laboratory. Nat Rev Cancer 2003;3:821–831.
29. Simpson ER. Aromatase: biologic relevance of tissue-specific expression. Semin Reprod Med 2004;22:11–23.
30. Simpson ER. Sources of estrogen and their importance. J Steroid Biochem Mol Biol 2003;86:225–230.
31. Speroff L, Vande Wiele RL. Regulation of the human menstrual cycle. Am J Obstet Gynecol 1971;109:234–247.
32. Grodin JM, Siiteri PK, MacDonald PC. Source of estrogen production in postmenopausal women. J Clin Endocrinol Metab 1973;36:207–214.
33. Ryan KJ, Engel LL. The interconversion of estrone and estradiol by human tissue slices. Endocrinology 1953;52:287–291.
34. Pundel JP. Die androgen abstrichbilder. Arch Gynaekol 1957;188:577.
35. Murad F, Kuret JA. Estrogens and progestins. In: Goodman LS, Gilman A, eds. The Pharmacological Basis of Therapeutics. New York: Pergamon Press, 1990:1384.
36. Clemons M, Goss P. Estrogen and the risk of breast cancer. N Engl J Med 2001;344:276–285.
37. Gruber DM, Huber JC. Tissue specificity: the clinical importance of steroid metabolites in hormone replacement therapy. Maturitas 2001;37:151–157.
38. Taioli E, Trachman J, Chen X, et al. A CYP1A1 restriction fragment length polymorphism is associated with breast cancer in African-American women. Cancer Res 1995;55:3757–3758.
39. Lavigne JA, Helzlsouer KJ, Huang HY, et al. An association between the allele coding for a low activity variant of catechol-O-methyltransferase and the risk for breast cancer. Cancer Res 1997;57:5493–5497.
40. Deghenghi R, Givner M. The female sex hormones and analogs. In: Wolff ME, ed. Burger's Medicinal Chemistry. Vol. 2. New York: Wiley-Liss, 1979:917.
41. Kutsky RJ. Estradiol. Handbook of Vitamins, Minerals, and Hormones. New York: Van Nostrand Reinhold, 1981:415.
42. Evans RM. The steroid and thyroid hormone receptor superfamily. Science 1988;240:889–895.
43. Shao W, Brown M. Advances in estrogen receptor biology: prospects for improvements in targeted breast cancer therapy. Breast Cancer Res 2004;6:39–52.
44. Yang NN, Venugopalan M, Hardikar S, et al. Identification of an estrogen response element activated by metabolites of 17beta-estradiol and raloxifene. Science 1996;273:1222–1225.
45. Speirs V, Carder PJ, Lane S, et al. Oestrogen receptor beta: what it means for patients with breast cancer. Lancet Oncol 2004;5:174–181.
46. Barkhem T, Carlsson B, Nilsson Y, et al. Differential response of estrogen receptor alpha and estrogen receptor beta to partial estrogen agonists/antagonists. Mol Pharmacol 1998;54:105–112.
47. Kuiper GG, Carlsson B, Grandien K, et al. Comparison of the ligand binding specificity and transcript tissue distribution of estrogen receptors alpha and beta. Endocrinology 1997;138:863–870.
48. Saunders FJ. Effects of norethynodrel combined with mestranol on the offspring when administered during pregnancy and lactation in rats. Endocrinology 1967;80:447–452.
49. Williams MT, Clark MR, Ling WY. Role of cyclic AMP in the action of luteinizing hormone on steroidogenesis in the corpus luteum. In: George WJ, Ignarro L, eds. Advances in Cyclic Nucleotide Research. Vol. 9. New York: Raven Press, 1978:573.
50. Weihua Z, Andersson S, Cheng G, et al. Update on estrogen signaling. FEBS Lett 2003;546:17–24.
51. Krege JH, Hodgin JB, Couse JF, et al. Generation and reproductive phenotypes of mice lacking estrogen receptor beta. Proc Natl Acad Sci USA 1998;95:15677–15682.
52. Porter W, Wang F, Wang W, et al. Role of estrogen receptor/Sp1 complexes in estrogen-induced heat shock protein 27 gene expression. Mol Endocrinol 1996;10:1371–1378.
53. Pace P, Taylor J, Suntharalingam S, et al. Human estrogen receptor beta binds DNA in a manner similar to and dimerizes with estrogen receptor alpha. J Biol Chem 1997;272:25832–25838.
54. McDonnell DP, Norris JD. Connections and regulation of the human estrogen receptor. Science 2002;296:1642–1644.
55. Xu L, Glass CK, Rosenfeld MG. Coactivator and corepressor complexes in nuclear receptor function. Curr Opin Genet Dev 1999;9:140–147.
56. Kamei Y, Xu L, Heinzel T, et al. A CBP integrator complex mediates transcriptional activation and AP-1 inhibition by nuclear receptors. Cell 1996;85:403–414.
57. Beato M, Candau R, Chavez S, et al. Interaction of steroid hormone receptors with transcription factors involves chromatin remodelling. J Steroid Biochem Mol Biol 1996;56:47–59.
58. Tremblay GB, Giguere V. Coregulators of estrogen receptor action. Crit Rev Eukaryot Gene Expr 2002;12:1–22.
59. Lannigan DA. Estrogen receptor phosphorylation. Steroids 2003;68:1–9.
60. Mueller H, Kueng W, Schoumacher F, et al. Selective regulation of steroid receptor expression in MCF-7 breast cancer cells by a novel member of the heregulin family. Biochem Biophys Res Commun 1995;217:1271–1278.
61. Pietras RJ, Arboleda J, Reese DM, et al. HER-2 tyrosine kinase pathway targets estrogen receptor and promotes hormone-independent growth in human breast cancer cells. Oncogene 1995;10:2435–2446.

62. El-Ashry D, Miller DL, Kharbanda S, et al. Constitutive Raf-1 kinase activity in breast cancer cells induces both estrogen-independent growth and apoptosis. Oncogene 1997;15:423–435.

63. Kato S, Masuhiro Y, Watanabe M, et al. Molecular mechanism of a cross-talk between oestrogen and growth factor signalling pathways. Genes Cells 2000;5:593–601.

64. Kato S, Endoh H, Masuhiro Y, et al. Activation of the estrogen receptor through phosphorylation by mitogen-activated protein kinase. Science 1995;270:1491–1494.

65. Ellis MJ. The insulin-like growth factor network and breast cancer. In: Bowcock AM, ed. Breast Cancer: Molecular Genetics, Pathogenesis, and Therapeutics. Totowa, NJ: Humana Press, 1999.

66. Lee AV, Jackson JG, Gooch JL, et al. Enhancement of insulin-like growth factor signaling in human breast cancer: estrogen regulation of insulin receptor substrate-1 expression in vitro and in vivo. Mol Endocrinol 1999;13:787–796.

67. McLeskey SW, Zhang L, El-Ashry D, et al. Tamoxifen-resistant fibroblast growth factor–transfected MCF-7 cells are cross-resistant in vivo to the antiestrogen ICI 182,780 and two aromatase inhibitors. Clin Cancer Res 1998;4:697–711.

68. Paech K, Webb P, Kuiper GG, et al. Differential ligand activation of estrogen receptors ERalpha and ERbeta at AP1 sites. Science 1997;277:1508–1510.

69. Barsalou A, Gao W, Anghel SI, et al. Estrogen response elements can mediate agonist activity of anti-estrogens in human endometrial Ishikawa cells. J Biol Chem 1998;273:17138–17146.

70. Ray P, Ghosh SK, Zhang DH, et al. Repression of interleukin-6 gene expression by 17 beta-estradiol: inhibition of the DNA-binding activity of the transcription factors NF-IL6 and NF-kappa B by the estrogen receptor. FEBS Lett 1997;409:79–85.

71. Levin ER. Cellular functions of plasma membrane estrogen receptors. Steroids 2002;67:471–475.

72. Segars JH, Driggers PH. Estrogen action and cytoplasmic signaling cascades, I: membrane-associated signaling complexes. Trends Endocrinol Metab 2002;13:349–354.

73. Pietras RJ, Szego CM. Specific binding sites for oestrogen at the outer surfaces of isolated endometrial cells. Nature 1977;265:69–72.

74. Pietras RJ, Szego CM. Partial purification and characterization of oestrogen receptors in subfractions of hepatocyte plasma membranes. Biochem J 1980;191:743–760.

75. Levin ER. Bidirectional signaling between the estrogen receptor and the epidermal growth factor receptor. Mol Endocrinol 2003;17:309–317.

76. Haddow A, Watkinson JM, Paterson E. Influence of synthetic estrogens on advanced malignant disease. Br Med J 1944;2:393–398.

77. Darbre P, Yates J, Curtis S, et al. Effect of estradiol on human breast cancer cells in culture. Cancer Res 1983;43:349–354.

78. Lippman M, Bolan G, Huff K. The effects of estrogens and antiestrogens on hormone-responsive human breast cancer in long-term tissue culture. Cancer Res 1976;36:4595–4601.

79. Soule HD, McGrath CM. Estrogen responsive proliferation of clonal human breast carcinoma cells in athymic mice. Cancer Lett 1980;10:177–189.

80. Reddel RR, Sutherland RL. Effects of pharmacological concentrations of estrogens on proliferation and cell cycle kinetics of human breast cancer cell lines in vitro. Cancer Res 1987;47:5323–5329.

81. Brunner N, Spang-Thomsen M, Cullen K. The T61 human breast cancer xenograft: an experimental model of estrogen therapy of breast cancer. Breast Cancer Res Treat 1996;39:87–92.

82. Santen RJ, Manni A, Harvey H, et al. Endocrine treatment of breast cancer in women. Endocr Rev 1990;11:221–265.

83. Tsutsui T, Maizumi H, McLachlan JA, et al. Aneuploidy induction and cell transformation by diethylstilbestrol: a possible chromosomal mechanism in carcinogenesis. Cancer Res 1983;43:3814–3821.

84. Ingle JN. Estrogen as therapy for breast cancer. Breast Cancer Res 2002;4:133–136.

85. Lonning PE, Taylor PD, Anker G, et al. High-dose estrogen treatment in postmenopausal breast cancer patients heavily exposed to endocrine therapy. Breast Cancer Res Treat 2001;67:111–116.

86. Mashchak CA, Lobo RA, Dozono-Takano R, et al. Comparison of pharmacodynamic properties of various estrogen formulations. Am J Obstet Gynecol 1982;144:511–518.

87. Rigg LA, Hermann H, Yen SS. Absorption of estrogens from vaginal creams. N Engl J Med 1978;298:195–197.

88. Nakamura K. Bioavailability, distribution and pharmacokinetics of diethylstilbestrol converted from diethylstilbestrol diphosphate in patients with prostatic cancer. Hiroshima J Med Sci 1986;35:325–338.

89. Liehr JG, DaGue BB, Ballatore AM, et al. Diethylstilbestrol (DES) quinone: a reactive intermediate in DES metabolism. Biochem Pharmacol 1983;32:3711–3718.

90. Herbst AL, Ulfelder H, Poskanzer DC. Adenocarcinoma of the vagina: association of maternal stilbestrol therapy with tumor appearance in young women. N Engl J Med 1971;284:878–881.

91. Henriksson P, Johansson SE. Prediction of cardiovascular complications in patients with prostatic cancer treated with estrogen. Am J Epidemiol 1987;125:970–978.

92. Henriksson P, Blomback M, Bratt G, et al. Activators and inhibitors of coagulation and fibrinolysis in patients with prostatic cancer treated with oestrogen or orchidectomy. Thromb Res 1986;44:783–791.

93. Agardh CD, Nilsson-Ehle P, Lundgren R, et al. The influence of treatment with estrogens and estramustine phosphate on platelet aggregation and plasma lipoproteins in non-disseminated prostatic carcinoma. J Urol 1984;132:1021–1024.

94. Carter AC, Sedransk N, Kelley RM, et al. Diethylstilbestrol: recommended dosages for different categories of breast cancer patients. Report of the Cooperative Breast Cancer Group. JAMA 1977;237:2079–2078.

95. Kennedy BJ. Massive estrogen administration in premenopausal women with metastatic breast cancer. Cancer 1962;15:641–648.

96. Surgically confirmed gallbladder disease, venous thromboembolism, and breast tumors in relation to postmenopausal estrogen therapy: a report from the Boston Collaborative Drug Surveillance Program, Boston University Medical Center. N Engl J Med 1974;290:15–19.

97. Ameriks JA, Thompson NW, Frey CF, et al. Hepatic cell adenomas, spontaneous liver rupture, and oral contraceptives. Arch Surg 1975;110:548–557.

98. Ziel HK, Finkle WD. Increased risk of endometrial carcinoma among users of conjugated estrogens. N Engl J Med 1975;293:1167–1170.

99. Bibbo M, Gill WB, Azizi F, et al. Follow-up study of male and female offspring of DES-exposed mothers. Obstet Gynecol 1977;49:1–8.

100. Melnick S, Cole P, Anderson D, et al. Rates and risks of diethylstilbestrol-related clear-cell adenocarcinoma of the vagina and cervix: an update. N Engl J Med 1987;316:514–516.

101. Marselos M, Tomatis L. Diethylstilboestrol, I: pharmacology, toxicology and carcinogenicity in humans. Eur J Cancer 1992;28A:1182–1189.

102. Marselos M, Tomatis L. Diethylstilboestrol, II: pharmacology, toxicology and carcinogenicity in experimental animals. Eur J Cancer 1992;29A:149–155.

103. Osborne CK. Tamoxifen in the treatment of breast cancer. N Engl J Med 1998;339:1609–1618.

104. Morgan LR Jr, Schein PS, Woolley PV, et al. Therapeutic use of tamoxifen in advanced breast cancer: correlation with biochemical parameters. Cancer Treat Rep 1976;60:1437–1443.

105. Rose C, Mouridsen HT. Treatment of advanced breast cancer with tamoxifen. Recent Results Cancer Res 1984;91:230–242.

106. Ingle JN, Krook JE, Green SJ, et al. Randomized trial of bilateral oophorectomy versus tamoxifen in premenopausal women with metastatic breast cancer. J Clin Oncol 1986;4:178–185.

107. Muss HB, Case LD, Atkins JN, et al. Tamoxifen versus high-dose oral medroxyprogesterone acetate as initial endocrine therapy for patients with metastatic breast cancer: a Piedmont Oncology Association study. J Clin Oncol 1994;12:1630–1638.

108. Jordan VC, Assikis VJ. Endometrial carcinoma and tamoxifen: clearing up a controversy. Clin Cancer Res 1995;1:467–472.

109. Uziely B, Lewin A, Brufman G, et al. The effect of tamoxifen on the endometrium. Breast Cancer Res Treat 1993;26:101–105.

110. Kavak ZN, Binoz S, Ceyhan N, et al. The effect of tamoxifen on the endometrium, serum lipids and hypothalamus pituitary axis in the postmenopausal breast cancer patient. Acta Obstet Gynecol Scand 2000;79:604–607.

111. Enck RE, Rios CN. Tamoxifen treatment of metastatic breast cancer and antithrombin III levels. Cancer 1984;53:2607–2609.

112. Love RR, Surawicz TS, Williams EC. Antithrombin III level, fibrinogen level, and platelet count changes with adjuvant tamoxifen therapy. Arch Intern Med 1992;152:317–320.

113. Barakat RR. The effect of tamoxifen on the endometrium. Oncology (Huntingt) 1995;9:129–134; discussion 139–140, 142.

114. Barni S, Lissoni P, Tancini G, et al. Effects of one-year adjuvant treatment with tamoxifen on bone mineral density in postmenopausal breast cancer women. Tumori 1996;82:65–67.

115. Schapira DV, Kumar NB, Lyman GH. Serum cholesterol reduction with tamoxifen. Breast Cancer Res Treat 1990;17:3–7.

116. Love RR, Newcomb PA, Wiebe DA, et al. Effects of tamoxifen therapy on lipid and lipoprotein levels in postmenopausal patients with node-negative breast cancer. J Natl Cancer Inst 1990;82:1327–1332.

117. Fromson JM, Pearson S, Bramah S. The metabolism of tamoxifen (I.C.I. 46,474), I: in laboratory animals. Xenobiotica 1973;3:693–709.

118. Lyman SD, Jordan VC. Metabolism of nonsteroidal antiestrogens. In: Jordan VC, ed. Estrogen/Antiestrogen Action and Breast Cancer Therapy. Madison: University of Wisconsin Press, 1986.

119. Bain RR, Jordan VC. Identification of a new metabolite of tamoxifen in patient serum during breast cancer therapy. Biochem Pharmacol 1983;32:373–375.

120. Robinson SP, Jordan VC. Metabolism of antihormonal anticancer agents. In: International Encyclopedia of Pharmacology and Therapeutics. Oxford: Pergamon Press, 1994.

121. Lonning PE, Lien EA, Lundgren S, et al. Clinical pharmacokinetics of endocrine agents used in advanced breast cancer. Clin Pharmacokinet 1992;22:327–358.

122. Adam HK, Douglas EJ, Kemp JV. The metabolism of tamoxifen in human. Biochem Pharmacol 1979;28:145–147.

123. Fromson JM, Pearson S, Bramah S. The metabolism of tamoxifen (I.C.I. 46,474), II: in female patients. Xenobiotica 1973;3:711–714.

124. Sutherland CM, Sternson LA, Muchmore JH, et al. Effect of impaired renal function on tamoxifen. J Surg Oncol 1984;27:222–223.

125. Langan-Fahey SM, Tormey DC, Jordan VC. Tamoxifen metabolites in patients on long-term adjuvant therapy for breast cancer. Eur J Cancer 1990;26:883–888.

126. Johnson MD, Zuo H, Lee KH, et al. Pharmacological characterization of 4-hydroxy-N-desmethyl tamoxifen, a novel active metabolite of tamoxifen. Breast Cancer Res Treat 2004;85:151–159.

127. Kemp JV, Adam HK, Wakeling AE, et al. Identification and biological activity of tamoxifen metabolites in human serum. Biochem Pharmacol 1983;32:2045–2052.

128. Bates DJ, Foster AB, Griggs LJ, et al. Metabolism of tamoxifen by isolated rat hepatocytes: anti-estrogenic activity of tamoxifen N-oxide. Biochem Pharmacol 1982;31:2823–2827.

129. Fabian C, Tilzer L, Sternson L. Comparative binding affinities of tamoxifen, 4-hydroxytamoxifen, and desmethyltamoxifen for estrogen receptors isolated from human breast carcinoma: correlation with blood levels in patients with metastatic breast cancer. Biopharm Drug Dispos 1981;2:381–390.

130. Fabian C, Sternson L, El-Serafi M, et al. Clinical pharmacology of tamoxifen in patients with breast cancer: correlation with clinical data. Cancer 1981;48:876–882.

131. Nicholson RI, Syne JS, Daniel CP, et al. The binding of tamoxifen to oestrogen receptor proteins under equilibrium and non-equilibrium conditions. Eur J Cancer 1979;15:317–329.

132. Wakeling AE, Slater SR. Estrogen-receptor binding and biologic activity of tamoxifen and its metabolites. Cancer Treat Rep 1980;64:741–744.

133. Daniel CP, Gaskell SJ, Bishop H, et al. Determination of tamoxifen and an hydroxylated metabolite in plasma from patients with advanced breast cancer using gas chromatography-mass spectrometry. J Endocrinol 1979;83:401–408.

134. Daniel P, Gaskell SJ, Bishop H, et al. Determination of tamoxifen and biologically active metabolites in human breast tumours and plasma. Eur J Cancer Clin Oncol 1981;17:1183–1189.

135. Wilkinson PM, Ribiero GG, Adam HK, et al. Tamoxifen (Nolvadex) therapy: rationale for loading dose followed by maintenance dose for patients with metastatic breast cancer. Cancer Chemother Pharmacol 1982;10:33–35.

136. Fabian C, Sternson L, Barnett M. Clinical pharmacology of tamoxifen in patients with breast cancer: comparison of traditional and loading dose schedules. Cancer Treat Rep 1980;64:765–773.

137. Ribeiro GG, Wilkinson PM. A clinical assessment of loading dose tamoxifen for advanced breast carcinoma. Clin Oncol 1984;10:363–367.

138. Noguchi S, Miyauchi K, Imaoka S, et al. Inability of tamoxifen to penetrate into cerebrospinal fluid. Breast Cancer Res Treat 1988;12:317–318.

139. Osborne CK, Wiebe VJ, McGuire WL, et al. Tamoxifen and the isomers of 4-hydroxytamoxifen in tamoxifen-resistant tumors from breast cancer patients. J Clin Oncol 1992;10:304–310.

140. Wolf DM, Langan-Fahey SM, Parker CJ, et al. Investigation of the mechanism of tamoxifen-stimulated breast tumor growth with nonisomerizable analogues of tamoxifen and metabolites. J Natl Cancer Inst 1993;85:806–812.

141. Jacolot F, Simon I, Dreano Y, et al. Identification of the cytochrome P450 IIIA family as the enzymes involved in the N-demethylation of tamoxifen in human liver microsomes. Biochem Pharmacol 1991;41:1911–1919.

142. Mani C, Gelboin HV, Park SS, et al. Metabolism of the antimammary cancer antiestrogenic agent tamoxifen, I: cytochrome P-450-catalyzed N-demethylation and 4-hydroxylation. Drug Metab Dispos 1993;21:645–656.

143. Mani C, Hodgson E, Kupfer D. Metabolism of the antimammary cancer antiestrogenic agent tamoxifen, II: flavin-containing monooxygenase-mediated N-oxidation. Drug Metab Dispos 1993;21:657–661.

144. Crewe HK, Lennard MS, Tucker GT, et al. The effect of selective serotonin re-uptake inhibitors on cytochrome P4502D6 (CYP2D6) activity in human liver microsomes. Br J Clin Pharmacol 1992;34:262–265.

145. Stearns V, Johnson MD, Rae JM, et al. Active tamoxifen metabolite plasma concentrations after coadministration of tamoxifen and the selective serotonin reuptake inhibitor paroxetine. J Natl Cancer Inst 2003;95:1758–1764.

146. Dowsett M, Pfister C, Johnston SR, et al. Impact of tamoxifen on the pharmacokinetics and endocrine effects of the aromatase inhibitor letrozole in postmenopausal women with breast cancer. Clin Cancer Res 1999;5:2338–2343.

147. Reid AD, Horobin JM, Newman EL, et al. Tamoxifen metabolism is altered by simultaneous administration of medroxyprogesterone acetate in breast cancer patients. Breast Cancer Res Treat 1992;22:153–156.

148. Fogarty PF, Rick ME, Swain SM. Tamoxifen and thrombosis: current clinical observations and treatment guidelines. In: Devita VT, Hellman S, Rosenberg SA, eds. Cancer: Principles and Practice of Oncology. 6th ed. Philadelphia: Lippincott Williams & Wilkins, 2002.

149. Fisher B, Costantino JP, Wickerham DL, et al. Tamoxifen for prevention of breast cancer: report of the National Surgical Adjuvant Breast and Bowel Project P-1 Study. J Natl Cancer Inst 1998;90:1371–1388.

150. Kaiser-Kupfer MI, Lippman ME. Tamoxifen retinopathy. Cancer Treat Rep 1978;62:315–320.

151. Kaiser-Kupfer MI, Kupfer C, Rodrigues MM. Tamoxifen retinopathy: a clinicopathologic report. Ophthalmology 1981;88:89–93.

152. McKeown CA, Swartz M, Blom J, et al. Tamoxifen retinopathy. Br J Ophthalmol 1981;65:177–179.

153. Gerner EW. Low-dose tamoxifen retinopathy. Can J Ophthalmol 1992;27:358.

154. Griffiths MF. Tamoxifen retinopathy at low dosage. Am J Ophthalmol 1987;104:185–186.

155. Bentley CR, Davies G, Aclimandos WA. Tamoxifen retinopathy: a rare but serious complication. BMJ 1992;304:495–496.

156. Pemberton KD, Melissari E, Kakkar VV. The influence of tamoxifen in vivo on the main natural anticoagulants and fibrinolysis. Blood Coagul Fibrinolysis 1993;4:935–942.

157. Fisher B, Costantino J, Redmond C, et al. A randomized clinical trial evaluating tamoxifen in the treatment of patients with node-negative breast cancer who have estrogen-receptor–positive tumors. N Engl J Med 1989;320:479–484.

158. Henderson ICI, et al., eds. Endocrine therapy in metastatic breast cancer. In: al HJRe, ed. Breast Diseases. Philadelphia: JB Lippincott, 1991:559.

159. Bruning PF, Bonfrer JM, Hart AA, et al. Tamoxifen, serum lipoproteins and cardiovascular risk. Br J Cancer 1988;58:497–499.

160. Ingram D. Tamoxifen use, oestrogen binding and serum lipids in postmenopausal women with breast cancer. Aust N Z J Surg 1990;60:673–675.

161. Jones AL, Powles TJ, Treleaven JG, et al. Haemostatic changes and thromboembolic risk during tamoxifen therapy in normal women. Br J Cancer 1992;66:744–747.

162. Gau TC. Letter to physicians. Stuart Pharmaceuticals, Pasadena, CA 1987.

163. Pathak DN, Bodell WJ. DNA adduct formation by tamoxifen with rat and human liver microsomal activation systems. Carcinogenesis 1994;15:529–532.

164. Turken S, Siris E, Seldin D, et al. Effects of tamoxifen on spinal bone density in women with breast cancer. J Natl Cancer Inst 1989;81:1086–1088.

165. Fornander T, Rutqvist LE, Sjoberg HE, et al. Long-term adjuvant tamoxifen in early breast cancer: effect on bone mineral density in postmenopausal women. J Clin Oncol 1990;8:1019–1024.

166. Gotfredsen A, Christiansen C, Palshof T. The effect of tamoxifen on bone mineral content in premenopausal women with breast cancer. Cancer 1984;53:853–857.

167. Planting AS, Alexieva-Figusch J, Blonk-vdWijst J, et al. Tamoxifen therapy in premenopausal women with metastatic breast cancer. Cancer Treat Rep 1985;69:363–368.

168. Kedar RP, Bourne TH, Powles TJ, et al. Effects of tamoxifen on uterus and ovaries of postmenopausal women in a randomised breast cancer prevention trial. Lancet 1994;343:1318–1321.

169. Bernstein L, Deapen D, Cerhan JR, et al. Tamoxifen therapy for breast cancer and endometrial cancer risk. J Natl Cancer Inst 1999;91:1654–1662.

170. Wysowski DK, Honig SF, Beitz J. Uterine sarcoma associated with tamoxifen use. N Engl J Med 2002;346:1832–1833.

171. Robinson SP, Jordan VC. Reversal of the antitumor effects of tamoxifen by progesterone in the 7,12-dimethylbenzanthracene–induced rat mammary carcinoma model. Cancer Res 1987;47:5386–5390.

172. Sherman BM, Chapler FK, Crickard K, et al. Endocrine consequences of continuous antiestrogen therapy with tamoxifen in premenopausal women. J Clin Invest 1979;64:398–404.

173. Manni A, Pearson OH. Antiestrogen-induced remissions in premenopausal women with stage IV breast cancer: effects on ovarian function. Cancer Treat Rep 1980;64:779–785.

174. Paterson AG, Turkes A, Groom GV, et al. The effect of tamoxifen on plasma growth hormone and prolactin in postmenopausal women with advanced breast cancer. Eur J Cancer Clin Oncol 1983;19:919–922.

175. Jordan VC, Fritz NF, Langan-Fahey S, et al. Alteration of endocrine parameters in premenopausal women with breast cancer during long-term adjuvant therapy with tamoxifen as the single agent. J Natl Cancer Inst 1991;83:1488–1491.

176. Szamel I, Vincze B, Hindy I, et al. Hormonal changes during a prolonged tamoxifen treatment in patients with advanced breast cancer. Oncology 1986;43:7–11.

177. Levin J, Markham MJ, Greenwald ES, et al. Effect of tamoxifen treatment on estrogen metabolism in postmenopausal women with advanced breast cancer. Anticancer Res 1982;2:377–380.

178. Ravdin PM, Fritz NF, Tormey DC, et al. Endocrine status of premenopausal node-positive breast cancer patients following adjuvant chemotherapy and long-term tamoxifen. Cancer Res 1988;48:1026–1029.

179. Wilking N, Carlstrom K, Skoldefors H, et al. Effects of tamoxifen on the serum levels of oestrogens and adrenocortical steroids in postmenopausal breast cancer patients. Acta Chir Scand 1982; 148:345–349.

180. Sakai F, Cheix F, Clavel M, et al. Increases in steroid binding globulins induced by tamoxifen in patients with carcinoma of the breast. J Endocrinol 1978;76:219–226.

181. Fex G, Adielsson G, Mattson W. Oestrogen-like effects of tamoxifen on the concentration of proteins in plasma. Acta Endocrinol (Copenh) 1981;97:109–113.

182. Gordon D, Beastall GH, McArdle CS, et al. The effect of tamoxifen therapy on thyroid function tests. Cancer 1986;58: 1422–1425.

183. Boccardo F, Bruzzi P, Rubagotti A, et al. Estrogen-like action of tamoxifen on vaginal epithelium in breast cancer patients. Oncology 1981;38:281–285.

184. Luciani L, Oriana S, Spatti G, et al. Hormonal and receptor status in postmenopausal women with endometrial carcinoma before and after treatment with tamoxifen. Tumori 1984;70: 189–192.

185. Namer M, Lalanne C, Baulieu EE. Increase of progesterone receptor by tamoxifen as a hormonal challenge test in breast cancer. Cancer Res 1980;40:1750–1752.

186. Fornander T, Rutqvist LE, Wilking N, et al. Oestrogenic effects of adjuvant tamoxifen in postmenopausal breast cancer. Eur J Cancer 1993;29A:497–500.

187. Lien EA, Johannessen DC, Aakvaag A, et al. Influence of tamoxifen, aminoglutethimide and goserelin on human plasma IGF-I levels in breast cancer patients. J Steroid Biochem Mol Biol 1992;41:541–543.

188. Pollak M, Costantino J, Polychronakos C, et al. Effect of tamoxifen on serum insulinlike growth factor I levels in stage I breast cancer patients. J Natl Cancer Inst 1990;82:1693–1697.

189. Dawson-Hughes B, Stern D, Goldman J, et al. Regulation of growth hormone and somatomedin-C secretion in postmenopausal women: effect of physiological estrogen replacement. J Clin Endocrinol Metab 1986;63:424–432.

190. Cullins SL, Pridjian G, Sutherland CM. Goldenhar's syndrome associated with tamoxifen given to the mother during gestation. JAMA 1994;271:1905–1906.

191. Clark S. Prophylactic tamoxifen. Lancet 1993;342:168.

192. Woo JC, Yu T, Hurd TC. Breast cancer in pregnancy: a literature review. Arch Surg 2003;138:91–98; discussion 99.

193. Halakivi-Clarke L, Cho E, Onojafe I, et al. Maternal exposure to tamoxifen during pregnancy increases carcinogen-induced mammary tumorigenesis among female rat offspring. Clin Cancer Res 2000;6:305–308.

194. Collinson MP, Hamilton DA, Tyrrell CJ. Two case reports of tamoxifen as a cause of impotence in male subjects with carcinoma of the breast. Breast Cancer Res 1998;2:48–49.

195. Fernando IN, Tobias JS. Priapism in patients on tamoxifen. Lancet 1989;1:436.

196. Anelli TF, Anelli A, Tran KN, et al. Tamoxifen administration is associated with a high rate of treatment-limiting symptoms in male breast cancer patients. Cancer 1994;74:74–77.

197. Traub AI, Thompson W. The effect of tamoxifen on spermatogenesis in subfertile men. Andrologia 1981;13:486–490.

198. Gooren LJ. Androgen levels and sex functions in testosterone-treated hypogonadal men. Arch Sex Behav 1987;16:463–473.

199. Plotkin D, Lechner JJ, Jung WE, et al. Tamoxifen flare in advanced breast cancer. JAMA 1978;240:2644–2646.

200. Beex L, Pieters G, Smals A, et al. Tamoxifen versus ethinyl estradiol in the treatment of postmenopausal women with advanced breast cancer. Cancer Treat Rep 1981;65:179–185.

201. Rossleigh MA, Lovegrove FT, Reynolds PM, et al. Serial bone scans in the assessment of response to therapy in advanced breast carcinoma. Clin Nucl Med 1982;7:397–402.

202. Vogel CL, Schoenfelder J, Shemano I, et al. Worsening bone scan in the evaluation of antitumor response during hormonal therapy of breast cancer. J Clin Oncol 1995;13:1123–1128.

203. Kaufman RJ, Escher GC. Rebound regression in advanced mammary carcinoma. Surg Gynecol Obstet 1961;113:635–640.

204. Howell A, Dodwell DJ, Anderson H, et al. Response after withdrawal of tamoxifen and progestogens in advanced breast cancer. Ann Oncol 1992;3:611–617.

205. Manson JE, Hsia J, Johnson KC, et al. Estrogen plus progestin and the risk of coronary heart disease. N Engl J Med 2003;349: 523–534.

206. O'Regan RM, Cisneros A, England GM, et al. Effects of the antie-strogens tamoxifen, toremifene, and ICI 182,780 on endometrial cancer growth. J Natl Cancer Inst 1998;90:1552–1558.

207. Lufkin EG, Whitaker MD, Nickelsen T, et al. Treatment of estab-lished postmenopausal osteoporosis with raloxifene: a random-ized trial. J Bone Miner Res 1998;13:1747–1754.

208. Buzdar AU, Marcus C, Holmes F, et al. Phase II evaluation of Ly156758 in metastatic breast cancer. Oncology 1988;45:344–345.

209. Ettinger B, Black DM, Mitlak BH, et al. Reduction of vertebral fracture risk in postmenopausal women with osteoporosis treated with raloxifene: results from a 3-year randomized clinical trial. Multiple Outcomes of Raloxifene Evaluation (MORE) Investigators. JAMA 1999;282:637–645.

210. Jordan VC. Targeted antiestrogens to prevent breast cancer. Trends Endocrinol Metab 1999;10:312–317.

211. Goldstein SR, Siddhanti S, Ciaccia AV, et al. A pharmacological review of selective oestrogen receptor modulators. Hum Reprod Update 2000;6:212–224.

212. Wijayaratne AL, Nagel SC, Paige LA, et al. Comparative analyses of mechanistic differences among antiestrogens. Endocrinology 1999;140:5828–5840.

213. Shang Y, Brown M. Molecular determinants for the tissue speci-ficity of SERMs. Science 2002;295:2465–2468.

214. Glasebrook A, Phillips DL, Sluka JP. Multiple binding sites for the antiestrogen raloxifene. J Bone Miner Res 1993;1(Suppl):268.

215. Morello KC, Wurz GT, DeGregorio MW. Pharmacokinetics of selective estrogen receptor modulators. Clin Pharmacokinet 2003;42:361–372.

216. Snyder KR, Sparano N, Malinowski JM. Raloxifene hydrochlo-ride. Am J Health Syst Pharm 2000;57:1669–1675; quiz 1676–1678.

217. Cummings SR, Eckert S, Krueger KA, et al. The effect of raloxifene on risk of breast cancer in postmenopausal women: results from the MORE randomized trial. Multiple Outcomes of Raloxifene Evaluation. JAMA 1999;281:2189–2197.

218. Hochner-Celnikier D. Pharmacokinetics of raloxifene and its clinical application. Eur J Obstet Gynecol Reprod Biol 1999;85:23–29.

219. Cauley JA, Norton L, Lippman ME, et al. Continued breast cancer risk reduction in postmenopausal women treated with raloxifene: 4-year results from the MORE trial. Multiple Outcomes of Raloxifene Evaluation. Breast Cancer Res Treat 2001;65:125–134.

220. Riggs BL, Hartmann LC. Selective estrogen-receptor modulators: mechanisms of action and application to clinical practice. N Engl J Med 2003;348:618–629.

221. Vogel CL. Phase II and III clinical trials of toremifene for metastatic breast cancer. Oncology (Huntingt) 1998;12:9–13.

222. Wiseman LR, Goa KL. Toremifene: a review of its pharmacologi-cal properties and clinical efficacy in the management of advanced breast cancer. Drugs 1997;54:141–160.

223. Wiebe VJ, Benz CC, Shemano I, et al. Pharmacokinetics of toremifene and its metabolites in patients with advanced breast cancer. Cancer Chemother Pharmacol 1990;25:247–251.

224. Howell A. Preliminary experience with pure antiestrogens. Clin Cancer Res 2001;7:4369s–4375s; discussion 4411s–4412s.

225. Johnston SR. Fulvestrant (AstraZeneca). Curr Opin Investig Drugs 2002;3:305–312.

226. Dauvois S, Danielian PS, White R, et al. Antiestrogen ICI 164,384 reduces cellular estrogen receptor content by increasing its turnover. Proc Natl Acad Sci USA 1992;89:4037–4041.

227. Dukes M, Miller D, Wakeling AE, et al. Antiuterotrophic effects of a pure antioestrogen, ICI 182,780: magnetic resonance imag-ing of the uterus in ovariectomized monkeys. J Endocrinol 1992;135:239–247.

228. Long BJ, Tilghman SL, Yue W, et al. The steroidal antiestrogen ICI 182,780 is an inhibitor of cellular aromatase activity. J Steroid Biochem Mol Biol 1998;67:293–304.

229. DeFriend DJ, Howell A, Nicholson RI, et al. Investigation of a new pure antiestrogen (ICI 182780) in women with primary breast cancer. Cancer Res 1994;54:408–414.

230. Ellis PA, Saccani-Jotti G, Clarke R, et al. Induction of apoptosis by tamoxifen and ICI 182780 in primary breast cancer. Int J Cancer 1997;72:608–613.

231. Thomas EJ, Walton PL, Thomas NM, et al. The effects of ICI 182,780, a pure anti-oestrogen, on the hypothalamic-pituitary-gonadal axis and on endometrial proliferation in pre-menopausal women. Hum Reprod 1994;9:1991–1996.

232. Howell A, DeFriend DJ, Robertson JF, et al. Pharmacokinetics, pharmacological and anti-tumour effects of the specific anti-oestrogen ICI 182780 in women with advanced breast cancer. Br J Cancer 1996;74:300–308.

233. Robertson JF, Harrison MP. Equivalent single-dose pharmacoki-netics of two different dosing methods of prolonged-release ful-vestrant ("Faslodex") in postmenopausal women with advanced breast cancer. Cancer Chemother Pharmacol 2003;52:346–348.

234. Faslodex [Info P. NDA 21–344]. Wilmington, DE: AstraZeneca;2002.

235. Gallagher A, Chambers TJ, Tobias JH. The estrogen antagonist ICI 182,780 reduces cancellous bone volume in female rats. Endocrinology 1993;133:2787–2791.

236. Howell A, Robertson JF, Abram P, et al. Comparison of fulves-trant versus tamoxifen for the treatment of advanced breast can-cer in postmenopausal women previously untreated with endocrine therapy: a multinational, double-blind, randomized trial. J Clin Oncol 2004;22:1605–1613.

237. Labrie F, Labrie C, Belanger A, et al. EM-652 (SCH 57068), a third generation SERM acting as pure antiestrogen in the mam-mary gland and endometrium. J Steroid Biochem Mol Biol 1999;69:51–84.

238. Santen RJ, Santner SJ, Pauley RJ, et al. Estrogen production via the aromatase enzyme in breast carcinoma: which cell type is responsible? J Steroid Biochem Mol Biol 1997;61:267–271.

239. Longcope C. Metabolic clearance and blood production rates of estrogens in postmenopausal women. Am J Obstet Gynecol 1971;111:778–781.

240. Abul-Hajj YJ, Iverson R, Kiang DT. Aromatization of androgens by human breast cancer. Steroids 1979;33:205–222.

241. Dowsett M, Lee K, Macaulay VM, et al. The control and biologi-cal importance of intratumoural aromatase in breast cancer. J Steroid Biochem Mol Biol 1996;56:145–150.

242. Lu Q, Nakmura J, Savinov A, et al. Expression of aromatase pro-tein and messenger ribonucleic acid in tumor epithelial cells and evidence of functional significance of locally produced estrogen in human breast cancers. Endocrinology 1996;137:3061–3068.

243. Brodie AM, Njar VC. Aromatase inhibitors and breast cancer. Semin Oncol 1996;23:10–20.

244. Griffiths CT, Hall TC, Saba Z, et al. Preliminary trial of aminog-lutethimide in breast cancer. Cancer 1973;32:31–37.

245. Samojlik E, Santen RJ, Wells SA. Adrenal suppression with aminoglutethimide, II: differential effects of aminoglutethimide on plasma androstenedione and estrogen levels. J Clin Endocrinol Metab 1977;45:480–487.

246. Santen RJ, Santner S, Davis B, et al. Aminoglutethimide inhibits extraglandular estrogen production in postmenopausal women with breast carcinoma. J Clin Endocrinol Metab 1978;47:1257–1265.

247. Goldhirsch A, Gelber RD. Endocrine therapies of breast cancer. Semin Oncol 1996;23:494–505.

248. Lawrence B, Santen RJ, Lipton A, et al. Pancytopenia induced by aminoglutethimide in the treatment of breast cancer. Cancer Treat Rep 1978;62:1581–1583.

249. Banting L. Inhibition of aromatase. Prog Med Chem 1996;33:147–184.

250. Evans TR, Di Salle E, Ornati G, et al. Phase I and endocrine study of exemestane (FCE 24304), a new aromatase inhibitor, in post-menopausal women. Cancer Res 1992;52:5933–5939.

251. Lonning P, Pfister C, Martoni A, et al. Pharmacokinetics of third-generation aromatase inhibitors. Semin Oncol 2003;30:23–32.

252. Scott LJ, Wiseman LR. Exemestane. Drugs 1999;58:675–680; dis-cussion 681–682.

253. Zilembo N, Noberasco C, Bajetta E, et al. Endocrinological and clinical evaluation of exemestane, a new steroidal aromatase inhibitor. Br J Cancer 1995;72:1007–1012.

254. Lonning PE, Paridaens R, Thurlimann B, et al. Exemestane expe-rience in breast cancer treatment. J Steroid Biochem Mol Biol 1997;61:151–155.

255. Di Salle E, Giudici D, Ornati G, et al. 4-Aminoandrostenedione derivatives: a novel class of irreversible aromatase inhibitors: comparison with FCE 24304 and 4-hydroxyandrostenedione. J Steroid Biochem Mol Biol 1990;37:369–374.

256. Buzzetti F, Di Salle E, Longo A, et al. Synthesis and aromatase inhibition by potential metabolites of exemestane (6-methylenandrosta-1,4-diene-3,17-dione). Steroids 1993;58:527–532.

257. Goss PE. Comparison of the effects of exemestane, 17-hydroxexemestane and letrozole on bone and lipid metabolism in the ovariectomized rat. Breast Cancer Res Treat 2002;76:415.

258. Goss PE, Strasser-Weippl K. Prevention strategies with aromatase inhibitors. Clin Cancer Res 2004;10:372S–379S.

259. Coombes RC, Hall E, Gibson LJ, et al. A randomized trial of exemestane after two to three years of tamoxifen therapy in postmenopausal women with primary breast cancer. N Engl J Med 2004;350:1081–1092.

260. Miller WR. Aromatase inhibitors: mechanism of action and role in the treatment of breast cancer. Semin Oncol 2003;30:3–11.

261. Boccardo F, Amoroso D, Iacobelli S, et al. Clinical efficacy and endocrine activity of vorozole in postmenopausal breast cancer patients: results of a multicentric phase II study. Ann Oncol 1997;8:745–750.

262. Plourde PV, Dyroff M, Dukes M. Arimidex: a potent and selective fourth-generation aromatase inhibitor. Breast Cancer Res Treat 1994;30:103–111.

263. Baum M, Buzdar A, Cuzick J, et al. Anastrozole alone or in combination with tamoxifen versus tamoxifen alone for adjuvant treatment of postmenopausal women with early-stage breast cancer: results of the ATAC (Arimidex, Tamoxifen Alone or in Combination) trial efficacy and safety update analyses. Cancer 2003;98:1802–1810.

264. Buzdar AU, Jones SE, Vogel CL, et al. A phase III trial comparing anastrozole (1 and 10 milligrams), a potent and selective aromatase inhibitor, with megestrol acetate in postmenopausal women with advanced breast carcinoma. Arimidex Study Group. Cancer 1997;79:730–739.

265. Buzdar A, Jonat W, Howell A, et al. Anastrozole, a potent and selective aromatase inhibitor, versus megestrol acetate in postmenopausal women with advanced breast cancer: results of overview analysis of two phase III trials. Arimidex Study Group. J Clin Oncol 1996;14:2000–2011.

266. Klein KO, Demers LM, Santner SJ, et al. Use of ultrasensitive recombinant cell bioassay to measure estrogen levels in women with breast cancer receiving the aromatase inhibitor, letrozole. J Clin Endocrinol Metab 1995;80:2658–2660.

267. Bajetta E, Zilembo N, Dowsett M, et al. Double-blind, randomised, multicentre endocrine trial comparing two letrozole doses, in postmenopausal breast cancer patients. Eur J Cancer 1999;35:208–213.

268. Bisagni G, Cocconi G, Scaglione F, et al. Letrozole, a new oral non-steroidal aromatase inhibitor in treating postmenopausal patients with advanced breast cancer: a pilot study. Ann Oncol 1996;7:99–102.

269. Brodie A, Lu Q, Yue W, et al. Intratumoral aromatase model: the effects of letrozole (CGS 20267). Breast Cancer Res Treat 1998;49(Suppl 1):S23–26; discussion S33–37.

270. Geisler J, Haynes B, Anker G, et al. Influence of letrozole and anastrozole on total body aromatization and plasma estrogen levels in postmenopausal breast cancer patients evaluated in a randomized, cross-over study. J Clin Oncol 2002;20:751–757.

271. Rose C, Vtoraya O, Pluzanska A, et al. An open randomised trial of second-line endocrine therapy in advanced breast cancer. Eur J Cancer 2003;39:2318–2327.

272. Dombernowsky P, Smith I, Falkson G, et al. Letrozole, a new oral aromatase inhibitor for advanced breast cancer: double-blind randomized trial showing a dose effect and improved efficacy and tolerability compared with megestrol acetate. J Clin Oncol 1998;16:453–461.

273. Goss PE, Ingle JN, Martino S, et al. A randomized trial of letrozole in postmenopausal women after five years of tamoxifen therapy for early-stage breast cancer. N Engl J Med 2003;349:1793–1802.

274. Ito Y, Fisher CR, Conte FA, et al. Molecular basis of aromatase deficiency in an adult female with sexual infantilism and polycystic ovaries. Proc Natl Acad Sci USA 1993;90:11673–11677.

275. Conte FA, Grumbach MM, Ito Y, et al. A syndrome of female pseudohermaphrodism, hypergonadotropic hypogonadism, and multicystic ovaries associated with missense mutations in the gene encoding aromatase (P450arom). J Clin Endocrinol Metab 1994;78:1287–1292.

276. Agarwal SK, Judd HL, Magoffin DA. A mechanism for the suppression of estrogen production in polycystic ovary syndrome. J Clin Endocrinol Metab 1996;81:3686–3691.

277. Santen RJ, Samojlik E, Wells SA. Resistance of the ovary to blockade of aromatization with aminoglutethimide. J Clin Endocrinol Metab 1980;51:473–477.

278. Celio L, Martinetti A, Ferrari L, et al. Premenopausal breast cancer patients treated with a gonadotropin-releasing hormone analog alone or in combination with an aromatase inhibitor: a comparative endocrine study. Anticancer Res 1999;19:2261–2268.

279. Dowsett M, Doody D, Miall S, et al. Vorozole results in greater oestrogen suppression than formestane in postmenopausal women and when added to goserelin in premenopausal women with advanced breast cancer. Breast Cancer Res Treat 1999;56:25–34.

280. Beard J. The span of gestation and the cause of birth. In: Fisher G, ed. Jena, 1897.

281. Fraenkel L. Die Funktion des Corpus Luteum. Arch Gynaekol 1905;68:483–545.

282. Corner GW, Allen WM. Physiology of the corpus luteum II: production of a special uterine reaction (progestational proliferation) by extracts of the corpus luteum. Am J Physiol 1929;88:326–339.

283. Van de Wiele RL, Gurpide E, Kelly WG. The secretory rate of progesterone and aldosterone in normal and abnormal late pregnancy. Acta Endocrinol [Suppl] (Copenh) 1960;51:159.

284. Fotherby K. Metabolism of synthetic steroids by animals and man. Acta Endocrinol [Suppl] (Copenh) 1974;185:119–147.

285. Gupta C, Osterman J, Santen R, et al. In vivo metabolism of progestins, V: the effect of protocol design on the estimated metabolic clearance rate and volume of distribution of medroxyprogesterone acetate in women. J Clin Endocrinol Metab 1979;48:816–820.

286. Janne O, Kontula K, Luukkainen T, et al. Oestrogen-induced progesterone receptor in human uterus. J Steroid Biochem 1975;6:501–509.

287. Allegra JC, Kiefer SM. Mechanisms of action of progestational agents. Semin Oncol 1985;12:3–5.

288. Blossey HC, Wander HE, Koeberling J, et al. Pharmacokinetic and pharmacodynamic basis for the treatment of metastatic breast cancer with high-dose medroxyprogesterone acetate. Cancer 1984;54:1208–1215.

289. Going JJ, Anderson TJ, Battersby S, et al. Proliferative and secretory activity in human breast during natural and artificial menstrual cycles. Am J Pathol 1988;130:193–204.

290. Michna H, Schneider MR, Nishino Y, et al. The antitumor mechanism of progesterone antagonists is a receptor mediated antiproliferative effect by induction of terminal cell death. J Steroid Biochem 1989;34:447–453.

291. Shi YE, Torri J, Yieh L, et al. Expression of 67 kDa laminin receptor in human breast cancer cells: regulation by progestins. Clin Exp Metastasis 1993;11:251–261.

292. Vignon F, Bardon S, Chalbos D. Antiproliferative effect of progestins and antiprogestins in human breast cancer cells. In: Klijn JGM, Paridaens R, Foekens JA, eds. Hormonal Manipulation of Cancer: Peptides, Growth Factors, and New (Anti) Steroidal Agents. Vol. 47. New York: Raven Press, 1987.

293. Sadoff L, Lusk W. The effect of large doses of medroxyprogesterone acetate (MPA) on urinary estrogen levels and serum levels of cortisol T4 LH and testosterone in patients with advanced cancer. Obstet Gynecol 1974;43:262–267.

294. Vesterinen E, Backas NE, Pesonen K, et al. Effect of medroxyprogesterone acetate on serum levels of LH, FSH, cortisol, and estrone in patients with endometrial carcinoma. Arch Gynecol 1981;230:205–211.

295. Hellman L, Yoshida K, Zumoff B, et al. The effect of medroxyprogesterone acetate on the pituitary-adrenal axis. J Clin Endocrinol Metab 1976;42:912–917.

296. van Veelen H, Willemse PH, Sleijfer DT, et al. Endocrine effects of medroxyprogesterone acetate: relation between plasma levels

and suppression of adrenal steroids in patients with breast cancer. Cancer Treat Rep 1985;69:977–983.

297. Antal EJ, Gillespie WR, Albert KS. The bioavailability of an orally administered medroxyprogesterone acetate suspension. Int J Clin Pharmacol Ther Toxicol 1983;21:257–259.

298. Neomto T, Patel J, Rosner D. Oral medroxyprogesterone acetate (NSC-26386) in metastatic breast cancer. Proc Am Assoc Cancer Res 1983;24.

299. Sikic BI, Scudder SA, Ballon SC, et al. High-dose megestrol acetate therapy of ovarian carcinoma: a phase II study by the Northern California Oncology Group. Semin Oncol 1986;13:26–32.

300. Willemse PH, van der Ploeg E, Sleijfer DT, et al. A randomized comparison of megestrol acetate (MA) and medroxyprogesterone acetate (MPA) in patients with advanced breast cancer. Eur J Cancer 1990;26:337–343.

301. Pannuti F, Martoni A, Di Marco AR, et al. Prospective, randomized clinical trial of two different high dosages of medroxyprogesterone acetate (MAP) in the treatment of metastatic breast cancer. Eur J Cancer 1979;15:593–601.

302. Crona N, Enk L, Samsioe G. Medroxyprogesterone acetate (MPA) in adjuvant treatment of endometrial carcinoma-changes in serum lipoproteins. Steroid Biochem 1983;195:198.

303. De Conno F, Martini C, Zecca E, et al. Megestrol acetate for anorexia in patients with far-advanced cancer: a double-blind controlled clinical trial. Eur J Cancer 1998;34:1705–1709.

304. Mantovani G, Maccio A, Lai P, et al. Cytokine involvement in cancer anorexia/cachexia: role of megestrol acetate and medroxyprogesterone acetate on cytokine downregulation and improvement of clinical symptoms. Crit Rev Oncog 1998;9: 99–106.

305. Quella SK, Loprinzi CL, Sloan JA, et al. Long term use of megestrol acetate by cancer survivors for the treatment of hot flashes. Cancer 1998;82:1784–1788.

306. Ovarian ablation in early breast cancer: overview of the randomised trials. Early Breast Cancer Trialists' Collaborative Group. Lancet 1996;348:1189–1196.

307. Taylor CW, Green S, Dalton WS, et al. Multicenter randomized clinical trial of goserelin versus surgical ovariectomy in premenopausal patients with receptor-positive metastatic breast cancer: an intergroup study. J Clin Oncol 1998;16: 994–999.

308. Harvey HA, Lipton A, Max DT, et al. Medical castration produced by the GnRH analogue leuprolide to treat metastatic breast cancer. J Clin Oncol 1985;3:1068–1072.

309. Klijn JG, de Jong FH, Lamberts SW, et al. LHRH-agonist treatment in clinical and experimental human breast cancer. J Steroid Biochem 1985;23:867–873.

310. Chrisp P, Goa KL. Goserelin: a review of its pharmacodynamic and pharmacokinetic properties, and clinical use in sex hormone–related conditions. Drugs 1991;41:254–288.

311. Cockshott ID. Clinical pharmacokinetics of goserelin. Clin Pharmacokinet 2000;39:27–48.

312. Jimenez-Gordo AM, de las Heras B, Zamora P, et al. Failure of goserelin ovarian ablation in premenopausal women with breast cancer: two case reports. Gynecol Oncol 2000;76:126–127.

313. Filicori M, Flamigni C, Cognigni G, et al. Comparison of the suppressive capacity of different depot gonadotropin-releasing hormone analogs in women. J Clin Endocrinol Metab 1993;77: 130–133.

314. Reichel RP, Schweppe KW. Goserelin (Zoladex) depot in the treatment of endometriosis. Zoladex Endometriosis Study Group. Fertil Steril 1992;57:1197–1202.

315. Winer EP, Hudis C, Burstein HJ, et al. American Society of Clinical Oncology technology assessment on the use of aromatase inhibitors as adjuvant therapy for women with hormone receptor-positive breast cancer: status report 2002. J Clin Oncol 2002;20:3317–3327.

316. Donnez J, Dewart PJ, Hedon B, et al. Equivalence of the 3-month and 28-day formulations of triptorelin with regard to achievement and maintenance of medical castration in women with endometriosis. Fertil Steril 2004;81:297–304.

317. Drieu K, Devissaguet JP, Duboistesselin R, et al. Pharmacokinetics of D-Trp6 LHRH in man: sustained release polymer microsphere study (I.M. route). Prog Clin Biol Res 1987;243A:435–437.

318. Muller FO, Terblanche J, Schall R, et al. Pharmacokinetics of triptorelin after intravenous bolus administration in healthy males and in males with renal or hepatic insufficiency. Br J Clin Pharmacol 1997;44:335–341.

319. Blamey RW, Jonat W, Kaufmann M, et al. Goserelin depot in the treatment of premenopausal advanced breast cancer. Eur J Cancer 1992;28A:810–814.

320. Devogelaer JP, Nagant DE, Deuxchaisnes C. Effect of goserelin implants, an LH-RH analogue, on lumbar and hip BMD as studied by deka technique [abstract 207]. Gynecol Endocrinol 1990;4:114.

321. Obhrai H, Samra JS, Brown P. Effects of medical oophorectomy on fasting lipids and lipoproteins in women with polycystic ovarian syndrome (PCOS) [abstract 123]. Gynecol Endocrinol 1990;4:72.

322. Varenhorst E, Svensson M, Hjertberg H, et al. Antithrombin III concentration, thrombosis, and treatment with luteinising hormone releasing hormone agonist in prostatic carcinoma. Br Med J [Clin Res] 1986;292:935–936.

323. Tonetti DA, Jordan VC. The role of estrogen receptor mutations in tamoxifen-stimulated breast cancer. J Steroid Biochem Mol Biol 1997;62:119–128.

324. Karnik PS, Kulkarni S, Liu XP, et al. Estrogen receptor mutations in tamoxifen-resistant breast cancer. Cancer Res 1994;54:349–353.

325. Fuqua SA, Chamness GC, McGuire WL. Estrogen receptor mutations in breast cancer. J Cell Biochem 1993;51:135–139.

326. Zhang QX, Borg A, Wolf DM, et al. An estrogen receptor mutant with strong hormone-independent activity from a metastatic breast cancer. Cancer Res 1997;57:1244–1249.

327. Roodi N, Bailey LR, Kao WY, et al. Estrogen receptor gene analysis in estrogen receptor-positive and receptor-negative primary breast cancer. J Natl Cancer Inst 1995;87:446–451.

328. Ali S, Coombes RC. Endocrine-responsive breast cancer and strategies for combating resistance. Nat Rev Cancer 2002;2:101–112.

329. Speirs V, Malone C, Walton DS, et al. Increased expression of estrogen receptor beta mRNA in tamoxifen-resistant breast cancer patients. Cancer Res 1999;59:5421–5424.

330. Iwase H, Zhang Z, Omoto Y, et al. Clinical significance of the expression of estrogen receptors alpha and beta for endocrine therapy of breast cancer. Cancer Chemother Pharmacol 2003; 52(Suppl 1):S34–38.

331. Zhang QX, Borg A, Fuqua SA. An exon 5 deletion variant of the estrogen receptor frequently coexpressed with wild-type estrogen receptor in human breast cancer. Cancer Res 1993;53:5882–5884.

332. Rea D, Parker MG. Effects of an exon 5 variant of the estrogen receptor in MCF-7 breast cancer cells. Cancer Res 1996;56: 1556–1563.

333. Webb P, Nguyen P, Shinsako J, et al. Estrogen receptor activation function 1 works by binding p160 coactivator proteins. Mol Endocrinol 1998;12:1605–1618.

334. Smith CL, Nawaz Z, O'Malley BW. Coactivator and corepressor regulation of the agonist/antagonist activity of the mixed antiestrogen, 4-hydroxytamoxifen. Mol Endocrinol 1997;11:657–666.

335. Schiff R, Massarweh S, Shou J, et al. Breast cancer endocrine resistance: how growth factor signaling and estrogen receptor coregulators modulate response. Clin Cancer Res 2003;9:447S–454S.

336. Wright C, Nicholson S, Angus B, et al. Relationship between c-erbB-2 protein product expression and response to endocrine therapy in advanced breast cancer. Br J Cancer 1992;65:118–121.

337. Leitzel K, Teramoto Y, Konrad K, et al. Elevated serum c-erbB-2 antigen levels and decreased response to hormone therapy of breast cancer. J Clin Oncol 1995;13:1129–1135.

338. Yamauchi H, O'Neill A, Gelman R, et al. Prediction of response to antiestrogen therapy in advanced breast cancer patients by pretreatment circulating levels of extracellular domain of the HER-2/c-neu protein. J Clin Oncol 1997;15:2518–2525.

339. van 't Veer LJ, Dai H, van de Vijver MJ, et al. Gene expression profiling predicts clinical outcome of breast cancer. Nature 2002; 415:530–536.

340. Gruvberger S, Ringner M, Chen Y, et al. Estrogen receptor status in breast cancer is associated with remarkably distinct gene expression patterns. Cancer Res 2001;61:5979–5984.

341. Cleator S, Ashworth A. Molecular profiling of breast cancer: clinical implications. Br J Cancer 2004;90:1120–1124.

342. Sgroi DC, Ma XJ, Ryan P, et al. Discovery of new gene expression predictors for adjuvant tamoxifen outcome for breast cancer patients [abstract 9503]. Proc Am Soc Clin Oncol 2004; 40:.

343. Frasor J, Stossi F, Danes JM, et al. Selective estrogen receptor modulators: discrimination of agonistic versus antagonistic activities by gene expression profiling in breast cancer cells. Cancer Res 2004;64:1522–1533.

344. Cunliffe HE, Ringner M, Bilke S, et al. The gene expression response of breast cancer to growth regulators: patterns and correlation with tumor expression profiles. Cancer Res 2003;63: 7158–7166.

Index

Page numbers followed by f indicate figures; page numbers followed t indicate tables.